ROGER STEVENSON
MARCH, 1994

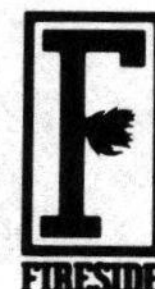
FIRESIDE

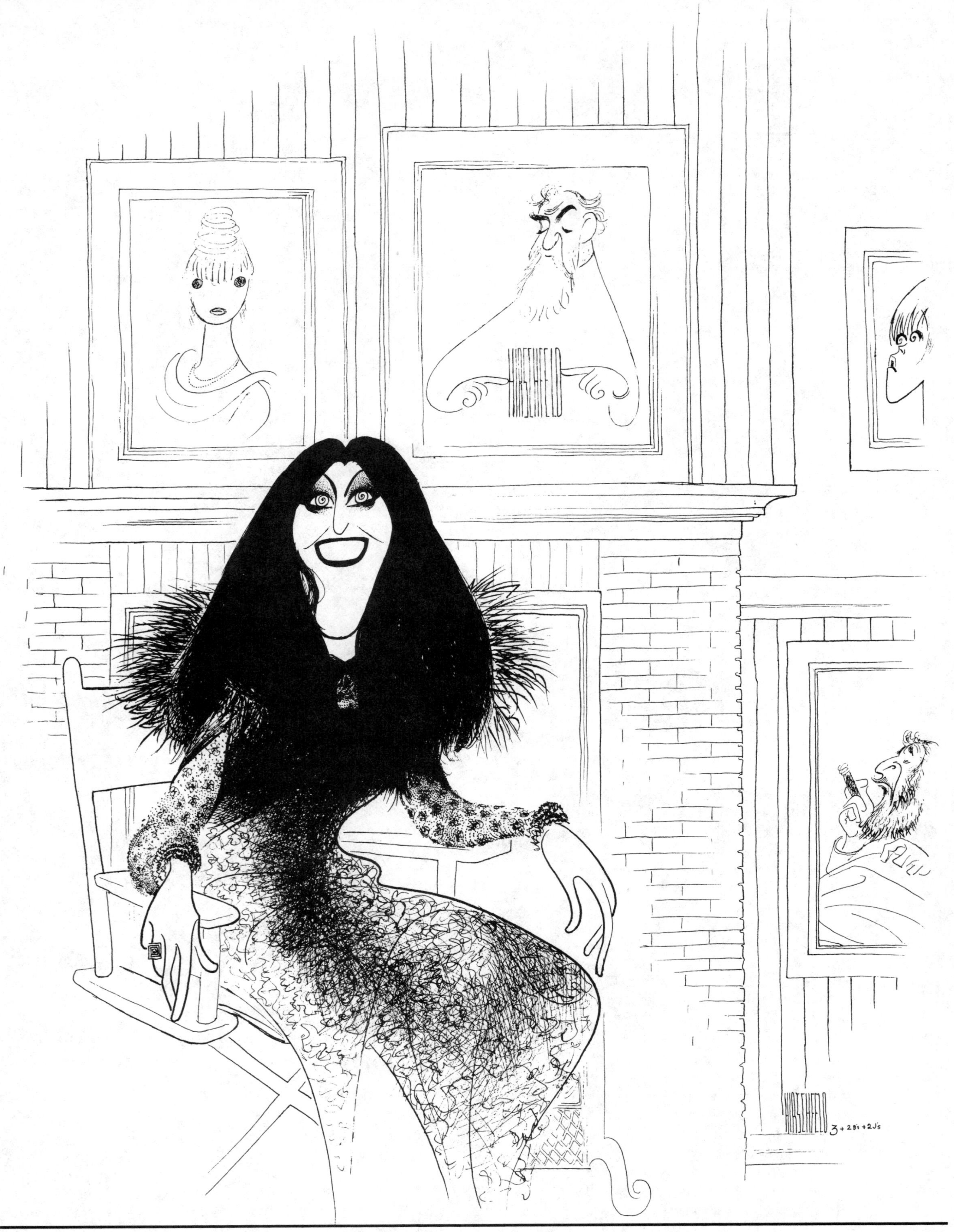
HIRSCHFELD
HIRSCHFELD

••• MARGO FEIDEN'S •••

THE CALORIE FACTOR

The Dieter's Companion

A Fireside Book
Published by Simon & Schuster Inc.
NEW YORK · LONDON · TORONTO · SYDNEY · TOKYO

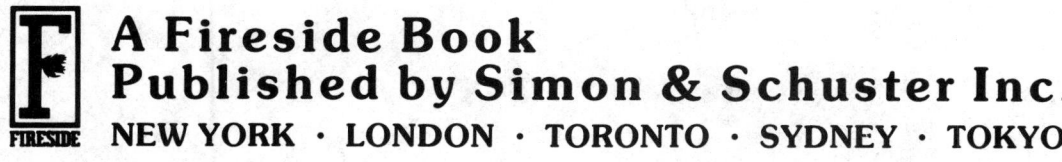

SIMON AND SCHUSTER/FIRESIDE
SIMON & SCHUSTER BUILDING
ROCKEFELLER CENTER
1230 AVENUE OF THE AMERICAS
NEW YORK, NEW YORK 10020

DESIGNED BY IRVING PERKINS ASSOCIATES
MANUFACTURED IN THE UNITED STATES OF AMERICA

10 9 8 7 6 5 4 3 2
10 9 8 7 6 5 4 3 PBK

LIBRARY OF CONGRESS CATALOGING IN PUBLICATION DATA

FEIDEN, MARGO.
MARGO FEIDEN'S THE CALORIE FACTOR: THE DIETER'S COMPANION.

INCLUDES INDEX.
1. FOOD—CALORIC CONTENT—TABLES. 2. FOOD—CARBOHYDRATE CONTENT—TABLES. I. TITLE.
TX551.F48 1985 641.1'042 85-11946
ISBN 0-671-43646-5
0-671-61800-8 (PBK.)

Margo Feiden gratefully acknowledges the three beautiful portraits by **AL HIRSCHFELD:**
Portrait of **MARGO FEIDEN, ART DEALER,** *including Hirschfeld's self-portrait, and portraits of his wife* **DOLLY, JANE FONDA,** *and* **PETER USTINOV;** *Portrait of* **MARGO FEIDEN** *and* **JULIUS COHEN;** *and Portrait of* **MARGO FEIDEN, AVIATRIX.**

• ACKNOWLEDGMENTS

To Al and Dolly Hirschfeld for their incalculable contribution to my life.

I would like to acknowledge a walking college—Richard Schmeidler. Thank you, Dick.

An art dealer by profession, when I began writing this book in 1977 my work divided itself in two: My Gallery, and The Calorie. Writing this book would not have been possible without key people on both fronts.

For their help in *The Gallery*:

Masha Fridman
Jay Geddis
Carla D. Heller
Eady Rickard
Lynn Surry

And thank you, Adam, Christopher Day, Richard Schmeidler, and Janet Lupoli.

For their help with *The Calorie*:

Carla D. Heller
Janet Lupoli
Eady Rickard
Joseph Williams

And thank you Ray Neinstein, Walter D. Glanze, Bill, Tina Viscardi, Cindy, Dan, Wendy, Jim, Laura, Jane, April, David, Brian, Carla, Laurel, Libby, Cherri, Ira, and Gloria. Thank you Linda Wasserman Zaccaro, Diane Engel, Jill Percival Wynns, and Gladys Katz.

I thank my lucky stars for Balducci's—a store specializing in, among other things, hard-to-find fruits and vegetables. There I would go, at the crack of dawn, to count and weigh berries and coconuts, fennel and fungi. Gus and Tony were always helpful. Richie Brennan picked me up at five in the morning to bring me to the fish markets. Nina and Andy Balducci were forever patient and encouraging. And Pop Balducci taught me how to tell a good melon.

The secret to a smooth-running life, I have found, lies in part in the quality of the professionals you have around you. I acknowledge the following individuals as doing the highest honors to their professions: John M. Schwartz, Marty Licht, and Perry Cohen of Herzfeld & Rubin, P.C.; Adil Antia, Susan Baisley, V. Judith Bowman, Bertha Caceres, Dave Frempong, Amy Hunter, John Roche, Alan Schlefman, Susan Turco, Susan Miller, and Mary P. Wilkinson of Citibank, N.A.; Lucille Mercurio of The Manhattan Savings Bank; and Laurence R. Marchini, Jr., of the Gotham Bank of New York.

Thank you Hank Trattner and Billy Marbit of "Reader's"; Cliff "Nice Man" Bareish, Michael Hecht, and Sam Diamond.

A special thanks to the late Michael Bennett. My heartfelt appreciation to Professor Richard Brown.

There was a constant exchange of information with the USDA. Particularly helpful were Jacob Exler, Ph.D.; Ruth Matthews, Supervisory Nutritionist; and Frank Hepburn, Chief, Nutrient Data Research Branch, Consumer Nutrition Center, Hyattsville, Maryland. Also of great help was Mrs. Reiko Ramsay of JETRO (Japan External Trade Organization), N.Y.

Thanksgiving to those hearts dear and true, who helped me to hold the fabric of my life together during the making of this book. They went the extra mile:

Julius Cohen
Richard Schmeidler
Margo Pollins Schab
William Shakespeare
Gilbert Leistner
Daria Enrick
Robert Fitch
Alan Kelman
Helga Tilton
Ludwig van Beethoven
Joseph Williams
Maximilian Schell
Daniel Rosen
Ilse and Henry Wolf
Cathy Hemming
Owen Laster, whose support of me and of this project never wavered.

To my very gifted parents who infused me with wonder: My Father, who sent me off to kindergarten with a slide rule, and my Mother, an actress who could recite from the telephone book and cause a roomful of men to cry.

And, of course, Bambi and Jeremy, who grew up with this book as a sibling for most of their lives (and I love You).

To JULIUS, belovéd companion on This Journey:

If I could write the beauty of your eyes
And in fresh numbers number all your graces,
The age to come would say "This poet lies!
Such heavenly touches ne'er touch'd earthly faces."

William Shakespeare
from Sonnet XVII
c. 1592

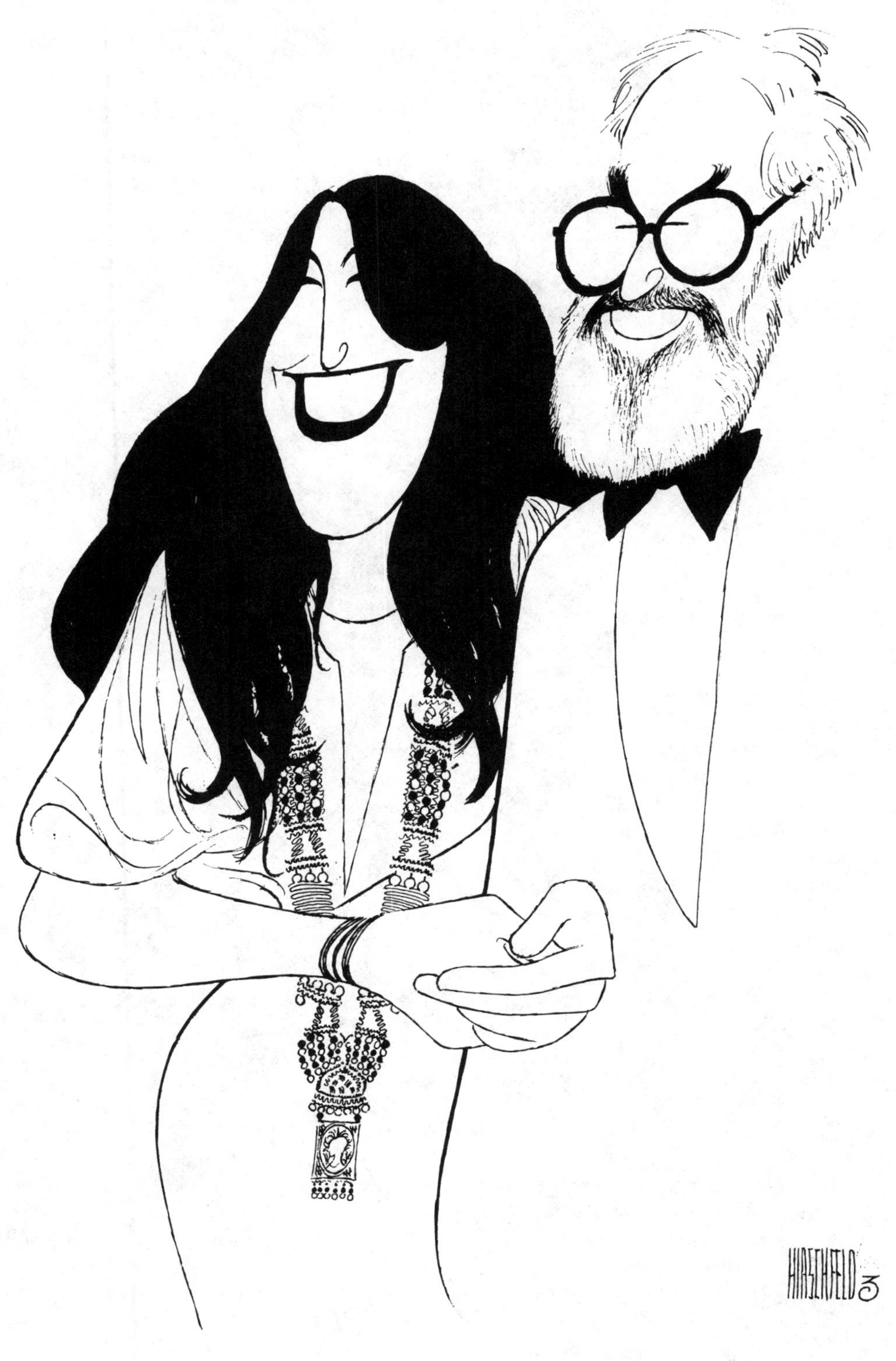

· CONTENTS

• PART III • THE CALORIELOGUE (The Data Pages)

• PART IV • EPILOGUE

• PART V • BIBLIOGRAPHY

• TO THE READER

English is a wonderful language, but it does have pronoun problems.

Fill in the following sentence with the appropriate pronoun:

Feed your child as much as ______ wants.

The incorrect way would be to say "it," the old-fashioned way would be to say "he," the currently current way would be to say "he or she."

I've solved the problem differently. I use a contraction, "s/he." I pronounce it sh'-he.

. . .

The **Prologue** and **Monologue** chapters of this book were written to be read together, in one, unhurried sitting.

Please do not read them now if you are in a rush. I think this is the only "Do Not!" in the book. Thank you.

. . .

I began writing ***THE CALORIE FACTOR*** in 1977. If I were beginning it now I would use my word processor and have a computerized data base. I didn't start out with either luxury, and resisted changing in midstream. By my own choosing, I never had the luxury of an editor, either. Whatever commas are out of place, there's no one to blame but, me.

. . .

THE CALORIE FACTOR has been ten years in the making. This means that it was not all written at the same time, and that data were gathered over a period of years. I have done what I could to add new data as they have come in, but . . .

. . . No matter when a book like this goes to press, events will overtake it. That venerated beverage, Coke, has been reformulated. Package sizes shrink and expand. Recently, Nutra-Sweet has widely supplanted saccharine. And so it goes. Some of the data in **The Calorielogue** are now out of date, and even more will be out of date before this book rolls off the presses.

I've done the best I could under very trying circumstances. I am not the only person to have had this problem, and I take comfort in quoting from an all–time master compiler:

". . . and believing that a repertory of which I had myself experienced the advantage might, when amplified, prove useful to others, I resolved to embark in an undertaking which, for the last three or four years, has given me incessant occupation, and has, indeed, imposed upon me an amount of labor very much greater than I had anticipated. Notwithstanding all the pains I have bestowed on its execution, I am fully aware of its numerous deficiencies and imperfections, and of its falling far short of the degree of excellence that might be attained. But, in a work of this nature, where perfection is placed at so great a distance, I have thought it best to limit my ambition to that moderate share of merit which it may claim in its present form; trusting to the indulgence of those for whose benefit it is intended, and to the candor of critics who, while they find it easy to detect faults, can at the same time duly appreciate difficulties."

P. M. Roget
April 29, 1852

I can only hope that my book will last as long, and prove as useful.

Margo Feiden
August 3, 1988

• PART I

PROLOGUE

MONOLOGUE

METHODOLOGY

• PROLOGUE

Everybody I know . . . everybody—my agent and his secretary; my landlord and my lawyer; my tailor, his wife, and their daughter; my doctor, my dentist, the druggist; my incredible manicurist; my best friend; my butcher and my baker, and believe it or not, yes, my candlestick maker; my compulsive accountants and countless other friends, relatives, and neighbors, among them: actors; artists and art dealers; oceanographers and explorers; chemical, electrical, and civil engineers; businessmen and babysitters; psychologists and psychiatrists; theatrical producers and theatrical professors; marvelous musicians, mathematicians, and even magicians' magicians—of my entire acquaintanceship with very few exceptions—everybody I know, no matter how successful s/he is at other endeavors, finds it just about impossible to succeed on a diet.

And so, as you might expect, everybody who knows me has asked how I lost weight. Everybody. It was one hundred and fifty pounds. Typically, the question is posed: "What is your secret?" The first hundred times I was asked, my reply was simply: "I have no secret. I count calories."

By the hundred and first time I had come to realize that I did have a secret, and I now understand why the most frequent response to "I count calories" was: "But . . . what else did you do?"

I counted calories, all right, and this is how I did it: So serious was I about losing weight that I measured, weighed, and kept a running calorie tally of every single thing I ate for fourteen months, to the teaspoonfuls of lettuce. In my own kitchen. At McDonald's. At "21." What I discovered is that, for all our experts, we have not known what causes people to become fat and stay fat. This was the beginning of ***THE CALORIE FACTOR.***

The book is called ***THE CALORIE FACTOR*** because it's very definitely a calorie book, and the message is a calorie message. In fact, the message is several calorie messages. The book rests on seven pillars.

I. Weight loss and weight gain depend upon calories.

II. If people do not have the figures they might like, it is not necessarily because they are undisciplined; they may be misinformed.

Everybody "knows" that people who are overweight overeat. Doctors know it. Diet writers know it. The lecturers at Weight Watchers know it. Everybody knows it. And so, if you are overweight, you probably know it, too.

But when I approached the problem mathematically the numbers didn't know it. And the numbers were clear. Boy, have we been wrong!

III. The calorie differences involved between gaining weight at a substantial clip, remaining stable, and losing weight at a substantial clip are a very small number of calories per day.

I computed that each pound of body fat is maintained by less than one extra calorie per hour. What does that mean in practical terms?

Well, let's say you're really overweight and not just trying to lose the same ten pounds that everybody else is. Let's say you are overweight by thirty-five pounds. Those thirty-five pounds are maintained by only 122,500 calories a year. Only?

Only. One hundred twenty-two thousand five hundred calories a year breaks down to one and a half glasses of milk a day and an extra meal about once a week.

Overeating?

If you are overweight by twenty-five pounds you won't need that extra meal. You will maintain those extra pounds by eating 87,000 calories a year. That's a glass of milk before bedtime, together with one cookie.

Overeating?

What all this means is that if you want to lose twenty-five pounds and continue to eat exactly the way you always have—including the bread, and the potatoes, and the binges—by cutting out the calorie equivalent of a glass of milk and a cookie a day, you could lose every one of those pounds.

IV. By making small changes in what you eat you can accomplish your entire diet.

Oh, a rose may be a rose—but to the dieter a hamburger is not a hamburger. If you eat only twenty-five burgers a year, but you have Whoppers at Burger King instead of Quarter Pounders at McDonald's, simply from that difference in calories alone, at the end of the year you can have gained more than one and one-half pounds.

Twenty-five hamburgers represent 2% of your yearly "allotment" of three meals a day. If you had the information that would enable you to make a comparable choice at every meal, in one year you could lose eighty-two pounds. Eighty-two pounds. In one year.

Right about now you're probably thinking, "This is the best diet book I have ever read. All I have to do is eat at McDonald's instead of Burger King." So you go to McDonald's, and you order a Big Mac.

Oh, a rose may be a rose—but a Quarter Pounder is not a Big Mac. A year's worth of meals, each increased by the same number of calories as the difference between the Quarter Pounder and the Big Mac, can make a thirty-eight Pounder difference in your weight. That's big, Mac.

And I know they aren't the same, but just for the record, if you reduced the number of calories in your meals for one year by the difference between the Whopper and a White Castle hamburger, you could end the year with 563,925 fewer calories, and 161 fewer pounds. I can't resist: The difference between the Whopper and a White Castle hamburger is Whopping. If you don't know what that difference is—you're getting rooked.

V. In the process of choosing what to eat, you can make perfectly acceptable choices among similar types of foods and save a lot of calories. And this will be true where you might least expect it.

Let's say you are a run-of-the-mill compulsive eater. Right now, pleasure can be found only in potatoes. You should know that the potatoes that come mashed and with gravy at Kentucky Fried Chicken have less than one-half the calories of potatoes that come fried and with catsup at McDonald's or at Burger King. That is, K.F.C. mashed potatoes have less than half the calories of the regular-size French fries. If your potato passion should become potatomania—if you were actually going to order the large French fries at McDonald's—you could go instead to the Colonel's and order four and one-quarter portions of gravy-gorged mashed potatoes. (Aren't you glad you bought this book?)

If you are considering two large portions of French fries, you could consider eight and a half portions of mashed potatoes with eight and a half portions' worth of gravy. (Now aren't you really glad you bought this book?)

By the way, while you are eating infinite portions of potatoes at Kentucky Fried Chicken, you should know that if you want chicken to go along with the potatoes, ordering "Extra Crispy" is ordering between 38 and 87 extra calories per piece.

And now for dessert. Yes, dessert. This book was written to be read by human beings, and so—of we two hundred million American human beings who watch our weight—one hundred and ninety-nine million of us will be faced from time to time with having to make the same decision, no matter what diet we have to break to do it: "Where should we stop for ice cream?"

You should know that for every two times you stop for a regular ice cream cone at Friendly's you can stop three times at Dairy Queen for a small ice cream cone—dipped in chocolate—without consuming one extra calorie. Once you know that, the third one feels like you're eating it for free. It is the consummate dieter's dream, the ice cream cone without calories.

Ice cream has a healthful mystique to it, and I've observed that parents who are resolute in restricting other sweets will still allow ice cream. Even if you think your child is overweight, it's likely that you may pass by the ice cream case and say "Yes."

You should know that if your child eats a half-cup of Good Humor's Royal Fudge ice cream instead of Good Humor's Vanilla Fudge Swirl ice cream every day from the time s/he's six to the time s/he's twelve, s/he can celebrate that twelfth birthday twelve pounds lighter.

Twelve pounds lighter, not from giving up ice cream, but simply from choosing one kind of Fudge ice cream instead of another. That's enough to put anyone into a good humor.

VI. Even people who know that calories matter don't know how to apply the calorie concept when they are sitting with fork in hand.

You're out to lunch with a client. You know s/he's on a diet when, without looking at the menu, s/he orders Chef's Salad. For the same reason, you've ordered Chef's Salad, too.

Automatically, your salad is served with melba toast instead of bread. You want the bread, but you're embarrassed to ask for it lest people doubt your fortitude. So you eat melba toast and feel worthy. Ounce for ounce, melba toast has more calories than bread. Oh.

But as you place your order you feel saintly. Certainly so virtuous a dieter deserves a little salad dressing. If you try steadfastly to maintain your present weight, making sure to eat only the same number of calories as you burn, just by adding three tablespoons of dressing to your salad every day for a year, you could gain more than twenty pounds. Oh!

But you can still be proud of your Chef's Salad. How fattening can anything be that is 90% lettuce? Take away the lettuce (which you weren't going to eat anyway) and, ounce for ounce, Chef's Salad is one of the highest-calorie meals you can eat.

Oh.

VII. Calories count, but we have not been able to count them until now.

The first problem has been specificity of measurement. It isn't enough to say, as so many calorie books do, that "½ a medium cantaloupe" is "60 calories." There is no such thing as a "medium" cantaloupe. That description covers just too broad a range. When I use the word "medium" (and I do), I tell you what "medium" means.

The second problem is that a calorie book must list many, many foods. Here we need specificity also, or we can run into trouble without knowing why. Take the olive.

In one of the glossiest books that lists calories, the poor olive isn't to be found at all. Then there are the books that list one olive. Or two. **The Calorielogue** of this book lists more than thirty olives by variety and size.

So what? How powerful can an olive be?

This is how powerful: You're a salad lover and you love olives in your salad. Every day at lunch and at dinner, you throw a handful of olives into your salad. Not list olives? The difference in calories between one kind of olive and another olive of the same size, but of a different style, can be so great that just by throwing in ten "Greek" olives instead of ten "Ripe" ones, at the end of the year you can have gained more than four pounds.

More than four pounds from the difference between handfuls of olives, identical in size. Never underestimate the power of an olive.

Never underestimate the power of a calorie.

Never underestimate the power of even one calorie. Fatness is not a condition maintained by overeating. Fatness is a condition brought about and maintained by eating a few too many calories, consistently.

If the information in this book helps Americans to reduce their daily intake by the number of calories that are in a cup of cottage cheese, without any other change in our diets—without diets altogether—by the end of two years we will no longer be fat.

• MONOLOGUE

According to statistics, once you are fat that is that. If such a small reduction in calories can make all the difference in the world, what, then, causes our sea of troubles when we try to lose weight?

I think I know. I think that we lack what's needed to solve any problem: Information.

Lack information? About dieting? Absurd! Why, more books and articles have been written about how to lose weight than there are stars visible from the middle of the Sahara desert on the clearest night of the year. How can it be that we lack information?

I state and rest my case on the following: Could you have told me which has fewer calories—the Quarter Pounder from McDonald's or the Whopper from Burger King?

You see, if you were unable to answer that question and its equivalents, then it doesn't matter how many books you've read on the subject, or what your friends have told you. It doesn't matter how many weight-loss organizations you've joined, and it doesn't matter how many magazines you've purchased because the cover story was "How To Lose Weight Sensibly, Easily, And In Time For That Next Big Affair." What does matter is being able to answer the Quarter-Pounder question, and all the questions like it.

If you're like many Americans, you will frequently have to make just such a choice as the one between the Quarter Pounder and the Whopper. Even if you are trying to stick to a structured diet, there will be those days when, having sat three times through a Disney movie and the accompanying giggling, cheering, shouting, trips to the bathroom, and popcorn fights, you will have the patience needed to unwrap seven hamburgers, but not enough patience to wrap up a sink full of dirty dishes.

Before it appears that I'm running for chairman of the "Ad Hoc Committee to Abolish the Whopper and Big Mac, and Urge to Ascendancy the Quarter Pounder," let me make my position clear. I don't advise you to eat the lowest-calorie hamburger, or to eat mashed potatoes instead of French fries, or to give up Greek olives for ripe ones. What I do advise is that you determine the calorie content of each of the choices available to you, and that you understand how important even small differences are in long-range weight control. Then you can decide which foods are worth their caloric cost.

That's not what we've been doing. We've been choosing our foods on the basis of reputation.

Let's talk turkey. Now there's a food with reputation. Except for one particular day in November, anybody who eats turkey is on a diet. To the dieter, turkey is sacred. But you're better off with sacrificial lamb. I know it seems impossible, but roasted leg of lamb has fewer calories than roasted leg of turkey.

And turkey is so much higher in calories than sweetbreads that you can sauté sweetbreads in butter and they will still have fewer calories. Yes, sauté them. Yes, in butter. Yes, fewer calories. I was thrilled to discover that turkey isn't the diet food it's cracked up to be. At last I could stop eating it.

Fish has a reputation for being diet food. Steak has a reputation for being fattening. . . . Salmon is higher in calories than many cuts of beef.

Yet we eat fish when we want meat, we eat Melba toast when we want bread, we eat Chef's Salad when we want something else, and turkey when we want anything else. Then we end up fatter because of it. What's going on here?

It's not for lack of trying. The fact is that we've spent far, far more money on our waistlines than we spent to put mankind on the moon. Yet imagine the physicists at NASA designing our space quest the way we design our diets—by popular myth. Think how it would have mucked up the works if they'd planned the moon landing for a surface made of green cheese.

The problem of putting a man on the moon was a matter of science. The problem of controlling one's weight is also a matter of science. Why, then, have we left our choices to folklore, instead of using objective data?

Because dealing with food subjectively is part of human nature.

Even before we were instructed to finish our cornflakes for the children starving in Europe, we were susceptible. When we endow Chef's Salad, high-calorie Chef's Salad, with a reputation for being "not fattening," we are behaving—well, we are behaving just like people. This is because—though food is material—eating it, my friends, is emotional.

It's always been so, always. Remember that all of mankind's problems started because some guy ate an apple that wasn't on his diet.

Since then, we've been ascribing special powers to food. Sometimes we're right. Take honey, for example. Honey is a food that does have special medicinal properties. It is an anti-inflammatory agent, a natural expectorant that works in much the same way as do Robitussin and other non-narcotic cough syrups.

Honey can soothe a sore throat, which is why many an actress keeps a jar backstage. Though she may not have a notion of why it works, she doesn't find it strange at all that a food can cure an illness.

In just the same way, the Kiganda people of Uganda find nothing strange about feeding their youngsters entrées of insects as the local cure for bedwetting. The belief that food can set things straight is found everywhere. As I was collecting calorie data from the four corners of the earth, I became fascinated with the dazzling array of uses and meanings that food can have. I want to detour for a few moments, and share some of these with you.

A little traveling music, please.

For centuries in China, brews made from dogs, snakes, and tortoises have been used to treat everything from bronchitis to palsy. Weak testicles, for example, may be treated with sheep wine. In Ecuador, toasted tomatoes are used to cure bruises, and the leaves of the plant are set on the stomach to cure indigestion. In Ethiopia, newborns are fed butter to grease the throat in preparation for mother's milk. In Andhra Pradesh, the Telugu-speaking people ingest onions to cure sunstroke, goats' milk for asthma, jambu fruit for diabetes, radishes for jaundice, and raw eggs for chest pain. In the United States of America, people drink orange juice to cure a cold.

But to endow food with power is not always to sing its praises. In parts of Central Asia, fish and eggplant are thought to aggravate skin diseases, and eating eggs in the summer causes boils. For adolescent girls in East and Southeast Asia, papaya, pineapple, and large bananas are taboo because they will cause sexual problems when a young woman is married. Among fishermen in Malaysia, ducks are poisonous if you have an itch, peanuts if you have an open sore, mutton if you have a cough, and cashews if you have scabies.

And while we Americans grab for Vitamin Citrus at the drop of a sniffle, that's not the case in other parts of the world. In East, Southeast, and Central Asia—in Pakistan, for example—citrus fruits are off-limits when you have a cold. Thousands of miles from Asia, in Central America, these fruits are proscribed in much the same way. Citrus fruits are forbidden to pregnant women, as they chill the body and cause respiratory illness in the unborn child. In Nicaragua, citrus fruits cause nasal obstruction in infants, while in the Philippines they curdle breastmilk and promote hemorrhage. Linus who?

Everybody knows that a sound maternal diet is essential to the health of the mother and to the child she carries. But exactly what constitutes a sound maternal diet varies strikingly from place to place. In Vietnam a pregnant woman may go hungry, believing that "excessive nourishment" will cause her fetus to grow too large. She will allow herself deer or peacock feet, which are reputed to increase lactation, while avoiding "sticky rice," pigeons, squid, and crabs, which cause a hard labor and delivery. In Indonesia, it's buffalo meat that causes difficult labor, while in Burma it's bananas. For the pregnant Waluguru tribeswoman in Tanzania, meat causes stillbirth and cowpeas stunt growth. A pregnant Wachaga woman must not eat in the company of women who have had miscarriages, and, since the fetus eats when the mother does, she must chew her food carefully to avoid choking her unborn child. The Isheg people of East Asia believe that eating twin bananas begets twins.

The diet of the growing child is also regulated by culture. When a newborn of the Waluguru tribe is not faring well, a drop of the mother's breastmilk is set on a tripod in the open air. Should a fly settle upon it, the breastmilk is presumed to be the cause of the illness and is withheld. In Malaysia and the Philippines, too much rice makes a child grow "wilted." In Indonesia, soybeans cause eye disease in infants. Tunisian children who eat the tail of an animal will be backward, and allowing children to eat the head of a fish or bird will encourage them to eat their father's head as well. Nigerian children who eat eggs become thieves.

The bias against eggs is widespread. In western Kenya, feeding eggs to children retards their ability to walk or talk. Eggs are taboo in Chad as well. The egg, being thought a "silent" thing, will forever keep a child from speaking. This is markedly similar to restrictions found in Asia. A widespread Buddhist belief holds that feeding eggs to children who have not yet learned to talk may prevent them from ever speaking of previous incarnations.

Not only the egg, but the chicken, too, is heir to tradition and lore. In Malaysia, chicken can be poisonous if you eat it when your stomach is upset, while for the rural Filipino, chicken gizzard is an aid to digestion. In Catigugan, a Filipino husband will feed his postpartum wife boiled chicken and unsalted corn porridge with a drop of blood from her placenta. To the north, in Ilocos Norte, chicken causes leprosy if it's cooked with squash and fruit.

Not that foul or fowl pharmacopoeia is confined to faraway places with strange sounding names. In regions of Austria, Russia, and Brooklyn—in fact, in generation after generation of my very own family—streptococcus has been laid low with chicken soup.

Tomato soup, on the other hand, has had a different history. The tomato was widely used for decoration, but believed to be deadly poisonous—not by aboriginal tribespeople, but by Englishmen. However, a French designation—*pomme d'amour*—gave the tomato a nickname, *love apple*. The tomato was reputed to be an aphrodisiac. It did wonders for sales.

The belief that you can eat your way to love forebodes one animal's extinction. In India and Sumatra, poachers gun down the rhinoceros, taking the horn and leaving the rest behind. The horn of the rhino has become one of the world's most precious commodities, more expensive by the ounce than platinum. Ground into a powder, it is sold for the most part to wealthy Chinese. The hope is that it will make the user, you should pardon the expression, horny.

And I even know of one culture—strange as this may sound—where teenage boys, hoping to make teenage girls horny, slipped aspirin into their Cokes.

Current fashion regarding our passion tells us to avoid garlic like the plague. Do you ever order salami on a date? "Of course not," you say, "but that's common sense, not fashion." No? Ask the French. We presume their expertise in matters amorous, and yet the French eat garlic, liberally, all the time. Just ride the Métro during rush hour—not just the evening, but the morning rush hour. Still, we Americans believe that eating garlic will ward off lovers, just as Central Europeans believed that wearing garlic would ward off vampires. In preparing this study I tried both eating garlic and wearing it, and found that only one of them worked.

Our attitude toward garlic is mild among American food taboos. Taboos? Taboos? Did she say "Taboos"? Well, if not for taboo, then for what other reason would McDonald's go out of business gracefully rather than announce: "In Order To Give You A Tastier, Less Expensive, Low-Calorie Burger, Our Main Ingredient Will Now Be Horsemeat"?

Our American distaste for horsemeat, which we share with several other Western cultures, actually is a vestigial religious taboo. It began with an eighth-century Pope, Gregory III, as an act of disassociation from the pagan tribes in Asia who ate horsemeat as part of their rituals. Horsemeat is still a favorite meal in Asia, as it has been at the Faculty Club of Harvard University.

There are people who would not be able to hold a meal down if they discovered that Roti de Cheval meant "Roasted Horsemeat," and not "Roasted Chicken." One man's meat can indeed be another man's poison. But there's an even better illustration of that, and it happens also to serve as the perfect example of how people endow what they eat with magic.

The example is the widely accepted explanation for ritual cannibalism. The presumed power in this food is the power that the cannibal ascribes to the person he is about to eat. The victor eats the heart or liver of his worthy opponent, incorporating the body parts of one whose virtues he would like to call his own. That which he ingests, the seats of wisdom, cunning, and bravery, adds to his self-esteem. The rest of the equation is easy to fill in. These virtues are now in the sole possession of the cannibal—at least until he runs into someone with an overwhelming respect for him.

"You are who you eat." A foreign myth.

"You are what you eat." The American counterpart.

Does that mean we urge fish on swimmers? No, but not so long ago fish had a reputation as brain food. People ate fish thinking it would make them smarter. In the same way, we urge children to eat carrots by saying they are good for the eyes. We tell them that eating spinach makes them stronger. (Awful riddle: What happens if you eat too many carrots and too much spinach at the same time? (You become Pop-eyed.)

Certainly, there are foods that do have special powers. Your morning cup of coffee really can wake you up. It's coffee's genuine power that helps sustain its reputation and its enormous commercial success. But, again, to endow a food with power is not always to sing its praises.

The year is 1951, and the food in question—the prune. Because of the prune's reputation, people limited its use. If you were eating prunes it could be for one reason only. Accordingly, people were embarrassed to eat them publicly. Order prunes in a restaurant? Serve them to guests at dinner? Carry them as snacks? Impossible. Prune growers, in despair, took their problem to Ernest Dichter, Ph.D. At that time, his company was called the Institute for Motivational Research. It's now called Ernest Dichter Motivations, Inc.

Sometimes Dr. Dichter is hired to find out why people buy things. Mostly he is hired to find out why they don't. When he considered the prune, for a consideration from the California Prune Advisory Board, he and his staff found that it had personality problems. Consumers were given word association tests. It wasn't surprising that people identified prunes with constipation, but for many people prunes also connoted stinginess, coldness, puritanism. People even associated the poor prune with boarding houses. As Dr. Dichter explains, "While peaches are juicy, the word 'peach' being used to describe young, attractive women, prunes bring to mind dried-up spinsters. My job was to take the wrinkles out of the prune."

And Dr. Dichter did. Ads became bright, colorful, glamorous. The prune was never shown by itself, but always in the company of other, more romantic fruits. What was once just a prune was now a super-ripe plum, super-ripe from soaking up the sunshine . . . ready, willing, and able to bestow its stored-up energy on you. The prune had become the California Wonder Fruit. We still knew it was a laxative, but now it was also first cousin to candy. By the late fifties, while crop values in this country were generally stable, prices paid to the prune grower rose by more than 50%.

So, possessing the power is secondary. It's possessing the reputation that makes a food a winner.

Making that very point, a Pakistani once told me that in his native country, a country bursting at its seams with overpopulation, women eat "pan," a confection made from shredded betel nuts, for the purpose of contraception. That may be difficult for us to understand. But I have a question for a pan-chewing Pakistani. Ask her if she understands why in America, a country also bursting at the seams, people eat Melba toast for the purpose of losing weight.

I do not know if pharmacies in Pakistan push the sale of betel-nut contraception. But for sure in America, restaurants promote the myth of Melba toast by forcing it on us every time we order a dish from that box marked "Dieter's Special."

It's marked "Dieter's Special" because the restaurant owner is also on a diet, and s/he picks his or her food the way anybody else would. Not based on the objective data that are, after all, available—but based on reputation.

In our American culture, dieting is so firmly linked with deprivation that we figure if a food doesn't taste too good it can't be all bad. Were you surprised that turkey and Melba toast have more calories than some delicious counterparts? Sure you were. Turkey and Melba toast don't taste fattening. That's because they don't taste at all.

There is a second route a food can take to acquire a reputation as "not fattening." In present-day America, the concept of being thin and the concept of being healthy are so closely associated that once we decide a food is good for us, we automatically assume it will help us diet as well. After all, how can anything healthy be fattening? Well . . .

You're on a diet, but your urge for rice pudding cannot be contained. Still, you're in contact with reality and you tell them to hold the whipped cream. But you don't tell them to hold the raisins. Of course you don't. Raisins are fruit. Raisins are natural. Raisins are healthy. Tablespoon for tablespoon, raisins have more calories than whipped cream.

If you love the raisins, then by all means indulge. But if you would no more eat rice pudding for its raisins than a hot fudge sundae for its cherry, it's better to pay the surcharge to have them picked out. If rice pudding is your obsession and you eat it every day, those few little raisins that get mixed into the pudding could make a two-and-a-half-pound difference in your weight for the year. Calories do show up in surprising places, don't they? A raisin is a surprising place to find a lot of calories. Where do they hide?

Now, as long as we're on the subject of rice, and as long as we're on the subject of natural, let's talk about brown rice. It's the perfect example of natural. It's the perfect example of healthy. People who wouldn't dream of eating the calories in white rice feel free to down the brown. Brown rice has more fiber than white rice does. It also has more calories.

Oh.

The word "healthy" has taken America by storm. The word's become so popular, it's changing the language. Foods cannot, in fact, be healthy. By the time they take on the character of food, they've long since forgotten any health of their own. Foods that impart health are properly called "healthful." But I bow to custom in keeping with the intent of these pages—"healthy" it is, and onward!

Let's look at honey again. It may make sense to use honey to relieve a sore throat. But does it make sense to use honey, as so many people do, because it's the bee's knees for a diet? Reputation has it that honey, a so-called natural sugar, is less fattening than refined sugar. That's objective, all right. It's dieting according to the principles of Euclidean geometry:

If A = B and B = C, then A = C.
If Honey = Healthy and Healthy = Thin, then Honey = Thin.

Tablespoon for tablespoon, honey has one-third more calories than ordinary table sugar. Another reputation bites the dust.

And where does all this reputation come from? Remember the prune?

In my experience, the foods that we consider special for dieters are special for those who want to keep dieting. Pick a food that always makes it into the Dieter's Box. Let's pick cottage cheese. People who don't really like it really eat it. They feel healthy when they do. The restaurant owner also feels healthy while s/he's eating cottage cheese, and Euclid strikes again. When you order the "Diet Hamburger" you get the same hamburger but it comes without the bun. The bun has been replaced by the cheese. The thin gentleman sitting three tables away gets his on the bun. Maybe that's why he's thin.

And then there's the "Dieter's Fresh Fruit Platter." Ah, yes. The Fresh and semi-Fresh Fruit Platter. We know it well. We order it to feed the soul. Order it, and your friends admire you. Order it, and you feel constructive. The aspiring actress sitting in the next booth feels so constructive when she eats it, that she eats it on her lunch hour every day. Unfortunately, she feels a little less comfortable about the sweetener she knows is in her diet soda. Yet she drinks that every day, too, because it makes her feel smaller—and when it comes to matters of vanity, what's a little discomfort here and there? So she chews away contentedly on her fruit, interspersing it with bites of Jell-O. Jell-O? Sure, you know, it's the red stuff they slip under the cottage cheese.

Now, before our friend drinks her soda, she squeezes in enough lemon to mask the taste. If you ask her when she had her last Coke, she'll answer right away. It was her birthday. After all, what could be higher-calorie than Coke? Jell-O could. One cup of Jell-O has more calories than one and a half cups of Coke.

How can that be, if you like Coke better?

And that's the way we diet. What we've been counting are subjective calories. No wonder people were surprised that calorie counting worked for me.

I've concluded that losing weight has something in common with learning Zen: It is said that when you know nothing of Zen, the rivers are rivers, the mountains are mountains, and the trees are trees. . . . When you know something of Zen, the rivers are no longer rivers, the mountains are no longer mountains, and the trees are no longer trees. . . . But when you know Zen, then rivers are truly rivers, mountains are truly mountains, and the trees are trees once more . . .

. . . One day in the fourth grade, Mrs. Greene explained to the class that what we weighed would depend upon the calories we took in and the ones we "gave out." I have at various times believed in carbohydrates, crazy combinations, and diet pills. I have investigated, but chickened out of, hypnosis and hormones. My hat is off to you, Mrs. Greene. It is the calorie, after all.

Surely into each life a Mrs. Greene must fall. Why, then, don't we just believe her?

The answer is that she has too much competition. And the competition that she has comes from the very people to whom we go for help, our experts: Our doctors. Our diet writers. Our diet clubs.

If you are overweight you've probably consulted all three. You try the first. You try the second when the first doesn't work. You try the third when the second doesn't work. You try the first when the third doesn't work. Which is more fattening, the chicken or the egg?

The doctor probably comes first. That's because you won't have to ask your doctor for advice. You will probably be given the advice whether you ask for it or not, and whether or not you want it.

I know, because when it comes to doctors and the way they deal with body weight, my first-hand experience is vast. Recollections of the dieting instructions given to me as a child are vague as to the specifics, but I remember well the all-pervasive message. How could I forget? It helped to form my earliest self-image.

The message was repeated to me by doctors with every check-up, with every injection of penicillin, with every weekly allergy shot. The message was given to me by the orthopedist who set my broken arm, and by the surgeon who took my tonsils out. While photographs of me taken before the second grade show a very pretty, perfectly normal-size youngster, I cannot remember a time in my life when I did not think of myself as fat.

I was fat, or so they said in their reprimands, because I gorged myself with cake and ice cream and candy. I was fat, or so they said in their reprimands, because I ate twice as much as I should. What a frightening thought to a child! But what frightened me more was the logical conclusion. I was a freak. I resigned myself to fatitude.

The first medical diet directive that I can quote word for word was given to me when I was fourteen, and in my junior year in high school. It was to "Eat as much beef as possible. Protein uses up 75% of its calories in the process of its own digestion." This advice was handed to me with a free sample of diet pills, and a prescription for more. Uppers. Speed. Habit forming. Fourteen.

I had requested neither the advice nor the pills, but I took both.

As for the advice, while it is true that protein may use more calories in its own digestion than carbohydrate does, or fat, the calories consumed in that process have already been accounted for in calorie tables. Values cited by the Department of Agriculture, and copied commercially, are net calories. The numbers tell you how much energy is available after a food has paid for its own digestion. A 300-calorie hamburger has 300 calories.

As for the diet pills, it was two years later during my first semester in college that I began to understand the implications of needing to take them although it had been ages since they affected my appetite. I locked myself in my room, a nice Jewish girl from Brooklyn, and went cold turkey at the age of sixteen.

When I was twenty, I heard it announced on the radio that a renowned institute for psychoanalysis was offering group therapy to people with weight problems. The psychiatrist who would lead the group was even renownder than the institute, having written profusely on obesity and self-improvement. "That's for me!" thought I. "What better way to get smaller than to go to a shrink?"

One of the things he told us repeatedly was that we did not merely overeat, we overate outrageously. I remember his admonishing us, and this I promise is verbatim: "You have to work very hard to be fat."

The group met for five years. Our famous psychiatrist left after about three years and was replaced by one who was not famous, but gorgeous. To the best of my recollection, at the last session of the group each one of us—each and every one of us—was fatter than when the group began.

But my most traumatic medical encounter was not at the hands of a psychiatrist. It took place in my obstetrician's office. More than my obstetrician, for many years he had been my friend. I was in my third month of pregnancy and the scale showed that I had gained weight. My friend became visibly upset. I was confused. I couldn't understand why I was gaining.

"You're anxious about being pregnant," he told me. "Stop bingeing!"

"That's not the answer," I said. "If I were bingeing I would know why I was gaining."

He insisted that I was eating and eating. I insisted that I was not.

It's difficult for me to describe what followed, although I remember it clearly, just as it can be difficult to describe a dream although you remember its every detail. "You're gorging yourself with cake and ice cream and candy," he shouted—a louder version of my childhood's reprimands. But this time I wasn't a defenseless kid. I refused to accept what he was saying.

He became furious. "You're lying!" he screamed at me. "You're going to kill yourself and you're lying!"

I was sobbing, but unyielding: "Ask my husband what I eat!"

When my husband came into the office he told the doctor I was right: "In the whole time she's been pregnant I haven't seen her eat one piece of anything like cake." And do you know what my obstetrician said to that? "Then she's been eating it in the closet!"

I was thunderstruck. I asked my friend if he realized that he was calling me a liar and a sneak. "Either that," he shouted, "or even you don't know that you're doing it!"

It was a valuable experience. It further confirmed my distrust of experts, and it fired my curiosity. I knew I wasn't eating cake. How had I gained weight?

When I began counting calories I realized exactly how.

I had been seen for one visit by my obstetrician's associate. I told him about my morning sickness, which began in the morning and continued on into the night. His prescription? He was hesitant to give me drugs, but instead suggested foods with medicinal properties. Goodly amounts of those tried and true folk remedies for an upset stomach: ginger ale, and concentrated Coca-Cola syrup. These, along with the extra milk that I was required to drink, were enough to account for every ounce I had gained—every last ounce. But I had never even given it a thought. How can anything healthy be fattening?

I can't quote verbatim all the lectures that doctors gave me, but I can tell you one I never had, but should have had. I was twenty-five pounds overweight in the sixth grade. If even one doctor had said to me then, "You know, Margo, you really don't have to cut out very much in order to be slim like the other kids. Maybe two hundred calories a day. If you cut down by only a little, it may take you longer to lose weight. But if you start now, you won't ever have to be a fat teenager." That is advice I can quote verbatim as never having had.

The advice I could not get from doctors was not available in bookstores either. At least, I never found it.

When I went to bookstores for the last word on losing weight, I was usually directed to the section called "Health." There I would find books telling me what foods to eat or not to eat to cure or prevent arthritis, multiple sclerosis, cancer, aging, typhoid fever, and fat. Buyer beware! Booksellers: Load a shopping cart with books about diet and pull them out of the "Health" section. Re-stack them where they belong. In "Magic."

Our shelves are filled with books that tell us that the best way to win the war against calories is to ignore them. Sometimes these books make it to the top of the bestseller list. Some twenty-five years ago, before its claims were refuted, the book *Calories Don't Count* caused a craze. On page 81 the author asks us, "Why, then, do people follow low-calorie diets?" We were answered: "Because dietary habits persist, regardless of logic."

I have the same answer in this book, but my question is different. Answer: "Because dietary habits persist, regardless of logic." Question: "Why will a dieter grin and bear Melba toast, although it has more calories than bread?"

One of the more popular anti-calorie crusades is an updated version of the old low-carbohydrate approach. It was brought to center stage this time around by Robert C. Atkins, M.D. I've known people who swear by the low-carbohydrate diet, and others who swear at it. Can it be that this diet works for some people, but not for others?

The Atkins low-carbohydrate diet allows you to eat some of the highest-calorie foods in the world—bacon, brisket, and duckling; mayonnaise and butter. The reason that these foods are high in calories is because of their high fat content. It takes more time to digest fat than to digest any other nutrient, so high-fat foods stay longer in the gut. Bacon "sticks to the ribs."

On the other hand, you begin to digest carbohydrates even before they leave your mouth. Enzymes in your salivary juices break down the starch and complex sugars into simple sugars, and these are absorbed very quickly once they hit the stomach. This helps to explain a common Chinese restaurant experience, and here the Cantonese cuisine has a well-earned reputation. We can consume gargantuan amounts of Chinese foods that are basically carbohydrate—rice, vegetables, noodles, and cornstarch gravy—only to feel hungry again in an hour.

We don't yet know all the factors that contribute to the feelings of satiety, either to its onset, or how long it will last. But aside from the fact that fat "sticks to the ribs" and stays there longer, there is another aspect of a low-carbohydrate diet that may affect caloric intake. By striking carbohydrates from your diet, the restricted variety of foods you can choose from may make the quantities self-limiting. How much corned beef can you eat before you lose your taste for pastrami?

Carbohydrates, fat, and protein are our sources of energy. Limiting any one of these in your diet accomplishes that same phenomenon. What do you think would likely happen if instead of limiting carbohydrates, you restricted your diet to mounds of it? Putting it another way—have you known many fat vegetarians?

What about a diet that restricts protein, but allows you all the carbohydrates and fat that you want? I'll invent one. Feiden's Fabulous Fudge Diet. Vitamin pills, plenty of water, and all the chocolate, double chocolate, Dutch chocolate, German chocolate, vanilla—and strawberry if you can find it—fudge you can eat. But absolutely nothing else. I submit that by the second week you will start losing weight. (I'll call that book *The Fudge Factor.*)

If carbohydrate counting works for you, this may be why it works. If you try counting your calories along with carbohydrates, you may discover that you've been on a low-calorie diet all along, and giving up some great food for no good reason.

Giving up food, both great food and otherwise, is the advice of yet another flock of diet books. Fasting. One jacket describes it as the "Ultimate Diet." I can't argue with that.

Fasting works, but only until you start to eat. If you lose weight by fasting, what have you learned about eating? You haven't learned to equate food with calories. If you don't know the numbers, how will you keep the weight off?

Still, as dieters going to our bookstores, we are confonted with an abundance of books that promise just that. They will teach us how to lose weight while avoiding the reality of the calorie. On their covers these books claim that what we will find inside is indeed, and at last, the definitive better mousetrap.

Book jackets promise us: "No calorie counting here." We are lured into taking drastic steps to change our figures, and as far-fetched as the theories are, we may lose weight by following the instructions of some of them. Problems arise when we try to maintain the loss. We haven't understood the real reason why these diets work, and how can we apply what we do not understand? The author has elaborated some new philosophy, but if you look behind the philosophy, there's likely to be a low-calorie diet lurking in the wings.

One book caught my eye, *Losing Weight While You Sleep.* You can't doubt the veracity of that one. How can you help but lose weight while you're sleeping? But why take 156 pages to tell us about it? Well, it turns out to be more complicated than sleeping. You "Reduce by Re-programming Your Mind." The cover admits that this "foolproof pounds-off revolution"—"Sounds like a miracle," but promises you right there that simply by using this method, called RRPM, you can "eat foods you enjoy without getting fat."

The appendix of this book is a collection of low-calorie menu plans, prefaced with the author's suggestion that you "purchase a companion volume—any one of those inexpensive books that list the number of calories in every common food."

I picked up the next book, *The Meditation Diet.* My hopes soared as high for this opus as they had for the one before it. No question about it, while you meditate you're losing weight. This jacket promises, meditate, and "Be Fat-Free Forever." Meditate, and you can "Lose Weight Without Drugs, Exercise, Calorie Counting and Crazy Gadgets." Note well: calorie counting is placed in line with drugs and crazy gadgets as though it were a soldier of equal rank, not even an officer, in the same nefarious army.

For more than one hundred pages we are taught about meditation. Then along about page 121, we are told that a new discussion is going to begin. Now we are going to talk about a "system of dieting that is specifically designed to help you achieve the weight control that you desire." The book tells us, finally, that "Reducing the kind of calories found in carbohydrate foods, such as sugar, bread, candy, cereal, milk, ice cream, pizza, spaghetti, and even alcohol, forces the body to turn to the reservoir of fat already within it." We're informed that "a diet that is too exaggerated in fat input results in too many calories, which can only be turned into unwanted layers of fat."

Then I came to *Dr. Siegal's Natural Fiber Permanent Weight-Loss Diet.* Was I more optimistic because its author was an M.D.? Nope. The books about sleeping and meditating your fat away were both written by M.D.'s. So was *Calories Don't Count,* by Dr. Herman Taller, a gynecologist.

Dr. Siegal's "Diet Discovery," says the cover, "is that you are not eating enough!" The cover proclaims that Dr. Siegal's breakthrough is "the most dramatic medical discovery of our times." This book promises to explain why "it is not what we are eating that is making us overweight and even killing us—it is what we aren't eating." Dr. Siegal takes 130 pages to explain what it is we aren't eating.

And then on page 131: "On this High-Fiber Reducing Diet, your breakfast will usually consist of a very high-fiber cereal only, or occasionally a low-calorie egg substitute, and you must not skip it. Lunch will be rather simple and quite low calorie. Dinner will be liberal and will prove quite adequate. Any intake between meals should be of a minimal nature . . . You should also use abnormally large amounts of very low-calorie foods to fill yourself up." When all is said and done, the "diet" part of the ". . . greatest breakthrough in dieting history," is a low-calorie diet.

Still, we should count our blessings. Luckily, no one is beating the drum for a low-water diet. If I found out tomorrow that an "expert" was writing *Weight Loss Through Dehydration,* I'd make papier-mâché from my shares of Perrier.

Am I being too cynical? Well, in 1961 when *Calories Don't Count* was published, people swarmed to their pharmacies to buy capsules of fat, of safflower oil. These they would swallow for the purpose of losing weight. Safflower oil is a whopping two hundred and fifty calories an ounce. Is there an entry in **The Calorielogue** that is higher in calories than safflower oil? Yes. Lard.

Books on "How to Lose Weight" go on and on and on, ad infinauseam. In this country alone, more than one dozen billion pages have gone into the printer's press blank and have come out discussing diet. Still I am asked the same question over, and over, and over again:

"What is your secret?"

Books that promote misinformation eclipse the useful information. Should the public be protected?

In his landmark opinion in Schenck v. United States, Justice Oliver Wendell Holmes addressed the question of whether limitations could be applied to the constitutional right to freedom of speech. What a man may write or say to the public, Justice Holmes decided, may under certain circumstances be restrained. The criterion he enunciated has become the now well-known test of "clear and present danger." Freedom of speech, he concluded, does not include the freedom to falsely shout FIRE! in a crowded theater.

Do I favor suppression of those books whose mythologies render us helpless when we attempt to combat our obesity?

No, I do not. I do believe these books represent a clear and present danger. I think they are very dangerous. But who is omniscient enough to make the censor's judgement? Members of the same profession that once ostracized a prescient obstetrician, Ignaz Philipp Semmelweiss?

In the mid-1800s, Dr. Semmelweiss tried to persuade his fellow physicians that they might reduce the many deaths in childbirth (puerperal fever) by disinfecting their hands between the dissecting room and their patients' beds. He met with unanimous opposition. When Semmelweiss finally ordered his medical students to use antiseptics, he was able to reduce childbirth mortality by over 90%. This courageous pioneer was promptly driven from Vienna by his jealous colleagues.

As a footnote to history, Justice Holmes's father was engaged in a similar struggle on this side of the Atlantic. My shelf-worn edition of the *Encyclopaedia Britannica* tells the story: "In 1843 he [Dr. Oliver Wendell Holmes] published his essay on the *Contagiousness of Puerperal Fever,* which brought upon him bitter personal abuse; but he maintained his position with dignity, temper, and judgement; and in time he was honoured as the discoverer of a beneficent truth."

So, I would fight to protect the dietmongers from censorship of any kind, but I'll not restrain my criticism. Sometimes I read a book that seems genuinely well-intentioned, however implausible its doctrine. But most of the time it seems that the author, whether motivated by money, or out for the fame, knows very well s/he's promoting nonsense. I think a whole bunch of diet books are written by people who don't mind shouting "Fire!" in a theater filled with susceptible crowds.

Susceptible. Vulnerable because what we weigh gets us where we sit. And misery, loving company, sends us finally to Weight Watchers, or forces us to Weigh of Life. Devotees of "Dear Abby" have been directed to Overeaters Anonymous.

And when we get there we are presented with a diet and a philosophy. Both come so well-disguised as wholesome that we dare not question their validity. When people fail at these diets they assume the failure is theirs. The failure, in fact, is in the concept. These organizations base their philosophies, and their diets, on the premise that human beings eat for fuel. But I know, and you know, too, that we want more from our food than that. For food may be material, but getting it, cooking it, tasting it, eating it, loving and remembering it—all these, my friends, are emotional.

Among popular diet organizations, the one with which I am most familiar is Weight Watchers.

The first thing Weight Watchers tells us is that we must revamp our style of eating. We must no longer eat sinfully; we must now eat sensibly. To make sure I understood the terminology, I called the headquarters of Weight Watchers International to find out what "sensible" means. I asked, "Why does your organization keep using that word?" The answer: "Because the Weight

Watchers diet is the most sensible diet that exists. Because its required foods provide the proper balance of nutrients, a balance of vitamins and minerals."

The plain fact about "required" foods is that all your required vitamins and minerals are obtainable in simple, over-the-counter, practically calorie-free capsules.

Vitamins in capsule form may offer an advantage over vitamins in food—the dose is more reliable. Let's suppose that you're relying on required vegetables for your vitamins and minerals. Let's say you're relying on spinach, that vegetable with a reputation. If so, you should realize this: Whatever nutrients have managed to survive the exposure to air, light, and heat as your spinach made its odyssey from farmer to fridge still have to face their Waterloo. It's a perilous journey from your refrigerator to your table. As you boil your spinach, water-soluble vitamins end up in the water—the B vitamins and Vitamin C.

What about iron? Have you heard that leafy green vegetables are high in iron? They are. But the iron that's in most vegetables, spinach included, is so difficult to absorb that it is essentially useless. And anyway, iron is water-soluble—and it ends up in the water, too. What about calcium? Yes, spinach has lots of calcium. But spinach also has oxalic acid, which binds the calcium and makes it difficult to absorb. Worse, the oxalic acid you eat in your spinach may bind the calcium you're getting from other foods as well. If you don't feel comfortable unless you think you've gotten your vitamin supply "naturally," then cook the spinach to death and drink the water.

But I say, take a vitamin pill and then eat spinach if you like spinach.

This doesn't mean that vitamin pills can or should replace food. For one thing, foods almost certainly contain important chemicals that haven't been promoted to vitaminship yet. For another thing, food tastes so good. But if you're eating spinach because some diet requires it, then as you chew please note that for every cup of required spinach you don't eat, you can have two cups of popcorn at the movies. For each cup of required carrots you don't eat, you could put a whole tablespoon of chocolate syrup into your required skim milk.

If you find that eating carrots and eating spinach is simply ingesting fuel, but that munching on popcorn and drinking chocolate-flavored milk is ingesting pleasure, ask yourself this: Is it possible that your ability to stay on any diet is in direct proportion to the entertainment value it holds for you?

If so, then why not eat for pleasure? If you get more pleasure from eating an apple in piecrust than from eating an apple in its original container then why eat an apple instead of apple pie? A 100-calorie portion of apple pie is no more or less fattening than a 100-calorie portion of apple, in exactly the same way as a ton of coal is neither heavier nor lighter than a ton of feathers. People think it is. The refined versus natural sugar myth again. Of course it can be argued, and with reason, that there is greater volume in a 100-calorie serving of fruit than in a 100-calorie serving of fruit pie. But experience teaches that in certain matters, especially in those emotional, fulfillment isn't found in quantity alone.

—This is some crazy book! First this woman advocates eight and a half portions of mashed potatoes, and now it's apple pie! Surely they should take her away! . . . Except for one thing. I lost one hundred and fifty pounds, and you can't argue with success.

My success came with learning to manipulate calories. But to shuffle the numbers, you have to know them first. Diet organizations readily acknowledge that calories count. What they're opposed to is your counting them for yourself. They say you'll get into trouble if you think.

That point was driven home to me a number of years ago at my local deli. A dieter was complaining to the counterman that he loved grilled cheese sandwiches for breakfast, but he was frustrated because he could only have one slice of American cheese on his one slice of bread. I'm a buttinsky, so I didn't hesitate to offer a ray of hope. "You could try the low-fat cheese," I suggested. "Then you could have two slices for exactly the same number of calories."

"I'm not allowed," he said.

"Not allowed?" I answered with surprise. "Not allowed by whom?"

He was a Weight Watcher, and subject to the law of No Substitutions. I tried reason. "Calorically, two ounces of one are identical to one ounce of the other," I pleaded. We discussed it for a quarter of an hour. He agreed to ask his lecturer's permission, but until then it was going to be one slice of the high-fat cheese. His devotion intrigued me. Was this his established way of life? Or was he new, and still overzealous? I asked him how long he had been a member. "This time?" he asked.

Since this encounter, Weight Watchers has come out with its own brand of reduced-calorie cheese. This would have solved my delicatessen friend's problem, but it doesn't change the point of the story: You're taught not to think in terms of calories.

Yet even if you intend to follow the W.W. diet to the letter, even then, understanding calories is vital. It could make all the difference to your weight. When I attended Weight Watchers, the program required me to choose my foods from specified groups such as "Fruits," "Vegetables," and "Poultry, Meat, Fish." Strange things can happen when you make one choice over another perfectly "equal" choice. For if there is no such thing as "a medium cantaloupe"—then I assure you there is no such thing as "Fruit."

Peaches, nectarines, cantaloupes, and grapefruit—all of these were choices under "Fruits." But where did they say that, ounce for ounce, nectarines have almost twice as many calories as peaches? Where did they say that the "½ small cantaloupe" they allowed would probably have twice as many calories as the "½ medium grapefruit" they allowed?

You know I won't advise against the cantaloupe. But I do advise you to know the difference between the two, so that you can eat half a cantaloupe only on days when half a cantaloupe is twice as appealing as half a grapefruit. When the cantaloupe is only one and a half times as appealing, you might decide to be stoic and stick to the grapefruit. Or, once you know that half a cantaloupe has the same calories as two half grapefruits, you could decide to have two half grapefruits instead. But don't ever simply call them "Fruit" and mistake one for the other. That would be like mixing apples and oranges.

Oh, you could follow the Weight Watchers diet as the night follows the day, but unknowingly make high-calorie choices within each group, even if you didn't prefer the higher-calorie foods. You could follow the diet as the night the day, but the difference between following it in one way and following it in another could make a one-pound difference in your weight every week.

That's fifty-two pounds a year.

Now that's all right if you're deriving an extra fifty-two pounds' worth of pleasure. Only you can judge that. It's an important judgement to make. You're supposed to follow the diet for the rest of your life.

If you do, you'll have exactly three meals a day, every day of every year, year in and year out, no less and no more. You aren't allowed more than three meals a day, and you aren't allowed fewer.

To me, the idea of telling people who want to lose weight that they should eat three meals a day, whether or not they are hungry, makes about as much sense as telling people on a budget to spend money three times a day, whether or not there's something they want to buy.

I've found nothing to convince me that eating three meals a day is natural to the human animal, or in itself beneficial to a dieter. I don't eat three meals a day, I'm sure of that. On days when I'm not particularly hungry, I'll often eat just two meals. When I spend my whole day writing I don't eat meals at all—I snack instead, whenever I'm hungry. I don't stop writing, so I choose my food for its portability. It has to be transferable from plate to mouth via left thumb and index finger. Bless you John Montagu, Fourth Earl of Sandwich!

The Weight Watchers program would have programmed me to eat three meals a day, and eat them at the same arbitrarily appointed hours. The same basic meals at the same basic times, when I know—and you know, too—that we have different appetites every day. Our needs for food are chameleon-like; they change with our surroundings.

Our appetites change with changes in our activity, changes in the weather, and changes in our mood. Food can function as an antidepressant. Food can function as a tranquilizer. That's a fact of life. Telling a human being to eat with his intellect and disregard his temperament is like telling a goldfish to breathe with his lungs instead of his gills. For food may be material, but eating it is—is and always has been, is and probably always will be—emotional.

By keeping track of my calories, by observing my own patterns over periods of time, I have learned about myself as an eater. I know that I will usually eat less on Monday than on any other day, because my stomach doesn't start the week until Tuesday. I know that I usually eat more when I eat with other people than when I eat alone. I expect that I will "over" eat when I eat with my family, for the starving children in Europe. And because I have learned to expect these patterns in my appetite, it no longer causes me anxiety if I eat ten courses when a grandmother is serving them.

It no longer causes me anxiety to eat ten courses because I've learned to predict, and because I've learned how to compensate. Compensation means knowing by how much you've gone overboard, then knowing how to go underboard.

Diets that are rigid doom us from the start. They require us to eat required food whether or not we are hungry. We can never have fewer calories to offset the times we will have more. And at times we will have more. Of course we will! Yes, if we are motivated enough we can stick to any diet for a while. But how long can we stay on a diet that is inflexible? And when we stray on organization diets, what then?

The Weight Watchers organization has added two words to the dictionary of diet terminology. Now you can eat in a way that is "legal" and in a way that is "illegal." The words suggest that the person who transgresses the limits of a diet is a criminal.

To be legal, you must eat sensibly. To be legal, you have to eat when you're not hungry. To be legal, you must eat on Friday basically what you ate on Thursday. To be legal, you must eat on Friday what everybody else ate on Thursday. To be legal, my chance acquaintance had to have one slice of high-fat cheese instead of two slices of low-fat cheese. To be legal, you must eat "2–3 servings" of bread each and every day if you're a woman, but "4–5 servings" a day if you're a man. I wonder, will they have to change the diet if the E.R.A. passes?

Anyone who would order millions of people to eat a specified amount of bread every day is a wolf in sheep's clothing, posing as a dietician, but behaving like a deity. Or behaving like Procrustes.

Procrustes lived in Greek mythology. He played host to weary travelers, offering them splendid food and inviting them to spend the night. Then he tailor-fit his visitors to the bed they slept in—stretching or slicing his guests to suit the mattress size. His accommodations became famous, as you can imagine, and the expression "procrustean bed" refers to forced and arbitrary conformity. The Weight Watchers version is "procrustean bread." I think they have a lot of crust.

As it took a lot of crust to tell us that we had to eat "at least three" fish meals a week, or even one.

Assuming that every one of us, we millions, liked fish, then it might be easy for us all to have eaten three fish meals every week. Easy, that is, as long as we were on the East Coast or the West Coast, or other areas where you could buy fresh seafood. But if you were not, it meant that somebody was ordering you to eat canned or frozen fish. If I had to choose between weekly meals of frozen fish or sawdust, I'd consider the sawdust. It's no doubt just as filling, and it has fewer calories. Millions of people for whom the diet was prescribed live between the Coasts in the heartland of America. Jean Nidetch, founder of Weight Watchers, comes from New York and then moved to California. Both are areas in which fresh fish abound.

But even where fresh fish is available, why did you have to eat it? Well, Weight Watchers said that you should eat fish "because it is high in polyunsaturated fats." If that concerns you, then by all means eat fish. If you like fish better, then by all means eat fish. Otherwise, why not eat steak?

Someone argues: "But to a dieter, fish is better than steak because it's lower in calories." Generally, that's true—but it may not matter. To reach the level of satisfaction to be had from five ounces of steak you may require eight ounces of fish. And the steak might be more entertaining. "Is it possible that your ability to stay on any diet is in direct proportion to the amount of entertainment value it holds for you?"

Entertainment, unlike calories, is subjective. Calories, unlike entertainment, are objective. In my experience, the only successful dieters are those who have learned to strike a balance between the two.

And that is why a diet must be designed by hand. Even in this day and age, a diet is not a commodity that can successfully be mass-produced.

How are mass-produced diets designed, anyway? Weight Watchers was founded in 1961. Their original menu plan, however, was drafted in 1929, by Norman Joliffe, M.D. Dr. Joliffe intended it as a weight-loss diet for patients who had coronary problems. He called it "The Prudent Diet." He advised his patients to cut down on eggs. I assume that Dr. Joliffe's reason for setting a limit on eggs was that egg yolks are high in cholesterol, and not because he agreed with the Bantu tribal belief that they would make a woman uncontrollable with passion.

The Weight Watchers people used the Joliffe diet intact. This is why, on the original Weight Watchers program, you were limited to "4–7 eggs per week" and "only at breakfast or luncheon, not at dinner."

Now, some researchers advise that all males and all post-menopausal females watch their cholesterol intake. But other researchers, even conservative ones, have said that healthy, menstruating females do not need to be on low-cholesterol diets. Since some 95% of the Weight Watchers membership is female, and between the ages of twenty-five and fifty, why should the diet limit cholesterol? If not to limit cholesterol, then why limit eggs? It must be the passion. Must be. Why else couldn't you eat them at night?

The Weight Watchers public relations office could offer no explanation for ever having imposed such a restriction. And yet there was a counterpart: Fruit. One serving had to be taken at the "Morning Meal."

And that's the way it is with mass-produced diets. They arbitrarily limit, they arbitrarily eliminate.

Mass-produced diets all but eliminate sugar. How silly! Sugar can be very helpful when you're trying to lose weight because it's so luxurious. And anyway, it isn't especially fattening. (Here she goes again!) Well, to say that sugar is more fattening than green beans because green beans are 113 calories a pound whereas sugar is 1,746 calories a pound doesn't tell the whole story. I know lots of people who can eat a pound of green beans.

Some experts would advise you to eliminate sugar even if it helps to provide the entertainment that keeps you on your diet. They would advise that sugar is unhealthy for body and mind. I do not agree. I do agree that sugar can contribute to dental problems. But tooth decay may prove the lesser of two evils, when all the truth about sugar substitutes is known.

During the first few months of my diet, I completely excluded sugar—reputation and all that. Then one day I made a bouillabaisse following the recipe in a Weight Watchers cookbook. I added a thing or two, changed a thing here and there, and deleted the required vegetable, string beans. But I never thought to use real sugar. When I tasted the finished soup, I thought, "This is heaven, but it misses nirvana by just that much." In this case, "just that much" was the difference between artificial sweetener and the real thing. I looked at the recipe again. Using sugar instead of artificial sweetener would have added 30 calories to a pot of fish stew meant to serve eight people: a 3¾-calorie difference per serving. From that point on I used only sugar in my kitchen.

Tell your Weight Watchers lecturess that you've put a teaspoonful of sugar (15 calories) in your morning coffee in exchange for one of the required servings of bread (75 calories). Will she say, "Congratulations!"? Or will she say, "You're cheating!"?

The idea that a person can cheat on a diet is a strange one, it seems to me. They make it clear who the cheater is, but who is the cheatee? Guilt is not an exercise that burns calories.

By now it probably seems that my diet consists of sugar, apple pie, popcorn, fudge and more fudge, and portions and portions of mashed potatoes with gravy. Right. And wrong.

I go in and out of popcorn passion, but I can't remember the last time I craved chocolate fudge. I love potatoes, but I can do without the gravy, thank you. And besides potatoes, I eat lots of other vegetables. But I eat only those fruits and vegetables that I like, and only when I want them. If I have the choice between prepackaged apple pie and a freshly harvested apple, I'll almost certainly take the apple. If my choice is between freshly baked apple pie and an apple in April, I'll probably take the pie. Freshly baked pie and a just-picked apple? Got a doggie bag?

Everything I eat must be worth it, now that I understand the power of every calorie. I have become, at long last, a fussy eater. If what I wanted were the two-humped variety of the "long-necked animal used in some desert regions as a beast of burden," then I would gladly walk a mile for a camel—but not one inch to eat a dromedary. We all have our camels; each of us, our dromedaries. And each of us, alone, knows which is which.

Am I recommending then that you eat "junk" food in order to lose weight? No. I recommend that if what you want is to lose weight but you can't give up junk food, you should be able to compare the calories in Junk A with the calories in Junk B.

Do I recommend that you give in to every emotional tug on the strings of your appetite? No. I recommend that if you're a person who needs to bracket every meal with snacks, then you should know which snacks have fewer calories. I say that if you want to lose weight, but can't refrain from having lost weekends where you eat in banquet proportions, then you should know which foods are best included in those banquets in order to keep the weekend from being lost altogether.

If you often need the banquets and you often need the snacks, I don't say that just by knowing calorie counts you will eventually look like a sylph. But knowing the difference between one snack and another might be the thing that keeps you from eventually looking like a sumo wrestler. And maybe, just maybe, as you find yourself becoming a little more like sylph and a little less like sumo, you may suddenly discover you prefer a "½ medium cantaloupe" to junk food after all.

We've been taught to feel ashamed after we eat "compulsively." We feel ashamed while we are eating, as well. We try to get it over with. We eat quickly. Well, there are better ways to deal with a binge than that . . .

. . . Having used three egg whites to make meringue for a dinner party on Tuesday, my friend Margo Schab (she's the *other* Margo who's a New York art dealer) had three extra egg yolks in the refrigerator on Wednesday. So she decided that rather than letting them go to waste (starving children in Europe), she would make crème caramel. If you had put all those ingredients in a line, then ordered Schab to eat them or walk the plank, she would ask you if a lifeguard were on duty. But if you could disguise the ingredients as a crème caramel, it becomes a different story. And the story is that she ate it all, the entire soufflé-pan-ful. All 5,000 calories, she thought.

Her diet was ruined.
Her day was ruined.
Her week was ruined.
Her life was ruined.

But then she sat down with the recipe and added up the calories. As it turned out, she was suffering 5,000 calories' worth of guilt for 1,600 calories' worth of food. She realized that by stopping there, she could have the perfect diet day. Schab had two glasses of water for dinner, and woke up a quarter-pound lighter in the morning.

The best way I know to deal with the aftermath of a binge is by after-math.

Sit down and figure out how many calories you've actually consumed, then plan to compensate for them. It could be as simple as having half a glass of orange juice instead of a whole one with your next dozen breakfasts.

Our anxiety-response to a binge doesn't take into account the importance of food as gratification, yet it's part and parcel of what makes us tick. Nature had to make food as tempting as possible, to make sure we would know what to do with it. So if you find yourself eating away, and what scares you is that you aren't hungry, take heart: You have centuries of history on your side. Before thin was in, people who could afford to would make elaborate preparations for eating when they weren't hungry. Just imagine the festivals in praise of Bacchus, or the feasts of Henry VIII. Picture in your mind's eye how much each guest would eat. Does it look like four ounces of white-meat turkey and two required vegetables?

From the beginning of recorded history, people have gorged themselves for days at a time and looked forward to it. Now we have the phrase "compulsive eating," and the same thing that people have done naturally for centuries has become neurotic.

We assume that being a compulsive eater is a bad thing. But have we ever asked, "Is being a compulsive eater a bad thing?"

In 1965, I went to Europe for the first time. I was like a brand-new sponge, thirsty to soak up the world around me. For this, I had purchased the all-inclusive railroad ticket, the Eurailpass, and traveled freely from city to city without any further expense. Weekdays I was in Paris, where I was taking a course at the Sorbonne. But come Friday afternoon I was off to one country or another for the weekend.

One Sunday evening in Amsterdam, with barely half an hour

to kill, I wandered into a coffee shop and ordered apple pancakes, pleading with the waiter to hurry because I had to catch the train to Paris. I think it was somewhere in Belgium that, having carefully sifted through a host of sensory memories, I decided that those pancakes were possibly the best things I had ever tasted. Was there any doubt I would return the next day for more?

Directly after class, I boarded the "Netherlands Express," having five hours in which to look forward to dinner. My train pulled into the Amsterdam station at 8:00 P.M. The train to Paris left at 8:30.

Taking the same seat I had left vacant exactly twenty-four hours earlier, I placed my order for the pancakes, once again urging the waiter to hurry—I had to catch the train to Paris.

Double take. "Weren't you catching that train to Paris last night?" he asked incredulously. "I was," I said, "and I still am."

There is a point here, but to make it I have to tell you Schab's story of a man she knew in Cincinnati named Sam.

Sam was a self-made multimillionaire. He was assertive in business, but socially shy. He had friends, but no lovers. He was surrounded by people, but very much alone. One afternoon a Tupperware lady came to his door, and between one thing and another he asked her to marry him. When Sam's friends heard about the proposed marriage they rallied en masse to protect him. The committee surrounded him—"Sam," they implored, "don't you realize that this woman is marrying you for your money?" But Sam didn't blink an eye: "If this woman is marrying me for my money," he answered, "boy, am I glad I have the money."

If being a compulsive eater means that I can find pancakes worth traveling 344 miles to have again, boy, am I glad I have the compulsion.

I was a compulsive eater, and I still am. But being a compulsive eater didn't stop me from losing 150 pounds. **The Calorielogue** contains the data that made the difference.

The statistics on successful weight control are discouraging, that's true. But remember that your interest is in what will be. A statistic tells you only what has been.

Now you have a tool that was not available before. This book.

But even with this book, with the data pages right at hand, one problem you face when you try to lose weight is that you've been fat. A "rose," you think, "is a rose, is a rose: I am fat, I will be fat." You create a "self-fulfilling prophecy." That is an expression brought into prominence by the research of Robert Rosenthal, Professor of Social Psychology at Harvard University.

In 1959, when Dr. Rosenthal was an associate professor at the University of North Dakota, he had what he thought was an interesting hypothesis and designed an experiment to check it out.

Psychology majors were divided into two groups. The students in Group A were given five very intelligent rats, selected from a colony that had been inbred for generations to produce genetically superior litters. These were "maze bright" rats and would learn quickly. The students in Group B were given five very unintelligent rats, selected from a colony that had been inbred for generations to produce genetically inferior litters. These were "maze dull" rats and would require more time in which to learn. The assignment was to train the rats to run through a maze, distinguishing correct turns from wrong ones. Correct turns were to be rewarded with food pellets, because even a rat will do outlandish things for oral gratification.

So far this looks like an everyday campus experiment. Similar experiments had been done at universities everywhere in "Introduction to Experimental Psychology."

But in this experiment the rats were just props. The students, not the rats, were the guinea pigs here. Rosenthal's real experimental question: When an experimenter expects a result, does s/he get it?

All the rats had come, in fact, from the very same colony. Yet at the end of the training period the students found that the performance of the "intelligent" rats far surpassed the performance of the "dull" ones.

How can that be?

This is how: the rats that had been labeled intelligent became intelligent rats. The ones that had been labeled unintelligent turned out very dull indeed.

Was the difference in the food pellets?

No. The difference was in the way the students treated the rats. As Dr. Rosenthal explains it: "In the eyes of the experimenters the allegedly bright rats were seen as brighter, more pleasant, and more likeable." The students who thought their rats were intelligent tended to handle them affectionately during the training periods, and may even have played with them in between sessions. The students with "smart" rats spoke to their animals during the experiment. The students with "dumb" ones figured, "Why bother?"

I asked Rosenthal, "Would you say that the "smart" rats had been treated as pets?" "Well," he said, "I wouldn't be at all surprised to find that a 'smart' rat or two had gotten to take a walk in the country on a leash."

The impact of the Rosenthal experiment immediately changed the methodology of experimental psychology. Self-fulfilling prophecy. You believe it, and all of a sudden an "intelligent" rat becomes an intelligent rat. One way to lose weight is to stop thinking of yourself as fat.

Something you've been taught as a fat person is that you can never hope to eat the way thin people do. You've heard it time and time again. But just how do thin people eat? Very much the way fat people do, even compulsively, except . . .

. . . Your present dilemma is donuts. You want them. Worse, they want you. You thought they were "doughnuts" but the sign says "Dunkin' Donuts," and you never were a speller. Neither Circe nor the Sirens did beckon with such a call. You wish your crew could tie you to a fire hydrant. You walk to the window and press your nose against the glass. Donuts. How have they managed to glaze them with bright subliminal neon?

Problem: Do you order the donut, which you really want, or do you go to the deli and force down something else?

Solution: A container of strawberry yogurt, you reason, will satisfy your taste for something sweet, even if it doesn't satisfy your compulsion for a donut.

Typically, the fat compulsee will eat the yogurt and then, still feeling unfulfilled, will reason this way: "I was going to eat the donut, which is much more fattening, but I was virtuous enough to eat a yogurt instead. So if I eat another yogurt it would be about the same as if I had eaten the donut to begin with." And as sure as a donut's hole will be gone before you can eat it—after having two yogurts, the compulsive eater must have the donut anyway.

The thin compulsive eater just sits down and eats the donut.

One Honey Dip glazed Dunkin' donut has fewer calories than almost any 8-ounce container of low-fat strawberry yogurt.

In a thoroughly unscientific survey taken among pre-Christmas shoppers at Bloomingdale's, I asked ninety-seven people to rank the relative caloric contents of an 8-ounce container of low-fat strawberry yogurt and a Honey Dip glazed Dunkin' donut. Every one of the people I asked—every one—told me that the yogurt was lower in calories. Which maybe, just maybe, helps to explain why . . .

Everybody I know . . . everybody—my agent and his secretary; my landlord and my lawyer; my tailor, his wife, and their daughter; my doctor, my dentist, the druggist; my incredible manicurist; my best friend; my butcher and my baker, and believe it or not, yes, my candlestick maker; my compulsive accountants and countless other friends, relatives, and neighbors, among them: actors; artists and art dealers; oceanographers and explorers; chemical, electrical, and civil engineers; businessmen and babysitters; psychologists and psychiatrists; theatrical producers and theatrical professors; marvelous musicians, mathematicians, and even magicians' magicians—of my entire acquaintanceship with very few exceptions—everybody I know, no matter how successful s/he is at other endeavors, finds it just about impossible to succeed on a diet.

• METHODOLOGY

How do you think a million numbers came to be sitting on your lap?

I would like to explain the concept of **The Calorielogue** and the Chapter Prefaces, what they are, and how they relate to calories. But before any more talk about calories, there's one more thing to discuss . . .

. . . What is a calorie?

Your car won't run on whipped cream, nor you on gasoline. There are only four materials that the human body can burn for fuel: carbohydrate, protein, fat, and alcohol. The calorie count of a food tells you one thing, and one thing only. It doesn't tell you how good a food tastes, and it has nothing to do with how "healthy" it is. The only thing a calorie count tells you is this: After that food has been digested, how much fuel will have been produced to keep the machinery running?

In round numbers for most (but not all) foods, every ounce of fat ingested provides 250 calories' worth of energy, every ounce of alcohol provides 200, and protein and carbohydrate both net 110 calories' worth of fuel per ounce. Carbohydrate, protein, fat, and alcohol each have their own distinct molecular structures, and all sorts of other characteristics. The calorie is simply a measure of one aspect of their existence.

Our bodies have elaborate mechanisms for hoarding fuel that isn't needed at the moment, and for calling upon that fuel when the need arises. It is evolution's protection—the human condition is often feast or famine. Three thousand five hundred calories' worth of fuel is stored in reserve as one pound of fat.

To help you keep track of your fuel consumption, to help you plan for your fuel needs in advance, **The Calorielogue** has 44 chapters' worth of calories. Adjacent to the columns for calories are columns for carbohydrates. In fact, looking through the data pages you might think it should be called **The Calorie- and Carbohydratelogue.** But it is called **The Calorielogue,** and that's not an accident. Carbohydrates are discussed only in their role as an energy contributor. This book is a hymn to the calorie.

To help you get a head start into the 44 data chapters there are 44 Chapter Prefaces. All of the Chapter Prefaces are together, rather than being attached to their chapters. This was done for two reasons. One was to keep them from getting lost. The other is that, together, they constitute a book within a book.

Every Chapter Preface has a title, and I usually start the Preface by defining the words in that title. Following this definition, the first two divisions in a Chapter Preface describe the boundary lines, that is—**What's in This Chapter,** and **What's Related, but Elsewhere.** Drawing those boundary lines—dividing **The Calorielogue** into 44 chapters—was a job in its own right. **Vegetables** is the first chapter. What's a vegetable?

The Oxford English Dictionary says (and other dictionaries pretty much agree) that a vegetable is "a plant cultivated for food; especially an edible herb or root used for human consumption and commonly eaten either cooked or raw."

Going by this definition, the **Vegetables** chapter could contain all the foods that we think of as fruits. But do we really want peaches in the thick of parsnips and peas? Resolved: Let's take all the fruits out, and give them a chapter of their own. But what exactly is a fruit? Back to the Oxford.

"Fruit" is the "edible product of a plant or tree, consisting of the seed and its envelope, especially the latter when it is of a juicy pulpy nature . . ."

Bye-bye, tomato! Biologically, the tomato would have to go to **Fruits,** since it's the part of the plant that houses the seed. Zucchini also gets sent to **Fruits,** and so does the cucumber. Eggplant goes too, and green beans with it. No. This simply won't do for the purposes of our book. Resolved: Those plants that are eaten as snacks or desserts go to **Fruits,** and those plants that are eaten as part of the main meal stay in **Vegetables.**

Terrific, and I hope pasta will be very happy there. Pasta? Well, pasta is all-vegetable and it's certainly eaten as part of the main meal. But Pasta? Between Parsnips and Peas? Please.

The fact is that if **Vegetables** included all the foods that started out as vegetables, the chapter would be hundreds of pages long, and lose its personality besides. It would include peanut butter, beer, Melba toast, soy sauce, potato chips, Life Savers . . .

Resolved: In this book, chapters will be divided sociologically, not biologically. And not by the world view, but with distinctions as seen through the American eye. Is the tomato a fruit or a vegetable? With that criterion, there's no doubt about it.

What to list, and where to list it? That was the question. When in doubt, I took this way out: I listed a food more than once. My feeling was that if I had difficulty figuring out where to put it, you might have difficulty finding it.

Chestnuts were that kind of fuzzy area. They're served as a vegetable, yet they retain their nutty character. They're snacked on just as other nuts are, but retain their vegetable quality. And so chestnuts are listed in **Vegetables** and again in **Nuts & Seeds.** These cross-listings are a matter of convenience, yes. But they also serve another function. If you're thinking of eating a vegetable, you'll see that a chestnut will be rather costly in terms of calories. If you're thinking of eating a nut, the chestnut is about the lowest-calorie nut you can eat.

Following **What's in This Chapter** and **What's Related, but Elsewhere,** is the third division, **The Arrangement of This Chapter.** Often this is a paragraph followed by a subsidiary table of contents. Its purpose is simple: to help you find what you're looking for.

The fourth division is **How to Read the Numbers.** Numbers are a subject that people find forbidding. I have to talk about them somewhere. "The time has come, the Walrus said . . ."

We have masses and masses of data here. No one, not even the United States Department of Agriculture, has ever published data of this scope or depth before.

All of the numbers in **The Calorielogue** are my numbers in the sense that I am publishing them. Many are very much my numbers, since they are appearing in their present form for the first time. But none of them are my numbers in the possible sense of my having performed the laboratory analyses that they represent. I want to make this as clear as I can from the beginning. I went at this project with pencils, not with test tubes.

The computations, on the other hand, are virtually all my own. At the outset, very few of the numbers looked the way you see them now. A number could find its way onto the data pages by any one of several routes. Here are the most common paths:

1. Thousands of numbers required simple conversion from grams to ounces and then on to the pound.
2. Thousands of numbers required more complicated conversions from grams or ounces to cups and tablespoons. Once in a blue moon, the conversion factors were provided with the data—but for the most part this was not the case.

   For **Breads,** as an example, you'll see a column headed "1 CUP CRUMBS—FINE, DRY." This column gives you breadcrumbs. But the information did not come from the bakers of prepackaged breads. All of these numbers needed to be calculated, and the conversion factor was the product of other published research.
3. Thousands of numbers required conversion where no factors were available. Publishing a full complement of numbers required quantitative analyses. Counting, weighing, crumbling all sorts of foods—cabbages, chicken, cheeses, blueberries, cookies and crackers, hamburgers and French fries . . .
4. Hundreds of prepared dishes were analyzed from their recipes. There are examples throughout the book, and an entire chapter—**Mess**—was constructed this way.
5. Thousands of numbers were calculated for one state of a food when other states were known. "Cooked" numbers were often calculated from "raw." For example, the entire *Beef* section of **Meats & Game** was computed this way. The Sharp programmable calculator I used held eighty steps; *Beef* used seventy-nine.
6. When the chemical composition of a food was reported in the literature, but no calories were given, energy values were calculated by using the classic Atwater formulae. (Atwater was the pioneer of calorie determination.) In round numbers, these figures are: grams of carbohydrate × 4, grams of protein × 4, and grams of fat × 9.

   The Calorielogue is so large that, relatively speaking, these computations were few. However, in some chapters —in **Fish** and in **Cheese,** for example—I had to use this method extensively.

But when all is said and done, computing numbers for the calories was simplicity itself compared to obtaining the underlying data. Where did the data come from?

Many of the data for raw foods came from governmental sources. Many of the data for prepackaged foods came from the manufacturers. It's easy to tell them apart.

Time and again, you will see listings for foods with no manufacturer's name attached. Sometimes you will see the word "Generic" hooked on. This does not mean that the Great Anonymous Generic Company is packaging it. Generic means that rather than having information for a product from a specific manufacturer, packager, or seller, I have only a general figure published at some time, based on a sample obtained somewhere, by somebody who did the research, and usually published by some government. And some of the information is extremely precise—species' names for fish—and some of the information is extremely general. Some of the information is new, and some of the information is old, which means the apple cited may have been harvested and analyzed before World War II. There's no telling how far that apple has fallen from the tree. Still, what we have here is the best generic information I could find, and I believe it's the best there is.

Of singular importance to this book were USDA publications that describe the composition of foods. (USDA means United States Department of Agriculture, not U.S. District Attorney.) Notable among these publications are *Nutritive Value of American Foods* (Agriculture Handbook No. 456) and *Composition of Foods* (Agriculture Handbook No. 8). However, "generic" is not synonymous with "USDA." In particular, if an entry says "Bamboo Shoots based on data from East Asia" you can be reasonably sure it did not come from the *Nutritive Value of American Foods.*

Often, information for any one food has been culled from a variety of sources. The calories may come from one set of analyses, the different stages of preparation from another, the weight/volume relationships from a third.

For example, potato skins. The USDA provided information for round potatoes and long potatoes, both of which are lovingly set out with explicit distinctions, such as pared or peeled (which really are different), and boiled, fried, and hash-browned. However, the USDA was not able to provide information for the potato still in its skin. To quote from *Composition of Foods:* "Unfortunately, data on composition were not available for all desired forms of foods, as, for example, the composition of cooked potato including skin." **The Calorielogue**'s data for baked potato still in its skin came from Canada.

The United States, being a country with two oceans outside, and thousands of lakes inside, gets its fish from a wide variety of places—and a wide variety of fish. Yet, there was relatively little information about the calories in fresh fish. We're primarily an agricultural country, and we pay less attention than we might to the variety of marine life around us. In order to complete the **Fish** chapter it was necessary to obtain analyses from Japan, East Asia, Africa, the Caribbean, Scandinavia, Great Britain, France, and India.

Sometimes I included foreign data for a food even when there was a good deal of information to be found within the United States. These, too, serve a useful purpose. It is interesting to see the variation in like foodstuffs grown in different parts of the world. And it's an indication that there will be variations around the United States, as well. One such variation is found among avocados. There are substantial differences in calories between avocados grown in California and those grown in Florida.

The data also suggest that it might be possible for meat and poultry breeders to breed with calories in mind. In the United States, the popular trend is to produce nice, high-calorie chickens. If you look at the data from Latin America, where chicken is also a popular dish, you can see that their chickens are popular, but not quite so fat.

With all these foreign data in hand, I had originally conceived ***THE CALORIE FACTOR*** to have two parts, one for American products, the other as a reference to foods found all around the world. But as the American section grew and grew and grew and grew, it became clear that I couldn't include any but a tiny fraction of the foreign data I had prepared.

What I did include virtually all of were the thousands upon thousands of data that I collected from American manufacturers.

When I started this book, let me admit, I had no idea what I was getting myself into. Mail didn't simply pour in, it arrived by avalanche. And I'd like to thank the United States Postal Service, which, maligned though it may be, really went through its paces on this one. And the Sanitation Department, too. The project was ongoing for more than ten years. The discarded envelopes, assorted drafts, outdated information, and used coffee cups filled two thousand 55-gallon garbage bags. If you were to prop two thousand 55-gallon garbage bags filled to capacity, one on top of the other, you would have a pile more than three Empire State Buildings high.

And some manufacturers were helpful; and some were super-helpful; and some weren't helpful at all:

5/4/79 RECEIVED

AMERICAN HOME FOODS

DIVISION OF AMERICAN HOME PRODUCTS CORPORATION

CHEF BOY-AR-DEE · G. WASHINGTON'S · DENNISON'S · FRANKLIN · JIFFY POP · GULDEN'S

EXECUTIVE OFFICES

685 THIRD AVENUE
NEW YORK, N. Y. 10017
PHONE YUKON 6-1000

May 2, 1979

Ms. Margo Feiden
Margo Feiden and Associates
51 East 10 Street
New York, NY 10003

Dear Ms. Feiden:

This is in reference to your letter of 4/27/79.

We are sorry but we continue to deny permission to anyone to publish our nutrition data.

Very truly yours,

William J. Hart, Jr.
Vice President
Research & Development

WJH/el

I was completely unprepared for the number of manufacturers who would say "No!" to my initial requests. Some manufacturers said they didn't have the information. Other manufacturers didn't want their data published. And one by one, by telephone or by mail, I tried to change their minds:

Chesebrough-Pond's Inc.

33 BENEDICT PLACE, GREENWICH, CONN.

1/19/79

January 17, 1979

KENNETH R. LIGHTCAP
DIRECTOR PUBLIC RELATIONS

Ms. Gloria Arnold
Margo Feiden and Associates
51 East 10th Street
New York, NY 10003

Dear Ms. Arnold:

Your letter of December 22nd addressed to Ragú Foods Inc. has been forwarded to me for response.

We would like to respond to all requests such as yours, but the volume of similar letters makes this quite impossible. Therefore we have to regretfully decline to take part in your book.

Thank you for thinking of Chesebrough-Pond's.

Sincerely,

Kenneth R. Lightcap

KRL:jd

Two months, and much communication, later:

RECEIVED

March 12, 1979

Ms. Margo Feiden
Margo Feiden and Associates
51 East 10 Street
New York, NY 10003

Dear Margo:

It was certainly a pleasure talking with you this morning. As a recap of our phone conversation regarding timing, we will have the information you requested sent to you no later than March 23. The information I will forward will be as follows:

1. Carbohydrate values per oz (wt)
2. Calorie values per oz (wt)
3. Weight per tablespoon
4. Weight per cup
5. All sizes of product

The product information will be forwarded for plain, meat and mushroom Traditional Spaghetti Sauce; plain, meat and mushroom Extra Thick and Zesty Spaghetti Sauce; Italian Cooking Sauce (four flavors); Adolph's Unseasoned and Seasoned Meat Tenderizers; and Adolph's Chicken and Meat Marinades.

Please do not hesitate to call me if further information is required.

Very truly yours,

CHESEBROUGH-POND'S INC.

Joseph A. Ricciardi
Manager, Product Development
Package Foods Division

JAR:lmb

SAFEWAY STORES, INCORPORATED

Oakland, California 94660 (4th and Jackson Streets)

Executive Offices FEB 26 1979

RECEIVED

February 21, 1979

Ms. Gloria Arnold,
Corresponding Secretary
Margo Feiden and Associates
51 East 10th Street
New York, New York 10003

Dear Ms. Arnold:

Thank you for inviting us to participate in an Encyclopedia of Calories and Carbohydrates.

Upon receipt of your letter, I circulated it among those having responsibility for this area of information and it was their decision to decline your invitation. We recognize that it should be a very worthwhile publication and wish you much success.

Thank you for including us in your invitation.

Sincerely yours,

C. P. Pond

CPP:lrs

Ten months, and much communication, later:

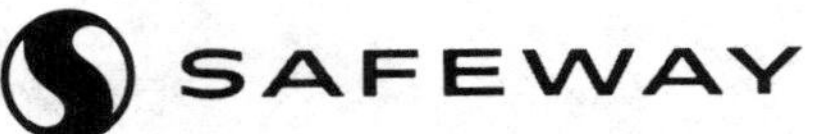

STORES, INCORPORATED

DEC 09 1979 RECEIVED

Mailing Address:
Safeway Stores, Incorporated
Dairy Division - Quality Control & Research Department
Oakland, California 94660

December 7, 1979

Margo Feiden
Margo Feiden & Associates
51 East 10 St.
New York, N.Y. 10003

Dear Ms. Feiden:

Thank you very much for your letter of November 29, 1979, concerning our Lucerne Vitamin D (whole) Milk, which has been forwarded to us by our Corporate Public Affairs Department.

The milkfat content of this particular product is 3.5% which amounts to 9 grams per one cup serving.

We are enclosing a copy of our recently revised booklet "Facts About Lucerne Diary and Delicatessen Products" which contains this information for our fluid milks, yogurt, cottage cheese, instant nonfat dry milk, instant breakfast, Cereal Blend and Coffee Tone (powdered and "Freezer Pack"). However, since this booklet has been revised, our Lucerne Cereal Blend has been re-formulated to contain partially hydrogenated soybean oil rather than hydrogenated coconut oil; thus, we are enclosing a photo copy of the label for the "new" product.

By the way, we are also sending along a photo copy of the nutrition information (label) for our various Safeway Brand foods, which are so labeled, in case this data will be of use to you. By copy of this letter, we are also asking that our Bakery Division forward any information they may have available which they feel might be of interest.

Ms. Feiden, we certainly appreciate your interest in our products and trust that you will feel free to call on us, if you should have other questions in the future.

Thank you very much again for writing and we wish you good luck and success in your project.

Sincerely,
DAIRY DIVISION

J. A. Bantly
Labels & Information Section Manager

Enc.
JAB:cs
cc: Bakery Division
Brookside Division
Brands Buying Division
Meat & Egg Division
Public Affairs Department

So one obvious problem with the listings is that the brand you're thinking of buying may not be in this book. On the other hand, a brand in this book may not be in your supermarket, or even sold in your part of the country. But there are other problems with the numbers that I must commend to your attention.

Green Giant, for example, has given us numbers for their French Style Green Beans that are lower in calories than everyone else's by just a little bit. Now, if someone were being a fastidious dieter, s/he might decide that what s/he needed to do was to switch to Green Giant. This may not be the case. . . . It could be that Green Giant is doing something different in its calculations. And different analytic techniques will produce different results. But it could also be that there are indeed fewer calories in the can.

One guaranteed inaccuracy is the error inherent in rounding off. I've rounded off, and there's no telling how many times a number had been rounded off before it got to me. So beware of tiny differences. Although even the smallest numbers of calories count, what looks like a calorie difference may be the result of one or more arithmetical inconsistencies.

This is not to say that I accepted any old number willy-nilly, and plopped it into the book. With the assistance of a tireless staff, I compared and scrutinized numbers. I wrote innumerable letters, and made innumerable phone calls asking for more information and clarification of data (see letters on pages 32 and 33):

As manufacturers' data flowed in, I sometimes noticed unanimity in calories among products where I would have expected a higher variation. It became apparent that some manufacturers had simply copied the USDA's statistics. When the numbers seemed plausible I accepted them. When they did not I questioned them. Such was the case with Goldenberg's Peanut Chews. The calories looked too low. When I asked Carl Goldenberg he said, "I looked up the ingredients in the USDA and my numbers are exact according to those." But he readily agreed to have his candy analyzed. When the lab results came back he corrected his figures to show the higher calories, a very honest thing to do. This means that any of Goldenberg's competitors who used USDA figures might show fewer calories, as would Goldenberg if he hadn't been so scrupulous.

It's important to understand the full range of inaccuracies that show up. Otherwise, you may be puzzled by what look like small arithmetical errors. For example, a box of 10 cookies, each 100 calories—with 1,050 calories in the box! So here's a list of common causes for inaccuracies, including a reason for the 1,050 calories! (See "Overfill.")

Nature's Changing Course There is no assurance that the cow, or the chicken, or the apple you are eating will match the calories of the foods whose analyses appear in these pages. If no two snowflakes are alike, what can you say about corn on the cob?

Rounding Errors Many companies round off their calorie figures to the nearest "10," and carbohydrates to the nearest whole number. In foods with a high calorie figure, this rounding does not have very serious consequences, although it does tend to obscure small differences between brands. For very low-calorie foods, rounding can have quite an impact on the figures, greatly reducing precision. And when small quantities are multiplied upward, inaccuracies become larger.

Estimated Data Many manufacturers do their own analysis. Many, however, take their figures wholesale from the USDA, even if the foods are not exactly comparable to those that the USDA analyzed. Somewhat more accurate, many companies will start with USDA data for a product's basic ingredients, and then re-calculate according to the company's recipe for the product.

Overfill Actual package weights will often be higher than what's stated on the package. Companies will overfill regularly to avoid coming up short, which could be publicly embarrassing and is illegal. Thus there may be more calories in a package than the stated package weight would suggest.

Manufacturers' Errors The nutrition information I received was regularly filled with typos, incorrect calculations, and other unlikely looking figures. These have been corrected as best I can. But only when I found them.

My Own Errors There are bound to be errors of my own making. Obviously I don't know where they are or they wouldn't be there.

Weight/Volume Relationships Often, a company will not make it clear whether its numbers are by weight or by volume. Yogurt, for example, is usually sold in a container that says 8 ounces. The "info" on the label may suggest that 8 ounces equals 1 cup, but this is not the case. The product is measured by weight and the cup conversion is only an approximation. In reality, an 8-ounce container of yogurt is slightly less than one full cup. (There is a further discussion of the relationship between weight and volume on page 35.)

Prepared? Unprepared? Often, label information for a product will give the calories without the addition of necessary preparation ingredients. For example, the nutrition information for some bread mixes gave only the calories for the flour mix, and not for the prepared bread for which shortening must be added. Wherever I could, I've given estimated figures that include all of the ingredients. (In these cases there is a separate line for the prepared product, and almost always the added ingredients are listed.)

Old Data Manufacturers are constantly revising, reformulating, and repackaging their products. In some industries (candy comes to mind), package sizes often change more than once a year. And every time you see the words, "NEW! IMPROVED!" on a box, it may mean the calories have changed from those I publish here—Higher? Lower? The same? Who knows?

Cheating Of course, it's conceivable that some manufacturers cheat. Although there, too, I looked at the numbers for consistency with what they were supposed to represent. Routinely, I multiplied the calorie components—fat, carbohydrate, and protein—by their energy values to double-check the submitted calorie counts for accuracy. All the numbers in this book have met that requirement.

*

In spite of this long list of possible errors, I recommend that you use the data pages as often as you can. They are by far the most useful, most complete, most accurate assemblage of calorie data that I know of anywhere in the world.

But in order for you to use the numbers, you have to understand them first. Actually, the numbers are easy to understand. It's the words that could use some explaining:

What are "As purchased," "Edible portion," and "Refuse"?
What does "Yield" mean?

argo Fei... and Associates
...treet, New York, N...

URGENT

February 12, 1979

New England Fish Company
Pier 89
Seattle, Washington 98119

Dear Sirs:

Thank you for the additional information which you sent for our Encyclopedia of Calories and Carbohydrates.

May I ask a question about one set of numbers? For your Icy Point Blue Back and Red Salmons, is the second column of figures, that is "Net Contents Per can" in grams, correct for the first three entries? I assume that the decimals are misplaced.

Also, I would be very interested in knowing how many shrimp, scallops, oysters, etc. are packed to the can.

Thank you for your cooperation.

Cordially,

Margo Feiden
Margo Feiden and Associates

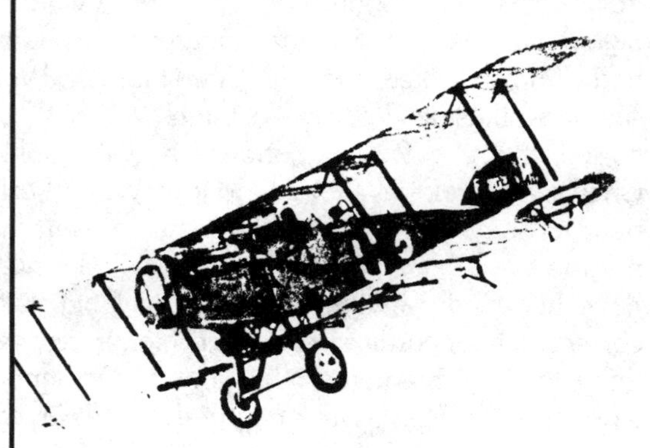

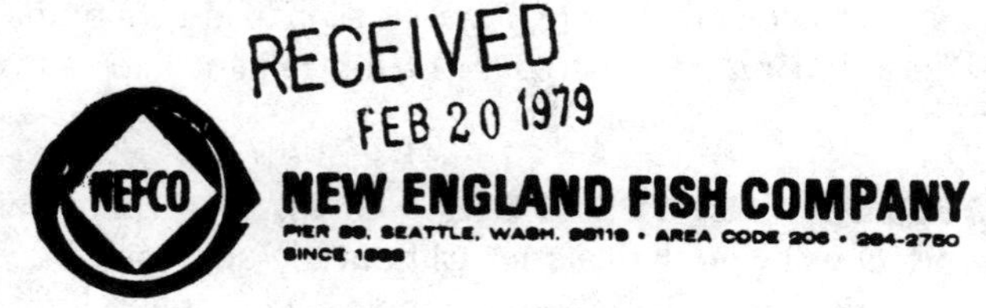

February 15, 1979

Margo Feiden and Associates
51 East 10 Street
New York, New York 10003

Dear Ms. Feiden:

This will acknowledge your letter of February 12, 1979.

You are quite correct in your assumption that the decimals are misplaced, in the net weight in grams column, for the first three entries. These should read 220,106 and 439, respectively.

With regard to your question as to how many shrimp, scallops and oysters are packed to the can, I regret I cannot give a specific precise answer. The count will vary with the size and since the size varies, seasonally, the count will also vary seasonally.

Incidentally, the calorie content per package column was also incorrectly stated. I am enclosing a corrected set of data.

Yours very truly,

NEW ENGLAND FISH COMPANY

R. E. Silver
Vice President

encl:

/jc

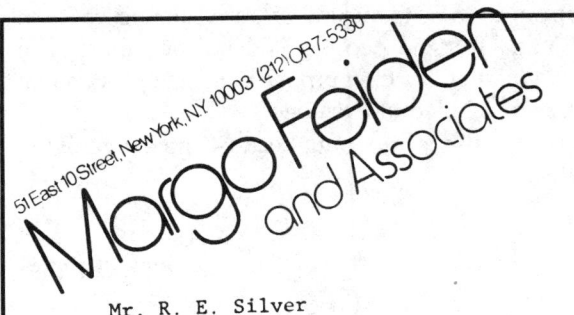

March 13, 1979

Mr. R. E. Silver
Vice President
New England Fish Company
Pier 89
Seattle, Washington 98119

Dear Mr. Silver:

Methinks the Post Office should provide us with a Watts line. I shall certainly telephone you the next time I'm in Seattle. In a previous letter (February 12, 1979) I asked if you could tell us how many shrimps, etc. were packed to a can. In your reply (February 15th) you answer that this count is variable and that a precise answer would be impossible.

By now you know my own penchant for precision. But sometimes precision is simply not available. Please, if you would, I would be most interested in knowing the counts and their variations, especially as they fluctuate with the seasons. I think that our readers would find this an interesting footnote.

Thank you again, and really, we must keep meeting this way.

Cordially,

Margo Feiden
Margo Feiden and Associates

MF/lr

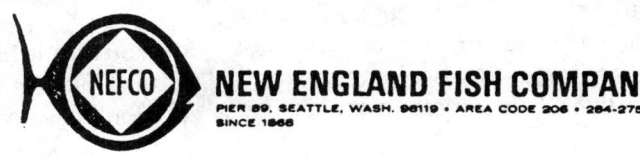

RECEIVED

March 16, 1979

Margo Feiden and Associates
51 East 10 Street
New York, New York 10003

Attention: Margo Feiden

Dear Ms. Feiden:

Responding to your persuasive letter of March 11, 1978- with further reference to your letter of February 12th:

(a) Our frozen products are packaged in polyethylene plastic bags (except for SHIP AHOY frozen OYSTERS, which are in cans).

(b) Can count range is as follows:

1. Shrimp - 100 to 200 shrimp per 8 oz. package (these are, of course the "tiny Alaskan shrimp").

2. Scallops - 15 to 30 per 10 oz. package.

3. Oysters - 20 to 50 per 10 oz. package.

With each product, while size may vary depending upon season, the contents of any given container should be fairly uniform in size and weight per individual unit.

I hope the foregoing will be of some help (and interest) to you and your readers.

Yours very truly,

NEW ENGLAND FISH COMPANY

R. E. Silver
Vice President

/jc

What is an "Ounce"?
What do I mean when I say "Weight/Volume Relationship"?
What is a "Tablespoon"?
What is the story on the column headings?
What do the parentheses around certain data mean?
And more . . .

Unit Column

For most of the chapters in **The Calorie-logue,** the first column of data is the "Unit" column.

For strawberries, as an example, when the descriptive line says "1 pound," the Unit is the pound. But another line for strawberries may read "1 small strawberry (approx. 0.4 oz.)," and in that case the Unit is that strawberry. Still another line may describe a commercially packaged container of strawberries, and the numbers in the Unit column will be for the calories in the entire container.

The Unit column is always "one" of whatever is being described on the data line.

The numbers in this column will vary widely, even for similar or identical products. It produces the widest range of comparison: A teaspoon of Peter Pan Peanut Butter has 32 calories; the 3-pound jar has 8,080.

As Purchased, Edible Portion, Refuse

In some of the chapters, including **Vegetables, Fruits,** and **Fish,** there is a trio of terms that occur so often that it is best for me to be precise as to exactly what they mean. The terms are "As purchased," "Edible portion," and "Refuse," and the need for all three arises from the fact that when you eat an apricot, you throw the pit away.

Let me sit back for a moment and take a breath, because I am just about to write the most important sentence in 44 chapters' worth of **How to Read the Numbers:**

All of the data in the tables of this book—every calorie figure, every carbohydrate figure, every fiber figure in the chapters that list fiber—pertain to those parts of the food that are "edible."

This is a very important thing to remember; otherwise there will be no end of confusion.

Bearing in mind that all the calorie figures pertain to that which is edible, the "trio of terms" refers to the particular form in which a food is being *measured:*

"Edible portion": The calorie value for cherries "Edible portion, 1 pound" is for a pound of cherry "meat" weighed without the pits and stems.

"As purchased": The weight specified on the "As purchased" lines will include those parts of a food that ordinarily come with your purchase but are not commonly eaten. The calories, however, will pertain only to the portion that is edible. The calorie value for cherries "As purchased, 1 pound" attempts to describe the calories that you will have left from a pound of cherries weighed with pits and stems, *after* you have thrown the pits and stems away. There is no figure in this book to tell you the calories in 1 pound of cherries if you were to eat the pits and stems as well.

Why do I say that "As purchased" *attempts* to describe what you will have left from that pound?

Because individual pounds of cherries are going to be different in their makeup. All we can do is make an educated guess, based on samples, as to what percentage of a pound of cherries, weighed as they are picked, will be edible by general standards.

"Refuse": That which is thrown away is the "refuse." Refuse is described explicitly on the line, and then expressed as a percentage. Why is it so important to describe the refuse explicitly, if it is only to be thrown away?

Well, moving from cherries to cucumbers, are cucumbers eaten with their skin? Yes, by some people. And no, by others. The refuse will tell you whether, for the purpose of the calories on that line, the skin is being included or excluded.

The percentage of refuse is important because the extent of the trim is also variable:

BEETS	**Unit Calories**	**1 oz. by wt. Calories**
RAW:		
As purchased:		
With tops (refuse: tops and parings, approx. 60%)		
1 pound	78	4.9
With part tops (refuse: part tops and parings, approx. 51%):		
1 pound	96	6.0
Without tops (refuse: parings, approx. 30%):		
1 pound	137	8.6

In this example of beets, the entry with the largest percentage of refuse (purchased "with tops," refuse approx. 60%) has the lowest calories for the Unit. That's just as you'd expect. After all, you're throwing more than half of it away.

The entry with the smallest percentage of refuse (purchased "without tops," refuse approx. 30%) has more calories for the Unit, and that's exactly as you would expect.

Wouldn't it have been simpler to have left out the "As purchased" figures altogether, and to have listed foods on an "Edible portion" basis only?

Simpler, yes, but not nearly so useful. That would have required you to weigh your food exactly the way you are going to eat it. You couldn't, for example, use this book in a butcher shop if you were buying a bone-in cut. And you couldn't weigh your food before you cooked it, since calories change in the cooking, too. You would have to weigh and measure everything at the table, exactly the way it goes onto your fork.

Still, it will always be best to measure food as closely as possible to the way you will be eating it, and then use the line of figures most appropriate. But sometimes that is not possible, or practical, or aesthetically appealing. That's why the "As purchased" figures are here for you.

Yield

The word "Yield" or "Yields" is closely related to "As purchased" and "Edible portion."

If the edible portion of a pound of vegetables "As purchased" is half a pound, then the pound "yields" 8 ounces. A pound of the edible portion is the "yield" of two pounds as purchased.

The word "yield" is also used to describe other changes that a food undergoes during preparation. What is taken into consideration are such factors as added ingredients, obviously, but also the evaporation of moisture, dripping, and the absorption of cooking mediums (the oils in frying).

"Yield" is also used to distinguish the final product of the cooking process. Cakes baked from mixes are a good example:

CAKE MIXES	**Unit Calories**	**1 oz. by wt. Calories**
German Chocolate Cake, Duncan Hines "Pudding Recipe," 18½-oz. box	2160	116.8
Prepared as package directs (yield: approx. 30 oz.)	3000	101.3

The first line for each cake mix describes the calories in the box of dry mix, without any additional ingredients.

The second line gives the "yield" of the box, that is, the weight of, and the calories in, the baked cake. The calories will often be higher for the "Unit" (that is, the entire cake) because of the added ingredients such as butter and eggs—but lower by the ounce because of the diluting effect of the added water.

An important point to remember about "yield" lines is that the next number on the line, the number following the word "yield," is the quantity being described on that line. When you see:

1 pound of raw sausage, cooked [yield: approx. 12 oz.] . . .

the numbers in the columns that follow this will describe 12 ounces of cooked food, not 1 pound of raw.

Drained

For manufactured goods we don't have "As purchased," "Edible portion," and "Refuse." The assumption is that you throw away the can, and everything inside of it is edible.

But sometimes the packing liquid is eaten, and sometimes it is thrown away.

One can see and one can taste that there is food value in the liquid, so there must be calories. The liquid in which a food is packed may be more caloric or less caloric than the food itself. The liquid for green beans, for example, is essentially water, and so the calories per ounce go up when you drain the contents of the can. But if what you're draining is the oil from a can of tuna, the calories per ounce will go down:

GREEN BEANS	**1 oz. by wt. Calories**
A & P Cut Green Beans, 8-oz. can	5.0
Drained solids (yield: approx. 4.8 oz.)	(6.3)

TUNA	**1 oz. by wt. Calories**
Chicken of the Sea Solid White Fancy Albacore Tuna, packed in Oil, solids and liquid, 10-oz. can	75.0
Drained solids (yield: approx. 8.5 oz.)	(47.1)

The Ounce Column

It's a peculiarity of the English language, but there are two units of measure called an "ounce." One is an ounce by weight, the other is an ounce by volume—a fluid ounce. The two, in fact, are different. An understanding of that difference can make or break your diet. This brings up the general issue of relationships between weight and volume. We'll return to "the ounce" shortly.

Weight/Volume, Continued

Materials of equal weight can fill varying amounts of space. Materials that fit into an identical space can have very different weights.

The classic embodiment of this weight/volume dichotomy is a well-known riddle: Which weighs more, a ton of coal or a ton of feathers? The answer, of course, is that a ton is a ton no matter what you are weighing.

But what if the question were: One ton of coal, one ton of feathers—which takes up more room?

Clearly it's going to be the feathers. Coal is a denser material (its molecules are closer together). So if you have to carry a shopping bag full of one or the other, feathers will be a much lighter load. A lighter load, yes, but less consistent. The quantity of feathers, hence the weight of feathers in your shopping bag, will depend on the way you pack them, whereas coal won't be subject to so much variation. The feathers are fluffier; there's more air between them.

Terrific information if you're a coal miner or a chicken plucker. But how will this help a dieter?

A borrowment from the **Frozen Confections** Chapter Preface:

The One Fluid Ounce column should not be confused with One Ounce by Weight. These are entirely different measurements, and for a great many of these products an ounce by weight will have considerably more calories than a fluid ounce. For example, Breyer's Coffee Ice Cream is 35 calories for a fluid ounce and 56.7 calories for an ounce by weight. The explanation is this: For the foods that characterize this chapter, air is a recognized and necessary ingredient. Air increases volume. However, because of the buoyancy of the atmosphere in which we weigh things, air will not affect the Ounce by Weight column. In other words, if two ice creams have otherwise identical ingredients—but one contains more air—the ice cream with more air will have fewer calories by the gallon, but the same number of calories by the pound.

As a further example of how air takes up space, but will not ordinarily affect weight, you have a roomful of air on your bathroom scale all the time. The scale reads "zero." (Then little you steps on it, and look what happens.)

Back to the Ounce

The existence of two kinds of ounces can cause confusion because it is not always obvious which kind of an ounce you are dealing with. It simply isn't true that solids are sold by weight, or that liquids are sold by "fluid" ounces. Rock-solid ice cream is sold by the fluid ounce (pints, quarts, gallons), and soup is commonly sold by weight. Yogurt is sold both ways—or shall I say "weighs"?

Whenever you see the word "ounce" in this book, whether as a column heading or as a descriptive, it is always an ounce by weight. An ounce by volume will always be referred to as a "fluid ounce." There are no exceptions. It is always true.

The Ounce by Weight column occurs very frequently in this book. It is the great leveler. A teaspoon of butter, 34 calories, and a pound of butter, 3,248 calories, both are equal here at 203 calories per ounce.

A related measure to the ounce by weight is the pound—always 16 ounces. The gram, which is referred to in some discussions, is a much smaller measure. There are 28.35 grams to the ounce. A more concrete example: there are about 1¼ M&Ms to a gram.

The fluid ounce is a volume measurement, always. Whereas an ounce by weight is a measurement pretty much confined to a scale, measurements by volume can be taken in a variety of ways. A measuring cup holds 8 fluid ounces, a measuring tablespoon holds ½ of a fluid ounce, a measuring teaspoon holds ⅙ of a fluid ounce. A pint is 16 fluid ounces, a quart is 32 fluid ounces, a gallon is 128.

For water, an ounce by weight will be a little less water than it takes to fill an ounce by volume. In other words, if you were to fill a laboratory-calibrated 8-fluid-ounce measuring cup to capacity, the water will weigh more than 8 ounces on a scale.

The difference is approximately 4%.

This weight/volume relationship will vary for different foods, according to whether they are more dense or less dense than water. Thus a fluid ounce of honey will weigh distinctly more than one ounce, and a fluid ounce of ice cream will weigh distinctly less. Ice cream floats in a soda. It would float even higher in honey.

The Cup Column

The Cup is invariably a measure of volume, always 8 fluid ounces. It is often the most accurate measuring device for liquids. For solids, the cup is inherently imprecise. Yet the Cup Column shows up in many "solid" chapters, including **Vegetables, Fruits,** and **Breakfast Cereals.** The cup shows up as a unit of measure in many other chapters, including **Meats, Poultry,** and **Nuts & Seeds,** to be used when these foods are chopped, sliced, diced, or cubed.

The Tablespoon Column

For water, a tablespoon will be ½ of a fluid ounce, always. For water, a tablespoon will be 1/16 of a cup, always.

I've printed all the tablespoon figures in this book as being 1/16 of a cup even though, for many foods, a tablespoon is not just a smaller version of a cup. Tablespoons pack differently than cups do. To the extent that it makes a difference how a spoon edge stirs up the flour, I haven't allowed for that here. This column does the arithmetic for you, but it doesn't do the physics.

So variations in packing will make a big difference. But not so much of a difference as if you use a "table" tablespoon instead of a measuring tablespoon. Spoons taken from the silverware drawer go all over the place size-wise, and bear no predictable relationship to the "tablespoon" figures I print here.

The Teaspoon Column

A teaspoon of water is 1/6 of a fluid ounce, 1/3 of a tablespoon, 1/48 of a cup. The packing problems described for the tablespoon apply to the teaspoon as well (only more so).

Other Column Headings

Other column headings include "One Slice" in chapters such as **Sausages & Cold Cuts, Cheese,** and **Breads.** In a slightly different use of the word, "One Slice" is a column heading for **Cakes** and for **Pies.** You'll find a "Jigger" in **Alcoholic Beverages** and a "1 Pinch" column in **Salts & Spices.**

For **Vegetables, Fruits, Nuts & Seeds,** and in sections of a few other chapters, you'll find a column headed "Fiber."

Fiber is not a unit of measure like the Cup or the Slice. Fiber is a different kind of column, and you'll find it discussed in greater detail, about four minutes from now.

Significant Figures

The number of decimal places I have elected to use is based on the concept of the number of significant figures.

The Unit column does not have a decimal place for calories. It has one decimal place for carbohydrates. The Ounce by Weight column has one decimal place for calories, and two for carbohydrates.

It may seem as though carbohydrates were being favored with the extra decimal place. In one sense, that's true. But in another sense it's the calories that are being favored: although the carbohydrates are taken one decimal place further, the numbers by which they are measured are smaller. Let me explain.

Suppose you walked into a room filled with adults. If the difference in weight between the lightest and the heaviest adult was seventy-five pounds, that would not be extraordinary. If you were to walk into a classroom of sixth graders, a difference of seventy-five pounds among the students would be surprising. And if you were to walk into a hospital's nursery of newborns, a difference of seventy-five pounds would be a shock.

In terms of the numbers that are used to measure them, calories are like adults and carbohydrates are like infants. It's not extraordinary to eat 2,500 calories in a day. But to eat 2,500 grams of carbohydrate would indeed be a feat. For one thing, to eat 2,500 grams of carbohydrate in a day would require you to eat at least 10,000 calories.

The number of decimal places chosen to go under each column heading was intended to provide a general accuracy of three significant figures. For example, in **Meats,** I considered that a typical "one ounce" figure for calories would be between 10 and 99. Therefore, one decimal place was chosen to provide three significant figures in that range.

Parentheses

In general, parentheses surrounding a number in the data tables mean that the number, for one reason or another, may not be as reliable as its neighbors. In rare instances, the parentheses will reflect an editorial opinion on my part that the number is suspect. However, the overwhelming majority of cases in which parentheses are used mean something completely different. They indicate estimates. Often an estimate will reflect a computation that was based on a related (and unparenthesized) number, such as estimating the calories per cup for a canned pie filling, when the calories for the ounce by weight were known. However, many computed values appear without parentheses where I was reasonably confident of the outcome.

I tried to use parentheses when I believed that my computed estimates might introduce an error in excess of 5%. This is not to say that the data that appear in this book without parentheses are perfectly reliable. You can compare the discussion of "overfill," which frequently exceeds 5%. And the same is true for the amount of sugar in any one apple, and all sorts of other things. . . .

Supplemental Numbers

Sprinkled throughout **The Calorielogue,** like raisins in rice pudding (or like NINAs in a Hirschfeld), you will find numbers in parentheses following the unit of measure for many generic entries. They provide additional nutrition information, this being for protein, carbohydrate, fat, moisture, and sodium content. These numbers are given only for American generic data, and then only for "Edible portion." As an example, a pound of shelled almonds bears these supplemental numbers: (5g/6g/15g/5%/1mg).

The first number gives you the grams of protein per ounce of edible portion.

The second gives you the grams of carbohydrate per ounce of edible portion. Note that this number is a rounded version of the carbohydrate figure given in the "1 Ounce by Weight" column on the right-hand side of the page. Its position here, between protein and fat, affords an immediate profile of the food with respect to its calorie contributors.

The third number gives you the grams of fat per ounce of edible portion.

The fourth tells you what percentage of the food is water. From a calorie standpoint, the percentage of water is highly significant. To the extent that a food has water in it, it doesn't have calories.

The fifth and last number gives you the milligrams of sodium per ounce of edible portion.

All the figures are rounded off to the nearest whole number. Numbers that would round off to zero—such as 0.3—are listed as "tr," meaning "trace." Sometimes not all of the data were available, and in such cases an "na" means "not available."

Fiber

For certain chapters—for **Vegetables, Fruits, Nuts & Seeds**—and in sections of other chapters such as **Breads, Cookies & Crackers,** and **Infant Formulas & Baby Foods**—you'll find the column "Fiber." The figures are given in grams of fiber per ounce of the food.

For most chapters, this column contains entries only for American generic listings, and then only on those lines that are described as "Edible portion." The decision to omit fiber figures on "As purchased" lines was made to facilitate quick and easy comparison between foods within a chapter, and from one chapter to another.

The numbers listed in this column were calculated almost exclusively from data found in the USDA's Handbook No. 8, *Composition of Foods,* which was published in 1963 and approved for reprinting in 1975. On page 165 of that book, the uncertainty of the fiber figures is discussed as follows:

> Nearly all of the values for fiber shown in table 1 were obtained by the Weende procedure. These values may be too low; values obtained by more recent procedures for fiber in some foods are three to four times higher.

Techniques of fiber analysis are constantly being developed and refined. Many sources for fiber information are available now, in 1988, that were nowhere in sight when I began this project in 1977. But I concluded that it was wiser to take all my fiber figures from one source—which will permit more reliable comparison within the covers of this book—than to use an updated figure for carrots, and leave zucchini behind. (Even for comparison purposes, the USDA's figures are not entirely reliable. It may turn out that the techniques that were used favored some forms of fiber and were not as effective for others.) Because of the diverse procedures used to analyze fiber, the figures in this book cannot be used for reliable comparison with fiber figures from other sources.

The amount of fiber in a food will affect its caloric potential. Humans cannot make full use of the energy content of a fibrous material. We can burn cellulose, as an example, for energy in a fireplace, but not in our own internal combustion machines.

Most foods have less than 1 gram of fiber per ounce. Fiber is likely to account for only 1% of the weight of a carrot.

The fiber you ingest by eating a carrot has a calorie effect on the steak you eat with it. This has actually been figured into the calories for steak. In other words, the presence of fiber has already been accounted for in the calorie figures I publish here. But even if it turns out, as the USDA indicates it might, that the fiber figures are imprecise, this does not invalidate the calorie values. ***THE CALORIE FACTOR***'s calories were calculated from analyses that did not depend upon the published numbers for fiber.

No matter by which methods the calorie analyses on any one food were performed, the values assigned to the nutrients—grams of carbohydrate × 4, grams of protein × 4, and grams of fat × 9—are based on "mixed" diets that contain fiber. But if you eat more fiber than the "mixed" diets included, this may have certain calorie advantages. The amount of fiber ingested in these mixed diets varied, yet looking at the data I can offer this conclusion: If you adopt a high-fiber diet as a way of eating, you may be able to get some sort of calorie discount on all your food in general.

Do you remember Mrs. Greene's equation (**Monologue,** page 17)—that what we weigh will depend on the difference between what we take in and what we give out? Fiber speeds the flow of food through the digestive tract, thereby decreasing the amount of time in which calories are absorbed. And that's one reason why fiber is important enough to have a column of its own.

*

The last eleven pages were concerned with **How to Read the Numbers,** a division in every Chapter Preface in this book. Following the discussion of **How to Read the Numbers,** the fifth and last division within a Chapter Preface is **How to Eat.** The philosophy of **How to Eat** has already been written. It's the **Prologue** and **Monologue** of this book. It comes first, up front.

Specific applications of this philosophy will be found in the individual Chapter Prefaces. "How to Eat" is not just a matter of looking down the calories per ounce column for something that is "low-calorie."

Three roomfuls of furniture—$399. To know whether that's a bargain, you have to see the furniture.

Three roomfuls of furniture—$300,000. That can still be a bargain, but again, you have to see the furniture.

What constitutes "low-calorie" is very much a matter of relativity—a matter of what you are comparing. One of the stars of the **Fast Foods** chapter turns out to be mashed potatoes—hardly a star of **Vegetables.** I might have called this the Theory of Relativity, but somebody thought of it first.

Omissions

Having described what you'll find in this book, it is only fair for me to list a few omissions.

Exercise is not mentioned in this book. It's not that I think exercise is unimportant. On the contrary, I think exercise is so important that unless I am prepared to do a comparable job (***THE EXERCISE FACTOR***?) I prefer to leave the subject alone. For now.

Also omitted from this book are "Suggested Daily Caloric Intake Tables for Men and Women." The uniqueness of the individual does not lend itself to such gross generalizations. Not in this book.

Another chart that you will search in vain to find is that old bugaboo, "Desirable Weights for Men and Women." Better to keep such things for fairy tales. In my opinion, the desirable weight for a man is the weight at which he is comfortable. The desirable weight for a woman is the weight at which she is comfortable. Period.

That about does it. This, being the introduction, has been written last. ***THE CALORIE FACTOR*** has been more than ten years in the making. It's unbelievable to me that tomorrow morning I can stay in bed past 4 or 5 A.M., and not get up to write **The Somethinglogue.**

And now I go to sleep, perchance to dream.

• PART II

THE CHAPTER PREFACES

1 VEGETABLES

What a vegetable is, What's in This Chapter, and **What's Related, but Elsewhere,** have already been discussed in the general introduction to the Chapter Prefaces—**Methodology,** beginning on page 26.

To recap, basically **What's in This Chapter** are those plants and plant products that are eaten as part of the main meal. **What's Related, but Elsewhere** includes many of the foods found in **Fruits, Nuts & Seeds, Pasta, Salty Snacks, Condiments, Basic Baking & Cooking Ingredients,** and **Breakfast Cereals & Breakfast Breads.**

Dehydrated vegetables are primarily in **Campers' Foods.** Another related chapter is **Vegetarian Foods,** but these are vegetables in highly specialized form—soybeans shaped like salami, and that sort of thing.

Oh, yes. One more word about what's in this chapter. To the best of my knowledge, this is the only calorie book to list figures for vegetables "steamed."

The Arrangement of This Chapter is best set forth by a display of vegetables in the order in which they appear in the data pages. Otherwise you might not be sure whether avocados were here, or in **Fruits** where they technically belong. And even for foods that you were absolutely sure were vegetables, there might be a confusion as to where to find them. Is spoon cabbage with the other cabbages, or—knowing this book—under *Silverware*?

So here's the list:

From Alfalfa Shoots to Zucchini—more than 100 vegetables in all, and bushels of data. Data "raw" and data "cooked." Data boiled, steamed, and baked. Data by the ounce, by the pound, by the package, by the cup. There are thousands of digits in the **Vegetables** chapter, which brings us to the doorstep of . . .

How to Read the Numbers. The column headings in this chapter are:

Unit
One Ounce by Weight
One Cup
Fiber, expressed in Grams per Ounce
(For a discussion of fiber, see **Methodology,** page 36.)

The Unit will frequently be one pound for fresh vegetables, frequently the can for canned vegetables, frequently the package for frozen vegetables. But the Unit can also be one celery stalk, or one cucumber, or one potato pancake.

The One Ounce by Weight column is exactly that. The numbers represent the calories in one ounce of the vegetable that is being described on the left-hand side of the page. In this chapter the Ounce by Weight column is the most reliable one, because most of the data from which these numbers originated were received in a weight format. The drawback to the Ounce by Weight column is that it cannot be used, in and of itself, for comparison purposes. You have to read the left-hand descriptives carefully to know exactly what the "ounce" describes. Is it corn weighed on the cob, or is it just the kernels? Is it a carrot weighed with its top still on? Or is it a carrot, trimmed, scraped, and topless?

The Cup column is 8 fluid ounces, as always. It is a measure of volume, not of weight. The cup is an inherently inexact way to measure most vegetables. Still, the cup is terribly important for this chapter. In a restaurant you might order a "¼-lb. Burger," or a "1-lb. Steak," but vegetables are likely to be served by the "scoop." You may not know how many fluid ounces the scoop holds, or how much the scoopful weighs, but still the Cup column will tell you how a scoop of green beans should compare to a scoop of green peas, and that may help you choose. The Cup column is especially useful for easy and quick comparisons in this chapter (and also in the **Fruits** chapter) because all the numbers in the Cup column are for the "Edible portion" lines.

The term "Edible portion" is elaborated upon in **Methodology,** page 34. Maybe you haven't read **Methodology** yet, so here's a quick review of some important terminology.

Edible Portion

The term "Edible portion" is used when the food that's being considered will be eaten in the same form in which it is being weighed. For some foods, what constitutes the "Edible portion" varies. For example, baked potatoes are eaten with or without their skins. So are cucumbers. You have to read the left-hand descriptives to know exactly what is being measured.

As Purchased

"As purchased" lines describe the calories present in the edible portion of the food, but include in all measures of weight the parts that will be discarded before the vegetable is eaten. The value of "As purchased" lines is that you can determine the calories you will have, for example, in an ear of corn weighed at the moment you purchase it.

Refuse

"Refuse" is that which is present at the time a vegetable is weighed, but discarded rather than eaten. The cob is refuse in corn on the cob.

Untrimmed

This is the same as "As purchased."

Trimmed

This generally implies a step mid-way between "As purchased" and "Edible portion." For Cabbage, "trimmed" means that the tough outer leaves have been removed but the core remains. Thus, the cabbage still has refuse, and the line is neither for the "Edible portion," nor does it describe the food "As purchased."

Whether or not your vegetable has been "manicured," there is still another distinction to be made. Is the vegetable raw or cooked? If it's cooked, how? Boiled? Fried? Steamed? The calories per ounce will change, depending on the answer. The effects of simple boiling can go either way. Some vegetables absorb moisture, and therefore gain weight when they are boiled. Others lose weight. (Brussels sprouts and cabbage go in opposite directions.) Rice and dried beans absorb large amounts of water in cooking and that can make a difference of over 70 calories per ounce!

A word about the numbers for steamed vegetables. You might be rather startled, when you look at the calories per ounce, to see that sometimes the calories are higher for steamed vegetables than they are for raw. This is because, even in steaming, a vegetable may lose some of its moisture. Such moisture loss will affect the numbers in the One Ounce by Weight column. However, the numbers in the Unit column will remain the same. A carrot neither gains nor loses calories in the steam room.

How to Eat Vegetables or Lettuce Entertain You: Nobody who's reading this book needs to be told that vegetables are a low-calorie food. Nobody needs to be told that some vegetables are lower-calorie than others. But what's worth saying right at the beginning of how to eat them is that even a high-calorie vegetable is likely to have fewer calories per ounce than the foods you serve it with. Ergo, the way to eat vegetables is to relax and enjoy them, knowing that you're saving calories over practically anything else in this book.

Where do a vegetable's calories come from, anyhow?

Members of the vegetable family, just like members of any family, are like each other in some ways, and in other ways they are entirely different. Some vegetables will have more protein than others; some will have more fat. After all, we do get corn oil from corn and soybean oil from soybeans—but asparagus oil from asparagus?

Be that as it may, neither protein nor fat provides the calories in this chapter. Even for corn, even for beans—with the striking exception of the avocado—most of the calories in the chapter come from carbohydrate. **Vegetables** are not unusual in this respect. **Breads; Breakfast Cereals; Confitures; Sugars, Sweeteners & Toppings,** and of course many candies and sodas, owe most of their calories to carbohydrate. Why, then, are vegetables so much lower in calories?

Is it the fiber?

No, not really. Most vegetables have less than half a gram of fiber per ounce. That's not enough to account for the difference between celery at 4.9 calories an ounce and a lollipop at 109. No, the principal difference between them isn't the roughage. You may look at celery and think you're seeing fiber, but what you are really looking at is water. Celery is 94.1% water. A lollipop is 1.4% water. That's the calorie difference between them. It's not that vegetable matter, per se, is a low-calorie food.

Is a salad really all that good for a diet, then? Or is another reputation about to go down the tubes?

To the tune of "Oh, Tannenbaum":

Oh Sá-lad,
Oh Sá-lad,
To You, I write this bál-lad,
Oh Sá-lad,
Oh Sá-lad,
Your reputation's
Vá-lid.

Because as things turn out, thanks to moisture, there are more than two dozen vegetables you can choose for less than ten calories an ounce:

Under 6 calories an ounce, raw	
Chinese cabbage	4.0
lettuce	4.0
cucumbers	4.3
radishes	4.8
zucchini	4.8
celery	4.9
New Zealand spinach	5.4
watercress	5.4
chicory greens	5.6
endive	5.7

6–9.9 calories an ounce, raw	
green peppers	6.2
tomatoes	6.2
arugula	6.4
cabbage	6.8
Savoy cabbage	6.8
Swiss chard	7.1
asparagus	7.4
spinach	7.4
cauliflower	7.6
wax or yellow beans	7.6
scallions (tops)	7.7
chives	7.9
fennel	7.9
mushrooms	7.9
mustard greens	8.8
red cabbage	8.8
red peppers	8.8
broccoli	9.1
garden cress	9.1
green or string beans	9.1
mung bean sprouts	9.9

10–15 calories an ounce, raw	
hot green chili peppers, excluding the seeds	10.5
carrots	11.9
parsley	12.5
leeks	14.8

16–30 calories an ounce, raw	
chervil	16.2
hot red chili peppers, excluding the seeds	18.4
green peas, pods and seeds together	23.8
hot red chili peppers, including the seeds	26.4

More than 30 calories an ounce	
avocados (grown in Florida)	36.2
avocados (grown in California)	48.6

So the way to eat salad is, yes, any way you like, deferring avocado for when you think it's worth it. But as high-calorie as the avocado is, it's chicken feed compared to the really high-calorie food that insinuates itself into salad. The Dressing.

While salad is about the lowest-calorie food you can eat, salad dressing runs about the same as chocolate:

Based on USDA data:	**Calories per Ounce**
French dressing	116
bittersweet chocolate	*135*
Russian dressing	140
Thousand Island dressing	142
blue cheese dressing	143
semisweet chocolate	*144*
milk chocolate	*147*
sweet chocolate	*150*
Italian dressing	157
mayonnaise	204

One ounce of salad dressing is roughly two tablespoons. A salad's worth might be 2 or 3 ounces—hundreds of calories—300, 400, 500 or more. Alternatives to traditional salad dressings are discussed in the Chapter Preface to **Condiments.** But here I ask a different question—where is it written that a salad has to get dressed?

Speaking of getting dressed, the next time you go to the movies consider bringing raw vegetables along. They're a crunchy finger food just like corn chips. One is a chip made out of corn, the other's a stick made out of carrot. The difference can be 148 calories an ounce.

Of course, some vegetables are never (never?) eaten raw. One of these is the potato. The potato is the American vegetable, especially French fried. It wouldn't surprise me one bit if Americans ate more potato-related calories than calories from all other vegetables combined. Potatoes have a bad reputation. The fact is this: The calories in a boiled potato or a baked potato are closer in calories to celery than they are to French fries:

	Calories per Ounce
celery	4.9
potato: boiled, skin removed before boiling	18.4
baked potato	25.8
French fries (McDonald's)	87.9

The calories in French fries come from the frying, not from the potato. If you ordered "French Fried Menu," it would still be a high-calorie meal.

How do potatoes compare with rice? With corn? With spaghetti?

Potatoes versus rice: Boiled white rice has 68% more calories than boiled potato, even with all that low-calorie water rice soaks up while you boil it. The message, of course, is not that you shouldn't eat rice, but that for the same number of calories you can eat 68% more potato.

Brown rice is going to be slightly higher in calories than white rice because the bran layer is less willing to soak up moisture. The message, of course, is not that you shouldn't eat brown rice—but that you shouldn't eat brown rice for the wrong reasons.

Potatoes versus corn: It's a close one. Corn, boiled, is in between boiled and baked potato. Corn is 25.8 calories an ounce if you boil it on the cob, and 23.5 calories an ounce if you cut the kernels off the cob before you cook them. Presumably, corn boiled off the cob will lose more of its sugar to the water. But friends, Romans, countrymen, lend me your ears: Canned cream-style corn—creamy, creamy, cream-style corn—has fewer calories than does corn right off the cob. That's because cream-style corn is moister. The calorie difference is tiny, less than a calorie an ounce, but there's still a message here. If you like your corn creamed, don't hesitate to eat it that way. The calories are on your side.

Popped corn, because it's so dry, is 109 calories an ounce. Remember 109 calories an ounce? It belonged to that nice, sweet, dry lollipop.

Potatoes versus spaghetti: Dry spaghetti is also about the same as a lollipop. One's a concentrated sugar, the other's a concentrated starch. But as spaghetti absorbs moisture from the cooking water, the calories per ounce go way down. The longer you cook it, the downer they go. Still, it's a relatively high-calorie alternative, even when compared to other starches:

	Calories per Ounce
spaghetti, boiled "al dente" 8–10 minutes	41.9
boiled until tender, 14–20 minutes	31.4
corn, boiled on the cob	25.8
boiled off the cob	23.5
potato, boiled	18.4
baked	25.8
white rice, boiled	30.9
brown rice, boiled	33.8

All forms and shapes of spaghetti and macaroni have the same calories per ounce, whether they're shells, ABC's, lasagne noodles, or elbows.

How do elbows compare with kidneys? Kidney beans, I means.

Foods called "beans" and foods called "peas" are at the highest and lowest ends of the vegetable calorie spectrum. Boiled green beans are 7.1 calories an ounce. Boiled red kidney beans are almost five times as high, at 33 calories an ounce, which puts them in the same neighborhood as creamed cottage cheese. The critical difference between green beans and kidney beans is the life stage at which the plant is eaten. The range of calories can be 6 to 1:

	Calories per Ounce Boiled, Drained
newly sprouted seeds:	
mung bean sprouts	7.9
soybean sprouts	10.8
immature pods:	
green beans	7.1
wax beans	6.3
immature seeds:	
lima beans	31.4
green peas	20.1
kidney beans	33.4
soybeans	33.5
mature seeds:	
dried lima beans	39.1
split peas	32.6
dried soybeans	36.9

Newly sprouted soybeans are but ⅓ the calories of their older cousins, the immature seeds. As you read through the Chapter Prefaces, you will see that one way to save calories in your diet as a whole is to eat "younger" food. In **Meats,** you can save calories by eating veal instead of adult cow; in **Poultry,** you can save calories by eating young birds rather than mature birds. Just like cows, just like chickens, the older a plant is the more time it's had to accumulate energy.

Not only will a vegetable age on the vine, but some vegetables also increase in calories while they sit in storage. Artichokes are a dramatic example. With the passage of time, inulin, a non-caloric substance within the choke, converts to sugar. A freshly harvested artichoke can have as little as 1 calorie per ounce. The same artichoke, after storage, can run 5 calories an ounce, an increase of 400%. Salsify is 3.7 calories an ounce when freshly harvested, but that number can jump six-fold while it's stored, to 23 plus.

In case the vegetable you're thinking of buying doesn't come with a birth certificate, here are two clues you can use: Generally speaking, the larger a vegetable is—let's say the larger a carrot is—the older it was when it was picked. Another sign of old age is wrinkles.

But whether you buy old vegetables or young ones, and whether you eat rice instead of potatoes, or red kidneys instead of golden corn, none of this is going to make the biggest difference to your diet. Because if you really want to know where the calories in vegetables come from, they come from butter, and cream sauce, and cheese sauce, and glazing. And our old friend, frying. Kidney beans may be higher-calorie than baked potato, but on which are you likely to put more sour cream?

How do the calories in sour cream compare to the potato you put it on? How many baked potatoes could you eat for, oh, two cups of sour cream? One potato? Two potatoes? Three potatoes? Four? Five potatoes? Six potatoes? Seven potatoes?

More. You can eat nine baked potatoes for the calories in two cups of sour cream. That's one whole baked potato for every 3½ tablespoons of sour cream.

And how do the other toppings compare? There is no end of things that can be put on vegetables, each with a different consequence. For cold vegetables there's salad dressing, and we already know that story. For vegetables served hot, butter is the classic topping at 203 calories an ounce, 34 a teaspoon. But note: If a teaspoon of butter is what it takes to persuade you to eat 4 ounces of string beans, it's still only about 15 calories an ounce for the dish.

A third category of toppings is what you sprinkle on:

	Representative Calories per Ounce
breadcrumbs (unseasoned)	111.1
croutons	100.0–132.0
grated Parmesan cheese	129.3
crumbled bacon	168.1
slivered almonds	169.8

A fourth category for vegetables is spices. Some are as high-calorie as salad dressing by the ounce, but less than one calorie by the portion. A "pinch" of thyme has about 0.35 calories.

Sauces are the other side of the calories-per-portion coin. You'll find commercially packaged sauces in the **Basic Baking & Cooking Ingredients** chapter, but here's a quick rundown on cheese sauce, cream sauce, scalloping, and glazing, based on USDA home recipes.

Glazing is accomplished with butter and a sugar. The other three recipes involve the use of a "white sauce." For creaming, scalloping, and the cheese sauce, the USDA provides data for recipes with four different versions of the white sauce: a standard thin sauce, a low-fat thin sauce, a standard medium sauce, and a low-fat medium sauce. Scalloping uses more fat and breadcrumbs than creaming does. The cheese sauce is made from a cup of white sauce and a cup of shredded cheddar.

A third of a cup of sauce is estimated to be sufficient for one cup of vegetables. From the lowest to highest, they are:

	Calories per ⅓ Cup of Sauce
cream sauce: low-fat thin	60
cream sauce: low-fat medium	82

	Calories per ⅓ Cup of Sauce
cream sauce: standard thin	97
scalloping: low-fat thin	127
glazing: syrup and butter sauce	133
glazing: sugar and butter sauce	133
glazing: sugar, butter, and orange juice	140
cheese sauce: low-fat thin	141
cream sauce: standard medium sauce	147
cheese sauce: low-fat medium	156
scalloping: low-fat medium	159
cheese sauce: standard thin	166
scalloping: standard thin	182
cheese sauce: standard medium	194
scalloping: standard medium	247

In general, the numbers say that cream sauce comes out lowest in calories. Scalloping and cheese sauce are highest. Glazing is in the middle position. However, there is a considerable overlap, so that the lowest-calorie scalloping recipe is lower than all the glazes. A typical value for a cup of vegetables might be 20 to 40 calories. The choice of what goes on top far outweighs your choice of vegetable.

I started off by saying that even a high-calorie vegetable is likely to have fewer calories per ounce than the food you serve with it. That's so as long as you don't fry them, or douse them in a rich sauce. With that qualification, I repeat: The way to eat vegetables is to relax and enjoy them—knowing that you're saving calories over practically anything else in this book.

2 FRUITS

What is a "fruit"? As per the *Oxford English Dictionary*, fruit is the "Edible product of a plant or tree, consisting of the seed and its envelope, especially the latter when it is of a juicy pulpy nature . . ."

But the question of "What is a fruit" is not simply answered by looking up "fruit" in the Oxford. Please see **Methodology,** page 26.

What's in This Chapter? What's in this chapter are dozens and dozens (and dozens) of fruits, thirty-one pages of fruits, from Acerolas to Zante Currants, with Loquats in between. In case you may wonder what in the world an acerola is, I'll tell you. Acerola is a fruit beginning with A.

But seriously, the acerola is a tiny red fruit, no larger than an inch in diameter. This fruit, also known as the Barbados, West Indian, or Puerto Rican cherry, is grown in the United States, in Hawaii. It is perhaps the most potent natural source of Vitamin C on earth. Ounce for ounce, these pretty little fruits have fifty times as much Vitamin C as a good orange.

What's Related, but Elsewhere are cucumbers, tomatoes, eggplant, zucchini, pumpkin, and avocados, all of which are technically fruits, and all of which are in **Vegetables.** The distinction between a fruit and a vegetable in this country is likely to hinge on sweetness.

Confitures are made almost entirely from fruit; **Nuts & Seeds** describes the seeds of fruits. Fruit juices and fruit drinks are in **Beverages,** with now-and-again examples here. Puréed fruits are in **Baby Foods.**

There are also fruit toppings, fruit cakes, fruit condiments, fruit pies, fruit breads, fruit soups, and fruit gelatins, all to be found in the chapters you would expect. Fruit rolls are in this chapter, as dried fruits. In **Sweet Little Nothings,** they're a candy.

The Arrangement of This Chapter: The **Fruits** chapter starts on page 226 with our old friend, Acerola. It's followed by an ancient friend, the Apple, without whose contribution to history his book would not have been written (see page 14, column 2 in the **Monologue,** if you need an explanation).

Considering the quantity of apples that we eat in this country, it's a shame that no calorie information is available for the different varieties such as Delicious, Macintosh, or Granny Smith. The data are averages. But you know by the taste that a Granny Smith doesn't have the same calories as a Red Delicious—they aren't equally sweet. And yet, even without the varieties, there's so much information that Apples may look forbidding when you first see them in **The Calorielogue.** I think a few words are in order, to help you find your way around. . . . As apples sit in storage their available carbohydrate increases, and calories increase along with it. So Apples are divided into three categories: Freshly Harvested, Stored, and then an Average of Freshly Harvested and Stored because you may not know how long ago your apple was picked. After the fresh apples come frozen apples, dried apples, dehydrated apples, applesauce, and then on page 228 you're in Apricots. Apricots come fresh, frozen, canned, dried, and dehydrated. Then Avocados are listed here, briefly, but mostly they're in **Vegetables.** Plantains or "cooking bananas" are also in **Vegetables,** but "common" Bananas and Red Bananas are here beginning on page 229. And then there are:

The cherimoya is a tropical fruit. Until I started working on this chapter, I had never eaten cherimoya. In fact, I had never heard of cherimoya.

Then one Saturday afternoon while I was working on this chapter preface, balancing five fruit and vegetable reference books on my knees, I became intrigued. The Hawaiian Agricultural Experimental Station, in the introduction to their data, described the cherimoya as "a green, heart-shaped fruit three to seven inches long, [with] a smooth custardlike consistency." The *Oxford English Dictionary* described the cherimoya as "highly esteemed on account of its delicious flavor" and quoted its praises through the centuries: "The cherimoya is universally allowed to be the most delicious of any known fruit"; "he who has not tasted the cherimoya has yet to learn what fruit is." In *FOOD,* Waverly Root called it luscious, and quoted Mark Twain—the cherimoya is "deliciousness itself." In the *Complete Book of Fruits and Vegetables,* Bianchini and Corbetta wrote, "In its native countries, it's considered one of the most delicate tropical fruits." The *World Atlas of Food* offered: "The texture and taste of a cherimoya is reminiscent of creamy ice-cream made from banana and pineapple."

I called Balducci's, the quintessential fruit market: "Becky—have you ever heard of 'cherimoya'? Have you ever had one in the store?"

"Of course. Cherimoya is my favorite fruit. I mean that. It's my absolute favorite fruit. It's the best-tasting food in the world!"

"What does it taste like?"

"A cross between a banana, a strawberry, a pineapple, a very ripe pear, and a little bit of mango."

"Where do you ship them from?"

"Italy, Mexico, and sometimes from Hawaii."

"Do you have any in the store now?"

"Not yet, they're a winter fruit. We'll be getting them in, in about three weeks."

"Are you sure you'll be getting them in?"

"I am sure."

"Really sure?"

"Really sure."

"How sure?"

"If Balducci's stops carrying cherimoya, I'll quit my job."

. . . Four days later, on December 23, 1981, my cherimoya arrived. It was the stuff that dreams are made of. Who needs hot fudge sundaes?

Hot fudge sundaes are topped with cherries. Cherries start on page 231, and follow the usual arrangement of fresh, then frozen, then canned. Then more cans, and more cans, and more cans, then dried, candied, and Maraschino—and suddenly you're in Citron.

Before I began this book, if you had played "dewberries" in Scrabble, I'd have challenged you. Nonetheless dewberries are here—fresh, frozen, and canned, packed in water, juice, light syrup, heavy syrup, and extra heavy syrup. And then you have the Elderberries:

The divisions and sub-divisions of Grapefruit get rather complex. As you might expect by now, the fresh grapefruit is distinct from the grapefruit in cans or jars. But within the "Fresh," there are two lists: one for "eating" grapefruit, and one for grapefruit that is cultivated for juice. For each of these, there are three further distinctions made: Place of Origin (California, Florida, Arizona, or Texas, and then a market-weighted average of the four); Color (pink, red, and white, and then a market-weighted average of the three); and, finally, "With seeds," and "Seedless."

Following the grapefruits are the grapes:

The Kiwi is a jewel to look at and a delight to eat. Hiding behind a fuzzy brown peel, not unlike a koala bear, the fruit inside looks as though a strawberry went out with a lime and wasn't careful. The kiwifruit data we have came from New Zealand, and were accompanied by this advice: "Hold the kiwifruit between the thumb and forefinger. If it is soft, it is ready to eat. Eating raw kiwifruit—cut in half across and lift out flesh with a small spoon. Or peel and slice across or long ways. Because the flesh is firm, it can be cut into wedges, segments, or a variety of shapes, which are so well suited to decorating and garnishing. The fruit is completely edible, even the brown skin, though it can also be used as a napkin to keep the fingers clean."

Mandarin Orange is a name applied to both tangerines and tangelos. None of the canned "mandarin oranges" specified which fruit was used, and so these are listed under Mandarin. Tangerines and tangelos are listed under "T."

After Oranges come Papaws and Papaya, and then Peaches begin on page 244. All analyses for fresh American peaches that I was able to find were done for the fruit with its skin removed. Perhaps it's because that's how peaches are commonly canned. And there is a tremendous variety in canned peaches, including what looks like practically an entire other fruit chapter. For as you look through the canned peaches, you will keep seeing peaches packed not only in their own juice, but packed in pear, apple, and grape juice; peaches packed in heavy syrup, in extra heavy syrup, in light syrup, in unsweetened fruit juice, and in water with no sugar added. It's not just "canned peaches," anymore.

After the Peaches come the Bartlett, Bosc, and D'Anjou Pears, then canned and candied pears. Persimmons are on page 246 and Pineapple, fresh, frozen, canned, and candied, begins on page 247.

The pineapple is not one fruit, it is many fruits. That tough prickly rind is really a collection of small hexagon-shaped fruits fused together, each one a different botanic individual. Siamese centuplets more or less. Unlike many other fruits, pineapples will not get sweeter as they age after harvesting.

Rhubarb is not biologically a fruit, but a vegetable. It's an edible stalk, just like celery. Rhubarb is here in **Fruits** because it's a dessert vegetable. It's seasoned with sugar, not cream sauce—and eaten like a baked apple, not like baked potato.

The Tangelo is a hybrid of the tangerine and grapefruit. It's a delicious fruit, having come from such exceptional parents.

And finally:

How to Read the Numbers: How to read the numbers for **Fruits** is first to read **How to Read the Numbers** for **Vegetables,** page 43, and then to come back here.

Go ahead, don't be lazy.

The column headings in **Fruits** are the same as they are for **Vegetables:**

Unit
One Ounce by Weight
One Cup
Fiber, expressed in Grams per Ounce
(For a discussion of fiber, see **Methodology,** page 36.)

The Unit column is particularly important for **Fruits.** Whereas vegetables generally aren't eaten so that you pick one up and eat the whole thing, fruit is. Fruit is eaten like candy, the portion size is frequently "one piece"—one apple, one peach, one Hershey Bar—in principle, it's the same thing.

The One Ounce by Weight column, as is true for **Vegetables,** cannot be used for quick glance-down-the-page comparisons. One line will reflect the banana as you eat it, another will be for a banana weighed in its peel.

The Cup column is important, but not as reliable as the Ounce. The Cup is subject to the uncertainties of packing, and to variations in the size of pieces.

The Fiber per Ounce column generally has lower numbers for **Fruits** than for **Vegetables.** The carbohydrate in fruit is more the sweet, digestible kind. By the ounce, dried fruit has substantially more fiber than fresh fruit does, and substantially more calories. But that's really more a subject for . . .

How to Eat Fruit: Strawberries are 10.5 calories an ounce. An entire pint container of strawberries, filled to overflowing, has about 120 calories. That's less than almost any candy bar—and filled to overflowing.

Like many candies in **Sweet Little Nothings,** the calories in fruit come from carbohydrate. This is true whether the fruit is fresh, canned, or dried. Protein plays a very small role, almost none. Fruits generally have so little fat that the calorie contribution from carbohydrate is often ten times, twenty times, fifty times as great.

The carbohydrate in fruit has as many calories as the carbohydrate in candy. The difference is that the sugar in candy is concentrated, and the sugar in a piece of fruit is diluted by all that nice, juicy, slurrrrrpy, fruit-flavored water.

How to eat fresh fruit is to enjoy it, because if ever a chapter had bargains, this is it.

What do ⅕ of a Big Mac, an ounce of French fries, ⅔ of an ounce of peanuts, and 70 acerolas have in common? They're all potential snacks, and they're each about 100 calories. If what you want is definitely French fries, then 70 acerolas won't do. But if you're open to suggestions, you should know that 100 calories—or less—can buy you any of the following:

an apple
5 apricots
a banana
a cup of blueberries
half a cantaloupe
3¾ ounces of cherimoya (*sigh)*
20 cherries
1 grapefruit
29 grapes
⅕ of a honeydew melon
½ of a mango
a nectarine
an orange or two
most of a papaya
a papaw
2 peaches
a pear
3 persimmons
⅐ of a pineapple
14 Damson plums
a pomegranate
a cup of raspberries
almost two cups of strawberries
2 or 3 tangelos
2 or 3 tangerines
10 ounces of watermelon, plus a little more

The lowest-calorie fresh fruits are the melons, 7.6 to 9.4 calories an ounce. Berries run 10.1 to 21.3 calories an ounce. Among the citrus fruits, lemon is 7.7 calories an ounce and oranges are 14.5. Grapefruit is smack in the middle, as you might expect by tasting it. The pulpy fruits, such as peaches, nectarines, and plums, run 10.8 to 18.7.

Typical analyses: Apples are about 16 calories an ounce, bananas are 24.1. Grapes are 19 calories an ounce, pears are 17.4. But fruit isn't necessarily eaten by the ounce—it's often eaten by "the piece." This is where you'll find the widest range of all. One blueberry is one calorie. One watermelon is 2,432.

So one way to save calories on fruit is to eat a blueberry instead of a watermelon. Another way to save, if you're going to eat "one," is to eat a smaller blueberry or a smaller watermelon.

Or a smaller apple. Take a guess. What would you think the calorie difference is between two apples, when one is 3 inches in diameter and the other is 4?

Twenty-five percent?

No. The difference is going to be greater than 100%. This is because, when you're talking about solid geometry, the relationship of a 3-inch diameter to a 4-inch diameter will not be 3 to 4. It is going to be $3 \times 3 \times 3$ as compared with $4 \times 4 \times 4$. In other words, the ratio is going to be 27 to 64. That means you can eat two 3-inch apples rather than one 4-inch apple, and save calories in the bargain. Thought you'd like to know.

For the equivalent in canned fruit, you'll have to pick a smaller can.

But there's a better way than that to save calories when you're buying canned fruit. A 16-ounce (1-pound) can of Libby's peaches in heavy syrup is 306 calories, the 8¾-ounce can is 167. A 16-ounce can of Balanced peaches packed in water is 99 calories. Substantially fewer calories in a pound of water-packed peaches than in half a pound of peaches packed in heavy syrup.

The impact of the syrup is such that it practically doesn't matter which fruit comes packed in it:

	Representative Calories per Ounce
apricots in heavy syrup	22.9
peaches in heavy syrup	22.1
pineapple in heavy syrup	21.1
fruit cocktail in heavy syrup	22.5

What happens if you buy fruit in heavy syrup, and drain the syrup off? According to the numbers, the syrup has soaked in, and draining isn't going to get most of those calories out:

	Representative Calories per Ounce Fruit and Syrup	Representative Calories per Ounce Drained Fruit
apricots in heavy syrup	22.9	22.9
peaches in heavy syrup	22.1	22.1
pineapple in heavy syrup	21.1	18.6
fruit cocktail in heavy syrup	22.5	22.3

The most effective way to drain canned fruit is to buy fresh fruit to begin with. But if you want canned fruit, you can still save lots of calories by choosing fruit that's packed in juice or light syrup: The numbers come down from the 20s to the teens:

	Representative Calories per Ounce Packed in Juice	Representative Calories per Ounce Packed in Light Syrup
apricots	13.6	18.7
peaches	12.5	16.4
pineapple	11.1	16.8
fruit cocktail	14.2	17.0

In defense of fruit packed in heavy syrup, I'd like to point out that it can be used as a topping at great savings when compared to syrups and confections sold for that purpose:

	Representative Calories per Ounce
canned apricots in heavy syrup	22.9
canned apricots in extra-heavy syrup	28.6
low-sugar Apricot Spread, Smuckers	39.5
Apricot Preserves, Kraft	69.8
Caramel Topping, Kraft	72.7
Apricot Syrup, Smuckers	74.6
honey	86.2
Chocolate Fudge Topping, Hersheys	90.0

The extreme in eating fruit without syrup is to eat dried fruits. Unfortunately, as a calorie-saving measure it doesn't work:

	Dried	Fresh	Canned in Heavy Syrup
apples	77.9	15.9	25.8 (sweetened applesauce)
apricots	73.7	14.4	22.9
figs	77.7	22.7	23.8
peaches	74.3	10.8	22.1
pears	76.0	17.4	21.6
prunes	72.3	18.7 (plums)	22.2 (plums)
raisins	81.9	19.0 (grapes)	21.8 (grapes)

So eat it moist, it you ve got the choist.

Perhaps the real question is how does dried fruit compare with candy? With nuts? With potato chips? Because in the situations where dried fruit is served, these are likely to be the competition:

	Representative Calories per Ounce
dried fruit	*70.0–104.0*
chocolate-covered raisins, Raisinets, Ward	90.0
popcorn	109.4
pretzels	110.0
carob-coated raisins, CaraCoa (El Molino)	130.0
M&Ms plain	138.0
M&Ms peanut	143.3
potato chips	150.0
cashews	159.0
peanuts	165.9

So dried fruit is substantially lower than an awful lot of other bite-size foods. And fruit pies can be lower still!

Based on USDA home recipes:	**Representative Calories per Ounce**
apple pie	72.6
cherry pie	74.0
peach pie	72.3

But fresh fruit is, of course, lowest of all:

apples	15.9
cherries	19.9
peaches	10.8

So the circle comes full round. Even cherries—nice, sweet, juicy, delicious cherries, a high-calorie fruit—are less than 20 calories an ounce.

In this chapter—no, in this book—fresh fruit is clearly in the limelight.

3 MEATS & GAME

The *Scribner Bantam English Dictionary* says:
Meat is "animal flesh used as food."
Game is "wild animals, birds, or fish pursued for sport or food."
Veal is "meat of the calf."
Lamb is "the flesh of a young sheep used as food."
Pork is "the flesh of swine used as food."

What's in This Chapter? This chapter is filled with the fresh meats you buy from a butcher—beef, veal, lamb, and pork. This chapter also includes a few canned and frozen versions of fresh meat—frozen Steak-Umms, for example.

In addition to beef, veal, lamb, and pork, the chapter also houses less familiar meats—rabbit, venison, beaver, whale, and still less familiar foods like snake, grasshopper, rice-hopper, and locust. They're in the book mostly for fun, but some of these you can find in restaurants. Even on the menu.

The lion's share of data for the less familiar meats came from Africa, the Orient, and Latin America.

What's Related, but Elsewhere? The most obvious related chapters are **Poultry & Game Birds, Fish, Eggs,** and **Cheese.**

Ham is here, but prepackaged sliced ham is not. It's in **Sausages & Cold Cuts.** Meat spreads and pâtés are half a book away, in **Hors D'Oeuvres, Dips & Spreads.**

Pork is not always in this chapter. Nope. Not when it's pork chow mein. Pork chow mein, beef stew, corned beef hash, and frozen meat dinners are all in **Combination Main Dishes.**

Meat soups—whether beef bouillon or Chunky Sirloin Burger—are in the **Soups** chapter.

"Strained Beef" and "Junior Lamb" are undeniably meats, but they're in **Baby Foods** nonetheless. The Big Mac. The Whopper. A Triple Burger with Cheese. They're all in **Fast Food.**

Airline Fare has a substantial meat component and the Army chapter, **Mess,** has half a ton of it. Other meats eaten away from home can be found in **Campers' Foods,** in **Boy Scouts,** and in **Foods for Space Travel.**

Imitations of meat are in **Vegetarian Foods.**

Meats for your pet have a chapter all their own. If you feed your dog or cat the scraps from this chapter, you might want to read the **Pet Foods** Chapter Preface first. Especially if your animal is overweight.

Another related chapter is **Three Frugal Repasts.** Look there, not here, for the calories in wildlife postage stamps.

Before we get into the arrangement of this chapter, I would like to address the arrangement of a cow. When it comes to beef, one picture is worth a thousand words. The following illustration, courtesy of the National Live Stock and Meat Board, shows a few dozen retail cuts, both by themselves and according to their anatomical origins.

There are innumerable names for the various cuts of beef, many of the fanciest names referring to chuck. The same cut may have a different name in a different butcher shop. Fortunately, the names used on the chart, and in this book, are widely known and accepted.

The Arrangement of This Chapter is as follows:

RETAIL CUTS OF BEEF

WHERE THEY COME FROM AND HOW TO COOK THEM

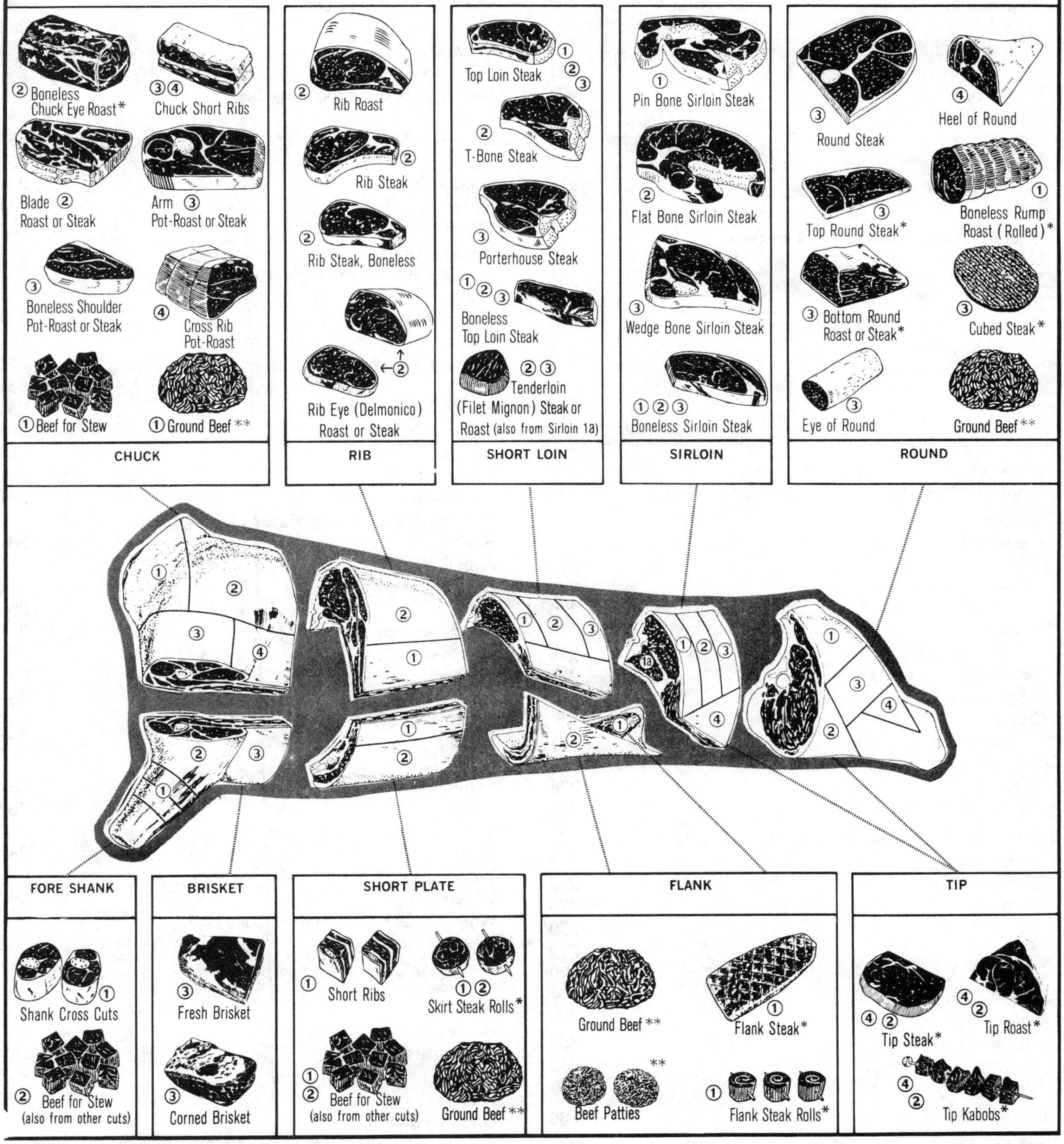

CHUCK

② Boneless Chuck Eye Roast*
③④ Chuck Short Ribs
Blade ② Roast or Steak
Arm ③ Pot-Roast or Steak
③ Boneless Shoulder Pot-Roast or Steak
④ Cross Rib Pot-Roast
① Beef for Stew
① Ground Beef**

RIB

② Rib Roast
② Rib Steak
② Rib Steak, Boneless
② Rib Eye (Delmonico) Roast or Steak

SHORT LOIN

①②③ Top Loin Steak
② T-Bone Steak
③ Porterhouse Steak
①②③ Boneless Top Loin Steak
②③ Tenderloin (Filet Mignon) Steak or Roast (also from Sirloin 1a)

SIRLOIN

① Pin Bone Sirloin Steak
② Flat Bone Sirloin Steak
③ Wedge Bone Sirloin Steak
①②③ Boneless Sirloin Steak

ROUND

③ Round Steak
④ Heel of Round
③ Top Round Steak*
① Boneless Rump Roast (Rolled)*
③ Bottom Round Roast or Steak*
③ Cubed Steak*
③ Eye of Round
Ground Beef**

FORE SHANK

① Shank Cross Cuts
② Beef for Stew (also from other cuts)

BRISKET

③ Fresh Brisket
③ Corned Brisket

SHORT PLATE

① Short Ribs
①② Skirt Steak Rolls*
①② Beef for Stew (also from other cuts)
Ground Beef**

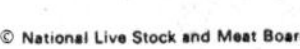

*May be Roasted, Broiled, Panbroiled or Panfried from high quality beef.
**May be Roasted, (Baked), Broiled, Panbroiled or Panfried.

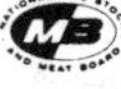

How to Read the Numbers for **Meats** is complicated, and will almost certainly require more than one read-through.

The column headings are:

Unit
One Ounce by Weight
One Cup, Diced, Not Packed

Almost without exception, the Unit will be one pound of meat. But that's not as simple as it sounds, because successive lines describe a succession of different kinds of pounds.

For most of the cuts of meat in this chapter, the descriptions follow a regular pattern. There are exceptions, of course. But the pattern is so common that it makes sense for us to look at an example together:

	UNIT		1 OZ., BY WT.		1 CUP DICED, NOT PACKED	
	Cal.	Carb.	Cal.	Carb.	Cal.	Carb.
BEEF						
LOIN OR SHORT LOIN						
T-BONE STEAK						
CHOICE GRADE						
BONE-IN						
1. One pound of Raw untrimmed meat (includes separable fat) with bone [55% lean, 34% fat, 11% bone]	1604	0.0	100.3	0.00	—	—
2. Cooked (broiled) [yield: approx. 12.2 oz, of which approx. 10.4 oz. are meat and approx. 1.8 oz. are bone]	1395	0.0	114.8	0.00	—	—
3. Trimmed of separable fat before cooking; Cooked (broiled) [yield: approx. 8.2 oz., of which approx. 6.4 oz. are meat and approx. 1.8 oz. are bone]	408	0.0	49.7	0.00	—	—
One pound of Cooked (broiled) meat (weight includes bone):						
4. Yield from approx. 21.1 oz. (1 lb. 5.1 oz.) of raw untrimmed meat with bone, which had **not** been trimmed of separable fat before cooking	1836	0.0	114.8	0.00	—	—
5. Yield from approx. 31.2 oz. (1 lb. 15.2 oz.) of raw untrimmed meat with bone, which **had** been trimmed of separable fat before cooking	795	0.0	49.7	0.00	—	—
BONELESS						
6. One pound of Raw untrimmed meat (includes separable fat) [62% lean, 38% fat]	1802	0.0	112.6	0.00	(518)	0.0
7. Cooked (broiled) [yield: approx. 11.7 oz.] (6g/0g/12g/36%/na)	1568	0.0	134.2	0.00	(617)	0.0
8. Trimmed of separable fat before cooking; Cooked (broiled) [yield: approx. 7.2 oz.] (9g/0g/3g/58%/na)	458	0.0	63.3	0.00	(291)	0.0
One pound of Cooked (broiled) meat:						
9. Yield from approx. 21.9 oz. (1 lb. 5.9 oz.) of raw untrimmed meat, which had **not** been trimmed of separable fat before cooking	2147	0.0	134.2	0.00	(617)	0.0
10. Yield from approx. 35.4 oz. (2 lbs. 3.4 oz.) of raw untrimmed meat, which **had** been trimmed of separable fat before cooking	1012	0.0	63.3	0.00	(291)	0.0

In the data pages, the lines are not numbered. I've added line numbers here for ease of reference.

The first five lines for a cut of meat will describe a pound weighed with the bone in. Of course, some cuts of meat are always boneless—for example, flank steak. But if the bone is sometimes present, the bone-in cut will always come first.

The first data line says, "One Pound of Raw untrimmed meat (includes separable fat) with bone." The description includes percentages for "lean," "fat," and "bone." Since every data line that follows will be a variation on one or more of these factors, let us take them up one at a time.

On **line 1**, "One pound" means one pound of the entire cut including the bone. An entire rib roast will obviously weigh much more than one pound, and a lamb chop will weigh less. But the calories in the Unit column will always be for one pound's worth.

The pound being described is "Raw." This means that all the calories are included, even those in the fat that usually drains away in cooking. For this reason, the first line is usually not a good one to take your calories from. There will be exceptions, however. This is the best line to use for a stew, or if all the drippings from the meat are to be used in a gravy.

This pound of meat is "untrimmed" and "includes separable fat." However, this does not mean that absolutely no fat was trimmed by the butcher; some certainly was. It does mean that the meat did not undergo a further careful trimming of all separable fat, either before or after it left the butcher shop. We will meet this trimming process again. It has the greatest impact on the calories.

Let me remind you once more that the meat is weighed with the bone, and that the pound measurement includes that bone.

But how much bone? The percentage that follows tells you how much. If the particular piece of meat that you buy contains either more or less bone than I've allowed for, the calories per pound, of course, will not be the same.

In addition to the percentage of bone, line 1 tells you the percentage of lean and the percentage of fat. But the terms "lean" and "fat" are not absolutes. "Separable lean" will, in fact, include some fat, notably as "marbling." The "separable fat" will include some meat and connective tissue.

The next two lines, **lines 2 and 3,** describe what happens when the pound of raw meat is cooked. The bone will still be there, but some of the meat will have been lost in the cooking process. The approximate yield is specified; this will always be less than the original 16 ounces. Of this yield, the approximate breakdown into meat and bone will also be given. (Following the lead of the USDA, my calculations assume that the weight of the bone does not change, so that all the weight loss comes from the meat.)

What about the calories? Calories in the Unit column go down, because fat is lost in the cooking process. The calories in the Ounce column, however, will usually go up. This is because it is common for even more water to be lost than fat. You wind up with cooked meat that is more "solid," and therefore has more calories per ounce. (Even after meat is cooked, water is still a substantial component. A cooked trimmed lamb chop is approximately 62% water.)

This second data line is the line to use when you're eating meat and all you know is what it weighed before cooking. (There will be a better line to use if you can weigh your meat after cooking.) Again, line 2 talks only about untrimmed bone-in meat.

The next data line, line 3, tells the story if the meat was trimmed of separable fat before cooking. Again the "pound" measurement is taken for one pound of raw untrimmed meat weighed with the bone—but this time the separable fat is trimmed off before the meat is cooked.

What happens to the calories?

The calories go way, way down. It is not uncommon for the calories per ounce to be cut in half if the meat is trimmed of separable fat before cooking.

The next two data lines, **lines 4 and 5,** describe the calories in one pound of cooked meat. The meat is weighed with the bone. Line 4 is for meat that had not been trimmed of separable fat before cooking, and line 5 is for meat that had been trimmed. In each case, the amount of raw meat with bone that was required to yield a pound of cooked meat with bone is specified. It will always take more than a pound of raw meat to yield a pound of cooked meat.

Lines 4 and 5 are the lines to use if you weigh your portion—with the bone—after cooking. The calories will be higher for a pound of cooked untrimmed meat than for a pound weighed raw.

Line 5 concludes the data for bone-in cuts. The same presentation is then given for the boneless form of the meat.

Line 6 is for raw untrimmed boneless meat. Indented under it, **lines 7 and 8** are the same two cooked versions we saw before: meat that had not been trimmed before cooking and meat that had been trimmed. All of these figures will be higher in calories per ounce than the corresponding figures for the bone-in cuts, because none of what you're weighing is bone. (For an explanation of the funny little numbers in parentheses on lines 7 and 8 (6g/0g/12g/36%/na) and (9g/0g/3g/58%/na), see **Supplemental Numbers** in **Methodology,** page 36.)

Lines 9 and 10 again describe one pound of cooked meat, but this time, of course, without the bone. Line 9 is for one pound of cooked meat that had not been trimmed of separable fat before cooking; line 10 is for one pound that had.

The boneless figures are bound to be more accurate than the bone-in because different servings will vary in their proportion of bone to meat. In fact it is a good general rule, in any chapter in this book, to measure your food in the form closest to the way in which you will be eating it. If you eat your food cooked, weigh your food cooked—or trimmed, or peeled, or with the shells taken off—just as long as this book has the figures you will need to use that weight in calculating calories.

With this mass of numbers, especially for beef, you might think that all these calorie figures are absolutely precise. Unfortunately, they aren't. There will always be variations in cutting and trimming. Fat content varies with the season of the year. Grading (which we're coming to) is not an exact science. Cooking time will make a big difference. But this is still a far more elaborate collection of data than you will find in almost any other chapter. The calorie content of vegetables and fruits and fish also varies with the season. Just as a cow does, a tuna fish has flesh of different sorts on different parts of its body—but you will search in vain for the counterpart of precision found here, in **Meats,** where calories are specified on a rib-by-rib basis.

Missing, however, from the *Beef* tables are figures for ground chuck, for ground round, and for ground sirloin. The reason they're missing is that there is no way of telling exactly what goes into any single pound of "ground sirloin." The extent of the trimming is much more difficult to determine than the extent of the trimming of a sirloin steak. Moreover, what are they calling sirloin? A pound of raw, choice "wedge and round-bone sirloin steak," untrimmed and boneless, is 1,421 calories. A pound of raw, choice "hipbone sirloin steak," untrimmed and boneless, is 1,870 calories. Both are certainly capable of becoming "ground sirloin," but the difference in calories can give you three free hamburger rolls—with room to spare.

We do have two "ground beef" figures in our tables, and both are quite lean. The "10% fat" ground beef is leaner than a choice round steak, and that is very lean indeed. The "20% fat" ground beef has about the same fat content as the average for the entire chuck portion of beef. What you find in your supermarket labeled as "ground beef" is likely to have substantially more fat than either of these. You can control what goes into your ground beef by having it ground to order from a cut that you specify. It's going to be more expensive. It's up to you to decide whether it's a good investment.

When we leave the territory of steaks, roasts, and chops, we turn to *Organ Meats,* and these include liver, sweetbreads, and tongue. The data lines are simpler. There's no bone to worry about, and the fat has been removed by the time the meat is purchased. Thus there are only two lines of data for each meat: "raw" and "cooked."

When it comes to *Game and Less Familiar Meats,* I don't have information in nearly such detail. There's raw walrus and cooked raccoon—in general, whatever data I could find.

How to Eat Meat: Meat has a reputation among dieters as being a very high-calorie food. To echo a phrase from *Porgy and Bess,* "It Ain't Necessarily So."

As with any food, when the question is how to eat meat, the answer is found in another question: Where do the calories come from?

Most of the calories in a pound of untrimmed meat come from fat. The calories in a pound of trimmed meat come from fat and from protein. An equal weight of fat and protein will not have an equal caloric impact. The ratio is approximately 9 to 4—or more than double for the fat. Moreover, most of the weight of "lean meat" is actually water, while most of the weight of "fat" is fat. A raw, untrimmed lamb chop that is "67% lean, 33% fat" will in fact have more than three times as many calories from fat as from protein.

The way to eat meat is to get rid of the fat.

Opportunity knocks three times: when you buy it, when you prepare it, and when you sit down to eat it at the table. Three different opportunities. Three different results.

Buying meat? Buying beef? Just look:

Choice grade, Trimmed and Cooked:	**Calories per Ounce**
round steak	54.2
chuck from the arm	54.8
rump roast	59.0
club steak	69.2
chuck from the fifth rib	70.7

The numbers tell the story here. If you eat a meat dinner every night, and it's half a pound of club steak instead of half a pound of round, at the end of a year you can have gained twelve. And one-half. Pounds. Zounds!

Good or Standard Grade meats are lower in fat and higher in protein than Choice. Choice is lower in fat and higher in protein than Prime. I don't mean the fat around the edges; there's fat in meat that can't be trimmed: Marbling.

	Calories per Ounce, Trimmed and Cooked		
	Choice	**Good**	**Standard**
round steak	54.2	49.7	46.8
chuck from the arm	54.8	50.8	47.7
rump roast	59.0	51.1	51.1
club steak	69.2	61.6	55.3
chuck from the fifth rib	70.7	62.1	58.5

One prominent exception to the higher-grade/higher-fat rule is chopped meat. There, the more you pay for it, the leaner it's likely to be—at least in theory.

If the idea of buying a lower grade is not appealing, there's another way to save calories. I would like to toss here some advice from Chaucer:

And bet(ter) than old beef is the tendre veel.

The data confirm what "The Merchant's Tale" advises. Even the finest milk-fed veal is substantially less fatty than beef. Trimmed figures for veal were not available and could not be calculated from the data I had. But this is how untrimmed veal compares with untrimmed beef, when both are cooked:

	Calories per Ounce, Untrimmed and Cooked
VEAL	
chuck cuts & boneless veal for stew	66.6
loin cuts	66.3
plate (breast of veal)	85.9
rib roast	76.3
round with rump (roasts and leg cutlets)	61.3
BEEF	
entire chuck (average of 1st–5th ribs, arm and neck)	92.8
loin or short loin:	
loin end or sirloin (wedge and round bone sirloin steak)	109.8
flatbone or hipbone steak	138.2
short plate including skirt steak	134.5
rib roast:	
entire rib (average of 6th–12th ribs) including rib eye or Delmonico cut	124.9
round:	
heel of round	74.1
rump roast	98.5

However, what holds true for the muscle meats doesn't necessarily follow for the organ meats. Here, veal can sometimes be higher-calorie than beef:

	Calories per Ounce, Cooked
Heart	
Beef	50.2
Lamb	39.7
Pork	40.8
Veal	43.4
Kidney	
Beef	39.1
Lamb	36.6
Pork	42.8
Veal	46.8
Liver	
Beef	38.8
Lamb	56.4
Pork	38.3
Veal	45.4
Lung	
Beef	34.0
Lamb	32.9
Pork	28.1
Veal	29.5
Pancreas	
Beef	76.8
Lamb	52.7
Pork	62.1
Veal	72.6
Spleen	
Beef	41.1
Lamb	42.5
Pork	42.2
Veal	35.4
Sweetbreads	
Beef	88.5
Veal	29.8
Tongue	
Beef	81.7
Lamb	78.5
Pork	76.6
Veal	53.0

If you've already decided on steak, then by far the most important advice on how to eat meat is to trim it before you cook it. Savings go over 50% in some cases. Even for the relatively leaner cuts, such as round steak, the savings are substantial. If you are a frequent meat eater, the effect of trimming your beef could be enough, by itself, to accomplish your entire diet. If you've decided to eat steak, **The Calorielogue** is there for you with many steaks to choose from. But regardless of which choice you make, the savings I quote for trimming are for meat trimmed before cooking. I have no figures for a steak trimmed of its separable fat while it's on your plate.

But even if you weren't able to trim your meat before it was cooked, you still have an opportunity to rid yourself of some of the fat. You can broil it out. The more "well done" you cook your meat, the more fat will melt away. This is not meant as epicurean advice, but it does get rid of calories.

If you're cooking chopped meat—a hamburger or a meat loaf—the finer you chop the meat, the more fat is likely to cook away. You're increasing the surface area, permitting more fat to drain out.

If you add breadcrumbs to chopped meat, you cannot simply figure in the calorie content of the bread, because the breadcrumbs will hold some of the fat that would otherwise have drained away.

A third opportunity to lower the calories in meat comes at the table. You can trim the fat from around the edges. Although I cannot say how much fat you can trim from each ounce of steak after it's cooked, I can say that each gram of fat you don't eat will save you about 9 calories. A gram is less than 1/28 of an ounce. (Of course, even the fattier part of cooked meat will not be pure fat but will include connective tissue, moisture, etc.)

I'll admit that by the time meat comes to the table, the selection of cut has pretty well been made; however, it may be possible, even then, to exercise a choice . . .

. . . You're invited to Aunt Tillie's for dinner, and she's also invited a big roast beef. The two side surfaces, obviously, are on different ribs. Six ounces of beef from the 11th to 12th rib has 818 calories. Six ounces from the 7th to 8th rib will have only 707. To put it another way, if looking at the data pages helps you pick the correct side, you can have your six ounces of roast beef —and then a scoop—3 fluid ounces—of Breyers Cherry Vanilla Ice Cream for free!

To make it just a little easier, have I got a list for you!

From out of the **Meats** data pages I have rounded up the "fork fulls." Here are the calories per ounce for every entry in *Beef, Veal, Lamb,* and *Pork.* There are calories for "trimmed" and "untrimmed," but only boneless, and only cooked. In other words, as you finally eat it:

	1 Oz. by Wt. Cooked		1 Oz. by Wt. Cooked		1 Oz. by Wt. Cooked	
	Choice		Good		Standard	
	Cal. Trim	Cal. Untrim	Cal. Trim	Cal. Untrim	Cal. Trim	Cal. Untrim
BEEF						
Brisket	62.9	116.8	56.5	105.8	53.1	99.3
Chuck Cuts:						
entire chuck (average of 1st–5th ribs, arm and neck)	60.7	92.8	—	—	—	—
1st–2nd ribs (short ribs) includes chuck eye	63.8	87.7	57.3	82.0	52.2	69.2
3rd–4th ribs (short ribs)	67.5	110.4	58.7	98.8	54.8	86.0
5th rib (short rib) includes chuck eye	70.7	121.2	62.1	107.0	58.5	90.5
arm	54.8	82.0	50.8	71.8	47.7	64.4
neck	55.6	83.1	52.2	79.7	50.8	74.3
Flank Steak	—	55.6	—	54.2	—	51.3
Foreshank (shin)	52.2	77.5	49.9	69.5	48.5	66.7
Hindshank	52.2	102.4	49.9	87.1	47.7	64.6
Loin or Short Loin: porterhouse steak	63.6	131.9	55.9	126.6	53.9	110.7
T-bone steak	63.3	134.2	56.5	125.4	55.9	108.4

	1 Oz. by Wt. Cooked		1 Oz. by Wt. Cooked		1 Oz. by Wt. Cooked	
	Choice		Good		Standard	
	Cal. Trim	Cal. Untrim	Cal. Trim	Cal. Untrim	Cal. Trim	Cal. Untrim
club steak (shell steak, top loin or New York State)	69.2	128.8	61.6	112.9	55.3	94.2
loin end or sirloin (wedge and round bone sirloin steak)	58.7	109.8	51.9	100.2	50.2	88.5
double-bone sirloin steak (pinbone steak)	61.3	115.8	53.9	103.6	49.7	89.1
flatbone or hipbone steak	68.1	138.2	59.3	125.1	57.9	111.8
short plate including skirt steak	63.0	134.5	56.5	122.6	53.1	109.0
Rib Roast: entire rib (average of 6th–12th ribs) including rib eye or Delmonico cut	68.4	124.9	—	—	—	—
6th (blade) rib	74.6	123.9	63.8	105.8	58.7	90.5
7th–8th ribs	67.2	117.8	60.2	104.1	58.2	90.2
9th–10th ribs includes rib eye or Delmonico cut	68.1	130.8	60.7	112.4	59.9	95.6
11th–12th ribs includes rib eye or Delmonico cut	68.1	136.5	61.0	118.3	58.2	99.9
Round: entire round	53.6	74.1	—	—	—	—
round steak	54.2	73.0	49.7	66.4	46.8	57.3
heel of round	51.1	74.1	49.4	67.0	46.0	55.6
rump roast	59.0	98.5	51.1	89.9	51.1	81.4

	Calories per Ounce, Cooked	
	Trimmed Before Cooking	Untrimmed
VEAL		
chuck cuts & boneless veal for stew	—	66.6
loin cuts	—	66.3
plate (breast of veal)	—	85.9
rib roast	—	76.3
round with rump (roasts and leg cutlets)	—	61.3
LAMB		
leg	52.8	79.1
loin chop	53.3	101.8
rib chops	59.8	115.4
shoulder	58.1	96.0
PORK		
ham (skinless)	61.5	106.0
loin (skinless)	72.0	102.6
loin chops (skinless)	76.5	110.8
shoulder cuts including Boston butt (skinless)	69.2	100.1
picnic (skinless)	60.1	106.0
spareribs	—	124.1
cured ham:		
dry, long cure, country-style, medium fatness	—	110.3
relatively lean	—	87.9
light cure, commercial (skinless)	53.0	81.9
cured, shoulder cuts, light cure commercial		
Boston butt (skinless)	68.9	93.6
picnic (skinless)	59.8	91.6
brains	36.9	—

And before you recover from that list, have I got another one for you!

Here are the calories per ounce and pound for common restaurant cuts of beef, veal, lamb, and pork—an average of choice to prime grades. This table is not drawn from **The Calorielogue.** Because the source of data for the list that follows is different than it was for the preceding list, comparisons between the two tables will not be as reliable as comparisons between two different cuts of meat within the same list. Almost all of the values were cited as for "lean meat including marbling, but with separable fat removed." The few exceptions are noted.

Common Restaurant Cuts	Calories per Pound, Raw	Calories per Ounce, Raw
Cuts of Beef: Choice to Prime Grades		
Lean (including marbling) with separable fat removed, except as indicated.		
STEAK:		
top loin	1271	79.4
flank	1067	66.6
Porterhouse	1099	68.6
rib	1189	74.3
round, bottom	1081	67.5
round, top	1040	65.0
sirloin	944	59.0
T-bone	1121	70.0
tenderloin	1017	63.5
ROAST:		
tip	844	52.7
rib	1294	80.8
POT-ROAST:		
arm	1194	74.6
blade	1353	84.5
heel of round	1003	62.6
boneless neck (rolled)	1117	69.8
standing rump	1067	66.6
OTHER CUTS:		
brisket, point half boneless	1380	86.2
brisket, flat half boneless	1416	88.5
ground beef (separable fat not removed)	1194	74.6
ground beef, extra lean (separable fat not removed)	740	46.2
short ribs	1830	114.3
stew meat, chuck (separable fat not removed)	1911	119.4
stew meat, round (separable fat not removed)	1180	73.7
Cuts of Veal		
Lean (including marbling) with separable fat removed, except as indicated.		
CHOP:		
loin (separable fat not removed)	940	58.7
rib (separable fat not removed)	976	61.0
STEAK:		
arm (all lean portion)	908	56.7
blade (all lean portion)	958	59.8
cutlet, round (all lean portion)	917	57.3
sirloin (all lean portion)	926	57.8
ROAST:		
rump	795	49.6
sirloin	799	49.9
STEW MEAT:		
breast (separable fat not removed)	1571	98.1

I guess that just about does it for fresh meat. We haven't discussed *Game,* but if you're game the numbers are there.

The last section of the **Meats & Game** chapter is *Insects.* **How to Eat Insects** is not within my bailiwick, but I can tell you where the calories come from.

"Waiter, waiter, there's a fly in my soup!"

"Protein, protein!" Except if it's fried.

4 SAUSAGES & COLD CUTS

What's a sausage? What is a "cold cut"? My *Webster's Collegiate* defines sausage as: "A highly seasoned minced meat (as pork) usually stuffed in casings of prepared animal intestine."

The same source defines cold cuts as "Sliced assorted cold meats."

What's in This Chapter: This chapter contains both fresh and canned sausages. Within these two broad categories, the sausages listed may be cooked or not cooked, dried or semi-dried, smoked or not smoked. Fresh sausages generally are seasoned, but must be cooked before eating. Among the fresh sausages are bockwurst, bratwurst, fresh pork sausage, and combination beef-pork sausages.

The dried sausages, such as pepperoni and the hard-style salamis, are frequently characterized by microbial fermentation, which produces the "tangy" taste. These sausages, and most sausages of Italian origin, are neither cooked nor smoked.

Summer sausage (cervelat; thuringer) is semi-dried. Like most Germanic sausages, it is generally smoked and cooked.

Most of the remaining sausages in the chapter are cured and cooked. They may or may not be smoked.

Certain of the sausages, such as bologna, frankfurters, knockwurst, and Vienna sausage, are restricted by federal regulation to a maximum of 30% fat based on cooked composition. The regulation permits these sausages to contain up to 10% added water, and also allows the inclusion of meat by-products and variety meats. Non-meat ingredients may include nonfat dry milk, soy flours, or cereal grains. The recipe for pork-veal bockwurst calls for milk and eggs.

Sausages can also be made from poultry—chicken franks, chicken bologna, and turkey pastrami are all here.

What's Related, but Elsewhere: There's no doubt about which chapter is most closely related—**Meats. Sausages & Cold Cuts** could, in fact, have been a sub-section there. But they have a chapter of their own because cold cuts function as the center of a sandwich, not as the center of a meal. Then, too, there were the chicken hot dogs and turkey bologna to consider.

Ham has its feet in two places. Canned ham that you cook and slice is both here and in **Meats.** But prepackaged ham sold for cold cuts clearly belonged only here.

Deviled ham and similar spreadable meat and poultry products are in **Hors D'Oeuvres.** So is pâté.

The primary listing for corned beef is here, but canned corned beef is in **Meats.** Corned beef hash is in **Combination Main Dishes.** (What is corned beef hash anyway, but a corned beef and potato sausage without the skin?) **Combination Main Dishes** also has a couple of franks. So does **Fast Food.**

This is the chapter from which to bring home the bacon—but for baconless bacon, see **Vegetarian Foods.** For bacon served on a large scale, see **Mess.** For a far-out bacon breakfast, see **Foods For Space Travel.**

The Arrangement of Sausages & Cold Cuts is alphabetical:

How to Read the Numbers: The column headings are:

Unit
One Slice or Link
One Ounce by Weight
One Pound

The Unit column will often be an entire package, when it comes to brand name products. For generic information, the Unit column will give the calories for one or more commonly marketed sizes, and possibly "one pound." In both cases, a slice will also frequently be specified as the Unit.

The One Slice column is provided for prepackaged, presliced sausages. You can find the lowest-calorie slice just by looking down this column—you won't have to look down the Unit column, and you won't have to look down the Ounce by Weight. But you should be aware that the least caloric slice may simply be the thinnest.

One thing to watch for is that the same product, sold in different size packages, may contain slices of different weights. For example, Kahn's "Thick Sliced Bologna" is actually thicker if you buy it in the 8-ounce package than if you buy it in the 12-ounce package.

The Ounce by Weight column is the old standard. The One Pound column is the ounce times 16.

Cold cuts are usually ready-to-eat. But sometimes, as with bacon, the numbers on alternate lines are for "raw" and "cooked." So if you're comparing bacon to bologna, please bear that difference in mind.

How to Eat Sausages & Cold Cuts: In this chapter, the range of calories is enormous.

The calories come overwhelmingly from fat, and because fat has an impact of approximately 9 calories per gram (a gram is less than 1⁄28 of an ounce), even a very small difference in fat content will make a big difference in the calories. The way to eat a sausage is to choose one with a higher proportion of its calories coming from protein or carbohydrate.

Protein, of course, is inherent in the meat or poultry ingredients. Carbohydrate will come from cereal fillers, and from sweeteners such as corn syrup and molasses. In liverwurst, some of the carbohydrate comes from liver.

Unfortunately, you cannot tell by the name of a sausage how many calories there will be. You can't even guess at it!

Based on USDA data:	**Calories per Ounce**
beef bologna	89.0
pork bologna	70.0
turkey bologna	57.0

I concede that at a guess, turkey bologna might be chosen as lower in calories than pork. But who could guess that pork bologna would have fewer calories than beef?

And look at this, also based on data from the USDA:

	Calories per Ounce
beef luncheon meat, thin-sliced	34.9
beef luncheon meat, loaved	87.0

How could you figure that the difference between "thin-sliced" and "loaved" would be better than two to one!

Well, wait a minute! Maybe the thing we should be looking for is consistently high calories among products called "Loaves"? According to the numbers, if there is any consistency to be found, it is that they are consistently inconsistent:

	Calories per Ounce
sliced Gourmet Loaf, Eckrich	35.0
sliced Luxury Loaf, Oscar Mayer	37.6
sliced Honey Loaf, Oscar Mayer	38.0
sliced Jellied Corned Beef Loaf, Oscar Mayer	39.7
Peppered Loaf, Eckrich	40.0
barbecue loaf, USDA	49.0
Old Fashioned Loaf, Oscar Mayer	65.8
picnic loaf, USDA	66.0
olive loaf, USDA	66.6
ham & cheese loaf, USDA	73.0
Banquet Loaf, Eckrich	75.0
mother's loaf, USDA	79.9

It's funny that "Gourmet" Loaf is the lowest. Mother's Loaf is the highest. (Must be a Jewish mother.)

Is there any way to determine calories for a cold cut, without this book in your hands?

Yes, there are some generalizations that can be made. I'm hesitant to give them though, because of course there will be exceptions. If you promise to keep that in mind, here they are. (If you haven't promised, skip the next 5 inches of text.)

In general, the poultry versions of cold cuts are lower than their red-meat counterparts—the chicken bologna, the turkey salami, the turkey pastrami, the chicken franks.

One exception will be the turkey hams. They range from 34.6 to 46 calories per ounce. The regular hams start even below that. In fact, as another general rule, one low-calorie way to eat cold cuts is to eat ham, believe it or not!

	Calories per Ounce
sliced Cooked Ham, Eckrich	33.3
Smoked Cooked Ham, Oscar Mayer	33.3
Ham, Hormel	35.0
sliced Jubilee Ham Steak, Oscar Mayer	35.0
sliced ham, extra lean, USDA	37.1
sliced Slender Smoked Ham, Eckrich	40.0
Chopped Ham, Eckrich	50.0
sliced Smoked Ham, A&P	50.0

One reason for ham's "low-calorie-ness" is that it's relatively moist. But again, generalizations won't always hold. Hormel's canned ham patties are 101.3 calories an ounce.

Consistently above 100 calories an ounce are the drier cold cuts—the hard salamis and the pepperonis:

	Calories per Ounce
sliced Hard Salami, Swift Premium	110.0
sliced Hard Salami, Oscar Mayer	113.0
sliced Dairy Hard Salami, Hormel	120.0
sliced Genoa Salami, Swift Premium	120.0
salami, dry roll, USDA	127.6
Genoa Salami, De Lusso	130.0
sliced Pepperoni, Hormel	140.0
pepperoni made with pork and beef, USDA	140.9
Pepperoni, Swift Premium	150.0

So there is a tremendous advantage in this chapter to picking and choosing, even among very similar foods. But even after you have made your decision: "Bologna or bust," you have a second chance. You can still choose your calories per slice:

	Calories per Slice
sliced Lebanon Beef Bologna, Oscar Mayer	46.0
thin-sliced Beef Bologna, Oscar Mayer	47.0
thin-sliced Bologna, Oscar Mayer	47.0
sliced German Bologna, Oscar Mayer	53.0
sliced Beef Bologna, Oscar Mayer	72.0
sliced Bologna and Cheese, Oscar Mayer	72.0
sliced Garlic Beef Bologna, Oscar Mayer	72.0
sliced Bologna, Oscar Mayer	75.0
thick-sliced Bologna, Oscar Mayer	120.0
thick-sliced Beef Bologna, Oscar Mayer	120.0

Question: If you are very hungry, do you do better calorie-wise to make a triple-decker with three slices of bread and two layers of cold cuts, or do you have two slices of bread with a lot of extra meat?

Answer: A typical slice of bread runs about 75 calories an ounce. So the answer is going to depend on which cold cut you're eating. If you're eating Oscar Mayer's Beef Bologna at 90.2 calories an ounce, the answer is to go for the triple-decker. If you are eating Oscar Mayer's "Lebanon" Beef Bologna at 57 calories an ounce, less bread and more meat is the answer.

But for heaven's sake don't stop here—go to the **Breads** chapter and see how much you can save by choosing a thinner slice of bread. The more you can save on the outside, the more you can put on the inside.

And further for people who like sandwiches I should say that:

a tablespoon of mustard has about 12 calories
a tablespoon of mayonnaise has 101 calories
a tablespoon of butter has 102 calories

an ounce of lettuce has 3.7 calories
an ounce of tomato has 6.3 calories

a 1-oz. slice of American cheese has about 106 calories
a 1-oz. slice of imported Swiss has about 112 calories
a 1-oz. slice of Muenster has about 104 calories

An order of potato salad might be anywhere from 125 to 185 calories for half a cup, depending on the recipe. Cole slaw made with mayonnaise might be 85 calories for half a cup. A large dill pickle, almost 5 ounces, has 15 calories.

The dill pickle has about 3 calories per ounce. The heavyweight in this chapter—bacon—can have 50 times that much!

	Calories per Ounce, Cooked
sliced Bacon, Range Brand	131.2
thick-sliced Hickory Smoked Bacon, Kahn's	142.5
Farm Hickory Smoked Bacon, Rudy's	146.0
Hickory Smoked Bacon, Kahn's	146.3
sliced Bacon, Black Label	161.3
Regular Bacon, Oscar Mayer	161.5
Thick Bacon Slices, Oscar Mayer	161.5
Wafer Thin Bacon Slices, Oscar Mayer	161.5
sliced Bacon, Lazy Maple	175.0
sliced Bacon, Swift Premium	175.0

An excellent alternative to the more familiar style of bacon is Canadian-style bacon:

	Calories per Ounce
Canadian-style bacon, USDA	78.5
Canadian-style Bacon, Oscar Mayer	73.5

With bacon running as high as 175 calories an ounce, and Canadian bacon as low as 73.5, the value of consulting the data becomes clear: If you eat one ounce of Canadian bacon instead of one ounce of "regular" bacon with your breakfast every morning—you could lose more than ten pounds a year.

5 POULTRY & GAME BIRDS

According to my Webster's Dictionary, poultry means "domesticated birds kept for eggs or meat."

Game birds, of course, are not domesticated.

What's in This Chapter: Chicken and turkey and duck and goose, and birds that are off the beaten quack: finch, grouse, partridge, pheasant, squab, and others. Much of the data for the less familiar game birds came from outside the United States. And the common domesticated chicken popped up in the literature from all over the world under its scientific name, *Gallus gallus.*

Certainly, we Americans eat more chicken than we do any other bird. Goose McNugget? Kentucky Fried Finch?

What's Related, but Elsewhere: In this book, the chicken comes first and the egg comes two chapters later.

Lots of fried chicken is in **Fast Food.**

Combination Main Dishes gets the chicken pot pies and the à la Kings, and the frozen chicken and turkey dinners. Chicken chow mein is also in **Combination Main Dishes.** Chicken of the Sea is in **Fish.**

Chicken roll and sliced turkey breast are in **Sausages & Cold Cuts.** Ditto for chicken hot dogs, turkey pastrami, and chicken bologna. Chicken spreads are in **Hors D'Oeuvres, Dips & Spreads,** and so is chicken liver pâté. There are bite-sized chicken sandwiches in **Foods For Space Travel.**

A great many **Soups** begin here in **Poultry.**

There are chicken and turkey dinners in **Baby Foods.** Chicken-flavored cat food is in **Pet Foods.** It all depends on who your baby is.

The Arrangement of This Chapter: First there's Chicken. On the heels of Chicken is Capon, and after Capon are the chickens from overseas.

Then comes Turkey, followed by Duck and Goose. The *Game And Less Familiar Birds* are in alphabetical order, Dusky Ouzel through Wood Sandpiper. *Frozen* and *Canned Poultry* close the chapter.

Back to fresh chicken. Within Chicken, there is a wealth of subdivision. There are full sets of data for broilers or fryers, for roasting chickens and for stewing chickens. Within each class, there are data for the entire bird, for the top and bottom quarters, and for the various chicken parts.

The Turkey subdivisions are similar, with separate listings for fryer-roasters, young hens, young toms, and a category called "Average, All Classes." The sizes of birds in these categories are rather strikingly different. For the "fryer-roasters," the data come from birds that have a ready-to-cook weight of 7 lb. 1 oz. with neck and giblets, or 6 lb. 7 oz. without. The "young hens" weigh almost twice as much at 12 lb. 9 oz. with neck and giblets, and "young toms" weigh almost twice as much again, at 23 lb. 1 oz.

The divisions and subdivisions of the chapter look like this:

CHICKEN

How to Read the Numbers: Let me say at the outset that all the numbers for cooked poultry in this chapter are based on birds that have been cooked with the skin still on. Calories listed for "cooked chicken without the skin" are for chicken that has had the skin removed *after* cooking. What we have for **Poultry,** then, is exactly the opposite of what we have for **Meats.** We have data for beef trimmed of separable fat before cooking, but no data for beef trimmed at the table. We have data for chicken trimmed of its skin at the table, but none for chicken with its skin removed before cooking.

I am certain that trimming separable fat from a steak at the table will reduce calories. I am certain that removing the skin from a chicken before it's stewed or roasted will do more good than removing the skin after the chicken's been cooked. (For frying, I'm not so certain; fried skinless chicken might pick up so much fat from the pan that a better result might be obtained by frying the chicken in its skin and then throwing the skin away.)

Thus we lack some important numbers for counting calories and are ignoring in our data pages some important ways of reducing calories. Still, what we have is a poultry chapter with the most comprehensive information available.

Most of the data lines follow a definite pattern. This pattern is most complete in *Chicken;* for other birds many of these lines had to be omitted for lack of information. For "Chicken Broilers or Fryers," the pattern begins with the raw form and continues for each of several different ways of cooking. For other kinds of chicken, for example—for "Roasting" or "Stewing" chickens, and for turkeys, there is only one method of cooking described. Roasting chickens, and all turkeys, ducks, and geese, are assumed to be roasted; stewing chickens are assumed to be stewed.

The column headings in this chapter are very simple: Unit, and One Ounce by Weight.

The Unit column is for "one" of whatever is being described. It may be one entire chicken or one single chicken wing. The wing may be raw, roasted, stewed, or fried. The Unit may be a pound of cooked wings with skin, or a pound of wings whose bones and skin have been removed after cooking.

The One Ounce by Weight column provides a common denominator for comparing these different units. However, it is still necessary to read the left-hand descriptives. If the lines says "One Chicken Wing," that ounce is going to include the bone. Thus, even the calories in the One Ounce by Weight column cannot be used without attention to what is being weighed.

As was true for **Meats,** reading the numbers for **Poultry** can be complicated. The most elaborate sets of data are for *Chicken;* The *Turkey* listings are like *Chicken,* but less detailed, and the quantities of data trail off sharply for the remaining birds.

Let's look at one set of data from *Chicken.* (I've added line numbers here. In the data pages, the lines are not numbered.)

	UNIT Cal.	UNIT Carb.	1 OZ., BY WT. Cal.	1 OZ., BY WT. Carb.
POULTRY				
CHICKEN				
BROILERS OR FRYERS				
DRUMSTICK				
Flour Coated, Fried				
Eaten with skin:				
Weighed with skin and bone (refuse: bones approx. 34%):				
1. One drumstick from a 3 lb. ready-to-cook chicken: approx. 2.6 oz. cooked	120	0.8	45.9	0.31
2. One pound of cooked drumsticks	734	4.9	45.9	0.31
3. Yield per pound of raw ready-to-cook chicken: approx. 0.9 oz. cooked	40	0.3	45.9	0.31
Weighing edible portion only:				
4. One pound of cooked meat with skin (8g/tr/4g/57%/25 mg)	1111	7.4	69.5	0.46
Fried with skin, but skin removed before eating:				
Weighed with skin and bone (refuse: bones approx. 34%, skin approx. 10%)				
5. One drumstick from a 3 lb. ready-to-cook chicken: approx. 2.6 oz. cooked	82	0.0	31.0	0.00
6. One pound of cooked drumsticks	496		31.0	
7. Yield per pound of raw ready-to-cook chicken: approx. 0.9 oz. cooked	27		31.0	
Weighing edible portion only:				
8. One pound of cooked meat without skin (8g/0g/2g/62%/27 mg)	885		55.3	

The first line of data will describe a poultry part eaten with the skin—for example, one drumstick from a 3-lb. ready-to-cook chicken. The part will always be described as "Weighed with skin and bones." The percentage of refuse will then be specified. For this line, refuse is the bones. The skin is not treated as refuse here. On the contrary, the calories cited on this line will always include the calories in the skin. The cooked weight of the part is specified on the line.

Line 2 is closely related. It describes the calories in one pound of these parts. For example, we can see that one pound of flour-coated fried drumsticks will have 734 calories. But remember—this pound is weighed with the bone.

Line 3 specifies the calories in the poultry part per pound of ready-to-cook bird. If you know how much your whole, raw, ready-to-cook chicken or turkey weighs, but it isn't the same weight as the chickens or turkeys on which the data are based, this will enable you to estimate how much your drumstick weighs. This is a better means of figuring calories than assuming that all drumsticks will be the same size. In the example shown, each of the two drumsticks from a 3-lb. bird weighs approximately 2.6 oz., cooked. Since the bird weighs 3 pounds, the weight of one drumstick—per pound of the uncooked bird—is 0.9 oz. (Of course, it will always be more accurate to weigh the individual drumstick before you eat it, and use line 1.)

Line 4 is the last of the data lines to describe the poultry eaten with skin. This is for "weighing edible portion only." It describes what happens if you weigh the meat and skin without the bones. The calories per ounce will be higher than if you had weighed it with the bones in, but the food is unchanged.

Of all the data lines, line 4 is likely to give the most accurate result. If you can weigh the meat (and skin, in this instance) after you have taken it from the bone, there will be less room for error.

This is one more illustration of the general rule: You should measure your food as closely as possible to the way you will be eating it. Estimating calories based simply on eating "one drumstick from a 3-lb.chicken" is not nearly as good as knowing how much your cooked drumstick actually weighs. And best of all would be to weigh the meat off the bone. (The cryptic numbers [8g/tr/4g/57%/25mg] represent additional nutrition analysis. See **Supplemental Numbers** in **Methodology,** page 36.)

For each part and method of cooking, our attention now turns to chicken without the skin.

The first of the skinless data lines, **line 5,** is for one poultry part. This is exactly the same part as was described above, on line 1, when the skin was going to be eaten. The weight that is specified is the weight including the skin and bones; this is how a chicken is likely to be served, even if you plan not to eat the skin. The calories, however, are for meat once the skin has been removed. They will invariably be lower than when the skin is eaten.

Line 6 describes the calories in one pound of these parts. Again, both the bones and the skin are weighed, but neither the bones nor the skin is eaten.

Line 7 is the yield of this part per pound of a ready-to-cook bird. Like line 3, this line can be used to find the weight and calorie content of a similar part from any size bird.

Line 8 is for one pound of meat with neither skin nor bone included in the weight. If you are cutting down on calories by leaving the skin on your plate, this is definitely the line to use. For some entries a 9th line will describe a measuring cup's worth of chopped or diced chicken, again, without its skin.

How to Eat Poultry: Where do the calories come from?

The skin. A pound of roasted chicken skin has enough calories to add more than half a pound of weight to your body.

The most important thing in this entire chapter is to take the skin off. You can choose your poultry without this book more securely than you can eat poultry skin, no matter how carefully you use this book.

For every food in this chapter—even for the skin—there will be calories from protein. For chicken liver, there will be calories from carbohydrate. But skin is mostly water and fat.

I am not going to tell you whether to eat your chicken with the skin or without it. It's not for me to say whether you should or shouldn't, any more than I would tell you to eat a chocolate cake and throw away the icing. If it makes you happy, you can eat the skin and throw the chicken away.

But do be aware that a little bit of skin can buy you a lot of chicken: Three ounces of roasted chicken skin, about the amount that covers one small breast, are equal in calories to 11½ ounces —almost three-quarters of a pound—of roasted breast meat.

And if you like barbecue sauce on your chicken, you can still take the skin off first. You may not be accustomed to the idea of barbecuing chicken that way, but why not? You do put barbecue sauce directly on steak, not on steak skin.

Shake 'N Bake in its various flavors can be used for chicken that has had its skin removed. Using Shake 'N Bake will add about 300 calories to 2½ pounds of chicken. But what looks like 300 additional calories can actually save you calories if the flavored coating mix adds enough zip to replace the skin.

So much for the skin, and I will try not to say any more about it. But I don't promise.

Second to removing the you-know-what, the way to eat chicken is to eat light meat rather than dark meat:

	Calories per Ounce
BROILERS/FRYERS	
Light meat without skin:	
stewed	45.1
roasted	49.1
fried	54.4
Dark meat without skin:	
stewed	54.4
roasted	58.1
fried	67.8
ROASTING CHICKEN	
Light meat without skin:	
roasted	43.4
Dark meat without skin:	
roasted	50.5
STEWING CHICKEN	
Light meat without skin:	
stewed	60.4
Dark meat without skin:	
stewed	73.1

And, as this chart also shows, the way to eat chicken is to avoid "stewing chickens." But as a cooking method, rather than a type of chicken, stewing is preferable. In fact, when it comes to "How to Cook" chicken, the answer is to stew it rather than roast it, and roast it rather than fry it. But if you must have it fried, the way to fry chicken is without dipping it into batter first:

	Calories per Ounce
BROILERS/FRYERS	
Flesh, skin, giblets, and neck:	
stewed	61.2
roasted	61.2
fried:	
flour-coated, then fried	77.1
batter-dipped, then fried	82.5
Flesh and skin:	
stewed	62.1
roasted	67.8
fried:	
flour-coated, then fried	76.3
batter-dipped, then fried	81.9
Flesh only:	
stewed	50.2
roasted	53.9
fried	62.1

But if you're a person who eats only the skin (Yuck!), in that case batter-dipped comes out way lower than flour-coated:

	Calories per Ounce
Skin only:	
stewed	102.9
roasted	128.7
fried:	
flour-coated, then fried	142.3
batter-dipped, then fried	111.7

What about eating turkey? The way to eat turkey is also to remove the skin, and, just as with chicken, to eat light meat rather than dark meat:

	Calories per Ounce
Turkey, average, all classes:	
light meat without skin, roasted	44.5
dark meat without skin, roasted	53.0

The way to eat duck is on special occasions:

Duck, domesticated	
average of all parts except the neck and giblets	
flesh without skin, roasted	57.0
flesh and skin, roasted	95.5

And just take a gander at goose:

Goose, domesticated	
average of all parts except the neck and giblets	
flesh without skin, roasted	67.5
flesh and skin, roasted	86.5

For **Poultry,** in general, the way to eat it is to select younger rather than older birds. The age of the bird can make a big difference, something that is unfortunately not apparent in **The Calorielogue.**

Most of the numbers for **Poultry** are based on brand new data from the USDA. These data are entirely for young birds, and do not show the effect of age on calories. Previous data from the USDA showed that, for example, a "fat mature turkey (more than 32 weeks old)" had 2.4 times the calories of "young turkeys." This seems like rather convincing information. It's also supported by data from other parts of the world, many of which make this kind of age distinction.

The age of the bird can be determined from its "As purchased" weight. The now out-dated USDA figures for chicken show that you can eat 7 ounces of light meat from a 1¾-pound bird for the same number of calories as are in 4 ounces of light meat from a 2½-pound bird.

The reason I've opted to use the newer data, although no distinctions by age or weight were included, is that the information is based on much more recent samples and there's been so much change in poultry breeding.

And now for the $64,000 question: everything considered, which is the better calorie choice—chicken or turkey? It goes without saying that chicken skin will be higher than turkey breast meat and turkey skin will be higher than chicken breast meat. But who comes out the winner in a contest between comparable parts of roast chicken and roast turkey?

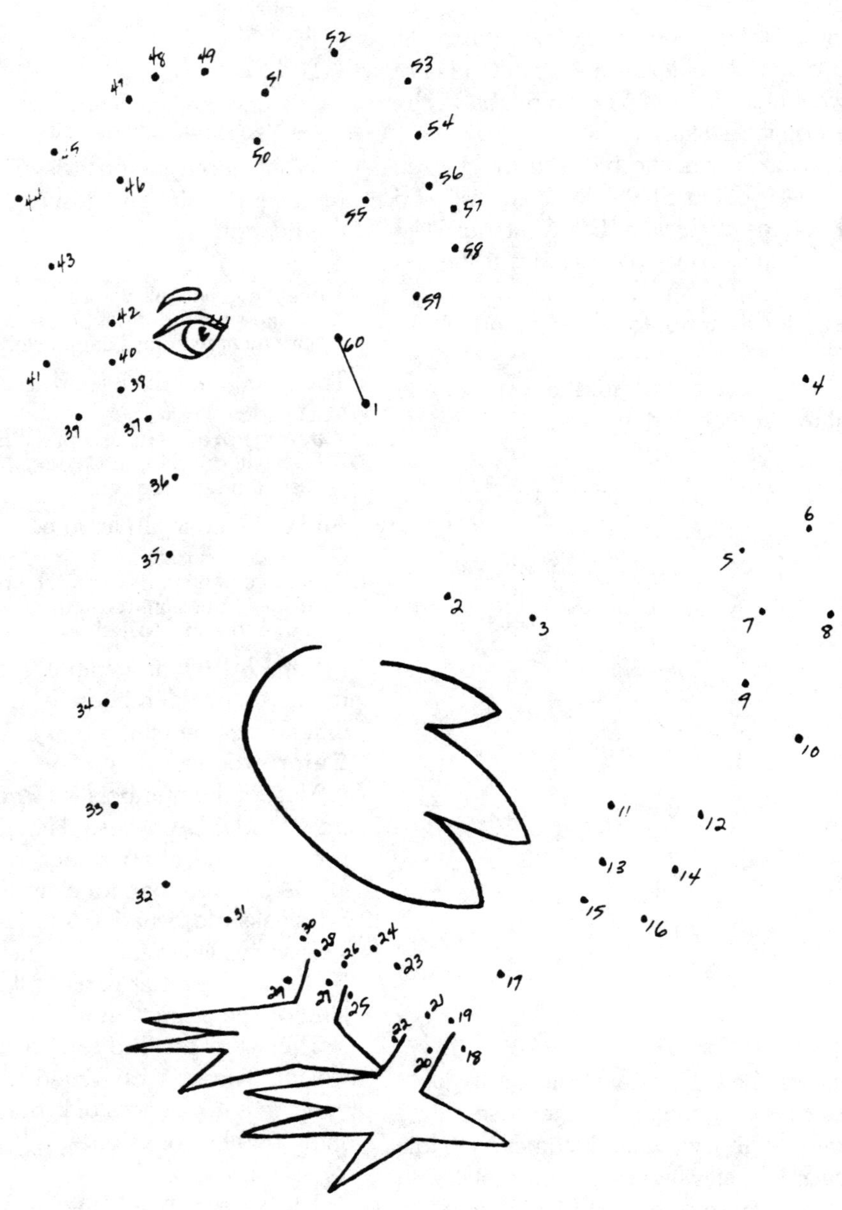

The *Gallus* wins the chalice. The turkey is a turkey.

Finding what you want in this chapter may indeed be a fishing expedition, for nowhere was the nomenclature more confusing. One fish can have many popular names. For example, some species of Lake Trout were listed in the literature under "W" for Whiting. Other Lake Trout were listed under "Trout," or under "Lake," or under "Herring."

Conversely, the same exact name—such as "Redfish"—can be applied to entirely different fish. If you can't find what you are looking for in the logical place, look elsewhere before giving up.

How to Read the Numbers: For *Fresh Fish and Shellfish,* there are only two column headings: Unit and One Ounce by Weight. The Unit is usually one pound.

This makes it sound easy, and it is easy, but only if you are careful in reading the descriptives. The words to watch out for are "As purchased," "Edible portion," "Refuse," and "Yield." These are discussed in **Methodology.** Go to page 34, please, and I'll wait till you come back.

These terms are needed in **Fish** because what one eats from this chapter is not the whole fish as it comes from the water. One can eat a candy bar or drink a glass of milk, but nobody eats a whole flounder, fins and all.

Back to the Unit column heading: Once you have read the descriptive material and determined what is being measured, the Unit column will tell you the calories in that amount of fish. If "refuse" is involved—such as the fins—there are certain to be calories in it. But these calories are ignored. As is true for every number in the book, the calories in the Unit column are for the edible part of what is being weighed.

The Ounce by Weight column gives the calories in a single ounce of the fish—whatever form of the fish is being described on that line. As with the Unit column, "refuse" may enter into the weighing, but only the edible parts are included into the calorie figures.

There are hundreds and hundreds of numbers for fresh fish. Yet there are reasons to doubt their absolute accuracy. While this is true for many of the chapters in the book, **Fish** seems a good place to once again point out the limitations of the data.

If you look in the **Meats** chapter, you will find the careful distinctions between chuck steak and sirloin steak. In **Poultry** you'll find those distinctions between wings and drumsticks. A tuna has the same sorts of variations in its body, but we have no data comparable to the distinctions we make for chickens and cows.

There are lots of variations for fish that simply do not show up in **The Calorielogue.** The same species of fish taken from different waters can have enormously different calorie values, but only a few of these variations are captured in our charts. The fat content of a fish will vary considerably with the seasons, but these distinctions are not generally shown. Finally, there is the question of size. The bigger—the older—a fish is, the higher its calories per ounce. Just look at the Lake Trout. And weep—

For "Lake Trout, Siscowet" we have data for a large and small trout. The data show the consequence of increased calories (presumably from increased fat) as a fish's size increases. For a trout weighing 6.5 pounds or more, the calories per ounce are more than double those of a smaller trout. Surely there is not a magical dividing line at 6.5 pounds. A bigger "small lake trout" will be higher in calories than a smaller "small lake trout." If a trout weighing "less than 6.5 pounds" has 68.4 calories per ounce and a trout weighing "6.5 pounds and over" has 148.7 calories per ounce, then I suspect that some lake trout will be 100 calories per ounce. But which?

Does this uncertainty mean that you should ignore the numbers in this chapter? No. You should use them. But it does mean that you cannot be absolutely sure that the fish you are eating will match the calorie figures printed here.

The same is true in **Vegetables.** Look at the variations within "Artichokes" and "Avocados," even before you leave the A's.

I wouldn't expect **Fish** to be that much more variable than the other chapters. But this seemed like a particularly suitable place to mention the inherent insecurity of all numbers for foods that have not undergone the leveling effect of human processing.

For the *Frozen Fish and Shellfish* section, the column headings remain the same—Unit, and One Ounce by Weight.

The Unit for *Frozen Fish and Shellfish* is not usually an entire fish, but an entire package. The Unit may additionally be one fish stick, one stuffed clam, one crab crêpe, one frozen flounder fillet. . . . How reliable these "one piece" figures are will depend on the uniformity (or lack of it) imposed by the manufacturing process.

For *Canned Fish and Shellfish* the column headings still are Unit, and One Ounce by Weight. Not surprisingly, a frequent Unit will be the entire can. But the Unit may also be a pound or a cup. It may be an individual shrimp or sardine.

Reading the numbers for canned fish requires special attention to what is being done with the packing liquid. If the fish is packed in oil, draining that oil will have an overwhelming effect on the calories. There's a short discussion of "Draining" in **Methodology**, page 35. Can I ask you to go to **Methodology** twice, in one chapter?

The One Ounce by Weight column will also include figures for solids and liquids, for drained solids, and for the packing liquid alone. In order to use the Ounce column, you must read the left-hand descriptives.

Unfortunately, you will not find drained figures for certain fish, including salmon, which really hurts. The oil, water, or broth these fish come packed in is always included in their calorie figures, as you'll see when you read the data lines. I tried over the course of almost eight years to find drained values for these. Could not. Sorry.

How to Eat Fresh Fish and Shellfish: Where do the calories come from? For raw, steamed, or broiled fish, most of the calories come from protein. This will be true except for the fattiest fish. Shellfish has carbohydrate. For other fish there's little or no calorie contribution from carbohydrate.

If a fish were all protein, it would be about 110 calories an ounce—the same, roughly, as granulated sugar. But a fish is mostly water, which is not surprising when you consider where it lives. The edible portion of a flounder may be 81% water, and the result is a food not with 110 calories per ounce—but with 21.1.

There are 117 examples on the list that follows. Sixty-four of them have fewer than 30 calories per ounce. From lowest to highest, they are:

	Representative Calories per Ounce of Edible Portion, Raw
Dover Sole	17.5
Eastern Oysters	18.7
Crayfish(Crawfish; Spiny Lobster)	20.4
Giant African Snail	20.7
Octopus	20.7
Hake	21.0
Flounder	21.1
Cusk	21.3
Cod	22.1
Haddock	22.4
King Crab	22.4
Tilefish	22.4
Red Drum (Redfish)	22.7
Scarlet Haws	22.7
Scallops (Bay and Sea)	23.0
Lemon Sole	23.1
Burbot	23.3
Soft Clams	23.3
Black Bullhead	23.8
Chain Pickerel	23.8
Lingcod	23.8
Sauger	23.8
Grouper	24.7
Northern Pike	25.0
Atlantic Ocean Perch (Redfish)	25.0
Green Turtle	25.2
Squid	25.2
Yellowfin Croaker	25.3
Tautog (Blackfish)	25.3
Blue Pike	25.5

Snail	25.5
English Sole	25.6
Shrimp	25.8
Yellow Perch	25.8
Northern Lobster	25.8
Pacific and Western Oysters	25.8
Walleye Pike	26.4
Black Sea Bass	26.4
Red and Gray Snapper	26.4
Sturgeon	26.7
Butterfish (Gulf Water)	26.9
Mussels (Atlantic/Pacific)	26.9
Ocean Perch (Pacific)	26.9
Pollack	27.0
Atlantic Croaker	27.2
Lake Herring	27.2
White Sea Bass	27.2
Halibut (California)	27.5
Rockfish (Black, Canary, Yellowtail, Rasphead, and Bocaccio)	27.5
Abalone	27.8
Redhorse (Silver)	27.8
Skate	27.8
Smelt (Atlantic Bay, Jack)	27.8
White Bass	27.8
Halibut (Atlantic/Pacific)	28.4
Brook Trout	28.7
Swordfish	29.1
Freshwater Catfish	29.2
Finnan Haddie (Smoked Haddock)	29.3
Bass (Smallmouth and Largemouth)	29.5
Suckers (including White and Mullet)	29.5
Lake Trout Herring	29.7
Kingfish (Whiting) (Southern, Gulf, and Northern)	29.8
Striped Bass	29.8
Scup	30.8
Muskellunge	30.9
Terrapin	31.4
Carp Sucker	31.5
Porgy	31.8
Atlantic Sheepshead	32.1
Barracuda	32.1
Buffalofish	32.1
Wreckfish	32.4
Carp	32.6
Bluefish	33.2
Euchalon	33.4
White Perch	33.4
Humpback Salmon	33.8
Freshwater Drum (Freshwater Sheepshead)	34.3
Weakfish (Sea Trout)	34.3
Alewife	36.0
Roe (including Carp, Cod, Haddock, Herring, and Shad)	36.9
Yellowfin Tuna	37.7
Yellowtail (Pacific Coast)	39.1
Chub	41.1
Bluefin Tuna	41.1
Greenland Halibut	41.4
Striped Mullet	41.4
Lake Whitefish	43.9
Spiny Dogfish (Grayfish)	44.3
Whale Meat	44.3
Pacific Herring	44.9
Pacific Sardines	45.4
Bonito	47.7
Butterfish (Northern Water)	47.9
Shad (American Shad)	48.2
Atlantic Herring	49.9
Spanish Mackerel	50.2
Sablefish	53.9
Atlantic Mackerel	54.2
Rainbow or Steelhead Trout	55.3
Smoked Herring Bloaters	55.6
Gizzard Shad	56.8
Roe (including Salmon, Sturgeon, and Turbot)	58.7
Smoked Kippered Herring	59.9
Atlantic Salmon	61.6
Salted or Brined Herring	61.9
Smoked Mackerel	62.1
Spot	62.1
Chinook (King) Salmon	63.0
Pickled Bismarck-type Herring	63.3
American Eel	66.1
Lake Trout, Siscowet (weighing less than 6.5 pounds when caught)	68.4
Sturgeon Caviar (Granular)	74.0
Smoked Herring (Hard)	85.1
Salted Mackerel	86.4
Sturgeon Caviar (Pressed)	90.0

You'd think I'd be able to end this chapter preface right here, but that's not the case. Those were the calories raw. A fried fish is a horse of a different color. This is what happens to bluefish if it's breaded and fried:

A. One ounce of raw bluefish contains 33.2 calories.

B. The breading for this one ounce of fish (including breadcrumbs, milk, and egg) weighs about 1/10 of an ounce and adds about 6.5 calories.

C. As the fish is fried in butter, evaporation and dripping will cause it to lose about 1/4 of an ounce in weight, and approximately 2 calories. The fish will absorb some butter, however, with a gain of about 12 calories from the 1/20 of an ounce of butter it can be expected to absorb.

D. We are now left with a piece of bluefish that weighs 4/5 of an ounce, and has gained about 16.5 calories per ounce of its original raw weight. That's an increase in calories of 50%. Holy mackerel!

One way to save calories when you cook fish is to steam it. Another is to broil it, using lemon juice and herbs instead of butter. Once you add the breadcrumbs, once you add the batter, once you cook it in oil—the fact that you are eating "fish" hardly seems to matter.

How much fat is picked up in the frying will depend, in part, on how much surface area is exposed. The thicker the cut of fish, the fewer calories per ounce it will pick up. Breadcrumbs will pick up more oil, and hold it. They're accessories after the fat.

Fish skin, just like chicken skin, contributes to the calories. You can save calories by taking the skin off, but not nearly as much as you might think from reading the **Poultry** Chapter Preface. That's because there's so much less fish skin than chicken skin per portion, and the layer of adhering fat is thinner. However, if the fish has been fried, then taking off the skin is bound to make a big difference. But be aware that removing the skin won't remove all the calories you've gained from the frying oil. Oil doesn't just sit on the frying surface, it gets in under the skin. You cannot, by simple subtraction, trim off the effect. You can only make a dent in it:

Avoid the oil. It's the fry in the ointment.

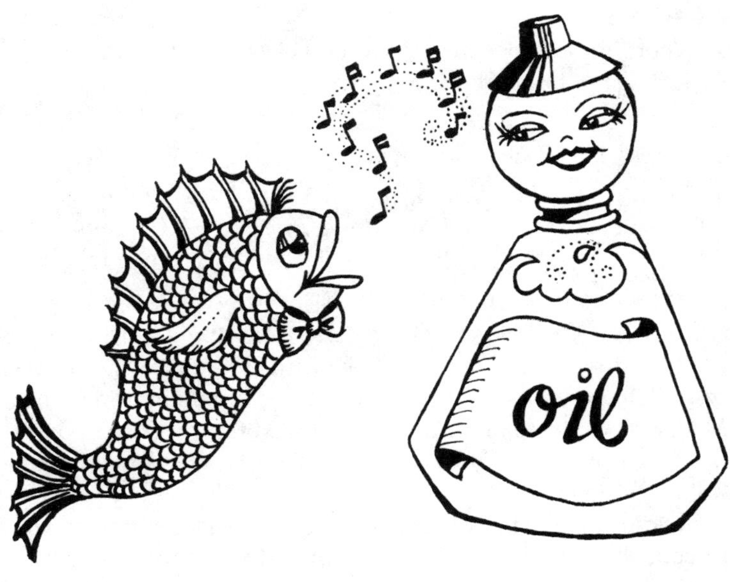

"I've got you under my skin..."

How to Eat Frozen Fish and Shellfish is to apply the same principles as with "Fresh." Calories will of course depend on which fish you choose, but mostly it will depend on what's been done to the fish.

If you're looking at plain frozen fish, almost anything you choose will be under 30 calories an ounce. Once the fish is breaded you've upped the calories—possibly by 50% or more:

	Calories per Ounce
Taste O'Sea:	
Cod Fillet	20.0
12 skinless Breaded Cod Fish Portions	30.0
Haddock Fillet	22.5
12 skinless Breaded Haddock Fish Portions	30.0
Whiting Fillet	20.0
12 Breaded Whiting Fish Portions	33.8

Impressive as the effect of breading is, it's the frying that really adds the calories:

	Calories per Ounce
12 Breaded Ocean Perch Fish Portions, Taste O'Sea	37.5
Fried Ocean Perch Fillets, Mrs. Paul's	62.5

(An aside: Fried ocean perch fillet is 62.5 calories an ounce. Broiled lamb chops are 59.8. One who believes that "fish" is Latin for "low-in-calories" is swallowing the bait.)

If the idea of plain frozen ocean perch doesn't enthrall you, there are other ways to skin this cat. Even fish prepared with butter, or with butter and cheese, is almost certain to be lower in calories than fried fish:

	Calories per Ounce
Mrs. Paul's:	
Flounder with Lemon Butter	43.3
Fried Flounder Fillets	55.0
Scallops with Butter and Cheese	37.1
Fried Scallops	60.0

Even "stuffing" is almost certain to be lower-calorie than frying:

	Calories per Ounce
Stuffed Clams, Matlaws	48.0
Fried Clams, Mrs. Paul's	108.0

Even crêpe-ing is better than frying:

	Calories per Ounce
Mrs. Paul's:	
Scallop Crêpes	40.0
Crab Crêpes	43.6
Shrimp Crêpes	45.5
Clam Crêpes	50.9

Where the calories in seafood crêpes end, the calories for fish sticks begin—but here we're in fried fish territory again:

	Calories per Ounce
Fish Sticks, Mrs. Paul's	50.0
Fishsticks, Booth Fisheries	55.0
14 Batter-dipped Fish Sticks, A&P	62.9
8 Golden Fried Fish Sticks (Cod), Taste O'Sea	63.5
8 Golden Fried Fish Sticks (Pollock), Taste O'Sea	63.5
Light Batter Fish Sticks, Mrs. Paul's	65.7
8 Batter-dipped Fish Sticks (Pollock), Mrs. Paul's	77.5

But even if you know the general rules, there's still an occasional surprise—Shrimp Scampi (Taste O'Sea) is in the data pages at 65.3 calories per ounce. I find that surprisingly high. Matlaw's "Oreganate Italian Style Stuffed Clams" are 68.6 calories an ounce, 20 calories more than their product labeled simply "Stuffed Clams."

So knowing the principles isn't always sufficient. It's always best to consult the numbers in **The Calorielogue**. But if you don't have your book with you and you have to resort to "principles," the principal principle for fresh or frozen fish is : Diet? Don't fry it.

The principal principle of **How to Eat Canned Fish and Shellfish** can be told in three numbers:

	Calories per Ounce
Tuna Fish, based on USDA data:	
packed in oil	81.6
packed in oil, drained	55.5
packed in water, drained	45.6

Throw away the oil, or buy water- or broth-packed fish to begin with. Shrimp, lobster, crab, and clams are commonly packed without oil:

	Calories per Ounce Drained Solids
Based on USDA data:	
lobster	26.9
clams	27.7
king crab	28.9
shrimp	32.9

Salmon is generally packed in its own juices, without added oil. But salmon is an oily fish to begin with, and so the packing liquid is bound to contain fat. As I've mentioned before, figures for drained salmon were nowhere to be found (nor was the composition of the liquid, which would have allowed me to compute the calories):

	Calories per Ounce Solids and Liquid
Salmon, based on USDA data:	
chum salmon	39.4
humpback (pink) salmon	40.0
coho	43.4
sockeye (red) salmon	48.5
Atlantic salmon	57.7
chinook (king) salmon	59.6

Sardines are frequently packed in oil, but they also come packed in mustard sauce or tomato sauce (very popular in Norway):

	Calories per Ounce
sardines, packed in oil, USDA	88.0
sardines, packed in oil, drained, USDA	57.5
Sardines in Mustard, Coastal Kitchen	42.5
Sardines in Tomato Sauce, Del Monte	44.0
Sardines in Tomato Sauce, Coastal Kitchen	50.0
Sardines in Mustard Sauce, King Oscar	64.0
Sardines in Tomato Sauce, King Oscar	64.0

I don't know why King Oscar's sardines are so much higher than the others. It may simply be that King Oscar puts in a higher proportion of sardine to sauce.

Sometimes packed in water, more often in a broth, is gefilte fish. "Gefilte" is Yiddish for "stuffed" or "filled." It's made of ground fish (carp, or whitefish and pike), eggs, and matzo meal or cracker crumbs. The mixture is poached in a broth made with carrots, celery, and onions. It's consistently a low-calorie choice:

	Calories per Ounce Solids and Liquid
Gefilte Fish in Redi-Jelled Broth, Rokeach	14.9
Gefilte Fish, Mrs. Adler's	16.7
Gefilte Fish in Redi-Jelled Broth, Rokeach "Old Vienna"	18.6
Whitefish & Pike Fish, Manischewitz	23.0
Gefilte Fish, Manischewitz	26.9

The USDA provided information for other canned fish and seafood that are less commonly eaten, although their names may be familiar:

	Calories per Ounce
abalone, solids and liquid	22.7
cod, drained solids	24.1

swordfish, solids and liquid	28.9
smoked haddock, drained solids	29.2
green turtle, solids and liquid	30.1
Pacific mussels, drained solids	32.3
alewife, solids and liquid	40.0
Atlantic mackerel, solids and liquid	51.9
rainbow and steelhead trout, solids and liquid	59.3

Fish is a food prescribed for dieters. To sum it up, how does this chapter compare with its competition, when the name of the game is "calories"?

Comparisons among the protein chapters are complicated. How does Chicken of the Sea compare with chicken from a barnyard? Well, what parts of a barnyard chicken? And are you comparing it with oil-packed or with water-packed Chicken of the Sea?

How does **Fish** compare to **Eggs?** Well, which fish, and how many eggs? Fried eggs or boiled eggs? Fried fish or broiled?

How does **Fish** compare to **Cheese?** There too, the question is "what are you comparing?" An 8-ounce swordfish steak for supper is not an extraordinary quantity, whereas half a pound of cheese in half an hour might very well be unusual.

So use discretion; but based strictly on calories per ounce, nothing can beat this chapter's stars as the protein centerpiece of a meal.

And now . . .

Surimi

In Japan, the word *surimi* is used to describe a "kneaded product." In the United States, the product "surimi" technically refers to mechanically deboned and washed fish flesh (a white fish, often pollock) to which sugar and sodium phosphates have been added. In the retail marketplace, however, "surimi" is used to describe a variety of analog seafood products such as mock crab, mock scallops, and mock shrimp.

A typical formulation for "surimi crab" might be: 55.2% deboned and washed fish flesh, 23% water, 5% natural king crab, 4.8% sugar, 4% egg white, 3% corn starch, 2.5% salt, 1% potato starch, 1% wheat starch, 0.5% monosodium glutamate (MSG), and 0.18% sodium phosphates.

Much of what is being sold in the United States as "seafood salad" is actually surimi. (If a restaurant or deli counter is selling "crab salad," they must indeed sell crab. But if they are selling "seafood salad," surimi crab is perfectly permissible. At the retail level, in supermarkets, genuine crab legs may cost upwards of $12-$15 a pound, weighed with the shell. Surimi crab has no shell, and is likely to cost the consumer between $3 and $5 a pound.)

As compared to the natural seafood products they are imitating, surimi products, at a very rough approximation, will have 20% more calories.

Sushi and Sashimi

The calories for sashimi are easy. A great many of the numbers in the **Fish** chapter—the numbers for the edible portion of many raw fish and shellfish—are the calories for sashimi. Period.

While the calories for sashimi can be summarized in a paragraph, the calories for sushi demand a profile in greater detail. The predominant ingredient of all sushi is sushi rice, which serves as the foundation for a second ingredient. This second ingredient is most commonly raw or cooked fish or shellfish, but it can also be a vegetable, such as cucumber, bean curd, or gourd. It can be the egg of a chicken or quail. It can be fish eggs (fish roe).

The two best-known forms of sushi are nigiri-zushi, popularly referred to simply as "sushi," and maki-zushi, which is rolled sushi. Nigiri-zushi usually consists of an oblong patty of sushi rice that is topped with the fish, vegetable, egg, or roe. (In Japanese, the second ingredient, or "topping," is called *tane.*) Nigiri-zushi may then be tied with a ribbon of nori seaweed, a staple of the sushi cuisine. (Nori seaweed is prepared commercially from fresh seaweed, usually purple laver, and is available in dried, paper-thin sheets with the texture of parchment.) Maki-zushi is made by rolling sushi rice together with pieces or strips of fish or vegetables in a sheet of the nori seaweed. The roll is then sliced crosswise. Most forms of sushi (and also sashimi) are traditionally served with soy sauce, pickled ginger, and wasabi—a tear-provoking Japanese horseradish that goes in your mouth and comes out your eyes.

The one ingredient common to all sushi is sushi rice (in Japanese, *shari* or *gohan*), which is made from short-grain Japanese white rice augmented with small amounts of sugar, rice vinegar, and salt. The proportions of these ingredients will vary, but a typical recipe might call for 2 cups of short-grain Japanese white rice (or short-grain American rice, if Japanese is not available), 2 cups of water, ¼ cup of rice vinegar, 1 tablespoon of sugar, and 2 teaspoons of salt. In this recipe, the calories for sushi rice are going to be approximately 32.4 per ounce. (The calories per ounce of short-grain American rice alone are approximately 30.9.)

Of course, different pieces of sushi will vary substantially in their proportion of fish to rice, and in the selection of fish or vegetable to be used. However, by a marvelous coincidence, the calories per ounce of most vegetables and many kinds of fish and shellfish are very close to, or lower than, the calories in the rice. This means that you can walk into a sushi restaurant with the figure "32.4" in mind, and then just relax and enjoy yourself.

Of course, the calories will be somewhat lower if you're eating cucumber sushi—and higher if you're eating a fatty fish. Salmon and mackerel are relatively high in calories, and some cuts of tuna can run as high as 89.9 calories an ounce. But looking at the mainstream of calories per ounce for popular sushi fish—the leaner cuts of tuna, shrimp, crab, sea bass, flounder, red snapper, conger eel, many varieties of clams, abalone, sea trout, squid, octopus, and scallops—all are below 35 calories an ounce.

For all its variability, I don't know of any other cuisine for which the mid-30s in calories per ounce will virtually allow you the run of the menu.

The menu itself takes some understanding, and a fuller grasp of the offerings can enrich the sushi experience, so I offer the following translations:

Aji—horse mackerel. The flesh is a translucent pink-gray. This fish is eaten raw, with its skin intact but without its scales. Books on sushi advise that the best season for horse mackerel is the spring.

Akagi—arkshell, a type of clam. This fish is described in Kinjiro Omae's book, *The Book of Sushi,* as being the monarch of sushi shellfish. It is peach-orange-red in color, and is often described as having a delicate taste, with a softer texture than that of most other shellfish. In the United States, however, it is likely that if you can find arkshell at all, it will have been frozen.

Amadai—tile fish, served raw. Although tile fish is available in Japan, it is commonly agreed that the very best tile fish is found in the United States, on the eastern seaboard.

Ama Ebi—a special variety of shrimp, served raw.

Anago—conger eel. The eel is first boiled, and then flavored with a mixture of soy sauce, sugar, eel broth, and possibly also sake or mirin (a sweet cooking wine made from rice). The eel is served with its skin intact, and I find the taste and texture to be similar to that of sardines.

Aoyagi—round clam. These clams may be brought in from Japan frozen. They are boiled before serving. One reference book suggested that in the United States, raw bay scallops may be substituted for clams.

Awabi—abalone. Prized in Japan. In the United States, abalone is found in Pacific waters off the West Coast. Awabi is served raw, boiled, or steamed.

California-Maki/California roll—crab and avocado. (Often, surimi crab is used instead of crab. See *Kani.*) Mayonnaise may also be used as an ingredient. California-maki indeed originated in California and has now, I am told, become popular in Tokyo. (Do they know that avocado and mayonnaise are two of the highest-calorie ingredients to be found at a sushi bar?)

Chirashi-zushi—literally translated from the Japanese, chirashi-zushi means "scattered sushi." Chirashi refers to the format in which the sushi is presented, rather than to a specific set of ingredients. Any or all of the ingredients that one can find in a sushi bar may be combined to make Chirashi. The chosen ingredients are arranged on a specially prepared mixture of sushi rice and seaweed. In other words, it's the sushi bar version of "Chef's Salad," with the sushi rice and seaweed serving as the "lettuce."

Chutoro—one of the fatty tunas. Chutoro has a "medium" amount of fat. Also see Maguro, Toro, and Otoro.

Ebi—prawn, or jumbo shrimp, usually served boiled.

Futo-Maki—a rolled sushi, with slices that are approximately 2 inches in diameter. Literally translated, *futo* means "fat." (Maki, again, means "roll.") The ingredients in futo-maki will vary, but typically will include vegetables, shellfish, egg, and a variety of other ingredients. The taste is on the sweet side, and I think of futo-maki as a dessert sushi, although that is my own idiosyncrasy.

Hamachi—yellowtail amberjack, sometimes referred to either as yellowtail or amberjack. Nobuko Tsuda's book, *Sushi Made Easy,* has the following interesting commentary: "Like the gizzard shad and sea bass, the yellowtail also changes its name during its lifetime and is known as 'success fish' in Japan. When it is young it is called *hamachi,* and when mature, *buri.* What is more, yellowtail goes by still other names depending on where it is caught." Hamachi is served raw.

Hirame—halibut. Hirame may also be made with other varieties of flat fishes, such as flounder or fluke. It is at its most flavorful in the winter months. The fishes used for hirame are in plentiful supply in American waters. Hirame is always served raw.

Hotategai—scallops, served raw.

Ika—squid, usually served raw. Squid eaten for sushi in the United States has generally been imported frozen from Japan. Some preparations call for boiling and/or grilling. The squid may be seasoned with a marinade similar to that used for anago.

Ikura—salmon roe. This is one of the most popular forms of sushi, certainly the most popular roe. The name ikura is said to derive from the Russian word, *ikra,* meaning fish roe.

Iwashi—sardine.

Kaibashira—scallops, served raw.

Kajiki—swordfish, served raw.

Kampyo-Maki—a rolled sushi made with seasoned dried gourd shavings.

Kani—crab, boiled. In most of the United States, what is used for kani starts out either as frozen king crab, or surimi—a processed crab analog. Surimi is sometimes referred to on a menu as Mock Crab Meat.

Surimi is described in this Chapter Preface, directly preceeding this discussion of "SUSHI AND SASHIMI."

Kappa-Maki—cucumber roll.

Katsuo—bonito. Also called skipjack tuna. This fish is prized in Japan because its coming into season heralds the arrival of Spring. Bonito does not freeze well, and for this reason it is most often available only where it can be caught locally.

Katsuo is served in sashimi; it is not commonly used in sushi.

Kazunoko—herring roe. A prized and expensive delicacy associated with feasts of celebration in Japan, especially for the New Year.

Kobashira—scallops, served raw.

Kohada—gizzard shad. The raw fish is cured with salt and vinegar.

Maguro—tuna, served raw. This is perhaps the most popular of sushi fish, at least in the United States. It is taken from the leaner part of the tuna. Also see Chutoro, Otoro, and Toro.

Maki-zushi—See: Futo-Maki
Kampyo-Maki
Kappa-Maki
Oshinko-Maki
Tekka-Maki

Masago—crab roe.

Oshinko-Maki—a rolled sushi made with pickled daikon radish.

Otoro—the fattiest of the fatty tunas, taken from the fattiest part of the belly. Otoro is considered a luxury and carries a luxurious price. It is also probably the highest-calorie sushi on any menu. It is served raw.

Saba—mackerel. Often salted and marinated for several days before serving. It has a strong, oily taste.

Sake—salmon, lightly smoked or cured. Although the spelling is identical to that of the famed rice wine, there is no similarity between the fish and the alcoholic beverage—except that they are both served at a bar.

Suzuki—sea bass, served raw.

Tai—in Japan, tai is sea bream. In the United States, where sea bream is not available, porgy and red snapper are used instead. All variations of tai are served raw.

Tako—boiled octopus.

Tamago—a sweet firm omelette made from chicken eggs.

Tekka-Maki—tuna roll. In Mia Detrick's book, *Sushi,* she notes that *tekka* is the word for gambling parlors in Japan, where the snack is said to have originated as a quick hand-held food that could be eaten without interrupting the game.

This story is of course similar to the traditional origin of our word "sandwich," named for the compulsive card player, the Earl of Sandwich. (The Earl of Tekka-Maki?)

Toro—fatty tuna belly, but not as fatty as chutoro or otoro. Served raw.

Umimasu—sea trout (weakfish).

Unagi—fresh water eel. A personal favorite of mine, unagi is broiled with the same or similar sauce as is used for anago.

Uni—sea urchin roe. So great is my love for uni sushi, that when I was preparing this book I said I could eat 50 pieces in one sitting. When my friend Elliott replied that he could do the same, we decided that upon completion of the manuscript, we'd celebrate by ordering 100 pieces of uni to share between the two of us. And we did.

For each of the fish named above, you'll find calories listed in **The Calorielogue.** However—as is true throughout this chapter—the fish that you are actually served may not come from the same waters as the fish of the same name in **The Calorielogue.** The fish that you are served may carry the same name, but may not even be of the same species. There are other uncertainties, such as size of the fish and the season in which the fish was caught—both of which influence the calories. Yet the "32.4" that I cited above seeks to describe all the fish in the ocean, as well as all the vegetables and other ingredients that go into sushi.

Using that estimated figure, it is interesting to see just what a meal of sushi might cost in calories. The following delights were ordered from the lunch menus of three Japanese restaurants here in Greenwich Village.

	Calories per Order, Applying Our Magic "32.4" per Ounce
One Order of Maki	
Anago-Maki (conger eel)	
Served at Japonica, 1 roll cut into 6 pieces, total weight 3.65 oz.	118
Served at Kaori Hana, 1 roll cut into 6 pieces, total weight 3.53 oz.	114
California-Maki (surimi crab and avocado roll)	
Served at Kaori Hana, 1 roll cut into 2 pieces, total weight 3.93 oz.	127
Futo-Maki (a "fat" roll of mixed ingredients, usually including vegetables, shellfish, and egg)	
Served at Japonica, 1 roll cut into 8 pieces, total weight 15.98 oz.	518
Served at Kaori Hana, 1 roll cut into 8 pieces, total weight 13.13 oz.	425
Served at New Tokyo, 1 roll cut into 8 pieces, total weight 14.66 oz.	475
Kani-Maki (surimi crab roll)	
Served at New Tokyo, 1 roll cut into 6 pieces, total weight 3.72 oz.	121
Kappa-Maki (cucumber roll)	
Served at Japonica, 1 roll cut into 6 pieces, total weight 3.13 oz.	101
Served at Kaori Hana, 1 roll cut into 6 pieces, total weight 3.54 oz.	115
Served at New Tokyo, 1 roll cut into 6 pieces, total weight 3.26 oz.	106
Tekka-Maki (tuna roll)	
Served at Japonica, 1 roll cut into 6 pieces, total weight 4.04 oz.	131
Served at Kaori Hana, 1 roll cut into 6 pieces, total weight 4.09 oz.	133
Served at New Tokyo, 1 roll cut into 6 pieces, total weight 3.75 oz.	122
Uni-Maki (sea urchin roll)	
Served at Japonica, 1 roll cut into 6 pieces, total weight 3.79 oz.	123
Served at Kaori Hana, 1 roll cut into 6 pieces, total weight 3.62 oz.	117
Served at New Tokyo, 1 roll cut into 6 pieces, total weight 3.76 oz.	122
One Order of Sushi, Regular	
Served at Japonica:	
1 Hamachi (yellowtail), 1.58 oz.	
1 Maguro (tuna), 1.62 oz.	
1 Hirame (fluke), 1.49 oz.	
1 Sake (salmon), 1.53 oz.	
1 Tai (red snapper), 1.53 oz.	
1 Kajiki (swordfish), 1.62 oz.	
1 Ebi (jumbo shrimp), 1.32 oz.	
1 Tamago (egg), without rice, 0.17 oz.	
8 pieces, total weight 10.86 oz.	352
Served at Kaori Hana:	
1 Tai (red snapper), 1.02 oz.	
1 Tai (red snapper), 1.09 oz.	
1 Hirame (flounder), 1.01 oz.	
1 Ebi (jumbo shrimp), 1.05 oz.	
1 Kani (surimi crab), 1.13 oz.	
1 Tobiko (flying fish roe), 0.86 oz.	
1 California-Maki (surimi crab and avocado roll), 3.83 oz.	
6 pieces plus 1 roll, total weight 9.99 oz.	324
Served at New Tokyo:	
1 Tai (red snapper), 0.84 oz.	
1 Tai (red snapper), 0.84 oz.	
1 Maguro (tuna), 0.91 oz.	
1 Kani (surimi crab), 1.02 oz.	
1 Ebi (jumbo shrimp), 0.91 oz.	
1 Saba (mackerel), 0.79 oz.	
1 Tamago (egg), 1.28 oz.	
½ Tekka-Maki (tuna roll), 1.86 oz.	
½ Kappa-Maki (cucumber roll), 1.63 oz.	
7 pieces plus 2 half rolls, total weight, 10.08 oz.	327
One Order of Sushi, Deluxe	
Served at Japonica:	
1 Maguro (tuna), 1.17 oz.	
1 Sake (salmon), 1.09 oz.	
1 Ebi (jumbo shrimp), 0.80 oz.	
1 Saba (mackerel), 1.01 oz.	
1 Amadai (tile fish), 1.17 oz.	
1 Hamachi (yellowtail), 1.08 oz.	
1 Hirame (fluke), 1.23 oz.	
1 Hirame (flounder), 1.00 oz.	
1 Kani (surimi crab), 1.11 oz.	
1 Tamago (egg), without rice, 0.17	
1 Tekka-Maki (tuna roll), 2.67 oz.	
10 pieces plus 1 roll, total weight 12.5 oz.	405
Served at Kaori Hana:	
1 Ikura (salmon roe), 0.97 oz.	
1 Kani (surimi crab), 0.96 oz.	
1 Ebi (jumbo shrimp), 1.08 oz.	
1 Maguro (tuna), 1.11 oz.	
1 Tai (red snapper), 1.04 oz.	
1 Tai (red snapper), 0.98 oz.	
1 Hirame (flounder), 0.95 oz.	
1 Tekka-Maki (tuna roll), 4.22 oz.	
1 California-Maki (surimi crab and avocado roll), 2.65 oz.	
7 pieces plus 2 rolls, total weight 13.96 oz.	452
Served at New Tokyo:	
1 Ebi (jumbo shrimp), 0.90 oz.	
1 Kani (surimi crab), 0.94 oz.	
1 Tobiko (flying fish roe), 0.78 oz.	
1 Maguro (tuna), 0.86 oz.	
1 Maguro (tuna), 0.80 oz.	
1 Hirame (flounder), 0.78 oz.	
1 Hirame (flounder), 0.89 oz.	
1 Hamachi (yellowtail), 0.88 oz.	

½ California-Maki (surimi crab and avocado roll), 1.89 oz.
½ Kappa-Maki (cucumber roll), 1.59 oz.
8 pieces plus 2 half rolls, total weight, 10.31 oz. 334

Of course it goes without saying that even in the same restaurant, portion sizes will vary. There will also be a substantial variation among restaurants in their proportions of rice to fish. Of the three restaurants I sampled, Kaori Hana and New Tokyo served smaller pieces of sushi, with the weight of the rice being just a bit more than the weight of the fish. At Japonica, the pieces of sushi were larger than at the other two restaurants. The fish itself weighed more, and the rice weighed substantially more—the proportion being approximately two parts rice to one part fish.

In the midst of enjoying all this sushi (naturally, after I weighed it, I ate it), a point came to mind that I feel I must address. Although I am an irrepressible fan of this cuisine, I cannot comfortably endorse the eating of any raw food, especially in restaurants, without a warning that potential contaminants may be present. But to balance this word of caution, it is an inarguable fact that the Japanese have been eating raw fish with obvious success for centuries.

And, of course, raw fish has been eaten in this country for quite some time, and is gaining in popularity with a tremendous momentum. In fact, I've heard a rumor that McDonald's will be carrying it, on a trial basis, at selected locations. The Big-Maki.

7 EGGS

What's an egg? The *Oxford English Dictionary* defines an egg as a ". . . spheroidal body produced by the female of birds and other animal species, and containing the germ of a new individual, enclosed within a shell or firm membrane."

What's in This Chapter? Most of the chapter is Chicken Eggs—raw, scrambled, omeletted, boiled, poached, and fried. We also have dried eggs, and egg substitutes.

Following the chicken eggs are all the other kinds. We have duck eggs, turkey eggs, and goose eggs. We have pigeon eggs, quail eggs, and turtle eggs. We have Chinese preserved eggs.

There are fish eggs listed here, borrowed from **Fish, Shellfish, & Waterlife.** Fish eggs do not really belong in this chapter, but then again, even turkey eggs are oddball entries—in the United States it's a chicken egg, or nothin'.

What's Related, but Elsewhere? "Egg Yolks" and "Cereal & Egg Yolk" are in **Baby Foods.** There are dehydrated eggs in **Campers' Foods**—and for other hikers, in **Foods For Space Travel.** If you want to see how eggs get served in the army, look in **Mess** under *Reveille.*

As a breakfast food, eggs compete with **Breakfast Cereals & Breakfast Breads,** and the Danishes and Donuts of **Cakes, Snack Cakes & Pastries.**

Seasoning mixes for eggs are in **Basic Baking & Cooking Ingredients.**

Egg McMuffins are in **Fast Food.**

Egg matzo is in **Breads.** Eggnog is in **Beverages**. There are egg noodles in **Pasta.** Eggplant, by the way, is in **Vegetables.**

The Arrangement of This Chapter is as follows:

How to Read the Numbers: The column headings are:

Unit
One Ounce by Weight
One Cup

The Unit may be a dozen eggs, a pound of eggs, a cup of eggs, or one single egg.

The Ounce by Weight column will have numbers for shelled eggs, and eggs weighed in their shell. The Cup column is for shelled eggs only.

In *Chicken Eggs* you will find the same egg listed in a number of different ways. This, to facilitate a multiplicity of comparisons. First we go through whole eggs in descending order of size. Then the white and the yolk are listed separately, because as cooking ingredients they are really two distinct foods.

The size or weight class for chicken eggs is based on a minimum weight per dozen. The size of single eggs will vary, one from the other, within the same carton—although each egg in the dozen must be within an acceptable weight range:

	Minimum Weight per Dozen Including Shell	Minimum Average Weight per Egg Including Shell
Jumbo	30 oz.	2.50 oz.
Extra Large	27 oz.	2.25 oz.
Large	24 oz.	2.00 oz.
Medium	21 oz.	1.75 oz.
Small	18 oz.	1.50 oz.
Peewee	15 oz.	1.25 oz.

The size/weight class for eggs should not be confused with the grade, which is dependent upon quality. The federal regulations for grading are lengthy. You would never forgive me if I asked you to read the rules in full, but let me quote a few of them:

To be graded AA . . .

1. Eggs from each flock must be packed separately. A flock must consist of birds which do not vary in age by more than 60 days.
2. Eggs must be gathered from the nest at least twice, but preferably three times every day.
3. Eggs must be cooled promptly after they are gathered to a temperature of 60° F or below and held at a relative humidity of approximately 70% except during washing and packaging operations, where the temperature may rise to 70°F provided that the eggs are moved promptly into a cooler with a temperature of 60°F or below.
4. Eggs must be transported and handled in such a way as to prevent sweating.
5. The temperature at which the eggs are kept and displayed in retail stores must not exceed 60°F.
6. Any flock which is excluded for failure to meet these requirements may be reinstated by the same procedures as are used to originally enter the flock as Grade AA.

How to Eat Eggs: There is no doubt about it, eggs are fairly high in calories per ounce. On the other hand, they are a very special kind of food, a highly concentrated source of nutrition. Not coincidentally, eggs are extremely satisfying for their size—you can eat two or three of them and feel as though you've eaten a meal.

Duck, goose, and turkey eggs are all higher-calorie than chicken eggs by the ounce. The difference is even more striking by the egg:

Type and Weight (Shelled)	Calories per Egg	Calories per Ounce
Chicken Egg (Medium), approx. 1.5 oz.	69	44.8
Duck egg, approx. 2.5 oz.	135	54.1
Turkey egg, approx. 2.9 oz.	138	48.5
Goose egg, approx. 4.3 oz.	233	52.3

Where do the calories in chicken eggs come from? In whole eggs, about 63% of the calories come from the fat in the yolk. About 35% of the calories come from protein, and about 2% from carbohydrate.

For the dieter, egg whites can be worth their weight in gold. They're 13.9 calories per ounce. The calories in an egg white come 94% from protein, and the rest come from carbohydrate. There are no calories from fat, none. Most of an egg white is water. In fact, 88% of an egg white is water, and water is virtually calorie-free. (For the calories in water, please see **Three Frugal Repasts,** page 666.)

The calories for chicken eggs look like this:

	Calories per Ounce
whole eggs	44.8
egg yolks	104.6
egg whites	13.9

One Large egg looks like this:

	Calories per Egg
one Large whole egg	79
one Large egg yolk	63
one Large egg white	16

So one good way to save calories when you are eating eggs is to decrease the amount of yolk and increase the amount of white. You can make perfectly good egg salad with, let's say, one whole hard-boiled egg and one or two hard-boiled egg whites. The same applies to scrambled eggs and omelets.

Another way to save calories is to use smaller eggs. Can two Large eggs take the place of two Extra Large eggs without your feeling deprived? If so, you should realize this: If you eat two eggs for breakfast every morning, simply by switching from Extra Large to Large eggs, you can lose more than two pounds a year.

Or instead of eating two Extra Large eggs, you can have three Small eggs. Eating an additional egg at breakfast, at no extra calories, may make it easier to do without the bacon—at a savings of 168 calories per ounce!

Because in this country, when you talk about eggs for breakfast you've got to talk about bacon, and ham and sausage, too. If you're going to have one of these meats with your eggs, the caloric impact of an egg breakfast will very much depend on which you choose:

	Calories per Ounce (Cooked)
extra-lean ham, USDA	37.1
Canadian-style Bacon, Oscar Mayer	73.5
pork sausage links, USDA	135.2
bacon, USDA	168.1

And don't forget the . . .

	Calories per Ounce
hashed brown potatoes, USDA	63.5
French fries, McDonald's	87.9

Poached eggs, hard-boiled eggs, soft-boiled eggs, medium-boiled eggs—all these eggs will have far fewer calories than fried eggs. How many calories you pick up in frying will depend on how large the egg is, because the larger it is the more surface area will be exposed to the cooking fat. Cooking with a little butter may add 50 to 100 calories for two eggs. This means that if you eat two eggs for breakfast every morning, by switching from fried eggs to poached eggs you could lose ten pounds a year.

But if you feel you must have fried eggs, don't despair. You can fry them without butter. There's a vegetable spray on the market called Pam, and it covers the cooking surface of a frying pan for a dozen calories or less. This also seems an appropriate spot to extoll the virtue of non-stick pots and pans. Extoll! Extoll! Eggstoll!

8 CHEESE

What is cheese? The USDA offers these informative paragraphs in *Cheese Varieties and Descriptions:*

"Natural" cheese is made directly from milk (or whey, in some instances). It is made by coagulating or curdling milk, stirring and heating the curd, draining off the whey, and collecting or pressing the curd. Desirable flavor and texture are obtained in many cheeses by curing the cheese, that is, holding it for a specified time at a specific temperature and humidity. Process cheese is made from a combination of one or more batches or kinds of natural cheese heated to pasteurization temperatures and packaged.

Cheese is made wherever animals are milked and produce more milk than the people use in fluid form. Most cheese is made from cow's milk, simply because cows are milked more generally throughout the world than other animals. Smaller quantities are made from the milk of goats and ewes. Cheese is also made in some countries from the milk of other animals, such as camels, asses, mares, buffaloes, and reindeer.

Many cheeses are named for the town or community in which they are made, or for a landmark of the community. Hence, many cheeses with different local names are practically the same in their characteristics. On the other hand, several different kinds are known by the same local name.

No one knows who made the first cheese, but according to an ancient legend it was made accidentally by an Arabian merchant. The merchant put his supply of milk into a pouch made of a sheep's stomach when he set out on a long day's journey across the desert. The rennet in the lining of the pouch combined with the heat of the sun caused the milk to separate into curd and whey. He found at nightfall that the whey satisfied his thirst and the cheese (curd) satisfied his hunger and had a delightful flavor. Thus, according to the legend, the making of one of our most useful foods was begun.

What's in This Chapter: This is the **Cheese** chapter, and boy do we have cheese! More than one hundred natural cheeses, and dozens and dozens of process cheeses, besides.

The USDA provided the calorie data for twenty-nine natural cheeses. Tracking down the additional hundred was a labor of love—I never met a cheese I didn't like. You'll find each one by name in "The Arrangement."

What's Related, but Elsewhere? Macaroni and cheese, and other prepared cheese dishes, are in **Combination Main Dishes.** So is cheese pizza. Cheese soup is in **Soups.** Cheese sauce is in **Basic Baking & Cooking Ingredients.** Cheesecake is in **Cakes.**

The cheeses in **Hors D'Oeuvres, Dips & Spreads** are taken directly from this chapter. Cheese-flavored crackers and crackers for cheese are in **Cookies & Crackers.** Cheese-flavored popcorn and Cheez Doodles are in **Salty Snacks.**

Functionally, the entire **Yogurt** chapter is related to cottage cheese (which at lunchtime is related to fruit salad and Jell-O. See the top of page 17 in the **Monologue,** if you don't know why.)

The Arrangement of This Chapter: Cheese is divided into *Natural Cheeses, Process Cheeses, Process Cheese Food, Process Cheese Products, Process Cheese Spreads,* and *Other Reduced-Calorie, Imitation, and Substitute Cheeses.* Within these lists, the arrangement is alphabetical.

NATURAL CHEESES:

How to Read the Numbers: The column headings are:

Unit
One Slice
One Ounce by Weight
One Pound

For the many cheeses that are sold by brand, the Unit is the package, and packages will come in all different shapes and sizes. For generics, the Unit column will almost always be for one pound of cheese. Moreover, the Unit column has slices and cups—and the cups can be of a cheese that's shredded, or diced, or crumbled.

The descriptives may also designate "Source A" or "Source B." "Source A" is *USDA Agriculture Handbook No. 8-1 (1976); "Source B"* is *USDA Agriculture Handbook No. 456 (1975),* which itself is based primarily on a 1963 compilation. These two excellent sets of data were obtained from analyses done years apart, and naturally they come from different sets of samples. Sometimes the numbers will differ, and this indicates a variation of which you should be aware. Sometimes the numbers are right on the nose. This is just as worth the noting. In both cases, it's what they call a "meaningful relationship."

The lowest figure in the Unit column is for Laughing Cow Cheesebits, where one bit is 13 calories. The highest figure is for Surchoix Roquefort cheese, where 60 lbs. is 100,800 calories. It's a range of 7,754 to 1.

The One Slice column has numbers for prepackaged sliced cheese only. Most frequently it is left blank. It's an important column, nonetheless. Manufacturers often sent their data for sliced cheeses on a "per-slice" basis, which means that for some cheeses this may be the most accurate column. Calories for any given cheese are frequently the same by the ounce from manufacturer to manufacturer, but vary—very—by the slice.

The Ounce by Weight column is its usual self. It is a good and accurate column for comparing cheeses to each other, and especially convenient for comparing cheeses with the foods in other chapters. The One Pound column is here for your convenience in measuring larger quantities.

The lowest figure in the Ounce column is for Lucerne Dry Curd Cottage Cheese at 20 calories per ounce. The highest figure is for Gjetost cheese at 132.3, a range of 6.5 to 1. It's a smaller variation than the Unit column, but for our purposes more significant. Overture completed, it's time for . . .

How to Eat Cheese: Curds and whey, and all I can say, is—Where do the calories come from?

The calories come from fat, with protein also a contributor. For most cheeses, the effect of carbohydrate is minor.

So, how do you eat cheese? The December 1980 issue of *Mademoiselle* offered this advice:

> "*Wine-and-cheese parties* are deceptive: It may not seem as though you're eating and drinking much, but the calories can mount up fast. Go for the harder cheeses (Cheddar, Swiss, Jarlsberg, Gouda): They contain less butterfat than softer varieties (Brie, Camembert) and may be eaten without crackers."

The advice to "go for the harder cheeses" is not startling—it's the commonly held view. Is it correct? Here are the six cheeses used by *Mademoiselle* magazine as examples. See how they run, see how they run!

	% Fat	Calories per Ounce
Cheddar, USDA Source A	33.14	114.4
Swiss, USDA Source A	27.45	106.7
Jarlsberg, Dorman's	—	107.0
Gouda, USDA Source A	27.44	101.0
Brie, USDA	27.68	94.8
Camembert, USDA Source A	24.26	85.1

Je regrette, Mademoiselle. The answer to how to eat cheese doesn't rest on whether it's a hard cheese or a soft cheese. Nor will it wholly depend on fat content. Brie has a slightly higher fat content than Swiss, but 11% fewer calories. It will often be true in this chapter that two lavish cheeses will be substantially different in their calories. And this will depend mostly on one thing . . .

. . . Moisture! Swiss cheese is 37.21% water; Brie is 48.42. And that's why Swiss and Brie have the calories they do.

Is there any way to classify the cheeses with calories in mind?

The USDA suggests a general classification of cheese into four categories—Very Hard, Hard, Semisoft, and Soft. This is a fine way to classify cheeses for some purposes, but unfortunately it doesn't work for calories:

Basic Cheese Category	Representative Cheese	Representative Calories per Ounce
Very Hard Cheese/ Grating Cheese	Skim-milk Sapsago	68.8
	Asiago Old	110.8
	Spalen	122.1
	Romano	127.5
	Parmesan	132.4
Hard Cheese	Caciocavallo	104.3
	Swiss	106.7
	Cheddar	112.8
	Gruyère	117.2
Semisoft Cheese	Trappist	94.1
	Limburger	97.8
	Port Salut	99.9
	Blue Cheese	104.3
	Muenster	104.4

Basic Cheese Category	Representative Cheese	Representative Calories per Ounce
	Roquefort	104.6
	Brick	105.3
	Gorgonzola	110.9
	Stilton	117.0
Soft Cheese	Low-fat (1% fat) Cottage Cheese	20.6
	Pot Cheese	25.0
	Whole Cottage Cheese	30.1
	Fresh Ricotta	49.4
	Neufchâtel, as made in the United States	73.8
	Camembert	85.1
	Brie	94.8
	Cream Cheese	106.0

This should dispel, once and for all, the notion that you can judge a cheese by its cover.

To set the calorie story straight, what follows is a list of the most common cheeses in ascending calorie order, plus some personal favorites that I had to include or they might never speak to me again:

	Representative Calories per Ounce or Range of Calories per Ounce
Cottage Cheese	20.0 to 33.0
Flavored Cottage Cheese	22.5 to 38.0
Pot Cheese	25.0
Ricotta Cheese	39.2 to 50.0
Mozzarella Cheese	63.2 to 90.3
Part Skim Milk Scamorze Cheese	70.0
Neufchâtel Cheese (as made in the U.S.)	73.8
Sheep's-Milk Feta Cheese	74.9
Tilsit Cheese	77.1 to 96.5
Sage Cheese	78.1 to 109.1
Weight Watchers Semisoft Skim Milk Cheese	80.0
Camembert Cheese	84.8 to 90.0
Edam Cheese	87.9 to 101.3
Limburger Cheese	92.8 to 100.0
Brie Cheese	94.8 to 100.0
Scamorze Cheese	95.9
Gouda Cheese	99.0 to 106.0
Regular or Whipped Cream Cheese	99.0 to 116.2
Port Salut Cheese	99.9
Provolone Cheese	100.0
Muenster Cheese	100.0 to 104.4
Monterey or Monterey Jack Cheese	100.0 to 106.0
Caraway Cheese	100.0 to 106.7
Swiss Cheese	100.0 to 112.8
Gruyère Cheese	100.0 to 117.2
Rondele Semisoft Cheese	103.0 to 109.0
Brick Cheese	104.1 to 110.0
Roquefort Cheese	104.6 to 105.0
Alouette Semisoft Cheese	105.5
Brick Cheese	106.0
Jarlsberg Cheese	107.0
Wensleydale Cheese	107.0 to 114.0
Derby or Sage Derby Cheese	107.8 to 112.0
Romano Cheese	109.6 to 127.5
Cheshire Cheese	109.8
Colby Cheese	110.0
Fontina Cheese	110.0 to 110.4
Gorgonzola Cheese	110.9
Parmesan Cheese	111.0 to 140.0
Cheddar Cheese	112.8
Smoked Swiss Cheese	117.0
Gjetost Cheese	132.3

The range of calories shown for certain of the cheeses—Ricotta, Mozzarella, Romano, and Parmesan, to pick a few—is not a matter of different sources, but of different forms of the cheese. Part skim milk Ricotta is 39.2 an ounce; whole milk Ricotta is 50. Parmesan cheese starts at 111.0, but if you buy the harder Parmesan cheese made for grating you're buying 140 calories an ounce.

When you get into cottage cheese, the variability is even greater—a range of more than 50%. Unflavored cottage cheese has a range of 20 to 33. When fruits and vegetables have been added, the range shifts upward. But you can have a flavored cottage cheese for fewer calories than plain cottage cheese, if you pick it right:

Plain	Calories per Ounce
USDA (Source A):	
low-fat cottage cheese (1% fat)	20.4
dry curd cottage cheese (0.42% fat)	24.0
low-fat cottage cheese (2% fat)	25.5
cream cottage cheese (4.51% fat)	29.2
Cottage Cheese Flavored with Fruit	
Yogurt Cottage Cheese with Blueberry, Zausner	23.0
Peach and Pineapple in Low-Fat Cottage Cheese, Light 'N Lively	25.0
Cottage Cheese Flavored with Fruit Salad, Friendship Calorie Meter	30.0
Cottage Cheese with Dutch Apple, Friendship	31.1
Cottage Cheese with Fruit Salad, Axelrod	35.0
Cottage Cheese with Pineapple, Friendship	35.0
Cottage Cheese with Fruit Salad, Lucerne	37.5
Cottage Cheese with Pineapple, Lucerne	37.5
Cottage Cheese Flavored with Vegetables	
Garden Salad in Low-fat Cottage Cheese, Light 'N Lively	22.5
Cottage Cheese with Garden Salad, Axelrod	28.0
Cottage Cheese with Garden Salad, Friendship	30.0
Cottage Cheese with Chives, Lucerne (Safeway)	30.0

An alternative to cottage cheese is pot cheese or pot-style cottage cheese. Friendship brand is a personal favorite—and an excellent buy at 25 calories for an ounce. Both cottage cheese and pot cheese are among the lowest-calorie sources of complete protein in the book.

Whipping right along, let's look at cream cheese:

	Calories per Ounce
cream cheese, USDA Source A	99.0
Whipped Cream Cheese, Lucerne	101.5
Pasteurized Process Cream Cheese Product, Philadelphia Light	60.0

Kraft's Philadelphia brand Light Cream Cheese is a product that I am happy to recommend. By the ounce it saves you forty calories compared to regular or whipped cream cheese. By the tablespoon, the relationship changes:

	Calories per Tablespoon
cream cheese, USDA Source A	51
Whipped Cream Cheese, Lucerne	35
Pasteurized Process Cream Cheese Product, Philadelphia Light	26

What this table doesn't show, however, is that whipped cream cheese is so "spreadable" that a tablespoon of it may go farther than a tablespoon of imitation cream cheese; whipped cream cheese may actually be a savings over the low-fat cream cheese depending on the application. Of course, the calories per tablespoon are lower because you're eating the air that's been whipped in. But if you ask me, air never tasted so good.

One more thing. What's the calories per ounce in cream cheese? About one hundred. What's the calories per ounce of fruit preserves? About seventy-seven. What happens if you add strawberry jam to your cream cheese sandwich? The calories per ounce go down. They go down even further if you use low-sugar fruit spreads. Smucker's makes an exciting assortment, at 39.5 calories an ounce. Fruit spreads are also excellent on pot cheese.

Roughly the equals of cream cheese, in calories per ounce, are the *Process Cheeses*.

There are three principal types of process cheeses on the market—pasteurized process cheese, cheese food, and cheese spreads. In contrast to the calorie chaos among natural cheeses, the process cheeses can be dealt with in a list of five lines:

	Calories per Ounce
USDA: (Source A):	
pasteurized process American cheese spread	82.3
pasteurized process American cheese food	94.0
pasteurized process Swiss cheese	94.8
pasteurized process American cheese	106.4
pasteurized process pimento cheese	106.4

Lower in calories per ounce than any of these are the reduced-calorie process cheeses and they certainly deserve attention. (But beware of the word "Imitation." It doesn't always mean reduced-calorie. For cheeses, "Imitation" often means low-cholesterol, which doesn't mean low-calorie.) There are many reduced-calorie process American cheeses on the market, and three of them are especially popular:

	Calories per Slice	Calories per Ounce
Borden's Lite Line (⅔-oz. slice)	33	50.0
Kraft Lite 'N Lively (¾-oz. slice)	53	70.0
Weight Watchers (1-oz. slice)	50	50.0

The three brands have distinctly different tastes, and so all three are worth trying if you are looking for a reduced-calorie cheese. As I told my chance acquaintance in the deli (**Monologue,** page 20) you can have two ounces of reduced-calorie American cheese for one ounce of regular American cheese. (On the other hand, you can have one ounce of regular American cheese for two ounces of reduced-calorie American cheese.)

Most reduced-calorie cheese is process cheese, but natural cheese can also be reduced-calorie. All it takes is for some of the fat to be removed. Nothing "unnatural" about that, any more than skim milk is an unnatural product.

But there's an even better way to reduce the calories per ounce in a cheese sandwich. Add cold cuts!

	Calories per Ounce
sliced Cooked Ham, Eckrich	33.3
Smoked Cooked Ham, Oscar Mayer	33.3
sliced Smoked Turkey Breast, Rich's	34.0
Ham, Hormel	35.0
sliced Slender Corned Beef, Eckrich	40.0
sliced Smoked Pastrami, A&P	45.0

There's no doubt about it, in a ham and cheese sandwich it's the cheese that provides the calories per ounce—more than the ham and more than the bread. (Bread ranges from approximately 65 to 80 calories per ounce.)

There are many ways to do calorie comparisons of foods—calories per ounce, certainly—calories per slice, calories per cup, and in some chapters we speak of calories per minute. But there is another comparison that can be made, and I think the **Cheese** chapter is just the place to do it: Calories per *sigh.* For how many feet of American cheese will it take to give you the flavor of an inch of Blue? . . . And in the same breath, I should also mention Limburger. Limburger.

9 PASTA

What is pasta? The *Scribner Bantam English Dictionary* says pasta is "thin, unleavened dough produced in a variety of shapes, usually boiled and served with a sauce."

What's in This Chapter/What's Related, but Elsewhere? What's in this chapter is dry pasta without sauce—and spaghetti sauce without the pasta. Spaghetti sauce is also in **Basic Baking & Cooking Ingredients.**

Canned spaghetti in tomato sauce is in **Combination Main Dishes,** as are spaghetti and meatballs, and macaroni and cheese. Boxed dry noodles that come with sauce mix are also in **Combination Main Dishes.** In other words, if it's dry it goes here, if it's wet it goes here, and once the wet and the dry get together, they go off someplace else.

Pasta dishes of a special sort are in **Baby Foods.**

The Arrangement of This Chapter is as follows:

How to Read the Numbers: First, for *Spaghetti Sauce,* the column headings are:

Entire Container
One Ounce by Weight
One Cup
One Tablespoon

The "Cup" is a measuring cup, of course, and the "Tablespoon" is a measuring spoon—tempted as you may be to use any spoon from the table.

The column headings for *Macaroni and Spaghetti* and the other noodle sections are:

Entire Box
One Ounce by Weight, Dry Form
One Ounce by Weight, Boiled
One Cup

The "uncooked" numbers in these columns apply only to prepackaged macaroni. Fresh pasta is a moister, heavier product.

In the Entire Box column, the numbers will be for the uncooked pasta or the yield from the box when its entire contents have been cooked. These two numbers are identical. All of the calories you put into the pot will still be calories when you take them out.

The calories per ounce, however, do change dramatically with cooking. Pasta will absorb two or three times its own weight in water. Hence there are separate columns for One Ounce by Weight, Dry Form, and One Ounce by Weight, Boiled.

For every kind of pasta, there are figures for "cooked medium." For some pastas there are also figures for two other cooked states. The description "al dente" refers to pasta that has been boiled less than "medium," and is still firm; "tender" has been cooked somewhat longer than "medium."

For spaghetti, al dente boiling time is 8–10 minutes; medium, 11–13 minutes; tender, 14–20 minutes. For other types of pasta, cooking times will of course be different.

The One Cup column has numbers for both the dry and cooked forms of pasta, and these values, for the most part, are estimated. The weight of a cup will depend on the shape of the pasta. And that's the perfect opening for . . .

How to Read the Noodle: All shapes of macaroni (of which spaghetti is one) are made from the same basic dough. The shape is what a noodle's name describes. Spaghetti is spaghetti, and here are descriptions of some of the rest (although there's by no means agreement among pasta authorities as to exactly what name applies to exactly what cut):

Acini (Acine) di Pepe—very small noodles, a pastina shaped like beads. The name means "pepper corns."
Alphabet (ABC's)—small, alphabet-shaped pastina.
Cannelloni—a smooth, tubular pasta about 2½ inches long and ¾ inch wide.
Cappellini—"Little Hairs," the thinnest grade of spaghetti, number 11.
Ditali—small, thimble-shaped pasta.
Ditalini—a round, smaller version of ditali (about one-quarter the size). Also, a round elbow about one-quarter the size of regular elbow macaroni.
Fideos—Spanish; a small cluster of very thin macaroni.
Fusilli—spiral-shaped macaroni.
Linguine—"Little Tongues," flattened spaghetti.
Manicotti—a tube for stuffing, about three inches long, ribbed on one side.
Margherite—a flat macaroni with a half twist.
Maruzelle—"Sea Shell," comes in several sizes.
Mezzani—a tubular pasta about half the size of ziti.
Mostaccioli—a long, straight, hollow tube about 1¼ inches wide, cut at an angle at both ends.
Occhio di Lupo—"the Eye of the Wolf," tubes of pasta.
Orzo—pastina about the same size and shape as rice, used for soup. Also called "Seme di Melone." This means "Melon Seeds."
Perciatelli—thin hollow pasta about the same length as spaghetti, but twice as thick.
Rigatoni—large, thick-ribbed pasta tubes (about 2 to 2½ inches in length).
Rotelle—"Wheels," flat, twisted pieces of macaroni, 1½ inches long, ¾ inch to 1 inch in diameter.
Rotini—small, round noodles shaped like corkscrews.
Tubetti—tiny tubes of pasta, similar in shape to ditali, but about half the size.
Vermicelli—very thin spaghetti.
Ziti—a tubular pasta about 1½ inches long.
Ziti Rigati—slightly larger, ribbed ziti, about 2 inches long.

EGG NOODLES:

Egg Bows—noodles shaped like bows.
Extra Wide Egg Noodles—½ inch wide.
Fettuccini—flat, narrow egg noodles the same length as spaghetti.
Kluski—long, very narrow noodles with a homemade appearance, whiter in color than egg noodles usually are.

How to Eat Pasta: Where do the calories come from? Most of the calories—about 83%—come from carbohydrate. Protein generally contributes 14%; fat, approximately 3%.

To look down the "uncooked" calories per ounce column, you might think that Simon & Schuster's printing press got stuck: 104.6, 104.6, 104.6, 104.6, 104.6, . . . Spaghetti is 104.6, alphabets are 104.6, cannelloni is 104.6, elbows are 104.6, lasagna is 104.6, shells are 104.6, and this is going to be true whether it comes from your corner deli or a merchant in Venice.

But one who looks at pasta hasta look at the calories, cooked. The pasta swells with water, and the calories per ounce go down. How much water will be absorbed depends on one thing: how long you boil it:

	Calories per Ounce	Approximate Moisture Content
dry form	104.6	10.4%
"al dente" 8 to 10 minutes	41.9	63.6%
"medium" 11 to 13 minutes	36.7	67.8%
"tender" 14 to 20 minutes	31.4	72.0%

Now one who looks at pasta hasta also look at sauce.

According to the data, the tomato sauces are the lowest in calories, and the clam sauces are the highest. Sauces flavored with meat are generally higher than "meatless" sauces, marinara sauces, or mushroom sauces. Consistently lower than their competition are the Ronzoni Lite 'n Natural sauces. The Lite 'n Natural Spaghetti Sauce flavored with Italian Sausage is lower in calories than the other brands of meatless or marinara sauces. That's impressive.

On a weight basis, all of the sauces in the list that follows range from 8.1 to 35 calories per ounce. But only the clam sauce at 35 calories per ounce comes close in calories to the pasta it goes on. That's impressive too—if the sauce is what you enjoy, don't force yourself to eat the pasta in order to finish the sauce:

		Calories per Cup	Calories per Tbsp.
Clam Sauce:	Buitoni Red Clam Sauce	227	14
	Buitoni White Clam Sauce	306	19
Marinara Sauce:	Ann Page Marinara Sauce	153	10
	Buitoni Marinara Sauce	149	9
	Ronzoni Lite 'n Natural Marinara Sauce	98	6
Meatless Sauce:	Ann Page Meatless Sauce, no mushrooms	153	10
	Ann Page Meatless Sauce with mushrooms	153	10
	Buitoni Meatless Sauce	166	10
	Ronzoni Lite 'n Natural All-Purpose Meatless Sauce	98	6
Flavored with Meat:	Ann Page Flavored with Meat	175	11
	Ragu Extra Thick and Zesty, Meat	235	15
	Ragu Homestyle, Meat	169	11
	Ragu Old World Style, Meat	169	11
	Ronzoni Lite 'n Natural Spaghetti Sauce Flavored with Meat	109	7
Flavored with Mushrooms:	Ragu Extra Thick and Zesty, Mushroom	258	16
	Ragu Homestyle, Mushroom	148	9
	Townhouse	160	10
Tomato Sauce:	Contadina Tomato Sauce	90	6
	Del Monte Tomato Sauce with Mushrooms	100	6
	Del Monte Tomato Sauce with Onions	100	6
	Del Monte Tomato Sauce with Tidbits	80	5
	Townhouse Spanish Style Tomato Sauce	84	5
	Stokely Tomato Sauce	70	4

Now one who looks at pasta hasta look at grated cheese:

	Calories per Ounce
Grated Parmesan, USDA	132.4
Grated Romano, USDA	127.5

To look at those numbers, grated cheese might seem deadly. But one ounce of a cheese that's been grated covers a huge surface area—yards and yards of spaghetti—because it's spoonful after spoonful to the ounce. A measuring tablespoon of grated cheese will add about 25 calories.

Putting it all together—pasta, sauce, and cheese—does the dish deserve its bad reputation? Well, that depends. Is it behaving like a main course, or like a vegetable?

Pasta Compared to Main Courses from Combination Main Dishes	Calories per Ounce
Chicken Chow Mein, La Choy	13.4
Canned Spaghetti in tomato sauce with cheese, USDA	*21.6*
Macaroni & Cheese, Franco-American	*24.8*
Beef Stew, Armour	26.3
Canned Spaghetti with meatballs and tomato sauce, USDA	*29.2*
Tangy Style Spaghetti Dinner, Kraft	*30.5*
Macaroni & Cheese Casserole, Betty Crocker	*31.0*
Chicken A La King, canned, Swanson	36.2
Cheese Enchilada Dinner, Banquet	38.3
Tuna Pot Pie, Morton	46.3
Eggplant Parmigiana, Buitoni	52.0
Corned Beef Hash, Armour	52.4
Mushroom Pizza, Stouffer's	56.7
Big Mac, McDonald's (borrowed from **Fast Food**)	83.3

Pasta Compared to Side Dishes from Vegetables	Calories per Ounce
Carrots, boiled	8.8
Ratatouille, Stouffer's	12.0
Broccoli, Cauliflower and Carrots in Cheese Sauce, Green Giant	15.6
Mixed Vegetables, Bird's Eye	18.6
Peas, boiled	20.1
Potato, baked	20.4
Canned Spaghetti in tomato sauce with cheese, USDA	*21.6*
Canned corn, creamed, USDA	23.3
Macaroni & Cheese, Franco American	*25.0*
Asparagus Souffle, Stouffer's	28.8
White rice, boiled	30.9
Macaroni & Cheese Casserole, Betty Crocker	*31.0*
Shells in Sauce, Buitoni	*34.0*
Candied Sweet Potatoes, Mrs. Paul's	45.0
Potato, French fried, McDonald's (borrowed from **Fast Food**)	87.9

So whether pasta deserves its bad reputation is relative, not absolute. It may be more obvious for pasta, but really, this is true throughout the book: One who looks at **Pasta** hasta use the old noodle.

10 COMBINATION MAIN DISHES

What are combination main dishes? See definition, **Fast Food.** These are the slower version.

What's in This Chapter is meat, fish, and poultry. It's eggs and pasta. It's vegetables. The foods in this chapter are none of these alone, and all of these together. For these are the frozen dinners, the pizzas, pot pies, pasta dinners, and stews. You could eat dinner in this chapter for a year, and never duplicate a single meal.

What's in this chapter is not always the entire dinner. Frozen fish sticks, which are also listed in **Fish,** are part of this chapter, too.

What's Related, but Elsewhere is basically the same as "What's in This Chapter." It's **Meats, Fish,** and **Poultry.** It's **Eggs** and **Pasta.** It's **Vegetables.**

Many of the entries in **Soups** are themselves combination main dishes. I mean, I'd hardly call bouillon a combination main dish—but when you're talking about clam chowders and Chunky Soups, the line becomes hair-thin. So when you're thinking of eating in this chapter, you might also want to look at **Soups.**

Along the highways of America, there are combination main dishes—and these are listed in **Vending** and **Fast Food.** Along the highways of the skies, combination main dishes are served in **Airline Fare** and **Foods For Space Travel.** Combination main dishes for footpaths can be found in **Campers' Foods, Mess,** and **The Boy Scouts.**

Baby Foods are combination main dishes for babies. **Pet Foods** are combination main dishes for pets. **Hors D'Oeuvres** are combination main dishes for Lilliputians.

The Arrangement of This Chapter is first by categories: *Frozen Dinners and Entrées, Frozen Pizza, Pizza Novelties, Pot Pies, Stews, One-Dish Meals in Cans or Jars* and *Boxes.* It's alphabetical by brand within each category. (If you have nothing to do one night, try alphabetizing the frozen dinners by flavor. Then try doing it as I did, with your head inside the freezer case. Someday, remind me to tell you how I almost got frostbite in Los Angeles.)

FROZEN DINNERS AND ENTRÉES

How to Read the Numbers is short. Good.

The column headings are Unit and One Ounce by Weight.

Most of the numbers in the Unit column are for an entire package. There may be an additional Unit—one cheese-filled manicotti, one cup of corned beef hash, one stuffed taco shell. For presliced pizza, there's a slice from the pie. For dishes that require preparation, there will be separate lines for both the unprepared and prepared states.

The only other column is the usual Ounce by Weight. It allows comparisons between very different foods—and in this chapter there are very different foods.

How Do You Eat Them? Even before we ask our usual first question, I want to begin by pointing out that, because of the nature of this chapter, everything here is a potential substitute for everything else. It's subject only to individual tastes. If you're in the supermarket, and it is all the same to you whether you eat a pot pie or a pizza pie, then you should be aware of the calorie differences between them. Pot pies average about 50 calories an ounce. Frozen pizzas average about 65. It's a difference you can take advantage of. Similarly, if it is all the same to you whether you eat a turkey pot pie or a turkey TV dinner, you can exercise a calorie choice there.

Then, too, pot pies come in all different flavors. Pizzas come in all different flavors. Pasta dishes come in all different flavors. And frozen dinners come in more flavors than anything else in the world.

In this chapter, asking "Where do the calories come from?" is like asking "Where do calories come from?"

It's the same old story. If the food has been fried—fried chicken, fried fish—the fat will have a substantial influence. There will also be fat in the meat or the chicken or the cheese. But often, there is actually very little meat, chicken, or cheese involved in these foods, because those ingredients are expensive. People who are selling "macaroni and cheese" are usually selling a lot more macaroni than cheese.

Of course, there will be a calorie contribution from protein, depending on the dish. But many of the calories in this chapter actually come from carbohydrate—the starch in the pot pie crust, the bread layer of the pizza, the pasta in the pasta dishes, and the flour that thickens the sauces and gravies. Carbohydrate also shows up as a major component of the desserts that sometimes come with frozen meals, in their own little compartments.

When it comes to the *Frozen Dinners,* just as you might guess, the calories in the entire package will vary enormously with the weight of the package.

But the package size by no means tells the entire story. The first data page entry for Banquet Frozen Dinners is the Beans & Frankfurters Dinner, a 10¼-ounce package. The second entry is the Beef Dinner, an 11-ounce package. The Beef Dinner has ¾ ounce more food, but is only about one-half the calories of Beans & Frankfurters—312 compared with 591. The calories per ounce are 55.0 and 28.4, respectively.

Banquet's Chopped Beef Dinner is an 11-ounce package; their Beef Chop Suey Dinner is 12 ounces. The Beef Chop Suey has one ounce more food—but one-third fewer calories.

The *Frozen Entrées* also show enormous variation. For Banquet's Chicken à la King Cookin' Bag Dinner, it's 27.6 calories an ounce. The Chop Suey Cookin' Bag Dinner, with no rice, comes in as low as 10.4 calories per ounce. A lot of the Cookin' Bag entrées are very low in calories per ounce, but remember, a Cookin' Bag means the cooking water's packed in it.

The highest-calorie frozen dinner is, of all things, a chicken dinner—Banquet's Chicken Man-Pleaser Dinner. It consists of chicken, mashed potatoes, carrots and peas, and apple cobbler. At 60.4 calories an ounce, it's 1,026 for the 17-ounce tray. Banquet's Turkey Dinner consists of turkey, gravy, dressing, mashed potatoes, and carrots. It's 26.6 calories an ounce—less than one-half the calories of the Chicken. So there are high ones, and there are low ones, and the only way to know which is which is to look them up in the book. I myself would be at a loss having to make a selection without the numbers in front of me. And, as of this writing, most of the brands on the market do not have the nutrition information printed on the label for you to compare.

Two brands of frozen dinners are always nutritionally labeled. These are Weight Watchers and Stouffer's Lean Cuisine. How do their calories compare?

Well, are you comparing calories per ounce or calories per package? Here they all are, in ascending order of calories per container:

	Calories per Container	Calories per Ounce
Weight Watchers, Flounder with Lemon Flavored Bread Crumbs, Vegetable Medley, 6½-oz. tray	140	21.5
Weight Watchers, Flounder Luncheon, 8½-oz. tray	162	19.1
Weight Watchers, Haddock Luncheon, 8¾-oz. tray	172	19.7
Stouffer's Lean Cuisine, Filet of Fish Florentine, 9-oz. tray	200	22.2
Weight Watchers, Sole in Lemon Sauce, Peas and Onions, 9¼-oz. tray	200	21.6
Weight Watchers, Perch Luncheon, 8½-oz. tray	202	23.8
Weight Watchers, Sole Dinner, 9½-oz. tray	210	22.1
Weight Watchers, Chicken Livers and Onions Luncheon, 10½-oz. tray	220	21.0
Weight Watchers, Chicken Parmigiana, Italian Cut Beans, 7¾-oz. tray	220	28.4
Stouffer's Lean Cuisine, Oriental Scallops and Vegetable with Rice, 11-oz. tray	230	20.9
Weight Watchers, Sole Luncheon, 9½-oz. tray	234	24.6
Weight Watchers, Turbot Luncheon, 8-oz. tray	234	29.3
Stouffer's Lean Cuisine, Beef and Pork Cannelloni with Mornay Sauce, 9⅝-oz. tray	240	24.9
Weight Watchers, Chicken à la King, 10-oz. tray	240	24.0
Stouffer's Lean Cuisine, Chicken Chow Mein with Rice, 11¼-oz. tray	240	21.3
Stouffer's Lean Cuisine, Filet of Fish Divan, 12⅜-oz. tray	240	19.4
Stouffer's Lean Cuisine, Meatball Stew, 10-oz. tray	240	24.0
Weight Watchers, Sliced Chicken Luncheon, 9-oz. tray	245	27.2
Weight Watchers, Chicken Creole Lunch Casserole, 13-oz. tray	250	19.3
Stouffer's Lean Cuisine, Salisbury Steak with Italian Style Sauce and Vegetables, 9½-oz. tray	260	27.4
Stouffer's Lean Cuisine, Zucchini Lasagna, 11-oz. tray	260	23.6
Weight Watchers, Flounder Dinner, 16-oz. tray	260	16.3
Stouffer's Lean Cuisine, Chicken and Vegetables with Vermicelli, 12¾-oz. tray	260	20.4
Stouffer's Lean Cuisine, Glazed Chicken with Vegetable Rice, 8½-oz. tray	270	31.8
Weight Watchers, Haddock Dinner, 16-oz. tray	270	16.9
Stouffer's Lean Cuisine, Oriental Beef with Vegetables and Rice, 8⅝-oz. tray	280	34.0
Stouffer's Lean Cuisine, Spaghetti with Beef and Mushroom Sauce, 11½-oz. tray	280	24.3
Weight Watchers, Chili Con Carne with Beans, 10-oz. tray	290	29.0
Weight Watchers, Perch Dinner, 16-oz. tray	311	19.4
Weight Watchers, Beef Steak and Peppers Luncheon, 10-oz. tray	321	32.1
Weight Watchers, Beef Steak (chopped and formed) in Green Pepper and Mushroom Sauce, Crinkle Cut Carrots, 9¾-oz. tray	340	34.9
Weight Watchers, Ziti Macaroni with Veal, Tomato Sauce and Cheese, 12½-oz. tray	340	27.2
Weight Watchers, Cheese Pizza Pie, 6-oz. tray	370	61.7
Weight Watchers, Lasagna with Veal, Tomato Sauce and Cheese, 12¾-oz. tray	380	29.8
Weight Watchers, Sliced Breast of Turkey Dinner, 19-oz. tray	380	20.0
Weight Watchers, Beef Steak and Mushrooms Dinner, 10-oz. tray	390	39.0
Weight Watchers, Sliced Turkey with Gravy and Stuffing, Carrots, Broccoli, 15¼-oz. tray	390	25.6
Weight Watchers, Turkey Tetrazzini with Cheese, Mushrooms and Red Peppers, 13-oz. tray	400	30.7
Weight Watchers, Sirloin of Beef (chopped and formed) in Mushroom Sauce, Cut Green Beans, Cauliflower, 13-oz. tray	410	31.5
Weight Watchers, Turbot Dinner, 16-oz. tray	416	26.0
Weight Watchers, Cannelloni Florentine Dinner, 13-oz. tray	450	34.6
Weight Watchers, Sirloin of Beef Dinner, 16-oz. tray	510	31.9
Weight Watchers, 2 Cheese and Tomato Pies, 12-oz. tray	760	63.3
Weight Watchers, 2 Sausage Cheese and Tomato Pies, 14-oz. tray	780	55.7

The calories per ounce, just among these two brands of frozen dinners, go from 16.3 to 63.3—a difference of almost 300%.

When it comes to the *Pot Pies,* the calories per ounce have a low of 32.9 for Swanson's Macaroni and Cheese Pot Pie. The highest entry is 58.8 calories per ounce—for Worthington's Vegetarian Pot Pie. (Not surprising, once you've read the Chapter Preface for **Vegetarian Foods.**)

Pot pies show a range of almost 80% in calories per ounce. But where you will find the really big difference is between one entire pie and another—a difference of almost 250%. From the lowest to the highest pie, they are:

	Calories per Pot Pie	Calories per Ounce
Macaroni and Cheese Pot Pie, Swanson's, 7 oz.	230	32.9
Beef Pot Pie, Morton, 8 oz.	320	40.0
Turkey Pot Pie, Morton, 8 oz.	320	40.0
Chicken Pot Pie, Morton, 8 oz.	350	43.8
Tuna Pot Pie, Morton, 8 oz.	370	46.3
Beef Pot Pie, Banquet, 8 oz.	409	51.1
Turkey Pot Pie, Banquet, 8 oz.	415	51.9
Chicken Pot Pie, Banquet, 8 oz.	427	53.4
Beef Pot Pie, Swanson's, 8 oz.	430	53.8
Tuna Pot Pie, Banquet, 8 oz.	434	54.3
Chicken Pot Pie, Swanson's, 8 oz.	450	56.3
Turkey Pot Pie, Swanson's, 8 oz.	450	56.3
Vegetarian Chicken-Like Pot Pie, Worthington, 8 oz.	450	56.3
Turkey Pot Pie, Stouffer, 10 oz.	460	46.0
Vegetarian Beef-Like Pot Pie, Worthington, 8 oz.	470	58.8
Chicken Pot Pie, Stouffer, 10 oz.	500	50.0
Beef Pot Pie, Stouffer, 10 oz.	550	55.0
Beef Pot Pie, Swanson's Hungry-Man, 16 oz.	770	48.1
Chicken Pot Pie, Swanson's Hungry-Man, 16 oz.	780	48.8

	Calories per Pot Pie	Calories per Ounce
Turkey Pot Pie, Swanson's Hungry-Man, 16 oz.	790	49.4
Sirloin Burger Pot Pie, Swanson's Hungry-Man, 16 oz.	800	50.0

If you ate two (t-w-o) Swanson's Macaroni and Cheese Pot Pies instead of one (o-n-e) Swanson's Hungry-Man Sirloin Burger Pot Pie every night for a year, you could lose 35 pounds!

The *Pot Pies* go up to 58.8 calories per ounce—just about where the *Frozen Pizzas* begin. (Caution: frozen pizza values cannot be applied to fresh-baked. They are different foods.) The One Ounce column for *Frozen Pizza* shows a surprising consistency in the calories per ounce. We have a low of 55.7 calories per ounce and a high of 76.5 calories per ounce, which represents a range of only 37%. This may sound like a lot, yet compared to most sections in the book, it's a very small range indeed. But once again, you cannot be led by a name:

	Calories per Ounce
Sausage Cheese and Tomato Pies, Weight Watchers	55.7
Cheese and Mushroom Pizza, Celeste	56.8
Cheese Pizza, La Pizzeria	58.0
Cheese Pizza, Tree Tavern	60.0
Cheese Pizza Pie, Weight Watchers	61.7
Combination Pizza, La Pizzeria	62.1
Pepperoni Pizza, La Pizzeria	62.9
Sausage and Mushroom Pizza, Celeste	63.2
Cheese and Tomato Pizza Pies, Weight Watchers	63.3
Regular Pizza, Appian Way	64.0
"Elegante" Pizza, Celentano	64.0
Cheese Pizza, Stouffer's	64.4
Cheese Pizza, Jeno's	64.6
Deluxe Pizza, Stouffer's	64.6
Hamburger Pizza, Jeno's	65.2
Sicilian Style Cheese Pizza, Celeste	65.8
Sausage Pizza, La Pizzeria	66.1
Deluxe Pizza, Celeste (the small size)	66.2
Thick Crust Cheese Pizza, La Pizzeria	66.5
Cheese Pizza, Appian Way	66.7
Sausage Pizza, Jeno's	66.7
Cheese Pizza, Celeste (the large size)	67.4
Sausage Pizza, Celeste (the large size)	68.1
Incredible Frozen Pizza, Lightstyle	68.3
Pepperoni Pizza, Jeno's	69.2
Cheese Pizza, Celeste (the small size)	70.0
Sausage Pizza, Celeste (the small size)	70.3
Pepperoni Pizza, Stouffer's	71.1
Pepperoni Pizza, Celeste (the large size)	71.2
Deluxe Sausage Pizza, Jeno's	71.4
Combination Pizza, Jeno's	72.7
Deluxe Cheese Pizza, Jeno's	73.1

There are cheese pizzas in the "fifties," the "sixties," and the "seventies" for calories per ounce—and no way to tell, by a name, which is which. Once again, in this chapter you need the book.

One of the virtues of Combination Main Dishes is that the meals are self-contained. If you have anxiety in planning the components of a meal, or in adding up the calories for multiple ingredients—if you're uncomfortable weighing and measuring food, this chapter may be a good place to start counting calories.

If you're a person for whom making a sandwich means putting two slices of bread in the toaster and one in your mouth, if cutting the family's barbecued chicken means cutting and tasting, the foods in this chapter may be a solution.

11 SOUPS

What's a soup? Traditionally, a soup is a liquid food made by boiling ingredients together in water.

What's in This Chapter:

																		B			■
	■																	E			
C	H	I	C	K	E	N	N	O	O	D	L	E	S	O	U	P	■	E			
	O																	F			
■	T	O	M	A	T	O	S	O	U	P	■							N			
	D									■			■					O			
D	O	Z	E	N	S	O	F	V	E	G	E	T	A	B	L	E	S	O	U	P	S
	G									A			L					D			
	S				■					Z			P					L			
■	O	R	A	N	G	E	S	O	U	P	■		H					E			
	U				I					A			A					S			
	P				G					C		■	B	E	A	N	S	O	U	P	S
	S				G					H			E					U			
	■				L		■			O			T					P			
		C			E		B			■		■	S	T	E	W	S	■			
		H			N		I						O			■		C			
	■	O	N	I	O	N	S	O	U	P	■	D	U	C	K	S	O	U	P	■	
		W			O		Q						P			C		R			
■		D			D		U						■			H		R			
B		E			L	■	E	S	C	A	R	O	L	E	■	A		Y			
R		R			E		S									V		S			
O		S			S		■									■		O			
T		■	■	B	O	R	S	C	H	T	■							U			
H					U													P			
S	P	L	I	T	P	E	A	W	I	T	H	H	A	M	■			■			

. . . and Watercress, which adds finesse—both "Vichyssoise" and "Potato" Soup, "Bacon, Lettuce, and Tomato" Soup. Yes, Bacon, Lettuce, and Tomato Soup.

What's Related, but Elsewhere: There are soups in other chapters, including **Baby Foods, Campers' Foods, Vending Machines,** and **Mess.** There's an example of chicken soup in **Pharmaceuticals.** But really, **Soups** is related to nearly every chapter in the book because practically anything can become a soup.

Garnishes for soup? Croutons are in **Condiments** and **Basic Baking & Cooking Ingredients.** Chinese-style hard noodles are in the *Oriental Noodles* section of **Pasta.** Grated Parmesan, grated Romano, and other grated cheeses are in **Cheese.** Lipton's dry Onion Soup Mix, prepared as California Onion Dip, is in **Hors D'Oeuvres, Dips & Spreads.**

The Arrangement of This Chapter is by brand; I gave up the attempt to arrange **Soups** by "flavor."

This is what I mean: For purposes of alphabetization, would you call "Chicken Noodle" a Chicken soup or a Noodle soup? . . . Is "Beef Noodle" a Beef soup or a Noodle soup?

If Chicken Noodle and Beef Noodle are Noodle soups, then is "Chicken 'N Stars" a Star soup?

If Chicken Noodle and Beef Noodle are Chicken and Beef soups, then is "Giggle Noodle" a Giggle soup?

So here's the arrangement:

Cup-a-Broth and Cup-a-Soup are both under Lipton; Soup Time is under Nestlé.

How to Read the Numbers: The column headings for **Soups** are:

Unit
One Ounce by Weight
One Fluid Ounce
One Cup

The Unit column will be for a can or package of soup as it is sold or prepared. Usually the soup will be prepared with water, but sometimes it will be prepared with milk or a mixture of milk and water. Occasionally it will be prepared with light cream.

One Ounce by Weight might seem a strange column to have in so wet a chapter, but canned soups are, in fact, typically sold by weight. For most of the soups in this chapter it was the Fluid Ounce column that had to be calculated by the use of conversion factors.

I'm going to skip out of order for a moment, passing by the One Fluid Ounce column and going directly on to One Cup. As always, the One Cup column is a measuring cup, not a kitchen cup or mug. It is usually not the same cup as is referred to on a manufacturer's label as a "one cup serving." Manufacturers often will use a hypothetical "6 fl. oz. cup" as their suggested serving size.

The Cup column measure is for condensed or prepared soup before it has been heated. When soup is heated it will gain in volume by expansion—but lose volume because of evaporation. In order to have a column for One Cup of Heated Soup, we would have to know how hot the soup is, and how long it had been cooking.

You will frequently see parentheses in the One Cup column. As I've said, volume measures in this chapter had to be estimated. Still, the figures in this column are relatively reliable. Indeed, there is no more uncertainty for these cup figures than there is for a cup of apples, or even for a pound of porterhouse steak.

Now let me return to the column I skipped. One Fluid Ounce. It's exactly 1/8 of the Cup, but the Fluid Ounce column serves two excellent functions that the Cup does not: First, it's a reminder that there is a difference between a weight and a fluid ounce. And second—unlike the Cup column, with its numbers for both condensed and prepared soups—the Fluid Ounce column includes numbers only for the soup as it's prepared. It is the best column, then, for comparing soups as you will actually eat them.

How to Eat Soup? Riddle. Penelope was taken by surprise when she found that she had finished all of her alphabet soup. Only seven noodles remained at the bottom of the bowl, but these letters expressed her thoughts exactly. What were they?

(O-I-C-U-R-M-T)

Now that the book is right-side-up again, where do the calories come from? Of course, it depends on the soup. But for most soups, carbohydrate is likely to be the dominant calorie contributor. For Campbell's Condensed Chicken Vegetable, as an example, carbohydrate contributes about one-half the calories in the bowl—with fat contributing just a little less than—and protein just a little more than—25% each.

What the numbers tell us about soups is that it may be possible to make painless substitutions and accomplish large savings:

	Calories per Can
Campbell's Condensed Soups:	
Chicken Gumbo, 10¾-oz. can	140
Chicken with Rice, 10½-oz. can	160
Chicken 'N Stars, 10½-oz. can	160
Chicken Noodle, 10¾-oz. can	180
Chicken Noodle O's, 10¼-oz. can	180
Chicken Vegetable, 10½-oz. can	180
Curly Noodle with Chicken, 10¾-oz. can	200
Chicken Alphabet, 10¾-oz. can	220

Or you can use the calorie difference to eat more soup. For example, for every can of Progresso Lentil Soup you eat, you could have one and one-half cans of Progresso Chickerina. For every can of Pepperidge Farm Hunters' Soup, you could have one and one-half cans of Pepperidge Farm Mushroom Soup, or almost two cans of Pepperidge Farm Gazpacho. If what you want is a vegetable soup, you can have three Crosse & Blackwell Gazpachos for one Crosse & Blackwell Minestrone.

The problem is that you can't infer the calories from the name on a label, and you can't determine calories from the list of ingredients. Celery, asparagus, and mushrooms all have fewer calories than potatoes—but look at this:

	Calories per Can
Campbell's Condensed Soups:	
Cream of Potato, 10¾-oz. can	180
Cream of Asparagus, 10¾-oz. can	200
Cream of Celery, 10¾-oz. can	220
Cream of Mushroom, 10¾-oz. can	300

Is there any way to tell calories then, when the cans are before you on the shelf? Yes. One way. Bring your book to the supermarket.

Without the numbers in hand, are there any generalizations at all that can be made in this chapter? Yes, there are. But beware —there will be exceptions.

The "Cream of" soups will certainly be among the highest. This is true even before you add the milk, because cream soups come to you with milk solids and starch as basic ingredients.

Broths, bouillons, and consommés will generally have the fewest calories per ounce, as few as 4 calories per cup. But do choose carefully—there's quite a range, and really no way to guess the calories from the flavor:

	Calories per Cup, as Prepared with Water
Beef Flavored Bouillon Cubes, Herb-Ox	6
Onion Flavored Bouillon Cubes, Herb-Ox	13
Chicken Flavored Broth, dry mix, MBT	16
Beef Broth, Condensed, Campbell's	28
Beef Consommé, Condensed, Campbell's	36
Mushroom Consommé, ready-to-serve, Pepperidge Farm	56
Scotch Broth, Condensed, Campbell's	80

The bean soups—Bean, Pea, Chili, Lentil—would have been the highest-calorie soups in the chapter, except that combination bean and meat soups beat them to it:

Based on USDA data for condensed or ready-to-serve soup:	Calories per Cup, as Prepared with Water
black bean	116
lentil with ham	140
green pea	164
chili beef	169
bean with bacon	173
bean with frankfurters	187
split pea with ham	189

As a general rule, a dehydrated soup, reconstituted, will have fewer calories than a condensed soup, prepared:

	Calories per Ounce, as Prepared with Water	
Based on USDA data:	CONDENSED	DEHYDRATED
cream of asparagus soup	9.9	6.5
bean with bacon	19.3	11.3
chicken noodle	8.8	6.0
minestrone	9.6	8.8
onion soup	6.8	3.1
tomato soup	9.9	11.1

You'll see that tomato soup is an exception to the rule. And that brings us back to the original conclusion: In this chapter you have to bring the numbers to the store.

There are some numbers, however, that are an open-and-shut case no matter which soup you choose: If you add a 10¾-oz. can of water to prepare your soup, you are adding 0.00 calories; a can of skimmed milk, about 110; if you add a can of whole milk you are adding about 200. If you add a can of light cream it's about 660. And these figures will not vary, no matter which flavor soup you choose.

But choosing a soup is more than choosing a flavor. Choosing a soup is choosing a brand. Campbell's Chicken Noodle is 72 calories per cup, prepared. Featherweight brand Chicken Noodle is 120. Isn't that something?

And I'll show you something else:

Campbell's:	Calories per Cup
Chicken Vegetable, condensed, prepared	72
Chicken Vegetable, semi-condensed, prepared	104
Chunky Chicken Vegetable, ready-to-serve	169

Same brand, same flavor, different treatment, different results.

Within any given flavor, Campbell's Chunky Soups will always be a high-calorie choice. If you've ever eaten a Chunky Soup you'll know why. Chunky Soups may be high when you compare them with the entries in **Soups**—but what about comparing them with **Combination Main Dishes?**

	Calories per Ounce
Chunky Chicken Vegetable Soup, Campbell's	20.0
Chicken à la King, Swanson	*36.2*
Chunky Chili Beef Soup, Campbell's	26.7
Chili with Beans, Hormel	*42.6*
Chunky Sirloin Burger Soup, Campbell's	22.1
Beef Stew, Dinty Moore	*24.0*
Chunky Turkey Soup, Campbell's	17.5
Turkey Pot Pie, Stouffer's	*46.0*

Even a high-calorie soup is going to be lower in calories than a good deal of the competition from other chapters.

Serving hint: Heat the bowl with hot water before you put the soup in, and serve the soup as piping hot as you can. The hotter the soup, the lower the calories per minute.

12 BEVERAGES

What's a beverage? According to the *Webster's New Collegiate Dictionary,* a beverage is defined as "a liquid for drinking; esp: one that is not water."

What's in This Chapter: The chapter begins with *Vegetable Juices.* Beetroot juice is the first entry. The chapter ends with *Tea.* Hundreds and hundreds of beverages come in between, including Buffalo milk, Carrot juice, and Ginger Beer.

What's Related, but Elsewhere: There are beverages in other chapters, too: **Fast Food, Vending, Mess, Campers' Foods**, and **Foods For Space Travel.** The most detailed listings for the juice of fresh oranges and fresh grapefruit are in **Fruits.** There are fruit juices in **Baby Foods. Alcoholic Beverages** have a chapter of their own. Soups are in **Soups.**

Whey is in this chapter; curds are in **Cheese**.

Beverages of a particular kind are in **Weight Loss and Weight Gain Preparations, Supplements & Boosters.**

Bottled water is here, but tap water is in **Three Frugal Repasts.**

To the extent that the foods in this chapter are taken as pick-me-ups, the other pick-me-up chapters are going to compete: **Sweet Little Nothings, Cookies & Crackers, Salty Snacks, Fruits, Frozen Confections,** and **Yogurt.**

The Arrangement of This Chapter is first by category:

Within the categories of *Vegetable Juices, Fruit Juices and Drinks,* and *Soda,* the arrangement is by the distinguishing name or flavor. This I did as best as I could. The best I could do for Dr. Pepper was to put it under Dr. Pepper, though it's neither pepper- nor doctor-flavored.

Most of the *Coffee* and *Tea* listings are alphabetized by brand, but the *Flavored Coffees* and *Flavored Teas* are alphabetized by flavor.

The arrangements for the other sections in this chapter should be self-evident at a glance or two.

How to Read the Numbers: The column headings are:

Unit
One Fluid Ounce
One Cup
One Tablespoon

The Unit is usually a bottle or a can, almost always holding a liquid that is ready to drink.

For dry mixes—both water-based like Kool-Aid and milk-based like cocoa—the Unit may be a package that will yield a much larger quantity of beverage. The lines will distinguish between the cocoa powder alone and cocoa plus milk.

Fruit juice concentrates have a line for the concentrated form and at least one line each for "reconstituted."

The One Cup column has no numbers for the dry or concentrated forms. This was an intentional omission that will allow you to scan and compare beverages as you will actually drink them.

The One Cup column is a standard measuring cup of 8 fluid ounces. In actual practice a glass of juice is likely to be smaller than a cup, and a glass of iced tea larger. And, too, if your cup is half filled with ice, you save half the calories per serving.

The One Fluid Ounce column is, of course, a volume measurement, ⅛ of a measuring cup. It is a "fluid" ounce even when it applies to dry mixes.

The One Tablespoon column is half the One Fluid Ounce column.

There is no Ounce by Weight column in this chapter, not even for unprepared Kool-Aid. (For an Ounce by Weight of packages sold by weight, simply divide the Unit column figures by the box size.) For most of the liquids in this chapter, a fluid ounce will weigh just a bit more than an ounce. (See "Back to the Ounce" in **Methodology,** page 35, for a discussion of the difference between weight and fluid ounces.)

How to Drink Beverages: Where do the calories come from? Let's start off with milk. Milk is a wonderful food. It has vitamins in it, it has minerals in it, it has protein in it. And, of course, it has calories in it, too—first from the fat, and then from the carbohydrate and protein. Milk has quite a lot of calories, which is why there are so many reduced-fat milks on the market.

Also there's an economic incentive to the dairy in selling reduced-fat milk. The less fat that goes into the milk, the more money can be made from selling cream and butter. Just compare the price of a quart of milk with that of a pint of heavy cream. From a purely economic standpoint, you are giving up a lot of what is commercially valuable in whole milk when you give up the butter-fat content. The calorie savings can be tremendous, but of this you are already thoroughly aware.

What you may not be aware of is that there are real differences among the brands—both in calories, and in taste. After the fat's been taken out, what's left is carbohydrate and protein. The particular mix used by a particular brand will affect the calories and the flavor.

The taste of milk will also vary from marketplace to marketplace. Milk is a highly localized product because of the expense of distance shipping and milk's perishability. The flavor—even of the same brand of milk—will vary at different times of the year because a cow's diet will vary with the season.

Most milks, perhaps all, are nutritionally labeled. You've got to look at the printed panel to know the calories. You can't just go by the label description, "skim," "low-fat," or even "whole" milk. Permissible levels of milk fat within those designations vary from place to place, and will be subject to different state regulations. But by law, as I understand it, all milk sold commercially must be labeled for fat content, and fat content will be the main, though by no means the only, determinant of caloric cost:

Based on USDA data:	**Calories per Cup**
reconstituted instantized nonfat dry milk (0.72% fat before reconstitution)	82
skim milk (.18% fat)	86
skim milk with nonfat milk solids added (.25% fat)	90
cultured buttermilk (.88% fat)	99
protein fortified skim milk (.25% fat)	100
low-fat milk (1% fat)	102
low-fat milk with nonfat milk solids added (1% fat)	104
reconstituted nonfat dry milk (0.77% fat before reconstitution)	109
protein fortified low-fat milk, (1% fat)	119
low-fat milk (2% fat)	121
low-fat milk with nonfat milk solids added (2% fat)	125
low-fat milk, protein fortified (2% fat)	137
low-sodium whole milk (3.5% fat)	149
whole milk (3.3% fat)	150
whole milk, producer (3.7% fat)	157
reconstituted whole dry milk (27.61% fat before reconstitution)	159
evaporated skim milk (.20% fat)	198
evaporated whole milk (7.6% fat)	338
condensed, sweetened, canned milk (8.7% fat)	982

Looking at the values for whole versus reduced-fat milk, what you add to milk—whether chocolate syrup or cocoa—is likely to have less of an impact than the milk fat you can reject. You do better calorie-wise to drink a low-fat milk with a tablespoon of chocolate syrup added to it than to drink the milk as it comes from the cow with no fat taken away:

	Calories per Cup
low-fat milk (1% fat)	102
low-fat milk (1% fat) with one tablespoon of Hershey's Chocolate Syrup	147
whole milk (3.3% fat)	150

We think of milk as coming from a cow, but there are other milks too:

	Calories per Cup
goat milk	168
human milk	171
Indian buffalo milk	237
sheep milk	265
reindeer milk	580

The numbers suggest that reindeer milk, at 580 calories a cup, is best avoided unless it's an absolute favorite. Or unless you can find it skimmed.

I've seen a lot of goat milk products on the market, and none of them have been skimmed. But that doesn't mean there isn't one or couldn't be one. Human breast milk is about 21 calories per fluid ounce, 171 calories per 8-ounce cup. Also without a skim-milk version, as far as I know.

What about vegetable-derived milk? Soybean milk runs about 129 calories a cup—less than whole milk, but more than most reduced-fat milks from a cow.

How does cow juice compare with orange juice? Milk has the disadvantage of calories from fat. Orange juice—for all of its sugar—is lower in calories per ounce.

For the vegetable juices and the fruit juices and drinks, all the calories come from sugar—pure carbohydrate. You can't buy them "skimmed." The way to save calories here is to dilute them.

Put them over ice. If you fill a 10-ounce glass with 7 ounces of juice and 3 ounces of ice, you will have 30% fewer calories per glassful, and it will also take longer to drink. Ice dilutes the calories, whether or not it melts.

And then there is the Feiden Fizz. The Feiden Fizz starts off with a chilled glass, adds about 2 ounces of ice, about 5 ounces of juice, about 3 ounces of seltzer, and slices of both lemon and lime. In the beginning, I drank my juice this way as a calorie-saving device. Very quickly I came to prefer the taste to that of straight undiluted juice.

Actually, I gave you last year's recipe. This year it's more like 3 ounces of juice to 5 ounces of seltzer. The preference for sweetness is very much a matter of habit.

Another way to save calories when drinking juice is to drink it still in its peel. An entire orange can have as few as 26 calories.

How do the juices compare among themselves? Here's the "Straw Poll":

	Calories per Cup
Tomato Juice, Campbell's	46
grapefruit juice, fresh, USDA	96
Lemonade, Minute Maid	99
orange juice, fresh, USDA	112
apple Juice, USDA	116
grape juice, USDA	155

Tomato juice is the best calorie buy in the section—tomato juice, and V-8. Comparing them to the calories in orange juice, the savings are better than 50%! Nice, rich, red, tomato juice. Tomato juice and V-8 both can be served hot, in mugs. Weight Watchers, in fact from the beginning of its diet, has suggested the use of tomato juice as a hot tomato soup.

Comparing the fruit juices, which are 100% fruit, with the fruit-flavored drinks that are partly fruit, and the fruit-flavored sodas, most of which are not fruit at all, this is what you'll find:

	Calories per Fluid Ounce
orange juice, fresh, USDA	13.9
orange soda, USDA	14.8
Orange Flavored Fruit Drink, Tang	15.0

It doesn't really matter, calorie-wise, where the sugar comes from. Orange juice is sweetened with the sugar produced by an orange tree. Orange soda is sweetened with the sugar from a sugar cane plant. The calories are very much the same.

Is grape soda higher-calorie than orange soda because grapes are higher-calorie than oranges? No, they run about the same.

How does Coke compare with Pepsi? Coca-Cola is 144 calories for the 12-fluid-ounce can. A 12-fluid-ounce can of Pepsi is 157. But both of them are relatively low among the sugar-sweetened sodas. A 12-ounce can of Dr. Brown's Cream Soda is 175, but that is not surprising. Cream soda is about the highest-calorie soda you can drink. (Maybe that's why they named it "Cream.")

Of course, the biggest differences in the *Soda* section are between the non-diet and the diet sodas. For people who like to drink diet soda, a lot of satisfaction can be had for very few calories. Until NutraSweet came along, I'd never finished a diet soda in my life. I can't say I had never started one, but I can tell you I had never finished one. And the "10% real fruit juices" diet sodas, such as Slice, were a welcome innovation, too.

Here, as elsewhere, I am not giving advice on what you should or shouldn't do. But be aware that the calorie consequences of sugar-sweetened sodas can be huge if you drink them in substantial quantity.

You may reason, if you are going to McDonald's to eat a Quarter Pounder, French fries, and a Coke, that you will get many more calories from the Quarter Pounder and the French fries than from the soda. But I think that depends on how you look at it. The 418 calories in a Quarter Pounder may last you until your next meal. The calories in a soda? If you look at it that way—calories per "staying power"—there are many more calories in a soda than in a Big Mac.

I think that a worthwhile comparison can be made here between soda and candy. A 12-ounce can of Coca-Cola is 144 calories, roughly the equivalent of the 1-ounce Chunky Bar. There are people who would much rather have the soda, and there are people who would much rather have the candy bar. If you are counting calories, it may or may not be unfortunate to have a soda. It may or may not be unfortunate to have a candy bar. But to have the one that you don't really want because of a misunderstanding—that is a tragedy.

What about non-diet soda compared to non-diet milk? A glass of soda has far fewer calories than a glass of whole milk.

Before I have nutritionists putting a price on my head for suggesting soda instead of milk, let me point out that milk is healthful for you when and if you need what's in it. If you are getting sufficient protein, and if you are eating or have stored sufficient vitamins, and if you have taken enough calcium (almost impossible without supplements), why not drink the soda for nearly one-third fewer calories?

An argument can be made against the soda that you are better off without the sugar. An argument can be made against the milk that you are better off without the fat. And while everybody else is arguing, all I am doing is making calorie comparisons. Making calorie comparisons, and reminding you that it is up to you to choose what you eat.

With that in mind, I introduce the next two sections of **Beverages**—*Coffee* and *Tea*.

Where do the calories come from? They come from the sugar and cream:

A standard restaurant packet of sugar has 26 calories.
A teaspoon of honey has 21 calories.
A standard-size lump of sugar has 15 calories.
A level measuring teaspoon of sugar has 15 calories.
Sugar substitutes vary from 0 to 4 calories for a suggested serving.

A tablespoon of skim milk has just less than 6 calories.
A tablespoon of low-fat milk has a bit more than 6 calories.
A tablespoon of whole milk has about 10 calories.
A tablespoon of half-and-half has about 20 calories.
A tablespoon of light table cream has about 32 calories.
A tablespoon of 25% fat medium cream has about 36 calories.
A tablespoon of heavy whipping cream has about 51 calories.

I should say that the calories per tablespoon do not, by themselves, tell the story. You might enjoy the taste of coffee with a little cream better than coffee with a lot of milk. If you use enough less (and possibly use less sugar because of it, too), then cream may be the lower-calorie choice.

If you're using milk, may I suggest that you try heating it first, as the French do when they make café au lait. The effect of heating milk is to cause its lactose, milk's natural sugar, to become more available to the taste buds. The result is sweeter coffee without any added sugar and without any additional calories. But even coffee with cream and sugar is likely to be about half the calories of an equal quantity of non-diet soda. As for the sugar, you may be able to save a significant percentage of calories by using superfine granulated, which dissolves more efficiently, and by putting the sugar into the coffee before you lower the coffee's temperature with milk.

Drinking-temperature will also have a significant effect on the perception of sweetness. Ever drink a room-temperature Coke? Even if you don't like the taste of hot coffee without sugar and cream, you might try drinking iced coffee without anything added to it but the ice. See if the coldness and the ice don't take some of the bitterness of black coffee away. The same thing goes for hot tea versus iced tea.

P.S.: A cup of fresh-brewed black coffee has about 2 calories. The calories in three cups of black coffee, few as they are, taken every day for a year can increase your body weight by more than half a pound. Never underestimate the power of a calorie.

Before we leave the chapter, there is one more beverage I would like to discuss. Believe it or not, water is a drink. It is a very low-calorie drink. It can also be prestigious if you pour it from a bottle.

If you want to try a bottled water, shop around—they're not all the same. Find one you like, squeeze fresh lemon and/or lime into it, and then toss in the peels. It makes a wonderful, delicious drink. I would never have believed it until I tried it, so I don't blame anyone who's reading this for not believing it either.

If you feel overindulgent spending money for bottled water, that's substantially what you're doing every time you buy a soda. Have you ever thought to yourself "If only they could bottle 'minus' calories!"? Well, they have. It's called H_2O, and it's minus calories every time you choose it over anything else.

13 FATS & OILS

Have you read Methodology? There are two discussions in that chapter that make good background reading for **Fats & Oils.** These are "What Is a Calorie?" which begins **Methodology,** and "Weight/Volume Continued" on page 35.

The word "fat" has a variety of meanings in our language—it can refer to animal tissue; to plumpness; idiomatically to smallness, as in "fat chance"; to best-ness, as in "fat city"; to conversation, as in "chew the fat."

In Nutritionese, the term "fat" is a loose one since it can be applied to several different types of compounds that are formed by the union of organic acids and glycerine. It refers generally to those components of food that do not mix with water and will dissolve in organic solvents. The term "fat" applies equally to material of animal or vegetable origin, saturated or unsaturated, with or without cholesterol, solid or liquid in state.

For the purposes of this chapter, I have used definitions that conform to general kitchen lingo—I've classified as *Fats* those fats that are solid at room temperature under ordinary circumstances. *Oils* are liquid at room temperature and come generally, but not necessarily, from the seeds of plants.

Both fats and oils are somewhat lighter than water. Oil will rise to the top of salad dressing, fat to the top of a stew.

What's in This Chapter/What's Related, but Elsewhere: What's in this chapter are fats and oils just by themselves. There are fats and oils scattered, or better, "splattered" throughout **The Calorielogue,** marbling the steaks in **Meats**, greasing the baking pans in **Breads,** frying the Kentucky Fried Chicken in **Fast Food,** and waiting under the skin in **Poultry.** Fat accounts for more than half the weight of most of the foods in **Nuts & Seeds.** But here, we have fats and oils in isolation.

Fats & Oils is rich with information from all over the world. To illustrate, there are entries for salt pork from the Far East and beef suet from France. This chapter has beef drippings from Great Britain, kidney fat from the Caribbean, fish liver oil and ghee from India, coconut oil from East Asia, and olive oil from Italy.

Every entry in this chapter is derived from another food. It seemed natural in some cases to cross-list the derived oil or fat of a product for comparison in other chapters, following the food from which it was obtained. If you want to know how almond oil compares with almonds turn to **Nuts & Seeds;** if you want to know how corn oil compares with corn turn to **Vegetables;** if you want to know how chicken fat compares with chicken turn to **Poultry.** But if you want to know how chicken fat compares with corn oil you're in the right place, because all the fats and oils listed anywhere in the book are listed together here.

This is also the chapter for substitutes for fats and oils, such as Pam Spray and of course the diet margarines.

Most salad dressings are principally oil. Whether mayonnaise, avocado, Caesar, or bleu, they are closely related to this chapter in use and in caloric impact. Salad dressings are often classified with fats in the literature, but in this book you'll find them with the other "sauces" in **Condiments.**

Butter-flavor extracts are in **Basic Cooking & Baking Ingredients.** Butter-flavor salt is in **Salts & Spices.**

Fat-soluble vitamins are in **Pharmaceuticals.**

The Arrangement of Fats & Oils is modeled after their use. The divisions are *Table Fats, Salad and Cooking Oils, Cooking and Baking Fats,* and *Cooking Sprays:*

Our next concern is **How to Read the Numbers.** The column headings are:

Unit
One Ounce by Weight
One Cup
One Tablespoon

The Unit column will frequently be one pound for generics, and an entire package for products by brand. The calorie range in the Unit column is 230,400 to 1: the 1¼-second spray of Pam has seven calories; the industrial-size drum (420 pounds) of Sterling soybean oil has 1,612,800 (one million, six hundred twelve thousand, eight hundred) calories and covers a lot of lettuce.

The second column of figures is our usual One Ounce by Weight. Here the relationship of Sterling to Pam is somewhat different. One ounce of soybean oil has 250 calories. One ounce of Pam has 248.

The third column is One Cup, which is 8 fluid ounces as it always is, but not necessarily 8 ounces by weight. A cup of most oils in this chapter weighs 7.68 ounces. A cup of non-whipped butter or margarine weighs almost precisely 8 ounces, but a cup of whipped butter or margarine weighs one-third less, or approximately 5⅓ ounces. The difference between 8 fluid ounces and 8 weight ounces of whipped butter is 544 calories.

The last column, One Tablespoon, is perhaps the most useful column for fats and oils. I remind you that this column is for a measuring, not an eating, tablespoon. A measuring tablespoon is half a fluid ounce or 1/16 of a cup. To find the calories in a measuring teaspoon, divide the tablespoon value by three.

You should be aware when reading these numbers that measuring the volume of solid fats—butter, margarine, shortening, and lard—can be tricky. To measure solid fats accurately by volume, you must pack firmly. Firm-packing two ounces of fat into an 8-ounce measuring cup is workable, but impractical. It's easier if you use as small a measuring cup as will suit your purpose, or use a tablespoon or teaspoon, again packing down firmly. Another technique for measuring solid fat is by displacement. If you want one-quarter cup of fat, fill a measuring cup three-quarters full of cold water. Add fat to the cup, pushing it down below the water line until the water level is at "one cup" exactly. Pour out the water, and what you have left is one-quarter cup of fat. Little beads of water will cling to the fat. No harm done—in restaurants we're often served butter on ice, which by mid-meal is butter in water. (Pat dry the fat you're going to use for baking, if the amount of liquid is critical.)

Compositionally, stick butter and margarine are identical to the butter or margarine that's sold in a tub. An advantage to the sticks is the built-in measuring device. If the sticks have been packaged four-to-the-pound, as they most frequently are, then each one is 4 ounces by weight, and 4 fluid ounces, too—one-half cup.

Whipped stick butter or margarine is generally packaged six-to-the-pound. Each stick is 2⅔ ounces by weight, 4 fluid ounces or one-half cup. Sticks will frequently have lines imprinted on the wrapper at 1-ounce and 1-tablespoon increments. For non-whipped butter or margarine each ounce will equal 2 tablespoons; for whipped, each ounce equals 3 tablespoons.

I'm making a fuss about measuring in this chapter because the ordinary margins for error simply do not apply here. In this chapter you can't afford to be casual about measuring your portions. And we're getting to why you cannot be casual, right now.

The question is **How to Eat** from this chapter, and the answer is this: A pound of raw potatoes has 345 calories; a pound of potato chips has 2,500 calories. The difference between them is **Fats & Oils.**

The calories in this chapter come from fat. The caloric contribution from protein and carbohydrate is practically nil. For this reason, and because the kinds of products we find here have a particularly low moisture content, this chapter surpasses all others for caloric density. The calories range from high to stupendous. Chocolate fudge pales by comparison.

Oil runs approximately 250 calories an ounce, or shall I say stampedes? One ounce of oil—two tablespoons' worth—is roughly the same calorically as four ounces of pumpkin pie. Oh, you can occasionally find a 2-digit number (50 calories for a tablespoon of diet margarine), but it seems clear than anyone who eats in quantity from this chapter is going to be consuming enormous numbers of calories.

And even though I've said it in the respective chapters, I think it's an important thing to repeat here: Any place where fat shows up—around the edges of meat, in the chicken skin, in the frying pan, wherever it is—even in small amounts, it will be a substantial factor in establishing the caloric content of a food. If you're thinking of skipping over this chapter because you don't use fats, spend a minute or two glancing down the One Ounce by Weight column. It will show you what you've been saving every time you trim your meat or skin your chicken.

For the most part, the suggestions for reducing calories in other chapters are suggestions for getting rid of the fat—discussions of trimming, optimum methods of cooking, guides to buying in the first place. In this chapter, where we need it the most, we can't trim the fat off and we can't cook the fat off. But what about when we buy fat?

There are huge differences in calories between products here, but they are for very different products; there are almost no differences among different brands of the same food. The Ounce column for corn oil is going to read "250," "250," "250," regardless of which company is making it.

Is margarine lower in calories than butter?

No.

No?

No! Margarine actually has about one more calorie per ounce. So much for General Knowledge and his troops.

A cup of whipped butter contains one-third fewer calories than a cup of non-whipped butter. This is because a cup of whipped butter contains one-third less butter.

What you have in a cup of whipped butter is two-thirds of a cup of butter and one-third cup of air. By weight, the calories for whipped and non-whipped butter are identical. The same is also true of whipped versus non-whipped margarine. In spite of this, the difference between whipped and non-whipped products is nothing to sneeze at. You can save calories by using whipped butter or margarine whenever your concern is with volume measurements. This doesn't just apply to a cup or tablespoon. Covering a slice of toast, for example, is a volume proposition, a problem of geometry, and the spreadability of whipped products may allow you to cover the same surface for less. Buttering vegetables is the same story. Another suggestion along these lines—spread your butter at room temperature and use a hot knife.

Diet margarine is a form of margarine with a lot more water in it. By the ounce it can save you half the calories of butter or non-diet margarine. Calorically, any brand of margarine is margarine, and any brand of butter is butter, but different brands of reduced-calorie spreads vary:

	Calories per Ounce	Calories per Tablespoon
Blue Bonnet diet margarine	100.0	50
Fleischmann's diet margarine	100.0	50
Parkay Light Spread margarine	142.2	70
Chiffon Lite Spread	153.0	70

Which has more calories, butter or mayonnaise? Mayonnaise, by a hair. But mayonnaise is an exception. Almost anything you use instead of butter or margarine is likely to save you calories:

The King asked
The Queen, and
The Queen asked
The Dairymaid:
"Could we have some butter for
The Royal slice of bread?"
The Queen asked
The Dairymaid,
The Dairymaid
Said, "Certainly,
I'll go and tell
The cow
Now
Before she goes to bed."

The Dairymaid
She curtsied,
And went and told
The Alderney:
"Don't forget the butter for
The Royal slice of bread."
The Alderney
Said sleepily
"You'd better tell
His Majesty
That many people nowadays
Like marmalade
Instead."

from "The King's Breakfast"
in *When We Were Very Young* by A. A. Milne

If the King had taken the Alderney's advice, he could have lost a lot of weight that year.

Butter is 203 calories per ounce, 102 calories per tablespoon. Here, in no particular order, are **Alternatives to butter on bread:**

Based on USDA generic data, unless specified:	Calories per Ounce	Calories per Tablespoon
jams, jellies, preserves	77.2 to 77.5	51 to 54
Smucker's low-sugar Apple, Apricot, Blackberry, Boysenberry, Cherry, Grape, Raspberry, and Strawberry Fruit Spreads	39.5	24
cream cheese	99.0	51
Philadelphia "Light" Pasteurized Process Cream Cheese Product	60.0	26
mustard	21.3	12
catsup	30.1	18
sweet relish	39.1	21
coleslaw	28.1	7
Horseradish, Gold's	12.5	6
Seafood Cocktail Sauce, Smither's	35.0	18
salad dressing	5.4 to 178.2	2.7 to 88
low-fat Plain Yogurt, Dannon	18.8	10.3
sour cream	60.7	31
imitation sour cream	59.9	30
Imitation Mayonnaise, Weight Watchers	80.0	40
cottage cheese	30.1	15
Pot Cheese, Friendship	25.0	8
Neufchâtel Cheese Spread with Onions, Kraft	70	37
chicken liver pâté	57.0	26
caviar, pressed	90.0	54
hummus; hommous (Middle East)	85.1	—
mashed banana	24.1	12

Based on USDA generic data, unless specified:	**Calories per Ounce**	**Calories per Tablespoon**
It isn't often that I get a chance to praise the calories in peanut butter, but at a saving of 35 calories an ounce over butter, here's my opportunity. Praise, peanut butter, praise!	167.0	95

However, I also have to say that if you spread it thick enough, peanut butter is going to be higher-calorie than butter. And if you spread it thin enough, butter would be a good substitute even for low-fat cream cheese.

Alternatives to butter on vegetables:

Look down the list of alternatives to butter on bread. Some of these also go well on vegetables. I can personally vouch for pot cheese. And if we put catsup on our French fries, why not on baked potato?

The French's Company makes a product called Butter-Flavored Salt, an entry in the **Salts & Spices** chapter. Butter-flavored salt has 63 calories an ounce, which may sound fairly high in calories for something labeled "salt." I call your attention to it for the same reason I'm going to single out Pam Spray, although it's over 200 calories an ounce: You don't eat it in "ounce" quantities.

Cooking with Fat: Diet margarines won't help you when you cook, and neither will whipped products, because to the extent that they are diluted with air or water you'll have to use more.

Whenever you put fat in a frying pan, be prepared for the fact that you're going to be eating some of it when the time comes. Another look at potatoes versus potato chips might remind you of this.

How much oil gets into the food when you deep fry? Some years ago, Crisco ran a popular television commercial that spoke to this issue: Two housewives are talking about French fries. "Look," one says, "I fried these French fries in one cup of Crisco Oil. And see? All the oil comes back except one tablespoon."

This is a very interesting point and a very important measurement. But it may not be that simple. Ask yourself—has any of the potato gotten into the cooking oil? If so, then the corresponding amount of cooking oil must have gone into the French fries—more than what simple addition and subtraction would indicate.

And there's an amount of oil lost to the air, too. The kitchen's going to smell of the oil cooking, even before you put food in it. That means some of the oil that simple arithmetic said was going into the potatoes actually went into the curtains. Whether the amount of potato that goes into the oil is more or less than the amount of oil that is lost to the room is going to require careful experimentation indeed—which I have not done. But simple arithmetic is just too simple to be counted on to give correct answers.

Alternatives to cooking in fat:

Cook with water: Steam, poach, boil. Frying an egg in a careful amount of butter is still likely to add between 25 and 50 calories to it. Poaching it adds none.

Broil: An open letter to my broiler: Dear Broiler, you've made it all possible. I thank you from the bottom of my heart. Loyally yours, Margo.

Barbecue: You can use a lot of barbecue sauce for a little bit of fat.

Cook in air: Hot-air popcorn poppers permit an oil-less popping process.

Use Pam Spray: It's about seven calories to cover the surface of a small frying pan.

Fry without fat: This is the Preface wherein to sing the praise of seasoned skillets and non-stick pots and pans. They permit cooking without reference to this chapter. You'll find seven different versions of how to season a skillet by consulting six different cookbooks.

If you still want to fry, don't cover your food with carbohydrate first. Flours and breadcrumbs have an impact above and beyond their own caloric value. They hold fat.

If you still want to fry, fry for less time (but long enough to cook the food thoroughly). The smaller a piece of food is, the more quickly it will cook. On the other hand, when you cut food into small pieces you increase the overall surface area, exposing more food to more oil and increasing absorption. If you want to fry, do it with the understanding that they don't call it "fat" for nothin'.

And if you still want to fry, have a cute one.

What's a cute fry?

Silly! It's a small fry, of course.

14 SUGARS, SWEETENERS & TOPPINGS

As was true for the previous Chapter Preface **Fats & Oils**, there are two discussions in **Methodology** that make good background reading for **Sugars, Sweeteners & Toppings.** These are "What Is a Calorie?" and "Weight/Volume Continued," on pages 26 and 35, respectively.

The following descriptions are excerpted (punctuation eccentricities, and all) from *Confectionary Facts,* published by the National Confectioners Association, The National Candy Wholesalers Association, and the Retail Confectioners International:

Sugar (Sucrose)

Sucrose is the refined or ordinary table sugar used in confections, comprising an *average* of just under 40% by weight of all ingredients used in all candy. It is a carbohydrate—a compound made up of carbon, hydrogen and oxygen. Sucrose is derived from sugar cane and the sugar beet, because these are the most economical sources. There is no qualitative difference in the final product derived from these two primary sources.

Raw sugar is a tan-brown coarse granulated solid obtained when sugar cane juice is evaporated. It is normally obtained from sugar cane at a sugar mill and then shipped to a refinery for further processing. It is about 96% sucrose and contains impurities, so it cannot legally be consumed without further refining.

Sugar Cane was raised in Asia or East Asia in prehistoric times. For over 2,500 years it has been obtained in India by crushing the cut cane stalks and boiling the juices to evaporate water; the dark brown sugar remaining is called "gur." The troops of Alexander the Great in India favored a Persian delicacy called "kand" or "qand," a sweet reed garnished with honey, spices and coloring, as far back as 325 B.C. Our current word "candy" is believed to have been derived from this Arab word.

Sugar cane is highly perishable and must be cut, and the syrup removed on the same day. It is planted from cuttings and only rarely re-seeds itself, but it has followed man in a tropical/subtropical pattern all over the world. In the fifteenth century, the Portuguese planted cane cuttings in Sicily and Madeira, and later in the Canary, Cape Verde, and Azores islands. Columbus took cuttings to plant in the New World, and others planted it on the islands off the African coast. By the eighteenth century, sugar had been planted all over the world.

Beet Sugar. Sugar was obtained exclusively from cane until 1747, when a chemist discovered that the same sugar could be obtained from what is now known as the sugar beet (Beta vulgaris). Beet sugar is chemically the same as cane sugar. Although the refining processes differ somewhat, the refined products from two sources are very similar.

Liquid Sugar is a solution of sucrose in water. The maximum possible concentration at room temperature is 67%; beyond this concentration, the sugar will begin to crystallize.

Granulated & Confectioners' (Powdered) Sugar is used for normal baking, canning and table use. Granulated sugar in a super-fine form also is used for extra-finely textured cakes, meringues, sweetening fruits and iced drinks. Powdered sugar is the same, but less *[sic]* finely granulated.

Brown Sugar or soft sugar, as it is called in the trade, is a fine-grained sugar covered with a thin layer of syrup (molasses). It is used for its distinguishing flavor as well as its light and darker colors. The darker the color, the higher the mineral ash content and the stronger the flavor. For example, brown sugars made from Hawaiian cane are stronger in flavor and darker in color than similar sugars made from American or Central American canes.

Molasses is the final liquid remaining after removal of the crystals from sugar cane or beet juice. Edible molasses contains about 55% total sugars and not more than 25% water; the remainder consists of mineral ash and other non-sugars.

Maple Sugar & Maple Syrup. Maple sugar contains 90.7%

sugar, 6.2% invert sugar and just under 1% ash; the solids in maple syrup consist of 95.1% sugar, 2.2% invert sugar and 1% ash. The characteristic flavor of maple products does not manifest itself until the raw sap from the maple tree has been boiled. These products primarily are used, like honey, as additions to other foods and food flavors.

Turbinado Sugar is a partially refined raw sugar that is washed in a centrifuge under sanitary conditions and that is closer to refined sugar than to raw sugar in total sugar content. It is edible (with a molasses flavor) when produced under the proper conditions and can be purchased by consumers in health stores; it also is used by some companies for the manufacture of food products.

Honey is essentially an invert sugar, formed by an enzyme, honey invertase, from the nectar gathered by bees. Honey contains an average of 38% fructose, 31% glucose, 1% sucrose, 9% other sugars, 17% water and .17% ash.

Invert Sugar is a mixture of dextrose and fructose or levulose, found naturally in fruits and honey. It also can be formed by the inversion of sucrose, which can be promoted with acids or enzymes.

Corn Syrups are the liquids containing dextrose, maltose and higher saccharides, obtained by treating corn starch with acids, enzymes or a combination of the two.

Fructose/Levulose, otherwise known as fruit sugar, occurs in invert sugar, honey, and many fruits. It has a sweetness value in the range of 1.7 to 1.8 relative to sucrose, which has a value of 1.0. High fructose corn syrup is a special corn sweetener composed primarily of dextrose and fructose. It is essentially as sweet as sucrose, but because it cannot duplicate the crystalline function of sucrose, it is not widely used in confectionery.

Maltose is a malt sugar, a disaccharide, composed of two dextrose units. It has a sweetness value of about one third that of sucrose, and has a pleasing, "malty" flavor.

Dextrose (Glucose), which is naturally present in grapes and is commercially prepared from corn starch, is also known as blood sugar (glucose). It is often used as an intravenous solution. It has a relative sweetness value of .7 in comparison to sucrose (1.0), and is the basic molecular unit of which starch, dextrins and glucose syrups are composed.

Lactose is milk sugar, so named because it occurs naturally in mammalian milk. It is a disaccharide composed of one unit of galactose and one unit of dextrose, and has a relative sweetness value of .15 compared to sucrose (1.0).

Sorbitol is a hexahydroxy sugar alcohol obtained from the mountain ash and other plants, and made industrially from glucose. It has a relative sweetness value of .60.

What's in This Chapter: There's sugar, as it comes sprinkling out of the sugar bowl. There's dextrose, fructose, honey, molasses, and maple syrup, all of which are sugars. There are calories listed here for cane juice, cane syrup, and sugar cane stalks.

This is also the chapter for sugar substitutes.

And then there are the toppings. "Toppings" include chocolate syrup, of course, and fruit syrups—apricot, blackberry, blueberry, boysenberry, etc.—butterscotch topping and caramel. There's marshmallow topping, nut topping, and whipped cream. You'll also find the cherry on top, which has become a figure of speech.

Still, this is a remarkably skinny chapter. It was very hard to get nutrition information for brand-name items here, and I thank those manufacturers who did supply it.

In defense of those who didn't, it is true that the foods from this chapter are not customarily eaten for their nutritional value. But I do think it's interesting that time and time again, manufacturers of honey declined to send the information. Luckily, the generic data should be pretty reliable for application to brand-name honey. It's all made by bees. Isn't it? . . . Still?

What's Related, but Elsewhere? The **Confitures**—jams, jellies, marmalades, and fruit spreads—are so closely related that they could have been a section here.

On the other hand, this entire chapter could have been a section in **Basic Baking & Cooking Ingredients.**

Inasmuch as sugars are used as flavorings rather than foods, **Salts & Spices** relate and compete. Extracts and flavorings are in the **Basic Baking** chapter.

All dessert chapters are related, for these provide the bottoms for the toppings. **Sweet Little Nothings** aren't usually served with whipped cream, but many candies are virtually 100% sugar. Every flavor of Lifesaver, for example. In the same way, **Beverages** is related. That chapter is mostly water, but what isn't water is sugar.

The Arrangement of This Chapter is as follows:

How to Read the Numbers: The column headings are:

Unit
One Ounce by Weight
One Cup
One Tablespoon

The Unit may be a pound of sugar, a packet of sweetener, or a bottle of pancake syrup.

The Ounce by Weight is its old self and, as always, a good column for comparisons with other chapters. Compare an ounce of pure sugar to an ounce of any candy to see what the chocolate and nuts contribute to its calorie count.

The Cup is a measuring cup, 8 fluid ounces. The Tablespoon is a measuring Tablespoon, ½ fluid ounce.

In this chapter there can be quite a difference between weight and fluid ounces. A fluid ounce of granulated sugar will weigh less than an ounce. A fluid ounce of sifted confectioners' sugar will weigh less than half an ounce.

That difference becomes important in . . .

How to Eat Sugars, Sweeteners and Toppings. If this book is ***THE CALORIE FACTOR,*** you might think this chapter is **The Calorie Factory.** Is it? Here's the scoop—

Where do the calories come from? The answer is in one word: Carbohydrate. With the exception of whipped cream and a few nut toppings, carbohydrate. Even for the chocolate-flavored syrups, carbohydrate.

In this chapter, it's usually a matter of the calories in sugar, and how much they are diluted by water.

You know from your own experience that syrups—let's say pancake syrups—have water in them. Syrup that's left over on a plate will dry out. So if you compare maple sugar at 8% moisture with maple syrup that is 33% moisture, but otherwise identical, you'll see that the liquid product has 27.6 fewer calories per ounce.

From highest to lowest, here are sixteen sugars:

Based on USDA data, unless specified:	Calories per Ounce
Fructose, Golden Harvest	120.0
granulated white sugar	109.1
Turbinado Sugar, Sugar-In-The-Raw	109.1
confectioners' sugar	109.1
Dextrose Cubes, Richter	106.3
brown sugar	105.8
Cinnamon Sugar, French's	105.5
maple sugar	99.0
honey	86.2
corn syrup, light or dark	82.2
cane syrup	80.6
concentrated cane juice	73.8
light molasses	71.4
maple syrup	71.4
medium molasses	65.8
blackstrap molasses	60.4

By the ounce, the lowest-calorie solid sugar is higher than the highest liquid. Fructose, you'll notice, is at the top. We'll get to that in a moment. First let me confirm that, yes, light and dark corn syrup are calorically the same; blackstrap molasses has fewer calories than light molasses; cinnamon sugar has fewer calories than granulated white.

I said I was going to talk about fructose. Actually, I'm going to talk about honey. Honey is about 38% fructose, and a sweetener with which we're all familiar. Counting calories? To bee or not to bee, that is the question.

But honey versus sugar is not a simple contest.

By the ounce, honey has 86.2 calories and granulated white sugar has 109.1. But is the ounce the most appropriate measurement? We spoon sugar into coffee; we spoon honey into tea; we spoon either one of them onto hot cereal. How do they compare by the spoonful? A tablespoon of honey has 64 calories, and a tablespoon of sugar has 46. Teaspoons are 21 and 15, respectively.

You see, honey happens to be a material with an especially high specific gravity. If you weigh a cup of honey, 8 fluid ounces, you won't get 8 ounces on the scale. You'll get 12 ounces. Twelve ounces of honey has 1,031 calories. Therefore one cup of honey has 1,031 calories, or 64 calories a tablespoon.

A cup of granulated white sugar, still 8 fluid ounces, weighs 7 ounces on a scale. Seven ounces of sugar has 770 calories. Therefore one cup of sugar has 770 calories. That's 46 calories a tablespoon.

So which is the lower-calorie sweetener? By the ounce, it's honey. By the spoonful, it's sugar. But what about by "sweetness"?

In honey's favor is that its flavor is strong. Analysis on a volume basis shows that one cup of honey can do the sweetening job of about 1.6 cups of sugar. Analysis by weight shows that one pound of honey has the sweetening potential of 0.94 pound of sugar.

A third analysis, which is by the calorie, shows that a calorie's worth of honey is about 5% sweeter than a calorie's worth of granulated white sugar.

Where does that leave us now?

With two choices: We can study for a Master of Honey degree, or we can remember this simple rule: It's not whether honey or sugar is better or worse, it's how much you use that counts.

What about sugar substitutes as substitutes for sugar? I don't use them, so I can't recommend one over another. But it's an odd fact that, by the ounce, some sugar substitutes have as many calories as sugar:

	Calories per Ounce
Featherweight Liquid Sweetening	0.0
Featherweight Saccharin	0.0
Pillsbury Sweet-10	0.0
Slim-ette Liquid Sugarless Sweetener	0.0
Sweet Magic Sugar Substitute	0.0
Zero-Cal Liquid Sweetener	0.0
Sweet 'n Low (brown or white)	99.2
Sprinkle Sweet	103.1
Sugar Twin (brown or white)	106.3
Sugar	*109.1*
Weight Watchers Granulated Sweetener	114.3

Some sugar substitutes are made primarily of sugar with a small amount of non-nutritive sweetener, such as sodium saccharin, added. Their calories come from the sugar, but most of the sweetness comes from the saccharin. What makes saccharin useful as a calorie-saving device is that it is so much sweeter than sugar. Can you imagine using two heaping teaspoons of saccharin in your coffee? Sodium saccharin is 300 times sweeter than sugar.

Just how does artificial sweetener work, anyhow? The attempt of the people who put these things together is to create a chemical that will activate the taste buds that respond to sugar. The key to sweetness lies in the shape of the sugar molecule, and the trick is to imitate the part of the molecular structure that says "SUGAR!" to the taste buds. The problem is that if you copy the structure exactly, you wind up with sugar. If you don't duplicate the structure, you don't quite duplicate the taste.

It's hard to offer suggestions from other chapters as alternatives for the foods here. It's not like the candy chapter, where I can suggest that you eat fruit instead. Even if you were inclined to try a peach in your coffee, a standard 6.2-ounce peach has more calories than three teaspoons of sugar. Not really surprising. A peach is mostly sugar and water, just as maple syrup is.

Jams, jellies, marmalades and preserves are all 69.8 to 79.9 calories an ounce, 48 to 60 calories a tablespoon. The fruit spreads are about half that much. On both a weight and a volume basis, these can all substitute for honey at a saving. But here again, the thickness of the layer is likely to make more of a difference than the printed calories per ounce. And that will be a matter of individual taste. If what you like is the stick-to-the-roof-of-your-mouth-ness of honey, you may be better off, calorie-wise, pampering yourself with smaller quantities of that which you really want.

The moral of this chapter is the moral of the bouillabaisse (**Monologue,** page 22). A small amount of sugar in the right place at the right time can add a great deal of flavor, more than the weight of it would suggest. If sugar is used as a spice in small quantities, rather than as a food, the calories are not that terribly great. It's "calories per dose" in this chapter all the way.

15 SALTS & SPICES

What is salt? What's a spice? The *Oxford English Dictionary* defines salt as "a substance, known chemically as sodium chloride (NaCl), very abundant in nature both in solution and in crystalline form, and extensively prepared for use as a condiment, a preservative of animal food, and in various industrial processes. Salt for domestic use is manufactured from Sea Salt (Marine salt, Bay-Salt), Rock-Salt (mineral salt, salt mineral) and now [ca. 1908–1914] from brine pumped up from rock-salt strata. Frequently called common salt."

The *Oxford* defines spice as "one or other of various strongly flavoured or aromatic substances of vegetable origin, obtained from tropical plants, commonly used as condiments or employed for other purposes on account of their fragrance or preservative qualities."

What's in This Chapter/What's Related, but Elsewhere: The chapter begins with salt—common table salt, butter-flavored salt, celery salt, and garlic salt, hickory-smoked and onion salt, sea salt—all kinds of salt, and salt substitutes.

And then come the spices—from Allspice to Turmeric, with dozens in between.

There are seasonings in other chapters—mustard, which is a spice, catsup, which is spicy, relish and horseradish—these are in **Condiments.** Grated Parmesan is in **Cheese.** Sauces and gravies are in **Basic Baking & Cooking Ingredients,** as are lemon juice, seasoning mixes, flavorings and extracts. Also related are these baking basics: nuts, chocolate chips, candied fruits, shredded coconut—for all of these foods are used to spice.

So are syrups and toppings. In fact, the whole of **Sugars, Sweeteners & Toppings** is closely akin to this chapter. "Sugar and spice and everything nice. . . ." The jams, jellies, and preserves of **Confitures** are also used to add flavor, but—

What makes this chapter unique is that its entries are going to be used in much smaller quantity—by the pinch as compared to the spoonful, and by spoons as compared to cupfuls. Yet as minute as these quantities are, there are people who would say that it is this chapter that makes food worth eating.

In that sense almost every chapter in the book is related, because those foods that aren't garnishes are garnishees.

The Arrangement of This Chapter is straightforward:

How to Read the Numbers: With one exception (China Bowl), all the spice merchants seemed to base their calorie figures on American Spice Trade Association data, and you will see the uniformity among them. The Trade Association data are relatively old. In this chapter, the USDA "generic" data are probably more accurate. Not that spices have changed recently, but analytic techniques have.

The column headings are:

Unit
One Pinch
One Ounce by Weight
One Teaspoon

This is a cooking-ingredients chapter, and you might have expected to find a column for One Cup. I didn't include a Cup because anyone who eats curry powder by the cup is likely to need a different kind of book.

The Unit column may be a pound or a tablespoon for generics; for spices sold by brand, the Unit will be an entire jar.

Since everything in this chapter is eaten as it's purchased, the

Ounce by Weight column can be used for comparison at a glance. The Teaspoon column can also be used this way.

A tablespoon of a spice will be roughly, but not exactly, three times a teaspoon.

A cup, however, cannot be inferred from the teaspoon measure simply by multiplying by 48. Except for questions of packing, a cup is 48 teaspoons, but packing is critical here. As we discuss in **The Tablespoon** on page 36 of **Methodology,** there is all the difference in the world between a cup of flour and 48 teaspoons of flour. The same rules will apply to mustard powder, which is not that dissimilar. So, if you're faced with large-scale cooking, your best bet is to weigh your spices and use the One Ounce column, or measure out the teaspoonfuls, one by one.

The One Pinch column is unique to this chapter, and is a calculated column if ever there was one. Five members of my staff, two males and three females, ranging in age from 20 to 30 years old and in height from 5′4″ to 6′, were asked to take "one pinch" of a spice as though they had been instructed to do so in a recipe. Everybody was asked to do this five times, which increased the number of samples to 25. However, there was no attempt to determine agreement between samples. It should be pointed out that, even if the size of a pinch varies two-fold, we are still talking about a very small number of calories. These may not be perfect numbers—but what can you do when you're in a pi . . . ? Never mind.

How to Eat Salts and Spices: Salts and spices have been with us since biblical times, and will probably outlast the Dead Sea. Lot's wife was turned into a pillar of salt, and if she wasn't iodized in the process, she ended up calorie-free.

Plain un-iodized table salt has no calories. This is true of the USDA data, and all the listings by brand. Diamond Crystal's Plain salt has no calories, Morton's Plain Salt has no calories. Then you get to butter-flavored salt, and you're running 1,000 calories a pound.

Where do the calories come from? For iodized salt, the one calorie per pound comes from the carbohydrate that is used to hold the iodine. For most of the flavored salts, most of the calories also come from carbohydrate.

Plain salt is all mineral.

The spices are all vegetable.

Within the vegetable kingdom, the spices in this chapter come from many different parts of the plant. There are fruits, seeds, bulbs or roots, buds or stigmas, barks and leaves. (Some spices that are botanically considered to be dried fruits are called "seeds.")

Fruits:
allspice
anise
caraway
cardamom
celery seed
coriander seed
cumin
dill seed
fennel seed
mace
paprika
pepper, black, white, and red

Leaves:
basil
bay leaf
chervil
coriander leaf
dill weed
marjoram
oregano
parsley
rosemary
sage
savory
tarragon
thyme

Seeds:
fenugreek
yellow mustard
nutmeg
poppy seed
sesame seed

Buds or Stigmas:
cloves
saffron

Bulbs or Roots:
garlic
ginger
onion
turmeric

Barks:
cassia
cinnamon

So spices are essentially dried foods, and have all of the calories that you would expect for dried foods.

The calories in most spices come primarily from carbohydrate, with some contribution from fat and protein. Some spices, especially the seeds, are oily and there will be a greater contribution from fat. In any case, all the foods in this chapter are very low in moisture and so the impact of the carbohydrate, protein, and fat is all the greater. The calories for spices run from below 75 to above 160 an ounce. In other words, some spices have more calories than sugar:

Based on USDA data:	**Calories per Ounce**
allspice	74.6
marjoram	76.8
tarragon	83.6
oregano	86.8
caraway seed	94.4
onion powder	98.4
turmeric	100.4
cumin seed	106.3
sugar	*109.1*
celery seed	111.0
mustard seed	133.0
nutmeg	148.9
poppy seed	151.1
sesame seed	166.7

But as a practical matter, the quantities you are likely to be eating in this chapter make the calorie contributions all but negligible. Compare the taste of a seeded versus a nonseeded rye, and yet the caraway seeds will contribute less than a calorie per slice. What the foods in this chapter really have in common is that they go a long, long way, at very few calories for the kick. One of the most important aspects of calorie counting is "How can I make a calorie go farther?" and this is the chapter where, indeed, it does go farther.

Not only that, but the spices in this chapter can have a calorie impact far beyond themselves. Seasoning a lean piece of meat—rubbing it down with mustard or garlic—may allow you to give up a fattier cut without feeling deprived. A squeeze of lemon, a sprinkling of spices—then fresh flounder, swordfish, gray or lemon sole can hold their heads high without butter.

To the extent that you can substitute the spices in this chapter for ingredients in other chapters—whether it is using a dried mustard powder from this chapter instead of prepared mustard (which is, of course, prepared with flour), or replacing half your sugar with a smaller quantity of cinnamon, or replacing butter with butter-flavored salt—any time you do that kind of exchange you are likely to show a calorie saving of virtually 100%. If you can take your bowl of tossed green salad and leave out half the oil because you are putting in parsley, sage, rosemary, and thyme—you are going to be saving lots of calories.

But perhaps the best comment about "How to Eat Salts and

Spices'' is made in this letter from Richard G. Sanders, president of China Bowl:

> In belated follow up to my letter of February 1, I'm enclosing data you requested in your letter of January 26th.
>
> I've shown calories and total carbohydrate including fiber per 100 grams, as reported in *Food Composition Table For Use In East Asia* jointly published by HEW and the UN in December 1972, for those of our products that are covered in this work.
>
> Sorry that figures aren't reported for a few of the spices, but a person who has to worry about the caloric content of Szechuan peppercorns is either in big trouble or a dragon.

16 NUTS & SEEDS

Is a coconut a nut? Or is it a fruit? Is a chestnut a nut or a vegetable? Are soybeans beans or nuts? Are peanuts nuts or peas?

Nuts: The *Oxford Dictionary* defines "nut" as "A fruit which consists of a hard and leathery (indehiscent) shell enclosing edible kernel; the kernel itself." The same source defines "indehiscent" as being "said of fruits that do not split open when they mature, but retain the seeds until they decay."

Now that you know that, is a coconut a nut or a fruit? The answer is, it's both. All nuts are fruits.

Seeds: The *Scribner-Bantam Dictionary* defines "seed" as "any small seedlike fruit." All seeds are fruits.

What's in This Chapter/What's Related, but Elsewhere: What's in this chapter are many things that botanically are nuts and seeds. However, common usage applies the word "nut" loosely—to nuts, to other fruits, and to vegetables. A peanut is really a pea, and a peanut shell is really a pea pod. But peanuts are not in **Vegetables,** they're here. This chapter is not a biological **Nuts & Seeds.** This is a cultural **Nuts & Seeds.**

Culture changes. Twenty years ago, the soybean, which is a bean, would have been an entry in **Vegetables.** It's still an entry in **Vegetables,** but soybeans are more and more commonly eaten as nuts, so we have them listed here as well—raw, barbecued, roasted, toasted, and garlicked.

The seeds that are in this chapter—sunflower seeds, squash seeds, sesame seeds, and such—are the seeds that we construe as nuts. Again, it is a social distinction. Poppy seeds, caraway seeds, and fennel seeds all are seeds, but they aren't here. They're in **Salts & Spices.** Sesame seeds, as you might expect, are listed in both chapters, with some fanciful treatments—sesame bars, halvah, and tahini—here in **Nuts & Seeds.**

Also in this chapter are foreign data for nuts and seeds that are familiar to us, although not many of us eat them. Examples are apricot kernels from East Asia and watermelon seeds from Africa.

It is to watermelon seeds that I owe great thanks. I used to munch on them as a child, and I was always curious as to their calories. When I began collecting nutrition data, I made watermelon-seed inquiries; no one could help. It seemed a good idea to write away to Africa, where, I had heard, watermelon seeds are a food. Having gotten that one piece of foreign information, I couldn't stop there. It was like a binge . . .

I list watermelon seeds here with great satisfaction at 160.7 calories an ounce—or 164.7, roasted.

Back to the business at hand. Peanut and other nut butters are in **Confitures & Nut Butters,** with a few representative samples in this chapter following their nut. To look at the ingredients, peanut butter has more in common with peanuts than it does with orange marmalade. But that's not how we consider it. Nuts that have been put through the grinder are treated like marmalade in our culture. On supermaket shelves, peanut butter competes for space with jam, while peanuts are in another part of the store. And most important from a dieter's point of view, peanut butter competes with jelly, not peanuts, for space in a sandwich.

There are close relationships, of course, between the peanuts in this chapter and the pretzels and potato chips in **Salty Snacks.** To be sure, they could have been together in one chapter. **Nuts & Seeds** might also have shared a chapter with **Sweet Little Nothings,** to the extent that we eat nuts and seeds like candy. Certain nut candies are cross-listed in this chapter for comparison with their prominent nut constituent. Goldenberg's Peanut Chews, Goobers, and Cracker Jack are under Peanuts. Jordan Almonds are under Almonds. How do they compare? We're getting there!

The nut and seed oils—peanut oil, coconut oil, sunflower-seed oil, etc.—are in **Fats & Oils.** There are examples here, following their respective nut or seed. There are some nut-flavored ice creams appearing here, too—butter almond, black walnut, butter pecan—courtesy of **Frozen Confections.**

Nut flavorings and extracts—almond, black walnut, coconut, pistachio—are in **Basic Baking & Cooking Ingredients.** A few nut flours and meals—peanut flour, chestnut flour, almond and pumpkin seed meal—are here as samples, but are basically in **Basic Baking.**

All flours—whether derived from nuts or not—are biologically related to this chapter. So is every breakfast cereal. A kernel of wheat is a seed. Ultimately, it is the part of the plant that carries life to the next generation. Post's well known cereal, Grape-Nuts, and Pillsbury's snack food, Wheat-Nuts, are both nut-like products, both made from wheat. Grape-Nuts are evaluated in **Breakfast Cereals,** but Wheat-Nuts—crunchy, roasted in oil, and sold on the shelf next to Planter's Mixed Cocktail Nuts—are evaluated here. Unfortunately, Wheat-Nuts won't save you any calories. They're among the highest-calorie foods in the chapter.

The Arrangement of This Chapter, despite botanical confusions, turns out to be simple:

Chocolate- and sugar-coated nuts follow the corresponding uncoated nut.

How to Read the Numbers: Throughout this chapter you'll see occasional slight differences in calories between one brand and another for the same nut. Although different soils and other variables affect all the nutritive values of foods grown in them, it is as likely that these differences are attributable to variations in individual analytic procedures, or the manner in which the numbers were rounded.

The column headings are:

Unit
One Ounce by Weight
One Pound
Fiber, expressed in Grams per Ounce

There's a discussion of fiber in **Methodology,** on page 36.

The descriptives make an enormous difference in this chapter. "In the Shell" means that the shells have been included in the measure of weight, or in the cup. "Shelled" means armor removed. It's not enough to see at a glance that one pound of peanuts is 1,769 calories. Are shells included in that pound?

The Unit will frequently be one pound for generics, and one package for nuts or seeds sold by brand. Sometimes, but not always, I was able to give "one nut" as a Unit, and I did this whenever I could. The "one nut" values are inherently less reliable, since nuts do vary so in size and weight, and therefore in calories. Still, it's useful information. Otherwise, what will happen when you encounter nuts as party food—and you stand there without a scale, picking them out of a bowl, one at a time?

Of course, if you know the size of the bowl, you may be able to use the cup values. The cup is a frequent Unit, but again, when you're talking about nuts, the descriptives are essential. Whereas, in **Vegetables,** a cup of sliced cauliflower is 23 calories and a cup of chopped cauliflower is 31 calories—the difference between two cups of almonds, one chopped and the other sliced, can be 209 calories!

The weight of—hence the calories in—a cupful will be subject to enormous variation depending on the size, shape, and treatment of the nuts. The relationships are not always apparent—a cupful of ground pecans actually has 20% fewer calories than a cupful of chopped pecans. To make matters worse, what exactly is "chopped"?

Because of the multiformity of nuts, the cup figures will give you less precision than will an ounce or a pound. This doesn't mean that the cup measure is less useful. If the recipe calls for "one cup of chopped pecans," and you don't have a scale, it's far better to have estimated cup values than none.

The One Ounce by Weight column should be relatively straightforward, bearing in mind the distinction between "In the Shell" and "Shelled." Ditto for the One Pound column.

The last column is a Fiber column. Values are expressed in grams per ounce, and given only on those lines that describe the nuts without their shells. As a practical matter, if you get a significant amount of your fiber from this chapter, you're going to be consuming enormous numbers of calories. Thus it may be a particularly useful column for those readers who are consulting **The Calorielogue** to gain weight. And that brings us to . . .

How to Eat Nuts and Seeds: A 6-ounce bag of almonds will buy you a hamburger, French fries, and a hot fudge sundae at McDonald's, with enough calories left over so that you can go back to the counter and take home their crispy apple pie. If you're trying to lose weight, the answer to "How to Eat Nuts and Seeds" is pretty much that you should eat them the way porcupines make love.

Nuts & Seeds is an important chapter in its own right, and even more so because the foods listed here are used as ingredients and ornaments for foods throughout the book. Nuts go into salads, and on top of vegetables. They almondine fish, decorate cakes, and show up like barnacles on cheese. Because they take a back seat ounce-wise, this is just the kind of thing that goes unnoticed and uncompensated for in a diet. I am simply pointing out what life has already taught you—a few nuts can make a big difference. Ten cashews are 90 calories. Eleven cashews, even more.

Where do the calories come from? Unlike most other fruits, in nuts and in seeds, carbohydrate takes a back seat. There is some calorie contribution from protein, but more than 50% of the weight of most nuts is oil. To add insult to injury, nuts are a food practically devoid of calorie-diluting moisture. The result is a chapter topped by only one for calories per ounce—**Fats & Oils.**

Anything you do to a nut is likely to reduce its calories. Anything you can coat it with, cover it with, or serve it with is likely to reduce the calories per ounce. One ounce of almonds is 170 calories. One ounce of chocolate-covered almonds is 161 calories. One ounce of sugar-coated almonds is 129 calories. But my best suggestion for how to eat nuts and seeds is how not to eat them. The best way I know to eat chocolate-covered peanuts is to eat chocolate-covered raisins.

Ward's Raisinets are 90 calories per ounce. But if you want something hard and crunchy, rather than soft and chewy, pretzels are about 111 calories per ounce. They save you more than 50 calories per ounce compared to peanuts.

Popcorn. For one cup of peanuts you can eat 36½ cups of popcorn; 20¼ cups, popped in oil. Or mix popcorn with peanuts. What are peanuts diluted with caramel-coated popcorn until they're 120 calories an ounce? They're Cracker Jack.

Cashews are a good choice among the popular nuts, at 159 per ounce. They are one of the few entries in this chapter with a fat content of less than 50% by weight. Also, cashews are 5.2% water in a chapter where moisture contents of 3 to 4% are not unusual. Chestnuts and fresh coconuts are relatively low in fat and relatively high in moisture. The calories reflect this at 55 and 98 an ounce, respectively. Dried unsweetened coconut, on the other hand, is a rousing 188 calories an ounce. Dried sweetened coconut is 155 calories, a saving of 17½% over unsweetened. Again, adding sugar reduces the calories.

Here's how the nuts line up, or Hail, hail, the gang's oil here!

Based on USDA, unless specified:	**Representative Calories per Ounce, Shelled**
chestnuts	55.0
acorns (Middle East)	76.0
Alfalfa Seeds, Natural Brand	98.0
coconuts	98.1
soybeans, dried	114.3
mixed nuts and fruit	130.0–160.0
apricot kernels (East Asia)	155.6
pinenuts	156.0
pumpkin and squash seeds	156.8
sunflower seeds	158.8
cashew nuts, roasted in oil	159.0
mixed nuts	160.0–190.0
watermelon seeds	160.7
beechnuts	161.1
peanuts	165.1
sesame seeds	166.7
pistachio nuts	169.0
almonds	169.8
safflower seeds	174.5
walnuts, black	178.1
butternuts	178.3
filberts (hazelnuts)	179.9
walnuts, persian	184.6
brazil nuts	185.4
pilinuts	189.8
hickory nuts	190.8
pecans	194.8
macadamia nuts	195.9
Wheat-Nuts, Pillsbury	200.0

Since nuts are fruits anyway, why not pick a fruit instead? If you want the crunchiness of nuts, then consider an apple, a nice, sweet, moist, crunchy apple.

How about cherries? Cherries aren't crunchy, but they are a finger food. They're relatively high in calories when reviewed in the **Fruits** chapter, but become a low-calorie snack when pitted against the competition here.

Breakfast Cereals is a chapter with good munchy-crunchy food. Cereal can substitute for, or dilute, nuts at a saving of about 50 to 85 calories an ounce, depending on which cereal is pinch-hitting for which nut. Good cereals for this purpose are Wheat Chex, Rice Chex, and Bran Chex, all 110 calories an ounce. Sweet and nutty is Kellogg's Honey & Nut Corn Flakes. It's made from milled corn, brown sugar, and peanuts in that order. At 120 calories an ounce, it is a fairly high-calorie breakfast cereal, but it still saves you plenty over peanuts. Captain Crunch is 121 calories an ounce, and tastes like corn chips made out of peanut butter.

A salad (Please don't close the book!) can be an alternative to nuts if it's made when the vegetables are fresh and crispy. A salad of crunchy raw carrots, celery, cauliflower, and apple, spiced with dill weed, lemon juice, black pepper, and freshly chopped onion, can go a long way toward satisfying an urge for nuts. Nuts do in fact function as salad vegetables, and if you want to eat nuts, salad is the best thing I can think of to dilute them with.

Just for the fun of it—how do nuts compare with butterscotch candy, which is practically pure sugar? Butterscotch is about 113 calories an ounce, so nuts are much higher. Despite their protein and their healthful reputation, the fact is they have many more calories per ounce.

But are nuts better for you? I'm not sure they are. What exactly is their virtue? To get the same amount of protein from peanuts as you would from 350 calories' worth of lean hamburger, you would have to eat more than 1,000 calories' worth of nuts. And then you would have to eat a food with complementary protein in order to utilize the protein in nuts.

Nuts have vitamins. Butterscotch does not. But whether these vitamins are beneficial depends on individual need at any particular time. And eating nuts for vitamins is, again, awfully expensive to a dieter. So I don't know that nuts are better for you, but I know they have more calories.

By the way, to get the same amount of fiber from peanuts as there is in 350 calories' worth of broccoli, you would have to eat more than 2,000 calories' worth of nuts.

Does dry roasting help to save calories? According to the numbers, the answer is that dry roasted nuts will sometimes be a little lower in calories—but will sometimes actually be higher in calories—than the same brand of nut roasted in oil!

Better than dry roasting, eat your nuts embedded in ice cream—almonds, pecans, and walnuts:

	Calories per Ounce
pecans	194.6
black walnuts	178.1
almonds	169.8
Butter Pecan Ice Cream, Breyers	72.9
Butter Almond Ice Cream, Breyers	68.8
Black Walnut Ice Cream, Meadow Gold	68.3
Caramel Nut Ice Milk, Light n' Lively	51.5
Caramel Pecan Frozen Yogurt, Johnston	33.3

But if you positively want nuts, and nothing but nuts will do, my suggestion is to buy them still in their shell. They're lower in calories per hour.

17 CONFITURES & NUT BUTTERS

What are confitures? What are nut butters?

Nut Butters: *The Oxford English Dictionary* says that "butter" is used "as a name for various substances resembling butter in appearance or consistence, as butter of almonds = Almond Butter."

Confitures: Distinctions are made among jams, jellies, marmalades, and preserves, but all of them are confitures—that is, confections made with preserved fruit.

USDA standards of identity (1978) specify that to be called a jam or preserve, a food must be at least 45% fruit, or in the case of a jelly, 45% fruit juice.

Jam: A fruit product made from fruit juice, a fruit pulp, and sugar.

Preserve: A fruit product made from fruit juice, fruit pulp, whole small fruits or slices of larger fruit, and sugar.

Jelly: A gel made from strained fruit juice and sugar.

Marmalade: A fruit product made from pulpy fruits with small pieces or slices suspended in the jelly-like moisture. Originally made from quinces, marmalade is now most commonly made from Seville oranges. (In 1524 it was recorded that Hull of Exeter's gift to Henry VIII was a box of marmalade—and wasn't that a tasty dish to set before a king?)

What's in This Chapter are strawberries; apricots and peaches; oranges, lemons, and grapefruits; blackberries, blueberries, boysenberries, and cherries—also guavas, currants, and quinces. These and other fruits, made into jellies, jams, marmalades, fruit butters, fruit spreads, and preserves. The co-stars of this chapter are peanuts, almonds, and cashews. Such is the stuff of nut butters. There's also a seed butter. The chapter closes with tahini, or as Ali Baba might have put it: "Close, sesame!"

You might not know it to look at them, but all the foods in this chapter are botanically very close. However, that's not why they share a chapter. The nut butters and fruit products are together because they are eaten in the same way—spooned out of a jar, then spread on bread and crackers. Together they make an excellent comparison between sugar and fat.

What's Related, but Elsewhere: The closest relatives to this chapter are **Fruits** and **Nuts & Seeds.** Peanut butter candies are officially in **Sweet Little Nothings,** but were invited here for comparison.

Fruit toppings and honey are in **Sugars, Sweeteners & Toppings. Yogurt** is a related chapter, for the overwhelming majority of yogurts have preserves at the bottom or mixed in. One glance at the difference in calories between plain and fruit-flavored yogurt will tell you just how related that chapter is.

The Arrangement of This Chapter is as follows:

How to Read the Numbers: The column headings are:

Unit
One Ounce by Weight
One Cup
One Tablespoon

For the *Confitures,* the Unit will always be an entire jar—usually a 10- or 12-ounce jar. Sometimes when a manufacturer produced more than one size, the numbers I received for the large and small jars didn't gel. The differences were small and probably due to errors in rounding. When this happened I used the data for the smaller jars, as these numbers most consistently corresponded with similar products of other brands, and with other flavors within the same brand.

For *Nut Butters,* the Unit column will have numbers for jars and for teaspoons. A 6-ounce jar of Peter Pan Peanut Butter has 1,010 calories. A teaspoonful has 32. You should have no trouble telling teaspoons from jars at a glance.

Tablespoons have their own column in this chapter, as well they might when the subject is jams, jellies, and nut butters.

But aside from providing a convenient measurement, there's another good reason for the Tablespoon column. Most of the numbers in this chapter were calculated from manufacturers' analysis "per serving." A "serving" was usually a teaspoon, two teaspoons, or a tablespoon. When multiplied by the "servings per container," this provided the calories in the entire jar. Dividing by the stated weight of the jar produced calories per ounce. The Tablespoon, then, is the most reliable column in this chapter. It is the best column to use for comparison between brands. Remember that it's a "measuring" tablespoon, and that it's level. When you are talking about peanut butter, the difference between a level and a heaping tablespoon can be 100 calories!

How to Eat Confitures and Nut Butters: Where do the calories come from? The calories in the confitures come exclusively from carbohydrate. Virtually all jams, jellies, preserves, and marmalades are 69.8 to 79.9 calories an ounce—48 to 60 calories per tablespoon—no matter what flavor they are, or who is making them. There are artificially sweetened fruit products in this chapter, and these have substantially fewer calories, as low as 10 calories an ounce. Some I've tried and didn't like. Others I have not tasted and can't evaluate.

And then there was Smucker's.

Smucker's makes an Apricot Spread, a Strawberry Spread, a Blackberry, a Boysenberry, and a Raspberry Spread, a Cherry Spread, a Grape Spread, and an Orange Marmalade. Smucker's Apple Spread is a personal favorite—but then again they all are, depending on my mood. Calories? About half the calories of preserves, and made without artificial sweetener.

What Smucker's has done with their fruit spreads is to leave out half the sugar and put in more fruit. Because these spreads contain more fruit and less sugar than the FDA's standards of identity for jams, jellies, or preserves allow, these products cannot be labeled "preserve," but must be labeled "spread," instead.

Fruit butters also have more fruit and less sugar than jams, jellies, or preserves. Here, the flavor you choose will make a difference. A tablespoon of apple butter can be as low as 30 calories; a tablespoon of apricot or prune is about 45. The fruit spreads and fruit butters are wonderful on bread, in sandwiches, mixed with yogurt or cottage cheese, as a topping for ice milk or ice cream. Fruit spreads and fruit butters taste good on crackers, and are especially good on saltines. Salt enhances the sensation of sweetness. It's like firecrackers going off in your mouth.

—Firecrackers remind me of the 4th of July, which reminds me of apple pie, which reminds me of peach pie, which reminds me of peaches, which reminds me that you can eat an awful lot of peach for every ounce of peach preserve. (You already know that, but I thought I'd remind you.)

How do peach preserves compare with peaches canned in syrup? Canned peaches are one-third the calories, dripping with heavy syrup. So, whereas in the **Fruits** chapter I told you to watch out for canned fruit packed in heavy syrup, here I say "dive right in."

In marked contrast to the confitures, the calories in nut butters come about 75% from fat, 15% from protein, and 10% from carbohydrate. Peanut butter made exclusively from peanuts will get all of its calories from peanuts. However, ordinary supermarket peanut butter contains added fat, sweeteners, and salt. The added sweeteners and salt will reduce the calories per ounce, but the added fat puts them right back in. The USDA says that peanut butter with "moderate amounts of" the added fat-sugar-salt combination is 167 calories an ounce. There are foods with more calories than peanut butter. For example—butter and mayonnaise. What America really needs is a good reduced-calorie peanut butter spread. (Smucker's, are you listening?)

As is true of jams, jellies, and preserves, there is virtual uniformity among flavors and brands of nut butters, crunchy or smooth:

	Range of Calories per Ounce	**Range of Calories per Tablespoon**
almond butter	168.0–180.0	95–102
cashew butter	168.3–180.0	95–102
peanut butter	165.0–180.0	94–102
sesame butter (tahini)	159.5–190.0	90–107

So sesame butter is both the winner and the loser, but not by very much. It's not like the **Salty Snacks** chapter where I will say "Eat pretzels instead of potato chips and save 39 calories an ounce." No. At 90-some-odd calories a tablespoon, I say eat the one you really like and compensate elsewhere. Choose a thinner slice of bread, which can actually save you more.

But even in *Nut Butters,* there's a product you should know about. It's called Goober Grape, and it's a peanut butter and grape jelly combination. It happens to be made by Smucker's. By virtue of its jelly component, Goober Grape has the lowest calories per ounce in the *Nut Butter* section. By virtue of its peanut butter component, Goober Grape has the highest calories per ounce among the *Confitures.* This may give you insight into the best way to eat a peanut butter and jelly sandwich.

It's ironic, but the impact of adding jelly—sweet, sweet jelly—to your peanut butter sandwich is to reduce the calories per ounce. (To lower the calories per sandwich, you have to take some of the peanut butter out before you put the jelly in.)

Do you like bananas? Bananas are a very high-calorie fruit, but a peanut butter and banana sandwich (thrilling!) is likely to have fewer calories, still, than peanut butter and jelly.

Peanut butter is a wonderful food in that practically anything you eat it with will lower its calories per ounce. Why, thanks to their chocolate coating, Reese's Peanut Butter Cups are "only" 158 calories an ounce.

Calories aside, isn't peanut butter high in protein?

Well, that depends. On paper, yes. Peanut butter has about 7.9 grams of protein per ounce (jelly has none). But the protein in peanut butter is incomplete, so peanut butter by itself won't provide you with the protein your body needs for growth and repair.

It does taste awfully good though—and if you add Smucker's Low-Sugar Red Raspberry Spread, it's almost decadent.

18 BASIC BAKING & COOKING INGREDIENTS

What's in This Chapter/What's Related, but Elsewhere: What's in this chapter are products that are obviously baking and cooking ingredients, such as flour and yeast. They couldn't go anywhere else. ("Home," wrote Robert Frost, "is the place where, when you have to go there, they have to take you in.") Baking chocolate also had no other place to go. It's not a candy.

What's also in **Basic Baking** are a slew of products gathered from other chapters: eggs, butter, milk and cream, shredded coconut, candied fruits. . . .

Although the raw ingredients are here, cake mixes and frostings are in **Cakes, Snack Cakes & Pastries.** Cookies and brownie mixes are in **Cookies & Crackers.** Bread and muffin mixes are in **Breads.** Pancake and waffle mixes are in **Breakfast Cereals & Breakfast Breads.** Pie mixes and pie fillings are in **Pies;** pie fillings are also listed in **Gelatins, Puddings & Custards.** Please refer to that chapter for unflavored gelatin as well.

Buttermilk and acidic juices are in **Beverages.** Bouillon cubes are in **Soups**. Miso and tofu are in **Vegetables.** You'll find dozens of fresh and dried fruits in **Fruits.** Nuts and seeds are in **Nuts & Seeds.**

This is the chapter for sauces and gravies, marinades, extracts, seasoning mixes, breadcrumbs, and extenders. **Condiments** has sauces, too. The general rule: sauces that are primarily used in cooking are here, but sauces added at the table are in **Condiments.** Examples: Barbecue sauce, clam sauce, and Gravy Master are in **Basic Baking;** catsup, chutney, and horseradish are in **Condiments.** There is an occasional overlap between these two chapters: croutons, grated Parmesan cheese, yogurt, and sour cream are in both chapters. So is butter.

Alcoholic Beverages is a related chapter, although cooking wines are here, not there.

Salt is not here; it's in **Salts & Spices.** So are spices.

The Arrangement of This Chapter, or the Cook's Tour:

How to Read the Numbers: The column headings for most of **Basic Baking** are:

Unit
One Ounce by Weight
One Cup
One Tablespoon

For *Extracts,* which are invariably fluid, a Fluid Ounce column has been substituted for the Ounce by Weight. Something else is unusual for *Extracts.* There are no figures for carbohydrate. I tried my best, but the lack of carbohydrate information was industry-wide. I couldn't extract it from anyone.

Back to the column headings. In this unusually diverse chapter, the Unit column produces numbers like these: 12,250 for a tub of shortening; 2 calories for a Kraft miniature marshmallow.

The Ounce by Weight column will be useful for comparing foods that come in different units.

The One Cup column was a natural in this chapter—cups are the language of recipes. A cup is always 8 fluid ounces, but the weight of a cup will vary even for the very same product. It will depend on how the cup is packed. Lightly, or tightly? This is a common concern in the baking process. That's why you will find frequent references in this chapter to the fashion in which the cup is filled. Is the flour sifted and spooned into the cup? Or is it unsifted flour, dipped with the cup?

The Tablespoon is a standard measuring spoon. Like the cup, it is a volume measure. All the tablespoons in this chapter were figured arithmetically at 1/16 the cup. But in actual practice a tablespoon will not necessarily pack the same way a cup does. Not in this chapter.

In **Beverages,** yes. Orange juice, for example, will "pack" the same way whether it's in a cup, tablespoon, thimble, or vat. Most baking and cooking ingredients will compress themselves by their own weight. The flour at the bottom of a cup will be pressed down by the weight of the flour above it. This cannot be said of a tablespoon, certainly not to the same degree.

The Ounce by Weight column is not affected by packing, which is another of its admirable qualities.

How to Eat Basic Baking and Cooking Ingredients: Where do the calories come from? Grains are carbohydrate, butter is fat, egg whites are protein. The extracts have calories from alcohol, but the alcohol evaporates in baking.

The amount of sugar used in a recipe will not have the greatest impact on calories per ounce and neither will the flour. (Sugar and flour are, calorically, about the same.) It's fat that will make the biggest difference. Adding fatty ingredients such as chocolate and nuts will increase the calories per ounce. Adding fresh fruits and fresh vegetables will reduce the calories per ounce.

Using ingredients that are high in fiber, such as whole wheat and bran, is another way to cut down on calories.

You see, all grains are seeds. Each seed contains three different layers—each with a different biological function and a different composition: the bran, the endosperm, and the germ. A chicken egg is also a seed. When we talk about bran, endosperm, and germ we can draw an analogy to eggshell, egg white, and egg yolk.

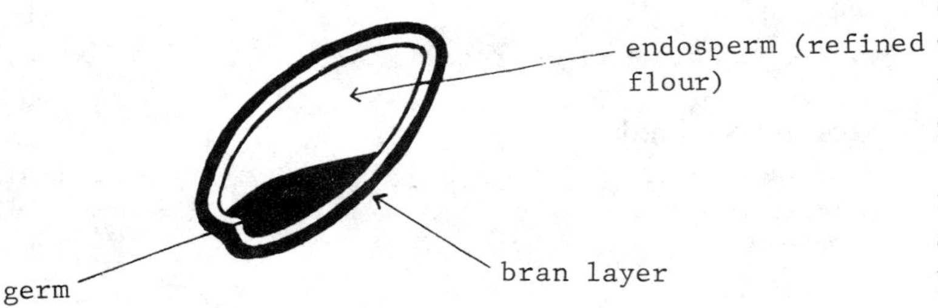

The germ is compositionally like the egg yolk—both are concentrated sources of energy, and relatively high in fat. If you squeeze wheat germ hard enough, you get wheat germ oil.

The endosperm—the middle layer—like the egg white, is very low in fat. Endosperm is what you are looking at in a bag of refined flour.

The bran, or outer layer, is like the eggshell. Like the eggshell, it serves a protective function for the seed within. Like the eggshell, it serves to maintain structural integrity. Bran is high in fiber. It's stiff, and it's tough. Some of it will pass through our system undigested. Good. That's why it's lower in calories. Wheat germ is up there at 100 to 110 calories per ounce; bran runs 60.4 to 100 calories per ounce.

And the endosperm? Flour is generally higher than bran, and slightly lower than germ:

Flours made from wheat, based on USDA data:	**Calories per Ounce**
whole wheat flour	94.6
patent flours:	
all-purpose family flour	103.3
bread flour	103.6
cake or pastry flour	103.2
gluten flour (45% gluten, 55% patent flour)	107.2
self-rising flour	99.9

The flours made from other grains are generally similar to wheat flours in their calories:

	Calories per Ounce
Barley flour, Featherweight	97.5
Buckwheat flour, Elam's	100.4
Buckwheat flour, Larrowe's	108.0
corn flour, USDA	104.3
cottonseed flour, USDA	100.9
Rice flour, Featherweight	100.0
rye flour, USDA	
light	101.3
medium	99.3
dark	92.9
soybean flour, USDA	
full-fat soybean flour	119.3
low-fat soybean flour	100.9
defatted soybean flour	92.4

We have other flours, too, with similar calories:

	Calories per Ounce
Banana flour	96.4
Grasshopper flour	119.1

The banana and grasshopper flours come from Africa. If you can't find them in your store, you can always make your own.

Just a step away from flour compositionally are the extenders and the breadcrumbs, coatings, croutons, and stuffings. These run from 81.5 for Shake 'N Bake Coating Mix for Hamburger to 140 for Pepperidge Farm Croutons.

But the printed calories—high as they are—are just the beginning. The calories in these foods really have to be viewed in light of what they're used for. All of these products are mechanisms by which your food will soak up fat. One function of a coating mix is to prevent fat from dripping to the bottom of the pan, so as to give you a nice, juicy, fatty crust.

One way out—at least it works with chicken—is to remove that fat before you put the coating mix on. I have said this 13 chapters ago in **Poultry,** but there is nothing wrong with saying something twice, especially when it's true. You can take the skin off the chicken first, and then coat it with Shake 'N Bake or glaze it with barbecue sauce.

Some of the highest-calorie teaspoons in ***THE CALORIE FACTOR*** are right here in this chapter. The *Extracts.* The following list was sent to us by the R. T. French Company, "French's" (whose return address is One Mustard Street, Rochester, N.Y.):

	Calories per Teaspoon
Almond, Pure Extract	10
Anise, Pure Extract	25
Banana, Imitation Extract	20
Black Walnut, Imitation Flavor	10
Brandy, Pure Flavor	15
Butter, Imitation Flavor	10
Cherry, Imitation Extract	15
Chocolate, Imitation Flavoring	10
Coconut, Imitation Flavor	15
Lemon, Pure Extract	30
Maple, Imitation Flavor	10
Orange, Pure Extract	30
Peach, Imitation Extract	25
Peppermint, Pure Extract	25
Pineapple, Imitation Extract	15
Pistachio, Imitation Flavor	15
Raspberry, Imitation Extract	15
Rum, Pure Flavor	20
Sherry, Pure Flavor	15
Strawberry, Imitation Extract	15
Vanilla, Imitation (Clear)	15
Vanilla, Pure Extract	10
Wintergreen, Pure Extract	25

At 30 calories a teaspoon, pure lemon extract has about twice the calories of pure sugar. But on a "per portion" basis, extracts are not among the highest-, but among the lowest-calorie foods in this book.

Also from French's:

> The normal use level for these flavorings is ½ to 1 teaspoon per four-serving recipe. If the flavoring is added to a recipe before cooking, the alcohol (which frequently contributes a major portion of the calories) will be evaporated and the calories reduced. Thus, the calories contributed by the above flavorings will usually be in the range of 1 to 8 calories per serving.

The marinades are that way, too. If you are basting a ham, for example, some of the sugar will "cook out." Unfortunately, you can't tell how much just by measuring what's left in the pan at the end. What's left in the pan will include other things—moisture, fat, and meat.

Meat tenderizers are 4.1 to 11.3 calories an ounce, but they save you calories every time you use them if they allow you to buy a less "tender"—i.e., less fatty—cut of meat to begin with.

When it comes to choosing among sauces and gravies, the difference in calories can be substantial:

	Calories per Cup Ready-to-Serve or Prepared
Sweet & Sour Sauce Mix, Durkee	230
Sweet & Sour Sauce Mix, French's	293
Sour Cream Sauce Gravy Mix, Durkee	321
Sour Cream Sauce Mix, French's	480
Beef Gravy, Franco American	123
Chicken Gravy, Franco American	210
Red Clam Sauce, Buitoni	227
White Clam Sauce, Buitoni	306
Light Soy Sauce, China Bowl	160
Dark Soy Sauce, China Bowl	249

There are alternatives to sauces and gravies outside of this chapter. Spices add flavor for virtually no calories per portion—although by the ounce, garlic is higher in calories than any tomato sauce in this book.

Salt can do wonders for the flavor of food, and it doesn't have any calories to speak of. But, as you know, salt can lead to water retention and a discouraging increase in body weight, if not in body fat.

The Potpourri

These "borrowed" data are included in this chapter for window shopping—not for efficient comparisons. There is a wealth of information for these foods that has not been reproduced in **Basic Baking.** If you're going to use the yolk from an Extra Large egg, the "Large" yolk reprinted here will not be the same. Go to **Eggs** for the calories.

The only butter cited in this chapter is unwhipped. A cup of whipped butter will not be the same. Go to **Fats & Oils.**

If you're using macadamias in a recipe, don't use the figures in this chapter for almonds, thinking "a nut is a nut." Go to **Nuts & Seeds.**

If you're going to go to the trouble of lugging this book around, you should get full benefit from its use. Look up the numbers. They're the light at the end of the funnel.

19 BREADS

STOP PRESS: There is a new bread on the market that wasn't on the shelves when the data for this book were collected. Now, in page proof time, it is my pleasure to commend this bread to you. It's Arnold's Bakery Light in three flavors, "Oatmeal," "Italian," and "Golden Wheat." All three flavors have just 40 calories for a full one-ounce slice. They compare favorably in taste and texture to breads in this chapter that run 75 calories an ounce. So when I say in ***HOW TO EAT BREAD*** that "You have very little flexibility in calories per ounce," this bread has become a welcome exception. And it does show what can be done by smart manufactuers with good intentions.

What is bread? The *Oxford English Dictionary* defines bread as "a well-known article of food prepared by moistening, kneading, and baking meal or flour, generally with the addition of yeast or leaven."

What's in This Chapter are breads made from scratch and breads made from mixes—Applesauce, Apricot, Banana through White. The bulk of the chapter is prepackaged breads: Black Bread, Bran Bread, Brown Bread, Buckwheat, Buttermilk, Butter Top . . . French Bread, and you have to go through Barbecue French, Brown 'n Serve French, Sour French, Sweet French, and Extra Sour French Bread before you get to Garlic. Leafing back and forth through the chapter, you'll find Pita and Potato Bread; Oatmeal, Corn, and Raisin Bread; Matzos, Tostadas, and Taco shells. There are over 500 breads in all, and that ain't hay. Of course the 500 also include the basic white breads, the rye breads, the whole wheat breads, and the pumpernickel. By the time you read this book, it may be pumperdime.

What's also included are hard rolls and soft rolls, hamburger and hot dog buns, popovers, muffins, biscuits, bagels, and croissants.

What's Related, but Elsewhere: The grains from which breads are made are in the **Basic Baking & Cooking Ingredients** chapter, as are prepackaged breadcrumbs. But there's a One Cup column here that will give you values for breadcrumbs from the bread of your choice.

Close to biscuits are things like Triscuits, and these are in **Cookies & Crackers.**

Croutons are in **Basic Baking & Cooking Ingredients,** and are listed again in **Condiments.**

French toast, pancakes, and waffles are in **Breakfast Cereals & Breakfast Breads.** Toaster pastries and Pop-Tarts are in **Cakes.** Honey rolls, honey buns, and other sweet rolls and buns are also in the **Cakes** chapter, although some may have sneaked in here. Bread pudding is in **Gelatins, Puddings & Custards.**

Taco shells, filled, are in **Combination Main Dishes.** So is pizza, although we do have pizza bagels here.

What's Related, but Not Elsewhere: There's a bread that is not in the data pages—communion wafers. Communion wafers may be white or whole wheat. The calories come predominantly from carbohydrate, with some contribution from protein and fat. From the recipe given to me by Sister Theresa in New York, wafers made with white flour will be approximately 54.6 calories per ounce; wafers made from a mixture of white and whole wheat flour will be approximately 59.5 calories per ounce. There will be approximately 16½ wafers per ounce when they are made from white flour, and approximately 18 wafers per ounce when they are made from the mixture of white and whole wheat. The difference in calories per ounce is offset by the difference in weight, and both types will have approximately 3.3 calories per wafer.

The Arrangement of This Chapter, or the Bread Line:

How to Read the Numbers: There are eight sections in the **Breads** chapter, and each one has a different set of column headings. Except for the Fiber column in *Prepackaged Breads and Rolls, based on generic data,* all the column headings in this chapter are variations on the headings for *Prepackaged Bread, by brand,* which is the largest section in the chapter. These column headings are:

Entire Loaf
One Slice
One Ounce by Weight
One Cup Crumbs, Fine, Dry

In *Prepackaged Buns and Rolls, by brand* the Entire Loaf has been replaced by a column for the Entire Package. The One Slice column becomes 1 Bun or Roll. For *Specialty Breads and Rolls,* there are columns for 1 Bagel, 1 Muffin, 1 Pita, 1 Croissant. . . . So an understanding of the column headings for *Prepackaged Bread, by brand,* gives a good understanding of the columns for the entire chapter. (For a discussion of fiber, see **Methodology,** page 36.)

The Entire Loaf and the One Slice columns are exactly that, but the arithmetic needs qualification: Often the weight of one slice when multiplied by the stated number of slices in a package did not equal the printed label weight. The printed label weight is a minimum weight, and many packages contain a bit more.

The One Cup figures are for breadcrumbs, and are based on a cup that is not packed. The numbers are estimates for dry—not fresh—crumbled breadcrumbs.

In this chapter, the One Ounce by Weight column is the most reliable: the Cup column figures are all estimates; the Slice column is only an average. (As we all know, end slices are generally smaller than slices taken from the middle of the loaf.) The Ounce figures, however, can be thrown off somewhat if you are using bread that's been in the bread box or refrigerator for a while. As bread loses moisture it becomes lighter—but still retains its original calories. For this reason, if you toast your bread weigh the slice beforehand.

A common belief is that toasting a slice of bread diminishes the calories. Is it true?

All is revealed in . . .

How to Eat Bread: As usual, our first question is—where do the calories come from? The answer is no surprise. Most of the calories in bread come from carbohydrate. Calories from fat and protein combined account for only about 30%. This is true for all kinds of bread, and therefore you can expect a high degree of calorie consistency:

Based on USDA data:	**Calories per Ounce**
Rye Bread	68.9
Whole Wheat Bread	68.9
White Bread	77.9

You have very little flexibility in the calories-per-ounce department. Almost all the breads in this book are within 10% of 72 calories an ounce, 65 to 80 calories any way you slice it. So the answer is—slice it thinner. The "slice" offers greater leeway, like spelling in Shakespeare's tyme.

Here is a virtually random selection of breads. The calories per ounce range only from 65 to 80, but the calories per slice range from 25 to 140:

	Calories per Slice	**Calories per Ounce**
Cocktail Rye, Rubschlager	25	68.8
Gluten Bread, Thomas' Glutogen	30	70.9
Very Thin Sandwich Bread, Dutch Hearth	35	70.0
Kommisbrot Country Bread, Rubschlager	40	80.0
Measure Up, White or Whole Wheat Bread, Arnold	40	75.0
Thin Sliced Whole Wheat Bread, Pepperidge Farm	40	70.0
Extra Thin Sliced (Sandwich) White Bread, Northridge	45	67.5
Old World Style Black Bread, Mrs. Wright's	50	69.1
Melba Thin Rye with Caraway Seeds, Arnold	50	68.8
100% Whole Wheat Bread, Thomas'	50	65.2
Brick Oven Whole Wheat Bread, Arnold	60	75.0
Swedish Limpa Rye, Rubschlager	65	73.1
Thin Sliced Wheat Germ Bread, Pepperidge Farm	65	65.0
Light Bread, Hollywood	70	70.0
Roman Meal Bread, Roman Meal	70	70.0
French Bread, Pepperidge Farm	75	75.0
Light Bread, Profile	75	75.0
Honey Wheat Berry Bread, Orowheat	85	70.8
Sprouted Stone Ground Wheat Bread, Pepperidge Farm	90	75.0
Dill Rye Bread, Mrs. Wright's	95	70.9
Raisin Whole Wheat Bread, Shiloh Farms	101	75.8
Hearty Wheat Bread, Bran'nola	105	78.8
Old Style White Bread, Bran'nola	105	78.8
Grain Belt Yogurt Oatmeal Bread, Mrs. Wright's	112	74.6
Sourdough Bread, Pioneer	140	70.0

Using the most extreme examples, what would happen if you switched from Pioneer's Sourdough Bread to Rubschlager's Cocktail Rye, assuming you ate 2 slices of bread a day? At the end of one year you could lose 23 pounds. I'm not suggesting that a 2-ounce slice of Sourdough bread can always be replaced by a .36-ounce slice of party rye. But be aware that for every 10 calories you save a day, it's a pound every year.

Shiloh Farms Date Nut Loaf, at 88.3 calories per ounce, is one of the few breads out of the usual 65–80 calories range. Another bread that doesn't conform to the general pattern is Fresh Horizons at 50 calories an ounce. Fresh Horizons has managed to reduce the calorie content of their bread by adding wood fiber to the recipe. Since wood is not a protein, a fat, a digestible carbohydrate, or an alcohol, its calorie content is zero for anyone reading this book. (I should point out, however, that Fresh Horizons bread, though it has one-third fewer calories for us, would be just what the doctor ordered for an anorectic termite.)

Wonder Light Bread—White or Wheat—is 50 calories per

ounce and 40 per slice. It's not made with sawdust, and can you ever taste the difference!

Arnold's Melba Thin Rye Bread with Caraway Seeds is 68.8 calories per ounce, and 50 calories per slice. Arnold has seen me through many a midnight. It has the chewiness, physical stability, and finger grip of a much thicker slice, plus the psychological satisfaction of eating rye. It also toasts well.

Bagel chips are another way to thin-slice your bread, and I think they are well worth knowing about. Bagel chips are ordinary John Q. Public bagels that have been cut into four slices so that they will fit easily into a toaster. The advantage for sandwiches is that two bagel chips have half the calories of one bagel sliced in two for the same purpose. "Chips" aren't of uniform diameter, thickness, or weight, and so the calories per slice are approximate. My data come from Balducci's, the pre-eminent Greenwich Village grocery. Their variety of chips include "rye," "whole wheat," "cinnamon-raisin," "sesame," and "poppy seed."

Another bread with a calories-per-sandwich advantage is the pita. There are pitas in the pages for only 80 calories apiece—replacing two slices of bread.

Still another way to save calories when you eat a sandwich is to eat it open-faced.

Open-faced, even on a roll. If you prefer the taste of a roll, it will usually—but not necessarily—cost you more calories than would an equal weight of bread. The rolls in this book range from a low of 50.6 calories per ounce to a high of 144 calories per ounce, with numbers all over the place in between. As with bread, the greatest variation will come from the differences in size; we have rolls in this chapter for 60 calories apiece, and rolls for 560. But it's interesting, I think, that there are many rolls that will accommodate a sandwich for fewer calories than two 1-ounce slices of bread. I'd like to give you some examples. Roll Call!

	Calories per Roll	Calories per Ounce
Petite Boule, Country French	70	58.3
Buttermilk Brown 'n Serve Rolls, Wonder	85	85.0
Brown & Serve Chef Rolls, Millbrook	85	85.0
Soft Family Rolls, Pepperidge Farm	90	73.5
French Style Rolls, Pepperidge Farm	110	82.5
Brown 'n' Serve Club Rolls, Pepperidge Farm	120	90.0
Egg Twist Dinner Rolls, Wenner's	140	84.0

There's another solution to the sandwich situation. Get thee to a bunnery:

	Calories per Bun	Calories per Ounce
Fun Buns, Millbrook	110	73.3
Hamburger Rolls, Jane Parker	120	80.0
Frankfurter Rolls, Pepperidge Farm	120	90.0
Hamburger Buns, Arnold	130	95.5
Multi-Meal Hamburger Buns, Mrs. Wright	130	80.0
Natural Hamburger Buns, Roman Meal	140	93.3
Natural, whole grain Hot Dog Buns, Roman Meal	140	89.7

Almost any bun that you choose is going to be lower in calories than two ounces of bread. Tuna fish sandwiches taste great on frankfurter rolls; hamburger buns are not just a hamburger's domain.

Muffins can also take the place of bread, especially at breakfast. How do they compare? English muffins are among the lowest-calorie foods in this chapter, almost always lower than bread when the comparison is made by the ounce:

	Calories per Muffin	Calories per Ounce
English Muffins, Newly Weds	153	61.1
Extra Crisp Muffins, Arnold	150	64.3
English Muffins, Jane Parker	130	65.0
English Muffins, Super-Value	130	65.0
English Muffins, Thomas'	130	64.7
English Muffins, Wonder	130	65.0
English Muffins, Morton	120	65.5
Seven Grain Wheat English Muffins, Ralph's	150	69.2
English Muffins, Pepperidge Farm	140	70.0
Bran'nola (Orowheat) Natural Muffins with Bran	160	68.6

The other muffins run all over the lot. You'll notice that we even have a muffin here for 55 calories an ounce. (How nice.):

	Calories per Muffin	Calories per Ounce
Bran with Honey Muffins, Pepperidge Farm	110	55.0
Cinnamon Apple Muffins, Pepperidge Farm	120	60.0
Orange with Honey, Pepperidge Farm	120	60.0
Raisin Muffin, Arnold	170	68.0
Granola Bran Muffins, Mrs. Wright's	160	68.6
Seven Grain Sprouted Wheat Raisin Muffins, Foods For Life Bakery	187	70.0
Bran'nola, (Orowheat), with Bran, Honey & Molasses	170	72.9
"Donut Shop" Toaster-Ready, Blueberry Muffin Rounds, Morton	110	73.3
"Donut Shop" Blueberry Muffins, Morton	120	75.9
"Donut Shop" Corn Muffins, Morton	130	78.3
"Donut Shop" Toaster-Ready Corn Muffin Rounds, Morton	130	86.7

You'll also notice that the corn muffins we have are at the higher end of the calories-per-ounce list.

Muffins are often served toasted. I promised a treatise on toast, so here it is: When you toast your bread or muffin the calories per ounce increase because some of the moisture is driven out.

In terms of the calories per slice, it is certainly true that what is burned in the toaster cannot be burned again by you. How many calories do you save? A guesstimate: perhaps a tenth of one percent of the bread gets burned away in standard toasting. If you eat one slice of toast rather than untoasted bread every day for the next three years, by the end of that time you'll be able to eat a slice for free. Toasted.

What is there left to say about bread? A Chapter Preface will often compare foods that its data chapter does not include. Cream Cheese, for example, is not an entry in **Fats & Oils,** yet it's discussed in the **Fats & Oils** Chapter Preface as an alternative to butter. For a list about what's eaten with bread, I have a suggestion to make: go to your book store and buy a book by Margo Feiden called ***THE CALORIE FACTOR.*** Disregard the chapters on **Pharmaceuticals** and **Pet Foods.** Almost everything else is eaten with bread.

20 BREAKFAST CEREALS & BREAKFAST BREADS

What are breakfast cereals and breakfast breads? The *Scribner-Bantam Dictionary* defines breakfast as "the first meal of the day." It defines cereal as "food made from grain."

"Breakfast Breads" is my own terminology, which allows this chapter to include French toast, pancakes, and waffles.

What's in This Chapter is oatmeal, farina, Wheatena . . . also the cold cereals: Alpha-Bits, Applejacks, Booberries . . . (I wonder how this will translate into French.)

What's also in this chapter are the aforementioned French toast, pancakes and waffles, two crepes, and one blintz.

Breakfast Bars and Breakfast Squares are in this chapter by default. By default? By de fault that I didn't know where else to put them. Included also are granola bars, Food Sticks, and Figurines. Granola bars and the rest are arguably more like a candy than a breakfast cereal. The decision to put granola bars, etc., in this chapter was based on the American merchandizing scheme. I see these bars in the breakfast aisle, not at the candy counter.

What's Related, but Elsewhere: Some granola bars are cross-listed in **Sweet Little Nothings.**

Breakfast cereals and breakfast breads are only a step removed from the grains in **Basic Baking & Cooking Ingredients** of which they're made.

There are little boxes of cereals in **Vending,** and cereals for littles in **Baby Foods.** There are breakfasts in **Fast Food, Campers' Foods, Boy Scouts,** and **Mess.**

The **Breads** chapter has the muffins and croissants; the **Cakes** chapter has the Danish pastries. Toaster pastries are in **Cakes** as well.

Pancake syrup is in **Sugars, Sweeteners & Toppings.** Coffee and orange juice are in **Beverages.**

The Arrangement of This Chapter is:

How to Read the Numbers depends on which numbers you are reading. Column headings are different for each of the sections—*Hot Cereals, Cold Cereals, Breakfast Breads,* and the *Breakfast Bars.* A flake of oatmeal, a corn flake, and a Downyflake waffle were too different to be treated in identical fashion.

Hot Cereals have column headings of:

Unit
One Ounce by Weight, Unprepared

One Ounce by Weight, Prepared
One Cup

The Unit is either an entire box of the dry cereal, or a single serving as suggested by the manufacturer. These vary in size from product to product.

The "One Ounce by Weight, Unprepared" column relates to the uncooked dry cereal, and provides a comparative figure independent of package size.

The "One Ounce by Weight, Prepared" column refers to cooked hot cereals. This ounce has substantially fewer calories because the water that is added in cooking has weight but no calories. Even for a few cereals cooked with milk, most of what is being added is still the water component of milk.

Finally, there is a One Cup column. This column has numbers for the cooked and the uncooked cereal. You can probably tell whether a number is for cooked or not, even without consulting the left-hand descriptives. A cup of cooked H-O Farina will be 120 calories. A cup of uncooked Farina is 160 calories. The difference is the moisture. A cup of uncooked cereal, when boiled, will yield at least two—but often three or more—cups of cooked cereal.

Conspicuous by its general absence is the ingredient milk. Milk is not included in these numbers (unless specifically stated), although you will sometimes see it included on the nutrition panel of a cereal box. So if the numbers in this book don't jibe with the printed numbers on the panel, this may be the reason why.

For *Cold Cereals*, the column headings are:

Unit
One Ounce by Weight
One Cup

The Unit is almost always a commercially packaged box of dry cereal. Often there are several box sizes for a single product.

If you're using the Ounce by Weight column, I should point out that comparisons between the hot and cold cereals are not so easy. An ounce of cooked oatmeal is mostly water, but the ounce for cold cereals is a very dry ounce, indeed.

The One Cup column for *Cold Cereals* is a fluid measurement that is being applied to a solid food. For most cold cereals, a cup will contain more air than cereal. This makes the cup, as well as the ounce, an uncertain mode of comparing cold and hot cereals with each other.

For both the *Breakfast Breads Made from Scratch* and the *Breakfast Breads Made from Mixes,* the column headings are:

Unit
One Pancake or Waffle (or One Crepe)
One Ounce by Weight
One Cup

For *Frozen French Toast, Pancakes, and Waffles,* the cup column has been omitted, and "One Pancake or Waffle" becomes "One Pancake, Waffle, or Slice." For *Frozen Blintzes*, the "One" is simply "One Blintz."

For the closing section of this chapter, *Breakfast Bars, Snack Bars and Food Sticks,* "One Blintz" has been replaced by "One Bar or Stick."

How to Eat Breakfast Cereals and Breakfast Breads: This chapter is predominantly breakfast cereals, but I am going to skip by them for a moment to talk about breakfast breads and also breakfast bars. (We'll get to the cereals Post haste.)

For most breakfast breads, the calories come primarily from the starch in the batter and from the sugar in the pancake syrup. If you use butter on your pancakes, there will be calories from fat.

How do pancakes stack up against waffles? Pancakes and waffles start out with identical batters, but they are cooked differently and the result is that waffles are a considerably drier product—by about 20%. Waffles are considerably higher in calories, not coincidentally, also by 20%. If you are making them at home, the USDA anticipates results something like this:

	Calories per Ounce
Pancakes made with enriched or unenriched flour	65.5
Waffles made with enriched or unenriched flour	79.1

By the piece, the difference between a waffle and a pancake is even more pronounced. While individual pancakes in this book may run 63 and 66 and 67 and 73 calories apiece, waffles made from those same mixes run 329 and 365 and 391 and 342 calories apiece.

I am not telling you to throw away your waffle iron, but maybe you should put it away for special occasions.

That is, if you are choosing between waffles and pancakes. If you are choosing between waffles and pastries, take that waffle iron right down out of the closet again. Either dry or overflowing with maple syrup, a waffle is still going to be lower in calories per ounce than almost anything in the **Cakes** chapter.

The *Breakfast Bars* are like candy, only higher-calorie. On the list that follows, the "candies" are in italics:

	Calories per Ounce
Mary Jane Bar	*72.0*
Raisinets, Ward's	*90.0*
Bonomo Turkish Taffy	*107.0*
Hi Energy Raisin Bran Bar	117.0
Hi Energy Granola Crunch Bar	119.0
Three Musketeers Bar	*123.3*
Snowcaps, Ward's	*124.0*
General Mills Chocolate Malt Bar	126.6
Pillsbury Chocolate Malt Food Stick	129.2
Pillsbury Peanut Butter Food Stick	129.2
Nature Valley Oats 'N Honey Granola Bar	132.0
Carnation Granola with Raisins Breakfast Bar	136.7
Carnation Granola with Peanut Crunch Breakfast Bar	137.0
Carnation Slender Cinnamon Bar	139.4
Crunchola Cinnamon Raisin Peanut Butter & Granola Bar	140.0
Crunchola Strawberry Yogurt & Granola Bar	140.0
Chunky Bar	*145.0*
Crunchola Chocolate Chip Peanut Butter & Granola Bar	150.0
Almond Joy	*151.0*
Hershey's Milk Chocolate Bar	*152.4*
Pillsbury Figurines Chocolate Bar	156.0
Pillsbury Figurines Raspberry Bar	156.0

So you may be better off starting the day with a candy bar and a vitamin pill.

Now if you want to gain weight, breakfast bars are probably a better choice than candy, so I can't be disparaging of them altogether. My heart belongs to Figurines? You might as well eat Almond Joy.

The breakfast bars are higher-calorie than breakfast cereals by virtue of their fat content. The calories in breakfast cereals come overwhelmingly from carbohydrate. As is usually the case when a chapter's energy factors come so single-mindedly from one source, the calories will reflect it in their consistency. Hot breakfast cereals look something like this:

	Calories per Ounce, Unprepared	Calories per Ounce, Prepared with Water
Cream of Wheat, Nabisco, Mix 'N Eat, "regular"	100.0	11.6
Enriched White Hominy Grits, Quaker, "quick"	100.0	15.4

	Calories per Ounce, Unprepared	Calories per Ounce, Prepared with Water
Enriched White Hominy Grits, Quaker, "regular"	100.0	15.4
Instant Oatmeal, H-O Bran & Raisin	100.0	21.1
100% Rolled Rye, Golden Harvest	100.0	16.1
Whole Wheat Hot Natural Cereal, Quaker	100.0	16.9
Farina, Creamed Enriched, H-O	103.1	14.0
Instant Oatmeal, H-O, Maple & Brown Sugar Flavors	105.5	28.1
Old Fashioned Oats, H-O	107.3	18.7
Scotch Style Oatmeal, Elam's	107.7	11.7
Instant Oatmeal, H-O "regular"	108.4	17.6
Steel Cut Oatmeal, Elam's	109.4	11.8
100% Rolled Oats, Golden Harvest	110.0	17.7
Quick Oats, A&P	110.0	20.4
Ralston, "Instant" Whole Wheat Cereal with added Wheat Germ	110.0	17.8
Ralston, "Regular" Whole Wheat Cereal with added Wheat Germ	110.0	17.8
Vermont Style Hot Oatmeal, Maypo	110.0	17.8
Wheatena, Standard Milling	120.0	14.0

Looking at the *Cold Cereals,* Kellogg's Frosted Flakes are Kellogg's Corn Flakes with sugar on them. You might expect that the Frosted Flakes would be higher in calories, but they're not. Both are 110 calories an ounce. Sugar and starch are equal from a calorie point of view. (Hot breakfast cereals are slightly lower than 110 calories in their dry form because they have more moisture than the cold cereals, even as they come out of the box.)

If breakfast cereals are so alike in composition, is there any way to save calories when you are eating them?

Yes—eat them by the bowl!

There are more than 200 cold cereals in this chapter. Almost all of them are within 20% of 110 calories an ounce. Whereas these cereals show an almost rigid uniformity by the ounce, the variety of shapes in which they are sold results in enormous differences in calories by the cupful.

Kellogg's Bran Flakes are 135 calories a cup; their Cracklin' Bran is 330.

Post's Alpha Bits are 110 calories for a cupful; their Family Style Cereal is 560. (Quite a family!)

General Mills Cheerios are 88 calories a cup; their Honey Nut Cheerios are 147.

Here's a list of 16 cold cereals. Every last one of them is 110 calories per ounce, but look at the variations by the cupful:

	Calories per Ounce	Calories per Cup
Puffed Rice, Quaker	110.0	74
Cheerios, General Mills	110.0	88
Special K, Kellogg's	110.0	88
Rice Chex, Ralston Purina	110.0	98
Alpha Bits, Post	110.0	110
Corn Flakes, Kellogg's	110.0	110
Fruit Loops, Kellogg's	110.0	110
Lucky Charms, General Mills	110.0	110
Wheaties, General Mills	110.0	110
Honey Nut Cheerios, General Mills	110.0	147
Buc Wheats, General Mills	110.0	147
Frosted Flakes, A&P	110.0	147
Product 19, Kellogg's	110.0	147
Sugar Smacks, Kellogg's	110.0	147
Bran Chex, Ralston Purina	110.0	165
Cracklin' Bran, Kellogg's	110.0	330

The so-called natural cereals consistently come out the highest by the ounce and by the cup. It's a fact of life. Eat them if you like, for any reason that you like, but not because you think that "natural" means "lower in calories." Just compare the cereals that follow to the list of cereals above:

	Calories per Ounce	Calories per Cup
Natural Cereal with Raisin, Alpen	110.0	440
Sprouted Seven Grain Natural Breakfast Cereal with Bananas & Honey, Health Valley	110.0	440
Apple Bran Granola, Golden Harvest	120.0	480
Vita Crunch Granola, Almond, Back-to-Nature	120.0	480
Natural High Protein Granola with Almonds & Seeds, Better Way	120.0	480
Country Morning with Coconut, Kellogg's	130.0	390
Country Morning with Raisins & Dates, Kellogg's	130.0	390
Crunchy Natural Cereal 'N Snack, Hearty Life	130.0	390
Fruit & Nut Natural 100 Cereal 'N Snack, Hearty Life	130.0	390
Unsweetened Granola, Good Shepherd	130.0	520
Proteinola, Golden Harvest	130.0	520
Vitagrain & Nuts, Lassen	130.0	520
100% Natural Cereal with Apple & Cinnamon, Quaker	135.0	640
100% Natural Cereal, Quaker	139.0	556

What happens when you mix raisins, at 82 calories an ounce, into cornflakes? The calories per ounce go down, but the calories per cupful go way up. A cup of cornflakes is about 110 calories; a cup of raisins is about 419. You know from your own experience that the 1-ounce box of cornflakes is a much bigger box than the familiar 1-ounce box of raisins. I am not intending to praise the grain and repudiate the raisin. I am just trying to tell it like it is.

And what of the other toppings—sugar, milk, and fruit?

Based on USDA data:	Calories
brown sugar, 1 tablespoon	34
white sugar, 1 tablespoon	46
maple syrup, 1 tablespoon	50
honey, 1 tablespoon	64
skim milk, ½ cup	43
whole milk, ½ cup	75
half-and-half, ½ cup	162
light table cream, ½ cup	253
strawberries, 2 oz. (approx. 3½ medium strawberries)	11
blueberries, ¼ cup	23
banana, ¼ cup, sliced	32
raisins, ¼ cup	105

What about wheat germ? Wheat germ is a full 100 to 110 calories per ounce, about the same as sugar or corn flakes. By the spoonful, at about 25 calories per tablespoon, wheat germ is lower in calories than granulated sugar and much higher than the corn flakes. Bran, by the tablespoon, has about half the calories of wheat germ.

So the way to eat breakfast cereals is to count what you put into the bowl, what you pour on top of what you put into the bowl, and what you sprinkle on top of what you pour on top of what you put into the bowl. I don't need to tell you that you can reduce calories by switching from whole milk to skim milk. But if you replace ¼ cup of raisins with ¼ cup of sliced strawberries AND ¼ cup of blueberries AND ¼ cup of sliced bananas, you will still save 34 calories per breakfast.

What's 34 calories a breakfast? Three and one-half pounds a year.

21 CAKES, SNACK CAKES & PASTRIES

What is cake? When I looked up "cake" in my *Roget's Thesaurus,* this is what I found:

> angel cake, angel food cake; chocolate cake, devil's food cake; white cake, yellow cake; spice cake; gingerbread; fruitcake, pound cake; marble cake; honey cake; sponge cake, génoise; shortcake; coffee cake, tea cake; cheesecake; layer cake, jumble; baba au rhum, savarin; Boston cream pie; upsidedown cake; jelly roll, bûche de Noël; baked Alaska.

What's in This Chapter is angel food cake, chocolate cake, devil's food cake, white cake, yellow cake, spice cake, gingerbread, fruitcake, pound cake, marble cake, honey cake, sponge cake, shortcake, coffee cake, cheesecake, layer cake, Boston cream pie, and pineapple upside-down cake.

Sorry, we don't have the génoise, tea cake, jumble, baba au rhum, savarin, jelly roll, bûche de Noël, or baked Alaska. And the only "angel cake" we have is angel food.

But we do have caramel cake, cottage pudding cake, applesauce raisin cake, chocolate macaroon Bundt cake, chocolate almond Snackin' Cake, chocolate pudding cake, milk chocolate cake, sour cream chocolate cake, Swiss chocolate cake, and—orange cupcakes, Sno Balls, Ding Dongs, Tiger Tails and Twinkies, Coconut Round cakes and Devil Square cakes; cake rolls and honey buns; apple dumplings, apple strudel, and apple pie tarts; apple turnovers, blueberry turnovers; cherry, peach, and raspberry turnovers; vanilla puffs and chocolate eclairs.

Frostings are also in this chapter.

What's Related, but Elsewhere? Although cakes made from scratch are in this chapter, the raw ingredients are listed in their own right in **Basic Baking & Cooking Ingredients.**

Other related chapters are **Pies, Gelatins, Puddings & Custards, Frozen Confections, Cookies & Crackers,** and **Sweet Little Nothings.**

Muffins are in **Breads.** Pancakes, waffles, French toast, Breakfast Bars, Breakfast Squares, and similar snack bars are in **Breakfast Cereals & Breakfast Breads.**

There are cakes from Chocolate through Upside Down in **Mess.**

The Arrangement of This Chapter is:

How to Read the Numbers: *Frostings* first. The column headings are:

Unit
Frosting for One Slice, 1/12 of Cake
One Ounce by Weight
One Cup

The Unit may be a can of ready-to-spread frosting, an entire box of unprepared frosting mix, or the yield when the entire box is prepared as the package directs.

The Frosting for One Slice of Cake is a column of very inexact figures. The nutrition information that I received for frostings was almost always expressed in terms of "one slice, 1/12 of a cake"—but how big is a cake?

Well, we don't know exactly. Pillsbury's Ready-To-Spread Frosting Supreme says that the "entire can" frosts "one 8- or 9-inch layer cake, one 13 × 9-inch cake or about 36 cupcakes."

Betty Crocker's Creamy White Frosting Mix says the entire box, when prepared, frosts "two 8- or 9-inch layers, a 13 × 9-inch rectangular or 3 dozen cupcakes."

What the Frosting for One Slice of Cake column really represents, between you and me, is simply 1/12 of an entire can or box of frosting, prepared.

For frostings that have been prepared from mixes, there were no good data for calculating an ounce of the finished product. Finished frostings were generally described by volume—hence the figures for "One Cup."

Now for the *Cakes*. The column headings are:

Unit
One Slice, Cupcake, or Pastry
One Ounce by Weight

The Unit column produces, on successive lines, numbers like 1,270 calories for an entire angel food cake and 8 calories for a cubic inch of the same cake.

The One Slice, Cupcake, or Pastry column is for comparison of individual servings. But in a chapter as varied as this, the nature and size of a serving will also vary greatly. It may be one slice from a cake, or one single cupcake, or one apple turnover.

Manufacturers' suggestions as to what constitutes a serving will vary from brand to brand and from cake to cake. For some cakes there are two slice sizes provided—figured at either 12 or 16 slices per cake.

"Calories per slice" is an important measurement in cakes. Cake is eaten by the slice, of course, and it is the size of a slice that may determine satisfaction rather than the calories per ounce. A larger slice from a fluffier cake may actually have considerably fewer calories than a smaller slice of a denser cake. And the fluffier cake is likely to win higher praise.

Cake mixes will frequently provide directions for baking either a cake or a batch of cupcakes. The cupcakes will generally have half the calories of the manufacturers' "suggested" slice for the same cake. So if one cupcake can substitute for one "suggested" slice of cake, baking cupcakes is an obvious suggestion for reducing calories. In fact, one reason for including the word "Cupcake" in the column heading is to remind you that cupcakes can be made from virtually any box of cake mix. Since both one slice and one cupcake represent a "portion" in a sense, I hope that rather than provoking confusion, this will provide a constant reminder of a calorie-conscious alternative.

The Ounce by Weight column for cakes made from mixes has many estimated values. These figures were calculated from the manufacturers' analyses, which almost always were based on "calories per slice." Weights for the slices were not usually given, and these had to be calculated from the estimated yield of the entire recipe. Does this make the Ounce column less reliable than the Slice? Well, maybe. But on the other hand, when one is talking about "calories per slice," the uncertainty in the size of a hand-cut slice is likely to be at least as significant.

The One Ounce by Weight column, as usual, provides a common basis for comparison within this chapter and without. It allows you to compare angel food to devil's food, and devil's food to Devil Dogs, and Devil Dogs to hot dogs.

And now for the fun. Lights! Camera! Action! It's time for . . .

How to Eat Cake:

How to eat cake? For pleasure, or not at all.

But first, where do the calories come from?

There are lots of different cakes in this chapter—angel food and fruitcake sharing a chapter with Boston cream pie. Although the calories will come from different sources for different cakes, predominantly they will come from the carbohydrate in the flour and sugar. But any chapter with butter and eggs in it is going to get some of its calories from fat. **Cakes** is no exception.

Some of the cakes in this chapter will contain a substantial amount of fat, and others will not. Angel food cake is virtually fat-free. It's 76.4 calories an ounce, or just about the same as white bread. On the other hand, when you are tempted to choose a pound cake (because "how fattening can plain cake be?") remember how it got its name. I think that the classic recipe started off with one pound of flour, one pound of sugar, one pound of eggs, and one pound of butter. Then you pound them together and it turns into pound cake, which in turn, turns into pounds. Pound cake is 134.9 calories an ounce, and it's the fat that does it.

But fat is not the only variable to look for. The effect of moisture can more than compensate for additional fat. Look at eclairs with custard filling and chocolate icing. Look at custard-filled cream puffs. They sound deadly, don't they? But thanks to their moisture content—they're almost twice as moist as angel food—eclairs and cream puffs are among the lowest-calorie pastries in the chapter.

Now that you've re-read that last sentence—how would you like to see a chart?

<u>Based on USDA home recipes:</u>

	% Moisture	% Fat	Calories per Ounce
Angel food cake	31.5	0.2	76.4
cream puffs	58.3	13.9	66.1
eclairs	56.2	13.6	67.8

A "standard size" cream puff—figured at 4.6 ounces—has 303 calories. The 3½-ounce eclair made from scratch has 239 calories. Three and a half ounces of pound cake would cost you about 470 calories.

This is a chapter in which, unquestionably, you can save calories by clever selection. Here are some comparisons:

	Calories per Ounce
<u>Cakes based on USDA home recipes:</u>	
without icing:	
sponge cake	83.8
gingerbread	92.9
cottage pudding cake	97.4
"plain" cake	101.0
yellow cake	103.2
chocolate devil's food cake	103.8
white cake	106.5
fruitcake, dark	107.4
caramel cake	109.1
fruitcake light	110.3
pound cake, modified	116.8
pound cake, old fashioned	134.9

Put icing on the cake, and you're going to add calories to it. But I think it's interesting to see that, although the calories per cake will go up, the calories per ounce generally go down:

	Calories per Ounce
Cakes based on USDA home recipes:	
yellow cake with icing:	
yellow cake with boiled white icing	85.3
yellow cake with uncooked white icing	93.0
yellow cake with coconut icing	95.8
yellow cake with caramel icing	102.2
yellow cake with chocolate icing	104.0

So if you like the icing, you can eat it knowing that it probably has fewer calories per ounce than the underlying cake. Of course, if what you like is the underlying cake, eat that, and forget about the icing. When you're eating in this chapter, what you're eating for is satisfaction, and the important thing is to get the maximum of satisfaction with the minimum number of calories. And if that means pulling the icing off the cake—or picking the cake off the icing—at these kinds of calories per ounce, you can afford to be choosy.

Be choosy. That's the way to eat cake.

If you're baking a cake from a mix rather than from scratch, you have two opportunities for choice. First, in selecting the basic kind of cake. Second, in selecting a brand:

	Calories per Ounce, Prepared
Banana Cake, Fearn Soya	86.8
Banana Walnut Snackin' Cake, Betty Crocker	90.0
Banana Cake, Pillsbury Plus	97.5
Apple Cinnamon Coffee Cake, Pillsbury	85.5
Coffee Cake, Aunt Jemima Easy Mix	102.2
Sour Cream Coffee Cake, Pillsbury	113.7
Devil's Food Cake, Duncan Hines "Deluxe"	85.7
Devil's Food Cake, Betty Crocker "Supermoist"	100.3
Whole Wheat Old Fashioned Gingerbread Mix, Vermont General Store and Grist Mill	70.0
Gingerbread Mix, Dromedary	80.0
Gingerbread Mix, Betty Crocker	94.5
Golden Yellow Cake, Jiffy	86.4
Yellow Cake, Pillsbury Plus	97.5

And when it comes time to frost the cake, you can be choosy there too:

	Estimated Calories per Cup, Ready-to-Spread or Prepared
Coconut Pecan Frosting Mix, Pillsbury	900
Milk Chocolate Frosting, Hershey's	950
Fudge Frosting Mix, Jiffy	1005
Caramel Frosting Mix, Jiffy	1014
Chiquita Banana Frosting Mix, Betty Crocker	1020
Dark Dutch Frosting, Betty Crocker	1097
Chocolate Nut Frosting, Betty Crocker	1162

In **Cakes,** as in every chapter, be skeptical when you see the word "dietetic." Batter-Lite's Dietetic White is 82.7 calories an ounce, prepared, as compared to an estimated 77.1 for Ann Page De Luxe. Batter-Lite's "per slice" figure is less than Ann Page's—99 calories as compared to 180—but that's because the suggested slice is only 1.2 ounces, the weight of a conventional cupcake. Sweet 'N Low's White Frost Mix is "sugar reduced"—and at about 130 calories an ounce, prepared, it's at the higher end of frostings. Hershey's Peanut Butter Creme Frosting is 10% less, at 116.4.

When it comes to the *Prepackaged Cakes,* calories per suggested slice range from 91 to 287. Since these cakes don't usually come with delineated slices, it's probably best to compare calories per ounce.

Between brands, and sometimes even within a brand, cakes with similar names aren't at all the same:

	Calories per Ounce
Bavarian Cake, Lemon, Sara Lee	92.7
Bavarian Cake, Chocolate, Sara Lee	101.2
Chocolate Cake, Pepperidge Farm	103.4
Chocolate Cake, Sara Lee	111.4
Old Fashioned Apple Walnut Pound Cake with Raisins, Pepperidge Farm	92.2
Pound Cake, Chock Full O' Nuts	104.9
Old Fashioned Carrot Pound Cake, Pepperidge Farm	112.3
Pound Cake, Sara Lee	115.1
Old Fashioned Pound Cake, Pepperidge Farm	120.9
Pound Cake, Stouffer	125.0

And as a special treat, I have some cheesecake for you. It's so luxurious, so creamy, so satisfying—and so low-calorie. That's right. Cheesecake is consistently lower in calories per ounce than the general run of its competition. I mean, Sara Lee's Cherry and Strawberry Cream Cheese Cakes are even lower in calories than the eclairs!

	Calories per Ounce
Cherry Cream Cheese Cake, Sara Lee	67.5
Strawberry Cream Cheese Cake, Sara Lee	67.5
Cherry Cheesecake, Morton "Great Little Desserts"	72.3
Pineapple Cheesecake, Morton "Great Little Desserts"	72.3
Cream Cheesecake, Morton "Great Little Desserts"	73.8
Strawberry Cheesecake, Morton "Great Little Desserts"	73.8
Cream Cheese Cake, Sara Lee	86.1
French Cream Cheese Cake, Sara Lee	93.3
Cheesecake, World's Best	98.6

But if sitting down with a cake means throwing away an empty box an hour later, there's a section of this chapter meant for you. The *Snack Cakes.* Pre-measured portions in all different sizes and shapes.

The snack cakes and the donuts, like the prepackaged cakes, run mostly around 100 to 120 calories per ounce. Pepperidge Farm Apple Strudel is 83.3 an ounce. Hostess Sno Balls are 93.3 an ounce. You might never guess how many of these things have fewer calories than two slices of American Cheese:

	Calories per Serving
Devil's Food Cake, Nabisco, 1 cake, .45 oz.	50
Sugar 'N Spice, mini-donuts, Morton, 1 donut, .55 oz.	60
Chocolate Cupcakes, Tastykake, 1 cupcake, .66 oz.	66
Crunch Donuts, Hostess, 1 donut, 1 oz.	100
Yankee Doodles, Drakes, 1 Yankee Doodle, 1 oz.	105
Cinnamon Donuts, Hostess, 1.1 oz.	110
Caramel Sticky Buns, Sara Lee, 1 bun, 1 oz.	118
Devil Twin Cakes, Little Debbie, 1 cake, approx. 1.09 oz.	120
Coffee Cake, Drakes, 1 cake, approx. 1.06 oz.	125
Cream Filled Koffee Kake, Tastykake, 1 Kake, 1 oz.	124
Crumb Cakes, Hostess, 1 cake, approx. 1¼ oz.	130
Chocolate Pinwheels Cakes, Nabisco, 1 cupcake, 1.1 oz.	140
Sno Balls, Hostess, 1 Sno Ball, approx. 1½ oz.	140
Coconut Rounds Cakes, Little Debbie, cake, approx. 1.09 oz.	148
Orange Cupcakes, Hostess, 1 cupcake, 1½ oz.	150
Blueberry Crumb Cakes, Sara Lee, 1 cake, 1¾ oz.	155
Chocolate Cupcakes, Hostess, 1 cupcake, approx. 1¾ oz.	160
Honey 'N Bran Cake, El Molino, 1½-oz. package	160
Ding Dongs, Hostess, 1 Ding Dong, approx. 1⅓ oz.	170
Big Wheels, Hostess, 1 Big Wheel, approx. 1⅓ oz.	170

	Calories per Serving
Oatmeal Creme Pies, Little Debbie, 1 cake, approx. 1.34 oz.	172
Yellow Cupcakes, Stouffer, 1 cupcake, 1 11/16 oz.	190
2 oz. of pasteurized process American Cheese	*212*

It's really surprising how non-disastrous these cakes are when eaten in limited quantities. You'd think after reading that line-up that you were looking at a list of the "10 Most Wanted Men." But as it turns out, these are not such dangerous criminals after all.

I think I would have to say that there are an awful lot of pleasant surprises in this chapter. You should look for them in the book instead of just settling for any ol' pastry that comes wrapped in cellophane.

But if it turns out that what you want is the highest-calorie item here, I say choose that. This is not the chapter in which to be sacrificial.

It's different in **Vegetables.** A vegetable can be delicious when seasoned in its own low-calorie aura. But there's no way you're going to be happy with a slice of cake you don't want because it's going to help your diet.

I think the best approach in this chapter is to pick exactly what you want to eat, and then try to save calories, if you can, by eating a little less of it. That way you can halve your cake, and eat it too.

22 • PIES

What is pie? *Webster's* defines pie as a "dessert consisting of a filling (as of fruit or custard) in a pastry shell or topped with pastry or both." The *Oxford English Dictionary* advises that no word related to pie is known outside the English language, with the exception of the Gaelic "pight."

What's in This Chapter? Simple Simon met a pieman going to the fair. Said Simple Simon to the pieman, let me taste your ware:

Apple Pie
Banana Pie
Banana Cream Pie
Banana Custard Pie
Blackberry Pie
Blueberry Pie
Butterscotch Pie
Cherry Pie
Chocolate Chiffon Pie
Chocolate Cream Pie
Chocolate Meringue Pie
Coconut Cream Pie
Coconut Custard Pie
Custard Pie
And many, many more.

What's in this chapter are pies made from scratch, pies made from mixes, and prepackaged pies.

What's Related, but Elsewhere are the **Cakes, Snack Cakes & Pastries; Cookies & Crackers;** and to a lesser extent the candies in **Sweet Little Nothings.** Pies have a long-standing relationship with **Frozen Confections.** You don't have to ask for vanilla ice cream—all you have to say is "à la mode."

This chapter is related to **Fruits** as in apple pie, to **Vegetables** as in sweet potato pie, to **Nuts & Seeds** as in pecan pie—and to **Gelatins, Puddings & Custards** with many pie fillings coming here directly from that chapter.

The pies in this chapter are all dessert pies. Pot pies are in **Combination Main Dishes.** The ingredients in Sweeney-Todd-type pies are touched upon, briefly, on page 16.

Pies eaten away from home are in the appropriate chapters. Snack pies are in **Cakes, Snack Cakes & Pastries,** but are listed in this chapter as well. They have not, however, been considered in the discussion of "How to Eat Pies."

The Arrangement of This Chapter is as follows:

How to Read the Numbers: The column headings for *Pies Made from Scratch* and *Prepackaged Pies* are:

Unit
One Slice
One Ounce by Weight

For *Pies Made from Scratch,* the Unit will be the entire pie (and, in the case of Apple Brown Betty, one cup).

The Slice column will be for ⅙ or ⅛ of the pie, as described on the left-hand side of the page. The approximate weight of the slice is given.

The One Ounce by Weight column is for an ounce of the finished pie, baked and cooled. A pie will be heavier if you weigh it directly out of the oven. As it sits there steaming, filling the room with fragrance as it cools, moisture leaves the pie. The other columns—the Unit and the One Slice columns—are not dependent upon cooling. They apply even before the pie is baked, in case you can't wait.

For *No-Bake Pie Mixes* the numbers in the Unit and the Ounce columns refer to both prepared and unprepared pies. So be careful when making comparisons. All the pies in this section are Pillsbury, and the Slice column is the manufacturer's "suggested" serving, always ⅙ of the prepared pie.

The *Prepackaged Pies* are ready to eat, of course, and you don't have to worry about distinguishing prepared from unprepared.

For *Pie Crusts Made from Scratch and from Mixes,* and for *Prepackaged Pie Crusts and Other Pastry Shells,* the column headings are:

Unit
Crust for One Slice
One Ounce by Weight

For those pie crusts that are made from mixes, the crust for one pie was based on the manufacturer's "suggested" serving.

For *Pie Fillings,* the column headings are:

Unit
Filling for One Slice
One Ounce by Weight
One Cup

The One Cup column is 8 fluid ounces as always, although what you are measuring does not appear to be a fluid food. For most of the pie fillings, either the One Ounce or the One Cup column had to be estimated, depending upon the format in which the original information was received.

All numbers in the Filling for One Slice column are estimated.

Important information about the numbers for pie fillings made from mixes is discussed in the **Gelatins, Puddings & Custards** chapter under the heading, **"What Else You Should Know About These Numbers"** (page 140).

How to Eat Pies, or Pie and Your Circumference: Where do the calories come from?

Most of the calories in pie filling will come from carbohydrate. Even when the filling has a relatively high fat content, the contribution from carbohydrate will still be higher. The calories in pie crust, on the other hand, come from fat. A pie crust is essentially fat-soaked flour. If what you like about a coconut custard pie is the coconut custard, you can eat twice as much custard as crust, for the same number of calories.

But if you like the crust go right ahead and eat it, because—crust and all—pies as a group are the lowest-calorie baked goods there are. The cakes and pastries in this book generally run about 90–130 calories an ounce. The cookies run about 90–175. Well, there are fruit pies in this chapter at 65 and 72 and 76 calories an ounce. Most of the cream pies—yes, the cream pies—are between 68 and 78 calories an ounce, depending on which you buy. There's a banana cream pie for 68.7 calories an ounce; a lemon cream pie for 71.4 calories an ounce. Even chocolate cream pie never rises above 77.1 calories an ounce. No matter which flavor or which brand you choose, cream pie will always be about the same as bread.

And you can have pumpkin pie for 60 calories an ounce.

And then, all of a sudden, in the middle of a chapter that didn't have anything much higher than 77 calories an ounce there is one for 117.7. That's pecan in the midst of peaches and pumpkins. Pecan pie has the highest calories per ounce in the pie section—117.7 calories for Frito Lay's and 118.5 for the pecan pie made from scratch. And who would have guessed it? Who would have thought that rich, nutty, luxurious, homemade pecan pie was 118.5 calories an ounce—only! And still, it's the highest-calorie figure in the Ounce column, for this entire chapter.

And what kind of pies will generally be the lowest? Guess. Because of their high moisture content, it's the custard pies.

Custard pie made from scratch is 62 calories an ounce. Banquet's coconut custard pie is 61. Morton's coconut custard pie is 56.9. And, again, who would have guessed it? I mean, the next time you threaten to hit someone in the face with a custard pie, ask him whether, to lose weight, he would rather it be a loaf of rye bread. See what he says.

So all in all, this is a marvelous chapter in which to have dessert, but even here there is variation. In the middle of a bunch of pies with calories in the 60s and 70s, Mrs. Smith's Banana Light Pie is 95.7 calories an ounce. Her Coconut Light Pie is 100!

So the way to eat pies is to compare brands; to favor fruit pies, cream pies, and custard pies; to avoid nut pies and—it would seem—pies that are called "chiffon."

Chiffon pies are generally less moist than their neighbors, and the calories per ounce show the result. An example: the "regular" pineapple pie made from scratch—with two crusts, already a handicap—still has fewer calories per ounce than the one-crust pineapple chiffon pie made from scratch.

Another example: lemon chiffon pie and lemon meringue pie are both one-crust pies. The meringue pie made from scratch is 72.4 calories an ounce as compared to the chiffon pie at 88.6.

Yet another example: chocolate chiffon pie and chocolate meringue pie are both one-crust pies. The meringue pie made from scratch is 71.7 calories an ounce as compared to the chiffon pie at 92.8. (Mrs. Smith's Chocolate Light Pie runs 108.7; I wonder how she does it.)

So now we've spoken about crusts—not comparing brands, but by now you pretty much know the pie crust story. We've spoken about the whole pie—what to avoid, and what to dive into. And now a word about pie fillings made from mixes. No, make that a list:

		Calories per Ounce, Prepared as Pie Filling
Chocolate:	Jell-O, Regular	31.0
	My-T-Fine	34.1
	Jell-Well, Instant	34.5
	Ann Page, Instant	35.3
	Ann Page, Regular	35.3
	Jell-Well, Regular	35.7
	Jell-O, Instant	36.4
	Royal, Instant	36.7
	Royal, Regular	37.9
Lemon:	Royal, Regular	26.6
	Ann Page, Regular	26.8
	My-T-Fine	27.5
	Jell-O, Regular	30.2
	Jell-Well, Regular	30.7
	Jell-O, Instant	33.8
	Jell-Well, Instant	33.8
	Royal, Instant	34.3
Key Lime:	Royal, Regular	26.6

The dry mixes, prepared as pie fillings, are consistently below 38 calories an ounce. Maybe Mrs. Smith should consider filling her pies with them.

I know I've been tough on Mrs. Smith. In all fairness, I think I should say that I've never tasted her pies. They may well be worth the extra calories. Certainly, many people will find pecan pie the one most worth the eating, even at 118.5 calories per ounce. And there will be lots of foods in this book that are worth eating although they're higher-calorie than their competition. That's why I put down the numbers, and leave the advice up to you.

23 COOKIES & CRACKERS

What's a cookie? What's a cracker? My *Webster's* provides us with the following definitions:

Cookie or Cooky: "Any of various small sweet flat or slightly raised cakes."

Cracker: "A thin crisp bakery product that may be leavened or unleavened and that is made in various shapes."

What's in This Chapter are certainly baked products and they certainly do come in various shapes. Some even look like elephants.

There are about three dozen cookies and brownies made from mixes, and a few made from scratch, but when it comes to the prepackaged section, this chapter has hundreds of different kinds. There are more than half a million calories' worth of prepackaged cookies in this chapter. Probably more than you and I could eat in an evening, together.

Crackers enjoy equal billing in this chapter. These are not in their own list, but are inter-alphabetized with the cookies, although they are not usually competitive foods. An Oreo cookie does not serve the function if you run out of oyster crackers for your soup.

Although I was philosophically in favor of separating the lists, I ran up against problems. Animal Crackers are an example. Would you look for them under "Crackers" or "Cookies"? What about Graham Crackers? What about Cinnamon Graham Crackers? Chocolate-covered Graham Crackers?

What's Related, but Elsewhere: There are cookies and biscuits in **Baby Foods.**

There's a "Cookies and Crackers" section in **Vended Foods.**

Cracker meal is in **Basic Baking & Cooking Ingredients.**

Granola Bars, which are like cookies—both in taste and in calories per ounce—are in the **Breakfast Cereals & Breakfast Breads** chapter, along with the Breakfast Bars, and such. Some granola bars are also listed in **Sweet Little Nothings.**

What's also related to cookies and crackers is any chapter whose foods are eaten as desserts or snacks. **Cakes, Snack Cakes & Pastries . . . Pies . . . Sweet Little Nothings . . . Salty Snacks . . .** all are potential substitutes. Conversely, cookies and crackers are potential substitutes for **Cakes** and the rest.

Fruits is also a related chapter, but not because we have Apple Crisp and Sunflower Raisin cookies. **Fruits** is related because Apple Crisp cookies have 132 calories an ounce, and apples have less than 16.

The Arrangement of This Chapter is as follows:

For *Prepackaged Cookies and Crackers, by brand,* an attempt was made to alphabetize by the key descriptive word. In some cases, this meant alphabetizing by flavor, e.g. "chocolate chip." In other cases, the most descriptive word was actually the brand name, e.g. "Hydrox." When I had a hard time deciding, I sometimes listed a cookie more than once.

How to Read the Numbers: The column headings vary somewhat from section to section within this chapter. The column headings for *Cookies and Brownies Made from Scratch* and *Cookies and Brownies Made from Mixes* are:

Unit
One Cookie
One Ounce by Weight

The columns are straightforward and should be easy to read, bearing in mind that some figures in the Unit and Ounce columns will be for prepared, and others for unprepared. All "One Cookie" values are for prepared.

For the *Prepackaged Cookies* and the *Prepackaged Crackers* that are based on USDA data, the column headings are:

Unit
One Cookie or Cracker
One Ounce by Weight
Fiber per Ounce, expressed in grams

The Unit for these generics will be a commonly marketed size package, or in some cases "one pound."

For *Prepackaged Cookies and Crackers, by brand,* the column headings are:

Entire Package
One Cookie or Cracker
One Ounce by Weight
One Cup, Crumbled

The One Ounce by Weight column is the most reliable, as most manufacturers sent data by the ounce (or by 100 grams, which was easily converted). The calories for the Entire Package were obtained by multiplying the ounce figure by the declared label weight. As is true in other chapters, the package will frequently weigh more than the stated weight. So if you are going to eat the boxful, weigh it first.

Fiber would have been a nice column to have in this section. Unfortunately, not enough fiber figures were available from the manufacturers to make such a column worthwhile.

I was undecided till very late in the game as to whether the fourth column should be for a cup of crumbled cookies or a pound. While bakery cookies do get purchased by the pound, they're not the cookies we're talking about here. The calorie figures for prepackaged cookies cannot be used for bakery cookies, which are almost certain to be higher.

A Cup column for crumbled cookies or crackers, on the other hand, could be useful in baking. And crumbled cookies taste so good on ice cream. Which brings us to the question of how to eat them.

First, the Cookies: As with any other food, knowing **How to Eat Cookies** begins with knowing where the calories come from. Is a cookie high in sugar or is a cookie high in fat?

A pound of "generic" chocolate chip cookies has 2136 calories. A pound of generic coconut bar cookies has 2241. The coconut cookies have about 8% less carbohydrate, yet they have more calories. The difference is the fat—the coconut cookies have about 17% more.

Fig bars are 1624 calories a pound. They are a full 27% lower in calories than the coconut bars. The fig bars have substantially more carbohydrate, but less fat. And that's the answer. Cookies may be "sweets," but what makes the difference is the fat.

So the way to eat cookies is to eat "sweeter" rather than "richer" cookies—and cookies with a high moisture content. But how can you tell which is which? The nine cookies in the list that follows are in alphabetical order. Guess which has the lowest calories per ounce, and which has the highest:

sugar-free, salt-free Angel Puffs, Stella D'Oro
Chocolate Chip Cookies, Chips Ahoy, Nabisco
Chocolate Hydrox Cookies, Sunshine
Date Nut Granola Cookies, Pepperidge Farm
Devil's Food Cakes, Nabisco
Ginger Snaps, Nabisco
Marshmallow Bars, Sunshine
Pirouette Cookies, Pepperidge Farm
Vanilla Hydrox Cookies, Sunshine

Devil's Food Cakes are the lowest-calorie cookie on the list.
Marshmallow Bars have fewer calories than Ginger Snaps.
Vanilla Hydrox have more calories than Chocolate Hydrox.
Date Nut Granola Cookies are identical in calories to the Chocolate Chip Cookies.

The sugar-free salt-free cookie, Angel Puffs, would be the highest on the list if it weren't for the Pirouettes.

Here's the list again, this time in ascending order of calories per ounce:

	Calories per Ounce
Devil's Food Cakes, Nabisco	105.0
Marshmallow Bars, Sunshine	107.8
Ginger Snaps, Nabisco	120.0
Chocolate Hydrox Cookies, Sunshine	134.9
Vanilla Hydrox Cookies, Sunshine	140.4
Chocolate Chip Cookies, Chips Ahoy, Nabisco	145.5
Date Nut Granola Cookies, Pepperidge Farm	145.5
sugar-free, salt-free Angel Puffs, Stella D'Oro	159.1
Pirouette Cookies, Pepperidge Farm	174.5

By the ounce, Pirouette is the highest-calorie cookie in the chapter; Devil's Food is one of the lowest. But if you're going to eat five of either of them, you'll save 43% by eating Pirouettes.

Recruiting our same nine cookies, it's a whole different list when ranked for calories per piece:

	Calories per Cookie
sugar-free, salt-free Angel Puffs, Stella D'Oro	18
Ginger Snaps, Nabisco	30
Pirouette Cookies, Pepperidge Farm	40
Chocolate Hydrox Cookies, Sunshine	49
Vanilla Hydrox Cookies, Sunshine	51
Chocolate Chip Cookies, Chips Ahoy, Nabisco	53
Date Nut Granola, Pepperidge Farm	53
Devil's Food Cakes, Nabisco	70
Marshmallow Bars, Sunshine	92

Five Devil's Food Cakes are 350. Five Pirouettes are 200 calories. The more you eat, the more you save by making a careful selection.

Cookies are a classic binge food. What if you're going to eat the entire box of whatever you bring home? Here's how they look, when you're looking at a box:

	Calories per Package
sugar-free, salt-free Angel Puffs, Stella D'Oro, 3-oz. package	477
Date Nut Granola, Pepperidge Farm, 5½-oz. package	800
Devil's Food Cakes, Nabisco, 8-oz. package	840
Pirouette Cookies, Pepperidge Farm, 5½-oz. package	960
Marshmallow Bars, Sunshine, 10-oz. package	1078
Ginger Snaps, Nabisco, 16-oz. (1-lb. package	1920
Chocolate Hydrox Cookies, Sunshine, 15-oz. package	2024
Vanilla Hydrox Cookies, Sunshine, 15-oz. package	2106
Chocolate Chip Cookies, Chips Ahoy, Nabisco, 21-oz. package	3040

If you have the urge for something sweet, you could try the chocolate chips without the cookies. Nestlé Tollhouse Morsels are only about 3 calories apiece, and if you suck on them like Life

Savers, they last a surprisingly long time. (What do you call chocolate chip cookies that remind you of your old neighborhood? . . . They're chips off the old block.)

And how do cookies compare with candy? Here are our same nine candidates running against some competition from **Sweet Little Nothings:**

	Calories per Ounce
Chuckles	95.0
Devil's Food Cakes, Nabisco	*105.0*
Marshmallow Bars, Sunshine	*107.8*
Life-Savers	110.0
Chocolate Tootsie Rolls	113.7
Bit O' Honey	117.0
Ginger Snaps, Nabisco	*120.0*
SnoCaps	124.0
Raisin & Cinnamon Granola Bar, Quaker	130.0
Chocolate Hydrox Cookies, Sunshine	*134.9*
old fashioned Peanut Candy Bar, Planters	140.0
Vanilla Hydrox Cookies, Sunshine	*140.4*
Peanut Chocolate Candies, M & M	143.3
Baby Ruth Bar	144.4
Chocolate Chip Cookies, Chips Ahoy, Nabisco	*145.5*
Date Nut Granola Cookies, Pepperidge Farm	*145.5*
Hershey's Chocolate Kisses	150.0
Rainbow Jordan Almonds, Schrafft's	151.9
sugar-free, salt-free Angel Puffs, Stella D'Oro	*159.1*
Pirouette Cookies, Pepperidge Farm	*174.5*

Even when compared to candy, Pirouettes and sugar-free Angel Puffs are still the highest on the list.

And how do cookies compare with **Cakes?** In the comparisons that follow, many of the "calories per ounce" for cakes had to be estimated from the yield of the recipe:

Applesauce Raisin Layer Cake, Duncan Hines, "suggested" serving
1/12 of cake is 190 calories; approximately 81 calories per ounce.
Apple Crisp Cookies, Nabisco,
50 calories a cookie; 132.0 calories per ounce.
3 4/5 cookies = one slice of cake

Chocolate Fudge Chip Cake, Betty Crocker Snackin' Cake, "suggested" serving
1/9 of cake is 190 calories; approximately 92 calories an ounce.
Chocolate Chip Cookies, Chips Ahoy, Nabisco,
53 calories a cookie; 145.5 calories an ounce.
3 1/2 cookies = 1 slice of cake

Sour Cream Chocolate Layer Cake, Duncan Hines, "suggested" serving
1/12 of cake is 200 calories; approximately 86 calories per ounce.
Oreo Cookies, Nabisco,
50 calories a cookie; 136.4 calories per ounce.
4 cookies = 1 slice of cake

Pound Cake, Dromedary, "suggested" serving
1/8 of cake is 320 calories; approximately 95 calories per ounce.
Shortbread Cookie, Lorna Doone,
40 calories a cookie; 144.0 calories per ounce.
8 cookies = 1 slice of cake

Lemon Pudding Cake, Betty Crocker, "suggested" serving
1/6 of cake is 230 calories; approximately 81 calories per ounce.
Lemon Coolers Cookies, Sunshine,
29 calories a cookie; 134.8 calories per ounce.
8 cookies = 1 slice of cake

Dietetic Lemon Sandwich Cookies, Estee,
60 calories a cookie; 144 calories per ounce.
3 5/6 cookies = 1 slice of cake

Did you notice—Estee's Dietetic Lemon Sandwich cookies are higher-calorie than Sunshine's Lemon Coolers? If that doesn't take the cake!

"Dietetic" reminds me—Melba toast is in this chapter, too. As with the cookies, the calories in crackers come from carbohydrate and fat; both are major contributors. The same is just as true for bread. The difference in calories between bread and crackers is the moisture. By the ounce, Melba toast is higher-calorie than any bread. That's **How to Eat Crackers:**

	Calories per Ounce
rye bread, USDA	68.9
whole wheat bread, USDA	68.9
white bread, USDA	77.9
Pumpernickel Melba Toast, Old London	100.0
Rye Toast, Devonsheer Melba	106.7
Sourdough Toast, Crisp Bread, Wasa Ry-King	108.3
Sesame Rounds, Old London	120.0
Wheat Toast, Keebler	157.5

Still, by the piece, crackers can save you calories over bread. Even thin-sliced and smaller-sized breads are usually—although not always—higher in calories than one single cracker:

	Calorie per Slice or Cracker
Cracker: Sesame Rounds, Old London	12
Cracker: Rye toast, Devonsheer Melba	16
Cracker: Pumpernickel Melba Toast, Old London	17
Bread: Party Rye, Pepperidge Farm	18
Cracker: Wheat Toast, Keebler	18
Bread: Party Pumpernickel, Pepperidge Farm	23
Bread: Cocktail Rye, Rubschlager	25
Bread: Cocktail Pumpernickel, Rubschlager	29
Bread: Extra Thin Sliced White Bread, Northridge	45
Cracker: Sourdough Toast, Crisp Bread, Wasa Ry-King	46
Bread: Melba Thin-Sliced Jewish Rye with Caraway Seeds, Arnold	50
Bread: One bagel chip (a thin-sliced bagel—it's discussed in the **Breads** Chapter Preface, page 118)	52
Bread: Thin Sliced Wheat Germ Bread, Pepperidge Farm	65

And when all is said and done, whether you do better by eating bread or eating crackers is likely to come down to this: on which will you spread more butter?

If you're going to be eating crackers right out of the box—"snacking" crackers like Triscuits or Ritz—then you should know how they compare to potato chips and other entries from the **Salty Snacks** chapter:

	Calories per Ounce
salty snack: Popcorn, Jolly Time	*109.4*
cracker: Whole Wheat Snack Sticks, Pepperidge Farm	110.0
cracker: Triscuits, Nabisco	127.3
cracker: Ritz Crackers, Nabisco	150.0
salty snack: Potato Chips, Wise	*150.0*
salty snack: Corn Chips, Fritos	*160.0*

Triscuits are 127.3 calories per ounce; potato chips are about 150. So if you're on a diet, how many calories do you save by eating Triscuits instead of potato chips? You save a lot by the ounce. You save a lot by the pound, that's certainly true. But how much do you save per afternoon?

Isn't that like asking "How long is a string?"

No, because there's a realistic answer to "The Triscuit-versus-potato-chip problem," although it's not an answer that's explicit in the charts: Some quantity of Triscuits will be enough to satisfy you, and some quantity of potato chips will be enough to satisfy you. That's the essential comparison.

24 SWEET LITTLE NOTHINGS—CANDY

What are Sweet Little Nothings? Well, they're sweet. For the most part they're little. And as to their being "nothings" . . .

What is candy? According to the *Scribner-Bantam Dictionary,* candy is a "confection of sugar, syrup, etc., often combined with other ingredients, as chocolate, nuts or fruits."

What is chocolate? Well, they take kind of a nut—the nut of the cacao tree—and grind it several times, and roast it, and grind it, and grind it, and grind it. Then they take the powder, moisten it, and grind it and grind it again. The cacao nut has oils in it—the stuff of cocoa butter—and oils are added and subtracted and multiplied and divided and processed, and other flavorings are included, too. Quantities of sugar are added because otherwise it's a very bitter food.

There are various treatments that chocolate can go through. "Alkali treating" gives you Dutch chocolate; milk is added to give you milk chocolate.

What's in This Chapter is candy. It's chocolate candies and nut candies and coconut candies and marshmallows. It's Baby Ruth and Mary Jane, Chocolate Babies and Mexican Hats. It's taffy and it's Tootsie Rolls, assorted Dots and lollipops. It's licorice and the classic after-dinner mint.

What's in this chapter is also halvah, and to my knowledge this is the first time that the calories for halvah are being published in this country. I called the Joyva people and told them that a childhood fantasy of mine was to get locked in their plant overnight, and if I had known that they were located in Brooklyn, and not in Istanbul . . .

. . . and while we were at it, would they be kind enough to send their various products to a laboratory for analysis?

The result is that we have Joyva's marble halvah, and vanilla halvah, and chocolate halvah and also their Sesame Bars, Sesame Crunch, Sesamettes, and Marshmallow Twists. But the pièce de résistance for me is their chocolate-covered Jell Bars—those Jell Bars you buy in candy stores. At 110 calories per ounce, it's one of the lowest-calorie candies in this chapter. And chocolate coated, besides.

What's Related, but Elsewhere: This chapter is related, of course, to **Sugars, Sweeteners & Toppings,** and, of course, to **Basic Baking & Cooking Ingredients** with its chocolate, and its coconut, and its so forth.

Cakes; Pies; Cookies & Crackers; Frozen Confections; Gelatins, Puddings & Custards; Yogurt; Nuts & Seeds, and **Fruits** all are related because that's where you'll find potential substitutes, whether higher or lower in calories, for the foods listed here. Another kindred chapter is **Beverages,** soda being candied water.

The Arrangement of Sweet Little Nothings:

Candy, by brand is alphabetical by what I considered the "best distinguishing word." A Reggie bar is under Reggie, not chocolate. Mounds bars are under Mounds, not Peter Paul or coconut. Halvah is under Halvah, not Joyva. So, if you're looking for a candy, and at first you don't succeed, try, try again.

However, three types of "candy" have been grouped together:

Gum, which is chewed but not eaten, has a separate list at the end of this chapter:

How to Read the Numbers: The column headings are:

Unit
One Ounce by Weight
One Pound

The Unit might be one candy bar, or a whole supermarket bagful of miniatures. The Unit might be one Chuckle or one M & M.

The Ounce by Weight column, of course, will show the same figure regardless of the Unit size. One M & M, by the ounce, is the same as one thousand M & Ms.

For lollipops, the Ounce and the Pound columns are for the weight of the lollipop without its stick. And speaking of sticks, *Gum* has only one column—the Unit.

As you look through the data pages for candy, you may see small discrepancies between the figures for the entire package, the ounce by weight, and the piece. It may look, for example, as though a "4½-ounce" candy bar has five 1-ounce pieces of candy in it. The reason this happens is that, industry-wide, the declared label weight of a candy bar is less than what the manufacturer actually does give you; s/he does this to avoid the possibility of shortweighting. As a result, the Ounce will be the most reliable column in this chapter.

It is true throughout the book, but it is especially true of candy, that package sizes will change frequently, even more than once a year. What's more, within three blocks of my home I was able to buy four different sizes of the same Hershey chocolate bar. If the candy bar you are thinking of eating is in this book, but the label weight is not the same, consult the One Ounce column and multiply up.

You will notice that I did not give you a Cup column in this chapter. For one cup of Clark Bars, you will have to do your own calculations.

The numbers for Almond Joy, Mounds, Milk Mounds, and Caravel bars are in this chapter although Peter Paul refused my request for nutrition information. The data for Peter Paul candies were given to me over the telephone as a consumer—I am a consumer, after all—and are therefore just telephone-relayed calorie numbers. I think this is important to say. Since I did not have a written analysis of the entire composition, I could not put their data through the normal rigors to check accuracy. I apologize, Peter, but I just couldn't do the book without Almond Joy. And now . . .

How in the world **to Eat Candy: Sweet Little Nothings** are more matters of the heart than matters of the mind. If you're eating a candy bar it's not for the same reason that you eat meat, and it's not for the same reason that you eat vegetables. It's customary to plan which meat and which vegetables to eat for dinner, sometimes before breakfast. But candy is oftentimes crave-food, and preferences are established along different lines, I think, than preferences in cuts of beef. You just aren't as likely to be haunted through the night by the broccoli you want, but can't have. This is a chapter where all you are getting for your calories is satisfaction, and if satisfaction is all you are getting, you might as well get it.

Still, it is important to know the relative calories of a This-Bar versus a That-Bar, when both bars are among the things that will satisfy your urge. So before you get ready for your shopping spree, let's ask the first question: Where do the calories come from?

The answer is that you might think the calories in this chapter come from sugar, and certainly they do. But first, if nuts are a substantial ingredient, much or most of the calorie impact is going to come from fat. Secondly, if you're eating chocolate, most of the calories will also come from fat. Of course there will be calories coming from the immense quantities of sugar in this chapter, pure carbohydrate at 110 calories per ounce. But you should be aware that sugar is not the worst villain in a Baby Ruth. Fat is 250 calories per ounce. One way to save calories when you buy candy, then, is to try to avoid the oils.

Mr. Goodbar bars are 161.5 calories an ounce. They are chocolate, and they have nuts in them. Heide's Jelly Eggs are 79.9 calories an ounce. They aren't chocolate, and they don't have nuts in them.

And this is one chapter where a raisin can be helpful. Raisins are a high-calorie choice if you're eating them in the **Fruits** chapter, but a good calorie buy if you're eating them here. Plain milk chocolate is about 147 calories an ounce. Chocolate-covered raisins, Ward's Raisinets, are 90.

Of course you can always eat the raisins without the chocolate. That way it's 82 calories an ounce.

Fruit can actually be a satisfying substitution for candy. Here I go talking substitutions, when you just heard me say that candy is a crave-food. That's true, but the question is—what exactly are you craving? Fruit and candy both are sweet. Fruit and candy both are finger foods—you eat them from hand to mouth without the intervention of a fork or spoon. If you're eating candy because you want something to do with your hands, what about cherries or grapes? You know that pound of cherries you've always wanted to eat but haven't, because you've been told that cherries are fattening? Well, here's your chance. M&M's are 138 calories an ounce, cherries are 19.9.

What about candy versus the possibilities in **Salty Snacks,** or **Nuts & Seeds?** Here's the situation:

	Calories per Ounce
Switzer's Licorice Stix	*94.0*
Chuckles	*95.0*
jelly beans, USDA	*104.1*
sugar-coated popcorn, USDA	108.6
popcorn popped without oil, USDA	109.4
Life Savers, Wild Cherry	*110.0*
Pretzels, Mr. Salty (Nabisco)	110.0
Tootsie Roll Bar, chocolate	*113.7*
Cracker Jack	*120.0*
Milky Way Bar	*126.7*
popcorn popped in oil, USDA	129.3
Clark Bar	*135.8*
Baby Ruth	*144.4*
Chunky Bar	*145.0*
Reggie Bar	*145.0*
Nestlé's Crunch Bar	*150.0*
Potato Chips, Wise	150.0
Hershey Bar	*152.4*
Potato Sticks, O & C	154.0
sunflower seeds, shelled, USDA	158.8
cashews, shelled, USDA	159.0
Cheez Doodles, Old London	160.0
Corn Chips, Frito Lay	160.0
Marble Halvah, Joyva	*160.0*
peanuts, shelled, USDA	165.1
pistachio nuts, shelled, USDA	169.0
almonds, shelled, USDA	169.8
Plantain Chips, Chiffles	176.0
Wheat-Nuts, Pillsbury	200.0

How does a candy bar compare with a Coke? By the ounce, Coke has the added advantage of added water and it shows in the calorie count. A 12-fluid-ounce can of Coke has 144 calories, about the same as one ounce of chocolate.

What about candy versus French fries? A pound of McDonald's French fries has about 1406 calories. A pound of Milky Way Bars has 2027. A 1.91-ounce Milky Way Bar has 242 calories. The regular-size portion of French fries at McDonald's has 211.

The McDonald's hamburger, roll and all, has 257.

How does candy compare to baked goods—the cakes, the pies, and the cookies?

If you're comparing one candy bar to one cookie, one cookie will almost always be lower. If you're making the comparison by the ounce, the range is about the same.

If you're comparing candy bars to pie, there is a clear winner. Just look down the numbers in the Ounce column, and you'll see that you can have a lot more pie than candy bar for the same calories. Not just apple pie—I mean banana custard and chocolate chiffon.

Cakes, by the ounce, generally run midway between pies and candy bars. But one candy bar versus one cupcake? Almost any cupcake you choose, almost any size and almost any flavor cupcake you choose, will have fewer calories than a candy bar.

Another winner over candy is ice cream and its companions from the **Frozen Confections** chapter. By the ounce, even "rich" chocolate ice cream has less than one-half the calories of plain milk chocolate. By the ounce, Light n' Lively Chocolate Ice Milk has less than one-third the calories of the milk chocolate.

How do ice cream bars compare with candy bars? A 1.8-oz. Baby Ruth bar has 260 calories. Good Humor's Chocolate Eclair Ice Cream Bar—3 ounces—has 220 calories. A 2½-fluid-ounce Fudgsicle has 102 calories. Popsicles are even lower, at 70 calories apiece—23.3 calories a fluid ounce, any flavor.

Or look to the **Condiments** chapter. It might not occur to you to eat a pickle instead of a Baby Ruth, but just because it wouldn't occur to you, this is the place to say it.

Pickles, popsicles, pies and fries aside, what if you still want candy?

In truth, what if you still want chocolate?

You may not be accustomed to the notion that there can be lower-calorie and higher-calorie chocolate, but there can be. Among the chocolates, and even among the chocolates with nuts, there are differences you can take advantage of. Something you might not have guessed is that rich, smooth, creamy chocolate fudge is lower in calories than milk chocolate. Fudge is a much moister food—it can have 10 times the water content of milk chocolate, and less than half the fat. The result is that a hunk of chocolate fudge can save you a hunk of calories:

Based on USDA data:	**Calories per Ounce**
chocolate-coated almonds	161.3
chocolate-coated peanuts	159.1
milk chocolate bar with peanuts	154.0
milk chocolate bar with almonds	150.8
sweet chocolate	149.7
milk chocolate	147.4
semi-sweet chocolate	144.0
bittersweet chocolate	135.3
chocolate fudge with nuts	120.8
vanilla fudge with nuts	120.2
chocolate fudge	113.4
vanilla fudge	112.8

And once again as a reminder, the lowest-calorie candies in this chapter will not be chocolate, and will not have nuts at all:

Based on USDA data:	**Calories per Ounce**
butterscotch	112.6
hard candies	109.4
jelly beans	104.1
candy corn	103.2
gum drops	98.5
marshmallows	90.4

Looking at the data from the USDA, marshmallows are about the lowest-calorie "candy" you can eat, with gum drops running a close second. Candy corn and jelly beans are in third and fourth place in the "generic" candy race. Yet the lowest-calorie entry in **Sweet Little Nothings** is not any of these. The star of this chapter is, in fact, a star of the entire book. Trumpets please!

Chewing gum. Low-calorie by the piece, by the package, by the hour, and by the chew. You can just go on and on all day, for no more than 10 calories per stick. There are no figures in the Ounce or Pound columns for chewing gum. Information was not provided by manufacturers on a weight basis, and for good reason. Most of the weight of a stick of gum gets thrown away when you've finished chewing it. The edible portion as compared to the refuse is very small. The calories may alter slightly if you swallow it.

Bubble gum generally has more calories than chewing gum does, even if you do burn more calories chewing it.

What about the sugarless gums? Artificially sweetened gums may save on cavities, but not on calories. The point of sugarless gum is not that it's "less fattening," but that it's sugar-free. It's another example of how something that is "dietetic" won't necessarily help your diet.

How does chewing on a piece of gum compare with sucking on a Life Saver? One Life Saver, one stick of chewing gum. The calories are about the same. Given that you'd like them equally, the question is—which lasts longer? With gum, that will depend on how quickly you discard it after the flavor is gone. With sucking candy, how long it will last is more complicated.

Sucking candies, even those of the same weight, will take different lengths of time to dissolve in your mouth. Life Savers, because they have a hole, will have a high surface area compared with other candies of the same approximate size. Life Savers dissolve more quickly than Charms do, at least for the same amount of weight. But we can't say that all sucking candies will operate according to their surface area, because there is more involved here than simple surface geometry would suggest. Physiological things go on when you pop something in your mouth, and they don't depend strictly on size. There's going to be an effect of sharp corners versus smooth edges. I think it is no accident that an all-day sucker is round. Then, too, two pieces will dissolve faster together than the two of them eaten separately, because several pieces rattling around in your mouth is a real perker-upper to salivation. When you chew on your sucking candy you increase the number of individual pieces in your mouth, and also the total surface area. Hence, you are going to part with it a lot sooner, original surface area aside. And sour sucking candy may stimulate salivation more than sweet or mild sucking candies do.

On the other hand, sour sucking candy may make the point with fewer pieces. The idea is to see how long a particular sucking candy lasts for you.

To make sucking candy out of a Milky Way, put it in the freezer first. The calories per ounce will be the same, but it will take much longer to eat. It also introduces an element of planning. Freezing is, after all, preparing your candy before eating it. This affords the added dignity of feeling that you are retaining control. If you like Milky Ways, frozen Milky Ways taste great. So do frozen Marshmallow Twists. (It doesn't work for all candies . . . frozen candy corn?)

And after all this, if you still want to eat the highest-calorie candy in **Sweet Little Nothings,** enjoy it. I won't advise you to discard it for something you don't really want. I'll offer only one word of advice. Once you are committed to it, eat it s-l-o-w-l-y.

25 FROZEN CONFECTIONS

What are frozen confections? The *Scribner-Bantam Dictionary* describes frozen as "congealed by cold," and confection as "something sweet, as candy, bonbons, or preserves."

What's in This Chapter is ice cream and ice milk, ice cream bars and ice cream sandwiches, soft and hard frozen yogurt, frozen yogurt bars, sherbet, ice pops, and a list of just-waiting-to-be-filled ice cream cones.

Also in this chapter is a list of concentrated flavorings used by manufacturers throughout the United States to give ice cream its many different tastes. The inside story, so to speak.

For the outside story, there's the chocolate ice cream bar coating, without any ice cream at all.

What's Related, but Elsewhere are the foods that are eaten for dessert or as snacks. That's all the candies in **Sweet Little Nothings;** all the goodies in **Cakes, Snack Cakes & Pastries; Pies; Gelatins, Puddings & Custards; Yogurt;** and even **Nuts & Seeds** and **Salty Snacks.**

Toppings for ice cream and ice milk are in **Sugars, Sweeteners & Toppings,** and fruit preserves are in **Confitures & Nut Butters.**

Cream and milk, from which ice cream, ice milk, and frozen yogurt are made, are in the **Beverages** chapter.

The Arrangement of This Chapter is unusual in that most of the entries have been listed at least twice. After an overview provided by the USDA data, the ice creams, ice milks, frozen yogurts, and other frozen desserts are listed together by flavor.

Containers with more than one flavor, such as Vanilla/Chocolate/Strawberry, are listed after the last flavor, which happens to be Wildberry Supreme. Yum.

Immediately following the list by flavor, everything is listed again, this time by brand. If you have a favorite brand of ice cream, you can go right to it and compare the possibilities.

There are several shorter lists, each focusing on different members of the **Frozen Confections** community. These are:

How to Read the Numbers: The column headings for the main body of this chapter are:

Unit
One Ounce by Weight
One Fluid Ounce
One Cup, Packed

For frozen confections sold on a stick, generally there were no data by weight available. For the bars, pops, and sandwiches the Ounce by Weight column has been replaced by One Bar.

The Unit may be an entire container as small as a single serving cup, as inviting as a box of ice cream bars, or as large as a three-gallon tub.

The One Fluid Ounce column is a volume measurement. This is an important column because ice cream, ice milk, the frozen yogurts, and so forth are sold by volume—pints, quarts, and gallons. There are 16 fluid ounces to a pint, 32 fluid ounces to a quart, 128 fluid ounces to a gallon. After that you are on your own.

For a tablespoon of ice cream, divide the fluid ounce figure in half.

The One Fluid Ounce column should not be confused with One Ounce by Weight. These are entirely different measurements, and for a great many of these products an ounce by weight will have considerably more calories than a fluid ounce. For example, Breyers Coffee Ice Cream is 35 calories for a fluid ounce and 56.7 calories for an ounce by weight. The explanation is this: For the foods that characterize this chapter, air is a recognized and necessary ingredient. Air increases volume. However, because of the buoyancy of the atmosphere in which we weigh things, air will not affect the Ounce by Weight column. In other words, if two ice creams have otherwise identical ingredients—but one contains more air—the ice cream with more air will have fewer calories by the gallon, but the same number of calories by the pound.

Between the effect of air, and the fact that ice cream, like ice, expands as it freezes, the volume measurements cannot be used for melted ice cream. The Ounce by Weight column is unaffected by melting. That's one good reason to have an Ounce by Weight column in this volume-oriented chapter.

The One Cup column is, of course, also a volume measurement. It's 8 Fluid Ounces just as it always is. But—and it's an important "but"—in this chapter the Cup column is a packed cup. In fact, it represents packing that can be achieved only by mechanical means. Unless you have a pile driver, it is very hard to duplicate at home. If you were to take a chisel to a big block of ice cream, and carve a cupful out of the block, and slide that cupful neatly into your measuring cup, that's the cup in this chapter.

The way I used to determine cups of ice cream when I started dieting was this: I would buy a half-gallon container of ice milk with its "16 one-half cup servings." I would take a felt tip pen and a ruler and draw my "half cups" on the outside, dividing the container into 16 equal parts. It helped me figure out how deep to scoop the scoop.

I would have included a One Scoop column, but when I looked into it I found that scoops don't come in a standard size.

How to Eat Frozen Confections:

> I shall never trust anyone who doesn't love ice cream. They probably hate the beach because of the sand, sleep in pajamas, never eat spareribs and kiss with their mouths closed. What deprivation. Give me rum raisin, give me butterscotch excess.
>
> Gael Greene
>
> *Time,* August 10, 1981

You can trust me, Gael. I love ice cream.

I love ice cream, I love ice milk, I love frozen yogurt, I love sherbet, I love ices. I eat something from this chapter almost every day, often more than once. I became a great fan of the foods in this chapter when I began dieting and realized what fantastic calorie-buys were to be had.

The delicious foods in this chapter are much lower in calories-per-ounce than the competition in **Cakes, Cookies & Crackers, Sweet Little Nothings, Salty Snacks,** or **Nuts & Seeds.** And why they are lower in calories becomes easy to understand as we answer our usual first question: Where do the calories come from?

Different brands and flavors will vary in their compositions. I make the following generalizations based on USDA data and conversations with manufacturers.

For Ice Cream:

For the rich ice creams, those with approximately 16% fat content, most of the calories will come from the fat. For ice cream with a 10% fat content, the calorie contribution from fat drops down to just below half. The rest of the calories will come almost entirely from carbohydrate, the contribution from protein being roughly 7%. But even assuming the richest ice cream, about 59% of what you are eating is water. The fats, the sugars, and the proteins are all minority ingredients compared to the water. All put together, they are still minority ingredients.

For Ice Milks:

Ice milk has less fat in it than ice cream, and more water—it's about 69% water. The calories usually come from carbohydrate, fat, and protein in that order.

For Hard & Soft Frozen Yogurt:

Approximately 54% of what you are eating in frozen yogurt is water. About two-thirds of the calories in frozen yogurt come from carbohydrate. Then comes the protein. Fat is in third place.

For Sherbet:

Sherbet is about 66% water. Approximately 84% of sherbet's calories come from carbohydrate. What calories are left come mostly from fat, with a minimal contribution from protein.

For Ices:

All of the calories come from carbohydrate. About 67% of what you're eating is water.

The consistently high moisture content gives us a chapter with very favorable calories per ounce when compared to the competition. In the whole of **Frozen Confections**—with its rich, rich ice creams from Häagen-Dazs, and its sundaes from Dairy Queen, and all the flavors of sherbet from Carvel—there are only two entries that are over 80 calories per ounce. One is Howard Johnson's vanilla ice cream at 85.0; the other is Howard Johnson's chocolate at 89.5. Well, the **Cakes** chapter just about starts at 80 calories per ounce. In **Sweet Little Nothings,** a Milky Way is at the lower end of the candy bars at 126.7 an ounce. But in this chapter you can choose among dozens and dozens of delicious desserts for less than 50 calories per ounce.

That's the good news.

The bad news is that when it comes to "how to eat," the **Frozen Confections** chapter poses a special problem. For many chapters, once you know the principles of where the calories come from, you can take a product that isn't listed and make a plausible guess as to what you have in your hands. It doesn't work with a handful of ice cream. What you have to have in your hands is this book: The way to eat **Frozen Confections** is to look up the numbers each and every time, because in this chapter it's one surprise after another.

Of course, almost every chapter has surprises. In **Cakes,** for example, it's surprising that eclairs and cream puffs are so low in calories. But once you have read the reasons for it, the cream puff need not come as a surprise any more. Unfortunately, that kind of advice just won't work here. And neither will reputation. There are ice milks that have more calories than ice cream. There are sherbets that have more calories than ice milk.

Finding your way amongst the **Frozen Confections** is particularly difficult in light of the names that some manufacturers have given to their creations. You might think that "Think Thin" brand Chocolate Ice Milk would have fewer calories by the cup than "Luxury" brand Chocolate Ice Cream. But no. Think Thin has more. You might think that Armel Vanilla Fudge Dietary Frozen Dessert would have fewer calories by the cup than Good Humor Toffee Fudge Swirl Ice Cream. But no. They are the same.

You can't divine calories by flavor either. You might think that a Danny-In-A-Cup hard-frozen boysenberry yogurt would have fewer calories than a Johnston hard-frozen caramel-pecan yogurt, but no. Boysenberry has more. And these examples are typical. They tell the story, I'm afraid.

(How does the frozen boysenberry compare with Dannon's non-frozen low-fat boysenberry yogurt? The frozen yogurt is almost one-third lower by the cup.)

All this talk about frozen confections entices me to have some. Excuse me for a moment.

Thank you. I have just returned with an ice cream cone, or shall I say an ice milk cone—at less than 100 calories for the whole kit and caboodle. A cone is a wonderful invention, an edible cup. And if you take a wafer cone instead of a sugar cone, they're only about 20 calories each. The sugar cones are about 40 calories each. It's not because sugar cones are "sugary" (sugar and starch are equally caloric by the ounce). The sugar cones have twice the calories because they weigh twice as much.

What's in my cone is Sealtest's Light 'n Lively Ice Milk. This time it happens to be Chocolate Marshmallow Twirl, and it's 30 calories per fluid ounce. All the flavors run between 100 and 120 calories for half a cup—or just a little less than cottage cheese!

	Calories per ½ Cup (4 Fluid Ounces), Packed
Cottage Cheese, 4.2% milk fat	130
Sealtest Light 'N Lively Ice Milk:	
Caramel Nut	120
Chocolate	100
Chocolate Marshmallow Twirl	120
Coffee	100
Heavenly Hash	120
Lemon Chiffon	120
Orange-Pineapple	100
Peach	100
Strawberry	100
Toffee Crunch	120
Vanilla	100
Vanilla Fudge	110

Fewer calories than cottage cheese! And how can you feel deprived when you're eating Chocolate Marshmallow Twirl?

Or drinking Toffee in your coffee. At 15 calories per tablespoon, there are several flavors of Light 'n Lively Ice Milk that are wonderful in coffee. Vanilla is a particular favorite of mine. It serves as both sugar and cream.

In competition with ice milks are the soft and hard frozen yogurts, and these range from 23.8 to 31.5 calories per fluid ounce, or approximately 90 to 126 calories per half cup.

Dannon's vanilla frozen yogurt bar, Danny-On-A-Stick, is 60 calories for 2½ fluid ounces. That's about as low-calorie a dessert as you can get—comparable to the calories of a 4-ounce apple. There are other frozen yogurt bars on the market with similar calories. I single out Danny-On-A-Stick for praise because Dannon says they invented the frozen yogurt bar. And besides, they do it so well.

I should caution that once you put the chocolate coating on, you can more than double the calories. The coating on a frozen yogurt bar can have more calories than all of the yogurt inside.

Carob coating? It doesn't save you any calories over chocolate.

How do frozen yogurt bars compare with ice cream sandwiches? With ice cream bars? With ices? Here are some examples, in ascending order of calories per unit. (Be aware that the bars you buy in the supermarket are not always the same size as the same-name bar sold by street vendors.)

	Calories per Unit
Blueberry frozen yogurt bar, Beautiful Day, 2½ fl. oz.	40
Grape Ice Whammy, Good Humor, 2½ oz. (net wt.)	50
Apple Sunshine Bar, Hood, 2 fl. oz.	50
Vanilla frozen yogurt bar, Danny-On-A-Stick, 2½ fl. oz.	60
Piña Colada frozen yogurt bar, Danny-On-A-Stick, 2½ fl. oz.	70
Dreamsicle, ice milk center, 2½ fl. oz.	70
Popsicles: Banana, Blue Grape, Blue Raspberry, Cherry, Chocolate, Grape, Lime, Orange, Raspberry, Root Beer, Strawberry, Vanilla, White Lemon; each 3 fl. oz.	70
Strawberry frozen yogurt bar, Tuscan, 2½ fl. oz.	70
Creamsicle, ice cream center, 2½ fl. oz.	78
Chocolate frozen yogurt bar, Tuscan, 2½ fl. oz.	85
Banana Pudding Pop, Jell-O, 1.65 fl. oz.	90
Chocolate Whammy Bar, Good Humor, 1.6 oz. (net wt.)	100
Chocolate Pudding Stix, Hood, 1.9 fl. oz.	100
Chocolate Pudding Pop, Jell-O, 2 fl. oz.	100
Chocolate Mint Treat frozen confection bar, Weight Watchers, 2.75 fl. oz.	100
Chocolate Fudgsicle, 2½ fl. oz.	102
Chip Crunch Whammy Bar, Good Humor, 1.6 oz. (net wt.)	110
Chocolate Bi-Sicle, Good Humor, 2½ oz. (net wt.)	112
Carob-coated Vanilla frozen yogurt bar, Danny-On-A-Stick, 2½ fl. oz.	120
Chocolate-coated Chocolate frozen yogurt bar, Danny-On-A-Stick, 2½ fl. oz.	130
Chocolate-coated Strawberry frozen yogurt bar, Tuscan, 2½ fl. oz.	130
Vanilla frozen dietary dessert bar, chocolate-flavor coated, Sweet 'N Low, 2½ fl. oz.	130
Carob-coated Boysenberry frozen yogurt bar, Danny-On-A-Stick, 2½ fl. oz.	140
Chocolate-coated Chocolate frozen yogurt bar, Colombo, 2½ fl. oz.	145
Chocolate-coated Chocolate frozen yogurt bar, Tuscan, 2½ fl. oz.	150
Chocolate-coated Vanilla Whammy Bar, Good Humor, 3 oz. (net wt.)	170
Toffee Ice Cream Bar, Heath, 3 fl. oz.	170
Strawberry Shortcake ice cream bar, Good Humor, 3 oz. (net wt.)	200
Vanilla ice cream sandwich, Good Humor, 2½ oz. (net wt.)	200
Ice cream sandwich with honey, Natural Nectar, 3 fl. oz.	206
Chocolate Eclair ice cream bar, Good Humor, 3 oz. (net wt.)	220
Toasted Almond ice cream bar, Good Humor, 3 oz. (net wt.)	220
Yulovit Ice Cream Pie, Natural Nectar, 4 fl. oz.	269
Nectar Ice Cream Pie, Natural Nectar, 4 fl. oz.	341
Mocha Ice Cream Pie, Natural Nectar, 4 fl. oz.	341

The ice cream sandwiches are the highest per piece and per fluid ounce. Uncoated frozen yogurt bars and ices are the lowest.

Sherbet is not included on this list. According to the USDA, it runs a little higher than ices. Generic sherbet is 39.7 calories per fluid ounce.

Next, to answer a question that almost every movie-going dieter has pondered: How many calories in a bon bon? There are about 24 calories in a one-third-ounce chocolate or vanilla ice cream or strawberry yogurt bon bon, which seems like an awfully long sentence for such a little thing. Although everything is relative. A little bon bon, when multiplied by 10 of them, has enough calories that you could eat an ice cream sundae instead:

	Calories per Sundae
Dairy Queen, small chocolate sundae, 3¾ oz.	190
McDonald's strawberry sundae, 5 oz.	229
McDonald's pineapple sundae, 5 oz.	230
10 bon bons, 3⅓ oz.	240

The ice cream sundaes in **Fast Food** range from a low of about 40.0 calories an ounce to a high of about 67.0. And which is the 40-calorie-an-ounce sundae? Is it Dull Ice Cream drenched in Boring Sauce? No, it's Dairy Queen's Banana Split.

At 13½ ounces, the entire Split will cost you 540 calories. On the other hand, it's only 270 calories apiece if you share it with a friend. A Banana Split, split.

What if you make your own sundae?

The subject of toppings is covered in **Sugars, Sweeteners & Toppings,** but do be aware of the relationship between the common toppings and ice cream:

	Calories per Tablespoon
The highest-calorie tablespoon of ice cream in this book	***33.5***
Marshmallow topping, Kraft	35
Caramel topping, Kraft	50
Strawberry topping, Kraft	50
chopped walnuts, USDA	52
preserves, all flavors, USDA	54
Chocolate-flavored syrup, Hershey's	60
Walnut topping, Kraft	90

Instead of topping your ice cream, you could bottom it. Put your ice cream in half a cantaloupe. By adding a hundred—or even fewer—extra calories, you can turn a frozen confection into a meal.

Everything considered, are **Frozen Confections** high-calorie foods? It depends on what you compare them to. Compared to **Fruits,** yes. Compared to **Cakes,** no. Compared to **Sweet Little Nothings,** no. Compared to **Salty Snacks,** no. Compared to **Nuts & Seeds,** no. Shall I compare them to a summer's day?

26 GELATINS, PUDDINGS & CUSTARDS

What are gelatins, puddings, and custards? The *Scribner-Bantam Dictionary* defines gelatin as a "whitish, tasteless, and odorless translucent substance extracted from animal tissues and also from vegetables; soluble in water, it forms a jellylike mass when cooked and is used in foods, confections, medicinal capsules, photographic films, etc."

Pudding is defined, by the same source, as a "soft dessert made of flour, milk, eggs, and various other ingredients."

Custard is defined, again by the same source, as "pudding or dessert made of eggs, milk, sugar, etc., baked or boiled."

What's in This Chapter are gelatins, puddings, and custards. Also rennin, tapioca, and flan. Many of the puddings and custards serve a dual function as pie fillings.

What's Related, but Elsewhere: There are puddings and custards in **Baby Foods.**

Puddings to serve a hundred are in **Mess.** Puddings to serve our astronauts are in **Foods for Space Travel.**

When puddings and custards have a shell around them they're in **Pies.** Eclairs and other custard-filled pastries are in **Cakes.**

Yogurt and **Frozen Confections** also have desserts with a creamy consistency.

The whipped cream and other dessert toppings are in **Sugars, Sweeteners & Toppings.**

The Arrangement of This Chapter: First come the data from the USDA, and the list includes custard, custard-filled pastries, gelatins, puddings, and rennin desserts. The rest of the chapter consists of products sold by brand, appearing in this order:

How to Read the Numbers: The column headings are:

Unit
One Ounce by Weight
One Cup
One Tablespoon

The Unit column will usually describe an entire box of mix, or a single envelope from within the box. Some numbers will be for the dry mix itself, while others will be for the mix prepared. Occasionally, the Unit will be a dessert that is ready-to-serve.

When water has been added to a dry mix, the calories in the Unit column remain unchanged, although calories per ounce will go down.

When milk has been added, calories for the Unit increase. The calories per ounce, however, will still go down because pudding in its dry form has many more calories per ounce than milk.

When a product may be prepared in two ways, as for either pudding or pie filling, both methods of preparation are listed.

The Ounce by Weight column, like the Unit column, has calories for both prepared and unprepared foods.

The Cup is 8 fluid ounces, as always. In this chapter, a cup of dessert is likely to weigh closer to 10 ounces than 8.

Unlike the Unit and Ounce columns, the Cup has no numbers for the dry mix. This was an intentional omission, so that the Cup column would allow comparisons at a glance between desserts as they will actually be eaten.

The Tablespoon column accomplishes the same purpose at one-sixteenth the calories.

What Else You Should Know About These Numbers: As I looked through the numbers for this chapter, I became aware that different manufacturers had different ideas of what the calories in whole milk are. When I compared Jell-O's Chocolate Pudding with Royal's Butterscotch I saw that both had listed 640 calories for one box of their pudding prepared with 2 cups of whole milk. In the case of Jell-O, the dry mix is 360 to start out with, but Royal submitted their calories for the box at 320. For both of them to end up at 640, "Jell-O whole milk" must be 140 calories per cup, and "Royal whole milk" must be 160.

The numbers you will see printed in the **Calorielogue** do not reflect this inconsistency. For calculating the prepared values in this chapter, I chose to use a constant value for milk, so that calorie differences would better reflect the true differences between products. I used 160 calories (and the associated carbohydrate value of 12.0 grams) when preparations called for whole milk, 121 calories for low-fat milk (carbohydrate, 11.7 grams), and 90 calories for skim milk and non-fat milk (carbohydrate, 12.3 grams).

There is one exception. Betty Crocker's Chocolate Mousse, also in this chapter, has a value that considers whole milk to be 200 calories a cup. They insisted the information was correct. All I can say is "Holy Cow!"

Milk was not the only ingredient that caused problems. Puddings prepared with ingredients other than milk also needed to be recalculated for accuracy, as I was not able to use the prepared numbers that I received from certain manufacturers. One such manufacturer was My-T-Fine. And this is why: When this book was in page proofs (an advanced stage in the publishing process, just prior to the actual press run), a review of the numbers in this chapter showed that the calories for My-T-Fine puddings seemed too low. A look at the nutrition analyses that My-T-Fine had sent revealed that there was less fat listed in a one-half cup serving of their puddings, prepared with whole milk, than there is in half a cup of whole milk alone. If these numbers had been accurate, it would have meant that My-T-Fine's dry pudding mix had "negative" fat. If that is true, it's the subject for a whole other book (and probably a Nobel Prize).

The people at My-T-Fine were very gracious when I called this error to their attention. They immediately agreed to recalculate their figures, and I agreed to keep the two chapters in which their products appeared (this chapter, and **Pies**) back from publication as long as I could, while awaiting their new analyses.

Imagine my joy when they called me to say that their numbers were ready, and would be sent to me by overnight express for receipt the next day.

Imagine my disappointment when I opened the envelope, and saw that some of their numbers were still obviously wrong.

In the examples that follow, photocopied directly from what My-T-Fine sent to me, you can see that their Chocolate Pudding in powder form is cited as having 100 calories. By adding a half cup of whole milk, the calories go from 100 to 170.

For My-T-Fine Chocolate Almond Pudding, the dry mix is also listed as 100 calories, but adding the same half cup of whole milk produces 180 calories for the pudding prepared:

MY-T-FINE PUDDING
CHOCOLATE

NUTRITION INFORMATION PER SERVING

	Dry mix To make 1 serving (25.7 g)	1/2 cup prepared pudding*
Calories	100	170
Protein	0	4
Carbohydrate	23	29
Fat	0	4
Sodium	135	190

MY-T-FINE PUDDING
CHOCOLATE ALMOND

NUTRITION INFORMATION PER SERVING

	Dry mix To make 1 serving (26.6 g)	1/2 cup prepared pudding*
Calories	100	180
Protein	0	5
Carbohydrate	23	29
Fat	1	5
Sodium	135	190

*Prepared using Vitamin D fortified whole milk.

In the case of My-T-Fine's Lemon Pudding, the consumer needs to add water, one-half cup of sugar and 2 egg yolks to a box that yields four servings. As you will see below, the information from My-T-Fine says that each of the four servings will equal 160 calories.

MY-T-FINE PUDDING
LEMON

NUTRITION INFORMATION PER SERVING

	Dry mix To make 1 serving (23 g)	1/2 cup prepared pudding*
Calories	60	160
Protein	0	1
Carbohydrate	15	34
Fat	0	2
Sodium	15	120

*Prepared according to directions for pie filling.

But when I added up the calories for the lemon pudding powder plus the sugar and the egg yolks, then divided by the 4 servings, my results were different:

	Calories
dry mix in the entire box	240
½ cup of granulated sugar	385
2 medium egg yolks	110
	735 ÷ 4 = 183.75, which rounds to 184 calories

The numbers you will see in the **Calorielogue** for My-T-Fine Lemon Pudding, prepared, are not their numbers, but my numbers. I used their dry mix calorie values and added my own values for the sugar and egg yolks. Of course, there is no guarantee that the calories that My-T-Fine sent me for their dry powder are any more reliable than the calories they attribute to the milk, sugar, and egg yolks.

There are two lessons to be learned from this experience:

(1) Reputable manufacturers can be absolutely incorrect when it comes to the nutritive content of their foods.

(2) I didn't catch the My-T-Fine mistake until page proof time. Although I've tried to scrutinize every number in this book, I can virtually promise you that some mistakes have remained.

How to Eat Gelatin, Puddings, and Custards: Where do the calories come from?

Unflavored gelatin is mostly protein, and that's where the calories come from. (Note: The protein in gelatin is not complete protein—that is, it does not contain all the essential amino acids.) But for most of the foods in this chapter—flavored gelatins, puddings, and custards—the calories come from carbohydrate.

The way to save calories when you eat gelatin is to eat the low-calorie ones, if you find a brand you like. I am always hesitant to recommend artifically sweetened products, not only because of the controversies, but because, generally, I feel they are not good substitutes. The calories per cup for a sugar-sweetened gelatin will be about 160. For the low-calorie gelatins, calories run anywhere from 2 to 80, so it's a big saving. But rather than recommend artifically sweetened gelatin, I would send you to the **Frozen Confections** chapter, with its Good Humor Ice Whammy for 50 calories.

I have a box of Jell-O Chocolate Pudding here. The calories in the entire package are 360. Prepared with milk as the package directs, it's 680. So more than half the calories in this prepared pudding come from the box, and the rest come out of a bottle. Royal's Butterscotch Pudding has 320 calories in the box, and 640 prepared. Here, it's exactly half in the box and half in the bottle.

How do the different brands of pudding compare, when they're prepared according to label directions—which in every case call for "whole milk"?

		Calories per Cup, Prepared
Chocolate:	Jell-O Regular	340
	My-T-Fine	360
	Ann Page Instant	380
	Ann Page Regular	380
	Jell-O Instant	380
	Jell-Well Instant	380
	Jell-Well Regular	380
	Royal Instant	400
	Royal Regular	400
Butterscotch:	Royal Regular	320
	My-T-Fine	340
	Ann Page Regular	360
	Jell-O Instant	360
	Jell-O Regular	360
	Jell-Well Instant	360
	Royal Instant	360
	Jell-Well Regular	380
Vanilla:	Jell-O Regular	320
	Royal Regular	320
	Ann Page Instant	340
	Ann Page Regular	340
	Jell-Well Regular	340
	My-T-Fine	340
	Jell-O Instant	360
	Jell-Well Instant	360
	Royal Instant	360

But how do these puddings turn out if you use skim milk instead of whole milk in the preparation?

Since half the calories in a prepared pudding come from milk, I wrote to the manufacturers to find out whether skim milk could be substituted for whole. There was considerable uniformity in their responses: the pudding mixes are formulated to be prepared with whole milk, fat and all. Jell-O does make a rather good sugar-free instant pudding that's meant to be prepared with low-fat milk. You'll find five flavors of sugar-free Jell-O listed in the data pages: Banana, Butterscotch, and Vanilla at 90 calories per half-cup serving, Chocolate at 95, and Chocolate Fudge at 100. That's 70–90 calories less per serving than Jell-O Instant—a savings of approximately 40–50%. Well, you can accomplish your whole diet on much less than a 40–50% savings, so, from that point of view, I'm willing to recommend it. On the other hand, when I tried their sugar-free Chocolate Pudding, I felt that those 95 calories went down awfully fast. I'd rather eat something that fights back a little more. Jell-O's Pudding Pops, which you'll find in the **Frozen Confections** chapter, are 90 calories for a 2-fluid-ounce bar. It almost certainly will take longer to eat, and it saves 5 calories, besides.

But whether you take your pudding on a pop or in a cup, what you're eating pudding for is the enjoyment. If one of the puddings in this chapter is a favorite, then you're in the right place. However, if you're undecided about how you want to enjoy yourself, you might want to look at these comparisons, from lowest to highest calories per cup:

	Calories per Cup
Vanilla Soft Frozen Yogurt, Johnston's	181
Vanilla Ice Milk, Light 'N Lively	200
Vanilla Low-fat Yogurt, Dannon	233
Vanilla Ice Cream, Hood	260
Vanilla Whole Milk Yogurt, Brown Cow Farm	290
Vanilla Pudding, Royal Regular	*320*
Royal Instant	*360*
Rich's Ready-To-Eat	*392*
Vanilla Ice Cream, Carvel	395
Vanilla Ice Cream, Häagen-Dazs	513

And, before we leave the chapter, you might also be interested in this assortment, all from **Gelatins, Puddings & Custards:**

	Calories per Cup, Prepared
Vanilla Rennin Dessert, based on generic data	238
Raspberry Currant Danish-Style Pudding, Junket Danish Dessert	260
Custard, Royal	267
Flan, Royal	280
apple tapioca, USDA home recipe	293
baked custard, USDA home recipe	305
Chocolate Tapioca, Ann Page	340
Vanilla Tapioca, My-T-Fine	340
Rice Pudding, Jell-O	360

So what's the conclusion?

I think it would be safe to say that this is one chapter where substitutes can result in substantial calorie savings. But then, who's to determine what a suitable substitute is? That decision will always be yours to make. Here, as elsewhere, the proof of the pudding is in the eating.

27 · YOGURT

What is yogurt? Timothy Metzger, Director of Planning and New Product Development of Dannon, gave this definition of **Yogurt:** Yogurt is a semi-solid custard-like dairy product, made by injecting milk with cultures from bacterial strains. (At Dannon, *Lactobacillus bulgaricus* and *Streptococcus thermophilus.*)

What's in This Chapter? Better than any description I could give, the flavor of this chapter can best be captured by a glimpse at the ABC's: Apple Yogurt, Apple Crisp Yogurt, Apple Yogurt with Granola, Dutch Apple Yogurt, French Apple Yogurt, Spiced Apple Yogurt, Apricot Yogurt, Apricot Fruit Yogurt, Apricot-Pineapple Yogurt, Banana Yogurt, Banana Colada Yogurt, Banana-Strawberry Yogurt, Blackberry Yogurt, Black Cherry Yogurt, Blueberry Yogurt, Blueberry Yogurt with Cottage Cheese, Blueberry Yogurt with Granola, Blueberry Ripple Yogurt, Boysenberry Yogurt, Caramel Nut Yogurt, Caramel Pecan Yogurt, Cherry Yogurt, Cherries Jubilee Yogurt, Cherry-Coconut Yogurt, Cherry Supreme Yogurt, Cherry Vanilla Yogurt, Dark Cherry Yogurt, Red Cherry Yogurt, Coffee Yogurt, Creamy Coffee Yogurt, Cottage Cheese with Plain Yogurt, Cottage Cheese with Blueberry Yogurt, Cottage Cheese with Pineapple Yogurt, Cottage Cheese with Raspberry Yogurt, Cottage Cheese with Strawberry Yogurt, and Cranberry-Apple Yogurt.

Now, try saying the list out loud. How far can you get on one breath?

What's Related, but Elsewhere: Frozen Yogurt is in **Frozen Confections,** not here.

As a creamy dessert, yogurt is related to **Gelatins, Puddings & Custards. Confitures** are related to the fruit-flavored yogurts. The fact is that, although their names come from **Fruits,** what we think of as a strawberry yogurt is not yogurt and strawberries—it's yogurt and strawberry preserves.

The dairy products most closely associated with plain yogurt are cottage cheese and sour cream. Cottage cheese is in **Cheese.** Sour cream is in **Basic Baking & Cooking Ingredients** and also in **Hors D'Oeuvres, Dips & Spreads.** Yogurt, too, is cross-listed there, as it can alternate with sour cream in a dip. Yogurt can take the place of mayonnaise in salad dressing, and a good thing too. The mayonnaise story is told in **Condiments.**

The Arrangement of This Chapter will ring a bell if you're acquainted with **Frozen Confections.** Every yogurt in this chapter is listed twice. First in alphabetical order according to flavor, so that all the "Apple" yogurts are together. But since yogurt is a food that inspires fierce brand loyalty, following the listings by flavor each entry is repeated—this time by brand. The chapter begins with "Plain" yogurt, based on generic data:

How to Read the Numbers: The column headings are:

One Container
One Ounce by Weight
One Cup
One Tablespoon

The usual Unit column has been replaced by One Container, as this will describe the first set of numbers throughout the chapter. The container of yogurt will often be a hand-held portion of 6 or 8 ounces, but it may be a much larger container of 16 or 32 ounces.

The Ounce by Weight column is its usual self, providing a means of ounce-to-ounce comparisons. This column also provides a standard basis of comparison with foods in other chapters.

The Cup column is not the cup of yogurt you balance on the palm of your hand—that's the Container. The Cup is a kitchen measuring cup of 8 fluid ounces.

What most manufacturers call an "8-ounce Cup," is not really a cup at all. An 8-ounce container, even if it's shaped like a cup —even if it says "One Cup" on the label—will in fact hold less than a measuring cupful of yogurt. The fact is that the majority of the Cup figures in this chapter had to be estimated. In cases where the weight/volume relationships (see **Methodology,** page 31) were not provided by the manufacturers, a general conversion figure was applied: the flavored yogurts were calculated as weighing 263 grams (9.28 ounces) per cup. Estimated values are indicated by parentheses, as usual.

The One Tablespoon column is one-half a fluid ounce, one-sixteenth of a measuring cup. It is a level kitchen tablespoon and not at all the same thing as what you may dig out from the container with one scoop of your spoon . . .

How to Read "Low-fat": The word "low-fat" is so much on our lips these days, that many manufacturers of yogurt and other dairy products have dropped the hyphen, adopting "lowfat" instead. Using both "low-fat" and "lowfat" would look really peculiar in the data pages. Therefore I have chosen to hyphenate the word throughout the chapter, whether or not it appears that way on the label.

Hyphen, schmyphen, it's time for **How to Eat Yogurt.**

Where do the calories come from?

Brands of yogurt will vary significantly in their compositions. But based on the sample yogurts cited by the USDA for unflavored low-fat yogurt, carbohydrates account for about 45% of the calories. Protein accounts for about 33% and fat about 22%.

For unflavored whole milk yogurt about one-half of the calories will come from fat, at the expense of both protein and carbohydrate.

For fruit- and extract-flavored low-fat yogurts the calories come primarily from the carbohydrate, with substantial contributions from protein and fat, in that order.

And how do these categories of yogurt compare in calories, one to the other? First let's look at "plain."

Based on USDA data:	**Calories per 8-Ounce Container**
Plain, skim milk yogurt (0.18% fat)	127
Plain, whole milk yogurt (3.25% fat)	139
Plain, low-fat yogurt (1.55% fat)	144

Low-fat versus whole milk yogurt? Surprise! Low-fat yogurt can actually be higher in calories than whole milk yogurt because of the milk solids that are added in:

	Calories per 8-Ounce Container
Blueberry, Brown Cow Farm whole milk yogurt	230
Blueberry, Light n' Lively low-fat yogurt	240
Lemon, Colombo whole milk yogurt	220
Lemon, Knudsen pre-stirred low-fat yogurt	250
Mandarin Orange, Breyers whole milk yogurt	240
Mandarin Orange, Meadow Gold Western sundae style skim milk yogurt	260
Peach, Brown Cow Farm whole milk yogurt	225
Peach, Dannon low-fat yogurt	260
Piña Colada, Colombo whole milk yogurt	240
Piña Colada, Knudsen pre-stirred low-fat yogurt	260

But the relationship of low-fat to whole milk yogurt is by no means steadfast:

	Calories per 8-Ounce Container
Blueberry, Knudsen Fruit-On-The-Bottom low-fat yogurt	270
Blueberry, Maya whole milk yogurt	280
Cherry, Johnston's low-fat yogurt	250
Cherry, Continental whole milk yogurt	310
Vanilla, Dannon low-fat yogurt	200
Vanilla, Brown Cow Farm whole milk yogurt	250

What's the resolution? You have to read the numbers.

Are there any generalizations that can be made in this chapter? Yes. The non-fat yogurts have substantially fewer calories per ounce. For low-fat yogurts, the extract flavors—that is, vanilla and coffee—tend to be lower in calories than the fruit-flavored yogurts within the same brand.

Strawberries are lower in calories than bananas. Is strawberry yogurt lower in calories than banana yogurt? Nope. Fruit-flavored yogurts aren't flavored with fruit, they're flavored with fruit preserves. Just as we saw in **Confitures,** fruit preserves are virtually uniform in their calories per ounce.

Manufacturers of yogurt tell me that "Strawberry" is, by far, the most popular flavor. Here are our Strawberry yogurts in ascending order of calories per container. Most of the containers are eight ounces, but there is an occasional 5-, 6-, or 12-ounce container as well. Still, the comparison by containers—even of different sizes—is perhaps the most practical one that can be made in this chapter.

	Calories per Container	Calories per Ounce
Sugar Lo non-fat Strawberry yogurt, 8-oz. container	130	16.3
Colombo sundae style whole milk Strawberry yogurt, 5-oz. container	140	28.0
Sippity non-fat Strawberry yogurt, 8-oz. container	150	18.8
Sweet 'n Low non-fat Strawberry yogurt, 8-oz. container	150	18.8
Sweet 'n Low non-fat Strawberry Banana yogurt, 8-oz. container	150	18.8
Dannon Mélangé low-fat Strawberry yogurt, 6-oz. container	180	30.0
Le Shake low-fat Strawberry yogurt, 8-oz. container	180	22.5
Chambourcy French style whole milk Strawberry yogurt, 6-oz. container	190	23.8
Colombo Lite non-fat Strawberry yogurt, 8-oz. container	190	23.8
Fresh 'N Fruity original style low-fat Strawberry yogurt, 8-oz. container	190	31.7
Ralph's low-fat Strawberry yogurt, 8-oz. container	190	23.8
Yoplait whole milk Strawberry yogurt, 6-oz. container	190	29.3
Europa whole milk Strawberry yogurt, 6-oz. container	210	35.0
Look-Fit (A&P) Swiss style low-fat Strawberry yogurt, 8-oz. container	220	27.5
Brown Cow Farm whole milk Strawberry yogurt, 8-oz. container	223	27.9
Colombo whole milk Strawberry yogurt, 8-oz. container	230	28.8
Friendship low-fat Strawberry yogurt, 8-oz. container	230	28.8
Bison low-fat Strawberry yogurt, 8-oz. container	250	31.3
Knudsen pre-stirred low-fat Strawberry yogurt, 8-oz. container	250	31.3
White Rose low-fat Strawberry yogurt, 8-oz. container	250	31.3
Breakstone parfait low-fat Strawberry yogurt, 8-oz. container	260	32.5
Dannon low-fat Strawberry yogurt, 8-oz. container	260	32.5
Knudsen Fruit-On-The-Bottom low-fat Strawberry yogurt, 8-oz. container	260	32.5
Knudsen Yogurt Plus low-fat Strawberry yogurt with Granola, 8-oz. container	260	32.5
Lucerne (Safeway) low-fat Strawberry yogurt, 8-oz. container	260	32.5
Breyers whole milk Strawberry yogurt, 8-oz. container	270	33.8
Knudsen low-fat Strawberry Daiquiri yogurt, 8-oz. container	270	33.8
Light n' Lively low-fat Strawberry Banana yogurt, 8-oz. container	260	32.5
Light n' Lively low-fat Strawberry Fruit Cup yogurt, 8-oz. container	250	31.3
Meadow Gold Western sundae style skim milk Strawberry yogurt, 8-oz. container	270	33.8
Zausners low-fat Strawberry with Cottage Cheese yogurt, 12-oz. container	276	23.0
Maya whole milk Strawberry yogurt, 8-oz. container	280	35.0

Since so many of the calories in a fruit-flavored yogurt come from the fruit flavoring, why not flavor it yourself? You can buy the plain yogurt of your choice, and mix in preserves to taste—if preserves are what you fancy. I would make a strong recommendation that you try mixing in a reduced-sugar fruit spread—Smucker's makes Apricot, Blackberry, Cherry, Strawberry, and others.

And of course, you can mix plain yogurt with fresh fruit.

Or eat your yogurt "frozen." Frozen yogurt is not simply a colder version of "What's in This Chapter." The formulation is different. Most frozen yogurts will have considerably fewer calories than their softer counterparts.

	Calories per Cup
Boysenberry Hard Frozen Yogurt, Dannon Danny-In-A-Cup	210
Boysenberry low-fat yogurt, Dannon	302
Piña Colada Frozen Yogurt, Colombo	220
Piña Colada whole milk yogurt, Colombo	279

How does yogurt compare with the other possibilities in **Frozen Confections**—ice cream, ice milk, sherbet, and ices?

	Calories per Cup
Caramel Nut Ice Milk, Light n' Lively	240
Caramel Nut Low-Fat Yogurt, Ralph's	256
Cherry Vanilla Ice Cream, Sealtest	260
Cherry Low-fat Yogurt, Lucerne	302
Coffee Ice Milk, Light n' Lively	200
Coffee Low-fat Yogurt, Dannon	233
Coffee Ice Cream, Häagen-Dazs	517
White Lemon Ice, Popsicle	187
Lemon Sherbet, Le Sorbet	192
Lemon Chiffon Ice Milk, Light n' Lively	240
Lemon Parfait Low-fat Yogurt, Breakstone's	296
Orange Sherbet, Meadow Gold	240
Mandarin Orange, Meadow Gold Western Sundae style skim milk yogurt	302
Peach Ice Cream, Breyers	260
Peach Whole Milk Yogurt, Breyers	314

And here's how yogurt generally compares with **Gelatins, Puddings & Custards:**

	Calories per Cup
Banana-Strawberry whole milk Yogurt, Colombo	273
Banana Pudding, Royal Regular	320
Cherry-Coconut low-fat yogurt, Lucerne	302
Coconut Cream Pudding, Jell-O Instant	360
Creamy Coffee whole milk yogurt, Brown Cow Farm	268
Coffee Pudding, Royal Instant	360

	Calories per Cup
Raspberry flavored gelatin, Jell-O	160
*Red Raspberry pre-stirred low-fat yogurt, Knudsen	290
Vanilla-Honey whole milk yogurt, Colombo	291
baked custard (USDA home recipe)	305

How does yogurt compare with cottage cheese?

Based on USDA data, unless specified:	Calories per 8-Ounce Container
plain whole milk yogurt (3.3% fat)	139
creamed cottage cheese (4.51% fat)	232
plain low-fat yogurt (1.55% fat)	144
low-fat cottage cheese (1% fat)	164
low-fat cottage cheese (2% fat)	205
Cottage Cheese with Dutch Apple, Friendship	248
Spiced Apple Fruit-On-The-Bottom low-fat yogurt, Knudsen	250
Dutch Apple low-fat yogurt, Dannon	260

And finally, how does yogurt compare with sour cream and mayonnaise?

Based on USDA data:	Calories per 8-Ounce Container
skim milk yogurt (0.18% fat)	127
whole milk yogurt (3.25% fat)	139
low-fat yogurt (1.55% fat)	144
sour cream	485
mayonnaise	1629

So whether or not yogurt is a high-calorie food depends on the company it keeps. Compared to **Frozen Confections,** it doesn't always fare well. Compared to mayonnaise, it's a godsend.

28 CONDIMENTS

What is a condiment? The *Webster's New Collegiate Dictionary* defines a condiment as "something used to enhance the flavor of food, esp: a pungent seasoning."

What's in This Chapter are foods that are very different, one from the other. As you can imagine, any chapter that contains pickles, mayonnaise, and croutons is more likely to be united by use than by composition. But they all have one thing in common: they're used to add relish to food.

What we have in this chapter are foods that go on top and to the side: pickles, olives, and relishes; potato salad and cole slaw; mustard, catsup, and horseradish; sauces; salad dressing (and salad dressing, and salad dressing, and more and more salad dressing); and salad toppings—croutons, bacon bits, and grated cheese. . . .

What's Related, but Elsewhere: One closely related chapter is **Basic Baking & Cooking Ingredients** with its marinades and seasoning mixes; its coating mixes and extenders; its bread-crumbs and a list of croutons, identical to this chapter's.

There are sauces in **Basic Baking & Cooking Ingredients.** A sauce is more likely to be there than here if:

1. It is used more commonly in cooking than at the table
2. It is applied hot rather than cold
3. It is served with a ladle, rather than a teaspoon

But these are not hard and fast rules. So if it's not in **Condiments,** try the *Sauces and Gravies* section of **Basic Baking & Cooking Ingredients**—especially if the word "Sauce" appears as part of the name.

Salts & Spices, the whole of it, is a related chapter. The whole of **Sugars, Sweeteners & Toppings** is related. **Confitures** are all related. **Hors D'Oeuvres, Dips & Spreads** are two-thirds related.

Fats & Oils are first cousins to salad dressings; **Soups** are first cousins to sauces.

Gelatins, when used for aspic rings, are fine examples of "things on the side." All sides.

The Arrangement of This Chapter Is:

How to Read the Numbers: The column headings are:

Unit
One Ounce by Weight

One Cup
One Tablespoon

This is one chapter where the Unit is thoroughly non-standardized—a jar of pickles and one pickle, a can of jumbo olives and one jumbo olive, a bottle of salad dressing or a teaspoon of bacon bits.

The Ounce by Weight column, however, is thoroughly standardized. It is also likely to be the most accurate column in this chapter. You may not know whether your olive is Jumbo or Colossal, but if a scale tells you how many ounces of olive you have, this column will tell you how many calories you have.

The One Cup and One Tablespoon columns both describe condiments measured by volume. The cup is a kitchen measuring cup. The tablespoon is a kitchen measuring tablespoon, not merely a table implement. Similarly, when a teaspoon is given as the Unit, it is a kitchen measuring teaspoon—not the flatware from a table setting.

How to Eat Things to the Side: For olives, the calories will vary with the ripeness and the type, but mostly the calories will depend on the fashion in which the olive is preserved. If it's cured in oil, you're eating oil.

If you like pickles, a sour pickle is as low-calorie a condiment as you could ask for. Fourteen calories for a large one. I mean, you can actually have a sour pickle for fewer calories than a cucumber! (Apparently, some of the carbohydrate is lost to the pickling water.)

For pickles and for relishes, the calories come from carbohydrate. There will be big differences between the "sweet" and the "sour." Sweet pickles have about fifteen times the calories of sour pickles. Yet that doesn't necessarily mean you should avoid them. Sweet pickles are lower in calories per ounce, for example, than cranberry sauce—and some people would say that an ounce of sweet pickle goes farther, besides.

For cole slaw and similar salads, the calories are in what's holding it together. The calories come from the glue. Potato salad, of course, is mostly potatoes. Yet most of the calories will come from the mayonnaise. Do you know how much potato you can have for one tablespoon of mayonnaise? Guess.

You can have an entire 5-ounce potato for one tablespoon of mayonnaise.

The following list is an assortment of pickles, relishes, and side salads. Here's how they look, in ascending caloric order:

Based on USDA data, unless specified:	**Calories per Ounce**
Cocktail Onions, Crosse & Blackwell	0.6
Kosher Pickles, Claussen	3.7
sauerkraut	5.1
Pimientos, Dromedary	10.0
Cucumber and Yogurt Salad (Middle East)	10.5
Cucumber Relish, Featherweight	10.6
unsweetened applesauce	11.6
Bread and Butter Pickles, Fanning's	13.6
Sweet-Sour Red Cabbage, Greenwood	20.3
Three-Bean Salad, Green Giant	21.3
Pickled Beets, Blue Boy	23.5
applesauce, sweetened	25.8
potato salad	28.1 to 41.1
Artichoke Hearts in Oil, Cara Mia	29.0
Three Bean Salad, Hanover	31.3
coleslaw	36.6
sweet pickle relish	39.1
Cranberry Sauce, Ocean Spray	45.0
cranberry-orange relish	50.5

Further on the subject of pickles and relishes, I should say that we don't have Heinz. They refused to assist me through four years' worth of telephone calls and request letters. Sorry, readers, I did my best.

How to Eat Things on Top: When it comes to the sauces in this chapter, most of them are used in small quantity. A discussion of one sauce versus another is not simply a discussion of calories per ounce. It's calories per "use." Even mayonnaise at 101 calories a tablespoon wouldn't have such an impact if you could use it in a small enough quantity.

I will give you an example. There's hardly a food in this book that can compete with Chinese hot oil for calories per ounce—250.4. But if you've ever tasted Chinese hot oil you'll know that an evening's worth of hot oil is bound to have fewer calories than an evening's worth of green beans.

Here's what the sauces and so forth look like, ranked strictly on the basis of calories per tablespoon. (Notice that hot oil is the last on the list.)

Based on USDA data, unless specified:	**Calories per Tablespoon**
Tabasco Sauce	2
cider vinegar	2
distilled vinegar	2
chili sauce	3
lemon juice	4
Horseradish, Gold's	6
Picante Sauce, Picante	6
Fish Sauce, China Bowl	8
whole milk yogurt	9
Worcestershire Sauce, Regular, French's,	10
Worcestershire Sauce, Smoky, French's	10
low-fat yogurt	10
Steak Sauce, A-1	12
yellow mustard	12
soy sauce	12
brown mustard	14
Oyster Sauce, China Bowl	16
catsup	18
Seafood Cocktail Sauce, Smithers	18
Steak Sauce, Steak Supreme	20
Taco Sauce, Ortega	22
Sweet and Sour Sauce, La Choy	28
imitation sour cream	30
sour cream	31
Plum Duck Sauce, China Bowl	38
Horseradish Sauce, Kraft	50
Avocado Sauce, Nickabood's Fisherman's Wharf	68
Big H Burger Sauce, Hellmann's	70
Tiger Sauce, Tulkoff's	70
tartar sauce	74
mayonnaise	101
butter	102
margarine	102
Hot Oil, China Bowl	120

Another kind of "sauce" that goes on top is salad dressing. The calories in salad dressing come from oil, plain and simple. If you use mayonnaise, it's the oil content of the mayonnaise. The range of calories for dressing is enormous:

	Range of Calories per Tablespoon for Salad Dressings Sold by Brand
Italian dressing	2.0–90.0
Russian dressing	4.0–81.0
French dressing	4.0–90.0
oil & vinegar dressing	6.0–70.0
blue or bleu cheese dressing	4.0–90.0
Thousand Island dressing	12.0–75.0
garlic dressing	14.0–90.0
Caesar salad dressing	10.6–80.0
green goddess dressing	51.2–80.0
mayonnaise	101.0

So you'll find salad dressings at 2 calories per tablespoon, and others at 90 calories per tablespoon. Putting it another way, you can have an entire 8-ounce bottle of Kraft's Low-Calorie Italian Dressing for two tablespoons of Kraft's Creamy Italian Dressing.

If you do use an imitation salad dressing, the taste will pretty much depend on how well they've managed to imitate the character of the oil or mayonnaise. And that will be a matter of preference, not just a matter of reading the numbers. I'm tempted to say, "Don't start a diet 'til you find a diet salad dressing that you like."

But don't rush out now to buy a "dietetic" dressing—not until you read this: The dressings intended as mayonnaise substitutes, though usually lower in calories than mayonnaise, are often higher in calories than regular salad dressings!

	Calories per Tablespoon
Tillie Lewis Tasti-Diet Low Calorie May-Lo-Naise	25
Mrs. Filbert's Imitation Mayonnaise	40
Weight Watchers Imitation Mayonnaise	40
Spredlite (Batter-Lite) Mayonnaise	44
Bright Day Imitation Mayonnaise Dressing	60
Saffola Imitation Mayonnaise	60
Hain Eggless Imitation Mayonnaise	85
Hollywood Eggfree Mayonnaise	85
Featherweight Low Sodium Soyamaise	100
Dia-Mel Mayonnaise	106

And as long as we're looking at salad dressings, let's look at salad toppings and seasonings:

	Calories per Ounce
Salad Lift, French's	47.3
No Sugar, No Oils, Sourdough Croutons, Pioneer	70.0
Salad Seasoning, Durkee	76.8
"Something Better than Croutons," NSB	88.9
Bacon Bits, Oscar Mayer	91.4
Imitation Bacon Crumbles, French's	106.3
Salad Crunchies, NSB	120.0
most prepackaged croutons	130.0–140.0
fresh grated Parmesan cheese	132.4
Imitation Bacon Bits, Durkee	139.6
Bac-Os, General Mills	147.7

But here again, the calories per ounce are only one side of the calorie coin. For a discourse on the virtues of grated Parmesan cheese—even at 132.4 calories an ounce—turn to the Chapter Preface for **Pasta,** page 85.

In this chapter it is certainly true that differences in flavor will, in some cases, more than counterbalance apparent differences in calories. As with the example of hot oil, you can not always look to the calories "per ounce" or "per tablespoon" as the one definitive guide. If two tablespoons of Italian Dressing—at 81.1 calories each—suit your personal taste as well as three tablespoons of French Dressing—at 64.1 calories each—you can save over 30 calories by choosing the Italian (although either choice has more calories than two pounds of iceberg lettuce).

29 SALTY SNACKS

What are salty snacks?/What's in This Chapter: Potato chips, corn chips, taco chips, tortilla chips, plantain chips, sesame chips, and yogurt chips. You'd think this was Las Vegas.

What's also in this chapter is an abundance of pretzels and popcorn.

What's Related, but Elsewhere: Dozens of salty snacks are not here. They have their own separate chapter—**Nuts & Seeds.**

Samplings from **Salty Snacks** are in the **Hor D' Oeuvres** chapter, and it's there that you'll find the dips and spreads that potato chips accompany.

Pretzels for babies are in **Baby Foods.** There are vended pretzels that are not in **Salty Snacks,** but in **Vending.** Goldfish Pretzels are in **Cookies & Crackers.**

In fact, all the crackers of **Cookies & Crackers** are pre-eminently related, and so are the candies in **Sweet Little Nothings.** This chapter is the "salty little nothings."

The Arrangement of This Chapter is a continuous alphabetical list, with major collections at:

How to Read the Numbers: The column headings are:

Entire Package
One Piece
One Quart
One Ounce by Weight

The Unit column will usually refer to a bag, but it also might be a box or a canister. In this chapter the Unit column takes on added importance, because salty snacks are often eaten by the bagful.

But there's a problem with the numbers in the Unit column.

The 8-ounce bag of Bachman Caramel Corn that I purchased weighed, in fact, 9 ounces. Wise's 4-ounce Natural Flavor Rippled Potato Chips weighed 4½. Frito Lay's 1¾-ounce bag of Chee · tos weighed in at 2 ounces.

Since I was not able to obtain and personally weigh every salty snack in this chapter, each value in the Unit column was calculated as though the bag held what the label says it does. This makes the Unit column reliably unreliable. Look to the Ounce for your most accurate numbers.

The second column of figures is for "One Piece," and it addresses the single potato chip or pretzel. Very appropriate. In its initial draft stages, this chapter's title was "Well, Just One . . ."

The Quart column, on the other hand, might seem a bit odd. "A quart of potato chips, please"??

The quart wasn't put in this chapter for measuring, although it can be used in that way. It's here for visualizing. A quart is the closest thing we have to a party bowl.

All of the One Quart figures and all of the One Piece figures are averages calculated by weighing, measuring, and counting the contents of dozens of bagfuls of chips.

The "One Piece" figure is about as inexact a number as you will find in this book. Pieces from the same bag are entirely different in size and weight. Then too, there were whole chips, broken chips, and chips stuck together like Siamese twins. All of these pieces were counted equally as "1." But when does a "small piece" become a "large crumb"?

In spite of this lack of homogeneity, if you eat a quantity of pieces, these variations should average out. In weighing sample lots of 25 pieces each, there was a gratifying consistency among them.

How to Eat Salty Snacks: All the foods in this chapter are high in calories, there's no doubt about it. But if you want to eat from this chapter, you have the opportunity to save a lot of calories by your selection. There's no doubt about that either. And the reason becomes clear as we ask our first question. Where do the calories come from?

Salty Snacks are starchy foods, and there's no way around that. What you do have control over are the calories from fat. Pretzels get most of their calories from carbohydrate. Pretzels are about 111 calories an ounce. Potato chips get their calories from carbohydrate and fat. Potato chips are about 150 calories an ounce. Eat pretzels instead of potato chips and save 39 calories an ounce.

Corn chips and popcorn both start out as corn. Popcorn is about 110 calories an ounce. Corn chips are about 160. The numbers speak for themselves.

Salty Snacks gives the impression of being a chapter where, once you know the basic principles, you can do pretty well without the book. To some extent this is true—potato chips are predictably a third higher in calories than pretzels, and pretzels run neck and neck with popcorn popped in air. Still, in a chapter filled with so many fanciful foods, you're not just choosing between popcorn and potato chips any more.

Can you guess the relative calories by looking at the names?

	Calories per Ounce
Cheez Waffles, Old London	140.0
Cheez Doodles, Old London	160.0
Corn Nuggets, Frito Lay	128.0
Corn Diggers, Nabisco	150.0
Corn Crunchies, Wise	160.0
Potato Chipsters, Nabisco	130.0
Potato Chips, Wise	150.0
Ridgies Rippled Potato Chips, Wise	170.0

And who would guess by their names that Chiffle's Plantain Chips would be 176 calories an ounce, and that Baken-ets' Pork Rinds would be only 150?

Still, if you're choosing chips without this book in hand there are a few guidelines you can follow.

Looking through the data pages you'll see that many snacks with the word "cheese" in their title are high in calories per ounce:

	Calories per Ounce
Cheese 'N Crunch, Nabisco	160.0
Cheez Doodles, Baked, Old London	160.0
Cheez Doodles Crunchy, Fried, Old London	160.0
Flings Cheese Flavored Curls, Nabisco	160.0
Cheese Nibbles, Granny Goose	167.6
Cheese Corn, Ann Page	180.0

And, time and time again, "tortilla chips" are lower in calories than "corn chips" when you're comparing them by the ounce:

		Calories per Ounce
Bachman:	Taco Flavor Tortilla Chips	138.0
	Toasted Tortilla Chips	143.0
	BBQ Corn Chips	150.0
	Indian Corn Chips	150.0
Granny Goose:	Tortilla Chips	139.8
	Barbecue Flavored Tortillas	140.3
	Stone Ground Tortillas	146.9
	American Style Corn Chips	155.4
	Corn Chips	158.8

And—time and time again—what holds true for an ounce-to-ounce comparison will not be the story when a different measurement is taken. The fact is, if what you want is a bowlful of something crunchy, then the Ounce column may not be the best place to look. Bachman's Corn Chips and Bachman's Jax Cheese Corn Twists are both 150 calories an ounce. But if you're eating them by the bowlful, just look at this:

	Calories per Ounce	Estimated Calories per Quart
Bachman's Jax Cheese Corn Twists	150	312
Bachman's Corn Chips	150	825

Why the difference by the bowl?

It's because the Corn Twists are a light, fluffy product. They're full of air. It's the same phenomenon we have in **Breakfast Cereals,** where a cup of cornflakes will weigh 1½ times as much as a cup of puffed rice. (And you thought air was just for breathing.)

In **Salty Snacks,** even more than in **Breakfast Cereals,** the variations by the bowlful are astonishing:

	Estimated Calories per Quart
Onion Flavored Rings, Wise	188
Pop Corn, Bachman	238
Jax Baked Cheese Corn Twists, Bachman	312
WheatTwists, Nacho Cheese Flavored, Spicer's	384
WheatTwists, Pizza Flavored, Spicer's	384
Twist Pretzels, Ann Page	396
Corn Diggers, Nabisco	450
Ruffles Potato Chips, Frito Lay	452
Ruffles Potato Chips, Bar-B-Q Flavor, Frito Lay	452
Barbecue Flavored Potato Chips, Wise	564
Doritos Nacho Cheese Flavor Tortilla Chips, Frito Lay	616
Baldies Pretzels, Anderson	768
Nacho Cheese Tortilla Chips, Bachman	769
Taco Flavor Tortilla Chips, Bachman	780
Potato Chips, Munchos	784
Bavarian Dutch Style Pretzels, Anderson	828
Corn Crunchies, Wise	832
Pretzel Nuggets, Wise	1032
Bavarian Thin Pretzels, Anderson	1072
Platanitas Plantain Chips, Chiffles	1180
Cheese Doodles, Wise	1244
Native American Style Corn Chips, Granny Goose	1380

You can have more than 6 quarts of Wise Onion Flavored Rings for one quart of Wise Cheese Doodles.

If you're measuring by the piece, the ratio is very different. By the piece, six Rings equal five Doodles:

	Estimated Calories per Piece
Pop Corn, Bachman	1
WheatTwists, Nacho Cheese Flavored, Spicer's	3
WheatTwists, Pizza Flavored, Spicer's	3
Corn Diggers, Nabisco	4
Onion Flavored Rings, Wise	5
Platanitas Plantain Chips, Chiffles	5
Corn Crunchies, Wise	6
Cheese Doodles, Wise	6
Jax Baked Cheese Corn Twists, Bachman	6
Ruffles Potato Chips, Frito Lay	6
Ruffles Potato Chips, Bar-B-Q Flavor, Frito Lay	6
Potato Chips, Munchos	7
Pretzel Nuggets, Wise	8
Barbecue Flavored Potato Chips, Wise	9
Doritos Nacho Cheese Flavor Tortilla Chips, Frito Lay	9
Nacho Cheese Tortilla Chips, Bachman	10
Taco Flavor Tortilla Chips, Bachman	10
Native American Style Corn Chips, Granny Goose	12
Bavarian Thin Pretzels, Anderson	22
Twist Pretzels, Ann Page	22
Baldies Pretzels, Anderson	64
Bavarian Dutch Style Pretzels, Anderson	64

Pretzels, at the lowest end in calories per ounce, are the highest in calories per piece.

Popcorn is the lowest in calories per piece, and in my opinion it's the star of this chapter. (You might say it's the movie star.) It is possible to have, for 100 calories, a bit more than a quart—yes, a bit more than a quart—of popcorn. You can sit there and eat it, and eat it, and eat it. Of course once you pour butter on, it becomes a sponge. You might as well eat potato chips.

I heartily recommend the popcorn poppers that can be used without oil. Practically all the stores have them—they're one of the appliance fads of the 80s. (After we had all bought our hair dryers, sales probably slowed down. So they mounted them slightly differently and changed the name.)

If butterless popcorn leaves you cold, you might try butter-flavored salt. Popcorn is also good with mustard. (That does it. Take her away!)

Do, but first let me tell you that practically anything in this chapter—even potato chips—will save you calories per ounce over practically anything in **Nuts & Seeds.**

Of course, you probably won't dunk your nuts in a party dip first—and dip can be hundreds of calories per cupful.

But if what you like is the dip, then dip with raw vegetables instead. The calories in the dip will remain the same, but because carrot sticks are so much thicker than potato chips you'll be eating a lot more carrot for every ounce of dip.

You can bring raw vegetables to the movies, too. They really are good substitutes for salty snacks—a tenth the calories of popcorn, even of unbuttered popcorn.

To sum up this chapter, these are high-calorie foods, all of them. There is considerable variation in calories, but also considerable consistency. The biggest variable in eating **Salty Snacks** is going to be the portion size. In contrast to an apple or a candy bar, there is often no telling just how big a "portion" of a salty snack will be—even if you do start out intending to eat "Well, just one. . . ."

30 HORS D'OEUVRES, DIPS & SPREADS

What's an hors d'oeuvre?/What's in This Chapter/What's Related, but Elsewhere: In French, it means "outside of the work." In English, as well as in French, "hors d'oeuvres" are served before and apart from the main body of the meal. Anything can be an hors d'oeuvre, and from that point of view nearly every chapter in the book is potentially related. Pineapple, salami, and cheese all become hors d'oeuvres if you add a toothpick.

The sister chapter to this one is **Salty Snacks.** In fact, sample entries from Salty Snacks—potato chips, pretzels, and popcorn—begin this chapter. There are samplings from **Nuts & Seeds,** and examples of crackers, cheese, and cold cuts. This chapter also has stuffed clams, egg rolls, shrimp rolls, pizza rolls, pickles, olives, crudités, and caviar.

We have deviled eggs and stuffed celery. These are G.I. issue and have been borrowed for the occasion from the United States Army.

Then there are the *Dips.* Baba gannuj, hummus, and tahini are in this chapter. The data come from the Middle East. The other dips are very American—Lipton's famous California onion dip, for example. Most of the dips are premixed, but others—like the onion dip—need to be blended. The principal listing for sour cream is here, in this chapter. Cream cheese, mayonnaise, and plain yogurt all have sample listings here as well.

Dips are followed by Spreads. Among them are a variety of Neufchâtel cheese spreads, deviled ham, vegetable spreads, and examples of goose- and chicken-liver pâtés.

The Arrangement of This Chapter: The arrangement of **Hors D'Oeuvres** looks like a tray of hors d'oeuvres—distinctly non-alphabetical.

Dips and *Spreads* are each alphabetical.

How to Read the Numbers: The column headings for *Hors D'Oeuvres* are:

Unit
One Ounce by Weight

One Unit may be one potato chip, one carrot stick, one egg roll, one fig.

For *Dips* and *Spreads* the column headings are:

Unit
One Ounce by Weight
One Cup
One Teaspoon

The Unit will be either an entire package or one tablespoon.

How to Eat Hors D'Oeuvres, Dips, and Spreads: For most of the Dips and Spreads, there is a large contribution of calories from fat.

But how much fat, and how many calories? One cup of Granny Goose Blue Cheese Dip is approximately 922 calories. Kraft's Blue Cheese Dip is 480. Light n' Lively Blue Cheese Dip is 360. Weight Watchers Blue Cheese Dressing and Chip Mix is 214. So the answer is that you have to look in the book.

If you manufacture the dip yourself, the first place to look is at sour cream, cream cheese, yogurt, and mayonnaise because that is where the calories are. Even a thickly flavored onion or clam dip is going to be mostly "dip," and not onions or clams:

Based on USDA data, unless specified:	**Calories per Cup**
skim-milk yogurt	139
whole milk yogurt	150
low-fat yogurt	158
half & half sour cream	320
Pasteurized Process Cream Cheese Product, Philadelphia "Light"	423
sour cream	492
Imitation Mayonnaise, Mrs. Filberts	640
cream cheese	812
mayonnaise	1580

One cup of whole milk yogurt has fewer calories than 4 tablespoons of mayonnaise. (The comparison of whole and low-fat yogurt—150 and 158 calories respectively—is not a misprint. According to the USDA, low-fat yogurt contains more milk solids than whole milk yogurt does.)

But as a practical matter, unless you design the dip yourself, the way to save calories is to use less of it—and on a carrot, not a potato chip. Skinny dipping, you might say.

When it comes to eating hors d'oeuvres, the Unit column shows just how wide a choice you have. A cubic inch of cheddar cheese is 69 calories. A blue-cheese-stuffed celery stalk has about 16 calories, and will probably take longer to eat. Certainly four blue-cheese-stuffed celery stalks will take longer to eat, and will still have fewer calories than, a cubic inch of cheese.

Perhaps more than any other chapter in this book, the foods here are impulse foods. You may go to a party having carefully thought out what you are going to eat. You may have called beforehand to ask what was going to be served. (Some readers may find this silly. Others will know exactly what I'm talking about.) In the extreme, you may even have brought your own food along. What a pity to exercise care and planning on dinner only to blow it on any Tom, Dick or Harry of an hors d'oeuvre that comes along, just because it's small.

31 ALCOHOLIC BEVERAGES

What is alcohol? *Webster's New Collegiate Dictionary* defines alcohol as:

1. A colorless volatile flammable liquid C_2H_6O that is the intoxicating agent in fermented and distilled liquors and is used as a solvent—also called ethyl alcohol.
2. Any of various compounds that are analogous to ethyl alcohol in constitution and that are hydroxyl derivatives of hydrocarbons.
3. Liquor (as whiskey) containing alcohol.

What's in This Chapter is beer, wine, liqueurs, and hard liquor. There are prepackaged cocktail mixes, and pre-mixed cocktails. Also in this chapter are garnishes, such as the olive, and mixers, such as ginger ale.

The recipes for mixed drinks will naturally vary from household to household and from bar to bar. Still, I wanted to include a sample of a Daiquiri, a sample of a Brandy Alexander, an example of a Sloe Gin Fizz. I called my friend Vincent Sardi, whose name it's a pleasure to drop, and he eagerly put me in the hands of Bartender Jack. As a result, we have sixty-four cocktails and mixed drinks as served at Sardi's.

What's Related, but Elsewhere: Cooking wine is in **Basic Baking & Cooking Ingredients** as are rum-, sherry-, and brandy-flavored extracts.

Non-alcoholic beverages are in **Beverages.**

The Arrangement of This Chapter is as follows:

How to Read the Numbers: Two column headings remain constant throughout most of the chapter:

Unit
One Fluid Ounce

For *Garnishes,* the Unit may be one olive, one cherry, one sprig of mint for the Julep. For the rest of the chapter the Unit is more likely to be a can of beer, a bottle of wine, a packet of cocktail mix. For Sardi's, the Unit column has been replaced by One Drink.

The Fluid Ounce column permits comparisons without regard to unit size.

The other column headings will vary according to the section of the chapter in which you find yourself. For *Hard Liquor* and *Cordials, Liqueurs, and Flavored Brandies,* the additional headings are:

One Jigger
One Tablespoon

The jigger reported in this chapter holds 1½ ounces. If the jigger you use is of a different size, you will not be able to apply this figure directly.

The Tablespoon, as always, is one-half of a fluid ounce. As always, it is a measuring tablespoon.

For the dry *Cocktail Mixes* there is an additional column, One Cocktail, for a drink prepared according to the label's directions.

For Sardi's cocktails and mixed drinks there are calories for the entire drink only. The Fluid Ounce column has been dropped. According to Jack's descriptions, the amount of soda water and ice is so variable the calories per ounce or per fluid ounce would be hardly more than a guess. By the ounce, calories will also depend on how much of your ice has melted by the time you finish your drink. And Jack wanted you to know that in actual practice he doesn't measure—he always mixes by feel.

How to Eat in This Chapter: Where do the calories come from? For straight hard liquor they come from alcohol, and the number of calories will depend upon the proof. The figures for gin, rum, vodka, and whiskey are given by the USDA as follows:

	Calories per Fluid Ounce
100-proof	83.0
94-proof	77.0
90-proof	74.0
86-proof	70.0
80-proof	65.0

In actual practice, there may be small calorie differences even among liquors of the same proof. To some extent, the calories will depend upon the other components that give the liquor its particular character. Pure alcohol is colorless, yet Scotch is yellow —and some brands of Scotch are yellower than others.

Most of the calories in beer and wine will also come from alcohol. But beer is a grain product, and wine is made from fruit, and so there will be a contribution from carbohydrate as well.

For mixed drinks there are the calories in the alcohol, and the rest will depend upon the mixture. When you add orange juice you're adding carbohydrate. When you add heavy cream you're adding fat.

So—How Do You Eat Drinks?

I am not an experienced drinker, yet as I look at the data pages I can't help but notice that a cocktail onion has fewer calories than an olive.

I also notice that most conventional White, Red, and Rosé dinner wines are approximately 19 to 27 calories per fluid ounce. The new light wines are lower in both calories and alcoholic content:

	Calories per Fluid Ounce
Taylor Light Rosé (alcohol content 8.6%)	17.2
Taylor Rosé (alcohol content 12.5%)	24.0
Taylor Light Chablis (alcohol content 8.2%)	15.7
Taylor Chablis (alcohol content 12.0%)	24.0

Dessert wines are higher in both alcohol content and calories than are dinner wines. Port runs as high as 48 calories per fluid ounce.

Beer has fewer calories than wine, and light beer has fewer calories still:

	Calories per Fluid Ounce
Coors Premium	12.0
Coors Light	*8.6*
Miller High Life	12.5
Miller Lite	*8.0*
Pabst Blue Ribbon	12.5
Pabst Extra Light	*5.8*

Unlike diet sodas, all of which are fairly uniform in their calories, light beers vary substantially according to the brand. In fact, the light beers listed in the data pages have a range of almost 2 to 1.

Also bound to vary among themselves are the cocktails and mixed drinks. This is how they rate per drink at Sardi's. Of course the drinks differ in size:

	Estimated Calories per Drink
Bloody Mary	86
Bull Shot	91
Mint Julep	115
Daiquiri	125
Black Russian	137
Old Fashioned	156
Sloe Gin Fizz	167
Gin and Tonic	175
Screwdriver	181
Planters Punch	184
Margarita	185
Martini	210
Irish Coffee	218
Brandy Alexander	253
Piña Colada	342

One more word about mixed drinks: I happened to mention at a social gathering that tonic water actually has more calories than ginger ale. This surprised a lot of people. I mention it here, in case it surprises you.

As I said, I'm not an experienced drinker. But I did have an experience in a bar. In a Cajun village in the bayous of Louisiana, I sought out the local watering hole in hopes of finding some water. I was astonished that out of the dozen strapping Cajun drinkers gathered at the bar, ten were drinking light beer. I wondered whether this was a calorie-related phenomenon, or perhaps some local ceremonial usage.

So I moseyed up to a man who was drinking Pabst Extra Light, sharing it sip for sip with a furry pet nutria that was sitting on his forearm. "Sir," I said, "why are you drinking light beer?"

He misunderstood my question, and replied, "My nutria is drinking light beer because his master drinks light beer."

"And why does his master drink light beer?" I pursued.

"Oh," he said, "his master drinks light beer because his master's on a diet."

32 VEGETARIAN FOODS

What is a vegetarian? The *Scribner-Bantam* defines a vegetarian as "one who eats no meat or fish, and sometimes also nothing derived from an animal, as milk or eggs."

What's in This Chapter: What's in this chapter are meatless imitations of hamburgers, sausages, bacon, corned beef, turkey, and chicken; there's meatless salami and meatless Swiss steak with gravy. I should mention that we also have Campbell's Vegetarian Vegetable Soup, but by no means does this characterize the chapter.

What's Related, but Elsewhere: Vegetables, of course. And **Fruits** and **Nuts & Seeds.** For Vegetarians who eat eggs and milk products (lacto-ovo-vegetarians) three major related chapters are **Cheese, Yogurt,** and **Eggs.** (Milk is in **Beverages.**)

The Arrangement of This Chapter: This is a very small chapter, alphabetized by brand:

How to Read the Numbers: The column headings are:

Unit
One Slice, Patty, or Piece
One Ounce by Weight
One Pound

All the basic data came from the manufacturers, usually in the form of nutrition labeling. In most cases, the labels were not explicit as to whether the numbers were for the food before or after preparation. My calculations assume that the nutrition labeling refers to the product as it is in the package. Unless otherwise specified, the calories are for the uncooked product.

For canned items, most of those packed in water have their drained weights recorded here. Many of the canned items are vacuum-packed, and thus there is no "drained" weight to list.

How to Eat Vegetarian Food: Where do the calories come from? Even without meat, you can still have a high-fat food.

This is especially true when nuts are used for the meat substitution. You might review the **Nuts & Seeds** Chapter Preface, and you'll see that these are not low-calorie foods. No way.

Ordinary hog-variety bacon is in the data pages at 168.1 calories per ounce, cooked. Morningstar Farms' Bacon-like Breakfast Strips, made without meat, are 198.2 calories an ounce, cooked. This may be a chapter to help save on cholesterol, but the calories per ounce can be whopping.

33 INFANT FORMULAS & BABY FOODS

What's an infant? What's a baby? "The Child is father of the Man" (William Wordsworth, "My Heart Leaps Up When I Behold," 1802).

What's in This Chapter: The *Infants'* section has breast milk and infant formulas. The *Strained* and *Junior Baby Foods* include meats, poultry, and vegetables, alone, and as "combination main dishes." There are sections for soups, for baked goods, for fruits and fruit juices, for puddings and custards.

There are a few international entries here—for example, Oxtail & Beef Casserole as sold in Great Britain. There are, however, no data in this chapter for the Beech-Nut, Gerber, and Heinz baby foods marketed abroad. These are made according to different formulations, even if the jars bear a familiar name.

The last section of this chapter isn't baby food at all. It's a listing of canned puréed vegetables. All of these are Featherweight brand, and are intended for people on soft diets.

What's Related, but Elsewhere: Strained and junior baby foods are practically ***THE CALORIE FACTOR*** in miniature.

The Arrangement of This Chapter is:

How to Read the Numbers: For the *Infants'* section, the column headings are:

Unit
One Fluid Ounce
One Cup
One Teaspoon

There is no One Ounce by Weight column in this section of the chapter, as information by weight was generally not provided by the manufacturers and did not lend itself to estimation. The One Teaspoon column is included because baby formula is so often mixed with dry cereal to make an infant's first solid meals.

For *Baby Foods,* the column headings are:

Unit
One Ounce by Weight
One Tablespoon
Fiber, expressed in Grams per Ounce

The Fiber column is here because it's information that I would want to have for baby food, and so I give it to you.

The calories for dry cereals are given for the unprepared state only. There will be great variation in the prepared cereal, depending on whether you're adding whole milk, non-fat milk, formula, or water.

Do be aware that babies' feeding spoons have no standard relationship to tablespoons or teaspoons. The two baby spoons that I measured held widely disparate amounts. One was roughly one-quarter of a teaspoon; the other, three times as much.

There were no fiber figures furnished for the *Puréed Vegetables,* and so the Fiber column has been replaced by One Cup.

How to Eat Infant Formulas and Baby Foods: Where do the calories come from? For breast milk and infant formulas, the calories come from protein, carbohydrate, and fat. For the meat and poultry dishes, the calories will come from fat and protein. For most of the other foods, most of the calories will come from carbohydrate.

How to eat baby foods depends on why you are eating them. To lose weight? To gain weight? To maintain weight? Because you're a baby? Whatever you're trying to accomplish, there are differences among brands of foods with similar names:

		Calories per Ounce
Strained Peaches	Heinz	13.3
Strained Peaches	Beech-Nut	20.0
Strained Peaches	Gerber	20.7
Junior Peaches	Heinz	13.3
Junior Peaches	Beech-Nut	20.0
Junior Peaches	Gerber	20.1
Strained Plums with Tapioca	Heinz	17.6
Strained Plums with Tapioca	Gerber	19.0
Strained Plums with Tapioca	Beech-Nut	20.0
Junior Sweet Potatoes	Beech-Nut	16.0
Junior Sweet Potatoes	Gerber	17.0
Junior Sweet Potatoes	Heinz	20.4
Strained Chicken & Chicken Broth	Beech-Nut	31.0
Strained Chicken & Chicken Broth	Heinz	37.7
Junior Chicken & Chicken Broth	Beech-Nut	31.0
Junior Chicken & Chicken Broth	Heinz	37.7

If you're buying prepared baby food, you may be interested in this assessment made by the USDA in 1978 in *Agriculture Handbook #8-3:*

> Since the 1963 Agriculture Handbook No. 8 was prepared, significant changes have occurred in the formulation of baby foods. The amount of added sugar has been reduced or eliminated in the fruit and dessert items, and the amount of salt has been reduced or eliminated in all food items. Monosodium glutamate, a flavor enhancer, has been removed altogether. Thus, the amount of added sodium has been reduced dramatically in processed baby foods.

Of course, you can always prepare the food yourself. Baby food can be whipped together in moments—all you need is a blender.

But the question of how to feed babies has answers that go beyond the food itself.

There are natural cycles to body weight in the ordinary course of maturing. Some babies are roly-poly before they learn to walk, and then as they walk they lose their premobile chubbiness. For some babies, movement will be a stimulant to appetite, signaling a child to eat more and perhaps to carry more weight.

The American tradition has been for round, chubby babies. There are those who speak disparagingly of this tradition, insisting that if you are corpulent as a child you are likely to have a weight problem as an adult.

Recent work on the subject questions this. It links the weight problems of adulthood with imposed dieting in childhood. Both views can be championed with sound, scientifically buttressed arguments.

I think that the best way to help your baby develop his or her own healthful pattern of eating is to: feed your baby when s/he is hungry, feed your baby as much as s/he wants to eat, never feed your baby more than s/he wants to eat. And, perhaps hardest of all—never use food as a reward nor withhold it as punishment.

34 WEIGHT LOSS AND WEIGHT GAIN PREPARATIONS, SUPPLEMENTS & BOOSTERS

What's in This Chapter are essentially special-purpose foods. They are mostly sold in health food stores. To say that these are mostly sold in health food stores describes them better in six words than I could possibly do otherwise. I would add that they are sometimes found in drugstores.

What's Related, but Elsewhere: Figurines and similar "one-bar meals," are in **Breakfast Cereals & Breakfast Breads.**

Vitamin supplements are in the **Pharmaceuticals** chapter.

The Arrangement of This Chapter is as follows:

How to Read the Numbers: The column headings throughout this chapter are:

Unit
One Ounce by Weight
One Fluid Ounce
One Cup

The Unit may be an entire can of protein powder, one tablespoon of yeast, or half a cup of Tiger's Milk.

How to Eat Weight Loss and Weight Gain Preparations, Supplements, & Boosters: I have had no personal experience with any of the foods in this chapter. If you are eating or drinking these foods, you are doing it neither on my advice nor against my advice. I list them to give you information about their calories, in a chapter of their own, without further comment.

35 PHARMACEUTICALS

What's a pharmaceutical? According to my *Webster's New International Dictionary*, the noun "pharmaceutical" means "A pharmaceutical preparation, especially a medicinal drug." *Webster's* further describes the adjectival use as "of or relating to pharmacy or pharmacists."

What's in This Chapter are products sold in drugstores. These are the tablets and capsules, the syrups and elixirs, the powders and the granules that we take for colds, headaches, indigestion, and the thousand natural shocks that flesh is heir to.

You can use this chapter not only in sickness, but in health, as the data begin with vitamins. It's thanks to the *Vitamins* section that I can say: "I give calories for Monsters in my book!" And Monsters with Iron, too.

What's Related, but Elsewhere: I suppose that the products in **Weight Loss and Weight Gain Preparations, Supplements & Boosters** are related in that they are sometimes sold in pharmacies. So are the infant formulas in Chapter 33. Aside from that, pharmaceutical products really don't relate to other chapters, except that **Sweet Little Nothings** has Life Savers, and this chapter has life savers.

The Arrangement of This Chapter is like this:

All the vitamins in the chapter are either capsules or tablets, but their special nature suggested a separate listing.

How to Read the Numbers: For *Vitamins* and for *Tablets and Capsules*, the column headings are:

Entire Bottle or Package
One Tablet or Capsule

Noticeably missing is a column for calories per ounce. An Ounce column for tablets would have been a misleading measure as these aren't sold by the ounce, or taken by the ounce. In fact, the stated weight on a bottle of medicine refers to the weight of the active ingredients only, and these are usually very small quantities within the tablet or capsule. Amnestrogen is the first drug listed in the section. One tablet is designated as .625 milligram. It would take 453.6 bottles of 100 tablets each to give you an ounce of the active ingredients.

For *Liquids—Syrups, Elixirs, Drops,* the column headings are:

Entire Bottle
One Teaspoon
One Tablespoon

Here—and your life may depend on it—it is important to remember that these are measuring spoons, not any old inhabitants of your silverware drawer.

At one point I thought about having a column for recommended dosage, but dosage instructions are more vague than specific—"Take 1 to 2 tablespoons 3 or 4 times daily." So there's no suggested dosage implied by these columns. The columns for One Teaspoon, One Tablespoon, One Tablet, and the rest are arbitrary choices for the sake of comparison.

For the *Powders and Granules,* the column headings are:

Entire Bottle
One Teaspoon
One Tablespoon
One Ounce by Weight

For *Lozenges and Cough Drops,* it's

Entire Package
One Lozenge or Cough Drop
One Ounce by Weight

How to Eat Pharmaceuticals: I received a letter from one drug manufacturer who refused to give me calorie information because, the letter read, selection of a drug should not be based on its caloric content. I assured the manufacturer that the purpose of this chapter is to inform, not to prescribe. For the serious dieter, knowing the calorie content of pharmaceuticals is important so that s/he may keep an accurate record, and compensate elsewhere if necessary.

And when it comes to selecting the form of a particular drug you are going to take, you may actually be able to exercise a calorie choice. Sumycin by Squibb is a good example. In the 250-mg dosage, a 100-capsule bottle is 61 calories. The 1,000-capsule bottle holds ten times as many capsules, and has ten times the calories, just as you would expect. But when you get up to the 500-mg capsule, something different has happened in the manufacture. There are only about one-quarter as many calories in these capsules as there are in the smaller dosage, an entire 100-capsule bottle having only 16 calories instead of 61. It could be a thinner coating, or perhaps an intrinsically less-caloric coating. The advantage of knowing this isn't so that you can take 500 mg of Sumycin instead of 250 mg. The advantage of knowing this is that if you're taking 500 mg worth anyway, you would be better off calorie-wise taking one 500-mg capsule rather than two 250-mg capsules.

There are advantages in knowing the calories for competing vitamins, too. Vitamins that have the same potency may have different amounts of sugar and starch.

The fact is that the calories in this chapter have to be respected in exactly the same way as the calories in a Milky Way have to be respected. I found that out for myself with a month's worth of Coca-Cola syrup. That story starts on page 18.

36 · PET FOODS

What is a pet? The *Scribner-Bantam Dictionary* describes a pet as a "tame animal, kept, treated kindly, and played with."

What's in This Chapter are foods sold for consumption by animals who commonly share the family home. And some who don't. If you are going to put your whole family on a diet, this chapter is the icing on the cake.

During the time that I was dieting, I noticed that my cat, Samantha, also needed to lose weight. While I was able to take measures for myself, I was helpless when it came to Sam. Hence, this chapter.

What's Not in This Chapter: I don't have grass for people's pet sheep, and I don't have tin cans for people's pet goats. Neither do I have garbage for people's pet hogs. If you want to put your cow on a diet, I recommend that you get a copy of *Composition of Cereal Grains & Forages,* Publication 585 of The National Academy of Sciences, Washington, D.C.

What's Related, but Elsewhere: Practically everything in every other chapter gets fed to cats and dogs, from baby foods to candy bars and ice cream—at least to some people's cats and dogs.

The Arrangement of This Chapter is by animal:

How to Read the Numbers: The first thing to say about how to read the numbers in this chapter, even before we talk about the column headings, is that you cannot use the calorie figures from other chapters for your pets. If your cat or dog is fed table scraps, please be aware that those numbers are based on human metabolism. In fact, even foods in this chapter may yield different calories for different species of animals. Thus the calories for cat food may apply only to cats; the calories for dog food may apply only to dogs. The same holds true for feeding lions and tigers and bears, oh my!

The column headings in this chapter are Unit and One Ounce by Weight.

The Unit will almost always be an entire can or package, but it might occasionally be a cup—or a day's recommended feeding portion.

How to Feed Pet Food: The usual way to influence a cat or dog to lose weight is to feed it less. This method doesn't work well with human beings, at least with adult human beings, because a hungry person will just go out and get more.

There is an alternative to feeding your pet less, once you are aware of the calories. There are calorie differences among brands, and there are differences among flavors within the same brand.

Dry pet foods will generally have more calories per ounce, because of their lower moisture content. But the calories per feeding are a different story, because once water gets added to dry food the calories per ounce go down.

For non-domestic animals the feeds listed in the data pages are most often supplementary to a diet that may also include fresh fruits or meats. For some animals, fresh foods predominate. Koala bears must have their fresh eucalyptus leaves, and platypuses their earthworms. There are species of birds and bats that eat only fruit, and most reptiles in captivity eat fruit and freshly killed mice.

Monkeys, true to their image, really do love bananas. And if you own a monkey, I have a message for you. The gentleman from Purina was anxious lest monkey-owning readers be misled. He emphasized that if a monkey is presented with its full recommended daily feeding at one time, it will become so excited that half of the food will be freely distributed around the room. He suggested that feeding the monkey half of its daily portion twice a day would be more economical.

37 FAST FOOD

What is fast food? *Scribner-Bantam:* fast'-food' adj specializing in the speedy preparation and service of hamburgers and the like

Webster's Collegiate: fast-food\fas(t)-fud\adj: specializing in the rapid preparation and service of food (as hamburgers or fried chicken) <a ~ restaurant chain>

There was no listing in the *Oxford.*

What's in This Chapter is McDonald's and McDonald's competitors.

What's Related, but Elsewhere: For a list of chapters related to this one, turn to ***THE CALORIE FACTOR***'s Table of Contents, and that's it.

The Arrangement of This Chapter is by vendor.

How to Read the Numbers: The two column headings are Unit and One Ounce by Weight.

The Unit is usually, but not always, a single serving. One hamburger. One order of French fries. One milk shake. One dessert. Sometimes the Unit is a whole meal. At Kentucky Fried Chicken, it may be one order of mashed potatoes, or perhaps a package intended to serve several people. (The terms "as purchased" and "edible portion" are used for Kentucky Fried Chicken to distinguish between chicken weighed on the bone and off the bone. Both of these terms are described in **Methodology** on page 34. Also note that Kentucky Fried Chicken uses the word "keel" for breast.)

In many chapters, the Units are commonly a pound or a cup or a standard-size can. Here the Units have only one thing in common: They're different.

The Ounce by Weight column provides a common denominator in this chapter as it does throughout the book.

Values for both the Unit and Ounce columns include all condiments and sauces that come on the burger or in the sandwich at the time of purchase, whether or not they are included in the description.

Just as the customer is likely to have little choice in what s/he orders, so I had little choice in which figures the fast food chains chose to disclose. If I've printed more complete information for some chains than for others, that's why.

How to Eat Fast Food:

James James
Morrison Morrison

Weatherby George Dupree
Took great
Care of his Mother,
Though he was only three.
James James
Said to his Mother,
"Mother," he said, said he:
"You must never go down to the end of the town,
if you don't go down with me."

James James
Morrison's Mother
Put on a golden gown,
James James
Morrison's Mother
Drove to the end of the town.
James James
Morrison's Mother
Said to herself, said she:
"I can get right down to the end of the town and be
back in time for tea."

King John
Put up a notice,
"LOST or STOLEN or STRAYED!
JAMES JAMES
MORRISON'S MOTHER
SEEMS TO HAVE BEEN MISLAID.
LAST SEEN
WANDERING VAGUELY:
QUITE OF HER OWN ACCORD,
SHE TRIED TO GET DOWN TO THE END
OF THE TOWN—FORTY SHILLINGS
REWARD!"

James James
Morrison Morrison
(Commonly known as Jim)
Told his
Other relations
Not to go blaming *him.*
James James
Said to his Mother,
"Mother," he said, said he:
"You must *never* go down to the end of the town
without consulting me."

James James
Morrison's mother
Hasn't been heard of since.
King John
Said he was sorry,
So did the Queen and Prince.
King John
(Somebody told me)
Said to a man he knew:
"If people go down to the end of the town, well,
what can *anyone* do?"
(Now then, very softly)
J. J.
M. M.
W. G. DuP.
Took great
C/o his M*****
Though he was only 3.
J. J.
Said to his M*****
"M*****," he said, said he:
"You-must-never-go-down-to-the-end-of-the-town-
if-you-don't-go-down-with ME!"

"Disobedience," from *When We Were Very Young,*
by A. A. Milne

You must *never* go to a Fast Food restaurant without this book.

Where do the calories in fast food come from? Fast foods are a microcosm of the American diet. The meats get top billing, and the vegetables get skimped. There's a lot of bread, pastry, ice cream, and soda, consistent with the American style. As usual, the higher-calorie foods will get their calories from fat. How do you get around the fat? You can't order your hamburger "lean"—and you can't order it "drained."

The way to order your hamburger is from this book.

And not just from the book at large, but from this very chapter. You cannot simply use the **Meats** and the **Fish** chapters when you're comparing a McDonald's hamburger with a McDonald's Filet of Fish.

The simple facts at McDonald's are that:

One: There is twice as much fat per ounce in the Fish as there is in the Hambuger.

Two: There is one and a half times as much fat per ounce in the Fish as in the Cheeseburger.

Three: There is about 41% more fat per ounce in the Fish than in the Quarter Pounder.

Four: There is 20% more fat per ounce in the Fish than in the Quarter Pounder with Cheese.

Five: It turns out that on an ounce-to-ounce basis the Filet of Fish is the highest-calorie sandwich on McDonald's menu.

Six: "You must **never** go down to the end of the town without consulting me."

If you have to make a choice without this book, are there any general principles that can be applied to fast foods? Let's see. Which one do you think is the lowest in calories per ounce within each group?

Arby's
- ☐ Ham & Cheese sandwich
- ☐ Turkey Deluxe
- ☐ Super Roast Beef

Arthur Treacher's
- ☐ Shrimp Platter
- ☐ Krunch Pup (batter-dipped hot dog)
- ☐ Krunch Pup & Chips (batter-dipped hot dog and French fries)

Burger King
- ☐ Whopper
- ☐ Whaler
- ☐ Steak Sandwich

Friendly's
- ☐ Chocolate Fribble
- ☐ Strawberry Fribble
- ☐ Vanilla Fribble

Hardee's
- ☐ Hamburger
- ☐ Fish Sandwich
- ☐ Hot Dog

Kentucky Fried Chicken
- ☐ All white meat 2-piece snack (1 rib, 1 keel)
- ☐ All dark meat 2-piece snack (1 drum, 1 thigh)
- ☐ All white meat 3-piece snack (2 ribs, 1 keel)
- ☐ All dark meat 3-piece snack (2 drums, 1 thigh)

Ponderosa
- ☐ Rib Eye & Shrimp Dinner
- ☐ T-Bone Dinner

Taco Bell
- ☐ Taco
- ☐ Tostada
- ☐ Burrito Supreme

ANSWERS:

When it comes to Turkey versus Roast Beef versus Ham & Cheese at a Fast Food Restaurant, there's nothing in this book that can tell you which will be lower in calories, except the number printed next to the name.

At Arby's, the Super Roast Beef is the winner at 63.6 calories per ounce, with Ham & Cheese a close second at 69.1. Turkey Deluxe is the highest-calorie sandwich on the entire menu, at 85.0 calories per ounce.

At Arthur Treacher's, the Krunch Pup is the highest at 101.5 calories per ounce. This batter-dipped hot dog is so high in calories that even French fries will bring the calories per ounce down. The Krunch Pup with fries is 82.0 calories per ounce. As high as that is, it's lower-calorie than the Shrimp Platter, which is 94.2.

At Burger King, the Whaler (which is not made from whales, but is a fish sandwich) is highest at 76.3 calories per ounce. The Steak Sandwich is lowest at 69.8 per ounce. The Whopper is in the middle, at 72.0.

At Friendly's, the Chocolate Fribble is lower-calorie than the Vanilla, at 39.9 and 42.7 calories per ounce, respectively. The Strawberry Fribble is the same as Vanilla.

At Hardee's, the Fish Sandwich, at 91.8 calories per ounce, is the highest. So what's new? The Hamburger is 78.2 and the Hot Dog is 82.4.

At Kentucky Fried Chicken, here are the results: the 2-piece white-meat snack is lowest, at 76.1 calories per ounce of edible portion, followed closely by the 3-piece dark-meat snack at 76.8 and the 2-piece dark-meat snack at 78.5. The 3-piece white-meat is 88.8. So neither white meat nor dark meat is the winner.

I don't want to leave the Colonel behind without mentioning his mashed potatoes. They're half the calories per ounce of everybody else's French fries. As of this writing, mashed potatoes are not available at most fast food stops. So this is a good place to remind you of them.

At Ponderosa, the Prime Rib Dinner is 31.8 calories per ounce; the Rib Eye & Shrimp dinner is 34.3.

At Taco Bell, the Taco has 63.5 calories per ounce. The Burrito Supreme is 57.6. The Tostada gotta 36.8.

About the only general rule to follow when you're eating fast food is that, time and time again, fried fish is sky-high by the ounce.

But the discussion of the Big Mac versus the Whopper versus Fried Fish cannot end with calories per ounce. These foods are eaten by the serving.

Hear ye, hear ye! Will all competitors please re-take their positions at the post! Now, which has the lowest calories per serving?

Arby's
- ☐ Ham & Cheese sandwich
- ☐ Turkey Deluxe
- ☐ Super Roast Beef

Arthur Treacher's
- ☐ Shrimp Platter
- ☐ Krunch Pup (batter-dipped hot dog)
- ☐ Krunch Pup & Chips (batter-dipped hot dog and French fries)

Burger King
- ☐ Whopper
- ☐ Whaler
- ☐ Steak Sandwich

Friendly's
- ☐ Chocolate Fribble
- ☐ Strawberry Fribble
- ☐ Vanilla Fribble

Hardee's
- ☐ Hamburger
- ☐ Fish Sandwich
- ☐ Hot Dog

Kentucky Fried Chicken
- ☐ All white meat 2-piece snack (1 rib, 1 keel)
- ☐ All dark meat 2-piece snack (1 drum, 1 thigh)
- ☐ All white meat 3-piece snack (2 ribs, 1 keel)
- ☐ All dark meat 3-piece snack (2 drums, 1 thigh)

Ponderosa
- ☐ Rib Eye & Shrimp Dinner
- ☐ T-Bone Dinner

Taco Bell
- ☐ Taco
- ☐ Tostada
- ☐ Burrito Supreme

Now we'll find the tables have turned, at least for some of the entries.

Arby's: The Super Roast Beef, which was lowest by the ounce, is highest at 620 calories per sandwich—but at 9.75 oz., that's quite a sandwich! Turkey Deluxe (6 oz.) is now in second place at 510, with Ham & Cheese (5.5 oz.) lowest of the three at 380.

Arthur Treacher's: The Krunch Pup alone (2 oz.) is 203 calories. The Krunch Pup & Chips (5 oz.) is 410. The Shrimp Platter (7.4 oz.) is the highest at 697.

Burger King: Now the Steak Sandwich is your best bet at 600 calories for 8.6 oz. The Whaler, at 8.65 oz., is 660. The Whopper at 9.2 oz. is 680.

Friendly's: The Fribbles line up this way: The Chocolate, which is lowest in calories per ounce, is the heaviest Fribble at 11.7 oz. —but it's still the lowest in calories per serving, at 420. The Vanilla and the Strawberry are both 11 oz., and both have 470 calories.

Hardee's: The Hamburger, at 3.9 oz., is 305 calories. The Hot Dog, at 4.2 oz., is 346. The Fish Sandwich, at 5.1 oz, is 468. So at Hardee's, these entries keep their relative positions.

At Kentucky Fried Chicken it is no surprise that the two 2-piece snacks are lower in calories than their 3-piece counterparts. The 2-piece dark-meat snack has forged into the lead, at 463 calories, compared to 525 calories for the 2-piece white-meat contestant. Being smaller—and lower in calories per ounce—the 3-piece dark-meat snack at 599 calories is substantially lower than the 817 calories of the 3-piece white-meat.

Ponderosa: The Prime Rib Dinner, which is 20.5 oz., has 653 calories. The Rib Eye & Shrimp Dinner, which is 22.3 oz., has 765.

At Taco Bell, the numbers tell that the Tostada is still in first place for lowest calories. It's 179 calories for 4.9 oz. The Taco is only 2.9 oz., and has 186. Burrito Supreme is 457 calories for 7.9 oz.

So what's the answer? The answer is that there is no answer except to look in the book.

"You must ***never*** go down to the end of the town without consulting me."

38 VENDING MACHINES

What are vending machines? Sub-stations of the Automat.

What's in This Chapter are peanut butter crackers and potato chips, and one-dish meals like Dinty Moore's Beef Stew, all in their special vended sizes. Vending machines used to be candy and soda. Now they're soup to nuts.

What's Related, but Elsewhere: Lots of chapters provide foods for vending machines, that's obvious. What may not be so obvious is that, functionally, nearly every chapter is related to **Vending Machines** because you can always pack your own snack. You can bring a sandwich. You can pack almost anything from **Fruits** or **Yogurt.** You can carry hard boiled eggs or a piece of cheese. This is not to say that yogurt or cheese or fruit will have fewer calories than what you'd find in a vending machine—only that it will be more predictable.

The Arrangement of This Chapter is, in fact, soup to nuts:

How to Read the Numbers: The column headings for most vended products are Unit and One Ounce by Weight.

For *Beverages,* the column headings are Unit and One Fluid Ounce.

When we eat foods from this chapter, we're likely to eat the whole thing. Yet you cannot blindly trust to the Unit column, because manufacturers do change their package sizes. For sizes other than what you find here, you will have to depend on the Ounce by Weight or One Fluid Ounce column and multiply accordingly.

How to Eat Vending Machines: Vending-machine foods are important beyond their size and scope because these are impulse items. They are eaten at the point of sale; they are purchased at the point of consumption.

Vending machines are associated with high-calorie foods. For the most part that's correct, for they intentionally provide a concentrated source of fuel. But even among these high-calorie foods, there will be a choice. An ounce of pretzels is still less than an ounce of nuts.

How to eat them, really, is to refer back to the Prefaces for the chapters in which these foods occur. But there's one thing I can say for all of them. They net fewer calories if you eat them standing up.

39

AIRLINE FARE

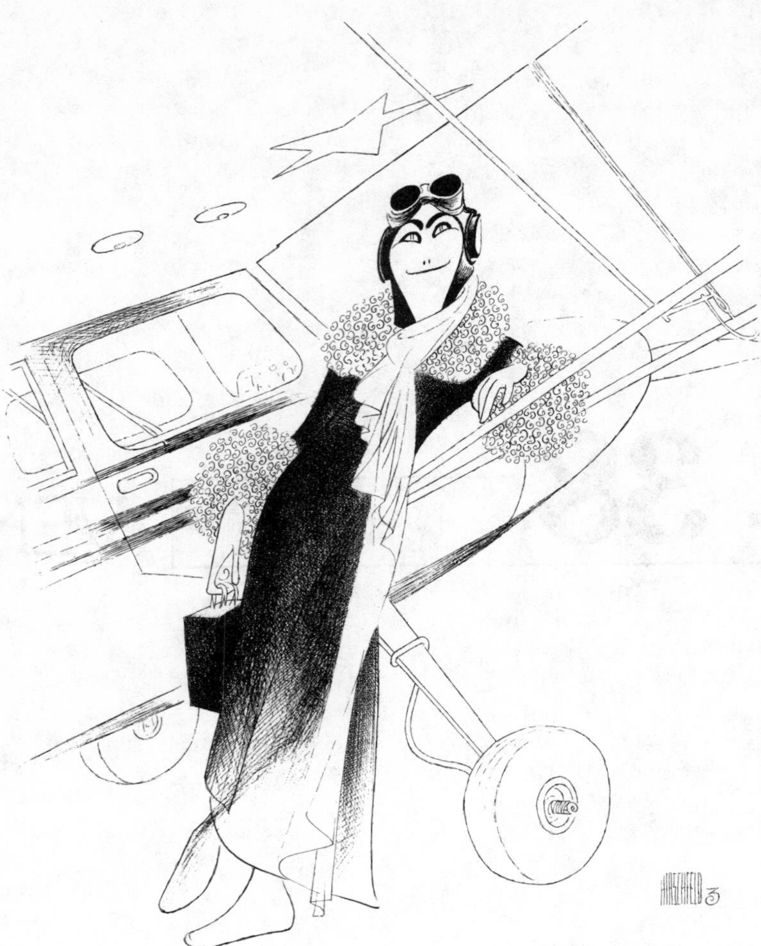

In plane geometry, a line is the shortest distance between two points. Airline Fare is what's served to us while we are trying to get from point A to point B on the earth's surface following an air line.

What's in This Chapter are the analyses of meals and snacks served on Braniff International, Lufthansa, Pan Am, TAP, and United Airlines.

What's in This Chapter Preface, in "How to Eat Airline Fare," is a list of 68 airlines with descriptions of the special meals that you can order. (If ordering a special meal is important to you, please check with the airline rather than hoping that this list is absolutely current.)

What's Related, but Elsewhere: What's related to **Airline Fare** is everything under the sun.

The Arrangement of This Chapter is alphabetical by airline:

How to Read the Numbers: There's only one column heading for this chapter, and that's the Unit.

In almost every instance, the Unit is "one serving." The exceptions are for Pan Am—and there you will find, in addition, the calories for the entire recipe. Pan Am's "Bird of Paradise," for example, starts off with 600 pounds of chicken and 65 gallons of chicken stock, seasoned with 4 gallons of soy sauce, 15 pounds of sugar, and 30 pounds of water chestnuts. It serves 1,800 passengers.

Almost all of the calories listed in the chapter are estimates, indicated as they usually are—by parentheses. Sometimes I was able to get calorie data directly from the airlines, but most often I was able to get hold of only the recipes. These numbers are my calculations based on those recipes.

Sometimes the numbers will include a premeasured portion of bread and butter, and sometimes I had no way of knowing how much bread was served with the meal. Sometimes the numbers are just for the entree and sometimes the numbers also include the vegetable. So you can't say, just by glancing down the Unit column, that one airline's menu is higher or lower in calories than another's. In this chapter you're talking about entirely different components.

The normal "leveler" of these differences—the Ounce column—does not appear in this chapter. The weight of these meals could not have been calculated accurately. To get an Ounce column, I would have had to send people up in airplanes with scales. Next edition.

How to Eat Airline Fare: Where the calories come from is going to depend on what's being served. What you may not know is that most airlines give you a choice, if you plan ahead. A list of airlines follows, with the alternative meals that are available and how much advance notice is needed to order them.

But there are some points to make beforehand, and the most important one is this: The meals that are designated as low-calorie may have more calories than regular in-flight meals!

This insight derives from the detailed figures that Braniff was so kind as to provide. Braniff was the only airline that presented the details for their special-diet meals. The numbers are shocking.

Based on estimations calculated from Braniff's recipes, their

Low-Calorie Lunch or Dinner had 557 calories. But the regular Beef Dinner had only 208 calories without the dessert; 307 calories with the fresh fruit dessert; or 342 with the brownie. Braniff's regular Seafood Platter had only 250 calories, and the Fresh Fruit Platter is estimated at between 164 and 205. Braniff's regular Fish Dinner had 408 calories including the brownie, or 288 calories without dessert. All were substantially lower in calories than the "Low-Calorie" meal. The Low-Carbohydrate Dinner also had fewer calories than the Low-Calorie Dinner, in fact about half. (As an aside, the Low-Carbohydrate Dinner had more than double the carbohydrates of the Fish Dinner.)

As an alternative to airline food, you can always bring your own food on to the plane. Don't forget to bring the popcorn for movie flights.

It's particularly important to carry with you any food or beverage that is essential. You cannot assume, as I once mistakenly did, that an airline will have sugar substitute on board. I had a fight with a man thousands of feet in the air about this. I don't use sugar substitute now, but during the time that I was following a low-carbohydrate diet, I did. I boarded TWA, only to be told by a customer relations man who was on the flight, that "customers on TWA are expected to provide for their own special dietary needs." I might add that he was nasty when he said it. That was several years ago, and TWA now officially carries artificial sweeteners aboard all its flights. But it's something to keep in mind with any airline. If you need it, carry it with you.

Unless noted, the airlines on the list that follows say they carry artificial sweeteners on board at all times. Remember as you read this list that "Low Calorie" may not mean low-calorie!

Aer Lingus serves dinner and breakfast on all its flights across the Atlantic. Dinner is served one hour after takeoff. Meals available: Low Calorie, Low Carbohydrate, Diabetic, Low Sodium, Low Cholesterol, Vegetarian, Kosher, and Moslem. Fresh fruits will be on board for you if you request them. Aer Lingus will make up other special meals to your particulars as well, but you must order them 24 hours prior to departure. Diet soda must also be ordered in advance, but juice and club soda are always available.

Aerolineas Argentinas, see Argentine Airlines.

Aeroméxico serves meals on all international flights. Special meals include: Low Calorie, Low Carbohydrate, Diabetic, Low Sodium, Low Cholesterol, Vegetarian, Kosher, and Moslem. These should be ordered at least 24 hours before flight time. Fresh fruit and diet soda are always on board.

Aero Peru says they do not have a Low Calorie meal available, but they do have: Diabetic, Low Sodium, Low Cholesterol, Vegetarian, and Kosher meals. They seem happy to prepare special requests if you tell them what you want. Requests should be made 72 hours prior to departure.

Aero Virgin Islands does not serve meals or snacks.

Air Afrique serves the following meals upon 48 hours' notice: Low Calorie, Low Carbohydrate, Diabetic, Low Sodium, Low Cholesterol. Meals can be prepared to your specifications if the airline is given the information a week in advance. Also with a week's notice you can get Vegetarian meals, Moslem meals, Kosher meals, or a Weight Watchers meal if you describe what you want. You can request fresh fruit in advance.

Air Bahama serves no food.

Air Canada offers only snacks—such as hero sandwiches. Snacks for the following diets are available with 24 hours' notice: Low Calorie, Diabetic, Low Sodium, Low Cholesterol, Vegetarian, Kosher, Moslem, Gluten-free, and Mormon. Diet sodas are on board, but not fresh fruit.

Air Florida serves cold snacks such as jelly sandwiches and salad. No special meals are available.

Air France serves dinner and breakfast over the Atlantic. Dinner is served 1½ hours after takeoff, and a continental breakfast one hour before you arrive in Paris. Meals available include: Low Calorie, Diabetic, Low Sodium, Vegetarian, and Kosher. These special meals can be ordered up to 24 hours in advance. Fresh fruit is always on board.

Air India serves meals on all its flights departing from JFK. Dinner is served 1½ hours after takeoff. Continental breakfast is served 45 minutes before landing. The following special meals are available: Low Calorie, Low Carbohydrate, Diabetic, Low Sodium, Low Cholesterol, Vegetarian, Kosher, and Moslem. Other special meals, including Weight Watchers, can be requested; give them at least 1 day's notice. Fruit will be provided if requested beforehand for "medical reasons."

Air Jamaica does not have a Low Calorie meal, but will provide: Diabetic, Vegetarian, Salt-free Vegetarian, Kosher, Bland, and Hindu meals. They will also honor other special food requests that are necessary to a diet. Fresh fruit will be available if requested beforehand. Special meals should be requested 3 days prior to departure, but orders placed 24 hours before will be accommodated.

Air Maroc, see Royal Air Maroc.

Air Mexico, see Aeroméxico.

Air New Zealand serves meals on all of its flights out of Los Angeles. Practically any food request will be honored with 24 hours' advance notice. Special meals include: Low Calorie, Low Carbohydrate, Diabetic, Low Sodium, Low Cholesterol, Vegetarian, Kosher, and Moslem. Weight Watchers meals will also be prepared if you tell them what you want. Fresh fruit can be requested beforehand.

Air Panama serves dinner on its 6 P.M. Miami–Panama flight. With 72 hours' notice (18 to 24 hours in a pinch) they will make the following special meals available: Low Calorie, Low Carbohydrate, Diabetic, Low Sodium, Low Cholesterol, Vegetarian, Kosher. Fresh fruit may also be ordered. Diet sodas are available.

Air Paraguay serves meals on all flights. Special meals available are: Low Calorie, Low Carbohydrate, Diabetic, Low Sodium, Low Cholesterol, Vegetarian, Kosher, or "anything." Just tell them 24 hours in advance. Fresh fruit and diet soda are always on hand.

Alaska Airlines serves meals on all flights. The following special meals are available: Low Calorie, Low Carbohydrate, Diabetic, Low Sodium, Vegetarian, Kosher, and Children's. Special meals should be requested at least 24 hours before departure. Fresh fruit is available in first class only. Tab diet soda is available.

Alitalia Airlines serves dinner, a snack, and breakfast on all its flights to Europe. The following special meals are available: Low Calorie, Low Carbohydrate, Diabetic, Low Sodium, Vegetarian, Kosher, and Moslem. These should be reserved no later than 24 hours before departure. Fresh fruit available in first class only. Diet sodas are available, and juice and club soda are always on board.

ALM-Antillean Airlines serves food on all of its flights. Special meals include: Low Calorie, Diabetic, Low Sodium, Low Cholesterol, Vegetarian, Kosher, and Moslem. These should be ordered 2 or 3 days before departure, but in a pinch the order can be placed 24 hours before. Fresh fruit platters can also be made available.

Aloha Airlines does not serve meals or snacks.

American Airlines serves meals on most flights of 2 hours or more. The following special meals are available on board: Low Calorie, Low Carbohydrate, Diabetic, Low Sodium, Low Cholesterol, Lacto-Vegetarian, Kosher, Seafood, and Fresh Fruit. They need at least 6 hours' notice. Tab and Diet Pepsi are available.

Argentine Airlines serves meals on all its dinner flights. The following special meals are available: Low Calorie, Low Carbohydrate, Diabetic, Low Sodium, Low Cholesterol, Vegetarian, Kosher, and Moslem. You can also request any specific foods you would like, but all special meals should be ordered 24 hours in advance, or 9 hours in a pinch. Fresh fruit is always on board. Diet sodas should be requested beforehand.

Austrian Airlines serves meals on most flights. The following special meals are available: Low Calorie, Diabetic, Low Sodium, Vegetarian, Kosher, Moslem, Hindu, and Fruit. They need at least 24 hours' notice. Diet sodas are available.

Balair Ltd. serves meals on all flights. Special meals include: Diabetic, Low Sodium, Vegetarian, and Kosher. These should be ordered when making your reservation. Fresh fruit is available. Bring your own diet soda and artificial sweetener.

British Airways serves breakfast and dinner on its morning and evening flights to London. The following special meals are available: Low Calorie, Low Carbohydrate, Diabetic, Low Sodium, Low Cholesterol, Vegetarian, Kosher, and Moslem. Special meals must be requested at least 24 hours in advance. Fresh fruit is available in first class only. Diet soda, juice, and club soda are always on board.

British West Indian Airways serves meals on all its flights. Special meals available include: Diabetic, Low Sodium, Vegetarian, Kosher, Moslem, Hindu, Oriental, and Seafood. These must be ordered 3 to 4 days in advance. Fresh fruit is sometimes on board. Diet soda is available.

Canadian Pacific Air serves dinner on their 6:25 P.M. flight and breakfast on the 11:25 A.M. flight. The following meals are available: Low Calorie, Diabetic, Low Sodium, Low Cholesterol, Vegetarian, Kosher, and Moslem. These meals should be ordered at least 24 hours prior to departure. Fresh fruit is available in first class only. The airline suggests you bring your own artificial sweetener.

Capitol International Airways serves meals on all its flights. Diabetic, Low Sodium, Vegetarian, and Kosher meals are available. The airline needs 24 hours' notice.

Continental Airlines serves meals on all flights. The following meals are available: Low Calorie, Low Carbohydrate, Diabetic, Low Sodium, Low Cholesterol, Lacto-Vegetarian, Kosher, and Moslem. Fruit plate and cottage cheese can be requested. No artificial sweetener is carried on board.

Costa Rica Airlines serves meals on all flights. They will arrange Low Calorie, Low Carbohydrate, Diabetic, Low Sodium, Low Cholesterol, Vegetarian, Kosher, and Moslem meals, or "whatever your heart desires." Just give them 24 hours' notice. Fresh fruit can also be made available. Diet soda, juice, and club soda are on board.

Czechoslovak Airlines serves Diabetic, Low Sodium, Vegetarian, Kosher, and Moslem meals. The airline needs 24 hours to fill a special food order. Artificial sweetener may not be available on board.

Delta Airlines serves meals on most flights of 2 hours or more. The following special meals are available on request: Low Calorie, Diabetic, Low Sodium, Low Cholesterol, Vegetarian, Kosher, and Moslem. Fresh fruit can also be made available for you.

East West Airlines of Australia offers Low Calorie, Low Carbohydrate, Diabetic, Low Sodium, Vegetarian, and Kosher meals. They need 2 weeks' notice. Fresh fruit can be ordered in advance. Artificial sweetener and diet sodas must also be requested beforehand.

Eastern Airlines (Domestic & Canada) serves meals on most flights of 2 hours or more. Breakfast is served from 8 to 9 A.M., lunch from 11 A.M. to 12 noon, and dinner from 5 to 7 P.M. The following special meals are available: Low Calorie, Hypoglycemic, Diabetic, Low Sodium, Low Cholesterol, Vegetarian, and Kosher. Fresh fruit is available. The airline would like to know 24 hours in advance, but can get you a special meal with as little as 4 hours' notice.

Eastern Airlines International serves meals on most flights of 2 hours or more. Breakfast is served from 8 A.M. to 12 noon, lunch from noon to 4 P.M., and dinner from 5 to 9 P.M. The following special meals are available: Low Calorie, Diabetic, Low Sodium, Low Cholesterol, Vegetarian, and Kosher.

Ecuatoriana Airlines serves meals on all its flights. Available are Low Calorie, Low Carbohydrate, Diabetic, Low Sodium, Low Cholesterol, Vegetarian, Kosher, and Moslem meals—or "whatever you wish." But you must tell them no later than 8 hours before departure. Fresh fruit as well as diet soda should be requested in advance.

El Al Israel Airlines serves dinner 1½ hours into the flight, and breakfast 1 hour before landing. All meals are Kosher. The following special meals are available: Low Calorie, Low Carbohydrate, Diabetic, Low Sodium, Low Cholesterol, Vegetarian. Basically, any meal that you want can be ordered. But they want to know 72 hours beforehand (24 hours, if necessary). Fresh fruit can be ordered as well. Diet soda, juice, and club soda are always on board.

Egyptair serves meals on all flights. All meals are made to Moslem dietary requirements. Diabetic and Vegetarian meals can be ordered. Fresh fruit will be made available upon prior request. Special meals require at least 4 or 5 days' notice before departure.

Finnair serves meals on all international flights. The following special meals are available: Low Calorie, Low Carbohydrate, Diabetic, Low Sodium, Low Cholesterol, Vegetarian, Kosher, and Moslem. They need 24 hours' notice. Fresh fruit is available in first class only. Club soda is always available.

Hawaiian Airlines travels locally within Hawaii and does not serve meals or snacks.

Iberia Airlines of Spain serves the following special meals: Low Calorie, Low Carbohydrate, Diabetic, Low Sodium, Low

Cholesterol, Vegetarian, and Kosher. Fresh fruit can be served as a meal. Let the airline know 24 hours in advance.

Icelandair serves meals on all flights. They don't have a Low Calorie meal but you can request Diabetic, Low Sodium, Vegetarian, Kosher, Moslem, and Seafood meals. They'd like to know 24 hours in advance of flight. No fresh fruit is available. Diet soda is carried on board.

Japan Airlines serves meals on all flights. They can provide Diabetic, Low Sodium, Vegetarian, Kosher, and Moslem meals —or "whatever you want." They ask that you order 24 hours before takeoff. Fresh fruit, diet soda, and artificial sweetener should also be ordered in advance.

JAT Yugoslavia serves meals on all its flights to and from the United States. The following special meals are served: Low Calorie, Low Carbohydrate, Diabetic, Low Sodium, Vegetarian, Kosher, and Moslem. They can make any special meal you request as long as you telephone 2 weeks in advance. Fresh fruit and diet soda should also be requested ahead of time.

KLM Royal Dutch Airlines serves dinner 2 hours after departure to Europe, and 3 hours later they serve breakfast. The following special meals are served: Low Calorie, Low Carbohydrate, Diabetic, Low Sodium, Low Cholesterol, Vegetarian, Kosher, and Moslem. These meals require 24 hours' notice, and any other special meal can be requested with 72 hours' notice.

Lan-Chile serves the following special meals: Low Calorie, Low Carbohydrate, Diabetic, Low Sodium, Low Cholesterol, Vegetarian, Kosher, and Moslem. Fresh fruit can also be requested. The airline needs at least 24 hours' notice.

Polish Airlines serves meals on all flights. Special meals available are: Low Calorie, Low Carbohydrate, Diabetic, Low Sodium, Low Cholesterol, Vegetarian, Kosher, and Moslem. They need a week's notice for special meals. Fresh fruit and diet soda are always available.

Lufthansa serves meals on all its flights. Special meals available include: Low Calorie, Low Carbohydrate, Diabetic, Low Sodium, Low Cholesterol, Vegetarian, Kosher, Moslem, Seafood, and Children's. The airline needs at least 24 hours' notice. Fresh fruit, diet soda, juice, and club soda are always available.

Northwest Orient (Domestic) serves meals on most flights of 2 hours or more. The following special meals are available: Low Calorie, Diabetic, Low Sodium, Low Cholesterol, Vegetarian, Kosher, Moslem, Seafood, and Children's. You must give them 24 hours' notice. Fresh fruit must be ordered in advance. Tab diet soda, juice, and club soda are always on board.

Northwest Orient (International) serves meals on all flights. They do not have a Low Calorie meal, but they serve the following special meals: Diabetic, Salt-free, Low Cholesterol, Dairy or Non-dairy Vegetarian, Kosher, Moslem, Seafood, Bland, Children's, and Baby. Special meals must be ordered at least 24 hours beforehand. No fresh fruit is available other than what may be served with meals. Tab and Diet Pepsi, juice, and club soda are always on hand.

Olympic Airways serves meals on all its international flights. The following special meals are available: Low Calorie, Low Carbohydrate, Diabetic, Low Sodium, Low Cholesterol, Vegetarian, and Moslem. They need 24 hours' notice. Fresh fruit and diet soda can be requested in advance. Juices are always available.

Ozark Airlines serves Kosher meals on request. They would like 24 to 48 hours' notice.

Pakistan International Airlines serves meals on all flights to Europe. Special meals include: Low Calorie, Low Carbohydrate, Diabetic, Low Sodium, Low Cholesterol, Vegetarian, Kosher, and Moslem. A special meal that you request can be provided. The airline would like to know a week in advance. Fresh fruit can be made available.

Pan Am (Domestic) serves meals on flights of 2½ hours or more. The following special meals are available: Diabetic, Low Sodium, Low Cholesterol, Vegetarian, Kosher, Moslem, Hindu, Oriental, Seafood, Bland, and a Fruit platter. They need 24 hours' notice. Fresh fruit is always on board.

Pan Am (International) serves meals on all its flights to Europe. They do not have a Low Calorie meal, but the following special meals are available: Diabetic, Low Sodium, Low Cholesterol, Non-dairy Vegetarian, Kosher, and Moslem. They need 24 hours' notice for special meals. Fresh fruit is not available. Diet soda, juice, and club soda are always on board.

Philippine Airlines serves meals on all flights. Special meals that can be requested are: Low Calorie, Low Carbohydrate, Diabetic, Low Sodium, Low Cholesterol, Vegetarian, Kosher, and Moslem. They would like a week's notice. Fruit is on board in first class and can be ordered on coach flights. Diet soda is available.

Piedmont Airlines serves meals on some flights depending on destination. Low Calorie, Diabetic, Low Sodium, and Kosher special meals can be requested but you must let them know at least 24 hours ahead of time. Fresh fruit can be ordered as well. Diet soda is available on board.

Qantas Airways serves meals on all its international flights. Special meals available are: Low Calorie, Low Carbohydrate, Diabetic, Low Sodium, Low Cholesterol, Vegetarian, Kosher, Moslem, or "anything." They need a minimum of 24 hours' notice. Fresh fruit, and Diet 7-Up and Shasta are always on hand.

Royal Air Maroc serves meals on all flights. Special meals available are: Low Calorie, Low Carbohydrate, Diabetic, Low Sodium, Low Cholesterol, Vegetarian, Kosher, and Moslem. They require 24 hours' notice for special meals. Fresh fruit is on board for first class, and can be ordered in coach. Diet soda should be ordered in advance.

Sabena Belgian World Airlines serves meals on all overseas flights. They'll serve the following special meals: Low Calorie, Low Carbohydrate, Diabetic, Low Sodium, Low Cholesterol, Vegetarian, Kosher, and Moslem; 1 week's advance notice is required. Fresh fruit and diet soda should be requested ahead of time.

Scandinavian Airlines serves meals on all transatlantic flights. Special meals they'll serve include: Low Calorie, Low Carbohydrate, Diabetic, Low Sodium, Low Cholesterol, Vegetarian, Kosher, Moslem, and "almost anything can be arranged." Four days' to a week's notice is required. Ask for fresh fruit or diet soda in advance.

Singapore Airlines serves meals on all flights. Low Calorie, Low Cholesterol, Diabetic, Low Sodium, Low Carbohydrate, Vegetarian, Kosher, Moslem, "any special meal" can be ordered. They'd like a minimum of 48 hours' notice for special meals. Fresh fruit can be ordered as well.

Swissair serves dinner on its evening flights to Europe. The following special meals are available: Low Calorie, Low Carbohydrate, Diabetic, Low Sodium, Low Cholesterol, Vegetarian, Kosher, and Moslem. These must be ordered at least 24 hours in advance of departure. Fresh fruit is always on board, as is diet soda.

TAP Airlines of Portugal serves meals on all flights. They can provide: Low Calorie, Low Carbohydrate, Diabetic, Low Sodium, Low Cholesterol, Vegetarian, Kosher, Moslem, Hindu, Oriental, Seafood, and Baby special meals. Special orders should be placed 24 hours in advance of flight. Fresh fruit can be specially ordered. Diet soda is not available.

Thai Airways International serves meals on all its flights. The following special meals are available: Low Calorie, Low Carbohydrate, Diabetic, Low Sodium, Low Cholesterol, Vegetarian, Kosher, Moslem, Seafood, and Children's. Special meals must be ordered at least 4 days before departure. Fresh fruit and diet soda are always on board.

TWA serves meals on all flights. Low Calorie, Low Carbohydrate, Diabetic, Low Sodium, Low Cholesterol, Vegetarian, Kosher, Moslem, Seafood, and Children's special meals are available. Special meals should be ordered 8 days prior to departure. Fresh fruit may be on board depending on the flight, but it can't be specially ordered. You may request diet soda at the airport just before leaving.

United Airlines serves meals on all its flights. Special meals available are: Low Calorie, Diabetic, Low Sodium, Vegetarian, Kosher, and Children's. Special meal orders must be placed at least 24 hours in advance. Fresh fruit is not available. Tab, juices, and club soda are always on board.

Varig Brazilian Airlines serves meals on its breakfast and dinner flights. You can request Diabetic, Low Sodium, Vegetarian, Kosher, Moslem, or any other special foods that you eat. They need 24 hours' advance notice of any special diet. Fresh fruit can also be ordered beforehand. They carry Tab on board.

Viasa Venezuelan International Airways serves meals on all flights. They serve special meals: Low Calorie, Low Carbohydrate, Diabetic, Low Sodium, Low Cholesterol, Vegetarian, and Kosher. They require a week's notice for special meals. Fresh fruit can be specially ordered. Diet soda is available.

World Airways serves meals on London and Frankfurt flights. No special meals are available, but "California Fruit Plate" is one of the menu selections. Diet 7-Up is available.

40 CAMPERS' FOODS

What's a camper? My *Webster's* defines camper as "one that camps."

What's in This Chapter are dry mixes that, when reconstituted, become breakfast foods, dinners with meat, meatless dinners, soups, vegetables, beverages, fruits, and even brownies.

The only brand represented in this chapter is Seidel's Trail Packets.

What's Related, but Elsewhere: There are dried foods in **Soups, Beverages,** and **Fruits.** But, what with variations in taste, and in styles of camping, practically anything anywhere in this book could be a camper's food.

The Arrangement of This Chapter is as follows:

How to Read the Numbers: The column headings for this chapter are:

Entire Package
One Ounce by Weight
One Suggested Portion
One Cup

The Entire Package column will always refer to a package of four portions. So if you have a different package size, be guided accordingly.

The Ounce by Weight column contains pairs of very different numbers. The point of bringing along foods in dry form is that they weigh less than the reconstituted product, whether it's a cereal, a vegetable, a dessert, or a drink. The calorie figure for One Ounce on the line that describes the four-portion pack, dry, will be substantially higher than the One Ounce figure for the reconstituted single portion.

In this chapter, the Suggested Portion is always exactly one-quarter of the entire package. The Suggested Portion is probably more carefully observed for campers' food than, for example, the suggested portion in **Cakes.** A cake mix manufacturer may suggest a serving of "one-twelfth" of the cake, but in actual practice —even if twelve people are sharing the cake—it's unlikely that they will all take slices of equal size. The exigencies of camping are such that a package that is intended to serve four will probably be used to serve four equally.

The One Cup column, like the Suggested Portion column, relates only to the reconstituted product. The Cup, as always, is a measuring cup of 8 fluid ounces.

If the suggestions for reconstitution are not followed exactly, the Cup and Ounce figures will be inaccurate, but the Suggested Portion figures won't be affected. Thus, although the Ounce and the Cup may be the most appropriate columns for comparison with other chapters, the Suggested Portion column may actually be the most reliable one in this chapter.

How to Eat Campers' Food: You eat what you brought with you, and then carry the wrappings out of the woods. Please.

• 41 • MESS—THE ARMY

What's in This Chapter are dishes that are served around the world to our uniformed service men and women. I put this chapter in the book for interest, and I put it in the book for fun, but really, an awful lot of people are eating this food. The Army, in fact, used to be the largest server of meats to Americans. Now, it's McDonald's.

Included in this chapter are the recipes that the Army uses—always for one hundred servings of the dish. The recipe for Pound Cake calls for 30 fresh eggs and 4 pounds of granulated sugar. You look at the quantity of ingredients, and they look enormous. But if you consider that, in the course of a year, you are likely to eat a hundred servings of something that you particularly like—that's only twice a week—then this chapter can well demonstrate how making the relatively small, relatively minor adjustments at the one-serving level will have a substantial impact.

What's Related, but Elsewhere: Nearly everything relates to **Mess**, I guess.

The Arrangement of This Chapter is as follows:

How to Read the Numbers: First off the bat, I have to say that the Army did not give me these recipes. I got them from Major "X." All the calories in this chapter were calculated by applying appropriate values for each of the ingredients. The column headings are Entire Recipe and One Serving.

The Entire Recipe is always for One Hundred servings.

There are no columns in this chapter for an ounce by weight, or for a cup.

How Not to Read the Numbers: When you read these numbers, please don't assume that the recipes will reflect the calories in any other recipe of the same name. For example, look at the Army's Chili Con Carne. There are 24 pounds of ground beef in it for every 8 pounds of beans—a ratio of 3-to-1. That is going to be one meaty chili. You'll find that Uncle Sam has more meat per bean in his recipe than Betty Crocker has in hers. You should be aware of this for comparison purposes.

Or take Uncle Sam's Beefburgers. The recipe starts off with 30 pounds of ground beef and a gallon of breadcrumbs. The Cheeseburgers start off with the same 30 pounds of ground beef, breadcrumbs, etc., and are served with 12½ pounds of processed Cheddar cheese. That's almost one ounce of cheese to every two ounces of meat, which is tremendously more cheese than you would ever expect to find in a restaurant. Once again, you can't look at the recipe and think it means "cheeseburgers" in general. Anyone can learn from studying this chapter: It shows the range of possibilities if you don't know what you are eating.

How to Eat in the Army, or What a Mess! Where the calories come from in the Army is naturally going to depend on which foods you are eating, but it's significant that even the peas are buttered by the time they reach you. I've heard it said that men in the Army, as they advance in rank and years, are prone to weight problems. It's not surprising. The recipes are geared for the caloric expenditure of a foot soldier.

There are always alternatives available in the mess hall, but they aren't low-calorie choices. According to one way of looking at it, the Army is really doing well by its soldiers when it puts all that meat in its chili. Certainly one can't say they are trying to skimp. Some years ago, I would have thought, "How wonderful of Uncle Samuel to do this for his nephews and nieces!" Now I'm not so sure—there was more fat in the Army's chili than in any of the chili recipes in the cookbooks I consulted. There was also a lot less fiber. Maybe it's time to rethink the Army's recipes.

42 THE BOY SCOUTS—A DAY AT CAMP PHILMONT

What's a Boy Scout? One who is clean in thought, word, and deed.

What's in This Chapter: This chapter is a calorie analysis of the first day's breakfast, lunch, and dinner at the Philmont Scout Ranch and Explorer Base in Cimarron, New Mexico. Camp Philmont is the largest Boy Scout camp in the United States.

What's Related, but Elsewhere: By ingredients, almost every chapter in the book is related; by function, any chapter in which food is served to eaters who cannot exert a choice. These include most notably **Mess** and **Airline Fare.** People eating **Foods for Space Travel** are in the same boat, so to speak.

The Arrangement of This Chapter is simple. It's Breakfast, Lunch, and Dinner.

How to Read the Numbers: The column headings are One Serving and One Ounce by Weight. Very straightforward.

How to Eat in Captivity: What is there to say when you're having a day at Camp Philmont? The Camp Philmont menu, the Army menu selections, and the foods for space travel represent a planned food intake based on the predicted calorie requirements of those eating it. These menus do not consider the person who wants to lose weight.

Still, someone at a Scout ranch doesn't have to eat everything on the plate, and certainly doesn't have to take all the bread that is allowed. And you can ask for a second serving of the mixed vegetables instead of eating the sweet potatoes. If they say "no," you can probably swap with your neighbor. If he says "no," take heart—hiking and biking and swimming are slimming.

43 FOODS FOR SPACE TRAVEL

What is space? Space is defined in the *Scribner-Bantam Dictionary* as "the limitless region beyond the earth's atmosphere containing the rest of the universe."

What's in This Chapter are foods that were developed for use on our Mercury, Gemini, and Apollo Space Missions. The problems in developing such foods were complex. There was, after all, no precedent.

In preparation for our flights into Space, there were three general theories with respect to anticipated caloric requirements.

One: That with prolonged periods of weightlessness, the calorie expenditure of the crew would be decreased—perhaps approaching the basal metabolic rate.

Two: Exactly the opposite prediction—that caloric requirements would increase because of the extra effort of working in a low-friction environment.

Three: That the caloric needs on board would essentially match those of moderately active men on Earth.

But there's no substitute for actually going out and seeing for oneself. The Skylab astronauts had their caloric intakes monitored both on the ground and in space. Their average daily preflight intake was 3128 calories. For flights lasting approximately one, two, and even three months, their average daily intake was 3130 calories. You couldn't hope for a closer equality than that.

About half of the foods carried on the early missions needed to be reconstituted before they were eaten. The other half were bite-size foods that would reconstitute in the mouth. A system of tube feeding was also developed, particularly for use outside the pressurized cabin. In other words, for use while walking in Space.

The development of nutritionally sound foods with acceptable taste took years. In addition to palatability and nutrition content, there were strict size and weight requirements. For the Gemini flights, the combined weight of food and packing was 1.7 pounds per person per day. For the Skylab, that figure rose to 4.2 pounds per person per day, but for the Space Shuttle, the weight was set at 2.9 pounds per person per day. Such constraints certainly encouraged the use of dried foods, and that was the basic approach of the American space program.

A typical breakfast for our Astronauts consisted of:

bacon squares
strawberry cereal cubes
Canadian bacon with apple sauce
chocolate pudding
orange drink

What's Related, but Elsewhere: A typical breakfast served by the Soviets on Vostok-Five consisted of:

a red caviar sandwich
coffee with milk
fresh lemons
a bon bon with vitamins

The Arrangement of This Chapter is as follows:

How to Read the Numbers: If you are using these numbers you don't need me to tell you how to read them.

How to Eat in Space: You eat what's set before you. The only alternative is to send out.

44 THREE FRUGAL REPASTS

What's in This Chapter? Air, water, and postage stamps.

What's Related, but Elsewhere is either everything or nothing, depending on how you look at it.

The Arrangement of This Chapter is alphabetical.

How to Read the Numbers: The only column heading is the Unit.

How to Eat Frugal Repasts: Where do the calories come from?

Absolutely pure water (H_2O) does not contain calories. Tap water may contain from one to five milligrams of natural organic matter per liter, which when metabolized may generate heat, i.e., calories.

Air may also be a source of these organic materials, but if there are calories in what you inhale, you exhale them too.

For postage stamps, the calories come from carbohydrate, a component of the glue. Stamps are backed with two types of adhesive, and you will see that there are differences in the calories. How to eat postage stamps is to hire someone else to do the work, or let a sponge get fat.

This is the last of the Chapter Prefaces. Venture beyond this point, and you're in **The Calorielogue.**

Good Luck!

Margo Feiden.

· PART III

THE CALORIELOGUE

1 VEGETABLES •

ALFALFA (based on data from Latin America)

	UNIT		1 OZ., BY WT.		1 CUP		Fiber per oz.
	Cal.	Carb.	Cal.	Carb.	Cal.	Carb.	(GMS.)
Tender Shoots							
RAW:							
Edible portion:							
1 pound (2g/3g/tr/83%/na)	235	43.0	14.7	2.89			0.88

AMARANTH

	UNIT		1 OZ., BY WT.		1 CUP		Fiber per oz.
	Cal.	Carb.	Cal.	Carb.	Cal.	Carb.	(GMS.)
RAW:							
As purchased [refuse: tough stems and rootlets, approx. 37%]:							
1 pound	103	18.6	6.4	1.16			
Edible portion:							
1 pound (1g/tr/2g/87%/na)	163	29.5	10.2	1.84			0.37

ARROWROOT (based on data from the Far East)

	UNIT		1 OZ., BY WT.		1 CUP		Fiber per oz.
	Cal.	Carb.	Cal.	Carb.	Cal.	Carb.	(GMS.)
RAW:							
Edible portion:							
1 pound (1g/8g/tr/67%/na)	566	133.8	35.4	8.36			0.57

ARTICHOKES

The energy value of artichokes increases during storage. In the course of time, inulin, a non-caloric substance within the artichoke, converts to sugars. This accounts for the increase in carbohydrates and therefore in calories.

	UNIT		1 OZ., BY WT.		1 CUP		Fiber per oz.
	Cal.	Carb.	Cal.	Carb.	Cal.	Carb.	(GMS.)
RAW:							
Average storage:							
As purchased [refuse: stem and inedible part of brachts and flower, approx. 60%]:							
1 pound	(94)	(17.9)	(5.9)	(1.12)			
Edible portion:							
1 pound (1g/3g/tr/86%/12mg)	(224)	(44.8)	(14.0)	(2.80)	(83)	(16.7)	(0.68)
COOKED:							
Boiled, drained:							
Freshest Artichokes:							
1 small bud or globe [refuse: stem and inedible parts of brachts and flower, approx. 60%], 8.6 oz.	(9)	(9.8)	(1.0)	(1.12)			
1 medium bud or globe [refuse: stem and inedible parts of brachts and flower, approx. 60%], 10.6 oz.	(11)	(11.9)	(1.0)	(1.12)			
1 large bud or globe [refuse: stem and inedible parts of brachts and flower, approx. 60%], 13.4 oz.	(13)	(15.0)	(1.0)	(1.12)			
1 pound [refuse: stem and inedible parts of brachts and flower, approx. 60%], (1g/3g/tr/87%/9mg)	(16)	(17.9)	(1.0)	(1.12)			
Longest stored:							
1 small bud or globe [refuse: stem and inedible parts of brachts and flower, approx. 60%], 8.6 oz.	(44)	(9.9)	(5.0)	(1.12)			
1 medium bud or globe [refuse: stem and inedible parts of brachts and flower, approx. 60%], 10.6 oz.	(53)	(11.9)	(5.0)	(1.12)			
1 large bud or globe [refuse: stem and inedible parts of brachts and flower, approx. 60%], 13.4 oz.	(67)	(15.0)	(5.0)	(1.12)			
1 pound [refuse: stem and inedible parts of brachts and flower, approx. 60%], (1g/1g/tr/87%/9mg)	(80)	(17.9)	(5.0)	(1.12)			
FROZEN, by brand:							
Birds Eye Artichoke Hearts, 9-oz. package	60	15.0	6.7	1.67	(40)	(10.0)	
Boiled, drained (yield: approx. 8½ oz.)	(60)	(15.0)	(7.1)	(1.76)	(42)	(10.5)	
1 cup (approx. 6 oz.)	(42)	(10.5)	(7.1)	(1.76)	(42)	(10.5)	
JARRED, by brand:							
Cara Mia Marinated Artichoke Hearts in oil, 6-oz. jar	(174)	(6.6)	(29.0)	(1.10)			

ARTICHOKES, JERUSALEM (also called Sunchokes) are not a species of artichoke, but an entirely different plant. They are listed under J.

ARUGULA

	UNIT		1 OZ., BY WT.		1 CUP		Fiber per oz.
	Cal.	Carb.	Cal.	Carb.	Cal.	Carb.	(GMS.)
RAW:							
Edible portion:							
1 pound	(102)	(21.6)	(6.4)	(1.35)			

ASPARAGUS

	UNIT		1 OZ., BY WT.		1 CUP		Fiber per oz.
	Cal.	Carb.	Cal.	Carb.	Cal.	Carb.	(GMS.)
RAW:							
As purchased [refuse: butt ends, approx. 44%]:							
1 pound	66	12.7	4.1	0.79			
Edible portion:							
1 cup, cut spears (approx. 4¾ oz.)	35	6.0	7.4	1.41	35	6.0	0.20
1 pound (approx. 3⅓ cups) (1g/1g/tr/92%/1mg)	118	22.7	7.4	1.41	35	6.8	0.20

	UNIT		1 OZ., BY WT.		1 CUP		Fiber per oz. (GMS.)
	Cal.	Carb.	Cal.	Carb.	Cal.	Carb.	
COOKED:							
Boiled, drained:							
1 spear:							
Small, 3/8" diameter at base (approx. 1/3 oz.)	2	0.3	5.7	1.01			0.20
Medium, 1/2" diameter at base (approx. 1/2 oz.)	3	0.5	5.7	1.01			0.20
Large, 3/4"–7/8" diameter at base (approx. 0.9 oz.)	5	0.9	5.7	1.01			0.20
1 cup							
Whole (approx. 6 1/3 oz.)	36	6.5	5.7	1.01	36	6.5	0.20
Cut pieces, 1 1/2–2" in length (approx. 5.1 oz.)	29	5.2	5.7	1.01	29	5.2	0.20
1 pound (approx. 2.5–3.1 cups)	91	16.3	5.7	1.01			0.20
Steamed:							
1 pound of raw asparagus, steamed (yield: approx. 14.9 oz.)	(118)	(22.7)	(7.9)	(1.53)			(0.22)
1 pound of steamed asparagus	(126)	(24.5)	(7.9)	(1.53)			(0.22)
FROZEN, by brand:							
Birds Eye Cut Asparagus, 10-oz. package	75	9.0	7.6	0.91			
Boiled, drained (yield: approx. 8 oz.)	(75)	(9.0)	(9.4)	(1.13)	(56)	(6.8)	
Jumbo Asparagus Spears, 10-oz. package	75	9.0	7.6	0.91			
Boiled, drained (yield: approx. 9 1/2 oz.)	(75)	(9.0)	(7.9)	(0.95)	(47)	(5.7)	
Seabrook Farms Asparagus Cuts & Tips, 10-oz. package	75	12.0	7.5	1.20			
Boiled, drained (yield: approx. 9 1/2 oz.)	(75)	(12.0)	(7.9)	(1.26)	(48)	(7.7)	
Asparagus Spears, 10-oz. package	75	12.0	7.5	1.20			
Boiled, drained (yield: approx. 9 1/2 oz.)	(75)	(12.0)	(7.9)	(1.26)	(45)	(7.1)	
Jumbo Asparagus Spears, 10-oz. package	75	12.0	7.5	1.20			
Boiled, drained (yield: approx. 9 1/2 oz.)	(75)	(12.0)	(7.9)	(1.26)	(45)	(7.1)	
Stouffer's Asparagus Soufflé, 12-oz. package	345	24.0	28.8	2.00			
CANNED, by brand:							
A & P Cut All Green Asparagus Spears, 14 1/2-oz. can	70	10.6	4.8	0.73	40	6.2	
Drained solids (yield: approx. 8.6 oz.)	(54)	(7.0)	(6.3)	(0.81)	(52)	(6.7)	
Balanced All Green Asparagus Cuts and Tips, packed in water, without added sugar or salt, 8-oz. can	(34)	(5.7)	(4.2)	(0.71)	35	6.0	
Drained solids (yield: approx. 5 oz.)	(24)	(3.5)	(5.0)	(0.72)	(42)	(6.1)	
Del Monte All Green Asparagus Spears and Tips, 8-oz. can	35	6.0	4.4	0.75	35	6.0	
Drained solids (yield: approx. 5 oz.)	(26)	(3.9)	(5.2)	(0.78)	(43)	(6.5)	
Green Tipped and White Asparagus Spears, 10 1/2-oz. can	46	9.1	4.4	0.87	35	7.0	
Drained solids (yield: approx. 6 1/2 oz.)	(33)	(6.5)	(5.2)	(1.03)	(43)	(8.5)	
Diet Delight All Green Asparagus Cut Spears, packed in water, low sodium, without added salt, 8-oz. can	32	4.0	4.0	0.50	(32)	(4.0)	
Drained solids (yield: approx. 4.7 oz.)	(23)	(2.2)	(4.6)	(0.44)	(38)	(3.7)	
Featherweight Cut Asparagus, no salt or sugar added, 8-oz. can	(32)	(6.0)	(4.0)	(0.75)	(34)	(6.3)	
Drained solids (yield: approx. 4.7 oz.)	(22)	(4.1)	(4.6)	(0.85)	(38)	(7.1)	
Green Giant Cut Asparagus Spears, 15-oz. can	64	7.2	4.3	0.48	40	5.0	
Drained solids (yield: approx. 8.9 oz.)	(46)	(3.0)	(5.1)	(0.33)	(42)	(2.7)	
Kounty Kist Cut Asparagus Spears, 14-oz. can	60	6.8	4.3	0.48	40	5.0	
Drained solids (yield: approx. 8.4 oz.)	(43)	(2.9)	(5.1)	(0.35)	(42)	(2.9)	
Stokely Cut All Green Asparagus Spears, 8-oz. can	38	5.7	4.7	0.71	40	6.0	
Drained solids (yield: approx. 4.7 oz.)	(28)	(3.4)	(6.0)	(0.72)	(49)	(5.9)	
10 1/2-oz. can	49	7.4	4.7	0.71	40	6.0	
Drained solids (yield: approx. 6.2 oz.)	(37)	(4.5)	(8.0)	(0.72)	(49)	(5.9)	
14 1/2-oz. can	68	10.3	4.7	0.71	40	6.0	
Drained solids (yield: approx. 8 1/2 oz.)	(51)	(6.1)	(6.0)	(0.72)	(49)	(5.9)	
JARRED, by brand:							
Featherweight Asparagus Purée, low sodium, 16 1/2-oz. jar	(100)	(14.0)	(6.1)	(0.85)	50	7.0	

AUBERGINE, see EGGPLANT

AVOCADO

	UNIT		1 OZ., BY WT.		1 CUP		Fiber per oz. (GMS.)
	Cal.	Carb.	Cal.	Carb.	Cal.	Carb.	
CALIFORNIA GROWN							
Primarily Fuerte, marketed in mid- and late winter:							
RAW:							
As purchased [refuse: seed and skin, approx. 24%]:							
1 medium avocado, 3 1/3" diameter (approx. 10 oz.)	369	12.9	36.9	1.30			
1 pound (approx. 1 2/3 medium avocados)	590	20.8	36.9	1.30			
Halved [refuse: skin, approx. 10%]:							
1 half of a medium avocado served in its skin (approx. 4 1/4 oz.)	185	6.6	43.5	1.55			
Edible portion:							
1 medium avocado (approx. 7.6 oz.)	369	12.9	48.6	1.70			0.43
1 cup:							
Cubed, 1/2" cubes (approx. 0.7 medium avocados, 5.3 oz.)	257	9.0	48.6	1.70	257	9.0	0.43
Pureed, mashed, or sieved (approx. 1.1 medium avocados, 8.1 oz.)	393	13.8	48.6	1.70	393	13.8	0.43
1 pound (approx. 3 cups cubed or 2 cups pureed, mashed, or sieved, 2.1 medium avocados) (1g/2g/5g/74%/1mg)	778	27.2	48.6	1.70			0.43
FLORIDA GROWN							
Marketed in late summer and fall:							
RAW:							
As purchased [refuse: seed and skin, approx. 33%]:							
1 medium avocado, 3 5/8" diameter (approx. 1 lb.)	389	26.7	24.3	1.67			
1 pound (approx. 1 medium avocado)	389	26.7	24.3	1.67			
Halved [refuse: skin, approx. 15%]:							
1 half of a medium avocado served in its skin (approx. 6.3 oz.)	196	13.5	31.1	2.14			
Edible portion:							
1 medium avocado (approx. 10.7 oz.)	389	26.7	36.2	2.49			(0.43)
1 cup:							
Cubed, 1/2" cubes (approx. 1/2 medium avocado, 5.3 oz.)	192	13.2	36.2	2.49	192	13.2	(0.43)
Pureed, mashed, or sieved (approx. 3/4 medium avocado, 8.1 oz.)	294	20.2	36.2	2.49	294	20.2	(0.43)
1 pound (approx. 3 cups cubed or 2 cups pureed, mashed, or sieved, 1 1/2 medium avocados) (tr/2g/3g/78%/1mg)	579	39.8	36.2	2.49			(0.43)
HAWAIIAN GROWN							
Beardslee Avocado							
RAW:							
As purchased [refuse: skin and seeds, approx. 35%]:							
1 small avocado (approx. 18 oz.)	778	19.4	42.9	1.07			
1 medium avocado (approx. 22 oz.)	942	23.4	42.9	1.07			
1 large avocado (approx. 27 oz.)	1160	28.9	42.9	1.07			
Edible portion:							
1 small avocado (approx. 11.8 oz.)	778	19.4	66.0	1.64			0.33
1 medium avocado (approx. 14.1 oz.)	942	23.4	66.0	1.64			0.33
1 large avocado (approx. 17.6 oz.)	1160	28.9	66.0	1.64			0.33
1 cup							
Cubed, 1/2" cubes (approx. 5.3 oz.)	350	8.7	66.0	1.64	350	8.7	0.33
Pureed, mashed, or sieved (approx. 8.1 oz.)	535	13.3	66.0	1.64	535	13.3	0.33
1 pound (approx. 3 cups cubed or 2 cups pureed, mashed, or sieved) (tr/2g/7g/67%/na)	1056	26.2	66.0	1.64			0.33
Hulumanu Avocado							
RAW:							
As purchased [refuse: skin and seed, approx. 24%]:							
1 medium avocado (approx. 20.6 oz.)	458	25.3	22.2	1.23			
Edible portion:							
1 medium avocado (approx. 15.7 oz.)	458	25.3	29.2	1.61			

	UNIT		1 OZ., BY WT.		1 CUP		Fiber per oz.
	Cal.	Carb.	Cal.	Carb.	Cal.	Carb.	(GMS.)
1 pound (approx. 2 cups cubed, or 3 cups pureed, mashed, or sieved, 1.1 medium avocados)	467	25.8	29.2	1.61			
Kahaluu Avocado							
RAW:							
As purchased [refuse: skin and seed, approx. 25%]:							
1 small avocado (approx. 12.3 oz.)	580	14.6	47.0	1.18			
1 medium avocado (approx. 14.3 oz.)	672	16.9	47.0	1.18			
1 large avocado (approx. 17.5 oz.)	822	20.7	47.0	1.18			
Edible portion:							
1 small avocado (approx. 9.2 oz.)	580	14.6	62.7	1.58			
1 medium avocado (approx. 10.7 oz.)	672	16.9	62.7	1.58			
1 large avocado (approx. 13.1 oz.)	822	20.7	62.7	1.58			
1 cup							
Cubed, approx., ½" cubes (approx. 5.3 oz.)	332	8.3	62.7	1.58	332	8.3	
Pureed, mashed, or sieved (approx. 8.1 oz.)	507	12.8	62.7	1.58	507	12.8	
1 pound (approx. 3 cups cubed, or 2 cups pureed, mashed, or sieved, 1.7 small, 1.5 medium, or 1.2 large avocados)	1003	25.3	62.7	1.58			
Nabal Avocado							
RAW:							
As purchased [refuse: skin and seed, approx. 30%]:							
1 medium avocado, (approx. 21.9 oz.)	908	27.5	41.5	1.25			
Edible portion:							
1 medium avocado (approx. 15.3 oz.)	908	27.5	59.3	1.79			
1 pound (approx. 1.1 medium avocados)	949	28.6	59.3	1.79			
AVERAGE OF CALIFORNIA AND FLORIDA GROWN *Figures weighted according to production, estimating 90% from California and 10% from Florida*							
RAW:							
As purchased [refuse: seed and skin, approx. 25%]:							
1 medium avocado (approx. 10⅔ oz.)	378	14.3	35.4	1.34			
1 pound (approx. 1½ medium avocados)	566	21.4	35.4	1.34			
Halved [refuse: skin, approx. 10%]:							
1 half of medium avocado served in its skin (approx. 4.4 oz.)	188	7.1	42.7	1.61			
Edible portion:							
1 medium avocado (approx. 7.9 oz.)	378	14.3	47.4	1.79			0.46
1 cup:							
Cubed, ½" cubes (approx. ⅔ medium avocado, 5.3 oz.)	251	9.5	47.4	1.79	251	9.5	0.46
Pureed, mashed, or sieved (approx. 1 medium avocado, 8.1 oz.)	384	14.5	47.4	1.79	384	14.3	0.46

BABA GHANOUJ, see under EGGPLANT

BAMBOO SHOOTS

	UNIT		1 OZ., BY WT.		1 CUP		Fiber per oz.
	Cal.	Carb.	Cal.	Carb.	Cal.	Carb.	(GMS.)
RAW:							
As purchased [refuse: sheaths, approx. 71%]:							
1 pound	36	6.8	2.3	0.43			
Edible portion							
1 cup, cut into 1" lengths (approx. 5.3 oz.)	(41)	(7.9)	7.7	1.47	(41)	(7.9)	0.20
1 pound (approx. 3 cups) (1g/1g/tr/91%/na)	123	23.6	7.7	1.47	(41)	(7.9)	0.20
CANNED, based on generic data:							
Solids and liquid:							
1 cup (approx. 8.6 oz.)	(48)	(7.3)	(5.6)	(0.86)	(48)	(7.3)	
1 pound (approx. 2 cups)	(94)	(13.8)	(5.6)	(0.86)	(48)	(7.3)	
1 can, 8½ oz. net wt.	(48)	(7.3)	(5.6)	(0.86)	(48)	(7.3)	
Drained solids:							
1 cup (approx. 5.4 oz.)	(40)	(5.2)	(7.4)	(0.98)	(40)	(5.2)	
1 pound (approx. 3 cups)	(118)	(15.7)	(7.4)	(0.98)	(40)	(5.2)	
1 can (approx. 5 oz.)	(37)	(4.9)	(7.4)	(0.98)	(40)	(5.2)	

	UNIT		1 OZ., BY WT.		1 CUP		Fiber per oz.
	Cal.	Carb.	Cal.	Carb.	Cal.	Carb.	(GMS.)
BAMBOO SHOOTS (based on data from East Asia)							
RAW:							
As purchased [refuse: sheaths, approx. 44%]:							
1 pound	71	13.5	4.4	0.84			
Edible portion:							
1 pound	127	24.0	7.9	1.50			0.34
COOKED (partly boiled):							
1 pound	91	15.8	5.7	0.99			0.34
CANNED:							
1 pound		23.5		1.47			
Pickled, 1 pound	394	25.9	24.6	1.62			0.34
DRIED:							
1 pound	862	172.0	53.9	10.75			2.10
SALTED:							
1 pound	259	43.0	16.2	2.69			0.79
STEEPED IN HOT OIL:							
1 pound	394	20.0	24.6	1.25			0.14

BAYO BEANS

	UNIT		1 OZ., BY WT.		1 CUP		Fiber per oz.
	Cal.	Carb.	Cal.	Carb.	Cal.	Carb.	(GMS.)
MATURE SEEDS, Dry							
RAW:							
1 cup (approx. 7.1 oz.)	678	122.4	96.1	17.35	678	122.4	1.25
1 pound (approx. 2.3 cups)	1538	277.6	96.1	17.35	678	122.4	1.25
COOKED:							
Boiled, drained:							
1 pound (yield from approx. 5.3 oz of raw bayo beans)	(513)	(92.5)	(32.1)	(5.78)			0.42

BEAN DISHES, MISCELLANEOUS (including Pork and Beans and Three Bean Salad)

	UNIT		1 OZ., BY WT.		1 CUP		Fiber per oz.
	Cal.	Carb.	Cal.	Carb.	Cal.	Carb.	(GMS.)
CANNED, by brand:							
Ann Page (A&P) Tender cooked Boston Style Beans with Pork and Molasses Sauce, 16-oz. (1-lb.) can	580	100.0	36.2	6.26	290	50.0	
Mexican Style Beans, 15-oz. can	431	67.5	28.7	4.50	(230)	(36.0)	
Pork and Beans in Tomato Sauce, 8-oz. can	240	42.0	30.0	5.25	(240)	(42.0)	
16-oz. (1-lb.) can	480	84.0	30.0	5.25	(240)	(42.0)	
Vegetarian Beans in Tomato Sauce, 16-oz. (1-lb.) can	460	88.0	28.8	5.50	(230)	(44.0)	
Blue Boy Chili Beans, 15.5-oz. can	499	46.0	32.2	2.97	290	26.7	
Campbell's Barbecued Beans, 15¾-oz. can	551	90.6	35.0	5.75	(276)	(45.3)	
Beans and Franks in Tomato and Molasses Sauce, 8-oz. can	370	40.0	46.3	5.00	(370)	(40.0)	
16-oz. (1-lb.) can	740	80.0	46.3	5.00	(370)	(40.0)	
Homestyle Beans, 16-oz. (1-lb.) can	600	104.0	37.5	6.50	(300)	(52.0)	
Old Fashioned Beans in Molasses and Brown Sugar Sauce, 16-oz. (1-lb.) can	580	98.0	36.3	6.13	(331)	(56.0)	
China Bowl Dried Spicy Bean Curd, 2-oz. package	262	8.4	130.7	4.22			
Bean Paste, 2½-oz. can	112	6.6	44.8	2.68			
Featherweight Bean Purée, 16-oz. (1-lb.) can	(140)	(30.0)	(8.8)	(1.88)	70	15.0	
Bean Purée, low sodium, 16-oz. (1-lb.) jar	(140)	(30.0)	(8.8)	(1.88)	70	15.0	
Green Giant Three Bean Salad, 17-oz. can	362	79.6	21.3	4.68	190	42.0	
Hanover Pork and Beans in Tomato Sauce, 28-oz. can	946	168.0	33.8	6.00	(300)	(53.1)	
40-oz. can	1352	240.0	33.8	6.00	(300)	(53.1)	
53-oz. can	1789	318.0	33.8	6.00	(300)	(53.1)	
Three Bean Salad, 8-oz. can	250	48.0	31.3	6.00	(270)	(51.0)	
52-oz. can	1628	312.0	31.3	6.00	(270)	(51.0)	
Libby's Deep Brown Pork And Beans in Molasses Sauce, 14-oz. can	(436)	(76.2)	(31.1)	(5.44)	280	49.0	
Deep Brown Pork And Beans in Tomato Sauce, 14-oz. can	(420)	(76.2)	(30.0)	(5.44)	270	49.0	
31-oz. can	(930)	(168.8)	(30.0)	(5.44)	270	49.0	
Deep Brown Vegetarian Beans in Tomato Sauce, 14-oz. can	(405)	(79.3)	(28.9)	(5.67)	260	51.0	
114-oz. can	(3295)	(646.4)	(28.9)	(5.67)	260	51.0	
Morton House Oven Baked Beans in Tomato Sauce, 16-oz. (1-lb.) can	540	90.0	33.8	5.68	(290)	(48.7)	
24-oz. can	810	135.0	33.8	5.68	(290)	(48.7)	

	UNIT Cal.	UNIT Carb.	1 OZ., BY WT. Cal.	1 OZ., BY WT. Carb.	1 CUP Cal.	1 CUP Carb.	Fiber per oz. (GMS.)
P & Q (A&P) Pork & Beans, 16-oz. (1-lb.) can	460	80.0	28.8	5.00	230	40.0	
Ralph's Chili Beans, 15-oz. can	460	76.0	30.7	5.07	230	38.0	
Great Northern Beans, 15-oz. can	330	60.0	22.0	4.00	330	60.0	
Pork & Beans, 15½-oz. can	480	100.0	31.0	6.45	240	50.0	
Vegetarian Beans, 15-oz. can	474	100.0	31.6	6.67	237	50.0	
Sultana Pork And Beans in Tomato Sauce, 52-oz. can	1560	273.0	30.0	5.25	(251)	(45.0)	
Van Camp Brown Sugar Beans, 16-oz. (1-lb.) can	611	106.4	38.2	6.65	350	61.0	
Mexican Style Chili Beans, 15½-oz. can	423	72.7	27.3	4.69	250	43.0	
Vegetarian Style Beans in Tomato Sauce, 31-oz. can	880	162.0	28.4	5.23	260	48.0	

BEAN SPROUTS, see MUNG BEAN SPROUTS

BEET GREENS

	UNIT Cal.	UNIT Carb.	1 OZ., BY WT. Cal.	1 OZ., BY WT. Carb.	1 CUP Cal.	1 CUP Carb.	Fiber per oz. (GMS.)
RAW:							
As purchased untrimmed [refuse: inedible leaves and stems, approx. 44%]:							
1 pound	61	11.7	3.8	0.73			
Edible portion:							
1 pound	109	20.9	6.8	1.30			0.40
COOKED:							
Steamed:							
1 pound of raw beet greens, steamed (yield: approx. 15.2 oz.)	109	20.9	7.2	1.38			0.42
1 pound of steamed beet greens	115	22.1	17.2	1.38			0.42

BEETROOT JUICE, see the BEVERAGES chapter

BEETS

	UNIT Cal.	UNIT Carb.	1 OZ., BY WT. Cal.	1 OZ., BY WT. Carb.	1 CUP Cal.	1 CUP Carb.	Fiber per oz. (GMS.)
RAW:							
As purchased:							
With tops [refuse: tops and parings, approx. 60%]:							
1 pound	78	18.0	4.9	1.13			
With part tops [refuse: part tops and parings, approx. 51%]:							
1 pound	96	22.0	6.0	1.38			
Without tops [refuse: parings, approx. 30%]:							
1 pound	137	31.4	8.6	1.96			
Edible portion:							
1 cup, diced (approx. 4.8 oz.)	58	13.4	12.2	2.81	58	13.4	0.23
1 pound (approx. 3.3 cups diced) (tr/3g/tr/87%/17mg)	195	44.9	12.2	2.81	58	13.4	0.23
COOKED:							
Boiled:							
1 whole beet, 2″ in diameter (approx. 1¾ oz.)	18	3.6	9.1	2.04	54	12.2	(0.17)
1 cup, sliced or diced (approx. 6 oz.)	54	12.2	9.1	2.04	54	12.2	(0.17)
1 pound (approx. 2⅔ cups sliced or diced) (tr/2g/tr/91%/12mg)	145	32.7	9.1	2.04	54	12.2	(0.17)
CANNED, based on generic data:							
Regular Pack:							
Solids and liquid:							
1 cup (approx. 8.8 oz.)	84	19.4	9.6	2.24	84	19.4	0.23
1 pound (approx. 1.8 cups)	154	35.8	9.6	2.24	84	19.4	0.23
1 #303 can, 16 oz. (1 lb.) net wt. (tr/2g/tr/90%/67mg)	154	35.8	9.6	2.24	84	19.4	0.23
Drained solids:							
1 cup (approx. 6 oz.)	63	14.9	10.5	2.49	63	14.9	0.14
1 pound (approx. 2.7 cups) (tr/2g/tr/89%/67mg)	168	39.9	10.5	2.49	63	14.9	0.14
Drained liquid:							
1 pound (approx. 1.9 cups) (tr/2g/tr/92%/67mg)	118	28.1	7.4	1.76	(61)	(14.6)	trace
Low-sodium pack:							
Solids and liquid:							
1 cup (approx. 8.7 oz.)	79	19.2	9.1	2.21	79	19.2	0.14
1 pound (approx. 1.8 cups)	145	35.4	9.1	2.21	79	19.2	0.14
1 #303 can. 16 oz. (1 lb.) net wt.	145	35.4	9.1	2.21	79	19.2	0.14
Drained solids:							
1 cup, diced (approx. 6 oz.)	63	14.8	10.5	2.47	63	14.8	0.23
1 pound (approx. 2⅔ cups)	168	39.5	10.5	2.47	63	14.8	0.23
1 #303 can, 16 oz. (1 lb.) net wt. (yield: approx. 10.4 oz.)	109	25.6	10.5	2.47	83	14.8	0.23
Drained liquid:							
1 cup (approx. 8.3 oz.)	(59)	(13.9)	7.1	1.68	(59)	(13.9)	trace
1 pound (approx. 1.9 cups)	113	26.8	7.1	1.68	(59)	(13.9)	trace
CANNED, by brand:							
A & P Sliced Beets, 8¼-oz. can	80	17.0	9.7	2.06	80	17.0	
Drained solids (yield: approx. 5.4 oz.)	(60)	(11.9)	(11.4)	(2.25)	(68)	(13.5)	
16-oz. (1-lb.) can	160	34.0	9.7	2.06	80	17.0	
Drained solids (yield: approx. 10.4 oz.)	(121)	(23.9)	(11.4)	(2.25)	(68)	(13.5)	
Balanced Sliced Beets, 8-oz. can	50	9.9	6.2	1.24	(54)	(10.8)	
Drained solid (yield: approx. 5.2 oz.)	(37)	(6.5)	(7.1)	(1.25)	(43)	(7.5)	
Blue Boy Beets, 8¼-oz. can	76	19.0	9.2	2.30	80	20.0	
Drained solid (yield: approx. 5.4 oz.)	56	13.8	10.4	2.57	65	15.9	
Harvard Beets, 16-oz. (1-lb.) can	368	84.6	23.0	5.29	200	46.0	
Drained solid (yield: approx. 10.4 oz.)	329	74.5	31.6	7.17	196	44.5	
Pickled Beets, 16-oz. (1-lb.) jar	376	84.6	23.5	5.29	200	45.0	
104-oz. can	2444	550.2	23.5	5.29	200	45.0	
Pickled Beets with Onions, 16-oz. (1-lb.) jar	376	84.6	23.5	5.29	200	45.0	
104-oz. can	2444	550.2	23.5	5.29	200	45.0	
Featherweight Sliced Beets, 8-oz. can	(80)	(20.0)	(10.0)	(2.50)	(80)	(20.0)	
Drained solids (yield: approx. 5.2 oz.)	(60)	(15.2)	(11.5)	(2.92)	(69)	(17.5)	
16-oz. (1-lb.) can	(160)	(40.0)	(10.0)	(2.50)	(80)	(20.0)	
Drained solids (yield: approx. 10.4 oz.)	(120)	(30.4)	(11.5)	(2.92)	(69)	(17.5)	
Golden Harvest Sliced Beets in Water, no sugar or salt added, 8-oz. can	80	18.0	10.0	2.25	80	18.0	
Drained solids (yield: approx. 5.2 oz.)	60	13.0	11.6	2.50	72	15.5	
Libby's Pickled Beets, 16-oz. (1-lb.) can	(278)	(68.8)	(17.4)	(4.30)	150	37.1	
Drained solids (yield: approx. 10¼ oz.)	(238)	(58.4)	(23.2)	(5.70)	(144)	(38.4)	
Shoestring Beets, 16-oz. (1-lb.) can	(93)	(22.3)	(5.8)	(1.40)	50	12.0	
Drained solids (yield: approx. 9¼ oz.)	(46)	(9.7)	(5.0)	(1.05)	(31)	(6.5)	
Whole Beets, 8¼-oz. can	(70)	(16.0)	(8.5)	(1.94)	70	16.0	
Drained solids (yield: approx. 5.5 oz.)	(51)	(11.0)	(9.3)	(2.00)	(56)	(12.0)	
Lohmann Pickled Beets, 16-oz. (1-lb.) can	250	40.0	15.6	2.50	(135)	(21.7)	
S & W Nutradiet Sliced Beets, no salt, no sugar, packed in water, 8-oz. can	70	18.0	8.8	2.30	(74)	(19.3)	
Drained solids (yield: approx. 5.2 oz.)	(50)	(13.0)	(9.6)	(2.50)	(54)	(14.0)	
Stokely Cut Beets, 16-oz. (1-lb.) can	166	35.2	10.4	2.20	90	19.0	
Drained solids (yield: approx. 10.4 oz.)	(127)	(25.1)	(12.2)	(2.41)	(73)	(14.5)	
Diced Beets, 8-oz. can	66	14.2	8.3	1.77	70	15.0	
Drained solids (yield: approx. 5.1 oz.)	(46)	(9.0)	(9.0)	(1.75)	(54)	(10.5)	
16-oz. (1-lb.) can	133	28.3	8.3	1.77	70	15.0	
Drained solids (yield: approx. 10¼ oz.)	(93)	(18.0)	(9.0)	(1.75)	(54)	(10.5)	
Sliced Beets, 8-oz. can	75	16.7	9.3	2.08	80	18.0	
Drained solids (yield: approx. 4¾ oz.)	(52)	(10.8)	(10.9)	(2.27)	(65)	(13.6)	
16-oz. (1-lb.) can	149	33.3	9.3	2.08	80	18.0	
Drained solids (yield: approx. 9½ oz.)	(103)	(21.6)	(10.9)	(2.27)	(65)	(13.6)	
Tillie Lewis "Tasti Diet" Diced Beets, 8-oz. can	70	16.0	8.8	2.00	70	16.0	
Drained solids (yield: approx. 5.1 oz.)	(50)	(10.8)	(5.1)	(2.11)	(58)	(12.7)	
Town House Fancy Pickled Sliced Beets, 16-oz. (1-lb.) can	280	68.0	17.5	4.25	280	68.0	
Drained solids (yield: approx. 10.4 oz.)	(241)	(57.9)	(23.2)	(5.57)	(144)	(34.6)	
JARRED, by brand:							
Del Monte 8¼-oz. jar	72	15.5	8.8	1.88	70	15.0	
Drained solids (yield: approx. 5½ oz.)	(53)	(10.5)	(9.7)	(1.90)	(58)	(11.4)	
Cut Beets, 16-oz. (1-lb.) jar	140	30.0	8.8	1.88	70	15.0	
Drained solids (yield: approx. 9¾ oz.)	(96)	(18.8)	(9.7)	(1.90)	(58)	(11.4)	

	UNIT Cal.	UNIT Carb.	1 OZ., BY WT. Cal.	1 OZ., BY WT. Carb.	1 CUP Cal.	1 CUP Carb.	Fiber per oz. (GMS.)
Pickled Crinkle Cut Beets, 16-oz. (1-lb.) jar	300	72.0	18.8	4.50	150	36.0	
Drained solids (yield: approx. 9¼ oz.)	(256)	(60.8)	(26.3)	(6.24)	(158)	(37.4)	
Sliced Beets, 8¼-oz. jar	72	15.5	8.8	1.88	70	15.0	
Drained solids (yield: approx. 5½ oz.)	(53)	(10.5)	(9.7)	(1.90)	(58)	(11.4)	
16-oz. (1-lb.) jar	140	30.0	8.8	1.88	70	15.0	
Drained solids (yield: approx. 9¾ oz.)	(96)	(18.8)	(9.7)	(1.90)	(58)	(11.4)	
Whole Beets, 8¼-oz. jar	72	15.5	8.8	1.88	70	15.0	
Drained solids (yield: approx. 5½ oz.)	(53)	(105)	(9.7)	(1.90)	(58)	(11.4)	
16-oz. (1-lb.) jar	140	30.0	8.8	1.88	70	15.0	
Drained solids (yield: approx. 9¾ oz.)	(96)	(18.8)	(9.7)	(1.90)	(58)	(11.4)	
Featherweight Beet Puree, low sodium, 16-oz. (1-lb.) jar	(200)	(40.0)	(12.5)	(2.50)	100	20.0	
Libby's Harvard Beets, 16-oz. (1-lb.) jar	(294)	(73.6)	(18.4)	(4.60)	160	40.0	
Drained solids (yield: approx. 10.4 oz.)	(255)	(61.0)	(24.5)	(5.87)	(147)	(35.2)	
Lohmann Pickled Beet Balls, 16-oz. (1-lb.) jar	250	50.0	15.6	3.13	(135)	(27.2)	
Drained solids (yield: approx. 10¼ oz.)	(210)	(39.6)	(20.5)	(3.86)	(123)	(23.2)	

BLACK BEANS

	UNIT Cal.	UNIT Carb.	1 OZ., BY WT. Cal.	1 OZ., BY WT. Carb.	1 CUP Cal.	1 CUP Carb.	Fiber per oz. (GMS.)
MATURE SEEDS, Dry							
RAW:							
1 cup (approx. 7.1 oz.)	678	122.4	96.1	17.35	678	122.4	1.25
1 pound (approx. 2.3 cups)	1538	277.6	96.1	17.35	678	122.4	1.25
COOKED:							
Boiled, drained: 1 pound (yield from approx. 5.3 oz. raw black beans)	(513)	(92.5)	(32.1)	(5.78)			0.42
CANNED, by brand:							
China Bowl, Fermented Black Beans, 2½-oz. can	112	6.6	44.8	2.64			

BLACK-EYE PEAS

	UNIT Cal.	UNIT Carb.	1 OZ., BY WT. Cal.	1 OZ., BY WT. Carb.	1 CUP Cal.	1 CUP Carb.	Fiber per oz. (GMS.)
MATURE SEEDS, Dry							
RAW:							
1 cup (approx. 6.0 oz.)	583	104.9	97.3	17.49	583	104.9	1.25
1 pound (approx. 2.7 cups)	1556	279.9	97.3	17.49	583	104.9	1.25
COOKED:							
Boiled, drained:							
1 cup (approx. 8.8 oz.)	(310)	(55.7)	(35.2)	(6.33)	(310)	(55.7)	0.45
1 pound (approx. 1.8 cups) (yield from approx. 5.8 oz. uncooked dry peas)	(564)	(101.2)	(35.2)	(6.33)	(310)	(55.7)	0.45
IMMATURE SEEDS							
RAW:							
1 cup (approx. 5.1 oz.)	184	31.6	36.0	6.18	184	31.6	0.51
1 pound (approx. 3.1 cups)	576	98.9	36.0	6.18	184	31.6	0.51
COOKED:							
Boiled, drained:							
1 cup (approx. 5.8 oz.)	178	29.9	30.6	5.13	178	29.9	0.43
1 pound (approx. 2.8 cups) (yield from approx. 13.6 oz. uncooked dry peas)	490	82.1	30.6	5.13	178	29.9	0.43
FROZEN, based on generic data:							
Measured when frozen:							
1 cup (approx. 5.6 oz.)	210	37.8	37.2	6.70	210	37.8	
1 pound (approx. 2.8 cups)	595	107.0	37.2	6.70	210	37.8	
1 container, 10 oz. net wt.	372	67.0	37.2	6.70	210	37.8	
Boiled, drained:							
1 cup (approx. 6.0 oz.)	221	40.0	36.9	6.66	221	40.0	
10-oz. container of frozen black-eye peas (yield: approx. 9.2 oz., 1½ cups)	338	61.1	36.9	6.66	221	40.0	
1 pound of frozen black-eye peas, boiled, drained, (approx. 14.8 oz., approx. 2½ cups)	546	98.7	36.9	6.66	221	40.0	
1 pound	590	106.6	36.9	6.66	221	40.0	
FROZEN, by brand:							
Bel-Air Black-Eye Peas, 20-oz. package	780	138.0	39.0	6.90			
Boiled, drained (yield: approx. 21.2 oz.)	(780)	(138.0)	(36.8)	(6.51)	(223)	(39.4)	
Birds Eye Black-Eye Peas, 10-oz. package	360	63.0	36.0	6.30			
Boiled, drained (yield: approx. 10.6 oz.)	(360)	(63.0)	(34.0)	(5.94)	(204)	(35.7)	
Green Giant Black-Eye Peas Southern Recipe, 10-oz. boil-in-bag	318	38.3	31.8	3.83	(280)	(32.0)	
Hopping John (a mixture of black-eye peas and rice), 10-oz. boil-in-bag	335	50.5	33.5	5.05	300	42.0	
Seabrook Farms Black-Eye Peas, 10-oz. package	390	69.0	39.0	6.90			
Boiled, drained (yield: approx. 10.6 oz.)	(390)	(69.0)	(36.8)	(6.51)	(223)	(39.4)	
Village Park Black-Eye Peas, 16-oz. (1-lb.)	600	110.0	37.5	6.88			
Boiled, drained (yield: approx. 17.0 oz.)	(600)	(110.0)	(35.4)	(6.49)	(215)	(39.3)	
CANNED, based on generic data:							
Solids and liquid:							
1 cup (approx. 9 oz.)	179	12.8	19.9	1.40	179	12.8	
1 pound (approx. 1.8 cups)	318	22.7	19.9	1.40	179	12.8	
1 #303 can, 16 oz. (1 lb.) net wt.	318	22.7	19.9	1.40	179	12.8	
CANNED, by brand:							
Ann Page (A&P) Black-Eye Peas with Pork, 15-oz. can	413	67.5	27.5	4.50	(247)	(40.5)	
Luck's Country Style Black-Eye Peas Seasoned with Pork, 17-oz. can	520	70.0	30.6	4.12	(275)	(37.1)	

BOK CHOY, see Spoon Cabbage under CABBAGE

BREADFRUIT

	UNIT Cal.	UNIT Carb.	1 OZ., BY WT. Cal.	1 OZ., BY WT. Carb.	1 CUP Cal.	1 CUP Carb.	Fiber per oz. (GMS.)
RAW:							
As purchased [refuse: skin, stem, and core, approx. 23%]:							
1 small breadfruit (approx. 4.1 oz.)	93	23.6	22.5	5.72			
1 pound	360	91.5	22.5	5.72			
Edible portion:							
1 cup, pulp (approx. 7.8 oz.)	227	57.7	29.2	7.43	227	57.7	0.341
1 pound (approx. 2.1 cups) (tr/7g/tr/71%/4mg)	467	118.9	29.2	7.43	227	57.7	0.34

BROAD BEANS

	UNIT Cal.	UNIT Carb.	1 OZ., BY WT. Cal.	1 OZ., BY WT. Carb.	1 CUP Cal.	1 CUP Carb.	Fiber per oz. (GMS.)
RAW:							
1 cup (approx. 5.1 oz.)	(152)	(25.7)	29.8	5.04	(152)	(25.7)	0.62
1 pound (approx. 3.1 cups)	476	80.7	29.8	5.04	(152)	(25.7)	0.62
COOKED:							
Boiled, drained:							
1 cup (approx. 5.8 oz.)	(147)	(24.9)	(25.3)	(4.25)	(147)	(24.9)	0.53
1 pound (approx. 2.8 cups) (yield from approx. 13.6 oz. uncooked dry beans)	(405)	(68.0)	(25.3)	(4.25)	(147)	(24.9)	0.53

BROCCOLI

	UNIT Cal.	UNIT Carb.	1 OZ., BY WT. Cal.	1 OZ., BY WT. Carb.	1 CUP Cal.	1 CUP Carb.	Fiber per oz. (GMS.)
RAW:							
As purchased untrimmed [refuse: large leaves, tough stalks, and trimmings, approx. 39%]:							
1 pound	89	16.3	5.6	1.02			
Edible portion:							
1 cup (approx. 5.5 oz.)	(50)	(9.3)	9.1	1.70	(50)	(9.3)	0.23
1 pound (approx. 2.9 cups)	145	26.8	9.1	1.70	(50)	(9.3)	0.23
COOKED:							
Boiled, drained:							
1 small stalk (approx. 4.9 oz.)	36	6.3	7.4	1.27	40	7.0	0.23
1 medium stalk (approx. 6.3 oz.)	47	8.1	7.4	1.27	40	7.0	0.23
1 large stalk (approx. 9.9 oz.)	73	12.6	7.4	1.27	40	7.0	0.23
1 pound (approx. 3.3 small stalks, 2.5 medium stalks, or 1.6 large stalks)	118	20.4	7.4	1.27	40	7.0	0.23
Cut into ½" pieces: 1 cup (approx. 5.4 oz.)	40	7.0	7.4	1.27	40	7.0	0.23
1 pound (approx. 3 cups)	118	20.4	7.4	1.27	40	7.0	0.23
Steamed:							
1 pound of raw broccoli, steamed (yield: approx. 15.2 oz.)	145	26.8	9.5	1.76			0.24
1 pound of steamed broccoli	152	28.2	9.5	1.76			0.24
FROZEN, based on generic data:							
Whole spears or stalks:							
Measured when frozen:							
1 medium stalk (approx. 4½"–5" long, 1.3 oz.)	10	1.8	7.9	1.44			0.31
1 pound (approx. 11–14 medium spears) (1g/1g/tr/91%/4mg)	127	23.1	7.9	1.44			0.31

	UNIT Cal.	UNIT Carb.	1 OZ., BY WT. Cal.	1 OZ., BY WT. Carb.	1 CUP Cal.	1 CUP Carb.	Fiber per oz. (GMS.)
1 package, 10 oz. net wt. (approx. 7–9 medium spears)	80	14.5	7.9	1.44			0.31
Boiled, drained:							
1 medium stalk	8	1.4	7.4	1.33			0.31
1 pound of boiled, drained broccoli (1g/1g/tr/91%/3mg)	118	21.3	7.4	1.33			0.31
1 10-oz. package boiled, drained (yield: approx. 8.8 oz.)	65	11.8	7.4	1.33			0.31
1 16-oz. (1-lb.) package boiled, drained (yield: approx. 14.1 oz.)	104	18.8	7.4	1.33			0.31
Chopped:							
Measured when frozen:							
1 pound (1g/1g/tr/91%/5mg)	82	14.8	8.2	1.48			0.31
1 package, 10 oz. net wt.	132	23.5	8.2	1.48			0.31
Boiled, drained:							
1 cup (approx. 6.5 oz.)	48	8.5	7.4	1.31	48	8.5	0.31
1 pound of boiled, drained broccoli (approx. 2.5 cups) (1g/1g/tr/92%/4mg)	118	20.9	7.4	1.31	48	8.5	0.31
1 package, 10 oz. net wt., boiled, drained (yield: approx. 8.8 oz.)	65	11.5	7.4	1.31	48	8.5	0.31
1 package, 16-oz. (1-lb.) net wt. boiled, drained (yield: approx. 14.1 oz.)	104	18.4	7.4	1.31	48	8.5	0.31
FROZEN, by brand:							
Bel-Air Chopped Broccoli, 10-oz. package	75	12.0	7.5	1.20			
Boiled, drained (yield: approx. 9.7 oz.)	75	12.0	7.7	1.24	51	8.2	
Broccoli Spears, 10-oz. package	100	12.0	10.0	1.20			
Boiled, drained (yield: approx. 8.9 oz.)	100	12.0	11.2	1.35	60	7.3	
Safeway Broccoli Spears, 10-oz. package	100	12.0	10.0	1.20			
Boiled, drained (yield: approx. 8.9 oz.)	(100)	(12.0)	(11.2)	(1.35)	(60)	(7.3)	
Seabrook Farms Broccoli Spears, 10-oz. package	90	12.0	9.0	1.20			
Boiled, drained (yield: approx. 8.9 oz.)	(90)	(12.0)	(10.1)	(1.35)	(66)	(8.8)	
Chopped Broccoli, 10-oz. package	75	12.0	7.5	1.20			
Boiled, drained (yield: approx. 9.7 oz.)	(75)	(12.0)	(7.7)	(1.24)	(51)	(8.2)	
Tender Broccoli Florets, 10-oz. package	90	12.0	9.0	1.20			
Boiled, drained (yield: approx. 9.7 oz.)	(90)	(12.0)	(9.3)	(1.24)	(62)	(8.2)	
Stouffer's Broccoli au Gratin, 10-oz. package	340	18.0	34.0	1.80			
Broccoli in Cheddar Cheese Sauce, 9-oz. package	260	16.0	28.9	1.78			
Village Park Broccoli cuts, 16-oz. (1-lb.) package	125	20.0	7.8	1.25			
Boiled, drained (yield: approx. 14.2 oz.)	(125)	(20.0)	(8.8)	(1.40)	(47)	(7.5)	
Broccoli Normandy, 16-oz. (1 lb.) package	150	25.0	9.4	1.56			

BROWN BEANS

MATURE SEEDS, Dry

	UNIT Cal.	UNIT Carb.	1 OZ., BY WT. Cal.	1 OZ., BY WT. Carb.	1 CUP Cal.	1 CUP Carb.	Fiber per oz. (GMS.)
RAW:							
1 cup (approx. 7.1 oz.)	678	122.4	96.1	17.35	678	122.4	1.25
1 pound (approx. 2.3 cups)	1538	277.6	96.1	17.35	678	122.4	1.25
COOKED:							
Boiled, drained:							
1 pound (yield from approx. 5.3 oz.)	(513)	(92.5)	(32.1)	(5.78)			0.42

BRUSSELS SPROUTS

	UNIT Cal.	UNIT Carb.	1 OZ., BY WT. Cal.	1 OZ., BY WT. Carb.	1 CUP Cal.	1 CUP Carb.	Fiber per oz. (GMS.)
RAW:							
As purchased, good quality [refuse: trimmings, approx. 8%]							
1 pound (approx. 24 sprouts, 1¼–1½" diameter)	188	34.6	11.8	2.16			
As purchased, fair quality [refuse: outer leaves and trimmings, approx. 26%]:							
1 pound (approx. 24 sprouts, 1¼–1½" diameter)	151	27.9	9.4	1.74			
Edible portion:							
1 pound	204	37.7	12.8	2.36			0.56
COOKED:							
Boiled, drained:							
1 sprout (approx. 1¼–1½" diameter, 0.74 oz.)	8	1.4	10.2	1.81	56	9.9	0.45
1 cup (approx. 7–8 sprouts, 5.5 oz.)	56	9.9	10.2	1.81	56	9.9	0.45
1 pound (approx. 21 sprouts, 2.9 cups) (1g/1g/tr/91%/3mg)	163	29.0	10.2	1.81	56	9.9	0.45
Steamed:							
1 pound of raw brussels sprouts, steamed (yield: approx. 16.8 oz.)	204	37.7	12.1	2.24			0.53
1 pound of steamed brussels sprouts	194	35.8	12.1	2.24			0.53
FROZEN, based on generic data:							
Measured when frozen:							
1 pound (1g/2g/tr/88%/5mg)	163	33.1	10.2	2.07			0.34
1 package, 10 oz. net wt.	102	20.7	10.2	2.07			0.34
Boiled, drained:							
1 cup (approx. 5.4 oz.)	51	10.1	9.4	1.85	51	10.1	0.34
1 10-oz. package, boiled, drained (yield: approx. 10.1 oz.)	94	18.5	9.4	1.85	51	10.1	0.34
1 pound of frozen brussels sprouts, boiled, drained (yield: approx. 16.1 oz. (1g/2g/tr/89%/4mg)	150	29.6	9.4	1.85	51	10.1	0.34
1 pound of boiled, drained brussels sprouts	149	29.5	9.4	1.85	51	10.1	0.34
FROZEN, by brand:							
Birds Eye Baby Brussels Sprouts, 10-oz. package	105	18.0	10.6	1.82			
Boiled, drained (yield: approx. 9.6 oz.)	(105)	(18.0)	(10.9)	(1.88)	(57)	(9.8)	
Brussels Sprouts, 10-oz. package	90	15.0	9.0	1.50			
Boiled, drained (yield: approx. 9.6 oz.)	(90)	(15.0)	(9.4)	(1.56)	(49)	(8.1)	
Green Giant Brussels Sprouts, 16-oz. (1-lb.) pouch	191	29.1	11.9	1.82			
Boiled, drained (yield: approx. 15.4 oz.)	(191)	(29.1)	(12.4)	(1.89)	50	8.0	
Brussels Sprouts in Butter Sauce, 10-oz. pouch	159	15.0	15.9	1.50	110	10.0	
Brussels Sprouts Halves in Cheese Sauce, 10-oz. pouch	182	19.9	18.2	1.99	170	19.0	
Hanover Brussels Sprouts, 16-oz. (1-lb.) polybag	174	30.1	10.9	1.88			
Boiled, drained (yield: approx. 15.4 oz.)	(174)	(30.1)	(11.3)	(1.95)	(58)	(10.1)	
Kounty Kist Brussels Sprouts, 20-oz. pouch	238	36.3	11.9	1.82			
Boiled, drained (yield: approx. 19.2 oz.)	(238)	(36.3)	(12.4)	(1.89)	(50)	(8.0)	
Stouffer's Brussels Sprouts au Gratin, 10⅞-oz. package	360	32.0	33.1	2.94			
Village Park Brussels Sprouts, 16-oz. (1-lb.) package	175	40.0	10.9	2.50			
Boiled, drained (yield: approx. 15.4 oz.)	(175)	(40.0)	(11.4)	(2.59)	(46)	(10.4)	

BUCKWHEAT, see Kasha under WHEAT

BUTTER BEANS

	UNIT Cal.	UNIT Carb.	1 OZ., BY WT. Cal.	1 OZ., BY WT. Carb.	1 CUP Cal.	1 CUP Carb.	Fiber per oz. (GMS.)
FROZEN, by brand:							
Birds Eye Baby Butter Beans, 10-oz. package	390	72.0	39.0	7.20			
Boiled, drained (yield: approx. 10 oz.)	(390)	(72.0)	(39.0)	(7.20)	(347)	(64.0)	
Green Giant Speckled Butter Beans, 10-oz. package, boil-in-bag	315	40.0	31.5	4.00			
Boiled, drained (yield: approx. 10 oz.)	(315)	(40.0)	(31.5)	(4.00)	(280)	(34.0)	
Seabrook Farms Baby Butter Beans, 10-oz. package	420	78.0	42.0	7.80			
Boiled, drained (yield: approx. 10 oz.)	(420)	(78.0)	(42.0)	(7.80)	(373)	(69.3)	
Butter Beans, 10-oz. package	390	66.0	39.0	6.60			
Speckled Butter Beans, 10-oz. package	390	72.0	39.0	7.20			
CANNED, by brand:							
Hanover Butter Beans, 16-oz. (1-lb.) can	480	84.0	30.0	5.25	(265)	(46.4)	
40-oz. can	1200	210.0	30.0	5.25	(265)	(46.4)	

CABBAGE

	UNIT		1 OZ., BY WT.		1 CUP		Fiber per oz. (GMS.)
	Cal.	Carb.	Cal.	Carb.	Cal.	Carb.	
CHINESE CABBAGE (Celery Cabbage, Petsai), Compact Heading Type							
RAW:							
As purchased, good quality [refuse: root base, approx. 3%]:							
1 medium head (approx. 1 lb. 12 oz.)	109	23.2	3.9	0.83			
As purchased, fair quality [refuse: root base and tough or wilted outer leaves, approx. 12%]:							
1 medium head (approx. 1¾ lb.)	98	21.0	3.5	0.75			
Edible portion:							
1 medium head (approx. 1 lb. 9 oz.)	98	21.0	4.0	0.85	11	2.3	0.17
1 cup, 1" pieces (approx. 2.6 oz.)	11	2.3	4.0	0.85	11	2.3	0.17
1 pound (approx. 6.2 cups) (tr/1g/tr/95%/7mg)	64	13.6	4.0	0.85	11	2.3	0.17
COOKED:							
Steamed:							
1 pound of raw Chinese cabbage, steamed (yield: 15.7 oz.)	64	13.6	4.1	0.87			0.17
1 pound of steamed Chinese cabbage	65	13.9	4.1	0.87			0.17
COMMON CABBAGE (Danish, domestic, and pointed types)							
RAW:							
As purchased untrimmed [refuse: outer leaves and core, approx. 21%]:							
1 medium head (approx. 2 lb. 13 oz.)	244	55.2	5.4	1.21			
As purchased trimmed [refuse: core approx. 10%]:							
1 medium head (approx. 2 lb. 8 oz.)	244	55.2	6.1	1.38			
1 pound (approx. 0.4 cabbages)	98	22.0	6.1	1.38			
Edible portion:							
1 medium head (approx. 2 lb. 4 oz.)	244	55.2	6.8	1.53			0.23
1 cup:							
Ground (approx. 5.3 oz.)	36	8.1	6.8	1.53	36	8.1	0.23
Shredded finely or chopped (approx. 3.2 oz.)	22	4.9	6.8	1.53	22	4.9	0.23
Shredded coarsely or sliced (approx. 2.5 oz.)	17	3.8	6.8	1.53	17	3.8	0.23
1 pound (approx. 3 cups of ground, or 6.5 cups of shredded coarsely or sliced, or 5 cups, shredded finely or chopped) (tr/1g/tr/92%/6mg)	109	24.5	6.8	1.53			0.23
COOKED:							
Boiled until tender, then drained:							
1 cup:							
Shredded, cooked in a small amount of water (approx. 5.1 oz.)	29	6.2	5.7	1.22	29	6.2	0.23
Wedges, cooked in a large amount of water (approx. 6 oz.)	31	6.8	5.1	1.13	31	6.8	0.23
1 pound:							
Shredded, cooked in a small amount of water (approx. 3.1 cups)	91	19.5	5.7	1.22	29	6.2	0.23
Wedges, cooked in a large amount of water (approx. 2.7 cups)	82	18.1	5.1	1.13	31	6.8	0.23
Steamed:							
1 pound of raw cabbage, steamed (yield: approx. 15.4 oz.)	109	24.5	7.1	1.60			0.24
1 pound of steamed cabbage	114	25.5	7.1	1.60			0.24
FROZEN, by brand:							
Green Giant Stuffed Cabbage Rolls with Beef in Tomato Sauce, 14-oz. package	417	32.9	29.8	2.35			0.23
DEHYDRATED, based on generic data:							
1 pound (4g/21g/4%/54mg)	1397	334.3	87.3	20.90			2.92
COLE SLAW, based on generic data:							
Prepared with homemade French dressing, based on USDA home recipe with ingredients as follows: 4 cups shredded cabbage, 4 Tbsp. oil, 1 Tbsp. vinegar, ½ tsp. sugar, and spices (yield: approx. 4 cups, approx. 17 oz.)	620	24.4	36.6	1.46	155	6.1	0.20
1 cup (approx. 4.2 oz.)	155	6.1	36.6	1.46	155	6.1	0.20
1 pound (approx. 3.8 cups) (tr/1g/3g/81%/37mg)	586	23.4	36.6	1.46	155	6.1	0.20

	UNIT		1 OZ., BY WT.		1 CUP		Fiber per oz. (GMS.)
	Cal.	Carb.	Cal.	Carb.	Cal.	Carb.	
Prepared with commercial French dressing:							
1 cup (approx. 4.2 oz.)	(114)	(9.1)	(26.9)	(2.15)	(114)	(9.1)	(0.20)
1 pound (approx. 3.8 cups) (tr/2g/2g/83%/76mg)	(430)	(34.4)	(26.9)	(2.15)	(114)	(9.1)	(0.20)
Prepared with mayonnaise:							
1 cup (approx. 4.2 oz.)	(173)	(5.8)	(42.1)	(1.37)	(173)	(5.8)	(0.20)
1 pound (approx. 3.8 cups) (tr/1g/4g/79%/56mg)	(674)	(21.9)	(42.1)	(1.37)	(173)	(5.8)	(0.20)
Prepared with salad dressing (mayonnaise type):							
1 cup (approx. 4.2 oz.)	(119)	(8.5)	(28.1)	(2.01)	(119)	(8.5)	(0.20)
1 pound (approx. 3.8 cups) (tr/2g/2g/83%/54mg)	(450)	(32.2)	(28.1)	(2.01)	(119)	(8.5)	(0.20)
SAUERKRAUT							
For SAUERKRAUT JUICE, also see the BEVERAGES chapter							
CANNED, based on generic data:							
1 cup:							
Solids and liquid (approx. 8.3 oz.)	42	9.4	5.1	1.13	42	9.4	0.20
Drained solids (yield: approx. 7.4 oz.)	(40)	(8.8)	(5.4)	(1.19)	(40)	(8.8)	(0.21)
Juice only (approx. 8.5 oz.)	24	5.6	2.8	0.66	24	5.6	trace
1 pound:							
Solids and liquid (approx. 1.9 cups) (1g/1g/tr/93%/212mg)	82	18.1	5.1	1.13	42	9.4	0.20
Drained solids (yield: 2.2 cups) (1g/1g/tr/na/na)	(86)	(19.0)	(5.4)	(1.19)	(40)	(8.8)	(0.21)
Juice only (approx. 1.9 cups) (tr/1g/tr/95%/223mg)	45	10.6	2.8	0.66	24	5.6	trace
1 Can, #303; 16 oz. (1 lb.) net wt.							
Solids and liquid, 16 oz. (1 lb.) (yield: approx. 1.9 cups)	82	18.1	5.1	1.13	42	9.4	0.20
Drained solids (yield: approx. 14.1 oz., 1.9 cup)	(77)	(16.8)	(5.4)	(1.19)	(40)	(8.8)	(0.21)
Juice only (approx. 1.9 oz.)	(5)	(1.3)	2.8	0.66	24	5.6	trace
1 Can, #10; 99 oz. (6 lb. 3 oz.) net wt.							
Solids and liquid, 99 oz. (approx. 11.9 cups)	505	112.3	5.1	1.13	42	9.4	0.20
Drained solids (yield: approx. 87.1 oz., 11.9 cups)	(472)	(103.6)	(5.4)	(1.19)	(40)	(8.8)	(0.21)
Juice only (approx. 11.9 oz.)	(33)	(8.7)	2.8	0.66	24	5.6	trace
CANNED OR JARRED, by brand:							
Blue Boy, 8-oz. can, solids and liquid	55	7.3	6.9	0.91	60	8.0	
16-oz. (1-lb.) can, solids and liquid	110	14.5	6.9	0.91	60	8.0	
99-oz. (6-lb. 3-oz.) can, solids and liquid	683	90.1	6.9	0.91	60	8.0	
Claussen, 32-fl.-oz. (2-lb.) jar (yield: 24.9 oz. drained solids)	141	26.1	5.7	1.05	(47)	(8.7)	
Stokely Bavarian Style Sauerkraut, 16-oz. (1-lb.) can	113	26.5	7.1	1.65	60	14.0	
Chopped Sauerkraut, 16-oz. (1-lb.) can	76	17.0	4.7	1.06	40	9.0	
Shredded Sauerkraut, 8-oz. can	38	8.5	4.7	1.06	40	9.0	
RED CABBAGE							
RAW:							
As purchased untrimmed [refuse: outer leaves, and core, approx. 21%]:							
1 small head (approx. 3 lb.)	331	73.9	6.9	1.54			
1 large head (approx. 5 lb.)	552	123.2	6.9	1.54			
1 pound (approx. 5.3 small heads or 3.2 large heads)	110	24.6	6.9	1.54			
As purchased trimmed [refuse: core, approx. 10%]:							
1 pound	127	28.2	7.9	1.76			
Edible portion:							
1 small head (approx. 2 lb. 6 oz.)	331	73.9	8.8	1.96			0.23
1 large head (approx. 3.9 oz.)	552	123.2	8.8	1.96			
1 cup:							
Shredded coarsely or sliced (approx. 2.5 oz.)	22	4.8	8.8	1.96	22	4.8	0.23
Shredded finely or chopped (approx. 3.2 oz.)	28	6.2	8.8	1.96	28	6.2	0.23
1 pound (approx. 6.5 cups of shredded coarsely or sliced, or 5 cups of shredded finely or chopped) (1g/1g/tr/90%/7mg)	141	31.3	8.8	1.96			0.23
JARRED, by brand:							
Greenwood Sweet-Sour Red Cabbage, 8-oz. jar, drained solids (yield: approx. 5.9 oz.)	120	25.0	20.3	4.24	120	25.0	
Lohmanns Red Cabbage, 32-oz. jar	450	90.0	14.1	2.80	113	23.0	
Drained solids (yield: approx. 24 oz.)	(426)	(85.2)	(17.8)	(3.55)			

	UNIT		1 OZ., BY WT.		1 CUP		Fiber per oz.
	Cal.	Carb.	Cal.	Carb.	Cal.	Carb.	(GMS.)
SAVOY CABBAGE							
RAW:							
As purchased untrimmed [refuse: outer leaves and core, approx. 21%]:							
1 medium head (approx. 2 lb. 6 oz.)	207	39.6	5.4	1.03			
1 pound (approx. 0.42 medium heads)	86	16.5	5.4	1.03			
As purchased trimmed [refuse: core, approx. 10%]							
1 medium head (approx. 2 lb. 2 oz.)	207	39.6	6.1	1.18			
1 pound (approx. 0.47 medium heads)	98	18.8	6.1	1.18			
Edible portion:							
1 medium head (approx. 1 lb. 14 oz.)	207	39.6	6.8	1.31			0.23
Shredded coarsely or sliced:							
1 cup (approx. 2½ oz.)	17	3.2	6.8	1.31	17	3.2	0.23
1 pound (approx. 6½ cups) (1g/1g/tr/92%/6mg)	109	20.9	6.8	1.31	17	3.2	0.23
SPOON CABBAGE (also called White Mustard Cabbage, Bok Choy, or Pak Choy), non-heading green leaf type							
Leaves and stems							
RAW:							
As purchased, good quality [refuse: root base, approx. 5%]:							
1 pound	69	12.5	4.3	0.78			
As purchased, fair quality [refuse: root base, and damaged leaves, approx. 20%]:							
1 pound	58	10.5	3.6	0.66			
Edible portion:							
1 cup, 1" pieces (approx. 2½ oz.)	11	2.0	4.6	0.83	11	2.0	0.02
1 pound (approx. 6.4 cups) (tr/1g/tr/94%/7mg)	73	13.2	4.6	0.83			0.02
COOKED:							
Boiled, drained:							
1 cup, 1" pieces (approx. 6 oz.)	24	4.1	4.0	0.68	24	4.1	0.02
1 pound (approx. 2.7 cups)	64	10.9	4.0	0.68			0.02
Steamed:							
1 pound of raw spoon cabbage, steamed (yield: approx. 14.9 oz.)	73	13.2	4.9	0.89			0.02
1 pound of steamed spoon cabbage (tr/1g/tr/95%/5mg)	78	14.2	4.9	0.89			0.02
CABBAGE, SWAMP, see SWAMP CABBAGE							
CALICO BEANS							
MATURE SEEDS, Dry							
RAW:							
1 cup (approx. 6.7 oz.)	663	121.0	98.9	18.06	663	121.0	1.22
1 pound (approx. 2.4 cups) (6g/18g/tr/8%/3mg)	1583	288.9	98.9	18.06	663	121.0	1.22
COOKED:							
Boiled, drained:							
1 cup (approx. 5.9 oz.)	(244)	(44.6)	(41.4)	(7.56)	(244)	(44.6)	0.51
1 pound (approx. 2.7 cups) (yield from approx. 6.7 oz. of uncooked dry beans) (3g/8g/tr/na/na)	(663)	(121.0)	(41.4)	(7.56)	(244)	(44.6)	0.51
CARROTS							
RAW:							
As purchased with full tops [refuse: tops and scrapings, approx. 41%]							
1 pound	112	26.0	7.0	1.63			
As purchased with part tops [refuse: part tops and scrapings, approx. 22%]							
1 pound	149	34.3	9.3	2.14			
As purchased (packaged without tops) [refuse: crowns, tips, and scrapings, approx. 11%]:							
1 medium carrot (approx. 1⅛" diameter, 7½" long, 2⅞ oz.)	30	7.0	10.6	2.45			
1 pound (approx. 5.6 carrots)	169	39.2	10.6	2.45			
1 package, declared net weight 16 oz. (1 lb.) (weight is actually approx. 20 oz., 7 carrots)	212	48.9	10.6	2.45			
Edible portion:							
1 medium carrot (approx. 2.5 oz.)	30	7.0	11.9	2.75			0.30
1 cup:							
Strips, ¼–⅜" wide, 2½–3" long (approx. 4.3 oz.)	51	12.0	11.9	2.75	51	12.0	0.30
Grated or shredded (approx. 3.9 oz.)	46	10.7	11.9	2.75	46	10.7	0.30
1 pound:							
Strips, ¼–⅜" wide, 2⅓–3" long (approx. 112 strips, 4 cups) (tr/3g/tr/88%/13mg)	191	44.0	11.9	2.75	51	12.0	0.30
Grated or shredded (approx. 4 cups)	191	44.0	11.9	2.75	46	10.7	0.30
COOKED:							
Boiled, drained:							
1 cup:							
Sliced crosswise, ¼–½" thick (approx. 5.5 oz.)	48	11.0	8.8	2.01	48	11.0	0.23
Diced, ¼–½" cubes (approx. 5.1 oz.) (tr/2g/tr/91%/9mg):	45	10.3	8.8	2.01	45	10.3	0.23
1 pound (approx. 3 cups of sliced or 3⅛ cups of diced carrots)	141	32.2	8.8	2.01			0.23
Steamed:							
1 pound of raw carrots, steamed (approx. 14.9 oz.)	191	44.0	12.8	2.96			0.32
1 pound of steamed carrots	205	47.4	12.8	2.96			0.32
FROZEN, by brand:							
Bel-Air Crinkle-Cut Carrots, 23-oz. package	280	56.0	12.2	2.43			
Boiled, drained (yield: approx. 22.5 oz.)	280	56.0	12.4	2.49	66	13.2	
Whole Baby Carrots, 17-oz. package	200	40.0	11.8	2.35			
Boiled, drained (yield: approx. 16.7 oz.)	200	40.0	12.0	2.40	67	13.4	
Birds Eye Carrots with Brown Sugar Glaze, 10-oz. package	240	45.0	24.2	4.55			
Green Giant Carrot Nuggets in Butter Sauce, 10-oz. boil-in-bag	139	18.2	13.9	1.82	100	12.0	
Hanover Sliced carrots, 16-oz. (1-lb.) polybag	174	40.0	10.9	2.50			
Boiled, drained (yield: approx. 15.7 oz.)	(174)	(40.0)	(11.1)	(2.54)	(58)	(13.3)	
Safeway Crinkle-Cut Carrots, 23-oz. package	280	56.0	12.2	2.43			
Boiled, drained (yield: approx. 22.5 oz.)	(280)	(56.0)	(12.4)	(2.49)	(66)	(13.2)	
Whole Baby Carrots, 17-oz. package	200	40.0	11.8	2.35			
Boiled, drained (yield: approx. 16.7 oz.)	(200)	(40.0)	(12.0)	(2.40)	(67)	(13.4)	
Seabrook Farms Whole Carrots, 10-oz. package	120	24.0	12.0	2.40			
Boiled, drained (yield: approx. 9.8 oz.)	(120)	(24.0)	(12.2)	(2.45)	(68)	(13.7)	
Village Park Whole Baby Carrots, 16-oz. (1-lb.) package	190	45.0	11.9	2.81			
Boiled, drained (yield: approx. 15.7 oz.)	(190)	(45.0)	(12.1)		(64)	(15.3)	
CANNED, based on generic data:							
Regular pack:							
Solids and liquid:							
1 cup (approx. 8.7 oz.)	69	16.0	7.9	1.84	69	16.0	0.17
1 pound (approx. 1.8 cups) (tr/2g/tr/92%/67mg)	127	29.5	7.9	1.84	69	16.0	0.17
1 #303 can, 16 oz. (1 lb.) net wt.	127	29.5	7.9	1.84	69	16.0	0.17
Drained solids:							
1 carrot, approx. .65 oz.	6	1.2	8.5	1.90			0.23
1 cup:							
Sliced crosswise, ¼–½" thick with a diameter of less than 1½" (approx. 5.5 oz.)	47	10.4	8.5	1.90	47	10.4	0.23
Diced, ¼" cubes (approx. 5.1 oz.)	44	9.7	8.5	1.90	44	9.7	0.23
1 pound (approx. 2.9 cups sliced or 3.1 cups diced) (tr/2g/tr/91%/67mg)	136	30.4	8.5	1.90			0.23
1 #303 can, when carrots inside are:							
Whole (yield: approx. 9¾ oz. solids (approx. 15 carrots, each approx. 2" long, ¾" diameter)	83	18.5	8.5	1.90			0.23
Sliced crosswise, ¼–½" thick with a diameter of less than 1½" (yield: approx. 10 oz., 1.8 cups)	85	19.0	8.5	1.90	47	10.4	0.23
Diced into ¼" cubes (yield: approx. 10½ oz., 2 cups)	89	20.0	8.5	1.90	44	9.7	0.23
Drained liquid:							
1 cup (approx. 8.3 oz.)	52	12.9	6.3	1.56	52	12.9	trace
1 pound (approx. 1.9 cups) (tr/2g/0g/93%/67mg)	100	24.9	6.3	1.56	52	12.9	trace

	UNIT		1 OZ., BY WT.		1 CUP		Fiber per oz.
	Cal.	Carb.	Cal.	Carb.	Cal.	Carb.	(GMS.)
Low-sodium pack:							
Solids and liquid:							
1 cup (approx. 8.7 oz.)	54	12.3	6.3	1.42	54	12.3	0.17
1 pound (approx. 1.8 cups) (tr/1g/tr/94%/11mg)	100	22.7	6.3	1.42	54	12.3	0.17
1 #303 can, 16 oz. (1 lb.) net wt.	100	22.7	6.3	1.42	54	12.3	0.17
Drained solids:							
1 cup (approx. 5.5 oz.)	39	8.7	7.1	1.59	39	8.7	0.23
1 pound (approx. 2.9 cups) (tr/1g/tr/93%/11mg)	113	25.4	7.1	1.59	39	8.7	0.23
1 #303 can, yield approx. 10 oz. (approx. 1.8 cups)	71	15.9	7.1	1.59	39	8.7	0.23
Drained liquid:							
1 cup (approx. 8.3 oz.)	(38)	(9.4)	4.6	1.13	(38)	(9.4)	trace
1 pound (approx. 1.9 cups) (tr/1g/0g/95%/11mg)	73	18.1	4.6	1.13	(38)	(9.4)	trace
1 #303 can (approx. 6 oz., approx. 0.7 cups)	(29)	(6.8)	4.6	1.13	(38)	(9.4)	trace
CANNED, by brand:							
Ann Page (A&P) Sliced Carrots, 16-oz. (1-lb.) can	120	28.0	7.5	1.75	60	14.0	
Drained solids (yield: approx. 10.4 oz.)	(86)	(19.0)	(8.3)	(1.83)	(45)	(10.0)	
Balanced Diced Carrots, packed in water, without added sugar or salt, 8¼-oz. can	59	11.6	7.1	1.41	(62)	(12.2)	
Drained (yield: approx. 5.4 oz.)	(45)	(8.4)	(8.3)	(1.56)	(42)	(8.0)	
Blue Boy Carrots, 8.5-oz. can	71	12.3	8.4	1.45	70	12.0	
Drained (yield: approx. 5.5 oz.)	53	7.5	9.7	1.37	53	7.4	
Del Monte Carrot Purée, low sodium, 17-oz. can	(140)	(30.0)	(8.3)	(1.76)	70	15.0	
Diced Carrots, 16-oz. (1-lb.) can	120	30.0	7.5	1.88	60	15.0	
Drained (yield: approx. 10.4 oz.)	(86)	(21.0)	(8.3)	(2.02)	(46)	(11.1)	
Sliced carrots, 16-oz. (1-lb.) can	120	30.0	7.5	1.88	60	15.0	
Drained solids (yield: approx. 10.4 oz.)	(86)	(21.0)	(8.3)	(2.02)	(46)	(11.1)	
Sliced Carrots, no salt or sugar added, 8-oz. can	(50)	(12.0)	(6.3)	(1.50)	50	12.0	
Drained solids (yield: approx. 5.2 oz.)	(36)	(8.9)	(6.9)	(1.71)	(38)	(9.4)	
16-oz. (1-lb.) can	(100)	(24.0)	(6.3)	(1.50)	50	12.0	
Drained solids (yield: approx. 10.4 oz.)	(72)	(17.8)	(6.9)	(1.71)	(38)	(9.4)	
Golden Harvest Sliced Carrots in Water, no sugar or salt added, 8-oz. can	50	13.0	6.3	1.63	50	13.0	
Drained solids (yield: approx. 5.2 oz.)	33	8.5	6.4	1.64	35	8.9	
Libby's Diced Carrots, 8¼-oz. can	(39)	(8.8)	(4.8)	(1.07)	40	9.0	
Drained solids (yield: approx. 5.4 oz.)	(22)	(4.2)	(4.2)	(0.78)	(22)	(4.2)	
16-oz. (1-lb.) can	(76)	(17.1)	(4.8)	(1.07)	40	9.0	
Drained solids (yield: approx. 10.4 oz.)	(43)	(8.1)	(4.2)	(0.78)	(22)	(4.2)	
Sliced carrots, 8¼-oz. can	(39)	(8.8)	(4.8)	(1.07)	40	9.0	
Drained solids (yield: approx. 5.4 oz.)	(22)	(4.2)	(4.2)	(0.78)	(22)	(4.2)	
16-oz. (1-lb.) can	(76)	(17.1)	(4.8)	(1.07)	40	9.0	
Drained solids (yield: approx. 10.4 oz.)	(43)	(8.1)	(4.2)	(0.78)	(22)	(4.2)	
S&W Fancy French Style Julienne Carrots, 8¼-oz. can	60	14.0	7.3	1.70	60	14.0	
Drained solids (yield: approx. 5.4 oz.)	(47)	(11.0)	(8.7)	(2.04)	(48)	(11.2)	
Fancy Tiny Whole Very Young Carrots, 16-oz. (1-lb.) can	120	14.0	7.5	0.88	60	14.0	
Drained solids (yield: approx. 10.8 oz.)	(89)	(8.3)	(8.2)	(0.77)	(45)	(4.2)	
For comparison: **S&W** Sweet Peas & Diced Carrots, 8½-oz. can	70	14.0	8.2	1.65	70	14.0	
Drained solids (yield: approx. 5.2 oz.)	(54)	(10.8)	(10.3)	(2.06)	(62)	(12.4)	
S&W Nutradiet Sliced Carrots, packed in water, no salt, 8¼-oz. can	60	14.0	7.3	1.70	60	14.0	
Drained solids (yield: approx. 3.9 oz.)	(43)	(10.9)	(11.1)	(2.02)	(61)	(11.1)	
Stokely Diced Carrots, 8-oz. can	46	11.1	6.9	1.39	50	12.0	
Drained solids (yield: approx. 5.1 oz.)	(29)	(6.3)	(5.7)	(1.22)	(30)	(6.4)	
16-oz. (1-lb.) can	93	22.2	5.8	1.39	50	12.0	
Drained solids (yield: approx. 10½ oz.)	(60)	(12.9)	(5.7)	(1.22)	(30)	(6.4)	
Sliced Carrots, 8¼-oz. can	43	9.5	5.2	1.16	45	10.0	
Drained solids (yield: approx. 5.2 oz.)	(25)	(4.3)	(4.8)	(0.83)	(25)	(4.4)	

	UNIT		1 OZ., BY WT.		1 CUP		Fiber per oz.
	Cal.	Carb.	Cal.	Carb.	Cal.	Carb.	(GMS.)
16-oz. (1-lb.) can	83	18.5	5.2	1.16	45	10.0	
Drained solids (yield: approx. 10.0 oz.)	(48)	(8.3)	(4.8)	(0.83)	(25)	(4.4)	
Tillie Lewis "Tasti Diet" Diced Carrots, sodium controlled, 8-oz. can	50	12.0	6.3	1.50	50	12.0	
Drained solids (yield: approx. 5.3 oz.)	(34)	(7.8)	(6.4)	(1.45)	(33)	(7.4)	
DEHYDRATED, based on generic data:							
1 pound	1547	367.9	96.7	22.99			

CARROT JUICE, see the BEVERAGES chapter

CAULIFLOWER

	UNIT		1 OZ., BY WT.		1 CUP		Fiber per oz.
	Cal.	Carb.	Cal.	Carb.	Cal.	Carb.	(GMS.)
RAW:							
As purchased untrimmed [refuse: jacket leaves, inner leaves, main stalk, base, and core, approx. 61%]:							
1 medium head (approx. 6-7" diameter, 4 lb. 13 oz.)	232	44.7	3.0	0.58			
1 pound (approx. ⅕ of a medium head)	48	9.2	3.0	0.58			
Edible portion:							
1 medium head (approx. 1 lb. 14 oz.)	232	44.7	7.6	1.48			0.28
1 cup:							
Whole flowerbuds (approx. 3.5 oz.)	27	5.2	7.6	1.48	27	5.2	0.28
Sliced (approx. 3 oz.)	23	4.4	7.6	1.48	23	4.4	0.28
Chopped (approx. 4.1 oz.)	31	6.0	7.6	1.48	31	6.0	0.28
1 pound (1g/1g/tr/91%/4mg) (approx. 4.6 cups whole, 4.4 cups sliced, or 3.9 cups chopped)	122	23.6	7.6	1.48			0.28
COOKED:							
Boiled, drained:							
1 cup (approx. 4.4 oz.)	28	5.1	6.3	1.16	28	5.1	(0.23)
1 pound (approx. 3.6 cups)	100	18.6	6.3	1.16	28	5.1	(0.23)
Steamed:							
1 pound of raw cauliflower, steamed (yield: approx. 15.5 oz.) (1g/1g/tr/93%/3mg)	122	23.6	7.9	1.52			0.29
1 pound of steamed cauliflower	126	24.3	7.9	1.52			0.29
RAW, by brand:							
Cel-A-Pak raw Cauliflower, pre-packaged, 1 head (approx. 30 oz.)	231	44.4	7.7	1.48			
Boiled, drained (approx. 29 oz.)	183	33.6	6.3	1.16			
FROZEN, by brand:							
Bel-Air Cauliflower, 10-oz. package	75	15.0	7.5	1.50			
Boiled, drained (yield: approx. 9.7 oz.)	75	15.0	7.7	1.55	46	9.8	
Birds Eye Cauliflower, 10-oz. package	75	12.0	7.6	1.21			
Boiled, drained (yield: approx. 9.3 oz.)	(75)	(12.0)	(8.1)	(1.29)	(51)	(8.1)	
Cauliflower with Cheese Sauce, 10-oz. package	330	24.0	33.0	2.40			
Green Giant Cauliflower, 18-oz. polybag	112	16.3	6.2	0.91			
Boiled, drained (yield: approx. 16.7 oz.)	(112)	(16.3)	(6.7)	(0.98)	(27)	(4.0)	
Cauliflower in Cheese Sauce, 10-oz. boil-in-bag	148	15.9	14.8	1.59	130	13.0	
Cauliflower in Cheese Sauce, 10-oz. oven Bake N' Serve	238	17.0	23.8	1.70	220	17.0	
Hanover Cauliflower Florets, 16-oz. (1-lb.) polybag	100	15.0	6.25	0.94	(39)	(5.9)	
Boiled, drained (yield: approx. 14.9 oz.)	(100)	(15.0)	(6.7)	(1.01)	(42)	(6.3)	
Kounty Kist Cauliflower, 20-oz. polybag	125	18.2	6.2	0.91			
Boiled, drained (yield: approx 18.6 oz.)	(125)	(18.2)	(6.7)	(0.98)	(27)	(4.0)	
Mrs. Paul's Light Batter Cauliflower and Cheese, 8-oz. package	370	46.2	46.2	5.78			
Safeway Cauliflower, 10-oz. package	75	15.0	7.5	1.50			
Boiled, drained (yield: approx. 9.7 oz.)	(75)	(15.0)	(7.7)	(1.55)	(46)	(9.8)	
Seabrook Farms Cauliflower, 10-oz. package	75	15.0	7.5	1.50	(39)	(7.8)	
Boiled, drained (yield: approx. 9.3 oz.)	(75)	(15.0)	(8.1)	(1.61)	(42)	(8.4)	
16-oz. (1-lb.) package	120	24.0	7.5	1.50			
Boiled, drained (yield: approx. 9.3 oz.)	(120)	(24.0)	(12.9)	(2.58)	(81)	(16.3)	

	UNIT Cal.	UNIT Carb.	1 OZ., BY WT. Cal.	1 OZ., BY WT. Carb.	1 CUP Cal.	1 CUP Carb.	Fiber per oz. (GMS.)
Stouffer's Cauliflower au Gratin, 10-oz. package	310	22.0	31.0	2.20			
Cauliflower in Cheddar Cheese Sauce, 9-oz. package	220	16.0	24.4	1.78			
Village Park Cauliflower Florets, 16-oz. (1-lb.) package	125	25.0	7.8	1.56			
Boiled, drained (yield: approx. 14.9 oz.)	(125)	(25.0)	(8.4)	(1.68)	(53)	(10.5)	

CELERIAC

	UNIT Cal.	UNIT Carb.	1 OZ., BY WT. Cal.	1 OZ., BY WT. Carb.	1 CUP Cal.	1 CUP Carb.	Fiber per oz. (GMS.)
RAW:							
As purchased [refuse: parings, approx. 14%]:							
1 pound	156	33.2	9.8	2.08			
Edible portion:							
1 cup (approx. 4.2 oz.)	(45)	(9.7)	10.8	2.31	(45)	(9.7)	0.37
1 pound (approx. 3.8 cups) (1g/2g/tr/88%/28mg)	173	36.9	10.8	2.31	(45)	(9.7)	0.37

CELERY

	UNIT Cal.	UNIT Carb.	1 OZ., BY WT. Cal.	1 OZ., BY WT. Carb.	1 CUP Cal.	1 CUP Carb.	Fiber per oz. (GMS.)
RAW:							
As purchased untrimmed [refuse: leaves, root ends, and trimmings, approx. 25%]:							
1 pound	58	13.3	3.6	0.83			
As purchased, prepackaged stalks trimmed of leaves [refuse: root end and trimmings, approx. 11%]:							
1 bunch (approx. 15¼" long, 11" diameter, 2 lb., approx. 14 stalks)	137	31.5	4.3	0.98			
1 pound	69	15.7	4.3	0.98			
Edible portion (trimmed stalks):							
1 small inner stalk (approx. 5" long, ¾" wide at root end, 0.6 oz.)	3	0.7	4.9	1.14			0.17
1 large outer stalk (approx. 8" long, 1½" wide at root end, 1.4 oz.)	7	1.6	4.9	1.14			0.17
1 cup, chopped or diced (approx. 4.2 oz.)	20	4.7	4.9	1.14	20	4.7	0.17
1 pound (approx. 3.8 cups) (tr/1g/tr/94%/36mg)	79	18.2	4.9	1.14			0.17
COOKED:							
Boiled, drained:							
1 cup (approx. 5.3 oz.)	21	4.7	4.0	0.88	21	4.7	0.17
1 pound (approx. 3 cups diced) (tr/1g/tr/95%/37mg)	64	14.1	4.0	0.88	21	4.7	0.17
Steamed:							
1 pound of raw celery, steamed (yield: approx. 14.6 oz.)	79	18.2	5.4	1.25			0.19
1 pound of steamed celery	86	20.0	5.4	1.25			0.19

CELERY JUICE, see the BEVERAGES chapter

CELERY SEED, see the SALTS & SPICES chapter

CHARD (SWISS CHARD)

	UNIT Cal.	UNIT Carb.	1 OZ., BY WT. Cal.	1 OZ., BY WT. Carb.	1 CUP Cal.	1 CUP Carb.	Fiber per oz. (GMS.)
RAW:							
As purchased untrimmed:							
Good quality [refuse: tough stem ends and damaged leaves, approx. 8%]:							
1 pound	111	20.5	7.0	1.28			
Fair quality [refuse: touch stem ends and wilted leaves, approx. 23%]:							
1 pound	87	16.1	5.5	1.01			
Edible portion:							
1 pound (1g/1g/tr/91%/42mg)	113	20.9	7.1	1.31			0.23
COOKED:							
Boiled, drained:							
1 cup:							
Leaves (approx. 6.2 oz.)	32	5.8	5.1	0.94	32	5.8	0.20
Leaves and stalks (approx. 5.1 oz.)	26	4.8	5.1	0.94	26	4.8	0.20
1 pound (1g/1g/tr/94%/24mg)	82	15.0	5.1	0.94			0.20
Steamed:							
1 pound of raw Swiss chard, steamed (yield: approx. 11.7 oz.)	113	20.9	9.7	1.79			0.31
1 pound of steamed Swiss chard	155	28.6	9.7	1.79			0.31

CHERRY TOMATOES, see TOMATOES, CHERRY

CHERVIL

	UNIT Cal.	UNIT Carb.	1 OZ., BY WT. Cal.	1 OZ., BY WT. Carb.	1 CUP Cal.	1 CUP Carb.	Fiber per oz. (GMS.)
RAW:							
All-edible:							
1 pound (1g/3g/tr/81%/na)	259	52.2	16.2	3.26			

CHERVIL, DRIED, see the SALTS & SPICES chapter

CHESTNUTS

	UNIT Cal.	UNIT Carb.	1 OZ., BY WT. Cal.	1 OZ., BY WT. Carb.	1 CUP Cal.	1 CUP Carb.	Fiber per oz. (GMS.)
RAW:							
Fresh:							
As purchased in shell [refuse: shells, approx. 19%]:							
1 small nut (approx. 0.18 oz., 5½ per oz.)	8	1.8	44.6	9.67	189	40.9	
1 large nut (approx. 1½" diameter, ⅓ oz., 3 per oz.)	15	3.2	44.6	9.67	189	40.9	
1 cup (approx. 13 large or 24 small chestnuts, 4¼ oz.)	189	40.9	44.6	9.67	189	40.9	
1 pound (approx. 50 large nuts or 89 small nuts; 3¾ cups)	713	154.7	44.6	9.67	189	40.9	
Shelled:							
1 cup (approx. 5.6 oz)	310	67.0	55.0	11.94	310	67.0	0.31
1 pound (approx. 2.8 cups) (1g/12g/tr/53%/2mg)	880	191.0	55.0	11.94	310	67.0	0.31
DRIED:							
As purchased in shell [refuse: shells, approx. 18%]:							
1 pound	377	78.6	23.6	4.91			
Shelled:							
1 cup (approx. 5.6 oz.)	310	67.0	55.0	11.94	310	67.0	0.71
1 pound (2g/22g/1g/8%/3mg)	880	191.0	55.0	11.94	310	67.0	0.71

Chestnut Products

	UNIT Cal.	UNIT Carb.	1 OZ., BY WT. Cal.	1 OZ., BY WT. Carb.	1 CUP Cal.	1 CUP Carb.	Fiber per oz. (GMS.)
Chestnut flour, 1 pound	1642	345.6	102.6	21.60			
Chestnut Paste (based on data from France), 1 pound	481	103.4	30.1	6.46			

CHICK-PEAS (Garbanzos)

	UNIT Cal.	UNIT Carb.	1 OZ., BY WT. Cal.	1 OZ., BY WT. Carb.	1 CUP Cal.	1 CUP Carb.	Fiber per oz. (GMS.)
RAW:							
1 cup (approx. 7.1 oz.)	(725)	(122.8)	102.1	17.29	(725)	(122.8)	1.42
1 pound (approx. 2.3 cups) (6g/17g/1g/11%/7mg)	1633	276.7	102.1	17.29	(725)	(122.8)	1.42
COOKED:							
Boiled, drained:							
1 cup (approx. 5.7 oz.)	(280)	(47.4)	(49.1)	(8.32)	(280)	(47.4)	0.68
1 pound (approx. 2.8 cups) (yield from approx. 7.7 oz. uncooked dry peas) (3g/8g/1g/na/na)	(786)	(133.0)	(49.1)	(8.32)	(280)	(47.4)	0.68

Chick-pea Products

	UNIT Cal.	UNIT Carb.	1 OZ., BY WT. Cal.	1 OZ., BY WT. Carb.	1 CUP Cal.	1 CUP Carb.	Fiber per oz. (GMS.)
FALAFEL							
Mashed and Fried Chick-pea Mixture (based on data from the Middle East), 1 pound	885	223.7	55.3	13.98			
HUMMUS							
Chick-pea salad dip (based on data from the Middle East), 1 pound	1361	95.5	85.1	5.97			

CHICORY (Witloof), Bleached Head (Forced), also called French or Belgian Endive

	UNIT Cal.	UNIT Carb.	1 OZ., BY WT. Cal.	1 OZ., BY WT. Carb.	1 CUP Cal.	1 CUP Carb.	Fiber per oz. (GMS.)
RAW:							
As purchased [refuse: root base and core, approx. 11%]:							
1 medium head (approx. 5-7" long, 2.1 oz.)	8	1.7	3.8	0.81			

	UNIT		1 OZ., BY WT.		1 CUP		Fiber per oz.
	Cal.	Carb.	Cal.	Carb.	Cal.	Carb.	(GMS.)
1 pound (approx. 29 medium heads)	61	12.9	3.8	0.81			
Edible portion:							
1 medium head (approx. 1.9 oz.)	8	1.7	4.3	0.81	14	2.9	
1 cup, chopped, ½" pieces (approx. 3.2 oz.)	14	2.9	4.3	0.91	14	2.9	
1 pound (approx. 5 cups) (tr/1g/tr/95%/2mg)	68	14.5	4.3	0.91	14	2.9	

CHICORY GREENS

	UNIT Cal.	UNIT Carb.	1 OZ. Cal.	1 OZ. Carb.	1 CUP Cal.	1 CUP Carb.	Fiber per oz. (GMS.)
RAW:							
As purchased [refuse: stems, approx. 18%]:							
1 pound	74	14.1	4.6	0.88			
Edible portion:							
1 cup (approx. 1.2 oz.)	7	1.3	5.6	1.08	7	1.3	0.23
1 pound (approx. 13 cups) (tr/1g/tr/93%/na)	90	17.2	5.6	1.08	7	1.3	0.23

CHILES, see under PEPPERS

CHINESE CABBAGE, see under CABBAGE

CHIVES

	UNIT Cal.	UNIT Carb.	1 OZ. Cal.	1 OZ. Carb.	1 CUP Cal.	1 CUP Carb.	Fiber per oz. (GMS.)
RAW:							
All edible:							
1 pound	127	26.3	7.9	1.64			
Chopped, ⅛" pieces:							
1 teaspoon (approx. 0.04 oz.)	trace	trace	7.9	1.64	16	3.2	0.31
1 tablespoon (approx. 0.1 oz.)	1	0.2	7.9	1.64	16	3.2	0.31
1 cup (approx. 2 oz., or 16 tablespoons or 50 teaspoons) (1g/2g/tr/91%/na)	16	3.2	7.9	1.64	16	3 2	0.31
FREEZE DRIED, by brand:							
Armanino Farms Chives, 2-oz. package	187	38.7	93.6	19.36			

COCOZELLE, see ZUCCHINI

COLE SLAW, see under CABBAGE

COLLARDS

	UNIT Cal.	UNIT Carb.	1 OZ. Cal.	1 OZ. Carb.	1 CUP Cal.	1 CUP Carb.	Fiber per oz. (GMS.)
RAW:							
As purchased:							
When only leaves are to be eaten: [refuse: stems, approx. 32%]:							
1 pound	139	23.1	8.7	1.44			
When leaves and stems are to be eaten:							
Good quality (all-edible):							
1 pound	181	32.7	11.3	2.04			
Fair quality [refuse: tough stems, approx. 26%]:							
1 pound	134	24.2	8.4	1.51			
Edible portion:							
Leaves only:							
1 pound (1g/2g/tr/87%/12mg)	203	32.7	12.7	2.04			0.31
Leaves and stems:							
1 pound	181	32.7	11.3	2.04			
COOKED:							
Boiled, drained:							
Leaves without stems:							
Cooked in a small amount of water:							
1 cup (approx. 6.7 oz.)	63	9.7	9.4	1.44	63	9.7	0.28
1 pound (approx. 2.4 cups) (1g/1g/tr/90%/na)	150	23.1	9.4	1.44	63	9.7	0.28
Cooked in a large amount of water:							
1 cup (approx. 6.7 oz.)	59	9.1	8.8	1.36	59	9.1	0.28
1 pound (approx. 2.4 cups)	141	21.8	8.8	1.36	59	9.1	0.28
Leaves and stems:							
Cooked in a small amount of water:							
1 cup (approx. 5.1 oz.)	42	7.1	8.3	1.39	42	7.1	0.23
1 pound (approx. 3.1 cups) (1g/1g/tr/91%/7mg)	132	22.2	8.3	1.39	42	7.1	0.23

	UNIT		1 OZ., BY WT.		1 CUP		Fiber per oz.
	Cal.	Carb.	Cal.	Carb.	Cal.	Carb.	(GMS.)
Steamed:							
Leaves without stems:							
1 pound of raw collards, steamed (yield: approx. 18.6 oz.)	203	32.7	10.9	1.76			0.27
1 pound of steamed collards	174	28.2	10.9	1.76			0.27
FROZEN, by brand:							
Birds Eye Chopped Collard Greens, 10-oz. package	90	12.0	9.1	1.21			
Boiled, drained (yield: approx. 8.9 oz.)	(90)	(12.0)	(10.1)	(1.35)	(61)	(8.2)	
Seabrook Farms Chopped Collards, 10-oz. package	75	12.0	7.5	1.20			
Boiled, drained (yield: approx. 8.9 oz.)	(75)	(12.0)	(8.4)	(1.35)	(50)	(8.1)	
16-oz. (1-lb.) package	120	19.2	7.5	1.20			
Boiled, drained (yield: approx. 14.2 oz)	(120)	(19.2)	(8.5)	1.35)			

CORN

(Succotash is listed separately under "S".)

SWEET, WHITE, OR YELLOW

	UNIT Cal.	UNIT Carb.	1 OZ. Cal.	1 OZ. Carb.	1 CUP Cal.	1 CUP Carb.	Fiber per oz. (GMS.)
RAW:							
As purchased:							
With husk [refuse: husk, silk, cob, and trimmings, approx. 64%]:							
1 medium ear (approx. 8 oz.)	78	18.1	9.8	2.26			
1 pound (approx. 2 medium ears)	157	36.1	9.8	2.26			
Without husk [refuse: cob, approx. 45%]:							
1 medium ear (approx. 5.3 oz.)	80	18.3	15.0	3.44			
1 pound (approx. 3 medium ears)	240	55.1	15.0	3.44			
Edible portion:							
1 pound of kernels (yield from approx. 5½ medium ears) (1g/5g/tr/73%/tr)	435	100.2	27.2	6.27	159	36.6	0.20
COOKED:							
Boiled, drained:							
Kernels cooked on the cob ("Corn on the Cob"):							
1 medium ear (approx. 5" long, 1¾" diameter, 4.9 oz.)	70	16.2	14.2	3.28			0.20
1 pound (approx. 3¼ 5" ears)	227	52.5	14.2	3.28			0.20
Kernels that have been cut from the cob before cooking:							
Kernels cut from 1 medium ear (yield: approx. 2.7 oz.)	70	16.2	23.5	5.33	137	31.0	0.20
1 cup (approx. 5.8 oz.)	137	31.0	23.5	5.33	137	31.0	0.20
1 pound (yield from approx. 5½ medium ears, 2.8 cups) (1g/5g/tr/76%/tr)	376	85.3	23.5	5.33	137	31.0	0.20
Kernels that have been cut from cob after cooking:							
Kernels cut from 1 medium ear (yield: approx. 2.7 oz.)	70	16.2	25.8	5.97			0.20
1 pound (yield from approx. 5½ medium ears, 2.8 cups)	413	95.5	25.8	5.97			0.20
FROZEN CORN ON THE COB, based on generic data:							
COOKED:							
Boiled, then drained:							
Ears approx. 5" long, weighing approx. 8 oz. each:							
1 ear trimmed to 3½" long (approx. 4 oz.)	59	13.5	14.7	3.37			
1 medium ear (approx. 5" long, 8 oz.)	118	27.2	14.7	3.37			
1 pound of ears (approx. 2 medium ears, or 4 ears that have been trimmed to 3½" long)	235	53.9	14.7	3.37			
1 package, approx. 32 oz. (2 lb.) net wt., containing 4 medium ears of corn	474	109.0	14.7	3.37			
1 package, approx. 48 oz. (3 lb.) net wt., containing 6 medium ears of corn	711	163.5	14.7	3.37			
FROZEN CORN ON THE COB, by brand:							
Birds Eye Corn on the Cob, 1 package, 4 ears (package weight varies)	(520)	(112.0)					
1 ear	(130)	(28.0)					

	UNIT		1 OZ., BY WT.		1 CUP		Fiber per oz. (GMS.)
	Cal.	Carb.	Cal.	Carb.	Cal.	Carb.	
Little Ears Cob Corn, 1 package, 8 ears (package weight varies)	(560)	(128.0)					
1 ear	(70)	(16.0)					
Green Giant Corn on the Cob 3" Nibbler, 1 package, 6 ears	(540)	(108.0)					
1 ear, approx. 3" long	(90)	(18.0)					
Golden Corn-on-Cob, 1 package, 4 ears, each approx. 5½" long	(640)	(132.0)					
1 ear, approx. 5½" long	(160)	(33.0)					
Ore-Ida Cob Corn, 1 package, 4 ears (package weight varies)	(560)	(108.0)					
1 ear	(140)	(27.0)					
Seabrook Farms Corn on Cob, 1 package, 4 ears (package weight varies)	(560)	(120.0)					
1 ear	(140)	(30.0)					
Village Park Corn on the Cob, 1 package, 4 ears (package weight varies)	560	120.0					
1 ear	140	30.0					
FROZEN KERNELS OFF THE COB, by brand:							
Birds Eye Sweet Whole Kernel Corn, 10-oz. package	210	54.0	21.0	5.40			
Boiled, drained (yield: approx. 9.6 oz.)	(210)	(54.0)	(21.9)	(5.63)	(121)	(31.1)	
Green Giant Whole Kernel Golden Corn, 20-oz. polybag	499	102.2	25.0	5.11			
Boiled, drained (yield: approx. 19.2 oz.)	(499)	(102.2)	(26.0)	(5.32)	(135)	(27.7)	
Whole Kernel White Corn, 20-oz. polybag	522	108.2	26.1	5.42			
Boiled, drained (yield: approx. 19.2 oz.)	(522)	(108.4)	(27.2)	(5.65)	(135)	(28.1)	
Cream-Style Golden Corn, 10-oz. boil-in-bag	218	45.9	21.8	4.59	180	40.0	
Mexicorn Golden Corn with Peppers in Butter Sauce, 10-oz. boil-in-bag	264	42.8	26.4	4.28	190	30.0	
Niblets Golden Corn in Butter Sauce, 10-oz. boil-in-bag	264	42.8	26.4	4.28	190	30.0	
Whole Kernel White Corn in Butter Sauce, 10-oz. boil-in-bag	270	46.0	27.0	4.60	190	30.0	
Hanover Golden Corn, 16-oz. (1-lb.) polybag	400	80.0	25.0	5.00	(138)	(27.5)	
White Shoepeg Corn, 16-oz. (1-lb.) polybag	(450)	(90.1)	(28.1)	(5.63)			
Boiled, drained (yield: approx. 15.4 oz.)	(450)	(90.1)	(29.2)	(5.85)	(162)	(32.5)	
For comparison: **Hanover** White Shoepeg Corn with Chef Cut Green Beans, 16-oz. (1-lb.) polybag	301	60.0	18.8	3.75			
Boiled, drained (yield: approx. 15.4 oz.)	(301)	(60.0)	(19.5)	(3.90)	(107)	(21.4)	
For comparison: **Hanover** White Shoepeg Corn with Fordhook Limas, 16-oz. (1-lb.) polybag	450	85.0	28.1	5.31			
Boiled, drained (yield: approx. 15.4 oz.)	(450)	(85.0)	(29.2)	(5.52)	(159)	(30.3)	
Golden Harvest Whole Kernel Corn, 16-oz. (1-lb.) package	320	74.0	20.0	4.63	160	37.0	
Kounty Kist Whole Kernel Golden Corn, 20-oz. polybag	522	107.8	26.1	5.39			
Boiled, drained (yield: approx. 19.2 oz.)	(522)	(107.8)	(27.2)	(5.61)	(146)	(30.1)	
Whole Kernel White Corn, 20-oz. polybag	522	107.8	26.1	5.39			
Boiled, drained (yield: approx. 19.2 oz.)	(522)	(107.8)	(27.2)	(5.61)	(146)	(30.1)	
Ore-Ida Whole Kernel Corn, 32-oz. (2-lb.) package	1000	200.0	31.3	6.25			
Boiled, drained (yield: approx. 30.7 oz.)	(1000)	(200.0)	(32.6)	(6.51)	(179)	(35.8)	
Seabrook Farms Cut Corn, 10-oz. package	270	60.0	27.0	6.00			
Boiled, drained (yield: approx. 9.6 oz.)	(270)	(60.0)	(28.1)	(6.23)	(155)	(34.3)	
16-oz. (1-lb.) polybag	432	96.0	27.0	6.00			
Boiled, drained (yield: approx. 15.4 oz.)	(432)	(96.0)	(28.1)	(6.23)	(155)	(34.3)	
32-oz. (2-lb.) polybag	864	192.0	27.0	6.00			
Boiled, drained (yield: approx. 30.7 oz.)	(864)	(192.0)	(28.1)	(6.23)	(155)	(34.3)	
Whole Kernel Sweet White Corn, 10-oz. box	225	45.0	22.5	4.50			
Boiled, drained (yield: approx. 9.6 oz.)	(225)	(45.0)	(23.4)	(4.69)	(129)	(25.8)	
Stouffer's Corn Souffle, 8-oz. package	310	38.0	38.8	4.75			

	UNIT		1 OZ., BY WT.		1 CUP		Fiber per oz. (GMS.)
	Cal.	Carb.	Cal.	Carb.	Cal.	Carb.	
CANNED, based on generic data							
Whole Kernel Corn:							
Vacuum pack, Yellow Corn:							
Solids and liquid:							
1 cup (approx. 7.4 oz.)	174	43.1	23.5	5.81	174	43.1	0.23
1 pound (approx. 2.2 cups) (1g/6g/tr/76%/67mg)	376	93.0	23.5	5.81	174	43.1	0.23
1 #2 Vacuum Can, 12 oz. net wt.	282	69.7	23.5	5.81	174	43.1	0.23
Regular wet pack, white and yellow corn:							
Solids and liquid:							
1 cup (approx. 9 oz.)	169	40.2	18.7	4.45	169	40.2	0.17
1 pound (approx. 1.8 cups) (1g/4g/tr/81%/67mg)	299	71.2	18.7	4.45	169	40.2	0.17
1 #303 can, 17 oz. net wt.	318	75.7	18.7	4.45	1.69	40.2	0.17
Drained solids:							
1 cup (approx. 5.8 oz.)	139	32.7	23.8	5.61	139	32.7	0.23
1 pound (approx. 2.7 cups) (1g/6g/tr/76%/67mg)	381	89.8	23.8	5.61	139	32.7	0.23
1 #303 can (yield: approx. 10½ oz. of drained corn, 1.8 cups)	250	59.0	23.8	5.61	139	32.7	0.23
Drained liquid:							
1 cup (approx. 8.3 oz.)	(87)	(21.3)	(10.5)	(2.57)	(87)	(21.3)	trace
1 pound (approx. 1.9 cups) (tr/2g/tr/92%/67mg)	(168)	(41.1)	(10.5)	(2.57)	(87)	(21.3)	trace
1 #303 can (yield: approx. 6½ oz. of liquid, 0.8 cups)	(68)	(16.7)	(10.5)	(2.57)	(87)	(21.3)	trace
Low-sodium wet pack, white and yellow corn:							
Solids and liquid:							
1 cup (approx. 9 oz.)	146	34.8	16.2	3.86	146	34.8	0.14
1 pound (approx. 1.8 cups) (1g/4g/tr/84%/1mg)	259	61.7	16.2	3.86	146	34.8	0.14
1 #303 can, 17 oz. net wt.	275	65.6	16.2	3.86	146	34.8	0.14
Drained solids:							
1 cup (approx. 7.1 oz.)	152	29.7	21.6	5.10	152	29.7	0.20
1 pound (approx. 2.3 cups) (1g/5g/tr/78%1mg)	345	81.6	21.6	5.10	152	29.7	0.20
1 #303 can (yield: approx. 10½ oz. of drained corn, 1.8 cups)	226	53.6	21.6	5.10	152	29.7	0.20
Drained liquid:							
1 cup (approx. 8.3 oz.)	(62)	(15.4)	(7.5)	(1.85)	(62)	(15.4)	trace
1 pound (approx. 1.9 cups) (tr/1g/tr/95%/1mg)	(121)	(29.6)	(7.5)	(1.85)	(62)	(15.4)	trace
1 #303 can (yield: approx. 6½ oz. of liquid, 0.8 cups)	(49)	(12.0)	(7.5)	(1.85)	(62)	(15.4)	trace
Cream-Style Corn, White and Yellow:							
Regular pack:							
Solids and liquid:							
1 cup (approx. 9 oz.)	215	51.2	23.3	5.67	215	51.2	0.14
1 pound (approx. 1.8 cups) (1g/6g/tr/76%/67mg)	372	90.7	23.3	5.67	215	51.2	0.14
1 #303 can, 17 oz. net wt.	395	96.4	23.3	5.67	215	51.2	0.14
Low-sodium pack:							
Solids and liquid:							
1 cup (approx. 9 oz.)	210	47.4	23.3	5.24	210	47.4	0.09
1 pound (approx. 1.8 cups) (1g/5g/tr/77%/1mg)	372	83.9	23.3	5.24	210	47.4	0.09
1 #303 can, 17 oz. net wt.	395	89.2	23.3	5.24	210	47.4	0.09
CANNED, by brand:							
Whole Kernel:							
A & P Whole Kernel Corn, 16½-oz. can	340	76.0	20.6	4.61	170	38.0	
Drained solids (yield: approx. 10.2 oz.)	(296)	(63.4)	(29.0)	(6.22)	(169)	(36.2)	
Ann Page (A&P) Whole Kernel Corn, 8½-oz. can	170	38.0	20.6	4.61	170	38.0	
Drained solids (yield: approx. 5.1 oz.)	(148)	(31.7)	(29.0)	(6.22)	(169)	(36.2)	
Vacuum Packed Whole Kernel Corn, 12-oz. can	300	64.5	25.0	5.38	200	43.0	
Drained solids (yield: approx. 10.8 oz.)	(300)	(64.5)	(27.8)	(5.97)	(162)	(34.7)	
Balanced Golden Sweet Whole Kernel Corn, packed in water, without added sugar or salt, 16-oz. (1-lb.) can	(336)	(67.3)	(21.0)	(4.21)	190	38.0	
Drained solids (yield: approx. 9.9 oz.)	(293)	(55.1)	(29.6)	(5.57)	(172)	(32.3)	
Blue Boy Whole Kernel Corn, 8½-oz. can	189	35.6	22.2	4.44	200	40.0	
Drained solids (yield: approx. 5.3 oz.)	166	29.1	31.5	5.93	177	33.3	

	UNIT Cal.	UNIT Carb.	1 OZ., BY WT. Cal.	1 OZ., BY WT. Carb.	1 CUP Cal.	1 CUP Carb.	Fiber per oz. (GMS.)
Del Monte Golden Family Style Corn, 8¾-oz. can	175	38.1	20.0	4.35	170	37.0	
Drained solids (yield: approx. 5.2 oz.)	(151)	(31.1)	(28.7)	(5.91)	(167)	(34.0)	
17-oz. can	340	74.0	20.0	4.35	170	37.0	
Drained solids (yield: approx. 10.2 oz.)	(293)	(60.5)	(28.7)	(5.91)	(167)	(34.4)	
Vacuum Packed Golden Corn, 12-oz. can	300	64.5	25.0	5.38	200	43.0	
Drained solids (yield: approx. 10.8 oz.)	(292)	(62.2)	(27.8)	(5.93)	(167)	(39.6)	
White Whole Kernel Corn, 16-oz. (1-lb.) can	300	66.0	18.8	4.13	150	33.0	
Drained solids (yield: approx. 10.5 oz.)	(262)	(55.0)	(24.9)	(5.24)	(145)	(30.5)	
Diet Delight Golden Sweet Corn, packed in water, low sodium without added sugar or salt, 8-oz. can	120	4.0	15.0	0.50	120	4.0	
Drained solids (yield: approx. 5 oz.)	(105)	(0.4)	(21.0)	(0.08)	(122)	(0.5)	
Featherweight Golden Whole Kernel Corn, no added salt or sugar, 8-oz. can	(140)	(32.0)	(17.5)	(4.00)	140	32.0	
Drained solids (yield: approx. 5 oz.)	(125)	(28.4)	(25.0)	(5.68)	(146)	(33.1)	
16-oz. (1-lb.) can	(280)	(64.0)	(17.5)	(4.00)	140	32.0	
Drained solids (yield: approx. 10 oz.)	(250)	(56.8)	(25.0)	(5.68)	(146)	(33.1)	
Green Giant Whole Kernel Golden Corn, liquid pack, 17-oz. can	309	63.2	18.2	3.72	160	33.0	
Drained solids (yield: approx. 10.5 oz.)	(263)	(50.2)	(25.0)	(4.78)	(153)	(29.2)	
Whole Kernel Mexicorn Golden Corn with Peppers, 7-oz. can	171	35.6	24.4	5.08	150	30.0	
Drained solids (yield: approx. 4.3 oz.)	(152)	(30.3)	(35.4)	(7.03)	(216)	(42.9)	
12-oz. can	293	60.9	24.4	5.08	150	30.0	
Drained solids (yield: approx. 7.4 oz.)	(261)	(51.7)	(35.4)	(7.03)	(216)	(42.9)	
Whole Kernel Niblets Golden Corn, vacuum pack, 7-oz. can	165	34.2	23.6	4.88	150	30.0	
Drained solids (yield: approx. 6.3 oz.)	(165)	(34.2)	(26.2)	(5.43)	(153)	(31.7)	
12-oz. can	283	58.6	23.6	4.88	150	30.0	
Drained solids (yield: approx. 10.8 oz.)	(283)	(58.6)	(26.2)	(5.43)	(153)	(31.7)	
Whole Kernel White Corn, vacuum pack, 7-oz. can	169	34.8	24.1	4.97	150	30.0	
Drained solids (yield: approx. 6.3 oz.)	(169)	(34.8)	(26.8)	(5.52)	(157)	(32.2)	
Golden Harvest Whole Kernel Corn, 16-oz. (1-lb.) can	320	74.0	20.0	4.63	(125)	(28.5)	
Drained solids (yield: approx. 10 oz.)	278	62.0	27.8	6.20	170	37.8	
Kounty Kist Whole Kernel Golden Corn, liquid pack, 17-oz. can	(327)	(68.9)	(20.4)	(4.31)	180	38.0	
Drained solids (yield: approx. 10.5 oz.)	(282)	(55.9)	(31.1)	(5.32)	(190)	(32.5)	
Whole Kernel Golden Corn, vacuum pack, 7-oz. can	185	38.7	26.4	5.53	160	35.0	
Drained solids (yield: approx. 6.3 oz.)	(185)	(38.7)	(29.4)	(6.14)	(171)	(35.6)	
Libby's Whole Kernel Sweet Corn, wet pack, 8¾-oz. can	(151)	(34.8)	(17.2)	(3.98)	(160)	(37.0)	
Drained solids (yield: approx. 5.3 oz.)	(126)	(27.8)	(23.6)	(5.25)	(144)	(32.0)	
17-oz. can	(292)	(67.7)	(17.2)	(3.98)	160	37.0	
Drained solids (yield: approx. 10.5 oz.)	(246)	(54.7)	(23.6)	(5.25)	(144)	(32.0)	
Lindy Whole Kernel Golden Corn, liquid pack, 17-oz. can	(327)	(68.9)	(20.4)	(4.31)	180	38.0	
Drained solids (yield: approx. 10.5 oz.)	(282)	(55.9)	(31.1)	(5.32)	(190)	(32.5)	
Whole Kernel Golden Corn, vacuum pack, 7-oz. can	185	38.7	26.4	5.53	160	35.0	
Drained solids (yield: approx. 6.3 oz.)	(185)	(38.7)	(29.4)	(6.14)	(171)	(35.6)	
P&Q (A&P) Whole Kernel Corn, 16½-oz. can	360	80.0	21.8	4.85	180	40.0	
Stokely Golden Corn, liquid pack, 8½-oz. can	170	36.9	20.0	4.34	180	39.0	
Drained solids (yield: approx. 5.3 oz.)	(147)	(30.4)	(28.0)	(5.80)	(171)	(35.4)	
17-oz. can	340	73.8	20.0	4.34	180	39.0	
Drained solids (yield: approx. 10.5 oz.)	(294)	(60.8)	(28.0)	(5.80)	(171)	(35.4)	
Golden Corn, vacuum pack, 12-oz. can	(326)	(72.0)	(27.2)	(6.01)	(240)	(53.0)	
Drained solids (yield: approx. 10 oz.)	(312)	(68.0)	(31.2)	(6.80)	(187)	(40.8)	

	UNIT Cal.	UNIT Carb.	1 OZ., BY WT. Cal.	1 OZ., BY WT. Carb.	1 CUP Cal.	1 CUP Carb.	Fiber per oz. (GMS.)
White Corn, 16-oz. (1-lb.) can	(338)	(73.0)	(21.1)	(4.56)	190	41.0	
Drained solids (yield: approx. 10 oz.)	(295)	(60.8)	(29.8)	(6.14)	(173)	(35.7)	
Whole Kernel White Corn, 17-oz. can	331	71.5	20.7	4.47	190	41.0	
Drained solids (yield: approx. 10.5 oz.)	(315)	(64.9)	(30.0)	(6.18)	(175)	(36.1)	
Tillie Lewis "Tasti Diet" Fancy Whole Kernel Golden Sweet Corn, sodium controlled, 8-oz. can	140	30.0	17.5	3.75	140	30.0	
Cream-Style:							
A & P Cream Style Corn, 16½-oz. can	440	102.0	26.7	6.18	220	51.0	
Ann Page (A&P) Cream Style Corn, 8½-oz. can	220	51.0	(26.0)	(6.00)	220	51.0	
17-oz. can	440	102.0	(26.0)	(6.00)	220	51.0	
Blue Boy Cream Style Corn, 8½-oz. can	198	45.3	23.3	5.33	210	48.0	
Del Monte Cream Style Golden Corn, 8¾-oz. can	216	47.4	24.7	5.41	210	46.0	
17-oz. can	420	92.0	24.7	5.41	210	46.0	
Cream Style White Corn, 8¾-oz. can	196	43.2	22.4	4.94	190	42.0	
17-oz. can	380	84.0	22.4	4.94	190	42.0	
Featherweight Cream Style Golden Corn, no added salt or sugar, 8-oz. can	(160)	(36.0)	(20.0)	(4.50)	160	36.0	
Green Giant Cream Style Golden Corn, 8½-oz. can	205	44.6	24.1	5.25	210	45.0	
17-oz. can	410	89.2	24.1	5.25	210	45.0	
Kounty Kist Cream Style Golden Corn, 8½-oz. can	210	46.3	24.7	5.45	230	50.0	
17-oz. can	420	92.6	24.7	5.45	230	50.0	
Libby's Cream Style Sweet Corn, 8½-oz. can	161	39.7	18.9	4.67	170	42.0	
16½-oz. can	312	77.1	18.9	4.67	170	42.0	
P&Q (A&P) Cream Style Corn, 16½-oz. can	440	102.0	26.7	6.18	220	51.0	
S & W Nutradiet Cream Style Fancy Corn, packed in water without salt or sugar, 8½-oz. can	200	42.0	23.5	4.94	200	42.0	
Stokely Cream Style Golden Corn, 8½-oz. can	198	44.4	23.3	5.22	210	47.0	
17-oz. can	396	88.7	23.3	5.22	210	47.0	
Cream Style White Corn, 17-oz. can	371	87.1	21.8	5.12	200	47.0	

Corn Products

	UNIT Cal.	UNIT Carb.	1 OZ., BY WT. Cal.	1 OZ., BY WT. Carb.	1 CUP Cal.	1 CUP Carb.	Fiber per oz. (GMS.)
CORN FRITTERS							
Based on USDA home recipe, made from 2 large eggs; 2 cups of flour; 2 cups of canned, drained corn; 1½ cups milk; 1 tsp. cooking fat; 1 tsp. salt (yield: approx. 21.94 oz., 17¾ fritters, each approx. 2″ in diameter, and 1½″ thick)	2345	246.9	106.9	11.25			0.20
1 fritter (approx. 1.2 oz.)	132	13.9	106.9	11.25			0.20
1 pound (approx. 13 fritters)	1710	180.1	106.9	11.25			0.20
Mrs. Paul's Corn Fritters, 12-oz. package, 6 fritters	780	93.0	65.0	7.75			
1 fritter, approx. 2 oz.	130	15.5	65.0	7.75			
8-oz. package, 4 fritters	520	62.0	65.0	7.75			
1 fritter, approx. 2 oz.	130	15.5	65.0	7.75			
CORN GRITS							
(Degermed, enriched or unenriched)							
Regular or quick-cooking, dry:							
1 cup (approx. 5.6 oz.)	579	125.0	103.4	22.32	579	125.0	
1 pound (approx. 2.8 cups) (tr/22g/2g/12%/tr)	1642	354.3	103.4	22.32	579	125.0	
Cooked:							
1 cup (approx. 8.6 oz.)	125	27.0	14.5	3.14	125	27.0	
1 pound (tr/3g/tr/87%/58mg)	231	49.9	14.5	3.14	125	27.0	
CORN OIL							
Arrowhead Mills Corn Oil, 1 pint (16-fl.-oz.) bottle	3840	0.0	250.0	0.00	1920	0.0	0.0
POPCORN							
Unpopped:							
1 cup (approx. 7¼ oz.)	742	147.8	102.6	20.44	742	147.8	0.60
1 pound (approx. 2¼ cups) (3g/20g/1g/10%/1mg)	1642	327.0	102.6	20.44	742	147.8	0.60
Popped, plain, large-kernel							
1 cup (approx. 0.2 oz.)	23	4.6	109.4	21.74	23	4.6	0.63
1 pound (approx. 76 cups) (4g/22g/1g/4%/1mg)	1751	347.9	109.4	21.74	23	4.6	0.63

	UNIT		1 OZ., BY WT.		1 CUP		Fiber per oz.
	Cal.	Carb.	Cal.	Carb.	Cal.	Carb.	(GMS.)
Popped with 1 tablespoon oil added per ¼ cup unpopped kernels, salt added:							
1 cup (approx. 0.3 oz.)	41	5.3	129.3	16.76	41	5.3	0.48
1 pound (approx. 53 cups) (3g/17g/6g/3%/550mg)	2068	268.1	129.3	16.76	41	5.3	0.48
COUSCOUS, see under WHEAT							
COWPEAS							
MATURE SEEDS, Dry							
RAW:							
1 cup (approx. 6.0 oz.)	583	104.9	97.3	17.49	583	104.9	1.25
1 pound (approx. 2.7 cups) (6g/17g/tr/11%/10mg)	1556	279.9	97.3	17.49	583	104.9	1.25
COOKED:							
Boiled, drained:							
1 cup (approx. 8.8 oz.)	(310)	(55.7)	(35.2)	(6.33)	(310)	(55.7)	0.45
1 pound (approx. 1.8 cups) (yield from approx. 5.8 oz. dry peas) (1g/6g/tr/80%/2mg)	(564)	(101.2)	(35.2)	(6.33)	(310)	(55.7)	0.45
IMMATURE SEEDS							
RAW:							
1 cup (approx. 5.1 oz.)	184	31.6	36.0	6.18	184	31.6	0.51
1 pound (approx. 3.1 cups (3g/6g/tr/67%/1mg)	576	98.9	36.0	6.18	184	31.6	0.51
COOKED:							
Boiled, drained							
1 cup (approx. 5.8 oz.)	178	29.9	30.6	5.13	178	29.9	0.43
1 pound (approx. 2.8 cups) (yield from approx. 13.6 oz. uncooked peas) (2g/5g/tr/72%/tr)	490	82.1	30.6	5.13	178	29.9	0.43
YOUNG PODS							
RAW:							
1 cup (approx. 3.2 oz.)	(36)	(7.8)	11.4	2.45	(36)	(7.8)	0.48
1 pound (approx. 5 cups) (1g/2g/tr/86%/1mg)	182	39.2	11.4	2.45	(36)	(7.8)	0.48
COOKED:							
Boiled, drained:							
1 cup (approx. 3.6 oz.)	(35)	(7.1)	9.8	1.98	(35)	(7.1)	0.40
1 pound (approx. 4.4 cups) (yield from approx. 13.5 oz. of uncooked pods) (1g/2g/tr/90%/1mg)	154	31.8	9.6	1.98	(35)	(7.1)	0.40
CRANBERRY SAUCE							
This is generic information. For information by brand, see the CONDIMENTS chapter.							
BASED ON USDA HOME RECIPE:							
Unstrained:							
1 cup (approx. 9.8 oz.)	493	126.0	53.0	12.86	493	126.0	0.20
1 pound (approx. 1.6 cups) (tr/13g/tr/54%/tr)	848	205.8	53.0	12.86	493	126.0	0.20
CANNED:							
Strained, sugar added							
1 cup (approx. 9.8 oz.)	404	103.9	41.4	10.63	404	103.9	0.06
1 pound (approx. 1.6 cups) (tr/11g/tr/52%/tr)	662	170.1	41.4	10.63	404	103.9	0.06
1 Can, #300, 16 oz. (1 lb.)	662	170.1	41.4	10.63	404	103.9	0.06
1 Can, #10, 117 oz. (7 lb. 5 oz.)	4843	1243.9	41.4	10.63	404	103.9	0.06
CRESS, see GARDEN CRESS and WATERCRESS							
CROWDER PEAS							
FROZEN, by brand:							
Seabrook Farms, Crowder Peas, 10-oz. package	390	63.0	39.0	6.30			
Boiled, drained (yield: approx. 9.3 oz.)	390	63.0	(41.9)	(6.77)	(247)	(39.9)	
CUCUMBERS							
RAW:							
As purchased [refuse: ends, approx. 3%]:							
1 small cucumber (approx. 1¾″ diameter, 6⅜″ long, 6.1 oz.)	25	5.8	4.1	0.93			
1 large cucumber (approx. 2⅛″ diameter, 8¼″ long, 10.9 oz.)	45	10.2	4.1	0.93			

	UNIT		1 OZ., BY WT.		1 CUP		Fiber per oz.
	Cal.	Carb.	Cal.	Carb.	Cal.	Carb.	(GMS.)
As purchased [refuse: parings, ends, and bruised spots, approx. 27%]:							
1 small cucumber (approx. 1¾″ diameter, 6⅜″ long (approx. 6.1 oz.)	22	5.1	3.6	0.84			
1 large cucumber (approx. 2⅛″ diameter, 8¼″ long, 10.9 oz.)	39	9.0	3.6	0.84			
Edible portion:							
Eaten with skins:							
1 cup of sliced cucumbers, each slice approx. ⅛″ thick (approx. 4.3 oz.)	16	3.6	4.3	0.96	16	3.6	0.17
1 pound (approx. 1½ large or 2⅔ small cucumbers, or 4⅓ cups of sliced cucumbers)	68	15.4	4.3	0.96	16	3.6	0.17
Eaten without skin:							
1 cup of sliced cucumbers, each slice approx. ⅛″ thick (approx. 4.9 oz.)	19	4.5	3.9	0.91	19	4.5	0.09
1 cup of diced cucumbers (approx. 5.1 oz.)	20	4.5	3.9	0.91	20	4.5	0.09
1 pound (approx. 1½ large or 2⅔ small cucumbers, or 3.3 cups of sliced or 3.1 cups of diced cucumber	62	14.6	3.9	0.91			0.09
CUCUMBER AND YOGURT SALAD (based on data from the Middle East)							
Prepared with 1 quart yogurt, 1¾ lb. sliced cucumber, garlic paste, and mint (yield: approx. 4 lbs. 64 oz.)	672	49.2	10.5	0.77			
1 pound	168	12.3	10.5	0.77			
Cucumbers, Pickled (pickles)							
This is generic information. For information by brand, see the CONDIMENTS chapter.							
BREAD AND BUTTER OR FRESH PICKLES (sugar added)							
Crosscut slices, each approx. 1½″ diameter, ¼″ thick:							
1 slice (approx. 0.3 oz.)	5	1.3	20.7	5.08	124	30.4	0.14
1 cup (approx. 23 slices, 6 oz.)	124	30.4	20.7	5.08	124	30.4	0.14
1 pound (approx. 2.7 cups) (tr/5g/tr/79%/192mg)	331	81.2	20.7	5.08	124	30.4	0.14
CHOWCHOW OR MUSTARD PICKLES (Cucumber with added cauliflower, onion, and mustard)							
Sour:							
1 cup (approx. 8.6 oz.)	70	9.8	8.3	1.16	70	9.8	0.17
1 pound (approx. 1.9 cups) (tr/1g/tr/88%/382mg)	132	18.6	8.3	1.16	70	9.8	0.17
Sweet:							
1 cup (approx. 8.4 oz.)	284	66.2	32.9	7.66	284	66.2	0.26
1 pound (approx. 1.9 cups) (tr/8g/tr/69%/151mg)	526	122.5	32.9	7.66	284	66.2	0.26
DILL PICKLES							
Whole:							
1 medium dill pickle (approx. 3¾″ long, 1¼″ diameter, 2.2 oz.)	7	1.4	3.1	0.63			0.14
1 large dill pickle (approx. 4″ long, 1¾″ diameter, 4.8 oz.)	15	3.0	3.1	0.63			0.14
1 pound (approx. 3.3 large or 7.3 medium pickles) (tr/1g/tr/93%/408mg)	50	10.0	3.1	0.63			0.14
Sliced:							
Sliced lengthwise with triangular-shaped cross section (spears or sticks) approx. 6″ long, 1″–1½″ across:							
1 slice (approx. 1.1 oz.)	3	0.7	3.1	0.63			0.14
1 pound (approx. 15 slices)	50	10.1	3.1	0.63			0.14
Sliced crosswise, 1½″ diameter, ¼″ thick:							
1 slice (approx. 0.22 oz.)	1	0.1	3.1	0.63	17	3.4	0.14
1 cup (approx. 23 slices, 5½ oz.)	17	3.4	3.1	0.63	17	3.4	0.14
1 pound (approx. 72 slices)	50	10.1	3.1	0.63			0.14
SOUR PICKLES							
1 medium sour pickle (approx. 3¾″ long, 1¼″ diameter, 2.3 oz.)	7	1.3	2.8	0.57			0.14
1 large sour pickle (approx. 4″ long, 1¾″ diameter, 4.8 oz.)	14	2.7	2.8	0.57			0.14
1 pound (approx. 3.3 large or 7 medium pickles) (tr/1g/tr/95%/386mg)	45	9.1	2.8	0.57			0.14

	UNIT		1 OZ., BY WT.		1 CUP		Fiber per oz. (GMS.)
	Cal.	Carb.	Cal.	Carb.	Cal.	Carb.	
SWEET PICKLES (sugar has been added)							
Whole:							
1 midget gherkin (approx. 2⅛" long, ⅜" diameter, 0.21 oz.)	9	2.2	41.4	10.35			
1 small gherkin (approx. 2½" long, ¾" diameter, 0.53 oz.)	22	5.5	41.4	10.35			
1 large gherkin (approx. 3" long, 1" diameter, 1.23 oz.)	51	12.8	41.4	10.35			
1 pound (approx. 13 large, 30 small, or 76 midget gherkins) (tr/10g/tr/61%/na)	662	165.6	41.4	10.35			
Sliced:							
Sliced lengthwise with triangular-shaped cross section, approx. 4½" long, 1½" across:							
1 slice, approx. 0.71 oz.	29	7.3	41.4	10.35			
1 pound (approx. 22½ slices)	662	165.6	41.4	10.35			
Chopped into ¼" cubes:							
1 cup (approx. 5.6 oz.)	234	58.4	41.4	10.35	234	58.4	
1 pound (approx. 2.9 cups)	662	165.6	41.4	10.35	234	58.4	
DANDELION GREENS							
RAW:							
As purchased fully trimmed (all-edible):							
1 pound (1g/3g/tr/86%/22mg)	204	41.7	12.8	2.61			
COOKED:							
Boiled, drained:							
1 cup:							
Not packed (approx. 3.7 oz.)	35	6.7	9.4	1.81	35	6.7	0.37
Packed (approx. 7.4 oz.)	70	13.4	9.4	1.81	70	13.4	0.37
1 pound (approx. 2.2 cups, packed; 4⅓ cups, not packed) (1g/2g/tr/90%/12mg)	150	29.0	9.4	1.81			0.37
DHAL, see under LENTILS							
DILL WEED, dried, see the SALTS & SPICES chapter							
DOCK (Curly or narrowleaf dock, broadleaf dock, and sheet sorrel)							
RAW:							
As purchased [refuse: stems, approx. 30%]:							
1 pound	89	17.8	5.6	1.11			
Edible portion:							
1 pound (1g/2g/tr/91%/1mg)	127	25.4	7.9	1.59			0.23
COOKED:							
Boiled, drained:							
1 pound (tr/1g/tr/94%/1mg)	86	17.7	5.4	1.11			0.20
EGGPLANT							
RAW:							
As purchased [refuse: ends, parings, and trimmings, approx. 19%]:							
1 pound	92	20.6	5.8	1.29			
Edible portion:							
1 pound	114	25.4	7.1	1.59			0.26
1 pound (based on data from the Middle East) (tr/2g/tr/92%/1mg)	145	23.1	9.1	1.45			
COOKED:							
Boiled, drained:							
1 cup, diced (approx. 7 oz.)	38	8.1	5.4	1.16	38	8.1	0.20
1 pound (approx. 2¼ cups diced) (tr/1g/tr/94%/tr)	86	18.6	5.4	1.16	38	8.1	0.20
Steamed:							
1 pound of raw eggplant, steamed (yield: approx. 15 oz.)	114	25.4	7.6	1.69			0.28
1 pound of steamed eggplant	122	27.1	7.6	1.69			0.28

	UNIT		1 OZ., BY WT.		1 CUP		Fiber per oz. (GMS.)
	Cal.	Carb.	Cal.	Carb.	Cal.	Carb.	
FROZEN, by brand:							
Mrs. Paul's Fried Eggplant Slices, 9-oz. package	690	66.0	76.7	7.33			
Fried Eggplant Sticks, 7-oz. package	520	54.0	74.3	7.71			
Tree Tavern Eggplant Parmigiana, 10-oz. box	370	25.0	37.0	2.50			
EGGPLANT DIP (Baba Ghanouj) (based on data from the Middle East)							
Prepared with 4½ lb. raw eggplant, 1 Tbsp. garlic, 1⅓ cups tahini sauce, 1 cup lemon juice, 3 fl. oz. water (yield: "10 servings")							
1 pound	481	66.2	30.1	4.14			
ENDIVE (Curly endive)							
RAW:							
As purchased:							
Good quality [refuse: ends, approx. 12%]:							
1 pound	80	16.4	5.0	1.03			
Fair quality [refuse: ends, outer leaves, and trimmings, approx. 25%]:							
1 pound	68	13.9	4.3	0.87			
Edible portion:							
1 cup, small pieces (approx. 1¾ oz.)	10	2.0	5.7	1.16	10	2.0	0.26
1 pound (approx. 9 cups) (tr/1g/tr/93%/4mg)	91	18.6	5.7	1.16	10	2.0	0.26
ENDIVE, FRENCH or BELGIAN, see CHICORY							
ESCAROLE							
RAW:							
As purchased:							
Good quality [refuse: ends, approx. 12%]:							
1 pound	80	16.4	5.0	1.03			
Fair quality [refuse: ends, outer leaves, trimmings, approx. 25%]:							
1 pound	68	13.9	4.3	0.87			
Edible portion:							
1 cup, small pieces (approx. 1¾ oz.)	10	2.0	5.7	1.16	10	2.0	0.26
1 pound (approx. 9 cups) (tr/1g/tr/93%/4mg)	91	18.6	5.7	1.16	10	2.0	0.26
FALAFEL, see under CHICK-PEAS							
FAVA BEANS (based on data from France)							
IMMATURE SEEDS							
RAW:							
1 pound	290	45.4	18.1	2.84			
COOKED:							
Boiled, drained:							
1 pound	200	22.7	12.5	1.42			
MATURE SEEDS, Dry							
RAW:							
1 pound	1556	267.6	97.2	16.73			
COOKED:							
Boiled, drained:							
1 pound	1016	133.8	63.5	8.36			
FENNEL							
COMMON LEAVES							
RAW:							
As purchased [refuse: trimmings, approx. 7%]:							
1 pound	118	21.5	7.4	1.34			
Edible portion:							
1 pound (1g/1g/tr/90%/na)	126	23.1	7.9	1.45			0.14

	UNIT		1 OZ., BY WT.		1 CUP		Fiber per oz.
	Cal.	Carb.	Cal.	Carb.	Cal.	Carb.	(GMS.)
FENNEL SEED, see the SALTS & SPICES chapter							
FIDDLEHEAD GREENS (based on data from Canada)							
FROZEN, based on generic data:							
Boiled, drained:							
1 pound	150	22.7	9.4	1.42			
GARBANZOS, see CHICK-PEAS							
GARDEN CRESS							
RAW:							
As purchased [refuse: stems, crowns, and spoiled leaves, approx. 29%]:							
1 pound	103	17.7	6.4	1.11			
Edible portion:							
1 pound (1g/2g/tr/89%/4mg)	145	24.9	9.1	1.56			0.31
COOKED:							
Boiled, drained:							
1 cup (approx. 4¾ oz.)	31	5.1	6.5	1.08	31	5.1	0.26
1 pound (approx. 3⅓ cups) (1g/1g/tr/93%/2mg)	104	17.2	6.5	1.08	31	5.1	0.26
GARLIC							
CLOVES							
RAW:							
As purchased [refuse: skins, approx. 12%]:							
1 pound	547	123.0	34.2	7.69			
Edible portion:							
1 clove (approx. 1/10 oz., 1¼ × ⅝ × ⅜")	4	0.9	38.8	8.73			0.43
1 pound (2g/9g/tr/61%/5mg)	621	139.7	38.8	8.73			0.43
GARLIC POWDER, see the SALTS & SPICES chapter							
GOOBER PEAS, see PEANUTS in the NUTS & SEEDS chapter							
GOURD, see TOWEL GOURD and WAX GOURD							
GRAPE LEAVES (based on data from the Middle East)							
RAW:							
Edible portion:							
1 pound	440	70.8	27.5	4.42			
STUFFED GRAPE LEAVES							
1 pound	508	(29.0)	31.8	(1.81)			
GREEN BEANS (String Beans, Snap Beans)							
RAW:							
As purchased [refuse: ends, strings, and trimmings, approx. 12%]:							
1 pound	128	28.3	8.0	1.77			
Edible portion:							
1 cup, pods, 1"–2" in length (approx. 3.9 oz.)	35	7.8	9.1	2.01	35	7.8	0.28
1 pound (approx. 4.1 cups) (yield: about 3⅔ cups cooked beans) (1g/2g/tr/90%/2mg)	145	32.2	9.1	2.01	35	7.8	0.28
COOKED:							
Boiled, drained:							
(Cups apply to regular-cut and French-cut beans)							
Cooked in a small amount of water for a short time:							
1 cup (approx. 4.4 oz.)	31	6.8	7.1	1.53	31	6.8	0.22
1 pound (approx. 3.6 cups) (tr/1g/tr/92%/1mg)	113	24.5	7.1	1.53	31	6.8	0.22
Cooked in a large amount of water for a long time:							
1 cup (approx. 4.4 oz.)	(31)	(6.8)	7.1	1.53	(31)	(6.8)	0.22
1 pound (approx. 3.6 cups) (tr/1g/tr/92%/1mg)	113	24.5	7.1	1.53	(31)	(6.8)	0.22
Steamed:							
1 pound of raw green beans, steamed (yield: approx. 15.7 oz.)	(145)	(32.2)	(9.2)	(2.05)			(0.29)
1 pound of steamed green beans	(148)	(32.9)	(9.2)	(2.05)			(0.29)
FROZEN, based on generic data:							
Cut crosswise:							
Measured when frozen:							
1 cup (approx. 4.4 oz.)	33	7.5	7.4	1.70	33	7.5	
1 pound (approx. 3.6 cups)	118	27.2	7.4	1.70	33	7.5	
1 container, 9 oz. net wt.	66	15.3	7.4	1.70	33	7.5	
1 container, 10 oz. net wt.	74	17.0	7.4	1.70	33	7.5	
Boiled, drained:							
1 cup (approx. 4.8 oz.)	34	7.7	7.1	1.62	34	7.7	0.28
1 pound of frozen green beans, boiled, then drained (yield: approx. 14.8 oz.)	105	23.9	7.1	1.62	34	7.7	0.28
1 pound of boiled, drained green beans (tr/2g/tr/92%/tr)	113	25.9	7.1	1.62	34	7.7	0.28
1 container, 9 oz., boiled, then drained (yield: approx. 8.3 oz.)	59	13.4	7.1	1.62	34	7.7	0.28
1 container, 10 oz., boiled, then drained (yield: approx. 9.2 oz.)	65	14.8	7.1	1.62	34	7.7	0.28
Cut French style:							
Measured when frozen:							
1 cup (approx. 3.5 oz.)	26	6.1	7.6	1.73	27	6.1	
1 pound (approx. 4.5 cups)	122	27.7	7.6	1.73	27	6.1	
1 container, 9 oz. net wt.	69	15.6	7.6	1.73	27	6.1	
1 container, 10 oz. net wt.	77	17.3	7.6	1.73	27	6.1	
Boiled, drained:							
1 cup (approx. 4.6 oz.)	34	7.8	7.4	1.70	34	7.8	0.31
1 pound of frozen green beans, boiled, then drained (yield: approx. 14.1 oz.)	104	23.9	7.4	1.70	34	7.8	0.31
1 pound of boiled, drained green beans (tr/29/tr/92%/tr)	118	27.2	7.4	1.70	34	7.8	0.31
1 container, 9 oz., boiled, then drained (yield: approx. 7.9 oz.)	59	13.5	7.4	1.70	34	7.8	0.31
1 container, 10 oz., boiled, then drained (yield: approx. 8.8 oz.)	65	15.0	7.4	1.70	34	7.8	0.31
FROZEN, by brand:							
Bel-Air Cut Green Beans, 9-oz. package	90	18.0	10.0	2.00			
Boiled, drained (yield: approx. 8.1 oz.)	90	18.0	11.1	2.22	61	12.2	
French Style Green Beans, 9-oz. package	90	18.0	10.0	2.00			
Boiled, drained (yield: approx. 8.1 oz.)	90	18.0	11.1	2.22	52	10.5	
Birds Eye Cut Green Beans, 9-oz. package	75	15.0	8.3	1.67			
Boiled, drained (yield: approx. 8.1 oz.)	(75)	(15.0)	(9.3)	(1.85)	(46)	(9.1)	
French Style Green Beans, 9-oz. package	90	18.0	10.0	2.00			
Boiled, drained (yield: approx. 8.1 oz.)	(90)	(18.0)	(11.1)	(2.22)	(47)	(9.5)	
Italian Green Beans, 9-oz. package	90	18.0	10.0	2.00			
Boiled, drained (yield: approx. 8.1 oz.)	(90)	(18.0)	(11.1)	(2.22)	(47)	(9.5)	
Whole Green Beans, 9-oz. package	75	15.0	8.3	1.67			
Boiled, drained (yield: approx. 9 oz.)	(75)	(15.0)	(8.3)	(1.67)	(40)	(8.0)	
Green Giant French Cut Green Beans, 9-oz. package, Boil-in-Bag	97	8.9	10.8	0.99			
Boiled, drained (yield: approx. 9 oz.)	97	8.9	10.8	0.99	70	7.0	
Hanover Blue Lake Cut Green Beans, 16-oz. (1-lb.) package	150	30.1	9.4	1.88			
Boiled, drained (yield: approx. 16 oz. (1 lb.)	150	30.1	9.4	1.88	(52)	(10.3)	

	UNIT		1 OZ., BY WT.		1 CUP		Fiber per oz.
	Cal.	Carb.	Cal.	Carb.	Cal.	Carb.	(GMS.)
Blue Lake French Style Green Beans, 16-oz. (1-lb.) package	100	20.0	6.3	1.25			
Boiled, drained (yield: approx. 16 oz.)	100	20.0		1.25	(30)	(5.9)	
Kounty Kist Cut Green Beans, 18-oz. package, poly bag	112	20.9	6.2	1.16			
Boiled, drained (yield: approx. 18 oz.)	112	20.9	6.2	1.16	30	6.0	
Seabrook Farms French Green Beans, 9-oz. package	90	18.0	10.0	2.00			
Boiled, drained (yield: approx. 8.1 oz.)	(90)	(18.0)	11.1	2.22	(47)	(9.5)	
Italian Green Beans, 9-oz. package	105	21.0	11.7	2.33			
Boiled, drained (yield: approx. 8.1 oz.)	(105)	(21.0)	13.0	2.59	(55)	(11.0)	
Whole Green Beans, 9-oz. package	90	18.0	10.0	2.00	(44)	(8.8)	
Village Park cut green beans, 16-oz. (1-lb.) package	150	30.0	9.4	1.88			
Boiled, drained (yield: approx. 14.4 oz.)	(150)	(30.0)	(10.4)	(2.08)	(57)	(11.4)	
GREEN BEANS AND . . . GREEN BEANS WITH							
Birds Eye French Green Beans with Toasted Almonds, 9-oz. package	150	24.0	16.7	2.67			
Boiled, drained (yield: approx. 8.1 oz.)	(150)	(24.0)	(18.5)	(2.96)	(102)	(16.3)	
French Green Beans with Sliced Mushrooms, 9-oz. package	90	18.0	10.0	2.00			
Boiled, drained (yield: approx. 8.1 oz.)	(90)	(18.0)	(11.1)	(2.22)	(61)	(12.2)	
Green Beans and Onions Flavored with Bacon Bits, 9-oz. package	94	10.7	10.5	1.19			
Boiled, drained (yield: approx. 8.1 oz.)	(94)	(10.7)	(11.1)	(1.32)	(61)	(7.3)	
Green Beans and Pearl Onions, 9-oz. package	90	18.0	10.0	2.00			
Boiled, drained (yield: approx. 8.1 oz.)	(90)	(18.0)	(11.1)	(2.96)	(61)	(16.3)	
Stouffer's Green Bean Mushroom Casserole, 9½-oz. package	300	24.0	31.6	2.53			
CANNED, based on generic data:							
Regular pack:							
Cut crosswise:							
Solids and liquid:							
1 cup (approx. 8.4 oz.)	43	10.0	5.1	1.19	43	10.0	0.17
1 pound (approx. 1.9 cups) (tr/1g/tr/94%/67mg)	82	19.1	5.1	1.19	43	10.0	0.17
1 #303 can, 15½ oz. net wt. (approx. 1.8 cups)	79	18.4	5.1	1.19	43	10.0	0.17
Drained solids:							
1 cup (approx. 4.7 oz.)	32	7.0	6.8	1.48	32	7.0	0.28
1 pound (approx. 3.4 cups) (tr/1g/tr/92%/67mg)	109	23.6	6.8	1.48	32	7.0	0.28
1 #303 can (yield: approx. 9¼ oz. of drained beans, approx. 2 cups)	63	13.6	6.8	1.48	32	7.0	0.28
Drained liquid:							
1 cup (approx. 8.3 oz.)	(21)	(6.4)	(2.6)	(0.77)	(21)	(6.4)	trace
1 pound (approx. 1.9 cups) (tr/1g/tr/96%/67mg)	42	12.3	(2.6)	(0.77)	(21)	(6.4)	trace
1 #303 can (yield: approx. 6¼ oz. of liquid, approx. ¾ cups)	(16)	(4.8)	(2.6)	(0.77)	(21)	(6.4)	trace
Low-sodium pack:							
Cut crosswise or French cut:							
Solids and liquid:							
1 cup (approx. 8.3 oz.)	38	8.6	4.6	102	38	8.6	0.17
1 pound (approx. 1.9 cups) (tr/1g/tr/95%/1mg)	73	16.3	4.6	1.02	38	8.6	0.17
1 #303 can, 15½ oz. net wt. (approx. 1.9 cups)	70	15.8	4.6	1.02	38	8.6	0.17
Drained solids:							
1 cup (approx. 4.8 oz.)	30	6.5	6.3	1.36	30	6.5	0.26
1 pound (approx. 3.3 cups) (tr/1g/tr/93%/1mg)	100	21.8	6.3	1.36	30	6.5	0.26
1 #303 can (yield: approx. 9¼ oz. of drained beans, approx. 1.9 cups)	58	12.6	6.3	1.36	30	6.5	0.26
Drained liquid:							
1 cup (approx. 8.3 oz.)	(16)	(4.3)	(1.9)	(0.51)	(16)	(4.3)	trace
1 pound (approx. 1.9 cups) (tr/1g/tr/97%/1mg)	(31)	(8.2)	(1.9)	(0.51)	(16)	(4.3)	trace
1 #303 can (yield: approx. 6¼ oz. of liquid, approx. ¾ cups)	(12)	(3.2)	(1.9)	(0.51)	(16)	(4.3)	trace

	UNIT		1 OZ., BY WT.		1 CUP		Fiber per oz.
	Cal.	Carb.	Cal.	Carb.	Cal.	Carb.	(GMS.)
CANNED, by brand:							
A&P Cut Green Beans, 8-oz. can	40	8.0	5.0	1.00	40	8.0	
Drained solids (yield: approx. 4.8 oz.)	(30)	(5.8)	(6.3)	(1.20)	(30)	(5.7)	
Whole Green Beans, 15½-oz. can	78	15.5	5.0	1.00	40	8.0	
Drained solids (yield: approx. 9.3 oz.)	(59)	(11.2)	(6.3)	(1.20)	(30)	(5.7)	
Ann Page (A&P) French-Style Stringless Green Beans, 8-oz. can	40	8.0	(5.0)	(1.00)	40	8.0	
Drained solids (yield: approx. 4.1 oz.)	(28)	(5.3)	(6.9)	(1.28)	(34)	(6.3)	
15½-oz. can	78	15.5	5.0	1.00	40	8.0	
Drained solids (yield: approx. 8 oz.)	(55)	(10.2)	(6.9)	(1.28)	(34)	(6.3)	
Balanced Cut Green Beans, packed in water, no added sugar or salt							
16-oz. (1-lb.) can	(114)	(22.7)	(7.1)	(1.42)	60	12.0	
Drained solids (yield: approx. 9.6 oz.)	(101)	(19.5)	(10.5)	(2.03)	(50)	(9.7)	
Blue Boy Green Beans, 8-oz. can	43	9.5	5.4	1.19	45	10.0	
Drained solids (yield: approx. 5.2 oz.)	35	7.5	6.7	1.45	30	6.4	
Del Monte Blue Lake Cut Green Beans, 8-oz. can	40	8.0	5.0	1.00	40	8.0	
Drained solids (yield: approx. 4 oz.)	(28)	(5.2)	(6.8)	(1.25)	(34)	(6.2)	
16-oz. (1-lb.) can	80	16.0	5.0	1.00	40	8.0	
Drained solids (yield: approx 8¾ oz.)	(58)	(10.9)	(6.8)	(1.25)	(34)	(6.2)	
Blue Lake French-Style Green Beans, 8-oz. can	40	7.0	5.0	0.88	40	7.0	
Drained solids (yield: approx. 4 oz.)	(28)	(4.2)	(6.8)	(1.04)	(34)	(5.2)	
16-oz. (1-lb.) can	80	14.0	5.0	0.88	40	7.0	
Drained solids (yield: approx. 8¾ oz.)	(58)	(9.1)	(6.8)	(1.04)	(34)	(5.2)	
Blue Lake French-Style Seasoned Green Beans, 8-oz. can	40	8.0	5.0	1.00	40	8.0	
Drained solids (yield: approx. 4 oz.)	(28)	(5.2)	(6.8)	(1.25)	(34)	(6.2)	
16-oz. (1-lb.) can	80	16.0	5.0	1.00	40	8.0	
Drained solids (yield: approx. 8¾ oz.)	(58)	(10.9)	(6.8)	(1.25)	(34)	(6.8)	
Italian Green Beans, 16-oz. (1-lb.) can	120	22.0	7.5	1.38	60	11.0	
Drained solids (yield: approx. 8¾ oz.)	(98)	(16.8)	(11.5)	(1.98)	(55)	(9.4)	
Seasoned Green Beans, 8-oz. can	(40)	(8.0)	5.0	1.00	50	8.0	
Drained solids (yield: approx. 4 oz.)	(28)	(5.2)	(6.8)	(1.25)	(34)	(6.2)	
16-oz. (1-lb.) can	(80)	(16.0)	5.0	1.00	50	8.0	
Drained solids (yield: approx. 8¾ oz.)	(58)	(10.9)	(6.8)	(1.25)	(34)	(6.2)	
Tiny Whole Green Beans, 16-oz. (1-lb.) can	80	14.0	5.0	0.88	40	7.0	
Drained solids (yield: approx. 9.6 oz.)	(61)	(9.5)	(6.4)	(0.99)	(28)	(4.4)	
Diet Delight Cut Green Beans, packed in water, 8-oz. can	40	6.0	5.0	0.75	40	6.0	
Drained solids (yield: approx. 4¼ oz.)	(30)	(3.8)	(6.3)	(0.78)	(30)	(3.7)	
Featherweight Cut Green Beans, no added sugar or salt, 8-oz. can	40	10.0	(5.0)	(1.25)	40	10.0	
Drained solids (yield: approx. 4.8 oz.)	(34)	(8.4)	(7.0)	(1.75)	(35)	(8.7)	
15½-oz. can	80	20.0	(5.0)	(1.25)	40	10.0	
Drained solids (yield: approx. 9.3 oz.)	(65)	(16.3)	(7.0)	(1.75)	(35)	(8.7)	
French-Style Green Beans, no added sugar or salt, 8-oz. can	(40)	(10.0)	(5.0)	(1.25)	(40)	(10.0)	
Drained solids (yield: approx. 4.8 oz.)	(34)	(8.4)	(7.0)	(1.75)	(35)	(8.6)	
Golden Harvest Green Beans, 15½-oz. can	80	18.0	5.2	1.16	40	9.0	
Drained solids (yield: approx. 8¾ oz.)	60	13.3	6.8	1.52	34	7.6	
Green Giant Whole Cut French-Style Green Beans, 8-oz. can	30	5.2	3.7	0.65	30	6.0	
Drained solids (yield: approx. 5.2 oz.)	(22)	(3.2)	(4.1)	(0.63)	(21)	(3.2)	
16-oz. (1-lb.) can	59	10.4	3.7	0.65	30	6.0	
Drained solids (yield: approx. 10.4 oz.)	(42)	(6.5)	(4.1)	(0.63)	(21)	(3.2)	

	UNIT Cal.	UNIT Carb.	1 OZ., BY WT. Cal.	1 OZ., BY WT. Carb.	1 CUP Cal.	1 CUP Carb.	Fiber per oz. (GMS.)
Hanover Blue Lake Cut Green Beans, 37-oz. can	207	41.8	5.6	1.13	(47)	(9.5)	
Drained solids (yield: approx. 22 oz.)	(162)	(31.3)	(7.3)	(1.48)	(37)	(7.4)	
50-oz. can	280	56.5	5.6	1.13	(47)	(9.5)	
Drained solids (yield: approx. 30 oz.)	(220)	(44.5)	(7.3)	(1.48)	(37)	(7.4)	
Cut Green Beans and Potatoes in Ham-Flavored Sauce, 39-oz. can	293	53.8	7.5	1.38			
Blue Lake French-Style Green Beans, 38½-oz. can	177	28.9	4.6	0.75	(39)	(6.3)	
Drained solids (yield: approx. 21.7 oz.)	(127)	(17.1)	(5.9)	(0.78)	(30)	(3.9)	
Libby's Blue Lake Cut Green Beans, 8-oz. can	(38)	(7.7)	(4.8)	(0.96)	40	8.0	
Drained solids (yield: approx. 4¼ oz.)	(27)	(5.1)	(6.3)	(1.20)	(32)	(6.0)	
16-oz (1-lb.) can	(77)	(15.4)	(4.8)	(0.96)	40	8.0	
Drained solids (yield: approx. 8¾ oz.)	(55)	(10.3)	(6.3)	(1.20)	(32)	(6.0)	
French-Style Green Beans, 8-oz. can	(34)	(7.8)	(4.3)	(0.97)	35	8.0	
Drained solids (yield: approx. 4.4 oz.)	(22)	(5.8)	(5.0)	(1.15)	(25)	(5.8)	
15½-oz. can	(67)	(15.0)	(4.3)	(0.97)	35	8.0	
Drained solids (yield: approx. 8 oz.)	(40)	(9.0)	(5.0)	(1.15)	(25)	(5.8)	
Whole Green Beans, 16-oz. (1-lb.) can	(69)	(15.7)	(4.3)	(0.98)	35	8.0	
Drained solids (yield: approx. 10.4 oz.)	(52)	(11.8)	(5.0)	(1.13)	(25)	(5.7)	
Lindy (Kounty Kist) Diagonal Cut Green Beans, 16-oz. (1-lb.) can	59	10.9	3.7	0.68	40	7.0	
Drained solids (yield: approx. 9.6 oz.)	(40)	(6.4)	(4.2)	(0.67)	(21)	(3.4)	
French-Style Green Beans, 16-oz. (1-lb.) can	59	10.9	3.7	0.68	40	7.0	
Drained solids (yield: approx. 9.6 oz.)	(40)	(6.4)	(4.2)	(0.67)	(21)	(3.4)	
Whole Green Beans, 16-oz. (1-lb.) can	59	10.9	3.7	0.68	40	7.0	
Drained solids (yield: approx. 9.6 oz.)	(40)	(6.4)	(4.2)	(0.67)	(21)	(3.4)	
P&Q (A&P) Cut Green Beans, 15½-oz. can	75	15.0	4.8	0.97	40	8.0	
Drained solids (yield: approx. 14.9 oz.)	(95)	(19.3)	(6.4)	(1.29)	(33)	(6.6)	
S&W Fancy Stringless Cut Green Beans, 8-oz. can	40	8.0	5.0	1.00	40	8.0	
Drained solids (yield: approx. 4.8 oz.)	(31)	(5.8)	(6.5)	(1.20)	(33)	(6.1)	
16-oz. (1-lb.) can	80	16.0	5.0	1.00	40	8.0	
Drained solids (yield: approx. 9.6 oz.)	(62)	(11.6)	(6.5)	(1.21)	(33)	(6.1)	
French-Style Julienne Green Beans, 8-oz. can	40	8.0	5.0	1.00	40	8.0	
Drained solids (yield: approx. 4.8 oz.)	(31)	(5.8)	(6.5)	(1.21)	(33)	(6.1)	
16-oz. (1-lb.) can	80	16.0	5.0	1.00	40	8.0	
Drained solids (yield: approx. 9.6 oz.)	(62)	(11.6)	(6.5)	(1.21)	(33)	(6.1)	
Whole Green Beans, vertically packed, 8-oz. can	40	8.0	5.0	1.00	40	8.0	
Drained solids (yield: approx. 4.8 oz.)	(31)	(5.8)	(6.5)	(1.21)	(33)	(6.1)	
16-oz. (1-lb.) can	80	16.0	5.0	1.00	40	8.0	
Drained solids (yield: approx. 9.6 oz.)	(62)	(11.6)	(6.5)	(1.21)	(33)	(6.1)	
S&W Nutradiet Cut Green Beans, packed in water without salt, 8-oz. can	40	8.0	5.0	1.00	40	8.0	
Drained solids (yield: approx. 4.8 oz.)	(31)	(5.8)	(6.5)	(1.21)	(33)	(6.1)	
Stokely Cut Green Beans, 8-oz. can	33	7.5	4.1	0.94	35	8.0	
Drained solids (yield: approx. 4.3 oz.)	(22)	(5.3)	(5.1)	(1.23)	(26)	(6.2)	
16-oz. (1-lb.) can	66	15.0	4.1	0.94	35	8.0	
Drained solids (yield: approx. 8½ oz.)	(44)	(10.5)	(5.1)	(1.23)	(26)	(6.2)	
French-Style Sliced Green Beans, 8-oz. can	33	7.5	4.1	0.94	35	8.0	
Drained solids (yield: approx. 4¼ oz.)	(27)	(4.9)	(6.5)	(1.15)	(33)	(5.8)	
16-oz (1-lb.) can	66	15.1	4.1	0.94	35	8.0	
Drained solids (yield: approx. 8½ oz.)	(55)	(9.8)	(6.5)	(1.15)	(33)	(5.8)	

	UNIT Cal.	UNIT Carb.	1 OZ., BY WT. Cal.	1 OZ., BY WT. Carb.	1 CUP Cal.	1 CUP Carb.	Fiber per oz. (GMS.)
Sliced Green Beans, 8-oz. can	37	7.4	4.6	0.93	40	8.0	
Drained solids (yield: approx. 4¼ oz.)	(26)	(4.8)	(6.1)	(1.13)	(31)	(5.7)	
16-oz. (1-lb.) can	74	14.9	4.6	0.93	40	8.0	
Drained solids (yield: approx. 8½ oz.)	(52)	(9.7)	(6.1)	(1.13)	(31)	(5.7)	
Whole Green Beans, 16-oz. (1-lb.) can	56	13.2	3.5	0.82	30	7.0	
Drained solids (yield: approx. 8½ oz.)	(54)	(8.0)	(6.3)	(0.94)	(32)	(4.7)	
Tillie Lewis "Tasti Diet" Fancy Blue Lake Cut Green Beans, for sodium-controlled diets, 8-oz. can	40	8.0	5.0	1.00	40	8.0	
Drained solids (yield: approx. 4.8 oz.)	(30)	(5.8)	(6.3)	(1.20)	(32)	(6.0)	
HUMMUS, see under CHICK-PEAS							
HYACINTH BEANS							
YOUNG PODS							
RAW:							
As purchased [refuse: ends, strings, and trimmings, approx. 12%] (1g/2g/tr/75%/1mg):							
1 pound	140	29.1	8.8	1.82			
Edible portion:							
1 cup, ½" pieces (approx. 3.2 oz.)	(28)	(5.8)	8.8	1.82	(28)	(5.8)	0.51
1 pound (approx. 5 cups) (1g/2g/tr/89%/1mg)	140	29.1	8.8	1.82	(28)	(5.8)	0.51
COOKED:							
Boiled, drained:							
1 cup, ½" pieces (approx. 3.6 oz.)	(34)	(6.9)	(9.4)	(1.93)	(34)	(6.9)	(0.54)
1 pound (approx. 4.4 cups) (yield from approx. 17 oz. of uncooked pods) (1g/2g/tr/na/na)	(150)	(30.9)	(9.4)	(1.93)	(34)	(6.9)	(0.54)
Steamed:							
1 pound of raw hyacinth beans, steamed (yield: approx. 15 oz.)	140	29.1	9.3	1.93			(0.54)
1 pound of steamed hyacinth beans	149	31.0	9.3	1.93			(0.54)
MATURE SEEDS, Dry							
RAW:							
1 cup (approx. 6.5 oz.)	(558)	(112.4)	85.8	17.29	(558)	(112.4)	2.00
1 pound (approx. 2.3 cups) (6g/17g/tr/12%/na)	1533	276.7	85.8	17.29	(558)	(112.4)	2.00
COOKED:							
Boiled, drained:							
1 cup (approx. 7.1 oz.)	(272)	(49.1)	38.3	6.92	(272)	(49.1)	0.89
1 pound (approx. 2.3 cups) (yield from approx. 7.1 oz. uncooked dry beans) (3g/7g/tr/na/na)	613	110.7	38.3	6.92	(272)	(49.1)	0.89
ITALIAN BEANS							
CANNED, by brand:							
Del Monte Italian Beans, 16-oz. (1-lb.) can	(90)	(20.0)	(5.6)	(1.25)	45	10.0	
Drained (yield: approx. 8 oz.)	(75)	(14.8)	(8.8)	(1.74)	(50)	(9.9)	
JELLY BEANS, see the SWEET LITTLE NOTHINGS chapter							
JERUSALEM ARTICHOKES (Sunchokes)							
RAW:							
As purchased [refuse: parings, approx. 31%]:							
1 pound	(129)	(52.3)	(8.0)	(3.27)			
Edible portion:							
1 pound (1g/5g/tr/80%/na)	(185)	(75.7)	(11.6)	(4.73)			
KALE							
RAW:							
As purchased:							
Untrimmed [refuse: stems, midribs, trimmings, and damaged leaves, approx. 36%]:							
1 pound	128	20.1	8.0	1.26			

	UNIT Cal.	UNIT Carb.	1 OZ., BY WT. Cal.	1 OZ., BY WT. Carb.	1 CUP Cal.	1 CUP Carb.	Fiber per oz. (GMS.)
Untrimmed [refuse: stem ends, tough stems, and tough part of midribs, approx. 26%]:							
1 pound	154	26.1	9.6	1.63			
Edible portion:							
Eaten with stems:							
1 pound (1g/2g/tr/88%/21mg)	172	27.2	10.8	1.70			0.37
Eaten without stems:							
1 cup (approx. 3.8 oz.)	(56)	(9.6)	15.0	2.55	(56)	(9.6)	
1 pound (approx. 4.3 cups) (2g/3g/tr/83%/21mg)	240	40.8	15.0	2.55	(56)	(9.6)	
COOKED:							
Boiled, drained:							
Leaves with stems:							
1 cup (approx. 3.9 oz.)	31	4.4	7.9	1.13	31	4.4	0.31
1 pound (approx. 4.1 cups) (1g/1g/tr/91%/12mg)	126	18.1	7.9	1.13	31	4.4	0.31
Leaves without stems, midribs:							
1 cup (approx. 3.9 oz.)	43	6.7	11.1	1.73	43	6.7	
1 pound (approx. 4.1 cups) (1g/2g/tr/88%/12mg)	177	27.7	11.1	1.73	43	6.7	
Steamed:							
Leaves with stems:							
1 pound of raw kale, steamed (yield: approx. 18.4 oz.)	263	27.2	14.3	1.48			
1 pound of steamed kale	229	23.7	14.3	1.48			
Leaves without stems:							
1 pound of raw kale, steamed (yield: approx. 18.4 oz.)	240	40.8	13.0	2.22			0.32
1 pound of steamed kale	208	35.5	13.0	2.22			0.32
FROZEN, by brand:							
Bel-Air Cut Leaf Kale, 10-oz. package	90	15.0	9.0	1.50			
Boiled, drained (yield: approx. 9 oz.)	90	15.0	10.0	1.67	48	8.0	
Birds Eye Chopped Kale, 10-oz. package	90	15.0	9.0	1.50			
Boiled, drained (yield: approx. 9 oz.)	(90)	(15.0)	(10.0)	(1.67)	(47)	(7.9)	
Safeway Cut Leaf Kale, 10-oz. package	90	15.0	9.0	1.50			
Boiled, drained (yield: approx. 9 oz.)	(90)	(15.0)	(10.0)	(1.67)	(48)	(8.0)	
Seabrook Farms Chopped Kale, 10-oz. package	90	15.0	9.0	1.50			
Boiled, drained (yield: approx. 9 oz.)	90	(15.0)	(10.0)	(1.67)	(47)	(7.9)	

KASHA (Buckwheat), see under WHEAT

KIDNEY BEANS

MATURE SEEDS, Dry

	UNIT Cal.	UNIT Carb.	1 OZ., BY WT. Cal.	1 OZ., BY WT. Carb.	1 CUP Cal.	1 CUP Carb.	Fiber per oz. (GMS.)
RAW:							
1 cup (approx. 6.5 oz.)	635	114.5	97.3	17.55	635	114.5	1.19
1 pound (approx. 2.5 cups) (6g/13g/tr/10%/3mg)	1556	280.8	97.3	17.55	635	114.5	1.19
COOKED:							
Boiled, drained:							
1 cup (approx. 6.5 oz.)	218	39.6	33.4	6.10	218	39.6	0.43
1 pound (approx. 2.5 cups) (yield from approx. 5.5 oz. of uncooked beans) (2g/6g/tr/69%/1mg)	535	97.1	33.4	6.10	218	39.6	0.43
CANNED, based on generic data:							
Solids and liquid:							
1 cup (approx. 9 oz.)	230	41.8	25.5	4.65	230	41.8	0.26
1 pound (approx. 1.8 cups) (2g/3g/tr/76%/1mg)	408	74.4	25.5	4.65	230	41.8	0.26
1 #2 can, 20 oz. net wt. (approx. 2.2 cups)	510	93.0	25.5	4.65	230	41.8	0.26
1 #3 cylinder can, 51 oz. (3 lb. 3 oz.) net wt. (approx. 5.7 cups)	1301	237.1	25.5	4.65	230	41.8	0.26
1 #10 can, 108 oz. (6 lb. 12 oz.) net wt. (approx. 12 cups)	2756	502.2	25.5	4.65	230	41.8	0.26
BOXED, by brand:							
Golden Harvest Red Kidney Beans, 16-oz. (1-lb.) box	1400	330.1	87.5	20.63	560	132.0	
1 cup, dry (approx. 6.4 oz.)	560	132.0	87.5	20.63	560	132.0	

	UNIT Cal.	UNIT Carb.	1 OZ., BY WT. Cal.	1 OZ., BY WT. Carb.	1 CUP Cal.	1 CUP Carb.	Fiber per oz. (GMS.)
CANNED, by brand:							
Ann Page (A&P) Red Kidney Beans, 8-oz. can	220	40.0	27.5	5.00	(248)	(45.1)	
Drained solids (yield: approx. 5.4 oz.)	(212)	(38.2)	(39.3)	(7.07)	(250)	(44.9)	
15½-oz. can	426	77.5	27.5	5.00	(248)	(45.1)	
Drained solids (yield: approx. 10½ oz.)	(413)	(74.2)	(39.3)	(7.07)	(250)	(44.9)	
Blue Boy Kidney Beans, 16-oz. (1-lb.)	462	71.0	28.9	4.44	260	40.0	
Hanover Red Kidney Beans, 8-oz. can	245	45.0	30.6	5.63	(275)	(50.6)	
Drained solids (yield: approx. 5.4 oz.)	(237)	(43.2)	(43.9)	(8.00)	(279)	(50.8)	
27-oz. can	826	152.0	30.6	5.63	(275)	(50.6)	
Drained solids (yield: approx. 18.4 oz.)	(808)	(147.2)	(43.9)	(8.00)	(279)	(50.8)	
Ralph's Kidney Beans, 15-oz. can	440	76.0	29.3	5.07	220	38.0	
Underwood Red Kidney Beans, 16-oz. (1-lb.) can	(490)	(67.6)	(30.6)	(4.23)	(276)	(38.2)	
Drained solids (yield: approx. 10.9 oz.)	(475)	(64.0)	(43.6)	(5.87)	(277)	(37.3)	
55-oz. can	(1688)	(232.5)	(30.6)	(4.23)	(276)	(38.2)	
Drained solids (yield: approx. 37.5 oz.)	(1635)	(220.0)	(43.6)	(5.87)	(277)	(37.3)	
Van Camp's Red Kidney Beans, New Orleans Style, 8-oz. can	186	33.8	23.3	4.22	210	38.0	
15-oz. can	350	63.3	23.3	4.22	210	38.0	

KOHLRABI

	UNIT Cal.	UNIT Carb.	1 OZ., BY WT. Cal.	1 OZ., BY WT. Carb.	1 CUP Cal.	1 CUP Carb.	Fiber per oz. (GMS.)
RAW:							
As purchased [refuse: leaves with stems, and parings, approx. 54%]:							
1 pound	61	13.8	3.8	0.86			
As purchased [refuse: stem ends and parings, approx. 27%]:							
1 pound	96	21.9	6.0	1.37			
Edible portion (stems only):							
1 cup, diced (approx. 4.9 oz.)	41	9.2	8.2	1.87	41	9.2	0.28
1 pound (approx. 3¼ cups) (1g/2g/tr/90%/2mg)	132	29.9	8.2	1.87	41	9.2	0.28
COOKED:							
Boiled, drained:							
1 cup (approx. 5.8 oz.)	40	8.7	6.8	1.50	40	8.7	(0.23)
1 pound (approx. 2¾ cups)	109	24.0	6.8	1.50	40	8.7	(0.23)

LADY FINGERS, see OKRA

LEEKS

	UNIT Cal.	UNIT Carb.	1 OZ., BY WT. Cal.	1 OZ., BY WT. Carb.	1 CUP Cal.	1 CUP Carb.	Fiber per oz. (GMS.)
RAW:							
As purchased [refuse: tops and rootlets, approx. 48%]:							
1 pound	123	26.4	7.7	1.65			
Edible portion:							
1 pound (1g/3g/tr/85%/1mg)	236	50.8	14.8	3.18			0.37
FREEZE DRIED, by brand:							
Armanino Farms Leeks, 1 pound	1634	351.6	102.1	21.97			

LENTILS

MATURE SEEDS, Dry

	UNIT Cal.	UNIT Carb.	1 OZ., BY WT. Cal.	1 OZ., BY WT. Carb.	1 CUP Cal.	1 CUP Carb.	Fiber per oz. (GMS.)
RAW:							
Whole:							
1 cup (approx. 6.7 oz.)	646	114.2	96.4	17.04	646	114.2	0.85
1 pound (approx. 2.4 cups) (7g/17g/tr/11%/9mg)	1542	272.6	96.4	17.04	646	114.2	0.85
Split, without seed coat:							
1 cup (approx. 6.7 oz.)	656	117.4	98.0	17.30	656	117.4	
1 pound (approx. 2.4 cups)	1567	280.5	98.0	17.30	656	117.4	
COOKED:							
Boiled, drained:							
1 cup (approx. 7.1 oz.)	(214)	(38.8)	30.1	5.47	(214)	(38.8)	0.26
1 pound (approx. 2.3 cups) (yield from approx. 5 oz. uncooked dry beans) (2g/5g/tr/72%/na)	482	87.6	30.1	5.47	(214)	(38.8)	0.26
BOXED, by brand:							
Near East Lentil Pilaf, 8-oz. box	800	152.0	100.0	19.00	(656)	(124.7)	
Prepared as package directs, without butter (yield: approx. 23 oz.)	(1208)	(152.4)	(52.5)	(6.63)	(302)	(38.1)	

	UNIT		1 OZ., BY WT.		1 CUP		Fiber per oz. (GMS.)
	Cal.	Carb.	Cal.	Carb.	Cal.	Carb.	
DHAL (based on data from Singapore)							
Red							
1 pound	1529	269.9	95.5	16.87			
Yellow							
1 pound	1510	271.7	94.4	16.98			
LETTUCE							
BUTTERHEAD VARIETIES (such as Boston types and Bibb)							
RAW:							
As purchased [refuse: outer leaves and core, approx. 26%]:							
1 head 5" diam (approx. 7¾ oz.)	23	4.1	3.0	0.53			
1 pound (approx. 2 heads)	48	8.5	3.0	0.53			
Edible portion:							
1 outer leaf, or two medium inner leaves, or three small heart leaves (approx. ½ oz.)	2	0.4	4.0	0.71	8	1.4	0.14
1 medium head (approx. 5.7 oz.)	23	4.1	4.0	0.71			0.14
1 cup, chopped or shredded (approx. 1.9 oz.)	8	1.4	4.0	0.71	8	1.4	0.14
1 pound (approx. 2.8 medium heads, approx. 8.4 cups, chopped or shredded) (tr/1g/tr/95%/3mg)	64	11.3	4.0	0.71			0.14
COS, see ROMAINE							
CRISPHEAD VARIETIES (such as Iceberg, New York, and Great Lakes)							
RAW:							
As purchased, good quality [refuse: core, approx. 5%]:							
1 medium head (approx. 1 lb. 4 oz.)	70	15.6	3.7	0.83			
1 pound (approx. ⅘ of 1 medium head)	59	13.2	3.7	0.83			
As purchased, fair quality [refuse: coarse leaves and core, approx. 26%]:							
1 medium head (approx. 1 lb. 4 oz.)	55	12.1	2.8	0.61			
1 pound (approx. ⅘ of 1 medium head)	44	9.7	2.8	0.61			
Edible portion:							
Piece:							
Portion of leaf, 5 × 4½" with edges curled (approx. 0.7 oz.)	3	0.6	3.7	0.83	(9)	(1.9)	0.14
1 medium head (approx. 14.8 oz.)	55	12.1	3.7	0.83	(9)	(1.9)	0.14
1 cup, chopped or shredded (approx. 2.4 oz.)	(9)	(1.9)	3.7	0.83	(9)	(1.9)	
1 pound (approx. 7 cups) (tr/1g/tr/96%/3mg)	59	13.3	3.7	0.83	(9)	(1.9)	0.14
Cut wedges:							
1 medium head cut into sixths:							
1 sixth of a good quality head (approx. 3.2 oz.)	12	2.7	3.7	0.83	(10)	(2.2)	0.14
1 sixth of a fair quality head (approx. 2.5 oz.)	9	2.1	3.7	0.83	(10)	(2.2)	0.14
1 medium head cut into quarters:							
1 quarter of a good quality head (approx. 4¾ oz.)	18	3.9	3.7	0.83	(10)	(2.2)	0.14
1 quarter of a fair quality head (approx. 3.7 oz.)	14	3.1	3.7	0.83	(10)	(2.2)	0.14
LOOSELEAF or BUNCH VARIETIES (Grand Rapids, Salad Bowl, Simpson)							
RAW:							
As purchased [refuse: outer leaves, core, and trimmings, approx. 36%]:							
1 pound	52	10.2	3.3	0.64			
Edible portion:							
1 cup, chopped or shredded (approx. 1.9 oz.)	10	1.9	5.1	0.99	10	1.9	0.20
1 pound (approx. 8.2 cups chopped or shredded) (tr/1g/tr/94%/3mg)	82	15.6	5.1	0.99	10	1.9	0.20
ROMAINE or COS (Dark Green and White Paris)							
RAW:							
As purchased [refuse: outer leaves, core, and trimmings, approx. 36%]:							
1 small head (approx. 12 oz.)	39	7.7	3.3	0.64			
1 large head (approx. 24 oz., 1½ lb.)	79	15.4	3.3	0.64			
1 pound	52	10.2	3.3	0.64			

	UNIT		1 OZ., BY WT.		1 CUP		Fiber per oz. (GMS.)
	Cal.	Carb.	Cal.	Carb.	Cal.	Carb.	
Edible portion:							
1 small head (approx. 7.6 oz.)	39	7.7	5.1	0.99			0.20
1 large head (approx. 15.4 oz.)	79	15.4	5.1	0.99			0.20
1 cup, chopped or shredded (approx. 1.9 oz.)	10	1.9	5.1	0.99	10	1.9	0.20
1 pound (approx. 8.4 cups chopped or shredded) (tr/1g/tr/94%/3mg)	82	15.9	5.1	0.99	10	1.9	0.20
LIMA BEANS							
MATURE SEEDS, Dry							
RAW:							
1 cup (approx. 6.3 oz.)	621	115.2	97.8	18.14	621	115.2	1.22
1 pound (approx. 2.5 cups) (6g/18g/tr/10%/1mg)	1565	290.3	97.8	18.14	621	115.2	1.22
COOKED:							
Boiled, drained:							
1 cup (approx. 6.7 oz.)	262	48.6	39.1	7.25	262	48.6	0.48
1 pound (approx. 2.4 cups) (yield from approx. 6.4 oz. uncooked dry beans) (2g/7g/tr/64%/1mg)	625	116.0	39.1	7.25	262	48.6	0.48
IMMATURE SEEDS							
RAW:							
1 cup (approx. 5.6 oz.)	191	34.3	34.9	6.26	191	34.3	0.51
1 pound (approx. 2.9 cups) (2g/6g/tr/68%/67mg)	558	100.2	34.9	6.26	191	34.3	0.51
COOKED:							
Boiled, drained:							
1 cup (approx. 6.0 oz.)	189	33.7	31.4	5.61	189	33.7	(0.46)
1 pound (approx. 2.7 cups) (2g/6g/tr/71%/67mg)	503	89.8	31.4	5.61	189	33.7	(0.46)
Steamed:							
1 pound of raw lima beans, steamed (yield: approx. 15.7 oz.)	(558)	(100.2)	(35.5)	(6.38)			(0.52)
1 pound of steamed lima beans	(568)	(102.1)	(35.5)	(6.38)			(0.52)
FROZEN, based on generic data:							
THICK-SEEDED TYPES, commonly called Fordhooks							
Measured when frozen:							
1 cup (approx. 5.8 oz.)	163	31.2	28.9	5.53	163	31.2	
1 pound (approx. 2.8 cups)	463	88.5	28.9	5.53	163	31.2	
1 container, 10 oz. net wt.	290	55.3	28.9	5.53	163	31.2	
Boiled, drained:							
1 cup (approx. 6.0 oz.)	168	32.5	28.1	5.41	168	32.5	0.45
1 pound of frozen lima beans, boiled, then drained (yield: approx. 16.1 oz.)	452	86.7	28.1	5.41	168	32.5	0.45
1 pound boiled, drained lima beans	449	86.6	28.1	5.41	168	32.5	0.45
1 container, 10 oz., boiled, then drained (yield: approx. 10.1 oz.)	283	54.3	28.1	5.41	168	32.5	0.45
THIN-SEEDED TYPES, commonly called Baby Limas							
Measured when frozen:							
1 cup (approx. 5.8 oz.)	201	38.0	34.6	6.53	201	38.0	
1 pound (approx. 2.8 cups)	553	104.3	34.6	6.53	201	38.0	
1 container, 10 oz. net wt.	346	65.3	34.6	6.53	201	38.0	
Boiled, drained:							
1 cup (approx. 6.3 oz.)	212	40.1	33.9	6.40	212	40.1	0.54
1 pound of frozen baby limas, boiled, then drained (yield: approx. 16 oz.)	541	102.2	33.9	6.40	212	40.1	0.54
1 pound of boiled, drained baby limas	535	101.2	33.9	6.40	212	40.1	0.54
1 container, 10 oz., boiled, then drained (yield: approx. 10 oz.)	339	64.0	33.9	6.40	212	40.1	0.54
FROZEN, by brand:							
Birds Eye Baby Lima Beans, 10-oz. package	360	66.0	36.4	6.67	(222)	(40.7)	
Boiled, drained (yield: approx. 10.5 oz.)	(360)	(66.0)	(34.3)	(6.29)	(209)	(38.4)	
Fordhook Lima Beans, 10-oz. package	300	54.0	30.3	5.45	(180)	(32.3)	
Boiled, drained (yield: approx. 10.3 oz.)	(300)	(54.0)	(29.1)	(5.24)	(174)	(31.3)	
Tiny Lima Beans, 10-oz. package	360	60.0	36.4	6.06	(222)	(37.0)	
Boiled, drained (yield: approx. 10.5 oz.)	(360)	(60.0)	(34.3)	(5.71)	(209)	(34.8)	
Blue Boy Lima Beans, 8.5-oz. package	274	48.9	32.2	5.75	280	50.0	
Boiled, drained (yield: approx. 6 oz.)	259	46.1	43.4	7.74	266	47.5	

	UNIT		1 OZ., BY WT.		1 CUP		Fiber per oz.
	Cal.	Carb.	Cal.	Carb.	Cal.	Carb.	(GMS.)
Golden Harvest Baby Lima Beans, 8-oz. package	150	33.5	18.7	4.19	150	33.5	
Boiled, drained (yield: approx. 4.5 oz.)	129	29.7	28.6	6.59	176	40.5	
Green Giant Baby Lima Beans, 16-oz. (1-lb.) package	499	89.4	31.2	5.59	150	28.0	
Boiled, drained (yield: approx. 16.8 oz.)	(499)	(89.4)	(29.7)	(5.32)	(181)	(32.4)	
Baby Lima Beans in Butter Sauce, 10-oz. boil-in-bag	323	47.4	32.3	4.74	220	32.0	
Boiled, drained (yield: approx. 10 oz.)	323	47.4	32.3	4.74	220	32.0	
Hanover Baby Lima Beans, 16-oz. (1-lb.) package	550	100.0	34.4	6.25	(210)	(38.1)	
Boiled, drained (yield: approx. 16.8 oz.)	(550)	(100.0)	(32.7)	(5.95)	(208)	(37.8)	
Fordhook Lima Beans, 16-oz. (1-lb.) package	501	85.0	31.3	5.31	(185)	(31.5)	
Boiled, drained (yield: approx. 16.5 oz.)	(501)	(85.0)	(30.4)	(5.16)	(189)	(32.1)	
Kounty Kist Baby Lima Beans, 20-oz. poly bag	772	137.3	38.6	6.87	190	35.0	
Boiled, drained (yield: approx. 20 oz.)	772	137.3	38.6	6.87	(190)	(35.0)	
Seabrook Farms Baby Lima Beans, 10-oz. package	390	72.0	39.0	7.20	(238)	(43.9)	
Boiled, drained (yield: approx. 10.5 oz.)	(390)	(72.0)	(37.1)	(6.86)	(236)	(43.6)	
Fordhook Lima Beans, 10-oz. package	300	54.0	30.0	5.40	(178)	(32.0)	
Boiled, drained (yield: approx. 10.3 oz.)	(300)	(54.0)	(29.1)	(5.24)	(174)	(31.3)	
Petite Lima Beans, 10-oz. package	330	60.0	33.0	6.00			
Boiled, drained (yield: approx. 10.5 oz.)	(330)	(60.0)	(31.4)	(5.71)	(192)	(34.8)	
Village Park Baby Lima Beans, 16-oz. (1-lb.) package	650	120.0	40.6	7.50			
Boiled, drained (yield: approx. 16.5)	(650)	(1200)	(39.4)	(7.27)	(241)	(44.5)	
CANNED, based on generic data:							
Regular pack:							
Solids and liquid: 1 cup (approx. 8.8 oz.)	176	33.2	20.1	3.80	176	33.2	0.37
1 pound (approx. 1.8 cups) (1g/4g/tr/81%/67 mg)	322	60.8	20.1	3.80	176	33.2	0.37
1 #303 can, 16 oz. (1 lb.) net wt.	322	60.8	20.1	3.80	176	33.2	0.37
1 #10 can, 105 oz. (6 lb. 9 oz.)	2114	389.9	20.1	3.80	176	33.2	0.37
Drained solids: 1 cup (approx. 6 oz.)	163	31.1	27.2	5.19	163	31.1	0.51
1 pound (approx. 2.7 cups) (1g/5g/tr/75%/67 mg)	435	83.0	27.2	5.19	163	31.1	0.51
1 #303 can (yield: approx. 11 oz.)	300	57.1	27.2	5.19	163	31.1	0.51
1 #10 can (yield: approx. 72 oz. [4 lb. 8 oz.])	1959	373.5	27.2	5.19	163	31.1	0.51
Drained liquid: 1 cup (approx. 8.3 oz.)	(37)	(6.1)	(4.4)	(0.74)	(37)	(6.1)	trace
1 pound (approx. 1.9 cups) (tr/1g/tr/93%/67 mg)	(70)	(11.8)	(4.4)	(0.74)	(37)	(6.1)	trace
1 #303 can (yield: approx. 5 oz., 0.6 cups)	(22)	(3.7)	(4.4)	(0.74)	(37)	(6.1)	trace
Low-sodium pack:							
Solids and liquid: 1 cup (approx. 8.7 oz.)	174	32.0	19.9	3.66	174	32.0	0.34
1 pound (approx. 1.8 cups) (1g/4g/tr/82%/1 mg)	318	58.5	19.9	3.66	174	32.0	0.34
1 #303 can, 16 oz. (1 lb.) net wt.	318	58.5	19.9	3.66	174	32.0	0.34
Drained solids: 1 cup (approx. 6.0 oz.)	162	30.1	26.9	5.02	162	30.1	0.51
1 pound (approx. 2.7 cups) (2g/5g/tr/76%/1 mg)	431	80.3	26.9	5.02	162	30.1	0.51
1 #303 can (yield: approx. 11 oz.)	296	55.2	26.9	5.02	162	30.1	0.51
Drained liquid: 1 cup (approx. 8.3 oz.)	(37)	(5.5)	(4.4)	(0.66)	(37)	(5.5)	trace
1 pound (approx. 1.9 cups) (tr/1g/tr/94%/1 mg)	(70)	10.6	(4.4)	(0.66)	(37)	(5.5)	trace
1 #303 can (yield: approx. 5 oz., 0.6 cups)	22	3.3	(4.4)	(0.66)	(37)	(5.5)	trace
CANNED, by brand:							
Ann Page (A&P) Lima Beans, medium green, 16-oz. (1-lb.) can	340	64.0	21.3	4.00	170	32.0	
Drained solids (yield: approx. 11 oz.)	(310)	(58.5)	(30.9)	(5.32)	(190)	(32.7)	
Del Monte Lima Beans, 17-oz. can	319	61.6	18.8	3.63	150	29.0	
Drained solids (yield: approx. 8½ oz.)	(268)	(52.3)	(31.5)	(6.15)	(193)	(37.7)	

	UNIT		1 OZ., BY WT.		1 CUP		Fiber per oz.
	Cal.	Carb.	Cal.	Carb.	Cal.	Carb.	(GMS.)
Lima Beans, seasoned, 16-oz. (1-lb.) can	320	58.0	20.0	3.63	160	29.0	
Drained solids (yield: approx. 11.2 oz.)	(290)	(52.7)	(25.9)	(4.70)	(159)	(28.8)	
Featherweight Green Lima Beans, no added salt or sugar, 8-oz. can	(146)	(32.0)	(18.3)	(4.00)	146	32.0	
Drained solids (yield: approx. 5.6 oz.)	(134)	(29.6)	(23.9)	(5.29)	(142)	(31.3)	
16-oz. (1-lb.) can	(292)	(64.0)	(18.3)	(4.00)	146	32.0	
Drained solids (yield: approx. 11.2 oz.)	(268)	(59.2)	(23.9)	(5.29)	(142)	(31.3)	
Libby's Lima Beans, 8½-oz. can	(155)	(29.0)	(18.2)	(3.41)	160	30.0	
Drained solids (yield: approx. 6 oz.)	(140)	(26.2)	(23.4)	(4.38)	(144)	(27.0)	
16-oz. (1-lb.) can	(291)	(54.6)	(18.2)	(3.41)	160	30.0	
Drained solids (yield: approx. 11.2 oz.)	(262)	(49.3)	(23.4)	(4.38)	(144)	(27.0)	
Stokely Green Lima Beans, 16-oz. (1-lb.) can	(309)	(61.7)	20.4	3.74	180	33.0	
Drained solids (yield: approx. 11.2 oz.)	(310)	(57.2)	(27.7)	(5.11)	(170)	(31.4)	
84-oz. can	(164)	(32.8)	(19.3)	(3.86)	170	34.0	
Drained solids (yield: approx. 5.6 oz.)	(155)	(28.6)	(27.7)	(5.11)	(170)	(31.4)	
Lima Bean Products							
LIMA BEAN FLOUR							
1 cup, sifted, spooned into the cup (approx. 4.4 oz.)	432	79.4	97.3	17.86	432	79.4	0.48
1 pound (approx. 3.6 cups of sifted flour, spooned into cup)	1556	285.8	97.3	17.86	432	79.4	0.48
MATAI, see WATER CHESTNUTS							
MEXICAN BEANS, Red							
MATURE SEEDS, Dry							
RAW: 1 cup (approx. 6.5 oz.)	663	121.0	98.9	18.06	663	121.0	1.22
1 pound (approx. 2.5 cups) (6g/18g/tr/8%/3mg)	1583	288.9	98.9	18.06	663	121.0	1.22
COOKED: Boiled, drained: 1 cup (approx. 6.5 oz.)	(273)	(49.9)	(42.0)	(7.67)	(273)	(49.9)	0.52
1 pound (approx. 2.5 cups) (yield from approx. 6.7 oz. uncooked beans) (3g/8g/tr/na/na)	(673)	(122.8)	(42.0)	(7.67)	(273)	(49.9)	0.52
MINT (based on data from the Middle East)							
RAW: 1 pound	295	35.8	18.4	2.24			
MIXED VEGETABLES are listed at the end of this chapter.							
MUNG BEANS							
MATURE SEEDS, Dry							
RAW: 1 cup (approx. 7.4 oz.)	714	126.6	96.4	17.07	714	126.6	1.25
1 pound (approx. 2.2 cups) (7g/17g/tr/11%/2mg)	1542	273.5	96.4	17.07	714	126.6	1.25
COOKED: Boiled, drained: 1 cup (approx. 7.4 oz.)	(299)	(52.9)	(40.4)	(7.15)	(299)	(52.9)	(0.52)
1 pound (approx. 2.2 cups) (yield from approx. 6.7 oz. uncooked dry beans) (3g/7g/tr/na/na)	(646)	(114.4)	(40.4)	(7.15)	(299)	(52.9)	(0.52)
MUNG BEAN SPROUTS (sprouted seeds)							
RAW: 1 cup (approx. 3.7 oz.)	37	6.9	9.9	1.87	37	6.9	0.20
1 pound (approx. 4.3 cups) (1g/2g/tr/89%/1mg)	159	29.9	9.9	1.87	37	6.9	0.20
COOKED: Boiled, drained: 1 cup (approx. 4.4 oz.)	35	6.5	7.9	1.48	35	6.5	(0.16)
1 pound (approx. 3.6 cups) (yield from approx. 13 oz. uncooked dry sprouts) (1g/1g/tr/91%/1mg)	127	23.6	7.9	1.48	35	6.5	(0.16)

	UNIT Cal.	UNIT Carb.	1 OZ., BY WT. Cal.	1 OZ., BY WT. Carb.	1 CUP Cal.	1 CUP Carb.	Fiber per oz. (GMS.)
CANNED, by brand:							
Chun King Bean Sprouts, 16-oz. (1-lb.) can	80	11.8	5.0	0.74			
Drained solids (yield: approx. 8 oz.)	(55)	(6.2)	(7.0)	(0.78)	(32)	(3.5)	
La Choy Bean Sprouts, 16-oz. (1-lb.) can drained (yield: approx. 8 oz.)	(23)	(2.2)	2.9	0.28	(13)	(1.3)	

MUSHROOMS

COMMONLY CULTIVATED MUSHROOM (Agaricus campeatris)

	UNIT Cal.	UNIT Carb.	1 OZ., BY WT. Cal.	1 OZ., BY WT. Carb.	1 CUP Cal.	1 CUP Carb.	Fiber per oz. (GMS.)
RAW:							
As purchased:							
Good quality [refuse: trimmings, mainly stem ends, approx. 3%]:							
1 pound	123	19.4	7.7	1.21			
Fair quality [refuse: peelings and trimmings, approx. 19%]:							
1 pound	103	16.2	6.4	1.01			
Edible portion:							
1 cup, sliced, chopped, or diced (approx. 2½ oz.)	20	3.1	7.9	1.25	20	3.1	0.23
1 pound (approx. 6½ cups) (1g/1g/tr/90%/4mg)	127	20.0	7.9	1.25	20	3.1	0.23
COOKED:							
Steamed:							
1 pound of raw mushrooms, steamed (yield: approx. 15.4 oz.)	127	20.0	8.3	1.30			0.18
1 pound of steamed mushrooms	132	20.8	8.3	1.30			0.18
OTHER EDIBLE SPECIES							
RAW:							
As purchased [refuse: trimmings, mainly stem ends, approx. 3%]:							
1 pound	154	28.6	9.6	1.79			
Edible portion:							
1 cup, sliced, chopped, or diced (approx. 2½ oz.)	25	4.6	9.9	1.84	25	4.6	0.31
1 pound (approx. 6½ cups) (1g/2g/tr/89%/na)	159	29.5	9.9	1.84	25	4.6	0.31
PREPACKAGED, by brand:							
Dole Sliced Mushrooms, 8-oz. bag	62	9.2	7.7	1.15	20	3.0	
1 cup (approx. 3 oz.)	20	3.0	7.7	1.15	20	3.0	
FROZEN, by brand:							
Green Giant Mushrooms in Butter Sauce, 6-oz. package	88	5.1	14.7	0.85			
Boiled, drained (yield: approx. 6 oz.)	88	5.1	14.7	0.85			
CANNED, based on generic data:							
Solids and liquid:							
1 cup (approx. 7.7 oz.)	(37)	(5.3)	4.8	0.68	(37)	(5.3)	0.17
1 pound (approx. 2.1 cups) (1g/1g/tr/93%/113mg)	77	10.9	4.8	0.68	(37)	(5.3)	0.17
CANNED, by brand:							
Green Giant Mushroom Stems and Pieces, 2½-oz. can	18	2.5	7.0	1.00	54	17.7	
4½-oz. can	32	4.5	7.0	1.00	54	17.7	
Sliced Mushrooms, 2½-oz. can	18	2.5	7.0	1.00	54	17.7	
4½-oz. can	32	4.5	7.0	1.00	54	17.7	
Whole Mushrooms, 2½-oz. can	18	2.5	7.0	1.00	54	17.7	
4½-oz. can	32	4.5	7.0	1.00	54	17.7	
Shady Oak Mushrooms, 2-oz. can	10	1.0	4.8	0.50	(37)	(3.9)	
4-oz. can	19	2.0	4.8	0.50	(37)	(3.9)	
DRIED, by brand:							
China Bowl Dried Black Mushrooms, 1-oz. package	(81)	(18.9)	(80.5)	(18.88)			
Dried Sliced Mushrooms, 1-oz. package	(72)	(10.5)	(71.7)	(10.50)			
Straw Mushrooms, 1-oz. package	(91)	(11.8)	(91.3)	(11.79)			
Tree Ear Mushrooms, ½-oz. package	(41)	(9.8)	(81.7)	(19.68)			

MUSTARD GREENS

	UNIT Cal.	UNIT Carb.	1 OZ., BY WT. Cal.	1 OZ., BY WT. Carb.	1 CUP Cal.	1 CUP Carb.	Fiber per oz. (GMS.)
RAW:							
As purchased [refuse: coarse leaves and stems, approx. 30%]:							
1 pound	98	17.8	6.1	1.10			
Edible portion:							
1 pound (1g/1g/tr/92%/na)	141	25.4	8.8	1.60			0.31
COOKED:							
Boiled, drained:							
1 cup (approx. 4.9 oz.)	32	5.6	6.5	1.10	32	5.6	0.26
1 pound (approx. 3.2 cups) (tr/1g/tr/95%/na)	104	18.1	6.5	1.10	32	5.6	0.26
Steamed:							
1 pound of raw mustard greens, steamed (yield: approx. 14.9 oz.)	141	25.4	9.5	1.71			0.33
1 pound of steamed mustard greens	152	27.3	9.5	1.71			0.33
FROZEN, based on generic data:							
Measured when frozen:							
1 pound (approx. 16 oz.)	91	14.5	5.7	0.91			
1 container, 10 oz. net wt.	57	9.1	5.7	0.91			
Boiled, drained:							
1 cup (approx. 5.3 oz.)	30	4.7	5.7	0.88	30	4.7	0.26
1 pound of frozen mustard greens, boiled, then drained (yield: approx. 12.0 oz.)	68	10.5	5.7	0.88	30	4.7	0.26
1 pound of boiled, drained mustard greens	91	14.1	5.7	0.88	30	4.7	0.26
1 container, 10 oz., boiled, then drained (yield: approx. 7.5 oz.)	42	6.6	5.7	0.88	30	4.7	0.26
FROZEN, by brand:							
Birds Eye Chopped Mustard Greens, 10-oz. package	54	9.0	5.5	0.90			
Boiled, drained (yield: approx. 9 oz.)	(54)	(9.0)	(6.0)	(1.00)	(29)	(4.9)	
Seabrook Farms Chopped Mustard Greens, 10-oz. package	75	9.0	7.5	0.90	(37)	(4.4)	
Boiled, drained (yield: approx. 9 oz.)	(75)	(9.0)	(8.3)	(1.00)	(41)	(4.9)	

MUSTARD SEED and MUSTARD POWDER, see the SALTS & SPICES chapter

MUSTARD SPINACH (Tendergreen)

	UNIT Cal.	UNIT Carb.	1 OZ., BY WT. Cal.	1 OZ., BY WT. Carb.	1 CUP Cal.	1 CUP Carb.	Fiber per oz. (GMS.)
RAW:							
All-edible:							
1 pound (1g/1g/tr/92%/na)	100	17.7	6.3	1.07			0.28
COOKED:							
Boiled, drained:							
1 pound (tr/1g/tr/95%/na)	73	12.7	4.6	0.79	29	5.0	0.23

NAVY BEANS, see PEA BEANS

NEW ZEALAND SPINACH (New Zealand Ice-plant)

	UNIT Cal.	UNIT Carb.	1 OZ., BY WT. Cal.	1 OZ., BY WT. Carb.	1 CUP Cal.	1 CUP Carb.	Fiber per oz. (GMS.)
RAW:							
All-edible:							
1 pound (1g/1g/tr/93%/45mg)	86	14.1	5.4	0.90			0.20
COOKED:							
Boiled, drained:							
1 cup (approx. 2½ oz.)	23	3.8	3.7	0.60	23	3.8	0.17
1 pound (approx. 6⅓ cups) (tr/1g/tr/95%/26mg)	59	9.5	3.7	0.60	23	3.8	0.17

OKRA

	UNIT Cal.	UNIT Carb.	1 OZ., BY WT. Cal.	1 OZ., BY WT. Carb.	1 CUP Cal.	1 CUP Carb.	Fiber per oz. (GMS.)
RAW:							
As purchased:							
Good quality [refuse: stem ends and tips, approx. 14%]:							
1 pound	140	29.6	8.6	1.85			
Fair quality [refuse: stem ends, tips, and culls, approx. 22%]:							
1 pound	127	26.9	7.9	1.68			
Edible portion:							
1 pound	144	30.6	9.0	1.91			0.30
COOKED:							
Boiled, drained:							
1 medium pod (approx. 3″ long, ⅝″ diameter ⅓ oz.)	(31)	(6.4)	8.3	1.70	46	9.6	0.28
1 cup, crosscut slices (approx. 5.6 oz.)	46	9.6	8.3	1.70	46	9.6	0.28
1 pound (approx. 2.8 cups crosscut slices, 48 medium pods)	132	27.2	8.3	1.70	46	9.6	0.28

	UNIT Cal.	UNIT Carb.	1 OZ., BY WT. Cal.	1 OZ., BY WT. Carb.	1 CUP Cal.	1 CUP Carb.	Fiber per oz. (GMS.)
Steamed:							
1 pound of raw okra, steamed (yield: approx. 14.7 oz. (1g/2g/tr/91%/1mg)	144	30.6	9.8	2.08			0.33
1 pound of steamed okra	157	33.3	9.8	2.08			0.33
FROZEN, based on generic data:							
Measured when frozen:							
1 pound	177	40.8	11.1	2.56			
1 container, 10 oz. net wt.	111	25.6	11.1	2.56			
Boiled, drained:							
1 cup (approx. 6.5 oz.)	70	16.3	10.8	2.49	70	16.3	0.27
1 pound of frozen okra, boiled, then drained (yield: approx. 14.4 oz.)	155	35.9	10.8	2.49	70	16.3	0.27
1 pound of boiled, drained okra (1g/2g/tr/91%/1mg)	172	39.9	10.8	2.49	70	16.3	0.27
1 container, 10 oz., boiled, then drained (yield approx. 9.0 oz.)	97	22.4	10.8	2.49	70	16.3	0.27
FROZEN, by brand:							
Birds Eye Cut Okra, 10-oz. package	76	15.0	7.6	1.50			
Boiled, drained (yield: approx. 8.2 oz.)	(75)	(15.0)	(9.3)	(1.83)	(60)	(11.9)	
Whole Okra, 10-oz. package	105	21.0	10.5	2.10			
Boiled, drained (yield: approx. 9.9 oz.)	(105)	(21.0)	(10.6)	(2.12)	(52)	(10.3)	
Green Giant Okra Gumbo, 10-oz. boil-in-bag	255	15.9	25.5	1.60	220	12.0	
Hanover Cut Okra, 16-oz. (1-lb.) polybag	125	20.8	7.8	1.30			
Boiled, drained (yield: approx. 13.1 oz.)	(125)	(20.0)	(9.5)	(1.53)	(62)	(9.9)	
Seabrook Farms Cut Okra, 10-oz. package	90	18.0	9.0	1.80			
Boiled, drained (yield: approx. 8.2 oz.)	(90)	(18.0)	(11.0)	(2.20)	(72)	(14.3)	
Whole Okra, 10-oz. package	105	21.0	10.5	2.10			
Boiled, drained (yield: approx. 9.9 oz.)	(105)	(21.0)	(10.6)	(2.12)	(52)	(10.5)	
Village Park Cut Okra, 16-oz. (1-lb.) package	150	30.0	9.4	1.88			
Boiled, drained (yield: approx. 13.1 oz.)	(150)	(30.0)	(11.5)	(2.29)	(75)	15.0	

OLIVES, see the CONDIMENTS chapter

ONIONS (also see SCALLIONS, and ONIONS, WELSH)

MATURE

	UNIT Cal.	UNIT Carb.	1 OZ., BY WT. Cal.	1 OZ., BY WT. Carb.	1 CUP Cal.	1 CUP Carb.	Fiber per oz. (GMS.)
RAW:							
As purchased [refuse: skins and ends, approx. 9%]:							
1 pound	157	35.9	9.8	2.24			
Edible portion:							
1 tablespoon:							
Chopped or minced (approx. 0.35 oz.)	4	0.9	10.8	2.47	65	14.8	0.17
1 cup:							
Chopped (approx. 6 oz.)	65	14.8	10.8	2.47	65	14.8	0.17
Grated or ground (approx. 8¼ oz.)	89	20.4	10.8	2.47	89	20.4	0.17
Sliced (approx. 4 oz.)	44	10.0	10.8	2.47	44	10.0	0.17
1 pound (approx. 6 cups chopped) (tr/2g/tr/89%/3mg)	172	39.5	10.8	2.47	65	14.8	0.17
COOKED:							
Boiled, drained:							
1 cup, whole or sliced (approx. 7.4 oz.)	61	13.7	8.3	1.80	61	13.7	(0.13)
1 pound (approx. 2.1 cups) (tr/2g/tr/92%/2mg)	132	29.5	8.3	1.80	61	13.7	(0.13)
Steamed:							
1 pound of raw onions, steamed (yield: approx. 13.6 oz.)	172	39.5	12.6	2.90			0.20
1 pound of steamed onions	202	46.4	12.6	2.90			0.20
DEHYDRATED (Flakes):							
1 cup (approx. 3.5 oz.)	350	82.1	99.2	23.28	350	82.1	1.24
1 pound (approx. 4.5 cups) (2g/23g/tr/4%/25mg)	1588	372.4	99.2	23.28	350	82.1	1.24
FROZEN, by brand:							
Birds Eye Chopped Onions, 12-oz. package	96	24.0	8.0	2.00			
Boiled, drained (yield: approx. 9.8 oz.)	(96)	(24.0)	(9.8)	(2.45)	(64)	(16.1)	
Small Whole Onions, 16-oz. (1-lb.) package	160	40.0	10.0	2.50			
Boiled, drained (yield: approx. 13.1 oz.)	(160)	(40.0)	(12.2)	(3.05)	(80)	(20.0)	
Durkee French Fried Onions, 3-oz. package	534	30.0	178.0	10.00			
Green Giant Onions in Creamy Cheese Flavor Sauce, 10-oz. package	148	15.3	14.8	1.53	140	14.0	
Moore's Onion Rings, 16-oz. (1-lb.) box	998	104.3	62.4	6.52			
Mrs. Paul's Fried Onion Rings, 5-oz. package	300	42.0	60.0	8.40			
Party Pak Fried Onion Rings, 16-oz. (1-lb.) package	960	136.0	60.0	8.50			
O&C Boiled Onions, 16-oz. (1-lb.) package	128	32.0	8.0	2.00			
Boiled, drained (yield: approx. 13.1 oz.)	(128)	(32.0)	(9.8)	(2.44)			
Onions in Cream Sauce, 15.5-oz. package	2217	263.5	143.0	17.00			
Ore-Ida Onion Ringers, 12-oz. package	960	102.0	80.0	8.50			
Chopped Onions, 12-oz. package	120	24.0	10.0	2.00			
Cooked (yield: approx. 9.8 oz.)	(120)	(24.0)	(12.2)	(2.45)	(80)	(16.1)	

ONIONS, PICKLED, see the CONDIMENTS chapter

ONION POWDER, see the SALTS & SPICES chapter

ONIONS, WELSH

	UNIT Cal.	UNIT Carb.	1 OZ., BY WT. Cal.	1 OZ., BY WT. Carb.	1 CUP Cal.	1 CUP Carb.	Fiber per oz. (GMS.)
RAW:							
As purchased [refuse: tops of leaves and roots, approx. 35%]:							
1 pound	100	19.2	6.3	1.20			
Edible portion:							
1 pound (1g/2g/tr/91%/2mg)	154	29.5	9.6	1.84			0.28

ORIENTAL RADISHES, see RADISHES

OYSTER PLANT, see SALSIFY

PAKCHOI, see SPOON CABBAGE under CABBAGE

PARSLEY

COMMON GARDEN and CURLED-LEAF VARIETIES

	UNIT Cal.	UNIT Carb.	1 OZ., BY WT. Cal.	1 OZ., BY WT. Carb.	1 CUP Cal.	1 CUP Carb.	Fiber per oz. (GMS.)
RAW:							
All-edible:							
1 sprig, approx. 2½" long, (approx. 0.03 oz.)	trace	0.1	12.5	2.41			0.43
1 pound of sprigs (1g/2g/tr/85%/13mg)	200	38.6	12.5	2.41			0.43
Chopped:							
1 tablespoon (approx. 0.1 oz.)	1	0.3	12.5	2.41	26	5.1	0.43
1 cup (approx. 2.1 oz.)	26	5.1	12.5	2.41	26	5.1	0.43
1 pound (approx. 7½ cups)	200	38.6	12.5	2.41	26	5.1	0.43

PARSLEY FLAKES, see the SALTS & SPICES chapter

PARSNIPS

	UNIT Cal.	UNIT Carb.	1 OZ., BY WT. Cal.	1 OZ., BY WT. Carb.	1 CUP Cal.	1 CUP Carb.	Fiber per oz. (GMS.)
RAW:							
As purchased:							
Good quality [refuse: parings, approx. 15%]:							
1 pound	293	67.5	18.3	4.22			
Fair quality [refuse: parings, trimmings, and pithy cores, approx. 30%]:							
1 pound	241	55.6	15.1	3.48			

	UNIT		1 OZ., BY WT.		1 CUP		Fiber per oz.
	Cal.	Carb.	Cal.	Carb.	Cal.	Carb.	(GMS.)
Trimmed, pre-packaged without tops [refuse: parings, approx. 15%]:							
1 pound	345	79.4	21.5	4.96			
Edible portion:							
1 pound (tr/5g/tr/79%/3mg)	419	96.4	26.2	6.03			0.57
COOKED:							
Boiled, drained:							
1 small parsnip (approx. 6" long, 1⅛" diameter, 1.2 oz.)	23	5.2	18.8	4.22			(0.41)
1 large parsnip (approx. 9" long, 2¼ diameter, 5.6 oz.)	106	23.8	18.8	4.22			(0.41)
1 cup:							
Diced or cut into 2" lengths (approx. 5½ oz.)	102	23.1	18.8	4.22	102	23.1	(0.41)
Mashed (approx. 7.4 oz.)	139	31.3	18.8	4.22	139	31.3	(0.41)
1 pound (approx. 3 cups diced, or 2⅞ cups mashed) (tr/4g/tr/82%/2mg)	299	67.6	18.8	4.22			(0.41)
Steamed:							
1 pound of raw parsnips, steamed (yield: approx. 15.8 oz.)	419	96.4	26.5	6.11			0.58
1 pound of steamed parsnips	424	97.8	26.5	6.11			0.58

PEA BEANS

	UNIT		1 OZ., BY WT.		1 CUP		Fiber per oz.
	Cal.	Carb.	Cal.	Carb.	Cal.	Carb.	(GMS.)
BOXED, by brand:							
Golden Harvest Navy Beans (Pea Beans), 16-oz. (1-lb.) box	1485	184.5	92.8	11.53	660	82.0	
1 cup, dry (approx. 7.1 oz.)	660	82.0	92.8	11.53	660	82.0	
CANNED, by brand:							
Underwood Pea Beans (Navy Beans), 16-oz. (1-lb.) can	672	102.4	42.0	6.40			
Drained solids (yield: approx. 10.9 oz.)	(663)	(99.7)	(60.8)	(9.15)			
55-oz. can	2310	352.0	42.0	6.40			
Drained solids (yield: approx. 37.4 oz.)	(2273)	(342.1)	(60.8)	(9.15)			

PEAS (Green Peas)

Peas and Carrots follows canned peas, and in turn is followed by other mixtures in which peas get top billing. Other peas are listed under their individual names, such as Chick-peas, Cowpeas, Pigeon Peas and Snow Peas.

	UNIT		1 OZ., BY WT.		1 CUP		Fiber per oz.
	Cal.	Carb.	Cal.	Carb.	Cal.	Carb.	(GMS.)
MATURE SEEDS, Dry, Whole							
RAW:							
1 cup (approx. 7.1 oz.)	680	120.6	96.4	17.09	680	120.6	1.39
1 pound (approx. 2.3 cups) (7g/17g/tr/12%/10 mg)	1542	273.5	96.4	17.09	680	120.6	1.39
COOKED:							
Boiled, drained:							
1 cup (approx. 7.1 oz.)	(278)	(49.2)	(39.2)	(6.94)	(278)	(49.2)	0.57
1 pound (approx. 2.3 cups) (yield from approx. 6.5 oz. dry peas) (2g/7g/tr/70%/4mg)	(627)	(111.1)	(39.2)	(6.94)	(278)	(49.2)	0.57
MATURE SEEDS, Dry, Split Without Seedcoat							
RAW:							
1 cup (approx. 7.1 oz.)	696	125.4	98.7	17.78	696	125.4	0.34
1 pound (approx. 2.3 cups) (7g/18g/tr/9%/11mg)	1579	284.4	98.7	17.78	696	125.4	0.34
COOKED:							
Boiled, drained:							
1 cup (approx. 7.1 oz.)	230	41.6	32.6	5.89	230	41.6	0.11
1 pound (approx. 2.3 cups) (yield from approx. 5.3 oz. uncooked dry peas) (2g/6g/tr/70%/4mg)	522	94.6	32.6	5.89	230	41.6	0.11
IMMATURE SEEDS							
RAW:							
1 cup (approx. 5.1 oz.)	122	20.9	23.8	4.08	122	20.9	0.57
1 pound (approx. 3.1 cups) (2g/14g/tr/78%/1mg)	381	65.3	23.8	4.08	122	20.9	0.57
COOKED:							
Boiled, drained:							
1 cup (approx. 5.6 oz.)	114	19.4	20.1	3.43	114	19.4	0.48
1 pound (approx. 2.9 cups) (yield from approx. 13.5 oz. uncooked peas) (2g/3g/tr/82%/tr)	322	54.9	20.1	3.43	114	19.4	0.48
Steamed:							
1 pound of raw peas, steamed (yield: approx. 15.5 oz.)	381	65.3	24.6	4.21			0.59
1 pound of steamed peas	394	67.4	24.6	4.21			0.59

	UNIT		1 OZ., BY WT.		1 CUP		Fiber per oz.
	Cal.	Carb.	Cal.	Carb.	Cal.	Carb.	(GMS.)
FROZEN, based on generic data:							
Measured when frozen:							
1 cup (approx. 5.1 oz.)	106	18.6	20.7	3.64	106	18.6	0.54
1 pound (approx. 3.1 cups)	331	58.1	20.7	3.64	106	18.6	0.54
1 container, 10 oz. net weight (approx. 2 cups)	207	36.4	20.7	3.64	106	18.9	0.54
Boiled, drained:							
1 cup (approx. 5.6 oz.)	109	18.9	19.2	3.33	109	18.9	0.54
1 pound of frozen peas, boiled, then drained (yield: approx. 14.3 oz., 2.5 cups)	275	47.7	19.2	3.33	109	18.9	0.54
1 pound of boiled, drained peas (approx. 2.8 cups)	308	53.5	19.2	3.33	109	18.9	0.54
1 container, 10 oz., boiled, drained (yield: approx. 8.9 oz.)	172	29.9	17.2	2.99	109	18.9	0.54
BOXED, by brand:							
Golden Harvest Whole Green Peas, 16-oz. (1-lb.) box, uncooked	2275	392.5	142.2	24.53	910	157.0	
1 cup, dry (approx. 6.4 oz.)	910	157.0	142.2	24.53	910	157.0	
FROZEN, by brand:							
Bel-Air Frozen Green Peas, 10-oz. package	240	39.0	24.0	3.90			
Boiled, drained (yield: approx. 8.8 oz.)	240	39.0	27.3	4.43	181	26.1	
Birds Eye Sweet Green Peas, 10-oz. package	210	33.0	21.0	3.30			
Boiled, drained (yield: approx. 9.3 oz.)	210	33.0	22.6	3.55	(135)	(21.3)	
Tender Tiny Peas, 10-oz. package	180	27.0	18.0	2.70			
Boiled, drained (yield: approx. 9.3 oz.)	(180)	(27.0)	(19.4)	(2.90)	(110)	(17.4)	
Green Giant Sweet Peas, 18-oz. package, polybag	342	56.2	19.0	3.12			
Boiled, drained (yield: approx. 18 oz.)	(342)	(56.2)	(19.0)	(3.12)	(100)	(16.0)	
Hanover Petite Pois Peas, 16-oz. (1-lb.) package	350	60.0	21.9	3.75			
Boiled, drained (yield: approx. 14.9 oz.)	(350)	(60.0)	(23.5)	(4.03)	(141)	(24.2)	
Sweet Peas, 16-oz. (1-lb.) package	350	60.0	21.9	3.75	(129)	(22.1)	
Boiled, drained (yield: approx. 14.9 oz.)	(350)	(60.0)	(23.5)	(4.03)	(141)	(24.2)	
Kounty Kist Peas, 20-oz. package	499	76.6	25.0	3.83			
Boiled, drained (yield: approx. 18.6 oz.)	(499)	(76.6)	(26.8)	(4.12)	(161)	(24.7)	
Seabrook Farms Green Peas, 10-oz. package	240	39.0	24.0	3.90			
Boiled, drained (yield: approx. 9.3 oz.)	(240)	(39.0)	(25.8)	(4.19)	(155)	(25.1)	
Petite Green Peas, 10-oz. package	180	30.0	18.0	3.00			
Boiled, drained (yield: approx. 9.3 oz.)	(180)	(30.0)	(19.4)	(3.23)	(116)	(19.4)	
Petite Green Peas, Extra Fancy, 10-oz. package	180	30.0	18.0	3.00			
Boiled, drained (yield: approx. 9.3 oz.)	(180)	(30.0)	(19.4)	(3.23)	(114)	(19.0)	
CANNED, based on generic data:							
ALASKA (Early or June Peas)							
Regular pack:							
Solids and liquid:							
1 cup (approx. 8.8 oz.)	164	31.1	18.7	3.54	164	31.1	0.43
1 pound (approx. 1.8 cups)	299	56.7	18.7	3.54	164	31.1	0.43
1 #303 can, or glass jar, 17 oz. net wt.	318	60.3	18.7	3.54	164	31.1	0.43
Drained solids:							
1 cup (approx. 6.0 oz.)	150	28.6	24.9	4.76	150	28.6	0.65
1 pound (approx. 2.7 cups)	399	76.2	24.9	4.76	150	28.6	0.65
1 #303 can, or glass jar, (yield: approx. 11 oz. drained peas)	275	52.6	24.9	4.76	150	28.6	0.65
Drained liquid:							
1 cup (approx. 8.3 oz.)	(60)	(10.7)	(7.2)	(1.28)	(60)	(10.7)	trace
1 pound (approx. 1.9 cups)	(115)	(20.5)	(7.2)	(1.28)	(60)	(10.7)	trace
1 #303 can, or glass jar, (yield: approx. 6 oz., 0.7 cups)	(43)	(7.7)	(7.2)	(1.28)	(60)	(10.7)	trace
Low-sodium pack:							
Solids and liquid:							
1 cup (approx. 8.8 oz.)	137	22.4	15.6	2.78	137	22.4	0.37
1 pound (approx. 1.8 cups)	249	44.5	15.6	2.78	137	22.4	0.37
1 #303 can, or glass jar, 17 oz. net wt.	265	47.2	15.6	2.78	137	22.4	0.37
Drained solids:							
1 cup (approx. 6.0 oz.)	133	24.3	22.1	4.06	133	24.3	0.57
1 pound (approx. 2.7 cups)	354	64.9	22.1	4.06	133	24.3	0.57
1 #303 can, or glass jar, (yield: approx. 11 oz.)	244	44.8	22.1	4.06	133	24.3	0.57

	UNIT		1 OZ., BY WT.		1 CUP		Fiber per oz. (GMS.)
	Cal.	Carb.	Cal.	Carb.	Cal.	Carb.	
Drained liquid:							
1 cup (approx. 8.3 oz.)	(29)	(3.3)	(3.5)	(0.40)	(29)	(3.3)	trace
1 pound (approx. 1.9 cups)	56	6.4	(3.5)	(0.40)	(29)	(3.3)	trace
1 #303 can, or glass jar, (yield: approx. 6 oz., 0.7 cups)	21	2.4	(3.5)	(0.40)	(29)	(3.3)	trace
SWEET WRINKLED PEAS (Sugar Peas)							
Regular pack:							
Solids and liquid:							
1 cup (approx. 8.8 oz.)	142	25.9	16.2	2.95	142	25.9	0.40
1 pound (approx. 1.8 cups)	259	47.2	16.2	2.95	142	25.9	0.40
1 #303 can, or glass jar, 17 oz. net wt.	275	50.1	16.2	2.95	142	25.9	0.40
Drained solids:							
1 cup (approx. 6.0 oz.)	136	25.5	22.7	4.25	136	25.5	0.62
1 pound (approx. 2.7 cups)	363	68.0	22.7	4.25	136	25.5	0.62
1 #303 can, or glass jar (yield: approx. 11 oz. of drained peas)	250	47.0	22.7	4.25	136	25.5	0.62
Drained liquid:							
1 cup (approx. 8.3 oz.)	(35)	(4.3)	(4.2)	(0.52)	(35)	(4.3)	trace
1 pound (approx. 1.9 cups)	(67)	(8.3)	(4.2)	(0.52)	(35)	(4.3)	trace
1 #303 can, or glass jar, (yield: approx. 6 oz., approx. 0.7 cups liquid)	(25)	(3.1)	(4.2)	(0.52)	(35)	(4.3)	
Low-sodium pack:							
Solids and liquid:							
1 cup (approx. 8.8 oz.)	117	0.7	13.3	0.09	117	0.7	0.37
1 pound (approx. 1.8 cups)	213	1.4	13.3	0.09	117	0.7	0.37
1 #303 can, or glass jar, 17 oz. net wt.	227	39.5	13.3	0.09	117	0.7	0.37
Drained solids:							
1 cup (approx. 6.0 oz.)	122	22.1	20.4	2.54	122	22.1	0.57
1 pound (approx. 2.7 cups)	327	59.0	20.4	2.54	122	22.1	0.57
1 #303 can, or glass jar, (yield: approx. 11 oz. of drained peas)	225	40.7	20.4	2.54	122	22.1	0.57
CANNED, by brand:							
A&P Small Early Peas, 8½-oz. can	130	25.0	15.3	2.94	(129)	(24.8)	
Drained solids (yield: approx. 5.3 oz.)	(108)	(20.2)	(20.3)	(3.81)	(122)	(22.9)	
16½-oz. can	252	48.5	15.3	2.94	(129)	(24.8)	
Drained solids (yield: approx. 10.3 oz.)	(209)	(39.2)	(20.3)	(3.81)	(122)	(22.9)	
Ann Page (A&P) Sweet Peas, mixed sizes, 8½-oz. can	130	25.0	15.3	2.94	(129)	(24.8)	
Drained solids (yield: approx. 5.3 oz.)	(108)	(20.2)	(20.3)	(3.81)	(122)	(22.9)	
16½-oz. can	(252)	(48.5)	15.3	2.94	(129)	(24.8)	
Drained solids (yield: approx. 10.3 oz.)	(209)	(39.2)	(20.3)	(3.81)	(122)	(22.9)	
April Showers Early Peas, 9.5-oz. can	121	21.2	14.2	2.49	120	22.0	
Drained solids (yield: approx. 5.3 oz.)	(98)	(16.4)	(18.5)	(3.09)	(111)	(18.5)	
Balanced Sweet Peas, packed in water, no added sugar or salt, 8-oz. can	84	12.7	10.5	1.59	(92)	(14.0)	
Drained solids (yield: approx. 5.2 oz.)	(67)	(9.3)	(12.9)	(1.79)	(77)	(10.7)	
Blue Boy Peas, 8.5-oz. can	155	29.1	18.2	3.42	160	30.0	
Drained solids (yield: approx. 5.5 oz.)	137	25.5	24.8	4.61	143	26.5	
Del Monte Early Garden Peas, 8½-oz. can	117	21.3	13.8	2.51	110	20.0	
Drained solids (yield: approx. 5.4 oz.)	(96)	(16.7)	(17.8)	(3.10)	(107)	(18.6)	
17-oz. can	234	42.5	13.8	2.51	110	20.0	
Drained solids (yield: approx. 10.4 oz.)	(185)	(32.2)	(17.8)	(3.10)	(107)	(18.6)	
Seasoned Peas, 8¼-oz. can	124	25.8	15.0	3.13	120	25.0	
Drained solids (yield: approx. 5.4 oz.)	(104)	(21.5)	(19.3)	(4.00)	(116)	(24.0)	
16-oz. (1-lb.) can	240	50.0	15.0	3.13	120	25.0	
Drained solids (yield: approx. 10.4 oz.)	(201)	(41.6)	(19.3)	(4.00)	(116)	(24.0)	
Sweet Tiny Peas, 16-oz. (1-lb.) can	200	36.0	12.5	2.25	100	18.0	
Drained solids (yield: approx. 10.25 oz.)	(166)	(29.1)	(16.2)	(2.83)	(97)	(17.0)	
Diet Delight Sweet Peas, packed in water, 8½-oz. can	100	8.0	11.8	0.94	(100)	(8.0)	
Drained solids (yield: approx. 5¼ oz.)	(84)	(4.8)	(16.0)	(0.90)	(96)	(5.4)	
Featherweight Peas, no added salt or sugar, 8-oz. can	124	24.0	15.5	3.00	(132)	(29.5)	
Drained solids (yield: approx. 5.2 oz.)	(104)	(19.2)	(20.0)	(3.68)	(120)	(22.1)	
16-oz. (1-lb.) can	248	48.0	15.5	3.00	(132)	(25.5)	
Drained solids (yield: approx. 10.4 oz.)	(208)	(38.3)	(20.0)	(3.68)	(120)	(22.1)	
Blended Sweet Peas, packed in water, no salt or sugar added 8-oz. can	124	24.0	15.5	3.00	(140)	(27.0)	
Drained solids (yield: approx. 5¼ oz.)	(105)	(19.3)	(20.0)	(3.68)	(120)	(22.1)	
Featherweight Pea Puree, 16-oz. (1-lb.) can	(280)	(58.0)	(17.5)	(3.63)	140	29.0	
Pea Puree, low sodium, 16-oz. (1-lb.) jar	(280)	(58.0)	(17.5)	(3.63)	140	29.0	
Golden Harvest Peas in Water, no sugar or salt added, 8-oz. can	120	24.0	15.0	3.00	120	24.0	
Drained solids (yield: approx. 5¼ oz.)	103	20.5	19.7	3.90	115	22.8	
Green Giant Sweet Peas, 8½-oz. can	104	16.9	12.2	1.99	110	17.0	
Drained solids (yield: approx. 5.5 oz.)	(86)	(13.3)	(15.5)	(2.41)	(93)	(14.5)	
17-oz. can	207	33.8	12.2	1.99	110	17.0	
Drained solids (yield: 11.1 oz.)	172	26.7	(15.5)	(2.41)	(93)	(14.5)	
Sweetlets Small Sweet Peas, 8½-oz. can	96	16.4	11.3	1.93	100	17.0	
Drained solids (yield: approx. 5.3 oz.)	(77)	(12.6)	(14.5)	(2.38)	(87)	(14.3)	
Le Sueur Small Early Peas, 8½-oz. can	104	18.3	12.2	2.15	110	19.0	
Drained solids (yield: approx. 5.3 oz.)	(82)	(13.5)	(15.5)	(2.55)	(93)	(15.3)	
Small Sweet Peas, 8½-oz. can	96	16.4	11.4	1.93	100	17.0	
Drained solids (yield: approx. 5.5 oz.)	(78)	(12.8)	(14.2)	(2.32)	(85)	(14.0)	
17-oz. can	193	32.8	11.4	1.93	100	17.0	
Drained solids (yield: approx. 11.1 oz.)	(158)	(25.7)	(14.2)	(2.32)	(85)	(14.0)	
Libby's Immature Sweet Green Peas, 8½-oz. can	(111)	(21.3)	(13.0)	(2.50)	120	23.0	
Drained solids (yield: approx. 5.3 oz.)	(88)	(16.4)	(16.9)	(3.15)	(101)	(18.9)	
17-oz. can	(221)	(42.6)	(13.0)	(2.50)	120	23.0	
Drained solids (yield: approx. 10.3 oz.)	(174)	(32.5)	(16.9)	(3.15)	(101)	(18.9)	
Lindy (Kounty Kist) Early Peas, 8½-oz. can	142	25.6	16.7	3.01	140	27.0	
Drained solids (yield: approx. 5.5 oz.)	(121)	(21.1)	(22.0)	(3.82)	(132)	(22.9)	
17-oz. can	285	51.1	16.7	3.01	140	27.0	
Drained solids (yield: approx. 11.1 oz.)	(244)	(42.2)	(22.0)	(3.82)	(132)	(22.9)	
Sweet Peas, 8½-oz. can	128	21.0	15.0	2.47	130	22.0	
Drained solids (yield: approx. 5.5 oz.)	(110)	(17.4)	(20.0)	(3.15)	(120)	(19.0)	
17-oz. can	256	42.0	15.0	2.47	130	22.0	
Drained solids (yield: approx. 11 oz.)	(221)	(34.9)	(20.0)	(3.15)	(120)	(19.0)	
Minnesota Valley Small Early Peas, 8⅕-oz. can	106	18.8	12.5	2.21	110	19.0	
Drained solids (yield: approx. 5.3 oz.)	(84)	(14.0)	(15.8)	(2.64)	(95)	(15.8)	
S&W Nutradiet Sweet Peas, no salt, packed in water, 8-oz. can	80	16.0	10.0	2.00	80	16.0	
Drained solids (yield: approx. 5.3 oz.)	(66)	(13.3)	(12.6)	(2.52)	(77)	(15.1)	
Stokely Early Peas, 8½-oz. can	116	24.1	13.6	2.84	120	25.0	
Drained solids (yield: approx. 5.1 oz.)	(92)	(19.0)	(18.1)	(3.73)	(109)	(22.4)	
17-oz. can	231	48.2	(13.6)	(2.84)	120	25.0	
Drained solids (yield: approx. 10¼ oz.)	(186)	(38.2)	(18.1)	(3.73)	(109)	(22.4)	
Honey Pod Sweet Peas, 8½-oz. can	(116)	(23.1)	(13.6)	(2.72)	120	24.0	
Sweet Peas, 8-oz. can	118	21.8	14.7	2.72	130	24.0	
Drained solids (yield: approx. 4.8 oz.)	(99)	(18.0)	(20.6)	(3.74)	(124)	(22.4)	
17-oz. can	250	46.2	14.7	2.72	130	24.0	
Drained solids (yield: approx. 10¼ oz.)	(210)	(38.1)	(20.6)	(3.74)	(124)	(22.4)	
Tillie Lewis "Tasti Diet" Sweet Peas, no added salt or sugar, 8-oz. can	80	16.0	10.0	2.00	80	16.0	
Drained solids (yield: approx. 5.2 oz.)	(63)	(12.6)	(12.1)	(2.42)	(73)	(14.5)	

Peas and Carrots

	UNIT Cal.	UNIT Carb.	1 OZ., BY WT. Cal.	1 OZ., BY WT. Carb.	1 CUP Cal.	1 CUP Carb.	Fiber per oz. (GMS.)
FROZEN, based on generic data:							
Measured when frozen:							
1 cup (approx. 4.9 oz.)	77	14.6	15.6	2.95	77	14.6	0.43
1 pound (approx. 3.2 cups)	249	47.2	15.6	2.95	77	14.6	0.43
1 container, 10 oz. net wt.	156	29.5	15.6	2.95	77	14.6	0.43
Boiled, drained:							
1 cup (approx. 5.6 oz.)	85	16.2	15.0	2.86	85	16.2	0.43
1 pound of frozen peas and carrots, boiled, drained (yield: approx. 15.7 oz.)	236	44.9	15.0	2.86	85	16.2	0.43
1 pound of boiled, drained peas and carrots (1g/3g/tr/86%/24mg)	240	45.8	15.0	2.86	85	16.2	0.43
1 container, 10 oz., boiled, drained (yield: approx. 9.8 oz.)	147	28.1	15.0	2.86	85	16.2	0.43
FROZEN, by brand:							
Birds Eye Peas and Carrots, 10-oz. package	150	27.0	15.0	2.70			
Boiled, drained (yield: approx. 9.9 oz.)	(150)	(27.0)	(15.3)	(2.73)	(88)	(15.8)	
Hanover Peas and Carrots, 16-oz (1-lb.) package	250	45.0	15.6	2.81			
Boiled, drained (yield: approx. 15.8 oz.)	(250)	(45.0)	(15.8)	(2.85)	(98)	(17.1)	
Kounty Kist Peas and Carrots, 20-oz. poly bag	510	73.8	25.5	3.69			
Boiled, drained (yield: approx. 20 oz.)	(510)	(73.8)	(25.5)	(3.69)	(160)	(22.9)	
Village Park Peas and Carrots, 16-oz. (1-lb.) package	300	55.0	18.8	3.44			
Boiled, drained (yield: approx. 15.8 oz.)	(300)	(55.0)	(19.0)	(3.48)	(109)	(19.9)	
CANNED, by brand:							
Balanced Peas and Carrots, no added sugar or salt, packed in water, 8-oz. can	(164)	(27.4)	(20.5)	(3.42)	180	30.0	
Drained solids (yield: approx. 5.2 oz.)	(147)	(23.5)	(28.3)	(4.52)	(162)	(25.8)	
Blue Boy Peas and Carrots, 8.5 oz.	117	19.6	13.8	2.30	120	20.0	
Drained solids (yield: approx. 5.5 oz.)	99	15.4	18.0	2.78	103	16.0	
Del Monte Peas and Carrots, 8½-oz. can	105	20.2	12.5	2.38	100	19.0	
Drained solids (yield: approx. 5½ oz.)	(88)	(16.0)	(15.8)	(2.90)	(91)	(16.7)	
16-oz (1-lb.) can	200	38.0	12.5	2.38	100	19.0	
Drained solids (yield: approx. 10.75 oz.)	(158)	(30.0)	(15.8)	(2.90)	(91)	(16.7)	
Diet Delight Sweet Peas and Diced Carrots, low sodium, no sugar, packed in water, 8½-oz. can	80	12.0	9.4	1.31	80	12.0	
Drained solids (yield: approx. 5¼ oz.)	(64)	(8.8)	(12.2)	(1.67)	(73)	(10.0)	
Freshlike Veg-All Sweet Peas and Carrots, 16-oz. (1-lb.) can	160	38.0	10.0	2.38	80	19.0	
Drained solids (yield: approx. 10¾ oz.)	(123)	(29.1)	(11.4)	(2.71)	(68)	(16.3)	
Golden Harvest Peas and Carrots, no sugar or salt added, in water, 8½-oz. can	100	20.0	11.8	2.35	100	20.0	
Drained solids (yield: approx. 5½ oz.)	82	15.4	14.9	2.80	85	16.4	
Peas and Carrots, no sugar or salt added, in water, 16-oz. (1-lb.) can	200	40.0	12.5	2.50	100	20.0	
Drained solids (yield: approx. 10.4 oz.)	166	32.2	16.0	3.10	91	17.8	
Libby's Peas and Carrots, 8½-oz. can	(98)	(19.5)	(11.5)	(2.30)	100	20.0	
Drained solids (yield: approx. 5.25 oz.)	(75)	(14.6)	(13.9)	(2.71)	(83)	(16.3)	
16-oz. (1-lb.) can	(184)	(36.8)	(11.5)	(2.30)	100	20.0	
Drained solids (yield: approx. 10.5 oz.)	(150)	(29.2)	(13.9)	(2.71)	(83)	(16.3)	
S&W Nutradiet Sweet Peas and Diced Carrots, 8½-oz. can	70	14.0	8.2	1.65	70	14.0	
Drained solids (yield: approx. 5¼ oz.)	(54)	(10.8)	(10.3)	(2.06)	(62)	(12.4)	
Stokely Peas and Carrots, 8½-oz. can	99	20.7	11.6	2.43	100	21.0	
Drained solids (yield: approx. 5.3 oz.)	(76)	(15.8)	(14.4)	(2.99)	(82)	(17.1)	
16-oz (1-lb.) can	186	38.9	11.6	2.43	100	21.0	
Drained solids (yield: approx. 10 oz.)	(144)	(29.9)	(14.4)	(2.99)	(82)	(17.1)	

Peas and . . . , Peas in . . . , Peas With . . .

	UNIT Cal.	UNIT Carb.	1 OZ., BY WT. Cal.	1 OZ., BY WT. Carb.	1 CUP Cal.	1 CUP Carb.	Fiber per oz. (GMS.)
FROZEN, by brand:							
Birds Eye Green Peas and Cauliflower with Cream Sauce, 10-oz. package	300	36.0	30.0	3.60			
Boiled (yield: approx. 9.9 oz.)	(300)	(36.0)	(30.3)	(3.64)	(267)	(32.1)	
Green Peas with Cream Sauce, 9-oz. package	360	42.0	40.0	4.67			
Boiled (yield: approx. 8.9 oz.)	(360)	(42.0)	40.4	4.72	(356)	(41.6)	
Green Peas and Pearl Onions, 10-oz. package	180	36.0	18.0	3.60			
Boiled (yield: approx. 9.9 oz.)	(180)	(36.0)	(18.2)	(3.63)	(108)	(21.8)	
Green Peas and Potatoes with Cream Sauce, 8-oz. package	420	45.0	52.5	5.63			
Boiled (yield: approx. 7.9 oz.)	(420)	(45.0)	(53.2)	(5.70)	(319)	(34.2)	
Green Giant Creamed Peas with Bread Crumb Topping Oven Bake 'N Serve, 10-oz. package	318	33.8	31.8	3.38	300	33.0	
Early Peas in Butter Sauce, 10-oz. package, boil-in-bag	216	29.2	21.6	2.92			
Boiled (yield: approx. 10 oz.)	216	29.2	21.6	2.92	150	20.0	
Early Peas with Onions, 17-oz. can	241	42.4	14.2	2.50	120	22.0	
Drained solids (yield: approx. 11.1 oz.)	(200)	(33.6)	(18.0)	(3.02)	(108)	(18.1)	
Sweet Peas in Butter Sauce, 10-oz. polybag	209	26.1	20.9	2.61			
Boiled (yield: approx. 10 oz.)	209	26.1	20.9	2.61	150	18.0	
Sweet Peas with Onions, 17-oz. can	207	33.8	12.2	1.99	110	17.0	
Drained solids (yield: approx. 11.1 oz.)	(166)	(25.0)	(15.0)	(2.25)	(90)	(13.5)	
Tiny Peas and Onions, Carrots in Butter Sauce, 10-oz. package, boil-in-bag	201	23.0	20.1	2.30			
Boiled (yield: approx. 10 oz.)	201	23.0	20.1	2.30	160	20.0	
Tiny Peas, Pea Pods and Water Chestnuts in Sauce, 10-oz. package, boil-in-bag	213	27.0	21.3	2.70			
Boiled (yield: approx. 10 oz.)	213	27.0	21.3	2.70	180	20.0	
Seabrook Farms Petite Peas & Cauliflower, 10-oz. package	135	21.0	13.5	2.10			
Boiled, drained (yield: approx. 9.3 oz.)	(135)	(21.0)	(14.5)	(2.26)			

PEPPERS (see also PIMIENTOS)

Sweet Peppers (Garden Varieties)

	UNIT Cal.	UNIT Carb.	1 OZ., BY WT. Cal.	1 OZ., BY WT. Carb.	1 CUP Cal.	1 CUP Carb.	Fiber per oz. (GMS.)
GREEN PEPPERS (Immature)							
RAW:							
As purchased [refuse: stem ends, seeds, and core, approx. 18%]:							
1 medium pepper:							
Fancy grade (approx. 3¾" long, 3" diameter, 7.1 oz.)	36	7.9	5.1	1.12			
No. 1 grade (approx. 2¾" long, 2½" diameter, 3.2 oz.)	16	3.5	5.1	1.12			
1 pound (approx. 2¼ fancy grade, or 5 No. 1 grade peppers)	82	17.9	5.1	1.12			
Edible portion:							
1 medium pepper:							
Fancy grade (approx. 5.8 oz.)	36	7.9	6.2	1.36			0.51
No. 1 grade (approx. 2.6 oz.)	16	3.5	6.2	1.36			0.51
1 pepper ring, 3" diameter, ¼" thick (approx. 0.35 oz.)	2	0.5	6.2	1.36			0.51
1 cup:							
Sliced (approx. 2.8 oz.)	18	3.8	6.2	1.36	18	3.8	0.51
Chopped or diced (approx. 5.3 oz.)	33	7.2	6.2	1.36	33	7.2	0.51
1 pound (approx. 3 cups of chopped or diced green pepper, or 5.7 cups of sliced green pepper) (tr/1g/tr/93%/4mg)	100	21.8	6.2	1.36			0.51
COOKED:							
Boiled, drained:							
1 medium pepper:							
Fancy grade A (approx. 5.6 oz.)	29	6.1	5.1	1.08			(0.42)
No. 1 grade (approx. 2.6 oz.)	13	2.8	5.1	1.08			(0.42)
1 cup, sliced, chopped, or diced (approx. 4.7 oz.)	24	5.2	5.1	1.08	24	5.2	(0.42)
1 pound (approx. 3.4 cups of chopped, diced, or sliced green peppers) (tr/1g/tr/95%/3mg)	82	17.2	5.1	1.08	24	5.2	(0.42)

	UNIT		1 OZ., BY WT.		1 CUP		Fiber per oz.
	Cal.	Carb.	Cal.	Carb.	Cal.	Carb.	(GMS.)
Steamed:							
1 pound of raw green peppers, steamed (yield: approx. 15.5 oz.)	100	21.8	6.4	1.40			0.53
1 pound of steamed green peppers	103	22.5	6.4	1.40			0.53
FROZEN, by brand:							
Green Giant Stuffed Green Peppers with Beef in Creole Sauce, 14-oz. package	400	36.1	28.6	2.58			
Stouffer's Stuffed Peppers, 15½-oz. package	450	36.0	29.0	2.32			
RED PEPPERS (Mature)							
RAW:							
As purchased [refuse: stem ends, seeds, and core, approx. 18%]:							
1 medium pepper:							
Fancy grade (approx. 3¾" long, 3" diameter, 7.1 oz.)	51	11.6	7.2	1.63			
No. 1 grade (approx. 2¾" long, 3" diameter, 3.2 oz.)	23	5.2	7.2	1.63			
1 pound (approx. 2¼ fancy grade, or 5 No. 1 grade peppers)	115	26.2	7.2	1.63			
Edible portion:							
1 medium pepper:							
Fancy grade (approx. 5.8 oz.)	51	11.6	8.8	2.01			0.48
No. 1 grade (approx. 2.6 oz.)	23	5.2	8.8	2.01			0.48
1 pepper ring, 3" diameter, ¼" thick (approx. 0.35 oz.)	3	0.7	8.8	2.01	47	10.7	0.48
1 cup:							
Sliced (approx. 2.8 oz.)	25	5.7	8.8	2.01	25	5.7	0.48
Chopped or diced (approx. 5.3 oz.)	47	10.7	8.8	2.01	47	10.7	0.48
1 pound (approx. 3 cups of chopped or diced red pepper or 5.7 cups of sliced red pepper) (tr/2g/tr/94%/na)	141	26.2	8.8	2.01			0.48
COOKED:							
Boiled, drained:							
1 medium pepper:							
Fancy grade A, (approx. 5.5 oz.)	(41)	(9.3)	(7.6)	(1.67)	(36)	(8.0)	(0.41)
No. 1 grade (approx. 2.5 oz.)	(19)	(4.2)	(7.6)	(1.67)	(36)	(8.0)	(0.41)
1 cup sliced, chopped, or diced (approx. 4.8 oz.)	(36)	(8.0)	(7.6)	(1.67)	(36)	(8.0)	(0.41)
1 pound (approx. 3.3 cups sliced, chopped, or diced) (tr/2g/tr/na/na)	(122)	(26.7)	(7.6)	(1.67)	(36)	(8.0)	(0.41)

Hot Chili Peppers

	UNIT		1 OZ., BY WT.		1 CUP		Fiber per oz.
	Cal.	Carb.	Cal.	Carb.	Cal.	Carb.	(GMS.)
GREEN CHILI PEPPERS (Immature)							
RAW:							
As purchased [refuse: stem ends, seeds, and core, approx. 27%]:							
1 pound	123	30.1	7.7	1.88			
Edible portion:							
1 pound (tr/3g/tr/89%/na)	168	41.3	10.5	2.58			0.51
RED CHILI PEPPERS (Mature)							
RAW:							
As purchased [refuse: stem ends, seeds, and core, approx. 27%]:							
1 pound	215	52.3	13.4	3.27			
As purchased [refuse: stem ends, approx. 4%]:							
1 pound	405	78.8	25.3	4.93			
Edible portion:							
1 pound, without seeds (1g/4g/tr/80%/7mg)	299	71.7	18.4	4.48			0.65
1 pound, with seeds (1g/5g/1g/74%/na)	422	82.1	26.4	5.13			2.55
DRIED, based on generic data:							
Pods							
1 pound (4g/17g/3g/13%/106mg)	1456	271.3	91.0	16.96			7.43
CANNED, by brand:							
Heublein Hot Peppers, 3.5-oz. can	28	5.5	8.0	1.58	(67)	(13.2)	
Diced Hot Peppers, 4-oz. can	32	6.3	8.0	1.58	(67)	(13.2)	
Ortega Chiles, diced, strips, or whole, 4-oz. can	24	4.4	6.0	1.10			
7-oz. can	42	7.7	6.0	1.10			
27-oz. can	162	29.7	6.0	1.10			
Diced Hot Peppers, 4-oz. can	32	6.3	8.0	1.58			
Green Chile Salsa, 7-oz. can	49	8.7	7.0	1.24			
28-oz. can	196	34.7	7.0	1.24			

	UNIT		1 OZ., BY WT.		1 CUP		Fiber per oz.
	Cal.	Carb.	Cal.	Carb.	Cal.	Carb.	(GMS.)
Hot Peppers, 3.5-oz. can	28	5.5	8.0	1.58			
6.5-oz. can	52	10.3	8.0	1.58			
Tomatoes & Hot Green Chiles, 10-oz. can	70	13.6	7.0	1.36			

GROUND CHILI PEPPER, see the SALTS & SPICES chapter

PETSAI, see Chinese Cabbage under CABBAGE

PIGEON PEAS

	UNIT		1 OZ., BY WT.		1 CUP		Fiber per oz.
	Cal.	Carb.	Cal.	Carb.	Cal.	Carb.	(GMS.)
MATURE SEEDS, Dry							
RAW:							
1 pound	1551	288.9	96.9	18.06			1.99
IMMATURE SEEDS							
RAW:							
1 cup (approx. 7.1 oz.) (yield: approx. 1 cup)	(92)	(16.7)	12.9	2.36	(92)	(16.7)	0.94
1 pound (approx. 2.3 cups) (yield: approx. 15.5 oz., 2.2 cups) (2g/2g/tr/70%/1mg)	207	37.7	12.9	2.36	(92)	(16.7)	0.94
COOKED:							
Steamed:							
1 cup (approx. 7 oz.)	(93)	(17.0)	13.3	(2.43)	(93)	(17.0)	0.97
1 pound (approx. 2–3 cups) (yield from approx. 16.5 oz. uncooked beans) (2g/2g/tr/na/na)	(213)	(38.9)	(13.3)	(2.43)	(93)	(17.0)	0.97

PIMIENTOS

	UNIT		1 OZ., BY WT.		1 CUP		Fiber per oz.
	Cal.	Carb.	Cal.	Carb.	Cal.	Carb.	(GMS.)
CANNED or JARRED, based on generic data:							
2-oz. jar	15	3.3	7.5	1.65			
4-oz. can	31	6.6	7.5	1.65			
JARRED, by brand							
Dromedary Pimientos, 4-oz. jar	40	8.0	10.0	2.00			

PINTO BEANS

	UNIT		1 OZ., BY WT.		1 CUP		Fiber per oz.
	Cal.	Carb.	Cal.	Carb.	Cal.	Carb.	(GMS.)
MATURE SEEDS, Dry							
RAW:							
1 cup (approx. 6.5 oz.)	663	121.0	98.9	18.10	663	121.0	1.22
1 pound (approx. 2.5 cups)	1583	288.9	98.9	18.10	663	121.0	1.22
COOKED:							
Boiled, drained:							
1 cup (approx. 6.5 oz.)	(269)	(49.3)	(41.4)	(7.58)	(269)	(49.3)	(0.51)
1 pound (approx. 2.5 cups) (yield from approx. 6.7 oz. uncooked beans)	(663)	(121.3)	(41.4)	(7.58)	(269)	(49.3)	(0.51)
BOXED, by brand:							
Golden Harvest Pinto Beans, 16-oz. (1-lb.) box	1500	270.1	93.8	16.88	600	108.0	
1 cup, dry (approx. 6.4 oz.)	600	108.0	93.8	16.88	600	108.0	
CANNED, by brand:							
Ralph's Pinto Beans, 15-oz. can	380	68.0	25.3	4.53	190	34.0	

PLANTAIN

	UNIT		1 OZ., BY WT.		1 CUP		Fiber per oz.
	Cal.	Carb.	Cal.	Carb.	Cal.	Carb.	(GMS.)
RAW:							
Medium (approx. 12.9 oz., 11" long along outer curvature, 1⅞" diameter, dimensions highly variable):							
As purchased [refuse: skin, approx. 28%] (Percent of refuse, dimensions, and weight are highly variable):							
1 medium plantain (approx. 12.9 oz.)	313	82.2	24.3	6.37			
1 pound (approx. 1¼ medium plantains)	389	101.9	24.3	6.37			
Edible portion:							
1 medium plantain (approx. 9⅓ oz.)	313	82.2	33.8	8.85			0.11
1 pound (approx. 1.7 medium plantains) (tr/9g/tr/66%/1mg)	540	141.6	33.8	8.85			0.11

	UNIT		1 OZ., BY WT.		1 CUP		Fiber per oz.
	Cal.	Carb.	Cal.	Carb.	Cal.	Carb.	(GMS.)
POKEBERRY (Poke) SHOOTS							
RAW:							
All-edible:							
1 pound (tr/1g/1g/92%/na)	104	16.8	6.5	1.05			
COOKED:							
Boiled, drained:							
1 cup (approx. 5.8 oz.)	33	5.1	5.7	0.88	33	5.1	
1 pound (approx. 2¾ cups) (tr/1g/1g/93%/na)	91	14.0	5.7	0.88	33	5.1	
POPCORN, see under CORN							
POTATOES							
LONG and ROUND TYPES							
RAW:							
As purchased [refuse: parings and trimmings. When pared by mechanical means, approx. 25%]:							
1 round potato, approx. 3" long, 1¾" diameter (approx. 5.3 oz.)	86	19.2	16.2	3.64			
1 long potato, approx. 4¾" long, 2⅓" diameter (approx. 8.8 oz.)	143	32.1	16.2	3.64			
1 pound (approx. 1.8 long potatoes or 3 round potatoes)	259	58.2	16.2	3.64			
As purchased [refuse: parings and trimmings. When pared with a split-knife peeler, approx. 10%]:							
1 round potato (approx. 5.3 oz.)	103	23.1	19.4	4.36			
1 long potato (approx. 8.8 oz.)	171	38.5	19.4	4.36			
1 pound (approx. 1.8 long potatoes or 3 round potatoes)	310	69.8	19.4	4.36			
Edible portion:							
1 round potato, pared by mechanical means (approx. 4.0 oz.)	86	19.2	21.6	4.85	114	25.7	0.14
1 long potato, pared by mechanical means (approx. 6.6 oz)	143	32.1	21.6	4.85	114	25.7	0.14
1 round potato, pared by split-knife peeler (approx. 4.8 oz.)	103	23.1	21.6	4.85	114	25.7	0.14
1 long potato, pared by split-knife peeler (approx. 7.9 oz.)	171	38.5	21.6	4.85	114	25.7	0.14
1 cup, chopped, diced, or sliced (approx. 5.3 oz.)	114	25.7	21.6	4.85	114	25.7	0.14
1 pound (approx. 3.3 round potatoes or 2 long potatoes, 3 cups) (1g/5g/tr/80%/1mg)	345	77.6	21.6	4.85	114	25.7	0.14
COOKED:							
Baked in skin [refuse: skins and adhering potato, approx. 23%]:							
1 round potato (approx. 4.1 oz.)	84	18.9	20.4	4.60			
1 long potato (approx. 7.1 oz.)	145	32.8	20.4	4.60			
1 pound weighed in skins but eaten without skins (approx. 2.2 long potatoes or 3.9 round potatoes) (1g/5g/tr/75%/1mg)	326	73.7	20.4	4.60			
Baked in skin, eaten with skin (based on data from Canada):							
1 round potato (approx. 4.1 oz.)	104	24.4	25.8	5.95			
1 long potato (approx. 7.1 oz.)	183	42.2	25.8	5.95			
1 pound (approx. 2.2 long potatoes or 3.9 round potatoes)	413	95.3	25.8	5.95			
Boiled in skin [refuse: skins and eyes, approx. 9%]:							
1 round potato (approx. 5.3 oz.)	104	23.3	19.6	4.42	118	26.5	
1 long potato (approx. 8.8 oz.)	173	38.9	19.6	4.42	118	26.5	
1 cup, diced or sliced (approx. 5.5 oz.)	118	26.5	19.6	4.42	118	26.5	
1 pound weighed in skins but eaten without skins (approx. 1.8 long potatoes or 3 round potatoes, 2.9 cups) (1g/4g/tr/80%/1mg)	314	70.6	19.6	4.42	118	26.5	
Boiled, pared before cooking:							
Pared by mechanical methods:							
1 round potato (approx. 4.0 oz.)	74	16.5	18.4	4.12	101	22.5	0.12
1 long potato (approx. 6.6 oz.)	122	27.3	18.4	4.12	101	22.5	0.12
1 cup, chopped, diced, or sliced (approx. 5.5 oz.)	101	22.5	18.4	4.12	101	22.5	0.12
1 pound (approx. 2.4 long potatoes or 4 round potatoes, 2.9 cups) (1g/4g/tr/83%/1mg)	295	65.9	18.4	4.12	101	22.5	0.12
Pared by split-knife peeler:							
1 round potato (approx. 4.8 oz.)	88	19.6	18.4	4.11	101	22.5	0.12
1 long potato (approx. 7.9 oz.)	146	32.6	18.4	4.11	101	22.5	0.12

	UNIT		1 OZ., BY WT.		1 CUP		Fiber per oz.
	Cal.	Carb.	Cal.	Carb.	Cal.	Carb.	(GMS.)
1 cup, chopped, diced, or sliced (approx. 5.5 oz.)	101	22.5	18.4	4.11	101	22.5	0.12
1 pound (approx. 2 long potatoes or 3⅓ round potatoes, 2.9 cups) (1g/4g/tr/83%/1mg)	295	65.8	18.4	4.11	101	22.5	0.12
French Fries (based on data from France):							
1 pound	1284	161.0	80.2	10.07			
Pared, steamed:							
1 pound of raw potatoes, steamed (yield: approx. 15.8 oz.)	345	77.6	21.8	4.91			0.14
1 pound of steamed potatoes	349	78.6	21.8	4.91			0.14
BOXED, by brand:							
Betty Crocker Creamed Potatoes, 4.75-oz. box	480	102.0	101.1	21.47			
Prepared as package directs, for saucepan or oven (yield: approx. 26 oz., 3 cups)	960	126.0	(36.9)	(4.85)	(320)	(42.0)	
Hash Browns Potatoes with Onion, 6-oz. box	600	132.0	100.0	22.00			
Prepared as package directs (yield: approx. 16.4 oz., 3 cups)	900	132.0	(54.9)	(8.05)	300	44.0	
Julienne Potatoes, 4.75-oz. box	480	96.0	101.1	20.21			
Prepared as package directs (yield: approx. 26 oz., 3 cups)	780	102.0	(30.9)	(3.94)	(267)	(34.0)	
Potatoes Au Gratin, 5.5-oz. box	540	114.0	98.2	20.73			
Prepared as package directs (yield: approx. 25.9 oz., 3 cups)	900	120.0	(34.7)	(4.63)	300	40.0	
Potato Buds, 16.5 oz. box	480	112.0	29.1	6.79	180	42.0	
Prepared as package directs (yield: approx. 28-oz.)	1040	120.0	(36.8)	(4.25)	260	30.0	
Potatoes with Sour Cream 'N Chives, 5.5-oz. box	540	102.0	98.2	18.55			
Prepared as package directs (yield: approx. 3 cups, 26 oz.)	840	108.0	(32.4)	(4.17)	(280)	(36.0)	
Scalloped Potatoes. 5.5-oz. box	540	114.0	98.2	20.73			
Prepared as package directs (yield: approx. 3 cups, approx. 26 oz.)	900	120.0	(34.7)	(4.63)	(300)	(40.0)	
French's Big Tate Hash Brown Potatoes with Seasoning, 5¾-oz. box	600	132.0	104.3	22.96			
Prepared as package directs (yield: approx. 3 cups)	990	132.0			330	44.0	
Big Tate Mashed Potatoes, 16-oz. (1-lb.) box	1686	360.0	105.0	22.50	(204)	(43.7)	
Prepared as package directs (yield: approx. 12 cups, 6 lb. 5 oz.)	3360	384.0	(33.4)	(3.82)	280	32.0	
28-oz. box	2800	600.0	105.0	22.50	(204)	(43.7)	
Prepared as package directs (yield: approx. 20 cups, 10 lb. 8 oz.)	5600	640.0	(33.4)	(3.82)	280	32.0	
Big Tate Potatoes Au Gratin, 5½-oz. box	650	105.0	118.2	19.09			
Prepared as package directs (yield: approx. 2½ cups, 22 oz.)	950	140.0	(44.0)	(6.48)	380	56.0	
Big Tate Potato Pancake Mix, 6-oz. box	560	136.0	93.3	22.67			
Prepared as package directs (yield: approx. 24 oz.)	1040	136.0	43.3	5.67			
1 pancake, approx. 1 oz.	43	5.7	43.3	5.67			
Big Tate Scalloped Potatoes, 5⅝-oz. box	575	125.0	102.2	22.22			
Prepared as package directs (yield: approx. 2½ cups, 22 oz.)	950	150.0	(44.0)	(6.94)	380	60.0	
Idaho Mashed Potatoes, 6½-oz. box	600	150.0	92.3	23.08	(179)	(44.8)	
Prepared as package directs (yield: approx. 5 cups, 42 oz.)	1200	160.0	(28.6)	(3.81)	240	32.0	
Hungry Jack Mashed (Flakes) Potatoes, 8-oz. box	840	180.0	105.0	22.50	(187)	(40.0)	
Prepared as package directs (yield: approx. 6 cups, 44 oz.)	1680	192.0	(37.8)	(4.32)	280	32.0	
"Suggested" serving, approx. ½ cup, 3.7 oz.	140	16.0	(37.8)	(4.32)	280	32.0	
Pride Pak Au Gratin Potatoes, 5½-oz. box	600	120.0	109.1	21.82			
Prepared as package directs (yield: approx. 3 cups, 24 oz.)	900	126.0	37.5	5.25	300	42.0	
Hash Brown Potatoes, 6-oz. box	600	126.0	100.0	21.00			
Prepared as package directs (yield: approx. 3 cups, 24 oz.)	900	126.0	37.5	5.25	300	42.0	
Instant Mashed Potato, 40-oz. box	4080	952	102.0	23.80	(240)	(56.0)	
Prepared as package directs (yield: approx. 34 cups, 17 lb.)	6120	1088.0	22.5	4.00	180	32.0	

	UNIT		1 OZ., BY WT.		1 CUP		Fiber per oz.
	Cal.	Carb.	Cal.	Carb.	Cal.	Carb.	(GMS.)
Mashed Potatoes, 16-oz. (1-lb.) box	1560	364.0	97.5	22.75	240	56.0	
Prepared as package directs (yield: approx. 13 cups, 6 lb. 8 oz.)	2860	416.0	27.5	4.00	220	32.0	
Scalloped Potatoes, 5½-oz. box	600	132.0	109.1	24.00			
Prepared as package directs (yield: approx. 3 cups, 24 oz.)	900	138.0	37.5	5.75	300	46.0	
Sour Cream & Chive Potatoes, 4¾-oz. box	540	114.0	113.7	24.00			
Prepared as package directs (yield: approx. 3 cups, 27.1 oz.)	840	120.0	(30.9)	(4.42)	280	40.0	
Rodgers Hash Brown Potatoes, 5½-oz. box	540	129.7	98.2	23.59			
Prepared as package directs (yield: approx. 2.4 oz., 3 cups)	(540)	(129.7)	(22.5)	(5.40)	180	58.0	
Potatoes Au Gratin, 5½-oz. box	540	144.0	98.2	26.18			
Prepared as package directs (yield: approx. 3 cups, 2.3 oz.)	(540)	(144.0)	(23.3)	(6.21)	(180)	(48.0)	
Potato Flakes, 14½-oz. box	1440	336.0	99.3	23.17			
Prepared as package directs (yield: approx. 12 cups, 4 lb. 9 oz.)	2640	384.0	(36.4)	(5.30)	220	32.0	
Scalloped Potatoes, 5½-oz. box	540	114.0	98.2	20.73			
Prepared as package directs (yield: approx. 3 cups, 25 oz.)	(540)	(114.0)	(21.4)	(4.52)	180	38.0	
Safeway Instant Mashed Potatoes, 13½-oz. box	1440	336.0	106.7	24.89	(207)	(48.3)	
Town House Instant Mashed Potatoes, 13½-oz. box	1440	336.0	106.7	24.89	207	48.3	
Prepared as package directs (yield: approx. 12 cups, 96.0 oz.)	2640	384.0	27.5	4.00	220	32.0	
FROZEN, based on generic data:							
1 cup:							
Crinkle Cut (approx. 3.9 oz.)	80	19.1	20.7	4.93	80	19.1	0.11
Diced (approx. 4.9 oz.)	101	24.2	20.7	4.93	101	24.2	0.11
1 pound (approx. 4.1 cups crinkle cut potatoes or 3.2 cups diced potatoes)	331	78.9	20.7	4.93			0.11
1 container, 12 oz. net wt. (approx. 3 cups crinkle cut potatoes or 2.4 cups diced potatoes)	248	59.2	20.7	4.93			0.11
1 container, 32 oz. (2 lb.) net wt. (approx. 8.2 cups crinkle cut potatoes or 6.5 cups diced potatoes)	662	157.8	20.7	4.93			0.11
COOKED:							
Hashed brown:							
1 cup (approx. 5.5 oz.)	347	45.0	63.5	8.22	347	45.0	0.40
1 pound (approx. 2.9 cups of hashed brown potatoes) (1g/8g/3g/56%/85mg)	1016	131.5	63.5	8.22	347	45.0	0.40
1 pound of frozen potatoes, hashed brown (yield: approx. 9.6 oz.)	611	79.1	63.5	8.22	347	45.0	0.40
1 12-oz. container of frozen raw potatoes, hashed brown (yield: approx. 7.2 oz., 1.3 cups)	459	59.5	63.5	8.22	347	45.0	0.40
1 32-oz. (2-lb.) container of frozen raw potatoes, hashed brown (yield: approx. 19.2 oz., 3.5 cups)	1221	158.1	63.5	8.22	347	45.0	0.40
French Fries (Straight-cut and crinkle-cut strips, with cross section approx. ½ × ½"):							
1 strip, 3½–4" long (approx. 0.35 oz. frozen)	17	2.6	48.2	7.40			0.17
Ovenheated (yield: approx. 0.28 oz.)	17	2.6	62.4	9.60	(300)	(46.1)	0.20
1 strip, 2–3½" long (approx. 0.23 oz. frozen)	11	1.7	48.2	7.40			0.17
Ovenheated (yield: approx. 0.18 oz.)	11	1.7	62.4	9.60	(300)	(46.1)	0.20
1 strip, 1–2" long (approx. 0.16 oz. frozen)	8	1.1	48.2	7.40			0.17
Ovenheated (yield: approx. 0.12 oz.)	8	1.1	62.4	9.60	(300)	(46.1)	0.20
1 container, 9 oz. net wt.	434	66.6	48.2	7.40			0.17
Ovenheated (yield: approx. 7 oz.)	434	66.6	62.4	9.60	(300)	(46.1)	0.20
1 container, 16 oz. (1 lb.) net wt.	771	118.4	48.2	7.40			0.17
Ovenheated (yield: 12.4 oz.)	771	118.4	62.4	9.60	(300)	(46.1)	0.20
1 container, 32 oz. (2 lb.) net wt.	1542	236.7	48.2	7.40			0.17
Ovenheated (yield: 28.8 oz. [1 lb. 8 oz.])	1542	236.7	62.4	9.60	(300)	(46.1)	0.20
1 pound (approx. 45 strips, 3½–4" in length, or 70 strips, 2–3½" in length, or 100 strips, 1–2" in length)	771	118.4	48.2	7.40			0.17
Ovenheated (yield: approx. 12.4 oz.) (1g/10g/4g/45%/2mg)	998	152.9	62.4	9.60	(300)	(46.1)	0.20

	UNIT		1 OZ., BY WT.		1 CUP		Fiber per oz.
	Cal.	Carb.	Cal.	Carb.	Cal.	Carb.	(GMS.)
FROZEN, by brand:							
Birds Eye Cottage Fried Potatoes, 14-oz. package	600	85.0	42.9	6.07	(232)	(32.8)	
Crinkle Cut Potatoes, 16-oz. (1-lb.) package	587	96.0	36.7	6.00	(176)	(28.8)	
French Fries, 16-oz. (1-lb.) package	587	90.7	36.7	5.67	(176)	(27.2)	
Hash Browns, 16-oz. (1-lb.) package	280	68.0	17.5	4.25	(77)	(18.6)	
Hash Brown O'Brien Potatoes, 24-oz. package	360	84.0	15.0	3.50	(66)	(15.3)	
Shredded Hash Browns, 12-oz. package	240	52.0	20.0	4.33	(88)	(18.9)	
Shoestring Potatoes, 20-oz. package	840	120.0	42.0	6.00			
Steak Fries, 24-oz. package	880	144.0	36.7	6.00	(176)	(28.8)	
Tasti Fries, 10-oz. package	560	680.0	56.0	6.80	(269)	(32.6)	
Tasti Puffs, 10-oz. package	760	76.0	76.0	7.60			
Tiny Taters, 16-oz. (1-lb.) package	1000	110.0	62.5	7.33			
Whole Peeled Potatoes, 32-oz. (2-lb.) package	600	130.0	18.8	4.06			
Golden Potato Pancakes, 12-oz. package, 8 pancakes	680	58.4	56.7	4.87			
1 pancake, approx. 1.5 oz.	85	7.3	56.7	4.87			
Green Giant Potatoes Au Gratin, 10-oz. package	426	36.6	42.6	3.66	390	32.0	
Potatoes in Sour Cream Sauce, Diced, 10-oz. package	318	102.1	31.8	10.21	270	36.0	
Potato Slices in Butter Sauce, 10-oz. package	227	32.9	22.7	3.29	210	27.0	
Potatoes and Sweet Peas in Bacon Cream Sauce, 10-oz. package	267	38.0	26.7	3.80	240	31.0	
Potatoes Vermicelli with Mushrooms & Cheese Sauce, 10-oz. package	409	43.4	40.9	4.34	390	42.0	
Shoestring Potatoes in Butter Sauce, 10-oz. package	366	44.5	36.6	4.45	310	37.0	
Stuffed Potatoes with Cheese Flavored Topping, 10-oz. package	473	59.8	47.3	5.98			
Stuffed Potatoes with Sour Cream and Chives, 10-oz. package	465	85.1	46.5	8.51			
Hanover Country Cut French Fries, 16-oz. (1-lb.) package	550	85.0	34.4	5.31	(165)	(25.5)	
"Suggested" serving, 3.2 oz.	110	17.0	34.4	5.31	(165)	(25.5)	
Crinkle Cut French Fries, 16-oz. (1-lb.) package	650	75.0	40.6	4.69	(195)	(22.5)	
Hash Brown Potatoes, 16-oz. (1-lb.) polybag	501	90.1	31.3	5.63	(138)	(24.8)	
"Suggested" serving, 3.2 oz.	100	18.0	31.3	5.63	(138)	(24.8)	
Hash Brown Potato Medley, 16-oz. (1-lb.) polybag	450	85.0	28.1	5.31	(124)	(23.4)	
"Suggested" serving, 3.2 oz.	90	17.0	28.1	5.31	(124)	(23.4)	
Home Fries, 16-oz. (1-lb.) polybag	501	80.0	31.3	5.00	(138)	(22.0)	
"Suggested" serving, 3.2 oz.	100	16.0	31.3	5.00	(138)	(22.0)	
Lamb's Frozen Steakhouse Potatoes, 24-oz. bag	1120	184.0	46.7	7.67	(225)	(36.8)	
Ore-Ida Cottage Fries, 32-oz. (2-lb.) package	1494	234.7	46.7	7.33	(205)	(32.3)	
Country Style Dinner Fries, 24-oz. package	960	144.0	40.0	6.00	(192)	(28.8)	
Crispers, 32-oz. (2-lb.) package	2454	277.4	76.7	8.67			
Golden Crinkles, 16-oz. (1-lb.) package	693	112.0	43.3	7.00	(208)	(33.6)	
Golden Fries, 16-oz. (1-lb.) package	693	112.0	43.3	7.33	(208)	(35.2)	
O'Brien Potatoes, 24-oz. package	480	112.0	20.0	4.67	(88)	(20.5)	
Pixie Crinkles, 20-oz. package	1134	166.6	56.7	8.33	(272)	(40.0)	
(Heinz) Self Sizzling Crinkles, 24-oz. package	1280	184.0	53.3	7.67	(256)	(36.8)	
(Heinz) Self Sizzling Fries, 24-oz. package	1280	192.0	53.3	8.00	(256)	(38.4)	
(Heinz) Self Sizzling Shoestrings, 12-oz. package	880	104.0	73.3	8.67	(323)	(38.1)	
Shoestrings, 20-oz. package	1134	166.6	56.7	8.33	(249)	(36.7)	
Shredded Hash Browns, 12-oz. package	240	48.0	20.0	4.00	(88)	(17.6)	
Small Whole Peeled Potatoes, 32-oz. (2-lb.) package	746	170.6	23.3	5.33	(126)	(28.8)	
Southern Style Hash Browns, 32-oz. (2-lb.) package	746	170.6	23.3	5.33	(103)	(23.5)	
Southern Style Hash Browns with Butter Sauce, 24-oz. package	960	120.0	40.0	5.00	(176)	(22.0)	
Tater Tots Potatoes, 16-oz. (1-lb.) package	853	106.7	53.3	6.67	(256)	(32.0)	
Tater Tots Potatoes with Bacon Flavor, 16-oz. (1-lb.) package	800	112.0	50.0	7.00	(240)	(33.6)	
Tater Tots Potatoes with Onions, 16-oz. (1-lb.) package	853	112.0	53.3	7.00	(256)	(33.6)	

	UNIT		1 OZ., BY WT.		1 CUP		Fiber per oz.
	Cal.	Carb.	Cal.	Carb.	Cal.	Carb.	(GMS.)
Seabrook Boiled White Whole Potatoes, 14-oz. package	280	60.0	20.0	4.29	(143)	(30.7)	
Stouffer's Creamed Potatoes and Peas, 10-oz. package	280	34.0	28.0	3.40			
Potatoes au Gratin, 7⅝-oz. package	270	26.0	35.4	3.41			
11½-oz. package	405	39.0	35.2	3.39			
Scalloped Potatoes, 8-oz. package	252	28.0	31.5	3.50			
12-oz. package	378	42.0	31.5	3.50			
Taterlan Crinkle Potatoes, 32-oz. (2-lb.) bag	1280	192.0	40.0	6.00	(192)	(28.8)	
Straight French Fries, 32-oz. (2-lb.) bag	1280	192.0	40.0	6.00	(192)	(28.8)	
Tater Puffs Potatoes, 32-oz. (2-lb.) bag	1707	224.0	53.3	7.00			
Village Park Small Whole Peeled Potatoes, 16-oz. (1-lb.) package	300	70.0	18.8	4.38			
CANNED, by brand:							
Ann Page (A&P) Whole Small White Potatoes, 16-oz. (1-lb.) can	180	40.0	11.3	2.50	90	20.0	
Drained solids (yield: approx. 9.5 oz.)	(180)	(38.0)	(18.8)	(4.17)	(188)	(26.2)	
Case Swayne Sliced New Potatoes, 15-oz. can	(200)	(44.0)	18.0	3.92	100	22.0	
Drained solids (yield: approx. 9 oz.)	(200)	(44.0)	(22.2)	(4.89)	(140)	(30.9)	
Whole New Potatoes, 15-oz. can	(220)	(48.0)	(17.4)	(3.80)	110	24.0	
Drained solids (yield: approx. 9 oz.)	(220)	(48.0)	24.4	5.33	(154)	(33.6)	
Del Monte New Potatoes, 16-oz. (1-lb.) can	180	38.0	11.3	2.38	90	19.0	
Drained solids (yield: approx. 9.6 oz.)	(180)	(38.0)	(18.8)	(3.95)	(188)	(24.9)	
Hanover Sliced White Potatoes, 16-oz. (1-lb.) can	180	38.0	11.3	2.38	(108)	(24.0)	
Drained solids (yield: approx. 9.6 oz.)	(165)	(36.4)	(17.2)	(3.79)	(108)	(23.9)	
Whole White Potatoes, 39-oz. can	441	97.5	11.3	2.50	(108)	(24.0)	
Drained solids (yield: approx. 23.4 oz.)	(403)	(88.8)	(17.2)	(3.79)	(108)	(23.9)	
16-oz. (1-lb.) can	180	40.4	11.3	2.50	(108)	(24.0)	
Drained solids (yield: approx. 9.6 oz.)	(165)	(36.4)	(17.2)	(3.79)	(108)	(23.9)	
Stokely Whole Potatoes, 17-oz. can	192	42.3	11.3	2.49	100	22.0	
Drained solids (yield: approx. 10.2 oz.)	(192)	(42.3)	(18.8)	(4.15)	(118)	(26.1)	
POTATO SALAD (based on USDA home recipe)							
Prepared with 4 boiled medium potatoes, 1 Tbsp. chopped onion, ¾ cup cooked salad dressing, and salt (yield: approx. 2¾ cups, 24.1 oz.) (1g/5g/1g/76%/150mg)	676	111.3	28.1	4.62	248	40.8	
1 cup (approx. 8.8 oz.)	248	40.8	28.1	4.62	248	40.8	
Prepared with 4 boiled medium potatoes, ½ cup celery, ¼ cup pickles, 1 Tbsp. chopped onion, ¼ cup French Dressing, ¼ cup mayonnaise, and salt (yield: approx. 3⅔ cups, 32.3 oz.) (1g/4g/3g/72%/136mg)	1328	122.7	41.1	3.80	363	33.5	
1 cup (approx. 8.8 oz.)	363	33.5	41.1	3.80	363	33.5	
POTATOES, SWEET, see SWEET POTATOES. Also see YAMS							
PUMPKIN							
RAW:							
As purchased [refuse: rind and seeds, approx. 30%]:							
1 medium pumpkin (approx. 5 lb.)	415	103.2	5.2	1.29			
1 pound (approx. 0.2 medium pumpkins)	83	20.6	5.2	1.29			
Edible portion:							
1 medium pumpkin (approx. 3.5 lb.)	414	103.0	7.4	1.84	64	15.8	0.31
1 cup (approx. 8.6 oz.)	64	15.8	7.4	1.84	64	15.8	0.31
1 pound (approx. 1.9 cups)	118	29.5	7.4	1.84	64	15.8	0.31
CANNED, by brand:							
Del Monte Pumpkin, 16-oz. (1-lb.) can	160	36.0	10.0	2.25	80	18.0	
29-oz. can	290	65.3	10.0	2.25	80	18.0	
Libby's Pumpkin, 16 oz. (1-lb.) can	(160)	(40.0)	(16.0)	(2.50)	80	20.0	
Stokely Pumpkin, 16-oz. (1-lb.) can	148	35.2	9.3	2.20	80	19.0	
1-lb. 13-oz. can	268	63.8	9.3	2.20	80	19.0	
1 Tablespoon	5	1.2	9.3	2.20	80	19.0	

	UNIT		1 OZ., BY WT.		1 CUP		Fiber per oz.
	Cal.	Carb.	Cal.	Carb.	Cal.	Carb.	(GMS.)
For comparison: **Stokely** Pumpkin Pie Filling, 18-oz. can	700	168.3	38.9	9.35	370	89.0	
1 Tablespoon	23	5.6	38.9	9.35	370	89.0	
PURSLANE							
RAW:							
All edible:							
1 pound	95	17.3	6.0	1.08			0.32
COOKED:							
Boiled, drained:							
1 pound (tr/1g/tr/95%/na)	68	12.7	4.3	0.79			0.23
Steamed:							
1 pound of raw purslane, steamed (yield: approx. 14.6 oz.)	95	17.3	6.5	1.18			0.35
1 pound of steamed purslane	104	19.0	6.5	1.18			0.35
RADISHES							
COMMON							
RAW:							
As purchased:							
With tops [refuse: tops, rootlets, and trimmings, approx. 37%]:							
1 pound (approx. 40 medium-large radishes)	49	10.3	3.1	0.64			
Without tops [refuse: stem ends, rootlets, and trimmings, approx. 10%]:							
1 pound (approx. 60 medium-large radishes)	69	14.7	4.3	0.92			
Prepackaged (round red radishes, packaged without tops) [refuse: stem ends, rootlets, and trimmings, approx. 10%]:							
1 package, 6 oz. net wt.	26	5.5	4.3	0.92			
1 pound (approx. 50 large radishes, or 91 medium radishes)	69	14.7	4.3	0.92			
Edible portion:							
1 medium radish (approx. ¾"–1" diameter, 0.2 oz.)	1	0.2	4.8	1.02			0.20
1 large radish (approx. 1"–1¼" diameter, 0.3 oz.)	1	0.3	4.8	1.02			0.20
1 cup, sliced (approx. 4.1 oz.)	20	4.2	4.8	1.02	20	4.2	0.20
1 pound (approx. 80 medium radishes or 53 large radishes) (tr/1g/tr/95%/5mg)	77	16.3	4.8	1.02			0.17
COOKED:							
Steamed:							
1 pound of raw radishes, steamed (yield: approx. 15 oz.)	77	16.3	5.1	1.09			0.21
1 pound of steamed radishes	82	17.4	5.1	1.09			0.21
ORIENTAL, including Chinese and Japanese, often called DAIKON							
RAW:							
As purchased:							
With tops [refuse: tops and parings, approx. 34%]:							
1 pound	57	12.6	3.6	0.79			
Without tops [refuse: parings, approx. 22%]:							
1 pound	67	14.9	4.2	0.93			
Edible portion:							
1 pound (tr/1g/tr/94%/na)	86	19.0	5.4	1.19			0.20
RATATOUILLE, see MIXED VEGETABLES (Stouffer's) at the end of this chapter							
RED BEANS							
Ann Page (A&P) Red Beans, 15½-oz. can	440	80.0	28.4	5.16	(256)	(46.4)	
Drained solids (yield: approx. 10.5 oz.)	(434)	(77.2)	(41.3)	(7.35)	(260)	(46.3)	
Van Camp's, 15½-oz. can	397	74.1	25.6	4.78	(230)	(43.0)	
Drained solids (yield: approx. 10.7 oz.)	(387)	(72.3)	(36.7)	(6.76)	(231)	(42.6)	
20-oz. can	512	95.6	25.6	4.78	(230)	(43.0)	
Drained solids (yield: approx. 13.6 oz.)	(499)	(92.0)	(36.7)	(6.76)	(231)	(42.5)	

	UNIT Cal.	UNIT Carb.	1 OZ., BY WT. Cal.	1 OZ., BY WT. Carb.	1 CUP Cal.	1 CUP Carb.	Fiber per oz. (GMS.)
RICE							
BROWN							
RAW:							
1 cup:							
Long grain (approx. 6.5 oz.)	666	143.2	102.1	21.94	666	143.2	0.26
Short grain (approx. 7.1 oz.)	720	154.8	102.1	21.94	720	154.8	0.26
1 pound (approx. 2.5 cups of long grain or 2.3 cups of short grain) (2g/22g/1g/12%/3mg)	1633	351.1	102.1	21.94			0.26
COOKED (cooked in the proportion of 1 cup rice to 1⅔ cups water):							
Long grain:							
1 cup:							
Hot rice (approx. 6.9 oz.)	232	49.7	33.8	7.23	232	49.7	0.09
Cold rice (approx. 5.1 oz.)	173	37.0	33.8	7.23	173	37.0	0.09
Short grain:							
1 cup:							
Hot rice (approx. 7.5 oz.)	(251)	(53.7)	33.8	7.23	(251)	(53.7)	0.09
Cold rice (approx. 5.5 oz.)	(187)	(40.0)	33.8	7.23	(187)	(40.0)	0.09
Long and Short Grain:							
1 pound (weighed hot: approx. 2.2 cups of long grain or 2.3 cups of short grain rice; weighed cold: 3.1 cups of long grain or 2.9 cups of short grain rice) (1g/7g/tr/70%/80mg)	540	115.7	33.8	7.23			0.09
WHITE (fully milled or polished)							
Enriched or unenriched (Enriching rice does not alter carbohydrate or caloric value.)							
RAW:							
1 cup:							
Long grain (approx. 6.5 oz.)	672	148.7	102.9	22.79	672	148.7	0.09
Medium grain (approx. 6.9 oz.)	708	156.8	102.9	22.79	708	156.8	0.09
Short grain (approx. 7.1 oz.)	726	160.8	102.9	22.79	726	160.8	0.09
1 pound (approx. 2.5 cups of long grain, or 2.3 cups of medium or short grain rice) (2g/23g/tr/10%/3mg)	1647	364.7	102.9	22.79			0.09
COOKED (cooked in the proportion of 1 cup rice to 2 cups water):							
Long grain:							
1 cup (moist, soft stage):							
Hot rice (approx. 7.2 oz.)	223	49.6	30.9	6.86	223	49.1	0.03
Cold rice (approx. 5.1 oz.)	158	35.1	30.9	6.86	158	35.1	0.03
Medium grain:							
1 cup (moist, soft stage):							
Hot rice (approx. 7.6 oz.)	(235)	(52.1)	30.9	6.86	(235)	(52.1)	0.03
Cold rice (approx. 5.4 oz.)	(167)	(37.0)	30.9	6.86	(167)	(37.0)	0.03
Short grain:							
1 cup (moist, soft stage):							
Hot rice (approx. 7.8 oz.)	(241)	(53.5)	30.9	6.86	(241)	(53.5)	0.03
Cold rice (approx. 5.6 oz.)	(173)	(38.4)	30.9	6.86	(173)	(38.4)	0.03
Long and short grain:							
1 pound moist, soft stage (weighed hot: approx. 2.2 cups of long grain, 2.1 cups of medium grain or 2 cups of short grain rice; weighed cold: 3.1 cups of long grain; 3 cups of medium grain or 2.9 cups of short grain rice) (1g/7g/tr/72%/106mg)	494	109.8	30.9	6.86			0.03
PARBOILED:							
DRY:							
1 cup (approx. 6.5 oz. of long grain rice)	683	150.4	104.6	23.05	683	150.4	0.06
1 pound (approx. 2.5 cups of long grain rice) (2g/23g/tr/10%/3mg)	1674	368.8	104.6	23.05	683	150.4	0.06
COOKED (cooked in the proportion of 1 cup rice to 1½ cups water):							
Long grain:							
1 cup:							
Hot rice (approx. 6.2 oz.)	186	40.8	30.1	6.61	186	40.8	0.03
Cold rice (approx. 5.1 oz.)	154	33.8	30.1	6.61	154	33.8	0.03
Long and short grain:							
1 pound (weighed hot: approx. 2.6 cups of long grain rice; weighed cold: 3.1 cups of long grain rice) (1g/7g/tr/73%/102mg)	481	105.7	30.1	6.61			0.03

	UNIT Cal.	UNIT Carb.	1 OZ., BY WT. Cal.	1 OZ., BY WT. Carb.	1 CUP Cal.	1 CUP Carb.	Fiber per oz. (GMS.)
PRECOOKED (INSTANT):							
DRY:							
1 cup (approx. 3.4 oz. of long grain rice)	355	78.4	106.0	23.39	355	78.4	0.11
1 pound (approx. 4.8 cups of long grain rice) (2g/24g/tr/10%/tr)	1696	374.2	106.0	23.39	355	78.4	0.11
READY-TO-SERVE, COOKED, FLUFFED (cooked in the proportion of 1 cup rice to 1 cup water):							
Long grain:							
1 cup:							
Hot rice (approx. 5.8 oz.)	180	39.9	30.9	6.86	180	39.9	0.03
Cold rice (approx. 4.6 oz.)	142	31.5	30.9	6.86	142	31.5	0.03
Long and short grain:							
1 pound (weighed hot: 2.8 cups of long grain rice; weighed cold: 3.5 cups of long grain rice) (1g/7g/tr/73%/77mg)	494	109.8	30.9	6.86			0.03
PACKAGED, by brand:							
A&P Long Grain enriched Rice, 2-lb. bag	3080	672.0	96.3	21.00	660	144.0	
Prepared as package directs (yield: approx. 4 lb. 14 oz., 14 cups)	3080	672.0	(39.3)	(8.57)	220	48.0	
3-lb. bag	4620	1008.0	96.3	21.00	660	144.0	
Prepared as package directs (yield: approx. 7 lb. 6 oz., 21 cups)	4620	1008.0	(39.3)	(8.57)	220	48.0	
5-lb. bag	7700	1680.0	96.3	21.00	660	144.0	
Prepared as package directs (yield: approx. 12 lb. 3 oz., 35 cups)	7700	1680.0	(39.3)	(8.57)	220	48.0	
10-lb. bag	15400	3360.0	96.3	21.00	660	144.0	
Prepared as package directs (yield: approx. 24 lb. 8 oz., 70 cups)	15400	3360.0	(39.3)	(8.57)	220	48.0	
Pre-cooked Long Grain enriched Instant Rice, 14-oz. package	1540	322.0	110.0	23.00	330	69.0	
Prepared as package directs (yield: approx. 3 lb. 1 oz., 9 cups)	1540	322.0	(31.4)	(6.57)	(171)	(35.7)	
28-oz. package	3080	644.0	110.0	23.00	330	69.0	
Prepared as package directs (yield: approx. 6 lb. 2 oz., 18 cups)	3080	644.0	(31.4)	(6.57)	(171)	(35.7)	
Canilla Fancy Extra Long Grain enriched Rice, 5-lb. bag	7700	1680.0	(96.3)	(21.00)	660	144.0	
Prepared as package directs, (yield: approx. 12 lb., 4 oz., 3 cups)	7700	1680.0	(39.2)	(8.56)	220	48.0	
Carolina Extra Long Grain enriched Rice, 3-lb. box	4800	1056.0	100.0	22.00	(677)	(150.0)	
Prepared as package directs (yield: approx. 9 lb. 4 oz., 26 cups)	4800	1056.0	(32.5)	(7.15)	(182)	(40.1)	
5-lb. bag	8000	1760.0	100.0	22.00	(677)	(150.0)	
Prepared as package directs (yield: approx. 15 lb. 6 oz., 44 cups)	8000	1760.0	(32.5)	(7.15)	(182)	(40.1)	
Long Grain and Wild Rice, 6-oz. box	540	120.0	90.0	20.00	(610)	(135.4)	
Prepared as package directs (yield: approx. 18.5 oz., 3 cups)	540	120.0	(29.2)	(6.49)	(164)	(36.4)	
Comstock ready-to-serve Spanish Rice, 15-oz. can	260	54.0	17.3	3.60			
Golden Harvest Natural Brown Long Grain Rice, 4-oz. package	400	92.0	100.0	23.00	(650)	(150.0)	
Prepared as package directs (yield: approx. 13.4 oz., 2.5 cups)	400	92.0	(29.9)	(6.87)	(206)	(47.4)	
16-oz. (1-lb.) box	1632	320.0	102.0	20.00	(660)	(130.0)	
Prepared as package directs (yield: approx. 3 lb. 6 oz., 10 cups)	1632	320.0	(30.4)	(5.97)	(164)	(32.2)	
48-oz. (3-lb.) package	4896	960.0	102.0	20.00	(660)	(130.0)	
Prepared as package directs (yield: approx. 10 lb. 1 oz., 30 cups)	4896	960.0	(30.4)	(5.97)	(164)	(32.2)	
Goya enriched Rice, 5-lb. bag	7780	1680.0	96.3	21.00	660	144.0	
Prepared as package directs (yield: approx. 12 lb. 6 oz., 35 cups)	7780	1680.0	(39.2)	(8.56)	220	48.0	
Green Giant Boil-in-Bag Rice Originals, frozen, Rice 'N Broccoli in cheese sauce, 11-oz. pouch	297	45.3	27.0	4.11	250	40.0	
Continental Rice With Green Beans & Almonds, 11-oz. pouch	275	108.9	25.0	9.90	230	35.0	
Medley-Rice With Sweet Peas & Mushrooms, 11-oz. pouch	268	47.4	24.4	4.31	200	35.0	

	UNIT		1 OZ., BY WT.		1 CUP		Fiber per oz.
	Cal.	Carb.	Cal.	Carb.	Cal.	Carb.	(GMS.)
Pilaf-Rice With Mushrooms & Onions, 11-oz. pouch	281	57.4	25.5	5.22	230	45.0	
Verdi-Rice With Bell Peppers & Parsley, 11-oz. pouch	337	64.0	30.6	5.82	270	47.0	
White & Wild Medley Rice With Peas, Celery, Mushrooms and Almonds, 11½-oz. pouch	388	55.8	33.8	4.85	320	47.0	
White & Wild Oriental Rice With Bean Sprouts, Pea Pods and Water Chestnuts, 12-oz. pouch	283	49.4	23.6	4.11	230	40.0	
White & Wild Rice, 11-oz. pouch	284	58.7	25.8	5.33	220	43.0	
Jello Rojo Enriched Rice, 10-lb. package	14600	3212.0	91.3	20.08	(600)	(132.0)	
Prepared as package directs (yield: approx. 35 lbs, 73 cups)	14600	3212.0	(25.9)	(5.69)	(200)	(43.9)	
Krasdale Long Grain enriched Rice, 5-lb. bag	7700	1680.0	96.3	21.00	660	144.0	
Prepared as package directs (yield: approx. 12 lb. 4 oz., 35 cups)	7700	1680.0	(39.2)	(8.56)	220	48.0	
La Choy Chicken Fried Rice, 12-oz. can	627	122.6	52.2	10.22	418	80.2	
Fried Rice, 12-oz. can	620	128.4	51.6	10.70	414	85.6	
Fried Rice & Pork, frozen, 12-oz. container	490	77.6	40.9	6.47			
Libby's Spanish Rice, ready to serve, 15-oz. can	(240)	(56.0)	(16.0)	(3.73)	120	28.0	
Minute Rice Drumstick Rice Mix, 7-oz. package	720	150.0	102.9	21.43			
Prepared as package directs (with butter yield: approx. 1 lb. 10 oz., 3 cups)	1020	150.0	(39.3)	(5.79)	340	50.0	
Fried Rice Mix, 7-oz. package	720	150.0	102.9	21.43			
Prepared as package directs (with oil, yield: approx. 1 lb. 10 oz., 3 cups)	960	150.0	(37.0)	(5.79)	320	50.0	
Minute Rice, 7-oz. package	360	81.0	51.4	11.57			
Prepared as package directs, without salt and butter (yield: approx. 10.9 oz., 2 cups)	360	81.0	(33.1)	(7.46)	180	40.5	
14-oz. package	720	162.0	51.4	11.57			
Prepared as package directs, without salt and butter (yield: approx. 1 lb. 6 oz., 4 cups)	720	162.0	(33.1)	(7.46)	180	40.5	
Rib Roast Rice Mix, 7-oz. package	720	140.0	102.9	21.43			
Prepared as package directs, with butter (yield: approx. 1 lb. 10 oz., 3 cups)	900	150.0	(34.7)	(5.79)	300	50.0	
Spanish Rice Mix, 6-oz. package	600	132.0	100.0	22.00			
Prepared as package directs, with butter and tomatoes (yield: approx. 1 lb. 10 oz., 3 cups)	900	150.0	(34.6)	(5.77)	300	50.0	
Near East Rice Pilaf, dry mix, 9-oz. box	900	190.0	100.0	21.11			
Prepared as package directs (yield: approx. 1 lb. 12 oz., 5 cups)	(1304)	(190.4)	(46.6)	(6.80)	(261)	(38.1)	
Spanish Rice Pilaf, 8-oz. box	800	168.0	100.0	21.00			
Prepared as package directs (yield: approx. 2 lb. 3 oz., 4 cups)	800	168.0	(23.1)	(4.86)	200	42.0	
R. M. Quigg Curry Rice, dry mix 7-oz. package	526	142.0	75.1	20.29	600	162.3	
Prepared as package directs (yield: approx 1 lb. 6½ oz., 3.8 cups)	730	165.0	32.4	7.33	194	44.0	
French Onion Rice, 7-oz. package	601	152.0	85.9	21.70	687	173.6	
Prepared as package directs (yield: approx. 1 lb. 6½ oz., 3¾ cups)	805	175.0	35.8	7.78	215	46.7	
Golden Paella Rice, 7-oz. package	526	142.0	75.1	20.29	601	162.3	
Prepared as package directs (yield: approx. 1 lb. 6½ oz., 3¾ cups)	730	165.0	32.4	7.33	194	44.0	
Herb Rice, 7-oz. package	546	142.0	78.0	20.29	624	162.3	
Prepared as package directs (yield: approx. 1 lb. 6½ oz., 3¾ cups)	750	165.0	33.0	7.33	200	44.0	
Long Grain & Wild Rice, 7-oz. package	541	142.0	77.3	20.29	618	162.3	
Prepared as package directs (yield: approx. 1 lb. 6½ oz., 3¾ cups)	745	165.0	33.1	7.33	199	44.0	
Original Yellow Rice, 7-oz. package	526	142.0	75.1	20.29	601	162.3	
Prepared as package directs (yield: approx. 1 lb. 6½ oz., 3¾ cups)	730	165.0	32.4	7.33	194	44.0	
Ranch Rice, 7-oz. package	526	142.0	75.1	20.29	601	162.3	
Prepared as package directs (yield: approx. 1 lb. 6½ oz., 3¾ cups)	730	165.0	32.4	7.33	194	44.0	

	UNIT		1 OZ., BY WT.		1 CUP		Fiber per oz.
	Cal.	Carb.	Cal.	Carb.	Cal.	Carb.	(GMS.)
Rice-A-Roni Beef Flavor Rice, dry mix 7.9-oz. box	780	162.0	98.7	20.51			
Prepared as package directs (yield: approx. 1 lb. 11 oz., 3 cups)	780	162.0	(28.9)	(6.00)	(260)	(54.0)	
Chicken Flavor Rice, 8-oz. box	800	165.0	100.0	20.63			
Prepared as package directs (yield: approx. 1 lb. 11 oz., 3¾ cups)	800	165.0	(29.6)	(6.11)	213	44.0	
Spanish Rice, 7½-oz. box	720	156.0	96.0	20.80			
Prepared as package directs (yield: approx. 2 lb. 7 oz., 4½ cups)	720	156.0	(18.5)	(4.01)	160	34.7	
Riceland Enriched rice, 10-lb. bag	17920	3328.0	(112.0)	(20.80)	(770)	(143.5)	
Prepared as package directs (yield: approx. 26 lb. 2 oz., 32 cups)	17920	3328.0	(42.9)	(9.45)	236	52.0	
River Enriched Rice, 16-oz. (1-lb.) bag	1600	352.0	100.0	22.00	(705)	(155.2)	
Prepared as package directs (yield: approx. 2 lb., 5.7 cups)	1600	352.0	(49.8)	(10.95)	(283)	(62.2)	
48-oz. (3-lb.) bag	4800	1056.0	100.0	22.00	(705)	(155.2)	
Prepared as package directs (yield: approx. 6 lb., 17 cups)	4800	1056.0	(49.8)	(10.95)	(283)	(62.2)	
Natural Long Grain Brown Rice, 12-oz. bag	1320	276.0	110.0	23.00	(715)	(150.0)	
Prepared as package directs (yield: approx. 2 lb. 1 oz., 6 cups)	1320	276.0	(40.0)	(8.36)	(220)	(46.0)	
Riviana Bake-It-Easy Beef Vermicelli-Rice Mix, 6-oz. box	660	138.0	110.0	23.00			
Prepared as package directs (yield: approx. 1 lb. 7 oz., 3 cups)	860	138.0	(37.4)	(6.00)	(287)	(46.0)	
Chicken Vermicelli-Rice Mix, 6-oz. box	660	138.0	110.0	23.00			
Prepared as package directs (yield: approx. 1 lb. 7 oz., 3 cups)	860	138.0	(37.4)	(6.00)	(287)	(46.0)	
Oriental Vermicelli-Rice Mix, 6-oz. box	720	150.0	120.0	25.00			
Prepared as package directs (yield: approx. 1 lb. 7 oz., 3 cups)	920	150.0	(40.0)	(6.52)	(307)	(50.0)	
Spanish Vermicelli-Rice Mix, 6-oz. box	660	144.0	110.0	24.00			
Prepared as package directs (yield: approx. 1 lb. 7 oz., 3 cups)	860	144.0	(37.4)	(6.26)	(287)	(48.0)	
Safeway Instant Rice, 20-oz. package	1320	300.0	(66.0)	(15.00)	220	50.0	
Prepared as package directs (yield: approx. 2 lb. 3 oz., 8 cups)	1320	300.0	(37.8)	(8.58)	165	32.5	
Long Grain Rice, 16-oz. (1-lb.) bag	1610	364.0	100.6	22.75	690	156.0	
Prepared as package directs (yield: approx. 2 lb. 7 oz., 7 cups)	(1610)	(364.0)	(41.0)	(9.27)	(230)	(52.0)	
Success Rice, 4-oz. boil-in-bag	440	92.0	110.0	23.00	(384)	(80.3)	
Prepared as package directs (yield: approx. 14 oz., 3¼ cups)	440	92.0	(31.4)	(6.57)	(137)	(28.7)	
8-oz. package	880	184.0	110.0	23.00	(384)	(80.3)	
Prepared as package directs (yield: approx. 1 lb. 12 oz., 6½ cups)	880	184.0	(31.4)	(6.57)	(137)	(28.7)	
Town House Instant Rice, 20-oz. package	1320	300.0	66.0	15.00			
Prepared as package directs (yield: approx. 35 oz.)	1320	300.0	37.8	8.58	220	50.0	
Long Grain Rice, 16-oz. (1-lb.) bag	1610	364.0	100.6	22.75			
Prepared as package directs (yield: approx. 39.3 oz.)	1610	364.0	41.0	9.27	230	52.0	
Uncle Ben's Beef Flavour'd Rice, dry mix, fast cooking, 6-oz. box	590	124.9	98.4	20.81	(669)	(141.5)	
Prepared as package directs:							
Without butter (yield: approx. 1 lb. 6 oz., 3 cups)	590	124.9	27.0	5.62	196	40.8	
With butter (yield: approx. 1 lb. 6 oz., 3 cups)	678	124.9	30.8	5.51	228	40.8	
Chicken Flavour'd Rice, dry mix, fast cooking, 6-oz. box	595	123.7	99.2	20.61	(675)	(140.1)	
Prepared as package directs:							
Without butter (yield: approx. 20 oz., 3 cups)	595	123.7	29.8	6.04	206	21.8	
With butter (yield: approx. 20 oz, 2.7 cups)	(742)	(123.7)	37.1	5.72	272	42.0	
Curried Rice, dry mix, fast cooking, 6-oz. box	570	124.4	95.0	20.73	(646)	(141.0)	
Prepared as package directs:							
Without butter (yield: approx. 20 oz., 3 cups)	570	124.4	29.6	6.46	192	41.8	
With butter (yield: approx. 20 oz., 2.3 cups)	(770)	(124.4)	(38.5)	(6.22)	230	41.8	

	UNIT Cal.	UNIT Carb.	1 OZ., BY WT. Cal.	1 OZ., BY WT. Carb.	1 CUP Cal.	1 CUP Carb.	Fiber per oz. (GMS.)
Long Grain Brown Rice, 16-oz. (1-lb.) box	1634	351.0	102.1	21.94	(694)	(149.2)	
Prepared as package directs:							
Without butter (yield: approx. 3 lb 2 oz., 8 cups)	1634	351.0	32.5	6.45	200	39.6	
With butter (yield: approx. 3 lb. 3 oz., 8 cups)	(1831)	(351.0)	35.9	6.24	228	39.6	
Long Grain White Enriched Rice, Converted, 16-oz. (1-lb.) package	1674	368.8	104.6	23.05	(708)	(156.1)	
Prepared as package directs:							
Without butter (yield: approx. 3 lb. 10 oz., 8.6 cups)	1674	368.8	28.4	6.35	194	43.4	
With butter (yield: approx. 3 lb. 11 oz., 8.4 cups)	(1864)	(368.8)	31.6	6.16	222	43.4	
Long Grain White Enriched Rice, Quick, 14-oz. package	1413	332.5	100.9	23.75	(352)	(81.2)	
Prepared as package directs:							
Without butter (yield: approx. 3 lb. 1 oz., 6.7 cups)	1413	332.5	(28.8)	(6.79)	(210)	(49.6)	
With butter (yield: approx. 3 lb 2 oz., 7.8 cups)	(1665)	(329.5)	33.3	6.59	(215)	(42.2)	
Long Grain & Wild Seasoned Rice, dry mix, fast cooking, 6-oz. package	601	127.4	100.1	21.24	(681)	(144.4)	
Prepared as package directs:							
Without butter (yield: approx. 1 lb. 7 oz., 3 cups)	601	127.4	26.2	5.56	194	41.2	
With butter (yield: approx. 1 lb. 7 oz., 3 cups)	(683)	(127.4)	29.7	5.41	226	41.2	
Pilaf Rice, dry mix, fast cooking, 6-oz. box	589	128.1	98.1	21.35	(667)	(145.2)	
Prepared as package directs:							
Without butter (yield: approx. 19 oz., or approx. 3 cups)	589	128.1	31.1	6.68	202	43.4	
With butter (yield: approx. 20 oz., or approx. 3 cups)	(790)	(128.1)	39.5	6.34	270	43.4	
Spanish Rice, dry mix, 5.5-oz. box	515	106.5	93.6	19.36	(636)	(131.6)	
Prepared as package directs:							
Without butter (yield: approx. 20 oz., or approx. 2½ cups)	515	106.5	25.9	5.39	212	44.0	
With butter (yield: approx. 20 oz., or 2.3 cups)	(600)	(106.5)	30.0	5.24	256	44.0	
Van Camp Spanish Rice, ready to serve, 8-oz. can	172	28.2	21.5	3.52	190	31.0	
15-oz. can	323	52.8	21.5	3.52	190	31.0	

RUTABAGAS

	UNIT Cal.	UNIT Carb.	1 OZ., BY WT. Cal.	1 OZ., BY WT. Carb.	1 CUP Cal.	1 CUP Carb.	Fiber per oz. (GMS.)
RAW:							
As purchased without tops [refuse: parings, approx. 15%]: 1 pound	177	42.4	11.1	2.65			
Edible portion:							
1 cup, cubed (approx. 4.9 oz.)	64	15.4	13.0	3.12	64	15.4	0.31
1 pound (approx. 3¼ cups (tr/3g/tr/87%/1mg)	208	49.9	13.0	3.12	64	15.4	0.31
COOKED:							
Steamed:							
1 pound of raw rutabagas, steamed (yield: approx. 14.9 oz.)	208	49.9	14.0	3.35			0.33
1 pound of steamed rutabagas	224	53.7	14.0	3.35			0.33
Boiled, drained:							
1 cup:							
Cubed or sliced (approx. 6.0 oz.)	60	13.9	9.9	2.33	60	13.9	(0.24)
Mashed (approx. 8.5 oz.)	84	19.7	9.9	2.33	84	19.7	(0.24)
1 pound (approx. 2.7 cups cubed or sliced, 1.9 cups mashed) (tr/2g/tr/90%/1mg)	159	37.2	9.9	2.33			(0.24)

SALSIFY (Oyster Plant)

Average of freshly harvested and stored:

	UNIT Cal.	UNIT Carb.	1 OZ., BY WT. Cal.	1 OZ., BY WT. Carb.	1 CUP Cal.	1 CUP Carb.	Fiber per oz. (GMS.)
RAW:							
As purchased:							
With tops [refuse: tops, scrapings, and rootlets, approx. 53%]: 1 pound	(77)	(38.4)	(4.8)	(2.40)			
Without tops [refuse: scrapings and rootlets, approx. 13%]:							
1 cup, diced (approx. 4.9 oz.)	(58)	(21.8)	(11.8)	(4.44)	(58)	(21.8)	
1 pound (approx. 3¼ cups diced)	(188)	(71.0)	(11.8)	(4.44)	(58)	(21.8)	
COOKED:							
Boiled, drained:							
1 cup (approx. 4¾ oz.)	(50)	(20.4)	(11.6)	(4.28)	(50)	(20.4)	(0.50)
1 pound (approx. 3⅓ cups) (1g/4g/tr/78%/na)	(186)	(68.5)	(11.6)	(4.28)	(50)	(20.4)	(0.50)

SAUERKRAUT, see under CABBAGE

SCALLIONS

YOUNG GREEN ONIONS (bunching varieties)

	UNIT Cal.	UNIT Carb.	1 OZ., BY WT. Cal.	1 OZ., BY WT. Carb.	1 CUP Cal.	1 CUP Carb.	Fiber per oz. (GMS.)
RAW:							
As purchased, when bulb and white portion of top are to be used [refuse: green tops and rootlets, approx. 9%]: 1 pound	76	17.6	4.7	1.10			
As purchased, when bulb and entire top are to be used [refuse: rootlets, approx. 4%]: 1 pound	157	35.7	9.8	2.23			
Edible portion:							
Bulb and entire top, 1 pound (tr/10g/tr/89%/1mg)	163	37.2	10.2	2.33			0.34
Bulb and white portion of top, 1 pound (tr/13g/tr/88%/1mg)	204	47.7	12.8	2.98			0.29
Tops only (green portion), 1 pound (tr/8g/tr/92%/1mg)	123	25.0	7.7	1.56			0.37

SEAWEED (based on data from East Asia and Japan)

	UNIT Cal.	UNIT Carb.	1 OZ., BY WT. Cal.	1 OZ., BY WT. Carb.	1 CUP Cal.	1 CUP Carb.	Fiber per oz. (GMS.)
RAW:							
Agar *(Gelidium spp.; Eucheuma spp.; Gracilarva spp.)*							
Dried, 1 pound	1416	378.7	88.5	23.67			1.13
Dried, soaked, drained, 1 pound	250	68.0	15.6	4.25			0.03
Green Laver							
Dried, 1 pound	(1504)	279.0	(94.0)	17.44			2.04
Purple Laver, (ordinary or superior quality)							
Dried, 1 pound	(1394)	179.7	(87.1)	11.23			1.33
Sea Lettuce							
Dried, 1 pound	(1221)	191.0	(76.3)	11.94			1.30
Seagirdle *(Laminaria spp.)*							
Edible portion, 1 pound	322	77.1	20.1	4.82			0.91
Dried, 1 pound	994	245.9	62.1	15.37			1.90
Dried, soaked, drained, 1 pound	163	38.1	10.2	2.38			
Dried, oiled, 1 pound	2445	119.8	152.8	7.49			2.41
Seahair *(Nastoc commune)*							
Dried, 1 pound	1179	265.6	73.7	16.60			0.57
Dried, soaked, drained, 1 pound	104	14.1	6.5	0.88			

SHELLIE BEANS

(Shellie beans are a combination of beans, approx. ¾ green beans and ¼ mature seeds, that is, pinto beans. The word SHELLIE originated from the description "shelled out.")

	UNIT Cal.	UNIT Carb.	1 OZ., BY WT. Cal.	1 OZ., BY WT. Carb.	1 CUP Cal.	1 CUP Carb.	Fiber per oz. (GMS.)
Stokely Shellie Beans, 8-oz. can	(65)	(13.9)	(8.1)	(1.74)	70	15.0	
16-oz. (1-lb.) can	(130)	(27.8)	(8.1)	(1.74)	70	15.0	
28-oz. can	(227)	(48.6)	(8.1)	(1.74)	70	15.0	

SNAP BEANS, see GREEN BEANS

SNOW PEAS

	UNIT Cal.	UNIT Carb.	1 OZ., BY WT. Cal.	1 OZ., BY WT. Carb.	1 CUP Cal.	1 CUP Carb.	Fiber per oz. (GMS.)
FROZEN, by brand:							
La Choy Pea Pods, 6-oz. package	90	20.4	15.0	3.41			
Drained solids (yield: approx. 5.6 oz.)	(90)	(20.4)	(16.1)	(3.64)	(97)	(21.9)	

SOYBEANS

MATURE SEEDS, Dry

	UNIT Cal.	UNIT Carb.	1 OZ., BY WT. Cal.	1 OZ., BY WT. Carb.	1 CUP Cal.	1 CUP Carb.	Fiber per oz. (GMS.)
RAW:							
1 cup (approx. 7.4 oz.)	846	70.3	114.3	9.50	846	70.4	1.39
1 pound (approx. 2.2 cups) (10g/10g/5g/10%/1mg)	1828	152.0	114.3	9.50	846	70.4	1.39
COOKED:							
Boiled, drained:							
1 cup (approx. 6.3 oz.)	234	19.4	36.9	3.06	234	19.4	0.45
1 pound (approx. 2.5 cups) (3g/3g/2g/71%/1mg)	590	49.0	36.9	3.06	234	19.4	0.45

	UNIT Cal.	UNIT Carb.	1 OZ., BY WT. Cal.	1 OZ., BY WT. Carb.	1 CUP Cal.	1 CUP Carb.	Fiber per oz. (GMS.)
SPROUTED SEEDS							
RAW:							
1 cup (approx. 3.7 oz.)	48	5.6	13.1	1.50	48	5.6	0.43
1 pound (approx. 4.4 cups) (2g/2g/tr/86%/na)	209	24.0	13.1	1.50	48	5.6	0.43
COOKED:							
Boiled, drained:							
1 cup (approx. 4.4 oz.)	48	4.6	10.8	1.05	48	4.6	(0.30)
1 pound (approx. 3.6 cups) (2g/1g/tr/89%/na)	172	16.8	10.8	1.05	48	4.6	(0.30)
IMMATURE SEEDS							
RAW:							
1 cup (approx. 5.5 oz.)	(209)	(20.6)	(38.0)	(3.74)	(209)	(20.6)	(0.40)
1 pound (approx. 2.9 cups) (3g/4g/1g/69%/na)	608	59.8	(38.0)	(3.74)	(209)	(20.6)	(0.40)
COOKED:							
Boiled, drained:							
1 cup (approx. 5.8 oz.)	194	16.6	33.5	2.86	194	16.6	(0.33)
1 pound (approx. 2.8 cups) (3g/3g/1g/74%/na)	536	45.8	33.5	2.86	194	16.6	(0.33)
CANNED or PACKAGED, by brand:							
Golden Harvest Whole Yellow Soy Beans, 32-oz. (2-lb.) package	3680	224.0	115.0	7.00	(702)	(42.7)	
Hollywood Health Foods, packed in water and sea salt Cooked Dried Green Soy Beans, 15-oz. can	448	20.0	29.9	1.33	(264)	(11.7)	
Soybean Products							
BEAN PASTE							
China Bowl Bean Paste, 2½ oz. can	112	6.6	44.8	2.68			
MISO							
1 cup (approx. 8.5 oz.)	(412)	(56.6)	48.5	6.66	(412)	(56.6)	0.65
1 pound (approx. 1.9 cups) (3g/4g/1g/53%/836mg)	776	106.6	48.5	6.66	(412)	(56.6)	0.65
NATTO							
1 cup (approx. 8.5 oz.)	(402)	(27.7)	47.3	3.26	(402)	(27.7)	0.91
1 pound (approx. 1.9 cups) (5g/3g/2g/63%/na)	758	52.2	47.3	3.26	(402)	(27.7)	0.91
OIL							
Arrowhead Mills Soybean Oil, 1-pint (16-fl.-oz.) bottle	3840	0.0	(250.0)	0.00	1920	0.0	0.00
TOFU (Soybean Curd)							
RAW:							
1 piece, 2½" × 2¾" × 1" (approx. 4.2 oz.)	86	2.9	20.4	0.68	(173)	(5.8)	0.03
1 pound (approx. 3.8 pieces, each 2½" × 2¾" × 1") (2g/1g/1g/85%/2mg)	327	10.9	20.4	0.68	(173)	(5.8)	0.03
Soy Dairy Tofu, 16-oz. (1-lb.) container	520	4.0	32.5	0.25	(276)	(2.1)	
1 portion (approx. 4 oz.)	130	1.0	32.5	0.25	(276)	(2.1)	
DRIED:							
China Bowl Dried Spicy Bean Curd, 2-oz. package	262	8.4	130.7	4.22			
Soybean Candies and Snacks							
El Molino Carob Coated Soy Beans, 4½-oz. package	653	54.0	145.0	12.00	(885)	(73.2)	
1-oz. package	145	12.0	145.0	12.00	(885)	(73.2)	
Golden Harvest Barbecue-Flavored Soy Beans, 12-oz. bag	1680	108.0	140.0	9.00	(854)	(54.9)	
Garlic-Flavored Soy Beans, 12-oz. bag	1680	108.0	140.0	9.00	(854)	(54.9)	
Onion-Flavored Soy Beans, 12-oz. bag	1680	108.0	140.0	9.00	(854)	(54.9)	
Toasted Soy Beans, Unsalted or With Sea Salt,							
¾-oz. bag	110	7.0	140.0	9.00	(854)	(54.9)	
2½-oz. bag	350	22.5	140.0	9.00	(854)	(54.9)	
12-oz. bag	1680	108.0	140.0	9.00	(854)	(54.9)	
SPINACH							
Mustard Spinach, New Zealand Spinach, and Vine Spinach are listed under M, N, and V, respectively.							

	UNIT Cal.	UNIT Carb.	1 OZ., BY WT. Cal.	1 OZ., BY WT. Carb.	1 CUP Cal.	1 CUP Carb.	Fiber per oz. (GMS.)
RAW:							
Untrimmed (bulk):							
As purchased:							
Good quality [refuse: large stems and roots, approx. 28%]: 1 pound	85	14.0	5.3	0.88			
Fair quality [refuse: stems, damaged leaves, and roots, approx. 39%]: 1 pound	72	11.9	4.5	0.74			
Trimmed (prepackaged):							
As purchased, fair quality [refuse: damaged leaves and trimmings, approx. 8%]:							
1 pound	109	17.9	6.8	1.12			
As purchased, good quality (all-edible):							
Container, 10 oz. net wt.	74	12.2	7.4	1.22			0.17
Container, 20 oz. net wt.	148	24.4	7.4	1.22			0.17
1 pound (1g/1g/tr/91%/20mg)	118	19.5	7.4	1.22			0.17
Chopped:							
1 cup (approx. 1.9 oz.)	14	2.4	7.4	1.22	14	2.4	
1 pound (approx. 8¼ cups) (1g/1g/tr/91%/20mg)	118	19.5	7.4	1.22	14	2.4	
COOKED:							
Boiled, drained:							
1 cup, leaves (approx. 6⅓ oz.)	41	6.5	6.5	1.02	41	6.5	(0.15)
1 pound (approx. 2½ cups) (1g/1g/tr/92%/14mg)	103	16.4	6.5	1.02	41	6.5	(0.15)
Steamed:							
1 pound of raw spinach, steamed (yield: approx. 14.9)	118	19.5	7.9	1.31			0.18
1 pound of steamed spinach	126	21.0	7.9	1.31			0.18
FROZEN, based on generic data:							
CHOPPED SPINACH							
Measured when frozen:							
1 pound	109	17.2	6.8	1.08			0.23
1 container, 10 oz. net wt.	68	10.8	6.8	1.08			0.23
Boiled, drained:							
1 cup (approx. 7.2 oz.)	47	7.6	6.5	1.05	47	7.6	0.23
1 pound of frozen spinach, boiled, then drained (yield: approx. 12.3 oz.)	81	13.0	6.5	1.05	47	7.6	0.23
1 pound boiled, drained spinach (1g/1g/tr/92%/15mg)	104	16.8	6.5	1.05	47	7.6	0.23
1 container, 10 oz., boiled, then drained (yield: approx. 7.8 oz.)	51	8.1	6.5	1.05	47	7.6	0.23
LEAF SPINACH							
Measured when frozen:							
1 pound	113	19.2	7.1	1.20			0.23
1 container, 10 oz. net wt.	71	11.9	7.1	1.20			0.23
Boiled, drained:							
1 cup (approx. 6.7 oz.)	46	7.4	6.8	1.11	46	7.4	0.23
1 pound of frozen spinach, boiled, drained (yield: approx. 12.3 oz.)	84	13.7	6.8	1.11	46	7.4	0.23
1 pound of boiled, drained spinach	109	17.8	6.8	1.11	46	7.4	0.23
1 container, 10 oz., boiled, drained (yield: approx. 7.8 oz.)	53	8.6	6.8	1.11	46	7.4	0.23
FROZEN, by brand:							
Birds Eye Chopped Spinach, 10-oz. package	60	9.0	6.1	0.91			
Boiled, drained (yield: approx. 6.6 oz.)	(60)	(9.0)	(9.1)	(1.36)	(59)	(8.9)	
Creamed Spinach, 9-oz. package	180	18.0	20.0	2.00	(180)	(18.0)	
Leaf Spinach, 10-oz. package	60	9.0	6.1	0.91			
Boiled, drained (yield: approx. 6.7 oz.)	(60)	(9.0)	(9.0)	(1.34)	(59)	(8.7)	
Green Giant Creamed Spinach, 10-oz. package	210	23.6	21.0	2.36	190	21.0	
Spinach in Butter Sauce, 10-oz. boil-in-bag	125	7.1	12.5	0.71	90	6.0	
Spinach Soufflé, 10-oz. package	329	24.7	32.9	2.47	300	27.0	
Seabrook Farms Chopped Spinach, 10-oz. package	75	9.0	7.5	0.90			
Boiled, drained (yield: approx. 6.6 oz.)	(75)	(9.0)	(11.4)	(1.36)	(74)	(8.8)	
Cut Spinach, 10-oz. package	75	9.0	7.5	0.90			
Boiled, drained (yield: approx. 6.6 oz.)	(75)	(9.0)	(11.4)	(1.36)			

	UNIT Cal.	UNIT Carb.	1 OZ., BY WT. Cal.	1 OZ., BY WT. Carb.	1 CUP Cal.	1 CUP Carb.	Fiber per oz. (GMS.)
Whole Leaf Spinach, 10-oz. package	75	9.0	7.5	0.90			
Boiled, drained (yield: approx. 6.7 oz.)	(75)	(9.0)	(11.2)	(1.34)	(73)	(8.7)	
Stouffer's Creamed Spinach, 9-oz. package	380	18.0	42.2	2.00			
Spinach Soufflé, 8-oz. package	270	24.0	33.8	3.00	(308)	(27.4)	
12-oz. package	405	36.0	33.8	3.00			
CANNED (whole leaf, cut leaf or sliced, chopped), based on generic data:							
Regular pack:							
Solids and liquid:							
1 cup (approx. 8 oz.)	44	7.0	5.4	0.85	44	7.0	0.20
1 pound (approx. 2 cups) ((1g/1g/tr/93%/67mg)	86	13.6	5.4	0.85	44	7.0	0.20
1 #303 can, 15 oz. net wt. (approx. 1.8 cups)	81	12.8	5.4	0.85	44	7.0	0.20
Drained solids:							
1 cup (approx. 7.2 oz.)	49	7.4	6.8	1.02	49	7.4	0.26
1 pound (approx. 1.4 cups) (1g/1g/tr/91%/67mg)	109	16.3	6.8	1.02	49	7.4	0.26
1 #303 can (yield: 10¼ oz. drained spinach)	70	10.5	6.8	1.02	49	7.4	0.26
Drained liquid:							
1 cup (approx. 8.3 oz.)	(19)	(4.0)	(2.3)	(0.48)	(19)	(4.0)	trace
1 pound (approx. 1.9 cups) (tr/tr/tr/96%/67mg)	(37)	(7.7)	(2.3)	(0.48)	(19)	(4.0)	trace
Low-sodium pack:							
Solids and liquid:							
1 cup (approx. 8 oz.)	49	7.7	5.9	0.94	49	7.7	0.20
1 pound (approx. 2 cups) (1g/1g/tr/93%/17mg)	95	15.0	5.9	0.94	49	7.7	0.20
1 #303 can, 15 oz. net wt. (approx. 1.8 cups)	89	14.0	5.9	0.94	49	7.7	0.20
Drained solids:							
1 cup (approx. 7.2 oz.)	53	8.2	7.4	1.13	53	8.2	0.26
1 pound (approx. 2.2 cups) (1g/1g/tr/91%/16mg)	118	18.1	7.4	1.13	53	8.2	0.26
1 #303 can (yield approx. 10¼ oz. drained spinach)	76	11.6	7.4	1.13	53	8.2	0.26
Drained liquid:							
1 cup (approx. 8.3 oz.)	(23)	(4.2)	(2.7)	(0.51)	(23)	(4.2)	trace
1 pound (approx. 1.9 cups) (tr/1g/tr/97%/16mg)	(44)	(8.2)	(2.7)	(0.51)	(23)	(4.2)	trace
CANNED, by brand:							
Ann Page (A&P) Young Tender Spinach, 7½-oz. can	50	8.0	6.7	1.07	50	8.0	
Drained solids (yield: approx. 4.7 oz.)	(44)	(6.9)	(9.4)	(1.47)	(74)	(11.6)	
15-oz. can	100	16.0	6.7	1.07	50	8.0	
Drained solids (yield: approx. 10 oz.)	(90)	(14.0)	(9.0)	(1.40)	(71)	(11.1)	
Balanced Foods Spinach packed in water, without added sugar or salt, 8-oz. can	46	5.4	5.7	0.68	(47)	(5.6)	
Drained solids (yield: approx. 5.5 oz.)	(41)	(4.4)	(7.5)	(0.82)	(54)	(5.9)	
Cellu Spinach Puree, low sodium, 16½-oz. can	90	14.0	5.5	0.85	45	7.0	
Del Monte Spinach, 7¾-oz. can	45	7.0	5.8	0.90	45	7.0	
Drained solids (yield: approx. 5 oz.)	(40)	(6.9)	(7.7)	(1.15)	(61)	(9.0)	
15-oz. can	87	13.5	5.8	0.90	45	7.0	
Drained solids (yield: approx. 10 oz.)	(77)	(11.5)	(7.7)	(1.15)	(61)	(9.0)	
Featherweight Spinach, 7¾-oz. can, no added salt or sugar,	(60)	(8.0)	(8.0)	(1.07)	60	8.0	
Drained solids (yield: approx. 5.1 oz.)	(55)	(6.5)	(10.5)	(1.24)	(85)	(10.1)	
15-oz. can	(120)	(16.0)	(8.0)	(1.07)	60	8.0	
Drained solids (yield: approx. 10.2 oz.)	(108)	(12.8)	(10.5)	(1.24)	(85)	(10.1)	
Libby's Spinach, 7¾-oz. can	(44)	(6.9)	(5.7)	(0.89)	45	7.0	
Drained solids (yield: approx. 5.3 oz.)	(39)	(5.9)	(7.4)	(1.12)	(58)	(8.8)	
15-oz. can	(86)	(13.4)	(5.7)	(0.89)	45	7.0	
Drained solids (yield: approx. 10.2 oz.)	(76)	(11.5)	(7.4)	(1.12)	(58)	(8.8)	
S&W Early Spring Whole Leaf Spinach, 7¾-oz. can	45	8.0	5.8	1.03	45	8.0	
Drained solids (yield: approx. 5.3 oz.)	(40)	(7.0)	(7.5)	(1.32)	(60)	(10.4)	
15-oz. can	87	15.5	5.8	1.03	45	8.0	
Drained solids (yield: approx. 10.3 oz.)	(78)	(13.6)	(7.6)	(1.32)	(60)	(10.4)	
JARRED, by brand:							
Featherweight Spinach Puree, low sodium, 16½-oz. jar	90	14.0	(5.5)	(0.85)	45	7.0	
SPOON CABBAGE, see under CABBAGE							
SQUASH (also see ZUCCHINI)							
ACORN SQUASH							
RAW:							
As purchased:							
1 medium acorn squash approx. 4″ diameter, 4⅓″ high, 1 lb. 4 oz.) [refuse: cavity contents and rind, 24%]	190	48.3	9.5	2.42			
1 pound	152	38.7	9.5	2.42			
Halved							
1 half of a medium acorn squash, cavity contents removed (approx. 8.6 oz.) [refuse: rind, approx. 10%]	97	24.6	11.3	2.86			
1 pound	180	45.7	11.3	2.86			
Edible portion:							
1 medium acorn squash (approx. 15.2 oz.)	190	48.3	12.5	3.18			0.40
1 pound (tr/3g/tr/8%/tr)	200	50.8	12.5	3.18			0.40
COOKED:							
Baked:							
1 cup mashed (approx. 7.2 oz.)	113	28.7	15.6	3.98	113	28.7	0.51
1 pound (approx. 2.2 cups mashed) (1g/4g/tr/83%/tr)	249	63.5	15.6	3.97	113	28.7	0.51
Boiled:							
1 cup, mashed (approx. 8.6 oz.)	83	20.6	9.6	2.39	83	20.6	(0.34)
1 pound (approx. 1.9 cups mashed) (tr/2g/tr/90%/tr)	154	38.1	9.6	2.39	83	20.6	(0.34)
Steamed:							
1 pound of acorn squash, steamed raw (yield: approx. 14.2 oz.)	172	41.7	12.1	2.94			0.45
1 pound of steamed acorn squash	194	47.0	12.1	2.94			0.45
BUTTERNUT SQUASH							
RAW:							
As purchased:							
1 medium butternut squash (approx. 2 lb. 4 oz.)	385	99.9	10.7	2.78			
1 pound [refuse: cavity contents, rind, and stem ends, approx. 30%]	171	44.4	10.7	2.78			
Edible portion:							
1 medium butternut squash (approx. 1 lb. 9 oz.)	385	99.9	15.3	3.96			0.40
1 pound (tr/4g/tr/84%/tr)	244	63.4	15.3	3.96			0.40
COOKED:							
Baked:							
1 cup, mashed (approx. 7.2 oz.)	139	35.9	19.2	4.97	139	35.9	0.51
1 pound (approx. 2.2 cups mashed) (1g/5g/tr/80%/tr)	308	79.5	19.2	4.97	139	35.9	0.51
Boiled:							
1 cup, mashed (approx. 8.6 oz.)	100	25.5	11.6	2.95	100	25.5	(0.30)
1 pound (approx. 1.9 cups mashed) (tr/3g/tr/88%/tr)	185	47.3	11.6	2.95	100	25.5	(0.30)
Steamed:							
1 pound of raw butternut squash, steamed (yield: approx. 14.2 oz.)	244	63.4	17.1	4.45			0.45
1 pound of steamed butternut squash	274	71.2	17.1	4.45			0.45
CROOKNECK AND STRAIGHT SQUASH							
RAW:							
As purchased:							
Good quality [refuse: stem ends, approx. 3%]:							
1 pound	88	18.8	5.5	1.18			
Fair quality [refuse: stem ends and blemishes, approx. 13%]:							
1 pound	79	17.0	4.9	1.06			
Edible portion:							
1 cup, sliced, cubed, or diced (approx. 4.6 oz.)	26	5.6	5.7	1.22	26	5.6	0.17
1 pound (approx. 3½ cups) (tr/1g/tr/94%/tr)	91	19.5	5.7	1.22	26	5.6	0.17

	UNIT		1 OZ., BY WT.		1 CUP		Fiber per oz. (GMS.)
	Cal.	Carb.	Cal.	Carb.	Cal.	Carb.	
COOKED:							
Boiled, drained:							
1 cup:							
Sliced (approx. 6.3 oz.)	27	5.6	4.3	0.88	27	5.6	0.17
Cubed or diced (approx. 7.4 oz.)	32	6.5	4.3	0.88	32	6.5	0.17
Mashed (approx. 8.5 oz.)	36	7.4	4.3	0.88	36	7.4	0.17
1 pound (approx. 2–2½ cups) (tr/1g/tr/95%/tr)	68	14.1	4.3	0.88			0.17
HUBBARD SQUASH							
RAW:							
As purchased:							
1 pound [refuse: cavity contents, rind, and stem ends, approx. 34%]	117	28.1	7.3	1.76			
Edible porion:							
1 pound (tr/3g/tr/88%/tr)	177	42.6	11.1	2.66			0.40
COOKED:							
Baked:							
1 cup, mashed (approx. 7.2 oz.)	103	24.0	14.3	3.32	103	24.0	0.51
1 pound (approx. 2.2 cups mashed) (1g/3g/tr/85%/tr)	228	53.2	14.3	3.32	103	24.0	0.51
Boiled, drained:							
1 cup, cubed or diced (approx. 8.3 oz.)	71	16.2	8.6	1.96	71	16.2	(0.31)
1 cup, mashed (approx. 8.6 oz.)	74	16.9	8.6	1.96	74	16.9	(0.31)
1 pound (approx. 1.9 cups) (tr/2g/tr/91%/tr)	137	31.3	8.6	1.96	71	16.2	(0.31)
SCALLOP VARIETIES, White and Pale Green							
RAW:							
As purchased:							
Good quality [refuse: stem ends, approx. 2%]:							
1 pound	95	23.1	5.9	1.44			
Fair quality [refuse: stem ends and blemishes, approx. 12%]:							
1 pound	80	17.2	5.0	1.08			
Edible portion:							
1 cup, sliced, cubed, or diced (approx. 4.6 oz.)	27	6.6	5.9	1.44	27	6.6	0.17
1 pound (approx. 3½ cups) (tr/1g/tr/93%/tr)	95	23.1	5.9	1.44	27	6.6	0.17
COOKED:							
Boiled, drained:							
1 cup:							
Sliced (approx. 6.3 oz.)	29	6.8	4.6	1.08	29	6.8	(0.13)
Cubed or diced (approx. 7.4 oz.)	34	8.0	4.6	1.08	34	8.0	(0.13)
Mashed (approx. 8.5 oz.)	38	9.1	4.6	1.08	38	9.1	(0.13)
1 pound (approx. 2–2½ cups) (tr/1g/tr/95%/tr)	73	17.2	4.6	1.08			(0.13)
SUMMER SQUASH, average of all varieties							
RAW:							
As purchased:							
Good quality [refuse: stem ends, approx. 30%]:							
1 pound	84	18.5	5.3	1.16			
Fair quality [refuse: stem ends and blemishes, approx. 12%]:							
1 pound	75	16.6	4.7	1.04			
Edible portion:							
1 cup, sliced, cubed, or diced (approx. 4.6 oz.)	25	5.5	5.4	1.19	25	5.5	0.17
1 pound (approx. 3½ cups) (tr/1g/tr/94%/tr)	86	19.1	5.4	1.19	25	5.5	0.17
COOKED:							
Boiled, drained:							
1 cup:							
Sliced (approx. 6.3 oz.)	25	5.6	4.0	0.88	25	5.6	(0.13)
Cubed or diced (approx. 7.4 oz.)	29	6.5	4.0	0.88	25	5.6	(0.13)
Mashed (approx. 8.5 oz.)	34	7.4	4.0	0.88	25	5.6	(0.13)
1 pound (approx. 2–2½ cups) (tr/1g/tr/96%/tr)	64	14.1	4.0	0.88			0.17
Steamed:							
1 pound of raw summer squash, steamed (yield: approx. 14.1 oz.)	86	19.1	6.1	1.35			0.18
1 pound of steamed summer squash	98	21.7	6.1	1.35			0.18

	UNIT		1 OZ., BY WT.		1 CUP		Fiber per oz. (GMS.)
	Cal.	Carb.	Cal.	Carb.	Cal.	Carb.	
WINTER SQUASH							
RAW:							
As purchased:							
1 squash (approx. 20 oz.) [refuse: cavity contents, rind, and stem ends, approx. 29%]	(154)	(37.0)	(7.7)	(1.85)			
1 pound (approx. 0.8 squash)	(123)	(29.6)	(7.7)	(1.85)			
Edible portion:							
1 pound (tr/3g/tr/85%/tr)	(172)	(41.7)	(10.8)	(2.61)			0.40
COOKED:							
Baked:							
1 cup, mashed (approx. 7.2 oz.)	129	31.6	127.9	4.39	129	31.6	0.57
1 pound (approx. 2.2 cups mashed) (1g/4g/tr/81%/tr)	286	69.9	17.9	4.37	129	31.6	0.57
Boiled, drained:							
1 cup, mashed (approx. 8.6 oz.)	93	22.5	10.8	2.61	93	22.5	0.40
1 pound (approx. 1.9 cups mashed) (tr/3g/tr/89%/tr)	172	41.7	10.8	2.61	93	22.5	0.40
FROZEN, based on generic data:							
Summer Squash, Yellow Crookneck							
1 pound, measured, when frozen:	95	21.3	5.9	1.33	(36)	(8.2)	0.17
1 pound, boiled, drained (tr/1g/tr/93%/47mg)	95	21.3	5.9	1.33	(37)	(8.4)	0.17
Winter Squash							
Measured when frozen:							
1 pound	172	41.7	10.8	2.61			0.34
1 container, 12 oz. net wt.	129	31.3	10.8	2.61			0.34
Boiled, drained:							
1 cup (approx. 8.5 oz.)	91	22.1	10.8	2.61	91	22.1	0.34
1 pound (approx. 1.9 cups) (tr/3g/tr/89%/59mg)	172	41.7	10.8	2.61	91	22.1	0.34
FROZEN, by brand:							
Birds Eye Cooked Squash, 12-oz. package	150	33.0	12.5	2.75			
Boiled, drained (yield: approx. 9.1 oz.)	(150)	(33.0)	(16.5)	(3.63)	(140)	(30.7)	
Sliced Summer Squash, 10-oz. package	54	9.0	5.5	0.91			
Boiled, drained (yield: approx. 7.8 oz.)	(54)	(5.0)	(6.9)	(1.15)	(58)	(9.7)	
Bel-Air Cooked Squash, 14-oz. package	160	40.0	11.4	2.86			
Boiled, drained (yield: approx. 13.2 oz.)	160	40.0	12.2	3.04			
Green Giant Summer Squash in Cheese Sauce, 10-oz. boil-in-bag	122	15.3	12.2	1.53	120	16.0	
Safeway Frozen Cooked Squash, 14-oz. package	160	40.0	11.4	2.86			
Boiled, drained (yield: approx. 13.2 oz.)	(160)	(40.0)	(12.2)	(3.04)			
Seabrook Farms Yellow Crookneck Squash, 10-oz. package	60	12.0	6.0	1.20			
Boiled, drained (yield: approx. 7.8 oz.)	(60)	(12.0)	(7.7)	(1.54)	(65)	(13.0)	
Village Park Sliced Yellow Squash, 16-oz. (1-lb.) package	100	20.0	6.3	1.25			
Boiled, drained (yield: approx. 12.5 oz.)	(100)	(20.0)	(8.0)	(1.60)	(67)	(13.5)	
CANNED, by brand:							
Cellu Squash Puree, low sodium, 16-oz. (1-lb.) can	(200)	(38.0)	(12.5)	(2.38)	100	19.0	
JARRED, by brand:							
Featherweight Squash Puree, low sodium, 16-oz. (1-lb.) jar	(200)	(38.0)	(12.5)	(2.38)	100	19.0	

STRING BEANS, see GREEN BEANS

SUCCOTASH (a mixture of corn and lima beans)

	UNIT		1 OZ., BY WT.		1 CUP		Fiber per oz. (GMS.)
	Cal.	Carb.	Cal.	Carb.	Cal.	Carb.	
FROZEN, based on generic data:							
Measured when frozen:							
1 cup (approx. 5.5 oz.)	150	33.3	27.5	6.09	150	33.3	0.26
1 pound (approx. 2.9 cups)	440	97.5	27.5	6.09	150	33.3	0.26
1 container, 10 oz. net wt. (approx. 1.8 cups)	275	61.1	27.5	6.09	150	33.3	0.26
Boiled, drained:							
1 cup (approx. 6 oz.)	158	34.9	26.4	5.81	158	34.9	0.26
1 pound boiled, drained (approx. 2.7 cups) (1g/6g/tr/74%/70mg)	422	93.0	26.4	5.81	158	34.9	0.26

	UNIT Cal.	UNIT Carb.	1 OZ., BY WT. Cal.	1 OZ., BY WT. Carb.	1 CUP Cal.	1 CUP Carb.	Fiber per oz. (GMS.)
FROZEN, by brand:							
Birds Eye Succotash, 10-oz. package	240	51.0	24.0	5.10			
Boiled, drained (yield: approx. 10 oz.)	(240)	(51.0)	(24.0)	(5.10)	(163)	(34.7)	
Blue Boy Cream Style Succotash, 8.5-oz. package	236	45.3	27.8	5.33	250	48.0	
Hanover Succotash, 16 oz. (1 lb.)	501	100.0	31.3	6.25			
Boiled, drained (yield: approx. 16 oz.)	(501)	(100.0)	(31.3)	(6.25)	(213)	(42.5)	
CANNED, by brand:							
Libby's Cream Style Succotash, 8¾-oz. can	(217)	(51.5)	(24.8)	(5.88)	190	45.0	
Whole Kernel Succotash, 16-oz. (1-lb.) can	(256)	(59.8)	(16.0)	(3.74)	150	35.0	
Drained solids (yield: approx. 11 oz.)	(224)	(52.3)	(20.4)	(4.75)	(123)	(28.6)	
Stokely Succotash, 17-oz. can	321	66.1	18.9	3.89	170	35.0	
Drained solids (yield: approx. 11.7 oz.)	(289)	(57.6)	(24.7)	(4.92)	(149)	(29.7)	

SUNCHOKES, see JERUSALEM ARTICHOKES

SWAMP CABBAGE

	UNIT Cal.	UNIT Carb.	1 OZ., BY WT. Cal.	1 OZ., BY WT. Carb.	1 CUP Cal.	1 CUP Carb.	Fiber per oz. (GMS.)
RAW:							
As purchased [refuse: inedible stems, and trimmings, approx. 19%]:							
1 pound	132	24.5	8.2	1.53			
Edible portion:							
1 pound (1g/1g/tr/90%/na)	132	24.5	8.2	1.53			0.31
COOKED:							
Boiled, drained:							
1 pound	95	17.7	5.9	1.11			0.26
Steamed:							
1 pound of raw swamp cabbage, steamed (yield: approx. 15.8 oz.)	132	24.5	8.3	1.55			0.31
1 pound of steamed swamp cabbage	133	24.8	8.3	1.55			0.31

SWEET POTATOES (see also YAMS)

	UNIT Cal.	UNIT Carb.	1 OZ., BY WT. Cal.	1 OZ., BY WT. Carb.	1 CUP Cal.	1 CUP Carb.	Fiber per oz. (GMS.)
FIRM FLESHED (Jersey types)							
RAW:							
As purchased [refuse: parings and trimmings. When pared by mechanical means, approx. 28%]:							
1 medium sweet potato (approx. 5″ long, 2″ diameter, 6.3 oz.)	148	34.1	23.3	5.36			
1 pound (approx. 2½ sweet medium potatoes)	372	85.9	23.3	5.36			
As purchased [refuse: parings, and trimmings. When pared with a split-knife peeler, approx. 10%]:							
1 medium sweet potato (approx. 5″ long, 2″ diameter, 6.3 oz.)	185	42.6	29.1	6.71			
1 pound (approx. 2½ medium sweet potatoes)	465	107.4	29.1	6.71			
Pared:							
1 medium sweet potato, pared by mechanical means (approx. 4.5 oz.)	148	34.1	33.2	7.74			
1 medium sweet potato, pared with split-knife peeler (approx. 5.6 oz.)	185	42.6	33.2	7.74			0.26
1 pound (approx. 2.8 medium sweet potatoes) (tr/8g/tr/74%/3mg)	531	123.8	33.2	7.74			0.26
SOFT FLESHED (mainly Puerto Rican variety)							
RAW:							
As purchased [refuse: parings and trimmings. When pared by mechanical means, approx. 28%]:							
1 medium sweet potato (approx. 5″ long, 2″ diameter, 6.3 oz.)	152	35.4	23.9	5.58			
1 pound (approx. 2½ medium sweet potatoes)	382	89.2	23.9	5.58			
As purchased [refuse: parings and trimmings. When pared with a split-knife peeler, approx. 10%]:							
1 medium sweet potato (approx. 5″ long, 2″ diameter, 6.3 oz.)	190	44.2	29.9	6.96			
1 pound (approx. 2½ medium sweet potatoes)	478	111.4	29.9	6.96			
Pared:							
1 medium sweet potato, pared by mechanical means (approx. 4.6 oz.)	152	35.4	33.2	7.74			
1 medium sweet potato, pared with split-knife peeler (approx. 5.7 oz.)	190	44.2	33.2	7.74			0.20
1 pound (approx. 2.8 medium sweet potatoes) (tr/8g/tr/70%/3mg)	531	123.8	33.2	7.74			0.20
ALL COMMERCIAL VARIETIES							
RAW:							
As purchased [refuse: parings and trimmings. When pared by mechanical means, approx. 28%]:							
1 medium sweet potato (approx. 5″ long, 2″ diameter, 6.3 oz.)	148	34.1	23.3	5.36			
1 pound (approx. 2½ medium sweet potatoes)	372	85.9	23.3	5.36			
As purchased [refuse: parings and trimmings. When pared with a split-knife peeler, approx. 28%]:							
1 medium sweet potato (approx. 5″ long, 2″ diameter, 6.3 oz.)	185	42.6	29.1	6.71			
1 pound (approx. 2½ medium sweet potatoes)	465	107.4	29.1	6.71			
Pared:							
1 medium sweet potato, pared by mechanical means (approx. 4.5 oz.)	185	42.6	33.2	7.74			
1 medium sweet potato, pared by split-knife peeler (approx. 5.7 oz.)	185	42.6	33.2	7.74			0.20
1 pound (approx. 2.8 medium sweet potatoes) (tr/8g/tr/71%/3mg)	531	123.8	33.2	7.74			0.20
COOKED:							
Baked in skin [refuse: skin, approx. 22%]:							
1 medium sweet potato (approx. 5″ long, 2″ diameter, 5.1 oz. before baking)	161	37.0	31.2	7.19			0.26
1 pound weighed in skins but eaten without skins (approx. 3.1 medium sweet potatoes)	499	115.0	31.2	7.19			0.26
1 pound weighed without skins (approx. 4 medium sweet potatoes) (tr/9g/tr/64%/3mg)	640	147.4	40.0	9.21			(0.31)
Boiled in skin [refuse: skins, approx. 16%]:							
1 medium sweet potato (approx. 5″ long, 2″ diameter, 6.3 oz. before cooking)	172	39.8	27.1	6.27			0.20
1 pound weighed in skins but eaten without skins (approx. 2½ medium sweet potatoes)	433	100.4	27.1	6.27			0.20
1 pound weighed without skins (approx. 3 medium sweet potatoes) (tr/7g/tr/71%/3mg)	517	119.3	32.3	7.45			0.20
Mashed:							
1 cup (approx. 9 oz.)	291	67.1	32.3	7.45	291	67.1	0.20
1 pound (approx. 1.8 cups) (tr/7g/tr/71%/3mg)	517	119.2	32.3	7.45	291	67.1	0.20
Candied:							
1 piece, 2½″ long, 2″ diameter before cooking:							
From sweet potato peeled mechanically, approx. 3 oz.	143	29.1	47.6	9.69			0.17
From sweet potato peeled with a split-knife peeler, approx. 3.7 oz.	176	35.9	47.6	9.69			0.17
1 pound (tr/10g/tr/60%/12mg)	762	155.1	47.6	9.69			0.17
Steamed in skin [refuse: skin, approx. 22%]:							
1 pound of raw sweet potatoes, steamed (yield: approx. 15.7 oz.)	465	107.4	29.6	6.84			
1 pound of steamed sweet potatoes weighed without skins	541	126.0	33.8	7.89			0.26
FROZEN, by brand:							
Green Giant Glazed Sweet Potatoes, 10-oz. package	363	68.7	36.3	6.87	340	65.0	
Mrs. Paul's Candied Sweet 'N' Apples Sweet Potatoes, 12-oz. package	480	111.0	40.0	9.25			
Candied Sweet Potatoes-Orange, 12-oz. package	540	132.0	45.0	11.00			
Family, 20-oz. package	900	220.0	45.0	11.00			
Candied Sweet Potatoes-Yellow, 12-oz. package	540	132.0	45.0	11.00			
Family, 20-oz. package	900	220.0	45.0	11.00			
CANNED, by brand:							
A&P Whole & Pieces Sweet Potatoes, vacuum packed, 18-oz. can	518	126.0	28.8	7.00	230	56.0	
Drained solids (yield: approx. 16.2 oz.)	(505)	(122.4)	(31.2)	(7.56)	(262)	(63.5)	

	UNIT Cal.	UNIT Carb.	1 OZ., BY WT. Cal.	1 OZ., BY WT. Carb.	1 CUP Cal.	1 CUP Carb.	Fiber per oz. (GMS.)
DEHYDRATED (Flakes), by brand:							
Dry:							
1 cup (approx. 4.2 oz.)	455	108.0	107.6	25.54	455	108.0	0.91
1 pound (approx. 3.8 cups) (1g/26g/tr/3%/51mg)	1721	408.6	107.6	25.54	455	108.0	0.91
Prepared with water:							
1 cup (approx. 9 oz.) (tr/6g/tr/76%/13mg)	242	57.6	26.9	6.41	242	57.6	0.23
SWISS CHARD, see CHARD							
TABOULEH, see under WHEAT							
TAROS							
Corms and Tubers							
RAW:							
As purchased [refuse: skin, approx. 16%]:							
1 pound	445	107.6	27.8	6.70			
Edible portion:							
1 pound (1g/7g/tr/73%/2mg)	373	107.0	23.3	6.69			0.23
Leaves and Stems							
RAW:							
All-edible:							
1 pound (1g/2g/tr/87%/na)	182	33.6	11.4	2.10			1.02
COOKED:							
Steamed:							
1 pound of raw taros, steamed (yield: approx. 1 lb.)	182	33.6	11.4	2.10			1.02
1 pound of steamed taros	182	33.6	11.4	2.10			1.02
TENDERGREEN, see MUSTARD SPINACH							
TIGER LILY BUDS							
China Bowl Tiger Lily Buds, dried, 1½-oz. package	(134)	(30.9)	(89.3)	(20.56)			
TOMATOES							
GREEN							
RAW:							
As purchased [refuse: cores and stem ends, approx. 9%]:							
1 pound	99	21.1	6.2	1.32			
Edible portion:							
1 pound (tr/1g/tr/93%/1mg)	109	23.1	6.8	1.45			0.14
RIPE							
Eaten with peel:							
Prepackaged:							
1 package, declared net weight 12 oz. (weight is actually approx. 14 oz.):							
As purchased: [refuse: core and stem ends, approx. 9%]:							
Three-tomato pack (each tomato approx. 2¾" diameter, 4¾ oz.)	80	17.1	5.7	1.22			
Edible portion:							
1 tomato (from three-tomato package, approx. 4⅓ oz.)	27	5.8	6.2	1.33			0.14
1 pound (approx. 3.7 tomatoes) (tr/1g/tr/94%/1mg)	99	21.3	6.2	1.33			0.14
As purchased [refuse: cores and stem ends, approx. 9%]:							
Bulk:							
1 medium tomato (approx. 3" diameter, 2⅛" high, 7 oz.)	40	8.6	5.7	1.22			
1 pound (approx. 2.3 medium tomatoes)	91	19.5	5.7	1.22			
Eaten without peel:							
Prepackaged:							
1 package, declared net weight 12 oz. (weight is actually approx. 14 oz):							
As purchased [refuse: skins, cores, stem ends, and trimmings, approx. 12%]							
Three-tomato pack (each tomato approx. 2¾" diameter, 4¾ oz.)	77	16.5	5.5	1.18			
Edible portion:							
1 tomato (from three-tomato package), approx. 4.1 oz.	26	5.6	6.3	1.36			0.14
1 pound (approx. 3.9 peeled tomatoes)	101	21.8	6.3	1.36			0.14
As purchased [refuse: skins, cores, stem ends, and trimmings, approx. 12%]:							
Bulk:							
1 medium tomato (approx. 3" diameter, 2⅛" high, 7 oz.)	39	8.3	5.5	1.18			
1 pound (approx. 2.3 medium tomatoes)	89	18.8	5.5	1.18			
COOKED:							
Boiled, drained:							
1 cup (approx. 8.5 oz.)	63	13.3	7.4	1.57	63	13.3	0.17
1 pound (approx. 1.9 cups) (tr/2g/tr/92%/1mg)	119	25.1	7.4	1.57	63	13.3	0.17
CANNED, based on generic data:							
Regular pack:							
Solids and liquids:							
1 cup (approx. 8.5 oz.)	51	10.4	5.9	1.22	51	10.4	0.06
1 pound (approx. 1.9 cups) (tr/1g/tr/94%/37mg)	95	19.5	5.9	1.22	51	10.4	0.06
1 #303 can, 16 oz. (1 lb.) net wt. (approx. 1.9 cups)	95	19.5	5.9	1.22	51	10.4	0.06
Low-sodium pack:							
Solids and liquid:							
1 cup (approx. 8.5 oz.)	48	10.1	5.7	1.19	48	10.1	0.06
1 pound (approx. 1.9 cups) (tr/1g/tr/94%/1mg)	91	19.1	5.7	1.19	48	10.1	0.06
1 #303 can, 16 oz. (1 lb.) net wt. (approx. 1.9 cups)	91	19.1	5.7	1.19	48	10.1	0.06
CANNED or JARRED, by brand:							
A&P Tomatoes, 16-oz. (1-lb.) can	100	22.0	6.3	1.38	50	11.0	
Drained solids (yield: approx. 9.6 oz.)	(62)	(15.6)	(6.5)	(1.63)			
28-oz. can	175	38.5	6.3	1.38	50	11.0	
Drained solids (yield: approx. 6.8 oz.)	(109)	(27.4)	(6.5)	(1.63)			
Ann Page (A&P) Stewed Tomatoes, 16-oz. (1-lb.) can	140	36.0	8.8	2.25	70	18.0	
Tomato Paste, 12-oz. can	240	51.0	20.0	4.25			
Balanced Tomatoes, packed in water without added sugar or salt, 8-oz. can	46	8.0	5.7	1.00	(48)	(8.4)	
Drained solids (yield: approx. 4.8 oz.)	(27)	(4.8)	(5.6)	(1.00)			
16-oz. (1-lb.) can	91	16.0	5.7	1.00	(48)	(8.4)	
Drained solids (yield: approx. 9.6 oz.)	(54)	(9.6)	(5.6)	(1.00)			
Tomato Paste, Dietetic, 6-oz. can	150	35.0	25.0	5.83	225	52.5	
Cellu Tomato Purée, low sodium, 19-oz. jar	(160)	(40.0)	(8.4)	(2.11)	80	20.0	
Claussen Tomatoes, Sour Green Kosher, 32-oz. (2-lb.) jar	(172)	(33.6)	(5.4)	(1.05)	(43)	(8.4)	
Drained solids (yield: approx. 18.5 oz.)	(92)	(25.5)	(4.9)	(1.38)			
Contadina Round and Pear Tomatoes, 14½-oz. can	86	18.8	5.9	1.29	50	11.0	
Drained solids (yield: approx. 9.6 oz.)	(58)	(13.9)	(6.0)	(1.45)			
Sliced Baby Tomatoes, 14½-oz. can	145	30.9	10.0	2.13	80	17.0	
Drained solids (yield: approx. 9.6 oz.)	(117)	(26.0)	(12.2)	(2.71)			
Stewed Tomatoes, 14½-oz. can	122	31.2	8.4	2.15	70	18.0	
Tomato Paste, 6-oz. can	150	35.0	25.0	5.83	200	46.7	
Tomato Paste, Heavy, 15-oz. can	204	45.9	13.6	3.06	120	27.0	
Del Monte Stewed Tomatoes, 16-oz. (1-lb.) can	140	32.0	8.8	2.00	70	16.0	
8-oz. can	70	16.0	8.8	2.00	70	16.0	
Tomato Paste, 6-oz. can	150	34.0	25.0	5.56	232	52.6	
Tomato Wedges, 16-oz. (1-lb.) can	120	28.0	1.75	60	14.0		
Drained solids (yield: approx. 10¼ oz.)	(86)	(24.6)	(8.4)	(2.40)			
Whole Peeled Tomatoes, 16-oz. (1-lb.) can	100	20.0	6.3	1.25	50	10.0	
Drained solids (yield: approx. 10½ oz.)	(67)	(16.7)	(6.4)	(1.60)			
Diet Delight California Tomatoes, packed in water, low sodium without added salt, 16-oz. (1-lb.) can	100	20.0	6.3	1.25	50	10.0	
Drained solids (yield: approx. 11 oz.)	(70)	(17.0)	(6.4)	(1.55)			

	UNIT		1 OZ., BY WT.		1 CUP		Fiber per oz.
	Cal.	Carb.	Cal.	Carb.	Cal.	Carb.	(GMS.)
Featherweight Stewed Tomatoes, no added sugar or salt, 8-oz. can	(70)	(18.0)	(8.8)	(2.25)	70	18.0	
Tomato Purée, low sodium, 19-oz. jar	(160)	(40.0)	(8.4)	(2.11)	80	20.0	
Tomatoes, no added salt or sugar, 10-oz. can	(60)	(12.0)	(6.0)	(1.20)	(40)	(8.0)	
Drained solids (yield: approx. 6 oz.)	(36)	(9.6)	(6.0)	(1.60)			
16-oz. (1-lb.) can	(96)	(19.2)	(6.0)	(1.20)	(40)	(8.0)	
Drained solids (yield: approx. 9.6 oz.)	(58)	(15.4)	(6.0)	(1.60)			
Tomatoes, packed in juice without added sugar or salt, 10-oz. can	40	4.0	4.0	0.40	40	4.0	
Golden Harvest Whole Tomatoes in Tomato Juice, no sugar or salt added, 16-oz. (1-lb.) can	100	22.0	6.3	1.38	50	11.0	
Drained solids (yield: approx. 11 oz.)	70	19.0	6.4	1.73			
Libby's Stewed Tomatoes, 16-oz. (1-lb.) can	(120)	(30.0)	7.5	(1.88)	60	15.0	
Whole Peeled Tomatoes, 16-oz. (1-lb.) can	(86)	(19.2)	(5.4)	(1.20)	45	10.0	
Drained solids (yield: approx. 9.6 oz.)	(54)	(16.0)	(5.6)	(1.67)			
Ortega Tomatoes and Hot Green Chiles, 10-oz. can	70	13.6	7.0	1.36			
P&Q (A&P) Tomatoes, 16-oz. (1-lb.) can	100	22.0	6.3	1.38			
S&W Peeled Whole Tomatoes, 16-oz. (1-lb.) can	98	21.3	6.1	1.33	50	11.0	
Drained solids (yield: approx. 9.6 oz.)	(61)	(14.9)	(6.4)	(1.55)			
8¼-oz. can	50	11.0	6.1	1.33	50	11.0	
Drained solids (yield: approx. 5 oz.)	(32)	(7.8)	(6.4)	(1.55)			
Whole Tomatoes in Thick Tomato Puree, 16-oz. (1-lb.) can	120	26.0	7.5	1.63	60	13.0	
S&W Nutradiet Peeled Whole Tomatoes, packed in Tomato Juice, no salt or sugar, 8¼-oz. can	50	10.0	6.1	1.21	50	10.0	
Drained solids (yield: approx. 5 oz.)	(31)	(6.8)	(6.2)	(1.35)			
Stokely Stewed Tomatoes, 16-oz. (1-lb.) can	133	28.3	8.3	1.77	70	15.0	
Whole Tomatoes, 16-oz. (1-lb.) can	140	18.0	8.8	1.13	70	9.0	
Drained solids (yield: approx. 9.6 oz.)	(103)	(11.5)	(10.7)	(1.21)			
Tillie Lewis "Tasti Diet" Whole Peeled Tomatoes, sodium controlled, 16-oz. (1-lb.) can	100	24.0	6.3	1.50	50	12.0	
Drained solids (yield: approx. 9.6 oz.)		17.6		1.83			
Town House Sliced Stewed Tomatoes, 16-oz. (1-lb.) can	140	36.0	8.8	1.13	70	18.0	
Whole Peeled Tomatoes, 16-oz. (1-lb.) can	100	22.0	6.3	0.69	50	11.0	
TOMATOES, CHERRY							
RAW (ripe):							
All-edible (refuse of stem tops is negligible):							
1 cherry tomato (approx. 0.7 oz.)	(4)	(0.9)	(6.2)	(1.33)			(0.14)
1 cup:							
whole (approx. 5.3 oz., 8 cherry tomatoes)	(33)	(7.0)	(6.2)	(1.33)			(0.14)
halves (approx. 6.5 oz., 9 cherry tomatoes)	(40)	(8.7)	(6.2)	(1.33)			(0.14)
1 pound (approx. 3 cups whole cherry tomatoes) (tr/1g/tr/94%/1mg)	(99)	(21.3)	(6.2)	(1.33)			(0.14)
1-pint container (approx. 12.5 oz.)	(78)	(16.7)	(6.2)	(1.33)			(0.14)
TOMATO JUICE, see the BEVERAGES chapter							
TOWEL GOURD							
RAW:							
As purchased [refuse: parings, approx. 15%]:							
1 pound	69	15.8	4.3	0.99			
Edible portion:							
1 pound (tr/1g/tr/95%/na)	82	18.6	5.1	1.16			0.14
COOKED:							
Steamed:							
1 pound of raw towel gourd (yield: approx. 14.1 oz.)	(82)	(18.6)	(5.8)	(1.32)			(0.16)
1 pound of steamed towel gourd	(93)	(21.1)	(5.8)	(1.32)			(0.16)

	UNIT		1 OZ., BY WT.		1 CUP		Fiber per oz.
	Cal.	Carb.	Cal.	Carb.	Cal.	Carb.	(GMS.)
TRUFFLES (based on data from the Middle East)							
RAW:							
All-edible:							
1 pound	458	68.5	28.6	4.28			
TURNIP GREENS							
RAW:							
As purchased untrimmed [refuse: discarded leaves, approx. 16%]:							
1 pound	107	19.0	6.7	1.19			
Edible portion:							
1 cup (approx. 5.1 oz.)	(40)	(7.2)	7.9	1.42	(40)	(7.2)	0.23
1 pound (approx. 3.1 cups) (1g/1g/tr/90%/na)	127	22.7	7.9	1.42	(40)	(7.2)	0.23
COOKED:							
Boiled, drained:							
In a small amount of water for a short time:							
1 cup (approx. 5.1 oz.)	29	5.2	5.7	1.02	29	5.2	0.20
1 pound (approx. 3.1 cups) (1g/1g/tr/93%/na)	91	16.3	5.7	1.02	29	5.2	0.20
In a large amount of water for a long time:							
1 cup (approx. 5.1 oz.)	28	4.8	5.5	0.94	28	4.8	(0.19)
1 pound (approx. 3.1 cups) (1g/1g/tr/94%/na)	88	15.0	5.5	0.94	28	4.8	(0.19)
FROZEN, based on generic data							
Chopped:							
Measured when frozen:							
1 pound	104	18.1	6.5	1.13			0.28
1 container, 10 oz. net wt.	65	11.4	6.5	1.13			0.28
Boiled, drained:							
1 cup (approx. 5.8 oz.)	38	6.4	6.5	1.11	38	6.4	0.28
1 pound of frozen turnip greens, boiled, drained (yield: approx. 12.4 oz.)	81	13.7	6.5	1.11	38	6.4	0.28
1 pound of boiled, drained turnip greens (1g/1g/tr/93%/5mg)	104	17.7	6.5	1.11	38	6.4	0.28
1 container, 10 oz., boiled, drained (yield: approx. 7.8 oz.)	51	8.6	6.5	1.11	38	6.4	0.28
FROZEN, by brand:							
Birds Eye Chopped Turnip Greens, 10-oz. package	60	6.0	6.0	0.60			
Boiled, drained (yield: approx. 9.7 oz.)	(60)	(6.0)	(6.2)	(0.62)	(34)	(3.4)	
Chopped Turnip Greens with Diced Turnips, 10-oz. package	60	9.0	6.0	0.90			
Boiled, drained (yield: approx. 9.7 oz.)	(60)	(9.0)	(6.2)	(0.93)	(34)	(5.0)	
Seabrook Farms Chopped Turnip Greens, 10-oz. package	60	9.0	6.0	0.90			
Boiled, drained (yield: approx. 9.7 oz.)	(60)	(9.0)	(6.2)	(0.93)	(34)	(5.1)	
CANNED, based on generic data:							
Solids and liquid:							
1 cup (approx. 8.2 oz.)	42	7.4	5.1	0.91	42	7.4	0.20
1 pound (approx. 2 cups)	82	14.5	5.1	0.91	42	7.4	0.20
1 #303 can, 15 oz. net wt. (approx. 1.8 cups) (tr/1g/tr/94%/67mg)	77	13.6	5.1	0.91	42	7.4	0.20
CANNED, by brand:							
Luck's Turnip Greens with Diced Turnips, seasoned with Pork, 15-oz. can	180	12.0	12.0	0.80			
Stokely Chopped Turnip Greens, 15-oz. can	63	10.8	4.2	0.72	35	6.0	
Drained solids (yield: approx. 10.8 oz.)	(55)	(9.1)	(5.1)	(0.84)	(29)	(4.7)	
TURNIPS							
RAW:							
As purchased:							
with tops							
Good quality [refuse: tops, rootlets, parings, and trimmings, approx. 35%]:							
1 pound	88	19.5	5.5	1.22			

	UNIT		1 OZ., BY WT.		1 CUP		Fiber per oz.
	Cal.	Carb.	Cal.	Carb.	Cal.	Carb.	(GMS.)
Fair quality [refuse: tops, rootlets, parings, and trimmings, approx. 45%]:							
1 pound	75	16.5	4.7	1.03			
As purchased:							
without tops							
Good quality [refuse: parings, rootlets, and trimmings, approx. 14%]:							
1 pound	117	25.7	7.3	1.61			
Fair quality [refuse: parings, rootlets, and trimmings, approx. 27%]:							
1 pound	99	21.9	6.2	1.40			
Edible portion:							
1 cup, cubed or sliced (approx. 4.6 oz.)	39	8.6	8.5	1.88	39	8.6	0.26
1 pound (approx. 3½ cups) (tr/2g/tr/92%/14mg)	136	30.0	8.5	1.88	39	8.6	0.26
COOKED:							
Boiled, drained:							
1 cup:							
Cubed (approx. 5½ oz.)	36	7.6	6.5	1.39	36	7.6	0.20
Mashed (approx. 8.1 oz.)	53	11.3	6.5	1.39	53	11.3	0.20
1 pound (approx. 2 cups mashed, or 3 cups cubed (tr/1g/tr/94%/10mg)	104	22.2	6.5	1.39	36	7.6	0.20
Steamed:							
1 pound of raw turnips steamed (yield: approx. 15.2 oz.)	136	30.0	8.9	1.98			0.27
1 pound of steamed turnips	143	31.7	8.9	1.98			0.27
FROZEN, by brand:							
Seabrook Farms Diced Turnip Roots, 10-oz. package	48	8.2	4.8	0.82	(27)	(4.6)	

VINE SPINACH (Basella)

	UNIT		1 OZ., BY WT.		1 CUP		Fiber per oz.
	Cal.	Carb.	Cal.	Carb.	Cal.	Carb.	(GMS.)
RAW:							
All-edible:							
1 pound (1g/1g/tr/93%/na)	86	15.4	5.4	0.96			

WATER BAMBOO, see WILD RICE

WATER CHESTNUTS (Matai, Waternuts)

	UNIT		1 OZ., BY WT.		1 CUP		Fiber per oz.
	Cal.	Carb.	Cal.	Carb.	Cal.	Carb.	(GMS.)
RAW:							
As purchased [refuse: skin, approx. 23%]:							
1 pound	272	66.4	17.0	4.15			
Edible portion:							
1 pound (tr/5g/tr/78%/6mg)	358	86.2	22.4	5.39	(125)	(30.0)	0.22
CANNED, by brand:							
Chun King Water Chestnuts, 8½-oz. can	119	27.0	14.0	3.18			
Drained solids (yield: approx. 5 oz.)	(109)	(24.9)	(21.8)	(4.98)	122	27.8	
La Choy Water Chestnuts, 8-oz. can	(76)	(17.1)	(9.5)	(2.14)			
Drained solids (yield: approx. 5 oz.)	(66)	(15.0)	12.9	2.92	(72)	(16.3)	

WATERCRESS

Leaves and Stems

	UNIT		1 OZ., BY WT.		1 CUP		Fiber per oz.
	Cal.	Carb.	Cal.	Carb.	Cal.	Carb.	(GMS.)
RAW:							
As purchased [refuse: stem ends, approx. 8%]:							
1 pound	79	12.5	4.9	0.78			
Edible portion:							
1 cup:							
Whole, or cut into ½"–¾" pieces (approx. 1¼ oz.)	7	1.1	5.4	0.85	7	1.1	0.20
Finely chopped (approx. 4.4 oz.)	24	3.8	5.4	0.85	24	3.8	0.20
1 pound (approx. 1.3 cups whole or 3.6 cups finely chopped) (1g/1g/tr/93%/15mg)	86	13.6	5.4	0.85			0.20
COOKED:							
Steamed:							
1 pound of steamed watercress	112	14.2	7.0	0.89			0.20

WATERNUTS, see WATER CHESTNUTS

WAX BEANS (Yellow Beans)

	UNIT		1 OZ., BY WT.		1 CUP		Fiber per oz.
	Cal.	Carb.	Cal.	Carb.	Cal.	Carb.	(GMS.)
RAW:							
1 cup (approx. 3.9 oz.)	30	6.6	7.6	1.70	30	6.6	0.28
1 pound (approx. 4.1 cups) (tr/2g/tr/91%/2mg)	122	27.2	7.6	1.70	30	6.6	0.28
COOKED:							
Boiled, drained							
1 cup (approx. 4.4 oz.)	28	5.8	6.3	1.31	28	5.8	0.23
1 pound (approx. 3.6 cups) (yield from approx. 13.2 oz. of uncooked dry beans) (tr/1g/tr/93%/1mg)	100	20.9	6.3	1.31	28	5.8	0.23
FROZEN, based on generic data:							
Cut unspecified:							
Measured when frozen:							
1 cup (approx. 4.4 oz.)	35	8.1	7.9	1.84	35	8.1	0.31
1 pound (approx. 3.6 cups)	127	29.5	7.9	1.84	35	8.1	0.31
1 container, 9 oz. net wt.	71	16.6	7.9	1.84	35	8.1	0.31
Boiled, drained:							
1 cup (approx. 4.7 oz.)	36	8.4	7.6	1.76	36	8.4	0.31
1 pound of frozen wax beans, boiled, drained (yield: approx. 14.8 oz.)	113	26.0	7.6	1.76	36	8.4	0.31
1 pound of boiled, drained wax beans (tr/2g/tr/92%/tr)	122	28.1	7.6	1.76	36	8.4	0.31
1 container, 9 oz., boiled, then drained (yield: approx. 8.3 oz.)	63	14.6	7.6	1.76	36	8.4	0.31
FROZEN, by brand:							
Birds Eye Cut Wax Beans, 9-oz. package	90	12.0	10.0	1.33			
Boiled, drained (yield: approx. 8.1 oz.)	(90)	(12.0)	(11.1)	(1.48)	(61)	(8.1)	
CANNED, based on generic data:							
Cut Crosswise:							
Regular pack:							
Solids and liquid:							
1 cup (approx. 8.4 oz.)	45	10.0	5.4	1.15	45	10.0	0.17
1 pound (approx. 1.9 cups) (tr/1g/tr/94%/67mg)	86	19.1	5.4	1.15	45	10.0	0.17
1 #303 can, 15½ oz. net wt.	83	18.4	5.4	1.15	45	10.0	0.17
Drained solids:							
1 cup (approx. 4.8 oz.)	32	7.0	6.8	1.48	32	7.0	0.26
1 pound (approx. 3.4 cups) (tr/1g/tr/92%/67mg)	109	23.6	6.8	1.48	32	7.0	0.26
1 #303 can (yield: approx. 9.2 oz. of drained wax beans)	63	13.6	6.8	1.48	32	7.0	0.26
Drained liquid:							
1 cup (approx. 8.3 oz.)	(26)	(5.9)	3.1	0.71	(26)	(5.9)	trace
1 pound (approx. 1.9 cups (tr/1g/tr/96%/67mg)	50	11.3	3.1	0.71	(26)	(5.9)	trace
Low-sodium pack:							
Solids and liquid:							
1 cup (approx. 8.4 oz.)	36	8.1	4.3	0.96	36	8.1	0.17
1 pound (approx. 1.9 cups) (tr/1g/tr/95%/1mg)	68	15.4	4.3	0.96	36	8.1	0.17
1 #303 can, 15½ oz. net wt.	66	14.9	4.3	0.96	36	8.1	0.17
Drained solids:							
1 cup (approx. 4.8 oz.)	28	6.3	5.9	1.33	28	6.3	0.26
1 pound (approx. 3.4 cups) (tr/1g/tr/94%/1mg)	95	21.3	5.9	1.33	28	6.3	0.26
1 #303 can (yield: approx. 9.2 oz. of drained wax beans)	55	12.3	5.9	1.33	28	6.3	0.26
Drained liquid:							
1 cup (approx. 8.3 oz.)	(17)	(3.3)	2.0	0.40	(17)	(3.3)	trace
1 pound (approx. 1.9 cups) (tr/tr/tr/98%/1mg)	32	6.4	2.0	0.40	(17)	(3.3)	trace
Cut lengthwise, or French-style cut:							
Regular pack:							
Solids and liquid:							
1 cup (approx. 8.4 oz.)	45	10.0	5.4	1.15	45	10.0	0.17
1 pound (approx. 1.9 cups) (tr/1g/tr/92%/67mg)	86	19.1	5.4	1.15	45	10.0	0.17
1 #303 can, 15½ oz. net wt.	83	18.4	5.4	1.15	45	10.0	0.17
Drained solids:							
1 cup (approx. 4.6 oz.)	31	6.8	6.8	1.48	31	6.8	0.26
1 pound (approx. 3.5 cups) (tr/1g/tr/92%/67mg)	109	23.6	6.8	1.48	31	6.8	0.26
1 #303 can (yield: approx. 8.7 oz. of drained French-style cut wax beans)	60	12.9	6.8	1.48	31	6.8	0.26

	UNIT Cal.	UNIT Carb.	1 OZ., BY WT. Cal.	1 OZ., BY WT. Carb.	1 CUP Cal.	1 CUP Carb.	Fiber per oz. (GMS.)
Drained liquid:							
1 cup (approx. 8.3 oz.)	26	5.9	3.1	0.71	26	5.9	trace
1 pound (approx. 1.9 cups) (tr/1g/tr/96%/67mg)	50	11.3	3.1	0.71	26	5.9	trace
CANNED, by brand:							
Ann Page (A&P) Wax Beans, 15½-oz. can	75	15.0	4.8	0.97	40	8.0	
Drained solids (yield: approx. 9.3 oz.)	(56)	(10.7)	(6.1)	(1.15)	(29)	(5.5)	
Balanced Cut Wax Beans, packed in water, no added sugar or salt, 8-oz. can	(57)	(10.4)	(7.1)	(1.30)	60	11.0	
Drained solids (yield: approx. 4.8 oz.)	(50)	(9.1)	(10.5)	(1.90)	(50)	(9.1)	
Blue Boy Wax Beans, 8-oz. can	43	9.5	5.4	1.19	45	10.0	
Drained solids (yield: approx. 5.2 oz.)	35	7.5	6.7	1.45	30	6.4	
Del Monte Cut Wax Beans, 16-oz. (1-lb.) can	70	14.0	4.4	0.88	37	7.0	
Drained solids (yield: approx. 8¾ oz.)	(48)	(8.9)	(5.5)	(1.02)	(26)	(4.9)	
French Cut Wax Beans, 16-oz. (1-lb.) can	70	14.0	4.4	0.88	35	7.0	
Drained solids (yield: approx. 8¾ oz.)	(48)	(8.9)	(5.5)	(1.02)	(26)	(4.9)	
Featherweight Cut Wax Beans, no added salt or sugar, 8-oz. can	(40)	(10.0)	(5.0)	(1.25)	40	10.0	
Drained solids (yield: approx. 4.8 oz.)	(34)	(8.4)	(7.0)	(1.75)	(33)	(8.3)	
15½-oz. can	(78)	(19.4)	(5.0)	(1.25)	40	10.0	
Drained solids (yield: approx. 9.3 oz.)	(65)	(16.3)	(7.0)	(1.75)	(33)	(8.3)	
Golden Harvest Cut Wax Beans in Water, no sugar or salt added, 8-oz. can	35	9.0	4.4	1.13	35	9.0	
Drained solids (yield: approx. 4¼ oz.)	24	6.4	5.6	1.51	32	8.6	
Libby's Wax Beans, 8-oz. can	(38)	8.7	4.8	1.08	40	9.0	
Drained solids (yield: approx. 5.2 oz.)	(30)	(6.7)	(5.8)	(1.30)	(27)	(6.2)	
16-oz. (1-lb.) can	(77)	(17.4)	(4.8)	(1.08)	40	9.0	
Drained solids (yield: approx. 10.4 oz.)	(60)	(13.5)	(5.8)	(1.30)	(27)	(6.2)	
Stokely Cut Wax Beans, 8-oz. can	42	7.4	5.2	0.93	45	8.0	
Drained solids (yield: approx. 4.25 oz.)	(31)	(4.8)	(7.3)	(1.14)	(35)	(5.4)	
16-oz. (1-lb.) can	83	14.9	5.2	0.93	45	8.0	
Drained solids (yield: approx. 8.5 oz.)	(62)	(9.7)	(7.3)	(1.14)	(35)	(5.4)	
French Style Sliced Wax Beans, 15½-oz. can	(63)	(12.6)	(4.1)	(0.81)	35	7.0	
Sliced Wax Beans, 16-oz. (1-lb.) can	74	13.0	4.6	0.81	40	7.0	
Drained solids (yield: approx. 9.6 oz.)	(56)	(8.5)	(5.8)	(0.89)	(28)	(4.2)	

WAX GOURD

	UNIT Cal.	UNIT Carb.	1 OZ., BY WT. Cal.	1 OZ., BY WT. Carb.	1 CUP Cal.	1 CUP Carb.	Fiber per oz. (GMS.)
RAW:							
As purchased [refuse: skin and cavity contents, approx. 31%]:							
1 pound	41	9.4	2.6	0.59			
Edible portion:							
1 pound (tr/1g/tr/96%/2mg)	59	13.6	3.7	0.85			0.14

WHEAT

	UNIT Cal.	UNIT Carb.	1 OZ., BY WT. Cal.	1 OZ., BY WT. Carb.	1 CUP Cal.	1 CUP Carb.	Fiber per oz. (GMS.)
BULGUR (Parboiled Wheat), Based on generic data							
Club Wheat, 1 cup (approx. 6.2 oz.)	628	139.1	101.3	22.44	628	139.1	
Hard Red Winter Wheat, 1 cup (approx. 6 oz.)	602	128.7	100.3	21.45	602	128.7	
White Wheat, 1 cup (approx. 5½ oz.)	553	121.8	100.5	22.14	553	121.8	
PACKAGED, by brand:							
Golden Harvest Bulgur, 16-oz. (1-lb.) package, dry	1800	396.0	112.5	24.75	600	132.0	
Boiled (yield: approx. 38.5 oz.)	1800	396.0	46.7	10.28	300	66.0	
Fried (yield: approx. 41.5 oz.)	2400	400.2	57.8	9.64	400	66.7	
Jolly Joan Bulghur Wheat, 1½-lb. box	2400	528.0	100.0	22.00	600	132.0	
1 cup (approx. 6 oz.)	600	132.0	100.0	22.00	600	132.0	
1 pound (approx. 2.7 cups)	1600	352.0	100.0	22.00	600	132.0	
COUSCOUS							
Near East Precooked Medium Grain, 16-oz. (1-lb.) box prepared as package directs without butter (yield: approx. 8 cups, 4 lb. 4 oz.)	1600	336.0	(23.5)	(4.94)	200	42.0	
1 cup, prepared (approx. 8.5 oz.)	200	42.0	(23.5)	(4.94)	200	42.0	
1 pound, prepared (approx. 1.9 cups)	(376)	(79.1)	(23.5)	(4.94)	200	42.0	
***KASHA* (Buckwheat)**							
Wolff's Whole Granulation, 13-oz. box, dry	1450	300.0	111.5	23.08	(580)	(120.0)	
1 cup of dry grain prepared as package directs with egg and butter (yield: approx. 3 cups, 1 lb. 4 oz.)	(860)	(121.5)	(43.0)	(6.08)	(287)	(40.5)	
1 cup, prepared (approx. 6.7 oz.)	(287)	(40.5)	(43.0)	(6.08)	(287)	(40.5)	
1 pound, prepared (approx. 2.4 cups)	(688)	(97.3)	(43.0)	(6.08)	(287)	(40.5)	
Medium Granulation, 13-oz. box, dry	1450	300.0	111.5	23.08	(580)	(120.0)	
1 cup of dry grain prepared as package directs with egg and butter (yield: approx. 3 cups, 1 lb. 4 oz.)	(860)	(121.5)	(43.0)	(6.08)	(287)	(40.5)	
1 cup, prepared (approx. 6.7 oz.)	(287)	(40.5)	(43.0)	(6.08)	(287)	(40.5)	
1 pound, prepared (approx. 2.4 cups)	(688)	(97.3)	(43.0)	(6.08)	(287)	(40.5)	
TABOULEH (based on data from the Middle East)							
Prepared with 6 oz. dry bulgur wheat, 2 oz. parsley, 1 Tbsp. mint, 2 oz. green onions, 28 oz. tomatoes, salt, pepper, ¾ cup lemon juice, 3½ oz. olive oil:							
1 pound	490		30.6				
Near East Tabouleh Wheat Salad Mix, 7-oz. box prepared as package directs (yield: approx. 4½ cups, 2 lb. 2 oz.)	880	192.0	(25.9)	(5.65)	147	32.0	
1 cup, prepared (approx. 8.5 oz.)	147	32.0	(25.9)	(5.65)	147	32.0	
1 pound, prepared (approx. 1.9 cups)	(414)	(90.4)	(25.9)	(5.65)	147	32.0	
WHEAT PILAF							
Near East, 8-oz. box prepared as package directs (yield: approx. 4 cups, 1 lb. 9 oz.)	800	160.0	(31.1)	(6.23)	200	40.0	
1 cup, prepared (approx. 6.4 oz.)	200	40.0	(31.1)	(6.23)	200	40.0	
1 pound, prepared (approx. 2.5 cups)	498	99.7	(31.1)	(6.23)	200	40.0	

WHITE BEANS

	UNIT Cal.	UNIT Carb.	1 OZ., BY WT. Cal.	1 OZ., BY WT. Carb.	1 CUP Cal.	1 CUP Carb.	Fiber per oz. (GMS.)
RAW:							
1 cup (approx. 7.2 oz.) (yield: approx. 3.1 cups)	697	125.7	96.4	17.30	697	125.7	1.22
1 pound (approx. 2.2 cups) (yield: approx. 2 lbs. 14 oz., 6.9 cups cooked) (6g/17g/tr/11%/5mg)	1542	278.1	96.4	17.30	697	125.7	1.22
COOKED:							
Boiled, drained:							
1 cup (approx. 6.7 oz.)	224	40.3	33.4	6.01	224	40.3	0.43
1 pound (approx. 2.4 cups) (yield from approx. 5.5 oz. uncooked dry beans) (2g/6g/tr/69%/2mg)	534	96.2	33.4	6.01	224	40.3	0.43

WILD RICE (WATER BAMBOO)

	UNIT Cal.	UNIT Carb.	1 OZ., BY WT. Cal.	1 OZ., BY WT. Carb.	1 CUP Cal.	1 CUP Carb.	Fiber per oz. (GMS.)
RAW:							
All-edible:							
1 cup (approx. 5.6 oz.)	565	120.5	100.2	21.37	565	120.5	
1 pound (approx. 2.8 cups) (4g/21g/tr/9%/2mg)	1603	341.9	100.2	21.37	565	120.5	

YAMBEANS

	UNIT Cal.	UNIT Carb.	1 OZ., BY WT. Cal.	1 OZ., BY WT. Carb.	1 CUP Cal.	1 CUP Carb.	Fiber per oz. (GMS.)
RAW:							
As purchased [refuse: parings, approx. 10%]:							
1 pound	225	52.2	14.1	3.26			
Edible portion:							
1 pound (tr/4g/tr/85%/na)	250	58.1	15.6	3.63			0.20
COOKED:							
Steamed:							
1 pound of raw yambeans, steamed (yield: approx. 16 oz.)	250	58.1	15.6	3.63			0.20
1 pound of steamed yambeans	250	58.1	15.6	3.63			0.20

	UNIT		1 OZ., BY WT.		1 CUP		Fiber per oz.
	Cal.	Carb.	Cal.	Carb.	Cal.	Carb.	(GMS.)
YAMS (also see SWEET POTATOES)							
RAW:							
As purchased [refuse: skin, approx. 14%]:							
1 medium yam (approx. 8 oz.)	196	45.3	24.6	5.66			
1 pound (approx. 2 medium yams)	394	90.5	24.6	5.66			
Edible portion:							
1 medium yam (approx. 6.9 oz.)	196	45.3	28.6	6.58			0.26
1 pound (approx. 2.3 medium yams) (1g/7g/tr/74%/na)	458	105.2	28.6	6.58			0.26
COOKED:							
Steamed:							
1 pound of raw yams, steamed (yield: approx. 15.8 oz.)	458	105.2	29.0	6.66			0.26
1 pound of steamed yams	464	106.5	29.0	6.66			0.26
CANNED, by brand:							
Ann Page (A&P) Cut Yams, Sweet Potatoes in Syrup, 40-oz. can	1304	317.6	32.6	7.94	230	56.0	
Yams, Whole Sweet Potatoes in Syrup, 16-oz. (1-lb.) can	518	126.0	32.4	7.88	230	56.0	
Case Swayne Fully Cooked Yams, 40-oz. can	(1050)	(240.0)	(25.0)	(5.71)	210	48.0	
16-oz. (1-lb.) can	(420)	(96.0)	(25.0)	(5.71)	210	48.0	
Mrs. Paul's Candied Yams, 12-oz. package	540	132.0	45.0	11.00			
Royal Prince Yams, Whole Sweet Potatoes in Heavy Syrup, 17-oz. can	588	140.0	34.6	8.24	294	70.0	
FROZEN, by brand:							
Stouffer's Yams and Apples, 10-oz. package	320	62.0	32.0	6.20			
YELLOW BEANS, see WAX BEANS							
YELLOW EYE BEANS							
Underwood Yellow Eye Beans, 55-oz. can	2475	346.5	45.0	6.30			
Drained solids (yield: approx. 37.4 oz.)	(2438)	(336.7)	(65.2)	(9.00)			
16-oz. (1-lb.) can	720	100.8	45.0	6.30			
Drained solids (yield: approx. 10.9 oz.)	(711)	(98.1)	(65.2)	(9.00)			
ZUCCHINI (Cocozelle)							
(ITALIAN NARROW-TYPE), GREEN							
RAW:							
As purchased:							
Good quality [refuse: stem ends, approx. 5%]:							
1 small zucchini (approx. 4.5 oz.)	21	4.3	4.6	0.97			
1 medium zucchini (approx. 9.6 oz.)	44	9.3	4.6	0.97			
1 pound	73	15.5	4.6	0.97			
Fair quality [refuse: stem ends and trimmings, approx. 18%]:							
1 small zucchini (approx. 4.5 oz.)	17	3.8	3.9	0.84			
1 medium zucchini (approx. 9.6 oz.)	37	8.1	3.9	0.84			
1 pound	63	13.4	3.9	0.84			
Edible portion:							
1 small good-quality zucchini (approx. 4.4 oz.)	21	4.3	4.8	1.02	22	4.7	0.17
1 medium good-quality zucchini (approx. 9.2 oz.)	44	9.3	4.8	1.02	22	4.7	0.17
1 cup, sliced (approx. 5.8 oz.)	22	4.7	4.8	1.02	22	4.7	0.17
1 pound (approx. 2.8 cups) (tr/1g/tr/95%/tr)	77	16.3	4.8	1.02	22	4.7	0.17
COOKED:							
Boiled, drained:							
1 cup:							
Sliced (approx. 6.3 oz.)	22	4.5	3.4	0.71	22	4.5	0.12
Cubed or diced (approx. 7.4 oz.)	25	5.3	3.4	0.71	25	5.3	0.12
Mashed (approx. 8.5 oz.)	29	6.0	3.4	0.71	29	6.0	0.12
1 pound (approx. 2–2½ cups) (tr/1g/tr/96%/tr)	54	11.3	3.4	0.71			0.12

	UNIT		1 OZ., BY WT.		1 CUP		Fiber per oz.
	Cal.	Carb.	Cal.	Carb.	Cal.	Carb.	(GMS.)
FROZEN, by brand:							
Birds Eye Zucchini Squash, 10-oz. package	48	9.0	5.5	0.91			
Boiled, drained (yield: approx. 7.3 oz.)	(48)	(9.0)	(6.6)	(1.23)	(56)	(10.4)	
Mrs. Paul's Light Batter Zucchini Sticks, 9-oz. package	540	69.0	60.0	7.67			
Safeway Frozen Crinkle Cut Zucchini Squash, 20-oz. package	108	18.0	5.4	0.90			
Boiled, drained (yield: approx. 14.6 oz.)	(108)	(18.0)	(7.4)	(1.23)	(48)	(7.9)	
Seabrook Farms Zucchini Squash, 10-oz. package	54	9.0	5.4	0.90			
Boiled, drained (yield: approx. 7.3 oz.)	(54)	(9.0)	(7.4)	(1.23)	(63)	(10.4)	
16-oz. (1-lb.) package	82	13.7	5.1	0.86			
Boiled, drained (yield: approx. 11.7 oz.)	(82)	(13.7)	(7.0)	(1.17)	(45)	(7.5)	
CANNED, by brand:							
Bel-Air Crinkle Cut Zucchini Squash, 20-oz. can	108	18.0	5.4	0.90			
Drained solids (yield: approx. 14.6 oz.)	108	18.0	7.4	1.23	48	7.9	
Del Monte Zucchini in Tomato Sauce, 16-oz. (1-lb.) can	120	32.0	7.5	2.00	60	16.0	
8-oz. can	60	16.0	7.5	2.00	60	16.0	
MIXED VEGETABLES							
Some vegetable mixtures are not in this list, but have their own headings:							
Succotash, a mixture of corn and lima beans, is listed under SUCCOTASH.							
Peas And Carrots is listed under Peas and Carrots.							
For other mixtures in which Peas get top billing, see Peas and . . . , Peas in . . . , and Peas with							
FROZEN, by brand:							
Birds Eye Bavarian Style Beans and Spaetzle, International Vegetables, 10-oz. package	150	30.0	15.0	3.00			
Cantonese Style Vegetables, 10-oz. package	150	30.0	15.2	3.00			
Chinese Style Vegetables, stir fry, 10-oz. package	105	21.0	10.5	2.10			
Chinese Style Vegetables with seasoned sauce, International Vegetables, 10-oz. package	60	15.0	6.0	1.50			
Danish Style Vegetables, International Vegetables, 10-oz. package	90	21.0	9.0	2.70			
Green Peas with Sliced Mushrooms, International Vegetables, 10-oz. package	210	33.0	21.0	3.30			
Hawaiian Style Vegetables with Pineapple, International Vegetables, 10-oz. package	120	36.0	12.0	3.60			
Italian Style Vegetables, International Vegetables, 10-oz. package	135	24.0	13.5	2.40			
Japanese Style Vegetables, 10-oz. package	120	27.0	12.0	2.70			
Mandarin Style Vegetables, 10-oz. package	90	18.0	9.0	1.80			
Mixed Vegetables, 10-oz. package	180	33.0	18.0	3.30			
Boiled, drained (yield: approx. 9.7 oz.)	(180)	(33.0)	(18.6)	(3.40)	(119)	(21.8)	
Mixed Vegetables with Onion Sauce, 8-oz. package	300	36.0	37.5	4.50	(241)	(28.9)	
New England Style Vegetables, Americana Recipe, 10-oz. package	180	33.0	18.0	3.30			
New Orleans Creole Style Vegetables, Americana Recipe, 10-oz. package	210	39.0	21.0	3.90			
Parisian Style Vegetables, International Vegetables, 10-oz. package	90	21.0	9.0	2.10			

	UNIT		1 OZ., BY WT.		1 CUP		Fiber per oz. (GMS.)
	Cal.	Carb.	Cal.	Carb.	Cal.	Carb.	
Pennsylvania Dutch Style Vegetables, Americana recipe, 10-oz. package	120	21.0	12.0	2.10			
Rice and Peas with Mushrooms, 7-oz. package	300	66.0	42.9	9.43			
San Francisco Style, Americana Recipe, 10-oz. package	135	18.0	13.5	1.80			
Vegetable Jubilee, 10-oz. package	360	51.0	36.0	5.10	(230)	(32.6)	
Wisconsin Country Style Vegetables, Americana Recipe, 10-oz. package	120	18.0	12.0	1.80			
Green Giant Broccoli, Cauliflower and Carrots in Cheese Sauce, 10-oz. polybag	156	18.2	15.6	1.82	140	17.0	
Chinese Style Vegetables, 10-oz. boil-in-bag	136	19.9	13.6	1.99			
Hawaiian Style Vegetables, 10-oz. boil-in-bag	204	34.6	20.4	3.46	200	33.0	
Japanese Style Vegetables, 10-oz. boil-in-bag	130	22.4	13.0	2.24			
Mexicorn Golden Corn/Peppers in Butter Sauce, 10-oz. boil-in-bag	204	85.1	26.4	8.51	190	60.0	
Mixed Vegetables (corn, peas, carrots, green beans, lima beans), 20-oz. polybag	341	64.1	17.0	3.21	90	16.0	
Boiled, drained (yield: approx. 19.4 oz.)	(341)	(64.1)	(17.6)	(3.30)	(113)	(21.1)	
Mixed Vegetables in Butter Sauce, 10-oz. boil-in-bag	184	25.5	18.4	2.55	130	17.0	
Okra Gumbo, 10-oz. boil-in-bag	255	15.9	25.5	1.59			
Hanover Garden Medley, 16-oz. (1-lb.) polybag	226	45.0	14.1	2.81			
Boiled, drained (yield: approx. 15.4 oz.)	(226)	(45.0)	(14.7)	(2.92)	(94)	(18.7)	
Harvest Vegetables, 16-oz. (1-lb.) polybag	350	65.0	21.9	4.00			
Boiled, drained (yield: approx. 15.5 oz.)	(350)	(65.0)	(22.6)	(4.19)	(122)	(22.6)	
Mixed Vegetables, 16-oz. (1-lb.) polybag	226	40.0	14.1	2.50			
Boiled, drained (yield: approx. 15.5 oz.)	(226)	(40.0)	(14.5)	(2.58)	(93)	(16.5)	
Summer Vegetables, 16-oz. (1-lb.) polybag	174	35.0	10.9	2.19	(70)	(14.1)	
White Shoepeg Corn with Chef Cut Green Beans, 16-oz. (1-lb) polybag	301	60.0	18.8	3.75			
Boiled, drained (yield: approx. 15.4 oz.)	(301)	(50.0)	(19.5)	(3.90)	(107)	(21.4)	
White Shoepeg Corn with Fordhook Limas, 16-oz. (1-lb.) polybag	450	85.0	28.1	5.31	(154)	(29.2)	
Boiled, drained (yield: approx. 15.4 oz.)	(450)	(85.0)	(29.2)	(5.52)	(160)	(30.3)	
Kounty Kist California Blend (broccoli, cauliflower & carrots), 18-oz. polybag	138	23.0	7.7	1.28	30	5.0	
Mixed Vegetables (corn, peas, carrots and green beans), 20-oz. polybag	335	63.0	16.7	3.15			
Boiled, drained (yield: approx. 19.4 oz.)	(335)	(63.0)	(17.2)	(3.25)	90	16.5	
La Choy Chinese Style Vegetables, 10-oz. package	72	10.5	7.2	1.05			
Japanese Vegetables, 10-oz. package	72	11.6	7.2	1.16			
Ore-Ida Stew Vegetables, 24-oz. package	480	104.0	20.0	4.33			
Boiled, drained (yield: approx. 23.3 oz.)	(480)	(104.0)	(20.0)	(4.33)	(128)	(27.7)	
Stouffer's Ratatouille, 10-oz. package	120	18.0	12.0	1.80			
Village Park Mediterranean Vegetables, 16-oz. (1-lb.)	150	30.0	9.4	1.88			
Boiled, drained (yield: approx. 15.5 oz.)	(150)	(30.0)	(9.7)	(1.94)			
Mixed Vegetables, 16-oz. (1-lb.) package	300	75.0	18.8	4.69			
Boiled, drained (yield: approx. 15.5 oz.)	(300)	(75.0)	(19.4)	(4.84)	(102)	(25.3)	
Oriental Vegetables, 16-oz. (1-lb.) package	150	30.0	9.4	1.88			
Boiled, drained (yield: approx. 15.5 oz.)	(150)	(30.0)	(9.7)	(1.94)			
Scandinavian Vegetables, 16-oz. (1-lb.) package	200	40.0	12.5	2.50			
Boiled, drained (yield: approx. 15.5 oz.)	(200)	(40.0)	(12.9)	(2.58)			
Stew Vegetables, 16-oz. (1-lb.) package	250	50.0	15.6	3.13			
Boiled, drained (yield: approx. 15.5 oz.)	(250)	(50.0)	(16.1)	(3.23)	(103)	(20.7)	
Winter Mix, 16-oz. (1-lb.) package	125	25.0	7.8	1.56			
Boiled, drained (yield: approx. 15.5 oz.)	(125)	(25.0)	(8.1)	(1.61)			
CANNED, by brand:							
Ann Page (A&P) Mixed Vegetables (carrots, potatoes, sweet peas, green beans, lima beans, whole kernel corn, celery), 8½-oz. can	96	17.0	11.3	2.00	90	16.0	
Drained solids (yield: approx. 5 oz.)	(71)	(11.1)	(14.1)	(2.22)	(81)	(12.8)	
16-oz. (1-lb.) can	180	32.0	11.3	2.00	90	16.0	
Drained solids (yield: approx. 10¼ oz.)	(145)	(22.8)	(14.1)	(2.22)	(81)	(12.8)	
Chun King Chow Mein Vegetables, 16-oz. (1-lb.) can	88	14.6	5.5	0.91	(44)	(7.3)	
Oriental Vegetables & Sauce Mix for Stir-Fry Pepper Steak, 28-oz. can	2291	430.2	77.3	14.46			
Del Monte Mixed Vegetables, 16-oz. (1-lb.) can	160	32.0	10.0	2.00	80	16.0	
Drained solids (yield: approx. 10¼ oz.)	(123)	(22.8)	(12.2)	(2.25)	(70)	(12.9)	
Featherweight Mixed Vegetables, no added salt or sugar, 8-oz. can	(70)	(16.0)	(8.8)	(2.00)	(70)	(16.0)	
Drained solids (yield: approx. 5.3 oz.)	(54)	(11.7)	(10.2)	(2.21)	(59)	(12.7)	
16-oz. (1-lb.) can	(140)	(32.0)	(8.8)	(2.00)	(70)	(16.0)	
Drained solids (yield: approx. 10.6 oz.)	(108)	(23.4)	(10.2)	(2.21)	(59)	(12.7)	
Freshlike Veg-All Mixed Vegetables (carrots, potatoes, celery, sweet peas, corn, green beans, lima beans) 8½-oz. can	(90)	(14.0)	(10.6)	(1.65)	90	14.0	
Drained solids (yield: approx. 5¼ oz.)	(74)	(9.6)	(14.1)	(1.83)	(80)	(10.4)	
16-oz. (1-lb.) can	(180)	(28.0)	(10.6)	(1.65)	90	14.0	
Drained solids (yield: approx. 10¼ oz.)	(145)	(18.8)	(14.1)	(1.83)	(80)	(10.4)	
Golden Harvest Mixed Vegetables in Water, no sugar or salt added, 8-oz. can	90	14.0	11.3	1.75	90	14.0	
Drained solids (yield: approx. 5.2 oz.)	73	10.6	14.1	2.05	81	11.8	
Hanover Garden Salad, 14.5-oz. can	236	58.0	16.3	4.00			
Drained solids (yield: approx. 14.1 oz.)	(236)	(58.0)	(16.7)	(4.11)			
Mixed Vegetables, 38.5-oz. can	435	86.6	11.3	2.25	(96)	(19.1)	
Drained solids (yield: approx. 26.2 oz.)	(349)	(65.7)	(13.3)	(2.51)	(76)	(14.4)	
Sweet and Sour Vegetable Salad, 14.5-oz. can	273	65.3	18.8	4.50	(150)	(36.0)	
La Choy Mixed Chinese Vegetables, 16-oz. (1-lb.) can	(59)	(4.6)	(3.7)	(0.29)			
Drained solids (yield: approx. 8 oz.)	(35)	(2.2)	4.3	0.28	(24)	(1.5)	
Sweet & Sour Vegetables with Chicken, 17-oz. can	680	142.4	40.0	8.38	427	89.3	
Sweet & Sour Vegetables with Pork, 17-oz. can	723	138.1	42.5	8.13	450	86.0	
Libby's Mixed Vegetables, 8½-oz. can	(96)	(20.3)	(11.3)	(2.39)	80	17.0	
Drained solids (yield: approx. 5.5 oz.)	(78)	(15.8)	(14.1)	(2.87)	(81)	(16.5)	
16-oz, (1-lb.) can	(181)	(38.2)	(11.3)	(2.39)	80	17.0	
Drained solids (yield: approx. 10.4 oz.)	(147)	(29.8)	(14.1)	(2.87)	(81)	(16.5)	
Stokely Mixed Vegetables, 8-oz. can	125	15.8	15.6	1.97	(132)	(16.6)	
Drained solids (yield: approx. 5.2 oz.)	(108)	(11.6)	(20.8)	(2.23)	(119)	(12.7)	
16-oz. (1-lb.) can	249	31.5	15.6	1.97	(132)	(16.6)	
Drained solids (yield: approx. 10.35 oz.)	(215)	(23.1)	(20.8)	(2.23)	(119)	(12.7)	
Townhouse Mixed Vegetables, 16-oz. (1-lb.)	180	28.0	11.3	1.75	90	14.0	
Drained solids (yield: 10 oz.)	168	23.8	16.8	2.38	108	15.3	
Worthington Veja-Bits, 13-oz. can	201	12.0	15.5	0.92			

2 FRUITS •

	UNIT		1 OZ., BY WT.		1 CUP		Fiber per oz.
	Cal.	Carb.	Cal.	Carb.	Cal.	Carb.	(GMS.)
ACEROLAS (Barbados-cherry or West Indian cherry)							
As purchased [refuse: stones, and stems, approx. 20%]:							
1 acerola (approx. 0.2 oz.)	2	0.4	7.1	1.74	31	7.5	
1 cup (approx. 4.3 oz., 20 acerolas)	31	7.5	7.1	1.74	31	7.5	
1 pound (approx. 76 acerolas)	113	2.78	7.1	1.74	31	7.5	
Edible portion:							
1 acerola (approx. 0.17 oz.)	2	0.4	9.1	2.18	31	7.5	
1 cup (approx. 3.4 oz., 20 acerolas)	31	7.5	9.1	2.18	31	7.5	
1 pound (approx. 94 acerolas) (tr/2g/tr/92%/2mg)	145	34.0	9.1	2.18	31	7.5	
ACEROLA JUICE, see the BEVERAGES chapter							
APPLES							
FRESHLY HARVESTED:							
As purchased [refuse: core and stem, approx. 8%]:							
1 small apple (2½" diameter, approx. 4 oz.)	59	14.9	14.6	3.68			
1 medium-small apple (2¾" diameter, approx. 5.3 oz.)	77	19.5	14.6	3.68			
1 medium-large apple (3" diameter, approx. 6.4 oz.)	93	23.3	14.6	3.68			
1 large apple (3¼" diameter, approx. 8 oz.)	118	29.8	14.6	3.68			
1 pound (approx. 4 small, 3 medium-small, 2.5 medium-large, or 2 large apples)	234	58.8	14.6	3.68			
Edible portion:							
Cored, but not peeled:							
1 small apple (approx. 3.7 oz.)	59	14.9	15.9	4.00			0.28
1 medium-small apple (approx. 4.9 oz.)	77	19.5	15.9	4.00			0.28
1 medium-large apple (approx. 5.8 oz.)	93	23.3	15.9	4.00			0.28
1 large apple (approx. 7.5 oz.)	118	29.8	15.9	4.00			0.28
1 cup, quartered (approx. 4.4 oz.)	70	17.6	15.9	4.00	70	17.6	0.28
1 cup, sliced (approx. 3.9 oz.)	62	15.5	15.9	4.00	62	15.5	0.28
1 pound (approx. 4.3 small, 3.3 medium-small, 2.8 medium-large, or 2.1 large apples) (tr/4g/tr/85%/tr)	254	68.6	15.9	4.00			0.28
Cored and pared:							
1 small apple (approx. 3.5 oz.)	52	13.7	15.0	3.94			0.17
1 medium-small apple (approx. 4.6 oz.)	68	17.9	15.0	3.94			0.17
1 medium-large apple (approx. 5.5 oz.)	82	21.5	15.0	3.94			0.17
1 large apple (approx. 7 oz.)	105	27.5	15.0	3.94			0.17
1 cup, quartered (approx. 4.4 oz.)	66	17.4	15.0	3.94	66	17.4	0.17
1 cup, sliced (approx. 3.9 oz.)	58	15.3	15.0	3.94	58	15.3	0.17
1 pound (approx. 4.6 small, 3.5 medium-small, 2.9 medium-large, or 2.3 large apples) (tr/4g/tr/85%/tr)	240	63.1	15.0	3.94			0.17
STORED:							
As purchased [refuse: core and stem, approx. 8%]:							
1 small apple (2½" diameter, approx. 4 oz.)	63	15.7	15.6	3.86			
1 medium-small apple (2¾" diameter, approx. 5.3 oz.)	83	20.4	15.6	3.86			
1 medium-large apple (3" diameter, approx. 6.4 oz.)	99	24.5	15.6	3.86			
1 large apple (3¼" diameter, approx. 8 oz.)	127	31.3	15.6	3.86			
1 pound (approx. 4 small, 3 medium-small, 2.5 medium-large, or 2 large apples)	250	61.8	15.6	3.86			
Edible portion:							
Cored, but not peeled:							
1 small apple (approx. 3.7 oz.)	63	15.7	17.0	4.19			0.28
1 medium-small apple (approx. 4.9 oz.)	83	20.4	17.0	4.19			0.28
1 medium-large apple (approx. 5.8 oz.)	99	24.5	17.0	4.19			0.28
1 large apple (approx. 7.5 oz.)	127	31.3	17.0	4.19			0.28
1 cup, quartered (approx. 4.3 oz.)	75	18.5	17.0	4.19	75	18.5	0.28
1 cup, sliced (approx. 3.9 oz.)	66	16.3	17.0	4.19	66	16.3	0.28
1 pound (approx. 4.3 small, 3.3 medium-small, 2.8 medium-large, or 2.1 large apples) (tr/4g/tr/84%/tr)	272	67.1	17.0	4.19	66	16.3	0.28
Cored and pared:							
1 small apple (approx. 3.5 oz.)	54	14.2	15.6	4.08			0.17
1 medium-small apple (approx. 4.6 oz.)	71	18.6	15.6	4.08			0.17
1 medium-large apple (approx. 5.5 oz.)	86	22.4	15.6	4.08			0.17
1 large apple (approx. 7 oz.)	109	28.5	15.6	4.08			0.17
1 cup, quartered (approx. 4.4 oz.)	69	18.0	15.6	4.08	69	18.0	0.17
1 cup, sliced (approx. 3.9 oz.)	61	15.8	15.6	4.06	61	15.8	0.17
1 pound (approx. 4.6 small, 3.5 medium-small, 2.9 medium-large, or 2.3 large apples) (tr/4g/tr/85%/tr)	249	65.3	15.6	4.08			0.17

	UNIT Cal.	UNIT Carb.	1 OZ., BY WT. Cal.	1 OZ., BY WT. Carb.	1 CUP Cal.	1 CUP Carb.	Fiber per oz. (GMS.)
AVERAGE OF COMMERCIAL VARIETIES, BOTH FRESHLY HARVESTED AND STORED:							
As purchased [refuse: core and stem, approx. 8%]:							
1 small apple (2½" diameter, approx. 4 oz.)	61	15.3	15.1	3.78			
1 medium-small apple (2¾" diameter, approx. 5.3 oz.)	80	20.0	15.1	3.78			
1 medium-large apple (3" diameter, approx. 6.4 oz.)	96	24.0	15.1	3.78			
1 large apple (3¼" diameter, approx. 8 oz.)	123	30.7	15.1	3.78			
1 pound (approx. 4 small, 3 medium-small, 2.5 medium-large, or 2 large apples)	242	60.5	15.1	3.78			
Edible portion:							
Cored, but not peeled:							
1 small apple (approx. 3.7 oz.)	61	15.3	16.4	4.11			0.28
1 medium-small apple (approx. 4.9 oz.)	80	20.0	16.4	4.11			0.28
1 medium-large apple (approx. 5.8 oz.)	96	24.0	16.4	4.11			0.28
1 large apple (approx. 7.5 oz.)	123	30.7	16.4	4.11			0.28
1 cup, quartered (approx. 4.4 oz.)	73	18.1	16.4	4.11	73	18.1	0.28
1 cup, sliced (approx. 3.9 oz.)	64	16.1	16.4	4.11	64	16.1	0.28
1 pound (approx. 4.3 small, 3.3 medium-small, 2.8 medium-large, or 2.1 large apples) (tr/4g/tr/84%/tr)	263	65.8	16.4	4.11			0.28
Cored and pared:							
1 small apple (approx. 3.5 oz.)	53	13.9	15.3	4.00			0.17
1 medium-small apple (approx. 4.6 oz.)	70	18.2	15.3	4.00			0.17
1 medium-large apple (approx. 5.5 oz.)	84	21.8	15.3	4.00			0.17
1 large apple (approx. 7 oz.)	107	27.9	15.3	4.00			0.17
1 cup, quartered (approx. 4.4 oz.)	68	17.6	15.3	4.00	68	17.6	0.17
1 cup, sliced (approx. 3.9 oz.)	59	15.9	15.3	4.00	59	15.9	0.17
1 pound (approx. 4.6 small, 3.5 medium-small, 2.9 medium-large, or 2.3 large apples) (tr/4g/tr/85%/tr)	245	64.0	15.3	4.00			0.17
FROZEN, based on generic data:							
Sweetened with sugar, sliced:							
1 pound (tr/7g/tr/74%/4mg)	422	110.2	26.4	6.89			0.20
FROZEN, by brand:							
Stouffer's Escalloped Apples, 12-oz. package	420	84.0	35.0	7.00			
DRIED RINGS, based on generic data:							
UNCOOKED:							
1 cup (approx. 3 oz.)	234	61.0	77.9	20.36	234	61.0	0.88
1 container, 8 oz.	624	163.0	77.9	20.36	234	61.0	0.88
1 pound (approx. 5⅓ cups) (tr/20g/tr/24%/1mg)	1247	325.7	77.9	20.36	234	61.0	0.88
COOKED:							
1 pound of dried apples to 5 cups of water:							
Without sugar:							
1 cup (approx. 9 oz.)	199	51.8	22.1	5.76	199	51.8	0.26
1 pound (approx. 1¾ cups) (tr/6g/tr/78%/tr)	354	92.1	22.1	5.76	199	51.8	0.26
With sugar added, 1 cup of sugar per pound of dried apples:							
1 cup (approx. 9.9 oz.)	314	81.8	31.8	8.28	314	81.8	0.23
1 pound (approx. 1⅔ cups) (tr/8g/tr/70%/tr)	508	132.5	31.8	8.28	314	81.8	0.23
DRIED, by brand:							
Del Monte Apples, Uncooked, Evaporated, 8-oz. package	560	148.0	70.0	18.50	(210)	(55.5)	
Fruit Pac Dried Apples, Honey Dipped, 4-oz. package	342	89.5	85.4	22.37			
Grocer's Choice Apple Fruit Roll, 1-oz. package	90	20.0	90.0	20.00			
Sonoma Dried Apples, soft, 4-oz. package	312	81.4	78.0	20.38			
Sun-Maid Selected Dried Apple Chunks for snacking or baking, 6-oz. foil package (equals 3¼ lb. of fresh apples)	450	120.0	75.0	20.00			
DEHYDRATED, based on generic data:							
UNCOOKED:							
1 cup (approx. 3½ oz.)	353	92.1	100.1	26.11	353	92.1	1.08
1 pound (approx. 4½ cups) (1g/20g/tr/3%/2mg)	1601	417.8	100.1	26.11	353	91.1	1.08

	UNIT Cal.	UNIT Carb.	1 OZ., BY WT. Cal.	1 OZ., BY WT. Carb.	1 CUP Cal.	1 CUP Carb.	Fiber per oz. (GMS.)
COOKED:							
1 cup of sugar per pound of dehydrated apples in 9 cups of water:							
1 cup (approx. 9 oz.)	194	50.0	21.6	5.56	194	50.0	0.26
1 pound (approx. 1¾ cups) (tr/6g/tr/80%/tr)	345	88.9	21.6	5.56	194	50.0	0.26
DEHYDRATED, by brand:							
Timber Crest Dehydrated Apples, hard, 5-lb. package	8008	2088.8	100.1	26.11	212	55.3	
Weight Watchers Apple Snack (Dehydrated Apples), ½-oz. foil package	50	13.0	100.0	26.00			
Fruit Snack, Artificially Cinnamon flavored Dehydrated Apples, ½-oz. foil package	50	13.0	100.0	26.00			
Fruit Snack, Artificially Peach flavored Dehydrated Apples, ½-oz. foil package	50	13.0	100.0	26.00			
Fruit Snack, Artificially Strawberry flavored Dehydrated Apples, ½-oz. foil package	50	13.0	100.0	26.00			
APPLESAUCE							
CANNED OR JARRED, based on generic data:							
Unsweetened:							
1 cup (approx. 8⅔ oz.)	100	26.4	11.6	3.06	100	26.4	0.17
1 pound (approx. 1.9 cups) (tr/4g/tr/89%/1mg)	186	49.0	11.6	3.06	100	26.4	0.17
Jar, 7½ oz. net wt. (approx. 9⁄10 cup)	87	23.0	11.6	3.06	100	26.4	0.17
Jar, 15 oz. net wt. (approx. 1¾ cups)	174	45.9	11.6	3.06	100	26.4	0.17
Can, 8Z Tall, Buffet; 8 oz. net wt. (approx. 9⁄10 cup)	93	24.5	11.6	3.06	100	26.4	0.17
Can, #303; 16 oz. (1 lb.) net wt. (approx. 1 9⁄10 cups)	186	49.0	11.6	3.06	100	26.4	0.17
Sugar added:							
1 cup (approx. 9 oz.)	232	60.7	25.8	6.72	232	60.7	0.14
1 pound (approx. 1¾ cups) (tr/4g/tr/76%/1mg)	413	108.0	25.8	6.72	232	60.7	0.14
Jar, 25 oz. (1 lb. 9 oz.) net wt. (approx. 2¾ cups)	645	168.7	25.8	6.72	232	60.7	0.14
Jar, 35 oz. (2 lb. 3 oz.) net wt. (approx. 3.9 cups)	903	236.1	25.8	6.72	232	60.7	0.14
Can, #303; 16½ oz. (1 lb. ½ oz.) net wt. (approx. 1⅘ cups)	426	111.4	25.8	6.72	232	60.7	0.14
Can, #10; 108 oz. (6 lb. 12 oz.) net wt. (approx. 11½ cups)	2786	728.8	25.8	6.72	232	60.7	0.14
CANNED OR JARRED, by brand:							
Additonal applesauces are in the CONDIMENTS chapter.							
Balanced Applesauce Prepared without added sugar or salt, 8-oz. can	90	20.5	11.3	2.56	(97)	(22.0)	
Country Pure Unsweetened Applesauce, 24-oz. package	330	87.0	13.8	3.63	125	32.9	
Del Monte Applesauce, 8½-oz. jar	181	49.9	21.3	5.88	170	47.0	
16-oz. (1-lb.) jar	340	94.0	21.3	5.88	170	47.0	
Diet Delight Unsweetened Applesauce, 15-oz. jar	173	44.9	11.5	3.00	100	26.0	
Featherweight Applesauce, prepared without added sugar or salt, 8-oz. can	100	24.0	12.5	3.00	100	24.0	
16-oz. (1-lb.) can	200	48.0	12.5	3.00	100	24.0	
Lucky Leaf Unsweetened Applesauce, 104-oz. (6 lb. 8 oz.) can	1300	338.0	12.5	3.25	(108)	(28.1)	
Mott's Natural Style Applesauce, 20-oz. jar	226	55.0	(10.4)	(2.55)	90	22.0	
30-oz. jar	339	82.5	(10.4)	(2.55)	90	22.0	
Musselman's Natural Style Applesauce, 16½-oz. jar	(200)	(48.0)	(12.1)	(2.91)	100	24.0	
25-oz. jar	(303)	(72.8)	(12.1)	(2.91)	100	24.0	
Regular Applesauce, 8-oz. jar	(170)	(41.5)	(21.3)	(5.18)	193	47.0	
15-oz. jar	(320)	(77.7)	(21.3)	(5.18)	193	47.0	
P&Q (A&P) Applesauce, 24-oz. jar	645	183.0	26.9	7.63	(241)	(68.7)	
Stokely Applesauce, 8½-oz. jar	170	42.5	20.0	5.00	180	45.0	
17-oz. jar	340	85.0	20.0	5.00	180	45.0	
Town House Gravenstein Applesauce, 16-oz. (1-lb.) jar)	340	94.0	21.3	5.89	193	53.4	

APPLE JUICE, see the BEVERAGES chapter

APRICOTS

	UNIT		1 OZ., BY WT.		1 CUP		Fiber per oz. (GMS.)
	Cal.	Carb.	Cal.	Carb.	Cal.	Carb.	
As purchased [refuse: pits, approx. 6%]:							
1 apricot (approx. 1⅓ oz.)	18	4.5	13.6	3.41			
1 pound (approx. 12 apricots)	217	54.6	13.6	3.41			
Edible portion:							
1 apricot (approx. 1¼ oz.)	18	4.5	14.4	3.63			
1 cup, halved (approx. 5½ oz., 8¾ apricot halves)	79	19.8	14.4	3.63	79	19.8	0.17
1 pound (approx. 2.9 cups, 13 apricots) (tr/4g/tr/85%/tr)	230	58.1	14.4	3.63	79	19.8	0.17
FROZEN, based on generic data:							
Sugar added:							
1 pound (tr/7g/tr/73%/tr)	445	113.9	27.8	7.12	(236)	(60.5)	0.17
FROZEN, by brand:							
Big Valley Individually Quick-Frozen Fresh Peeled Apricot Halves, 20-oz. polybag	244		12.2		(104)		
Thawed, drained (yield: approx. 13 oz.)	(244)		(18.8)		(160)		
CANNED, based on generic data:							
Packed in water, with or without artificial sweetener:							
Solids and Liquid:							
Halved (pits removed):							
1 half apricot with ½ Tbsp. of liquid (approx. 1 oz.)	11	2.7	10.8	2.72	93	23.6	0.11
1 cup (approx. 8⅔ oz.)	93	23.6	10.8	2.72	93	23.6	0.11
1 pound (approx. 1.9 cups) (tr/3g/tr/89%/tr)	172	43.5	10.8	2.72	93	23.6	0.11
Can, 8Z Tall, Buffet; 8 oz. net wt. (contents: 6–12 halves and approx. 5 Tbsp. of drained liquid)	86	21.8	10.8	2.72	93	23.6	0.11
Can, #303, 16 oz. (1 lb.) net wt. (contents: 12–20 halves and approx. 9½ Tbsp. of drained liquid)	172	43.5	10.8	2.72	93	23.6	0.11
Can, #10, 103 oz. (6 lb. 7 oz.) net wt. (contents: 85–108 halves and approx. 4 cups of drained liquid)	1110	280.3	10.8	2.72	93	23.6	0.11
Packed in juice:							
Halved (pits removed), with skin:							
3 apricot halves with 1¾ Tbsp. of drained liquid (approx. 2.9 oz.)	40	10.4	13.6	3.50	119	30.6	0.11
1 cup (approx. 8.7 oz.)	119	30.6	13.6	3.50	119	30.6	0.11
1 pound (approx. 1.8 cups) (tr/4g/tr/87%/tr)	218	56.0	13.6	3.50	119	30.6	0.11
Packed in extra light syrup:							
Halved (pits removed) with skin:							
3 apricot halves with 1¾ Tbsp. of drained liquid (approx. 2.9 oz.)	41	10.5	13.9	3.54	121	30.9	0.11
1 cup (approx. 8.6 oz.)	121	30.9	13.9	3.54	121	30.9	0.11
1 pound (approx. 1.9 cups) (tr/4g/tr/86%/tr)	222	56.8	13.9	3.54	121	30.9	0.11
Packed in light syrup:							
Halved (pits removed):							
1 cup (approx. 9.7 oz.)	181	46.2	18.7	4.76	181	46.2	0.11
1 pound (approx. 1⅔ cups) (tr/5g/tr/82%/tr)	299	76.2	18.7	4.76	181	46.2	0.11
Packed in heavy syrup:							
Whole:							
1 apricot with 1 Tbsp. of liquid (approx. 1.7 oz.)	39	10.0	22.9	5.86	222	56.9	
1 cup [refuse: pits, approx. 6%] (approx. 9.7 oz.)	222	56.9	22.9	5.86	222	56.9	
1 pound [refuse: pits, approx. 6%] (approx. 1⅔ cups) (tr/6g/tr/77%/tr)	367	93.8	22.9	5.86	222	56.9	
Can, #303, 17 oz. (1 lb. 1 oz.) net wt. (contents: 8–14 apricots and approx. 10 Tbsp. of drained liquid) [refuse: pits, approx. 6%]	390	99.7	22.9	5.86	222	56.9	
Drained solids (yield: approx. 12 oz.)	(275)	(69.7)	(22.9)	(5.81)	(174)	(44.3)	
Can, #2½, 30 oz. (1 lb. 14 oz.) net wt. (contents: 15–18 apricots and approx. 18 Tbsp. of drained liquid) [refuse: pits, approx. 6%]	688	176.0	22.9	5.86	222	56.9	
Drained solids (yield: approx. 1 lb. 5 oz.)	(481)	(122.0)	(22.9)	(5.81)	(174)	(44.3)	
Halved (pits removed):							
1 half apricot with ½ Tbsp. liquid (approx. 1 oz.)	24	6.0	24.4	6.24	222	56.8	0.11
1 cup (approx. 9.1 oz.)	222	56.8	24.4	6.24	222	56.8	0.11
1 pound (approx. 1¾ cups)	390	99.8	24.4	6.24	222	56.8	0.11
Can, 8Z Tall, Buffet; 8¾ oz. net wt. (contents: 6–12 halves and approx. 5½ Tbsp. of drained liquid)	213	54.6	24.4	6.24	222	56.8	0.11
Drained solids (yield: approx. 6 oz.)	(153)	(38.1)	(25.0)	(6.34)	(208)	(53.3)	
Can, #303, 17 oz. (1 lb. 1 oz.) net wt. (contents: 12–20 halves and approx. 10⅔ Tbsp. of drained liquid)	415	106.0	24.4	6.24	222	56.8	0.11
Drained solids (yield: approx. 11.7 oz.)	(292)	(74.0)	(25.0)	(6.34)	(208)	(53.3)	
Can, #2½, 30 oz. (1 lb. 14 oz.) net wt. (contents: 26–35 halves and approx. 19 Tbsp. of drained liquid)	732	187.2	24.4	6.24	222	56.8	0.11
Drained solids (yield: approx. 20.5 oz.)	(513)	(130.0)	(25.0)	(6.34)	(208)	(53.3)	
Solids only:							
1 half apricot (approx. ⅔ oz.)	(17)	(4.2)	(25.0)	(6.34)	(208)	(53.3)	
1 cup (approx. 8.3 oz.)	(208)	(53.3)	(25.0)	(6.34)	(208)	(53.3)	
1 pound (approx. 1.9 cups)	(400)	(101.4)	(25.0)	(6.34)	(208)	(53.3)	
Liquid only:							
1 tablespoon	(13)	(3.4)	(23.0)	(6.00)	(209)	(54.6)	
1 cup (approx. 9.1 oz.)	(209)	(54.6)	(23.0)	(6.00)	(209)	(54.6)	
1 pound (approx. 1.8 cups)	(368)	(96.0)	(23.0)	(6.00)	(209)	(54.6)	
Packed in extra heavy syrup:							
Halved (pits removed):							
1 cup (approx. 9.4 oz.)	269	69.3	28.6	7.37	269	69.3	0.11
1 pound (approx. 1.7 cups) (tr/7g/tr/73%/tr)	458	117.9	28.6	7.37	269	69.3	0.11
CANNED, by brand:							
Ann Page (A&P) Unpeeled Apricot Halves, packed in heavy syrup, 8¾-oz. can	220	56.0	25.1	6.40			
16-oz. (1-lb.) can	402	102.4	25.1	6.40			
Balanced Unpeeled Apricot Halves, packed in water, without added sugar or salt, 8-oz. can	89	20.4	11.1	2.55	(96)	(22.1)	
Drained solids (yield: approx. 4.8 oz.)	(66)	(14.2)	(13.4)	(2.89)	(112)	(24.1)	
16-oz. (1-lb.) can	178	40.8	11.1	2.55	(96)	(22.1)	
Drained solids (yield: approx. 9.8 oz.)	(131)	(28.3)	(13.4)	(2.89)	(112)	(24.1)	
Del Monte Unpeeled Apricot Halves, packed in heavy syrup, 8¾-oz. can	206	53.5	23.5	6.11	200	52.0	
Drained solids (yield: approx. 4.5 oz.)	(174)	(45.0)	(38.8)	(10.10)			
17-oz. can	400	(105.0)	23.5	6.11	200	52.0	
Drained solids (yield: approx. 8.7 oz.)	(338)	(88.4)	(38.8)	(10.10)			
Diet Delight Unpeeled Apricot Halves, packed in white grape juice, 8-oz. can	110	27.4	13.7	3.43			
16-oz. (1-lb.) can	219	54.9	13.7	3.43			
Unpeeled Apricot Halves, packed in water, 8-oz. can	70	18.0	8.8	2.25	70	18.0	
16-oz. (1-lb.) can	140	36.0	8.8	2.25	70	18.0	
Featherweight Apricot Halves, packed in juice without added sugar, 8-oz. can	(100)	(24.0)	(12.5)	(3.00)	100	24.0	
16-oz. (1-lb.) can	(200)	(48.0)	(12.5)	(3.00)	100	24.0	
Apricot Halves, packed in water without added sugar, 8-oz. can	(60)	(18.0)	(7.5)	(2.25)	60	18.0	
16-oz. (1-lb.) can	(120)	(36.0)	(7.5)	(2.25)	60	18.0	
Golden Harvest California Unpeeled Apricots in Water, no sugar or salt added, 16-oz. (1-lb.) can	140	36.0	8.8	2.25	70	18.0	
Libby's Apricots, packed in heavy syrup, 8¾-oz. can	(201)	(54.3)	(23.0)	(6.21)	200	54.0	
Drained solids (yield: approx. 5.7 oz.)	(131)	(36.3)	(23.0)	(6.35)	(191)	(52.9)	
16-oz. (1-lb.) can	200	56.0	12.5	3.50	100	28.0	
17-oz. can	(391)	(105.6)	(23.0)	(6.21)	200	54.0	
Drained solids (yield: approx. 11.1 oz.)	(255)	(70.2)	(23.0)	(6.35)	(191)	(52.9)	
Stokely Apricot Halves, 8¾-oz. can	210	51.5	24.0	5.89	220	54.0	
16-oz. (1-lb.) can	384	94.2	24.0	5.89	220	54.0	
Tillie Lewis "Tasti Diet" Apricot Halves Unpeeled, no sugar added, packed in unsweetened fruit juices from concentrates and water, 8-oz. can	100	26.0	12.5	3.25	100	26.0	
16-oz. (1-lb.) can	200	52.0	12.5	3.25	100	26.0	
Town House Apricot Halves, Unpeeled (in heavy syrup), 17-oz.	440	112.0	25.9	6.59	220	56.0	
Boiled, drained (yield: approx. 10½ oz.)	291	66.5	27.7	6.33	231	52.7	

	UNIT Cal.	UNIT Carb.	1 OZ., BY WT. Cal.	1 OZ., BY WT. Carb.	1 CUP Cal.	1 CUP Carb.	Fiber per oz. (GMS.)
DRIED, based on generic data:							
Medium Halves (approx. 1⅓″ diameter):							
UNCOOKED:							
1 medium apricot half (approx. 0.13 oz.)	9	2.3	73.7	18.85	338	86.5	0.85
1 cup (approx. 4.6 oz., 37 medium halves)	338	86.5	73.7	18.85	338	86.5	0.85
1 pound (approx. 3½ cups, 130 medium halves)	1179	301.6	73.7	18.85	338	86.5	0.85
Container, 11 oz. net wt. (approx. 2.4 cups, 90 medium halves)	811	207.5	73.7	18.85	338	86.5	0.85
COOKED without sugar:							
1 cup (approx. 8.8 oz.)	213	54.0	24.1	6.13	213	54.0	0.28
1 pound (approx. 1.8 cups) (tr/6g/tr/76%/2mg)	386	98.0	24.1	6.13	213	54.0	0.28
COOKED, with sugar:							
(1 pound of medium apricot halves cooked in 9 cups of water with 1 cup of sugar)							
1 cup (approx. 9½ oz.)	329	84.8	34.6	8.90	329	84.8	0.26
1 pound (approx. 1⅔ cups) (tr/9g/tr/66%/2mg)	553	142.4	34.6	8.90	329	84.8	0.26
Large Halves (approx. 1½″ diameter):							
UNCOOKED:							
1 large dried apricot half (approx. 0.17 oz.)	13	3.2	73.7	18.85	338	86.5	0.85
1 cup (approx. 4.6 oz., 28 large halves)	338	86.5	73.7	18.85	338	86.5	0.85
1 pound (approx. 3½ cups, 95 large halves) (tr/19g/1g/25%/7mg)	1179	301.6	73.7	18.85	338	86.5	0.85
Container, 11 oz. net wt. (approx. 2.4 cups, 65 large halves)	811	207.5	73.7	18.85	338	86.5	0.85
COOKED:							
1 pound of apricot halves cooked in 5 cups of water:							
Without sugar:							
1 cup (approx. 8.8 oz.)	213	54.0	24.1	6.13	213	54.0	0.28
1 pound (approx. 1.8 cups) (tr/6g/tr/76%/2mg)	386	98.0	24.1	6.13	213	54.0	0.28
With sugar added, 1 cup of sugar per pound of dried apricots:							
1 cup (approx. 9.5 oz.)	329	84.8	34.6	8.90	329	84.8	0.26
1 pound (approx. 1⅔ cups) (tr/9g/tr/66%/2mg)	553	142.4	34.6	8.90	329	84.8	0.26
DRIED, by brand:							
Del Monte Apricots, 6-oz. package	420	105.0	70.0	17.50	(314)	(78.4)	
Cooked, drained (yield: approx. 10.7 oz.)	(420)	(105.0)	(39.3)	(9.81)	(345)	(86.2)	
11-oz. package	770	192.5	70.0	17.50	(314)	(78.4)	
Cooked, drained (yield: approx. 19.7 oz.)	(770)	(192.5)	(39.3)	(9.81)	(345)	(86.2)	
Fruit Pac Dried Apricots, Honey Dipped, 8-oz. package	656	168.1	82.0	21.01	367	94.1	
Grocer's Choice Apricot Fruit Roll, 1-oz. package	90	21.0	90.0	21.00			
Sonoma Dried Apricots, Soft, 8-oz. package	590	150.8	73.7	18.85	330	84.5	
Sun Land California Apricots, 6-oz. package	420	105.0	70.0	17.50	(314)	(78.4)	
Cooked, drained (yield: approx. 10.7 oz.)	(420)	(105.0)	(39.3)	(9.81)	(345)	(86.2)	
Sun-Maid California Sun-Dried Apricots for snacking or baking, 6-oz. foil package (equals 2½ lb. of fresh apricots)	420	105.0	70.0	17.50			
Sunsweet California Apricots, 11-oz. box	770	192.5	70.0	17.50	(314)	(78.4)	
Cooked, Drained (yield: approx. 19.7 oz.)	(770)	(192.5)	(39.3)	(9.81)	(345)	(86.2)	
DEHYDRATED, based on generic data:							
Nugget-Type and Pieces:							
UNCOOKED:							
1 cup (approx. 3½ oz.)	332	84.6	94.1	23.98	332	84.6	1.08
1 pound (approx. 4½ cups) (2g/24g/tr/4%/9mg)	1506	383.7	94.1	23.98	332	84.6	1.08
COOKED:							
1 pound of dehydrated apricots cooked in 9 cups of water with 1 cup of sugar:							
1 cup (approx. 10½ oz.)	337	91.5	33.8	8.64	337	91.5	0.26
1 pound (approx. 1½ cups) (tr/9g/tr/67%/2mg)	540	138.3	33.8	8.64	337	91.5	0.26

	UNIT Cal.	UNIT Carb.	1 OZ., BY WT. Cal.	1 OZ., BY WT. Carb.	1 CUP Cal.	1 CUP Carb.	Fiber per oz. (GMS.)
DEHYDRATED, by brand:							
Timber Crest Dehydrated Apricots, 5-lb. package	7528	1919.2	94.1	23.99	445	113.4	
APRICOT NECTAR, see the BEVERAGES chapter							
AVOCADO							
For more complete information, see AVOCADO in the VEGETABLES chapter							
California Grown							
Primarily Fuerte, marketed in midwinter and late winter							
As purchased [refuse: seed and skin, approx. 24%]:							
1 avocado (approx. 10 oz., 3⅓″ diameter)	369	12.9	36.9	1.30			
1 pound (approx. 1⅔ avocados)	590	20.8	36.9	1.30			
Florida Grown							
Marketed in late summer and fall							
As purchased [refuse: seed and skin, approx. 33%]:							
1 avocado (approx. 16 oz., 3⅝″ diameter)	389	26.7	24.3	1.67			
1 pound (approx. 1 avocado)	389	26.7	24.3	1.67			
BANANAS							
COMMON BANANAS							
As purchased [refuse: skin, approx. 32%. Percent of refuse, dimensions and weight will vary widely]:							
1 small banana (approx. 4.9 oz., 7¾″ long along outer curvature, 1¹¹⁄₃₂″ diameter, highly variable)	81	21.1	16.4	4.28			
1 medium banana (approx. 6.2 oz., 8¾″ long along outer curvature, 1¹³⁄₃₂″ diameter, highly variable)	101	26.4	16.4	4.28			
1 large banana (approx. 7.1 oz., 9¾″ long along outer curvature, 1⁷⁄₁₆″ diameter, highly variable)	116	30.2	16.4	4.28			
1 pound (approx. 3¼ small, 2⅔ medium or 2¼ large bananas)	262	68.5	16.4	4.28			
Edible portion:							
1 small banana (approx. 3.3 oz.) (tr/6g/tr/76%/tr)	81	21.1	24.1	6.29	128	33.3	0.14
1 medium banana (approx. 4.2 oz.)	101	26.4	24.1	6.29	128	33.3	0.14
1 large banana (approx. 4.8 oz.)	116	30.2	24.1	6.29	128	33.3	0.14
1 cup:							
Sliced or chunks (approx. 1.6 small, 1¼ medium or 1.1 large bananas) (approx. 5.3 oz.)	128	33.3	24.1	6.29	128	33.3	0.14
Mashed (approx. 2.4 small, 1.9 medium or 1⅔ large bananas) (approx. 7.9 oz.)	191	50.0	24.1	6.29	191	50.0	0.14
1 pound (approx. 4¾ small, 3.8 medium, or 3⅓ large bananas)	386	100.6	24.1	6.29	128	33.3	0.14
By brand:							
Dole, 7″ banana As purchased, approx. 4.7 oz.	77	20.1	(16.4)	(4.27)			
Edible portion, approx. 3 oz. (approx. ⅔ cups, sliced)	77	20.1	24.1	6.28	114	29.7	
DRIED (based on data from France):							
1 pound	1325	299.4	82.8	18.70			
DEHYDRATED BANANA FLAKES, based on generic data:							
1 tablespoon (approx. 2 oz.)	21	5.5	96.0	25.10	340	88.6	0.57
1 cup (approx. 3½ oz.)	340	88.6	96.0	25.10	340	88.6	0.57
1 pound (approx. 4½ cups)	1536	401.6	96.0	25.10	340	88.6	0.57
BANANA FLOUR (based on data from France):							
1 pound	1551	366.5	97.0	22.90			0.71
PLANTAIN, see the VEGETABLES chapter							
RED BANANAS							
Data based on Red Bananas of "fair" quality.							
As purchased [refuse: skin, approx. 32%. Percent of refuse, dimensions and weight, will vary widely]							
1 banana (approx. 6.8 oz.)	118	30.7	17.3	4.51			

	UNIT Cal.	UNIT Carb.	1 OZ., BY WT. Cal.	1 OZ., BY WT. Carb.	1 CUP Cal.	1 CUP Carb.	Fiber per oz. (GMS.)
1 pound (approx. 2⅓ medium red bananas)	277	72.2	17.3	4.51			
Edible portion:							
1 red banana (approx. 4.6 oz.)	118	30.7	25.5	6.62	135	35.1	0.11
1 cup, sliced or chunks (approx. 1.1 red bananas, 5.3 oz.)	135	35.1	25.5	6.62	135	35.1	0.11
1 pound (approx. 3½ red bananas) (tr/7g/tr/74%/tr)	408	106.1	25.5	6.62	135	35.1	0.11

BARBADOS-CHERRY, see ACEROLAS

BLACKBERRIES

	UNIT Cal.	UNIT Carb.	1 OZ., BY WT. Cal.	1 OZ., BY WT. Carb.	1 CUP Cal.	1 CUP Carb.	Fiber per oz. (GMS.)
As purchased [refuse: caps and damaged berries, approx. 5%]:							
1 pound (approx. 305 berries)	251	55.6	15.7	3.48	84	18.6	
Edible portion:							
1 berry (approx. 0.05 oz.)	1	0.2	16.5	3.66	84	18.6	1.16
1 cup (approx. 5 oz., 100 berries)	84	18.6	16.5	3.66	84	18.6	1.16
1 pound (approx. 3.2 cups, 320 berries) (tr/4g/tr/85%/tr)	267	58.6	16.5	3.66	84	18.6	1.16
FROZEN, based on generic data:							
Unsweetened:							
1 cup (approx. 4.4 oz.)	60	14.4	13.6	3.23	60	14.4	0.77
1 pound (approx. 3.6 cups) (tr/3g/tr/87%/tr)	218	51.7	13.6	3.23	60	14.4	0.77
Container, 10 oz. net (approx. 2¼ cups)	136	32.4	13.6	3.23	60	14.4	0.77
Sweetened with sugar:							
1 cup (approx. 5 oz.)	137	34.9	27.2	6.90	137	34.9	0.51
1 pound (approx. 3.2 cups) (tr/7g/tr/74%/tr)	435	110.7	27.2	6.90	137	34.9	0.51
Container, 10 oz. net wt. (approx. 2 cups)	273	69.3	27.2	6.90	137	34.9	0.51
CANNED, based on generic data:							
Solids and liquid:							
Packed in water, with or without artificial sweetener:							
1 cup (approx. 8⅔ oz.)	98	22.0	11.3	2.55	98	22.0	0.79
1 pound (approx. 1.9 cups) (tr/3g/tr/89%/tr)	181	40.8	11.3	2.55	98	22.0	0.79
Packed in juice:							
1 pound (tr/3g/tr/86%/tr)	245	54.9	15.3	3.43	(133)	(29.7)	0.77
Packed in light syrup:							
1 cup (approx. 8¾ oz.)	179	43.0	20.4	4.91	179	43.0	0.77
1 pound (approx. 1.8 cups) (tr/5g/tr/81%/tr)	327	78.5	20.4	4.91	179	43.0	0.77
Packed in heavy syrup:							
1 cup (approx. 9 oz.)	233	56.8	25.8	6.29	233	56.8	0.73
1 pound (approx. 1¾ cups) (tr/6g/tr/76%/tr)	413	100.7	25.8	6.29	233	56.8	0.73
Can, #303, 16 oz. (1 lb.) net wt.	413	100.7	25.8	6.29	233	56.8	0.73
Packed in extra heavy syrup:							
1 cup (approx. 9⅓ oz.)	291	71.7	31.2	7.68	291	71.7	0.73
1 pound (approx. 1.7 cups) (tr/8g/tr/71%/tr)	499	122.9	31.2	7.68	291	71.7	0.73
CANNED, by brand:							
Oregon Blackberries, packed in heavy syrup, 17-oz. can	404	101.0	23.8	5.95	(218)	(54.5)	
Drained solids (yield: approx. 9 oz.)	(220)	(53.0)	(24.4)	(5.89)	(151)	(36.4)	

BLUEBERRIES

	UNIT Cal.	UNIT Carb.	1 OZ., BY WT. Cal.	1 OZ., BY WT. Carb.	1 CUP Cal.	1 CUP Carb.	Fiber per oz. (GMS.)
As purchased [refuse: stems and soft or withered berries, approx. 8%]:							
1 pound (approx. 295 berries)	259	63.8	16.2	3.99	81	19.9	
Edible portion:							
1 berry (approx. 0.05 oz.)	1	0.2	17.6	4.34	90	22.2	0.43
1 cup (approx. 5 oz. berries)	90	22.2	17.6	4.34	90	22.2	0.43
1 pound (approx. 3.2 cups, 320 berries) (tr/4g/tr/83%/tr)	281	69.4	17.6	4.34	90	22.2	0.43
1-pint container, filled to overflowing (approx. 14½ oz. net wt.)	254	62.7	17.6	4.34	90	22.2	0.43
FROZEN, based on generic data:							
Unsweetened:							
1 cup thawed (approx. 5.8 oz.)	91	22.4	15.6	3.90	91	22.4	0.43
Container, 10 oz. net wt. (approx. 1¾ cups)	156	38.6	15.6	3.90	91	22.4	0.43
1 pound (approx. 2¾ cups) (tr/4g/tr/85%/tr)	249	61.7	15.6	3.90	91	22.4	0.43
Sweetened with sugar:							
1 cup (approx. 8.1 oz.)	242	61.0	29.8	7.50	242	61.0	0.26
Container, 10 oz. net wt. (approx. 1¼ cups)	298	74.3	29.8	7.50	242	61.0	0.26
1 pound (approx. 2 cups) (tr/8g/tr/72%/tr)	476	120.2	29.8	7.50	242	61.0	0.26
CANNED, based on generic data:							
Solids and liquid:							
Packed in water, with or without artificial sweetener:							
1 cup (approx. 8.8 oz.)	(98)	(24.5)	11.1	2.78	(98)	(24.5)	0.29
1 pound (approx. 1.8 cups) (tr/3g/tr/89%/tr)	177	44.5	11.1	2.78	(98)	(24.5)	0.29
Packed in heavy syrup:							
1 cup (approx. 9 oz.)	225	56.5	25.0	6.26	225	56.5	0.26
1 pound (approx. 1.8 cups) (tr/6g/tr/77%/tr)	400	100.2	25.0	6.26	225	56.5	0.26
Packed in extra heavy syrup:							
1 cup (approx. 8.8 oz.)	257	66.3	28.6	7.37	257	66.3	
1 pound (approx. 1.8 cups) (tr/8g/tr/73%/tr)	458	117.9	28.6	7.37	(252)	(65.0)	
For comparison: Blueberry Yogurt, **Knudsen** Fruit-On-The-Bottom, low-fat, 8-oz. container	270	49.0	33.8	6.13	314	57.0	

BOYSENBERRIES

	UNIT Cal.	UNIT Carb.	1 OZ., BY WT. Cal.	1 OZ., BY WT. Carb.	1 CUP Cal.	1 CUP Carb.	Fiber per oz. (GMS.)
FROZEN, based on generic data:							
Unsweetened:							
1 cup (approx. 4.4 oz.)	60	14.4	13.6	3.23	60	14.4	0.77
1 pound (approx. 3.6 cups) (tr/3g/tr/87%/tr)	218	51.4	13.6	3.23	60	14.4	0.77
Container, 10 oz. net wt. (approx. 2⅓ cups)	136	32.4	13.6	3.23	60	14.4	0.77
Sweetened with sugar:							
1 cup (approx. 5 oz.)	137	34.9	27.2	6.90	137	34.9	0.51
1 pound (approx. 3.2 cups) (tr/7g/tr/74%/tr)	435	110.7	27.2	6.90	137	34.9	0.51
Container, 10 oz. net wt. (approx. 2 cups)	273	69.3	27.2	6.90	137	34.9	0.51
CANNED, based on generic data:							
Solids and liquid:							
Packed in water, with or without artificial sweetener:							
1 cup (approx. 8.6 oz.)	88	22.2	10.2	2.58	88	22.2	0.54
1 pound (approx. 1.9 cups) (tr/3g/tr/90%/tr)	163	41.3	10.2	2.58	88	22.2	0.54
Packed in heavy syrup:							
1 cup (approx. 9 oz.)	225	57.1	25.0	6.33	225	57.1	0.54
1 pound (approx. 1.8 cups) (tr/6g/tr/76%/tr)	400	101.3	25.0	6.33	225	57.1	0.54
CANNED, by brand:							
Oregon Boysenberries, packed in heavy syrup, 17-oz. can	404	101.0	23.8	5.94	(204)	(50.9)	
Drained solids (yield: approx. 10.5 oz.)	(254)	(62.0)	(24.2)	(5.90)	(186)	(45.4)	

BREADFRUIT, see the VEGETABLES chapter

BULLOCKS-HEART, see CUSTARD-APPLES

CACTUS FRUIT (based on data from Hawaii)

	UNIT Cal.	UNIT Carb.	1 OZ., BY WT. Cal.	1 OZ., BY WT. Carb.	1 CUP Cal.	1 CUP Carb.	Fiber per oz. (GMS.)
As purchased [refuse: skin, stem, and bud ends, approx. 5%]:							
1 medium cactus fruit (3½″ diameter, approx. 5.3 oz.)	76	19.7	14.3	3.71			
1 pound (approx. 3 medium cactus fruits)	229	59.4	14.3	3.71			
Edible portion:							
1 medium cactus fruit (approx. 5.0 oz.)	76	19.7	15.0	3.90			
1 pound (approx. 3.2 medium cactus fruits)	240	62.4	15.0	3.90			

CANTALOUPE

	UNIT Cal.	UNIT Carb.	1 OZ., BY WT. Cal.	1 OZ., BY WT. Carb.	1 CUP Cal.	1 CUP Carb.	Fiber per oz. (GMS.)
As purchased [refuse: rind and cavity contents, approx. 50%]:							
1 medium cantaloupe (approx. 5″ diameter, approx. 2⅓ lb.)	159	39.8	4.3	1.07			

	UNIT		1 OZ., BY WT.		1 CUP		Fiber per oz.
	Cal.	Carb.	Cal.	Carb.	Cal.	Carb.	(GMS.)
1 half of a medium cantaloupe (weighed with rind, approx. 16.8 oz.) [refuse: rind, approx. 43%]	82	20.4	4.9	1.21			
Edible portion:							
1 medium cantaloupe (approx. 1 lb. 2 oz.)	159	39.8	8.5	2.13			
Cubed, diced, or cut into melon balls:							
1 melon ball (approx. 0.3 oz.)	2	0.6	8.5	2.13	48	12.0	0.09
1 cup (approx. 5.6 oz., 20 melon balls)	48	12.0	8.5	2.13	48	12.0	0.09
1 pound (approx. 2.8 cups, 56 melon balls)	136	34.0	8.5	2.13	48	12.0	0.09
FROZEN, based on generic data:							
In syrup, solids and liquid:							
1 cup (approx. 8.1 oz.)	143	36.1	17.6	4.40	143	36.1	0.09
1 pound (approx. 2 cups)	281	71.2	17.6	4.40	143	36.1	0.09
FROZEN, by brand:							
Big Valley Sliced Cantaloupe Melon Chunks, 20-oz. polybag	178		8.9		(65)		0.09
1 cup (approx. 7.3 oz.)	(65)		8.9		(65)		0.09
1 pound (approx. 2.2 cups)	142		8.9		(65)		0.09
Seabrook Cantaloupe Balls, 16-oz. (1-lb.) polybag	155	34.7	9.7	2.17	(71)	(15.8)	0.09
1 cup (approx. 7.3 oz.)	(71)	(15.8)	9.7	2.17	(71)	(15.8)	0.09
CAPE-GOOSEBERRIES, see GROUNDCHERRIES and POHA							
CARAMBOLA (Starfruit)							
SMALL:							
As purchased [refuse: skin and seeds, approx. 19%]:							
1 small carambola (approx. 2½ oz.)	20	4.5	8.1	1.82			
1 pound (approx. 6½ small carambolas)	128	28.8	8.1	1.82			
Edible portion:							
1 small carambola (approx. 2 oz.)	20	4.5	10.0	2.25			0.26
1 pound (approx. 8 small carambolas) (tr/2g/tr/90%/1mg)	160	36.0	10.0	2.25			0.26
MEDIUM (based on data from Hawaii):							
As purchased [refuse: skin and seeds, approx. 19%]:							
1 medium carambola (approx. 8.4 oz.)	71	14.5	8.5	1.73			
1 pound (approx. 1.9 medium carambolas)	136	27.7	8.5	1.73			
Edible portion:							
1 medium carambola (approx. 6.8 oz.)	71	14.5	10.4	2.13			
1 pound (approx. 2.4 medium carambolas) (tr/2g/tr/90%/na)	166	34.1	10.4	2.13			
CARISSA (Natalplum)							
SMALL:							
As purchased [refuse: skin and seeds, approx. 14%]:							
1 small carissa (approx. ⅘ oz.)	14	3.2	17.3	3.94			
1 pound (approx. 19¾ small carissas)	277	63.0	17.3	3.94			
Edible portion:							
1 cup, sliced to ⅛" thick (approx. 5.3 oz.)	105	24.0	20.1	4.59	105	24.0	0.26
1 pound (approx. 23 small carissas) (tr/5g/tr/82%/na)	322	73.4	20.1	4.59	105	24.0	0.26
CASABA MELON (Golden Beauty Melon)							
As purchased [refuse: rind and cavity contents, approx. 50%]:							
1 medium casaba melon (approx. 6½" diameter, 7¾" long, 6 lb.)	367	88.5	3.8	0.92			
1 wedge, ⅒ of a 6-lb. melon (approx. 7¾" long, 2" wide at center, 9.6 oz. weighed with rind) [refuse: rind, approx. 43%]	38	9.1	4.4	1.05			

	UNIT		1 OZ., BY WT.		1 CUP		Fiber per oz.
	Cal.	Carb.	Cal.	Carb.	Cal.	Carb.	(GMS.)
Edible portion:							
1 medium casaba melon (approx. 3 lb.)	367	88.5	7.6	1.84	46	11.1	0.14
1 cup (approx. 6 oz.)	46	11.1	7.6	1.84	46	11.1	0.14
1 pound (approx. 2.7 cups) (tr/2g/tr/92%/3mg)	122	29.5	7.6	1.84	46	11.1	0.14
CHERIMOYA							
As purchased [refuse: skin and seeds, approx. 42%]:							
1 medium cherimoya (approx. 1.9 lb.)	459	117.2	15.4	3.94			
1 pound (approx. 3⅞" high, 5" diameter)	246	63.0	15.4	3.94			
Edible portion:							
1 medium cherimoya (approx. 1.1 lb.)	459	117.2	26.6	6.79			0.62
1 pound (tr/7g/tr/74%/na)	426	108.6	26.6	6.79			0.62
CHERRIES							
SOUR, RED CHERRIES							
As purchased [refuse: pits and stems, approx. 10%]:							
1 cherry (approx. 0.27 oz.)	4	0.9	14.8	3.65	60	14.7	
1 cup (approx. 4 oz., 15 cherries)	60	14.7	14.8	3.65	60	14.7	
1 pound (approx. 4 cups, 60½ cherries)	237	58.4	14.8	3.65	60	14.7	
1-quart container, filled to overflowing (approx. 27¾ oz., 105 cherries)	411	101.3	14.8	3.65	60	14.7	
Edible portion:							
1 cherry (approx. 0.24 oz.)	4	1.0	16.4	4.05	90	22.2	0.06
1 cup (approx. 4.9 oz., 20¾ cherries)	90	22.2	16.4	4.05	90	22.2	0.06
1 pound (approx. 2.9 cups, 64 cherries) (tr/4g/tr/84%/1mg)	263	64.9	16.4	4.05	90	22.2	0.06
FROZEN, based on generic data:							
Measured when frozen:							
Unsweetened:							
1 cup (approx. 9.1 oz.)	142	34.6	15.6	3.80	142	34.6	0.09
1 pound (approx. 1¾ cups)	249	60.8	15.6	3.80	142	34.6	0.09
Sugar added:							
1 cup (approx. 9.1 oz.)	289	71.0	31.8	7.80	289	71.0	0.06
1 pound (approx. 1¾ cups) (tr/8g/tr/71%/1mg)	508	126.1	31.8	7.90	289	71.0	0.06
FROZEN, by brand:							
Big Valley Pitted Sweet Cherries, 20-oz. polybag	397		19.9		(147)		
Thawed, drained (yield: approx. 14 oz.)	(397)		(28.4)		(210)		
CANNED, based on generic data:							
Packed in water, with or without artificial sweetener:							
Pits removed:							
1 cup (approx. 8.6 oz.)	105	26.1	12.2	3.03	105	26.1	0.03
1 pound (approx. 1.9 cups) (tr/3g/tr/88%/1mg)	195	48.5	12.2	3.03	105	26.1	0.03
Can, #303, 16 oz. (1 lb.) net wt. (contents: approx. 1¾ cups of drained solids and 9½ Tbsp. of drained liquid)	195	48.5	12.2	3.03	105	26.1	0.03
Can, #10, 103 oz. (6 lb. 7 oz.) net wt. (contents: approx. 11¼ cups of drained solids and 3¾ cups of drained liquid)	1256	312.4	12.2	3.03	105	26.1	0.03
Packed in light syrup:							
Pits removed:							
1 cup (approx. 8.8 oz.)	189	48.6	21.3	5.48	189	48.6	0.03
1 pound (approx. 1.8 cups) (tr/5g/tr/80%/2mg)	341	87.6	21.3	5.48	189	48.6	0.03
Packed in heavy syrup:							
Pits removed:							
1 cup (approx. 9 oz.)	232	59.6	25.8	6.60	232	59.6	0.03
1 pound (approx. 1.8) (tr/7g/tr/76%/2mg)	413	105.6	25.8	6.60	232	59.6	0.03
Packed in extra heavy syrup:							
Pits removed:							
1 cup (approx. 9.1 oz.)	297	76.3	32.3	8.29	297	76.3	0.03
1 pound (approx. 1.8 cups) (tr/8g/tr/87%/tr)	518	132.7	32.3	8.29	297	76.3	0.03

	UNIT		1 OZ., BY WT.		1 CUP		Fiber per oz.
	Cal.	Carb.	Cal.	Carb.	Cal.	Carb.	(GMS.)
SWEET CHERRIES (light or dark)							
As purchased [refuse: pits and stems, approx. 10%]:							
1 cherry (approx. 0.27 oz.)	5	1.1	17.9	4.43	82	20.4	
1 cup (approx. 4.6 oz., 17⅓ cherries)	82	20.4	17.9	4.43	82	20.4	
1 pound (approx. 3.5 cups, 60½ cherries)	286	71.0	17.9	4.43	82	20.4	
Edible portion:							
1 cherry (approx. 0.24 oz.)	5	1.2	19.9	4.93	102	25.2	0.11
1 cup (approx. 4.6 oz., 19⅓ cherries)	102	25.2	19.9	4.93	102	25.2	0.11
1 pound (approx. 3.5 cups, 67 cherries) (tr/5g/tr/80%/1mg)	318	78.9	19.9	4.93	102	25.2	0.11
CANNED, based on generic data:							
Packed in water, with or without artificial sweetener:							
With pits:							
1 cup (approx. 9.8 oz.)	208	52.7	21.1	5.34	208	52.7	0.09
1 pound (approx. 1⅗ cups)	338	85.5	21.1	5.34	208	52.7	0.09
Can, #8Z Tall, Buffet; 8¾ oz. net wt. (contents: approx. ¾ cup of drained solids and 5 Tbsp. of drained liquid)	185	46.8	21.1	5.34	208	52.7	0.09
Can, #303, 16 oz. (1 lb.) net wt. (contents: approx. 1⅓ cups of drained solids and 9 Tbsp. of drained liquid)	338	85.5	21.1	5.34	208	52.7	0.09
Can, #10, 108 oz. (6 lb. 12 oz.) net wt. (contents: approx. 9 cups of drained solids and 3⅔ cups of drained liquid)	2282	577.5	21.1	5.34	208	52.7	0.09
Pits Removed:							
1 cup (approx. 9.1 oz.)	208	52.7	22.9	5.81	208	52.7	0.09
1 pound (approx. 1.7 cups) (tr/5g/tr/87%/tr)	367	93.0	22.9	5.81	208	52.7	0.09
Can, #303, 16 oz. (1 lb.) net wt. (contents: approx. 1⅓ cups of drained solids and 9⅔ Tbsp. of drained liquid)	367	93.0	22.9	5.81	208	52.7	0.09
Packed in juice:							
Pits removed:							
1 cup (approx. 8.8 oz.)	136	34.5	15.3	3.92	136	34.5	0.06
1 pound (approx. 1.8 cups) (tr/4g/tr/85%/1mg)	245	62.7	15.3	3.92	136	34.5	0.06
Packed in light syrup:							
With pits [refuse: pits, approx. 8%]:							
1 cup (approx. 9.6 oz.)	168	42.6	17.5	4.44	168	42.6	0.09
1 pound (approx. 1.7 cups)	280	71.1	17.5	4.44	168	42.6	0.09
Pits removed:							
1 cup (approx. 8.8 oz.)	163	41.2	18.4	4.68	163	41.2	0.09
1 pound (approx. 1.8 cups) (tr/5g/tr/82%/tr)	295	74.8	18.4	4.68	163	41.2	0.09
Packed in heavy syrup:							
With pits [refuse: pits, approx. 8%]:							
1 cup (approx. 9.6 oz.)	209	53.0	21.8	5.52	209	53.0	0.09
1 pound (approx. 1.7 cups)	349	88.3	21.8	5.52	209	53.0	0.09
Pits removed:							
1 cup (approx. 9.1 oz.)	208	52.9	22.9	5.81	208	52.9	0.09
1 pound (approx. 1¾ cups) (tr/6g/tr/78%/tr)	367	93.0	22.9	5.81	208	52.9	0.09
Packed in extra heavy syrup:							
With pits [refuse: pits, approx. 8%]:							
1 cup (approx. 10.1 oz.)	272	69.1	26.9	6.89	272	69.1	0.09
1 pound (approx. 1.6 cups)	431	110.3	26.9	6.89	272	69.1	0.09
Pits removed:							
1 cup (approx. 9.3 oz.)	264	67.5	28.4	7.26	264	67.5	0.09
1 pound (approx. 1.9 cups) (tr/7g/tr/72%/tr)	454	116.1	28.4	7.26	264	67.5	0.09
CANNED, by brand:							
Balanced Dark Sweet Cherries, packed in water, without added sugar or salt, 8-oz. can	(118)	(29.4)	(14.7)	(3.68)	140	35.0	
Royal Anne Cherries, packed in water, without added sugar or salt, 16-oz. (1-lb.) can	200	50.4	12.5	3.15	(115)	28.9)	
Blue Tag Dark Sweet Cherries, Unpitted, packed in water, 16-oz. (1-lb.) can	280	70.0	17.5	4.38	(140)	(35.0)	
Dark Sweet Cherries, Pitted, packed in water, 16-oz. (1-lb.) can	280	70.0	17.5	4.38	(140)	35.0	
Dark Sweet Cherries, 16-oz. (1-lb.) can	280	70.0	17.5	4.38	140	35.0	
Fancy Dark Sweet Cherries, 16-oz. (1-lb.) can	280	70.0	17.5	4.38	140	35.0	
Fancy Royal Anne Cherries, 16-oz. (1-lb.) can	280	70.0	17.5	4.38	140	35.0	
Royal Anne Cherries, Unpitted, packed in water, 16-oz. (1-lb.) can	280	70.0	17.5	4.38	(140)	(35.0)	
Del Monte Dark Sweet Cherries with Pits, 17-oz. can	360	96.0	21.2	5.65	180	48.0	
Light Sweet Royal Anne Cherries with Pits, 17-oz. can	380	100.0	22.4	5.88	190	50.0	
Diet Delight Light Sweet Royal Anne Cherries, packed in water, 8-oz. can	120	34.0	15.0	4.25	(120)	(34.0)	
Featherweight Dark Cherries, Pitted, packed in water, with no sugar added, 16-oz. (1-lb.) can	(228)	(52.0)	(14.3)	(3.25)	114	26.0	
Light Cherries, Pitted, packed in water, with no sugar added, 16-oz. (1-lb.) can	(192)	(44.0)	(12.0)	(2.75)	96	22.0	
Libby's Dark Sweet Cherries, packed in heavy syrup, 8¾-oz. can	(206)	(54.6)	(23.5)	(6.24)	200	53.0	
Drained solids (yield: approx. 4.5 oz.)	(108)	(29.1)	(24.0)	(6.47)	(162)	(43.6)	
17-oz. can	400	106.0	(23.5)	(6.24)	200	53.0	
Drained solids (yield: approx. 8.7 oz.)	(209)	(56.3)	(24.0)	(6.47)	(162)	(43.6)	
Light Sweet Cherries, packed in heavy syrup, 8¾-oz. can	(206)	(54.6)	(23.5)	(6.24)	200	53.0	
17-oz. can	400	106.0	(23.5)	(6.24)	200	53.0	
Oregon Dark Sweet Cherries, Unpitted, packed in heavy syrup, 16-oz. (1-lb.) can	(380)	(95.0)	(23.8)	(5.94)	(202)	(50.5)	
Drained solids (yield: approx. 9.3 oz.)	(226)	(54.8)	(24.3)	(5.89)	(164)	(39.7)	
Dark Sweet Bing Cherries, Pitted, packed in heavy syrup, 16½-oz. can	392	98.0	23.8	5.94	(202)	(50.5)	
Drained solids (yield: approx. 9.6 oz.)	(233)	(56.6)	(24.3)	(5.90)	(154)	(37.5)	
Royal Anne Cherries, Pitted, packed in heavy syrup, 16-oz. (1-lb.) can	380	95.0	23.8	5.94	(202)	(50.5)	
Drained solids (yield: approx. 9.3 oz.)	(226)	(54.8)	(24.3)	(5.89)	(154)	(37.4)	
Red Tag Dark Sweet Cherries, Unpitted, packed in heavy syrup, 16-oz. (1-lb.) can	(460)	(112.0)	(28.8)	(7.00)	230	56.0	
Drained solids (yield: approx. 8.2 oz.)	(226)	(49.6)	(27.6)	(6.05)	(185)	(40.5)	
Stokely Red Sour Pitted Cherries, packed in water, 16-oz. (1-lb.) can	(170)	(39.9)	(10.6)	(2.49)	90	21.0	
Tillie Lewis "Tasti Diet" Light Sweet Cherries, Unpitted, packed in fruit juices with no sugar added, 8-oz. can	120	30.0	15.0	3.75	120	30.0	
DRIED, by brand:							
Grocer's Choice Cherry Fruit Roll, 1-oz. package	90	20.0	90.0	20.00			
CANDIED, based on generic data:							
1 cup (approx. 5.3 oz.)	511	130.7	96.0	24.60	511	130.7	0.14
1 pound (approx. 3 cups, 130 cherries) (tr/25g/tr/12%/na)	1536	393.6	96.0	24.60	511	130.7	0.14
1 cherry (approx. 0.12 oz.)	12	3.0	96.0	24.60	511	130.7	0.14
MARASCHINO (Bottled), based on generic data:							
Solids and liquid:							
1 cup (approx. 10.7 oz.)	352	89.2	32.9	8.34	352	89.2	0.09
1 pound (approx. 1.5 cups (tr/33g/tr/70%/na)	526	133.4	32.9	8.34	352	89.2	0.09
Drained:							
1 medium maraschino cherry (approx. 0.2 oz.)	(6)	(1.4)	32.9	8.34			

CHINESE DATE, see JUJUBE

CHINESE GOOSEBERRIES, see KIWIFRUIT

CITRON

	UNIT Cal.	UNIT Carb.	1 OZ. Cal.	1 OZ. Carb.	1 CUP Cal.	1 CUP Carb.	Fiber
Edible portion (based on data from Latin America):							
1 pound	181	46.3	11.3	2.89			

	UNIT		1 OZ., BY WT.		1 CUP		Fiber per oz. (GMS.)
	Cal.	Carb.	Cal.	Carb.	Cal.	Carb.	
CANDIED, based on generic data:							
1 tablespoon (approx. ⅓ oz.)	33	8.4	89.0	22.70	525	133.9	0.40
1 cup (approx. 5.9 oz.)	525	133.9	89.0	22.70	525	133.9	0.40
1 pound (approx. 2.7 cups) (tr/23g/tr/18%/82mg)	1424	363.2	89.0	22.70	525	133.9	0.40
COCONUTS							
As purchased: [refuse: shell, brown skin, and water, approx. 48%]:							
1 medium coconut (approx. 4⅝" diameter, 4⅞" high, 1⅔ lb.)	1373	37.3	51.5	1.40			
1 pound	816	22.2	51.5	1.40			
Edible portion:							
1 medium coconut (approx. 14 oz.)	1373	37.3	98.1	2.66			1.14
1 piece, approx. 2" x 2" x ½" (approx. 1.6 oz)	156	4.2	98.1	2.66			1.14
1 pound (1g/3g/10g/51%/7mg)	1569	42.6	98.1	2.66			1.14
1 cup, shredded or grated:							
Not packed (approx. 2.8 oz.)	277	7.5	98.1	2.66	277	7.5	1.14
Packed (approx. 4.6 oz.)	450	12.2	98.1	2.66	450	12.2	1.14
1 pound (approx. 5.7 cups not packed, or 3.5 cups packed)	1569	42.6	98.1	2.66			1.14
DRIED, based on generic data:							
Unsweetened, shredded:							
1 pound (2g/7g/18g/4%/na)	3003	104.3	187.7	6.52	(596)	(20.7)	1.11
Sweetened, shredded:							
1 cup (3.2 oz.)	(596)	(20.7)	187.7	6.52	(596)	(20.7)	1.11
1 cup (approx. 3.4 oz.)	528	51.3	155.4	15.08	528	51.3	1.16
1 pound (approx. 4.71 cups) (1g/15g/11g/3%/na)	2486	241.3	155.4	15.08	528	51.3	1.16
COCONUT CREAM (liquid expressed from grated coconut meat)							
1 tablespoon (approx. 0.5 oz.)	50	1.2	94.4	2.34	802	19.9	
1 cup (approx. 8.5 oz.)	802	19.9	94.4	2.34	802	19.9	
1 pound (approx. 1.9 cups) (1g/2g/9g/54%/1mg)	1510	37.4	94.4	2.34	802	19.9	
COCONUT MILK (liquid expressed from mixture of grated coconut meat and coconut water)							
1 cup (approx. 8.5 oz.)	605	12.5	71.2	1.47	605	12.5	
1 pound (approx. 1.9 cups) (1g/1g/7g/66%/na)	1132	23.5	71.2	1.47	605	12.5	
COCONUT WATER (liquid from coconuts)							
1 cup (approx. 8.5 oz.)	53	11.3	6.2	1.34	53	11.3	
1 pound (approx. 1.9 cups) (tr/1g/tr/94%/na)	100	21.3	6.2	1.34	53	11.3	
SHREDDED COCONUT, by brand:							
The primary listing for shredded coconut is in the BASIC BAKING & COOKING INGREDIENTS chapter.							
Durkee Shredded Coconut, 8-oz. package	277	8.0	34.6	1.00			
CRAB APPLES							
As purchased [refuse: cores and stems, approx. 8%]:							
1 pound	309	80.8	19.3	5.05			
Edible portion:							
1 cup, sliced (approx. 3.9 oz.)	81	21.3	21.0	5.49	81	21.3	0.17
1 pound (approx. 4.1 cups, sliced) (tr/5g/tr/81%/tr)	366	87.8	21.0	5.49	81	21.3	0.17
CRANBERRIES							
As purchased [refuse: stems and damaged berries, approx. 4%]:							
1 cup (approx. 3.4 oz.)	44	10.3	12.5	2.94	44	10.3	
1 pound (approx. 4.7 cups)	200	47.0	12.5	2.94	44	10.3	
Edible portion:							
1 cup, chopped (approx. 3.9 oz.)	51	11.9	13.1	3.05	51	11.9	0.40
1 pound (approx. 4.1 cups) (tr/3g/tr/88%/1mg)	209	48.8	13.1	3.05	51	11.9	0.40
CRANBERRIES, by brand							
Ocean Spray Fresh Fruit Cranberries, 16-oz. (1-lb.) poly bag	200	48.0	12.5	3.00	50	12.0	
DEHYDRATED, based on generic data:							
As purchased, all-edible:							
1 pound (1g/24g/2g/5%/5mg)	1669	382.4	104.3	23.90			

	UNIT		1 OZ., BY WT.		1 CUP		Fiber per oz. (GMS.)
	Cal.	Carb.	Cal.	Carb.	Cal.	Carb.	
CANNED, based on generic data:							
Strained, sugar added:							
1 cup (approx. 9.8 oz.)	404	103.9	41.4	10.63	404	103.9	0.06
1 pound (approx. 1.6 cups) (tr/11g/tr/62%/tr)	662	170.1	41.4	10.63	404	103.9	0.06
Can, #300, 16 oz. (1 lb.)	662	170.1	41.4	10.63	404	103.9	0.06
Can, #10, 117 oz. (7 lb. 5 oz.)	4843	1243.9	41.4	10.63	404	103.9	0.06
CRANBERRY SAUCE							
For more information on CRANBERRY SAUCE, see the CONDIMENTS chapter.							
Based on USDA Home Recipe:							
1 cup, not strained (approx. 9.8 oz.) (tr/13g/tr/54%/tr)	493	126.0	53.0	12.86	493	126.0	0.20
CANNED, by brand							
Town House Jellied Cranberry Sauce, 16-oz. (1-lb.) can	800	200.0	50.0	12.50	478	119.4	
CRANBERRY JUICE COCKTAIL, see the BEVERAGES chapter							
CURRANTS							
BLACK, EUROPEAN							
As purchased [refuse: stems, approx. 2%]:							
1 cup (approx. 4.6 oz.)	69	16.7	15.0	3.64	69	16.7	
1 pound (approx. 3.5 cups)	240	58.3	15.0	3.64	69	16.7	
Edible portion:							
1 cup (approx. 4.6 oz.)	70	17.1	15.3	3.72	70	17.1	0.68
1 pound (approx. 3.5 cups) (tr/4g/tr/84%/1mg)	245	59.5	15.3	3.72	70	17.1	0.68
RED AND WHITE							
As purchased [refuse: stems, approx. 3%]:							
1 cup (approx. 4.6 oz.)	63	15.3	13.8	3.33	63	15.3	
1 pound (approx. 3.5 cups)	220	53.3	13.8	3.33	63	15.3	
Edible portion:							
1 cup (approx. 4.6 oz.)	65	15.8	14.2	3.43	65	15.8	0.96
1 pound (approx. 3.5 cups) (tr/3g/tr/86%/1mg)	277	54.9	14.2	3.43	65	15.8	0.96
RED (based on data from France)							
Edible portion:							
1 pound	172	39.0	10.8	2.44			
WHITE (based on data from France)							
Edible portion:							
1 pound	204	44.0	12.8	2.75			
CURRANT JUICE, see the BEVERAGES chapter							
CUSTARD-APPLES							
As purchased [refuse: skin and seeds, approx. 42%]:							
1 pound	266	66.3	16.6	4.14			
Edible portion:							
1 pound (tr/7g/tr/72%/na)	459	114.3	28.7	7.14			0.96
DATES							
Edible portion (based on data from France):							
1 pound	1384	332.1	86.5	20.75			
MOISTURIZED or HYDRATED, based on generic data:							
As purchased [refuse: pits, approx. 13%]:							
1 date (approx. ⅓ oz.)	21	5.8	67.6	17.98			0.56
1 cup (approx. 6.4 oz., approx. 21 dates)	433	115.1	67.6	17.98	433	115.1	0.56
1 pound (approx. 49⅓ dates)	1081	287.7	67.6	17.98			0.56
1 container, 12 oz. net wt. (approx. 37 dates)	810	215.6	67.6	17.98			0.56
Edible portion:							
1 date (approx. ¼ oz.)	21	5.8	77.7	20.67			0.65
1 cup, whole (approx. 5¾ oz., 21 dates)	447	119.0	77.7	20.67	447	119.0	0.65
1 cup, chopped (approx. 6.3 oz., 25 dates)	490	129.8	77.7	20.67	490	129.8	0.65

	UNIT		1 OZ., BY WT.		1 CUP		Fiber per oz.
	Cal.	Carb.	Cal.	Carb.	Cal.	Carb.	(GMS.)
1 pound (approx. 57 dates) (tr/21g/1g/23%/tr)	1243	330.7	77.7	20.67			0.65
1 container, 8 oz. net wt. (approx. 28½ dates)	622	165.5	77.7	20.67			0.65
1 container, 10 oz. net wt (approx. 35½ dates)	778	207.0	77.7	20.67			0.65
1 container, 16 oz. (1 lb.) net wt. (approx. 57 dates)	1243	330.7	77.7	20.67			0.65
DATES, by brand:							
Dromedary Chopped Dates, 8-oz. package	832	198.4	104.0	24.80	520	124.0	
Pitted Dates, 16-oz. (1-lb.) package	1600	368.0	100.0	23.00			
Sonoma Dried, Soft Dates, 16-oz. (1-lb.) package	(1243)	(330.7)	(77.7)	(20.67)			
Sun Giant Chopped Dates, 8-oz. carton	(622)	(165.4)	(77.7)	(20.67)	(469)	(124.7)	
Chopped Dates, 10-oz. container	(777)	(206.7)	(77.7)	(20.67)	(469)	(124.7)	
Macerated Dates, 16-oz. (1-lb.) brick pack	(1243)	(330.7)	(77.7)	(20.67)			
Natural sliced pitted Dates, 5-oz. pouch	(389)	(103.3)	(77.7)	(20.67)	(447)	(118.8)	
Whole, pitted Dates, 8-oz. carton	(622)	(165.4)	(77.7)	(20.67)	(447)	(118.8)	
10-oz. tray	(777)	(206.7)	(77.7)	(20.67)	(447)	(118.8)	
16-oz. (1-lb.) carton or bag	(1243)	(330.7)	(77.7)	(20.67)	(447)	(118.8)	
Whole, unpitted Dates, 8-oz. tray	(540)	(143.8)	(67.5)	(17.97)			
12-oz. tray	(810)	(215.6)	(67.5)	(17.97)			
24-oz. bag	(1620)	(431.3)	(67.5)	(17.97)			
DEHYDRATED, by brand:							
Timber Crest Dehydrated, hard Dates, 5-lb. package	(7712)	(2055.2)	(96.4)	(25.69)			
For comparison: **El Molino** Carob Coated Dates, 1-oz. bar	125	18.0	125.0	18.00			
Fruit Pac Dried, Honey Dipped Dates, 16-oz. (1-lb.) package	1344	357.9	84.0	22.37	(483)	(128.6)	

DATE, CHINESE, see JUJUBE

DEWBERRIES

	UNIT		1 OZ., BY WT.		1 CUP		Fiber per oz.
	Cal.	Carb.	Cal.	Carb.	Cal.	Carb.	(GMS.)
As purchased [refuse: caps and damaged berries, approx. 5%]:							
1 pound (approx. 217 berries)	250	55.7	15.6	3.48	82	17.7	
Edible portion:							
1 berry (approx. 0.07 oz.)	1	0.3	16.4	3.66	84	18.6	1.16
1 cup (approx. 5.1 oz., 73 berries)	84	18.6	16.4	3.66	84	18.6	1.16
1 pound (approx. 3.1 cups, 230 berries) (tr/4g/tr/85%/tr)	262	58.6	16.4	3.66	84	18.6	1.16
FROZEN, based on generic data:							
Unsweetened:							
1 cup (approx. 4.4 oz.)	60	14.4	13.6	3.23	60	14.4	0.77
1 container, 10 oz.	136	32.4	13.6	3.23	60	14.4	0.77
1 pound (approx.) (tr/3g/tr/87%/tr)	218	51.7	13.6	3.23	60	14.4	0.77
Sugar added:							
1 cup (approx. 5.0 oz.)	137	34.9	27.2	6.90	137	34.9	0.51
1 container, 10 oz.	273	69.3	27.2	6.90	137	34.9	0.51
1 pound (approx. 2.9 cups) (tr/7g/tr/74%/tr)	435	110.7	27.2	6.90	137	34.9	0.51
CANNED, based on generic data:							
Solids and liquid:							
Packed in water, with or without artificial sweetener:							
1 cup (approx. 8.6 oz.)	98	22.0	11.3	2.75	98	22.0	0.79
1 pound (approx. 1.9 cups) (tr/3g/tr/89%/tr)	181	40.8	11.3	2.55	98	22.0	0.79
Packed in juice:							
1 cup (approx. 8.6 oz.)	132	29.5	15.3	3.43	132	29.5	0.76
1 pound (approx. 1.9 cups) (tr/3g/tr/86%/tr)	245	54.9	15.3	3.43	132	29.5	0.76
Packed in light syrup:							
1 cup (approx. 9.2 oz.)	(187)	(45.0)	20.4	4.91	(187)	(45.0)	0.77
1 pound (approx. 1.7 cups)	326	76.8	20.4	4.91	(187)	(45.0)	0.77
Packed in heavy syrup:							
1 cup (approx. 9.0 oz.)	233	56.8	25.9	6.38	233	56.8	0.74
1 pound (approx. 1.8 cups)	413	100.7	25.8	6.29	233	56.8	0.74
1 can, #303, 16 oz. (1 lb.)	413	100.7	25.8	6.29	233	56.8	0.74
Packed in extra heavy syrup:							
1 cup (approx. 9.2 oz.)	(286)	(70.4)	31.2	7.68	(286)	(70.4)	0.74
1 pound (approx. 1.7 cups)	499	122.9	31.2	7.68	(286)	(70.4)	0.74

ELDERBERRIES

	UNIT		1 OZ., BY WT.		1 CUP		Fiber per oz.
	Cal.	Carb.	Cal.	Carb.	Cal.	Carb.	(GMS.)
As purchased [refuse: stems, approx. 6%]:							
1 pound	307	69.9	19.2	4.37			
Edible portion:							
1 cup (approx. 5.1 oz.)	104	23.8	20.4	4.65	104	23.8	0.26
1 pound (approx. 3.1 cups) (tr/5g/1g/80%/na)	327	74.4	20.4	4.65			0.26

FIGS

	UNIT		1 OZ., BY WT.		1 CUP		Fiber per oz.
	Cal.	Carb.	Cal.	Carb.	Cal.	Carb.	(GMS.)
All-edible:							
1 small fig (approx. 1.4 oz., 1½" diameter)	32	8.1	22.7	5.76			0.34
1 medium fig (approx. 1.8 oz., 2¼" diameter)	40	10.2	22.7	5.76			0.34
1 large fig (approx. 2.3 oz., 2½" diameter)	52	13.2	22.7	5.76			0.34
1 pound (approx. 11 small figs, 9 medium figs, or 7 large figs) (tr/6g/tr/78%/1mg)	363	92.2	22.7	5.76			0.34
(Based on data from the Middle East) 1 pound	399	81.2	25.0	5.08			0.37
CANNED OR JARRED, based on generic data:							
Packed in water, with or without artificial sweetener:							
1 fig with approx. ½ Tbsp. of liquid	24	6.2	13.6	3.51	119	30.8	0.20
1 cup (approx. 8.7 oz.)	119	30.8	13.6	3.51	119	30.8	0.20
1 pound (approx. 1.8 cups) (tr/4g/tr/87%/1mg)	218	56.2	13.6	3.51	119	30.8	0.20
Can, #303, 16 oz. (1 lb.) net wt. (contents: approx. 12–20 figs and approx. 9½ Tbsp. of drained liquid)	218	56.2	13.6	3.51	119	30.8	0.20
Packed in light syrup:							
1 cup (approx. 8.9 oz.)	164	42.4	18.4	4.76	164	42.4	0.20
1 pound (approx. 1.8 cups) (tr/5g/tr/82%/1mg)	294	76.2	18.4	4.76	164	42.4	0.20
Packed in heavy syrup:							
1 fig with approx. ½ Tbsp. of liquid	24	6.2	23.8	6.18	218	56.5	0.20
1 cup (approx. 9.1 oz.)	218	56.5	23.8	6.18	218	56.5	0.20
1 pound (approx. 1.8 cups) (tr/6g/tr/77%/1mg)	381	98.9	23.8	6.18	218	56.5	0.20
Can, #8Z Tall, Buffet; 8¾ oz. (contents: 6–12 figs and approx. 5 Tbsp. of drained liquid)	208	54.1	23.8	6.18	218	56.5	0.20
Can, #303, 17 oz. (1 lb. 1 oz.) net wt. (contents: 12–20 figs and approx. 10 Tbsp. of drained liquid)	405	105.1	23.8	6.18	218	56.5	0.20
Packed in extra heavy syrup:							
1 cup (approx. 9.3 oz.)	272	70.4	29.2	7.57	272	70.4	0.17
1 pound (approx. 1.7 cups) (tr/8g/tr/72%/1mg)	467	121.1	29.2	7.57	272	70.4	0.17
CANNED OR JARRED, by brand:							
Balanced Kadota Figs, packed in water, without added sugar or salt, 16-oz. (1-lb.) can	181	41.3	11.3	2.58	(99)	(22.6)	
Del Monte Whole Figs, 17-oz. jar	420	110.0	24.7	6.47	210	55.0	
Featherweight Figs, packed in water, with no sugar added, 8-oz. can	(120)	(30.0)	(15.0)	(3.75)	120	30.0	
Oregon Whole, Split Kadota Figs, packed in heavy syrup, 17-oz. can	(460)	(115.0)	(27.1)	(6.76)	(242)	(60.3)	
Drained solids (yield: approx. 9.9 oz.)	(297)	(72.4)	(30.0)	7.31	220	53.6	
DRIED, based on generic data:							
1 fig (approx. 0.5 oz.)	41	10.4	77.7	19.61	474	119.6	0.65
1 cup (approx. 6.1 oz, 11.5 figs)	474	119.6	77.7	19.61	474	119.6	0.65
1 pound (approx. 2.6 cups, 30 figs) (tr/20g/1g/23%/10mg)	1243	313.7	77.7	19.61	474	119.6	0.65
(based on data from the Middle East) 1 pound	1374	284.0	85.9	17.70			0.48
DRIED, by brand:							
Blue Ribbon California Mission Figs, 12-oz. box	840	200.0	70.0	16.67	420	100.0	
Fruit Pac Honey Dipped Calimyrna Figs, 12-oz. package	(1013)	(256.4)	(84.4)	(21.37)	(515)	(130.4)	
Honey Dipped Mission Figs, 12-oz. package	(1013)	(256.4)	(84.4)	(21.37)	(515)	(130.4)	
Sonoma Soft Calimyrna Figs, 12-oz. package	(932)	(235.1)	(77.7)	(19.59)	(474)	(119.5)	
Soft Mission Figs, 12-oz. package	(932)	(235.1)	(77.7)	(19.59)	(474)	(119.5)	

	UNIT Cal.	UNIT Carb.	1 OZ., BY WT. Cal.	1 OZ., BY WT. Carb.	1 CUP Cal.	1 CUP Carb.	Fiber per oz. (GMS.)
Sun-Maid California Sun-Dried Calimyrna Figs for snacking or baking, 8-oz. foil package (equals 1½ lb. of fresh figs)	575	135.7	71.9	16.96			
California Sun-Dried Mission Figs for snacking or baking, 8-oz. foil package (equals 1½ lb. of fresh figs)	567	135.0	70.9	16.88			
For comparison: **Tom's** Fig Bar. 1.8-oz. package	180	39.0	100.0	21.67			
DEHYDRATED, HARD, by brand:							
Timber Crest Calimyrna Figs. 5-lb. package	(7776)	(1960)	(97.2)	(24.50)			
Mission Figs, 5-lb. package	(7776)	(1960)	(97.2)	(24.50)			
CANDIED, based on generic data:							
1 fig (approx. 1.2 oz.)	104	25.7	84.8	20.90	534	131.7	
1 cup (approx. 6.3 oz., 5 figs)	534	131.7	84.8	20.90	534	131.7	
1 pound (approx. 2.5 cups, 13 figs) (tr/21g/1g/21%/na)	1357	334.4	84.8	20.90	534	131.7	
FRUIT COCKTAIL and FRUIT SALAD, see MIXED FRUITS at the end of this chapter							
GOOSEBERRIES							
1 cup (approx. 5.3 oz.)	59	14.6	11.2	2.76	59	14.6	
1 pound (approx. 3 cups) (tr/3g/tr/89%/tr)	179	44.2	11.2	2.76	59	14.3	
CANNED, based on generic data:							
Solids and liquid:							
Packed in water, with or without artificial sweetener:							
1 cup (approx. 8.6 oz.)	64	15.9	7.4	1.85	64	15.9	0.37
1 pound (approx. 1.9 cups) (tr/2g/tr/93%/tr)	118	29.6	7.4	1.85	64	15.9	0.37
Packed in heavy syrup:							
1 cup (approx. 9.1 oz.)	232	59.3	25.5	6.52	232	59.3	0.34
1 pound (approx. 1.8 cups) (tr/7g/tr/76%/tr)	408	104.3	25.5	6.52	232	59.3	0.34
Packed in extra heavy syrup:							
1 cup (approx. 9.3 oz.)	309	79.1	33.2	8.51	309	79.1	0.34
1 pound (approx. 1.7 cups) (tr/9g/tr/76%/tr)	531	136.2	33.2	8.51	309	79.1	0.34
CANNED, by brand:							
Oregon Gooseberries, packed in light syrup, 16-oz. (1-lb.) can	(328)	(82.0)	(19.3)	(4.82)	(177)	(44.3)	
GRANADILLA, PURPLE (Passion Fruit)							
As purchased [refuse: shells, approx. 48%]:							
1 pound	212	50.0	13.3	3.13			
Edible portion (pulp and seeds):							
1 pound (1g/6g/tr/75%/8mg)	408	96.2	25.5	6.01			
GRAPEFRUIT							
Grown for Eating							
GROWN IN ARIZONA AND CALIFORNIA, Marsh Seedless							
As purchased [refuse: peel, membranes, and handling loss, approx. 57%]:							
1 medium grapefruit (approx. 14.1 oz., 3¾" diameter, size 40; packed 40 grapefruits to a 7/10-bushel container, net wt. approx. 35 lb.)	76	19.8	5.4	1.41			
1 pound (approx. 0.6-0.8 grapefruit)	86	22.5	5.4	1.41			
Halved [refuse: peel and membranes, approx. 57%]:							
1 half grapefruit, served in skin (approx. 7.0 oz., 3¾" diameter)	38	9.9	5.4	1.41			
Edible portion:							
Sections:							
Served with juice:							
1 cup (approx. 7.8 oz.)	97	21.3	12.5	2.74	97	21.3	0.06
1 pound (approx. 2.1 cups) (tr/3g/tr/88%/tr)	200	43.8	12.5	2.74	97	21.3	0.06

	UNIT Cal.	UNIT Carb.	1 OZ., BY WT. Cal.	1 OZ., BY WT. Carb.	1 CUP Cal.	1 CUP Carb.	Fiber per oz. (GMS.)
Drained sections:							
1 cup (approx. 6.7 oz.)	84	21.9	12.5	3.08	84	21.9	0.06
1 pound (approx. 2.4 cups) (tr/3g/tr/88%/tr)	200	49.3	12.5	3.08	84	21.9	0.06
Cut into bite-size pieces, approx. 55 pieces, ½"–¾" in length, 1 cup, lightly packed (approx. 6.2 oz.)	77	17.0	12.5	2.74	77	20.1	0.06
GROWN IN FLORIDA, average of all colors and varieties							
As purchased [refuse: peel, seeds, core, membranes, and handling loss, approx. 50%]:							
1 grapefruit (approx. 14.1 oz., 3⁹⁄₁₆" diameter, size 48; packed 48 grapefruits to a ⅘-bushel container, net weight approx. 42½ lb.)	76	19.8	5.4	1.40			
1 pound (approx. 1.1 grapefruits)	86	22.5	5.4	1.40			0.06
Halved [refuse: peel, seeds, core, membranes, and handling loss, approx. 50%]:							
1 half grapefruit, served in skin (approx. 7.0 oz., 3⁹⁄₁₆" diameter)	38	9.9	5.4	1.40			0.06
Edible portion:							
Sections:							
Served with juice:							
1 cup (approx. 8.1 oz.)	87	22.8	10.7	2.81	87	22.8	0.06
1 pound (approx. 2.0 cups) (tr/3g/tr/89%/tr)	171	44.6	10.7	2.81	87	22.8	0.06
Drained sections:							
1 cup (approx. 7.1 oz.)	76	19.8	10.7	2.79	76	19.8	0.06
1 pound (approx. 2.3 cups) (tr/3g/tr/89%/tr)	171	44.6	10.7	2.79	76	19.8	
Cut into bite-size pieces, approx. 55 pieces, ½"–¾" in length, 1 cup, lightly packed	67	17.3	10.7	2.79	67	17.3	
GROWN IN TEXAS, average of all colors and varieties							
As purchased: [refuse: peel, seeds, core, membranes, and handling loss, approx. 50%]:							
1 grapefruit (approx. 13.4 oz., 3⅜" diameter, size 48; packed 48 grapefruits to a ⅘-bushel container, net wt. approx. 42½ lb.)	82	21.5	6.1	1.61			
1 pound (approx. 1.2 grapefruits)	98	25.7	6.1	1.61			
Halved [refuse: peel, seeds, core, membranes, and handling loss, approx. 50%]:							
1 half grapefruit, served in skin (approx. 6.7 oz., 3⅜" diameter)	41	10.7	6.1	1.61			
Edible portion:							
Sections:							
Served with juice:							
1 cup (approx. 8.1 oz.)	99	26.0	12.2	3.18	99	26.0	0.06
1 pound (approx. 2.0 cups) (tr/3g/tr/88%/tr)	195	50.9	12.2	3.18	99	26.0	0.06
Drained sections:							
1 cup (approx. 7.1 oz.)	86	22.6	12.1	3.18	86	22.6	0.06
1 pound (approx. 2.3 cups) (tr/3g/tr/88%/tr)	194	50.9	12.1	3.18	86	22.6	0.06
Cut into bite-size pieces, approx. 55 pieces, ½"–¾" in length, 1 cup, lightly packed (approx. 6.2 oz.)	75	19.8	12.1	3.18	75	19.8	0.06
AVERAGES OF ALL REGIONS:							
Pink or Red							
VARIETIES WITH SEEDS (including Foster Pink):							
As purchased [refuse: peel, seeds, core, membranes, and handling loss, approx. 52%]:							
1 small grapefruit (approx. 18.9 oz., 3¹⁵⁄₁₆" diameter, size 36; packed 36 grapefruits to a ⅘-bushel container, net wt. 42½ lb.)	103	26.8	5.4	1.42			
1 medium grapefruit (approx. 21.2 oz., 4³⁄₁₆" diameter, size 32; packed 32 grapefruits to a ⅘-bushel container, net wt. 42½ lb.)	116	30.1	5.4	1.42			
1 large grapefruit (approx. 25.2 oz., 4⅜" diameter, size 27; packed 27 grapefruits to a ⅘-bushel container, net wt. 42½ lb.)	137	35.6	5.4	1.42			
1 pound (approx. 0.6–0.8 grapefruit)	87	22.6	5.4	1.42			

	UNIT Cal.	UNIT Carb.	1 OZ., BY WT. Cal.	1 OZ., BY WT. Carb.	1 CUP Cal.	1 CUP Carb.	Fiber per oz. (GMS.)
Halved [refuse: peel, seeds, core, membranes and handling loss, approx. 52%]:							
1 half small grapefruit, served in skin (approx. 9.4 oz., 3 15/16" diameter)	51	13.4	5.4	1.42			
1 half medium grapefruit, served in skin (approx. 10.6 oz., 4 3/16" diameter)	58	15.0	5.4	1.42			
1 half large grapefruit, served in skin (approx. 12.6 oz., 4 3/8" diameter)	68	17.8	5.4	1.42			
Edible portion:							
Served with juice:							
1 pound (tr/3g/tr/83%/tr)	182	47.2	11.4	2.95	92	23.9	0.06
1 cup (approx. 8.1 oz.)	92	23.9	11.4	2.95	92	23.9	0.06
Drained sections:							
1 cup (approx. 7.1 oz.)	80	20.8	11.3	2.93	80	20.8	0.06
1 pound (approx. 2.3 cups) (tr/3g/tr/83%/tr)	180	46.9	11.3	2.93	80	20.8	0.06
Cut into bite-size pieces without juices, approx. 55 pieces, ½"–¾" in length, 1 cup, lightly packed, (approx. 6.2 oz.)	70	18.2	11.3	2.93	70	18.2	0.06
SEEDLESS (including Pink Marsh, Redblush):							
As purchased [refuse: peel, membranes, and handling loss, approx. 49%]:							
1 small grapefruit (approx. 14.2 oz., 3 9/16" diameter, size 48, packed 48 grapefruits to a 4/5-bushel container, net wt. 42½ lb.)	82	21.3	5.8	1.51			
1 medium grapefruit (approx. 17.0 oz., 3 3/4" diameter, size 40, packed 40 grapefruits to a 4/5-bushel container, net wt. 42½ lb.)	98	25.6	5.8	1.51			
1 large grapefruit (approx. 18.9 oz., 3 15/16" diameter, size 36, packed 36 grapefruits to a 4/5-bushel container, net wt. 42½ lb.)	109	28.4	5.8	1.51			
1 pound (approx. 0.8–1.1 grapefruit)	92	24.1	5.8	1.51			
Halved [refuse: peel, membranes, and handling loss, approx. 49%]:							
1 half small grapefruit, served in skin (approx. 7.1 oz., 3 9/16" diameter)	41	10.7	5.8	1.51			
1 half medium grapefruit, served in skin (approx. 8.4 oz., 3 3/4" diameter)	49	12.8	5.8	1.51			
1 half large grapefruit, served in skin (approx. 9.5 oz., 3 15/16" diameter)	55	14.2	5.8	1.51			
Edible portion:							
Sections:							
Served with juice (2 Tbsp. per cup)							
1 cup (approx. 8.1 oz.)	92	23.9	11.4	2.95	92	23.9	0.06
1 pound (approx. 2 cups) (tr/3g/tr/89%/tr)	182	47.2	11.4	2.95	92	23.9	0.06
Drained sections:							
1 cup (approx. 7.1 oz.)	80	20.8	11.0	2.85	78	20.2	0.06
1 pound (approx. 2.3 cups) (tr/3g/tr/89%/tr)	176	45.6	11.0	2.85	78	20.2	0.06
Cut into bite-size pieces, approx. 55 pieces, ½"–¾" in length, 1 cup, lightly packed, (approx. 6.4 oz.)	70	18.2	11.0	2.85	70	18.2	0.06
White							
VARIETIES WITH SEEDS (Including Duncan, other varieties):							
As purchased [refuse: peel, seeds, core, membranes, and handling loss, approx. 55%]:							
1 small grapefruit (approx. 19.0 oz., 3 15/16" diameter, size 36, packed 36 grapefruits to a 4/5-bushel container, net wt. 42½ lb.)	99	26.0	5.2	1.38			
1 medium grapefruit (approx. 23 oz., 4 3/16" diameter, size 32, packed 32 grapefruits to a 4/5-bushel container, net wt. 42½ lb.)	111	29.3	5.2	1.38			
1 large grapefruit (approx. 25.4 oz., 4 3/8" diameter, size 27, packed 27 grapefruits to a 4/5-bushel container, net wt. 42½ lb.)	132	34.7	5.2	1.38			
1 pound (approx. 0.6–0.8 grapefruit)	83	22.1	5.2	1.38			
Halved [refuse: peel, seeds, core, membranes, and handling loss, approx. 55%]:							
1 half small grapefruit, served in skin (approx. 9.5 oz., 3 5/16" diameter)	49	13.0	5.2	1.38			
1 half medium grapefruit, served in skin (approx. 11.5 oz., 4 3/16" diameter)	56	14.7	5.2	1.38			
1 half large grapefruit, served in skin (approx. 12.7 oz., 4 3/8" diameter)	66	17.4	5.2	1.38			
Edible portion:							
Sections:							
Served with juice:							
1 cup (approx. 8.1 oz.)	94	24.8	11.6	3.06	94	24.8	0.06
1 pound (approx. 2 cups) (tr/3g/tr/88%/tr)	186	49.0	11.6	3.06	94	24.8	0.06
Drained sections:							
1 cup (approx. 7.1 oz.)	78	20.2	11.0	2.85	78	20.2	0.06
1 pound (approx. 2.3 cups) (tr/3g/tr/88%/tr)	176	45.6	11.0	2.85	78	20.2	0.06
Cut into bite-size pieces, approx. 55 pieces, ½"–¾" in length, 1 cup, lightly packed (approx. 6.5 oz.)	72	18.9	11.0	2.85	72	18.9	0.06
SEEDLESS (Marsh seedless):							
As purchased [refuse: peel, membranes, and handling loss, approx. 51%]:							
1 small grapefruit (approx. 14.3 oz., 3 9/16" diameter, size 48, packed 48 grapefruits to a 4/5-bushel container, net wt. 42½ lb.)	77	19.9	5.4	1.40			
1 medium grapefruit (approx. 17.0 oz., 3 3/4" diameter, size 40, packed 40 grapefruits to a 4/5-bushel container, net wt. 42½ lb.)	92	23.9	5.4	1.40			
1 large grapefruit (approx. 18.9 oz., 3 15/16" diameter, size 36, packed 36 grapefruits to a 4/5-bushel container, net wt. 42½ lb.)	102	26.5	5.4	1.40			
1 pound (approx. 0.6–0.8 grapefruits)	86	22.4	5.4	1.40			
Halved [refuse: peel and membranes, approx. 51%]:							
1 half small grapefruit, served in skin (approx. 7.0 oz., 3 9/16" diameter)	38	9.9	5.4	1.40			
1 half medium grapefruit, served in skin (approx. 8.5 oz., 3 3/4" diameter)	46	11.9	5.4	1.40			
1 half large grapefruit, served in skin (approx. 9.4 oz., 3 15/16" diameter)	51	13.3	5.4	1.40			
Edible portion:							
Sections:							
Served with juice:							
1 cup (approx. 8.1 oz.)	94	24.8	11.6	3.10	94	24.8	0.06
1 pound (approx. 2 cups) (tr/3g/tr/89%/tr)	186	49.6	11.6	3.10	94	24.8	0.06
Drained sections:							
1 cup (approx. 7.1 oz.)	78	19.9	11.0	2.80	78	19.9	0.06
1 pound (approx. 2.3 cups) (tr/3g/tr/89%/tr)	176	45.6	11.0	2.85	78	19.9	0.06
AVERAGE OF ALL REGIONS, COLORS, AND VARIETIES:							
As purchased [refuse: peel, seeds, core, membranes, and handling loss, approx. 51%]:							
1 grapefruit (approx. 14.1 oz., 3 9/16" diameter)	80	20.8	5.7	1.48			
1 pound (approx. 1.1 grapefruits)	91	23.6	5.7	1.48			
Halved [refuse: peel, seeds, core, membranes, and handling loss, approx. 51%]:							
1 half grapefruit, served in skin (approx. 7.1 oz., 3 9/16" diameter)	40	10.4	5.7	1.48			
Edible portion:							
Sections:							
Served with juice:							
1 cup (approx. 8.1 oz.)	94	24.4	11.6	3.01	94	24.4	0.06
1 pound (approx. 2.0 cups) (tr/3g/tr/88%/tr)	186	48.1	11.6	3.01	94	24.4	0.06
Drained sections:							
1 cup (approx. 7.1 oz.)	84	21.2	11.8	2.99	84	21.2	0.06
1 pound (approx. 2.3 cups) (tr/3g/tr/88%/tr)	189	47.8	11.8	2.99	84	21.2	0.06
Cut into bite-size pieces, approx. 55 pieces, ½"–¾" in length, 1 cup, lightly packed (approx. 6.1 oz.)	72	18.6	11.8	2.99	72	18.6	0.06
CANNED OR JARRED, based on generic data:							
Sections:							
Packed in water, with or without artificial sweetener:							
1 can, solids and liquid, 16 oz. (1 lb.)	136	34.4	8.5	2.15	73	18.5	

	UNIT		1 OZ., BY WT.		1 CUP		Fiber per oz. (GMS.)
	Cal.	Carb.	Cal.	Carb.	Cal.	Carb.	
Drained solids (yield: approx. 9.3 oz.)	(96)	(24.3)	(10.3)	(2.62)	(70)	(17.8)	
Packed in juice:							
1 cup (approx. 8.7 oz.)	93	22.9	10.5	2.61	93	22.9	0.05
1 pound (approx. 1.8 cups) (tr/3g/tr/90%/2mg)	168	41.8	10.5	2.61	93	22.9	0.05
Packed in light syrup:							
1 cup (approx. 9.0 oz.)	152	39.2	17.0	4.38	152	39.2	0.09
1 pound (approx. 1.8 cups) (tr/4g/tr/84%/1mg)	272	70.1	17.0	4.38	152	39.2	0.09
1 can, solids and liquid, 8.5 oz.	145	37.2	17.0	4.38	152	39.2	0.09
16-oz. (1-lb.) can	272	70.1	17.0	4.38	152	39.2	0.09
50-oz. can	850	219.0	17.0	4.38	152	39.2	0.09
CANNED OR JARRED, by brand:							
Balanced Grapefruit Sections, packed in water, without added sugar or salt, 8 oz.-can	68	17.2	8.5	2.15	(73)	(18.5)	
Drained solids (yield: approx. 4.4 oz.)	(47)	(11.8)	(10.6)	(2.68)	(72)	(18.3)	
16-oz. (1-lb.) can	136	34.4	8.5	2.15	(73)	(18.5)	
Drained solids (yield: approx. 8.8 oz.)	(93)	(23.6)	(10.6)	(2.68)	(72)	(14.3)	
Del Monte Grapefruit Sections, packed in juice, 16-oz. (1-lb.) can	180	42.0	11.3	2.63	90	21.0	
Drained solids (yield: approx. 8.8 oz.)	(94)	(21.8)	(10.7)	(2.48)	(73)	(17.0)	
Grapefruit Sections, packed in syrup, 16-oz. (1-lb.) can	280	70.0	17.5	4.38	140	35.0	
Diet Delight Grapefruit Sections, packed in grapefruit juice, with no sugar added, 8-oz. can	90	18.0	11.3	2.25	90	18.0	
Drained solids (yield: approx. 4.4 oz.)	(43)	(7.2)	(9.8)	(1.64)			
16-oz. (1-lb.) can	180	36.0	11.3	2.25	90	18.0	
Drained solids (yield: approx. 8.8 oz.)	(86)	(14.4)	(9.8)	(1.64)			
Featherweight Grapefruit Sections, packed in juice, with no sugar added, 8-oz. can	(80)	(18.0)	(10.0)	(2.25)	80	18.0	
Drained solids (yield: approx. 4.4 oz.)	(33)	(7.2)	(7.5)	(1.64)			
16-oz. (1-lb.) can	(160)	(36.0)	(10.0)	(2.25)	80	18.0	
Drained solids (yield: approx. 8.8 oz.)	(66)	(14.4)	(7.5)	(1.64)			
Kraft Pure Unsweetened Grapefruit Sections, 16-oz. jar	240	56.0	15.0	3.50	120	28.0	
Drained solids (yield: approx. 8.8 oz.)	(154)	(35.8)	(17.5)	(4.07)	(119)	(27.8)	
32-oz. (2-lb.) jar	480	112.0	15.0	3.50	120	28.0	
Drained solids (yield: approx. 17.6 oz.)	(308)	(71.6)	(17.5)	(4.07)	(119)	(27.8)	
Libby's Grapefruit, 16-oz. (1-lb.) can	180	44.0	11.3	2.75	90	22.0	
Tillie Lewis "Tasti Diet" Grapefruit Sections, packed in fruit juice, with no added sugar, 16-oz. (1-lb.) can	180	44.0	11.3	2.75	90	22.0	
Drained solids (yield: approx. 8.8 oz.)	(97)	(23.8)	(11.0)	2.70	92	22.6	

Peel, Candied

	UNIT Cal.	UNIT Carb.	1 OZ. Cal.	1 OZ. Carb.	1 CUP Cal.	1 CUP Carb.	Fiber per oz. (GMS.)
1 pound (tr/23g/tr/17%/nd)	1433	365.6	89.6	22.85			0.65

Cultivated for Juice

	UNIT Cal.	UNIT Carb.	1 OZ. Cal.	1 OZ. Carb.	1 CUP Cal.	1 CUP Carb.	Fiber per oz. (GMS.)
GROWN IN ARIZONA AND CALIFORNIA							
Marsh Seedless:							
As purchased [refuse: peel, seeds, membranes, and handling loss, approx. 57%]:							
1 medium grapefruit (approx. 14.1 oz., 3¾″ diameter, size 40; packed 40 grapefruits to a 7/10-bushel container, net wt. approx. 35 lb.) (yield: juice approx. 6.1 oz., ⅔ cup)	72	17.5	5.1	1.24			
1 pound (approx. 0.6–0.8 grapefruits (yield: juice, approx. 6.9 oz., 0.8 cup)	82	19.9	5.1	1.24			
Juice:							
1 cup (approx. 8.7 oz.)	104	25.2	11.9	2.89	104	25.2	trace
1 pound (approx. 1.8 cups) (tr/3g/tr/89%/tr)	191	46.3	11.9	2.89	104	25.2	trace

	UNIT		1 OZ., BY WT.		1 CUP		Fiber per oz. (GMS.)
	Cal.	Carb.	Cal.	Carb.	Cal.	Carb.	
GROWN IN FLORIDA, average of all colors and varieties							
As purchased [refuse: peel, seeds, core, membranes, and handling loss, approx. 50%]:							
1 grapefruit (approx. 14.1 oz., 3 9/16″ diameter, size 48; packed 48 grapefruits to a ⅘-bushel container, net wt. approx. 42½ lb.) (yield: juice, approx. 7.1 oz., 0.8 cup)	74	17.6	5.3	1.25			
1 pound (approx. 1.1 grapefruits) (yield: juice, approx. 8.0 oz., 0.9 cup)	84	20.0	5.3	1.25			
Juice:							
1 cup (approx. 8.7 oz.)	91	21.6	10.5	2.49	91	21.6	trace
1 pound (approx. 1.8 cups) (tr/2g/tr/90%/tr)	168	39.9	10.5	2.49	91	21.6	trace
GROWN IN TEXAS, average of all colors and varieties							
As purchased [refuse: peel, seeds, core, membranes, and handling loss, approx. 50%]:							
1 grapefruit (approx. 13.4 oz., 3⅜″ diameter, size 48; packed 48 grapefruits to a ⅘-bushel container, net wt. approx. 42½ lb.)	80	19.0	5.9	1.42			
1 pound (approx. 1.2 grapefruits) (yield: juice, approx. 8.0 oz., 0.9 cup)	95	22.7	5.9	1.42			
Juice:							
1 cup (approx. 8.7 oz.)	104	24.8	11.9	2.84	104	24.8	trace
1 pound (approx. 1.8 cups) (tr/3g/tr/89%/tr)	191	45.4	11.9	2.84	104	24.8	trace
AVERAGE OF ALL REGIONS							
Pink and Red							
VARIETIES WITH SEEDS (including Foster Pink):							
As purchased [refuse: peel, seeds, core, membranes, and handling loss, approx. 52%]:							
1 small grapefruit (approx. 18.9 oz., 3 15/16″ diameter, size 36; packed 36 grapefruits to a ⅘-bushel container, net wt. 42½ lb.) (yield: juice, approx. 9.1 oz., 1.0 cups)	98	23.4	5.2	1.24			
1 medium grapefruit (approx. 21.2 oz., 4 3/16″ diameter, size 32; packed 32 grapefruits to a ⅘-bushel container, net wt. 42½ lb.) (yield: juice, approx. 10.2 oz., 1.2 cups)	110	26.3	5.2	1.24			
1 large grapefruit (approx. 25.2 oz., 4⅜″ diameter, size 27; packed 27 grapefruits to a ⅘-bushel container, net wt. 42½ lb.) (yield: juice, approx. 12.1 oz., 1.4 cups)	130	31.2	5.2	1.24			
1 pound (approx. 0.6–0.8 grapefruits) (yield: juice, approx. 7.7 oz., 0.9 cup)	83	19.8	5.2	1.24			
Juice:							
1 cup (approx. 8.7 oz.)	93	22.4	10.8	2.58	93	22.4	trace
1 pound (approx. 1.8 cups) (tr/3g/tr/89%/tr)	172	41.3	10.8	2.58	93	22.4	trace
SEEDLESS (including Pink Marsh, Redblush):							
As purchased [refuse: peel, membranes, and handling loss, 49%]:							
1 small grapefruit (approx. 14.3 oz., 3 9/16″ diameter, size 48, packed 48 grapefruits to a ⅘-bushel container, net wt. 42½ lb.) (yield: juice, approx. 7.2 oz., 0.8 cup)	80	19.1	5.6	1.34			
1 medium grapefruit (approx. 17.1 oz., 3¾″ diameter, size 40, packed 40 grapefruits to a ⅘-bushel container, net wt. 42½ lb.) (yield: juice, approx. 8.7 oz., 1.0 cup)	96	22.9	5.6	1.34			
1 large grapefruit (approx. 19.1 oz., 3 15/16″ diameter, size 36, packed 36 grapefruits to a ⅘-bushel container, net wt. 42½ lb.) (yield: juice, approx. 9.6 oz., 1.1 cup)	107	25.4	5.6	1.34			
1 pound (approx. 0.8 grapefruits) (yield: juice, approx. 8.1 oz., 0.9 cup)	90	21.5	5.6	1.34			
Juice:							
1 cup (approx. 8.7 oz.)	96	22.9	11.1	2.64	96	22.9	trace

	UNIT Cal.	UNIT Carb.	1 OZ., BY WT. Cal.	1 OZ., BY WT. Carb.	1 CUP Cal.	1 CUP Carb.	Fiber per oz. (GMS.)
1 pound (approx. 1.8 cups) (tr/3g/tr/90%/tr)	177	42.2	11.1	2.64	96	22.9	trace
White							
VARIETIES WITH SEEDS (including Duncan, other varieties):							
As purchased [refuse: peel, seeds, core, membranes, and handling loss, approx. 55%]:							
1 small grapefruit (approx. 18.8 oz., 3 15/16" diameter, size 36, packed 36 grapefruits to a 4/5-bushel container, net wt. 42½ lb.) (yield: juice, approx. 8.5 oz., 1.0 cup)	96	22.9	5.1	1.21			
1 medium grapefruit (approx. 21.2 oz., 4 3/16" diameter, size 32, packed 32 grapefruits to a 4/5-bushel container, net wt. 42½ lb.) (yield: juice, approx. 9.6 oz., 1.1 cup)	108	25.7	5.1	1.21			
1 large grapefruit (approx. 25.3 oz., 4 3/8" diameter, size 27, packed 27 grapefruits to a 4/5-bushel container, net wt. 42½ lb.) (yield: juice, approx. 11.3 oz., 1.3 cup)	129	30.5	5.1	1.21			
1 pound (approx. 0.6–0.8 grapefruits) (yield: juice, approx. 7.3 oz., 0.8 cup)	82	19.4	5.1	1.21			
Juice:							
1 cup (approx. 8.7 oz.)	98	23.4	11.3	2.69	98	23.4	trace
1 pound (approx. 1.8 cups) (tr/3g/tr/90%/tr)	181	43.1	11.3	2.69	98	23.4	trace
SEEDLESS (Marsh seedless):							
As purchased [refuse: peel, membranes, and handling loss, approx. 51%]:							
1 small grapefruit (approx. 13.8 oz., 3 9/16" diameter, size 48, packed 48 grapefruits to a 4/5-bushel container, net wt. 42½ lb.) (yield: juice, approx. 6.9 oz., 0.8 cup)	73	17.7	5.3	1.25			
1 medium grapefruit (approx. 17.0 oz., 3¾" diameter, size 40, packed 40 grapefruits to a 4/5-bushel container, net wt. 42½ lb.) (yield: juice, approx. 8.3 oz., 1.0 cup)	90	21.3	5.3	1.25			
1 large grapefruit (approx. 18.9 oz., 3 15/16" diameter, size 36, packed 36 grapefruits to a 4/5-bushel container, net wt. 42½ lb.) (yield: juice, approx. 9.3 oz., 1.1 cup)	100	23.6	5.3	1.25			
1 pound (approx. 0.6–0.8 grapefruits) (yield: juice, approx. 7.8 oz., 0.9 cup)	84	20.0	5.3	1.25			
Juice:							
1 cup (approx. 8.7 oz.)	93	22.1	10.8	2.55	93	22.1	trace
1 pound (approx. 1.8 cups) (tr/3g/tr/90%/tr)	172	40.8	10.8	2.55	93	22.1	trace
AVERAGE OF ALL REGIONS, COLORS, AND VARIETIES							
As purchased [refuse: peel, seeds, core, membranes, and handling loss, approx. 51%]:							
1 grapefruit (approx. 14.1 oz., 3 9/16" diameter) (yield: juice, approx. 6.9 oz., 0.8 cup)	76	18.0	5.4	1.28			
1 pound (approx. 1.1 grapefruits)	86	20.5	5.4	1.28			
Juice:							
1 cup (approx. 8.7 oz.)	96	22.6	11.0	2.60	96	22.6	trace
1 pound (approx. 1.8 cups) (tr/3g/tr/90%/tr)	176	41.6	11.0	2.60	96	22.6	trace

GRAPEFRUIT JUICE, see also the BEVERAGES chapter

GRAPES

	UNIT Cal.	UNIT Carb.	1 OZ., BY WT. Cal.	1 OZ., BY WT. Carb.	1 CUP Cal.	1 CUP Carb.	Fiber per oz. (GMS.)
AMERICAN TYPE (slip skin), such as Concord, Delaware, Niagara, Catawba, Scuppernong:							
As purchased [refuse: seeds and skins, approx. 34%]:							
1 grape (approx. ¾" diameter, ¾" high. 0.14 oz.)	2	0.4	12.8	2.91	70	15.9	
1 cup (approx. 5.4 oz., 38 grapes)	70	15.9	12.8	2.91	70	15.9	
1 pound (approx. 3 cups, 114 grapes)	207	47.0	12.8	2.91	70	15.9	
Edible portion, halved, with seeds removed, 1 pound (approx. 5.3 cups, 75 grapes) (tr/5g/tr/81%/1mg)	(314)	(71.2)	19.6	4.45	(110)	(25.1)	0.17
EUROPEAN TYPE (adherent skin) with seeds, such as Emperor, Flame Tokay, Ribier:							
As purchased [refuse: seeds, approx. 5%]:							
1 grape (approx. 7/8" diameter, 7/8" high, 0.21 oz.)	4	1.0	18.1	4.66	102	26.3	
1 cup (approx. 5.6 oz., 23 Ribier or 27 Tokay or Emperor grapes)	102	26.3	18.1	4.66	102	26.3	
1 pound (approx. 2.9 cups, 65 Ribier or 76 Tokay or Emperor grapes)	289	74.6	18.1	4.66	102	26.3	
Edible portion, halved with seeds removed:							
1 grape (cut from Tokay or Emperor grape ¾" diameter, 7/8" high, approx. 0.12 oz., cut from Ribier grape 7/8" diameter, 7/8" high, approx. 0.11 oz.)	2	(0.6)	19.0	4.91	107	27.7	0.17
1 cup (approx. 5.6 oz., 58 Tokay or Emperor halves, or 50 Ribier halves)	107	27.7	19.0	4.91	107	27.7	0.17
1 pound (approx. 2.6 cups, approx. 151 Tokay or Emperor halves, or 130 Ribier halves) (tr/5g/tr/81%/1mg)	304	78.5	19.0	4.91	107	27.7	0.17
EUROPEAN TYPE (adherent skin) seedless, such as Thompson Seedless							
All-edible:							
1 grape (approx. 5/8" diameter, 7/8" high, 0.18 oz.)	3	0.9	19.0	4.91	107	27.7	0.14
1 cup (approx. 5.6 oz., 32 grapes)	107	27.7	19.0	4.91	107	27.7	0.14
1 pound (approx. 2.9 cups, 91 grapes) (tr/5g/tr/81%/1mg)	304	78.5	19.0	4.91	107	27.7	0.14
Halved:							
½ grape (cut from grape 5/8" diameter, 7/8" high)	2	0.4	19.0	4.91	117	30.3	0.14
1 cup (approx. 6.2 oz., 70 grape halves)	117	30.3	19.0	4.91	117	30.3	0.14
1 pound (approx. 2.6 cups, 183 grape halves)	304	78.5	19.0	4.91	117	30.3	0.14
CANNED OR JARRED, based on generic data:							
THOMPSON SEEDLESS							
Solids and liquid:							
Packed in water, with or without artificial sweetener:							
1 cup (approx. 8.6 oz.)	125	33.3	14.4	3.86	125	33.3	0.06
1 pound (approx. 1.9 cups (tr/4g/tr/86%/1mg)	231	61.7	14.4	3.86	125	33.3	0.06
Packed in heavy syrup:							
1 cup (approx. 9 oz.)	197	51.2	21.8	5.67	197	51.2	0.06
1 pound (approx. 1.8 cups) (tr/6g/tr/79%/1mg)	349	90.7	21.8	5.67	197	51.2	0.06
Can, #8Z Tall, Buffet; 8¾ oz. net wt. (approx. 1 cup)	191	49.6	21.8	5.67	197	51.2	0.06
CANNED OR JARRED, by brand:							
Featherweight Seedless Grapes, packed in water, with no sugar added, 8-oz. can	(100)	(26.0)	(12.5)	(3.25)	100	26.0	
Drained solids (yield: approx. 5 oz.)	(82)	(21.5)	(16.4)	(4.30)	(109)	(28.5)	
Oregon Light Seedless Thompson Grapes, packed in heavy syrup, 16-oz. (1-lb.) can	364	91.0	22.8	5.69	(197)	(49.2)	
Drained solids (yield: approx. 9.9 oz.)	(224)	(54.4)	(22.6)	(5.49)	(150)	(36.4)	
DRIED, by brand:							
Grocer's Choice Grape Fruit Roll, 1-oz. package	90	21.0	90.0	21.00			

GRAPE JUICE, see the BEVERAGES chapter

GRAPE LEAVES, see the VEGETABLES chapter

GROUNDCHERRIES (Cape-Gooseberries), (see also POHA)

	UNIT Cal.	UNIT Carb.	1 OZ., BY WT. Cal.	1 OZ., BY WT. Carb.	1 CUP Cal.	1 CUP Carb.	Fiber per oz. (GMS.)
(Based on data from Hawaii)							
As purchased [refuse: husks, approx. 8%]:							
1 cup (approx. 4.9 oz.)	68	14.3	13.8	2.92	68	14.3	
1 pound (approx. 3.3 cups)	221	46.7	13.8	2.92	68	14.3	

	UNIT Cal.	UNIT Carb.	1 OZ., BY WT. Cal.	1 OZ., BY WT. Carb.	1 CUP Cal.	1 CUP Carb.	Fiber per oz. (GMS.)
Edible portion:							
1 cup (approx. 4.9 oz.)	74	15.7	15.0	3.18	74	15.7	0.79
1 pound (approx. 3.3 cups) (tr/3g/tr/84%/na)	240	50.8	15.0	3.18	74	15.7	0.79
GUAVAS							
COMMON GUAVA							
As purchased [refuse: stems and blossom ends, approx. 3%]:							
1 medium guava (approx. 4.0 oz.)	68	16.5	17.1	4.13			
1 pound (approx. 4 medium guavas)	274	66.1	17.1	4.13			
Edible portion:							
1 medium guava (approx. 3.9 oz.)	68	16.5	17.6	4.26			1.59
1 pound (approx. 4.1 medium guavas) (tr/4g/tr/83%/1mg)	281	68.1	17.6	4.26			1.59
STRAWBERRY GUAVA							
As purchased [refuse: stems and blossom ends, approx. 2%]:							
1 medium strawberry guava (approx. 0.17 oz.)	3	0.7	18.0	4.39			
1 pound (approx. 94 medium strawberry guavas)	288	70.2	18.0	4.39			
Edible portion:							
1 medium strawberry guava (approx. 0.16 oz.)	3	0.7	18.4	4.48			1.82
1 pound (approx. 96 medium strawberry guavas) (tr/4g/tr/82%/1mg)	295	71.7	18.4	4.48			1.82
GUAVA DRINK, see the BEVERAGES chapter							
HONEYDEW							
As purchased [refuse: rind and cavity contents, approx. 37%]:							
1 medium honeydew melon (approx. 6½" diameter, 7" long, 5¼ lb.)	495	115.5	5.9	1.37			
1 wedge, 1/10 of a 5¼-lb. melon (approx. 7" long, 2" wide at center, 8.4 oz. weighed with rind) [refuse: rind approx. 34%]	49	11.5	6.1	1.44			
Edible portion:							
1 medium honeydew (approx. 3 lb. 4 oz.)	495	115.5	9.4	2.18	56	13.1	0.17
1 melon ball (approx. 0.3 oz.)	3	0.7	9.4	2.18	56	13.1	0.17
1 cup (approx. 6 oz., 20 melon balls)	56	13.1	9.4	2.18	56	13.1	0.17
1 pound (approx. 2.7 cups, 53.3 melon balls)	150	34.9	9.4	2.18	56	13.1	0.17
FROZEN, based on generic data:							
Packed in syrup:							
Solids and liquid:							
1 cup (approx. 8.1 oz.)	143	36.1	17.6	4.50	143	36.1	0.09
1 pound (approx. 2 cups)	281	71.2	17.6	4.40	143	36.1	0.09
FROZEN, by brand:							
Big Valley Sliced Honeydew Melon Chunks (Individually Quick Frozen), 20-oz. polybag	216		10.8		(79)		0.17
1 cup (approx. 7.3 oz.)	(79)		10.8		(79)		0.17
1 pound (approx. 2.2 cups)	73		10.8		(79)		0.17
Seabrook Honeydew Melon Balls, 16-oz. (1-lb.) polybag	164	37.1	10.2	2.32	(75)	(16.9)	0.17
1 cup (approx. 7.3 oz.)	(75)	(16.9)	10.2	2.32	(75)	(16.9)	0.17
JACKFRUIT							
As purchased [refuse: seeds and skin, approx. 72%]:							
1 pound	125	32.3	7.8	2.02			
Edible portion:							
1 pound (tr/7g/tr/72%/1mg)	445	115.3	27.8	7.21			0.28
JAMBOLAN, see JAVA PLUM							
JAVA PLUM (based on data from Hawaii)							
As purchased [refuse: pits, approx. 6%]:							
1 medium plum (approx. 1½" diameter, 1.1 oz.)	21	5.6	20.0	5.25			

	UNIT Cal.	UNIT Carb.	1 OZ., BY WT. Cal.	1 OZ., BY WT. Carb.	1 CUP Cal.	1 CUP Carb.	Fiber per oz. (GMS.)
1 pound (approx. 14½ medium plums)	320	84.0	20.0	5.25			
Edible portion:							
1 cup (approx. 4.8 oz.)	73	19.2	15.3	4.03	73	19.2	
1 pound (approx. 3.3 cups) (tr/4g/tr/85%/na)	245	64.5	15.3	4.03	73	19.2	
JUJUBE (Chinese Date)							
COMMON							
As purchased [refuse: seeds, approx. 7%]:							
1 pound	443	116.5	27.7	7.28			
Edible portion:							
1 pound (tr/8g/tr/70%/1mg)	477	125.2	29.8	7.83			0.40
DRIED, based on generic data:							
As purchased [refuse: seeds, approx. 11%]:							
1 pound	1158	297.3	72.4	18.58			
Edible portion:							
1 pound (tr/21g/1g/20%/na)	1303	334.1	81.4	20.88			0.85
KETAMBILLA (based on data from Hawaii)							
All-edible:							
1 cup:							
Whole (approx. 4.5 oz.)	60	14.6	13.3	3.24	60	14.6	
Mashed (approx. 8.3 oz.)	110	26.7	13.3	3.24	110	26.7	
1 pound (approx. 3.6 cups whole or 1.9 cups mashed) (tr/3g/tr/86%/na)	213	51.8	13.3	3.24			
KIWIFRUIT (based on data from New Zealand)							
All-edible:							
1 medium kiwifruit (approx. 3.0 oz.)	56	10.2	18.6	3.40			
1 pound (approx. 5⅓ kiwis)	298	54.4	18.6	3.40			
KUMQUATS							
As purchased [refuse: seeds, approx. 7%]:							
1 medium kumquat (approx. 0.7 oz.)	12	3.2	17.0	4.54			
1 pound (approx. 22½ medium kumquats)	272	72.6	17.0	4.54			
Edible portion:							
1 medium kumquat (approx. 0.65 oz.)	12	3.2	18.3	4.88			
1 pound (approx. 23 medium kumquats) (tr/5g/tr/81%/2mg)	293	78.1	18.3	4.88			1.05
Rind (based on data from Japan), 1 pound	422	90.7	26.4	5.67			
LEMONS							
As purchased [refuse: peel and seeds, approx. 33%]:							
1 medium lemon (approx. 3.9 oz.)	20	6.0	5.2	1.55			
1 large lemon (approx. 4.5 oz.)	24	7.1	5.2	1.55			
1 pound (approx. 4.1 medium lemons or 3.6 large lemons)	83	24.8	5.2	1.55			
Quartered [refuse: peel, approx. 32%]:							
Cut from 1 medium lemon (approx. 1⅝" arc., 1 oz.)	5	1.5	5.2	1.55			
Cut from 1 large lemon (approx. 1⅞" arc., 1.4 oz.)	7	2.2	5.2	1.55			
Wedge [refuse: peel, approx. 32%]:							
1 wedge, approx. ⅙ of medium lemon (approx. 1⅛" arc, 0.6 oz.)	3	1.0	5.2	1.55			
1 wedge, approx. ⅙ of large lemon (approx. 1¼" arc. 0.9 oz.)	5	1.5	5.2	1.55			
Sliced "Cartwheels" [refuse: peel, approx. 32%]:							
1 slice, approx. 1/10 of a medium lemon (approx. ⅓ oz.)	2	0.5	5.2	1.55			
1 slice, approx. 1/10 of a large lemon (approx. ⅓ oz.)	2	0.5	5.2	1.55			

	UNIT		1 OZ., BY WT.		1 CUP		Fiber per oz.
	Cal.	Carb.	Cal.	Carb.	Cal.	Carb.	(GMS.)
Edible portion:							
Lemon eaten with the peel [refuse: seeds, approx. 1%]:							
1 medium lemon (approx. 2⅛" diameter, 3.9 oz.)	22	11.7	5.7	3.02			
1 large lemon (approx. 2¼" diameter, 4.6 oz.)	24	7.1	5.2	1.54			
1 large lemon (approx. 2⅜" diameter, 5.6 oz.)	29	8.7	5.2	1.55			
1 pound (approx. 4.1 medium lemons) (tr/2g/tr/87%/1mg)	91	48.3	5.7	3.02			
1 pound (approx. 3 large lemons)	83	24.9	5.2	1.55			
Pulp only:							
1 pound (yield from approx. 6–6½ medium lemons or 4½–5 large lemons)	123	37.1	7.7	2.32			0.11
Juice only:							
Juice of 1 medium lemon (approx. 3 Tbsp., approx. 1.7 oz.)	(12)	(3.8)	7.1	2.27	61	19.5	
Yield from 1 pound of lemons [refuse: seeds, central axis, and segment membranes, approx. 57%], approx. ¾ cup juice (tr/2g/tr/91%/tr)	49	15.6	7.1	2.27	61	19.5	trace
Peel only, grated fresh:							
1 teaspoon (approx. 0.1 oz.)	(2)	0.3	(18.9)	4.73	(64)	16.1	
1 tablespoon (approx. 0.2 oz.)	(4)	1.0	(18.9)	4.73	(64)	16.1	
1 cup (approx. 3.4 oz.)	(64)	16.1	(18.9)	4.73	(64)	16.1	
1 pound (approx. 4.7 cups) (tr/5g/tr/82%/2mg)	(303)	75.7	(18.9)	4.73	(64)	16.1	
For information about bottled lemon peel, see the SALTS & SPICES chapter.							
CANDIED, based on generic data:							
1 pound (tr/23g/tr/17%/na)	1440	366.4	90.0	22.90	720	183.2	0.65

LEMON JUICE (and LEMONADE), see also the BEVERAGES chapter

LIMES

	UNIT		1 OZ., BY WT.		1 CUP		Fiber per oz.
	Cal.	Carb.	Cal.	Carb.	Cal.	Carb.	(GMS.)
As purchased [refuse: peel and seeds, approx. 16%]:							
1 medium lime (approx. 2.8 oz.)	19	6.4	6.7	2.27			
1 pound (approx. 5.7 medium limes)	108	36.3	6.7	2.27			
Quartered [refuse: rind and seeds, approx. 16%]:							
Cut from a medium lime (approx. 0.7 oz.)	5	1.6	6.7	2.27			
Edible portion:							
Pulp only:							
Pulp of 1 medium lime (approx. 2.4 oz.)	19	6.4	8.0	2.70			
1 pound (approx. 6¾ medium limes) (tr/3g/tr/89%/tr)	128	43.2	8.0	2.70			0.14
Peel only (based on data from Latin America):							
Peel of 1 lime (approx. 0.4 oz.)	(15)	(3.5)	36.6	8.34			
1 pound (peel from approx. 40 medium limes)	586	133.4	36.6	8.34			

LIME JUICE (and LIMEADE), see the BEVERAGES chapter

LITCHIS, see LYCHEES

LOGANBERRIES

	UNIT		1 OZ., BY WT.		1 CUP		Fiber per oz.
	Cal.	Carb.	Cal.	Carb.	Cal.	Carb.	(GMS.)
As purchased [refuse: caps and damaged berries, approx. 5%]:							
1 pound (approx. 305 berries)	267	64.3	16.7	4.02	85	20.5	
Edible portion:							
1 berry (approx. 0.05 oz.)	1	0.2	17.6	4.23	89	21.5	0.85
1 cup (approx. 5.1 oz., 100 berries)	89	21.5	17.6	4.23	89	21.5	0.85
1 pound (approx. 3.1 cups, 320 berries) (tr/4g/tr/83%/tr)	281	67.6	17.6	4.23	89	21.5	0.85
CANNED, based on generic data:							
Solids and liquid:							
Packed in water: with or without artificial sweetener:							
1 cup (approx. 9.2 oz.)	104	24.4	11.3	2.66	104	24.4	0.85
1 pound (approx. 1.7 cups) (tr/3g/tr/89%/tr)	181	42.6	11.3	2.66	104	24.4	0.85
Packed in juice:							
1 cup (approx. 9.2 oz.)	140	33.0	15.3	3.60	140	33.0	0.57
1 pound (approx. 1.7 cups) (tr/4g/tr/86%/tr)	245	57.6	15.3	3.60	140	33.0	0.57
Packed in light syrup:							
1 cup (approx. 9.2 oz.)	183	44.8	19.9	4.88	183	44.8	0.57
1 pound (approx. 1.7 cups) (tr/5g/tr/81%/tr)	318	78.0	19.9	4.88	183	44.8	0.57
Packed in heavy syrup:							
1 cup (approx. 9.2 oz.)	232	57.7	25.3	6.29	232	57.7	0.54
1 pound (approx. 1.7 cups) (tr/6g/tr/77%/tr)	404	100.7	25.3	6.29	232	57.7	0.54
Packed in extra heavy syrup:							
1 cup (approx. 9.2 oz.)	281	70.7	30.6	7.71	281	70.1	0.54
1 pound (approx. 1.7 cups) (tr/8g/tr/72%/tr)	490	123.4	30.6	7.71	281	70.1	0.54

LONGANS

	UNIT		1 OZ., BY WT.		1 CUP		Fiber per oz.
	Cal.	Carb.	Cal.	Carb.	Cal.	Carb.	(GMS.)
As purchased [refuse: shell and seeds, approx. 47%]:							
1 pound	147	38.0	9.2	2.37			
Edible portion:							
1 pound (tr/4g/tr/82%/tr)	277	71.7	17.3	4.48			0.11
DRIED, based on generic data:							
As purchased [refuse: shell and seeds, approx. 64%]:							
1 pound	467	121.0	29.2	7.56			
Edible portion:							
1 pound (tr/21g/1g/18%/tr)	1298	336.0	81.1	21.00			0.57

LOQUATS

	UNIT		1 OZ., BY WT.		1 CUP		Fiber per oz.
	Cal.	Carb.	Cal.	Carb.	Cal.	Carb.	(GMS.)
As purchased [refuse: seeds, approx. 23%]:							
1 medium loquat (approx. ½ oz.)	6	1.4	10.5	2.71			
1 pound (approx. 28½ medium loquats)	168	43.4	10.5	2.71			
Edible portion:							
1 medium loquat (approx. 0.4 oz.)	6	1.5	13.6	3.52			
1 pound (approx. 37 medium loquats) (tr/4g/tr/87%/na)	218	56.3	13.6	3.52			0.14

LYCHEES

	UNIT		1 OZ., BY WT.		1 CUP		Fiber per oz.
	Cal.	Carb.	Cal.	Carb.	Cal.	Carb.	(GMS.)
As purchased [refuse: thin shell and seeds, approx. 40%]:							
1 medium lychee (approx. ½ oz.)	5	1.4	10.9	2.79			
1 pound (approx. 30 medium lychees)	174	44.6	10.9	2.79			
Edible portion:							
1 medium lychee (approx. ⅓ oz.)	6	1.5	18.1	4.65	122	31.2	0.09
1 cup (approx. 6.7 oz., 21 lychees)	122	31.2	18.1	4.65	122	31.2	0.09
1 pound (approx. 2.4 cups, 50 medium lychees) (tr/5g/tr/82%/1mg)	290	74.4	18.1	4.65	122	31.2	0.09
DRIED, based on generic data:							
As purchased [refuse: thin shell and seeds, approx. 54%]:							
1 medium lychee (approx. 0.16 oz.)	6	1.5	36.1	9.20			
1 pound (approx. 96 dried lychees)	578	147.5	36.1	9.20			
Edible portion:							
1 medium lychee (approx. 0.08 oz.)	6	1.5	78.5	20.05			0.40
1 pound (approx. 210 dried lychees) (tr/20g/1g/22%/1mg)	1256	320.7	78.5	20.05			0.40

MAMMEE APPLES (Mameys) (also see SAPOTES)

	UNIT		1 OZ., BY WT.		1 CUP		Fiber per oz.
	Cal.	Carb.	Cal.	Carb.	Cal.	Carb.	(GMS.)
As purchased [refuse: skin and seeds, approx. 38%]:							
1 medium mammee apple (approx. 49¾ oz., 3.1 lb.)	446	109.3	9.0	2.20			
1 pound (approx. ⅓ mammee apple)	144	35.2	9.0	2.20			
Edible portion:							
1 medium mammee apple (approx. 31 oz., 1.9 lb.)	446	109.3	14.5	3.54			0.28
1 pound (approx. ½ medium mammee apple) (tr/4g/tr/86%/6mg)	232	56.7	14.5	3.54			0.28

	UNIT Cal.	UNIT Carb.	1 OZ., BY WT. Cal.	1 OZ., BY WT. Carb.	1 CUP Cal.	1 CUP Carb.	Fiber per oz. (GMS.)
MANDARIN ORANGES							
(Mandarin Orange is the commonly used name for canned tangerines. It may also be applied to tangelos.)							
CANNED, by brand:							
A&P Whole Segments Mandarin Oranges, packed in light syrup, 11-oz. can	200	50.0	18.2	4.55			
Del Monte Mandarin Oranges, 11-oz. can	200	50.0	18.2	4.55	100	25.0	
Featherweight Mandarin Oranges, packed in water with no sugar added, 10.5-oz. can	70	16.0	6.7	1.52			
Geisha Mandarin Orange Sections, 11-oz. can	(200)		(18.2)				
Town House Fancy Mandarin Orange Segments, in light syrup, 11-oz. can	200	50.0	18.2	4.55	158	39.6	
MANGOS							
As purchased [refuse: seeds and skin, approx. 38%]:							
1 medium mango (approx. 10.6 oz.)	152	38.8	14.3	3.66			
1 pound (approx. 1½ medium mangos)	229	58.6	14.3	3.66			
Edible portion:							
1 medium mango (approx. 6.6 oz.)	152	38.8	23.1	5.90	134	34.2	0.26
1 cup, sliced or diced (approx. 5.8 oz., ⅘ medium mango)	134	34.2	23.1	5.90	134	34.2	0.26
1 pound (approx. 2⅓ medium mangos, 2.8 cups) (tr/5g/tr/82%/3mg)	370	94.5	23.1	5.90	134	34.2	0.26
MARIONBERRIES							
CANNED, by brand:							
Oregon Marionberries, 16½-oz. can	392	98.0	23.8	5.94	(204)	(50.9)	
MARMALADE PLUMS, see SAPOTES (also see MAMMEE APPLES)							
MELONS, see CANTALOUPE, CASABA, HONEYDEW, and WATERMELON							
MOUNTAIN APPLES (based on data from Hawaii)							
As purchased [refuse: seeds and stem ends, approx. 13%]:							
1 medium mountain apple (approx. 2.3 oz.)	17	4.4	7.5	1.94			
1 pound (approx. 7 medium mountain apples)	120	31.0	7.5	1.94			
Edible portion:							
1 medium mountain apple (approx. 2.0 oz.)	17	4.4	8.6	2.22	44	11.5	
1 cup, ½" cubes (approx. 5.2 oz., 2.6 mountain apples)	44	11.5	8.6	2.22	44	11.5	
1 pound (approx. 8.1 mountain apples, 3 cups) (tr/2g/tr/92%/na)	137	35.6	8.6	2.22	44	11.5	
MULBERRIES (based on data from Hawaii)							
All-edible:							
1 cup (approx. 4.9 oz.)	64	14.8	13.0	3.00	64	14.8	
1 pound (approx. 3.2 cups) (tr/3g/tr/87%/na)	208	48.0	13.0	3.00	64	14.8	
MULBERRY JUICE, see the BEVERAGES chapter							

	UNIT Cal.	UNIT Carb.	1 OZ., BY WT. Cal.	1 OZ., BY WT. Carb.	1 CUP Cal.	1 CUP Carb.	Fiber per oz. (GMS.)
MUSKMELONS, see CANTALOUPE, CASABA, and HONEYDEW							
NATALPLUM, see CARISSA							
NECTARINES							
As purchased [refuse: pits, approx. 8%]:							
1 medium nectarine (approx. 5⅓ oz.)	88	23.6	16.6	4.46			
1 pound (approx. 3 medium nectarines)	266	71.4	16.6	4.46			
Edible portion:							
1 medium nectarine (approx. 4.9 oz.)	88	23.6	18.0	4.85			0.11
1 pound (approx. 3⅓ medium nectarines) (tr/5g/tr/82%/2mg)	289	77.6	18.0	4.85			0.11
OHELO BERRIES (based on data from Hawaii)							
All-edible:							
1 cup (approx. 4.9 oz.)	50	12.7	10.1	2.57	50	12.7	
1 pound (approx. 3.2 cups) (tr/3g/tr/90%/na)	162	41.1	10.1	2.57	50	12.7	
ORANGES							
Eating Oranges Used for Peeled Fruit							
GROWN IN CALIFORNIA							
NAVEL (WINTER ORANGES)							
As purchased [refuse: peel and navel, approx. 32%]:							
1 small navel orange (approx. 4.6 oz., 2⅜" diameter, size 138; packed 138 oranges to a 7/10-bushel container, 40 lb. net wt.)	45	11.3	9.8	2.45			
1 medium navel orange (approx. 7.2 oz., 2⅞" diameter, size 88; packed 88 oranges to a 7/10-bushel container, 40 lb. net wt.)	71	17.8	9.8	2.45			
1 large navel orange (approx. 8.9 oz., 3 1/16" diameter, size 72; packed 72 oranges to a 7/10-bushel container, 40 lb. net wt.)	87	21.8	9.8	2.45			
1 pound (approx. 3.5 small, 2.2 medium, or 1.8 large navel oranges)	156	39.2	9.8	2.45			
Wedge [refuse: peel and navel, approx. 32%]:							
1 wedge, approx. ⅙ of a medium orange (approx. 1½" arc, 1.2 oz.)	12	2.9	10.0	2.42			
1 wedge, approx. ¼ of a medium orange (approx. 2¼" arc, 1.8 oz.)	18	4.5	10.0	2.50			
Edible portion:							
Sections with membranes:							
1 cup (approx. 5.3 oz.)	77	19.1	14.5	3.61	77	19.1	0.14
1 pound (approx. 3 cups) (tr/4g/tr/86%/tr)	233	57.8	14.5	3.61	77	19.1	0.14
Sections without membranes:							
1 cup (approx. 5.8 oz.)	84	21.0	14.5	3.61	84	21.0	(0.14)
1 pound (approx. 2.8 cups) (tr/4g/tr/85%/tr)	232	57.9	14.5	3.61	84	21.0	(0.14)
Cut into bite-size pieces, approx. 24 pieces, ½"–⅝" in length, lightly packed:							
With membranes:							
1 cup (approx. 5.3 oz.)	77	19.1	14.5	3.61	77	19.1	0.14
1 pound (approx. 3 cups)	232	57.6	14.5	3.61	77	19.1	0.14
Without membranes:							
1 cup (approx. 5.8 oz.)	82	20.3	14.5	3.61	82	20.3	0.14
1 pound (approx. 2.8 cups)	226	56.0	14.5	3.61	82	20.3	0.14

	UNIT		1 OZ., BY WT.		1 CUP		Fiber per oz.
	Cal.	Carb.	Cal.	Carb.	Cal.	Carb.	(GMS.)
Diced, small pieces:							
1 cup (approx. 7.4 oz.)	107	26.7	14.5	3.61	107	26.7	0.14
1 pound (approx. 2.2 cups)	234	57.8	14.5	3.61	107	26.7	0.14
Sliced "Cartwheels":							
1 slice (approx. 2¼" diameter, ¼" thick, 0.6 oz.)	9	2.3	14.5	3.61			0.14
1 slice (approx. 2½" diameter, ¼" thick, 0.7 oz.)	11	2.7	14.5	3.61			0.14
VALENCIAS (SUMMER ORANGES)							
As purchased [refuse: peel and seeds, approx. 25%]:							
1 small Valencia orange (approx. 4.6 oz., 2⅜" diameter, size 138; packed 138 oranges to a 1/10-bushel container, 40 lb. net wt.)	50	12.2	10.8	2.64			
1 medium Valencia orange (approx. 5.7 oz., 2⅝" diameter, size 113; packed 113 oranges to a 7/10-bushel container, 40 lb. net wt.)	62	15.0	10.9	2.64			
1 large Valencia orange (approx. 8.9 oz., 3 1/16" diameter, size 72; packed 72 oranges to a 1/10-bushel container, 40 lb. net wt.)	96	23.4	10.8	2.64			
1 pound (approx. 3.5 small, 2.8 medium, or 1.8 large Valencia oranges)	175	42.3	10.9	2.64			
Wedge served with peel [refuse: peel and seeds, approx. 25%]:							
1 wedge, approx. ¼ of a medium orange (approx. 2⅙" arc, 1.4 oz.)	15	3.7	10.0	2.64			
1 wedge, approx. ⅙ of a medium orange (approx. 1⅜" arc, 1.0 oz.)	10	2.5	10.0	2.50			
Edible portion:							
Sections without membranes:							
1 cup (approx. 6.3 oz.)	92	22.3	14.5	3.52	92	22.3	(0.14)
1 pound (approx. 2.5 cups) (tr/4g/tr/86%/tr)	232	56.2	14.5	3.52	92	22.3	(0.14)
Cut into bite-size pieces, approx. 24 pieces, ½"–⅝" in length, lightly packed:							
With membranes:							
1 cup (approx. 5.5 oz.)	79	19.2	14.5	3.49	79	19.2	(0.14)
1 pound (approx. 2.9 cups) (tr/4g/tr/86%/tr)	230	55.8	14.5	3.49	79	19.2	(0.14)
Without membranes:							
1 cup (approx. 5.8 oz.)	84	20.5	14.5	3.52	84	20.5	(0.14)
1 pound (approx. 2.8 cups)	232	56.3	14.5	3.52	84	20.5	(0.14)
Diced, small pieces:							
1 cup (approx. 7.4 oz.)	107	26.0	14.5	3.52	107	26.0	(0.14)
1 pound (approx. 2.2 cups)	232	56.2	14.5	3.52	107	26.0	(0.14)
Sliced "Cartwheels" ¼" thick (approx. 5–9 slices from a medium-size orange):							
1 slice (approx. 2" diameter, 0.5 oz.)	8	1.9	14.5	3.52			(0.14)
1 slice (approx. 2⅜" diameter, 0.7 oz.)	10	2.5	14.5	3.52			(0.14)
GROWN IN FLORIDA, average of all varieties							
As purchased [refuse: peel and seeds, approx. 26%]:							
1 small Florida orange (approx. 5.7 oz., 2½" diameter, size 138; packed 138 oranges to a ⅘-bushel container, 45 lb. net wt.)	56	14.4	9.9	2.52			
1 medium Florida orange (approx. 7.2 oz., 2 11/16" diameter, size 100; packed 113 oranges to a ⅘-bushel container, 45 lb. net wt.)	71	18.1	9.9	2.52			
1 large Florida orange (approx. 9 oz., 2 15/16" diameter, size 80; packed 80 oranges to a ⅘-bushel container, 45 lb. net wt.)	89	22.9	9.9	2.52			
1 pound (approx. 2.8 small, 2.2 medium, or 1.8 large oranges)	158	40.4	9.9	2.52			
Wedge served with peel [refuse: peel and seeds, approx. 26%]:							
1 wedge, approx. ⅙ of a medium orange (approx. 1⅜" arc, 1.2 oz.)	12	3.0	10.0	2.50			
1 wedge, approx. ¼ of a medium orange (approx. 2⅛" arc, 1.8 oz.)	18	4.5	10.0	2.50			
Edible portion:							
Sections without membranes:							
1 cup (approx. 6.5 oz.)	87	22.2	13.4	3.40	87	22.2	(0.14)
1 pound (approx. 2.5 cups) (tr/3g/tr/86%/tr)	214	54.5	13.4	3.40	87	22.2	(0.14)
Cut into bite-size pieces, approx. 24 pieces, ½"–⅝" in length, lightly packed:							
1 cup (approx. 5.8 oz.)	78	19.8	13.4	3.41	78	19.8	(0.14)
1 pound (approx. 2.8 cups)	214	54.6	13.4	3.41	78	19.8	(0.14)
Diced, small pieces:							
1 cup (approx. 7.4 oz.)	99	25.2	13.4	3.41	99	25.2	(0.14)
1 pound (approx. 2.2 cups)	214	54.6	13.4	3.41	99	25.2	(0.14)
Sliced "Cartwheels" ¼" thick (approx. 5–9 slices from a medium orange):							
1 slice (approx. 2" diameter, 0.5 oz.)	7	1.8	13.4	3.41			(0.14)
1 slice (approx. 2½" diameter, 0.7 oz.)	10	2.5	13.4	3.41			(0.14)
GROWN IN HAWAII							
As purchased [refuse: peel, seeds and membranes, approx. 49%]:							
1 small orange (2¾" diameter, approx. 6.6 oz.)	36	9.3	5.4	1.40			
1 medium orange (3" diameter, approx. 9.3 oz.)	50	13.0	5.4	1.40			
1 large orange (3⅝" diameter, approx. 15.1 oz.)	81	21.2	5.4	1.40			
1 pound (approx. 2.4 small, 1.7 medium or 1.1 large oranges)	86	22.4	5.4	1.40			
Edible portion:							
Sections without membranes:							
1 cup (approx. 6.7 oz.)	70	18.4	10.5	2.74	168	43.8	
1 pound (approx. 2.4 cups) (tr/3g/tr/89%/na)	168	43.8	10.5	2.74	168	43.8	

Eating Oranges Eaten with Peel (California Valencias)

	UNIT		1 OZ., BY WT.		1 CUP		Fiber per oz.
	Cal.	Carb.	Cal.	Carb.	Cal.	Carb.	(GMS.)
As purchased [refuse: seeds, approx. 1%]:							
1 medium orange (approx. 2⅝" diameter, 5.7 oz.)	64	24.7	11.3	4.40			
1 cup chopped into small pieces (approx. 6 oz.)	68	26.4	11.3	4.40	68	26.4	
1 pound (approx. 2.8 medium oranges, 2.6 cups) (tr/3g/tr/82%/1mg)	181	70.4	11.3	4.40	68	26.4	

Peel Only

	UNIT		1 OZ., BY WT.		1 CUP		Fiber per oz.
	Cal.	Carb.	Cal.	Carb.	Cal.	Carb.	(GMS.)
GRATED FRESH							
1 teaspoon (approx. 0.1 oz.)	(2)	0.5	(33.6)	7.09	(113)	23.8	
1 tablespoon (approx. 0.2 oz.)	(7)	1.5	(33.6)	7.09	(113)	23.8	
1 cup (approx. 3.4 oz.)	(113)	23.8	(33.6)	7.09	(113)	23.8	
1 pound (approx. 4.7 cups) (tr/8g/tr/73%/1mg)	(538)	113.4	(33.6)	7.09	(113)	23.8	
(For information about bottled orange peel, see the SALTS & SPICES chapter.)							
CANDIED, based on generic data:							
1 pound (tr/23g/tr/17%/na)	1433	356.6	89.6	22.84	720	183.2	

Oranges Cultivated for Juice

	UNIT		1 OZ., BY WT.		1 CUP		Fiber per oz.
	Cal.	Carb.	Cal.	Carb.	Cal.	Carb.	(GMS.)
AVERAGE OF ALL COMMERCIAL VARIETIES							
As purchased [refuse: peel, membranes, seeds, core, and handling loss, approx. 52%]:							
1 orange (approx. 6.3 oz., 2⅝" diameter) [yield: juice, approx. 3.0 oz., ⅓ cup]	66	16.9	9.9	2.52			
1 pound (approx. 2.5 oranges)	158	40.4	9.9	2.52			
Juice:							
1 cup (approx. 8.7 oz.)	112	25.8	12.8	2.97	112	25.8	(0.03)
1 pound (approx. 1.8 cups) (tr/3g/tr/88%/tr)	205	47.5	12.8	2.97	112	25.8	(0.03)
GROWN IN CALIFORNIA							
NAVEL (WINTER ORANGES)							
As purchased [refuse: peel, membranes, seeds, and handling loss, approx. 59%]:							
1 small navel orange (approx. 4.6 oz., 2⅜" diameter, size 138; packed 138 oranges to a 7/10-bushel container, 40 lb. net wt.) (yield: juice, approx. 1.9 oz., 0.2 cup)	26	6.1	5.6	1.32			

	UNIT		1 OZ., BY WT.		1 CUP		Fiber per oz.
	Cal.	Carb.	Cal.	Carb.	Cal.	Carb.	(GMS.)
1 medium navel orange (approx. 7.2 oz., 2⅞″ diameter, size 88; packed 88 oranges to a 7/10-bushel container, 40 lb. net wt.) (yield: juice, approx. 3.0 oz., ⅓ cup)	41	9.5	5.6	1.32			
1 large navel orange (approx. 8.9 oz., 3 1/16″ diameter, size 72; packed 72 oranges to a 7/10-bushel container, 40 lb. net wt.) (yield: juice, approx. 3.6 oz., 0.4 cup)	50	11.7	5.6	1.32			
Juice:							
1 cup (approx. 8.8 oz.)	120	28.1	13.6	3.21	120	28.1	(0.03)
1 pound (approx. 1.8 cups) (tr/3g/tr/87%/tr)	218	51.3	13.6	3.21	120	28.1	(0.03)
VALENCIAS (SUMMER ORANGES)							
As purchased [refuse: peel, membrane, seeds, and handling loss, approx. 59%]:							
1 small Valencia orange (approx. 4.6 oz., 2⅜″ diameter, size 138; packed 138 oranges to a 7/10-bushel container, 40 lb. net wt.) (yield: juice approx. 2.3 oz., ¼ cup)	30	6.7	6.5	1.46			
1 medium Valencia orange (approx. 5.7 oz., 2⅝″ diameter, size 113; packed 113 oranges to a 7/10-bushel container, 40 lb. net wt.) (yield: juice, approx. 2.8 oz., 0.3 cup)	37	8.3	6.5	1.46			
1 large Valencia orange (approx. 8.9 oz., 3 1/16″ diameter, size 72; packed 72 oranges to a 7/10-bushel container, 40 lb. net wt.) (yield: juice, approx. 4.3 oz. ½ cup)	58	13.0	6.5	1.46			
Juice:							
1 cup (approx. 8.7 oz.)	117	26.0	13.3	2.98	117	26.0	(0.03)
1 pound (approx. 1.8 cups) (tr/3g/tr/86%/tr)	213	47.6	13.3	2.98	117	26.0	(0.03)
GROWN IN FLORIDA							
AVERAGE OF ALL VARIETIES:							
As purchased [refuse: peel, membrane, seeds, and handling loss, approx. 50%]:							
1 medium Florida orange (approx. 6.7 oz., 2⅝″ diameter) (yield: juice, approx. 3.4 oz., 0.4 cup)	41	9.5	6.1	1.42			
Juice:							
1 cup (approx. 8.7 oz.)	106	24.7	12.2	2.84	106	24.7	(0.03)
1 pound (approx. 1.8 cups) (tr/3g/tr/86%/tr)	195	45.4	12.2	2.84	106	24.7	(0.03)
As purchased [refuse: peel, membranes, seeds, and handling loss, approx. 52%]:							
1 small Florida orange (approx. 5.7 oz., 2½″ diameter, size 122; packed 122 oranges to a ⅘-bushel container, 45 lb. net wt.) (yield: juice, approx. 2.8 oz., 0.3 cup)	31	7.3	5.4	1.26			
1 medium Florida orange (approx. 7.2 oz., 2 11/16″ diameter, size 98; packed 98 oranges to a ⅘-bushel container, 45 lb. net wt) (yield: juice, approx. 3.5 oz., 0.4 cup)	39	9.1	5.4	1.26			
1 large Florida orange (approx. 9.0 oz., 2 15/16″ diameter, size 78; packed 78 oranges to a ⅘-bushel container, 45 lb. net wt.) (yield: juice, approx. 4.3 oz., ½ cup)	49	11.4	5.4	1.26			
Juice:							
1 cup (approx. 8.7 oz.)	98	22.9	11.3	2.64	98	22.9	(0.03)
1 pound (approx. 1.8 cups)	181	42.2	11.3	2.64	98	22.9	(0.03)
LATE-SEASON (VALENCIA):							
As purchased refuse peel, membranes, seeds, and handling loss, approx. 48%]:							
1 small Florida orange (approx. 5.7 oz., 2½″ diameter, size 125; packed 125 oranges to a ⅘-bushel container, 45 lb. net wt.) (yield: juice, approx. 3.0 oz., ⅓ cup)	38	8.9	6.6	1.55			
1 medium Florida orange (approx. 7.2 oz. 2 11/16″ diameter, size 100; packed 100 oranges to a ⅘-bushel container, 45 lb. net wt.) (yield: juice, approx. 3.7 oz., 0.4 cup)	48	11.1	6.6	1.55			
1 large Florida orange (approx. 9.0 oz., 2 15/16″ diameter, size 80; packed 80 oranges to a ⅘-bushel container, 45 lb. net wt.) (yield: juice, approx. 4.7 oz., ½ cup)	60	13.9	6.6	1.55			
Juice:							
1 cup (approx. 8.7 oz.)	112	26.0	12.8	2.98	112	26.0	(0.03)
1 pound (approx. 1.8 cups) (tr/3g/tr/86%/tr)	204	47.6	12.8	2.98	112	26.0	(0.03)

	UNIT		1 OZ., BY WT.		1 CUP		Fiber per oz.
	Cal.	Carb.	Cal.	Carb.	Cal.	Carb.	(GMS.)
TEMPLE:							
As purchased [refuse: peel, membranes, seeds, and handling loss, approx. 48%]:							
1 small Florida orange (approx. 6.0 oz., 2 9/16″ diameter, size 120; packed 120 oranges to a ⅘-bushel container, 45 lb. net wt.) (yield: juice, 3.1 oz., ⅓ cup)	48	11.4	7.9	1.90			
1 medium Florida orange (approx. 8.1 oz., 2⅞″ diameter, size 90; packed 90 oranges to a ⅘-bushel container, 45 lb. net wt.) (yield: juice, 4.2 oz., ½ cup)	65	15.4	7.9	1.90			
1 large Florida orange (approx. 10.9 oz., 3⅛″ diameter, size 66; packed 66 oranges to a ⅘-bushel container, 45 lb. net wt.) (yield: juice, approx. 5.7 oz., ⅔ cup)	87	20.7	7.9	1.90			
Juice:							
1 cup (approx. 8.7 oz.)	134	32.0	15.3	3.66	134	32.0	(0.03)
1 pound (approx. 1.8 cups)	245	58.5	15.3	3.66	134	32.0	(0.03)

ORANGE JUICE, also see the BEVERAGES chapter

PAPAWS (Pawpaws)

	UNIT		1 OZ., BY WT.		1 CUP		Fiber per oz.
	Cal.	Carb.	Cal.	Carb.	Cal.	Carb.	(GMS.)
COMMON, NORTH AMERICAN							
As purchased [refuse: rind and seeds, approx. 25%]:							
1 medium papaw (approx. 4.6 oz)	83	16.4	18.1	3.58			
1 pound (approx. 35 medium papaws)	289	57.2	18.1	3.58			
Edible portion:							
1 medium papaw (approx. 3.5 oz.)	83	16.4	24.1	4.76	213	41.9	
1 cup, mashed (approx. 8.8 oz.)	213	41.9	24.1	4.76	213	41.9	
1 pound (approx. 1.8 cups, 4.6 medium papaws) (1g/5g/tr/77%/na)	386	76.2	24.1	4.76	213	41.9	

PAPAYA

	UNIT		1 OZ., BY WT.		1 CUP		Fiber per oz.
	Cal.	Carb.	Cal.	Carb.	Cal.	Carb.	(GMS.)
COMMON, NORTH AMERICAN							
As purchased [refuse: skin and seeds, approx. 33%]:							
1 medium papaya (approx. 16.0 oz.)	119	30.4	7.4	1.90			
1 pound (approx. 1 medium papaya)	119	30.4	7.4	1.90			
Edible portion:							
1 medium papaya (approx. 10.7 oz.)	119	30.4	11.2	2.85			0.26
1 pound (approx. 1.5 medium papayas) (tr/3g/tr/89%/13mg)	179	45.6	11.2	2.85			0.26
SOLO, HERMAPHRODITE (based on data from Hawaii)							
As purchased [refuse: skin and seeds, approx. 44%]:							
1 small papaya (approx. 12.2 oz.)	90	23.6	7.4	1.93			
1 medium papaya (approx. 17.8 oz.)	132	35.0	7.4	1.93			
1 large papaya (approx. 25.1 oz.)	186	49.2	7.4	1.93			
1 pound (approx. 0.7 large, 0.9 medium, or 1.3 small papayas)	118	30.9	7.4	1.93			
Edible portion:							
1 small papaya (approx. 6.8 oz.)	90	23.6	13.1	3.45			
1 medium papaya (approx. 10.1 oz.)	132	35.0	13.1	3.45			
1 large papaya (approx. 14.2 oz.)	186	49.2	13.1	3.45			
1 cup:							
Cubed, ½″ pieces (approx. 4.9 oz.)	64	17.1	13.6	3.45	64	17.1	
Mashed (approx. 8.2 oz.)	107	28.3	13.6	3.45	107	28.3	
1 pound (approx. 2 cups mashed, or 3.2 cups cubed) (tr/3g/tr/87%/na)	218	55.3	13.6	3.45			
SOLO, PISTILLATE (based on data from Hawaii)							
As purchased [refuse: skin and seeds, approx. 37%]:							
1 medium papaya (approx. 25.7 oz.)	220	58.4	8.6	2.27			
1 pound (approx. 0.6 medium papayas)	138	36.3	8.6	2.27			
Edible portion:							
1 medium papaya (approx. 16.2 oz.)	220	58.4	13.6	3.60			
1 pound (approx. 1 medium papaya)	218	57.6	13.6	3.60			

	UNIT Cal.	UNIT Carb.	1 OZ., BY WT. Cal.	1 OZ., BY WT. Carb.	1 CUP Cal.	1 CUP Carb.	Fiber per oz. (GMS.)
PAPAYA JUICE, see the BEVERAGES chapter							
PASSION FRUIT, see GRANADILLA							
PASSION FRUIT JUICE, see the BEVERAGES chapter							
PEACHES							
(All analyses of American peaches that I was able to find were done on peaches with the skin removed):							
As purchased [refuse: thin skin and pits, approx. 13%]:							
1 medium-small peach (approx. 4.1 oz.)	38	9.7	9.4	2.39			
1 medium-large peach (approx. 6.2 oz.)	58	14.8	9.4	2.39			
1 pound (approx. 3.9 medium-small or 2.6 medium-large peaches)	150	38.3	9.4	2.39			
As purchased [refuse: parings with some adherent flesh and pits, approx. 24%]:							
1 medium-small peach (approx. 4.1 oz.)	33	8.5	8.2	2.09			
1 medium-large peach (approx. 6.2 oz.)	51	12.9	8.2	2.09			
1 pound (approx. 3.9 medium-small or 2.6 medium-large peaches)	130	33.6	8.2	2.09			
Edible portion:							
1 medium-small peach (approx. 3.1 oz.)	33	8.5	10.8	2.75			0.17
1 medium-large peach (approx. 4.7 oz.)	51	12.9	10.8	2.75			0.17
Sliced (approx. 6 oz.)	65	16.5	10.8	2.75	65	16.5	0.17
Diced (approx. 6½ oz.)	70	17.9	10.8	2.75	70	17.9	0.17
1 pound (approx. 2.5 cups sliced or 2.7 cups diced) (tr/11g/tr/89%/tr)	173	44.0	10.8	2.75			0.17
FROZEN, based on generic data:							
Sugar added, sliced:							
1 cup, thawed (approx. 8.8 oz.)	220	56.5	25.0	6.42	220	56.5	0.17
1 pound (approx. 1.8 cups) (tr/6g/tr/77%/1mg)	339	102.5	21.2	6.41	220	56.5	0.17
Container, 10 oz. net wt. (approx. 1.1 cups)	250	64.2	25.0	6.42	220	56.5	0.17
FROZEN, by brand:							
Big Valley Fresh Sliced Freestone Peaches, 20-oz. package	239		12.0		(102)		
Drained solids (yield: approx. 19 oz.)	(239)		(12.6)		(107)		
Birds Eye Frozen Peaches, 10-oz. package	260	68.0	26.0	6.80	(229)	(60.0)	
Drained solids (yield: approx. 9.5 oz.)	(260)	(68.0)	(27.4)	(7.16)	(233)	(60.9)	
Seabrook Frozen Sliced Peaches, 16-oz (1-lb.) package	(205)	(46.6)	12.8	2.91	(103)	(23.4)	
Drained solids (yield: approx. 15.2 oz.)	(205)	(46.6)	(13.7)	(3.07)	(116)	(26.1)	
CANNED, based on generic data:							
Solids and liquid:							
Packed in water with or without artificial sweetener:							
Clingstones, halved or sliced, pitted:							
1 small peach half with 1⅔ Tbsp. of liquid	24	6.2	8.8	2.30	76	19.8	0.11
1 large peach half with 2 Tbsp. of liquid, 3.2 oz.	28	7.4	8.8	2.30	76	19.8	0.11
1 cup, slices or halves (approx. 8.6 oz.)	76	19.8	8.8	2.30	76	19.8	0.11
1 pound (approx. 1.9 cups) (tr/2g/tr/91%/1mg)	141	36.7	8.8	2.30	76	19.8	0.11
Can, 8Z Tall, Buffet; 8 oz. net wt. (halved)	70	18.4	8.8	2.30	76	19.8	0.11
Can, #10, 103 oz. (6 lb. 7 oz.) net wt. (contents: 30–35 large or 35–40 small peach halves and approx. 4 cups of drained liquid)	905	236.5	8.8	2.30	76	19.8	0.11
Packed in juice (values based on data for clingstone peaches):							
1 peach half with 1⅔ Tbsp. of liquid (approx. 2.7 oz.)	34	8.9	12.5	3.28	109	28.7	0.07
1 cup, slices or halves (approx. 8.7 oz.)	109	28.7	12.5	3.28	109	28.7	0.07
1 pound (approx. 1.8 cups) (tr/3g/tr/87%/1mg)	200	52.5	12.5	3.28	109	28.7	0.07
Packed in extra light syrup (values based on data for clingstone peaches):							
1 peach half with 1⅔ Tbsp. of liquid (approx. 2.7 oz.)	32	8.6	11.9	3.15	104	27.4	0.06
1 cup, slices or halves (approx. 8.6 oz.)	104	27.4	11.9	3.15	104	27.4	0.06
1 pound (approx. 1.9 cups) (tr/3g/tr/88%/1mg)	191	50.4	11.9	3.15	104	27.4	0.06
Packed in light syrup:							
Clingstones, halved or sliced, pitted:							
1 pound (tr/4g/tr/84%/1mg)	263	68.5	16.4	4.28	(141)	(36.8)	0.11
Packed in heavy syrup:							
Halved or sliced, pitted:							
1 peach half with 1⅔ Tbsp. of liquid (approx. 2.7 oz.)	59	15.3	22.1	5.70	200	51.5	0.11
Can, 8Z Tall, Buffet; 8¾ oz. net wt. (contents: approx. ¾ cup of drained slices and 5½ Tbsp. of drained liquid) (tr/6g/tr/79%/1mg)	193	49.8	22.1	5.70	200	51.5	0.11
Can #303, 16 oz. (1 lb.) net wt. (contents: 5–8 halves and approx. 10 Tbsp. of drained liquid or approx. 1¼ cups of drained slices and 10 Tbsp. of drained liquid)	354	91.2	22.1	5.70	200	51.5	0.11
Can, #2½, 29 oz. (1 lb. 13 oz.) net wt. (contents: 7 halves and approx. 1¼ cups of drained liquid or 2¼ cups of drained slices (or chunks) and approx. 1⅛ cups of drained liquid)	641	165.2	22.1	5.70	200	51.5	0.11
One peach, half with 2⅔ Tbsp. of liquid	91	23.5	22.1	5.70	200	51.5	0.11
Can, #10, 108 oz. (6 lb. 12 oz.) net wt. (contents: 25–30 large, or 30–35 medium, or 35–40 small peach halves, and approx. 4¼ cups of drained liquid, or approx. 8½ cups of drained slices and 4¼ cups of drained liquid)	2388	615.5	22.1	5.70	200	51.5	0.11
1 small peach half (35–40 per can) with 1¾ Tbsp. of liquid	63	16.3	22.1	5.70	200	51.5	0.11
1 medium peach half (30–35 per can) with 2⅛ Tbsp. of liquid	75	19.3	22.1	5.70	200	51.5	0.11
1 large peach half (25–30 per can) with 2½ Tbsp. of liquid	85	21.9	22.1	5.70	200	51.5	0.11
1 cup (approx. 9 oz.)	200	51.5	22.1	5.70	200	51.5	0.11
1 pound (approx. 1¾ cups)	354	91.2	22.1	5.70	200	51.5	0.11
Packed in extra heavy syrup:							
Clingstones, halved, pitted:							
1 cup (approx. 9⅓ oz.)	257	66.5	27.5	7.12	257	66.5	(0.11)
1 pound (approx. 1¾ cups) (tr/7g/tr/74%/1mg)	440	113.9	27.5	7.12	257	66.5	(0.11)
CANNED, by brand:							
Ann Page (A&P) Yellow Cling Peaches, Sliced, packed in heavy syrup, 8¾-oz. can	200	50.0	22.9	5.71	(200)	(50.0)	
16-oz. (1-lb.) can	400	100.0	(25.0)	(6.25)	(200)	(50.0)	
Yellow Cling Peaches, Sliced, packed in extra heavy syrup, 30-oz. can	910	238.0	30.3	7.93	(242)	(63.3)	
Yellow Cling Peaches, Halved, packed in heavy syrup, 16-oz. can	380	100.0	23.8	6.25	(190)	(50.0)	
29-oz. can	618	162.5	21.3	5.60	(170)	(44.7)	
Balanced Yellow Cling Peaches, Sliced, packed in water without added sugar or salt, 16-oz (1-lb.) can	99	23.5	6.2	1.47	(53)	(12.7)	
Del Monte Freestone Halves or Slices, 16-oz. (1-lb.) can	340	90.0	21.3	5.63	170	45.0	
29-oz. can	616	163.1	21.3	5.63	170	45.0	
Diet Delight Yellow Cling Peaches, Halved, packed in juice, 16-oz. (1-lb.) can	200	56.0	12.5	3.50	(100)	(27.9)	
Yellow Cling Peaches, packed in water, Halved, 16-oz. (1-lb.) can	120	28.0	7.5	1.75	(60)	(14.0)	
Yellow Cling Peaches, Sliced, packed in juice of white grapes, 8-oz. can	100	28.0	12.5	3.50	(100)	(28.0)	
16-oz. (1-lb.) can	200	56.0	12.5	3.50	(100)	(28.0)	
Yellow Cling Peaches, Sliced, packed in water, 8-oz. can	60	16.0	7.5	2.00	(60)	(16.0)	
16-oz. (1-lb.) can	120	32.0	7.5	2.00	(60)	(16.0)	
Yellow Freestone Elberta Peaches, Halved, packed in juice from concentrate of white grapes, 8-oz. can	100	28.0	12.5	3.50	(100)	(28.0)	
16-oz. (1-lb.) can	200	56.0	12.5	7.00	(100)	(28.0)	

	UNIT Cal.	UNIT Carb.	1 OZ., BY WT. Cal.	1 OZ., BY WT. Carb.	1 CUP Cal.	1 CUP Carb.	Fiber per oz. (GMS.)
Yellow Freestone and Elberta Peaches, Sliced, packed in juice, 16-oz. (1-lb.) can	200	56.0	12.5	7.00	(100)	(28.0)	
Featherweight Peach Halves, packed in water, no sugar added, 8-oz. can	(120)	(32.0)	(15.0)	(4.00)	120	32.0	
16-oz (1-lb) can	(240)	(64.0)	(15.0)	(4.00)	120	32.0	
Peaches, Sliced, packed in water, 8-oz. can	(120)	(16.0)	(15.0)	(2.00)	60	16.0	
Peaches, Sliced, packed in water 16-oz. (1-lb.) can	(240)	(2.0)	(15.0)	(2.00)	60	16.0	
Cling Peaches, Halved, packed in juice, 8-oz. can	(100)	(24.0)	(12.5)	(3.00)	100	24.0	
16-oz. (1-lb) can	(200)	(48.0)	(15.0)	(2.00)	100	24.0	
Cling Peaches, Peeled Halved Yellow, packed in pear, apple and grape juices from concentrate, 8-oz. can	100	24.0	12.5	3.00	(100)	(24.0)	
16-oz. (1-lb.) can	200	48.0	12.5	3.00	(100)	(24.0)	
Cling Peaches, Sliced, packed in juice, 8-oz. can	(100)	(24.0)	(12.5)	(3.00)	100	24.0	
16-oz. (1-lb.) can	(200)	(48.0)	(12.5)	(3.00)	100	24.0	
Freestone Peaches, Halved, packed in juice, 16-oz. (1-lb.) can	(200)	(48.0)	(12.5)	(3.00)	100	24.0	
Freestone Peaches, Sliced, packed in juice, 8-oz. can	(100)	(24.0)	(12.5)	(3.00)	100	24.0	
Fruitcup Yellow Cling Peaches, Diced, 5-oz. can	110	28.0	22.0	5.60	(175)	(44.4)	
Yellow Cling Peaches Spiced with Pits, Whole, 17-oz. can	352	93.8	20.7	5.52			
29-oz. can	600	160.0	20.7	5.52			
Golden Harvest California Yellow Cling Peach Halves in Water, no sugar or salt added, 16-oz. (1-lb.) can	120	30.0	7.5	1.88	60	15.0	
Drained solids (yield, approx. 10.5 oz.)	87	22.1	8.3	2.10	66	16.6	
California Yellow Cling Peach Slices in Water, no sugar or salt added, 16-oz. (1-lb.) can	120	30.0	7.5	1.88	60	15.0	
Drained solids (yield: approx. 10.75 oz.)	89	22.1	8.2	2.06	63	15.8	
Libby's Cling Peaches, packed in heavy syrup, 8¾ oz. can	(167)	(44.3)	(19.1)	(5.06)	170	45.0	
16-oz. (1-lb.) can	(306)	(81.0)	(19.1)	(5.06)	170	45.0	
29-oz. can	(554)	(146.7)	(19.1)	(5.06)	170	45.0	
P&Q (A&P) Yellow Cling Peaches, Sliced, in light syrup, 16-oz. (1-lb.) can	280	72.0	17.5	4.50	140	36.0	
Stokely Finast California Yellow Cling Peach Halves, 16-oz. (1-lb.) can	355	87.1	22.2	5.44	200	49.0	
29-oz. can	644	157.8	21.5	5.56	190	49.0	
California Yellow Cling Sliced Peaches, 8¾-oz. can	175	46.7	20.0	5.34	(175)	(46.7)	
16-oz. (1-lb.) can	320	85.4	20.0	5.34	(175)	(46.7)	
29-oz.can	580	154.9	20.0	5.34	(175)	(46.7)	
Tillie Lewis "Tasti Diet" Yellow Cling Peaches, Sliced, packed in unsweetened fruit juice, 8-oz. can	100	26.0	12.5	3.25	100	26.0	
16-oz. (1-lb.) can	200	52.0	12.5	3.25	100	26.0	
Yellow Cling Peaches, Halved, packed in unsweetened fruit juices, 16-oz. (1-lb.) can	200	52.0	12.5	3.25	100	26.0	
Town House Yellow Elberta Peaches in heavy syrup, 1-lb. 13-oz. can	700	1820	24.1	6.28	200	52.0	
Drained solids (yield: approx. 19 oz.)	470	112.0	24.7	5.89	195	46.5	
Yellow Sliced Cling Peaches in heavy syrup, 1-lb. 13-oz. can	665	175.0	22.9	6.03	190	50.0	
Drained solids (yield: approx. 19 oz.)	435	105.0	22.9	5.53	176	42.5	
DRIED, based on generic data:							
Uncooked:							
1 medium-large half (approx. ½-oz.)	38	9.9	74.3	19.36	419	109.3	0.88
1 cup of loosely packed halves (approx. 5.6 oz.)	419	109.3	74.3	19.36	419	109.3	0.88
1 pound (approx. 2.8 cups) (tr/19g/1g/25%/5mg)	1188	309.8	74.3	19.36	419	109.3	0.88
Container, 11–12 oz. net wt. (approx. 2 cups)	(854)	(222.7)	74.3	19.36	419	109.3	0.88
Cooked (1 pound of dried peaches, cooked in 5 cups of water):							
Without sugar:							
1 cup (approx. 8.8 oz.)	(205)	(53.5)	23.3	6.07	(205)	(53.5)	0.28
1 pound (approx. 1.8 cups) (tr/6g/tr/77%/1mg)	372	97.1	23.3	6.07	(205)	(53.5)	0.28

	UNIT Cal.	UNIT Carb.	1 OZ., BY WT. Cal.	1 OZ., BY WT. Carb.	1 CUP Cal.	1 CUP Carb.	Fiber per oz. (GMS.)
With sugar (1 cup of sugar per pound of dried peaches):							
1 cup (approx. 9½ oz.)	321	83.2	33.8	8.73	321	83.2	0.16
1 pound (approx. 1.7 cups) (tr/9g/tr/67%/1mg)	540	139.7	33.8	8.73	321	83.2	0.26
DRIED, by brand:							
Del Monte Dried Uncooked Peaches, 8-oz. can	560	140.0	70.0	17.50			
11-oz. can	770	192.5	70.0	17.50			
17-oz. can	1190	297.5	70.0	17.50			
Fruit Pac Dried Peaches, Honey Dipped, 8-oz. package	660	172.4	82.5	21.55			
Sonoma Dried Peaches, soft, 8-oz. package	594	154.9	74.3	19.36	461	120.2	
Sun-Maid California Sun-Dried Peaches for snacking or baking, 8-oz. foil package (equals 3½ lb. of fresh peaches)	560	140.0	70.0	17.50			
DEHYDRATED:							
Nugget-Type and Pieces:							
Uncooked:							
1 cup (approx. 3½ oz.)	340	88.0	96.4	24.95	340	88.0	(1.14)
1 pound (approx. 4½ cups) (tr/25g/1g/3%/6mg)	1542	399.2	96.4	24.95	340	88.0	(1.14)
Cooked (one cup of sugar per pound of dehydrated peaches, cooked in 9 cups of water):							
1 cup (approx. 10.2 oz.)	351	90.8	34.4	8.90	351	90.8	(0.26)
1 pound (approx. 1.6 cups) (tr/9g/tr/67%/1mg)	549	142.0	34.3	8.89	351	90.8	(0.26)
DEHYDRATED, by brand:							
Timber Crest Dehydrated Peaches, hard, 5-lb. package	7712	1996.0	96.4	24.95	384	99.4	

PEACH JUICE and PEACH NECTAR, see the BEVERAGES chapter

PEARS

	UNIT Cal.	UNIT Carb.	1 OZ., BY WT. Cal.	1 OZ., BY WT. Carb.	1 CUP Cal.	1 CUP Carb.	Fiber per oz. (GMS.)
BARTLETT							
As purchased [refuse: stem and core, approx. 9%]:							
1 medium Bartlett pear (2½" diameter, 3½" high, approx. 6⅓ oz.)	100	25.1	15.8	3.96			
1 pound (approx. 2½ medium Bartlett pears)	252	63.3	15.8	3.96			
Edible portion:							
1 medium Bartlett pear (approx. 5¾ oz.)	100	25.0	17.4	4.35	101	25.2	0.40
1 cup, sliced or cubed (approx. 5.8 oz., 1 medium Bartlett pear)	101	25.2	17.4	4.35	101	25.2	0.40
1 pound (approx. 2.8 cups, 2¾ medium Bartlett pears) (tr/4g/tr/83%/1mg)	278	69.6	17.4	4.35	101	25.2	0.40
BOSC							
As purchased [refuse: stem and core, approx. 9%]:							
1 medium Bosc pear (2½" diameter, 3½" high, approx. 5½ oz.)	86	21.6	15.7	3.95			
1 pound (approx. 2.9 medium Bosc pears)	252	63.3	15.7	3.95			
Edible portion:							
1 medium Bosc pear (approx. 5 oz.)	87	21.7	17.3	4.34			0.40
1 pound (approx. 3.2 cups, 3.2 medium Bosc pears) (tr/4g/tr/83%/1mg)	277	69.4	17.3	4.34			0.40
D'ANJOU							
As purchased [refuse: stem and core, approx. 9%]:							
1 medium D'Anjou pear (3" diameter, 3½" high, approx. 7¾ oz.)	122	30.6	15.7	3.95			
1 pound (approx. 2.1 medium D'Anjou pears)	252	63.1	15.7	3.95			
Edible portion:							
1 medium D'Anjou pear (approx. 7.1 oz.)	123	30.8	17.3	4.34	100	25.2	0.40
1 cup, sliced or cubed (approx. 5.8 oz., 0.8 medium D'Anjou pears)	100	25.2	17.3	4.34	100	25.2	0.40
1 pound (approx. 2.8 cups, 2¼ medium D'Anjou pears) (tr/4g/tr/83%/1mg)	277	69.4	17.3	4.34	100	25.2	0.40

	UNIT		1 OZ., BY WT.		1 CUP		Fiber per oz.
	Cal.	Carb.	Cal.	Carb.	Cal.	Carb.	(GMS.)
CANNED, based on generic data:							
Packed in water, with or without artificial sweetener:							
Halved or sliced, pitted:							
1 pear half with 2 Tbsp. of liquid, 3.2 oz.	29	7.6	9.1	2.35	78	20.3	0.20
1 cup, slices or halves (approx. 3.6 oz.)	78	20.3	9.1	2.35	78	20.3	0.20
1 pound (approx. 1.9 cups) (tr/2g/tr/91%/tr)	145	37.6	9.1	2.35	78	20.3	0.20
Can, 8Z Tall, Buffet: 8 oz. net wt. (approx. 1 cup scant)	73	18.8	9.1	2.35	78	20.3	0.20
Can, #10, 103 oz. (6 lb. 7 oz.) net wt. (contents: approx. 35 pear halves and 4 cups of drained liquid)	934	242.4	9.1	2.35	78	20.3	0.20
Packed in extra light syrup:							
1 pear half with 1⅔ Tbsp. liquid (approx. 2.7 oz.)	36	9.4	13.3	3.46	116	30.1	0.17
1 cup, halves (approx. 8.6 oz.)	116	30.1	13.3	3.46	116	30.1	0.17
1 pound (approx. 1.9 cups) (tr/3g/tr/87%/tr)	213	55.4	13.3	3.46	116	30.1	0.17
Packed in light syrup:							
Halved or sliced, pitted:							
1 cup (approx. 8¾ oz.)	(151)	(38.8)	17.3	4.43	(151)	(38.8)	0.20
1 pound (approx. 1.8 cups) (tr/4g/tr/84%/tr)	277	70.8	17.3	4.43	(151)	(38.8)	0.20
Packed in heavy syrup:							
Halved or sliced, cored:							
1 small pear half with 1¾ Tbsp. of liquid	60	15.5	21.6	5.56	194	50.0	0.17
1 medium pear half with 2⅛ Tbsp. of liquid	71	18.4	21.6	5.56	194	50.0	0.17
1 large pear half with 2½ Tbsp. of liquid	81	21.0	21.6	5.56	194	50.0	0.17
1 cup medium-sized pear halves and liquid (approx. 9 oz.)	194	50.0	21.6	5.56	194	50.0	0.17
1 pound of pear halves and liquid (approx. 1¾ cups) (tr/6g/tr/80%/tr)	346	88.9	21.6	5.56	194	50.0	0.17
Can, 8Z Tall, Buffet; 8½ oz. net wt. (contents: approx. 5 pear halves and 5 Tbsp. of drained liquid or approx. ⅝ cup of drained slices and 5 Tbsp. of drained liquid)	183	47.2	21.6	5.56	194	50.0	0.17
1 pear half, with 1 Tbsp. of liquid	36	9.4	21.6	5.56	194	50.0	0.17
Can, #303, 16 oz. (1 lb.) net wt. (contents: 5–8 halves and approx. 10 Tbsp. of drained liquid or approx. 1⅓ cups of drained slices and 10 Tbsp. of drained liquid)	345	88.9	21.6	5.56	194	50.0	0.17
1 pear half, with 1⅔ Tbsp. of liquid (approx. 2.0 oz.)	58	14.9	21.6	5.56	194	50.0	0.17
Can, #2½, 29 oz. (1 lb. 13 oz.) net wt. (contents: 6–9 halves and approx. 1¼ cups of drained liquid)	625	161.1	21.6	5.56	194	50.0	0.17
1 pear half with 2¼ Tbsp. of liquid	78	20.2	21.6	5.56	194	50.0	0.17
Can, #10, 103 oz. (6 lb. 7 oz.) net wt. (contents: 25–30 large, or 30–35 medium, or 35–40 small pear halves, and approx. 4⅛ cups of drained liquid)	2284	589.0	21.6	5.56	194	50.0	0.17
Packed in extra heavy syrup:							
1 cup (approx. 9⅓ oz.)	243	62.2	26.1	6.69	243	62.2	0.17
1 pound (approx. 1.7 cups scant) (tr/7g/tr/76%/tr)	417	107.0	26.1	6.69	243	62.2	0.17
CANNED, by brand:							
Ann Page (A&P) Bartlett Pears, packed in heavy syrup, 8½-oz. can	190	49.0	22.4	5.76	(190)	(49.0)	
Drained solids (yield: approx. 5.1 oz.)	(112)	(25.1)	(22.0)	(4.93)	(176)	(39.4)	
29-oz. can	650	167.0	22.4	5.76	(190)	(49.0)	
Drained solids (yield: approx. 17.4 oz.)	(383)	(85.8)	(22.0)	(4.93)	(176)	(39.4)	
Balanced Bartlett Pears Halves, packed in water without added sugar or salt, 8-oz. can	(65)	(17.7)	(8.1)	(2.21)	70	19.0	
Blue Tag Bartlett Pears, packed in heavy syrup, 16-oz. (1-lb.) can	(380)	(98.0)	(23.8)	(6.13)	190	49.0	
Bartlett Pears, packed in water, 16-oz. (1-lb.) can	(160)	(40.0)	(10.0)	(2.50)	80	20.0	
Del Monte Halves or Slices, Bartlett Pears, 8½-oz. can	170	45.7	20.0	5.38	160	43.0	
Featherweight Pear Halves, no sugar added, packed in water, 8-oz. can	(74)	(18.0)	(9.3)	(2.25)	74	18.0	
Bartlett Pears, Halved, packed in juice, 8-oz. can	(114)	(28.0)	(14.3)	(3.50)	114	28.0	
Golden Harvest California Pear Halves in Water, no sugar or salt added, 16-oz. (1-lb.) can	140	38.0	8.8	2.38	70	19.0	
Drained solids (yield: approx. 9¾ oz.)	99	31.8	10.2	3.26	82	26.1	
Green Tag Halved Bartlett Pears, packed in light syrup, 16 oz. (1-lb.) can	(320)	(80.0)	(20.0)	(5.00)	160	40.0	
Libby's Pears, 8½-oz. can	128	63.8	15.0	7.50	120	30.0	
16-oz. (1-lb.) can	(296)	(77.0)	(18.5)	(4.81)	150	39.0	
Pears, packed in heavy syrup, 8½-oz. can	(179)	(46.2)	(21.0)	(5.43)	170	44.0	
Drained solids (yield: approx. 5 oz.)	(99)	(21.7)	(19.7)	(4.34)	(158)	(34.7)	
16-oz. (1-lb.) can	(336)	(86.9)	(21.0)	(5.43)	170	44.0	
Drained solids (yield: approx. 9.75 oz.)	(192)	(42.3)	(19.7)	(4.34)	(158)	(34.7)	
Pears, packed in light syrup, 8½-oz. can	(157)	(40.9)	(18.5)	(4.81)	150	39.0	
P&Q (A&P) Halved Pears in light syrup, 16-oz. (1-lb.) can	280	76.0	17.5	4.75	140	38.0	
Stokely Bartlett Pear Halves, 8½-oz. can	189	47.2	22.2	5.35	200	50.0	
16-oz. (1-lb.) can	356	88.9	22.2	5.55	200	50.0	
29-oz. can	644	161.1	22.2	5.55	200	50.0	
1 Slice with liquid (approx. 2.7 oz.)	(60)	(15.0)	22.2	5.55	200	50.0	
Sliced Pears, 16-oz. (1-lb.) can	338	83.6	21.1	5.22	190	47.0	
29-oz. can	644	151.7	22.2	5.23	200	47.0	
Tillie Lewis "Tasti Diet" Peeled Halved Bartlett Pears, packed in unsweetened fruit juices from concentrates and water, no sugar added, 16-oz. (1-lb.) can	180	48.0	11.3	3.00	90	24.0	
Town House, Halves Bartlett Pears in heavy syrup, 1-lb. 13-oz. can	665	171.5	22.9	5.91	190	49.0	
Drained solids (yield: approx. 19 oz.)	435	101.5	22.9	5.34	183	42.7	
Sliced Bartlett Pears in heavy syrup, 16-oz. (1-lb.) can	380	98.0	23.8	6.13	190	49.0	
Drained solids (yield: approx. 10¼ oz.)	248	57.8	24.2	5.63	194	45.0	
DRIED, based on generic data:							
Uncooked:							
1 half (approx. ⅔ oz.)	47	11.8	76.0	19.08	428	121.1	1.76
1 cup, loosely packed halves (approx. 6⅓ oz.)	482	121.1	76.0	19.08	428	121.1	1.76
1 pound (approx. 2.5 cups, 26 halves) (tr/19g/1g/26%/2mg)	1212	305.3	76.0	19.08	428	121.1	1.76
Cooked (1 pound of dried pears cooked in 3 cups of water):							
Without sugar:							
1 cup (approx. 9 oz.)	321	80.8	35.7	8.99	321	80.8	0.82
1 pound (approx. 1¾ cups) (tr/9g/tr/65%/1mg)	572	143.8	35.7	8.99	321	80.8	0.82
With sugar added (½ cup of sugar per pound of dried pears):							
1 cup (approx. 9.9 oz.)	423	106.4	42.8	10.78	423	106.4	0.73
1 pound (approx. 1.6 cups) (tr/11g/tr/59%/1mg)	685	172.4	42.8	10.78	423	106.4	0.73
DRIED, by brand:							
Del Monte Pears, Uncooked, 11-oz. container	825	220.0	75.0	20.00			
16-oz. (1-lb.) container	1200	320.0	75.0	20.00			
Fruit Pac Dried Pears, Honey Dipped, 12-oz. package	1021	257.5	85.1	21.46	541	136.3	
Sonoma Dried Pears, soft, 12-oz. package	912	229.0	76.0	19.08	428	121.1	
DEHYDRATED, by brand:							
Timber Crest Dehydrated Pears, hard, 5-lb. package	7896	1982.4	98.7	24.78	400	100.5	
CANDIED, based on generic data:							
1 pound (tr/22g/tr/21%/na)	1374	344.3	85.9	21.52	(456)	(114.3)	

PEAR NECTAR, see the BEVERAGES chapter

PERSIMMONS

	UNIT		1 OZ., BY WT.		1 CUP		Fiber per oz.
	Cal.	Carb.	Cal.	Carb.	Cal.	Carb.	(GMS.)
As purchased [refuse: seeds and calyx, approx. 18%]:							
1 medium persimmon (approx. 1.1 oz.)	31	8.2	29.5	7.79			
1 pound (approx. 15.1 medium persimmons)	472	124.6	29.5	7.75			

	UNIT		1 OZ., BY WT.		1 CUP		Fiber per oz.
	Cal.	Carb.	Cal.	Carb.	Cal.	Carb.	(GMS.)
Edible portion:							
1 medium persimmon (approx. 0.9 oz.)	31	8.2	36.0	9.50			0.43
1 pound (approx. 18 medium persimmons) (tr/10g/tr/64%/tr)	576	152.0	36.0	9.50			0.43
HACHINA (based on data from Hawaii)							
As purchased [refuse: skin, approx. 18%]:							
1 medium persimmon (approx. 5.9 oz.)	103	27.6	17.6	4.72			
1 pound (approx. 2.7 medium persimmons)	282	75.5	17.6	4.72			
Edible portion:							
1 medium persimmon (approx. 4.8 oz.)	103	27.6	21.5	5.75			
1 pound (approx. 3.3 medium persimmons) (tr/6g/tr/79%/na)	344	92.0	21.5	5.75			
JAPANESE (Kaki)							
VARIETIES WITH SEEDS:							
As purchased [refuse: seeds, calyx, and skin, approx. 18%]:							
1 medium persimmon (approx. 7.1 oz.)	(127)	(32.5)	17.9	4.58			
1 pound (approx. 2.3 medium persimmons)	286	73.3	17.9	4.58			
Edible portion:							
1 medium persimmon (approx. 5.8 oz.)	(127)	(32.5)	21.8	5.59			0.45
1 pound (approx. 2.8 medium persimmons) (tr/6g/tr/79%/2mg)	349	89.4	21.8	5.59			0.45
SEEDLESS VARIETIES:							
As purchased [refuse: calyx and skin, approx. 16%]:							
1 medium persimmon (approx. 7.1 oz.)	129	33.1	18.3	4.69			
1 pound (approx. 2.7 medium persimmons)	293	75.1	18.3	4.69			
Edible portion:							
1 medium persimmon (approx. 6.0 oz.)	129	33.1	21.8	5.59			0.45
1 pound (approx. 2.7 medium persimmons) (tr/6g/tr/79%/2mg)	349	89.4	21.8	5.59			0.45
DRIED, based on generic data:							
As purchased [refuse: stems, approx. 8%]:							
1 medium persimmon (approx. 1.3 oz.)	93	25.0	71.5	19.20			
1 pound (approx. 12.3 medium persimmons)	1144	307.2	71.5	19.20			
Edible portion:							
1 medium persimmon (approx. 1.2 oz.)	93	25.0	77.7	20.82			1.03
1 pound (approx. 13.3 medium persimmons) (tr/21g/tr/23%/tr)	1244	332.2	77.7	20.82			1.03

PINEAPPLE

	UNIT		1 OZ., BY WT.		1 CUP		Fiber per oz.
	Cal.	Carb.	Cal.	Carb.	Cal.	Carb.	(GMS.)
As purchased [refuse: crown, core, skin, and defects, approx. 48%]:							
1 pound	123	32.3	7.7	2.01			
Edible portion:							
1 slice 3½" diameter, ¾" thick (approx. 3.0 oz.)	44	11.5	14.8	3.88	81	21.2	0.11
1 cup, diced (approx. 5.5 oz.)	81	21.2	14.8	3.88	81	21.2	0.11
1 pound (approx. 2.9 cups) (tr/4g/tr/85%/tr)	236	62.1	14.8	3.88	81	21.2	0.11
(Based on data from Hawaii)							
As purchased [refuse: skin, crown, and core, approx. 44%]:							
1 medium pineapple, 7½" high, 5½" diameter, approx. 75 oz. (6 lb. 3 oz.)	616	159.9	8.3	2.14			
1 pound (approx. 0.2 medium pineapple)	133	34.2	8.3	2.14			
Edible portion:							
1 medium pineapple, approx. 41.8 oz. (2 lb. 9.8 oz.)	616	159.9	14.7	3.83	88	23.0	0.14
1 slice, ⅝" thick, 5½" diameter (approx. 5.6 oz.)	83	21.5	14.7	3.83	88	23.0	0.14
1 cup, ½" cubes (approx. 6.0 oz.)	88	23.0	14.7	3.83	88	23.0	0.14
1 pound (approx. 2.7 cups) (tr/4g/tr/86%/na)	235	61.3	14.7	3.83	88	23.0	0.14
By brand:							
Dole Fresh Pineapple, 28-oz. (1 lb. 12 oz.)	832	219.3	29.5	7.77	104	27.4	

	UNIT		1 OZ., BY WT.		1 CUP		Fiber per oz.
	Cal.	Carb.	Cal.	Carb.	Cal.	Carb.	(GMS.)
FROZEN, based on generic data:							
Measured when frozen:							
Chunks, sugar added:							
1 pound (approx. 1.9 cups) (tr/6g/tr/77%/1mg)	386	100.7	24.1	6.30	208	54.4	0.09
CANNED, based on generic data:							
Solids and liquid:							
Packed in water:							
1 slice (3" diameter, 5⁄16" thick) with 1¼ Tbsp. of liquid (approx. 2 oz.)	19	4.8	9.1	2.36	79	20.4	0.13
1 cup, tidbits (approx. 8.6 oz.)	79	20.4	9.1	2.36	79	20.4	0.13
1 pound (approx. 1.9 cups) (tr/2g/tr/91%/tr)	145	37.7	9.1	2.36	79	20.4	0.13
Packed in juice:							
Tidbits:							
1 cup (approx. 8.7 oz.)	96	25.1	11.1	2.90	96	25.1	0.09
1 pound (approx. 1.8 cups) (tr/3g/tr/84%/tr)	177	46.3	11.1	2.90	96	25.1	0.09
Packed in light syrup:							
1 pound (tr/4g/tr/84%/tr)	268	69.9	16.8	4.37	145	37.8	0.09
Packed in heavy syrup:							
Tidbits:							
9 small tidbits and 1¼ Tbsp. of liquid (approx. 2.0 oz.)	43	11.3	21.0	5.50	189	49.5	0.09
17 small tidbits and 2¼ Tbsp. of liquid (approx. 3.7 oz.)	78	20.4	21.0	5.50	189	49.5	0.09
Chunks:							
4 chunks and 1¼ Tbsp. of liquid (approx. 2.0 oz.)	43	11.3	21.0	5.50	189	49.5	0.09
8 chunks and 2¼ Tbsp. of liquid (approx. 3.7 oz.)	78	20.4	21.0	5.50	189	49.5	0.09
Slices:							
1 medium slice and 1¼ Tbsp. of liquid (approx. 2.0 oz.)	43	11.3	21.0	5.50	189	49.5	0.09
1 large slice and 2¼ Tbsp. of liquid (approx. 3.7 oz.)	78	20.4	21.0	5.50	189	49.5	0.09
All Styles:							
1 cup, chunk or tidbit, crushed (approx. 9 oz.)	189	49.5	21.0	5.50	189	49.5	0.09
1 pound, chunk or tidbit, crushed, (approx. 1.8 cups) (tr/6g/tr/80%/tr)	336	88.0	21.0	5.50	189	49.5	0.09
Can, #1 Flat, 8¼ oz. net wt. (contents: 4 medium slices and approx. 5 Tbsp. of drained liquid or 1 cup [scant] of crushed pineapple)	173	45.4	21.0	5.50	189	49.5	0.09
Can, #211 Cylinder, 13¼ oz. net wt. (contents: approx. 1½ cups of crushed pineapple, or 1⅓ cups of drained chunks or small tidbits and 8 Tbsp. of drained liquid)	278	72.9	21.0	5.50	189	49.5	0.09
Can, #2, 20 oz. (1 lb. 4 oz.) net wt. (contents: approx. 2¼ cups of crushed pineapple, or 10 medium slices and approx. 10 Tbsp. of drained liquid, or 2 cups of drained chunks or small tidbits and approx. 12 Tbsp. of drained liquid)	420	110.0	21.0	5.50	189	49.5	0.09
Can, #2½, 29½ oz. (1 lb. 13½ oz.) net wt. (contents: 8 large slices and approx. 18 Tbsp. of drained liquid)	619	162.2	21.0	5.50	189	49.5	0.09
Packed in extra heavy syrup:							
Chunks:							
4 chunks with 1¼ Tbsp. of liquid (approx. 2.0 oz.)	52	13.8	25.4	6.61	234	60.8	0.09
8 chunks with 2⅓ Tbsp. of liquid (approx. 3.7 oz.)	95	24.6	25.4	6.61	234	60.8	0.09
Slices:							
1 medium slice with 1¼ Tbsp. of drained liquid (approx. 2.0 oz.)	52	13.6	26.0	6.80			0.09
1 large slice with 2⅓ Tbsp. of drained liquid (approx. 3.7 oz.)	95	24.6	25.7	6.65			0.09
All Styles:							
1 cup, chunk or crushed pineapple (approx. 8.9 oz.) (tr/7g/tr/76%/tr)	234	60.8	25.4	6.61	234	60.8	0.09
1 pound (approx. 1.8 cups) (tr/7g/tr/76%/tr)	408	106.1	25.4	6.61	234	60.8	0.09
Can, 8Z Tall, Buffet; 8¾ oz. net wt. (contents: approx. 1 cup [scant] of crushed pineapple)	223	58.0	25.5	6.63	208	54.4	0.09
Can, #2, 20½ oz. (1 lb. 4½ oz.) net wt. (contents: 10 medium slices and approx. 13 Tbsp. of drained liquid)	523	136.0	25.5	6.63	208	54.4	0.09

	UNIT Cal.	UNIT Carb.	1 OZ., BY WT. Cal.	1 OZ., BY WT. Carb.	1 CUP Cal.	1 CUP Carb.	Fiber per oz. (GMS.)
Can, #2½, 30 oz. (1 lb. 14 oz.) net wt. (contents: 8 large slices and approx. 19 Tbsp. of drained liquid, or approx. 3¼ cups of chunk pineapple and liquid)	766	199.1	25.5	6.63	208	54.4	0.09
CANNED, by brand:							
A & P Pineapple Chunks, packed in heavy syrup, 20-oz. can	475	122.5	23.8	6.13	190	49.0	
Drained solids (yield: approx. 14 oz.)	(337)	(86.5)	(24.1)	(6.18)	(157)	(40.3)	
Pineapple Chunks, packed in its own juice, no sugar, 20-oz. can	350	87.5	17.5	4.38	140	35.0	
Drained solids (yield: approx. 14 oz.)	(248)	(62.3)	(17.7)	(4.45)	(116)	(29.0)	
Pineapple, Crushed, packed in unsweetened pineapple juice, no sugar added, 20-oz. can	350	87.5	17.5	4.38	140	35.0	
Drained solids (yield: approx. 14 oz.)	(248)	(62.3)	(17.7)	(4.45)	(116)	(29.0)	
Pineapple, Sliced, packed in heavy syrup, 20-oz. can	475	122.5	23.8	6.13	190	49.0	
Drained solids (yield: approx. 14 oz.)	(337)	(86.5)	(24.1)	(6.18)	(157)	(40.3)	
Pineapple, Sliced, packed in unsweetened juice, no sugar, 20-oz. can	350	87.5	17.5	4.38	140	35.0	
Drained solids (yield: approx. 14 oz.)	(248)	(62.3)	(17.7)	(4.45)	(116)	(29.0)	
Balanced Pineapple, Sliced, packed in water without added sugar or salt, 8.5-oz. can	159	37.8	18.7	4.45	(162)	(38.6)	
20-oz. can	374	89.0	18.7	4.45	(162)	(3.6)	
Del Monte Pineapple Chunks, packed in juice, 8¼-oz. can	144	36.1	17.5	4.38	140	35.0	
Drained solids (yield: approx. 5.8 oz.)	(102)	(25.6)	(17.6)	(4.41)	(117)	(29.4)	
Pineapple, Chunked, packed in syrup, 15½-oz. can	368	94.9	23.7	6.12	190	49.0	
Drained solids (yield: approx. 10.8 oz.)	(227)	(57.3)	(21.1)	(5.31)	(140)	(35.0)	
Pineapple, Chunked, packed in syrup, 20-oz. can	475	122.4	23.7	6.12	190	49.0	
Drained solids (yield: approx. 14 oz.)	(295)	(74.4)	(21.1)	(5.31)	(140)	(35.0)	
Pineapple, Crushed, packed in juice, 8¼-oz. can	144	36.1	17.5	4.38	140	35.0	
Drained solids (yield: approx. 5.8 oz.)	(102)	(25.6)	(17.6)	(4.41)	(117)	(29.4)	
Pineapple, Crushed, packed in juice, 15½-oz. can	271	67.8	17.5	4.38	140	35.0	
Drained solids (yield: approx. 10.9 oz.)	(192)	(48.1)	(17.6)	(4.41)	(117)	(29.4)	
Pineapple, Crushed, packed in syrup, 15½-oz. can	368	94.9	23.7	6.12	190	49.0	
Drained solids (yield: approx. 10.8 oz.)	(227)	(57.3)	(21.1)	(5.31)	(140)	(35.0)	
Pineapple, Crushed, packed in syrup, 20-oz. can	475	22.4	23.7	6.12	190	49.0	
Drained solids (yield: approx. 14 oz.)	(295)	(74.4)	(21.1)	(5.31)	(140)	(35.0)	
Pineapple Slices, packed in juice, 8¼-oz. can	144	36.1	17.5	4.38	140	35.0	
Drained solids (yield: approx. 5.8 oz.)	(102)	(25.6)	(17.6)	(4.41)	(117)	(29.4)	
Pineapple Slices, packed in juice, 15½-oz. can	271	67.8	17.5	4.38	140	35.0	
Drained solids (yield: approx. 10.9 oz.)	(192)	(48.1)	(17.6)	(4.41)	(117)	(29.4)	
Pineapple Slices, Medium, packed in syrup, 15½-oz. can	368	94.9	23.7	6.12	190	49.0	
Drained solids (yield: approx. 10.8 oz.)	(227)	(57.3)	(21.1)	(5.31)	(140)	(35.0)	
Pineapple Slices, Medium, packed in syrup, 20-oz. can	475	122.4	23.7	6.12	190	49.0	
Drained solids (yield: approx. 14 oz.)	(295)	(74.4)	(21.1)	(5.31)	(140)	(35.0)	
Diet Delight Pineapple Chunks, packed in pineapple juice, 15¼-oz. can	263	67.5	17.2	4.43	140	36.0	
Drained solids (yield: approx. 10.5 oz.)	(182)	(47.5)	(17.3)	(4.52)	(113)	(29.5)	
Pineapple, Fancy Hawaiian Sliced, packed in pineapple juice, 15¼-oz. can	263	67.5	17.2	4.43	140	36.0	
Drained solids (yield: approx. 10.5 oz.)	(182)	(47.5)	(17.3)	(4.52)	(113)	(29.5)	
Pineapple Tidbits, packed in pineapple juice, 8-oz. can	140	36.0	17.5	4.50	140	36.0	
Drained solids (yield: approx. 5.3 oz.)	(93)	(24.5)	(17.5)	(4.67)	(116)	(30.5)	
Dole Pineapple Chunks, packed in juice, 8¼-oz. can	133	34.2	16.1	4.14	128	33.0	
Drained solids (yield: approx. 5¼ oz.)	(87)	(22.8)	(16.4)	(4.32)	(107)	(28.2)	
Pineapple Chunks, packed in juice, 20-oz. can	321	82.9	16.1	4.14	128	33.0	
Drained solids (yield: approx. 14 oz.)	(228)	(60.1)	(16.4)	(4.32)	(107)	(23.2)	
Pineapple Chunks, packed in heavy syrup, 8¼-oz. can	174	45.5	21.1	5.52	168	44.0	
Drained solids (yield: approx. 5¼ oz.)	(96)	(27.5)	(18.6)	(5.30)	(121)	(34.6)	
Pineapple Chunks, packed in heavy syrup, 20-oz. can	421	110.4	21.1	5.52	168	44.0	
Drained solids (yield: approx. 14 oz.)	(265)	(74.4)	(18.6)	(5.30)	(121)	(34.6)	
Pineapple, Crushed, packed in pineapple juice, 8¼-oz. can	133	34.2	16.1	4.14	128	33.0	
Drained solids (yield: approx. 5.3 oz.)	(87)	(22.8)	(16.4)	(4.32)	(107)	(23.2)	
Pineapple, Crushed, packed in pineapple juice, 20-oz. can	321	82.9	16.1	4.14	128	33.0	
Drained solids (yield: approx. 14 oz.)	(228)	(60.1)	(16.4)	(4.32)	(107)	(23.2)	
Pineapple, Crushed, packed in heavy syrup, 8¼-oz. can	174	45.5	21.1	5.52	168	44.0	
Drained solids (yield: approx. 5¼ oz.)	(96)	(27.6)	(18.6)	(5.30)	(121)	(34.6)	
Pineapple, Crushed, packed in heavy syrup, 20-oz. can	421	110.4	21.1	5.52	168	44.0	
Drained solids (yield: approx. 14 oz.)	(265)	(74.4)	(18.6)	(5.30)	(121)	(34.6)	
Pineapple, Sliced, packed in pineapple juice, 8¼-oz. can	133	34.2	16.1	4.14	128	33.0	
Drained solids (yield: approx. 5.3 oz.)	(87)	(22.8)	(16.4)	(4.32)	(107)	(28.2)	
Pineapple, Sliced, packed in pineapple juice, 20-oz. can	321	82.9	16.1	4.14	128	33.0	
Drained solids (yield: approx. 14 oz.)	(228)	(60.1)	(16.4)	(4.32)	(107)	(23.2)	
Pineapple, Sliced, packed in heavy syrup, 8¼-oz. can	174	45.5	21.1	5.52	168	44.0	
Drained solids (yield: approx. 5¼ oz.)	(96)	(27.5)	(18.6)	(5.30)	(121)	(34.6)	
Pineapple, Sliced, packed in heavy syrup, 20-oz. can	421	110.4	21.1	5.52	168	44.0	
Drained solids (yield: approx. 14 oz.)	(265)	(74.4)	(18.6)	(5.30)	(121)	(34.6)	
Pineapple Tidbits, packed in heavy syrup, 8¼-oz. can	174	45.5	21.1	5.52	168	44.0	
Drained solids (yield: approx. 5¼ oz.)	(96)	(27.6)	(18.6)	(5.30)	(121)	(34.6)	
Pineapple Tidbits, packed in heavy syrup, 20-oz. can	421	110.4	21.1	5.52	168	44.0	
Drained solids (yield: approx. 14 oz.)	(265)	(74.4)	(18.6)	(5.30)	(121)	(34.6)	
Enchanted Elsie Pineapple Chunks in unsweetened pineapple juice, 20 oz. can	350	87.5	17.5	4.38	140	35.0	
Drained solids (yield: approx. 14 oz.)	248	62.3	17.7	4.45	116	29.2	
Pineapple, in unsweetened pineapple juice, Crushed, 20-oz. can	350	87.5	17.5	4.38	140	35.0	
Drained solids (yield: approx. 14 oz.)	248	62.3	17.7	4.45	159	39.9	
Pineapple Slices (in unsweetened pineapple juice), 20-oz. can	350	87.5	17.5	4.38	140	35.0	
Drained solids (yield: approx. 14 oz.)	248	62.3	17.7	4.45	116	29.2	
Featherweight Pineapple Chunks, packed in juice, no sugar added, 8-oz. can	(140)	(36.0)	(17.5)	(4.50)	140	36.0	
Drained solids (yield: approx. 5.2 oz.)	(92)	(24.2)	(17.8)	(4.67)	(116)	(30.4)	
Pineapple, Crushed, packed in juice, 8-oz.	(140)	(36.0)	(17.5)	(4.50)	140	36.0	
Drained solids (yield: approx. 5.2 oz.)	(92)	(24.2)	(17.8)	(4.67)	(116)	(30.4)	
Pineapple, Sliced, packed in juice, 8-oz. can	(140)	(36.0)	(17.5)	(4.50)	140	36.0	
Drained solids (yield: approx. 5.2 oz.)	(92)	(24.2)	(17.8)	(4.67)	(116)	(30.4)	
Pineapple, Sliced, packed in juice, 20-oz. can	(350)	(90.0)	(17.5)	(4.50)	140	36.0	
Drained solids (yield: approx. 13 oz.)	(231)	(60.6)	(17.8)	(4.67)	(116)	(30.4)	
Pineapple, Sliced, packed in pineapple juice, 8-oz. can	(140)	(36.0)	(17.5)	(4.50)	140	36.0	

	UNIT		1 OZ., BY WT.		1 CUP		Fiber per oz.
	Cal.	Carb.	Cal.	Carb.	Cal.	Carb.	(GMS.)
Drained solids (yield: approx. 5.2 oz.)	(92)	(24.2)	(17.8)	(4.67)	(116)	(30.4)	
Pineapple, Sliced, packed in water, 8-oz. can	(120)	(30.0)	(15.0)	(3.75)	120	30.0	
Pineapple Tidbits, packed in juice, 8½-oz. can	(140)	(36.0)	(16.5)	(4.24)	(140)	(36.0)	
Drained solids (yield: approx. 5.5 oz.)	(89)	(23.4)	(16.2)	(4.25)	(106)	(27.7)	
Golden Harvest Pineapple Chunks in Pineapple Juice, 8-oz. can	140	36.0	17.5	4.50	140	36.0	
Pineapple Slices in Water, no salt or sugar added, 8-oz. can	140	36.0	17.5	4.50	140	36.0	
Libby's Pineapple, 20-oz. can	300	80.0	15.0	4.00	120	32.0	
Tillie Lewis "Tasti Diet" Pineapple Chunks, packed in fruit juice, 20-oz. can	350	90.0	17.5	4.50	140	36.0	
Drained solids (yield: approx. 13 oz.)	(248)	(64.8)	(17.7)	(4.63)	(115)	(30.2)	
Pineapple, Sliced, packed in unsweetened pineapple juice, 8-oz. can	140	36.0	17.5	4.50	140	36.0	
Drained solids (yield: approx. 5.2 oz.)	(92)	(24.2)	(17.8)	(4.66)	(116)	(30.4)	
Pineapple Tidbits, packed in unsweetened pineapple juice, 8-oz. can	140	36.0	17.5	4.50	140	36.0	
Drained solids (yield: approx. 5.2 oz.)	(92)	(24.2)	(17.8)	(4.66)	(116)	(30.4)	
Town House Fancy Hawaiian Pineapple Chunks in heavy syrup, 13¼-oz. can	285	73.5	21.5	5.55	190	49.0	
Drained solids (yield: approx. 9.25 oz.)	193	49.5	20.9	5.35	140	34.9	
Fancy Hawaiian Pineapple, Crushed, in unsweetened pineapple juice, 20-oz. can	350	87.5	17.5	4.38	140	35.0	
Drained solids (yield: approx. 14 oz.)	248	62.3	17.7	4.45	159	39.9	
Fancy Hawaiian Pineapple Slices in heavy syrup, 16¼-oz. can	380	98.0	23.4	6.03	190	49.0	
Fancy Hawaiian Pineapple Slices in unsweetened pineapple juice, 20-oz. can	350	87.5	17.5	4.38	140	35.0	
Drained solids (yield: approx. 14 oz.)	248	62.3	17.7	4.45	116	29.2	
DRIED, by brand:							
Fruit Pac Dried Pineapple, Honey Dipped, 8-oz. package	675	178.1	84.4	22.26			
Sonoma Dried Pineapple, soft, 8-oz. package	618	162.8	77.2	20.35			
DEHYDRATED, by brand:							
Timber Crest Dehydrated Pineapple, hard, 5-lb. package	7760	2046.4	97.0	25.58			
CANDIED, based on generic data:							
1 pound (tr/23g/tr/18%/na)	1433	362.9	89.6	22.68	714	180.8	0.23

PINEAPPLE JUICE, see the BEVERAGES chapter

PITANGAS (also see SURINAM CHERRIES)

	UNIT		1 OZ., BY WT.		1 CUP		Fiber per oz.
	Cal.	Carb.	Cal.	Carb.	Cal.	Carb.	(GMS.)
As purchased [refuse: stem, blossom ends, and seeds, approx. 19%]:							
1 medium pitanga (approx. 0.2 oz.)	3	0.6	11.8	2.84			
1 pound (approx. 76 medium pitangas)	189	45.4	11.8	2.84			
Edible portion:							
1 medium pitanga (approx. 0.2 oz.)	3	0.6	14.5	3.56	87	21.3	0.17
1 cup (approx. 6 oz., 35 medium pitangas)	87	21.3	14.5	3.56	87	21.3	0.17
1 pound (approx. 2.7 cups, 94 pitangas) (tr/4g/tr/86%/na)	232	56.9	14.5	3.56	87	21.3	0.17

PLANTAIN, see the VEGETABLES chapter

PLUMS

The PLUMS listed here are the fresh fruit. For the dried fruit, see PRUNES.

	UNIT		1 OZ., BY WT.		1 CUP		Fiber per oz.
	Cal.	Carb.	Cal.	Carb.	Cal.	Carb.	(GMS.)
DAMSON							
As purchased [refuse: pits and clinging pulp, approx. 9%]:							
1 medium plum (approx. 1" diameter, ⅔ oz.)	7	1.8	17.0	4.59	87	23.5	
1 cup (approx. 5.1 oz.)	87	23.5	17.0	4.59	87	23.5	
1 pound (approx. 3.1 cups, 41 medium plums)	272	73.5	17.0	4.59	87	23.5	
Edible portion:							
1 medium plum (approx. ⅓ oz.)	7	1.8	18.7	5.04	112	30.3	0.11
1 cup, halved (approx. 6 oz.)	112	30.3	18.7	5.04	112	30.3	0.11
1 pound (approx. 2.7 cups, 45½ plums) (tr/5g/tr/81%/1mg)	299	80.7	18.7	5.04	112	30.3	0.11
JAPANESE AND HYBRID							
As purchased [refuse: pits approx. 6%]:							
1 medium plum (approx. 2⅛" diameter, 2.5 oz.)	32	8.1	12.8	3.28			
1 pound (approx. 6½ medium plums)	205	52.4	12.8	3.28			
Edible portion:							
1 medium plum (approx. 2.3 oz.)	32	8.1	13.7	3.50	89	22.8	0.17
1 cup:							
halved (approx. 6½ oz.)	89	22.8	13.7	3.50	89	22.8	0.17
sliced or diced (approx. 5⅘ oz.)	79	20.3	13.7	3.50	79	20.3	0.17
1 pound (approx. 2.5 cups halved or 2.8 cups sliced or diced, 7 medium plums) (tr/4g/tr/87%/tr)	218	56.0	13.7	3.50	89	22.8	0.17
MIRABELLE PLUM (based on data from France)							
Edible portion:							
1 pound	304	70.3	19.0	4.39			
PRUNE TYPE							
As purchased [refuse: pits, approx.6%]							
1 plum (approx. 1½" diameter, 1.1 oz.)	21	5.6	19.0	5.10			
1 pound (approx. 15.1 plums)	320	84.0	19.0	5.10			
Edible portion:							
1 plum (approx. 1 oz.)	21	5.6	21.4	5.60			
1 cup, halved (approx. 5.8 oz.)	124	32.5	21.4	5.60	124	32.5	
1 pound (approx. 2.8 cups, 15.9 plums) (tr/6g/tr/79%/tr)	340	89.4	21.4	5.60	124	32.5	
PURPLE (Italian Prunes)							
CANNED, based on generic data:							
Solids and liquid:							
Packed in water, with or without artificial sweetener:							
Whole [refuse: pits, approx. 4%]:							
1 cup (approx. 9.2 oz.)	114	29.6	12.4	3.21	114	29.6	
1 pound (approx. 1.7 cups)	198	51.4	12.4	3.21	114	29.6	
Can, #303, 16 oz. (1 lb.) net wt. (contents: 10–14 plums and 9 Tbsp. of drained liquid)	198	51.3	12.4	3.21	114	29.6	
Halved (pits removed):							
1 pound (tr/3g/tr/87%/2mg)	209	53.9	13.0	3.37	(120)	(31.0)	0.09
Packed in juice:							
Pits removed:							
3 plums with 2 Tbsp. of liquid (approx. 3.3 oz.)	55	14.4	16.5	4.30	263	68.8	0.07
1 cup (approx. 8.8 oz.)	146	38.2	16.5	4.30	263	68.8	0.07
1 pound (approx. 1.8 cups) (tr/4g/tr/84%/tr)	263	68.8	16.5	4.30	263	68.8	0.07
Packed in light syrup:							
Whole [refuse: pits, approx. 4%]							
1 cup (approx. 9.3 oz.)	159	42.0	17.1	4.52	159	42.0	
1 pound (approx. 1¾ cups)	274	72.3	17.1	4.52	159	42.0	
Halved (pits removed):							
1 pound (tr/5g/tr/82%/tr)	285	4.9	17.8	4.71	159	42.0	0.09
Packed in heavy syrup:							
Whole [refuse: pits, approx. 4%]:							
1 cup (approx. 9.6 oz.)	214	55.8	22.2	5.77	214	55.8	
1 pound (approx. 1½ cups)	358	92.3	22.2	5.77	214	55.8	
Can, #303, 16¾–17 oz. net wt. (contents: approx. 10–14 plums and 9 Tbsp. of drained liquid)	377	98.1	22.2	5.77	214	55.8	
Can, #2½, 30 oz. (1 lb. 14 oz.) net wt. (contents: 12–20 plums and 17 Tbsp. of drained liquid)	671	174.6	22.2	5.77	214	55.8	
Halved (pits removed):							
1 pound (tr/6g/tr/77%/tr)	376	98.0	23.5	6.12	(226)	(58.8)	0.09
Packed in extra heavy syrup:							
Whole [refuse: pits, approx. 4%]:							
1 cup (approx. 9.9 oz.)	275	72.0	27.8	7.27	275	72.0	
1 pound (approx. 1.6 cups)	444	116.3	27.8	7.27	275	72.0	
Halved (pits removed):							
1 pound (tr/8g/tr/72%/tr)	463	121.1	28.9	7.57	(286)	(74.9)	0.09

	UNIT		1 OZ., BY WT.		1 CUP		Fiber per oz.
	Cal.	Carb.	Cal.	Carb.	Cal.	Carb.	(GMS.)
CANNED, by brand:							
Balanced Whole Purple Plums, packed in water without sugar or salt 16-oz. (1-lb.) can	200	49.9	12.5	3.12	(103)	(25.8)	
Del Monte Purple Plums With Pits, 8-oz. can	179	49.0	22.4	6.12	190	52.0	
Diet Delight Halved Purple Plums, packed in water and grape juice concentrate, 8-oz. can	140	38.0	17.5	4.75	(148)	(40.3)	
Whole Purple Plums, packed in water, 8½-oz. can	96	23.1	11.3	2.72	(100)	(24.0)	
16-oz. (1-lb.) can	181	43.5	11.3	2.72	(100)	(24.0)	
Featherweight Purple Plums, packed in water, 8-oz. can	(78)	(18.0)	(9.8)	(2.25)	78	18.0	
Whole Purple Plums, packed in pear juice, 8-oz. can	(134)	(18.0)	(16.8)	(2.25)	(134)	(18.0)	
16-oz. (1-lb.) can	(268)	(36.0)	(16.8)	(2.25)	(134)	(18.0)	
Golden Harvest Purple Plum Halves in Water, no sugar or salt added, 16-oz. (1-lb.) can	220	68.0	13.8	4.25	110	34.0	
Libby's Plums, packed in heavy syrup, 8½-oz. can	(217)	(57.7)	(25.5)	(6.79)	210	56.0	
17-oz. can	(434)	(115.0)	(25.5)	(6.79)			
Oregon Whole Purple Plums, packed in heavy syrup, 16-oz. can	380	95.0	23.8	5.94	(196)	(49.0)	
Stokely Purple Plums, 16-oz. (1-lb.) can	419	104.6	26.2	6.54	240	60.0	
30-oz. can	786	196.2	26.2	6.54	240	60.0	
DRIED, by brand:							
Grocer's Choice Plum Fruit Roll, 1-oz. package	90	20.0	90.0	20.00			
POHA (also see GROUNDCHERRIES)							
As purchased [refuse: husk, approx. 9%]:							
1 pound	266	63.9	16.6	3.99			
Edible portion:							
1 cup (approx. 4.9 oz.)	90	21.7	18.2	4.39	90	21.7	
1 pound (approx. 3.2 cups) (tr/4g/tr/82%/na)	291	70.3	18.2	4.39	90	21.7	
POMEGRANATES							
As purchased [refuse: skin and seeds, approx. 44%]:							
1 medium pomegranate, approx. 3⅜" diameter, 2¾" high, 9.7 oz.)	97	25.3	10.0	2.61			
1 pound (approx. 1⅔ medium pomegranates)	160	41.8	10.0	2.61			
Edible portion:							
1 medium pomegranate (approx. 5.4 oz.)	97	25.3	17.9	4.67			0.06
1 pound (approx. 3 medium pomegranates) (tr/5g/tr/82%/1mg)	286	74.6	17.9	4.67			0.06
POMEGRANATE JUICE, see the BEVERAGES chapter							
PRICKLY PEARS							
As purchased [refuse: rind and seeds, approx. 56%]:							
1 pound	84	21.8	5.3	1.36			
Edible portion:							
1 pound (tr/3g/tr/88%/1mg)	191	49.4	11.9	3.09			0.45
PRUNES							
CANNED, based on generic data:							
Solids and liquid:							
Packed in heavy syrup:							
Pits removed:							
5 prunes with 2 Tbsp. of liquid (approx. 3 oz.)	90	23.9	29.8	7.89	245	65.1	0.20
1 cup (approx. 8.2 oz.)	245	65.1	29.8	7.89	245	65.1	0.20
1 pound (approx. 2 cups) (tr/89/tr/71%/1mg)	477	126.2	29.8	7.89	245	65.1	0.20
DEHYDRATED, SULFURED, based on generic data:							
Nugget-Type and Pieces:							
Uncooked:							
1 cup (approx. 3½ oz.)	344	91.3	97.5	25.89	344	91.3	(0.62)
1 pound (approx. 4½ cups) (tr/13g/1g/3%/3mg)	1560	414.1	97.5	25.89	344	91.3	(0.62)
Cooked:							
1 pound of dehydrated prunes cooked in 3 cups of water with 1 cup sugar:							
1 cup (approx. 9.9 oz.)	504	131.9	51.0	13.35	504	131.9	(0.23)
1 pound (approx. 1.6 cups) (tr/13g/tr/51%/1mg)	816	213.6	51.0	13.35	504	131.9	(0.23)
DRIED, "SOFTENIZED" (28% moisture), based on generic data:							
Uncooked:							
As purchased [% refuse varies greatly with size]:							
Small (approx. 80 per lb.) [refuse: pits, approx. 18%]:							
1 small prune (approx. ⅕ oz.)	(12)	(3.1)	(59.3)	(15.67)	(385)	(101.9)	
1 cup (approx. 6½ oz., 32½ small prunes)	(385)	(101.9)	(59.3)	(15.67)	(385)	(101.9)	
1 pound (approx. 2.5 cups, 80 small prunes)	(949)	(250.7)	(59.3)	(15.67)	(385)	(101.9)	
Medium (approx. 60 per lb.) [refuse: pits, approx. 15%]:							
1 medium prune (approx. ¼ oz.)	16	4.4	62.2	16.43	404	106.8	
1 cup (approx. 6½ oz., 26 medium prunes)	404	106.8	62.2	16.43	404	106.8	
1 pound (approx. 2.5 cups, 60 medium prunes)	995	262.9	62.2	16.43	404	106.8	
1 container, 32 oz. net wt. (approx. 120 medium prunes)	1990	525.8	62.2	16.43	404	106.8	
Large (approx. 50 per lb.) [refuse: pits, approx. 12%]:							
1 large prune (approx. ⅓ oz.)	22	5.7	62.9	16.63	409	108.1	
1 cup (approx. 6½ oz., 19½ large prunes)	409	108.1	62.9	16.63	409	108.1	
1 pound (approx. 2.5 cups, 50 large prunes)	1006	266.0	62.9	16.63	409	108.1	
Extra large (approx. 40 per lb.) [refuse: pits, approx. 12%]:							
1 extra large prune (approx. 0.43 oz.)	27	7.2	63.6	16.82	411	108.5	
1 cup (approx. 6½ oz., 15 extra large prunes)	411	108.5	63.6	16.82	411	108.5	
1 pound (approx. 2.5 cups, 40 extra large prunes)	1018	269.1	63.6	16.82	411	108.5	
1 container, 16 oz. net wt. (approx. 40 extra large prunes)	1018	269.1	63.6	16.82	411	108.5	
Edible portion:							
1 small prune (approx. 0.17 oz.)	(12)	(3.1)	72.3	19.11	(459)	(121.3)	0.45
1 medium prune (approx. ¼ oz.)	16	4.4	72.3	19.11	(459)	(121.3)	0.45
1 large prune (approx. 0.3 oz.)	22	5.7	72.3	19.11	(459)	(121.3)	0.45
1 extra large prune (approx. ⅓ oz.)	27	7.2	72.3	19.11	(459)	(121.3)	0.45
1 cup:							
Whole (approx. 6⅓ oz.)	459	121.3	72.3	19.11	459	121.3	0.45
Chopped, not packed (approx. 5.6 oz.)	408	107.8	72.3	19.11	408	107.8	0.45
Chopped, packed (approx. 9.2 oz.)	663	175.2	72.3	19.11	663	175.2	0.45
1 pound (tr/19g/1g/28%/2mg)	1157	305.7	72.3	19.11			0.45
1 container, 12 oz. net wt.	868	229.3	72.3	19.11			0.45
Cooked, with pits [refuse: pits, 15%, variable with size]:							
Cooked without sugar (served cold):							
1 cup (approx. 8.8 oz.)	253	66.7	28.7	7.57	253	66.7	
1 pound (approx. 1.8 cups) (tr/8g/tr/66%/1mg)	459	121.1	28.7	7.57	253	66.7	
Cooked with sugar, 1 pound dried prunes cooked in 3 cups of water with 1 cup sugar (served cold):							
1 cup (approx. 9.9 oz.)	409	107.3	41.4	10.87	409	107.3	
1 pound (approx. 1.6 cups) (tr/11g/tr/53%/1mg)	663	173.9	41.4	10.87	409	107.3	
Edible portion:							
Cooked without sugar (served cold), 1 pound	539	142.4	33.7	8.90			0.23
Cooked with sugar (served cold), 1 pound	780	204.6	48.8	12.79			0.17
Prune Whip (based on USDA home recipe) prepared with ¾ cup of cooked prune pulp, 3 Tbsp. of sugar, 3 medium egg whites, 1 Tbsp. of lemon juice [yield: approx. 4 cups (loss of 20% applied for evaporation in cooking)] (1g/10g/tr/51%/46mg)	(560)	(132.8)	44.1	10.46	140	33.2	0.17

	UNIT Cal.	UNIT Carb.	1 OZ., BY WT. Cal.	1 OZ., BY WT. Carb.	1 CUP Cal.	1 CUP Carb.	Fiber per oz. (GMS.)
CANNED, by brand:							
Del Monte Stewed Prunes with Pits, 16-oz. (1-lb.) can	460	120.0	28.8	7.50	230	60.0	
Pits removed (yield: approx. 13.3 oz.)	460	120.0	34.6	9.02			
32-oz. (2-lb.) can	920	240.0	28.8	7.50	230	60.0	
Pits removed (yield: approx. 26.6 oz.)	(920)	(240.0)	(34.6)	(9.02)			
Featherweight Stewed Prunes, packed in water, 8-oz. can	(260)	(70.0)	(32.5)	(8.75)	260	70.0	
Drained solids (yield: approx. 6.4 oz.)	(250)	(67.6)	(39.1)	(10.56)	(218)	(70.8)	
16-oz. (1-lb.) can	(520)	(140.0)	(32.5)	(8.75)	260	70.0	
Drained solids (yield: approx. 12.8 oz.)	(500)	(135.2)	(39.1)	(10.56)	(218)	(70.8)	
RTS Cooked Prunes, packed in heavy syrup, 16-oz. can	384	96.0	24.0	6.00	240	60.0	
Drained solids (yield: approx. 10.1 oz.)	(248)	(60.5)	(24.6)	(6.00)	(165)	(40.2)	
25-oz. can	600	150.0	24.0	6.00	240	60.0	
Drained solids (yield: approx. 15.8 oz.)	(387)	(94.5)	(24.6)	(6.00)	(165)	(40.2)	
DRIED, by brand:							
Del Monte Dried Uncooked with Pits, 16-oz. (1-lb.) can	960	240.0	60.0	15.00	(396)	(99.0)	
32-oz. (2-lb.) can	1920	480.0	60.0	15.00	(396)	(99.0)	
Dried Pitted Prunes, 12-oz. can	840	216.0	70.0	18.00			
24-oz. can	1680	432.0	70.0	18.00			
Fruit Pac Dried Breakfast Prunes, Honey Dipped, 16-oz. (1-lb.) package	1325	351.0	82.8	21.94	546	144.7	
Dried Jumbo Prunes, Honey Dipped, 16-oz. (1-lb.) package	1325	351.0	82.8	21.94	546	144.7	
Dried Large Prunes, Honey Dipped, 16-oz. (1-lb.) package	1325	351.0	82.8	21.94	546	144.7	
Dried Petite Prunes, Honey Dipped, 16-oz. (1-lb.) package	1325	351.0	82.8	21.94	546	144.7	
Sonoma Dried Breakfast Prunes, soft, 16-oz. (1-lb.) package	1157	305.8	72.3	19.11	434	114.6	
Dried Jumbo Prunes, soft, 16-oz. (1-lb.) package	1157	305.8	72.3	19.11	434	114.6	
Dried Large Prunes, soft, 16-oz. (1-lb.) package	1157	305.8	72.3	19.11	434	114.6	
Sunsweet California Large Prunes, 32-oz. (2-lb.) box	1920	512.0	60.0	16.00			
California Pitted Prunes, 12-oz. box (equals 3 lb. of fresh plums)	840	216.0	70.0	18.00			
Large Prunes, 16-oz. (1-lb.) box (equals 3½ lb. of fresh plums)	960	248.0	60.0	15.50			
32-oz. (2-lb.) box (equals 7 lb. of fresh plums)	1920	496.0	60.0	15.50			
Pitted Prunes, 12-oz. box	840	216.0	70.0	18.00			
24-oz. box	1680	432.0	70.0	18.00			
DEHYDRATED, by brand:							
Timber Crest Dehydrated Breakfast Prunes, hard, 5-lb. package	7800	2071.2	97.5	25.89	403	106.8	
Dehydrated Jumbo Prunes, hard, 5-lb. package	7800	2071.2	97.5	25.89	403	106.8	
Dehydrated Large Prunes, hard, 5-lb. package	7800	2071.2	97.5	25.89	403	106.8	

PRUNE JUICE, see the BEVERAGES chapter

PUMMELOS (Shaddocks) (based on data from Hawaii)

	UNIT Cal.	UNIT Carb.	1 OZ., BY WT. Cal.	1 OZ., BY WT. Carb.	1 CUP Cal.	1 CUP Carb.	Fiber per oz. (GMS.)
As purchased [refuse: skin, seeds, and membranes, approx. 44%]:							
1 medium pummelo (approx. 2 lb. 6.4 oz.)	207	53.5	5.4	1.39			
1 pound (approx. 0.4 medium pummelos)	86	22.3	5.4	1.39			
Edible portion:							
1 medium pummelo (approx. 1 lb. 5.4 oz.) (tr/2g/tr/90%/na)	207	53.5	9.6	2.49			
1 cup, sections (approx. 6.7 oz.)	65	16.7	9.6	2.49	65	16.7	
1 pound (approx. 2.4 cups, 0.7 medium pummelos)	154	39.8	9.6	2.49	65	16.7	

QUINCES

	UNIT Cal.	UNIT Carb.	1 OZ., BY WT. Cal.	1 OZ., BY WT. Carb.	1 CUP Cal.	1 CUP Carb.	Fiber per oz. (GMS.)
As purchased [refuse: parings, core, and seeds, approx. 39%]:							
1 pound	158	42.3	9.9	2.64			
Edible portion:							
1 pound (tr/4g/tr/84%/1mg)	259	69.5	16.2	4.34			0.48

RAISINS

	UNIT Cal.	UNIT Carb.	1 OZ., BY WT. Cal.	1 OZ., BY WT. Carb.	1 CUP Cal.	1 CUP Carb.	Fiber per oz. (GMS.)
"NATURAL" (UNBLEACHED) SEEDLESS, based on generic data:							
(Averages taken primarily on Thompson seedless)							
All-edible:							
UNCOOKED:							
1 pound (approx. 3⅛ cups whole raisins, not packed, or 2¾ cups packed) (tr/22g/1g/18%/8mg)	1311	351.1	81.9	21.91	419	112.2	0.26
1 package, ½ oz. net wt. (approx. 1½ Tbsp.)	40	10.8	81.9	21.91	419	112.2	0.26
1 package, 1½ oz. net wt. (approx. ⅓ cup, not packed)	124	33.3	81.9	21.91	419	112.2	0.26
1 package, 15 oz. net wt. (approx. 3 cups, not packed, or 2½ cups packed)	1228	329.0	81.9	21.91	419	112.2	0.26
1 cup							
Whole:							
Not packed (approx. 5.1 oz.)	419	112.2	81.9	21.91	419	112.2	0.26
Packed (approx. 5.8 oz.)	477	127.7	81.9	21.91	477	127.7	0.26
Chopped:							
Not packed (approx. 4.8 oz.)	393	105.2	81.9	21.91	393	105.2	0.26
Packed (approx. 6.7 oz.)	549	146.8	81.9	21.91	549	146.8	0.26
Ground:							
Not packed (approx. 7.1 oz.)	581	155.6	81.9	21.91	581	155.6	0.26
Packed (approx. 9½ oz.)	778	208.1	81.9	21.91	778	208.1	0.26
COOKED:							
1 pound of seedless raisins cooked in 3 cups of water with 1 cup of sugar:							
1 cup (approx. 10.4 oz.)	628	166.4	60.4	16.00	628	166.4	0.26
1 pound (approx. 1½ cups) (tr/16g/tr/41%/4mg)	966	256.0	60.4	16.00	628	166.4	0.26
NATURAL THOMPSON SEEDLESS, based on data from California Raisin Advisory Board:							
15-oz. package	1250	330.0	83.3	22.00	500	132.0	
PREPACKAGED, by brand:							
A & P Seedless Raisins, 11-oz. box	925	244.2	84.1	22.00	500	132.0	
15-oz. box	1250	330.0	83.3	22.00			
Bonner Golden Raisins, 15-oz. box	1250	330.0	83.3	22.00	500	132.0	
Del Monte Golden Seedless Raisins, 8-oz. box	694	181.3	86.7	22.67	520	136.0	
15-oz. box	1300	340.0	86.7	22.67	(520)	(136.0)	
Muscat Raisins, 15-oz. box	1250	330.0	83.3	22.00	(500)	(132.0)	
Thompson Seedless Raisins, 8-oz. box	693	176.0	86.7	22.00	(520)	(132.0)	
15-oz. box	1300	330.0	86.7	22.00	(520)	(132.0)	
Fruit Pac Dried Monukka Raisins, Honey Dipped, 16-oz. (1-lb.) package	1379	369.8	86.2	23.11	438	117.4	
Dried Thompson Raisins, Honey Dipped, 16-oz. (1-lb.) package	1379	369.8	86.2	23.11	438	117.4	
Sonoma Dried Monukka Raisins, soft, 16-oz. (1-lb.) package	1310	351.0	81.9	21.94	416	111.5	
Dried Thompson Raisins, soft, 16-oz. (1-lb.) package	1310	351.0	81.9	21.94	416	111.5	
Sun-Maid Puffed Seeded Muscat Raisins, 15-oz. package	1250	330.0	83.3	22.00	(500)	(132.0)	
DEHYDRATED, by brand:							
Timber Crest Dehydrated Monukka Raisins, hard, 5-lb. package	8192	2196.0	102.4	27.45			
Dehydrated Thompson Raisins, hard, 5-lb. package	8192	2196.0	102.4	27.45			
For comparison: Raisinets, **WARD,** 8-oz. box	720	112.0	90.0	14.00			

RASPBERRIES

	UNIT Cal.	UNIT Carb.	1 OZ., BY WT. Cal.	1 OZ., BY WT. Carb.	1 CUP Cal.	1 CUP Carb.	Fiber per oz. (GMS.)
BLACK RASPBERRIES							
As purchased [refuse: stems, caps and damaged berries, approx. 3%]:							
1 pound (approx. 215 small berries or 135 large berries)	331	71.7	20.7	4.45	(98)	(21.0)	
Edible portion:							
1 small berry (approx. 0.07 oz.)	2	0.3	21.3	4.59	101	21.6	1.48
1 large berry (approx. 0.12 oz.)	3	0.5	21.3	4.59	101	21.6	1.48
1 cup (approx. 4.7 oz., 67 small berries or 39 large berries)	101	21.6	21.3	4.59	101	21.6	1.48

	UNIT		1 OZ., BY WT.		1 CUP		Fiber per oz.
	Cal.	Carb.	Cal.	Carb.	Cal.	Carb.	(GMS.)
1 pound (approx. 3.4 cups, 228 small berries or 133 large berries) (tr/4g/tr/81%/tr)	341	73.9	21.3	4.59	101	21.6	1.48
RED RASPBERRIES							
As purchased [refuse: stems, caps, damaged berries, approx. 3%]:							
1 pound (approx. 215 small berries or 135 large berries)	259	61.7	16.2	3.86	70	16.7	
Edible portion:							
1 small berry (approx. 0.07 oz.)	1	0.3	16.7	3.98	72	17.1	0.85
1 large berry (approx. 0.12 oz.)	2	0.5	16.7	3.98	72	17.1	0.85
1 cup (approx. 4.3 oz., 61 small berries or 36 large berries)	72	17.1	16.7	3.98	72	17.1	0.85
1 pound (approx. 3.7 cups, 229 small berries or 133 large berries) (tr/4g/tr/84%/tr)	267	63.7	16.7	3.98	72	17.1	0.85
1 pint container, filled to overflowing (11.5 oz. net wt., approx. 164 small berries or 96 large berries)	192	45.8	16.7	3.98	72	17.1	0.85
FROZEN, by brand:							
Birds Eye Red Raspberries, 10 oz. package	280	70.0	28.0	7.00	(215)	(53.8)	
Drained solids (yield: approx. 5 oz.)	(280)	(70.0)	56.0	14.00			
CANNED, based on generic data:							
Packed in heavy syrup:							
1 cup (approx. 9.0 oz.)	234	59.8	25.8	6.60	234	59.8	
1 pound (approx. 1.8 cups) (tr/7g/tr/75%/1mg)	413	106.1	25.8	6.60	234	59.8	
CANNED, by brand:							
Oregon Red Raspberries, packed in heavy syrup, 16-oz. (1-lb.) can	416	104.0	26.0	6.50	(223)	(55.7)	
Drained solids (yield: approx. 8.3 oz.)	(216)	(50.1)	(26.0)	(6.04)	(200)	(46.0)	
DRIED, by brand:							
Grocer's Choice Raspberry fruit roll, 1-oz. package	90	21.0	90.0	21.00			
RASPBERRY JUICE, see the BEVERAGES chapter							
RHUBARB							
As purchased, freshly harvested with full tops [refuse: ends and full leaves, approx. 55%]:							
1 pound	33	7.6	2.1	0.48			
As purchased, partially trimmed [refuse: ends and trimmings, approx. 14%]:							
1 pound (approx. 3.7 cups)	62	14.4	3.9	0.90			
Edible portion:							
1 cup, diced (approx. 4.3 oz.)	20	4.5	4.7	1.05	20	4.5	0.20
1 pound (approx. 3.7 cups) (tr/1g/tr/95%/1mg)	75	16.8	4.7	1.05	20	4.5	0.20
COOKED:							
2 cups of diced rhubarb cooked in 2 Tbsp. of water with ½ cup of sugar (yield: approx. 10.2 oz.; 1.1 cups)	408	104.1	40.0	10.21	381	97.2	0.17
1 cup (approx. 9½ oz.)	381	97.2	40.0	10.21	381	97.2	0.17
1 pound (approx. 1.7 cups) (tr/10g/tr/63%/1mg)	641	163.0	40.0	10.21	381	97.2	0.17
FROZEN, based on generic data:							
Measured when frozen:							
All-edible, pre-sweetened:							
1 package, 10 oz. net wt.	213	52.5	21.3	5.25	340	83.9	0.26
1 pound (tr/5g/tr/80%/1mg)	340	83.9	21.3	5.25	340	83.9	0.26
Boiled, drained:							
2 cups of pre-sweetened frozen rhubarb cooked in 2½ Tbsp. of water with an additional ½ cup of sugar: Yield from 10 oz. package (approx. 12 oz., 1¼ cups)	486	123.1	40.5	10.26	386	97.7	0.23
1 cup (approx. 9½ oz.)	386	97.7	40.5	10.26	386	97.7	0.23
1 pound (approx. 1.7 cups)	650	165.0	40.5	10.26	386	97.7	0.23
ROSEAPPLES							
As purchased [refuse: caps and seeds, approx. 33%]:							
1 pound	170	43.2	10.6	2.70			
Edible portion:							
1 pound (tr/4g/tr/85%/na)	254	64.5	15.9	4.00			0.31

	UNIT		1 OZ., BY WT.		1 CUP		Fiber per oz.
	Cal.	Carb.	Cal.	Carb.	Cal.	Carb.	(GMS.)
ROSELLE (based on data from Hawaii)							
As purchased [refuse: seed pods and stems, approx. 39%]							
1 cup (approx. 2 oz.)	12	2.4	6.0	1.22	12	2.4	
1 pound (approx. 8 cups)	96	19.5	6.0	1.22	12	2.4	
Edible portion:							
1 pound (tr/2g/tr/91%/na)	157	32.0	9.8	2.00			
SAPODILLA							
As purchased [refuse: skin and seeds, approx. 20%]:							
1 pound	323	79.1	20.2	4.94			
Edible portion:							
1 pound (tr/6g/tr/76%/3mg)	404	99.0	25.3	6.19			0.40
SAPOTES (Marmalade Plums) (also see MAMMEE APPLES)							
As purchased [refuse: skin and seeds, approx. 24%]:							
1 pound	431	108.9	26.9	6.81			
Edible portion:							
1 pound (tr/9g/1g/6%/na)	567	143.3	35.4	8.96			0.31
(Based on data from Hawaii)							
Edible portion:							
1 medium sapote (approx. 7.9 oz.)	241	60.7	30.5	7.68			
1 pound (approx. 2 medium sapotes)	488	122.9	30.5	7.68			
SHADDOCKS, see PUMMELOS							
SOURSOP (based on data from Hawaii)							
As purchased [refuse: skin and seeds, approx. 34%]:							
1 medium soursop (approx. 44.1 oz.)	586	150.4	13.3	3.41			
1 pound (approx. 0.4 medium soursops)	213	54.6	13.3	3.41			
Edible portion:							
1 medium soursop (approx. 29.1 oz.)	586	150.4	20.2	5.17	160	41.0	
1 cup (approx. 7.9 oz.)	160	41.0	20.2	5.17	160	41.0	
1 pound (approx. 0.55 medium soursops, 2 cups) (tr/5g/tr/80%/na)	323	82.7	20.2	5.17	160	41.0	
Juice only:							
Juice of 1 medium soursop [yield: approx. 22.0 oz. (17.6 fl. oz., 2.2 cups) of juice]	444	113.9	(20.2)	(5.17)	(198)	(50.7)	
SOURSOP JUICE, see also the BEVERAGES chapter							
1 cup (approx. 9.8 oz.)	(198)	(50.7)	(20.2)	(5.17)	(198)	(50.7)	
1 pound (approx. 1.6 cups) (tr/5g/tr/82%/na)	(323)	(82.7)	(20.2)	(5.17)	(198)	(50.7)	
STARFRUIT, see CARAMBOLA							
STRAWBERRIES							
Based on strawberries of good quality:							
As purchased [refuse: caps and stems, approx. 4%]							
1 pound (approx. 40 small; 28 medium; 34 mixed, small and medium; or 10 very large strawberries)	161	36.6	10.1	2.29	(55)	(12.5)	
1-pint container, filled to overflowing (approx. 12 oz. net wt., Approx. 30 small; 20 medium; 24 mixed, small and medium; or 7½ very large strawberries)	121	27.4	10.1	2.29	(55)	(12.5)	

	UNIT Cal.	UNIT Carb.	1 OZ., BY WT. Cal.	1 OZ., BY WT. Carb.	1 CUP Cal.	1 CUP Carb.	Fiber per oz. (GMS.)
1-quart container, filled to overflowing (approx. 24 oz. net wt., Approx. 60 small; 40 medium; 48 mixed, small and medium; or 15 very large strawberries)	242	54.8	10.1	2.29	(55)	(12.5)	
Edible portion:							
1 small strawberry (approx. 0.4 oz.)	4	1.0	10.5	2.38	55	12.5	0.37
1 medium strawberry (approx. 0.6 oz.)	6	1.4	10.5	2.38	55	12.5	0.37
1 very large strawberry (approx. 1.6 oz.)	17	3.8	10.5	2.38	55	12.5	0.37
1 cup (approx. 5¼ oz. Approx. 13 small; 8¾ medium; 10½ mixed, small and medium; or 3¼ very large strawberries)	55	12.5	10.5	2.38	55	12.5	0.37
1 pound (approx. 40 small; 28 medium; 34 mixed, small and medium; or 10 very large strawberries)	168	38.1	10.5	2.38	55	12.5	0.37
Based on strawberries of fair quality:							
As purchased [refuse: caps, stems, green berries and damaged berries, approx. 13%]:							
1 pound (approx. 38 medium or 10 very large strawberries)	146	33.1	9.1	2.07	(56)	(12.6)	
1-pint container, filled to overflowing (approx. 12 oz. net wt. Approx. 21 medium or 8 very large strawberries)	109	24.8	9.1	2.07	(56)	(12.6)	
1-quart container, filled to overflowing (approx. 24 oz. net wt. Approx. 42 medium or 15 very large strawberries)	218	49.7	9.1	2.07	(56)	(12.6)	
Edible portion:							
1 medium strawberry (approx. 0.57 oz.)	6	1.4	10.5	2.38	56	12.6	0.37
1 very large strawberry (approx. 0.63 oz.)	7	1.5	10.5	2.38	56	12.6	0.37
1 cup (approx. 5.3 oz., 9.3 medium or 8.4 very large strawberries)	56	12.6	10.5	2.38	56	12.6	0.37
1 pound (approx. 3 cups, 28 medium or 10 very large strawberries)	168	38.1	10.5	2.38	56	12.6	0.37
FROZEN, by brand:							
Big Valley Fresh Whole Frozen Strawberries, 20-oz. package	210		10.5		(94)		
Drained solids (yield: approx. 18 oz.)	(210)		(11.7)		(105)		
Birds Eye Frozen Strawberries, 10-oz. package	220	60.0	22.0	6.00	(158)	(43.2)	
Drained solids (yield: approx. 6 oz.)	(220)	(60.0)	(36.7)	(10.00)	(264)	(72.0)	
Frozen Strawberry Halves, 16-oz. (1-lb.) package	510	144.0	31.9	9.00	(269)	(80.0)	
Drained solids (yield: approx. 9.6 oz.)	(510)	(144.0)	(53.1)	(15.00)	(382)	(108.0)	
Frozen Strawberries, Sliced, 10-oz. package	360	96.0	36.0	9.60	(302)	(80.6)	
Drained solids (yield: approx. 6.0 oz.)	(360)	(96.0)	(60.0)	(16.00)	(432)	(115.2)	
Frozen Whole Strawberries, 16-oz. (1-lb.) package	280	80.0	17.5	5.00	(126)	(36.0)	
Drained solids (yield: approx. 14.4 oz.)	(280)	(80.0)	(19.4)	(5.56)	(140)	(40.0)	
Brady's Unsweetened Whole Frozen Strawberries, 16-oz. (1-lb.) package	148	36.0	9.3	2.25	(67)	(16.2)	
Drained solids (yield: approx. 14.4 oz.)	(148)	(36.0)	(10.3)	(2.50)	(148)	(18.0)	
Ralph's Whole Strawberries frozen with no added sugar, 16-oz. (1-lb.) package	180	48.0	11.3	3.00	90	24.0	
CANNED, based on generic data:							
Solids and liquids:							
Packed in heavy syrup:							
1 cup, whole (approx. 8.9 oz.)	234	59.8	26.1	6.68	234	59.8	
1 pound (approx. 1.8 cups) (tr/7g/tr/73%/1mg)	418	106.8	26.1	6.68	234	59.8	
CANNED, by brand:							
Oregon Strawberries, packed in heavy syrup, 17-oz. can	440	110.6	25.9	6.47	(210)	(52.0)	
Drained solids (10.2 oz.)	(248)	(69.2)	(27.8)	(6.78)			
DRIED, by brand:							
Grocer's Choice Strawberry Fruit Roll, 1-oz. package	100	22.0	100.0	22.00			
For comparison: Strawberry Jam, **Kraft,** 32-oz. (2-lb.) jam	2233	558.4	69.8	17.45	768	192.0	

	UNIT Cal.	UNIT Carb.	1 OZ., BY WT. Cal.	1 OZ., BY WT. Carb.	1 CUP Cal.	1 CUP Carb.	Fiber per oz. (GMS.)
SUGARAPPLES							
These are USDA data. For data from Hawaii, see SWEETSOPS.							
As purchased [refuse: skin and seeds, approx. 55%]:							
1 pound	192	48.4	12.0	3.03			
Edible portion:							
1 pound (1g/7g/tr/73%/3mg)	427	107.7	20.7	6.73	(183)	(59.3)	0.48
SURINAM CHERRIES (based on data from Hawaii) (also see PITANGAS)							
As purchased [refuse: seeds, stems, and blossom ends, approx. 22%]:							
1 medium surinam cherry (approx. 0.3 oz.)	2	0.61	8.6	2.26			
1 pound (approx. 63 medium surinam cherries)	138	36.2	8.6	2.26			
Edible portion:							
1 medium surinam cherry (approx. 0.2 oz.)	2	0.6	11.0	2.90	67	17.6	
1 cup (approx. 6.1 oz., 30.5 medium surinam cherries)	67	17.6	11.0	2.90	67	17.6	
1 pound (approx. 2.6 cups, 80 medium surinam cherries) (tr/3g/tr/89%/na)	177	46.4	11.0	2.90	67	17.6	
SWEETSOPS (based on data from Hawaii)							
For USDA data, see SUGARAPPLES.							
As purchased [refuse: skin and seeds, approx. 45%]:							
1 medium sweetsop (approx. 9.9 oz.)	133	32.3	13.4	3.26			
1 pound (approx. 1.6 medium sweetsops)	215	52.2	13.4	3.26			
Edible portion:							
1 medium sweetsop (approx. 5.5 oz.)	133	32.3	24.3	5.91			
1 cup (approx. 8.8 oz., 1.6 sweetsops)	215	52.1	24.3	5.91	215	52.1	
1 pound (approx. 1.8 cups, 2.9 medium sweetsops) (1g/6g/tr/76%/na)	389	94.5	24.3	5.91	215	52.1	
TAMARINDS							
As purchased [refuse: pods and seeds, approx. 52%]:							
1 pound	520	136.1	32.5	8.51			
Edible portion:							
1 pound (1g/18g/tr/34%/14mg)	1085	283.8	67.8	17.72			1.45
TANGELOS							
No data were available for the whole fruit; this information pertains to the juice only.							
SMALL (approx. 2¼" diameter, 4.3 oz. net wt., size 168):							
As purchased [refuse: peel, membranes, and seeds, approx. 44%]:							
1 small tangelo (approx. 4.3 oz.)	28	6.6	6.5	1.54			
1 pound (approx. 3¾ small tangelos)	105	24.7	6.5	1.54			
Edible portion:							
Juice of 1 small tangelo (approx. 2.4 oz.)	28	6.6	11.6	2.75	101	24.1	trace
1 cup (juice of approx. 3.6 small tangelos)	101	24.1	11.6	2.75	101	24.1	trace
1 pound of juice (juice of approx. 6⅔ small tangelos)	186	44.0	11.6	2.75	101	24.1	trace
MEDIUM (approx. 2$\frac{9}{16}$" diameter, 6 oz. net wt., size 120):							
As purchased [refuse: peel, membranes, and seeds, approx. 44%]:							
1 medium tangelo (approx. 6 oz.)	39	9.2	6.5	1.54			
1 pound (approx. 2⅔ medium tangelos)	105	24.7	6.5	1.54			

	UNIT		1 OZ., BY WT.		1 CUP		Fiber per oz.
	Cal.	Carb.	Cal.	Carb.	Cal.	Carb.	(GMS.)
Edible portion:							
1 medium tangelo (approx. 3⅓ oz.)	39	9.2	11.6	2.75	101	24.1	trace
1 cup (juice of approx. 2.6 medium tangelos)	101	24.1	11.6	2.75	101	24.1	trace
1 pound of juice (juice of approx. 4¾ medium tangelos)	186	44.0	11.6	2.75	101	24.1	trace
LARGE (approx. 2¾" diameter, 7.2 oz. net wt., size 100):							
As purchased [refuse: peel, membranes, and seeds, approx. 44%]:							
1 large tangelo (approx. 7.2 oz.)	47	11.1	6.5	1.54			
1 pound (approx. 2.2 large tangelos)	105	24.7	6.5	1.54			
Edible portion:							
Juice of 1 large tangelo (approx. 4 oz.)	47	11.1	11.6	2.75	101	24.1	trace
1 cup (juice of approx. 2.2 large tangelos)	101	24.1	11.6	2.75	101	24.1	trace
1 pound of juice (juice of approx. 4 large tangelos)	186	44.0	11.6	2.75	101	24.1	trace
TANGERINES							
DANCY VARIETY							
SMALL (approx. 2¼" diameter, 3.4 oz. net wt., size 210):							
As purchased [refuse: peel and seeds, approx. 26%]:							
1 small tangerine (approx. 3.4 oz.)	33	8.3	9.6	2.43			
1 pound (approx. 4.7 small tangerines)	154	38.9	9.6	2.43			
Edible portion:							
1 small tangerine (approx. 2½ oz.)	33	8.3	13.0	3.28			0.14
1 pound (approx. 6⅓ small tangerines) (tr/3g/tr/87%/1mg)	208	52.5	13.0	3.28			0.14
Sections, without membranes:							
1 cup (approx. 6.9 oz.)	90	22.6	13.0	3.28	90	22.6	0.14
1 pound (approx. 2⅓ cups) (tr/3g/tr/87%/1mg)	208	52.5	13.0	3.28	90	22.6	0.14
MEDIUM (approx. 2⅜" diameter, 4 oz. net wt., size 176):							
As purchased [refuse: peel and seeds, approx. 26%]:							
1 medium tangerine (approx. 4 oz.)	39	10.0	9.6	2.43			
1 pound (approx. 4 medium tangerines)	154	38.9	9.6	2.43			
Edible portion:							
1 medium tangerine (approx. 3 oz.)	39	10.0	13.0	3.28			0.14
1 pound (approx. 5⅓ medium tangerines) (tr/3g/tr/87%/1mg)	208	52.5	13.0	3.28			0.14
LARGE (approx. 2½" diameter, 4.8 oz. net wt., size 150):							
As purchased [refuse: peel and seeds, approx. 26%]:							
1 large tangerine (approx. 4.8 oz.)	46	11.7	9.6	2.43			
1 pound (approx. 3⅓ large tangerines)	154	38.9	9.6	2.43			
Edible portion:							
1 large tangerine (approx. 3.5 oz.)	46	11.7	13.0	3.28			
1 pound (approx. 5 large tangerines) (tr/3g/tr/87%/1mg)	208	52.5	13.0	3.28			
CANNED, based on generic data:							
Solids and liquid:							
Packed in juice:							
1 cup (approx. 8.7 oz.)	92	23.8	10.5	2.72	92	23.8	0.03
1 pound (approx. 1.8 oz.) (tr/3g/tr/90%/1mg)	168	43.4	10.5	2.72	92	23.8	0.03
Packed in light syrup:							
1 cup (approx. 8.8 oz.)	153	40.8	17.3	4.59	153	40.8	0.04
1 pound (approx. 1.8 cups) (tr/5g/tr/83%/2mg)	277	73.5	17.3	4.59	153	40.8	0.04
TANGERINE JUICE, see the BEVERAGES chapter							
WATERMELON							
As purchased [refuse: rind, seeds, and cutting loss, approx. 48%]:							
Whole:							
1 medium watermelon (approx. 16" long, 10" diameter, 32⅔ lb.)	2432	553.9	4.6	1.06			

	UNIT		1 OZ., BY WT.		1 CUP		Fiber per oz.
	Cal.	Carb.	Cal.	Carb.	Cal.	Carb.	(GMS.)
Cut:							
1 wedge, 1/16 of 32⅔-lb. melon, approx. 4" arc, 8" radius (approx. 33 oz., 2 lb. 1 oz.)	152	34.6	4.6	1.06			
1 Slice, approx. 10" diameter, 1" thick (approx. 33 oz., 2 lb. 1 oz.)	152	34.6	4.6	1.06			
Edible portion:							
1 medium watermelon (approx. 16 lb., 11.2 oz.)	2432	553.9	9.1	2.04	50	11.5	
1 cup, diced (approx. 5.6 oz.)	50	11.5	9.1	2.04	50	11.5	0.09
1 pound (approx. 2.8 cups diced) (tr/2g/tr/92%/tr)	145	32.6	9.1	2.04	50	11.5	0.09
WEST INDIAN CHERRY, see ACEROLAS							
WI-APPLE (based on data from Hawaii)							
As purchased [refuse: skin, seed, and fibers, approx. 34%]:							
1 wi-apple (approx. 5.2 oz.)	48	12.3	9.4	2.40			
1 pound (approx. 3.1 medium wi-apples)	150	38.3	9.4	2.40			
Edible portion:							
1 medium wi-apple (approx. 3.4 oz.)	48	12.3	14.2	3.63			
1 pound (approx. 4.7 medium wi-apples) (tr/4g/tr/86%/na)	227	58.1	14.2	3.63			
YOUNGBERRIES							
As purchased [refuse: caps and damaged berries, approx. 5%]:							
1 pound (approx. 305 berries)	251	55.6	15.7	3.48	84	18.3	
Edible portion:							
1 berry (approx. 0.05 oz.)	1	0.2	16.5	3.66	84	18.3	
1 cup (approx. 5 oz., 100 berries)	84	18.3	16.5	3.66	84	18.3	
1 pound (approx. 3.2 cups, 320 berries) (tr/4g/tr/85%/tr)	281	58.6	16.5	3.66	84	18.3	
CANNED, based on generic data							
Solids and liquid:							
Packed in water, with or without artificial sweetener:							
1 cup (8.6 oz.)	97	21.9	11.3	2.55	97	21.9	0.79
1 pound (approx. 1.9 cups) (tr/3g/tr/89%/tr)	181	40.8	11.3	2.55	97	21.9	0.79
Packed in juice:							
1 cup (8.7 oz.)	(133)	(29.7)	15.3	3.43	(133)	(29.7)	0.77
1 pound (approx. 1.8 cups) (tr/3g/tr/86%/tr)	245	54.9	15.3	3.43	(133)	(29.7)	0.77
Packed in light syrup:							
1 cup (8.7 oz.)	179	43.0	20.4	4.91	179	43.0	0.77
1 pound (approx. 1.8 cups) (tr/5g/tr/81%/tr)	327	78.5	20.4	4.91	179	43.0	0.77
Packed in heavy syrup:							
1 cup (9.0 oz.)	233	56.8	25.8	6.29	233	56.8	0.74
1 pound (approx. 1.8 cups) (tr/6g/tr/76%/tr)	413	100.7	25.8	6.29	233	56.8	0.74
Packed in extra heavy syrup:							
1 cup (9.3 oz.)	291	71.7	31.2	7.68	291	71.7	0.74
1 pound (approx. 1.7 cups) (tr/8g/tr/71%/tr)	499	122.9	31.2	7.68	291	71.7	0.74
ZANTE CURRANTS							
(Zante currants are dried black Corinth grapes. They are not related to European black, red, or white currants.)							
DRIED, based on generic data:							
1 cup (approx. 5.0 oz.)	407	106.7	80.3	21.02	407	106.7	0.45
1 pound (approx. 3.2 cups) (1g/21g/tr/19%/2mg)	1285	336.3	80.3	21.02	407	106.7	0.45
DRIED, by brand:							
Del Monte Zante Currants, 8-oz. package	1287	325.3	80.5	20.33			
11-oz. package	885	223.6	80.5	20.33	380	96.0	

MIXED FRUITS

FRUIT COCKTAIL

	UNIT		1 OZ., BY WT.		1 CUP		Fiber per oz.
	Cal.	Carb.	Cal.	Carb.	Cal.	Carb.	(GMS.)
CANNED, based on generic data:							
Solids and liquid:							
Packed in water, with or without artificial sweetener:							
1 cup (approx. 8.6 oz.)	91	23.8	10.5	2.75	91	23.8	0.11
1 pound (approx. 1.8 cups) (tr/3g/tr/90%/1mg)	168	44.0	10.5	2.75	91	23.8	0.11
Can, 8Z Tall, Buffet; 8 oz. net wt.	84	22.0	10.5	2.75	91	23.8	0.11
Can, #303, 16 oz. (1 lb.) net wt.	168	44.0	10.5	2.75	91	23.8	0.11
Packed in juice (Mixture includes peaches, pears, apricots, pineapples, and cherries):							
1 cup (approx. 8.7 oz.)	125	32.5	14.2	3.70	125	32.5	0.10
1 pound (approx. 1.8 cups) (tr/4g/tr/86%/1mg)	227	59.2	14.2	3.70	227	32.5	0.10
Packed in light syrup:							
1 cup (approx. 8¾ oz.)	(149)	(38.9)	17.0	4.45	(149)	(38.9)	0.11
1 pound (approx. 1.8 cups) (tr/4g/tr/84%/1mg)	272	71.2	17.0	4.45	(149)	(38.9)	0.11
Packed in extra light syrup (Mixture includes peaches, pineapples, and cherries):							
1 cup (approx. 8.6 oz.)	110	28.6	12.8	3.30	110	28.6	0.13
1 pound (approx. 1.9 cups) (tr/3g/tr/88%/1mg)	204	52.8	12.8	3.30	110	28.6	0.13
Packed in heavy syrup:							
1 cup (approx. 9 oz.)	194	50.2	21.6	5.59	194	50.2	0.11
1 pound (approx. 1¾ cups) (tr/6g/tr/80%/1mg)	345	89.4	21.6	5.59	194	50.2	0.11
Can, #303, 17 oz. net wt.	366	95.0	21.5	5.59	194	50.2	0.11
Can, #2½, 30 oz. (1 lb. 14 oz.) net wt.	647	167.6	21.6	5.59	194	50.2	0.11
Can, #10, 108 oz. (6 lbs. 12 oz.) net wt.	2327	603.2	21.6	5.59	194	50.2	0.11
Packed in extra heavy syrup:							
1 cup (approx. 9⅓ oz.)	(244)	(62.7)	26.1	6.72	(244)	(62.7)	0.11
1 pound (approx. 1¾ cups) (tr/7g/tr/76%/1mg)	418	107.5	26.1	6.72	(244)	(62.7)	0.11
CANNED, by brand:							
A&P Fruit Cocktail, packed in extra heavy syrup, 17-oz. can	480	124.0	28.0	7.23	240	62.0	
30-oz. can	840	217.0	28.0	7.23	240		
Ann Page (A&P) Fruit Cocktail, packed in heavy syrup, 17-oz. can	350	89.4	20.6	5.26	180	46.0	
8¾-oz. can	180	46.0	20.6	5.26	180	46.0	
Balanced Fruit Cocktail, packed in water, 8-oz. can	73	17.9	9.1	2.24	(79)	(19.4)	
Del Monte Fruit Cocktail, 8¾-oz. can	175	46.3	20.0	5.29	170	45.0	
30-oz. can	600	158.8	20.0	5.29	170	45.0	
Diet Delight Fruit Cocktail, packed in juice of white grapes, 8-oz. can	100	28.0	12.4	3.50	100	28.0	
16-oz. (1-lb.) can	200	56.0	12.4	3.50	100	28.0	
Fruit Cocktail, packed in water, 8-oz. can	80	20.0	10.0	2.50	80	20.0	
16-oz. (1-lb.) can	160	40.0	10.0	2.50	80	20.0	
Featherweight Fruit Cocktail, packed in pear and pineapple juices, 8-oz. can	(100)	(24.0)	(12.5)	(3.00)	100	24.0	
16-oz. (1-lb.) can	(200)	(48.0)	(12.5)	(3.00)	100	24.0	
Fruit Cocktail, packed in water, 8-oz. can	(80)	(20.0)	(10.0)	(2.50)	80	20.0	
16-oz. (1-lb.) can	(160)	(40.0)	(10.0)	(2.50)	80	20.0	
Golden Harvest no sugar or salt added Fruit Cocktail in Water, 16-oz. (1-lb.) can	160	42.0	10.0	2.63	80	21.0	
Libby's Fruit Cocktail, packed in heavy syrup, 8¾-oz. can	(165)	(43.8)	(18.9)	(5.00)	170	45.0	
17-oz. can	(321)	(85.0)	(18.9)	(5.00)	170	45.0	
Fruit Cocktail, 8½-oz. can	106	55.3	12.5	6.50	100	26.0	
Fruit Cocktail, packed in light syrup, 8¾-oz. can	(145)	(37.8)	(16.6)	(4.32)	150	39.0	
17-oz. can	(282)	(73.4)	(16.6)	(4.32)	150	39.0	
P&Q (A&P) Fruit Cocktail in light syrup, 16-oz. (1-lb.) can	300	78.0	18.8	4.88	150	39.0	
Stokely Fruit Cocktail, 8¾-oz. can	185	44.7	21.1	5.11	190	40.0	
17-oz. can	359	86.9	21.5	5.11	190	40.0	

	UNIT		1 OZ., BY WT.		1 CUP		Fiber per oz.
	Cal.	Carb.	Cal.	Carb.	Cal.	Carb.	(GMS.)
Tillie Lewis "Tasti Delight" Fruit Cocktail, packed in unsweetened fruit juice, 8-oz. can	90	24.0	11.3	3.00	90	24.0	
16-oz. (1-lb.) can	180	48.0	11.3	3.00	90	24.0	
Town House, Fruit Cocktail in heavy syrup, 28-oz. can	630	168.0	22.5	6.00	180	48.0	
Drained solids (yield: approx. 20¾ oz.)	463	117.3	22.3	5.65	168	42.4	
FRUIT SALAD							
CANNED, based on generic data:							
Solids and liquid:							
Packed in water with or without artificial sweetener:							
1 cup (approx. 8.6 oz.)	86	22.3	9.9	2.59	86	22.3	0.11
1 pound (approx. 1.8 cups) (tr/3g/tr/90%/tr)	159	41.3	9.9	2.59	86	22.3	0.11
Can, 8Z Tall, Buffet, 8 oz. net wt.	79	20.7	9.9	2.59	86	22.3	0.11
Can, #303, 16 oz. (1 lb.) net wt.	159	41.3	9.9	2.59	86	22.3	0.11
Packed in juice (Mixture includes peaches, pears, apricots, pineapples, and cherries):							
1 cup (approx. 8.7 oz.)	125	32.5	14.2	3.70	125	32.5	0.10
1 pound (approx. 1.8 cups) (tr/4g/tr/86%/1mg)	227	59.2	14.2	3.70	227	32.5	0.10
Packed in light syrup:							
1 cup (approx. 8¾ oz.)	(147)	(38.4)	16.8	4.39	(147)	(38.4)	0.11
1 pound (approx. 1.8 cups) (tr/4g/tr/84%/tr)	268	70.3	16.8	4.39	(147)	(38.4)	0.11
Packed in heavy syrup:							
1 cup (approx. 9 oz.)	191	49.5	21.3	5.50	191	49.5	0.11
1 pound (approx. 1¾ cups) (tr/6g/tr/80%/tr)	340	88.0	21.3	5.50	191	49.5	0.11
Can, 8Z Tall, Buffet; 8¾ oz. net wt.	186	48.1	21.3	5.50	191	49.5	0.11
Can, #303, 17 oz. net wt.	362	93.5	21.3	5.50	191	49.5	0.11
Can, #10, 108 oz. (6 lbs. 12 oz.) net wt.	2297	594.0	21.3	5.50	191	49.5	0.11
Packed in extra heavy syrup:							
1 cup (approx. 9⅓ oz.)	(238)	(61.9)	25.5	6.63	(238)	(61.9)	0.11
1 pound (approx. 1¾ cups) (tr/7g/tr/76%/tr)	408	106.1	25.5	6.63	(238)	(61.9)	0.11
CANNED, by brand:							
A & P Fruits For Salad, packed in heavy syrup, 8¾-oz. can	219	54.7	25.0	6.25	(200)	(50.0)	
16-oz. (1-lb.) can	400	100.0	25.0	6.25	(200)	(50.0)	
Del Monte Fruits For Salad, 8¾-oz. can	175	47.3	20.0	5.41	170	46.0	
29-oz. can	580	156.9	20.0	5.41	170	46.0	
Tropical Fruit Salad, 8¾-oz. can	219	57.4	25.0	6.56	200	52.0	
16-oz. (1-lb.) can	400	105.0	25.0	6.56	200	52.0	
Diet Delight Fruits For Salad, packed in juice of white grapes, 8-oz. can	120	32.0	15.0	4.00	120	32.0	
16-oz. (1-lb.) can	240	64.0	15.0	4.00	120	32.0	
Featherweight Fruits For Salad, packed in juice, 8-oz. can	(100)	(24.0)	(12.5)	(3.00)	100	24.0	
Fruits For Salad, packed in pear and pineapple juices, 8-oz. can	100	24.0	12.5	3.00	(100)	(24.0)	
Fruit Salad, packed in water, 8-oz. can	(140)	(40.0)	(17.5)	(5.00)	70	20.0	
16-oz. can	(280)	(80.0)	(17.5)	(5.00)	70	20.0	
Libby's Fruits For Salad, 16-oz. (1-lb.) can	240	60.8	15.0	3.75	120	30.0	
Fruits For Salad, packed in heavy syrup, 8¾-oz. can	(175)	(46.6)	(20.0)	(5.33)	180	48.0	
17-oz. can	(340)	(90.6)	(20.0)	(5.33)	180	48.0	
Stokely Fruits For Salad, 16-oz. (1-lb.) can	338	78.2	21.1	4.89	190	44.0	
MIXED FRUIT							
FROZEN (sweetened), based on generic data:							
(Mixture includes peaches, sweet cherries, red sour cherries, red raspberries, boysenberries, and grapes.)							
Thawed:							
1 cup (approx. 8.8 oz.)	245	60.6	27.8	6.88	245	60.6	
1 pound (approx. 1.8 cups) (tr/7g/tr/74%/1mg)	445	110.1	27.8	6.88	245	60.6	
CANNED (heavy syrup), based on generic data:							
(Mixture includes peaches, pears, and pineapple)							
1 cup (approx. 8.9 oz.)	184	47.8	20.4	5.32	184	47.8	0.11

	UNIT Cal.	UNIT Carb.	1 OZ., BY WT. Cal.	1 OZ., BY WT. Carb.	1 CUP Cal.	1 CUP Carb.	Fiber per oz. (GMS.)
1 pound (approx. 1.8 cups) (tr/5g/tr/81%/1mg)	327	85.2	20.4	5.32	184	47.8	0.11
DRIED, based on generic data:							
Pits removed:							
(Mixture includes 50% prunes, 20% peaches, 15% apples, and 15% pears)							
1 pound (1g/17g/tr/31%/5mg)	1036	273.0	64.7	17.06			0.82
FROZEN, by brand:							
Big Valley Fresh Mixed Fruit, 20-oz. package	250		12.5		(107)		
Birds Eye Frozen Mixed Fruit, 10-oz. package	260	68.0	26.0	6.80	(205)	(53.7)	
CANNED, by brand:							
Fruit Cup Mixed Fruit, 5-oz. can	100	27.0	20.0	5.40			
Libby's Chunky Mixed Fruits, 16-oz. (1-lb.) can	200	52.0	12.5	3.25	100	26.0	

	UNIT Cal.	UNIT Carb.	1 OZ., BY WT. Cal.	1 OZ., BY WT. Carb.	1 CUP Cal.	1 CUP Carb.	Fiber per oz. (GMS.)
Scotch Buy Fruit Mix in light syrup, 29-oz. can	525	136.5	18.1	4.71	150	39.0	
DRIED, by brand:							
Fruit Pac Dried Mixed Fruit, Honey Dipped, 12-oz. package	1249	324.5	104.1	27.04	680	176.4	
Golden Harvest Tropical Fruit Mix, 4-oz. package	440	80.0	110.0	20.00			
Sonoma Dried Mixed Fruit, soft, 12-oz. package	884	229.2	73.7	19.10	442	114.5	
Sun-Maid California Dried Fruits & Raisins for snacking or baking, 6-oz. foil package	450	120.0	75.0	20.00			
DEHYDRATED, by brand:							
Timber Crest Dehydrated Mixed Fruit, hard, 5-lb. package	7744	2008.0	96.8	25.10	393	101.8	

3 MEATS & GAME •

	UNIT		1 OZ., BY WT.		1 CUP, DICED, NOT PACKED	
	Cal.	Carb.	Cal.	Carb.	Cal.	Carb.
BEEF						
Brisket						
CHOICE GRADE:						
Bone-in						
1 pound of Raw untrimmed meat (includes separable fat) with bone [58% separable lean, 26% separable fat, 16% bone]	1284	0.0	80.3	0.00		
Cooked (braised) [yield: approx. 11.1 oz., of which approx. 8.5 oz. are meat and approx. 2.6 oz. are bone]	1014	0.0	91.5	0.00		
Trimmed of separable fat before cooking; Cooked (braised) [yield: approx. 8.5 oz., of which approx. 5.9 oz. are meat and approx. 2.6 oz. are bone]	371	0.0	43.9	0.00		
1 pound of Cooked (braised) meat (weight includes bone):						
Yield from approx. 23.0 oz. (1 lb. 7.0 oz.) of raw untrimmed meat (weighed with the bone) that had ***not*** been trimmed of separable fat before cooking	1464	0.0	91.5	0.00		
Yield from approx. 30.1 oz. (1 lb. 14.1 oz.) of raw untrimmed meat (weighed with the bone) that ***had*** been trimmed of separable fat before cooking	703	0.0	43.9	0.00		
Boneless						
1 pound of Raw untrimmed meat (includes separable fat) [69% separable lean, 31% separable fat]	1528	0.0	95.5	0.00	(439)	0.0
Cooked (braised) [yield: approx. 10.7 oz.] (6g/0g/10g/45%/na)	1245	0.0	116.8	0.00	(538)	0.0
Trimmed of separable fat before cooking; Cooked (braised) [yield: approx. 7.5 oz.] (8g/0g/3g/61%/na)	534	0.0	62.9	0.00	(289)	0.0
1 pound of Cooked (braised) meat:						
Yield from approx. 23.9 oz. (1 lb. 7.9 oz.) of raw untrimmed meat that had ***not*** been trimmed of separable fat before cooking	1869	0.0	116.8	0.00	(538)	0.0
Yield from approx. 34.3 oz. (2 lb. 2.3 oz.) of raw untrimmed meat that ***had*** been trimmed of separable fat before cooking	1006	0.0	62.9	0.00	(289)	0.0
GOOD GRADE:						
Bone-in						
1 pound of Raw untrimmed meat (includes separable fat) with bone [60% separable lean, 23% separable fat, 17% bone]	1123	0.0	70.2	0.00		
Cooked (braised) [yield: approx. 11.6 oz., of which approx. 8.9 oz. are meat and approx. 2.7 oz. are bone]	941	0.0	81.1	0.00		
Trimmed of separable fat before cooking; Cooked (braised) [yield: approx. 9.1 oz., of which approx. 6.4 oz. are meat and approx. 2.7 oz. are bone]	362	0.0	39.6	0.00		

	UNIT		1 OZ., BY WT.		1 CUP, DICED, NOT PACKED	
	Cal.	Carb.	Cal.	Carb.	Cal.	Carb.
1 pound of Cooked (braised) meat (weight includes bone):						
Yield from approx. 22.0 oz. (1 lb. 6.0 oz.) of raw untrimmed meat (weighed with the bone) that had ***not*** been trimmed of separable fat before cooking	1297	0.0	81.1	0.00		
Yield from approx. 28.1 oz. (1 lb. 12.1 oz.) of raw untrimmed meat (weighed with the bone) that ***had*** been trimmed of separable fat before cooking	634	0.0	39.6	0.00		
Boneless						
1 pound of Raw untrimmed meat (includes separable fat) [71% separable lean, 29% separable fat]	1353	0.0	84.6	0.00	(389)	0.0
Cooked (braised) [yield: approx. 10.7 oz.] (7g/0g/9g/45%/na)	1135	0.0	105.8	0.00	(487)	0.0
Trimmed of separable fat before cooking; Cooked (braised) [yield: approx. 7.7 oz.] (9g/0g/2g/61%/na)	436	0.0	56.5	0.00	(260)	0.0
1 pound of Cooked (braised) meat:						
Yield from approx. 23.9 oz. (1 lb. 7.9 oz.) of raw untrimmed meat that had ***not*** been trimmed of separable fat before cooking	1693	0.0	105.8	0.00	(487)	0.0
Yield from approx. 33.2 oz. (2 lbs. 1.2 oz.) of raw untrimmed meat that ***had*** been trimmed of separable fat before cooking	903	0.0	56.5	0.00	(260)	0.0
STANDARD GRADE:						
Bone-in						
1 pound of Raw untrimmed meat (includes separable fat) with bone [60% separable lean, 22% separable fat, 18% bone]	1035	0.0	64.7	0.00		
Cooked (braised) [yield: approx. 11.7 oz., of which approx. 8.8 oz. are meat and approx. 2.9 oz. are bone]	873	0.0	74.8	0.00		
Trimmed of separable fat before cooking; Cooked (braised) [yield: approx. 9.3 oz., of which approx. 6.4 oz. are meat and approx. 2.9 oz. are bone]	340	0.0	36.6	0.00		
1 pound of Cooked (braised) meat (weight includes bone):						
Yield from approx. 21.9 oz. (1 lb. 5.9 oz.) of raw untrimmed meat (weighed with the bone) that had ***not*** been trimmed of separable fat before cooking	1197	0.0	74.8	0.00		
Yield from approx. 27.5 oz. (1 lb. 11.5 oz.) of raw untrimmed meat (weighed with the bone) that ***had*** been trimmed of separable fat before cooking	586	0.0	36.6	0.00		
Boneless						
1 pound of Raw untrimmed meat (includes separable fat) [73% separable lean, 27% separable fat]	1262	0.0	78.9	0.00	(363)	0.0
Cooked (braised) [yield: approx. 10.7 oz.] (7g/0g/8g/47%/na)	1065	0.0	99.3	0.00	(457)	0.0

	UNIT Cal.	UNIT Carb.	1 OZ., BY WT. Cal.	1 OZ., BY WT. Carb.	1 CUP, DICED, NOT PACKED Cal.	1 CUP, DICED, NOT PACKED Carb.
Trimmed of separable fat before cooking; Cooked (braised) [yield: approx. 7.8 oz.] (9g/0g/2g/62%/na)	415	0.0	53.1	0.00	(244)	0.0
1 pound of Cooked (braised) meat:						
Yield from approx. 23.9 oz. (1 lb. 7.9 oz.) of raw untrimmed meat that had ***not*** been trimmed of separable fat before cooking	1589	0.0	99.3	0.00	(457)	0.0
Yield from approx. 32.7 oz. (2 lbs. 0.7 oz.) of raw untrimmed meat that ***had*** been trimmed of separable fat before cooking	849	0.0	53.1	0.00	(244)	0.0

Chuck Cuts

ENTIRE CHUCK (1ST–5TH RIBS, ARM, AND NECK)

	UNIT Cal.	UNIT Carb.	1 OZ., BY WT. Cal.	1 OZ., BY WT. Carb.	1 CUP, DICED, NOT PACKED Cal.	1 CUP, DICED, NOT PACKED Carb.
CHOICE GRADE:						
Bone-in						
1 pound of Raw untrimmed meat (includes separable fat) with bone [69% separable lean, 15% separable fat, 16% bone]	980	0.0	61.3	0.00		
Cooked (braised) [yield: approx. 11.6 oz., of which approx. 9.0 oz. are meat and approx. 2.6 oz. are bone]	836	0.0	72.2	0.00		
Trimmed of separable fat before cooking; Cooked (braised) [yield: approx. 10 oz., of which approx. 7.4 oz. are meat and approx. 2.6 oz. are bone]	448	0.0	45.1	0.00		
1 pound of Cooked (braised) meat (weight includes bone):						
Yield from approx. 22.1 oz. (1 lb. 6.1 oz.) of raw untrimmed meat (weighed with the bone) that had ***not*** been trimmed of separable fat before cooking	1156	0.0	72.2	0.00		
Yield from approx. 26.0 oz. (1 lb. 10.0 oz.) of raw untrimmed meat (weighed with the bone) that ***had*** been trimmed of separable fat before cooking	721	0.0	45.1	0.00		
Boneless						
1 pound of Raw untrimmed meat (includes separable fat) [81% separable lean, 19% separable fat]	1167	0.0	72.9	0.00	(335)	0.0
Cooked (braised) [yield: approx. 10.7 oz.] (7g/0g/7g/49%/na)	995	0.0	92.8	0.00	(427)	0.0
Trimmed of separable fat before cooking; Cooked (braised) [yield: approx. 8.8 oz.] (9g/0g/3g/60%/na)	534	0.0	60.7	0.00	(279)	0.0
1 pound of Cooked (braised) meat:						
Yield from approx. 23.9 oz. (1 lb. 7.9 oz.) of raw untrimmed meat that had ***not*** been trimmed of separable fat before cooking	1485	0.0	92.8	0.00	(427)	0.0
Yield from approx. 29.1 oz. (1 lb. 13.1 oz.) of raw untrimmed meat that ***had*** been trimmed of separable fat before cooking	972	0.0	60.7	0.00	(279)	0.0

1ST–2ND RIBS (SHORT RIBS)

	UNIT Cal.	UNIT Carb.	1 OZ., BY WT. Cal.	1 OZ., BY WT. Carb.	1 CUP, DICED, NOT PACKED Cal.	1 CUP, DICED, NOT PACKED Carb.
CHOICE GRADE:						
Bone-in						
1 pound of Raw untrimmed meat (includes separable fat) with bone [74% separable lean, 11% separable fat, 15% bone]	930	0.0	58.1	0.00		
Cooked (braised) [yield: approx. 11.5 oz., of which approx. 9.1 oz. are meat and approx. 2.4 oz. are bone]	799	0.0	69.4	0.00		
Trimmed of separable fat before cooking; Cooked (braised) [yield: approx. 10.2 oz., of which approx. 7.8 oz. are meat and approx. 2.4 oz. are bone]	505	0.0	49.8	0.00		
1 pound of Cooked (braised) meat (weight includes bone):						
Yield from approx. 22.2 oz. (1 lb. 6.2 oz.) of raw untrimmed meat (weighed with the bone) that had ***not*** been trimmed of separable fat before cooking	1110	0.0	69.4	0.00		
Yield from approx. 25.2 oz. (1 lb. 9.2 oz.) of raw untrimmed meat (weighed with the bone) that ***had*** been trimmed of separable fat before cooking	797	0.0	49.8	0.00		
Boneless (Chuck Eye)						
1 pound of Raw untrimmed meat (includes separable fat) [85% separable lean, 15% separable fat]	1094	0.0	68.4	0.00	(315)	0.0
Cooked (braised) [yield: approx. 10.7 oz.] (8g/0g/6g/51%/na)	940	0.0	87.7	0.00	(403)	0.0
Trimmed of separable fat before cooking; Cooked (braised) [yield: approx. 9.3 oz.] (8g/0g/3g/59%/na)	595	0.0	63.8	0.00	(293)	0.0
1 pound of Cooked (braised) meat:						
Yield from approx. 23.9 oz. (1 lb. 7.9 oz.) of raw untrimmed meat that had ***not*** been trimmed of separable fat before cooking	1403	0.0	87.7	0.00	(403)	0.0
Yield from approx. 27.4 oz. (1 lb. 11.4 oz.) of raw untrimmed meat that ***had*** been trimmed of separable fat before cooking	1022	0.0	63.8	0.00	(293)	0.0
GOOD GRADE:						
Bone-in						
1 pound of Raw untrimmed meat (includes separable fat) with bone [73% separable lean, 13% separable fat, 14% bone]	871	0.0	54.4	0.00		
Cooked (braised) [yield: approx. 11.4 oz., of which approx. 9.2 oz. are meat and approx. 2.2 oz. are bone]	756	0.0	66.0	0.00		
Trimmed of separable fat before cooking; Cooked (braised) [yield: approx. 10 oz., of which approx. 7.8 oz. are meat and approx. 2.2 oz. are bone]	449	0.0	44.6	0.00		
1 pound of Cooked (braised) meat (weight includes bone):						
Yield from approx. 22.3 oz. (1 lb. 6.3 oz.) of raw untrimmed meat (weighed with the bone) that had ***not*** been trimmed of separable fat before cooking	1056	0.0	66.0	0.00		
Yield from approx. 25.4 oz. (1 lb. 9.4 oz.) of raw untrimmed meat (weighed with the bone) that ***had*** been trimmed of separable fat before cooking	713	0.0	44.6	0.00		
Boneless (Chuck Eye)						
1 pound of Raw untrimmed meat (includes separable fat) [85% separable lean, 15% separable fat]	1012	0.0	63.3	0.00	(291)	0.0
Cooked (braised) [yield: approx. 10.7 oz.] (8g/0g/5g/53%/na)	879	0.0	82.0	0.00	(377)	0.0
Trimmed of separable fat before cooking; Cooked (braised) [yield: approx. 9.1 oz.] (9g/0g/2g/61%/na)	522	0.0	57.3	0.00	(264)	0.0
1 pound of Cooked (braised) meat:						
Yield from approx. 23.9 oz. (1 lb. 7.9 oz.) of raw untrimmed meat that had ***not*** been trimmed of separable fat before cooking	1312	0.0	82.0	0.00	(377)	0.0
Yield from approx. 28.1 oz. (1 lb. 12.1 oz.) of raw untrimmed meat that ***had*** been trimmed of separable fat before cooking	917	0.0	57.3	0.00	(264)	0.0
STANDARD GRADE:						
Bone-in						
1 pound of Raw untrimmed meat (includes separable fat) with bone [75% separable lean, 9% separable fat, 16% bone]	702	0.0	43.9	0.00		
Cooked (braised) [yield: approx. 11.6 oz., of which approx. 9.0 oz. are meat and approx. 2.6 oz. are bone]	623	0.0	53.9	0.00		
Trimmed of separable fat before cooking; Cooked (braised) [yield: approx. 10.6 oz., of which approx. 8.0 oz. are meat and approx. 2.6 oz. are bone]	418	0.0	39.6	0.00		
1 pound of Cooked (braised) meat (weight includes bone):						
Yield from approx. 22.1 oz. (1 lb. 6.1 oz.) of raw untrimmed meat (weighed with the bone) that had ***not*** been trimmed of separable fat before cooking	863	0.0	53.9	0.00		
Yield from approx. 24.2 oz. (1 lb. 8.2 oz.) of raw untrimmed meat (weighed with the bone) that ***had*** been trimmed of separable fat before cooking	633	0.0	39.6	0.00		
Boneless (Chuck Eye)						
1 pound of Raw untrimmed meat (includes separable fat) [89% separable lean, 11% separable fat]	835	0.0	52.2	0.00	(240)	0.0
Cooked (braised) [yield: approx. 10.7 oz.] (8g/0g/4g/57%/na)	742	0.0	69.2	0.00	(558)	0.0
Trimmed of separable fat before cooking; Cooked (braised) [yield: approx. 9.5 oz.] (9g/0g/2g/63%/na)	498	0.0	52.2	0.00	(240)	0.0
1 pound of Cooked (braised) meat:						
Yield from approx. 23.9 oz. (1 lb. 7.9 oz.) of raw untrimmed meat that had ***not*** been trimmed of separable fat before cooking	1108	0.0	69.2	0.00	(558)	0.0
Yield from approx. 26.8 oz. (1 lb. 10.8 oz.) of raw untrimmed meat that ***had*** been trimmed of separable fat before cooking	835	0.0	52.2	0.00	(240)	0.0

	UNIT Cal.	UNIT Carb.	1 OZ., BY WT. Cal.	1 OZ., BY WT. Carb.	1 CUP, DICED, NOT PACKED Cal.	1 CUP, DICED, NOT PACKED Carb.
3RD–4TH RIBS (SHORT RIBS)						
CHOICE GRADE:						
Bone-in						
1 pound of Raw untrimmed meat (includes separable fat) with bone [65% separable lean, 21% separable fat, 14% bone]	1230	0.0	76.9	0.00		
Cooked (braised) [yield: approx. 11.4 oz., of which approx. 9.2 oz. are meat and approx. 2.2 oz. are bone]	1018	0.0	88.8	0.00		
Trimmed of separable fat before cooking; Cooked (braised) [yield: approx. 9.1 oz., of which approx. 6.9 oz. are meat and approx. 2.2 oz. are bone]	467	0.0	51.0	0.00		
1 pound of Cooked (braised) meat (weight includes bone):						
Yield from approx. 22.3 oz. (1 lb. 6.3 oz.) of raw untrimmed meat (weighed with the bone) that had ***not*** been trimmed of separable fat before cooking	1421	0.0	88.8	0.00		
Yield from approx. 28.0 oz. (1 lb. 12.0 oz.) of raw untrimmed meat (weighed with the bone) that ***had*** been trimmed of separable fat before cooking	816	0.0	51.0	0.00		
Boneless (Chuck Eye)						
1 pound of Raw untrimmed meat (includes separable fat) [74% separable lean, 26% separable fat]	1430	0.0	89.4	0.00	(411)	0.0
Cooked (braised) [yield: approx. 10.7 oz.] (7g/0g/9g/44%/na)	1183	0.0	110.4	0.00	(508)	0.0
Trimmed of separable fat before cooking; Cooked (braised) [yield: approx. 8.0 oz.] (8g/0g/4g/57%/na)	543	0.0	67.5	0.00	(311)	0.0
1 pound of Cooked (braised) meat:						
Yield from approx. 23.9 oz. (1 lb. 7.9 oz.) of raw untrimmed meat that had ***not*** been trimmed of separable fat before cooking	1766	0.0	110.4	0.00	(508)	0.0
Yield from approx. 31.8 oz. (1 lb. 15.8 oz.) of raw untrimmed meat that ***had*** been trimmed of separable fat before cooking	1081	0.0	67.5	0.00	(311)	0.0
GOOD GRADE:						
Bone-in						
1 pound of Raw untrimmed meat (includes separable fat) with bone [66% separable lean, 20% separable fat, 14% bone]	1082	0.0	67.6	0.00		
Cooked (braised) [yield: approx. 11.4 oz., of which approx. 9.2 oz. are meat and approx. 2.2 oz. are bone]	910	0.0	79.4	0.00		
Trimmed of separable fat before cooking; Cooked (braised) [yield: approx. 9.3 oz., of which approx. 7.1 oz. are meat and approx. 2.2 oz. are bone]	417	0.0	44.6	0.00		
1 pound of Cooked (braised) meat (weight includes bone):						
Yield from approx. 22.3 oz. (1 lb. 6.3 oz.) of raw untrimmed meat (weighed with the bone) that had ***not*** been trimmed of separable fat before cooking	1271	0.0	79.4	0.00		
Yield from approx. 27.4 oz. (1 lb. 11.4 oz.) of raw untrimmed meat (weighed with the bone) that ***had*** been trimmed of separable fat before cooking	714	0.0	44.6	0.00		
Boneless (Chuck Eye)						
1 pound of Raw untrimmed meat (includes separable fat) [76% separable lean, 24% separable fat]	1258	0.0	78.6	0.00	(362)	0.0
Cooked (braised) [yield: approx. 10.7 oz.] (7g/0g/8g/47%/na)	1059	0.0	98.8	0.00	(454)	0.0
Trimmed of separable fat before cooking; Cooked (braised) [yield: approx. 8.3 oz.] (9g/0g/2g/60%/na)	485	0.0	58.7	0.00	(270)	0.0
1 pound of Cooked (braised) meat:						
Yield from approx. 23.9 oz. (1 lb. 7.9 oz.) of raw untrimmed meat that had ***not*** been trimmed of separable fat before cooking	1580	0.0	98.8	0.00	(454)	0.0
Yield from approx. 31.0 oz. (1 lb. 15.0 oz.) of raw untrimmed meat that ***had*** been trimmed of separable fat before cooking	940	0.0	58.7	0.00	(270)	0.0
STANDARD GRADE:						
Bone-in						
1 pound of Raw untrimmed meat (includes separable fat) with bone [67% separable lean, 16% separable fat, 17% bone]	889	0.0	55.6	0.00		
Cooked (braised) [yield: approx. 11.6 oz., of which approx. 8.9 oz. are meat and approx. 2.7 oz. are bone]	765	0.0	65.8	0.00		
Trimmed of separable fat before cooking; Cooked (braised) [yield: approx. 9.9 oz., of which approx. 7.2 oz. are meat and approx. 2.7 oz. are bone]	395	0.0	39.8	0.00		
1 pound of Cooked (braised) meat (weight includes bone):						
Yield from approx. 22.0 oz. (1 lb. 6.0 oz.) of raw untrimmed meat (weighed with the bone) that had ***not*** been trimmed of separable fat before cooking	1054	0.0	65.8	0.00		
Yield from approx. 25.8 oz. (1 lb. 9.8 oz.) of raw untrimmed meat (weighed with the bone) that ***had*** been trimmed of separable fat before cooking	636	0.0	39.8	0.00		
Boneless (Chuck Eye)						
1 pound of Raw untrimmed meat (includes separable fat) [81% separable lean, 19% separable fat]	1071	0.0	67.0	0.00	(308)	0.0
Cooked (braised) [yield: approx. 10.7 oz.] (8g/0g/6g/52%/na)	922	0.0	86.0	0.00	(396)	0.0
Trimmed of separable fat before cooking; Cooked (braised) [yield: approx 8.7 oz.] (9g/0g/2g/62%/na)	476	0.0	54.8	0.00	(252)	0.0
1 pound of Cooked (braised) meat:						
Yield from approx. 23.9 oz. (1 lb. 7.9 oz.) of raw untrimmed meat that had ***not*** been trimmed of separable fat before cooking	1376	0.0	86.0	0.00	(396)	0.0
Yield from approx. 29.5 oz. (1 lb. 13.5 oz.) of raw untrimmed meat that ***had*** been trimmed of separable fat before cooking	876	0.0	54.8	0.00	(252)	0.0
5TH RIB (SHORT RIB)						
CHOICE GRADE:						
Bone-in						
1 pound of Raw untrimmed meat (includes separable fat) with bone [59% separable lean, 25% separable fat, 16% bone]	1342	0.0	83.9	0.00		
Cooked (braised) [yield: approx. 11.6 oz., of which approx. 9.0 oz. are meat and approx. 2.6 oz. are bone]	1091	0.0	94.3	0.00		
Trimmed of separable fat before cooking; Cooked (braised) [yield: approx. 8.9 oz., of which approx. 6.3 oz. are meat and approx. 2.6 oz. are bone]	445	0.0	50.2	0.00		
1 pound of Cooked (braised) meat (weight includes bone):						
Yield from approx. 22.1 oz. (1 lb. 6.1 oz.) of raw untrimmed meat (weighed with the bone) that had ***not*** been trimmed of separable fat before cooking	1509	0.0	94.3	0.00		
Yield from approx. 28.9 oz. (1 lb. 12.9 oz.) of raw untrimmed meat (weighed with the bone) that ***had*** been trimmed of separable fat before cooking	803	0.0	50.2	0.00		
Boneless (Chuck Eye)						
1 pound of Raw untrimmed meat (includes separable fat) [69% separable lean, 31% separable fat]	1598	0.0	99.9	0.00	(460)	0.0
Cooked (braised) [yield: approx. 10.7 oz.] (6g/0g/10g/40%/na)	1299	0.0	121.2	0.00	(558)	0.0
Trimmed of separable fat before cooking; Cooked (braised) [yield: approx. 7.5 oz.] (8g/0g/4g/57%/na)	530	0.0	70.7	0.00	(325)	0.0
1 pound of Cooked (braised) meat:						
Yield from approx. 23.9 oz. (1 lb. 7.9 oz.) of raw untrimmed meat that had ***not*** been trimmed of separable fat before cooking	1939	0.0	121.2	0.00	(558)	0.0
Yield from approx. 34.1 oz. (2 lbs. 2.1 oz.) of raw untrimmed meat that ***had*** been trimmed of separable fat before cooking	1130	0.0	70.7	0.00	(325)	0.0
GOOD GRADE:						
Bone-in						
1 pound of Raw untrimmed meat (includes separable fat) with bone [62% separable lean, 22% separable fat, 16% bone]	1156	0.0	72.2	0.00		
Cooked (braised) [yield: approx. 11.6 oz., of which approx. 9.0 oz. are meat and approx. 2.6 oz. are bone]	963	0.0	83.3	0.00		
Trimmed of separable fat before cooking; Cooked (braised) [yield: approx. 9.3 oz., of which approx. 6.7 oz. are meat and approx. 2.6 oz. are bone]	414	0.0	44.9	0.00		
1 pound of Cooked (braised) meat (weight includes bone):						
Yield from approx. 22.1 oz. (1 lb. 6.1 oz.) of raw untrimmed meat (weighed with the bone) that had ***not*** been trimmed of separable fat before cooking	1333	0.0	83.3	0.00		

	UNIT		1 OZ., BY WT.		1 CUP, DICED, NOT PACKED	
	Cal.	Carb.	Cal.	Carb.	Cal.	Carb.
Yield from approx. 28.0 oz. (1 lb. 12.0 oz.) of raw untrimmed meat (weighed with the bone) that ***had*** been trimmed of separable fat before cooking	718	0.0	44.9	0.00		
Boneless (Chuck Eye)						
1 pound of Raw untrimmed meat (includes separable fat) [73% separable lean, 27% separable fat]	1376	0.0	86.0	0.00	(396)	0.0
Cooked (braised) [yield: approx. 10.7 oz.] (7g/0g/9g/45%/na)	1147	0.0	107.0	0.00	(492)	0.0
Trimmed of separable fat before cooking; Cooked (braised) [yield: approx. 7.9 oz.] (8g/0g/3g/59%/na)	492	0.0	62.1	0.00	(286)	0.0
1 pound of Cooked (braised) meat:						
Yield from approx. 23.9 oz. (1 lb. 7.9 oz.) of raw untrimmed meat that had ***not*** been trimmed of separable fat before cooking	1712	0.0	107.0	0.00	(492)	0.0
Yield from approx. 32.3 oz. (2 lbs. 0.3 oz.) of raw untrimmed meat that ***had*** been trimmed of separable fat before cooking	994	0.0	62.1	0.00	(286)	0.0
STANDARD GRADE:						
Bone-in						
1 pound of Raw untrimmed meat (includes separable fat) with bone [64% separable lean, 17% separable fat, 19% bone]	919	0.0	57.5	0.00		
Cooked (braised) [yield: approx. 11.7 oz., of which approx. 8.7 oz. are meat and approx. 3.0 oz. are bone]	786	0.0	67.0	0.00		
Trimmed of separable fat before cooking; Cooked (braised) [yield: approx. 9.9 oz., of which approx. 6.9 oz. are meat and approx. 3.0 oz. are bone]	406	0.0	40.7	0.00		
1 pound of Cooked (braised) meat (weight includes bone):						
Yield from approx. 21.8 oz. (1 lb. 5.8 oz.) of raw untrimmed meat (weighed with the bone) that had ***not*** been trimmed of separable fat before cooking	1073	0.0	67.0	0.00		
Yield from approx. 25.6 oz. (1 lb. 9.6 oz.) of raw untrimmed meat (weighed with the bone) that ***had*** been trimmed of separable fat before cooking	651	0.0	40.7	0.00		
Boneless (Chuck Eye)						
1 pound of Raw untrimmed meat (includes separable fat) [80% separable lean, 20% separable fat]	1135	0.0	70.9	0.00	(326)	0.0
Cooked (braised) [yield: approx. 10.7 oz.] (7g/0g/7g/50%/na)	970	0.0	90.5	0.00	(416)	0.0
Trimmed of separable fat before cooking; Cooked (braised) [yield: approx. 8.6 oz.] (9g/0g/2g/60%/na)	501	0.0	58.5	0.00	(269)	0.0
1 pound of Cooked (braised) meat:						
Yield from approx. 23.9 oz. (1 lb. 7.9 oz.) of raw untrimmed meat that had ***not*** been trimmed of separable fat before cooking	1448	0.0	90.5	0.00	(416)	0.0
Yield from approx. 29.9 oz. (1 lb. 13.9 oz.) of raw untrimmed meat that ***had*** been trimmed of separable fat before cooking	935	0.0	58.5	0.00	(269)	0.0
ARM						
CHOICE GRADE:						
Bone-in						
1 pound of Raw untrimmed meat (includes separable fat) with bone [77% separable lean, 12% separable fat, 11% bone]	901	0.0	56.3	0.00		
Cooked (braised) [yield: approx. 11.3 oz., of which approx. 9.5 oz. are meat and approx. 1.8 oz. are bone]	782	0.0	69.2	0.00		
Trimmed of separable fat before cooking; Cooked (braised) [yield: approx. 10.0 oz., of which approx. 8.2 oz. are meat and approx. 1.8 oz. are bone]	449	0.0	45.1	0.00		
1 pound of Cooked (braised) meat (weight includes bone):						
Yield from approx. 22.7 oz. (1 lb. 6.7 oz.) of raw untrimmed meat (weighed with the bone) that had ***not*** been trimmed of separable fat before cooking	1108	0.0	69.2	0.00		
Yield from approx. 25.7 oz. (1 lb. 9.7 oz.) of raw untrimmed meat (weighed with the bone) that ***had*** been trimmed of separable fat before cooking	721	0.0	45.1	0.00		
Boneless						
1 pound of Raw untrimmed meat (includes separable fat) [83% separable lean, 17% separable fat]	1012	0.0	63.3	0.00	(291)	0.0
Cooked (braised) [yield: approx. 10.7 oz.] (7g/0g/5g/53%/na)	879	0.0	82.0	0.00	(377)	0.0

	UNIT		1 OZ., BY WT.		1 CUP, DICED, NOT PACKED	
	Cal.	Carb.	Cal.	Carb.	Cal.	Carb.
Trimmed of separable fat before cooking; Cooked (braised) [yield: approx. 9.1 oz.] (9g/0g/2g/62%/na)	505	0.0	54.8	0.00	(252)	0.0
1 pound of Cooked (braised) meat:						
Yield from approx. 23.9 oz. (1 lb. 7.9 oz.) of raw untrimmed meat that had ***not*** been trimmed of separable fat before cooking	1312	0.0	82.0	0.00	(377)	0.0
Yield from approx. 27.8 oz. (1 lb. 11.8 oz.) of raw untrimmed meat that ***had*** been trimmed of separable fat before cooking	876	0.0	54.8	0.00	(252)	0.0
GOOD GRADE:						
Bone-in						
1 pound of Raw untrimmed meat (includes separable fat) with bone [79% separable lean, 10% separable fat, 11% bone]	772	0.0	48.2	0.00		
Cooked (braised) [yield: approx. 11.3 oz., of which approx. 9.5 oz. are meat and approx. 1.8 oz. are bone]	684	0.0	60.6	0.00		
Trimmed of separable fat before cooking; Cooked (braised) [yield: approx. 10.3 oz., of which approx. 8.5 oz. are meat and approx. 1.8 oz. are bone]	431	0.0	42.1	0.00		
1 pound of Cooked (braised) meat (weight includes bone):						
Yield from approx. 22.7 oz. (1 lb. 6.7 oz.) of raw untrimmed meat (weighed with the bone) that had ***not*** been trimmed of separable fat before cooking	970	0.0	60.6	0.00		
Yield from approx. 25.0 oz. (1 lb. 9.0 oz.) of raw untrimmed meat (weighed with the bone) that ***had*** been trimmed of separable fat before cooking	673	0.0	42.1	0.00		
Boneless						
1 pound of Raw untrimmed meat (includes separable fat) [88% separable lean, 12% separable fat]	867	0.0	54.2	0.00	(249)	0.0
Cooked (braised) [yield: approx. 10.7 oz.] (8g/0g/4g/56%/na)	770	0.0	71.8	0.00	(330)	0.0
Trimmed of separable fat before cooking; Cooked (braised) [yield: approx. 9.5 oz.] (9g/0g/1g/63%/na)	485	0.0	50.8	0.00	(234)	0.0
1 pound of Cooked (braised) meat:						
Yield from approx. 23.9 oz. (1 lb. 7.9 oz.) of raw untrimmed meat that had ***not*** been trimmed of separable fat before cooking	1149	0.0	71.8	0.00	(330)	0.0
Yield from approx. 26.8 oz. (1 lb. 10.8 oz.) of raw untrimmed meat that ***had*** been trimmed of separable fat before cooking	813	0.0	50.8	0.00	(234)	0.0
STANDARD GRADE:						
Bone-in						
1 pound of Raw untrimmed meat (includes separable fat) with bone [80% separable lean, 8% separable fat, 12% bone]	675	0.0	42.2	0.00		
Cooked (braised) [yield: approx. 11.3 oz., of which approx. 9.4 oz. are meat and approx. 1.9 oz. are bone]	608	0.0	53.5	0.00		
Trimmed of separable fat before cooking; Cooked (braised) [yield: approx. 10.5 oz., of which approx. 8.6 oz. are meat and approx. 1.9 oz. are bone]	409	0.0	39.0	0.00		
1 pound of Cooked (braised) meat (weight includes bone):						
Yield from approx. 22.5 oz. (1 lb. 6.5 oz.) of raw untrimmed meat (weighed with the bone) that had ***not*** been trimmed of separable fat before cooking	856	0.0	53.5	0.00		
Yield from approx. 24.4 oz. (1 lb. 8.4 oz.) of raw untrimmed meat (weighed with the bone) that ***had*** been trimmed of separable fat before cooking	623	0.0	39.0	0.00		
Boneless						
1 pound of Raw untrimmed meat (includes separable fat) [91% separable lean, 9% separable fat]	767	0.0	48.0	0.00	(221)	0.0
Cooked (braised) [yield: approx. 10.7 oz.] (8g/0g/3g/59%/na)	690	0.0	64.4	0.00	(296)	0.0
Trimmed of separable fat before cooking; Cooked (braised) [yield: approx. 9.8 oz.] (9g/0g/1g/64%/na)	465	0.0	47.7	0.00	(219)	0.0
1 pound of Cooked (braised) meat:						
Yield from approx. 23.9 oz. (1 lb. 7.9 oz.) of raw untrimmed meat that had ***not*** been trimmed of separable fat before cooking	1031	0.0	64.4	0.00	(296)	0.0
Yield from approx. 26.2 oz. (1 lb. 10.2 oz.) of raw untrimmed meat that ***had*** been trimmed of separable fat before cooking	763	0.0	47.7	0.00	(219)	0.0

	UNIT		1 OZ., BY WT.		1 CUP, DICED, NOT PACKED	
	Cal.	Carb.	Cal.	Carb.	Cal.	Carb.
NECK						
CHOICE GRADE:						
Bone-in						
1 pound of Raw untrimmed meat (includes separable fat) with bone [68% separable lean, 12% separable fat, 20% bone]	821	0.0	51.3	0.00		
Cooked (braised) [yield: approx. 11.8 oz., of which approx. 8.6 oz. are meat and approx. 3.2 oz. are bone]	712	0.0	60.5	0.00		
Trimmed of separable fat before cooking; Cooked (braised) [yield: approx. 10.5 oz., of which approx. 7.3 oz. are meat and approx. 3.2 oz. are bone]	405	0.0	38.6	0.00		
1 pound of Cooked (braised) meat (weight includes bone):						
Yield from approx. 21.7 oz. (1 lb. 5.7 oz.) of raw untrimmed meat (weighed with the bone) that had ***not*** been trimmed of separable fat before cooking	969	0.0	60.5	0.00		
Yield from approx. 24.4 oz. (1 lb. 8.4 oz.) of raw untrimmed meat (weighed with the bone) that ***had*** been trimmed of separable fat before cooking	618	0.0	38.6	0.00		
Boneless						
1 pound of Raw untrimmed meat (includes separable fat) [83% separable lean, 17% separable fat]	1026	0.0	64.1	0.00	(295)	0.0
Cooked (braised) [yield: approx. 10.7 oz.] (8g/0g/6g/53%/na)	891	0.0	83.1	0.00	(382)	0.0
Trimmed of separable fat before cooking; Cooked (braised) [yield: approx. 9.1 oz.] (9g/0g/2g/62%/na)	507	0.0	55.6	0.00	(256)	0.0
1 pound of Cooked (braised) meat:						
Yield from approx. 23.9 oz. (1 lb. 7.9 oz.) of raw untrimmed meat that had ***not*** been trimmed of separable fat before cooking	1330	0.0	83.1	0.00	(382)	0.0
Yield from approx. 28.1 oz. (1 lb. 12.1 oz.) of raw untrimmed meat that ***had*** been trimmed of separable fat before cooking	890	0.0	55.6	0.00	(256)	0.0
GOOD GRADE:						
Bone-in						
1 pound of Raw untrimmed meat (includes separable fat) with bone [67% separable lean, 13% separable fat, 20% bone]	785	0.0	49.0	0.00		
Cooked (braised) [yield: approx. 11.7 oz., of which approx. 8.5 oz. are meat and approx. 3.2 oz. are bone]	684	0.0	58.1	0.00		
Trimmed of separable fat before cooking; Cooked (braised) [yield: approx. 10.4 oz., of which approx. 7.2 oz. are meat and approx. 3.2 oz. are bone]	376	0.0	36.2	0.00		
1 pound of Cooked (braised) meat (weight includes bone):						
Yield from approx. 21.7 oz. (1 lb. 5.7 oz.) of raw untrimmed meat (weighed with the bone) that had ***not*** been trimmed of separable fat before cooking	929	0.0	58.1	0.00		
Yield from approx. 24.6 oz. (1 lb. 8.6 oz.) of raw untrimmed meat (weighed with the bone that ***had*** been trimmed of separable fat before cooking	578	0.0	36.2	0.00		
Boneless						
1 pound of Raw untrimmed meat (includes separable fat) [84% separable lean, 16% separable fat]	981	0.0	61.3	0.00	(282)	0.0
Cooked (braised) [yield: approx. 10.7 oz.] (8g/0g/5g/54%/na)	855	0.0	79.7	0.00	(367)	0.0
Trimmed of separable fat before cooking; Cooked (braised) [yield: approx. 9.0 oz.] (9g/0g/2g/63%/na)	470	0.0	52.2	0.00	(240)	0.0
1 pound of Cooked (braised) meat:						
Yield from approx. 23.9 oz. (1 lb. 7.9 oz.) of raw untrimmed meat that had ***not*** been trimmed of separable fat before cooking	1276	0.0	79.7	0.00	(367)	0.0
Yield from approx. 28.4 oz. (1 lb. 12.4 oz.) of raw untrimmed meat that ***had*** been trimmed of separable fat before cooking	835	0.0	52.2	0.00	(240)	0.0
STANDARD GRADE:						
Bone-in						
1 pound of Raw untrimmed meat (includes separable fat) with bone [66% separable lean, 12% separable fat, 22% bone]	696	0.0	43.5	0.00		
Cooked (braised) [yield: approx. 12 oz., of which approx. 8.3 oz. are meat and approx. 3.7 oz. are bone]	614	0.0	51.4	0.00		

	UNIT		1 OZ., BY WT.		1 CUP, DICED, NOT PACKED	
	Cal.	Carb.	Cal.	Carb.	Cal.	Carb.
Trimmed of separable fat before cooking; Cooked (braised) [yield: approx. 10.7 oz., of which approx. 7.0 oz. are meat and approx. 3.7 oz. are bone]	356	0.0	33.3	0.00		
1 pound of Cooked (braised) meat (weight includes bone):						
Yield from approx. 21.5 oz. (1 lb. 5.5 oz.) of raw untrimmed meat (weighed with the bone) that had ***not*** been trimmed of separable fat before cooking	823	0.0	51.4	0.00		
Yield from approx. 23.9 oz. (1 lb. 7.9 oz.) of raw untrimmed meat (weighed with the bone) that ***had*** been trimmed of separable fat before cooking	533	0.0	33.3	0.00		
Boneless						
1 pound of Raw untrimmed meat (includes separable fat) [85% separable lean, 15% separable fat]	903	0.0	56.5	0.00	(260)	0.0
Cooked (braised) [yield: approx. 10.7 oz.] (8g/0g/4g/55%/na)	797	0.0	74.3	0.00	(342)	0.0
Trimmed of separable fat before cooking; Cooked (braised) [yield: approx. 9.1 oz.] (9g/0g/2g/63%/na)	544	0.0	50.8	0.00	(234)	0.0
1 pound of Cooked (braised) meat:						
Yield from approx. 23.9 oz. (1 lb. 7.9 oz.) of raw untrimmed meat that had ***not*** been trimmed of separable fat before cooking	1189	0.0	74.3	0.00	(342)	0.0
Yield from approx. 28.1 oz. (1 lb. 12.1 oz.) of raw untrimmed meat that ***had*** been trimmed of separable fat before cooking	813	0.0	50.8	0.00	(234)	0.0

Flank Steak

Flank steak is boneless, and has no separable fat.

	UNIT		1 OZ., BY WT.		1 CUP, DICED, NOT PACKED	
	Cal.	Carb.	Cal.	Carb.	Cal.	Carb.
CHOICE GRADE:						
Boneless						
1 pound of Raw untrimmed meat (100% separable lean, 0% separable fat]	1025	0.0	64.1	0.00	(295)	0.0
Cooked (braised) [yield: approx. 10.7 oz.] (9g/0g/2g/61%/na)	596	0.0	55.6	0.00	(256)	0.0
1 pound of Cooked (braised) meat:						
Yield from approx. 23.9 oz. (1 lb. 7.9 oz.) of raw untrimmed meat	889	0.0	55.6	0.00	(256)	0.0
GOOD GRADE:						
Boneless						
1 pound of Raw untrimmed meat [100% separable lean, 0% separable fat]	630	0.0	39.4	0.00	(181)	0.0
Cooked (braised) [yield: approx. 10.6 oz.] (9g/0g/2g/62%/na)	572	0.0	54.2	0.00	(249)	0.0
1 pound of Cooked (braised) meat:						
Yield from approx. 24.2 oz. (1 lb. 8.2 oz.) of raw untrimmed meat	866	0.0	54.2	0.00	(249)	0.0
STANDARD GRADE:						
Boneless						
1 pound of Raw untrimmed meat [100% separable lean, 0% separable fat]	594	0.0	37.1	0.00	(171)	0.0
Cooked (braised) [yield: approx. 10.7 oz.] (9g/0g/2g/63%/na)	550	0.0	51.3	0.00	(236)	0.0
1 pound of Cooked (braised) meat:						
Yield from approx. 23 oz. (1 lb. 7 oz.) of raw untrimmed meat	821	0.0	51.3	0.00	(236)	0.0

Foreshank (Shin)

	UNIT		1 OZ., BY WT.		1 CUP, DICED, NOT PACKED	
	Cal.	Carb.	Cal.	Carb.	Cal.	Carb.
CHOICE GRADE:						
Bone-in						
1 pound of Raw untrimmed meat (includes separable fat) with bone [47% separable lean, 9% separable fat, 44% bone]	531	0.0	33.2	0.00		
Cooked (braised) [yield: approx. 13.0 oz., of which approx. 6.0 oz. are meat and approx. 7.0 oz. are bone]	465	0.0	35.7	0.00		
Trimmed of separable fat before cooking; Cooked (braised) [yield: approx. 12 oz., of which approx. 5.0 oz. are meat and approx. 7.0 oz. are bone]	263	0.0	21.8	0.00		
1 pound of Cooked (braised) meat (weight includes bone):						
Yield from approx. 19.6 oz. (1 lb. 3.6 oz.) of raw untrimmed meat (weighed with the bone) that had ***not*** been trimmed of separable fat before cooking	570	0.0	35.7	0.00		
Yield from approx. 21.2 oz. (1 lb. 5.2 oz.) of raw untrimmed meat (weighed with the bone) that ***had*** been trimmed of separable fat before cooking	349	0.0	21.8	0.00		

	UNIT Cal.	UNIT Carb.	1 OZ., BY WT. Cal.	1 OZ., BY WT. Carb.	1 CUP, DICED, NOT PACKED Cal.	1 CUP, DICED, NOT PACKED Carb.
Boneless						
1 pound of Raw untrimmed meat (includes separable fat) [84% separable lean, 16% separable fat]	949	0.0	59.3	0.00	(273)	0.0
Cooked (braised) [yield: approx. 10.7 oz.] (8g/0g/5g/54%/na)	830	0.0	77.5	0.00	(366)	0.0
Trimmed of separable fat before cooking; Cooked (braised) [yield: approx. 9.0 oz.] (9g/0g/2g/63%/na)	470	0.0	52.2	0.00	(240)	0.0
1 pound of Cooked (braised) meat:						
Yield from approx. 23.9 oz. (1 lb. 7.9 oz.) of raw untrimmed meat that had ***not*** been trimmed of separable fat before cooking	1239	0.0	77.5	0.00	(366)	0.0
Yield from approx. 28.4 oz. (1 lb. 12.4 oz.) of raw untrimmed meat that ***had*** been trimmed of separable fat before cooking	835	0.0	52.2	0.00	(240)	0.0
GOOD GRADE:						
Bone-in						
1 pound of Raw untrimmed meat (includes separable fat) with bone [48% separable lean, 8% separable fat, 44% bone]	470	0.0	29.4	00.0		
Cooked (braised) [yield: approx. 13.0 oz., of which approx. 6.0 oz. are meat and approx. 7.0 oz. are bone]	417	0.0	32.0	0.00		
Trimmed of separable fat before cooking; Cooked (braised) [yield: approx. 12.1 oz., of which approx. 5.1 oz. are meat and approx. 7.0 oz. are bone]	255	0.0	21.0	0.00		
1 pound of Cooked (braised) meat (weight includes bone):						
Yield from approx. 19.6 oz. (1 lb. 3.6 oz.) of raw untrimmed meat (weighed with the bone) that had ***not*** been trimmed of separable fat before cooking	512	0.0	32.0	0.00		
Yield from approx. 21.1 oz. (1 lb. 5.1 oz.) of raw untrimmed meat (weighed with the bone) that ***had*** been trimmed of separable fat before cooking	335	0.0	21.0	0.00		
Boneless						
1 pound of Raw untrimmed meat (includes separable fat) [85% separable lean, 15% separable fat]	840	0.0	52.5	0.00	(242)	0.0
Cooked (braised) [yield: approx. 10.7 oz.] (8g/0g/4g/57%/na)	745	0.0	69.5	0.00	(561)	0.0
Trimmed of separable fat before cooking; Cooked (braised) [yield: approx. 9.1 oz.] (9g/0g/1g/63%/na)	455	0.0	49.9	0.00	(230)	0.0
1 pound of Cooked (braised) meat:						
Yield from approx. 23.9 oz. (1 lb. 7.9 oz.) of raw untrimmed meat that had ***not*** been trimmed of separable fat before cooking	1112	0.0	69.5	0.00	(561)	0.0
Yield from approx. 28.1 oz. (1 lb. 12.1 oz.) of raw untrimmed meat that ***had*** been trimmed of separable fat before cooking	799	0.0	49.9	0.00	(230)	0.0
STANDARD GRADE:						
Bone-in						
1 pound of Raw untrimmed meat (includes separable fat) with bone [46% separable lean, 8% separable fat, 46% bone]	431	0.0	27.0	0.00		
Cooked (braised) [yield: approx. 13.2 oz., of which approx. 5.8 oz. are meat and approx. 7.4 oz. are bone]	386	0.0	29.4	0.00		
Trimmed of separable fat before cooking; Cooked (braised) [yield: approx. 12.3 oz., of which approx. 4.9 oz. are meat and approx. 7.4 oz. are bone]	239	0.0	19.4	0.00		
1 pound of Cooked (braised) meat (weight includes bone):						
Yield from approx. 19.5 oz. (1 lb. 3.5 oz.) of raw untrimmed meat (weighed with the bone) that had ***not*** been trimmed of separable fat before cooking	470	0.0	29.4	0.00		
Yield from approx. 20.8 oz. (1 lb. 4.8 oz.) of raw untrimmed meat (weighed with the bone) that ***had*** been trimmed of separable fat before cooking	311	0.0	19.4	0.00		
Boneless						
1 pound of Raw untrimmed meat (includes separable fat) [85% separable lean, 15% separable fat]	799	0.0	49.9	0.00	(230)	0.0
Cooked (braised) [yield: approx. 10.7 oz.] (8g/0g/3g/58%/na)	715	0.6	66.7	0.00	(307)	0.0
Trimmed of separable fat before cooking; Cooked (braised) [yield: approx. 9.1 oz.] (9g/0g/1g/64%/na)	442	0.0	48.5	0.00	(223)	0.0

	UNIT Cal.	UNIT Carb.	1 OZ., BY WT. Cal.	1 OZ., BY WT. Carb.	1 CUP, DICED, NOT PACKED Cal.	1 CUP, DICED, NOT PACKED Carb.
1 pound of Cooked (braised) meat:						
Yield from approx. 23.9 oz. (1 lb. 7.9 oz.) of raw untrimmed meat that had ***not*** been trimmed of separable fat before cooking	1067	0.0	66.7	0.00	(307)	0.0
Yield from approx. 28.1 oz. (1 lb. 12.1 oz.) of raw untrimmed meat that ***had*** been trimmed of separable fat before cooking	776	0.0	48.5	0.00	(223)	0.0
Hindshank						
CHOICE GRADE:						
Bone-in						
1 pound of Raw untrimmed meat (includes separable fat) with bone [31% separable lean, 15% separable fat, 54% bone]	604	0.0	37.7	0.00		
Cooked (braised) [yield: approx. 13.5 oz., of which approx. 4.9 oz. are meat and approx. 8.6 oz. are bone]	505	0.0	37.2	0.00		
Trimmed of separable fat before cooking; Cooked (braised) [yield: approx. 11.9 oz., of which approx. 3.3 oz. are meat and approx. 8.6 oz. are bone]	173	0.0	14.4	0.00		
1 pound of Cooked (braised) meat (weight includes bone):						
Yield from approx. 18.9 oz. (1 lb. 2.9 oz.) of raw untrimmed meat (weighed with the bone) that had ***not*** been trimmed of separable fat before cooking	596	0.0	37.2	0.00		
Yield from approx. 21.4 oz. (1 lb. 5.4 oz.) of raw untrimmed meat (weighed with the bone) that ***had*** been trimmed of separable fat before cooking	231	0.0	14.4	0.00		
Boneless						
1 pound of Raw untrimmed meat (includes separable fat) [67% separable lean, 33% separable fat]	1312	0.0	82.0	0.00	(377)	0.0
Cooked (braised) [yield: approx. 10.7 oz.] (7g/0g/8g/46%/na)	1098	0.0	102.4	0.00	(471)	0.0
Trimmed of separable fat before cooking; Cooked (braised) [yield: approx. 7.1 oz.] (9g/0g/2g/63%/na)	369	0.0	52.2	0.00	(240)	0.0
1 pound of Cooked (braised) meat:						
Yield from approx. 23.9 oz. (1 lb. 7.9 oz.) of raw untrimmed meat that had ***not*** been trimmed of separable fat before cooking	1639	0.0	102.4	0.00	(471)	0.0
Yield from approx. 36.2 oz. (2 lb. 4.2 oz.) of raw untrimmed meat that ***had*** been trimmed of separable fat before cooking	835	0.0	52.2	0.00	(240)	0.0
GOOD GRADE:						
Bone-in						
1 pound of Raw untrimmed meat (includes separable fat) with bone [31% separable lean, 13% separable fat, 56% bone]	477	0.0	29.8	0.00		
Cooked (braised) [yield: approx. 13.7 oz., of which approx. 4.7 oz. are meat and approx. 9.0 oz. are bone]	411	0.0	30.0	0.00		
Trimmed of separable fat before cooking; Cooked (braised) [yield: approx. 12.3 oz., of which approx. 3.3 oz. are meat and approx. 9.0 oz. are bone]	167	0.0	13.6	0.00		
1 pound of Cooked (braised) meat (weight includes bone):						
Yield from approx. 18.7 oz. (1 lb. 2.7 oz.) of raw untrimmed meat (weighed with the bone) that had ***not*** been trimmed of separable fat before cooking	481	0.0	30.0	0.00		
Yield from approx. 20.8 oz. (1 lb. 4.8 oz.) of raw untrimmed meat (weighed with the bone) that ***had*** been trimmed of separable fat before cooking	217	0.0	13.6	0.00		
Boneless						
1 pound of Raw untrimmed meat (includes separable fat) [71% separable lean, 29% separable fat]	1085	0.0	67.8	0.00	(312)	0.0
Cooked (braised) [yield: approx. 10.7 oz.] (8g/0g/6g/51%/na)	934	0.0	87.1	0.00	(401)	0.0
Trimmed of separable fat before cooking; Cooked (braised) [yield: approx. 7.6 oz.] (9g/0g/1g/63%/na)	380	0.0	49.9	0.00	(230)	0.0
1 pound of Cooked (braised) meat:						
Yield from approx. 23.9 oz. (1 lb. 7.9 oz.) of raw untrimmed meat that had ***not*** been trimmed of separable fat before cooking	1394	0.0	87.1	0.00	(401)	0.0
Yield from approx. 33.6 oz. (2 lbs. 1.6 oz.) of raw untrimmed meat that ***had*** been trimmed of separable fat before cooking	799	0.0	49.9	0.00	(230)	0.0

	UNIT Cal.	UNIT Carb.	1 OZ., BY WT. Cal.	1 OZ., BY WT. Carb.	1 CUP, DICED, NOT PACKED Cal.	1 CUP, DICED, NOT PACKED Carb.
STANDARD GRADE:						
Bone-in						
1 pound of Raw untrimmed meat (includes separable fat) with bone [29% separable lean, 10% separable fat, 61% bone]	372	0.0	23.2	0.00		
Cooked (braised) [yield: approx. 14 oz., of which approx. 4.2 oz. are meat and approx. 9.8 oz. are bone]	325	0.0	23.3	0.00		
Trimmed of separable fat before cooking; Cooked (braised) [yield: approx. 12.9 oz., of which approx. 3.1 oz. are meat and approx. 9.8 oz. are bone]	149	0.0	11.6	0.00		
1 pound of Cooked (braised) meat (weight includes bone):						
Yield from approx. 18.4 oz. (1 lb. 2.4 oz.) of raw untrimmed meat (weighed with the bone) that had ***not*** been trimmed of separable fat before cooking	373	0.0	23.3	0.00		
Yield from approx. 19.9 oz. (1 lb. 3.9 oz.) of raw untrimmed meat (weighed with the bone) that ***had*** been trimmed of separable fat before cooking	185	0.0	11.6	0.00		
Boneless						
1 pound of Raw untrimmed meat (includes separable fat [75% separable lean, 25% separable fat]	953	0.0	59.6	0.00	(274)	0.0
Cooked (braised) [yield: approx. 10.7 oz.] (8g/0g/5g/54%/na)	833	0.0	64.6	0.00	(297)	0.0
Trimmed of separable fat before cooking; Cooked [yield: approx. 8.0 oz.]	383	0.0	47.7	0.00	(219)	0.0
1 pound of Cooked (braised) meat:						
Yield from approx. 19.9 oz. (1 lb. 3.9 oz.) of raw untrimmed meat that had ***not*** been trimmed of separable fat before cooking (9g/0g/1g/64%/na)	1034	0.0	64.6	0.00	(297)	0.0
Yield from approx. 31.8 oz. (1 lb. 15.8 oz.) of raw untrimmed meat that ***had*** been trimmed of separable fat before cooking	763	0.0	47.7	0.00	(219)	0.0

Loin or Short Loin Cuts

	UNIT Cal.	UNIT Carb.	1 OZ., BY WT. Cal.	1 OZ., BY WT. Carb.	1 CUP, DICED, NOT PACKED Cal.	1 CUP, DICED, NOT PACKED Carb.
PORTERHOUSE STEAK						
CHOICE GRADE:						
Bone-in						
1 pound of Raw untrimmed meat (includes separable fat) with bone [57% separable lean, 33% separable fat, 9% bone]	1611	0.0	100.7	0.00		
Cooked (broiled) [yield: approx. 12 oz., of which approx. 10.6 oz. are meat and approx. 1.4 oz. are bone]	1402	0.0	116.2	0.00		
Trimmed of separable fat before cooking; Cooked (broiled) [yield: approx. 8.1 oz., of which approx. 6.7 oz. are meat and approx. 1.4 oz. are bone]	426	0.0	52.3	0.00		
1 pound of Cooked (broiled) meat (weight includes bone):						
Yield from approx. 21.2 oz. (1 lb. 5.2 oz.) of raw untrimmed meat (weighed with the bone) that had ***not*** been trimmed of separable fat before cooking	1859	0.0	116.2	0.00		
Yield from approx. 31.5 oz. (1 lb. 15.5 oz.) of raw untrimmed meat (weighed with the bone) that ***had*** been trimmed of separable fat before cooking	837	0.0	52.3	0.00		
Boneless						
1 pound of Raw untrimmed meat (includes separable fat) [63% separable lean, 37% separable fat]	1771	0.0	110.7	0.00	(509)	0.0
Cooked (broiled) [yield: approx. 11.7 oz.] (6g/0g/12g/37%/na)	1541	0.0	131.9	0.00	(607)	0.0
Trimmed of separable fat before cooking; Cooked (broiled) [yield: approx. 7.4 oz.] (9g/0g/3g/58%/na)	468	0.0	63.6	0.00	(293)	0.0
1 pound of Cooked (broiled) meat:						
Yield from approx. 21.9 oz. (1 lb. 5.9 oz.) of raw untrimmed meat that had ***not*** been trimmed of separable fat before cooking	2111	0.0	131.9	0.00	(607)	0.0
Yield from approx. 34.8 oz. (2 lbs. 2.8 oz.) of raw untrimmed meat that ***had*** been trimmed of separable fat before cooking	1017	0.0	63.6	0.00	(293)	0.0
GOOD GRADE:						
Bone-in						
1 pound of Raw untrimmed meat (includes separable fat) with bone [58% separable lean, 33% separable fat, 9% bone]	1528	0.0	95.5	0.00		
Cooked (broiled) [yield: approx. 12 oz., of which approx. 10.6 oz. are meat and approx. 1.4 oz. are bone]	1345	0.0	111.5	0.00		
Trimmed of separable fat before cooking; Cooked (broiled) [yield: approx. 8.2 oz., of which approx. 6.8 oz. are meat and approx. 1.4 oz. are bone]	380	0.0	46.1	0.00		
1 pound of Cooked (broiled) meat (weight includes bone):						
Yield from approx. 21.2 oz. (1 lb. 5.2 oz.) of raw untrimmed meat (weighed with the bone) that had ***not*** been trimmed of separable fat before cooking	1783	0.0	111.5	0.00		
Yield from approx. 31.1 oz. (1 lb. 15.1 oz.) of raw untrimmed meat (weighed with the bone) that ***had*** been trimmed of separable fat before cooking	738	0.0	46.1	0.00		
Boneless						
1 pound of Raw untrimmed meat (includes separable fat) [64% separable lean, 36% separable fat]	1680	0.0	105.0	0.00	(483)	0.0
Cooked (broiled) [yield: approx. 11.7 oz.] (6g/0g/11g/39%/na)	1478	0.0	126.6	0.00	(582)	0.0
Trimmed of separable fat before cooking; Cooked (broiled) [yield: approx. 7.4 oz.] (9g/0g/2g/60%/na)	418	0.0	55.9	0.00	(257)	0.0
1 pound of Cooked (broiled) meat:						
Yield from approx. 21.9 oz. (1 lb. 5.9 oz.) of raw untrimmed meat that had ***not*** been trimmed of separable fat before cooking	2025	0.0	126.6	0.00	(582)	0.0
Yield from approx. 34.2 oz. (2 lbs. 2.2 oz.) of raw untrimmed meat that ***had*** been trimmed of separable fat before cooking	894	0.0	55.9	0.00	(257)	0.0
STANDARD GRADE:						
Bone-in						
1 pound of Raw untrimmed meat (includes separable fat) with bone [63% separable lean, 26% separable fat, 11% bone]	1277	0.0	79.8	0.00		
Cooked (broiled) [yield: approx. 12.2 oz., of which approx. 10.4 oz. are meat and approx. 1.8 oz. are bone]	1150	0.0	94.6	0.00		
Trimmed of separable fat before cooking; Cooked (broiled) [yield: approx. 9.2 oz., of which approx. 7.4 oz. are meat and approx. 1.8 oz. are bone]	398	0.0	43.5	0.00		
1 pound of Cooked (broiled) meat (weight includes bone):						
Yield from approx. 21.1 oz. (1 lb. 5.1 oz.) of raw untrimmed meat (weighed with the bone) that had ***not*** been trimmed of separable fat before cooking	1514	0.0	94.6	0.00		
Yield from approx. 28.0 oz. (1 lb. 12.0 oz.) of raw untrimmed meat (weighed with the bone) that ***had*** been trimmed of separable fat before cooking	697	0.0	43.5	0.00		
Boneless						
1 pound of Raw untrimmed meat (includes separable fat) [71% separable lean, 29% separable fat]	1435	0.0	89.7	0.00	(413)	0.0
Cooked (broiled) [yield: approx. 11.7 oz.] (7g/0g/9g/44%/na)	1293	0.0	110.7	0.00	(509)	0.0
Trimmed of separable fat before cooking; Cooked (broiled) [yield: approx. 8.3 oz.] (9g/0g/2g/61%/na)	447	0.0	53.9	0.00	(248)	0.0
1 pound of Cooked (broiled) meat:						
Yield from approx. 21.9 oz. (1 lb. 5.9 oz.) of raw untrimmed meat that had ***not*** been trimmed of separable fat before cooking	1771	0.0	110.7	0.00	(509)	0.0
Yield from approx. 30.9 oz. (1 lb. 14.9 oz.) of raw untrimmed meat that ***had*** been trimmed of separable fat before cooking	863	0.0	53.9	0.0	(248)	0.0
T-BONE STEAK						
CHOICE GRADE:						
Bone-in						
1 pound of Raw untrimmed meat (includes separable fat) with bone [55% separable lean, 34% separable fat, 11% bone]	1604	0.0	100.3	0.00		
Cooked (broiled) [yield: approx. 12.2 oz., of which approx. 10.4 oz. are meat and approx. 1.8 oz. are bone]	1395	0.0	114.8	0.00		
Trimmed of separable fat before cooking; Cooked (broiled) [yield: approx. 8.2 oz., of which approx. 6.4 oz. are meat and approx. 1.8 oz. are bone]	408	0.0	49.7	0.00		
1 pound of Cooked (broiled) meat (weight includes bone):						
Yield from approx. 21.1 oz. (1 lb. 5.1 oz.) of raw untrimmed meat (weighed with the bone) that had ***not*** been trimmed of separable fat before cooking	1836	0.0	114.8	0.00		

	UNIT Cal.	UNIT Carb.	1 OZ., BY WT. Cal.	1 OZ., BY WT. Carb.	1 CUP, DICED, NOT PACKED Cal.	1 CUP, DICED, NOT PACKED Carb.
Yield from approx. 31.2 oz. (1 lb. 15.2 oz.) of raw untrimmed meat (weighed with the bone) that ***had*** been trimmed of separable fat before cooking	795	0.0	49.7	0.00		
Boneless						
1 pound of Raw untrimmed meat (includes separable fat) [62% separable lean, 38% separable fat]	1802	0.0	112.6	0.00	(518)	0.0
Cooked (broiled) [yield: approx. 11.7 oz.] (6g/0g/12g/36%/na)	1568	0.0	134.2	0.00	(617)	0.0
Trimmed of separable fat before cooking; Cooked (broiled) [yield: approx. 7.2 oz.] (9g/0g/3g/58%/na)	458	0.0	63.3	0.00	(291)	0.0
1 pound of Cooked (broiled) meat:						
Yield from approx. 21.9 oz. (1 lb. 5.9 oz.) of raw untrimmed meat that had ***not*** been trimmed of separable fat before cooking	2147	0.0	134.2	0.00	(617)	0.0
Yield from approx. 35.4 oz. (2 lbs. 3.4 oz.) of raw untrimmed meat that ***had*** been trimmed of separable fat before cooking	1012	0.00	63.3	0.00	(291)	0.0
GOOD GRADE:						
Bone-in						
1 pound of Raw untrimmed meat (includes separable fat) with bone [56% separable lean, 32% separable fat, 12% bone]	1462	0.0	91.4	0.00		
Cooked (broiled) [yield: approx. 12.2 oz., of which approx. 10.3 oz. are meat and approx. 1.9 oz. are bone]	1289	0.0	105.7	0.00		
Trimmed of separable fat before cooking; Cooked (broiled) [yield: approx. 8.5 oz., of which approx. 6.6 oz. are meat and approx. 1.9 oz. are bone]	371	0.0	43.7	0.00		
1 pound of Cooked (broiled) meat (weight includes bone):						
Yield from approx. 21.0 oz. (1 lb. 5.0 oz.) of raw untrimmed meat (weighed with the bone) that had ***not*** been trimmed of separable fat before cooking	1691	0.0	105.7	0.00		
Yield from approx. 30.1 oz. (1 lb. 14.1 oz.) of raw untrimmed meat (weighed with the bone) that ***had*** been trimmed of separable fat before cooking	699	0.0	43.7	0.00		
Boneless						
1 pound of Raw untrimmed meat (includes separable fat) [64% separable lean, 36% separable fat]	1662	0.0	103.9	0.00	(478)	0.0
Cooked (broiled) [yield: approx. 11.7 oz.] (6g/0g/11g/39%/na)	1465	0.0	125.4	0.00	(577)	0.0
Trimmed of separable fat before cooking; Cooked (broiled) [yield: approx. 7.5 oz.] (9g/0g/2g/60%/na)	422	0.0	56.5	0.00	(260)	0.0
1 pound of Cooked (broiled) meat:						
Yield from approx. 21.9 oz. (1 lb. 5.9 oz.) of raw untrimmed meat that had ***not*** been trimmed of separable fat before cooking	2007	0.0	125.4	0.00	(577)	0.0
Yield from approx. 34.2 oz. (2 lbs. 2.2 oz.) of raw untrimmed meat that ***had*** been trimmed of separable fat before cooking	903	0.0	56.5	0.00	(260)	0.0
STANDARD GRADE:						
Bone-in						
1 pound of Raw untrimmed meat (includes separable fat) with bone [61% separable lean, 25% separable fat, 14% bone]	1203	0.0	75.2	0.00		
Cooked (broiled) [yield: approx. 12.3 oz., of which approx. 10.1 oz. are meat and approx. 2.2 oz. are bone]	1089	0.0	88.6	0.00		
Trimmed of separable fat before cooking; Cooked (broiled) [yield: approx. 9.3 oz., of which approx. 7.1 oz. are meat and approx. 2.2 oz. are bone]	399	0.0	42.5	0.00		
1 pound of Cooked (broiled) meat (weight includes bone):						
Yield from approx. 20.8 oz. (1 lb. 4.8 oz) of raw untrimmed meat (weighed with the bone) that had ***not*** been trimmed of separable fat before cooking	1418	0.0	88.6	0.00		
Yield from approx. 27.3 oz. (1 lb. 11.3 oz.) of raw untrimmed meat (weighed with the bone) that ***had*** been trimmed of separable fat before cooking	681	0.0	42.5	0.00		
Boneless						
1 pound of Raw untrimmed meat (includes separable fat) [71% separable lean, 29% separable fat]	1398	0.0	87.4	0.00	(402)	0.0
Cooked (broiled) [yield: approx. 11.7 oz.] (7g/0g/9g/44%/na)	1266	0.0	108.4	0.00	(499)	0.0
Trimmed of separable fat before cooking; Cooked (broiled) [yield: approx. 8.3 oz.] (9g/0g/2g/60%/na)	464	0.0	55.9	0.00	(257)	0.0

	UNIT Cal.	UNIT Carb.	1 OZ., BY WT. Cal.	1 OZ., BY WT. Carb.	1 CUP, DICED, NOT PACKED Cal.	1 CUP, DICED, NOT PACKED Carb.
1 pound of Cooked (broiled) meat:						
Yield from approx. 21.9 oz. (1 lb. 5.9 oz.) of raw untrimmed meat that had ***not*** been trimmed of separable fat before cooking	1734	0.0	108.4	0.00	(499)	0.0
Yield from approx. 30.9 oz. (1 lb. 14.9 oz.) of raw untrimmed meat that ***had*** been trimmed of separable fat before cooking	894	0.0	55.9	0.00	(257)	0.0
CLUB STEAK (SHELL STEAK, TOP LOIN, OR NEW YORK STEAK)						
CHOICE GRADE:						
Bone-in						
1 pound of Raw untrimmed meat (includes separable fat) with bone [54% separable lean, 30% separable fat, 16% bone]	1449	0.0	90.6	0.00		
Cooked (broiled) [yield: approx. 12.4 oz., of which approx. 9.8 oz. are meat and approx. 2.6 oz. are bone]	1264	0.0	102.1	0.00		
Trimmed of separable fat before cooking; Cooked (broiled) [yield: approx. 8.9 oz., of which approx. 6.3 oz. are meat and approx. 2.6 oz. are bone]	435	0.0	49.2	0.00		
1 pound of Cooked (broiled) meat (weight includes bone):						
Yield from approx. 20.7 oz. (1 lb. 4.7 oz.) of raw untrimmed meat (weighed with the bone) that had ***not*** been trimmed of separable fat before cooking	1634	0.0	102.1	0.00		
Yield from approx. 29.0 oz. (1 lb. 13.0 oz.) of raw untrimmed meat (weighed with the bone) that ***had*** been trimmed of separable fat before cooking	787	0.0	49.2	0.00		
Boneless						
1 pound of Raw untrimmed meat (includes separable fat) [64% separable lean, 36% separable fat]	1725	0.0	107.8	0.00	(496)	0.0
Cooked (broiled) [yield: approx. 11.7 oz.] (6g/0g/12g/38%/na)	1505	0.0	128.8	0.00	(592)	0.0
Trimmed of separable fat before cooking; Cooked (broiled) [yield: approx. 7.4 oz.] (8g/0g/4g/56%/na)	518	0.0	69.2	0.00	(318)	0.0
1 pound of Cooked (broiled) meat:						
Yield from approx. 21.9 oz. (1 lb. 5.9 oz.) of raw untrimmed meat that had ***not*** been trimmed of separable fat before cooking	2016	0.0	128.8	0.00	(592)	0.0
Yield from approx. 34.2 oz. (2 lbs. 2.2 oz.) of raw untrimmed meat that ***had*** been trimmed of separable fat before cooking	1108	0.0	69.2	0.00	(318)	0.0
GOOD GRADE:						
Bone-in						
1 pound of Raw untrimmed meat (includes separable fat) with bone [58% separable lean, 24% separable fat, 18% bone]	1206	0.0	75.4	0.00		
Cooked (broiled) [yield: approx. 12.5 oz., of which approx. 9.6 oz. are meat and approx. 2.9 oz. are bone]	1083	0.0	86.8	0.00		
Trimmed of separable fat before cooking; Cooked (broiled) [yield: approx. 9.6 oz., of which approx. 6.7 oz. are meat and approx. 2.9 oz. are bone]	413	0.0	43.1	0.00		
1 pound of Cooked (broiled) meat (weight includes bone):						
Yield from approx. 20.5 oz. (1 lb. 4.5 oz.) of raw untrimmed meat (weighed with the bone) that had ***not*** been trimmed of separable fat before cooking	1389	0.0	86.8	0.00		
Yield from approx. 26.7 oz. (1 lb. 10.7 oz.) of raw untrimmed meat (weighed with the bone) that ***had*** been trimmed of separable fat before cooking	689	0.0	43.1	0.00		
Boneless						
1 pound of Raw untrimmed meat (includes separable fat) [70% separable lean, 30% separable fat]	1471	0.0	91.9	0.00	(423)	0.0
Cooked (broiled) [yield: approx. 11.7 oz.] (7g/0g/9g/43%/na)	1319	0.0	112.9	0.00	(519)	0.0
Trimmed of separable fat before cooking; Cooked (broiled) [yield: approx. 8.2 oz.] (9g/0g/3g/59%/na)	503	0.0	61.6	0.00	(283)	0.0
1 pound of Cooked (broiled) meat:						
Yield from approx. 21.9 oz. (1 lb. 5.9 oz.) of raw untrimmed meat that had ***not*** been trimmed of separable fat before cooking	1807	0.0	112.9	0.00	(519)	0.0
Yield from approx. 31.3 oz. (1 lb. 15.3 oz.) of raw untrimmed meat that ***had*** been trimmed of separable fat before cooking	985	0.0	61.6	0.00	(283)	0.0

	UNIT Cal.	UNIT Carb.	1 OZ., BY WT. Cal.	1 OZ., BY WT. Carb.	1 CUP, DICED, NOT PACKED Cal.	1 CUP, DICED, NOT PACKED Carb.
STANDARD GRADE:						
Bone-in						
1 pound of Raw untrimmed meat (includes separable fat) with bone [61% separable lean, 20% separable fat, 19% bone]	1022	0.0	63.9	0.00		
Cooked (broiled) [yield: approx. 12.5 oz., of which approx. 9.5 oz. are meat and approx. 3.0 oz. are bone]	891	0.0	71.3	0.00		
Trimmed of separable fat before cooking; Cooked (broiled) [yield: approx. 10.2 oz., of which approx. 7.2 oz. are meat and approx. 3.0 oz. are bone]	398	0.0	38.9	0.00		
1 pound of Cooked (broiled) meat (weight includes bone):						
Yield from approx. 20.5 oz. (1 lb. 4.5 oz.) of raw untrimmed meat (weighed with the bone) that had ***not*** been trimmed of separable fat before cooking	1141	0.0	71.3	0.00		
Yield from approx. 25.0 oz. (1 lb. 9.0 oz.) of raw untrimmed meat (weighed with the bone) that ***had*** been trimmed of separable fat before cooking	622	0.0	38.9	0.00		
Boneless						
1 pound of Raw untrimmed meat (includes separable fat) [76% separable lean, 24% separable fat]	1262	0.0	78.9	0.00	(363)	0.0
Cooked (broiled) [yield: approx. 11.7 oz.] (7g/0g/7g/49%/na)	1100	0.0	94.2	0.00	(433)	0.0
Trimmed of separable fat before cooking; Cooked (broiled) [yield: approx. 8.9 oz.] (9g/0g/2g/61%/na)	491	0.0	55.3	0.00	(254)	0.0
1 pound of Cooked (broiled) meat:						
Yield from approx. 21.9 oz. (1 lb. 5.9 oz.) of raw untrimmed meat that had ***not*** been trimmed of separable fat before cooking	1507	0.0	94.2	0.00	(433)	0.0
Yield from approx. 28.8 oz. (1 lb. 12.8 oz.) of raw untrimmed meat that ***had*** been trimmed of separable fat before cooking	885	0.0	55.3	0.00	(254)	0.0

Loin End or Sirloin

	UNIT Cal.	UNIT Carb.	1 OZ., BY WT. Cal.	1 OZ., BY WT. Carb.	1 CUP, DICED, NOT PACKED Cal.	1 CUP, DICED, NOT PACKED Carb.
WEDGE AND ROUND BONE SIRLOIN STEAK						
CHOICE GRADE:						
Bone-in						
1 pound of Raw untrimmed meat (includes separable fat) with bone [68% separable lean, 25% separable fat, 7% bone]	1322	0.0	82.6	0.00		
Cooked (broiled) [yield: approx. 12.0 oz., of which approx. 10.9 oz. are meat and approx. 1.1 oz. are bone]	1193	0.0	99.5	0.00		
Trimmed of separable fat before cooking; Cooked (broiled) [yield: approx. 9.0 oz., of which approx. 7.9 oz. are meat and approx. 1.1 oz. are bone]	466	0.0	51.5	0.00		
1 pound of Cooked (broiled) meat (weight includes bone):						
Yield from approx. 21.4 oz. (1 lb. 5.4 oz.) of raw untrimmed meat (weighed with the bone) that had ***not*** been trimmed of separable fat before cooking	1593	0.0	99.5	0.00		
Yield from approx. 28.3 oz. (1 lb. 12.3 oz.) of raw untrimmed meat (weighed with the bone) that ***had*** been trimmed of separable fat before cooking	823	0.0	51.5	0.00		
Boneless						
1 pound of Raw untrimmed meat (includes separable fat) (73% separable lean, 27% separable fat]	1421	0.0	88.8	0.00	(408)	0.0
Cooked (broiled) [yield: approx. 11.7 oz.] (7g/0g/9g/44%/na)	1283	0.0	109.8	0.00	(505)	0.0
Trimmed of separable fat before cooking; Cooked (broiled) [yield: approx. 8.5 oz.] (9g/0g/2g/59%/na)	500	0.0	58.7	0.00	(270)	0.0
1 pound of Cooked (broiled) meat:						
Yield from approx. 21.9 oz. (1 lb. 5.9 oz.) of raw untrimmed meat that had ***not*** been trimmed of separable fat before cooking	1757	0.0	109.8	0.00	(505)	0.0
Yield from approx. 30.0 oz. (1 lb. 14.0 oz.) of raw untrimmed meat that ***had*** been trimmed of separable fat before cooking	940	0.0	58.7	0.00	(207)	0.0
GOOD GRADE:						
Bone-in						
1 pound of Raw untrimmed meat (includes separable fat) with bone [69% separable lean, 23% separable fat, 8% bone]	1174	0.0	73.4	0.00		
Cooked (broiled) [yield: approx. 12.0 oz., of which approx. 10.7 oz. are meat and approx. 1.3 oz. are bone]	1076	0.0	89.5	0.00		
Trimmed of separable fat before cooking; Cooked (broiled) [yield: approx. 9.3 oz., of which approx. 8.0 oz. are meat and approx. 1.3 oz. are bone]	418	0.0	44.8	0.00		
1 pound of Cooked (broiled) meat (weight includes bone):						
Yield from approx. 21.3 oz. (1 lb. 5.3 oz.) of raw untrimmed meat (weighed with the bone) that had ***not*** been trimmed of separable fat before cooking	1432	0.0	89.5	0.0		
Yield from approx. 27.4 oz. (1 lb. 11.4 oz.) of raw untrimmed meat (weighed with the bone) that ***had*** been trimmed of separable fat before cooking	717	0.0	44.8	0.00		
Boneless						
1 pound of Raw untrimmed meat (includes separable fat) [75% separable lean, 25% separable fat]	1276	0.0	79.7	0.00	(367)	0.0
Cooked (broiled) [yield: approx. 11.7 oz.] (7g/0g/8g/47%/na)	1170	0.0	100.2	0.00	(461)	0.0
Trimmed of separable fat before cooking; Cooked (broiled) [yield: approx. 8.8 oz.] (9g/0g/2g/62%/na)	455	0.0	51.9	0.00	(239)	0.0
1 pound of Cooked (broiled) meat:						
Yield from approx. 21.9 oz. (1 lb. 5.9 oz.) of raw untrimmed meat that had ***not*** been trimmed of separable fat before cooking	1603	0.0	100.2	0.00	(461)	0.0
Yield from approx. 29.2 oz. (1 lb. 13.2 oz.) of raw untrimmed meat that ***had*** been trimmed of separable fat before cooking	831	0.0	51.9	0.00	(239)	0.0
STANDARD GRADE:						
Bone-in						
1 pound of Raw untrimmed meat (includes separable fat) with bone [72% separable lean, 19% separable fat, 9% bone]	1004	0.0	62.7	0.00		
Cooked (broiled) [yield: approx. 12 oz., of which approx. 10.6 oz. are meat and approx. 1.4 oz. are bone]	941	0.0	78.0	0.00		
Trimmed of separable fat before cooking; Cooked (broiled) [yield: approx. 9.9 oz., of which approx. 8.5 oz. are meat and approx. 1.4 oz. are bone]	427	0.0	43.0	0.00		
1 pound of Cooked (broiled) meat (weight includes bone):						
Yield from approx. 21.2 oz. (1 lb. 5.2 oz.) of raw untrimmed meat (weighed with the bone) that had ***not*** been trimmed of separable fat before cooking	1247	0.0	78.0	0.00		
Yield from approx. 25.7 oz. (1 lb. 9.7 oz.) of raw untrimmed meat (weighed with the bone) that ***had*** been trimmed of separable fat before cooking	687	0.0	43.0	0.00		
Boneless						
1 pound of Raw untrimmed meat (includes separable fat) [80% separable lean, 20% separable fat]	1103	0.0	69.0	0.00	(317)	0.0
Cooked (broiled) [yield: approx. 11.7 oz.] (8g/0g/6g/50%/na)	1034	0.0	88.5	0.00	(407)	0.0
Trimmed of separable fat before cooking; Cooked (broiled) [yield: approx. 9.3 oz.] (9g/0g/1g/62%/na)	469	0.0	50.2	0.00	(231)	0.0
1 pound of Cooked (broiled) meat:						
Yield from approx. 21.9 oz. (1 lb. 5.9 oz.) of raw untrimmed meat that had ***not*** been trimmed of separable fat before cooking	1416	0.0	88.5	0.00	(407)	0.0
Yield from approx. 27.4 oz. (1 lb. 11.4 oz.) of raw untrimmed meat that ***had*** been trimmed of separable fat before cooking	804	0.0	50.2	0.00	(231)	0.0
DOUBLE-BONE SIRLOIN STEAK (PINBONE STEAK)						
CHOICE GRADE:						
Bone-in						
1 pound of Raw untrimmed meat (includes separable fat) with bone [59% separable lean, 23% separable fat, 18% bone]	1240	0.0	77.5	0.00		
Cooked (broiled) [yield: approx. 12.5 oz., of which approx. 9.6 oz. are meat and approx. 2.9 oz. are bone]	1109	0.0	89.0	0.00		
Trimmed of separable fat before cooking; Cooked (broiled) [yield: approx. 9.8 oz., of which approx. 6.9 oz. are meat and approx. 2.9 oz. are bone]	423	0.0	43.2	0.00		

	UNIT		1 OZ., BY WT.		1 CUP, DICED, NOT PACKED	
	Cal.	Carb.	Cal.	Carb.	Cal.	Carb.
1 pound of Cooked (broiled) meat (weight includes bone):						
Yield from approx. 20.5 oz. (1 lb. 4.5 oz.) of raw untrimmed meat (weighed with the bone) that had ***not*** been trimmed of separable fat before cooking	1424	0.0	89.0	0.00		
Yield from approx. 26.2 oz. (1 lb. 10.2 oz.) of raw untrimmed meat (weighed with the bone) that ***had*** been trimmed of separable fat before cooking	692	0.0	43.2	0.00		
Boneless						
1 pound of Raw untrimmed meat (includes separable fat) [72% separable lean, 28% separable fat]	1512	0.0	94.5	0.00	(435)	0.0
Cooked (broiled) [yield: approx. 11.7 oz.] (6g/0g/10g/42%/na)	1352	0.0	115.8	0.00	(533)	0.0
Trimmed of separable fat before cooking; Cooked (broiled) [yield: approx. 8.4 oz.] (9g/0g/3g/59%/na)	515	0.0	61.3	0.00	(282)	0.0
1 pound of Cooked (broiled) meat:						
Yield from approx. 21.9 oz. (1 lb. 5.9 oz.) of raw untrimmed meat that had ***not*** been trimmed of separable fat before cooking	1852	0.0	115.8	0.00	(533)	0.0
Yield from approx. 30.4 oz. (1 lb. 14.4 oz.) of raw untrimmed meat that ***had*** been trimmed of separable fat before cooking	981	0.0	61.3	0.00	(282)	0.0
GOOD GRADE:						
Bone-in						
1 pound of Raw untrimmed meat (includes separable fat) with bone [60% separable lean, 21% separable fat, 19% bone]	1077	0.0	67.3	0.00		
Cooked (broiled) [yield: approx. 12.5 oz., of which approx. 9.5 oz. are meat and approx. 3.0 oz. are bone]	980	0.0	78.4	0.00		
Trimmed of separable fat before cooking; Cooked (broiled) [yield: approx. 10.1 oz., of which approx. 7.1 oz. are meat and approx. 3.0 oz. are bone]	383	0.0	37.7	0.00		
1 pound of Cooked (broiled) meat (weight includes bone):						
Yield from approx. 20.5 oz. (1 lb. 4.5 oz.) of raw untrimmed meat (weighed with the bone) that had ***not*** been trimmed of separable fat before cooking	1254	0.0	78.4	0.00		
Yield from approx. 25.3 oz. (1 lb. 9.3 oz.) of raw untrimmed meat (weighed with the bone) that ***had*** been trimmed of separable fat before cooking	604	0.0	37.7	0.00		
Boneless						
1 pound of Raw untrimmed meat (includes separable fat) [75% separable lean, 25% separable fat]	1330	0.0	83.1	0.00	(428)	0.0
Cooked (broiled) [yield: approx. 11.7 oz.] (7g/0g/8g/46%/na)	1210	0.0	103.6	0.00	(477)	0.0
Trimmed of separable fat before cooking; Cooked (broiled) [yield: approx. 8.8 oz.] (9g/0g/2g/61%/na)	472	0.0	53.9	0.00	(248)	0.0
1 pound of Cooked (broiled) meat:						
Yield from approx. 21.9 oz. (1 lb. 5.9 oz.) of raw untrimmed meat that had ***not*** been trimmed of separable fat before cooking	1657	0.0	103.6	0.00	(477)	0.0
Yield from approx. 29.2 oz. (1 lb. 13.2 oz.) of raw untrimmed meat that ***had*** been trimmed of separable fat before cooking	863	0.0	53.9	0.00	(248)	0.0
STANDARD GRADE:						
Bone-in						
1 pound of Raw untrimmed meat (includes separable fat) with bone [63% separable lean, 17% separable fat, 20% bone]	886	0.0	55.4	0.00		
Cooked (broiled) [yield: approx. 12.5 oz., of which approx. 9.3 oz. are meat and approx. 3.2 oz. are bone]	833	0.0	66.4	0.00		
Trimmed of separable fat before cooking; Cooked (broiled) [yield: approx. 10.6 oz., of which approx. 7.4 oz. are meat and approx. 3.2 oz. are bone]	367	0.0	34.6	0.00		
1 pound of Cooked (broiled) meat (weight includes bone):						
Yield from approx. 20.4 oz. (1 lb. 4.4 oz.) of raw untrimmed meat (weighed with the bone) that had ***not*** been trimmed of separable fat before cooking	1062	0.0	66.4	0.00		
Yield from approx. 24.2 oz. (1 lb. 8.2 oz.) of raw untrimmed meat (weighed with the bone) that ***had*** been trimmed of separable fat before cooking	554	0.0	34.6	0.00		

	UNIT		1 OZ., BY WT.		1 CUP, DICED, NOT PACKED	
	Cal.	Carb.	Cal.	Carb.	Cal.	Carb.
Boneless						
1 pound of Raw untrimmed meat (includes separable fat) [79% separable lean, 21% separable fat]	1108	0.0	69.2	0.00	(318)	0.0
Cooked (broiled) [yield: approx. 11.7 oz.] (7g/0g/6g/50%/na)	1041	0.0	89.1	0.00	(410)	0.0
Trimmed of separable fat before cooking; Cooked (broiled) [yield: approx. 9.2 oz.] (9g/0g/1g/62%/na)	458	0.0	49.7	0.00	(229)	0.0
1 pound of Cooked (broiled) meat:						
Yield from approx. 21.9 oz. (1 lb. 5.9 oz.) of raw untrimmed meat that had ***not*** been trimmed of separable fat before cooking	1426	0.0	89.1	0.00	(410)	0.0
Yield from approx. 27.7 oz. (1 lb. 11.7 oz.) of raw untrimmed meat that ***had*** been trimmed of separable fat before cooking	795	0.0	49.7	0.00	(229)	0.0
FLATBONE OR HIPBONE STEAK						
CHOICE GRADE:						
Bone-in						
1 pound of Raw untrimmed meat (includes separable fat) with bone [52% separable lean, 33% separable fat, 15% bone]	1590	0.0	99.4	0.00		
Cooked (broiled) [yield: approx. 12.3 oz., of which approx. 9.9 oz. are meat and approx. 2.4 oz. are bone]	1372	0.0	111.3	0.00		
Trimmed of separable fat before cooking; Cooked (broiled) [yield: approx. 8.5 oz., of which approx. 6.1 oz. are meat and approx. 2.4 oz. are bone]	412	0.0	48.8	0.00		
1 pound of Cooked (broiled) meat (weight includes bone):						
Yield from approx. 20.8 oz. (1 lb. 4.8 oz.) of raw untrimmed meat (weighed with the bone) that had ***not*** been trimmed of separable fat before cooking	1781	0.0	111.3	0.00		
Yield from approx. 30.3 oz. (1 lb. 14.3 oz.) of raw untrimmed meat (weighed with the bone) that ***had*** been trimmed of separable fat before cooking	780	0.0	48.8	0.00		
Boneless						
1 pound of Raw untrimmed meat (includes separable fat) [61% separable lean, 39% separable fat]	1870	0.0	116.9	0.00	(538)	0.0
Cooked (broiled) [yield: approx. 11.7 oz.] (5g/0g/13g/35%/na)	1614	0.0	138.2	0.00	(636)	0.0
Trimmed of separable fat before cooking; Cooked (broiled) [yield: approx. 7.1 oz.] (8g/0g/4g/56%/na)	485	0.0	68.1	0.00	(!313)	0.0
1 pound of Cooked (broiled) meat:						
Yield from approx. 21.9 oz. (1 lb. 5.9 oz.) of raw untrimmed meat that had ***not*** been trimmed of separable fat before cooking	211	0.0	138.2	0.00	(636)	0.0
Yield from approx. 35.9 oz. (2 lbs. 3.9 oz.) of raw untrimmed meat that ***had*** been trimmed of separable fat before cooking	1090	0.0	68.1	0.00	(313)	0.0
GOOD GRADE:						
Bone-in						
1 pound of Raw untrimmed meat (includes separable fat) with bone [54% separable lean, 30% separable fat, 16% bone]	1400	0.0	87.5	0.00		
Cooked (broiled) [yield: approx. 12.4 oz., of which approx. 9.8 oz. are meat and approx. 2.6 oz. are bone]	1228	0.0	99.2	0.00		
Trimmed of separable fat before cooking; Cooked (broiled) [yield: approx. 8.9 oz., of which approx. 6.3 oz. are meat and approx. 2.6 oz. are bone]	372	0.0	42.1	0.00		
1 pound of Cooked (broiled) meat (weight includes bone):						
Yield from approx. 20.7 oz. (1 lb. 4.7 oz.) of raw untrimmed meat (weighed with the bone) that had ***not*** been trimmed of separable fat before cooking	1588	0.0	99.2	0.00		
Yield from approx. 29.0 oz. (1 lb. 13.0 oz.) of raw untrimmed meat (weighed with the bone) that ***had*** been trimmed of separable fat before cooking	674	0.0	42.1	0.00		
Boneless						
1 pound of Raw untrimmed meat (includes separable fat) [64% separable lean, 36% separable fat]	1666	0.0	104.1	0.00	(479)	0.0
Cooked (broiled) [yield: approx. 11.7 oz.] (6g/0g/11g/39%/na)	1462	0.0	125.1	0.00	(575)	0.0
Trimmed of separable fat before cooking; Cooked (broiled) [yield: approx. 7.5 oz.] (9g/0g/2g/59%/na)	443	0.0	59.3	0.00	(273)	0.0

	UNIT		1 OZ., BY WT.		1 CUP, DICED, NOT PACKED	
	Cal.	Carb.	Cal.	Carb.	Cal.	Carb.
1 pound of Cooked (broiled) meat:						
Yield from approx. 21.9 oz. (1 lb. 5.9 oz.) of raw untrimmed meat that had ***not*** been trimmed of separable fat before cooking	2002	0.0	125.1	0.00	(575)	0.0
Yield from approx. 34.2 oz. (2 lb. 2.2 oz.) of raw untrimmed meat that ***had*** been trimmed of separable fat before cooking	949	0.0	59.3	0.00	(273)	0.0
STANDARD GRADE:						
Bone-in						
1 pound of Raw untrimmed meat (includes separable fat) with bone [57% separable lean, 25% separable fat, 18% bone]	1191	0.0	74.5	0.00		
Cooked (broiled) [yield: approx. 12.5 oz., of which approx. 9.6 oz. are meat and approx. 2.9 oz. are bone]	1071	0.0	86.0	0.00		
Trimmed of separable fat before cooking; Cooked (broiled) [yield: approx. 9.5 oz., of which approx. 6.6 oz. are meat and approx. 2.9 oz. are bone]	383	0.0	40.3	0.00		
1 pound of Cooked (broiled) meat (weight includes bone):						
Yield from approx. 20.5 oz. (1 lb. 4.5 oz.) of raw untrimmed meat (weighed with the bone) that had ***not*** been trimmed of separable fat before cooking	1375	0.0	86.0	0.00		
Yield from approx. 27.0 oz. (1 lb. 11.0 oz.) of raw untrimmed meat (weighed with the bone) that ***had*** been trimmed of separable fat before cooking	645	0.0	40.3	0.00		
Boneless						
1 pound of Raw untrimmed meat (includes separable fat) [69% separable lean, 31% separable fat]	1453	0.0	90.8	0.00	(418)	0.0
Cooked (broiled) [yield: approx. 11.7 oz.] (7g/0g/9g/43%/na)	1306	0.0	111.8	0.00	(514)	0.0
Trimmed of separable fat before cooking; Cooked (broiled) [yield: approx. 8.1 oz.] (9g/0g/2g/60%/na)	467	0.0	57.9	0.00	(266)	0.0
1 pound of Cooked (broiled) meat:						
Yield from approx. 21.9 oz. (1 lb. 5.9 oz.) of raw untrimmed meat that had ***not*** been trimmed of separable fat before cooking	1789	0.0	111.8	0.00	(514)	0.0
Yield from approx. 31.8 oz. (1 lb. 15.8 oz.) of raw untrimmed meat that ***had*** been trimmed of separable fat before cooking	926	0.0	57.9	0.00	(266)	0.0

Short Plate

	UNIT		1 OZ., BY WT.		1 CUP, DICED, NOT PACKED	
	Cal.	Carb.	Cal.	Carb.	Cal.	Carb.
CHOICE GRADE:						
Bone-in						
1 pound of Raw untrimmed meat (includes separable fat) with bone [52% separable lean, 37% separable fat, 11% bone]	1616	0.0	101.0	0.00		
Cooked (braised) [yield: approx. 11.3 oz., of which approx. 9.5 oz. are meat and approx. 1.8 oz. are bone]	1283	0.0	113.6	0.00		
Trimmed of separable fat before cooking; Cooked (braised) [yield: approx. 7.4 oz., of which approx. 5.6 oz. are meat and approx. 1.8 oz. are bone]	355	0.0	48.0	0.00		
1 pound of Cooked (braised) meat (weight includes bone):						
Yield from approx. 22.7 oz. (1 lb. 6.7 oz.) of raw untrimmed meat (weighed with the bone) that had ***not*** been trimmed of separable fat before cooking	1817	0.0	113.6	0.00		
Yield from approx. 34.6 oz. (2 lbs. 2.6 oz.) of raw untrimmed meat (weighed with the bone) that ***had*** been trimmed of separable fat before cooking	768	0.0	48.0	0.00		
Boneless (Skirt Steak)						
1 pound of Raw untrimmed meat (includes separable fat) [59% separable lean, 41% separable fat]	1816	0.0	113.5	0.00	(522)	0.0
Cooked (braised) [yield: approx. 10.7 oz.] (6g/0g/12g/36%/na)	1442	0.0	134.5	0.00	(619)	0.0
Trimmed of separable fat before cooking; Cooked (braised) [yield: approx. 6.3 oz.] (8g/0g/3g/59%/na)	398	0.0	63.0	0.00	(290)	0.0
1 pound of Cooked (braised) meat:						
Yield from approx. 23.9 oz. (1 lb. 7.9 oz.) of raw untrimmed meat that had ***not*** been trimmed of separable fat before cooking	2152	0.0	134.5	0.00	(619)	0.0
Yield from approx. 40.5 oz. (2 lbs. 8.5 oz.) of raw untrimmed meat that ***had*** been trimmed of separable fat before cooking	1008	0.0	63.0	0.00	(290)	0.0

	UNIT		1 OZ., BY WT.		1 CUP, DICED, NOT PACKED	
	Cal.	Carb.	Cal.	Carb.	Cal.	Carb.
GOOD GRADE:						
Bone-in						
1 pound of Raw untrimmed meat (includes separable fat) with bone [54% separable lean, 33% separable fat, 13% bone]	1406	0.0	87.9	0.00		
Cooked (braised) [yield: approx. 11.4 oz., of which approx. 9.3 oz. are meat and approx. 2.1 oz. are bone]	1143	0.0	100.2	0.00		
Trimmed of separable fat before cooking; Cooked (braised) [yield: approx. 7.9 oz., of which approx. 5.8 oz. are meat and approx. 2.1 oz. are bone]	327	0.0	41.5	0.00		
1 pound of Cooked (braised) meat (weight includes bone):						
Yield from approx. 22.4 oz. (1 lb. 6.4 oz.) of raw untrimmed meat (weighed with the bone) that had ***not*** been trimmed of separable fat before cooking	1604	0.0	100.2	0.00		
Yield from approx. 32.6 oz. (2 lb. 0.6 oz.) of raw untrimmed meat (weighed with the bone) that ***had*** been trimmed of separable fat before cooking	664	0.0	41.5	0.00		
Boneless (Skirt Steak)						
1 pound of Raw untrimmed meat (includes separable fat) [64% separable lean, 36% separable fat]	1616	0.0	101.0	0.00	(465)	0.0
Cooked (braised) [yield: approx. 10.7 oz.] (6g/0g/11g/40%/na)	1314	0.0	122.6	0.00	(564)	0.0
Trimmed of separable fat before cooking; Cooked (braised) [yield: approx. 6.6 oz.] (9g/0g/2g/61%/na)	375	0.0	56.5	0.00	(260)	0.0
1 pound of Cooked (braised) meat:						
Yield from approx. 23.9 oz. (1 lb. 7.9 oz.) of raw untrimmed meat that had ***not*** been trimmed of separable fat before cooking	1961	0.0	122.6	0.00	(564)	0.0
Yield from approx. 38.5 oz. (2 lb. 6.5 oz.) of raw untrimmed meat that ***had*** been trimmed of separable fat before cooking	903	0.0	56.5	0.00	(260)	0.0
STANDARD GRADE:						
Bone-in						
1 pound of Raw untrimmed meat (includes separable fat) with bone [57% separable lean, 28% separable fat, 15% bone]	1200	0.0	75.0	0.00		
Cooked (braised) [yield: approx. 11.5 oz., of which approx. 9.1 oz. are meat and approx. 2.4 oz. are bone]	993	0.0	86.2	0.00		
Trimmed of separable fat before cooking; Cooked (braised) [yield: approx. 8.5 oz., of which approx. 6.1 oz. are meat and approx. 2.4 oz. are bone]	324	0.0	38.1	0.00		
1 pound of Cooked (braised) meat (weight includes bone):						
Yield from approx. 22.2 oz. (1 lb. 6.2 oz.) of raw untrimmed meat (weighed with the bone) that had ***not*** been trimmed of separable fat before cooking	1380	0.0	86.2	0.00		
Yield from approx. 30.1 oz. (1 lb. 14.1 oz.) of raw untrimmed meat (weighed with the bone) that ***had*** been trimmed of separable fat before cooking	609	0.0	38.1	0.00		
Boneless (Skirt Steak)						
1 pound of Raw untrimmed meat (includes separable fat) [67% separable lean, 33% separable fat]	1412	0.0	88.2	0.00	(406)	0.0
Cooked (braised) [yield: approx. 10.7 oz.] (7g/0g/9g/44%/na)	1168	0.0	109.0	0.00	(501)	0.0
Trimmed of separable fat before cooking; Cooked (braised) [yield: approx. 7.1 oz.] (9g/0g/2g/62%/na)	381	0.0	53.1	0.00	(244)	0.0
1 pound of Cooked (braised) meat:						
Yield from approx. 23.9 oz. (1 lb. 7.9 oz.) of raw untrimmed meat that had ***not*** been trimmed of separable fat before cooking	1743	0.0	109.0	0.00	(501)	0.0
Yield from approx. 35.6 oz. (2 lbs. 3.6 oz.) of raw untrimmed meat that ***had*** been trimmed of separable fat before cooking	849	0.0	53.1	0.00	(244)	0.0

Rib Roast

	UNIT		1 OZ., BY WT.		1 CUP, DICED, NOT PACKED	
	Cal.	Carb.	Cal.	Carb.	Cal.	Carb.
ENTIRE RIB (6TH–12TH RIBS)						
CHOICE GRADE:						
Bone-in						
1 pound of Raw untrimmed meat (includes separable fat) with bone [59% separable lean, 33% separable fat, 8% bone]	1675	0.0	104.7	0.00		
Cooked (roasted) [yield: approx. 12.0 oz., of which approx. 10.7 oz. are meat and approx. 1.3 oz. are bone]	1342	0.0	111.6	0.00		

	UNIT		1 OZ., BY WT.		1 CUP, DICED, NOT PACKED	
	Cal.	Carb.	Cal.	Carb.	Cal.	Carb.
Trimmed of separable fat before cooking; Cooked (roasted) [yield: approx. 8.2 oz., of which approx. 6.9 oz. are meat and approx. 1.3 oz. are bone]	470	0.0	57.7	0.00		
1 pound of Cooked (roasted) meat (weight includes bone):						
Yield from approx. 21.3 oz. (1 lb. 5.3 oz.) of raw untrimmed meat (weighed with the bone) that had ***not*** been trimmed of separable fat before cooking	1785	0.0	111.6	0.00		
Yield from approx. 31.4 oz. (1 lb. 15.4 oz.) of raw untrimmed meat (weighed with the bone) that ***had*** been trimmed of separable fat before cooking	922	0.0	57.7	0.00		
Boneless (Rib Eye or Delmonico Cut)						
1 pound of Raw untrimmed meat (includes separable fat) [64% separable lean, 36% separable fat]	1821	0.0	113.8	0.00	(523)	0.0
Cooked (roasted) [yield: approx. 11.7 oz.] (6g/0g/11g/40%/na)	1458	0.0	124.9	0.00	(575)	0.0
Trimmed of separable fat before cooking; Cooked (roasted) [yield: approx. 7.5 oz.] (8g/0g/4g/57%/na)	511	0.0	68.4	0.00	(315)	0.0
1 pound of Cooked (roasted) meat:						
Yield from approx. 21.9 oz. (1 lb. 5.9 oz.) of raw untrimmed meat that had ***not*** been trimmed of separable fat before cooking	1998	0.0	124.9	0.00	(575)	0.0
Yield from approx. 34.2 oz. (2 lbs. 2.2 oz.) of raw untrimmed meat that ***had*** been trimmed of separable fat before cooking	1094	0.0	68.4	0.00	(315)	0.0
6TH (BLADE) RIB						
CHOICE GRADE:						
Bone-in						
1 pound of Raw untrimmed meat (includes separable fat) with bone [66% separable lean, 27% separable fat, 7% bone]	1641	0.0	102.6	0.00		
Cooked (braised) [yield: approx. 11.1 oz., of which approx. 10.0 oz. are meat and approx. 1.1 oz. are bone]	1279	0.0	115.2	0.00		
Trimmed of separable fat before cooking; Cooked (braised) [yield: approx. 8.2 oz., of which approx. 7.1 oz. are meat and approx. 1.1 oz. are bone]	569	0.0	69.4	0.00		
1 pound of Cooked (braised) meat (weight includes bone):						
Yield from approx. 23.1 oz. (1 lb. 7.1 oz.) of raw untrimmed meat (weighed with the bone) that had ***not*** been trimmed of separable fat before cooking	1844	0.0	115.2	0.00		
Yield from approx. 31.2 oz. (1 lb. 15.2 oz.) of raw untrimmed meat (weighed with the bone) that ***had*** been trimmed of separable fat before cooking	1110	0.0	69.4	0.00		
Boneless						
1 pound of Raw untrimmed meat (includes separable fat) [71% separable lean, 29% separable fat]	1765	0.0	110.3	0.00	(474)	0.0
Cooked (braised) [yield: approx. 10.7 oz.] (6g/0g/11g/39%/na)	1326	0.0	123.9	0.00	(570)	0.0
Trimmed of separable fat before cooking; Cooked (braised) [yield: approx. 7.6 oz.] (8g/0g/4g/55%/na)	567	0.0	74.6	0.00	(343)	0.0
1 pound of Cooked (braised) meat:						
Yield from approx. 23.9 oz. (1 lb. 7.9 oz.) of raw untrimmed meat that had ***not*** been trimmed of separable fat before cooking	1982	0.0	123.9	0.00	(570)	0.0
Yield from approx. 33.6 oz. (2 lbs. 1.6 oz.) of raw untrimmed meat that ***had*** been trimmed of separable fat before cooking	1193	0.0	74.6	0.00	(343)	0.0
GOOD GRADE:						
Bone-in						
1 pound of Raw untrimmed meat (includes separable fat) with bone [71% separable lean, 21% separable fat, 8% bone]	1253	0.0	78.3	0.00		
Cooked (braised) [yield: approx. 11.2 oz., of which approx. 9.9 oz. are meat and approx. 1.3 oz. are bone]	1044	0.0	93.7	0.00		
Trimmed of separable fat before cooking; Cooked (braised) [yield: approx. 8.9 oz., of which approx. 7.6 oz. are meat and approx. 1.3 oz. are bone]	485	0.0	54.6	0.00		
1 pound of Cooked (braised) meat (weight includes bone):						
Yield from approx. 23.0 oz. (1 lb. 7.0 oz.) of raw untrimmed meat (weighed with the bone) that had ***not*** been trimmed of separable fat before cooking	1499	0.0	93.7	0.00		
Yield from approx. 28.8 oz. (1 lb. 12.8 oz.) of raw untrimmed meat (weighed with the bone) that ***had*** been trimmed of separable fat before cooking	874	0.0	54.6	0.00		
Boneless						
1 pound of Raw untrimmed meat (includes separable fat) [77% separable lean, 23% separable fat]	1362	0.0	85.1	0.00	(391)	0.0
Cooked (braised) [yield: approx. 10.7 oz.] (7g/0g/8g/45%/na)	1135	0.0	105.8	0.00	(487)	0.0
Trimmed of separable fat before cooking; Cooked (braised) [yield: approx. 8.3 oz.] (8g/0g/3g/59%/na)	527	0.0	63.8	0.00	(293)	0.0
1 pound of Cooked (braised) meat:						
Yield from approx. 23.9 oz. (1 lb. 7.9 oz.) of raw untrimmed meat that had ***not*** been trimmed of separable fat before cooking	1693	0.0	105.8	0.00	(487)	0.0
Yield from approx. 31.0 oz. (1 lb. 15.0 oz.) of raw untrimmed meat that ***had*** been trimmed of separable fat before cooking	1022	0.0	63.8	0.00	(293)	0.0
STANDARD GRADE:						
Bone-in						
1 pound of Raw untrimmed meat (includes separable fat) with bone [75% separable lean, 16% separable fat, 9% bone]	1033	0.0	64.6	0.00		
Cooked (braised) [yield: approx. 11.2 oz., of which approx. 9.8 oz. are meat and approx. 1.4 oz. are bone]	883	0.0	78.9	0.00		
Trimmed of separable fat before cooking; Cooked (braised) [yield: approx. 9.5 oz., of which approx. 8.1 oz. are meat and approx. 1.4 oz. are bone]	476	0.0	49.9	0.00		
1 pound of Cooked (braised) meat (weight includes bone):						
Yield from approx. 22.9 oz. (1 lb. 6.9 oz.) of raw untrimmed meat (weighed with the bone) that had ***not*** been trimmed of separable fat before cooking	1262	0.0	78.9	0.00		
Yield from approx. 26.8 oz. (1 lb. 10.8 oz.) of raw untrimmed meat (weighed with the bone) that ***had*** been trimmed of separable fat before cooking	798	0.0	49.9	0.00		
Boneless						
1 pound of Raw untrimmed meat (includes separable fat) [83% separable lean, 17% separable fat]	1135	0.0	70.9	0.00	(326)	0.0
Cooked (braised) [yield: approx. 10.7 oz.] (7g/0g/7g/50%/na)	970	0.0	90.5	0.00	(416)	0.0
Trimmed of separable fat before cooking; Cooked (braised) [yield: approx. 8.9 oz.] (9g/0g/3g/60%/na)	523	0.0	58.7	0.00	(270)	0.0
1 pound of Cooked (braised) meat:						
Yield from approx. 23.9 oz. (1 lb. 7.9 oz.) of raw untrimmed meat that had ***not*** been trimmed of separable fat before cooking	1448	0.0	90.5	0.00	(416)	0.0
Yield from approx. 28.8 oz. (1 lb. 12.8 oz.) of raw untrimmed meat that ***had*** been trimmed of separable fat before cooking	940	0.0	58.7	0.00	(270)	0.0
7TH–8TH RIBS						
CHOICE GRADE:						
Bone-in						
1 pound of Raw untrimmed meat (includes separable fat) with bone [62% separable lean, 30% separable fat, 8% bone]	1562	0.0	97.6	0.00		
Cooked (roasted) [yield: approx. 12.0 oz., of which approx. 10.7 oz. are meat and approx. 1.3 oz. are bone]	1265	0.0	105.2	0.00		
Trimmed of separable fat before cooking; Cooked (roasted) [yield: approx. 8.5 oz., of which approx. 7.2 oz. are meat and approx. 1.3 oz. are bone]	484	0.0	57.1	0.00		
1 pound of Cooked (roasted) meat (weight includes bone):						
Yield from approx. 21.3 oz. (1 lb. 5.3 oz.) of raw untrimmed meat (weighed with the bone) that had ***not*** been trimmed of separable fat before cooking	1684	0.0	105.2	0.00		
Yield from approx. 30.2 oz. (1 lb. 14.2 oz.) of raw untrimmed meat (weighed with the bone) that ***had*** been trimmed of separable fat before cooking	914	0.0	57.1	0.00		
Boneless (Rib Eye or Delmonico Cut)						
1 pound of Raw untrimmed meat (includes separable fat) [67% separable lean, 33% separable fat]	1698	0.0	106.1	0.00	(488)	0.0
Cooked (roasted) [yield: approx. 11.7 oz.] (6g/0g/10g/42%/na)	1375	0.0	117.8	0.00	(542)	0.0

	UNIT		1 OZ., BY WT.		1 CUP, DICED, NOT PACKED	
	Cal.	Carb.	Cal.	Carb.	Cal.	Carb.
Trimmed of separable fat before cooking; Cooked (roasted) [yield: approx. 7.8 oz.] (8g/0g/4g/58%/na)	526	0.0	67.2	0.00	(309)	0.0
1 pound of Cooked (roasted) meat:						
Yield from approx. 21.9 oz. (1 lb. 5.9 oz.) of raw untrimmed meat that had ***not*** been trimmed of separable fat before cooking	1884	0.0	117.8	0.00	(542)	0.0
Yield from approx. 32.7 oz. (2 lbs. 0.7 oz.) of raw untrimmed meat that ***had*** been trimmed of separable fat before cooking	1076	0.0	67.2	0.00	(309)	0.0
GOOD GRADE:						
Bone-in						
1 pound of Raw untrimmed meat (includes separable fat) with bone [65% separable lean, 25% separable fat, 10% bone]	1324	0.0	82.7	0.00		
Cooked (roasted) [yield: approx. 12.1 oz., of which approx. 10.5 oz. are meat and approx. 1.6 oz. are bone]	1095	0.0	90.4	0.00		
Trimmed of separable fat before cooking; Cooked (roasted) [yield: approx. 9.2 oz., of which approx. 7.6 oz. are meat and approx. 1.6 oz. are bone]	455	0.0	49.7	0.00		
1 pound of Cooked (roasted) meat (weight includes bone):						
Yield from approx. 21.1 oz. (1 lb. 5.1 oz.) of raw untrimmed meat (weighed with the bone) that had ***not*** been trimmed of separable fat before cooking	1446	0.0	90.4	0.00		
Yield from approx. 27.9 oz. (1 lb. 11.9 oz.) of raw untrimmed meat (weighed with the bone) that ***had*** been trimmed of separable fat before cooking	795	0.0	49.7	0.00		
Boneless (Rib Eye or Delmonico Cut)						
1 pound of Raw untrimmed meat (includes separable fat) [72% separable lean, 28% separable fat]	1471	0.0	91.9	0.00	(423)	0.0
Cooked (roasted) [yield: approx. 11.7 oz.] (7g/0g/8g/46%/na)	1216	0.0	104.1	0.00	(479)	0.0
Trimmed of separable fat before cooking; Cooked (roasted) [yield: approx. 8.4 oz.] (8g/0g/3g/60%/na)	506	0.0	60.2	0.00	(277)	0.0
1 pound of Cooked (roasted) meat:						
Yield from approx. 21.9 oz. (1 lb. 5.9 oz.) of raw untrimmed meat that had ***not*** been trimmed of separable fat before cooking	1666	0.0	104.1	0.00	(479)	0.0
Yield from approx. 30.4 oz. (1 lb. 14.4 oz.) of raw untrimmed meat that ***had*** been trimmed of separable fat before cooking	962	0.0	60.2	0.00	(277)	0.0
STANDARD GRADE:						
Bone-in						
1 pound of Raw untrimmed meat (includes separable fat) with bone [69% separable lean, 20% separable fat, 11% bone]	1099	0.0	68.7	0.00		
Cooked (roasted) [yield: approx. 12.2 oz., of which approx. 10.4 oz. are meat and approx. 1.8 oz. are bone]	938	0.0	77.2	0.00		
Trimmed of separable fat before cooking; Cooked (roasted) [yield: approx. 9.9 oz., of which approx. 8.1 oz. are meat and approx. 1.8 oz. are bone]	472	0.0	47.8	0.00		
1 pound of Cooked (roasted) meat (weight includes bone):						
Yield from approx. 21.1 oz. (1 lb. 5.1 oz.) of raw untrimmed meat (weighed with the bone) that had ***not*** been trimmed of separable fat before cooking	1235	0.0	77.2	0.00		
Yield from approx. 25.9 oz. (1 lb. 9.9 oz.) of raw untrimmed meat (weighed with the bone) that ***had*** been trimmed of separable fat before cooking	765	0.0	47.8	0.00		
Boneless (Rib Eye or Delmonico Cut)						
1 pound of Raw untrimmed meat (includes separable fat) [78% separable lean, 22% separable fat]	1235	0.0	77.2	0.00	(355)	0.0
Cooked (roasted) [yield: approx. 11.7 oz.] (7g/0g/7g/51%/na)	1054	0.0	90.2	0.00	(415)	0.0
Trimmed of separable fat before cooking; Cooked (roasted) [yield: approx. 9.1 oz.] (8g/0g/3g/61%/na)	530	0.0	58.2	0.00	(268)	0.0
1 pound of Cooked (roasted) meat:						
Yield from approx. 21.9 oz. (1 lb. 5.9 oz.) of raw untrimmed meat that had ***not*** been trimmed of separable fat before cooking	1444	0.0	90.2	0.00	(415)	0.0

	UNIT		1 OZ., BY WT.		1 CUP, DICED, NOT PACKED	
	Cal.	Carb.	Cal.	Carb.	Cal.	Carb.
Yield from approx. 28.1 oz. (1 lb. 12.1 oz.) of raw untrimmed meat that ***had*** been trimmed of separable fat before cooking	931	0.0	58.2	0.00	(268)	0.0
9TH–10TH RIBS						
CHOICE GRADE:						
Bone-in						
1 pound of Raw untrimmed meat (includes separable fat) with bone [55% separable lean, 37% separable fat, 8% bone]	1763	0.0	110.2	0.00		
Cooked (roasted) [yield: approx. 12.0 oz., of which approx. 10.7 oz. are meat and approx. 1.3 oz. are bone]	1406	0.0	116.9	0.00		
Trimmed of separable fat before cooking; Cooked (roasted) [yield: approx. 7.7 oz., of which approx. 6.4 oz. are meat and approx. 1.3 oz. are bone]	439	0.0	56.8	0.00		
1 pound of Cooked (roasted) meat (weight includes bone):						
Yield from approx. 21.3 oz. (1 lb. 5.3 oz.) of raw untrimmed meat (weighed with the bone) that had ***not*** been trimmed of separable fat before cooking	1870	0.0	116.9	0.00		
Yield from approx. 33.1 oz. (2 lbs. 1.1 oz.) of raw untrimmed meat (weighed with the bone) that ***had*** been trimmed of separable fat before cooking	909	0.0	56.8	0.00		
Boneless (Rib Eye or Delmonico Cut)						
1 pound of Raw untrimmed meat (includes separable fat) [60% separable lean, 40% separable fat]	1916	0.0	119.7	0.00	(551)	0.0
Cooked (roasted) [yield: approx. 11.7 oz.] (5g/0g/12g/38%/na)	1528	0.0	130.8	0.00	(602)	0.0
Trimmed of separable fat before cooking; Cooked (roasted) [yield: approx. 7.0 oz.] (8g/0g/4g/57%/na)	477	0.0	68.1	0.00	(313)	0.0
1 pound of Cooked (roasted) meat:						
Yield from approx. 21.9 oz. (1 lb. 5.9 oz.) of raw untrimmed meat that had ***not*** been trimmed of separable fat before cooking	2093	0.0	130.8	0.00	(602)	0.0
Yield from approx. 36.5 oz. (2 lbs. 4.5 oz.) of raw untrimmed meat that ***had*** been trimmed of separable fat before cooking	1090	0.0	68.1	0.00	(313)	0.0
GOOD GRADE:						
Bone-in						
1 pound of Raw untrimmed meat (includes separable fat) with bone [61% separable lean, 30% separable fat, 9% bone]	1302	0.0	81.4	0.00		
Cooked (roasted) [yield: approx. 10.9 oz., of which approx. 9.5 oz. are meat and approx. 1.4 oz. are bone]	1194	0.0	99.0	0.00		
Trimmed of separable fat before cooking; Cooked (roasted) [yield: approx. 7.7 oz., of which approx. 6.3 oz. are meat and approx. 1.4 oz. are bone]	432	0.0	50.5	0.00		
1 pound Cooked (roasted) meat (weight includes bone):						
Yield from approx. 23.5 oz. (1 lb. 7.5 oz.) of raw untrimmed meat (weighed with the bone) that had ***not*** been trimmed of separable fat before cooking	1583	0.0	99.0	0.00		
Yield from approx. 32.9 oz. (2 lbs. 0.9 oz.) of raw untrimmed meat (weighed with the bone) that ***had*** been trimmed of separable fat before cooking	808	0.0	50.5	0.00		
Boneless (Rib Eye or Delmonico Cut)						
1 pound of Raw untrimmed meat (includes separable fat) [67% separable lean, 33% separable fat]	1607	0.0	100.4	0.00	(462)	0.0
Cooked (roasted) [yield: approx. 11.7 oz.] (6g/0g/10g/44%/na)	1312	0.0	112.4	0.00	(517)	0.0
Trimmed of separable fat before cooking; Cooked (roasted) [yield: approx. 7.8 oz.] (8g/0g/3g/60%/na)	475	0.0	60.7	0.00	(279)	0.0
1 pound of Cooked (roasted) meat:						
Yield from approx. 21.9 oz. (1 lb. 5.9 oz.) of raw untrimmed meat that had ***not*** been trimmed of separable fat before cooking	1798	0.0	112.4	0.00	(517)	0.0
Yield from approx. 32.7 oz. (2 lbs. 0.7 oz.) of raw untrimmed meat that ***had*** been trimmed of separable fat before cooking	972	0.0	60.7	0.00	(279)	0.0
STANDARD GRADE:						
Bone-in						
1 pound of Raw untrimmed meat (includes separable fat) with bone [67% separable lean, 22% separable fat, 11% bone]	1180	0.0	73.7	0.00		

	UNIT		1 OZ., BY WT.		1 CUP, DICED, NOT PACKED	
	Cal.	Carb.	Cal.	Carb.	Cal.	Carb.
Cooked (roasted) [yield: approx. 12.2 oz., of which approx. 10.4 oz. are meat and approx. 1.8 oz. are bone]	994	0.0	81.8	0.00		
Trimmed of separable fat before cooking; Cooked (roasted) [yield: approx. 9.6 oz., of which approx. 7.8 oz. are meat and approx. 1.8 oz. are bone]	467	0.0	48.8	0.00		
1 pound of Cooked (roasted) meat (weight includes bone):						
Yield from approx. 21.1 oz. (1 lb. 5.1 oz.) of raw untrimmed meat (weighed with the bone) that had ***not*** been trimmed of separable fat before cooking	1308	0.0	81.8	0.00		
Yield from approx. 26.8 oz. (1 lb. 10.8 oz.) of raw untrimmed meat (weighed with the bone) that ***had*** been trimmed of separable fat before cooking	782	0.0	48.8	0.00		
Boneless (Rib Eye or Delmonico Cut)						
1 pound of Raw untrimmed meat (includes separable fat) [75% separable lean, 25% separable fat]	1326	0.0	82.9	0.00	(381)	0.0
Cooked (roasted) [yield: approx. 11.7 oz.] (7g/0g/7g/49%/na)	1117	0.0	95.6	0.00	(440)	0.0
Trimmed of separable fat before cooking; Cooked (roasted) [yield: approx. 8.8 oz.] (8g/0g/3g/60%/na)	524	0.0	59.9	0.00	(276)	0.0
1 pound of Cooked (roasted) meat:						
Yield from approx. 21.9 oz. (1 lb. 5.9 oz.) of raw untrimmed meat that had ***not*** been trimmed of separable fat before cooking	1530	0.0	95.6	0.00	(440)	0.0
Yield from approx. 29.2 oz. (1 lb. 13.2 oz.) of raw untrimmed meat that ***had*** been trimmed of separable fat before cooking	958	0.0	59.9	0.00	(276)	0.0
11TH–12TH RIBS						
CHOICE GRADE:						
Bone-in						
1 pound of Raw untrimmed meat (includes separable fat) with bone [51% separable lean, 41% separable fat, 8% bone]	1854	0.0	115.9	0.00		
Cooked (roasted) [yield: approx. 12.0 oz., of which approx. 10.7 oz. are meat and approx. 1.3 oz. are bone]	1467	0.0	122.0	0.00		
Trimmed of separable fat before cooking; Cooked (roasted) [yield: approx. 7.2 oz., of which approx. 5.9 oz. are meat and approx. 1.3 oz. are bone]	402	0.0	56.0	0.00		
1 pound of Cooked (roasted) meat (weight includes bone):						
Yield from approx. 21.3 oz. (1 lb. 5.3 oz.) of raw untrimmed meat (weighed with the bone) that had ***not*** been trimmed of separable fat before cooking	1951	0.0	122.0	0.00		
Yield from approx. 35.6 oz. (2 lbs. 3.6 oz.) of raw untrimmed meat (weighed with the bone) that ***had*** been trimmed of separable fat before cooking	896	0.0	56.0	0.00		
Boneless (Rib Eye or Delmonico Cut)						
1 pound of Raw untrimmed meat (includes separable fat) [55% separable lean, 45% separable fat]	2016	0.0	126.0	0.00	(580)	0.0
Cooked (roasted) [yield: approx. 11.7 oz.] (5g/0g/13g/36%/na)	1594	0.0	136.5	0.00	(628)	0.0
Trimmed of separable fat before cooking; Cooked (roasted) [yield: approx. 6.4 oz.] (8g/0g/4g/57%/na)	437	0.0	68.1	0.00	(313)	0.0
1 pound of Cooked (roasted) meat:						
Yield from approx. 21.9 oz. (1 lb. 5.9 oz.) of raw untrimmed meat that had ***not*** been trimmed of separable fat before cooking	2184	0.0	136.5	0.00	(628)	0.0
Yield from approx. 39.9 oz. (2 lbs. 7.9 oz.) of raw untrimmed meat that ***had*** been trimmed of separable fat before cooking	1090	0.0	68.1	0.00	(313)	0.0
GOOD GRADE:						
Bone-in						
1 pound of Raw untrimmed meat (includes separable fat) with bone [56% separable lean, 34% separable fat, 10% bone]	1536	0.0	96.0	0.00		
Cooked (roasted) [yield: approx. 12.1 oz., of which approx. 10.5 oz. are meat and approx. 1.6 oz. are bone]	1244	0.0	102.7	0.00		
Trimmed of separable fat before cooking; Cooked (roasted) [yield: approx. 8.2 oz., of which approx. 6.6 oz. are meat and approx. 1.6 oz. are bone]	404	0.0	49.1	0.00		

	UNIT		1 OZ., BY WT.		1 CUP, DICED, NOT PACKED	
	Cal.	Carb.	Cal.	Carb.	Cal.	Carb.
1 pound of Cooked (roasted) meat (weight includes bone):						
Yield from approx. 21.1 oz. (1 lb. 5.1 oz.) of raw untrimmed meat (weighed with the bone) that had ***not*** been trimmed of separable fat before cooking	1643	0.0	102.7	0.00		
Yield from approx. 31.1 oz. (1 lb. 15.1 oz.) of raw untrimmed meat (weighed with the bone) that ***had*** been trimmed of separable fat before cooking	786	0.0	49.1	0.00		
Boneless (Rib Eye or Delmonico Cut)						
1 pound of Raw untrimmed meat (includes separable fat) [63% separable lean, 37% separable fat]	1707	0.0	106.7	0.00	(491)	0.0
Cooked (roasted) [yield: approx. 11.7 oz.] (6g/0g/10g/42%/na)	1382	0.0	118.3	0.00	(544)	0.0
Trimmed of separable fat before cooking; Cooked (roasted) [yield: approx. 7.4 oz.] (8g/0g/3g/60%/na)	449	0.0	61.0	0.00	(281)	0.0
1 pound of Cooked (roasted) meat:						
Yield from approx. 21.9 oz. (1 lb. 5.9 oz.) of raw untrimmed meat that had ***not*** been trimmed of separable fat before cooking	1893	0.0	118.3	0.00	(544)	0.0
Yield from approx. 34.8 oz. (2 lbs. 2.8 oz.) of raw untrimmed meat that ***had*** been trimmed of separable fat before cooking	976	0.0	61.0	0.00	(281)	0.0
STANDARD GRADE:						
Bone-in						
1 pound of Raw untrimmed meat (includes separable fat) with bone [63% separable lean, 25% separable fat, 12% bone]	1227	0.0	76.7	0.00		
Cooked (roasted) [yield: approx. 12.2 oz., of which approx. 10.3 oz. are meat and approx. 1.9 oz. are bone]	1027	0.0	84.2	0.00		
Trimmed of separable fat before cooking; Cooked (roasted) [yield: approx. 9.2 oz., of which approx. 7.3 oz. are meat and approx. 1.9 oz. are bone]	425	0.0	46.1	0.00		
1 pound of Cooked (roasted) meat (weight includes bone):						
Yield from approx. 21.0 oz. (1 lb. 5.0 oz.) of raw untrimmed meat (weighed with the bone) that had ***not*** been trimmed of separable fat before cooking	1347	0.0	84.2	0.00		
Yield from approx. 27.8 oz. (1 lb. 11.8 oz.) of raw untrimmed meat (weighed with the bone) that ***had*** been trimmed of separable fat before cooking	737	0.0	46.1	0.00		
Boneless (Rib Eye or Delmonico Cut)						
1 pound of Raw untrimmed meat (includes separable fat) [71% separable lean, 29% separable fat]	1394	0.0	87.1	0.00	(401)	0.0
Cooked (roasted) [yield: approx. 11.7 oz.] (7g/0g/8g/48%/na)	1167	0.0	99.9	0.00	(460)	0.0
Trimmed of separable fat before cooking; Cooked (roasted) [yield: approx. 8.3 oz.] (8g/0g/3g/61%/na)	482	0.0	58.2	0.00	(268)	0.0
1 pound of Cooked (roasted) meat:						
Yield from approx. 21.9 oz. (1 lb. 5.9 oz.) of raw untrimmed meat that had ***not*** been trimmed of separable fat before cooking	1598	0.0	99.9	0.00	(460)	0.0
Yield from approx. 30.9 oz. (1 lb. 14.9 oz.) of raw untrimmed meat that ***had*** been trimmed of separable fat before cooking	931	0.0	58.2	0.00	(268)	0.0
Round						
ENTIRE ROUND						
CHOICE GRADE:						
Bone-in						
1 pound of Raw untrimmed meat (includes separable fat) with bone [86% separable lean, 11% separable fat, 3% bone]	868	0.0	54.2	0.00		
Cooked (broiled) [yield: approx. 11.8 oz., of which approx. 11.3 oz. are meat and approx. 0.5 oz. are bone]	839	0.0	71.0	0.00		
Trimmed of separable fat before cooking; Cooked (broiled) [yield: approx. 10.6 oz., of which approx. 10.1 oz. are meat and approx. 0.5 oz. are bone]	541	0.0	51.2	0.00		
1 pound of Cooked (broiled) meat (weight includes bone):						
Yield from approx. 21.7 oz. (1 lb. 5.7 oz.) of raw untrimmed meat (weighed with the bone) that had ***not*** been trimmed of separable fat before cooking	1137	0.0	71.0	0.00		

	UNIT Cal.	UNIT Carb.	1 OZ., BY WT. Cal.	1 OZ., BY WT. Carb.	1 CUP, DICED, NOT PACKED Cal.	1 CUP, DICED, NOT PACKED Carb.
Yield from approx. 24.0 oz. (1 lb. 8.0 oz.) of raw untrimmed meat (weighed with the bone) that ***had*** been trimmed of separable fat before cooking	819	0.0	51.2	0.00		
Boneless						
1 pound of Raw untrimmed meat (includes separable fat) [89% separable lean, 11% separable fat]	894	0.0	55.9	0.00	(257)	0.0
Cooked (broiled) [yield: approx. 11.7 oz.] (8g/0g/4g/55%/na)	865	0.0	74.1	0.00	(341)	0.0
Trimmed of separable fat before cooking; Cooked (broiled) [yield: approx. 10.4 oz.] (9g/0g/2g/61%/na)	557	0.0	53.6	0.00	(247)	0.0
1 pound of Cooked (broiled) meat:						
Yield from approx. 21.9 oz. (1 lb. 5.9 oz.) of raw untrimmed meat that had ***not*** been trimmed of separable fat before cooking	1185	0.0	74.1	0.00	(341)	0.0
Yield from approx. 24.6 oz. (1 lb. 8.6 oz.) of raw untrimmed meat that ***had*** been trimmed of separable fat before cooking	858	0.0	53.6	0.00	(247)	0.0
ROUND STEAK						
CHOICE GRADE:						
Bone-in						
1 pound of Raw untrimmed meat (includes separable fat) with bone [87% separable lean, 9% separable fat, 4% bone]	846	0.0	52.8	0.00		
Cooked (broiled) [yield: approx. 11.8 oz., of which approx. 11.2 oz. are meat and approx. 0.6 oz. are bone]	818	0.0	69.0	0.00		
Trimmed of separable fat before cooking; Cooked (broiled) [yield: approx. 10.7 oz., of which approx. 10.1 oz. are meat and approx. 0.6 oz. are bone]	547	0.0	51.0	0.00		
1 pound of Cooked (broiled) meat (weight includes bone):						
Yield from approx. 21.6 oz. (1 lb. 5.6 oz.) of raw untrimmed meat (weighed with the bone) that had ***not*** been trimmed of separable fat before cooking	1104	0.0	69.0	0.00		
Yield from approx. 23.9 oz. (1 lb. 7.9 oz.) of raw untrimmed meat (weighed with the bone) that ***had*** been trimmed of separable fat before cooking	815	0.0	51.0	0.00		
Boneless						
1 pound of Raw untrimmed meat (includes separable fat) [90% separable lean, 10% separable fat]	881	0.0	55.0	0.00	(253)	0.0
Cooked (broiled) [yield: approx. 11.7 oz.] (8g/0g/4g/55%/na)	852	0.0	73.0	0.00	(336)	0.0
Trimmed of separable fat before cooking; Cooked (broiled) [yield: approx. 10.5 oz.] (9g/0g/2g/61%/na)	570	0.0	54.2	0.00	(249)	0.0
1 pound of Cooked (broiled) meat:						
Yield from approx. 21.9 oz. (1 lb. 5.9 oz.) of raw untrimmed meat that had ***not*** been trimmed of separable fat before cooking	1167	0.0	73.0	0.00	(336)	0.0
Yield from approx. 24.4 oz. (1 lb. 8.4 oz.) of raw untrimmed meat that ***had*** been trimmed of separable fat before cooking	867	0.0	54.2	0.00	(249)	0.0
GOOD GRADE:						
Bone-in						
1 pound of Raw untrimmed meat (includes separable fat) with bone [87% separable lean, 9% separable fat, 4% bone]	754	0.0	47.1	0.00		
Cooked (broiled) [yield: approx. 11.8 oz., of which approx. 11.2 oz. are meat and approx. 0.6 oz. are bone]	745	0.0	62.8	0.00		
Trimmed of separable fat before cooking; Cooked (broiled) [yield: approx. 10.8 oz., of which approx. 10.2 oz. are meat and approx. 0.6 oz. are bone]	507	0.0	46.7	0.00		
1 pound of Cooked (broiled) meat (weight includes bone):						
Yield from approx. 21.6 oz. (1 lb. 5.6 oz.) of raw untrimmed meat (weighed with the bone) that had ***not*** been trimmed of separable fat before cooking	1005	0.0	62.8	0.00		
Yield from approx. 23.6 oz. (1 lb. 7.6 oz.) of raw untrimmed meat (weighed with the bone) that ***had*** been trimmed of separable fat before cooking	748	0.0	46.7	0.00		
Boneless						
1 pound of Raw untrimmed meat (includes separable fat) [91% separable lean, 9% separable fat]	785	0.0	49.1	0.00	(226)	0.0
Cooked (broiled) [yield: approx. 11.7 oz.] (8g/0g/3g/57%/na)	776	0.0	66.4	0.00	(305)	0.0

	UNIT Cal.	UNIT Carb.	1 OZ., BY WT. Cal.	1 OZ., BY WT. Carb.	1 CUP, DICED, NOT PACKED Cal.	1 CUP, DICED, NOT PACKED Carb.
Trimmed of separable fat before cooking; Cooked (broiled) [yield: approx. 10.6 oz.] (9g/0g/1g/62%/na)	528	0.0	49.7	0.00	(229)	0.0
1 pound of Cooked (broiled) meat:						
Yield from approx. 21.9 oz. (1 lb. 5.9 oz.) of raw untrimmed meat that had ***not*** been trimmed of separable fat before cooking	1062	0.0	66.4	0.00	(305)	0.0
Yield from approx. 24.1 oz. (1 lb. 8.1 oz.) of raw untrimmed meat that ***had*** been trimmed of separable fat before cooking	795	0.0	49.7	0.00	(229)	0.0
STANDARD GRADE:						
Bone-in						
1 pound of Raw untrimmed meat (includes separable fat) with bone [89% separable lean, 6% separable fat, 5% bone]	626	0.0	39.1	0.00		
Cooked (broiled) [yield: approx. 11.9 oz., of which approx. 11.1 oz. are meat and approx. 0.8 oz. are bone]	637	0.0	53.5	0.00		
Trimmed of separable fat before cooking; Cooked (broiled) [yield: approx. 11.2 oz., of which approx. 10.4 oz. are meat and approx. 0.8 oz. are bone]	488	0.0	43.5	0.00		
1 pound of Cooked (broiled) meat (weight includes bone):						
Yield from approx. 21.5 oz. (1 lb. 5.5 oz.) of raw untrimmed meat (weighed with the bone) that had ***not*** been trimmed of separable fat before cooking	855	0.0	53.5	0.00		
Yield from approx. 22.8 oz. (1 lb. 6.8 oz.) of raw untrimmed meat (weighed with the bone) that ***had*** been trimmed of separable fat before cooking	696	0.0	43.5	0.00		
Boneless						
1 pound of Raw untrimmed meat (includes separable fat) [94% separable lean, 6% separable fat]	658	0.0	41.1	0.00	(189)	0.0
Cooked (broiled) [yield: approx. 11.7 oz.] (9g/0g/2g/60%/na)	669	0.0	57.3	0.00	(264)	0.0
Trimmed of separable fat before cooking; Cooked (broiled) [yield: approx. 11.0 oz.] (9g/0g/1g/63%/na)	514	0.0	46.8	0.00	(215)	0.0
1 pound of Cooked (broiled) meat:						
Yield from approx. 21.9 oz. (1 lb. 5.9 oz.) of raw untrimmed meat that had ***not*** been trimmed of separable fat before cooking	917	0.0	57.3	0.00	(264)	0.0
Yield from approx. 23.3 oz. (1 lb. 7.3 oz.) of raw untrimmed meat that ***had*** been trimmed of separable fat before cooking	749	0.0	46.8	0.00	(215)	0.0
HEEL OF ROUND						
CHOICE GRADE:						
Boneless						
1 pound of Raw untrimmed meat (includes separable fat) [84% separable lean, 16% separable fat]	967	0.0	60.4	0.00	(278)	0.0
Cooked (roasted) [yield: approx. 11.7 oz.] (8g/0g/5g/56%/na)	865	0.0	74.1	0.00	(341)	0.0
Trimmed of separable fat before cooking; Cooked (roasted) [yield: approx. 9.8 oz.] (9g/0g/2g/63%/na)	501	0.0	51.1	0.00	(235)	0.0
1 pound of Cooked (roasted) meat:						
Yield from approx. 21.9 oz. (1 lb. 5.9 oz.) of raw untrimmed meat that had ***not*** been trimmed of separable fat before cooking	1185	0.0	74.1	0.00	(341)	0.0
Yield from approx. 26.1 oz. (1 lb. 10.1 oz.) of raw untrimmed meat that ***had*** been trimmed of separable fat before cooking	817	0.0	51.1	0.00	(235)	0.0
GOOD GRADE:						
Boneless						
1 pound of Raw untrimmed meat (includes separable fat) [87% separable lean, 13% separable fat]	854	0.0	53.3	0.00	(248)	0.0
Cooked (roasted) [yield: approx. 11.7 oz.] (8g/0g/4g/58%/na)	782	0.0	67.0	0.00	(308)	0.0
Trimmed of separable fat before cooking; Cooked (roasted) [yield: approx. 10.2 oz.] (9g/0g/1g/64%/na)	502	0.0	49.4	0.00	(227)	0.0
1 pound of Cooked (roasted) meat:						
Yield from approx. 21.9 oz. (1 lb. 5.9 oz.) of raw untrimmed meat that had ***not*** been trimmed of separable fat before cooking	1071	0.0	67.0	0.00	(308)	0.0
Yield from approx. 25.2 oz. (1 lb. 9.2 oz.) of raw untrimmed meat that ***had*** been trimmed of separable fat before cooking	790	0.0	49.4	0.00	(227)	0.0

	UNIT Cal.	UNIT Carb.	1 OZ., BY WT. Cal.	1 OZ., BY WT. Carb.	1 CUP, DICED, NOT PACKED Cal.	1 CUP, DICED, NOT PACKED Carb.
STANDARD GRADE:						
Boneless						
1 pound of Raw untrimmed meat (includes separable fat) [92% separable lean, 8% separable fat]	667	0.0	41.7	0.00	(192)	0.0
Cooked (roasted) [yield: approx. 11.7 oz.] (8g/0g/2g/62%/na)	650	0.0	55.6	0.00	(256)	0.0
Trimmed of separable fat before cooking; Cooked (roasted) [yield: approx. 10.7 oz.] (9g/0g/1g/65%/na)	494	0.0	46.0	0.00	(211)	0.0
1 pound of Cooked (roasted) meat:						
Yield from approx. 21.9 oz. (1 lb. 5.9 oz.) of raw untrimmed meat that had ***not*** been trimmed of separable fat before cooking	890	0.0	55.6	0.00	(256)	0.0
Yield from approx. 23.8 oz. (1 lb. 7.8 oz.) of raw untrimmed meat that ***had*** been trimmed of separable fat before cooking	735	0.0	46.0	0.00	(211)	0.0
RUMP ROAST						
CHOICE GRADE:						
Bone-in						
1 pound of Raw untrimmed meat (includes separable fat) with bone [63% separable lean, 22% separable fat, 15% bone]	1169	0.0	73.1	0.00		
Cooked (roasted) [yield: approx. 12.3 oz., of which approx. 9.9 oz. are meat and approx. 2.4 oz. are bone]	978	0.0	79.3	0.00		
Trimmed of separable fat before cooking; Cooked (roasted) [yield: approx. 9.8 oz., of which approx 7.4 oz. are meat and approx. 2.4 oz. are bone]	439	0.0	44.6	0.00		
1 pound of Cooked (roasted) meat (weight includes bone):						
Yield from approx. 20.7 oz. (1 lb. 4.7 oz.) of raw untrimmed meat (weighed with the bone) that had ***not*** been trimmed of separable fat before cooking	1269	0.0	79.3	0.00		
Yield from approx. 26.0 oz. (1 lb. 10.0 oz.) of raw untrimmed meat (weighed with the bone) that ***had*** been trimmed of separable fat before cooking	714	0.0	44.6	0.00		
Boneless						
1 pound of Raw untrimmed meat (includes separable fat) [75% separable lean, 25% separable fat]	1376	0.0	86.0	0.00	(396)	0.0
Cooked (roasted) [yield: approx. 11.7 oz.] (7g/0g/8g/48%/na)	1150	0.0	98.5	0.00	(453)	0.0
Trimmed of separable fat before cooking; Cooked (roasted) [yield: approx. 8.8 oz.] (8g/0g/3g/60%/na)	517	0.0	59.0	0.00	(271)	0.0
1 pound of Cooked (roasted) meat:						
Yield from approx. 21.9 oz. (1 lb. 5.9 oz.) of raw untrimmed meat that had ***not*** been trimmed of separable fat before cooking	1575	0.0	98.5	0.00	(453)	0.0
Yield from approx. 29.2 oz. (1 lb. 13.2 oz.) of raw untrimmed meat that ***had*** been trimmed of separable fat before cooking	944	0.0	59.0	0.00	(271)	0.0
GOOD GRADE:						
Bone-in						
1 pound of Raw untrimmed meat (includes separable fat) with bone [64% separable lean, 20% separable fat, 16% bone]	1033	0.0	64.6	0.00		
Cooked (roasted) [yield: approx. 12.4 oz., of which approx. 9.8 oz. are meat and approx. 2.6 oz. are bone]	883	0.0	71.3	0.00		
Trimmed of separable fat before cooking; Cooked (roasted) [yield: approx. 10.1 oz., of which approx. 7.5 oz. are meat and approx. 2.6 oz. are bone]	381	0.0	38.0	0.00		
1 pound of Cooked (roasted) meat (weight includes bone):						
Yield from approx. 20.7 oz. (1 lb. 4.7 oz.) of raw untrimmed meat (weighed with the bone) that had ***not*** been trimmed of separable fat before cooking	1141	0.0	71.3	0.00		
Yield from approx. 25.6 oz. (1 lb. 9.6 oz.) of raw untrimmed meat (weighed with the bone) that ***had*** been trimmed of separable fat before cooking	608	0.0	38.0	0.00		
Boneless						
1 pound of Raw untrimmed meat (includes separable fat) [76% separable lean, 24% separable fat]	1230	0.0	76.9	0.00	(354)	0.0
Cooked (roasted) [yield: approx. 11.7 oz.] (7g/0g/7g/51%/na)	1051	0.0	89.9	0.00	(414)	0.0
Trimmed of separable fat before cooking; Cooked (roasted) [yield: approx. 8.9 oz.] (8g/0g/2g/62%/na)	453	0.0	51.1	0.00	(235)	0.0
1 pound of Cooked (roasted) meat:						
Yield from approx. 21.9 oz. (1 lb. 5.9 oz.) of raw untrimmed meat that had ***not*** been trimmed of separable fat before cooking	1439	0.0	89.9	0.00	(414)	0.0
Yield from approx. 28.8 oz. (1 lb. 12.8 oz.) of raw untrimmed meat that ***had*** been trimmed of separable fat before cooking	817	0.0	51.1	0.00	(235)	0.0
STANDARD GRADE:						
Bone-in						
1 pound of Raw untrimmed meat (includes separable fat) with bone [65% separable lean, 17% separable fat, 18% bone]	893	0.0	55.8	0.00		
Cooked (roasted) [yield: approx. 12.5 oz., of which approx. 9.6 oz. are meat and approx. 2.9 oz. are bone]	780	0.0	62.6	0.00		
Trimmed of separable fat before cooking; Cooked (roasted) [yield: approx. 10.5 oz., of which approx. 7.6 oz. are meat and approx. 2.9 oz. are bone]	386	0.0	37.0	0.00		
1 pound of Cooked (roasted) meat (weight includes bone):						
Yield from approx. 20.5 oz. (1 lb. 4.5 oz.) of raw untrimmed meat (weighed with the bone) that had ***not*** been trimmed of separable fat before cooking	1002	0.0	62.6	0.00		
Yield from approx. 24.5 oz. (1 lb. 8.5 oz.) of raw untrimmed meat (weighed with the bone) that ***had*** been trimmed of separable fat before cooking	592	0.0	37.0	0.00		
Boneless						
1 pound of Raw untrimmed meat (includes separable fat) [79% separable lean, 21% separable fat]	1090	0.0	68.1	0.00	(313)	0.0
Cooked (roasted) [yield: approx. 11.7 oz.] (7g/0g/6g/53%/na)	951	0.0	81.4	0.00	(374)	0.0
Trimmed of separable fat before cooking; Cooked (roasted) [yield: approx. 9.2 oz.] (9g/0g/2g/63%/na)	471	0.0	51.1	0.00	(235)	0.0
1 pound of Cooked (roasted) meat:						
Yield from approx. 21.9 oz. (1 lb. 5.9 oz.) of raw untrimmed meat that had ***not*** been trimmed of separable fat before cooking	1303	0.0	81.4	0.00	(374)	0.0
Yield from approx. 27.7 oz. (1 lb. 11.7 oz.) of raw untrimmed meat that ***had*** been trimmed of separable fat before cooking	817	0.0	51.1	0.00	(235)	0.0

Ground Beef

	UNIT Cal.	UNIT Carb.	1 OZ., BY WT. Cal.	1 OZ., BY WT. Carb.	1 CUP, DICED, NOT PACKED Cal.	1 CUP, DICED, NOT PACKED Carb.
10% fat:						
Raw, 1 pound	812	0.0	50.8	0.00		
Raw, 1 cup, packed	405	0.0	50.8	0.00		
Cooked (well done; oven broiled, pan broiled, or sauteed) [yield from 1 pound: approx. 12 oz.] (8g/0g/3g/60%/19 mg)	745	0.0	62.1	0.00		
Cooked, 1 cup (approx. 4 oz.)	(680)	0.0	62.1	0.00		
Cooked, 1 pound [yield from approx. 21 oz. (1 lb. 5 oz.) raw meat]	993	0.0	62.1	0.00		
20% fat:						
Raw, 1 pound	1216	0.0	76.0	0.00		
Raw, 1 cup, packed	606	0.0	76.0	0.00		
Cooked (well done; oven broiled, pan broiled, or sauteed) [yield from 1 pound: approx. 12 oz.] (5g/0g/5g/54%/13mg)	932	0.0	81.0	0.00		
Cooked, 1 cup (approx. 4 oz.)	(533)	0.0	81.0	0.00		
Cooked, 1 pound [yield from approx. 21 oz. (1 lb. 5 oz.) raw meat]	1297	0.0	81.0	0.00		
1 pound	4192	0.0	262.0	0.00		

Beef Organ Meats

A list that compares the organ meats of Beef, Lamb, Pork, and Veal begins on page 278.

All cooked values are for lean meat, both measured and cooked after all separable fat has been removed.

	UNIT Cal.	UNIT Carb.	1 OZ., BY WT. Cal.	1 OZ., BY WT. Carb.	1 CUP, DICED, NOT PACKED Cal.	1 CUP, DICED, NOT PACKED Carb.
BRAINS:						
Raw, 1 pound	554	3.6	34.6	0.23		
Cooked:						
1 pound of cooked brains (3g/tr/3g/78%/na)	590	3.6	36.9	0.23		

	UNIT		1 OZ., BY WT.		1 CUP, DICED, NOT PACKED	
	Cal.	Carb.	Cal.	Carb.	Cal.	Carb.
HEART:						
Raw, 1 pound	499	3.2	31.2	0.20		
Cooked:						
1 pound of raw heart, cooked [yield: approx. 9.3 oz.]	466	1.9	50.2	0.20		
1 pound of cooked heart (9g/tr/2g/61%/na)	804	3.2	50.2	0.20		
KIDNEYS:						
Raw, 1 pound	454	0.5	28.4	0.03		
Cooked:						
1 pound of raw kidneys, cooked [yield: approx. 8 oz.]	313	2.1	39.1	0.26	353	1.1
1 pound of cooked kidneys (9g/tr/3g/53%/na)	626	4.1	39.1	0.26	353	1.1
LIVER:						
Raw, 1 pound	595	24.0	37.1	1.50		
Cooked:						
1 pound of raw liver, cooked [yield: approx. 11.8 oz.]	459	17.8	38.8	1.50		
1 pound of cooked liver (7g/2g/3g/56%/na)	622	24.0	38.8	1.50		
LUNG:						
Raw, 1 pound	458	0.0	28.6	0.00		
Cooked:						
1 pound of cooked lung (6g/0g/1g/78%/na)	545	0.0	34.0	0.00		
PANCREAS (Sweetbreads):						
Raw, 1 pound	935	0.0	58.4	0.00		
Cooked:						
1 pound of cooked sweetbreads (8g/0g/3g/62%/na)	1230	0.0	76.8	0.00		
SPLEEN:						
Raw, 1 pound	468	0.0	29.2	0.00		
Cooked:						
1 pound of cooked spleen (8g/0g/1g/68%/na)	658	0.0	41.1	0.00		
THYMUS (Sweetbreads):						
Raw, 1 pound	1117	0.0	69.7	0.00		
Cooked:						
1 pound of raw thymus, cooked [yield: approx. 9.3 oz.]	821	0.0	88.5	0.00		
1 pound of cooked thymus (7g/0g/7g/50%/na)	1416	0.0	88.5	0.00		
TONGUE:						
Raw, 1 pound	1035	1.4	64.6	0.09		
Cooked:						
1 pound of raw tongue, cooked [yield: approx. 12.5 oz.]	1020	1.4	81.7	0.11		
1 pound of cooked tongue (6g/tr/5g/61%/na)	1307	1.8	81.7	0.11		
TRIPE:						
Raw, 1 pound	536	0.0	33.4	0.00		
Beef Drippings (based on data from Great Britain)	4178	0.0	261.1	0.00		
VEAL						
CHUCK CUTS AND BONELESS VEAL FOR STEW						
Bone-in						
1 pound of Raw untrimmed meat (includes separable fat) with bone [69% separable lean, 11% separable fat, 20% bone]	628	0.0	39.3	0.00		
Cooked (braised, pot-roasted or stewed) [yield: approx. 11.6 oz., of which approx. 8.4 oz. are meat and approx. 3.2 oz. are bone]	564	0.0	48.6	0.00		
1 pound of Cooked (braised, pot-roasted or stewed) meat (weight includes bone):						
Yield from approx. 22 oz. (1 lb. 6 oz.) of raw untrimmed meat (weighed with the bone) that had ***not*** been trimmed of separable fat before cooking	778	0.0	48.6	0.00		
Boneless						
1 pound of Raw untrimmed meat (includes separable fat) [86% separable lean, 14% separable fat]	785	0.0	49.1	0.00		
Cooked (braised, pot-roasted or stewed) [yield: approx. 10.6 oz.] (8g/0g/4g/59%/14 mg)	703	0.0	66.6	0.00	329	0.0
1 pound of Cooked (braised, pot-roasted or stewed) meat:						
Yield from approx. 24 oz. (1 lb. 8 oz.) of raw untrimmed meat that had ***not*** been trimmed of separable fat before cooking	1066	0.0	66.6	0.00	329	0.0

	UNIT		1 OZ., BY WT.		1 CUP, DICED, NOT PACKED	
	Cal.	Carb.	Cal.	Carb.	Cal.	Carb.
LOIN CUTS						
Bone-in						
1 pound of Raw untrimmed meat (includes separable fat) with bone [71% separable lean, 12% separable fat, 17% bone]	681	0.0	42.6	0.00		
Cooked (braised or broiled) [yield: approx. 12.2 oz., of which approx. 9.5 oz. are meat and approx. 2.7 oz. are bone]	629	0.0	51.6	0.00		
1 pound of Cooked (braised or broiled) meat (weight includes bone):						
Yield from approx. 21 oz. (1 lb. 5 oz.) of raw untrimmed meat (weighed with the bone) that had ***not*** been trimmed of separable fat before cooking	825	0.0	51.6	0.00		
Boneless						
1 pound of Raw untrimmed meat (includes separable fat) [85% separable lean, 15% separable fat]	821	0.0	51.3	0.00		
Cooked (braised or broiled) [yield: approx. 11.4 oz.] (7g/0g/4g/59%/18 mg)	758	0.0	66.3	0.00	328	0.0
1 pound of Cooked (braised or broiled) meat:						
Yield from approx. 22 oz. (1 lb. 6 oz.) of raw untrimmed meat that had ***not*** been trimmed of separable fat before cooking	1061	0.0	66.3	0.00	328	0.0
PLATE (Breast of Veal)						
Bone-in						
1 pound of Raw untrimmed meat (includes separable fat) with bone [58% separable lean, 21% separable fat, 21% bone]	828	0.0	51.8	0.00		
Cooked (braised or stewed) [yield: approx. 11.7 oz., of which approx. 8.3 oz. are meat and approx. 3.4 oz. are bone]	718	0.0	61.4	0.00		
1 pound of Cooked (braised or stewed) meat (weight includes bone):						
Yield from approx. 22 oz. (1 lb. 6 oz.) of raw untrimmed meat (weighed with the bone) that had ***not*** been trimmed of separable fat before cooking	981	0.0	61.4	0.00		
Boneless						
1 pound of Raw untrimmed meat (includes separable fat) [74% separable lean, 26% separable fat]	1048	0.0	65.5	0.00		
Cooked (braised or stewed) [yield: approx. 10.6 oz.] (7g/0g/6g/52%/13 mg)	906	0.0	85.9	0.00	329	0.0
1 pound of Cooked (braised or stewed) meat:						
Yield from approx. 24 oz. (1 lb. 8 oz.) of raw untrimmed meat that had ***not*** been trimmed of separable fat before cooking	1374	0.0	85.9	0.00	329	0.0
RIB ROAST						
Bone-in						
1 pound of Raw untrimmed meat (includes separable fat) with bone [63% separable lean, 14% separable fat, 23% bone]	723	0.0	45.2	0.00		
Cooked (roasted) [yield: approx. 12.2 oz., of which approx. 8.5 oz. are meat and approx. 3.7 oz. are bone]	648	0.0	53.1	0.00		
1 pound of Cooked (roasted) meat (weight includes bone):						
Yield from approx. 21 oz. (1 lb. 5 oz.) of raw untrimmed meat (weighed with the bone) that had ***not*** been trimmed of separable fat before cooking	850	0.0	53.1	0.00		
Boneless						
1 pound of Raw untrimmed meat (includes separable fat) [82% separable lean, 18% separable fat]	939	0.0	58.7	0.00		
Cooked (roasted) [yield: approx. 11 oz.] (8g/0g/5g/55%/19mg)	842	0.0	76.3	0.00	377	0.0
1 pound of Cooked (roasted) meat:						
Yield from approx. 23 oz. (1 lb. 7 oz.) of raw untrimmed meat that had ***not*** been trimmed of separable fat before cooking	1220	0.0	76.3	0.00	377	0.0
ROUND WITH RUMP (Roasts and Leg Cutlets)						
Bone-in						
1 pound of Raw untrimmed meat (includes separable fat) with bone [67% separable lean, 10% separable fat, 23% bone]	573	0.0	35.8	0.00		
Cooked (braised or broiled) [yield: approx. 12.4 oz., of which approx. 8.7 oz. are meat and approx. 3.7 oz. are bone]	534	0.0	43.1	0.00		

	UNIT Cal.	UNIT Carb.	1 OZ., BY WT. Cal.	1 OZ., BY WT. Carb.	1 CUP, DICED, NOT PACKED Cal.	1 CUP, DICED, NOT PACKED Carb.
1 pound of Cooked (braised or broiled) meat (weight includes bone):						
Yield from approx. 21 oz. (1 lb. 5 oz.) of raw untrimmed meat (weighed with the bone) that had ***not*** been trimmed of separable fat before cooking	689	0.0	43.1	0.00		
Boneless						
1 pound of Raw untrimmed meat (includes separable fat) [87% separable lean, 13% separable fat]	744	0.0	46.5	0.00		
Cooked (braised or broiled) [yield: approx. 11.3 oz.] (8g/0g/3g/60%/19mg)	693	0.0	61.3	0.00	302	0.0
1 pound of Cooked (braised or broiled) meat:						
Yield from approx. 23 oz. (1 lb. 7 oz.) of raw untrimmed meat that had ***not*** been trimmed of separable fat before cooking	980	0.0	61.3	0.00	302	0.0

Veal Organ Meats

A list that compares the organ meats of Beef, Lamb, Pork, and Veal begins on page 278.

All cooked values are for lean meat, both measured and cooked after all separable fat has been removed.

	UNIT Cal.	UNIT Carb.	1 OZ., BY WT. Cal.	1 OZ., BY WT. Carb.	1 CUP Cal.	1 CUP Carb.
BRAINS:						
Raw, 1 pound	477	3.6	29.8	0.23		
Cooked:						
1 pound of cooked brains (3g/tr/2g/80%/na)	504	(3.6)	31.5	(0.23)		
HEART:						
Raw, 1 pound	495	8.2	30.9	0.51		
Cooked:						
1 pound of raw heart, cooked [yield: approx. 9.4 oz.]	410	6.8	43.4	0.72		
1 pound of cooked heart (8g/1g/3g/60%/na)	695	11.5	43.4	0.72		
KIDNEYS:						
Raw, 1 pound	472	0.5	29.5	0.03		
Cooked:						
1 pound of raw kidneys, cooked [yield: approx. 8.0 oz.]	374	0.2	69.5	0.03		
1 pound of cooked kidneys (7g/tr/1g/70%/na)	749	0.5	69.5	0.03		
LIVER (Calf's liver):						
Raw, 1 pound	636	18.6	39.7	1.16		
Cooked:						
1 pound of raw liver, cooked [yield: approx. 10.2 oz.]	465	11.6	45.4	1.13		
1 pound of cooked liver (8g/1g/4g/51%/na)	726	18.1	45.4	1.13		
LUNG:						
Raw, 1 pound	418	0.0	26.1	0.00		
Cooked:						
1 pound of cooked lung (5g/0g/1g/79%/na)	472	0.0	29.5	0.00		
PANCREAS (Sweetbreads):						
Raw, 1 pound	931	0.0	58.1	0.00		
Cooked:						
1 pound of cooked (8g/0g/5g/52%/na)	1162	0.0	72.6	0.00		
SPLEEN:						
Raw, 1 pound	449	0.0	28.1	0.00		
Cooked:						
1 pound of cooked spleen (7g/tr/1g/74%/na)	567	0.0	35.4	0.00		
THYMUS (Sweetbreads):						
Raw, 1 pound	445	0.0	27.8	0.00		
Cooked:						
1 pound of raw thymus, cooked [yield: approx. 9.3 oz.]	277	0.0	29.8	0.00		
1 pound of cooked thymus (9g/0g/1g/73%/na)	477	0.0	29.8	0.00		
TONGUE:						
Raw, 1 pound	604	3.1	37.7	0.19		
Cooked:						
1 pound of raw tongue, cooked [yield: approx. 11.1 oz.]	590	3.1	53.0	0.28		
1 pound of cooked tongue (7g/tr/2g/69%/na)	849	4.5	53.0	0.28		
TRIPE:						
Raw, 1 pound	672	0.0	42.0	0.00		

LAMB

LEG

	UNIT Cal.	UNIT Carb.	1 OZ., BY WT. Cal.	1 OZ., BY WT. Carb.	1 CUP, DICED, NOT PACKED Cal.	1 CUP, DICED, NOT PACKED Carb.
Bone-in						
1 pound of Raw untrimmed meat (includes separable fat) with bone (70% separable lean, 14% separable fat, 16% bone]	845	0.0	52.8	0.00		
Cooked (roasted) [yield: approx. 12 oz., of which approx. 9.4 oz. are meat and approx. 2.6 oz. are bone]	745	0.0	62.1	0.00		
Trimmed of separable fat before cooking; Cooked (roasted) [yield: approx. 10.4 oz., of which approx. 7.8 oz. are meat and approx. 2.6 oz. are bone]	411	0.0	39.5	0.00		
1 pound of Cooked (roasted) meat (weight includes bone):						
Yield from approx. 21 oz. (1 lb. 5 oz.) of raw untrimmed meat (weighed with the bone) that had ***not*** been trimmed of separable fat before cooking	994	0.0	62.1	0.00		
Yield from approx. 25 oz. (1 lb. 9 oz.) of raw untrimmed meat with bone that ***had*** been trimmed of separable fat before cooking	632	0.0	39.5	0.00		
Boneless						
1 pound of Raw untrimmed meat (includes separable fat) [83% separable lean, 17% separable fat]	1007	0.0	62.9	0.00		
Cooked (roasted) [yield: approx. 11.2 oz] (7g/0g/5g/54%/18mg)	887	0.0	79.1	0.00	391	0.0
Trimmed of separable fat before cooking; Cooked (roasted) [yield: approx. 9.3 oz.] (8g/0g/2g/62%/20mg)	491	0.0	52.8	0.00	260	0.0
1 pound of Cooked (roasted) meat:						
Yield from approx. 23 oz. (1 lb. 7 oz.) of raw untrimmed meat that had ***not*** been trimmed of separable fat before cooking	1266	0.0	79.1	0.00	391	0.0
Yield from approx. 28 oz. (1 lb. 12 oz.) of raw untrimmed meat that ***had*** been trimmed of separable fat before cooking	844	0.0	52.8	0.00	260	0.0

LOIN CHOPS

	UNIT Cal.	UNIT Carb.	1 OZ., BY WT. Cal.	1 OZ., BY WT. Carb.	1 CUP Cal.	1 CUP Carb.
Bone-in						
1 pound of Raw untrimmed meat (includes separable fat) with bone [62% separable lean, 24% separable fat, 14% bone]	1146	0.0	71.6	0.00		
Cooked (roasted) [yield: approx. 12.3 oz., of which approx. 10.1 oz. are meat and approx. 2.2 oz. are bone]	1023	0.0	83.2	0.00		
Trimmed of separable fat before cooking; Cooked (roasted) [yield: approx. 9.1 oz., of which approx. 6.9 are meat and approx. 2.2 oz. are bone]	368	0.0	40.4	0.00		
1 pound of Cooked (roasted) meat (weight includes bone):						
Yield from approx. 21 oz. (1 lb. 5 oz.) of raw untrimmed meat (weighed with the bone) that had ***not*** been trimmed of separable fat before cooking	1331	0.0	83.2	0.00		
Yield from approx. 28 oz. (1 lb. 12 oz.) of raw untrimmed meat (weighed with the bone) that ***had*** been trimmed of separable fat before cooking	647	0.0	40.4	0.00		
1 chop (3 to the pound), Raw untrimmed meat (includes separable fat) with bone [62% separable lean, 24% separable fat, 14% bone] approx. 5.3 oz.	382	0.0	71.6	0.00		
Cooked (roasted) [yield: approx. 4.1 oz., of which approx. 3.4 oz. are meat and approx. 0.7 oz. are bone]	341	0.0	83.2	0.00		
Trimmed of separable fat before cooking; Cooked (roasted) [yield: approx. 3 oz., of which 2.3 oz. are meat and 0.7 oz. are bone]	122	0.0	40.7	0.00		
Boneless						
1 pound of Raw untrimmed meat (includes separable fat) [72% separable lean, 28% separable fat]	1328	0.0	83.0	0.00		
Cooked (roasted) [yield: approx. 11.7 oz.] (6g/0g/8g/47%/15mg)	1191	0.0	101.8	0.00	(501)	0.0
Trimmed of separable fat before cooking; Cooked (roasted) [yield: approx. 8 oz.] (8g/0g/2g/62%/20mg)	426	0.0	53.3	0.00	(262)	0.0
1 pound of Cooked (roasted) meat:						
Yield from approx. 22 oz. (1 lb. 6 oz.) of raw untrimmed meat that had ***not*** been trimmed of separable fat before cooking	1629	0.0	101.8	0.00	(501)	0.0
Yield from approx. 32 oz. (2 lbs.) of raw untrimmed meat that ***had*** been trimmed of separable fat before cooking	853	0.0	53.3	0.00	(262)	0.0

	UNIT		1 OZ., BY WT.		1 CUP, DICED, NOT PACKED	
	Cal.	Carb.	Cal.	Carb.	Cal.	Carb.
1 chop (4 to the pound), Raw untrimmed meat (includes separable fat) [72% separable lean, 28% separable fat] approx. 4.2 oz.	382	0.0	83.0	0.00		
Cooked (roasted) [yield: approx. 3.4 oz.]	341	0.0	101.8	0.00	(501)	0.0
Trimmed of separable fat before cooking; Cooked (roasted) [yield: approx. 2.3 oz.]	122	0.0	53.3	0.00	(262)	0.0
RIB CHOPS						
Bone-in						
1 pound of Raw untrimmed meat (includes separable fat) with bone [54% separable lean, 26% separable fat, 20% bone]	1229	0.0	76.8	0.00		
Cooked (broiled) [yield: approx. 12.7 oz., of which approx. 9.5 oz. are meat and approx. 3.2 oz. are bone]	1091	0.0	85.9	0.00		
Trimmed of separable fat before cooking; Cooked (broiled) [yield: approx. 9.2 oz., of which approx. 6 oz. are meat and approx. 3.2 oz. are bone]	361	0.0	39.2	0.00		
1 chop (3 to the pound), Raw untrimmed meat (includes separable fat) with bone [54% separable lean, 26% separable fat, 20% bone] approx. 5.3 oz.	407	0.0	76.8	0.00		
Cooked (broiled) [yield: approx. 4.2 oz., of which approx. 3.1 oz. are meat and approx. 1.1 oz. are bone]	362	0.0	85.9	0.00		
Trimmed of separable fat before cooking; Cooked (broiled) [yield: approx. 3.1 oz., of which approx. 2 oz. are meat and approx. 1.1 oz. are bone]	120	0.0	39.2	0.00		
1 chop (4 to the pound), Raw untrimmed meat (includes separable fat) with bone [54% lean, 26% fat, 20% bone] approx. 4 oz.	307	0.0	76.8	0.00		
Cooked (broiled) [yield: approx. 3.2 oz., of which approx. 2.4 oz. are meat and approx. 0.8 oz. are bone]	273	0.0	85.9	0.00		
Trimmed of separable fat before cooking; Cooked (broiled) [yield: approx. 2.3 oz., of which approx. 1.5 oz. are meat and approx. 0.8 oz. are bone]	91	0.0	39.2	0.00		
1 pound of Cooked (broiled) meat (weight includes bone):						
Yield from approx. 20 oz. (1 lb. 4 oz.) of raw untrimmed meat (weighed with the bone) that had ***not*** been trimmed of separable fat before cooking	1374	0.0	85.9	0.00		
Yield from approx. 28 oz. (1 lb. 12 oz.) of raw untrimmed meat (weighed with the bone) that ***had*** been trimmed of separable fat before cooking	628	0.0	39.2	0.00		
Boneless						
1 pound of Raw untrimmed meat (includes separable fat) [67% separable lean, 33% separable fat]	1536	0.0	96.0	0.00		
Cooked (broiled) [yield: approx. 11.9 oz.] (6g/0g/10g/43%/14mg)	1373	0.0	115.4	0.00	(570)	0.0
Trimmed of separable fat before cooking; Cooked (broiled) [yield: approx. 7.5 oz.] (8g/0g/3g/60%/19mg)	449	0.0	59.8	0.00	(295)	0.0
1 chop (4 to the pound), Raw untrimmed meat (includes separable fat) [67% separable lean, 33% separable fat] approx. 4.2 oz.	407	0.0	96.0	0.00		
Cooked (broiled) [yield: approx. 3.1 oz.]	362	0.0	115.4	0.00	(570)	0.0
Trimmed of separable fat before cooking; Cooked (broiled) [yield: approx. 2 oz.]	120	0.0	59.8	0.00	(295)	0.0
1 chop (5 to the pound), Raw untrimmed meat (includes separable fat) [67% separable lean, 33% separable fat] approx. 3.2 oz.	307	0.0	96.0	0.00		
Cooked (broiled) [yield: approx. 2.4 oz.]	273	0.0	115.4	0.00	(570)	0.0
Trimmed of separable fat before cooking; Cooked (broiled) [yield: approx. 15 oz.]	91	0.0	59.8	0.00	(295)	0.0
1 pound of Cooked (broiled) meat:						
Yield from approx. 22 oz. (1 lb. 6 oz.) of raw untrimmed meat that had ***not*** been trimmed of separable fat before cooking	1846	0.0	115.4	0.00	(570)	0.0
Yield from approx. 34 oz. (2 lb. 2 oz.) of raw untrimmed meat that ***had*** been trimmed of separable fat before cooking	957	0.0	59.8	0.00	(295)	0.0
SHOULDER						
Bone-in						
1 pound of Raw untrimmed meat (includes separable fat) with bone [63% separable lean, 22% separable fat, 15% bone]	1082	0.0	67.6	0.00		
Cooked (roasted) [yield: approx. 11.9 oz., of which approx. 9.5 oz. are meat and approx. 2.4 oz. are bone]	913	0.0	76.7	0.00		

	UNIT		1 OZ., BY WT.		1 CUP, DICED, NOT PACKED	
	Cal.	Carb.	Cal.	Carb.	Cal.	Carb.
Trimmed of separable fat before cooking; Cooked (roasted) [yield: approx. 9.4 oz., of which approx. 7 oz. are meat and approx. 2.4 oz. are bone]	410	0.0	43.6	0.00		
1 pound of Cooked (roasted) meat (weight includes bone):						
Yield from approx. 22 oz. (1 lb. 6 oz.) of raw untrimmed meat (weighed with the bone) that had ***not*** been trimmed of separable fat before cooking	1228	0.0	76.7	0.00		
Yield from approx. 27 oz. (1 lb. 11 oz.) of raw untrimmed meat (weighed with the bone) which ***had*** been trimmed of separable fat before cooking	698	0.0	43.6	0.00		
Boneless						
1 pound of Raw untrimmed meat (includes separable fat) [74% separable lean, 26% separable fat]	1275	0.0	79.7	0.00		
Cooked (roasted) [yield: approx. 11.2 oz.] (6g/0g/8g/50%/15mg)	1075	0.0	96.0	0.00	473	0.0
Trimmed of separable fat before cooking; Cooked (roasted) [yield: approx. 8.3 oz.] (8g/10g/3g/61%/19mg)	482	0.0	58.1	0.00	287	0.0
1 pound of Cooked (roasted) meat:						
Yield from approx. 23 oz. (1 lb. 7 oz.) of raw untrimmed meat that had ***not*** been trimmed of separable fat before cooking	1533	0.0	96.0	0.00	473	0.0
Yield from approx. 31 oz. (1 lb. 15 oz.) of raw untrimmed meat that ***had*** been trimmed of separable fat before cooking	930	0.0	58.1	0.00	287	0.0

Lamb Organ Meats

A list that compares the organ meats of Beef, Lamb, Pork, and Veal begins on page 278.

All cooked values are for lean meat, both measured and cooked after all separable fat has been removed.

	UNIT		1 OZ., BY WT.		1 CUP, DICED, NOT PACKED	
	Cal.	Carb.	Cal.	Carb.	Cal.	Carb.
BRAINS:						
Raw, 1 pound	540	3.6	33.7	0.23		
Cooked:						
1 pound of cooked brains (4g/tr/3g/76%/na)	622	(3.6)	38.8	(0.23)		
HEART:						
Raw, 1 pound	567	4.5	35.4	0.28		
Cooked:						
1 pound of raw heart, cooked [yield: approx. 9.0 oz.]	356	2.5	39.7	0.28		
1 pound of cooked heart (9g/tr/2g/61%/na)	636	4.5	39.7	0.28		
KIDNEYS:						
Raw, 1 pound	476	4.2	29.8	0.26		
Cooked:						
1 pound of raw kidneys cooked [yield: approx. 8.0 oz.]	293	3.2	36.6	0.40		
1 pound of cooked kidneys (6g/tr/1g/72%/na)	586	6.2	36.6	0.40		
LIVER:						
Raw, 1 pound	717	13.2	44.8	0.83		
Cooked:						
1 pound of raw liver, cooked [yield: approx. 9.8 oz.]	550	8.9	56.4	0.91		
1 pound of cooked liver (9g/1g/4g/54%/na)	903	14.5	56.4	0.91		
LUNG:						
Raw, 1 pound	441	0.0	27.5	0.00		
Cooked:						
1 pound of cooked lung (5g/0g/3g/78%/na)	527	0.0	32.9	0.00		
PANCREAS (Sweetbreads):						
Raw, 1 pound	713	0.0	44.5	0.00		
Cooked:						
1 pound of cooked pancreas (7g/0g/1g/76%/na)	844	0.0	52.7	0.00		
SPLEEN:						
Raw, 1 pound	463	0.0	28.9	0.00		
Cooked:						
1 pound of cooked spleen (8g/0g/1g/65%/na)	681	0.0	42.5	0.00		
TONGUE:						
Raw, 1 pound	1012	1.7	63.2	0.11		
Cooked:						
1 pound of raw tongue, cooked [yield: approx. 12.8 oz.]	1005	1.7	78.5	0.14		
1 pound of cooked tongue (6g/tr/5g/60%/na)	1258	2.3	78.5	0.14		
TRIPE:						
Raw, 1 pound	567	0.0	35.4	0.00		

	UNIT		1 OZ., BY WT.		1 CUP, DICED, NOT PACKED	
	Cal.	Carb.	Cal.	Carb.	Cal.	Carb.
PORK						
Fresh Pork						
HAM						
Bone-in, with skin						
1 pound of Raw untrimmed meat (includes separable fat) with bone and skin [63% separable lean, 22% separable fat, 15% bone and skin]	1188	0.0	74.2	0.00		
Cooked (baked or roasted) [yield: approx. 11.6 oz., of which approx. 9.2 oz. are meat and approx. 2.4 oz. are bone and skin]	980	0.0	84.5	0.00		
Trimmed of separable fat before cooking; Cooked (baked or roasted) [yield: approx. 9.2 oz., of which approx. 6.8 oz. are meat and approx. 2.4 oz. are bone and skin]	421	0.0	45.8	0.00		
1 pound of Cooked (baked or roasted) meat (weight includes bone and skin)						
Yield from approx. 22 oz. (1 lb. 6 oz.) of raw untrimmed meat (weighed with the bone and skin) that had ***not*** been trimmed of separable fat before cooking	1352	0.0	84.5	0.00		
Yield from approx. 28 oz. (1 lb. 12 oz.) of raw untrimmed meat (weighed with the bone and skin) that ***had*** been trimmed of separable fat before cooking	732	0.0	45.8	0.00		
Boneless, skinless						
1 pound of Raw untrimmed meat (includes separable fat) [74% separable lean, 26% separable fat]	1397	0.0	87.3	0.00		
Cooked (baked or roasted) [yield: approx. 10.9 oz.] (7g/0g/9g/49%/16mg)	1152	0.0	106.0	0.00	524	0.0
Trimmed of separable fat before cooking; Cooked (baked or roasted) [yield: approx. 8.1 oz.] (8g/0g/13g/59%/21mg)	495	0.0	61.5	0.00	304	0.0
1 pound of Cooked (baked or roasted) meat:						
Yield from approx. 23 oz. (1 lb. 7 oz.) of raw untrimmed meat that had ***not*** been trimmed of separable fat before cooking	1696	0.0	106.0	0.00	524	0.0
Yield from approx. 32 oz. (2 lbs.) of raw untrimmed meat that ***had*** been trimmed of separable fat before cooking	984	0.0	61.5	0.00	304	0.0
1 cup of Cooked (baked or roasted) meat, with separable fat:						
Chopped or diced (approx. 4.9 oz.)	524	0.0	106.0	0.00	524	0.0
Ground (approx. 3.9 oz.)	411	0.0	106.0	0.00		
1 cup of Cooked (baked or roasted) meat, trimmed of separable fat:						
Chopped or diced (approx. 4.9 oz.)	304	0.0	61.5	0.00	304	0.0
Ground (approx. 3.9 oz.)	0.0	0.0	61.5	0.00		
LOIN						
Bone-in, with skin						
1 pound of Raw untrimmed meat (includes separable fat) with bone and skin [63% separable lean, 16% separable fat, 21% bone and skin]	1065	0.0	66.6	0.00		
Cooked (baked or roasted) [yield: approx. 12 oz., of which approx. 8.6 oz. are meat and approx. 3.4 oz. are bone and skin]	883	0.0	73.6	0.00		
Trimmed of separable fat before cooking; Cooked (baked or roasted) [yield: approx. 10.3 oz., of which approx. 6.9 oz. are meat and approx. 3.4 oz. are bone and skin]	495	0.0	48.1	0.00		
1 pound of Cooked (baked or roasted) meat (weight includes bone and skin)						
Yield from approx. 21 oz. (1 lb. 5 oz.) of raw untrimmed meat (weighed with the bone and skin) that had ***not*** been trimmed of separable fat before cooking	1177	0.0	73.6	0.00		
Yield from approx. 25 oz. (1 lb. 9 oz.) of raw untrimmed meat (weighed with the bone and skin) that ***had*** been trimmed of separable fat before cooking	769	0.0	48.1	0.00		
Boneless, skinless						
1 pound of Raw untrimmed meat (includes separable fat) [80% separable lean, 20% separable fat]	1352	0.0	84.5	0.00		
Cooked (baked or roasted) [yield: approx. 10.9 oz.] (7g/0g/8g/46%/17mg)	1115	0.0	102.6	0.00	507	0.0
Trimmed of separable fat before cooking; Cooked (baked or roasted) [yield: approx. 8.7 oz.] (8g/0g/4g/55%/20mg)	627	0.0	72.0	0.00	356	0.0
1 pound of Cooked (baked or roasted) meat:						
Yield from approx. 23 oz. (1 lb. 7 oz.) of raw untrimmed meat that had ***not*** been trimmed of separable fat before cooking	1642	0.0	102.6	0.00	507	0.0

	UNIT		1 OZ., BY WT.		1 CUP, DICED, NOT PACKED	
	Cal.	Carb.	Cal.	Carb.	Cal.	Carb.
Yield from approx. 29 oz. (1 lb. 13 oz.) of raw untrimmed meat that ***had*** been trimmed of separable fat before cooking	1152	0.0	72.0	0.00	356	0.0
LOIN CHOPS						
Bone-in, with skin						
1 pound of Raw untrimmed meat (includes separable fat) with bone and skin [63% separable lean, 16% separable fat, 21% bone and skin]	1065	0.0	66.6	0.00		
Cooked (baked or roasted) [yield: approx. 11.6 oz., of which approx. 8.2 oz. are meat and approx. 3.4 oz. are bone and skin]	911	0.0	78.5	0.00		
Trimmed of separable fat before cooking; Cooked (baked or roasted) [yield: approx. 9.3 oz., of which approx. 5.9 oz. are meat and approx. 3.4 oz. are bone and skin]	454	0.0	48.8	0.00		
1 chop, Raw untrimmed meat (includes separable fat) with bone and skin [63% separable lean, 16% separable fat, 21% bone and skin] approx. 5.3 oz.	353	0.0	66.6	0.00		
Cooked (baked or roasted) [yield: approx. 3.8 oz., of which approx. 2.7 oz. are meat and approx. 1.1 oz. are bone and skin]	305	0.0	78.5	0.00		
Trimmed of separable fat before cooking; Cooked (baked or roasted) [yield: approx. 3.1 oz., of which approx. 2 oz. are meat and approx. 1.1 oz. are bone and skin]	151	0.0	48.8	0.00		
1 chop, Raw untrimmed meat (includes separable fat) with bone and skin [63% separable lean, 16% separable fat, 21% bone and skin] approx. 4 oz.	266	0.0	66.6	0.00		
Cooked (baked or roasted) [yield: approx. 2.8 oz., of which approx. 2 oz. are meat and approx. 0.8 oz. are bone and skin]	227	0.0	78.5	0.00		
Trimmed of separable fat before cooking; Cooked (baked or roasted) [yield: approx. 2.3 oz., of which approx. 1.5 oz. are meat and approx. 0.8 oz. are bone and skin]	113	0.0	48.8	0.00		
1 pound of Cooked (baked or roasted) meat (weight includes bone and skin)						
Yield from approx. 22 oz. (1 lb. 6 oz.) of raw untrimmed meat (weighed with the bone and skin) that had ***not*** been trimmed of separable fat before cooking	1257	0.0	78.5	0.00		
Yield from approx. 28 oz. (1 lb. 12 oz.) of raw untrimmed meat (weighed with the bone and skin) that ***had*** been trimmed of separable fat before cooking	781	0.0	48.8	0.00		
Boneless, skinless						
1 pound of Raw untrimmed meat (includes separable fat) [80% separable lean, 20% separable fat]	1352	0.0	84.5	0.00		
Cooked (baked or roasted) [yield: approx. 10.4 oz.] (7g/0g/9g/42%/17mg)	1153	0.0	110.8	0.00	(550)	0.0
Trimmed of separable fat before cooking; Cooked (baked or roasted) [yield: approx. 7.5 oz.] (9g/0g/4g/53%/21mg)	572	0.0	76.5	0.00	(380)	0.0
1 chop, Raw untrimmed meat (includes separable fat) [80% separable lean, 20% separable fat] approx. 4.2 oz.	353	0.0	84.5	0.00		
Cooked (baked or roasted) [yield: approx. 2.7 oz.]	305	0.0	110.8	0.00	(550)	0.0
Trimmed of separable fat before cooking; Cooked (baked or roasted) [yield: approx. 2 oz.]	151	0.0	76.5	0.00	(380)	0.0
1 chop, Raw untrimmed meat (includes separable fat) [80% separable lean, 20% separable fat] approx. 3.2 oz.	266	0.0	84.5	0.00		
Cooked (baked or roasted) [yield: approx. 2 oz.]	227	0.0	110.8		(550)	0.0
Trimmed of separable fat before cooking; Cooked (baked or roasted) [yield: approx. 1.5 oz.]	113	0.0	76.5	0.00	(380)	0.0
1 pound of Cooked (baked or roasted) meat:						
Yield from approx. 25 oz. (1 lb. 9 oz.) of raw untrimmed meat that had ***not*** been trimmed of separable fat before cooking	1773	0.0	110.8	0.00	(550)	0.0
Yield from approx. 34 oz. (2 lb. 2 oz.) of raw untrimmed meat that ***had*** been trimmed of separable fat before cooking	1224	0.0	76.5	0.00	(380)	0.0
SHOULDER CUTS						
BOSTON BUTT:						
Bone-in, with skin						
1 pound of Raw untrimmed meat (includes separable fat) with bone and skin [74% separable lean, 20% separable fat, 6% bone and skin]	1220	0.0	76.3	0.00		

	UNIT		1 OZ., BY WT.		1 CUP, DICED, NOT PACKED	
	Cal.	Carb.	Cal.	Carb.	Cal.	Carb.
Cooked (roasted) [yield: approx. 11.2 oz., of which approx. 10.2 oz. are meat and approx. 1 oz. bone and skin]	1024	0.0	91.4	0.00		
Trimmed of separable fat before cooking; Cooked (roasted) [yield: approx. 9.1 oz., of which approx. 8.1 oz. are meat and approx. 1 oz. bone and skin]	559	0.0	61.4	0.00		
1 pound of Cooked (roasted) meat (weight includes bone and skin):						
Yield from approx. 23 oz. (1 lb. 7 oz.) of raw untrimmed meat (weighed with the bone and skin) that had ***not*** been trimmed of separable fat before cooking	1463	0.0	91.4	0.00		
Yield from approx. 28 oz. (1 lb. 12 oz.) of raw untrimmed meat (weighed with the bone and skin) that ***had*** been trimmed of separable fat before cooking	983	0.0	61.4	0.00		
Boneless, skinless						
1 pound of Raw untrimmed meat (includes separable fat) [79% separable lean, 21% separable fat]	1302	0.0	81.4	0.00		
Cooked (roasted) [yield: approx. 10.9 oz.] (6g/0g/8g/48%/16mg)	1087	0.0	100.1	0.00	494	0.0
Trimmed of separable fat before cooking; Cooked (baked or roasted) [yield: approx. 8.6 oz.] (8g/0g/4g/58%/19mg)	595	0.0	69.2	0.00	342	0.0
1 pound of Cooked (roasted) meat:						
Yield from approx. 23 oz. (1 lb. 7 oz.) of raw untrimmed meat that had ***not*** been trimmed of separable fat before cooking	1601	0.0	100.1	0.00	494	0.0
Yield from approx. 30 oz. (1 lb. 14 oz.) of raw untrimmed meat that ***had*** been trimmed of separable fat before cooking	1107	0.0	69.2	0.00	342	0.0
1 cup of Cooked (roasted) meat, including separable fat:						
Chopped or diced (approx. 4.9 oz.)	494	0.0	100.1	0.00	494	0.0
Ground (approx. 3.9 oz.)	388	0.0	100.1	0.00		
1 cup of Cooked (roasted) meat, trimmed of separable fat:						
Chopped or diced (approx. 4.9 oz.)	342	0.0	69.2	0.00	342	0.0
Ground (approx. 3.9 oz.)	268	0.0	69.2	0.00		
PICNIC:						
Bone-in, with skin						
1 pound of Raw untrimmed meat (includes separable fat) with bone and skin [61% separable lean, 22% separable fat, 17% bone and skin]	1083	0.0	67.7	0.00		
Cooked (simmered) [yield: approx. 11.3 oz., of which approx. 8.4 oz. are meat and approx. 2.9 oz. are bone and skin]	890	0.0	78.8	0.00		
Trimmed of separable fat before cooking; Cooked (simmered) [yield: approx. 9.1 oz., of which approx. 6.2 oz. are meat and approx. 2.9 oz. are bone and skin]	373	0.0	41.0	0.00		
1 pound of Cooked (simmered) meat (weight includes bone and skin):						
Yield from approx. 23 oz. (1 lb. 7 oz.) of raw untrimmed meat (weighed with the bone and skin) that had ***not*** been trimmed of separable fat before cooking	1261	0.0	78.8	0.00		
Yield from approx. 28 oz. (1 lb. 12 oz.) of raw untrimmed meat (weighed with the bone and skin) that ***had*** been trimmed of separable fat before cooking	656	0.0	41.0	0.00		
Boneless, skinless						
1 pound of Raw untrimmed meat (includes separable fat) [74% separable lean, 26% separable fat]	1315	0.0	82.2	0.00		
Cooked (simmered) [yield: approx. 10.2 oz.] (7g/0g/9g/46%/12mg)	1085	0.0	106.0	0.00	524	0.0
Trimmed of separable fat before cooking; Cooked (simmered) [yield: approx. 7.6 oz.] (8g/0g/3g/60%/14mg)	456	0.0	60.1	0.00	297	0.0
1 pound of Cooked (simmered) meat:						
Yield from approx. 25 oz. (1 lb. 9 oz.) of raw untrimmed meat that had ***not*** been trimmed of separable fat before cooking	1696	0.0	106.0	0.00	524	0.0
Yield from approx. 34 oz. (2 lb. 2 oz.) of raw untrimmed meat that ***had*** been trimmed of separable fat before cooking	962	0.0	60.1	0.00	297	0.0
SPARERIBS						
Bone-in						
1 pound of Raw untrimmed meat (includes separable fat) with bone [refuse: bone, approx. 40%]	976	0.0	61.0	0.00		
Cooked (braised) [yield: approx. 12.7 oz., of which approx. 6.3 oz. are meat and approx. 6.4 oz. are bone]	782	0.0	61.6	0.00		

	UNIT		1 OZ., BY WT.		1 CUP, DICED, NOT PACKED	
	Cal.	Carb.	Cal.	Carb.	Cal.	Carb.
1 pound of cooked (braised) meat (weight includes bone):						
Yield from approx. 20 oz. (1 lb. 4 oz.) of raw untrimmed meat (weighed with the bone) that had ***not*** been trimmed of separable fat before cooking	986	0.0	61.6	0.00		
Boneless						
1 pound of Raw untrimmed meat (includes separable fat)	1627	0.0	101.7	0.00		
Cooked (braised) [yield: approx. 10.5 oz.] (6g/0g/11g/40%/10mg)	1303	0.0	124.1	0.00		
1 pound of cooked (braised) meat:						
Yield from approx. 24 oz. (1 lb. 8 oz.) of raw untrimmed meat that had ***not*** been trimmed of separable fat before cooking	1986	0.0	124.1	0.00		
Spareribs, lean (based on data from East Asia)						
Bone-in						
1 pound of cooked spareribs [refuse: bone, approx. 27%]	885	0.0	55.3	0.00		
Boneless						
1 pound of cooked spareribs	1216	0.0	76.0	0.00		

Cured Pork

CURED HAM

	UNIT		1 OZ., BY WT.		1 CUP, DICED, NOT PACKED	
	Cal.	Carb.	Cal.	Carb.	Cal.	Carb.
Dry, long cure, country style:						
Bone-in, with skin						
1 pound of Raw untrimmed meat (medium fatness, includes separable fat) with bone and skin [87% meat and separable fat, 13% bone and skin]	1535	1.2	95.9	0.07		
1 pound of Raw untrimmed meat (relatively lean, includes some separable fat) with bone and skin [86% meat and separable fat, 14% bone and skin]	1209	1.2	75.6	0.07		
Boneless, skinless						
1 pound of untrimmed meat (medium fatness, includes separable fat) (5g/tr/10g/42%/na)	1764	1.4	110.3	0.09		
1 pound of untrimmed meat (relatively lean, includes some separable fat) (6g/tr/7g/49%/na)	1406	1.4	87.9	0.09		
Light cure, commercial:						
Bone-in, with skin						
1 pound of Raw untrimmed meat (includes separable fat) with bone and skin [65% separable lean, 21% separable fat, 14% bone and skin]	1100	0.0	68.8	0.00		
Cooked (baked or roasted) [yield: approx. 13.5 oz., of which approx. 11.3 oz. are meat and approx. 2.2 oz. are bone and skin]	925	0.0	68.5	0.00		
Trimmed of separable fat before cooking; Cooked (baked or roasted) [yield: approx. 10.9 oz., of which approx. 8.7 oz. are meat and approx. 2.2 oz. are bone and skin]	460	0.0	42.2	0.00		
1 pound of Cooked (baked or roasted) meat (weight includes bone and skin):						
Yield from approx. 19 oz. (1 lb. 3 oz.) of raw untrimmed meat (weighed with the bone and skin) that had ***not*** been trimmed of separable fat before cooking	1096	0.0	68.5	0.00		
Yield from approx. 24 oz. (1 lb. 8 oz.) of raw untrimmed meat (weighed with the bone and skin) that had ***not*** been trimmed of separable fat before cooking	675	0.0	42.2	0.00		
Boneless, skinless						
1 pound of Raw untrimmed meat (includes separable fat) [76% separable lean, 24% separable fat]	1279	0.0	79.9	0.00		
Cooked (baked or roasted) [yield: approx. 13.1 oz.] (6g/0g/6g/54%/212mg)	1075	0.0	81.9	0.00	405	0.0
Trimmed of separable fat before cooking; Cooked (baked or roasted) [yield: approx. 10.2 oz.] (7g/0g/2g/62%/257mg)	539	0.0	53.0	0.00	262	0.0
1 pound of Cooked (baked or roasted) meat:						
Yield from approx. 20 oz. (1 lb. 4 oz.) of raw untrimmed meat that had ***not*** been trimmed of separable fat before cooking	1311	0.0	81.9	0.00	405	0.0
Yield from approx. 25 oz. (1 lb. 9 oz.) of raw untrimmed meat that ***had*** been trimmed of separable fat before cooking	848	0.0	53.0	0.00	262	0.0
1 cup of Cooked (baked or roasted) meat, trimmed of separable fat:						
Chopped or diced (approx. 4.9 oz.)	262	0.0	81.9	0.00	262	0.0
Ground (approx. 3.9 oz.)	206	0.0	53.0	0.00		

	UNIT Cal.	UNIT Carb.	1 OZ., BY WT. Cal.	1 OZ., BY WT. Carb.	1 CUP, DICED, NOT PACKED Cal.	1 CUP, DICED, NOT PACKED Carb.
CURED SHOULDER CUTS (Light cure, commercial)						
BOSTON BUTT:						
Bone-in, with skin						
1 pound of Raw untrimmed meat (includes separable fat) with bone and skin [70% separable lean, 23% separable fat, 7% bone and skin]	1227	0.0	76.7	0.00		
Cooked (baked or roasted) [yield: approx. 12.1 oz., of which approx. 11 oz. are meat and approx. 1.1 oz. are bone and skin]	1030	0.0	85.1	0.00		
Trimmed of separable fat before cooking; Cooked (baked or roasted) [yield: approx. 10.2 oz., of which approx. 9.1 oz. are meat and approx. 1.1 oz. are bone and skin]	629	0.0	52.0	0.00		
1 pound of Cooked (baked or roasted) meat (weight includes bone and skin):						
Yield from approx. 21 oz. (1 lb. 5 oz.) of raw untrimmed meat (weighed with the bone and skin) that had ***not*** been trimmed of separable fat before cooking	1362	0.0	85.1	0.00		
Yield from approx. 25 oz. (1 lb. 9 oz.) of raw untrimmed meat (weighed with the bone and skin) that ***had*** been trimmed of separable fat before cooking	832	0.0	52.0	0.00		
Boneless, skinless						
1 pound of Raw untrimmed meat (includes separable fat) [75% separable lean, 25% separable fat]	1320	0.0	82.5	0.00		
Cooked (baked or roasted) [yield: approx. 11.8 oz.] (6g/0g/7g/48%/233mg)	1109	0.0	93.6	0.00	462	0.0
Trimmed of separable fat before cooking; Cooked (baked or roasted) [yield: approx. 9.8 oz.] (8g/0g/4g/54%/282mg)	678	0.0	68.9	0.00	340	0.0
1 pound of Cooked (baked or roasted) meat:						
Yield from approx. 22 oz. (1 lb. 6 oz.) of raw untrimmed meat that had ***not*** been trimmed of separable fat before cooking	1497	0.0	93.6	0.00	462	0.0
Yield from approx. 26 oz. (1 lb. 10 oz.) of raw untrimmed meat that ***had*** been trimmed of separable fat before cooking	1102	0.0	68.9	0.00	340	0.0
1 cup of Cooked (baked or roasted) meat, trimmed of separable fat:						
Chopped or diced (approx. 4.9 oz.)	340	0.0	68.9	0.00	340	0.0
Ground (approx. 3.9 oz.)	267	0.0	68.9	0.00		
PICNIC:						
Bone-in, with skin						
1 pound of Raw untrimmed meat (includes separable fat) with bone and skin [57% separable lean, 25% separable fat, 18% bone and skin]	1060	0.0	66.3	0.00		
Cooked (baked or roasted) [yield: approx. 12.6 oz., of which approx. 9.7 oz. are meat and approx. 2.9 oz. are bone and skin]	888	0.0	70.5	0.00		
Trimmed of separable fat before cooking; Cooked (baked or roasted) [yield: approx. 9.7 oz., of which approx. 6.8 oz. are meat and approx. 2.9 oz. are bone and skin]	405	0.0	41.8	0.00		
1 pound of Cooked (baked or roasted) meat (weight includes bone and skin):						
Yield from approx. 20 oz. (1 lb. 4 oz.) of raw untrimmed meat (weighed with the bone and skin) that had ***not*** been trimmed of separable fat before cooking	1128	0.0	70.5	0.00		
Yield from approx. 26 oz. (1 lb. 10 oz.) of raw untrimmed meat (weighed with the bone and skin) that ***had*** been trimmed of separable fat before cooking	668	0.0	41.8	0.00		
Boneless, skinless						
1 pound of Raw untrimmed meat (includes separable fat) [70% separable lean, 30% separable fat]	1293	0.0	80.0	0.00		
Cooked (baked or roasted) [yield: approx. 11.8 oz.] (6g/0g/7g/49%/227mg)	1085	0.0	91.6	0.00	452	0.0
Trimmed of separable fat before cooking; Cooked (baked or roasted) [yield: approx. 8.3 oz.] (8g/0g/3g/57%/288mg)	496	0.0	59.8	0.00	295	0.0
1 pound of Cooked (baked or roasted) meat:						
Yield from approx. 22 oz. (1 lb. 6 oz.) of raw untrimmed meat that had ***not*** been trimmed of separable fat before cooking	1465	0.0	91.6	0.00	452	0.0
Yield from approx. 31 oz. (1 lb. 15 oz.) of raw untrimmed meat that ***had*** been trimmed of separable fat before cooking	957	0.0	59.8	0.00	295	0.0
1 cup of Cooked (baked or roasted) meat, trimmed of separable fat:						
Chopped or diced (approx. 4.9 oz.)	295	0.0	59.8	0.00	295	0.0
Ground (approx. 3.9 oz.)	232	0.0	59.8	0.00		

Pork Organ Meats

A list that compares the organ meats of Beef, Lamb, Pork, and Veal begins below.

All cooked values are for lean meat, both measured and cooked after all separable fat has been removed.

	UNIT Cal.	UNIT Carb.	1 OZ., BY WT. Cal.	1 OZ., BY WT. Carb.	1 CUP, DICED, NOT PACKED Cal.	1 CUP, DICED, NOT PACKED Carb.
BRAINS:						
Raw, 1 pound	567	3.6	35.4	0.23		
Cooked:						
1 pound of cooked brains (4g/tr/3g/76%/na)	590	(3.6)	36.9	(0.23)		
CHITTERLINGS:						
Raw, 1 pound	1021	0.0	63.8	0.00		
HEART:						
Raw, 1 pound	522	1.8	32.6	0.11		
Cooked:						
1 pound of raw heart, cooked [yield: approx. 9.0 oz.]	366	0.8	40.8	0.09		
1 pound of cooked heart (9g/tr/2g/61%/na)	654	1.4	40.8	0.09		
KIDNEYS:						
Raw, 1 pound	454	5.0	28.4	0.31		
Cooked:						
1 pound of raw kidneys, cooked [yield: approx. 8.0 oz.]	342	3.8	42.8	0.47		
1 pound of cooked kidneys (7g/tr/1g/69%/na)	685	7.5	42.8	0.47		
LIVER:						
Raw, 1 pound	586	11.8	36.6	0.74		
Cooked:						
1 pound of raw liver, cooked [yield: approx. 10.6 oz.]	404	7.5	38.3	0.71		
1 pound of cooked liver (8g/1g/3g/54%/na)	613	11.3	38.3	0.71		
LUNG:						
Raw, 1 pound	377	0.0	23.5	0.00		
Cooked:						
1 pound of cooked lung (5g/0g/1g/78%/na)	449	0.0	28.1	0.00		
PANCREAS (Sweetbreads):						
Raw, 1 pound	840	0.0	52.4	0.00		
Cooked:						
1 pound of cooked pancreas (8g/0g/3g/62%/na)	994	0.0	62.1	0.00		
SPLEEN:						
Raw, 1 pound	454	0.0	28.4	0.00		
Cooked:						
1 pound of cooked spleen (8g/0g/1g/65%/na)	676	0.0	42.2	0.00		
TONGUE:						
Raw, 1 pound	1008	1.7	63.0	0.11		
Cooked:						
1 pound of raw tongue, cooked [yield: approx. 10.4 oz.]	797	1.4	76.6	0.14		
1 pound of cooked tongue (6g/tr/5g/59%/na)	1226	2.3	76.6	0.14		

ORGAN MEATS OF BEEF, LAMB, PORK, AND VEAL

All cooked values are for lean meat, both measured and cooked after all separable fat has been removed.

	UNIT Cal.	UNIT Carb.	1 OZ., BY WT. Cal.	1 OZ., BY WT. Carb.	1 CUP, DICED, NOT PACKED Cal.	1 CUP, DICED, NOT PACKED Carb.
BRAINS						
Average, all common kinds (beef, calf, hog, sheep), 1 pound (3g/tr/3g/74%/na)	567	3.6	35.4	0.23		
BEEF BRAINS:						
Raw, 1 pound	554	3.6	34.6	0.23		
Cooked:						
1 pound of cooked beef brains (3g/tr/3g/78%/na)	590	(3.6)	36.9	(0.23)		
LAMB BRAINS:						
Raw, 1 pound	540	3.6	33.7	0.23		
Cooked:						
1 pound of cooked lamb brains (4g/tr/3g/76%/na)	622	(3.6)	38.8	(0.23)		
PORK BRAINS:						
Raw, 1 pound	567	3.6	35.4	0.23		
Cooked:						
1 pound of cooked pork brains (4g/tr/3g/76%/na)	590	(3.6)	36.9	(0.23)		

	Unit Cal.	Unit Carb.	1 Oz., by Wt. Cal.	1 Oz., by Wt. Carb.	1 Cup, Diced, Not Packed Cal.	1 Cup, Diced, Not Packed Carb.
VEAL BRAINS:						
Raw, 1 pound	477	3.6	29.8	0.23		
Cooked:						
1 pound of cooked veal brains (3g/tr/2g/80%/na)	504	(3.6)	31.5	(0.23)		
CHITTERLINGS						
PORK:						
Raw, 1 pound	1021	0.0	63.8	0.00		
HEART						
BEEF HEART:						
Raw, 1 pound	499	3.2	31.2	0.20		
Cooked:						
1 pound of raw beef heart, cooked [yield: approx. 9.3 oz.]	468	1.9	50.2	0.20		
1 pound of cooked beef heart (9g/tr/2g/61%/na)	804	3.2	50.2	0.20		
LAMB HEART:						
Raw, 1 pound	567	4.5	35.4	0.28		
Cooked:						
1 pound of raw lamb heart, cooked [yield: approx. 9.0 oz.]	356	2.5	39.7	0.28		
1 pound of cooked lamb heart (9g/tr/2g/61%/na)	636	4.5	39.7	0.28		
PORK HEART:						
Raw, 1 pound	522	1.8	32.6	0.11		
Cooked:						
1 pound of raw pork heart, cooked [yield: approx. 9.0 oz.]	368	0.8	40.8	0.09		
1 pound of cooked pork heart (9g/tr/2g/61%/na)	654	1.4	40.8	0.09		
VEAL HEART:						
Raw, 1 pound	495	8.2	30.9	0.51		
Cooked:						
1 pound of raw veal heart, cooked [yield: approx. 9.4 oz.]	410	6.8	43.4	0.72		
1 pound of cooked veal heart (8g/1g/3g/60%/na)	695	11.5	43.4	0.72		
KIDNEYS						
BEEF KIDNEYS:						
Raw, 1 pound	454	0.5	28.4	0.03		
Cooked:						
1 pound of raw beef kidneys, cooked [yield: approx. 8.0 oz.]	313	2.1	39.1	0.26		
1 pound of cooked beef kidneys (9g/tr/3g/53%/na)	626	4.1	39.1	0.26		
LAMB KIDNEYS:						
Raw, 1 pound	436	4.1	27.2	0.26		
Cooked:						
1 pound of raw lamb kidneys, cooked [yield: approx. 8.0 oz.]	293	3.2	36.6	0.40		
1 pound of cooked lamb kidneys (6g/tr/1g/62%/na)	586	6.2	36.6	0.40		
PORK KIDNEYS:						
Raw, 1 pound	454	5.0	28.4	0.31		
Cooked:						
1 pound of raw pork kidneys, cooked [yield: approx. 8.0 oz.]	342	3.8	42.8	0.47		
1 pound of cooked pork kidneys (7g/tr/1g/69%/na)	685	7.5	42.8	0.47		
VEAL KIDNEYS:						
Raw, 1 pound	472	0.5	29.5	0.03		
Cooked:						
1 pound of raw veal kidneys, cooked [yield: approx. 8.0 oz.]	374	0.2	46.8	0.03		
1 pound of cooked veal kidneys (7g/tr/1g/70%/na)	749	(0.5)	46.8	(0.03)		
LIVER						
BEEF LIVER:						
Raw, 1 pound	595	24.0	37.1	1.50		
Cooked:						
1 pound of raw beef liver, cooked [yield: approx. 11.8 oz.]	459	17.8	38.8	1.50		
1 pound of cooked beef liver (7g/2g/3g/56%/na)	622	24.0	38.8	1.50		
LAMB LIVER:						
Raw, 1 pound	717	13.2	44.8	0.83		
Cooked:						
1 pound of raw lamb liver, cooked [yield: approx. 9.8 oz.]	550	8.9	56.4	0.91		
1 pound of cooked lamb liver (9g/1g/4g/54%/na)	903	14.5	56.4	0.91		
PORK LIVER:						
Raw, 1 pound	586	11.8	36.6	0.74		
Cooked:						
1 pound of raw pork liver, cooked [yield: approx. 10.6 oz.]	404	7.5	38.3	0.71		
1 pound of cooked pork liver (8g/1g/3g/54%/na)	613	11.3	38.3	0.71		
VEAL (CALF'S) LIVER:						
Raw, 1 pound	636	18.6	39.7	1.16		
Cooked:						
1 pound of raw veal liver, cooked [yield: approx. 10.2 oz.]	465	11.6	45.4	1.13		
1 pound of cooked veal liver (8g/1g/4g/51%/na)	726	18.1	45.4	1.13		
LUNG						
BEEF LUNG:						
Raw, 1 pound	458	0.0	28.6	0.00		
Cooked:						
1 pound of cooked beef lung (6g/0g/1g/78%/na)	545	0.0	34.0	0.00		
LAMB LUNG:						
Raw, 1 pound	441	0.0	27.5	0.00		
Cooked:						
1 pound of cooked lamb lung (5g/0g/3g/78%/na)	527	0.0	32.9	0.00		
PORK LUNG:						
Raw, 1 pound	377	0.0	23.5	0.00		
Cooked:						
1 pound of cooked pork lung (5g/0g/1g/78%/na)	449	0.0	28.1	0.00		
VEAL LUNG:						
Raw, 1 pound	418	0.0	26.1	0.00		
Cooked:						
1 pound of cooked veal lung (5g/0g/1g/79%/na)	472	0.0	29.5	0.00		
PANCREAS (Sweetbreads)						
BEEF PANCREAS:						
Raw, 1 pound	935	0.0	58.4	0.00		
Cooked:						
1 pound of cooked beef pancreas (8g/0g/3g/62%/na)	1230	0.0	76.8	0.00		
LAMB PANCREAS:						
Raw, 1 pound	713	0.0	44.5	0.00		
Cooked:						
1 pound of cooked lamb pancreas (7g/0g/1g/76%/na)	844	0.0	52.7	0.00		
PORK PANCREAS:						
Raw, 1 pound	840	0.0	52.4	0.00		
Cooked:						
1 pound of cooked pork pancreas (8g/0g/3g/62%/na)	994	0.0	62.1	0.00		
VEAL PANCREAS:						
Raw, 1 pound	931	0.0	58.1	0.00		
Cooked:						
1 pound of cooked veal pancreas (8g/0g/5g/52%/na)	1162	0.0	72.6	0.00		
SPLEEN						
BEEF SPLEEN:						
Raw, 1 pound	468	0.0	29.2	0.00		
Cooked:						
1 pound of cooked beef spleen (8g/0g/1g/68%/na)	658	0.0	41.1	0.00		
LAMB SPLEEN:						
Raw, 1 pound	463	0.0	28.9	0.00		
Cooked:						
1 pound of cooked lamb spleen (8g/0g/1g/65%/na)	681	0.0	42.5	0.00		
PORK SPLEEN:						
Raw, 1 pound	454	0.0	28.4	0.00		
Cooked:						
1 pound of cooked pork spleen (8g/0g/1g/65%/na)	676	0.0	42.2	0.00		
VEAL SPLEEN:						
Raw, 1 pound	449	0.0	28.1	0.00		
Cooked:						
1 pound of cooked veal spleen (7g/tr/1g/75%/na)	567	0.0	35.4	0.00		

	UNIT		1 OZ., BY WT.		1 CUP, DICED, NOT PACKED	
	Cal.	Carb.	Cal.	Carb.	Cal.	Carb.
THYMUS (Sweetbreads)						
BEEF THYMUS:						
Raw, 1 pound	1117	0.0	69.7	0.00		
Cooked:						
1 pound of raw beef thymus, cooked [yield: approx. 9.3 oz.]	821	0.0	88.5	0.00		
1 pound of cooked beef thymus (7g/0g/7g/50%/na)	1416	0.0	88.5	0.00		
VEAL THYMUS:						
Raw, 1 pound	445	0.0	27.8	0.00		
Cooked:						
1 pound of raw veal thymus, cooked [yield: approx. 9.3 oz.]	277	0.0	29.8	0.00		
1 pound of cooked veal thymus (9g/0g/1g/73%/na)	477	0.0	29.8	0.00		
TONGUE						
BEEF TONGUE:						
Raw, 1 pound	1035	1.4	64.6	0.09		
Cooked:						
1 pound of raw beef tongue, cooked [yield: approx. 12.5 oz.]	1020	1.4	81.7	0.11		
1 pound of cooked beef tongue (6g/tr/5g/61%/na)	1307	1.8	81.7	0.11		
LAMB TONGUE:						
Raw, 1 pound	1012	1.7	63.2	0.11		
Cooked:						
1 pound of raw lamb tongue, cooked [yield: approx. 12.8 oz.]	1005	1.7	78.5	0.14		
1 pound of cooked lamb tongue (6g/tr/5g/60%/na)	1258	2.3	78.5	0.14		
PORK TONGUE:						
Raw, 1 pound	1008	1.7	63.0	0.11		
Cooked:						
1 pound of raw pork tongue, cooked [yield: approx. 10.4 oz.]	797	1.4	76.6	0.14		
1 pound of cooked pork tongue (6g/tr/5g/59%/na)	1226	2.3	76.6	0.14		
VEAL TONGUE:						
Raw, 1 pound	604	3.1	37.7	0.19		
Cooked:						
1 pound of raw veal tongue, cooked [yield: approx. 11.1 oz.]	590	3.1	53.0	0.28		
1 pound of cooked veal tongue (7g/tr/2g/69%/na)	849	4.5	53.0	0.28		
TRIPE						
BEEF TRIPE:						
Raw, 1 pound	536	0.0	33.4	0.00		
LAMB TRIPE:						
Raw, 1 pound	567	0.0	35.4	0.00		
VEAL TRIPE:						
Raw, 1 pound	672	0.0	42.0	0.00		

FROZEN MEATS

	Cal.	Carb.	Cal.	Carb.	Cal.	Carb.
BEEF						
Table Treats all beef Handyburgers, 30-oz. package, approx. 10 burgers	2200	0.0	73.3	0.00		
1 burger, approx. 3 oz.	220	0.0	73.3	0.00		
Steak-Umm flaked, chopped, formed, thinly sliced Sandwich Steaks, 10-oz. box	800	0.00	80.0	0.00		
14-oz. box, approx. 7 slices	1120	0.0	80.0	0.00		
1 slice, approx. 2 oz.	160	0.0	80.0	0.00		
32-oz. (2-lb.) box, approx. 16 slices	2560	0.0	80.0	0.00		
1 slice, approx. 2 oz.	160	0.0	80.0	0.00		
VEAL						
Table Treats flaked, chopped, and formed, beef added, breaded Veal Steaks, frozen, 16-oz. (1-lb.) box, approx. 4 steaks	880	72.0	55.0	4.50		
1 veal steak, approx. 4 oz.	220	18.0	55.0	4.50		
PORK						
Swift Premium fully cooked Ham Patties, 120-oz. (7½-lb.) carton, approx. 76 patties	19048	76.2	119.0	0.48		
1 patty, approx. 2.1 oz.	250	1.0	119.0	0.48		

CANNED, JARRED, OR PREPACKAGED MEATS

	Cal.	Carb.	Cal.	Carb.	Cal.	Carb.
BEEF						
Armour Chopped Beef, 12-oz. container	1160	12.0	96.6	1.00		
Armour sliced Dried Beef, 2½-oz. jar	120	1.0	48.0	0.40		
5-oz. jar	240	2.0	48.0	0.40		
Hormel creamed Dried Beef, Short Orders, 7½-oz. can	160	9.0	21.3	1.20		
Swift Premium chunked and formed, wafer thin sliced Dried Beef, 3-oz. package	140	0.0	46.7	0.00		
CORNED BEEF						
(Corned Beef has its primary listing in the SAUSAGES & COLD CUTS chapter.)						
Dinty Moore Corned Beef, 12-oz. can	1260	0.0	105.0	0.00		
Libby's Corned Beef, 7-oz. can	476	4.0	68.7	0.57		
12-oz. can	815	6.5	67.0	0.54		
CORNED BEEF HASH and ROAST BEEF HASH, see the COMBINATION MAIN DISHES chapter						
HAM						
(HAM has its primary listing in the SAUSAGES & COLD CUTS chapter.)						
WHOLE HAM:						
Cure/81 Whole Ham, 16-oz. (1-lb.) package	773	0.0	48.3	0.00		
Curemaster Whole Ham, 2- to 3-lb. plastic bag	1120-1680	10.7-16.0	35.0	0.33		
Hormel Whole Ham, 3-lb. can	2360	0.0	49.2	0.00		
Bone-in Ham, 16- to 18-lb. package	(7610)-(8562)	0.0	51.7	0.00		
Oscar Mayer Whole Ham, boneless Jubilee, 1½-lb. can	840	0.0	35.0	0.00		
10-lb. can	5600	0.0	35.0	0.00		
SECTIONED AND FORMED HAM:						
Oscar Mayer Ham, sectioned & formed Jubilee, 3-lb. can	1624	2.7	33.8	0.06		
10-lb. can	5413	9.1	33.8	0.06		
CHOPPED HAM:						
Armour Chopped Ham, 12-oz. can	720	0.0	60.0	1.00		
Hormel Chopped Ham, 6-oz. can	540	0.0	90.0	0.00		
12-oz. can	840	0.0	90.0	0.00		
8-lb. can	11520	0.0	90.0	0.00		
PORK, see Sliced Pork and Gravy and Pork Brains in Milk Gravy in the COMBINATION MAIN DISHES chapter						
TRIPE						
Armour Beef Tripe, 24-oz. can	1240	12.0	51.7	0.50		
Libby's Tripe, 24-oz. can	1181	4.3	49.2	0.18		

GAME AND LESS FAMILIAR MEATS

	Cal.	Carb.	Cal.	Carb.	Cal.	Carb.
Alligator (based on data from Latin America)						
Semi-Dried edible portion, 1 pound	1052	0.0	65.8	0.00		
Antelope (based on data from Africa)						
Raw, edible portion, 1 pound	680	0.0	42.5	0.00		
Antelope, Royal (based on data from Ghana)						
Raw, edible portion, 1 pound	490	0.0	30.6	0.00		
Armadillo (based on data from Latin America)						
Raw, edible portion, 1 pound	780	0.0	48.8	0.00		
Bear, see Polar Bear						
Beaver (United States)						
Roasted, edible portion, 1 pound	1125	0.0	70.3	0.00		
Boar (based on data from East Asia)						
Raw, edible portion, 1 pound	667	0.0	41.7	0.00		
Boar (based on data from Japan)						
Raw, edible portion, 1 pound	667	0.0	41.7	0.00		
Buffalo (based on data from India)						
Raw, edible portion, 1 pound	481	9.1	30.1	0.57		
Bull-Frog (based on data from India)						
Raw, edible portion, 1 pound	372	0.0	23.2	0.00		
Bush Buck (based on data from Ghana)						
Raw, edible portion, 1 pound	535	0.0	33.5	0.00		
Camel (based on data from Africa)						
Raw, edible portion, 1 pound	1211	0.0	75.7	0.00		
Camel (based on data from the Middle East)						
Raw, edible portion, 1 pound	876	0.0	54.7	0.00		
Carabao or Water Buffalo (based on data from East Asia)						
Raw, edible portion, 1 pound	544	0.0	34.0	0.00		

	UNIT		1 OZ., BY WT.		1 CUP, DICED, NOT PACKED	
	Cal.	Carb.	Cal.	Carb.	Cal.	Carb.
Carabao or Water Buffalo (based on data from the Far East)						
Very lean meat, all visible fat removed, edible portion, 1 pound	481	9.1	30.1	0.57		
Caribou (based on data from Canada)						
Raw, edible portion, 1 pound	485	0.0	30.3	0.00		
Cooked, edible portion, 1 pound	798	0.0	49.9	0.00		
Cowhide (based on data from Ghana)						
Raw, edible portion, 1 pound	449	0.0	28.1	0.00		
Crocodile, narrow snouted (based on data from India)						
Edible portion, 1 pound	395	1.4	24.7	0.09		
Dhauns, see Bull-Frog						
Dog (based on data from East Asia)						
Raw, edible portion, 1 pound	1244	0.0	77.8	0.00		
Elephant (based on data from Ghana)						
Meat, raw, edible portion, 1 pound	1325	0.0	82.8	0.00		
Skin, raw, edible portion, 1 pound	1370	0.0	85.6	0.00		
Goat (based on data from East Asia)						
Raw:						
Lean:						
As purchased [refuse: bones, approx. 14%], 1 pound	745	0.0	46.5	0.00		
Edible portion, 1 pound	812	0.0	50.8	0.00		
Medium fat:						
As purchased [refuse: bones and trimming, approx. 19%], 1 pound	1312	0.0	101.3	0.00		
Edible portion, 1 pound	1621	0.0	101.3	0.00		
Fat:						
Edible portion, 1 pound	2461	0.0	153.7	0.00		
Goat (based on data from Japan)						
Raw, edible portion, 1 pound	558	0.5	34.9	0.03		
Goat Blood (based on data from East Asia)						
Coagulated, uncooked:						
As purchased, 1 pound	445	4.5	27.8	0.28		
Goat Brain (based on data from East Asia)						
Raw, edible portion, 1 pound	680	2.3	42.5	0.14		
Guinea Pig (based on data from Latin America)						
Raw, edible portion, 1 pound	436	0.0	27.3	0.00		
Hare (based on data from East Asia)						
Raw, edible portion, 1 pound	644	0.0	40.3	0.00		
Hare (based on data from France)						
Raw, edible portion, 1 pound	513	0.0	32.0	0.00		
Cooked (method unspecified), edible portion, 1 pound	667	0.0	41.7	0.00		
Hartebeest (based on data from Ghana)						
Raw, edible portion, 1 pound	608	0.0	38.0	0.00		
Hippopotamus (based on data from Africa)						
Dried, edible portion, 1 pound	1669	0.0	104.3	0.00		
Smoked, edible portion, 1 pound	1747	0.0	109.2	0.00		
Hog, see Red River Hog						
Horse (based on data from East Asia)						
Raw, edible portion, 1 pound	549	0.0	39.3	0.00		
Horse (based on data from Far East)						
Raw, lean, edible portion, 1 pound	536	4.1	33.5	0.26		
Horse (based on data from Japan)						
Raw, average, all cuts: Edible portion, 1 pound	568	4.4	35.5	0.28		
Horse Feathers (based on data from the Marx Bros.)						
Any amount	0	0.0	0.0	0.00		
Iguana (based on data from Africa)						
Raw, edible portion, 1 pound	513	0.0	32.1	0.00		
Iguana (based on data from Latin America)						
Raw, edible portion, 1 pound	508	0.0	31.8	0.00		
Monkey, Green (based on data from Ghana)						
Raw, edible portion, 1 pound	376	0.0	23.5	0.00		
Moose (based on data from Canada)						
Raw, edible portion, 1 pound	463	0.0	28.9	0.00		
Muskrat (United States)						
Roasted, edible portion, 1 pound	695	0.0	43.4	0.00		

	UNIT		1 OZ., BY WT.		1 CUP, DICED, NOT PACKED	
	Cal.	Carb.	Cal.	Carb.	Cal.	Carb.
Muskrat Porcupine (based on data from Canada)						
Raw, edible portion, 1 pound	472	0.0	29.5	0.00		
Cooked, edible portion, 1 pound	594	0.0	37.1	0.00		
Mutton (based on data from France)						
Chop						
Raw, edible portion, 1 pound	1021	0.0	63.8	0.00		
Leg						
Raw, edible portion, 1 pound	1061	0.0	66.3	0.00		
Shoulder						
Raw, edible portion, 1 pound	1311	0.0	81.9	0.00		
Opossum (United States)						
Roasted, edible portion, 1 pound	1003	0.0	62.7	0.00		
Polar Bear (based on data from Canada)						
Raw, edible portion, 1 pound	530	0.0	33.2	0.00		
Porcupine, see Muskrat Porcupine						
Rabbit (United States)						
Raw, edible portion, 1 pound	735	0.0	46.0	0.00		
Stewed, 1 pound of raw, ready-to-cook rabbit, cooked (yield: approx. 8.6 oz.)	529	0.0	61.5	0.00		
Rabbit (based on data from Australia)						
Baked, edible portion, 1 pound	926	0.0	57.9	0.00		
Stewed, edible portion, 1 pound	854	9.1	53.4	0.57		
Rabbit or Hare (based on data from Canada)						
Cooked, steamed, edible portion, 1 pound	880	0.0	55.0	0.00		
Rabbit (based on data from Denmark)						
Raw, edible portion, 1 pound	454	0.0	28.4	0.00		
Rabbit, Domesticated (based on data from East Asia)						
Raw, edible portion, 1 pound	594	0.0	37.1	0.00		
Rabbit, Domesticated (based on data from France)						
Raw, edible portion, 1 pound	699	2.7	43.7	0.17		
Rabbit, Wild (United States)						
Raw:						
Drawn [refuse: head, skin, feet, and bones, approx. 40%], 1 pound	367	0.0	22.9	0.00		
Ready-to-Cook [refuse: bones, approx. 20%], 1 pound	490	0.0	30.6	0.00		
Flesh only, raw, 1 pound	613	0.0	38.8	0.00		
Raccoon (United States)						
Cooked, edible portion, 1 pound	1157	0.0	72.3	0.00		
Rat, Cane (based on data from Ghana)						
Raw, edible portion, 1 pound	612	0.0	38.3	0.00		
Smoked, edible portion, 1 pound	608	45.4	38.0	2.84		
Rat, Common field (based on data from India)						
Raw, edible portion, 1 pound	472	0.5	29.5	0.03		
Red River Hog (based on data from Ghana)						
Raw, edible portion, 1 pound	585	0.0	36.6	0.00		
Reindeer (United States)						
Raw:						
Side:						
Weighed with bone [refuse: bones, approx. 20%], 1 pound	787	0.0	49.2	0.00		
Edible portion (84% lean, 16% fat), 1 pound	985	0.0	61.6	0.00		
Forequarter:						
Weighed with bone [refuse: bones, approx. 26%], 1 pound	597	0.0	37.3	0.00		
Edible portion, 1 pound	808	0.0	50.5	0.00		
Hindquarter:						
Weighed with bone [refuse: bones, approx. 14%], 1 pound	999	0.0	62.4	0.00		
Edible portion (78% lean, 22% fat), 1 pound	1162	0.0	72.6	0.00		
Roebuck (based on data from France)						
Raw, edible portion, 1 pound	535	0.0	33.5	0.00		
Cooked (method unspecified), edible portion, 1 pound	689	0.0	43.1	0.00		
Seal (based on data from Canada)						
Raw, edible portion, 1 pound	599	0.0	37.4	0.00		
Cooked, edible portion, 1 pound	612	0.0	38.3	0.00		

	UNIT		1 OZ., BY WT.		1 CUP, DICED, NOT PACKED	
	Cal.	Carb.	Cal.	Carb.	Cal.	Carb.
Snake, small, Mehilia (based on data from Africa)						
Raw, edible portion, 1 pound	427	3.6	26.7	0.23		
Squirrel (based on data from East Asia)						
Raw:						
As purchased [refuse: bones, approx. 40%], 1 pound	313	0.0	19.6	0.00		
Edible portion, 1 pound	527	0.0	32.9	0.00		
Squirrel, Palm (based on data from Africa)						
Raw, edible portion, 1 pound	427	0.0	26.6	0.00		
Stag (based on data from France)						
Raw, edible portion, 1 pound	508	0.0	31.8	0.00		
Cooked (method unspecified), edible portion, 1 pound	658	0.0	41.1	0.00		
Terrapin, Diamondback (United States)						
Raw:						
As purchased [refuse: shell, approx. 79%], 1 pound	106	0.0	6.6	0.00		
Edible portion, 1 pound	503	0.0	31.4	0.00		
Turtle, Green (United States)						
Raw:						
As purchased [refuse: shell, approx. 76%], 1 pound	97	0.0	6.1	0.00		
Edible portion, 1 pound	404	0.0	25.2	0.00		
Turtle, Labi (based on data from Singapore)						
Raw:						
As purchased [refuse: approx. 11%], 1 pound	367	0.0	23.0	0.00		
Edible portion, 1 pound	413	0.0	25.8	0.00		
Turtle, Snapping (based on data from East Asia)						
Raw, edible portion, 1 pound	313	0.0	19.6	0.00		
Venison (United States)						
Lean meat only, raw, edible portion, 1 pound	572	0.0	35.8	0.00		
Venison (based on data from Canada)						
Raw, lean meat, edible portion, 1 pound	516	0.0	32.0	0.00		
Venison (based on data from India)						
Raw, edible portion, 1 pound	440	8.6	27.5	0.54		
Venison (based on data from Latin America)						
Roasted, edible portion, 1 pound	663	0.0	41.4	0.00		
Semi-dried, salted, edible portion, 1 pound	645	0.0	40.3	0.00		
Walrus (based on data from Canada)						
Raw, edible portion, 1 pound	476	0.0	29.8	0.00		
Warthog (based on data from Ghana)						
Raw, edible portion, 1 pound	485	0.0	30.3	0.00		
Waterbuck (based on data from Ghana)						
Raw, edible portion, 1 pound	558	0.0	34.9	0.00		
Water Buffalo, see Carabao						
Whale (United States)						
Raw, edible portion, 1 pound	708	0.0	44.3	0.00		
Whale (based on data from East Asia)						
Raw:						
Lean, edible portion, 1 pound	454	0.0	28.3	0.00		
Tail, edible portion, 1 pound	1198	0.0	74.8	0.00		
Bacon, edible portion, 1 pound	1238	0.0	77.4	0.00		
Cured:						
Blubber, edible portion, 1 pound	504	0.0	31.5	0.00		
Lean, edible portion, 1 pound	726	0.0	45.3	0.00		
Ventral grooves:						
Fat, edible portion, 1 pound	2093	0.0	130.8	0.00		
Lean, edible portion, 1 pound	1348	0.0	84.2	0.00		
Canned:						
"Yamatoni" (Japan), 1 pound	730	34.5	4.5	9.78		

	UNIT		1 OZ., BY WT.		1 CUP, DICED, NOT PACKED	
	Cal.	Carb.	Cal.	Carb.	Cal.	Carb.
Whale (based on data from Japan)						
Cured:						
Lean, edible portion, 1 pound	731	0.5	45.6	0.03		
Ventral grooves:						
Fat, edible portion, 1 pound	2038	1.3	127.3	0.36		
Lean, edible portion, 1 pound	1353	1.3	84.5	0.36		
Blubber, edible portion, 1 pound	508	0.9	31.7	0.25		
Frozen:						
Tail, edible portion, 1 pound	1117	1.4	69.8	0.36		
Lean, edible portion, 1 pound	577	1.4	36.0	0.36		
Fluke, edible portion, 1 pound	1289	0.9	80.5	0.25		
Canned:						
"Yamatoni," 1 pound	863	34.5	53.9	9.78		

INSECTS AND WORMS

There is no refuse for insects and worms. They are eaten in their entirety.

	UNIT		1 OZ., BY WT.		1 CUP, DICED, NOT PACKED	
	Cal.	Carb.	Cal.	Carb.	Cal.	Carb.
Ants (based on data from India)						
Pregnant Red Ants						
Raw: 1 pound	595	14.3	37.1	2.57		
Winged White Ants ("Boordood")						
Raw, 1 pound	2715	0.0	169.7	0.00		
Beetles (based on data from Africa)						
Raw, 1 pound	872	50.8	54.5	3.18		
Caterpillars (based on data from Africa)						
Raw, 1 pound	390	19.1	24.4	1.19		
Dried, 1 pound	1952	76.7	122.0	4.79		
Smoked, 1 pound	1512	29.5	94.5	1.84		
Smoked, dried, 1 pound	1930	71.7	120.6	4.48		
Crickets (based on data from Africa)						
Raw, 1 pound	531	13.2	33.2	0.82		
Flies, Lake (based on data from Africa)						
Cake, 1 pound	1734	96.2	108.4	6.02		
Grasshoppers (based on data from Africa)						
Raw, 1 pound	772	25.0	48.2	1.56		
Grilled Grasshopper Flour: 1 pound	1907	71.7	119.1	4.48		
Larvae, see Caterpillars and **Weevils**						
Locusts (based on data from Africa)						
Flour, 1 pound	1979	30.9	123.7	1.93		
Maggots, Bee (based on data from India)						
Canned, 1 pound	1049	89.4	65.6	5.59		
Mopanie Worms, see Worms						
Rice-Hoppers (based on data from East Asia)						
Raw, 1 pound	1262	0.0	78.9	0.00		
Silkworms, see Worms						
Termites (based on data from Africa)						
Raw, 1 pound	1616	19.1	101.0	1.19		
Dried, 1 pound	2978	15.9	186.1	1.00		
Smoked, 1 pound	2629	26.8	164.3	1.67		
Fried, 1 pound	2461	26.3	153.8	1.65		
Weevils, Palm (based on data from Africa)						
Raw, 1 pound	390	19.1	24.4	1.19		
Dried, 1 pound	1952	76.7	122.0	4.80		
Smoked, 1 pound	1512	29.5	94.5	1.84		
Smoked, dried, 1 pound	1930	71.7	120.6	4.48		
Worms, Mopanie (based on data from Africa)						
Dried, 1 pound	2016	62.7	126.0	3.92		
Worms, Silkworms (based on data from India)						
Raw, 1 pound	1040	2.3	65.0	0.14		

4 SAUSAGES & COLD CUTS •

	UNIT		1 SLICE OR LINK		1 OZ., BY WT.		1 POUND	
	Cal.	Carb.	Cal.	Carb.	Cal.	Carb.	Cal.	Carb.
BACON, based on generic data								
Cured Bacon, 1 pound, raw	3016	4.5			188.5	0.28	3016	4.5
Cooked (yield: approx. 5.1 oz.)	860	4.5			168.1	0.90	2690	14.3
Thick slice, cooked, approx. 0.4 oz.	72	0.4	72	0.4	168.1	0.90	2690	14.3
Medium slice, cooked, approx. 0.3 oz.	43	0.3	43	0.3	168.1	0.90	2690	14.3
Thin slice, cooked, approx. 0.1 oz.	30	0.2	30	0.2	168.1	0.90	2690	14.3
Canadian-Style Bacon, 1 pound, before browning	980	1.4			61.2	0.09	980	1.4
1 pound, browned	1256	1.4			78.5	0.09	1256	1.4
BACON, by brand								
Black Label Sliced Bacon, 16-oz. (1-lb.) package, 18–22 slices, raw	2526	3.0			157.9	0.19	2526	3.0
Cooked (yield: approx. 4.1 oz.)	(665)	(0.9)			161.3	0.23	2582	3.6
1 slice (based on 19 slices per package), approx. 0.8 oz., raw	133	0.2	133	0.2	157.9	0.19	2526	3.0
Cooked (yield: approx. 0.2 oz.)	(35)	(0.1)	(35)	(0.1)	161.3	0.23	2582	3.6
12-oz. package, 14–16 slices, raw	1895	2.2			157.9	0.19	2526	3.0
Cooked (yield: approx. 3.1 oz.)	(499)	(0.7)			161.3	0.23	2582	3.6
1 slice (based on 14 slices per package), approx. 0.8 oz., raw	(133)	(0.2)	(133)	(0.2)	157.9	0.19	2526	3.0
Cooked (yield: approx. 0.2 oz.)	(35)	trace	(35)	trace	161.3	0.23	2582	3.6
Eckrich Canadian Style Bacon, 6-oz. package, 5 slices, before browning	300	10.0			50.0	1.67	800	26.7
1 slice, approx. 1.2 oz. before browning	60	2.0	60	2.0	50.0	1.67	800	26.7
Kahn's Hickory Smoked Bacon, 16-oz. (1-lb.) package, 16–18 slices	(2340)	0.0			(146.3)	0.00	(2340)	0.0
Cooked, 16-oz. (1-lb.) package	(630)	0.0						
1 slice (based on 17 slices per package), approx. 0.9 oz.)	138	0.0	138	0.0	(146.3)	0.00	(2340)	0.0
1 slice, cooked	35	0.0	35	0.0				
Hickory Smoked Bacon, Thick sliced, 16-oz. (1-lb.) package, 12 slices, raw	(2280)	0.0			(142.5)	0.00	(2280)	0.0
Cooked, 16-oz. (1-lb.) package	(600)	0.0						
1 slice, approx. 1.3 oz.	190	0.0	190	0.0	(142.5)	0.00	(2280)	0.0
1 slice, cooked	50	0.0	50	0.0				
Lazy Maple Sliced Bacon, 16-oz. (1-lb.) package, 20 slices cooked (yield: approx. 4.6 oz.)	(812)	0.0			(175.0)	0.00	(2800)	0.0
1 slice, approx. 0.7 oz., cooked (yield: approx. 0.2 oz.)	40	0.0	40	0.0	(175.0)	0.00	2800	0.0
Oscar Mayer Canadian Style Bacon, 6-oz. package, 6 slices, cooked (yield: approx. 3.4 oz.)	246	0.7			(73.5)	(0.20)	(1174)	(3.2)
Regular Bacon, 16-oz. (1-lb.) package, 18–26 slices, raw	2658	7.7			166.1	0.48	2658	7.7
Cooked (yield: approx. 4.6 oz.)	749	3.0			161.5	0.65	2584	10.4
1 slice (based on 22 slices per package), approx. 0.7 oz., raw	(121)	(0.4)	(121)	(0.4)	166.1	0.42	2658	7.7
Cooked (yield: approx. 0.2 oz.)	(34)	(0.1)	(34)	(0.1)	161.5	0.65	2584	10.4
Thick Bacon Slices (1/8"), 16-oz. (1-lb.) package (11–14 slices)	2658	7.7			166.1	0.42	2658	7.7
Cooked (yield: approx. 4.8 oz.)	(780)	(3.1)			161.5	0.65	2584	10.4
1 slice (based on 12 slices per package), approx. 1.3 oz., raw	216	0.5	216	0.5	166.1	0.42	2658	7.7
Cooked (yield: approx. 0.4 oz.)	65	0.3	65	0.3	161.5	0.65	2584	10.4
Wafer Thin Sliced Bacon, 12-oz. package (23–33 slices)	1993	5.0			166.1	0.42	2658	7.7
Cooked (yield: approx. 3.5 oz.)	(560)	(2.3)			161.5	0.65	2584	10.4
1 slice (based on 28 slices per package), approx. 0.4 oz., raw	71	0.2	71	0.2	166.1	0.42	2658	7.7
Cooked (yield: approx. 0.1 oz.)	20	0.1	20	0.1	161.5	0.65	2584	10.4
1 slice, approx. 1 oz., cooked (yield: approx. 0.6 oz.)	41	0.1	41	0.1	(73.5)	(0.20)	(1174)	(3.2)
Range Brand Sliced Bacon, 32-oz. (2-lb.) package, 22–30 slices, raw	5542	8.6			173.2	0.27	2771	4.3
Cooked (yield: approx. 9.3 oz.)	1170	(0.0)			131.2	(0.00)	2000	(0.0)

	UNIT		1 SLICE OR LINK		1 OZ., BY WT.		1 POUND	
	Cal.	Carb.	Cal.	Carb.	Cal.	Carb.	Cal.	Carb.
1 slice (based on 27 slices per package), approx. 1.2 oz., raw	205	0.3	205	0.3	173.2	0.27	2771	4.3
Cooked (yield: approx. 0.4 oz.)	45	(0.0)	45	(0.0)	131.2	(0.00)	2000	(0.0)
Rudy's Farm Hickory Smoked Bacon, 16-oz. (1-lb.) package, 16–18 slices (based on 17 slices per package)	2340	0.0			146.0	0.00	2340	0.0
Cooked, 16-oz. (1-lb.) package	(630)	0.0						
1 slice, approx. 0.9 oz., raw	138	0.0	138	0.0	146.0	0.00	2340	0.0
Cooked	35	0.0	35	0.0				
Swift Premium Bacon 'N Sausage (bacon-flavored sausage), 8-oz. package, 10 links Cooked (yield: approx. 7 oz.)	700	5.0			100.0	0.71	1600	11.4
1 link, approx. 0.8 oz., cooked (yield: approx. 0.7 oz.)	70	0.5	70	0.5	100.0	0.71	1600	11.4
Sliced Bacon, 16-oz. (1-lb.) package, 22 slices Cooked (yield: approx. 4.6 oz.)	(812)	0.0			175.0	0.00	2800	0.0
1 slice, approx. 0.7 oz., cooked (yield: approx. 0.2 oz.)	40	0.0	40	0.0	175.0	0.00	2800	0.0

BACON, IMITATION, by brand

	UNIT		1 SLICE OR LINK		1 OZ., BY WT.		1 POUND	
	Cal.	Carb.	Cal.	Carb.	Cal.	Carb.	Cal.	Carb.
Oscar Mayer Lean 'n Tasty Breakfast Strips, 12-oz. package, 14 strips, raw	1260	7.0			105.0	0.58	1680	9.3
Cooked (yield: approx. 5.6 oz.)	700	7.0			(116.3)	(1.16)	(1861)	(18.6)
1 strip, approx. 0.9 oz., raw	90	0.5	90	0.5	105.0	0.58	1680	9.3
Cooked (yield: approx. 0.4 oz.)	50	0.5	50	0.5	(116.3)	(1.16)	(1861)	(18.6)
Swift Sizzlean Breakfast Strips, 12-oz. package, 18–20 strips, cooked (yield: approx. 7.7 oz.)	(950)	0.0			(125.0)	0.00	(2000)	0.0
1 strip (based on 19 slices per package), approx. 0.4 oz., cooked	50	0.0	50	0.0	(125.0)	0.00	(2000)	0.0
Worthington Foods frozen Stripples, 5-oz. package, precooked, 18 strips	425	12.8			85.0	2.55	1360	40.8
1 strip, approx. 0.28 oz.	25	0.8	25	0.8	85.0	2.55	1360	40.8

BARBECUE LOAF, see LOAVES

BEEF

Corned Beef is under CORNED; Beef Bologna is under BOLOGNA; Beef Franks are under FRANKFURTERS; and so forth.

BEEF, SLICED, by brand

	UNIT		1 SLICE OR LINK		1 OZ., BY WT.		1 POUND	
	Cal.	Carb.	Cal.	Carb.	Cal.	Carb.	Cal.	Carb.
A & P Smoked Beef, Sliced, 3-oz. package, 3 slices	105	3.0			35.0	1.00	560	16.0
1 slice, approx. 1 oz.	35	1.0	35	1.0	35.0	1.00	560	16.0
Smoked Spicy Beef, Sliced, 3-oz. package, 3 slices	120	3.0			40.0	1.00	640	16.0
1 slice, approx. 1 oz.	40	1.0	40	1.0	40.0	1.00	640	16.0
Carl Buddig Beef, 2.5-oz. package	100	0.0			40.0	0.00	640	0.0
Eckrich Sliced Slender Beef, 3-oz. package, 3 slices	120	2.0			40.0	0.67	640	10.7
1 slice, approx. 1 oz.	40	0.7	40	0.7	40.0	0.67	640	10.7
Oscar Mayer Thin Sliced Beef, 3-oz. package, 18–23 slices	118	1.1			39.4	0.37	630	5.9
1 slice, approx. 0.14 oz.	6	0.1	6	0.1	39.4	0.37	630	5.9

BEEF JERKY, by brand

	UNIT		1 SLICE OR LINK		1 OZ., BY WT.		1 POUND	
	Cal.	Carb.	Cal.	Carb.	Cal.	Carb.	Cal.	Carb.
Big Horn As sold individually: Beef Jerky, 3.75″ long, approx. 0.13 oz.	14	0.5	14	0.5	107.7	3.96	1723	63.4
5.00″ long, approx. 0.17 oz.	18	0.7	18	0.7	107.7	3.96	1723	63.4
6.00″ long, approx. 0.21 oz.	23	0.8	23	0.8	107.7	3.96	1723	63.4
7.25″ long, approx. 0.26 oz.	28	1.0	28	1.0	107.7	3.96	1723	63.4
8.50″ long, approx. 0.30 oz.	32	1.2	32	1.2	107.7	3.96	1723	63.4
4-Pak (4 3.75″ long sticks, each approx. 0.13 oz.), approx. 0.52 oz.	56	2.0			107.7	3.98	1723	63.4
1 stick, approx. 0.13 oz.	14	0.5	14	0.5	107.7	3.98	1723	63.4
Beef Jerky, 4¼-oz. cylinder, 20 jerkies	444	16.3			107.7	3.96	1723	63.4
1 jerky, approx. 0.21 oz.	23	0.8	23	0.8	107.7	3.96	1723	63.4
3-oz. cylinder, 23 jerkies	323	11.9			107.7	3.96	1723	63.4
1 jerky, approx. 0.13 oz.	14	0.5	14	0.5	107.7	3.96	1723	63.4
1¼-oz. bag	135	5.0			107.7	3.96	1723	63.4
Lowrey's As sold individually: Beef Jerky, 3.75″ long, approx. 0.13 oz.	14	0.5	14	0.5	107.7	3.96	1723	63.4
5.00″ long, approx. 0.17 oz.	18	0.7	18	0.7	107.7	3.96	1723	63.4
6.00″ long, approx. 0.21 oz.	23	0.8	23	0.8	107.7	3.96	1723	63.4
7.25″ long, approx. 0.26 oz.	28	1.0	28	1.0	107.7	3.96	1723	63.4
8.50″ long, approx. 0.30 oz.	32	1.2	32	1.2	107.7	3.96	1723	63.4
4-Pak (4 3.75″ long sticks, each approx. 0.13 oz.), approx. 0.52 oz.	56	2.0			107.7	3.98	1723	63.4
1 stick, approx. 0.13 oz.	14	0.5	14	0.5	107.7	3.98	1723	63.4
Spicy Sticks, 4.83″ long stick, approx. 0.33 oz.	54	0.2	54	0.2	160.5	0.67	2568	10.7
1 stick, approx. 0.25 oz.	40	0.2	40	0.2	160.5	0.67	2568	10.7
Beef Jerky, 4¼-oz. cylinder, 20 jerkies	444	16.3			107.7	3.96	1723	63.4
1 jerky, approx. 0.21 oz.	23	0.8	23	0.8	107.7	3.96	1723	63.4
3-oz. cylinder, 23 jerkies	323	11.9			107.7	3.96	1723	63.4
1 jerky, approx. 0.13 oz.	14	0.5	14	0.5	107.7	3.96	1723	63.4
1¼-oz. bag	135	5.0			107.7	3.96	1723	63.4
Beef Stick, 4.83″ long, approx. 0.33 oz.	53	0.2	53	0.2	160.5	0.67	2568	10.7
7.25″ long, approx. 0.5 oz.	80	0.3	80	0.3	160.5	0.67	2568	10.7
9.67″ long, approx. 0.66 oz.	106	0.4	106	0.4	160.5	0.67	2568	10.7
"Old Fashioned" Beef Stick, 5-Pak, approx. 1.25 oz.	201	0.8			160.5	0.67	2568	10.7
1 stick, approx. 0.25 oz.	40	0.2	40	0.2	160.5	0.67	2568	10.7
Pemmican Tender Beef Jerky Tomahawk Stick, 4¼″ stick, approx. 0.25 oz.	22	0.5	22	0.5	85.9	2.18	1374	34.9
1-oz. package (4 sticks)	86	2.2			85.9	2.18	1374	34.9
Slim Jim Beef Jerky, 3-stick pouch, approx. 0.5 oz.	49	1.7			94.1	3.23	1506	51.7
1 stick, 4¼″ long, approx. 0.2 oz.	16	0.6	16	0.6	94.1	3.23	1506	51.7
Spicy Smoked Meat Snack, 3¹⁵⁄₁₆″ stick, approx. 0.32 oz.	51	0.4	51	0.4	157.9	1.19	2527	19.1

BEERWURST (Beer Salami), based on generic data

	UNIT		1 SLICE OR LINK		1 OZ., BY WT.		1 POUND	
	Cal.	Carb.	Cal.	Carb.	Cal.	Carb.	Cal.	Carb.
Made with Beef:								
1 pound (4g/tr/8g/54%/264 mg)	1470	7.9			91.9	0.49	1470	7.9
1 slice, 2¾″ diameter × 1⁄16″ thick, approx. 0.2 oz.	19	0.1	19	0.1	91.9	0.49	1470	7.9
1 slice, 4″ diameter × ⅛″ thick, approx. 0.8 oz.	75	0.4	75	0.4	91.9	0.49	1470	7.9
Made with Pork:								
1 pound (4g/1g/5g/61%/352mg)	1080	9.4			67.5	0.58	1080	9.4
1 slice, 2¾″ diameter × 1⁄16″ thick, approx. 0.2 oz.	14	0.1	14	0.1	67.5	0.58	1080	9.4
1 slice, 4″ diameter × ⅛″ thick, approx. 0.8 oz.	55	0.5	55	0.5	67.5	0.58	1080	9.4

	UNIT		1 SLICE OR LINK		1 OZ., BY WT.		1 POUND	
	Cal.	Carb.	Cal.	Carb.	Cal.	Carb.	Cal.	Carb.
BERLINER, made with pork and beef, based on generic data								
1 pound (4g/1g/5g/61%/368mg)	1040	11.8			65.0	0.74	1040	11.8
1 slice, 2½" diameter × ¼" thick, approx. 0.8 oz.	53	0.6	53	0.6	65.0	0.74	1040	11.8
BLOOD SAUSAGE (Blood Pudding), based on generic data								
1 pound (4g/tr/10g/47%/na)	1712	5.8			107.0	0.36	1712	5.8
1 slice, 5" × 4⅝" × 1/16" thick, approx. 0.9 oz.	95	0.3	95	0.3	107.0	0.36	1712	5.8
BLOOD AND TONGUE SAUSAGE, based on generic data								
1 pound	1797	1.8			112.3	0.11	1797	1.8
1 slice, loaf shape, 5" x 4⅝" x 1/16", approx. 0.9 oz.	99	0.1	99	0.1	112.3	0.11	1797	1.8
BOCKWURST, based on generic data								
1 pound, 7 links (4g/tr/8g/56%/na)	1392	2.2			87.0	0.14	1392	2.2
1 link, approx. 2.3 oz.	200	0.3	200	0.3	87.0	0.14	1392	2.2
BOLOGNA, based on generic data								
(Lebanon Bologna is under LEBANON)								
Made with Beef:								
1 pound (3g/1g/8g/55%/284mg)	1424	8.8			89.0	0.55	1424	8.8
1 slice, 4" diameter × ⅛" thick, approx. 0.8 oz.	72	0.5	72	0.5	89.0	0.55	1424	8.8
1 slice, 4½" diameter × ⅛" thick, approx. 1 oz.	89	0.6	89	0.6	89.0	0.55	1424	8.8
Made with Beef and Pork:								
1 pound (3g/1g/8g/54%/289mg)	1424	12.6			89.0	0.79	1424	12.6
1 slice, 4" diameter × ⅛" thick, approx. 0.8 oz.	73	0.6	73	0.6	89.0	0.79	1424	12.6
1 slice, 4½" diameter × ⅛" thick, approx. 1 oz.	89	0.8	89	0.8	89.0	0.79	1424	12.6
Made with Pork:								
1 pound (4g/tr/6g/61%/336mg)	1120	3.4			70.0	0.21	1120	3.4
1 slice, 4" diameter × ⅛" thick, approx. 0.8 oz.	57	0.2	57	0.2	70.0	0.21	1120	3.4
1 slice, 4½" diameter × ⅛" thick, approx. 1 oz.	70	0.2	70	0.2	70.0	0.21	1120	3.4
Made with Turkey:								
1 pound (4g/tr/4g/65%/249mg)	912	4.3			57.0	0.27	912	4.3
1 slice, approx. 1 oz.	57	0.3	57	0.3	57.0	0.27	912	4.3
Made without binders (meat ingredient not specified)								
Prepackaged, Not Presliced:								
Chub:								
1 package, cylindrical, approx. 8¾" long, 3" diameter, 32 oz. (2 lb.) net wt.	2512	33.6			78.5	1.05	1256	16.8
Ring:								
1 ring, 15" long × 1⅜" diameter, 12 oz. net wt.	942	12.6			78.5	1.05	1256	16.8
Prepackaged, Presliced:								
Package, 4½" diameter (4⅜"–4½"); slices, approx. 1⅛" thick:								
1 package, 16 oz. (1 lb.) net wt., 16 slices	1256	16.8			78.5	1.05	1256	16.8
1 slice, approx. 1 oz.	79	1.0	79	1.0	78.5	1.05	1256	16.8

	UNIT		1 SLICE OR LINK		1 OZ., BY WT.		1 POUND	
	Cal.	Carb.	Cal.	Carb.	Cal.	Carb.	Cal.	Carb.
1 package, 8 oz. net wt., 8 slices	629	8.4			78.5	1.05	1256	16.8
1 slice, approx. 1 oz.	79	1.0	79	1.0	78.5	1.05	1256	16.8
1 package, 6 oz. net wt., 6 slices	471	6.3			78.5	1.05	1256	16.8
1 slice, approx. 1 oz.	79	1.0	79	1.0	78.5	1.05	1256	16.8
Package, 4" diameter (3⅞"–4⅓"); slices, approx. ⅛" thick:								
1 package, 16 oz. (1 lb.) net wt., 20 slices	1256	16.8			78.5	1.05	1256	16.8
1 slice, approx. 0.8 oz.	61	0.8	61	0.8	78.5	1.05	1256	16.8
1 package, 8 oz. net wt., 10 slices	629	8.4			78.5	1.05	1256	16.8
1 slice, approx. 0.8 oz.	61	0.8	61	0.8	78.5	1.05	1256	16.8
1 package, 6 oz. net wt., 8 slices	471	6.3			78.5	1.05	1256	16.8
1 slice, approx. ¾ oz.	61	0.8	61	0.8	78.5	1.05	1256	16.8
Made with cereal (meat ingredient not specified):								
Prepackaged, Not Presliced:								
Chub:								
1 package, cylindrical, 8¾" long × 3" diameter, 32 oz. (2 lb.) net wt.	2376	35.4			74.3	1.11	1188	17.7
Ring:								
1 ring, 15" long × 1⅜" diameter, 12 oz. net wt.	891	13.3			74.3	1.11	1188	17.7
Prepackaged, Presliced:								
Package, 4½" diameter (4⅜"–4½"); slices approx. ⅛" thick:								
1 package, 16 oz. (1 lb.) net wt., 16 slices	1188	17.7			74.3	1.11	1188	17.7
1 slice, approx. 1 oz.	74	1.1	74	1.1	74.3	1.11	1188	17.7
1 package, 8 oz. net wt., 8 slices	595	8.9			74.3	1.11	1188	17.7
1 slice, approx. 1 oz.	74	1.1	74	1.1	74.3	1.11	1188	17.7
1 package, 6 oz. net wt., 6 slices	445	6.6			74.3	1.11	1188	17.7
1 slice, approx. 1 oz.	74	1.1	74	1.1	74.3	1.11	1188	17.7
Package, 4" diameter (3⅞"–4⅛"); slices approx. ⅛" thick:								
1 package, 16 oz. (1 lb.) net wt., 20 slices	1188	17.7			74.3	1.11	1188	17.7
1 slice, approx. 0.8 oz.	58	0.9	58	0.9	74.3	1.11	1188	17.7
1 package, 8 oz. net wt., 10 slices	595	8.9			74.3	1.11	1188	17.7
1 slice, approx. 0.8 oz.	58	0.9	58	0.9	74.3	1.11	1188	17.7
1 package, 6 oz. net wt., 8 slices	445	6.6			74.3	1.11	1188	17.7
1 slice, approx. ¾ oz.	58	0.9	58	0.9	74.3	1.11	1188	17.7
AVERAGE, ALL VARIETIES								
(Includes kinds made with and without binders and meat by-products or variety meats)								
Prepackaged, Not Presliced:								
Chub:								
1 package, cylindrical, 8¾" long × 3" diameter, 32 oz. (2 lb.) net wt.	2757	10.0			86.2	0.31	1379	5.0
Ring:								
1 ring, 15" long × 1⅜" diameter, 12 oz. net wt.	1034	3.7			86.2	0.31	1379	5.0
Prepackaged, Presliced:								
Package, 4½" diameter (4⅜"–4½"); slices approx. ⅛" thick:								
1 package, 16 oz. (1 lb.) net wt. 16 slices	1379	5.0			86.2	0.31	1379	5.0
1 slice, approx. 1 oz.	86	0.3	86	0.3	86.2	0.31	1379	5.0
1 package, 8 oz. net wt., 8 slices	690	2.5			86.2	0.31	1379	5.0
1 slice, approx. 1 oz.	86	0.3	86	0.3	86.2	0.31	1379	5.0
1 package, 6 oz. net wt., 6 slices	517	1.9			86.2	0.31	1379	5.0
1 slice, approx. 1 oz.	86	0.3	86	0.3	86.2	0.31	1379	5.0
Package, 4" diameter (3⅞"–4⅛"); slices approx. ⅛" thick:								
1 package, 16 oz. (1 lb.) net wt., 20 slices	1379	5.0			86.2	0.31	1379	5.0
1 slice, approx. 0.8 oz.	69	0.2	69	0.2	86.2	0.31	1379	5.0
1 package, 8 oz. net wt., 10 slices	690	2.5			86.2	0.31	1379	5.0
1 slice, approx. 0.8 oz.	69	0.2	69	0.2	86.2	0.31	1379	5.0
1 package, 6 oz. net wt., 8 slices	517	1.9			86.2	0.31	1379	5.0
1 slice, approx. ¾ oz.	69	0.2	69	0.2	86.2	0.31	1379	5.0

BOLOGNA, by brand

	UNIT Cal.	UNIT Carb.	1 SLICE OR LINK Cal.	1 SLICE OR LINK Carb.	1 OZ., BY WT. Cal.	1 OZ., BY WT. Carb.	1 POUND Cal.	1 POUND Carb.
Eckrich Bologna, Sliced, 16-oz. (1-lb.) package, 16 slices	1520	24.0			95.0	1.50	1520	24.0
1 slice, approx. 1 oz.	95	1.5	95	1.5	95.0	1.50	1520	24.0
Bologna, Sliced, 12-oz. package, 12 slices	1140	18.0			95.0	1.50	1520	24.0
1 slice, approx. 1 oz.	95	1.5	95	1.5	95.0	1.50	1520	24.0
Bologna, Sliced, 8-oz. package, 8 slices	760	12.0			95.0	1.50	1520	24.0
1 slice, approx. 1 oz.	95	1.5	95	1.5	95.0	1.50	1520	24.0
Bologna, Thick sliced, 16-oz. (1-lb.) package, 9 slices	1530	27.0			95.6	1.69	1530	27.0
1 slice, approx. 1.8 oz.	170	3.0	170	3.0	95.6	1.69	1530	27.0
Bologna, Thick sliced, 12-oz. package, 7 slices	1129	21.2			94.0	1.77	1506	28.2
1 slice, approx. 1.7 oz.	160	3.0	160	3.0	94.0	1.77	1506	28.2
Bologna, Thin sliced, 12-oz. package, 7–8 slices	1050	21.0			87.5	1.75	1400	28.0
1 slice (based on 7 slices per package), approx. 1.7 oz.	150	3.0	150	3.0	87.5	1.75	1400	28.0
Beef Bologna, Sliced, 8-oz. package, 8 slices	760	12.0			95.0	1.50	1520	24.0
1 slice, approx. 1 oz.	95	1.5	95	1.5	95.0	1.50	1520	24.0
12-oz. package, 12 slices	1140	18.0			95.0	1.50	1520	24.0
1 slice, approx. 1 oz.	95	1.5	95	1.5	95.0	1.50	1520	214.0
Garlic Bologna, Sliced, 8-oz. package, 8 slices	760	12.0			95.0	1.50	1520	24.0
1 slice, approx. 1 oz.	95	1.5	95	1.5	95.0	1.50	1520	24.0
German Brand Bologna, Chub, 12-oz. package, 12 slices	1020	12.0			85.0	1.00	1360	16.0
1 slice, approx. 1 oz.	85	1.0	85	1.0	85.0	1.00	1360	16.0
German Brand Bologna, Sliced, 8-oz. package, 8 slices	640	8.0			80.0	1.00	1280	16.0
1 slice, approx. 1 oz.	80	1.0	80	1.0	80.0	1.00	1280	16.0
Pickled Ring Bologna, 13-oz. package	1235	19.5			95.0	1.50	1520	24.0
Ring Bologna, 13-oz. package	1300	19.5			100.0	1.50	1600	24.0
Sandwich Bologna, Sliced, 8-oz. package, 8 slices	720	12.0			90.0	1.50	1440	24.0
1 slice, approx. 1 oz.	90	1.5	90	1.5	90.0	1.50	1440	24.0
Smoky Tang Bologna, Chub, 12-oz. package, 12 slices	960	6.0			80.0	0.50	1280	8.0
1 slice, approx. 1 oz.	80	0.5	80	0.5	80.0	0.50	1280	8.0
Hormel Bologna, Coarse ground, 16-oz. (1-lb.) package	1200	0.0			75.0	0.00	1200	0.0
Bologna, Fine ground, 16-oz. (1-lb.) package	1280	0.0			80.0	0.00	1280	0.0
Meat Bologna, 8-oz. package	680	0.0			85.0	0.00	1360	0.0
Kahn's Bologna, 8-oz. package	700	11.4			87.5	1.42	1400	22.8
Bologna, Thick sliced, 8-oz. package, 5 slices	700	11.4			87.5	1.42	1400	22.8
1 slice, approx. 1.6 oz.	140	2.3	140	2.3	87.5	1.42	1400	22.8
Bologna, Thick sliced, 12-oz. package, 10 slices	1050	17.0			87.5	1.42	1400	22.8
1 slice, approx. 1.2 oz.	105	1.7	105	1.7	87.5	1.42	1400	22.8
Bologna, Thin sliced, 8-oz. package, 13 slices	700	11.4			87.5	1.42	1400	22.8
1 slice, approx. 0.6 oz.	54	0.8	54	0.8	87.5	1.42	1400	22.8
DeLuxe Club Bologna, Sliced, 12-oz. package, 15 slices	1050	10.2			87.5	0.85	1400	13.6
1 slice, approx. 0.8 oz.	70	0.7	70	0.7	87.5	0.85	1400	13.6
DeLuxe Club Bologna, Thick sliced, 8-oz. package, 5 slices	700	6.8			87.5	0.85	1400	13.6
1 slice, approx. 1.6 oz.	140	1.4	140	1.4	87.5	0.85	1400	13.6
DeLuxe Club Bologna, Thin sliced, 8-oz. package, 13 slices	700	6.8			87.5	0.85	1400	13.6
1 slice, approx. 0.6 oz.	54	0.5	54	0.5	87.5	0.85	1400	13.6
Giant Beef Bologna, Sliced, 12-oz. package, 15 slices	1050	17.0			87.5	1.42	1400	22.8
1 slice, approx. 0.8 oz.	70	1.1	70	1.1	87.5	1.42	1400	22.8
Longacre Chicken Bologna, 6-oz. package, 6 slices	390	0.0			65.0	0.00	1040	0.0
1 slice, approx. 1 oz.	65	0.0	65	0.0	65.0	0.00	1040	0.0
Oscar Mayer Bologna, Sliced, 8-oz. package, 10 slices	723	5.0			90.4	0.62	1446	9.9
1 slice, approx. 0.8 oz.	75	0.5	75	0.5	90.4	0.62	1446	9.9
Bologna, Thick sliced, 12-oz. package, 8–10 slices (based on 9 slices per package)	1085	7.4			90.4	0.62	1446	9.9
1 slice, approx. 1.3 oz.	120	0.8	120	0.8	90.4	0.62	1446	9.9
Bologna, Thin sliced, 12-oz. package, 21–25 slices (based on 23 slices per package)	1085	7.5			90.4	0.62	1446	9.9
1 slice, approx. 0.5 oz.	47	0.3	47	0.3	90.4	0.62	1446	9.9
Bologna and Cheese, Sliced, 8-oz. package, 10 slices	723	5.0			90.4	0.62	1446	9.92
1 slice, approx. 0.8 oz.	72	0.5	72	0.5	90.4	0.62	1446	9.92
Beef Bologna, Sliced, 8-oz. package, 10 slices	722	4.3			90.2	0.54	1443	8.6
1 slice, approx. 0.8 oz.	72	0.4	72	0.4	90.2	0.54	1446	8.6
Beef Bologna, Thick sliced, 12-oz. package, 8–10 slices (based on 9 slices per package)	1082	6.5			90.2	0.54	1443	8.6
1 slice, approx. 1.3 oz.	120	0.7	120	0.7	90.2	0.54	1446	8.6
Beef Bologna, Thin sliced, 12-oz. package, 21–25 slices (based on 23 slices per package)	1082	6.5			90.2	0.54	1443	8.6
1 slice, approx. 0.5 oz.	47	0.3	47	0.3	90.2	0.54	1443	8.6
Garlic Beef Bologna, Sliced, 8-oz. package, 10 slices	722	4.3			90.2	0.54	1443	8.6
1 slice, approx. 0.8 oz.	72	0.4	72	0.4	90.2	0.54	1443	8.6
German Bologna, Sliced, 8-oz. package, 10 slices	529	2.7			66.1	0.34	1058	5.4
1 slice, approx. 0.8 oz.	53	27.2	53	27.2	66.1	0.34	1058	4.3
Lebanon Beef Bologna, Sliced, 8-oz. package, 10 slices	456	6.8			57.0	0.85	912	13.6
1 slice, approx. 0.8 oz.	46	0.7	46	0.7	57.0	0.85	912	13.6
Ring Bologna, coarse ground, 12-oz. ring	986	3.4			82.2	0.28	1315	4.5
Ring Bologna, Wisconsin Made, coarse ground, 12-oz. ring	983	4.1			81.9	0.34	1310	5.4
Ring Bologna, Wisconsin Made, fine ground, 12-oz. ring	1062	7.8			88.5	0.65	1416	10.4
Rich's Turkey Bologna, 8-oz. package, 8 slices	560	4.0			70.0	0.50	1120	8.0
1 slice, approx. 1 oz.	70	0.5	70	0.5	70.0	0.50	1120	8.0
Swift Premium Bologna, Sliced, 6-oz. package, 6 slices	570	9.0			95.0	1.50	1520	24.0
1 slice, approx. 1 oz.	95	1.5	95	1.5	95.0	1.50	1520	24.0
12-oz. package, 12 slices	1140	18.0			95.0	1.50	1520	24.0
1 slice, approx. 1 oz.	95	1.5	95	1.5	95.0	1.50	1520	24.0
16-oz. (1-lb.) package, 16 slices	1520	24.0			95.0	1.50	1520	24.0
1 slice, approx. 1 oz.	95	1.5	95	1.5	95.0	1.50	1520	24.0
Weaver Chicken Bologna, Sliced, 8-oz. package, 12 slices	581	7.9			72.6	0.99	1182	15.8
1 slice, approx. ⅔ oz.	48	0.7	48	0.7	72.6	0.99	1182	15.8

BRATWURST, cooked, made with pork, based on generic data

	UNIT Cal.	UNIT Carb.	1 SLICE OR LINK Cal.	1 SLICE OR LINK Carb.	1 OZ., BY WT. Cal.	1 OZ., BY WT. Carb.	1 POUND Cal.	1 POUND Carb.
1 pound (4g/2g/7g/56%/158mg)	1360	9.4			85.0	0.59	1360	9.4
1 link, approx. 3 oz.	256	1.8	256	1.8	85.0	0.59	1360	9.4

BRATWURST, by brand

	UNIT Cal.	UNIT Carb.	1 SLICE OR LINK Cal.	1 SLICE OR LINK Carb.	1 OZ., BY WT. Cal.	1 OZ., BY WT. Carb.	1 POUND Cal.	1 POUND Carb.
Oscar Mayer Cured Bratwurst, 12-oz. package, 4 links	1109	8.9			92.4	0.74	1478	11.8
1 link, approx. 3 oz.	277	2.2	277	2.2	92.4	0.74	1478	11.8

BRAUNSCHWEIGER (Smoked Liverwurst), made with pork, based on generic data

	UNIT Cal.	UNIT Carb.	1 SLICE OR LINK Cal.	1 SLICE OR LINK Carb.	1 OZ., BY WT. Cal.	1 OZ., BY WT. Carb.	1 POUND Cal.	1 POUND Carb.
1 pound (4g/1g/9g/48%/324 mg)	1632	14.2			102.0	0.89	1632	14.2
1 slice, approx. 0.6 oz.	65	0.6	65	0.6	102.0	0.89	1632	14.2

	UNIT		1 SLICE OR LINK		1 OZ., BY WT.		1 POUND	
	Cal.	Carb.	Cal.	Carb.	Cal.	Carb.	Cal.	Carb.
Prepackaged, Not Presliced:								
Roll:								
1 package, 6½" long, 2½" diameter, 16 oz. (1 lb.) net wt.	1447	10.4			90.4	0.65	1447	10.4
1 package, 5½" long, 2" diameter; 8 oz. net wt.	724	5.2			90.4	0.65	1447	10.4
Prepackaged, Presliced:								
1 package, 3⅛" diameter; 6 oz. net wt.; slices, approx. ¼" thick	542	3.9			90.4	0.65	1447	10.4
1 slice, approx. 1 oz.	90	0.7	90	0.7	90.4	0.65	1447	10.4
BRAUNSCHWEIGER (Smoked Liverwurst), by brand								
Oscar Mayer Braunschweiger, 8-oz. Chub	800	5.2			100.0	0.65	1600	10.4
Sliced Braunschweiger, 8-oz. package, 8 slices	824	2.7			103.0	0.34	1648	5.4
1 slice, approx. 1 oz.	103	0.3	103	0.3	103.0	0.34	1648	5.4
BROTWURST, made with pork, beef, and nonfat milk, based on generic data								
1 pound, 7 links (4g/2g/8g/51%/315mg)	1472	13.4			92.0	0.84	1472	13.4
1 link, approx. 2.5 oz.	226	2.1	226	2.1	92.0	0.84	1472	13.4
BROWN-AND-SERVE SAUSAGE, based on generic data								
These generic data did not specify ingredients. Other Brown and Serve Sausages (by brand) can be found throughout the chapter. For example, Hormel's Brown 'N Serve Pork Sausage is under PORK, and Jones' Brown 'N Serve Minute Breakfast Links are with SAUSAGES, OTHER.								
Prepackaged Links:								
Before browning: 1 package, 8 oz. net wt.; 10–11 links	892	6.1			111.5	0.76	1783	12.2
Browned: Yield from 1 8-oz. package, 10–11 links, approx. 6.3 oz.	760	5.0			119.7	0.79	1915	12.6
1 link, 3⅞" long, ⅝" diameter (based on 10 links per package), approx. 0.8 oz.	83	0.6	83	0.6	111.5	0.76	1783	12.2
Browned: Yield from 1 link, 3⅞" long, ⅝" diameter (based on 10 links per package), approx. 0.8 oz.	72	0.5	72	0.5	119.7	0.79	1915	12.6
Prepackaged Patties:								
Before browning: 1 package, 8 oz. net wt.; 8–9 oval patties	892	6.1			111.5	0.76	1783	12.2
Browned: Yield from 1 8-oz. package, 8–9 oval patties, approx. 6.3 oz.	760	5.0			119.7	0.79	1915	12.6
Before browning: 1 patty, 2⅜" × 1⅞" x ½" thick, (based on 8 patties per package), approx. 1 oz.	111	0.8	111	0.8	111.5	0.76	1783	12.2
Browned: Yield from 1 patty, 2⅜" × 1⅞" × ½" thick (based on 8 patties per package), approx. 0.8 oz.	97	0.6	97	0.6	119.7	0.79	1915	12.6
CANADIAN BACON, see BACON								
CAPICOLA or CAPACOLA, based on generic data								
1 package, 4¼" × 4¼", 4½ oz. net wt., approx. 6 slices, 1⁄16" thick	639	0.0			141.4	0.00	2263	0.0
1 slice, approx. ¾ oz.	105	0.0	105	0.0	141.4	0.00	2263	0.0
1 pound, approx. 21½ slices	2263	0.0			141.4	0.00	2263	0.0
CERVELAT, see SUMMER SAUSAGE								
CHEESEFURTER (Cheese Smokie), made with pork and beef, based on generic data								
1 pound (4g/1g/8g/52%/307mg)	1488	6.9			93.0	0.43	1488	6.9
1 cheesefurter, approx. 1.5 oz.	141	0.6	141	0.6	93.0	0.43	1488	6.9
CHICKEN								
Chicken Bologna is under BOLOGNA; Chicken Franks are under FRANKFURTERS; and so forth.								
CHICKEN, SLICED, by brand								
A & P Sliced Chicken, 3-oz. package, 3 slices	180	0.0			60.0	0.00	960	0.0
1 slice, approx. 1 oz.	60	0.0	60	0.0	60.0	0.00	960	0.0
Carl Buddig Chicken, "The Original Ready-to-Eat," 2.5-oz. package	113	0.0			45.0	0.00	720	0.0
Eckrich Sliced Slender Chicken, 3-oz. package, 3 slices	140	4.0			46.7	1.33	747	21.3
1 slice, approx. 1 oz.	47	1.3	47	1.3	46.7	1.33	747	21.3
Rich's Sliced Chicken Breast, 6-oz. package, 6 slices	270	0.0			45.0	0.00	720	0.0
1 slice, approx. 1 oz.	45	0.0	45	0.0	45.0	0.00	720	0.0
Safeway Chicken, Smoked/Pressed/Sliced, 3-oz. package, 3 slices	135	0.0			45.0	0.00	720	0.0
1 slice, approx. 1 oz.	45	0.0	45	0.0	45.0	0.00	720	0.0
CHICKEN ROLL, made with light meat, based on generic data								
6 oz. package (6g/1g/2g/69%/166mg)	271	4.2			45.1	0.69	721	11.1
1 pound	721	11.1			45.1	0.69	721	11.1
1 slice, approx. 1 oz.	45	0.7	45	0.7	45.1	0.69	721	11.1
CHICKEN ROLL, by brand								
Swift Premium Boneless Chicken Roll, 5-lb. package	4114	0.0			51.4	0.00	822	0.0
Weaver Sliced Chicken Roll, 8-oz. package, 14 slices	320	4.8			40.0	0.60	640	9.6
1 slice, approx. 0.6 oz.	23	0.3	23	0.3	40.0	0.60	640	9.6
CORNED BEEF, by brand								
A & P Corned Beef, Sliced, 3-oz. package, 3 slices	120	3.0			40.0	1.00	640	16.0
1 slice, approx. 1 oz.	40	1.0	40	1.0	40.0	1.00	640	16.0
Carl Buddig Corned Beef, 2.5-oz. package	100	0.0			40.0	0.00	640	0.0
Eckrich Jellied Corned Beef, Sliced, 8-oz. package, 8 slices	240	4.0			30.0	0.50	480	8.0
1 slice, approx. 1 oz.	30	0.5	30	0.5	30.0	0.50	480	8.0
Slender Corned Beef, Sliced, 3-oz. package, 3 slices	120	4.0			40.0	1.33	640	21.3
1 slice, approx. 1 oz.	40	1.3	40	1.3	40.0	1.33	640	21.3
Featherweight Corned Beef Loaf, 7-oz. package	270	0.0			38.6	0.00	618	0.0
Safeway Corned Beef, Sliced/Chopped/Pressed, 3-oz. package, 3 slices	135	0.0			45.0	0.00	720	0.0
1 slice, approx. 1 oz.	45	0.0	45	0.0	45.0	0.00	720	0.0
Swift Premium Corned Beef, 16-oz. (1-lb.) package	1234	0.0			77.1	0.00	1234	0.0

	UNIT		1 SLICE OR LINK		1 OZ., BY WT.		1 POUND	
	Cal.	Carb.	Cal.	Carb.	Cal.	Carb.	Cal.	Carb.
CORNED BEEF LOAF, see LOAVES								
COUNTRY-STYLE SAUSAGE, based on generic data								
1 pound	1565	0.0			97.8	0.00	1565	0.0
FISH SAUSAGE (based on data from Japan)								
1 pound	653	27.7			40.8	1.70		
FRANKFURTERS AND HOT DOGS, based on generic data (see also WIENERS)								
As Made from Different Types of Meat:								
Made with Beef:								
1 pound, 10 frankfurters (3g/1g/8g/54%/290mg)	1461	10.8			91.0	0.68	1461	10.8
1 frankfurter, 5″ long × ¾″ diameter, approx. 1.6 oz.	145	1.1	145	1.1	91.0	0.68	1461	10.8
1 pound, 8 frankfurters	1461	10.8			91.0	0.68	1461	10.8
1 frankfurter, 5″ long × ⅞″ diameter, approx. 2 oz.	184	1.4	184	1.4	91.0	0.68	1461	10.8
Made with Beef and Pork:								
1 pound, 10 frankfurters (3g/1g/8g/54%/318mg)	1452	11.6			90.7	0.72	1452	11.6
1 frankfurter, 5″ long × ¾″ diameter, approx. 1.6 oz.	144	1.2	144	1.2	90.7	0.72	1452	11.6
1 pound, 8 frankfurters	1452	11.6			90.7	0.72	1452	11.6
1 frankfurter, 5″ long × ⅞″ diameter, approx. 2 oz.	183	1.5	183	1.5	90.7	0.72	1452	11.6
Made with Chicken:								
1 pound (4g/2g/6g/57%/388mg)	1168	31.4			73.0	1.96	1168	31.4
1 frankfurter, approx. 1.6 oz.	116	3.1	116	3.1	73.0	1.96	1168	31.4
Made with Turkey:								
1 pound (4g/tr/5g/63%/404mg)	1024	6.7			64.0	0.42	1024	6.7
1 frankfurter, approx. 1.6 oz.	102	0.7	102	0.7	64.0	0.42	1024	6.7
By style of manufacture without regard to the type of meat used:								
Made without binders:								
NOT SMOKED:								
1 package, 5½ oz. net wt., 16 frankfurters	462	3.9			83.9	0.70	1343	11.3
1 frankfurter, 1¾″ long, ½″ diameter, approx. ⅓ oz.	30	0.3	30	0.3	83.9	0.70	1343	11.3
1 package, 16 oz. (1 lb.) net wt., 8 frankfurters	1343	11.3			83.9	0.70	1343	11.3
1 frankfurter, 5″ long, ⅞″ diameter, approx. 2 oz.	169	1.4	169	1.4	83.9	0.70	1343	11.3
1 package, 16 oz. (1 lb.) net wt., 10 frankfurters	1343	11.3			83.9	0.70	1343	11.3
1 frankfurter, 5″ long, ¾″ diameter, approx. 1.6 oz.	133	1.1	133	1.1	83.9	0.70	1343	11.3
HALF SMOKED:								
1 package, 11 oz. net wt., 5 frankfurters	924	7.8			83.9	0.70	1343	11.3
1 frankfurter, 5″ long, 1″ diameter, approx. 2.2 oz.	184	1.6	184	1.6	83.9	0.70	1343	11.3
SMOKED:								
1 package, 5 oz. net wt., 16 frankfurters	420	3.6			83.9	0.70	1343	11.3
1 frankfurter, 1¾″ long, ⅝″ diameter, approx. 0.3 oz.	27	0.2	27	0.2	83.9	0.70	1343	11.3
1 package, 12 oz. net wt., 8 frankfurters	1006	8.5			83.9	0.70	1343	11.3
1 frankfurter, 4¾″ long, ¾″ diameter, approx. 1.5 oz.	124	1.1	124	1.1	83.9	0.70	1343	11.3
1 package, 12 oz. net wt., 10 frankfurters	1006	8.5			83.9	0.70	1343	11.3
1 frankfurter, 4½″ long, ¾″ diameter, approx. 1.2 oz.	101	0.9	101	0.9	83.9	0.70	1343	11.3

	UNIT		1 SLICE OR LINK		1 OZ., BY WT.		1 POUND	
	Cal.	Carb.	Cal.	Carb.	Cal.	Carb.	Cal.	Carb.
Made with non-fat dry milk:								
1 package, 16 oz. (1 lb.) net wt., 8 frankfurters	1361	15.4			85.1	0.95	1361	15.4
1 frankfurter, 5″ long, ⅞″ diameter, approx. 2 oz.	171	1.9	171	1.9	85.1	0.95	1361	15.4
1 package, 16 oz. (1 lb.) net wt., 10 frankfurters	1361	15.4			85.1	0.95	1361	15.4
1 frankfurter, 5″ long, ¾″ diameter, approx. 1.6 oz.	135	1.5	135	1.5	85.1	0.95	1361	15.4
Made with cereal:								
1 package, 16 oz. (1 lb.) net wt., 8 frankfurters	1125	0.9			70.3	0.06	1125	10.9
1 frankfurter, 5″ long, ⅞″ diameter, approx. 2 oz.	141	0.9	141	0.1	70.3	0.06	1125	0.9
1 package, 16 oz. (1 lb.) net wt., 10 frankfurters	1125	0.9			70.3	0.06	1125	0.9
1 frankfurter, 5″ long, ¾″ diameter, approx. 1.6 oz.	112	0.1	112	0.1	70.3	0.06	1125	0.9
AVERAGE, ALL STYLES OF MANUFACTURE								
Including kinds made with and without binders and meat by-products or variety meats.								
UNCOOKED:								
1 package, 16 oz. (1 lb.) net wt., 8 frankfurters	1402	8.2			87.6	0.51	1402	8.2
1 frankfurter, 5″ long, ⅞″ diameter, approx. 2 oz.	176	1.0	176	1.0	87.6	0.51	1402	8.2
COOKED (reheated):								
1 package, 16 oz. (1 lb.) net wt. (yield: approx. 15.7 oz.)	1353	7.1			86.2	0.45	1379	7.2
1 frankfurter, 5″ long, ⅞″ diameter, approx. 2 oz.	170	0.9	170	0.9	86.2	0.45	1379	7.2
1 package, 16 oz. (1 lb.) net wt., 10 frankfurters	1402	8.2			87.6	0.51	1402	8.2
1 frankfurter, 5″ long, ¾″ diameter, approx. 1.6 oz.	139	0.8	139	0.8	87.6	0.51	1402	8.2
COOKED (reheated):								
1 package, 16 oz. (1 lb.) net wt. (yield: approx. 15.7 oz.)	1353	7.1			86.2	0.45	1379	7.2
1 frankfurter, 5″ long, ¾″ diameter, approx. 1.6 oz.	134	0.7	134	0.7	86.2	0.45	1379	7.2
FRANKFURTERS AND HOT DOGS, by brand (see also WIENERS)								
Ball Park Beef Franks, 16-oz. (1-lb.) package, 8 frankfurters	1304	0.8			81.5	0.05	1304	0.8
1 frankfurter, approx. 2 oz.	163	0.1	163	0.1	81.5	0.05	1304	0.8
Meat Franks, 16-oz. (1-lb.) package, 8 frankfurters	1376	0.8			86.0	0.05	1376	0.8
1 frankfurter, approx. 2 oz.	172	0.1	172	0.1	86.0	0.05	1376	0.8
Best's Kosher Frankfurters, "Lower Fat Beef," 12-oz. package, 8 frankfurters	880	16.0			73.3	0.00	1173	0.0
1 frankfurter, approx. 1.5 oz.	110	2.0	110	2.0	73.3	0.00	1173	0.0
Eckrich Franks, 16-oz. (1-lb.) package, 10 frankfurters	1500	30.0			93.8	1.88	1500	30.0
1 frankfurter, approx. 1.6 oz.	150	3.0	150	3.0	93.8	1.88	1500	30.0
Franks, 12-oz. package, 10 frankfurters	1200	20.0			75.0	1.25	1200	20.0
1 frankfurter, approx. 1.2 oz.	120	2.0	120	2.0	75.0	1.25	1200	20.0
Beef Franks, 16-oz. (1-lb.) package, 10 frankfurters	1500	30.0			93.8	1.88	1500	30.0
1 frankfurter, approx. 1.6 oz.	150	3.0	150	3.0	93.8	1.88	1500	30.0
Beef Franks, 12-oz. package, 10 frankfurters	1200	30.0			100.0	2.50	1600	40.0
1 frankfurter, approx. 1.2 oz.	120	3.0	120	3.0	100.0	2.50	1600	40.0
Jumbo Franks, 16-oz. (1-lb.) package, 8 frankfurters	1520	24.0			95.0	1.50	1520	24.0
1 frankfurter, approx. 2 oz.	190	3.0	190	3.0	95.0	1.50	1520	24.0
Jumbo Beef Franks, 16-oz. (1-lb.) package, 8 frankfurters	1520	24.0			95.0	1.50	1520	24.0
1 frankfurter, approx. 2 oz.	190	3.0	190	3.0	95.0	1.50	1520	24.0
Skinless Franks, 16-oz. (1-lb.) package, 10 frankfurters	1500	30.0			93.8	1.88	1500	30.0
1 frankfurter, approx. 1.6 oz.	150	3.0	150	3.0	93.8	1.88	1500	30.0

	UNIT		1 SLICE OR LINK		1 OZ., BY WT.		1 POUND	
	Cal.	Carb.	Cal.	Carb.	Cal.	Carb.	Cal.	Carb.
Empire Kosher Chicken Franks, 16-oz. (1-lb.) package, 8 frankfurters	1120	8.0			70.0	0.50	1120	8.0
1 frankfurter, approx. 2 oz.	140	1.0	140	1.0	70.0	0.50	1120	8.0
Featherweight Frankfurters, low sodium, 4.9-oz. package. 4 frankfurters	360	0.0			73.5	0.00	1176	0.0
1 frankfurter, approx. 1.2 oz.	90	0.0	90	0.0	73.5	0.00	1176	0.0
Hygrade Beef Franks, 16-oz. (1-lb.) package, 10 frankfurters	1500	14.0			93.8	0.88	1500	14.0
1 frankfurter, approx. 1.6 oz.	150	1.4	150	1.4	93.8	0.88	1500	14.0
Meat Franks, 16-oz. (1-lb.) package, 10 frankfurters	1500	14.0			93.8	0.88	1500	14.0
1 frankfurter, approx. 1.6 oz.	150	1.4	150	1.4	93.8	0.88	1500	14.0
Kahn's Beef Franks, 16-oz. (1-lb.) package, 10 frankfurters	1400	20.0			87.5	1.25	1400	20.0
1 frankfurter, approx. 1.6 oz.	140	2.0	140	2.0	87.5	1.25	140	20.0
Jumbo Franks, 16-oz. (1-lb.) package, 8 frankfurters	1496	14.6			94.0	0.91	1496	14.6
1 frankfurter, approx. 2 oz.	187	1.8	187	1.8	94.0	0.91	1496	14.6
Jumbo Beef Franks, 16-oz. (1-lb.) package, 8 frankfurters	1424	16.0			89.0	1.00	1424	16.0
1 frankfurter, approx. 2 oz.	174	2.0	174	2.0	89.0	1.00	1424	16.0
Longacre Chicken Franks, "Lower Fat," 16-oz. (1-lb.) package, 8 frankfurters	960	0.0			60.0	0.00	960	0.0
1 frankfurter, approx. 2 oz.	120	0.0	120	0.0	60.0	0.00	960	0.0
Turkey Franks, 16-oz. (1-lb.) package, 10 frankfurters	1100	0.0			68.8	0.00	1101	0.0
1 frankfurter, approx. 1.6 oz.	110	0.0	110	0.0	68.8	0.00	1101	0.0
Longmont Turkey Franks, 12-oz. package, 10 frankfurters	786	18.7			65.5	1.56	1048	25.0
1 frankfurter, approx. 1.2 oz.	79	1.9	79	1.9	65.5	1.56	1048	25.0
16-oz. (1-lb.) package, 10 frankfurters	1048	25.0			65.5	1.56	1048	25.0
1 frankfurter, approx. 1.6 oz.	105	2.5	105	2.5	65.5	1.56	1048	25.0
Louis Rich Turkey Franks, 12-oz. package, 8 frankfurters	800	8.0			66.7	0.67	1067	10.7
1 frankfurter, approx. 1.5 oz.	100	1.0	100	1.0	66.7	0.67	1067	10.7
Turkey Franks, "33⅓% Lower Fat," 12-oz. package, 8 frankfurters	1040	16.0			65.0	1.00	1040	16.0
1 frankfurter, approx. 1.5 oz.	130	2.0	130	2.0	65.0	1.00	1040	16.0
Machiaeh Brand Beef Franks, 16-oz. (1-lb.) package, 8 frankfurters	1456	9.9			91.0	0.62	1456	9.9
1 frankfurter, approx. 2 oz.	182	1.2	182	1.2	91.0	0.62	1456	9.9
Moore's Corn Dogs "Batter-Coated Frankfurters on a Stick," 10⅔-oz. package, 4 corn dogs	923	72.5			86.5	6.80	1384	108.9
1 corn dog, approx. 2⅔ oz.	231	18.1	231	18.1	86.5	6.80	1384	108.9
Oscar Mayer Beef Franks, 16-oz. (1-lb.) package, 8 frankfurters	1451	10.9			90.7	0.68	1451	10.9
1 frankfurter, approx. 2 oz.	191	1.4	191	1.4	90.7	0.68	1451	10.9
16-oz. (1-lb.) package, 10 frankfurters	1451	10.9			90.7	0.68	1451	10.9
1 frankfurter, approx. 1.6 oz.	145	1.1	145	1.1	90.7	0.68	1451	10.9
Weaver Chicken Hot Dogs, 16-oz. (1-lb.) package, 10 Hot Dogs	1200	20.0			75.0	1.25	1200	20.0
1 Hot Dog, approx. 1.6 oz.	120	2.0	120	2.0	75.0	1.25	1200	20.0
Wranglers Smoked Franks, 16-oz. (1-lb.) package, 8 frankfurters	1280	16.0			80.0	0.00	1280	0.0
1 frankfurter, approx. 2 oz.	160	2.0	160	2.0	80.0	0.00	1280	0.0

FRANKFURTERS, CANNED, based on generic data

	UNIT		1 SLICE OR LINK		1 OZ., BY WT.		1 POUND	
	Cal.	Carb.	Cal.	Carb.	Cal.	Carb.	Cal.	Carb.
1 can, 12 oz. net wt. drained, 7 frankfurters	751	0.7			62.5	0.08	1002	0.9
1 frankfurter, 4⅞" long, ⅞" diameter, approx. 1.7 oz.	106	0.1	106	0.1	62.5	0.08	1002	0.9

HAM, based on generic data

	UNIT		1 SLICE OR LINK		1 OZ., BY WT.		1 POUND	
	Cal.	Carb.	Cal.	Carb.	Cal.	Carb.	Cal.	Carb.
BOILED HAM:								
Prepackaged, Presliced:								
1 package, 8 oz. net wt., 8 slices	531	0.0			66.3	0.00	1061	0.0
1 slice, 6¼" × 4" × 1/16", approx. 1 oz.	66	0.0	66	0.0	66.3	0.00	1061	0.0
1 package, 6 oz. net wt., 8 slices	398	0.0			66.3	0.00	1061	0.0
1 slice, 4¼" × 4¼" × 1/16", approx. ¾ oz.	49	0.0	49	0.0	66.3	0.00	1061	0.0
CHOPPED HAM, PREFORMED, SLICED:								
Canned:								
1 pound (5g/tr/5g/61%/387mg)	1088	1.3			68.0	0.08	1088	1.3
1 slice, 4¼" × 4¼" × 1/16" thick, approx. ¾ oz.	50	0.1	50	0.1	68.0	0.08	1088	1.3
Not Canned:								
1 pound (5g/0g/5g/64%/389mg)	1040	0.0			65.0	0.00	1040	0.0
1 slice, 4" × 4" × 3/32" thick, approx. ¾ oz.	48	0.0	48	0.0	65.0	0.00	1040	0.0
1 slice, 4¼" × 4¼" × 1/16" thick, approx. 1 oz.	65	0.0	65	0.0	65.0	0.00	1040	0.0
DEVILED HAM:								
Canned:								
1 can, 2¼ oz. net wt.	225	0.0			99.8	0.00	1597	0.0
1 can, 3 oz. net wt.	298	0.0			99.8	0.00	1597	0.0
1 can, 4½ oz. net wt.	449	0.0			99.8	0.00	1597	0.0
MINCED HAM, PREFORMED, SLICED:								
1 pound, (5g/1g/6g/57%/353mg)	1200	8.3			75.0	0.52	1200	8.3
1 slice, 4¼" × 4¼" × 1/16" thick, approx. ¾ oz.	55	0.4	55	0.4	75.0	0.52	1200	8.3
SLICED HAM:								
Extra Lean (approx. 5% fat), 1 pound (6g/tr/1g/71%/405mg)	594	4.4			37.1	0.27	594	4.4
1 slice, 6¼" × 4" × 1/16" thick, approx. 1 oz.	37	0.3	37	0.3	37.1	0.27	594	4.4
Regular (approx. 11% fat), 1 pound (5g/1g/3g/65%/373mg)	826	14.1			51.6	0.88	826	14.1
1 slice, 6¼" × 4" × 1/16" thick, approx. 1 oz.	52	0.9	52	0.9	51.6	0.88	826	14.1

HAM, by brand

	UNIT		1 SLICE OR LINK		1 OZ., BY WT.		1 POUND	
	Cal.	Carb.	Cal.	Carb.	Cal.	Carb.	Cal.	Carb.
A & P Sliced Smoked Ham, 3-oz. package, 3 slices	150	3.0			50.0	1.00	800	16.0
1 slice, approx. 1 oz.	50	1.0	50	1.0	50.0	1.00	800	16.0
Armour Chopped Ham, 12-oz. can	720	0.0			60.0	1.00		
Carl Buddig Ham, 2½-oz. package	100	0.0			40.0	0.00	640	0.0
Turkey Ham, 2½-oz. package	113	0.0			45.0	0.00	720	0.0
Cure/81 Whole Ham, 16-oz. (1-lb.) package	773	0.0			48.3	0.00		
Curemaster Whole Ham, 2-to-3-lb. plastic bag	1120-1680	10.7-16.0			35.0	0.33		
Eckrich Chopped Ham, 8-oz. package	400	4.0			50.0	0.50	800	8.0
1 slice, approx. 1 oz.	50	0.5	50	0.5	50.0	0.50	800	8.0
Cooked Ham, Sliced, 6-oz. package, 5 slices	200	5.0			33.3	0.83	533	13.3
1 slice, approx. 1.2 oz.	40	1.0	40	1.0	33.3	0.83	533	13.3
Slender Smoked Ham, Sliced, 3-oz. package, 3 slices	120	2.0			40.0	0.67	640	10.7
1 slice, approx. 1 oz.	40	0.7	40	0.7	40.0	0.67	640	10.7
Featherweight Ham, low sodium, 16-oz. (1-lb.) package	550	0.0			34.4	0.00	550	0.0
Hormel Ham, 4-oz. package	140	0.0			35.0	0.00	560	0.0
Bone-in Ham, 16–18-lb. package	(7610)-(8562)	0.0			(51.7)	0.00		
Chopped Ham, 8-lb. can	11520	0.0			90.0	0.00		
12-oz. can	840	0.0			70.0	0.00		
6-oz. can	540	0.0			90.0	0.00		

	Unit Cal.	Unit Carb.	1 Slice or Link Cal.	1 Slice or Link Carb.	1 Oz., by Wt. Cal.	1 Oz., by Wt. Carb.	1 Pound Cal.	1 Pound Carb.
Ham Patties, 12-oz. can, 6 patties	1215	3.0			101.3	0.25	1621	4.0
1 patty, approx. 2 oz.	203	0.5	203	0.5	101.3	0.25	1621	4.0
Whole Ham, 3-lb. can	2360	0.0			49.2	0.00		
Land O'Lakes Turkey Ham, 1¾-lb. roll	1120	14.0			46.0	0.50	736	8.0
Longacre Turkey Ham, baked, 6-oz. package, 8 slices	240	0.0			40.0	0.00	640	0.0
1 slice, approx. 0.8 oz.	30	0.0	30	0.0	40.0	0.00	640	0.0
Longmont Turkey Ham, 2½-lb. package	1600	11.0			40.0	0.28	640	4.5
Turkey Ham, Sliced, 8-oz. package, 10 slices	320	2.2			40.0	0.28	640	4.5
1 slice, approx. 0.8 oz.	32	0.2	32	0.2	40.0	0.28	640	4.5
Louis Rich Turkey Ham, 8-oz. package, 8 slices	360	4.0			45.0	0.50	720	8.0
1 slice, approx. 1 oz.	45	0.5	45	0.5	45.0	0.50	720	8.0
Oscar Mayer Chopped Ham, Sliced, 8-oz. package, 8 slices	513	7.3			64.1	0.91	1025	14.6
1 slice, approx. 1 oz.	64	0.9	64	0.9	64.1	0.91	1025	14.6
Ham, Thin sliced, 3-oz. package, 8–12 slices	113	0.1			37.7	0.03	603	0.5
1 slice, approx. 0.3 oz.	11	0.0	11	0.0	37.7	0.03	603	0.5
Ham Roll Sausage, Sliced, 8-oz. package, 10 slices	352	5.2			44.0	0.68	702	10.9
1 slice, approx. 0.8 oz.	35	0.5	35	0.5	44.0	0.68	702	10.9
Jubilee Ham Slice, Smoked, 8-oz. package	280	2.0			35.0	0.25	560	4.0
Jubilee Ham Steaks, Sliced, 16-oz. (1-lb.) package, 8 slices	560	8.0			35.0	0.50	560	8.0
1 slice, approx. 2 oz.	70	1.0	70	1.0	35.0	0.50	560	8.0
Minced Ham, Sliced, 8-oz. package, 10 slices	549	3.2			68.6	0.40	1098	6.4
1 slice, approx. 0.8 oz.	55	0.3	55	0.3	68.6	0.40	1098	6.4
Sectioned & Formed Jubilee, 10-lb. can	5413	9.1			33.8	0.06		
3-lb. can	1624	2.7			33.8	0.06		
Smoked Cooked Ham, 6-oz. package	200	6.0			33.3	1.00	533	16.0
Whole Ham, boneless Jubilee, 1½-lb. can	840	0.0			35.0	0.00		
10-lb. can	56000	0.0			35.0	0.00		
Ralph's Ham, Cooked (Danish), 4-oz. package, 4 slices	120	4.0			30.0	1.00	480	16.0
1 slice, approx. 1 oz.	30	1.0	30	1.0	30.0	1.00	480	16.0
Rich's Cured and Smoked Turkey Ham, 8-oz. package, 8 slices	320	4.0			40.0	0.50	640	8.0
1 slice, approx. 1 oz.	40	0.5	40	0.5	40.0	0.50	640	8.0
Safeway Ham, Pressed/Smoked, 3-oz. package, 3 slices	135	0.0			45.0	0.00	720	0.0
1 slice, approx. 1 oz.	45	0.0	45	0.0	45.0	0.00	720	0.0
Swift Premium Ham, 48-oz. (3-lb.) can, drained	3017	13.7			62.9	0.29	1006	4.6
Suggested slice, approx. 1¾ oz.	110	0.5	110	0.5	62.9	0.29	1006	4.6
Ham Patties, 160-oz. (10-lb.) institutional carton, 76 patties	19068	76.2			119.0	0.48	1904	10.9
1 patty, approx. 2.1 oz.	250	1.0	250	1.0	119.0	0.48	1904	10.9
Hostess Ham, 32-oz. (2-lb.) package	1371	9.1			42.9	0.29	686	4.6
64-oz. (4-lb.) package	3840	27.4			40.0	0.29	640	4.6
Suggested slice, approx. 1¾ oz.	140	1.0	140	1.0	40.0	0.29	640	4.6
Weaver Turkey Ham, Sliced, 6-oz. package, 9 slices	208	1.4			34.6	0.23	554	3.6
1 slice, approx. ⅔ oz.	23	0.2	23	0.2	34.6	0.23	554	3.6

HEADCHEESE, based on generic data

	Unit Cal.	Unit Carb.	1 Slice or Link Cal.	1 Slice or Link Carb.	1 Oz., by Wt. Cal.	1 Oz., by Wt. Carb.	1 Pound Cal.	1 Pound Carb.
Prepackaged, Presliced:								
1 package, 8-oz. net wt., 8 slices	608	2.3			76.0	0.29	1218	4.5
1 slice, 4″ × 4″, 3/32″ thick, approx. 1 oz.	76	0.3	76	0.3	76.0	0.29	1216	4.5
Made with pork:								
1 pound, 16 slices (5g/tr/4g/65%/356mg)	960	1.6			60.0	0.10	960	1.6
1 slice, 4″ × 4″ × 3/32″ thick, approx. 1 oz.	60	0.1	60	0.1	60.0	0.10	960	1.6

HEADCHEESE, by brand

	Unit Cal.	Unit Carb.	1 Slice or Link Cal.	1 Slice or Link Carb.	1 Oz., by Wt. Cal.	1 Oz., by Wt. Carb.	1 Pound Cal.	1 Pound Carb.
Oscar Mayer Sliced Head Cheese, 8-oz. package, 8 slices	415	10.4			51.9	1.30	830	20.8
1 slice, approx. 1 oz.	52	1.3	52	1.3	51.9	1.30	830	20.8

HONEY LOAF, see LOAVES

HONEY ROLL SAUSAGE, made with beef, based on generic data

	Unit Cal.	Unit Carb.	1 Slice or Link Cal.	1 Slice or Link Carb.	1 Oz., by Wt. Cal.	1 Oz., by Wt. Carb.	1 Pound Cal.	1 Pound Carb.
1 pound (5g/1g/3g/65%/375mg)	832	9.9	42	0.5	52.0	0.62	832	9.9
1 slice, 4″ diameter × ⅛″ thick, approx. 0.81 oz.			42	0.5	52.0	0.62	832	9.9

HOT DOGS, see FRANKFURTERS AND HOT DOGS (see also WIENERS)

ITALIAN SAUSAGE, made with pork, based on generic data

	Unit Cal.	Unit Carb.	1 Slice or Link Cal.	1 Slice or Link Carb.	1 Oz., by Wt. Cal.	1 Oz., by Wt. Carb.	1 Pound Cal.	1 Pound Carb.
RAW:								
1 pound, 5 sausages (4g/1g/9g/51%/207mg)	1570	10.4			98.1	0.65	1570	10.4
1 sausage, approx. 3.2 oz.	315	0.6	315	0.6	98.1	0.65	1570	10.4
1 pound, 4 sausages	1570	10.4			98.1	0.65	1570	10.4
1 sausage, approx. 4 oz.	391	0.7	391	0.7	98.1	0.65	1570	10.4
COOKED:								
1 pound of raw sausage, cooked (yield: approx. 12 oz.), 5 sausages (6g/tr/7g/50%/261mg)	1080	5.0			91.6	0.43	1465	6.8
1 sausage, cooked, approx. 2.4 oz.	216	1.0	216	1.0	91.6	0.43	1465	6.8
1 pound of raw sausage, cooked (yield: approx. 12 oz.), 4 sausages	1072	4.8			91.6	0.43	1465	6.8
1 sausage, cooked, approx. 2.9 oz.	268	1.2	268	1.2	91.6	0.43	1465	6.8

KIELBASA (Polish Sausage), made with pork, beef, and non-fat milk, based on generic data

	Unit Cal.	Unit Carb.	1 Slice or Link Cal.	1 Slice or Link Carb.	1 Oz., by Wt. Cal.	1 Oz., by Wt. Carb.	1 Pound Cal.	1 Pound Carb.
Kielbasa or Kolbassy, 1 pound (4g/1g/8g/54%/305mg)	1408	9.8			88.0	0.61	1408	9.8
1 slice, 6″ × 3¾″ × 1/16″ thick, approx. 0.9 oz.	81	0.6	81	0.6	88.0	0.61	1408	9.8
Prepackaged Links:								
1 package, 16-oz. (1-lb.) net wt., 2 sausages	1379	5.4			86.2	0.34	1379	5.4
1 sausage, 10″ long, 1¼″ diameter, approx. 8 oz.	690	2.7	690	2.7	86.2	0.34	1379	5.4
1 package, 16-oz. (1-lb.) net wt., 6 sausages	1379	5.4			86.2	0.34	1379	5.4
1 sausage, 5⅜″ long, 1″ diameter, approx. 2.7 oz.	231	0.9	231	0.9	86.2	0.34	1379	5.4

KIELBASA (Polish Sausage), by brand

	Unit Cal.	Unit Carb.	1 Slice or Link Cal.	1 Slice or Link Carb.	1 Oz., by Wt. Cal.	1 Oz., by Wt. Carb.	1 Pound Cal.	1 Pound Carb.
Eckrich Polska Kielbasa, 19-oz. package, 1–2 links	1900	9.5			100.0	0.50	1600	8.0
1 link (based on 2 links per package), approx. 9.5 oz.	950	4.8	950	4.8	100.0	0.50	1600	8.0

	UNIT Cal.	UNIT Carb.	1 SLICE OR LINK Cal.	1 SLICE OR LINK Carb.	1 OZ., BY WT. Cal.	1 OZ., BY WT. Carb.	1 POUND Cal.	1 POUND Carb.
Skinless Polska Kielbasa, 16-oz. (1-lb.) package, 8 links	1520	16.0			95.0	1.00	1520	16.0
1 link, approx. 2 oz.	190	2.0	190	2.0	95.0	1.00	1520	16.0
Hormel Kolbase Polish Sausage, 12-oz. package, 4 links	960	12.0			80.0	1.00	1280	16.0
1 link, approx. 3 oz.	240	3.0	240	3.0	80.0	1.00	1280	16.0
Kahn's Big Bucs Kielbasa Links, 16-oz. (1-lb.) package, 8 links	1470	13.6			91.9	0.85	1470	13.6
1 link, approx. 2 oz.	184	1.7	184	1.7	91.9	0.85	1470	13.6
Polska Kielbasa, 16-oz. (1-lb.) package, 8 sausages	1470	13.6			91.9	0.85	1470	13.6
1 sausage, approx. 2 oz.	184	1.7	184	1.7	91.9	0.85	1470	13.6
KNOCKWURST or KNACKWURST, made with pork and beef, based on generic data								
Knockwurst, 1 pound (3g/1g/8g/56%/286mg)	1392	8.0			87.0	0.50	1392	8.0
1 link, 4" long × 1⅛" diameter, approx. 2.4 oz.	209	1.2	209	1.2	87.0	0.50	1392	8.0
Prepackaged:								
1 package, 12 oz. net wt., 5 links	945	7.5			78.8	0.63	1261	10.0
1 link, 4" long × 1⅛" diameter, approx. 2.4 oz.	189	1.5	189	1.5	78.8	0.63	1261	10.0
KNOCKWURST or KNACKWURST, by brand								
Oscar Mayer Knackwurst Sausage Chubbies, 12-oz. package, 5 links	1068	7.4			89.0	0.62	1424	9.9
1 link, approx. 2.4 oz.	214	1.5	214	1.5	89.0	0.62	1424	9.9
LEBANON BOLOGNA, made with beef, based on generic data								
1 pound (6g/1g/4g/59%/359mg)	1024	9.6			64.0	0.60	1024	9.6
1 slice, 4" diameter × ⅛" thick, approx. 0.8 oz.	52	0.5	52	0.5	64.0	0.60	1024	9.6
LIVER CHEESE, made with pork, based on generic data								
1 pound (4g/1g/7g/54%/347mg)	1376	9.4			86.0	0.59	1376	9.4
1 slice, approx. 1.3 oz.	115	0.8	115	0.8	86.0	0.59	1376	9.4
LIVER CHEESE, by brand								
Oscar Mayer Liver Cheese, Sliced, 8-oz. package, 6 slices	689	2.9			86.1	0.37	1378	5.9
1 slice, approx. 1.3 oz.	115	0.5	115	0.5	86.1	0.37	1378	5.9
LIVER SAUSAGE (Liverwurst), made with pork, based on generic data								
1 pound (4g/1g/8g/52%/na)	1488	10.1			93.0	0.63	1488	10.1
1 slice, 2½" diameter × ¼" thick, approx. 0.6 oz.	59	0.4	59	0.4	93.0	0.63	1488	10.1
LIVERWURST, FRESH (not smoked), based on generic data								
1 pound	1488	10.1			93.0	0.63	1488	10.1
LIVERWURST, SMOKED, see BRAUNSCHWEIGER								

	UNIT Cal.	UNIT Carb.	1 SLICE OR LINK Cal.	1 SLICE OR LINK Carb.	1 OZ., BY WT. Cal.	1 OZ., BY WT. Carb.	1 POUND Cal.	1 POUND Carb.
LOAVES, based on generic data (see also MEAT LOAF and under LUNCHEON MEAT)								
Barbecue Loaf made with pork and beef, 1 pound (4g/2g/3g/65%/378mg)	784	29.1			49.0	1.82	784	29.1
1 slice, 5⅞" × 3½" × 1/16" thick, approx. 0.8 oz.	40	1.5	40	1.5	49.0	1.82	784	29.1
Corned Beef Loaf, jellied, 1 pound (7g/0g/2g/67%/294mg)	736	0.0			46.0	0.00	736	0.0
1 slice, 4" × 4" × 3/32" thick, approx. 1 oz.	46	0.0	46	0.0	46.0	0.00	736	0.0
Dutch Brand Loaf made with pork and beef, 1 pound (4g/2g/5g/59%/354mg)	1088	25.3			68.0	1.58	1088	25.3
1 slice, 4" × 4" × 3/32" thick, approx. 1 oz.	68	1.6	68	1.6	68.0	1.58	1088	25.3
Ham & Cheese Loaf or Roll, 1 pound (5g/tr/6g/58%/381mg)	1168	6.4			73.0	0.40	1168	6.4
1 slice, 4" × 4" × 3/32" thick, approx. 1 oz.	73	0.4	73	0.4	73.0	0.40	1168	6.4
Honey Loaf made with pork and beef, 1 pound (4g/2g/1g/70%/374mg)	576	24.2			36.0	1.51	576	24.2
1 slice, 4" × 4" × 3/32" thick, approx. 1 oz.	36	1.5	36	1.5	36.0	1.51	576	24.2
Luxury Loaf made with pork, 1 pound (5g/1g/1g/68%/347mg)	644	22.2			40.0	1.39	640	22.2
1 slice, 4" × 4" × 3/32" thick, approx. 1 oz.	40	1.4	40	1.4	40.0	1.39	640	22.2
Mother's Loaf made with pork, 1 pound (3g/2g/6g/55%/320mg)	1280	34.2			79.9	2.14	1278	34.2
1 slice, 4¼" × 4¼" × 1/16" thick, approx. 0.7 oz.	59	1.6	59	1.6	79.9	2.14	1278	34.2
Olive Loaf made with pork, 1 pound (4g/3g/5g/58%/421mg)	1072	41.6			66.6	2.60	1065	41.6
1 slice, 4" × 4" × 3/32" thick, approx. 1 oz.	67	2.6	67	2.6	66.6	2.60	1065	41.6
Peppered Loaf made with pork and beef, 1 pound (5g/1g/2g/71%/296mg)	672	20.8			42.0	1.30	672	20.8
1 slice, 4" × 4" × 3/32" thick, approx. 0.5 oz.	42	1.3	42	1.3	42.0	1.30	672	20.8
Pickle & Pimiento Loaf made with pork, 1 pound (3g/1g/6g/57%/394mg)	1184	26.7			74.0	1.67	1184	26.7
1 slice, 4" × 4" × 3/32" thick, approx. 1 oz.	74	1.7	74	1.7	74.0	1.67	1184	26.7
Picnic Loaf made with pork and beef, 1 pound (4g/1g/5g/60%/330mg)	1056	21.6			66.0	1.35	1056	21.6
1 slice, 4" × 4" × 3/32" thick, approx. 1 oz.	66	1.4	66	1.4	66.0	1.35	1056	21.6
LOAVES, by brand								
Eckrich Banquet Loaf, Sliced, 8-oz. package, 8 slices	600	12.0			75.0	1.50	1200	24.0
1 slice, approx. 1 oz.	75	1.5	75	1.5	75.0	1.50	1200	24.0
Bar B Loaf, Sliced, 8-oz. package, 8 slices	320	8.0			40.0	1.00	640	16.0
1 slice, approx. 1 oz.	40	1.0	40	1.0	40.0	1.00	640	16.0
Gourmet Loaf, Sliced, 8-oz. package, 8 slices	280	16.0			35.0	2.00	560	32.0
1 slice, approx. 1 oz.	35	2.0	35	2.0	35.0	2.00	560	32.0
Ham Loaf, Sliced, 8-oz. package, 8 slices	640	4.0			80.0	0.50	1280	8.0
1 slice, approx. 1 oz.	80	0.5	80	0.5	80.0	0.50	1280	8.0
Ham and Cheese Loaf, Sliced, 8-oz. package, 8 slices	560	8.0			70.0	1.00	1120	16.0
1 slice, approx. 1 oz.	70	1.0	70	1.0	70.0	1.00	1120	16.0
Honey Style Loaf, Sliced, 8-oz. package, 8 slices	320	16.0			40.0	2.00	640	32.0
1 slice, approx. 1 oz.	40	2.0	40	2.0	40.0	2.00	640	32.0
Macaroni Cheese Loaf, Sliced, 8-oz. package, 8 slices	560	20.0			70.0	2.50	1120	40.0
1 slice, approx. 1 oz.	70	2.5	70	2.5	70.0	2.50	1120	40.0

	UNIT Cal.	UNIT Carb.	1 SLICE OR LINK Cal.	1 SLICE OR LINK Carb.	1 OZ., BY WT. Cal.	1 OZ., BY WT. Carb.	1 POUND Cal.	1 POUND Carb.
Old Fashion Loaf, Sliced, 8-oz. package, 8 slices	600	16.0			75.0	2.00	1200	32.0
1 slice, approx. 1 oz.	75	2.0	75	2.0	75.0	2.00	1200	32.0
Olive Loaf, Sliced, 8-oz. package, 8 slices	680	12.0			85.0	1.50	1360	24.0
1 slice, approx. 1 oz.	85	1.5	85	1.5	85.0	1.50	1360	24.0
Peppered Loaf, Sliced, 8-oz. package, 8 slices	320	8.0			40.0	1.00	640	16.0
1 slice, approx. 1 oz.	40	1.0	40	1.0	40.0	1.00	640	16.0
Pickle Loaf, Sliced, 8-oz. package, 8 slices	680	12.0			85.0	1.50	1360	24.0
1 slice, approx. 1 oz.	85	1.5	85	1.5	85.0	1.50	1360	24.0
Oscar Mayer Bar-B-Q Loaf, Sliced, 8-oz. package, 8 slices	400	15.2			50.0	1.90	800	30.4
1 slice, approx. 1 oz.	50	1.9	50	1.9	50.0	1.90	800	30.4
Cocktail Loaf, Sliced, 8-oz. package, 8 slices	517	23.4			64.6	2.92	1034	46.7
1 slice, approx. 1 oz.	65	2.9	65	2.9	64.6	2.92	1034	46.7
Jellied Corned Beef Loaf, Sliced, 8-oz. package, 8 slices	318	0.0			39.7	0.00	635	0.0
1 slice, approx. 1 oz.	40	0.0	40	0.0	39.7	0.00	635	0.0
Ham And Cheese Loaf, Sliced, 8-oz. package, 8 slices	572	5.0			71.4	0.31	1142	5.0
1 slice, approx. 1 oz.	71	0.3	71	0.3	71.4	0.31	1142	5.0
Honey Loaf, Sliced, 8-oz. package, 8 slices	304	7.9			38.0	0.99	608	15.8
1 slice, approx. 1 oz.	38	1.0	38	1.0	38.0	0.99	608	15.8
Luxury Loaf, Sliced, 8-oz. package, 8 slices	302	11.8			37.6	1.47	603	23.5
1 slice, approx. 1 oz.	38	1.5	38	1.5	37.6	1.47	603	23.5
Old Fashioned Loaf, Sliced, 8-oz. package, 8 slices	526	17.2			65.8	2.15	1053	34.4
1 slice, approx. 1 oz.	66	2.2	66	2.2	65.8	2.15	1053	34.4
Olive Loaf, Sliced, 8-oz. package, 8 slices	519	20.9			64.9	2.61	1038	41.8
1 slice, approx. 1 oz.	65	2.6	65	2.6	64.9	2.61	1038	41.8
Peppered Loaf, Sliced, 8-oz. package, 8 slices	372	12.5			46.5	1.56	744	25.0
1 slice, approx. 1 oz.	47	1.6	47	1.6	46.5	1.56	744	25.0
Pickle & Pimiento Loaf, Sliced, 8-oz. package, 8 slices	517	23.4			64.6	2.92	1034	46.7
1 slice, approx. 1 oz.	65	2.9	65	2.9	64.6	2.92	1034	46.7
Picnic Loaf, Sliced, 8-oz. package, 8 slices	494	10.9			61.8	1.36	989	21.8
1 slice, approx. 1 oz.	62	1.4	62	1.4	61.8	1.36	989	21.8

LUNCHEON MEAT, based on generic data

	UNIT Cal.	UNIT Carb.	1 SLICE OR LINK Cal.	1 SLICE OR LINK Carb.	1 OZ., BY WT. Cal.	1 OZ., BY WT. Carb.	1 POUND Cal.	1 POUND Carb.
Loaf, Made with Beef:								
1 pound (52.5% water) (4g/1g/7g/52%/377mg)	1392	13.1			87.0	0.82	1392	13.1
1 slice, 4″ × 4″ × 3/32″ thick, approx. 1 oz.	87	0.8	87	0.8	87.0	0.82	1392	13.1
Thin sliced, Made with Beef:								
1 pound (70% water) (6g/tr/1g/70%/470mg)	560	1.4			34.9	0.09	557	1.4
1 slice, approx. 0.2 oz.	5	trace	5	trace	34.9	0.09	557	1.4
Made with Pork and Beef:								
1 pound (4g/1g/9g/49%/367mg)	1600	10.6			100.0	0.66	1601	10.6
1 slice, 4″ × 4″ × 3/32″ thick, approx. 1 oz.	100	0.7	100	0.7	100.0	0.66	1601	10.6
Canned, Made with Pork:								
1 pound (4g/1g/9g/52%/365mg)	1520	9.3			95.0	0.58	1517	9.3
1 slice, 4¼″ × 4¼″ × 1/16″ thick, approx. 0.7 oz.	70	0.4	70	0.4	95.0	0.58	1517	9.3

LUNCHEON MEAT, by brand

	UNIT Cal.	UNIT Carb.	1 SLICE OR LINK Cal.	1 SLICE OR LINK Carb.	1 OZ., BY WT. Cal.	1 OZ., BY WT. Carb.	1 POUND Cal.	1 POUND Carb.
Armour Treet, 12-oz. container	1200	12.0			100.0	1.00	1600	16.0
Hormel Spiced Luncheon Meat, 8-oz. package	640	8.0			80.0	1.00	1280	16.0
Oscar Mayer Sliced Luncheon Meat, 8-oz. package, 8 slices	747	5.9			95.8	0.74	1533	11.8
1 slice, approx. 1.0 oz.	96	0.7	96	0.7	95.8	0.74	1533	11.8

LUNCHEON SAUSAGE, made with pork and beef, based on generic data

	UNIT Cal.	UNIT Carb.	1 SLICE OR LINK Cal.	1 SLICE OR LINK Carb.	1 OZ., BY WT. Cal.	1 OZ., BY WT. Carb.	1 POUND Cal.	1 POUND Carb.
1 pound (4g/tr/6g/59%/335mg)	1184	7.2			73.8	0.45	1181	7.2
1 slice, 4″ diameter × 1/8″ thick, approx. 0.9 oz.	60	0.4	60	0.4	73.8	0.45	1181	7.2

MEAT LOAF, based on generic data

	UNIT Cal.	UNIT Carb.	1 SLICE OR LINK Cal.	1 SLICE OR LINK Carb.	1 OZ., BY WT. Cal.	1 OZ., BY WT. Carb.	1 POUND Cal.	1 POUND Carb.
Ingredients Not Specified:								
1 pound	907	15.0			56.7	0.94	907	15.0

MORTADELLA, based on generic data

	UNIT Cal.	UNIT Carb.	1 SLICE OR LINK Cal.	1 SLICE OR LINK Carb.	1 OZ., BY WT. Cal.	1 OZ., BY WT. Carb.	1 POUND Cal.	1 POUND Carb.
Ingredients Not Specified:								
1 pound	1429	2.7			89.3	0.17	1429	2.7
1 slice, 4⅞″ diameter, 3/32″ thick, approx. 0.9 oz.	79	0.2	79	0.2	89.3	0.17	1429	2.7
Made with Beef and Pork:								
1 pound (5g/1g/7g/52%/353mg)	1408	13.9			88.2	0.87	1411	13.9
1 slice, approx. 0.5 oz.	47	0.5	47	0.5	88.2	0.87	1411	13.9

MOTHER'S LOAF, see LOAVES

NEW ENGLAND BRAND SAUSAGE, made with pork and beef, based on generic data

	UNIT Cal.	UNIT Carb.	1 SLICE OR LINK Cal.	1 SLICE OR LINK Carb.	1 OZ., BY WT. Cal.	1 OZ., BY WT. Carb.	1 POUND Cal.	1 POUND Carb.
1 pound (5g/1g/2g/67%/346mg)	736	21.9			45.6	1.37	730	21.9
1 slice, 4″ diameter × 1/8″ thick, approx. 0.8 oz.	37	1.1	37	1.1	45.6	1.37	730	21.9

NEW ENGLAND BRAND SAUSAGE, by brand

	UNIT Cal.	UNIT Carb.	1 SLICE OR LINK Cal.	1 SLICE OR LINK Carb.	1 OZ., BY WT. Cal.	1 OZ., BY WT. Carb.	1 POUND Cal.	1 POUND Carb.
Eckrich New England Brand Sausage, Sliced, 8-oz package, 8 slices	280	8.0			35.0	1.00	560	16.0
1 slice, approx. 1 oz.	35	1.0	35	1.0	35.0	1.00	560	16.0
Oscar Mayer New England Brand Sausage, Sliced, 8-oz. package, 10 slices	329	4.5			41.1	0.57	658	9.1
1 slice, approx. 0.8 oz.	33	0.5	33	0.5	41.1	0.57	658	9.1

PASTRAMI, by brand

	UNIT Cal.	UNIT Carb.	1 SLICE OR LINK Cal.	1 SLICE OR LINK Carb.	1 OZ., BY WT. Cal.	1 OZ., BY WT. Carb.	1 POUND Cal.	1 POUND Carb.
A & P Smoked Pastrami, Sliced, 3-oz. package, 3 slices	135	3.0			45.0	1.00	720	16.0
1 slice, approx. 1 oz.	45	1.6	45	1.6	45.0	1.00	720	16.0
Carl Buddig Pastrami, 2.5-oz. package	100	0.0			40.0	0.00	640	0.0
Eckrich Slender Pastrami, Sliced, 3-oz. package, 3 slices	140	4.0			46.7	1.33	747	21.3
1 slice, approx. 1 oz.	47	1.3	47	1.3	46.7	1.33	747	21.3
Longacre Turkey Pastrami, Sliced, 6-oz. package, 8 slices	240	0.0			40.0	0.00	640	0.0
1 slice, approx. 0.8 oz.	30	0.0	30	0.0	40.0	0.00	640	0.0
Longmont Turkey Pastrami, Sliced, 8-oz. package, 10 slices	309	100.0			38.6	0.26	618	4.2
1 slice, approx. 0.8 oz.	31	10.0	31	10.0	38.6	0.26	618	4.2
Rich's Smoked Turkey Pastrami, Sliced, 8-oz. package, 8 slices	280	0.0			35.0	0.00	560	0.0
1 slice, approx. 1 oz.	35	0.0	35	0.0	35.0	0.00	560	0.0
Safeway Smoked Pastrami, Chopped-Pressed-Cooked, Sliced, 3-oz. package, 3 slices	135	0.0			45.0	0.00	720	0.0
1 slice, approx. 1 oz.	45	0.0	45	0.0	45.0	0.00	720	0.0

	UNIT		1 SLICE OR LINK		1 OZ., BY WT.		1 POUND	
	Cal.	Carb.	Cal.	Carb.	Cal.	Carb.	Cal.	Carb.
PEPPERONI, made with pork and beef, based on generic data								
1 pound	2255	12.9			140.9	0.81	2255	12.9
1 sausage, 10¼″ long × 1⅜″ diameter, approx. 8.9 oz.	1248	7.1			140.9	0.81	2255	12.9
1 slice, 1⅜″ diameter × ⅛″ thick, approx. 0.2 oz.	27	0.2	27	0.2	140.9	0.81	2255	12.9
PEPPERONI, by brand								
Hormel Pepperoni, Sliced, 3½-oz. package	490	0.0			140.0	0.00	2240	0.0
Lowrey's Pepperoni Sticks, 16½-oz. jar, 25 sticks	2648	11.0			161.0	0.67	2576	10.7
26.4-oz. jar, 40 sticks	4250	17.6			161.0	0.67	2576	10.7
1 stick, approx. ⅔ oz.	107	0.5	107	0.5	161.0	0.67	2576	10.7
Pepperoni Stick, 1 stick, approx. ¼ oz.	40	0.2	40	0.2	161.0	0.67	2576	10.7
Swift Premium Pepperoni, 5-oz. package	750	5.0			150.0	1.00	2400	16.0
POLISH SAUSAGE, based on generic data (see also KIELBASA)								
Polish Sausage made with pork, 1 pound (4g/tr/8g/53%/248mg)	1472	7.4			92.0	0.46	1472	7.4
1 sausage, 10″ long × 1¼″ diameter, approx. 8 oz.	739	3.7	739	3.7	92.0	0.46	1472	7.4
PORK, cured ham or shoulder, chopped, spiced or unspiced, based on generic data								
CANNED:								
1 can, rectangular piece, 3½″ long × 2″ wide × 3″ high, 12 oz. net wt.	1000	4.4			83.4	2.56	1334	5.9
1 slice, 3″ × 2″ × ½″, ⅙ of piece, approx. 2.1 oz.	176	0.8	176	0.8	83.4	2.56	1334	5.9
1 can, rectangular piece, 3½″ long × 2″ wide × 1¾″ high, 7 oz. net wt.	582	2.6			83.4	2.56	1334	5.9
1 slice, 3″ × 2″ × ½″, approx. 2.1 oz.	176	0.8	176	0.8	83.4	2.56	1334	5.9
PORK, by brand								
Eckrich Slender Smoked Pork, Sliced, 3-oz. package, 3 slices	140	2.0			46.7	0.67	747	10.7
1 slice, approx. 1 oz.	47	0.7	47	0.7	46.7	0.67	747	10.7
PORK SAUSAGE, based on generic data								
RAW:								
Fresh, 1 pound (3g/tr/11g/45%/228mg)	1892	4.6			118.2	0.29	1892	4.6
1 link, 4″ long × ⅞″ diameter, approx. 1.0 oz.	118	0.3	118	0.3	118.2	0.29	1892	4.6
1 patty, 3⅞″ diameter × ¼″ thick, approx. 2 oz.	238	0.6	238	0.6	118.2	0.29	1892	4.6
COOKED:								
Fresh, (yield from 1 lb. raw: approx. 7.6 oz., cooked) (6g/tr/9g/45%/367mg)	793	2.2			104.6	0.29	1674	4.7
1 link, 4″ long × ⅞″ diameter, approx. 0.5 oz.	48	0.1	48	0.1	104.6	0.29	1674	4.7
1 patty, 3⅞″ diameter × ¼″ thick, approx. 1 oz.	100	0.3	100	0.3	104.6	0.29	1674	4.7
1 pound, cooked	1674	4.7			104.6	0.29	1674	4.7

	UNIT		1 SLICE OR LINK		1 OZ., BY WT.		1 POUND	
	Cal.	Carb.	Cal.	Carb.	Cal.	Carb.	Cal.	Carb.
Prepackaged:								
Roll:								
RAW:								
1 package, 5⅞″ long × 2¼″ diameter, 16 oz. (1 lb.) net wt. (3g/tr/15g/38%/211mg)	2259	trace			141.2	trace	2259	trace
1 package, 5⅜″ long × 2½″ diameter, 16 oz. (1 lb.) net wt.	2259	trace			141.2	trace	2259	trace
COOKED:								
Yield from 1 pound: approx. 7.5 oz. (5g/tr/13g/35%/274mg)	1014	trace			135.2	trace	2263	trace
Brick:								
RAW:								
1 package, 5⅛″ × 3″ × 1⅞″, 16 oz. (1 lb.) net wt. (3g/tr/15g/38%/211mg)	2259	trace			141.2	trace	2259	trace
COOKED:								
Yield from 1 pound: approx. 7.5 oz. (5g/tr/13g/35%/274mg)	1014	trace			135.2	trace	2163	trace
Rope Form:								
RAW:								
1 package, 20″ long × 1¼″ diameter, 16 oz. (1 lb.) net wt. (3g/tr/15g/38%/211mg)	2259	trace			141.2	trace	2259	trace
COOKED:								
Yield from 1 pound: approx. 7.5 oz. (5g/tr/13g/35%/274 mg)	1014	trace			135.2	trace	2163	trace
Links:								
RAW:								
1 package, 16 oz. (1 lb.) net wt., 16 links, approx. 1 oz.) (3g/tr/15g/38%/214mg)	2259	trace			141.2	trace	2259	trace
1 link 4″ long, ⅞″ diameter, approx. 1 oz.	141	trace	141	trace	141.2	trace	2259	trace
COOKED:								
Yield from 1 pound: approx. 7.5 oz. (5g/tr/13g/35%/274mg)	1014	trace			135.2	trace	2163	trace
1 link, approx. 0.5 oz.	62	trace	62	trace	135.2	trace	2163	trace
RAW:								
1 package, 8 oz. net wt., 8 links (3g/tr/15g/38%/211mg)	1130	trace			141.2	trace	2259	trace
1 link, 4″ long, ⅞″ diameter, approx. 1 oz.	141	trace	141	trace	141.2	trace	2259	trace
COOKED:								
Yield from 8 oz.: approx. 3.8 oz. (5g/tr/13g/35%/274mg)	509	trace			135.2	trace	2163	trace
1 link	62	trace	62	trace	135.2	trace	2163	trace
CANNED:								
1 can, 8 oz. net wt., 14 sausage links. Solids and liquid, approx. 1 cup (4g/1g/11g/42%/na)	942	5.4			117.8	0.68	1884	10.8
Drained solids (approx. 5.7 oz.) (5g/1g/9g/43%/na)	617	3.1			108.0	0.54	1728	8.7
1 link, 3″ long × ½″ diameter, approx. 0.4 oz.	46	0.2	46	0.2	108.0	0.54	1728	8.7
PORK SAUSAGE, by brand								
Hormel Brown 'N Serve Pork Sausage, 8-oz. package, 10 sausages	775	0.0			96.9	0.00	1550	0.0
1 sausage, approx. 0.8 oz.	78	0.0	78	0.0	96.9	0.00	1550	0.0
Little Sizzlers Pork Sausage, 12-oz. package, 10 sausages	1325	2.5			110.4	0.21	1766	3.4
1 sausage, approx. 1.2 oz.	133	0.3	133	0.3	110.4	0.21	1766	3.4
Midget Link Pork Sausage, 16-oz. (1-lb.) package, 16 sausages	1800	4.0			112.5	0.25	1800	4.0
1 sausage, approx. 1 oz.	113	0.3	113	0.3	112.5	0.25	1800	4.0
Smoked Pork Sausage, 16-oz. (1-lb.) package	1547	0.0			96.7	0.00	1547	0.0
Smokies, 12-oz. package, 12 sausages	1110	6.0			92.5	0.58	1480	8.0
1 sausage, approx. 1 oz.	93	0.5	93	0.5	92.5	0.58	1480	8.0

	UNIT		1 SLICE OR LINK		1 OZ., BY WT.		1 POUND	
	Cal.	Carb.	Cal.	Carb.	Cal.	Carb.	Cal.	Carb.
Jones Dinner Pork Sausages, 16-oz. (1-lb.) box, 8 links (cooked yield: approx. 10.6 oz.)	1464	trace			(125.8)	trace	(2012)	trace
1 link, approx. 2 oz. raw (cooked yield: approx. 1.3 oz.)	183	trace	183	trace	(125.8)	trace	(2012)	trace
Little Pork Sausages, 8-oz. box, 8 links (cooked yield: approx. 5.3 oz.)	664	trace			(125.8)	trace	(2012)	trace
1 link, approx. 1 oz. raw (cooked yield: approx. 0.7 oz.)	83	trace	83	trace	(125.8)	trace	(2012)	trace
Oscar Mayer Bulk Tube Pork Sausage, 16-oz. (1-lb.) tube (yield: approx. 8 oz. cooked)	880	2.7			109.4	0.34	1750	5.4
1 patty, approx. 1 oz. (yield: approx. 0.5 oz. cooked)	55	0.2	55	0.2	109.4	0.34	1750	5.4
Little Friers Pork Sausage, 12-oz. package, 12 links (yield: approx. 7.9 oz. cooked)	780	5.1			99.2	0.65	1588	10.4
1 link, approx. 1 oz. (yield: approx. 0.7 oz. cooked)	65	0.4	65	0.4	99.2	0.65	1588	10.4

PORK & BEEF SAUSAGE, based on generic data

	UNIT		1 SLICE OR LINK		1 OZ., BY WT.		1 POUND	
	Cal.	Carb.	Cal.	Carb.	Cal.	Carb.	Cal.	Carb.
Fresh (yield from 1 lb. raw: approx. 7.6 oz., cooked) (4g/1g/10g/44%/228mg)	853	5.9			112.3	0.77	1796	12.3
1 link, cooked, 4″ long × ⅞″ diameter, approx. 0.5 oz.	52	0.4	52	0.4	112.3	0.77	1796	12.3
1 patty, cooked, 3⅞″ diameter × ¼″ thick, approx. 1 oz.	107	0.7	107	0.7	112.3	0.77	1796	12.3
1 pound, cooked	1796	12.3			112.3	0.77	1796	12.3

POTTED MEAT, based on generic data

	UNIT		1 SLICE OR LINK		1 OZ., BY WT.		1 POUND	
	Cal.	Carb.	Cal.	Carb.	Cal.	Carb.	Cal.	Carb.
CANNED:								
1 can, 3 to 3¼ oz. net wt.	(211-229)	0.0			70.4	0.00	1126	0.0
1 can, 5½ oz. net wt.	387	0.0			70.4	0.00	1126	0.0
1 cup (approx. 7.9 oz.)	558	0.0			70.4	0.00	1126	0.0
1 tablespoon (approx. 0.5 oz.)	32	0.0			70.4	0.00	1126	0.0

SALAMI, based on generic data

	UNIT		1 SLICE OR LINK		1 OZ., BY WT.		1 POUND	
	Cal.	Carb.	Cal.	Carb.	Cal.	Carb.	Cal.	Carb.
DRY:								
Roll								
Prepackaged, Not Presliced:								
1 package, 5¾″ long × 1¾″ diameter, 8¼ oz. net wt.	1053	2.8			127.6	0.34	2042	5.4
Prepackaged, Presliced:								
1 package, 3⅛″ diameter, 4 oz., 12 slices	509	1.4			127.6	0.34	2042	5.4
1 slice, 1/16″ thick, approx. ⅓ oz.	45	0.1	45	0.1	127.6	0.34	2042	5.4
1 package, 2¾″ diameter, 4 oz., 12 slices	504	1.4			127.6	0.34	2042	5.4
1 slice, 3/32″ thick, approx. ⅓ oz.	45	0.1	45	0.1	127.6	0.34	2042	5.4
COOKED:								
Made with Beef:								
1 pound (4g/1g/6g/59%/328mg)	1152	11.4			72.0	0.71	1152	11.4
1 slice, 4″ diameter × ⅛″ thick, approx. 0.8 oz.	58	0.6	58	0.6	72.0	0.71	1152	11.4
Made with Beef and Pork:								
1 pound (4g/1g/6g/60%/302mg)	1136	10.2			71.0	0.64	1136	10.2
1 slice, 4″ diameter × ⅛″ thick, approx. 0.8 oz.	57	0.5	57	0.5	71.0	0.64	1136	10.2
Turkey Salami:								
1 pound (5g/tr/4g/66%/287mg)	891	2.5			55.7	0.16	889	2.5
8-oz. package, 8 slices	446	1.2			55.7	0.16	889	2.5
1 slice, approx. 1 oz.	56	0.2	56	0.2	55.7	0.16	889	2.5

SALAMI, by brand

	UNIT		1 SLICE OR LINK		1 OZ., BY WT.		1 POUND	
	Cal.	Carb.	Cal.	Carb.	Cal.	Carb.	Cal.	Carb.
Best's Salami, "Lower Fat Beef," Kosher, 6-oz. package, 8 slices	400	8.0			66.7	1.33	1067	21.3
1 slice, approx. ¾ oz.	50	1.0	50	1.0	66.7	1.33	1067	21.3
De Lusso Genoa Salami, 6-lb. stick	12480	96.0			130.0	1.00	2080	16.0
Hormel Dairy Hard Salami, Sliced, 4-oz. package, 15 slices	480	0.0			120.0	0.00	1920	0.0
1 slice, approx. 0.3 oz.	32	0.0	32	0.0	120.0	0.00	1920	0.0
Longacre Turkey Salami, 6-oz. package, 8 slices	240	0.0			40.0	0.00	640	0.0
1 slice, approx. 0.8 oz.	30	0.0	30	0.0	40.0	0.00	640	0.0
Turkey Salami, cooked, 6-oz. package, 8 slices	280	8.0			46.7	1.33	747	21.3
1 slice, approx. 0.8 oz.	35	0.5	35	0.5	46.7	1.33	747	21.3
Longmont Turkey Salami, Sliced, 16-oz. (1-lb.) package, 10 slices	653	5.9			40.8	0.37	656	5.9
1 slice, approx. 1.6 oz.	66	0.6	66	0.6	40.8	0.37	656	5.9
12-oz. package, 12 slices	490	4.4			40.8	0.37	656	5.9
1 slice, approx. 1 oz.	41	0.4	41	0.4	40.8	0.37	656	5.9
Oscar Mayer Beef Cotto Salami, Sliced, 8-oz. package, 10 slices	492	4.8			61.5	0.60	984	9.6
1 slice, approx. 0.8 oz.	49	0.6	49	0.6	61.5	0.60	984	9.6
Cotto Salami, Sliced, 8-oz. package, 10 slices	528	5.0			66.1	0.62	1058	9.9
1 slice, approx. 0.8 oz.	53	0.5	53	0.5	66.1	0.62	1058	9.9
Hard Salami, Sliced, 8-oz. package, 22–26 slices	900	2.5			113.0	0.31	1808	5.0
1 slice, approx. 0.3 oz. (based on 24 slices per package)	38	0.1	38	0.1	113.0	0.31	1808	5.0
Salami for Beer, Sliced, 8-oz. package, 10 slices	503	3.6			62.9	0.45	1006	7.2
1 slice, approx. 0.8 oz.	50	0.4	50	0.4	62.9	0.45	1006	7.2
Rich's Smoked Turkey Salami, Sliced, 8-oz. package, 8 slices	440	4.0			55.0	0.50	880	8.0
1 slice, approx. 1 oz.	55	0.1	55	0.1	55.0	0.50	880	8.0
Swift Premium Genoa Salami, Sliced, 4-oz. package	480	0.0			120.0	0.00	1920	0.0
Hard Salami, Sliced, 4-oz. package	440	4.0			110.0	1.00	1760	16.0

SAUSAGES, OTHER, by brand

	UNIT		1 SLICE OR LINK		1 OZ., BY WT.		1 POUND	
	Cal.	Carb.	Cal.	Carb.	Cal.	Carb.	Cal.	Carb.
Armour Banner Sausage, 10½-oz. container, 2 sausages	620	5.9			59.1	0.57	946	9.1
1 sausage, approx. 5¼ oz.	310	3.0	310	3.0	59.1	0.57	946	9.1
24-oz. container, 6 sausages	1440	12.0			60.0	0.50	960	8.0
1 sausage, approx. 4 oz.	240	2.0	240	2.0	60.0	0.50	960	8.0
Eckrich Minced Sausage Roll, Sliced, 8-oz. package, 8 slices	640	8.0			80.0	1.00	1280	16.0
1 slice, approx. 1 oz.	80	1.0	80	1.0	80.0	1.00	1280	16.0
Smoked Beef Sausage, 16-oz. (1-lb.) package, approx. 8 sausages	1520	8.0			95.0	0.50	1520	8.0
1 link, approx. 2 oz.	190	1.0	190	1.0	95.0	0.50	1520	8.0
Smoked Skinless Sausage Links, 12-oz. package, 10 links	1150	10.0			95.8	0.83	1533	13.3
1 link, approx. 1.2 oz.	115	1.0	115	1.0	95.8	0.83	1533	13.3
16-oz. (1-lb.) package, 8 links	1520	16.0			95.0	1.00	1520	16.0
1 link, approx. 2 oz.	190	2.0	190	2.0	95.0	1.00	1520	16.0
Smok-Y-Links, Beef, 10-oz. package, 12 links	900	12.0			90.0	1.20	1440	19.2
1 link, approx. 0.8 oz.	75	1.0	75	1.0	90.0	1.20	1440	19.2
Smok-Y-Links, Natural Maple Flavored, 10-oz. package, 12 links	900	12.0			90.0	1.20	1440	19.2
1 link, approx. 0.8 oz.	75	1.0	75	1.0	90.0	1.20	1440	19.2
Smok-Y-Links, Skinless, 10-oz. package, 12 links	1020	12.0			102.0	1.20	1632	19.2
1 link, approx. 0.8 oz.	85	1.0	85	1.0	102.0	1.20	1632	19.2
Jones Brown 'N Serve Minute Breakfast Links, 8-oz. box, 10 links	625				78.1	trace	1250	
1 link, approx. 0.8 oz.	63	trace	63	trace	78.1	trace	1250	

	UNIT		1 SLICE OR LINK		1 OZ., BY WT.		1 POUND	
	Cal.	Carb.	Cal.	Carb.	Cal.	Carb.	Cal.	Carb.
Brown 'N Serve Minute Breakfast Links with Bacon, 8-oz. box, 10 links	625				78.1	trace	1250	
1 link, approx. 0.8 oz.	63	trace	63	trace	78.1	trace	1250	
Kahn's Big Red Smokeys Sausage, 16-oz. (1-lb.) package, 8 sausages	1453	9.1			90.8	0.57	1453	9.1
1 sausage, approx. 2 oz.	182	1.1	182	1.1	90.8	0.57	1453	9.1
Endless Sausage, 16-oz. (1-lb.) package	1451	9.0			90.7	0.57	1451	9.0
Jumbo Smokeys Sausage, 16-oz. (1-lb.) package, 8 sausages	1453	9.1			90.8	0.57	1453	9.1
1 sausage, approx. 2 oz.	182	1.1	182	1.1	90.8	0.57	1453	9.1
Reds Rookies Smoked Sausage, 10-oz. package, 5 sausages	908	5.7			90.7	0.57	1451	9.0
1 sausage, approx. 2 oz.	182	1.1	182	1.1	90.7	0.57	1451	9.0
Smoked Sausage and Hot Metts, 16-oz. (1-lb.) package, 8 sausages	1453	9.1			90.8	0.57	1453	9.1
1 sausage, approx. 2 oz.	182	1.1	182	1.1	90.8	0.57	1453	9.1
Louis Rich Turkey Breakfast Sausage, 16-oz. (1-lb.) package, 8 patties, raw	880	8.0			55.0	0.50	880	8.0
Cooked (yield: approx. 10.4 oz.)	624	7.8			60.0	0.75	960	12.0
1 patty, approx. 2 oz., raw	110	1.0	110	1.0	55.0	0.50	880	8.0
Cooked, (yield: approx. 1.3 oz.)	80	1.0	80	1.0	60.0	0.75	960	12.0
Turkey Sausage Links, 8-oz. package, 8 links	440	4.0			55.0	0.50	880	8.0
1 link, approx. 1 oz.	55	0.5	55	0.5	55.0	0.50	880	8.0
Oscar Mayer Beef Honey Hill Sausage, Sliced, 8-oz. package, 10 slices	395	5.4			49.3	0.68	789	10.9
1 slice, approx. 0.8 oz.	40	0.5	40	0.5	49.3	0.68	789	10.9
Little Smokie Links Sausage, 5-oz. package, 16 links	481	2.3			96.2	0.45	1538	7.2
1 link, approx. 0.3 oz.	30	0.1	30	0.1	96.2	0.45	1538	7.2
Minced Sausage Roll, Sliced, 8-oz. package, 10 slices	542	5.4			67.8	0.68	1085	10.9
1 slice, approx. 0.8 oz.	54	0.5	54	0.5	67.8	0.68	1085	10.9
Smoked Breakfast Sausage, 5-oz. package, 7 links	481	2.3			96.1	0.45	1538	7.2
1 link, approx. 0.7 oz.	69	0.3	69	0.3	96.1	0.45	1538	7.2
Smokie Links Sausage, 12-oz. package, 8 links	1061	4.1			88.5	0.34	1416	5.4
1 link, approx. 1.5 oz.	133	0.5	133	0.5	88.5	0.34	1416	5.4
Swift Premium Brown 'N Serve Bacon 'N Sausage, 8-oz. carton, 10 links (yield: approx. 7 oz. cooked)	700	5.0			99.2	0.71	1588	11.3
1 link, 0.8 oz. (yield: approx. 0.7 oz. cooked)	70	0.5	70	0.5	99.2	0.71	1588	11.3
Brown 'N Serve Sausage, 8-oz. carton, 8 links (yield: approx. 7 oz. cooked)	750	5.0			107.1	0.71	1714	11.4
1 link, approx. 0.8 oz. (yield: approx. 0.7 oz. cooked)	75	0.5	75	0.5	107.1	0.71	1714	11.4

SCRAPPLE, based on generic data

	UNIT		1 SLICE OR LINK		1 OZ., BY WT.		1 POUND	
	Cal.	Carb.	Cal.	Carb.	Cal.	Carb.	Cal.	Carb.
Prepackaged Loaf:								
1 package, 4½" × 2¾" × 2⅛", 16 oz. (1 lb.) net wt.	975	66.2			60.9	4.14	975	66.2

SMOKED LINK SAUSAGE, made with pork, based on generic data

	UNIT		1 SLICE OR LINK		1 OZ., BY WT.		1 POUND	
	Cal.	Carb.	Cal.	Carb.	Cal.	Carb.	Cal.	Carb.
1 pound (6g/1g/9g/39%/429mg)	1765	9.5			110.3	0.60	1765	9.5
1 "little" link, 2" long × ¾" diameter, approx. 0.6 oz.	62	0.3	62	0.3	110.3	0.60	1765	9.5
1 link, 4" long × 1⅛" diameter, approx. 2.4 oz.	265	1.4	265	1.4	110.3	0.60	1765	9.5

SOUSE, based on generic data

	UNIT		1 SLICE OR LINK		1 OZ., BY WT.		1 POUND	
	Cal.	Carb.	Cal.	Carb.	Cal.	Carb.	Cal.	Carb.
Prepackaged, Presliced:								
1 package, 3⅞" × 3⅞", 6 oz. net wt., 6 slices	308	2.0			51.3	0.05	821	0.8
1 slice, approx. 1 oz.	51	0.3	51	0.3	51.3	0.05	821	0.8

SUMMER SAUSAGE (Thuringer, Cervelat), dry, based on generic data

	UNIT		1 SLICE OR LINK		1 OZ., BY WT.		1 POUND	
	Cal.	Carb.	Cal.	Carb.	Cal.	Carb.	Cal.	Carb.
Prepackaged:								
Roll, not presliced:								
1 package 5" long × 1½" diameter roll, approx. 5⅓ oz. net wt.	465	2.4			87.1	0.46	1393	73.0
Roll, presliced:								
1 package 4⅜" diameter, 8 oz. net wt., 8 slices	697	3.5			87.1	0.46	1393	73.0
1 slice, approx. 1 oz.	87	0.5	87	0.5	87.1	0.46	1393	73.0
1 package, 4⅛" diameter, 8 oz. net wt., 10 slices	697	3.6			87.1	0.46	1393	73.0
1 slice, approx. ¾ oz.	70	0.4	70	0.4	87.1	0.46	1393	73.0
1 package, 2⅞" diameter, 4 oz. net wt., 15 slices	347	1.8			87.1	0.46	1393	73.0
1 slice, approx. ¼ oz.	23	0.1	23	0.1	87.1	0.46	1393	73.0

SUMMER SAUSAGE (Thuringer, Cervelat), by brand

	UNIT		1 SLICE OR LINK		1 OZ., BY WT.		1 POUND	
	Cal.	Carb.	Cal.	Carb.	Cal.	Carb.	Cal.	Carb.
Big Horn Summer Sausage, 4.9-oz. can	608	2.6			124.0	0.52	1980	8.3
Louis Rich Turkey Summer Sausage, 8-oz. package, 8 slices	440	0.0			55.0	0.00	720	0.0
1 slice, approx. 1 oz.	55	0.0	55	0.0	55.0	0.00	720	0.0
Old Smokehouse Thuringer, Sliced, 4-oz. package, 15 slices	400	0.0			100.0	0.00	1600	0.0
1 slice, approx. ¼ oz.	27	0.0	27	0.0	100.0	0.00	1600	0.0
11-oz. stick	1100	0.0			100.0	0.00	1600	0.0
Oscar Mayer Thuringer Cervelat, Sliced, 8-oz. package, 10 slices	719	2.3			89.9	0.28	1438	4.5
1 slice, approx. 0.8 oz.	72	0.2	72	0.2	89.9	0.28	1438	4.5
Beef Thuringer Cervelat, Sliced, 8-oz. package, 10 slices	674	4.1			84.3	0.51	1347	8.2
1 slice, approx. 0.8 oz.	67	0.4	67	0.4	84.3	0.51	1347	8.2
Slim Jim Summer Sausage, 6" stick, 0.9 oz.	130	1.9	130	1.9	140.3	2.04	2246	32.7
Swift Premium Summer Sausage, 4-lb. package	5760	64.0			90.0	1.00	1440	16.0

THURINGER, see SUMMER SAUSAGE

TONGUE, by brand

(Tongue has its primary listing in the MEATS & GAME chapter.)

	UNIT		1 SLICE OR LINK		1 OZ., BY WT.		1 POUND	
	Cal.	Carb.	Cal.	Carb.	Cal.	Carb.	Cal.	Carb.
Armour Lunch Tongue, 6-oz. container	380	2.0			63.3	0.33	1013	5.3

TURKEY

Turkey Bologna is under BOLOGNA; Turkey Franks are under FRANKFURTERS; Turkey Ham is under HAM; and so forth.

TURKEY, SLICED, based on generic data

	UNIT		1 SLICE OR LINK		1 OZ., BY WT.		1 POUND	
	Cal.	Carb.	Cal.	Carb.	Cal.	Carb.	Cal.	Carb.
Turkey Roll, light and dark meat, 1 pound (5g/1g/2g/70%/166mg)	672	9.6			42.2	0.60	672	9.6
1 slice, approx. 1 oz.	42	0.6	42	0.6	42.2	0.60	672	9.6
light meat, 1 pound (5g/1g/2g/72%/139mg)	667	2.4			41.7	0.15	667	2.4
1 slice, approx. 1 oz.	42	0.2	42	0.2	41.7	0.15	667	2.4

TURKEY, SLICED, by brand

	UNIT		1 SLICE OR LINK		1 OZ., BY WT.		1 POUND	
	Cal.	Carb.	Cal.	Carb.	Cal.	Carb.	Cal.	Carb.
A & P Smoked Turkey, Sliced, 3-oz. package, 3 slices	150	3.0			50.0	1.00	800	16.0
1 slice, approx. 1 oz.	50	1.0	50	1.0	50.0	1.00	800	16.0
Carl Buddig Turkey, 2.5-oz. package	113	0.0			45.0	0.00	720	0.0
Eckrich Slender, Smoked Turkey, Sliced, 3-oz. package, 4 slices	160	4.0			53.3	1.33	853	21.3
1 slice, approx. ¾ oz.	80	2.0	80	2.0	53.3	1.33	853	21.3
Longacre Turkey Breast Roll, Baked, 6-oz. package, 8 slices	200	4.0			33.3	0.67	533	10.7
1 slice, approx. 0.8 oz.	25	0.5	25	0.5	33.3	0.67	533	10.7
Smoked Turkey Breast, 6-oz. package, 8 slices	180	4.0			30.0	0.67	480	10.7
1 slice, approx. 0.8 oz.	23	0.5	23	0.5	30.0	0.67	480	10.7
Louis Rich Barbecued Boneless Turkey Breast Portion, 16-oz. (1-lb.) package	640	0.0			40.0	0.00	640	0.0
Hickory Smoked Boneless Turkey Breast Portion, 16-oz. (1-lb.) package	720	0.0			45.0	0.00	720	0.0
Natural Hickory Smoked Turkey Drumsticks, 16-oz. (1-lb.) package	600	0.0			37.5	0.00	600	0.0
Edible portion, 12 oz.	600	0.0			50.0	0.00	800	0.0
Natural Hickory Smoked Turkey Wing Drumettes, 16-oz. (1-lb.) package	587	0.0			36.7	0.00	587	0.0
Edible portion, 12 oz.	0.0			55.0	0.00	880	0.0	
Oven Roasted Boneless Turkey Breast Portion, 16-oz. (1-lb.) package	800	0.0			50.0	0.00	800	0.0
Smoked Turkey, 8-oz. package, 8 slices	360	4.0			45.0	0.50	720	8.0
1 slice, approx. 1 oz.	45	0.5	45	0.5	45.0	0.50	720	8.0
Oscar Mayer Turkey Breast, Sliced, 6-oz. package, 8 slices	167	0.0			27.8	0.00	445	0.0
1 slice, approx. ¾ oz.	21	0.0	21	0.0	27.8	0.00	445	0.0
Park Lane Frozen All White Young Turkey Roll with Broth, 10-lb. container	6400	182.8			40.0	1.14	640	18.2
Frozen Boneless White and Dark Young Turkey Roll with Broth, 10-lb. roll	6400	137.2			40.0	0.86	640	13.8
Rich's Turkey Breast, Sliced, 6-oz. package, 6 slices	210	0.0			35.0	0.00	560	0.0
1 slice, approx. 1 oz.	35	0.0	35	0.0	35.0	0.00	560	0.0
Smoked Turkey Breast, Sliced, 4-oz. package, 6 slices	135	3.0			34.0	0.75	541	12.0
1 slice, approx. ⅔ oz.	23	0.5	23	0.5	34.0	0.75	541	12.0
Safeway Turkey, Smoked/Sliced/Pressed, 3-oz. package, 3 slices	120	0.0			40.0	0.00	640	0.0
1 slice, approx. 1 oz.	40	0.0	40	0.0	40.0	0.00	640	0.0
Weaver Deli Delight Turkey Combination, 7½-lb. roll	4680	34.5			39.0	0.29	624	4.6
Deli Flavor White Meat Turkey Roll, 6-lb. roll	3562	22.1			37.1	0.23	594	3.6

VIENNA SAUSAGE, based on generic data

	UNIT		1 SLICE OR LINK		1 OZ., BY WT.		1 POUND	
	Cal.	Carb.	Cal.	Carb.	Cal.	Carb.	Cal.	Carb.
CANNED:								
Water Pack (stated label weight is for drained solids):								
1 can, 4 oz., 7 sausages	271	0.3			67.8	0.08	1084	1.2
Broth Pack:								
1 can, 5 oz., 7 sausages	(278)	(0.9)			(55.6)	(0.18)	(890)	(2.9)
Drained solids (yield: approx. 4 oz.)	271	0.3			67.8	0.08	1084	1.2
1 sausage, water or broth packed, 2″ long × ⅞″ diameter, approx. 0.6 oz.	38	trace	38	trace	67.8	0.08	1084	1.2
Made with beef and pork (3g/2g/7g/60%/272mg)								
1 5-oz. can, drained solids (yield: approx. 4 oz., 7 sausages)	315	2.3			79.1	2.04	1266	32.6
1 sausage, 2″ long × ⅞″ diameter, approx. 0.6 oz.	45	0.3	45	0.3	79.1	2.04	1266	32.6

VIENNA SAUSAGE, by brand

	UNIT		1 SLICE OR LINK		1 OZ., BY WT.		1 POUND	
	Cal.	Carb.	Cal.	Carb.	Cal.	Carb.	Cal.	Carb.
CANNED:								
Armour Vienna Sausage in Barbecue Sauce, 5-oz. can (7 sausages)	380	10.0			76.0	2.00	1216	32.0
1 sausage, with ⅐ of the sauce, approx. 0.7 oz.	54	1.4	54	1.4	76.0	2.00	1216	32.0
Vienna Sausage, in Beef Stock, 5-oz. can (7 sausages)	(347)	(2.6)			(69.4)	(0.52)	(1110)	(8.3)
Drained solids (yield: approx. 4 oz.)	340	2.0			85.0	0.50	1360	8.0
1 sausage, approx. 0.6 oz.	49	0.3	49	0.3	85.0	0.50	1360	8.0
9-oz. can (12 sausages)	(625)	(4.7)			(69.4)	(0.52)	(1110)	(8.3))
Drained solids (yield: approx. 7.2 oz.)	(612)	(3.6)			85.0	0.50	1360	8.0
1 sausage, approx. 0.6 oz.	49	0.3	49	0.3	85.0	0.50	1360	8.0
Vienna Sausage, Smoked, 5-oz. can (7 sausages)	450	2.5			90.0	0.50	1440	8.0
Drained solids (yield: approx. 4 oz.)	368	3.5			73.5	0.70	1176	11.2
1 sausage, approx. 0.6 oz.	53	0.5	53	0.5	73.5	0.70	1176	11.2
Hormel Vienna Sausage, 5-oz. can, 7 sausages	368	3.5			73.5	0.70	1176	11.2
1 sausage, approx. 0.7 oz.	55	0.5	55	0.5	73.5	0.70	1176	11.2
Libby's Vienna Sausage in Beef Broth, 5-oz. can, 7 sausages	322	2.1			64.4	0.42	1030	6.7
Drained solids (yield: approx. 4 oz.)	(315)	(1.5)			(78.8)	(0.38)	(1260)	(6.0)
1 link, approx. 0.6 oz.	45	0.2	45	0.2	(78.8)	(0.38)	(1260)	(6.0)
9-oz. can, 13 sausages	580	3.8			64.4	0.42	1030	6.7
Drained solids (yield: approx. 7.2 oz.)	(567)	(2.7)			(78.8)	(0.38)	(1260)	(6.0)
1 link, approx. 0.6 oz.	45	0.2	45	0.2	(78.8)	(0.38)	(1260)	(6.0)
Vienna Sausage, Barbeque Sauce, 5-oz. can, 7 sausages	359	3.7			71.9	0.74	1150	18.4
1 link with ⅐ of the sauce, approx. 0.7 oz.	51	0.5	51	0.5	71.9	0.74	1150	18.4

WIENERS, by brand

	UNIT		1 SLICE OR LINK		1 OZ., BY WT.		1 POUND	
	Cal.	Carb.	Cal.	Carb.	Cal.	Carb.	Cal.	Carb.
Hormel Beef Wieners, 12-oz. package, 10 wieners	1050	5.0			87.5	0.42	1400	6.7
1 wiener, approx. 1.2 oz.	105	0.5	105	0.5	87.5	0.42	1400	6.7
16-oz. (1-lb.) package, 10 wieners	1400	10.0			87.5	0.63	1400	10.0
1 wiener, approx. 1.6 oz.	140	1.0	140	1.0	87.5	0.63	1400	10.0
Meat Wieners, 12-oz. package, 10 wieners	1050	5.0			87.5	0.42	1400	6.7
1 wiener, approx. 1.2 oz.	105	0.5	105	0.5	87.5	0.42	1400	6.7
16-oz. (1-lb.) package, 10 wieners	1400	10.0			87.5	0.63	1400	10.0
1 wiener, approx. 1.6 oz.	140	1.0	140	1.0	87.5	0.63	1400	10.0
Kahn's Jumbo Wieners, 16-oz. (1-lb.) package, 8 wieners	1496	14.6			93.5	0.91	1496	14.6
1 wiener, approx. 2 oz.	187	1.8	187	1.8	93.5	0.91	1496	14.6
Wieners, 16-oz. (1-lb.) package, 10 wieners	1500	20.0			93.8	1.25	1500	20.0
1 wiener, approx. 1.6 oz.	150	1.8	150	1.8	93.8	1.25	1500	20.0
Oscar Mayer Wieners, 16-oz. (1-lb.) package, 10 wieners	1450	(20.0)			90.6	(1.25)	1450	(20.0)
1 wiener, approx. 1.6 oz.	145	(2.0)	145	(2.0)	90.6	(1.25)	1450	(20.0)

	UNIT Cal.	UNIT Carb.	1 SLICE OR LINK Cal.	1 SLICE OR LINK Carb.	1 OZ., BY WT. Cal.	1 OZ., BY WT. Carb.	1 POUND Cal.	1 POUND Carb.
Imperial Size Wieners, 16-oz. (1-lb.) package, 8 wieners	1438	9.1			89.9	0.57	1438	9.1
1 wiener, approx. 2 oz.	180	1.1	180	1.1	89.9	0.57	1438	9.1
Little Wieners, 5½-oz. package, 16 wieners	499	3.4			90.7	0.62	1451	9.9
1 wiener, approx. 0.3 oz.	31	0.2	31	0.2	90.7	0.62	1451	9.9

PREPACKAGED COLD CUT ASSORTMENTS

	UNIT Cal.	UNIT Carb.	1 SLICE OR LINK Cal.	1 SLICE OR LINK Carb.	1 OZ., BY WT. Cal.	1 OZ., BY WT. Carb.	1 POUND Cal.	1 POUND Carb.
Eckrich, Smorgas Pac, 16-oz. (1-lb.) package, 16 slices	1180	28.0			73.8	1.75	1180	28.0
consisting of:								
Bologna, 4 oz., 4 slices	360	6.0			90.0	1.50	1440	24.0
1 slice, approx. 1 oz.	90	1.5	90	1.5	90.0	1.50	1440	24.0
Honey Style Loaf, 4 oz., 4 slices	180	8.0			45.0	2.00	720	32.0
1 slice, approx. 1 oz.	45	2.0	45	2.0	45.0	2.00	720	32.0
Old Fashioned Loaf, 4 oz., 4 slices	300	8.0			75.0	2.00	1200	32.0
1 slice, approx. 1 oz.	75	2.0	75	2.0	75.0	2.00	1200	32.0
Pickle Loaf, 4 oz., 4 slices	340	6.0			85.0	1.50	1360	24.0
1 slice, approx. 1 oz.	85	1.5	85	1.5	85.0	1.50	1360	24.0
Beef Smorgas Pac, 12-oz. package, 12 slices	880	19.0			73.3	1.58	1173	25.3
consisting of:								
Banquet Loaf, 3 oz., 4 slices	225	4.5			75.0	1.50	1200	24.0
1 slice, approx. ¾ oz.	56	1.1	56	1.1	75.0	1.50	1200	24.0
Beef Bologna, 3 oz., 4 slices	280	4.0			93.3	1.33	1493	21.3
1 slice, approx. ¾ oz.	70	1.0	70	1.0	93.3	1.33	1493	21.3
Beef Pickle Loaf, 3 oz., 4 slices	255	4.5			85.0	1.50	1360	24.0
1 slice, approx. ¾ oz.	64	1.1	64	1.1	85.0	1.50	1360	24.0
Gourmet Loaf, 3 oz., 4 slices	120	6.0			40.0	2.00	640	32.0
1 slice, approx. ¾ oz.	30	1.5	30	1.5	40.0	2.00	640	32.0

5 POULTRY & GAME BIRDS •

CHICKEN

Broilers or Fryers

	UNIT Cal.	UNIT Carb.	1 OZ., BY WT. Cal.	1 OZ., BY WT. Carb.
ENTIRE CHICKEN (with neck and giblets):				
RAW:				
With skin:				
Weighed with skin and bones [refuse: bones, approx. 31%]:				
1 3-lb. 5-oz. ready-to-cook chicken	2223	1.4	41.6	0.03
1 pound of raw bird, average all parts	665	0.4	41.6	0.03
Weighing edible portion only:				
1 pound of raw meat with skin	966	0.6	60.4	0.04
Without skin:				
Weighed with skin and bones [refuse: bones, approx. 31%; skin, approx. 10%]:				
1 3-lb. 5-oz. ready-to-cook chicken	(1673)	(1.4)	(31.4)	(0.03)
1 pound of raw bird, average all parts	(502)	(0.5)	(31.4)	(0.03)
Weighing edible portion only:				
1 pound of raw meat without skin	(858)	(0.6)	(53.6)	(0.04)
ROASTED				
Eaten with skin:				
Weighed with skin and bones [refuse: bones, approx. 33%]:				
1 3-lb. 5-oz. ready-to-cook chicken: approx. 2 lb. 7 oz. cooked	1625	0.4	41.1	0.01
1 pound of cooked bird, average all parts	658	0.2	41.1	0.01
Yield per pound of raw ready-to-cook chicken: approx. 11.9 oz. cooked	487	0.1	41.1	0.01
Weighing edible portion only:				
1 pound of cooked meat with skin (8g/tr/4g/60%/22mg)	980	0.3	61.2	0.02
Cooked with skin but skin removed before eating:				
Weighed with skin and bones [refuse: bones, approx. 33%; skin, approx. 10%]				
1 3-lb. 5-oz. ready-to-cook chicken: approx. 2 lb. 7 oz. cooked	(1117)	(0.4)	(28.3)	(0.01)
1 pound of cooked bird, average all parts	(453)	(0.2)	(28.3)	(0.01)
Yield per pound of raw ready-to-cook chicken: approx. 11.9 oz. cooked	(335)	(0.1)	(28.3)	(0.01)
Weighing edible portion only:				
1 pound of cooked meat without skin	(794)	(0.3)	(49.6)	(0.02)
FLOUR COATED, FRIED				
Eaten with skin:				
Weighed with skin and bones [refuse: bones, approx. 28%]:				
1 3-lb. 5-oz. ready-to-cook chicken: approx. 2 lb. 3 oz. cooked	1928	23.2	55.6	0.67
1 pound of cooked bird, average all parts	890	10.7	55.6	0.67
Yield per pound of raw ready-to-cook chicken: approx. 10.6 oz. cooked	587	7.1	55.6	0.67
Weighing edible portion only:				
1 pound of cooked meat with skin (8g/1g/4g/52%/24mg)	1234	14.8	77.1	0.93
Fried with skin, but skin removed before eating:				
Weighed with skin and bones [refuse: bones, approx. 28%; skin, approx. 14%]				
1 3-lb. 5-oz. ready-to-cook chicken: approx. 2 lb. 3 oz. cooked	(1366)	(12.7)	(25.0)	(0.24)
1 pound of cooked bird, average all parts	(410)	(3.8)	(25.6)	(0.24)
Yield per pound of raw ready-to-cook chicken: approx. 10.6 oz. cooked	(410)	(3.8)	(25.6)	(0.24)
Weighing edible portion only:				
1 pound of cooked meat without skin	(1038)	(9.6)	(64.9)	(0.60)
BATTER DIPPED, FRIED				
Eaten with skin:				
Weighed with skin and bones [refuse: bones, approx. 21%]:				
1 3-lb. 5-oz. ready-to-cook chicken: approx. 2 lb. 14 oz. cooked	2987	92.8	64.7	2.01
1 pound of cooked bird, average all parts	1035	32.2	64.7	2.01
Yield per pound of raw ready-to-cook chicken: approx. 13.9 oz. cooked	895	27.8	64.7	2.01
Weighing edible portion only:				
1 pound of cooked meat with skin (6g/3g/5g/49%/81mg)	1320	41.0	82.5	2.56
Fried with skin, but skin removed before eating:				
Weighed with skin and bones [refuse: bones, approx. 21%; skin, approx. 29%]				
1 3-lb. 5-oz. ready-to-cook chicken: approx. 2 lb. 14 oz. cooked	(1491)		(32.4)	
1 pound of cooked bird, average all parts	(518)		(32.4)	
Yield per pound of raw ready-to-cook chicken: approx. 13.9 oz. cooked	(447)		(32.4)	
Weighing edible portion only:				
1 pound of cooked meat without skin	(732)		(45.7)	
STEWED				
Eaten with skin:				
Weighed with skin and bones [refuse: bones, approx. 33%]:				
1 3-lb. 5-oz. ready-to-cook chicken: approx. 2 lb. 7 oz. cooked	1625	0.4	41.1	0.01
1 pound of cooked bird, average all parts	658	0.2	41.1	0.01
Yield per pound of raw ready-to-cook chicken: approx. 11.8 oz. cooked	484	0.1	41.1	0.01
Weighing edible portion only:				
1 pound of cooked meat with skin (7g/tr/4g/64%/19mg)	980	0.3	61.2	0.02
Stewed with skin, but skin removed before eating:				
Weighed with skin and bones [refuse: bones, approx. 33%; skin, approx. 7%]:				
1 3-lb. 5-oz. ready-to-cook chicken: approx. 2 lb. 2 oz. cooked	(1103)	(0.4)	(32.4)	(0.01)
1 pound of cooked bird, average all parts	(518)	(0.2)	(32.4)	(0.01)
Yield per pound of raw ready-to-cook chicken: approx. 10 oz. cooked	(333)	(0.1)	(32.4)	(0.01)

	UNIT		1 OZ., BY WT.	
	Cal.	Carb.	Cal.	Carb.
Weighing edible portion only:				
1 pound of cooked meat without skin	(836)	(0.3)	(52.3)	(0.02)
ENTIRE CHICKEN (without neck and giblets):				
RAW				
With skin:				
Weighed with skin and bones [refuse: bones, approx. 32%]:				
1 3-lb. ready-to-cook chicken	1980	0.0	41.5	0.00
1 pound of raw bird, average all parts	664	0.0	41.5	0.00
Weighing edible portion only:				
1 pound of raw meat with skin	975	0.0	61.0	0.00
Without skin:				
Weighed with skin and bones [refuse: bones, approx. 32%; skin, approx. 12%]:				
1 3-lb. ready-to-cook chicken	784	0.0	16.3	0.00
1 pound of raw bird, average all parts	259	0.0	16.3	0.00
Weighing edible portion only:				
1 pound of raw meat without skin	540	0.0	33.7	0.00
ROASTED				
Eaten with skin:				
Weighed with skin and bones [refuse: bones, approx. 33%]:				
1 3-lb. ready-to-cook chicken: approx. 2 lb. cooked	1530	0.0	45.4	0.00
1 pound of cooked bird, average all parts	727	0.0	45.4	0.00
Yield per pound of raw ready-to-cook chicken: approx. 10.4 oz. cooked	510	0.0	45.4	0.00
Weighing edible portion only:				
1 pound of cooked meat with skin (8g/0g/4g/59%/23mg)	1084	0.0	67.8	0.00
Roasted with skin, but skin removed before eating:				
Weighed with skin and bones [refuse: bones, approx. 33%; skin, approx. 13%]:				
1 3-lb. ready-to-cook chicken: approx. 2 lb. cooked	918	0.0	29.1	0.00
1 pound of cooked bird, average all parts	466	0.0	29.1	0.00
Yield per pound of raw ready-to-cook chicken: approx. 10.4 oz. cooked	306	0.0	29.1	0.00
Weighing edible portion only:				
1 pound of cooked meat without skin (8g/0g/2g/64%/24mg)	862	0.0	53.9	0.00
1 cup, chopped or diced (approx. 4.9 oz.)	266	0.0	53.9	0.00
FLOUR COATED, FRIED				
Eaten with skin:				
Weighed with skin and bones [refuse: bones, approx. 29%]:				
1 3-lb. ready-to-cook chicken: approx. 1 lb. 15 oz. cooked	1688	19.8	54.1	0.63
1 pound of cooked bird, average all parts	865	10.1	54.1	0.63
Yield per pound of raw ready-to-cook chicken: approx. 10.3 oz. cooked	563	6.6	54.1	0.63
Weighing edible portion only:				
1 pound of cooked meat with skin (8g/1g/4g/52%/24mg)	1220	14.3	76.3	0.89
Fried with skin, but skin removed before eating:				
Weighed with skin and bones [refuse: bones, approx. 29%; skin, approx. 13%]:				
1 3-lb. ready-to-cook chicken: approx. 1 lb. 15 oz. cooked	1127	8.8	36.4	0.28
1 pound of cooked bird, average all parts	582	4.5	36.4	0.28
Yield per pound of raw ready-to-cook chicken: approx. 10.3 oz. cooked	376	2.9	36.4	0.28
Weighing edible portion only:				
1 pound of cooked meat without skin	993	7.7	62.1	0.48
1 cup, chopped or diced (approx. 4.9 oz.)	307	2.4	62.1	0.48
BATTER DIPPED, FRIED				
Eaten with skin:				
Weighed with skin and bones [refuse: bones, approx. 22%]:				
1 3-lb. ready-to-cook chicken: approx. 2 lb. 10 oz. cooked	2694	87.8	63.9	2.08
1 pound of cooked bird, average all parts	1023	33.3	63.9	2.08
Yield per pound of raw ready-to-cook chicken: approx. 14 oz. cooked	810	26.4	63.9	2.08
Weighing edible portion only:				
1 pound of cooked meat with skin (6g/0g/5g/49%/82mg)	1311	42.7	81.9	2.67
Fried with skin, but skin removed before eating:				
Weighed with skin and bones [refuse: bones, approx. 22%; skin, approx. 35%]:				
1 3-lb. ready-to-cook chicken: approx. 2 lb. 10 oz. cooked	1127	8.8	26.8	0.21
1 pound of cooked bird, average all parts	429	3.4	26.8	0.21
Yield per pound of raw ready-to-cook chicken: approx. 14 oz. cooked	376	2.9	26.8	0.21
Weighing edible portion only:				
1 pound of cooked meat without skin (9g/tr/3g/58%/26mg)	(993)	(7.7)	(62.1)	(0.48)
1 cup, chopped or diced (approx. 4.9 oz.)	(307)	(2.4)	(62.1)	(0.48)

	UNIT		1 OZ., BY WT.	
	Cal.	Carb.	Cal.	Carb.
STEWED				
Eaten with skin:				
Weighed with skin and bones [refuse: bones, approx. 34%]:				
1 3-lb. ready-to-cook chicken: approx. 2 lb. 4 oz. cooked	1460	0.0	40.9	0.00
1 pound of cooked bird, average all parts	655	0.0	40.9	0.00
Yield per pound of raw ready-to-cook chicken: approx. 12 oz. cooked	487	0.0	40.9	0.00
Weighing edible portion only:				
1 pound of cooked meat with skin (7g/0g/4g/64%/19mg)	993	0.0	62.1	0.00
Stewed with skin, but skin removed before eating:				
Weighed with skin and bones [refuse: bones, approx. 34%; skin, approx. 14%]				
1 3-lb. ready-to-cook chicken: approx. 2 lb. 4 oz. cooked	937	0.0	26.1	0.00
1 pound of cooked bird, average all parts	418	0.0	26.1	0.00
Yield per pound of raw ready-to-cook chicken: approx. 12 oz. cooked	312	0.0	26.1	0.00
Weighing edible portion only:				
1 pound of cooked meat without skin	803	0.0	50.2	0.00
1 cup, chopped or diced (approx. 4.9 oz.)	248	0.0	50.2	0.00
TOP QUARTER (Breast and Wing—Light Meat):				
RAW				
With skin:				
Weighed with skin and bones [refuse: bones, approx. 28%]:				
1 top quarter from a 3-lb. ready-to-cook chicken: approx. 9.6 oz.	362	0.0	38.1	0.00
1 pound of raw top quarters	609	0.0	38.1	0.00
Weighing edible portion only:				
1 pound of raw meat with skin	844	0.0	52.7	0.00
Without skin:				
Weighed with skin and bones [refuse: bones, approx. 28%; skin, approx. 13%]:				
1 top quarter from a 3-lb. ready-to-cook chicken: approx. 9.6 oz.	168	0.0	17.8	0.00
1 pound of raw top quarters	284	0.0	17.8	0.00
Weighing edible portion only:				
1 pound of raw meat without skin (9g/0g/2g/60%/23mg)	517	0.0	32.3	0.00
ROASTED				
Eaten with skin:				
Weighed with skin and bones [refuse: bones, approx. 29%]:				
1 top quarter from a 3-lb. ready-to-cook chicken: approx. 6.5 oz. cooked	293	0.0	44.6	0.00
1 pound of cooked top quarters	714	0.0	44.6	0.00
Yield per pound of raw ready-to-cook chicken: approx. 2.2 oz. cooked	98	0.0	44.6	0.00
Weighing edible portion only:				
1 pound of cooked meat with skin	1007	0.0	62.9	0.00
Roasted with skin, but skin removed before eating:				
Weighed with skin and bones [refuse: bones, approx. 29%; skin, approx. 13%]:				
1 top quarter from a 3-lb. ready-to-cook chicken: approx. 6.5 oz. cooked	242	0.0	28.4	0.00
1 pound of cooked top quarters	454	0.0	28.4	0.00
Yield per pound of raw ready-to-cook chicken: approx. 2.2 oz. cooked	81	0.0	28.4	0.00
Weighing edible portion only:				
1 pound of cooked meat without skin (9g/0g/1g/65%/22mg)	785	0.0	49.1	0.00
1 cup, chopped or diced (approx. 4.9 oz.)	242	0.0	49.1	0.00
FLOUR COATED, FRIED				
Eaten with skin:				
Weighed with skin and bones [refuse: bones, approx. 28%]:				
1 top quarter from a 3-lb. ready-to-cook chicken: approx. 6.3 oz. cooked	320	2.4	50.3	0.37
1 pound of cooked top quarters	804	6.0	50.3	0.37
Yield per pound of raw ready-to-cook chicken: approx. 2.1 oz. cooked	107	0.8	50.3	0.37
Weighing edible portion only:				
1 pound of cooked meat with skin	1116	8.3	69.7	0.52
Fried with skin, but skin removed before eating:				
Weighed with skin and bones [refuse: bones, approx. 28%; skin, approx. 13%]:				
1 top quarter from a 3-lb. ready-to-cook chicken: approx. 6.3 oz. cooked	268	0.6	42.2	0.09
1 pound of cooked top quarters	675	1.5	42.2	0.09
Yield per pound of raw ready-to-cook chicken: 2.1 oz. cooked	89	0.2	42.2	0.09
Weighing edible portion only:				
1 pound of cooked meat without skin (9g/tr/2g/60%/23mg)	871	1.9	54.4	0.12
1 cup, chopped or diced (approx. 4.9 oz.)	268	0.6	54.4	0.12

	UNIT Cal.	UNIT Carb.	1 OZ., BY WT. Cal.	1 OZ., BY WT. Carb.
BATTER DIPPED, FRIED				
Eaten with skin:				
Weighed with skin and bones [refuse: bones, approx. 21%]:				
1 top quarter from a 3-lb. ready-to-cook chicken: approx. 8.4 oz. cooked	520	17.9	61.9	2.13
1 pound of cooked top quarters	991	34.0	61.9	2.13
Yield per pound of raw ready-to-cook chicken: approx. 2.8 oz. cooked	173	6.0	61.9	2.13
Weighing edible portion only:				
1 pound of cooked meat with skin	1257	43.1	78.5	2.69
Fried with skin, but skin removed before eating:				
Weighed with skin and bones [refuse: bones, approx. 21%; skin, approx. 20%]:				
1 top quarter from a 3-lb. ready-to-cook chicken: approx. 8.4 oz. cooked	268	2.6	32.1	0.07
1 pound of cooked top quarters	513	1.1	32.1	0.07
Yield per pound of raw ready-to-cook chicken: approx. 2.8 oz. cooked	89	0.9	32.1	0.07
Weighing edible portion only:				
1 pound of cooked meat without skin	871	1.9	54.4	0.12
1 cup, chopped or diced (approx. 4.9 oz.)	268	0.6	54.4	0.12
STEWED				
Eaten with skin:				
Weighed with skin and bones [refuse: bones, approx. 29%]:				
1 top quarter from a 3-lb. ready-to-cook chicken: approx. 7.5 oz. cooked	302	0.0	40.6	0.00
1 pound of cooked top quarters	649	0.0	40.6	0.00
Yield per pound of raw ready-to-cook chicken: approx. 2.5 oz. cooked	101	0.0	40.6	0.00
Weighing edible portion only:				
1 pound of cooked meat with skin (7g/0g/3g/65%/18mg)	912	0.0	57.0	0.00
Stewed with skin, but skin removed before eating:				
Weighed with skin and bones [refuse: bones, approx. 29%; skin, approx. 15%]:				
1 top quarter from a 3-lb. ready-to-cook chicken: approx. 7.5 oz. cooked	223	0.0	25.3	0.00
1 pound of cooked top quarters	405	0.0	25.3	0.00
Yield per pound of raw ready-to-cook chicken: approx. 2.5 oz. cooked	74	0.0	25.3	0.00
Weighing edible portion only:				
1 pound of cooked meat without skin (8g/0g/1g/68%/18mg)	721	0.0	45.1	0.00
1 cup, chopped or diced (approx. 4.9 oz.)	223	0.0	45.1	0.00
BOTTOM QUARTER (Drumstick, Thigh, and Back—Dark Meat):				
RAW				
With skin:				
Weighed with skin and bones [refuse: bones, approx. 35%]:				
1 bottom quarter from a 3-lb. ready-to-cook chicken: approx. 14.4 oz.	630	0.0	43.6	0.00
1 pound of raw bottom quarters	698	0.0	43.6	0.00
Weighing edible portion only:				
1 pound of raw meat with skin	1075	0.0	67.2	0.00
Without skin:				
Weighed with skin and bones [refuse: bones, approx. 35%; skin, approx. 21%]:				
1 bottom quarter from a 3-lb. ready-to-cook chicken: approx. 14.4 oz.	227	0.0	15.6	0.00
1 pound of raw bottom quarters	249	0.0	15.6	0.00
Weighing edible portion only:				
1 pound of raw meat without skin	567	0.0	35.4	0.00
ROASTED				
Eaten with skin:				
Weighed with skin and bones [refuse: bones, approx. 36%]:				
1 bottom quarter from a 3-lb. ready-to-cook chicken: approx. 9.2 oz. cooked	423	0.0	45.9	0.00
1 pound of cooked bottom quarters	735	0.0	45.9	0.00
Yield per pound of raw ready-to-cook chicken: approx. 3.1 oz. cooked	141	0.0	45.9	0.00
Weighing edible portion only:				
1 pound of cooked meat with skin (7g/0g/4g/59%/25mg)	1148	0.0	71.7	0.00
Roasted with skin, but skin removed before eating:				
Weighed with skin and bones [refuse: bones, approx. 36%; skin, approx. 12%]:				
1 bottom quarter from a 3-lb. ready-to-cook chicken: approx. 9.2 oz. cooked	279	0.0	30.2	0.00
1 pound of cooked bottom quarters	483	0.0	30.2	0.00
Yield per pound of raw ready-to-cook chicken: approx. 3.1 oz. cooked	93	0.0	30.2	0.00

	UNIT Cal.	UNIT Carb.	1 OZ., BY WT. Cal.	1 OZ., BY WT. Carb.
Weighing edible portion only:				
1 pound of cooked meat without skin	930	0.0	58.1	0.00
1 cup, chopped or diced (approx. 4.9 oz.)	286	0.0	58.1	0.00
FLOUR COATED, FRIED				
Eaten with skin:				
Weighed with skin and bones [refuse: bones, approx. 30%]:				
1 bottom quarter from a 3-lb. ready-to-cook chicken: approx. 9.3 oz. cooked	523	7.5	56.4	0.81
1 pound of cooked bottom quarters	903	13.0	56.4	0.81
Yield per pound of raw ready-to-cook chicken: approx. 3.1 oz. cooked	174	2.5	56.4	0.81
Weighing edible portion only:				
1 pound of cooked meat with skin (8g/1g/5g/51%/25mg)	1293	18.5	80.8	1.16
Fried with skin, but skin removed before eating:				
Weighed with skin and bones [refuse: bones, approx. 30%; skin, approx. 12%]:				
1 bottom quarter from a 3-lb. ready-to-cook chicken: approx. 9.3 oz. cooked	366	4.0	39.3	0.43
1 pound of cooked bottom quarters	628	6.8	39.3	0.43
Yield per pound of raw ready-to-cook chicken: approx. 3.1 oz. cooked	122	1.3	39.3	0.43
Weighing edible portion only:				
1 pound of cooked meat without skin	1084	11.7	67.8	0.73
1 cup, chopped or diced (approx. 4.9 oz.)	334	3.6	67.8	0.73
BATTER DIPPED, FRIED				
Eaten with skin:				
Weighed with skin and bones [refuse: bones, approx. 23%]:				
1 bottom quarter from a 3-lb. ready-to-cook chicken: approx. 12.6 oz. cooked	828	26.1	65.0	2.11
1 pound of cooked bottom quarters	1040	32.8	65.0	2.11
Yield per pound of raw ready-to-cook chicken: approx. 4.2 oz. cooked	276	8.7	65.0	2.11
Weighing edible portion only:				
1 pound of cooked meat with skin (6g/3g/5g/49%/84mg)	1352	42.6	84.5	2.66
Fried with skin, but skin removed before eating:				
Weighed with skin and bones [refuse: bones, approx. 23%; skin, approx. 12%]:				
1 bottom quarter from a 3-lb. ready-to-cook chicken: approx. 12.6 oz. cooked	366	4.0	29.0	0.32
1 pound of cooked bottom quarters	628	6.8	29.0	0.32
Yield per pound of raw ready-to-cook chicken: approx. 4.2 oz. cooked	111	1.2	29.0	0.32
Weighing edible portion only:				
1 pound of cooked meat without skin	1084	11.7	67.8	0.73
1 cup, chopped or diced (approx. 4.9 oz.)	334	3.6	67.8	0.73
STEWED				
Eaten with skin:				
Weighed with skin and bones [refuse: bones, approx. 38%]:				
1 bottom quarter from a 3-lb. ready-to-cook chicken: approx. 10.5 oz. cooked	428	0.0	40.9	0.00
1 pound of cooked bottom quarters	654	0.0	40.9	0.00
Yield per pound of raw ready-to-cook chicken: approx. 3.5 oz. cooked	143	0.0	40.9	0.00
Weighing edible portion only:				
1 pound of cooked meat with skin (7g/0g/4g/63%/20mg)	1057	0.0	66.1	0.00
Roasted with skin, but skin removed before eating:				
Weighed with skin and bones [refuse: bones, approx. 38%; skin, approx. 14%]:				
1 bottom quarter from a 3-lb. ready-to-cook chicken: approx. 10.5 oz. cooked	273	0.0	26.1	0.00
1 pound of cooked bottom quarters	418	0.0	26.1	0.00
Yield per pound of raw ready-to-cook chicken: approx. 3.5 oz. cooked	91	0.0	26.1	0.00
Weighing edible portion only:				
1 pound of cooked meat without skin	871	0.0	54.4	0.00
1 cup, chopped or diced (approx. 4.9 oz.)	269	0.0	54.4	0.00
CHICKEN PARTS:				
BACK:				
RAW				
With skin:				
Weighed with skin and bones [refuse: bones, approx. 44%]:				
½ back from a 3-lb. ready-to-cook chicken: approx. 6.2 oz.	316	0.0	50.7	0.00
1 pound of raw backs	811	0.0	50.7	0.00
Weighing edible portion only:				
1 pound of raw meat with skin	1447	0.0	90.4	0.00

	UNIT Cal.	UNIT Carb.	1 OZ., BY WT. Cal.	1 OZ., BY WT. Carb.
Without skin:				
Weighed with skin and bones [refuse: bones, approx. 44%; skin, approx. 27%]:				
½ back from a 3-lb. ready-to-cook chicken: approx. 6.2 oz.	70	0.0	11.3	0.00
1 pound of raw backs	180	0.0	11.3	0.00
Weighing edible portion only:				
1 pound of raw meat without skin	625	0.0	38.8	0.00
ROASTED				
Eaten with skin:				
Weighed with skin and bones [refuse: bones, approx. 47%]:				
½ back from a 3-lb. ready-to-cook chicken: approx. 3.5 oz. cooked	159	0.0	45.1	0.00
1 pound of cooked backs	721	0.0	45.1	0.00
Yield per pound of raw ready-to-cook chicken: approx. 1.2 oz. cooked	53	0.0	45.1	0.00
Weighing edible portion only:				
1 pound of cooked meat with skin (7g/0g/6g/54%/25mg)	1361	0.0	85.1	0.00
Roasted with skin, but skin removed before eating:				
Weighed with skin and bones [refuse: bones, approx. 47%; skin, approx. 13%]:				
½ back from a 3-lb. ready-to-cook chicken: approx. 3.5 oz. cooked	96	0.0	27.1	0.00
1 pound of cooked backs	434	0.0	27.1	0.00
Yield per pound of raw ready-to-cook chicken: approx. 1.2 oz. cooked	32	0.0	27.1	0.00
Weighing edible portion only:				
1 pound of cooked meat without skin (8g/0g/4g/59%/29mg)	1084	0.0	67.8	0.00
FLOUR COATED, FRIED				
Eaten with skin:				
Weighed with skin and bones [refuse: bones, approx. 33%]:				
½ back from a 3-lb. ready-to-cook chicken: approx. 3.8 oz. cooked	238	4.7	62.9	1.24
1 pound of cooked backs	1006	19.8	62.9	1.24
Yield per pound of raw ready-to-cook chicken: approx. 1.3 oz. cooked	79	1.6	62.9	1.24
Weighing edible portion only:				
1 pound of cooked meat with skin (8g/2g/6g/44%/26mg)	1502	29.5	93.8	1.84
Fried with skin, but skin removed before eating:				
Weighed with skin and bones [refuse: bones, approx. 33%; skin, approx. 13%]:				
½ back from a 3-lb. ready-to-cook chicken: approx. 3.8 oz. cooked	167	3.3	44.1	0.87
1 pound of cooked backs	706	13.9	44.1	0.87
Yield per pound of raw ready-to-cook chicken: approx. 1.3 oz. cooked	56	1.1	44.1	0.87
Weighing edible portion only:				
1 pound of cooked meat without skin (9g/2g/4g/48%/28mg)	1306	25.8	81.7	1.61
BATTER DIPPED, FRIED				
Eaten with skin:				
Weighed with skin and bones [refuse: bones, approx. 23%]:				
½ back from a 3-lb. ready-to-cook chicken: approx. 5.5 oz. cooked	397	12.3	72.3	2.24
1 pound of cooked backs	1156	35.8	72.3	2.24
Yield per pound of raw ready-to-cook chicken: approx. 1.8 oz. cooked	132	4.1	72.3	2.24
Weighing edible portion only:				
1 pound of cooked meat with skin (6g/3g/6g/45%/90mg)	1502	46.5	93.8	2.91
Fried with skin, but skin removed before eating:				
Weighed with skin and bones [refuse: bones, approx. 23%; skin, approx. 40%]:				
½ back from a 3-lb. ready-to-cook chicken: approx. 5.5 oz. cooked	167	3.3	30.4	0.60
1 pound of cooked backs	487	9.6	30.4	0.60
Yield per pound of raw ready-to-cook chicken: approx. 1.8 oz. cooked	56	1.1	30.4	0.60
Weighing edible portion only:				
1 pound of cooked meat without skin	1306	25.8	81.7	1.61
STEWED				
Eaten with skin:				
Weighed with skin and bones [refuse: bones, approx. 48%]:				
½ back from a 3-lb. ready-to-cook chicken: approx. 4.2 oz. cooked	158	0.0	38.1	0.00
1 pound of cooked backs	610	0.0	38.1	0.00
Yield per pound of raw ready-to-cook chicken: 1.4 oz. cooked	53	0.0	38.1	0.00
Weighing edible portion only:				
1 pound of cooked meat with skin (6g/0g/5g/61%/18mg)	1170	0.0	73.1	0.00

	UNIT Cal.	UNIT Carb.	1 OZ., BY WT. Cal.	1 OZ., BY WT. Carb.
Stewed with skin, but skin removed before eating:				
Weighed with skin and bones [refuse: bones, approx. 48%; skin, approx. 16%]:				
½ back from a 3-lb. ready-to-cook chicken: approx. 4.2 oz. cooked	88	0.0	21.3	0.00
1 pound of cooked backs	341	0.0	21.3	0.00
Yield per pound of raw ready-to-cook chicken: approx. 1.4 oz. cooked	29	0.0	21.3	0.00
Weighing edible portion only:				
1 pound of cooked meat without skin (7g/0g/3g/64%/19mg)	948	0.0	59.3	0.00
BREAST:				
RAW				
With skin:				
Weighed with skin and bones [refuse: bones, approx. 20%]:				
½ breast from a 3-lb. ready-to-cook chicken: approx. 6.4 oz.	250	0.0	39.1	0.00
1 pound raw breasts	626	0.0	39.1	0.00
Weighing edible portion only:				
1 pound of cooked meat with skin (6g/0g/3g/69%/18mg)	780	0.0	48.8	0.00
Without skin:				
Weighed with skin and bones [refuse: bones, approx. 20%; skin, approx. 9%]:				
½ breast from a 3-lb. ready-to-cook chicken: approx. 6.4 oz. cooked	129	0.0	20.3	0.00
1 pound of raw breasts	324	0.0	20.3	0.00
Weighing edible portion only:				
1 pound of raw meat without skin (7g/0g/tr/75g/18mg)	499	0.0	31.2	0.00
ROASTED				
Eaten with skin:				
Weighed with skin and bones [refuse: bones, approx. 19%]:				
½ breast from a 3-lb. ready-to-cook chicken: approx. 6.8 oz. cooked	196	0.0	45.3	0.00
1 pound of cooked breasts	725	0.0	45.3	0.00
Yield per pound of raw ready-to-cook chicken: approx. 2.3 oz. cooked	65	0.0	45.3	0.00
Weighing edible portion only:				
1 pound of cooked meat with skin (8g/0g/2g/62%/20mg)	894	0.0	55.9	0.00
Roasted with skin, but skin removed before eating:				
Weighed with skin and bones [refuse: bones, approx. 19%; skin, approx. 9%]:				
½ breast from a 3-lb. ready-to-cook chicken: approx. 6.8 oz. cooked	142	0.0	33.6	0.00
1 pound of cooked breasts	538	0.0	33.6	0.00
Yield per pound of raw ready-to-cook chicken: approx. 2.3 oz. cooked	47	0.0	33.6	0.00
Weighing edible portion only:				
1 pound of cooked meat without skin (9g/0g/1g/65%/21mg)	749	0.0	46.8	0.00
FLOUR COATED, FRIED				
Eaten with skin:				
Weighed with skin and bones [refuse: bones, approx. 17%]:				
½ back from a 3-lb. ready-to-cook chicken: approx. 4.2 oz. cooked	218	1.6	52.3	0.39
1 pound of cooked breasts	837	6.2	52.3	0.39
Yield per pound of raw ready-to-cook chicken: approx. 1.4 oz. cooked	73	0.5	52.3	0.39
Weighing edible portion only:				
1 pound of cooked meat with skin	1007	7.4	62.9	0.46
Cooked with skin, but skin removed before eating:				
Weighed with skin and bones [refuse: bones, approx. 17%; skin, approx. 10%]:				
½ breast from a 3-lb. ready-to-cook chicken: approx. 4.2 oz. cooked	161	0.4	38.8	0.11
1 pound of cooked breasts	620	1.7	38.8	0.11
Yield per pound of raw ready-to-cook chicken: approx. 1.4 oz. cooked	54	0.1	38.8	0.11
Weighing edible portion only:				
1 pound of cooked meat without skin	848	2.3	53.0	0.14
BATTER DIPPED, FRIED				
Eaten with skin:				
Weighed with skin and bones [refuse: bones, approx. 12%]:				
½ breast from a 3-lb. ready-to-cook chicken: approx. 5.6 oz. cooked	364	12.6	64.8	2.24
1 pound of cooked breasts	1037	35.9	64.8	2.24
Yield per pound of raw ready-to-cook chicken: approx. 1.9 oz. cooked	121	4.2	64.8	2.24
Weighing edible portion only:				
1 pound of cooked meat with skin (7g/3g/4g/52%/78mg)	1179	40.8	73.7	2.55

	UNIT Cal.	UNIT Carb.	1 OZ., BY WT. Cal.	1 OZ., BY WT. Carb.
Fried with skin, but skin removed before eating:				
Weighed with skin and bones [refuse: bones, approx. 12%; skin, approx. 33%]:				
½ breast from a 3-lb. ready-to-cook chicken: approx. 5.6 oz. cooked	161	0.4	28.5	0.07
1 pound of cooked breasts	456	1.1	28.5	0.07
Yield per pound of raw ready-to-cook chicken: approx. 1.9 oz. cooked	54	0.1	28.5	0.07
Weighing edible portion only:				
1 pound of cooked meat without skin (9g/tr/1g/60%/23mg)	848	2.3	53.0	0.14
STEWED				
Eaten with skin:				
Weighed with skin and bones [refuse: bones, approx. 18%]:				
½ breast from a 3-lb. ready-to-cook chicken: approx. 4.8 oz. cooked	202	0.0	42.8	0.00
1 pound of cooked breasts	684	0.0	42.8	0.00
Yield per pound of raw ready-to-cook chicken: approx. 1.6 oz. cooked	67	0.0	42.8	0.00
Weighing edible portion only:				
1 pound of cooked meat with skin (8g/0g/2g/66%/18mg)	835	0.0	52.2	0.00
Stewed with skin, but skin removed before eating:				
Weighed with skin and bones [refuse: bones, approx. 18%; skin, approx. 12%]:				
½ breast from a 3-lb. ready-to-cook chicken: approx. 4.8 oz. cooked	144	0.0	30.0	0.00
1 pound of cooked breasts	480	0.0	30.0	0.00
Yield per pound of raw ready-to-cook chicken: approx. 1.6 oz. cooked	48	0.0	30.0	0.00
Weighing edible portion only:				
1 pound of cooked meat without skin (8g/0g/1g/68%/18mg)	685	0.0	42.8	0.00
DRUMSTICK:				
RAW				
With skin:				
Weighed with skin and bones [refuse: bones, approx. 33%]:				
1 drumstick from a 3-lb. ready-to-cook chicken: approx. 3.9 oz.	117	0.0	30.5	0.00
1 pound of raw drumsticks	488	0.0	30.5	0.00
Weighing edible portion only:				
1 pound of raw meat with skin (5g/0g/2g/72%/24mg)	730	0.0	45.6	0.00
Without skin:				
Weighed with skin and bones [refuse: bones, approx. 33%; skin, approx. 9%]:				
1 drumstick from a 3-lb. ready-to-cook chicken: approx. 3.9 oz.	74	0.0	18.9	0.00
1 pound of raw drumsticks	302	0.0	18.9	0.00
Weighing edible portion only:				
1 pound of raw meat without skin (6g/0g/1g/76%/25mg)	540	0.0	33.7	0.00
ROASTED				
Eaten with skin:				
Weighed with skin and bones [refuse: bones, approx. 35%]:				
1 drumstick from a 3-lb. ready-to-cook chicken: approx. 2.9 oz. cooked	112	0.0	39.8	0.00
1 pound of cooked drumsticks	637	0.0	39.8	0.00
Yield per pound of raw ready-to-cook chicken: approx. 1 oz. cooked	40	0.0	39.8	0.00
Weighing edible portion only:				
1 pound of cooked meat (8g/0g/3g/63%/26mg)	980	0.0	61.2	0.00
Roasted with skin, but skin removed before eating:				
Weighed with skin and bones [refuse: bones, approx. 35%; skin, approx. 11%]:				
1 drumstick from a 3-lb. ready-to-cook chicken: approx. 2.9 oz. cooked	76	0.0	26.3	0.00
1 pound of cooked drumsticks	421	0.0	26.3	0.00
Yield per pound of raw ready-to-cook chicken: approx. 1 oz. cooked	26	0.0	26.3	0.00
Weighing edible portion only:				
1 pound of cooked meat without skin (8g/0g/2g/67%/27mg)	780	0.0	48.8	0.00
FLOUR COATED, FRIED				
Eaten with skin:				
Weighed with skin and bones [refuse: bones, approx. 34%]:				
1 drumstick from a 3-lb. ready-to-cook chicken: approx. 2.6 oz. cooked	120	0.8	45.9	0.31
1 pound of cooked drumsticks	734	4.9	45.9	0.31
Yield per pound of raw ready-to-cook chicken: approx. 0.9 oz. cooked	40	0.3	45.9	0.31
Weighing edible portion only:				
1 pound of cooked meat with skin (8g/tr/4g/57%/25mg)	1111	7.4	69.5	0.46

	UNIT Cal.	UNIT Carb.	1 OZ., BY WT. Cal.	1 OZ., BY WT. Carb.
Fried with skin, but skin removed before eating:				
Weighed with skin and bones [refuse: bones, approx. 34%; skin, approx. 10%]:				
1 drumstick from a 3-lb. ready-to-cook chicken: approx. 2.6 oz. cooked	82	0.0	31.0	0.00
1 pound of cooked drumsticks	496	0.0	31.0	0.00
Yield per pound of raw ready-to-cook chicken: approx. 0.9 oz. cooked	27	0.0	31.0	0.00
Weighing edible portion only:				
1 pound of cooked meat without skin (8g/0g/2g/62%/27mg)	885	0.0	55.3	0.00
BATTER DIPPED, FRIED				
Eaten with skin:				
Weighed with skin and bones [refuse: bones, approx. 26%]:				
1 drumstick from a 3-lb. ready-to-cook chicken: approx. 3.4 oz. cooked	193	6.0	56.2	1.74
1 pound of cooked drumsticks	899	27.8	56.2	1.74
Yield per pound of raw ready-to-cook chicken: approx. 1.1 oz. cooked	64	2.0	56.2	1.74
Weighing edible portion only:				
1 pound of cooked meat with skin	1216	37.6	76.0	2.35
Fried with skin, but skin removed before eating:				
Weighed with skin and bones [refuse: bones, approx. 26%; skin, approx. 26%]:				
1 drumstick from a 3-lb. ready-to-cook chicken: approx. 3.4 oz. cooked	82	0.0	24.0	0.00
1 pound of cooked drumsticks	383	0.0	24.0	0.00
Yield per pound of raw ready-to-cook chicken: approx. 1.1 oz. cooked	27	0.0	24.0	0.00
Weighing edible portion only:				
1 pound of cooked meat without skin	885	0.0	55.3	0.00
STEWED				
Eaten with skin:				
Weighed with skin and bones [refuse: bones, approx. 36%]:				
1 drumstick from a 3-lb. ready-to-cook chicken: approx. 3.1 oz. cooked	116	0.0	37.0	0.00
1 pound of cooked drumsticks	592	0.0	37.0	0.00
Yield per pound of raw ready-to-cook chicken: approx. 1 oz. cooked	39	0.0	37.0	0.00
Weighing edible portion only:				
1 pound of cooked meat with skin (7g/0g/3g/65%/22mg)	925	0.0	57.8	0.00
Stewed with skin, but skin removed before eating:				
Weighed with skin and bones [refuse: bones, approx. 36%; skin, approx. 12%]:				
1 drumstick from a 3-lb. ready-to-cook chicken: approx. 3.1 oz. cooked	78	0.0	24.9	0.00
1 pound of cooked drumsticks	399	0.0	24.9	0.00
Yield per pound of raw ready-to-cook chicken: approx. 1 oz. cooked	26	0.0	24.9	0.00
Weighing edible portion only:				
1 pound of cooked meat without skin (8g/0g/2g/68%/23mg)	767	0.0	47.9	0.00
LEG (Drumstick and Thigh):				
RAW				
With skin:				
Weighed with skin and bones [refuse: bones, approx. 27%]:				
1 leg from a 3-lb. ready-to-cook chicken: approx. 8.1 oz. cooked	312	0.0	38.6	0.00
1 pound of raw legs	618	0.0	38.6	0.00
Weighing edible portion only:				
1 pound of raw meat with skin (5g/0g/3g/70%/23mg)	848	0.0	53.0	0.00
Without skin:				
Weighed with skin and bones [refuse: bones, approx. 27%; skin, approx. 11%]:				
1 leg from a 3-lb. ready-to-cook chicken: approx. 8.1 oz. cooked	156	0.0	19.4	0.00
1 pound of raw legs	311	0.0	19.4	0.00
Weighing edible portion only:				
1 pound of raw meat without skin (6g/0g/1g/76%/24mg)	544	0.0	34.0	0.00
ROASTED				
Eaten with skin:				
Weighed with skin and bones [refuse: bones, approx. 29%]:				
1 leg from a 3-lb. ready-to-cook chicken: approx. 5.7 oz. cooked	265	0.0	46.8	0.00
1 pound of cooked legs	748	0.0	46.8	0.00
Yield per pound of raw ready-to-cook chicken: approx. 1.9 oz. cooked	88	0.0	46.8	0.00
Weighing edible portion only:				
1 pound of cooked meat with skin (7g/0g/4g/61%/25mg)	1052	0.0	65.8	0.00

	UNIT Cal.	UNIT Carb.	1 OZ., BY WT. Cal.	1 OZ., BY WT. Carb.
Roasted with skin, but skin removed before eating:				
Weighed with skin and bones [refuse: bones, approx. 29%; skin, approx. 12%]:				
1 leg from a 3-lb. ready-to-cook chicken: approx. 5.7 oz. cooked	182	0.0	32.0	0.00
1 pound of cooked legs	512	0.0	32.0	0.00
Yield per pound of raw ready-to-cook chicken: approx. 1.9 oz. cooked	61	0.0	32.0	0.00
Weighing edible portion only:				
1 pound of cooked meat without skin (8g/0g/2g/65%/26mg)	866	0.0	54.2	0.00
FLOUR COATED, FRIED				
Eaten with skin:				
Weighed with skin and bones [refuse: bones, approx. 28%]:				
1 leg from a 3-lb. ready-to-cook chicken: approx. 5 oz. cooked	285	2.8	51.9	0.51
1 pound of cooked legs	831	8.2	51.9	0.51
Yield per pound of raw ready-to-cook chicken: approx. 1.7 oz. cooked	95	0.9	51.9	0.51
Weighing edible portion only:				
1 pound of cooked meat with skin (8g/1g/4g/55%/28mg)	1152	11.3	72.0	0.71
Fried with skin, but skin removed before eating:				
Weighed with skin and bones [refuse: bones, approx. 28%; skin, approx. 12%]				
1 leg from a 3-lb. ready-to-cook chicken: approx. 5 oz. cooked	195	0.6	35.3	0.11
1 pound of cooked legs	565	1.8	35.3	0.11
Yield per pound of raw ready-to-cook chicken: approx. 1.7 oz. cooked	65	0.2	35.3	0.11
Weighing edible portion only:				
1 pound of cooked meat without skin (8g/tr/3g/61%/27mg)	944	2.9	59.0	0.18
BATTER DIPPED, FRIED				
Eaten with skin:				
Weighed with skin and bones [refuse: bones, approx. 22%]:				
1 leg from a 3-lb. ready-to-cook chicken: approx. 7.2 oz. cooked	431	30.8	60.3	1.93
1 pound of cooked legs	964	30.8	60.3	1.93
Yield per pound of raw ready-to-cook chicken: approx. 2.4 oz. cooked	144	10.3	60.3	1.93
Weighing edible portion only:				
1 pound of cooked meat with skin (6g/2g/4g/52%/79mg)	1238	39.6	77.4	2.47
Fried with skin, but skin removed before eating:				
Weighed with skin and bones [refuse: bones, approx. 22%; skin, approx. 32%]:				
1 leg from a 3-lb. ready-to-cook chicken: approx. 7.2 oz. cooked	195	0.6	27.1	0.08
1 pound of cooked legs	432	1.3	27.1	0.08
Yield per pound of raw ready-to-cook chicken: approx. 2.4 oz. cooked	65	0.2	27.1	0.08
Weighing edible portion only:				
1 pound of cooked meat without skin	944	2.9	59.0	0.18
STEWED				
Eaten with skin:				
Weighed with skin and bones [refuse: bones, approx. 30%]:				
1 leg from a 3-lb. ready-to-cook chicken: approx. 6.3 oz. cooked	275	0.0	43.6	0.00
1 pound of cooked legs	698	0.0	43.6	0.00
Yield per pound of raw ready-to-cook chicken: approx. 2.1 oz. cooked	92	0.0	43.6	0.00
Weighing edible portion only:				
1 pound of cooked meat with skin (7g/0g/4g/64%/21mg)	998	0.0	62.4	0.00
Stewed with skin, but skin removed before eating:				
Weighed with skin and bones [refuse: bones, approx. 30%; skin, approx. 13%]:				
1 leg from a 3-lb. ready-to-cook chicken: approx. 6.3 oz. cooked	187	0.0	29.9	0.00
1 pound of cooked legs	478	0.0	29.9	0.00
Yield per pound of raw ready-to-cook chicken: approx. 2.1 oz. cooked	62	0.0	29.9	0.00
Weighing edible portion only:				
1 pound of cooked meat without skin (7g/0g/2g/66%/22mg)	839	0.0	52.5	0.00
THIGH:				
RAW				
With skin:				
Weighed with skin and bones [refuse: bones, approx. 21%]:				
1 thigh from a 3-lb. ready-to-cook chicken: approx. 4.2 oz.	199	0.0	47.3	0.00
1 pound of raw thighs	757	0.0	47.3	0.00

	UNIT Cal.	UNIT Carb.	1 OZ., BY WT. Cal.	1 OZ., BY WT. Carb.
Weighing edible portion only:				
1 pound of raw meat with skin (5g/0g/4g/68%/22mg)	957	0.0	59.8	0.00
Without skin:				
Weighed with skin and bones [refuse: bones, approx. 21%; skin, approx. 22%]:				
1 thigh from a 3-lb. ready-to-cook chicken: approx. 4.2 oz.	82	0.0	19.3	0.00
1 pound of raw thighs	308	0.0	19.3	0.00
Weighing edible portion only:				
1 pound of raw meat without skin (6g/0g/1g/76%/24mg)	540	0.0	33.7	0.00
ROASTED				
Eaten with skin:				
Weighed with skin and bones [refuse: bones, approx. 23%]:				
1 thigh from a 3-lb. ready-to-cook chicken: 2.9 oz. cooked	153	0.0	53.9	0.00
1 pound of cooked thighs	862	0.0	53.9	0.00
Yield per pound of raw ready-to-cook chicken: approx. 1 oz. cooked	51	0.0	53.9	0.00
Weighing edible portion only:				
1 pound of cooked meat with skin (7g/0g/4g/59%/24mg)	1120	0.0	70.0	0.00
Roasted with skin, but skin removed before eating:				
Weighed with skin and bones [refuse: bones, approx. 23%; skin, approx. 12%]:				
1 thigh from a 3-lb. ready-to-cook chicken: approx. 2.9 oz. cooked	109	0.0	38.5	0.00
1 pound of cooked thighs	616	0.0	38.5	0.00
Yield per pound of raw ready-to-cook chicken: approx. 1 oz. cooked	36	0.0	38.5	0.00
Weighing edible portion only:				
1 pound of cooked meat without skin (7g/0g/3g/63%/25mg)	948	0.0	59.3	0.00
FLOUR COATED, FRIED				
Eaten with skin:				
Weighed with skin and bones [refuse: bones, approx. 23%]:				
1 thigh from a 3-lb. ready-to-cook chicken: approx. 2.9 oz. cooked	162	2.0	57.1	0.69
1 pound of cooked thighs	914	11.1	57.1	0.69
Yield per pound of raw ready-to-cook chicken: approx. 1 oz. cooked	54	0.7	57.1	0.69
Weighing edible portion only:				
1 pound of cooked meat with skin (8g/1g/4g/54%/25mg)	1189	14.4	74.3	0.90
Fried with skin, but skin removed before eating:				
Weighed with skin and bones [refuse: bones, approx. 23%; skin, approx. 13%]:				
1 thigh from a 3-lb. ready-to-cook chicken: approx. 2.9 oz. cooked	113	0.6	39.5	0.21
1 pound of cooked thighs	632	3.4	39.5	0.21
Yield per pound of raw ready-to-cook chicken: approx. 1 oz. cooked	38	0.2	39.5	0.21
Weighing edible portion only:				
1 pound of cooked meat without skin (8g/tr/3g/59%/27mg)	989	5.4	61.8	0.33
BATTER DIPPED, FRIED				
Eaten with skin:				
Weighed with skin and bones [refuse: bones, approx. 19%]:				
1 thigh from a 3-lb. ready-to-cook chicken: approx. 3.7 oz. cooked	238	7.8	63.5	2.09
1 pound of cooked thighs	1016	33.4	63.5	2.09
Yield per pound of raw ready-to-cook chicken: approx. 1.2 oz. cooked	79	2.6	63.5	2.09
Weighing edible portion only:				
1 pound of cooked meat with skin (6g/12g/4g/51%/82mg)	1257	41.2	78.5	2.57
Fried with skin, but skin removed before eating:				
Weighed with skin and bones [refuse: bones, approx. 19%; skin, approx. 33%]:				
1 thigh from a 3-lb. ready-to-cook chicken: approx. 3.7 oz. cooked	(113)	(0.6)	(30.2)	(0.16)
1 pound of cooked thighs	(484)	(2.6)	(30.2)	(0.16)
Yield per pound of raw ready-to-cook chicken: approx. 1.2 oz. cooked	(38)	(0.2)	(30.2)	(0.16)
Weighing edible portion only:				
1 pound of cooked meat without skin	989	5.4	61.8	0.33
STEWED				
Eaten with skin:				
Weighed with skin and bones [refuse: bones, approx. 24%]:				
1 thigh from a 3-lb. ready-to-cook chicken: approx. 3.2 oz. cooked	158	0.0	50.1	0.00
1 pound of cooked thighs	801	0.0	50.1	0.00
Yield per pound of raw ready-to-cook chicken: approx. 1.1 oz. cooked	53	0.0	50.1	0.00

	UNIT		1 OZ., BY WT.	
	Cal.	Carb.	Cal.	Carb.
Weighing edible portion only:				
1 pound of cooked meat with skin (7g/0g/4g/63%/20mg)	1052	0.0	65.8	0.00
Stewed with skin, but skin removed before eating:				
Weighed with skin and bones [refuse: bones, approx. 24%; skin, approx. 15%]:				
1 thigh from a 3-lb. ready-to-cook chicken: approx. 3.2 oz. cooked	107	0.0	33.8	0.00
1 pound of cooked thighs	540	0.0	33.8	0.00
Yield per pound of raw ready-to-cook chicken: approx. 1.1 oz. cooked	36	0.0	33.8	0.00
Weighing edible portion only:				
1 pound of cooked meat without skin (7g/0g/3g/66%/22mg)	885	0.0	55.3	0.00
WING:				
RAW				
With skin:				
Weighed with skin and bones [refuse: bones, approx. 46%]:				
1 wing from a 3-lb. ready-to-cook chicken: approx. 3.2 oz.	109	0.0	34.0	0.00
1 pound of raw wings	544	0.0	34.0	0.00
Weighing edible portion only:				
1 pound of raw meat with skin (5g/0g/4g/66%/21mg)	1007	0.0	62.9	0.00
Without skin:				
Weighed with skin and bones [refuse: bones, approx. 46%; skin, approx. 22%]:				
1 wing from a 3-lb. ready-to-cook chicken: approx. 3.2 oz.	36	0.0	11.4	0.00
1 pound of raw wings	183	0.0	11.4	0.00
Weighing edible portion only:				
1 pound of raw meat without skin (6g/0g/1g/25%/23mg)	572	0.0	35.7	0.00
ROASTED				
Eaten with skin:				
Weighed with skin and bones [refuse: bones, approx. 48%]:				
1 wing from a 3-lb. ready-to-cook chicken: approx. 2.3 oz. cooked	99	0.0	42.8	0.00
1 pound of cooked wings	685	0.0	42.8	0.00
Yield per pound of raw ready-to-cook chicken: approx. 0.8 oz. cooked	33	0.0	42.8	0.00
Weighing edible portion only:				
1 pound of cooked meat with skin (8g/0g/5g/55%/23mg)	1316	0.0	82.2	0.00
Roasted with skin, but skin removed before eating:				
Weighed with skin and bones [refuse: bones, approx. 48%; skin, approx. 20%]:				
1 wing from a 3-lb. ready-to-cook chicken: approx. 2.3 oz. cooked	43	0.0	18.4	0.00
1 pound of cooked wings	295	0.0	18.4	0.00
Yield per pound of raw ready-to-cook chicken: approx. 0.8 oz. cooked	14	0.0	18.4	0.00
Weighing edible portion only:				
1 pound of cooked meat without skin (9g/0g/2g/63%/23mg)	921	0.0	57.6	0.00
FLOUR COATED, FRIED				
Eaten with skin:				
Weighed with skin and bones [refuse: bones, approx. 47%]:				
1 wing from a 3-lb. ready-to-cook chicken: approx. 2.2 oz. cooked	103	0.8	48.2	0.36
1 pound of cooked wings	771	5.7	48.2	0.36
Yield per pound of raw ready-to-cook chicken: approx. 0.7 oz. cooked	34	0.3	48.2	0.36
Weighing edible portion only:				
1 pound of cooked meat with skin (7g/1g/6g/49%/22mg)	1456	10.8	91.0	0.68
Fried with skin, but skin removed before eating:				
Weighed with skin and bones [refuse: bones, approx. 47%; skin, approx. 19%]:				
1 wing from a 3-lb. ready-to-cook chicken: approx. 2.2 oz. cooked	42	0.0	20.4	0.00
1 pound of cooked wings	326	0.0	20.4	0.00
Yield per pound of raw ready-to-cook chicken: approx. 0.7 oz. cooked	14	0.0	20.4	0.00
Weighing edible portion only:				
1 pound of cooked meat without skin (9g/0g/3g/60%/26mg)	957	0.0	59.8	0.00
BATTER DIPPED, FRIED				
Eaten with skin:				
Weighed with skin and bones [refuse: bones, approx. 38%]:				
1 wing from a 3-lb. ready-to-cook chicken: approx. 2.8 oz. cooked	159	5.4	56.9	1.92
1 pound of cooked wings	911	30.8	56.9	1.92
Yield per pound of raw ready-to-cook chicken: approx. 0.9 oz. cooked	53	1.8	56.9	1.92
Weighing edible portion only:				
1 pound of cooked meat with skin (6g/3g/6g/46%/91mg)	1470	49.6	91.9	3.10

	UNIT		1 OZ., BY WT.	
	Cal.	Carb.	Cal.	Carb.
Fried with skin, but skin removed before eating:				
Weighed with skin and bones [refuse: bones, approx. 38%; skin, approx. 37%]:				
1 wing from a 3-lb. ready-to-cook chicken: approx. 2.8 oz. cooked	42	0.0	14.9	0.00
1 pound of cooked wings	238	0.0	14.9	0.00
Yield per pound of raw ready-to-cook chicken: approx. 0.9 oz. cooked	14	0.0	14.9	0.00
Weighing edible portion only:				
1 pound of cooked meat without skin	957	0.0	59.8	0.00
STEWED				
Eaten with skin:				
Weighed with skin and bones [refuse: bones, approx. 48%]:				
1 wing from a 3-lb. ready-to-cook chicken: approx. 2.7 oz. cooked	100	0.0	36.7	0.00
1 pound of cooked wings	587	0.0	36.7	0.00
Yield per pound of raw ready-to-cook chicken: approx. 0.9 oz. cooked	33	0.0	36.7	0.00
Weighing edible portion only:				
1 pound of cooked meat with skin (7g/0g/5g/62%/19mg)	1130	0.0	70.6	0.00
Stewed with skin, but skin removed before eating:				
Weighed with skin and bones [refuse: bones, approx. 48%; skin, approx. 20%]:				
1 wing from a 3-lb. ready-to-cook chicken: approx. 2.7 oz. cooked	43	0.0	16.4	0.00
1 pound of cooked wings	263	0.0	16.4	0.00
Yield per pound of raw ready-to-cook chicken: approx. 0.9 oz. cooked	14	0.0	16.4	0.00
Weighing edible portion only:				
1 pound of cooked meat without skin (8g/0g/2g/67%/21mg)	821	0.0	51.3	0.00
GIBLETS (1 each gizzard, heart, and liver):				
RAW				
Giblets from a 3-lb. 5-oz. chicken: approx. 2.6 oz.	93	1.4	35.2	0.51
1 pound of giblets	563	8.2	35.2	0.51
FLOUR COATED, FRIED				
Giblets from a 3-lb. 5-oz. chicken: approx. 1.6 oz. cooked	(126)	(2.0)	78.5	1.23
1 pound of giblets (9g/1g/4g/48%/32mg)	1257	19.7	78.5	1.23
1 cup (approx. 5.1 oz.)	402	6.3	78.5	1.23
SIMMERED				
Giblets from a 3-lb. 5-oz. chicken: approx. 1.6 oz. cooked	(71)	(0.4)	44.5	0.27
1 pound of giblets (7g/tr/1g/68%/16mg)	712	4.3	44.5	0.27
1 cup (approx. 5.1 oz.)	228	1.4	44.5	0.27
GIZZARD:				
RAW				
Gizzard from a 3-lb. 5-oz. chicken: approx. 1.3 oz.	44	0.2	33.5	0.16
1 pound of gizzards	535	2.6	33.5	0.16
SIMMERED				
Gizzard from a 3-lb. 5-oz. chicken: approx. 0.8 oz. cooked	(35)	(0.3)	43.4	0.32
1 pound of gizzards (8g/tr/1g/67%/19mg)	694	5.2	43.4	0.32
1 cup (approx. 5.1 oz.)	222	1.7	43.4	0.32
HEART:				
RAW				
Heart from a 3-lb. 5-oz. chicken: approx. 0.2 oz.	9	trace	43.4	0.20
1 pound of hearts	694	3.2	43.4	0.20
SIMMERED				
Heart from a 3-lb. 5-oz. chicken: approx. 0.1 oz. cooked	(6)	trace	52.5	0.03
1 pound of hearts (8g/tr/2g/65%/14mg)	839	0.5	52.5	0.03
1 cup (approx. 5.1 oz.)	268	0.2	52.5	0.03
LIVER:				
RAW				
Liver from a 3-lb. 5-oz. chicken: approx. 1.1 oz.	40	1.1	35.4	0.97
1 pound of livers	567	15.5	35.4	0.97
SIMMERED				
Liver from a 3-lb. 5-oz. chicken: approx. 0.7 oz. cooked	(31)	(0.2)	44.5	0.25
1 pound of livers (7g/tr/2g/68%/14mg)	712	4.0	44.5	0.25
1 cup (approx. 4.9 oz.)	219	1.2	44.5	0.25
NECK:				
RAW				
With skin:				
Weighed with skin and bones [refuse: bones, approx. 36%]:				
1 neck from a 3-lb. 5-oz. ready-to-cook chicken: approx. 2.8 oz.	148	0.0	53.8	0.00
1 pound of raw necks	861	0.0	53.8	0.00
Weighing edible portion only:				
1 pound of raw meat with skin (4g/0g/7g/60%/18mg)	1347	0.0	84.2	0.00

	UNIT Cal.	UNIT Carb.	1 OZ., BY WT. Cal.	1 OZ., BY WT. Carb.
Without skin:				
Weighed with skin and bones [refuse: bones, approx. 36%; skin, approx. 39%]:				
1 neck from a 3-lb. 5-oz. ready-to-cook chicken: approx. 2.8 oz.	31	0.0	10.9	0.00
1 pound of raw necks	175	0.0	10.9	0.00
Weighing edible portion only:				
1 pound of raw meat without skin (5g/0g/3g/71%/23mg)	699	0.0	43.7	0.00
FLOUR COATED, FRIED				
Eaten with skin:				
Weighed with skin and bones [refuse: bones, approx. 29%]:				
1 neck from a 3-lb. 5-oz. ready-to-cook chicken: approx. 1.8 oz. cooked	119	1.5	66.8	0.85
1 pound of cooked necks	1069	13.6	66.8	0.85
Yield per pound of raw ready-to-cook chicken: approx. 0.5 oz. cooked	40	0.5	66.8	0.85
Weighing edible portion only:				
1 pound of cooked meat with skin (7g/1g/7g/48%/23mg)	1506	19.2	94.1	1.20
Fried with skin, but skin removed before eating:				
Weighed with skin and bones [refuse: bones, approx. 29%; skin, approx. 27%]:				
1 neck from a 3-lb. 5-oz. ready-to-cook chicken: approx. 1.8 oz. cooked	50	0.4	28.6	0.22
1 pound of cooked necks	457	3.5	28.6	0.27
Yield per pound of raw ready-to-cook chicken: approx. 0.5 oz. cooked	15	0.1	28.6	0.27
Weighing edible portion only:				
1 pound of cooked meat without skin (8g/tr/3g/59%/28mg)	1039	8.0	64.9	0.50
BATTER DIPPED, FRIED				
Eaten with skin:				
Weighed with skin and bones [refuse: bones, approx. 25%]:				
1 neck from a 3-lb. 5-oz. ready-to-cook chicken: approx. 2.5 oz. cooked	172	4.5	70.3	1.85
1 pound of cooked necks	1124	29.6	70.3	1.85
Yield per pound of raw ready-to-cook chicken: approx. 0.8 oz. cooked	52	1.4	70.3	1.85
Weighing edible portion only:				
1 pound of cooked meat with skin (6g/2g/7g/47%/78mg)	1497	39.5	93.6	2.47
Fried with skin, but skin removed before eating:				
Weighed with skin and bones [refuse: bones, approx. 25%; skin, approx. 39%]:				
1 neck from a 3-lb. 5-oz. ready-to-cook chicken: approx. 2.5 oz. cooked	50	0.4	20.3	0.16
1 pound of cooked necks	325	2.6	20.3	0.16
Yield per pound of raw ready-to-cook chicken: approx. 0.8 oz. cooked	15	0.1	20.3	0.16
Weighing edible portion only:				
1 pound of cooked meat without skin	1039	8.0	64.9	0.50
SIMMERED				
Eaten with skin:				
Weighed with skin and bones [refuse: bones, approx. 32%]:				
1 neck from a 3-lb. 5-oz. ready-to-cook chicken: approx. 2 oz. cooked	94	0.0	47.6	0.00
1 pound of cooked necks	762	0.0	47.6	0.00
Yield per pound of raw ready-to-cook chicken: approx. 0.7 oz. cooked	28	0.0	47.6	0.00
Weighing edible portion only:				
1 pound of cooked meat with skin (6g/0g/5g/62%/15mg)	1120	0.0	70.0	0.00
Simmered with skin, but skin removed before eating:				
Weighed with skin and bones [refuse: bones, approx. 32%; skin, approx. 35%]:				
1 neck from a 3-lb. 5-oz. ready-to-cook chicken: approx. 2 oz. cooked	32	0.0	16.7	0.00
1 pound of cooked necks	267	0.0	16.7	0.00
Yield per pound of raw ready-to-cook chicken: approx. 0.7 oz. cooked	10	0.0	16.7	0.00
Weighing edible portion only:				
1 pound of cooked meat without skin (7g/0g/2g/67%/18mg)	812	0.0	50.8	0.00
SKIN (not including neck skin):				
RAW				
Skin from a 3-lb. chicken: approx. 5.6 oz.	550	0.0	99.0	0.00
1 pound of skin	1583	0.0	99.0	0.00
BATTERED DIPPED, FRIED				
Skin from a 3-lb. chicken: approx. 13 oz. cooked (3g/7g/8g/36%/165mg)	1496	88.0	111.7	6.56
1 pound of skin	1787	105.0	111.7	6.56

	UNIT Cal.	UNIT Carb.	1 OZ., BY WT. Cal.	1 OZ., BY WT. Carb.
FLOUR COATED, FRIED				
Skin from a 3-lb. chicken: approx. 3.9 oz. cooked (5g/3g/12g/29%/15mg)	562	10.5	142.3	2.65
1 pound of skin	2276	42.4	142.3	2.65
ROASTED				
Skin from a 3-lb. chicken: approx. 3.9 oz. cooked (6g/0g/12g/40%/18mg)	508	0.0	128.7	0.00
1 pound of skin	2060	0.0	128.7	0.00
STEWED				
Skin from a 3-lb. chicken: approx. 5.1 oz. cooked (4g/0g/9g/53%/16mg)	522	0.0	102.9	0.00
1 pound of skin	1647	0.0	102.9	0.00
SEPARABLE FAT:				
RAW				
Fat from a 3-lb. chicken: approx. 3.7 oz.	654	0.0	178.3	0.00
1 pound of chicken fat (1g/0g/19g/29%/9mg)	2853	0.0	178.3	0.00
Roasters				
ENTIRE CHICKEN (with neck and giblets):				
RAW				
With skin:				
Weighed with skin and bones [refuse: bones, approx. 27%]:				
1 4-lb. 9-oz. ready-to-cook chicken	3210	1.3	44.0	0.02
1 pound of raw bird, average all parts	704	0.3	44.0	0.02
Weighing edible portion only:				
1 pound of raw meat with skin (5g/tr/4g/66%/20mg)	966	0.4	60.4	0.03
Without skin:				
Weighed with skin and bones [refuse: bones, approx. 27%; skin, approx. 20%]:				
1 4-lb. 9-oz. ready-to-cook chicken	(1254)	(1.3)	(17.2)	(0.02)
1 pound of raw bird, average all parts	(275)	(0.3)	(17.2)	(0.02)
Weighing edible portion only:				
1 pound of raw meat without skin	(518)	(0.5)	(32.4)	(0.03)
ROASTED				
Eaten with skin:				
Weighed with skin and bones [refuse: bones, approx. 29%]:				
1 4-lb. 9-oz. ready-to-cook chicken: approx. 3 lb. 5 oz. cooked	2363	0.6	44.4	0.01
1 pound of cooked bird, average all parts	710	0.6	44.4	0.01
Yield per pound of raw ready-to-cook chicken: approx. 11.7 oz. cooked	518	0.1	44.4	0.01
Weighing edible portion only:				
1 pound of cooked meat with skin (7g/tr/4g/62%/20mg)	998	0.2	62.4	0.01
Roasted with skin, but skin removed before eating:				
Weighed with skin and bones [refuse: bones, approx. 29%; skin, approx. 7%]:				
1 4-lb. 9-oz. ready-to-cook chicken: approx. 3 lb. 5 oz. cooked	(1444)	(0.6)	(21.0)	(0.01)
1 pound of cooked bird, average all parts	(336)	(0.1)	(21.0)	(0.01)
Yield per pound of raw ready-to-cook chicken: approx. 11.7 oz. cooked	(317)	(0.1)	(21.0)	(0.01)
Weighing edible portion only:				
1 pound of cooked meat without skin	(434)	(0.7)	(27.1)	(0.01)
ENTIRE CHICKEN (without neck and giblets):				
RAW				
With skin:				
Weighed with skin and bones [refuse: bones, approx. 28%]:				
1 4-lb. 2-oz. ready-to-cook chicken	2888	0.0	44.1	0.00
1 pound of raw bird, average all parts	706	0.0	44.1	0.00
Weighing edible portion only:				
1 pound of raw meat with skin	980	0.0	61.2	0.00
Without skin:				
Weighed with skin and bones [refuse: bones, approx. 28%; skin, approx. 21%]:				
1 4-lb. 2-oz. ready-to-cook chicken	1060	0.0	16.1	0.00
1 pound of raw bird, average all parts	257	0.0	16.1	0.00
Weighing edible portion only:				
1 pound of raw meat without skin	504	0.0	31.5	0.00
ROASTED				
Eaten with skin:				
Weighed with skin and bones [refuse: bones, approx. 30%]:				
1 4-lb. 2-oz. ready-to-cook chicken: approx. 3 lb. 1 oz. cooked	2142	0.0	44.3	0.00
1 pound of cooked bird, average all parts	708	0.0	44.3	0.00
Yield per pound of raw ready-to-cook chicken: approx. 11.9 oz. cooked	519	0.0	44.3	0.00
Weighing edible portion only:				
1 pound of cooked meat with skin	1012	0.0	63.2	0.00

	UNIT Cal.	UNIT Carb.	1 OZ., BY WT. Cal.	1 OZ., BY WT. Carb.
Roasted with skin, but skin removed before eating:				
Weighed with skin and bones [refuse: bones, approx. 30%; skin, approx. 13%]:				
1 4-lb. 2-oz. ready-to-cook chicken: approx. 3 lb. 1 oz. cooked	1300	0.0	26.9	0.00
1 pound of cooked bird, average all parts	431	0.0	26.9	0.00
Yield per pound of raw ready-to-cook chicken: approx. 11.9 oz. cooked	315	0.0	26.9	0.00
Weighing edible portion only:				
1 pound of cooked meat without skin	758	0.0	47.3	0.00
TOP QUARTER (Breast and Wing—Light Meat):				
RAW				
Without skin:				
Weighed with skin and bones [refuse: bones, approx. 26%; skin, approx. 17%]:				
1 top quarter from a 4-lb. 2-oz. ready-to-cook chicken: approx. 13.5 oz.	241	0.0	17.7	0.00
1 pound of raw top quarters	283	0.0	17.7	0.00
Weighing edible portion only:				
1 pound of raw meat without skin	494	0.0	30.9	0.00
ROASTED				
Roasted with skin, but skin removed before eating:				
Weighed with skin and bones [refuse: bones, approx. 24%; skin, approx. 16%]:				
1 top quarter from a 4-lb. 2-oz. ready-to-cook chicken: approx. 10.4 oz. cooked	214	0.0	25.9	0.00
1 pound of cooked top quarters	415	0.0	25.9	0.00
Yield per pound of raw ready-to-cook chicken: 2.5 oz. cooked	52	0.0	25.9	0.00
Weighing edible portion only:				
1 pound of cooked meat without skin	694	0.0	43.4	0.00
1 cup, chopped or diced (approx. 4.9 oz.)	214	0.0	43.4	0.00
BOTTOM QUARTER (Drumstick, Thigh, and Back—Dark Meat):				
RAW				
Without skin:				
Weighed with skin and bones [refuse: bones, approx. 30%; skin, approx. 23%]:				
1 bottom quarter from a 4-lb. 2-oz. ready-to-cook chicken: approx. 1 lb. 3.3 oz.	290	0.0	15.0	0.00
1 pound of raw bottom quarters	240	0.0	15.0	0.00
Weighing edible portion only:				
1 pound of raw meat without skin	513	0.0	32.0	0.00
ROASTED				
Roasted with skin, but skin removed before eating:				
Weighed with skin and bones [refuse: bones, approx. 35%; skin, approx. 11%]:				
1 bottom quarter from a 4-lb. 2-oz. ready-to-cook chicken: approx. 13.9 oz. cooked	250	0.0	27.3	0.00
1 pound of cooked bottom quarters	436	0.0	27.3	0.00
Yield per pound of raw ready-to-cook chicken: approx. 3.4 oz. cooked	61	0.0	27.3	0.00
Weighing edible portion only:				
1 pound of cooked meat without skin	807	0.0	50.5	0.00
1 cup, chopped or diced (approx. 4.9 oz.)	250	0.0	50.5	0.00
GIBLETS (1 each gizzard, heart, and liver):				
RAW				
Giblets from a 4-lb. 9-oz. chicken: approx. 4 oz. (5g/tr/1g/75%/22mg)	288	1.3	36.0	0.32
1 pound of giblets	576	5.2	36.0	0.32
SIMMERED:				
Giblets from a 4-lb. 9-oz. chicken: approx. 2.4 oz. cooked (8g/tr/2g/66%/17mg)	(112)	(0.5)	46.8	0.24
1 pound of giblets	749	3.9	46.8	0.24
1 cup (approx. 5.1 oz.)	239	1.2	46.8	0.24
Stewing Chickens				
ENTIRE CHICKEN (with neck and giblets):				
RAW				
With skin:				
Weighed with skin and bones [refuse: bones and separable fat, approx. 31%]:				
1 2-lb. 15-oz. ready-to-cook chicken	2275	1.7	48.4	0.04
1 pound of raw bird, average all parts	775	0.6	48.4	0.04
Weighing edible portion only:				
1 pound of raw meat with skin (5g/tr/6g/63%/20mg)	1139	0.9	71.2	0.05
Without skin:				
Weighed with skin and bones [refuse: bones, approx. 31%; skin, approx. 12%]:				
1 2-lb. 15-oz. ready-to-cook chicken	(1059)	(1.7)	(22.6)	(0.04)
1 pound of raw bird, average all parts	(362)	(0.6)	(22.6)	(0.04)
Weighing edible portion only:				
1 pound of raw meat without skin	(634)	(1.0)	(39.6)	(0.06)

	UNIT Cal.	UNIT Carb.	1 OZ., BY WT. Cal.	1 OZ., BY WT. Carb.
STEWED				
Weighed with skin and bones [refuse: bones, approx. 31%]:				
1 2-lb. 15-oz. ready-to-cook chicken: approx. 1 lb. 14 oz. cooked	1636	trace	54.0	trace
1 pound of cooked bird, average all parts	864	trace	54.0	trace
Yield per pound of raw ready-to-cook chicken: approx. 10.3 oz. cooked	557	trace	54.0	trace
Weighing edible portion only:				
1 pound of cooked meat with skin (9g/tr/5g/54%/20mg)	1252	0.1	78.3	trace
Stewed with skin, but skin removed before eating:				
Weighed with skin and bones [refuse: bones, approx. 31%; skin, approx. 34%]:				
1 2-lb. 15-oz. ready-to-cook chicken: approx. 1 lb. 14 oz. cooked	(1091)	trace	(23.2)	trace
1 pound of cooked bird, average all parts	(371)	trace	(23.2)	trace
Yield per pound of raw ready-to-cook chicken: approx. 10.3 oz. cooked	(371)	trace	(23.2)	trace
Weighing edible portion only:				
1 pound of cooked meat without skin	(1056)	trace	(66.0)	trace
ENTIRE CHICKEN (without neck and giblets):				
RAW				
With skin:				
Weighed with skin and bones [refuse: bones, approx. 30%]:				
1 2-lb. 8-oz. ready-to-cook chicken	2056	0.0	51.3	0.00
1 pound of raw bird, average all parts	820	0.0	51.3	0.00
Weighing edible portion only:				
1 pound of raw meat with skin (5g/0g/6g/62%/20mg)	1170	0.0	73.1	0.00
Without skin:				
Weighed with skin and bones [refuse: bones, approx. 30%; skin, approx. 20%]:				
1 2-lb. 8-oz. ready-to-cook chicken	840	0.0	20.9	0.00
1 pound of raw bird, average all parts	335	0.0	20.9	0.00
Weighing edible portion:				
1 pound of raw meat without skin (6g/0g/2g/76%/22mg)	671	0.0	42.0	0.00
STEWED				
Eaten with skin:				
Weighed with skin and bones [refuse: bones, approx. 32%]:				
1 2-lb. 8-oz. ready-to-cook chicken: approx. 1 lb. 11 oz. cooked	1488	0.0	54.9	0.00
1 pound of cooked bird, average all parts	879	0.0	54.9	0.00
Yield per pound of raw ready-to-cook chicken: approx. 10.8 oz. cooked	595	0.0	54.9	0.00
Weighing edible portion only:				
1 pound of cooked meat with skin (8g/0g/5g/53%/21mg)	1293	0.0	80.8	0.00
Stewed with skin, but skin removed before eating:				
Weighed with skin and bones [refuse: bones, approx. 32%; skin, approx. 16%]:				
1 2-lb. 8-oz. ready-to-cook chicken: approx. 1 lb. 11 oz. cooked	1396	0.0	34.9	0.00
1 pound of cooked bird, average all parts	559	0.0	34.9	0.00
Yield per pound of raw ready-to-cook chicken: approx. 10.8 oz. cooked	558	0.0	34.9	0.00
Weighing edible portion only:				
1 pound of cooked meat without skin	1075	0.0	67.2	0.00
1 cup, chopped or diced (approx. 4.9 oz.)	332	0.0	67.2	0.00
TOP QUARTER (Breast and Wing—Light Meat):				
RAW				
Without skin:				
Weighed with skin and bone [refuse: bones, approx. 26%; skin, approx. 18%]:				
1 top quarter from a 2-lb. 8-oz. ready-to-cook chicken: approx. 8.2 oz.	178	0.0	21.7	0.00
1 pound of raw top quarters	347	0.0	21.7	0.00
Weighing edible portion only:				
1 pound of raw meat without skin	621	0.0	38.8	0.00
STEWED				
Stewed with skin, but skin removed before eating:				
Weighed with skin and bones [refuse: bones, approx. 26%; skin, approx. 16%]:				
1 top quarter from a 2-lb. 8-oz. ready-to-cook chicken: approx. 5.9 oz. cooked	204	0.0	34.4	0.00
1 pound of cooked top quarters	551	0.0	34.4	0.00
Yield per pound of raw ready-to-cook chicken: approx. 2.4 oz. cooked	82	0.0	34.4	0.00
Weighing edible portion only:				
1 pound of cooked meat without skin	966	0.0	60.4	0.00
1 cup, chopped or diced (approx. 4.9 oz.)	298	0.0	60.4	0.00

	UNIT Cal.	UNIT Carb.	1 OZ., BY WT. Cal.	1 OZ., BY WT. Carb.
BOTTOM QUARTER (Drumstick, Thigh, and Back—Dark Meat):				
RAW				
Without skin:				
Weighed with skin and bones [refuse: bones, approx. 33%; skin, approx. 21%]:				
1 bottom quarter from a 2-lb. 8-oz. ready-to-cook chicken: approx. 11.9 oz.	242	0.0	20.5	0.00
1 pound of raw bottom quarters	328	0.0	20.5	0.00
Weighing edible portion only:				
1 pound of raw meat without skin (6g/0g/2g/72%/29mg)	712	0.0	44.5	0.00
STEWED				
Stewed with skin, but skin removed before eating:				
Weighed with skin and bones [refuse: bones, approx. 36%; skin, approx. 15%]:				
1 bottom quarter from a 2-lb. 8-oz. ready-to-cook chicken: approx. 7.8 oz. cooked	361	0.0	35.9	0.00
1 pound of cooked bottom quarters	574	0.0	35.9	0.00
Yield per pound of raw ready-to-cook chicken: approx. 3.1 oz. cooked	144	0.0	35.9	0.00
Weighing edible portion only:				
1 pound cooked meat without skin (8g/0g/4g/55%/27mg)	1170	0.0	73.1	0.00
1 cup, chopped or diced (approx. 4.9 oz.)	361	0.0	73.1	0.00
GIBLETS (1 each gizzard, heart, and liver):				
RAW				
Giblets from a 2-lb. 15-oz. chicken: approx. 2.9 oz. (5g/1g/3g/70%/22mg)	136	1.7	47.6	0.60
1 pound of giblets	762	9.7	47.6	0.60
SIMMERED				
Giblets from a 2-lb. 15-oz. chicken: approx. 1.8 oz. cooked (7g/tr/3g/64%/16mg)	(99)	(0.1)	55.0	0.03
1 pound of giblets	880	0.5	55.0	0.03
1 cup (approx. 5.1 oz.)	281	0.2	55.0	0.03

Capon

	UNIT Cal.	UNIT Carb.	1 OZ., BY WT. Cal.	1 OZ., BY WT. Carb.
ENTIRE CAPON (with neck and giblets):				
RAW				
With skin:				
Weighed with skin and bones [refuse: bones, approx. 27%]:				
1 6-lb. 8-oz. ready-to-cook chicken	4987	1.6	47.9	0.02
1 pound of raw bird, average all parts	767	0.3	47.9	0.02
Weighing edible portion only:				
1 pound of raw meat with skin (5g/tr/4g/64%/13mg)	1052	0.4	65.8	0.02
ROASTED				
Eaten with skin:				
Weighed with skin and bones [refuse: bones, approx. 28%]:				
1 6-lb. 8-oz. ready-to-cook chicken: approx. 4 lb. 6 oz. cooked	3211	0.5	46.2	0.01
1 pound of cooked bird, average all parts	739	0.1	46.2	0.01
Yield per pound of raw ready-to-cook chicken: approx. 10.8 oz. cooked	494	0.1	46.2	0.01
Weighing edible portion only:				
1 pound of cooked meat with skin (8g/tr/3g/59%/14mg)	1025	0.2	64.1	0.01
ENTIRE CAPON (without neck and giblets):				
RAW				
With skin:				
Weighed with skin and bones [refuse: bones, approx. 28%]:				
1 5-lb. 14-oz. ready-to-cook chicken	4514	0.0	47.8	0.00
1 pound of raw bird, average all parts	765	0.0	47.8	0.00
Weighing edible portion only:				
1 pound of raw meat with skin (5g/0g/5g/63%/13mg)	1062	0.0	66.3	0.00
ROASTED				
Eaten with skin:				
Weighed with skin and bones [refuse: bones, approx. 29%]:				
1 5-lb. 14-oz. ready-to-cook chicken: approx. 4 lb. cooked	2914	0.0	46.1	0.00
1 pound of cooked bird, average all parts	737	0.0	46.1	0.00
Yield per pound of raw ready-to-cook chicken: approx. 10.9 oz. cooked	496	0.0	46.1	0.00
Weighing edible portion only:				
1 pound of cooked meat with skin	1039	0.0	64.9	0.00
GIBLETS (1 each gizzard, heart, and liver):				
RAW (All-edible)				
Giblets from a 6-lb. 8-oz. chicken: approx. 4.1 oz. (5g/tr/2g/74%/22mg)	151	1.6	36.9	0.40
1 pound of giblets	590	6.4	36.9	0.40
SIMMERED (All-edible)				
Giblets from a 6-lb. 8-oz. chicken: approx. 0.4 oz. cooked (8g/tr/2g/67%/16mg)	18	0.1	46.6	0.22
1 pound of giblets	745	3.5	46.6	0.22
1 cup (approx. 5.1 oz.)	238	1.1	46.6	0.22

Foreign Chickens, Domesticated Breeds

	UNIT Cal.	UNIT Carb.	1 OZ., BY WT. Cal.	1 OZ., BY WT. Carb.
(Based on data from Africa)				
RAW, average all parts				
Edible portion, 1 pound	663	0.0	41.4	0.00
(Based on data from the Caribbean)				
DRESSED, Ready-to-cook, raw				
Young Birds, average all parts:				
Edible portion, 1 pound	772	0.0	48.3	0.00
Mature Bird, average all parts:				
Edible portion, 1 pound	1117	0.0	69.8	0.00
(Based on data from East Asia)				
RAW				
Very Young Birds (live weight under 3½ pounds), average all parts:				
As purchased:				
Live, 1 pound [refuse, approx. 51%: bones, feathers, head, feet, inedible viscera, blood]	336	0.0	21.0	0.00
Dressed, 1 pound [refuse, approx. 45%: feet, inedible viscera, bones)	377	0.0	23.6	0.00
Ready-to-cook, 1 pound [refuse: approx., bones 25%]	518	0.0	32.4	0.00
Edible portion, 1 pound	686	0.0	42.9	0.00
Young Birds (live weight over 3½ pounds), average all parts:				
As purchased:				
Live, 1 pound [refuse, approx. 46%: blood, feathers, head, feet, inedible viscera, bones]	490	0.0	30.6	0.00
Dressed, 1 pound [refuse, approx. 39%: head, feet, inedible viscera, bones]	554	0.0	34.6	0.00
Ready-to-cook, 1 pound [refuse: approx. bones 23%]	699	0.0	43.7	0.00
Edible portion, 1 pound	908	0.0	56.8	0.00
Mature Birds, average all parts:				
As purchased:				
Live, 1 pound [refuse, approx. 42%: blood, feathers, head, feet, inedible viscera, bones]	1795	0.0	49.7	0.00
Dressed, 1 pound [refuse, approx. 36%: head, feet, inedible viscera, bones]	876	0.0	54.8	0.00
Ready-to-cook, 1 pound [refuse: bones approx. 20%]	1099	0.0	68.7	0.00
Edible portion, 1 pound	1371	0.0	85.7	0.00
(Based on data from Ethiopia)				
RAW, average all parts				
Edible portion, 1 pound	545	22.3	34.1	1.39
(Based on data from Japan)				
RAW				
Young Birds, average all parts:				
Edible portion, 1 pound	554	0.0	34.6	0.00
Mature Birds, average all parts:				
Edible portion, 1 pound	613	0.0	38.3	0.00
(Based on data from Latin America)				
RAW				
Young Birds, average all parts:				
Edible portion, 1 pound	772	0.0	48.3	0.00
Mature Birds, average all parts:				
Edible portion, 1 pound	1117	0.0	69.8	0.00
(Based on data from Pakistan)				
RAW, average all kinds and classes				
Edible portion, 1 pound	558	0.9	34.9	0.06

TURKEY

Fryer-Roaster

	UNIT Cal.	UNIT Carb.	1 OZ., BY WT. Cal.	1 OZ., BY WT. Carb.
ENTIRE TURKEY (with neck and giblets):				
RAW				
With skin:				
Weighed with skin and bones [refuse: bones, approx. 25%]:				
1 7-lb. 1-oz. ready-to-cook turkey	3207	1.2	28.3	0.01
1 pound of raw bird, average all parts	453	0.2	28.3	0.01

	UNIT Cal.	UNIT Carb.	1 OZ., BY WT. Cal.	1 OZ., BY WT. Carb.
Weighing edible portion only:				
1 pound of raw meat with skin (6g/tr/1g/73%/17mg)	603	0.2	37.7	0.01
Without skin:				
Weighed with skin and bones [refuse: bones, approx. 25%; skin, approx. 8%]:				
1 7-lb. 1-oz. ready-to-cook turkey	(2385)	(1.2)	(21.1)	(0.01)
1 pound of raw bird, average all parts	(338)	(0.2)	(21.1)	(0.01)
Weighing edible portion only:				
1 pound of raw meat without skin	(504)	(0.2)	(31.5)	(0.01)
ROASTED				
Eaten with skin:				
Weighed with skin and bones [refuse: bones, approx. 25%]:				
1 7-lb. 1-oz. ready-to-cook turkey: approx. 5 lb. 3 oz. cooked	3029	0.8	36.4	0.01
1 pound of cooked bird, average all parts	582	0.2	36.4	0.01
Yield per pound of raw ready-to-cook turkey: approx. 11.8 oz. cooked	429	0.1	36.4	0.01
Weighing edible portion only:				
1 pound of cooked meat with skin (8g/tr/2g/66%/18mg)	776	0.2	48.5	0.01
Roasted with skin, but skin removed before eating:				
Weighed with skin and bones [refuse: bones, approx. 25%; skin, approx. 11%]:				
1 7-lb. 1-oz. ready-to-cook turkey: approx. 5 lb. 3 oz. cooked	(2275)	(0.8)	(30.7)	(0.01)
1 pound of cooked bird, average all parts	(491)	(0.2)	(30.7)	(0.01)
Yield per pound of raw ready-to-cook turkey: approx. 11.8 oz. cooked	(322)	(0.2)	(30.7)	(0.01)
Weighing edible portion only:				
1 pound of cooked meat without skin	(685)	(0.2)	(42.8)	(0.02)
ENTIRE TURKEY (without neck and giblets):				
RAW				
With skin:				
Weighed with skin and bones [refuse: bones, approx. 25%]:				
1 6-lb. 7-oz. ready-to-cook turkey	2926	0.0	28.4	0.00
1 pound of raw bird, average all parts	455	0.0	28.4	0.00
Weighing edible portion only:				
1 pound of raw meat with skin (6g/0g/1g/73%/16mg)	608	0.0	38.0	0.00
Without skin:				
Weighed with skin and bones [refuse: bones, approx. 25%; skin, approx. 9%]:				
1 6-lb. 7-oz. ready-to-cook turkey	2104	0.0	20.5	0.00
1 pound of raw bird, average all parts	328	0.0	20.5	0.00
Weighing edible portion only:				
1 pound of raw meat without skin (6g/0g/1g/75%/17mg)	499	0.0	31.2	0.00
ROASTED				
Eaten with skin:				
Weighed with skin and bones [refuse: bones, approx. 25%]:				
1 6-lb. 7-oz. ready-to-cook turkey: approx. 4 lb. 12 oz. cooked	2784	0.0	36.6	0.00
1 pound of cooked bird, average all parts	586	0.0	36.6	0.00
Yield per pound of raw ready-to-cook turkey: approx. 11.8 oz. cooked	432	0.0	36.6	0.00
Weighing edible portion only:				
1 pound of cooked meat with skin (8g/0g/2g/66%/19mg)	780	0.0	48.8	0.00
Roasted with skin, but skin removed before eating:				
Weighed with skin and bones [refuse: bones, approx. 25%; skin, approx. 11%]:				
1 6-lb. 7-oz. ready-to-cook turkey: approx. 4 lb. 12 oz. cooked	2071	0.0	27.2	0.00
1 pound of cooked bird, average all parts	435	0.0	27.2	0.00
Yield per pound of raw ready-to-cook turkey: approx. 11.8 oz. cooked	322	0.0	27.2	0.00
Weighing edible portion only:				
1 pound of cooked meat without skin (19g/0g/1g/68%/19mg)	680	0.0	42.5	0.00
1 cup, chopped or diced (approx. 4.9 oz.)	210	0.0	42.5	0.00
TOP QUARTER (Breast and Wing—Light Meat):				
RAW				
With skin:				
Weighed with skin and bones [refuse: bones, approx. 19%]:				
1 top quarter from a 6-lb. 7-oz. ready-to-cook turkey: approx. 1 lb. 5 oz.	746	0.0	30.5	0.00
1 pound of raw top quarter	488	0.0	30.5	0.00
Weighing edible portion only:				
1 pound of raw meat with skin	603	0.0	37.7	0.00
Without skin:				
Weighed with skin and bones [refuse: bones, approx. 19%; skin, approx. 12%]:				
1 top quarter from a 6-lb. 7-oz. ready-to-cook turkey: approx. 1 lb. 5 oz.	518	0.0	21.1	0.00
1 pound of raw top quarter	337	0.0	21.1	0.00

	UNIT Cal.	UNIT Carb.	1 OZ., BY WT. Cal.	1 OZ., BY WT. Carb.
Weighing edible portion only:				
1 pound of raw meat without skin (7g/0g/tr/75%/15mg)	490	0.0	30.6	0.00
ROASTED				
Eaten with skin:				
Weighed with skin and bones [refuse: bones, approx. 19%]:				
1 top quarter from a 6-lb. 7-oz. ready-to-cook turkey: approx. 1 lb. 3 oz. cooked	711	0.0	37.7	0.00
1 pound of cooked top quarter	603	0.0	37.7	0.00
Yield per pound of raw ready-to-cook turkey: approx. 3 oz. cooked	110	0.0	37.7	0.00
Weighing edible portion only:				
1 pound of cooked meat with skin	744	0.0	46.5	0.00
Roasted with skin, but skin removed before eating:				
Weighed with skin and bones [refuse: bones, approx. 19%; skin, approx. 12%]:				
1 top quarter from a 6-lb. 7-oz. ready-to-cook turkey: approx. 1 lb. 3 oz. cooked	516	0.0	27.3	0.00
1 pound of cooked top quarter	437	0.0	27.3	0.00
Yield per pound of raw ready-to-cook turkey: approx. 3 oz. cooked	80	0.0	27.3	0.00
Weighing edible portion only:				
1 pound of cooked meat without skin (9g/0g/tr/69%/16mg)	635	0.0	39.7	0.00
1 cup, chopped or diced (approx. 4.9 oz.)	195	0.0	39.7	0.00
BOTTOM QUARTER (Drumstick, Thigh, and Back—Dark Meat):				
RAW				
With skin:				
Weighed with skin and bones [refuse: bones, approx. 30%]:				
1 bottom quarter from a 6-lb. 7-oz. ready-to-cook turkey: approx. 1 lb. 11 oz.	685	0.0	25.6	0.00
1 pound of raw bottom quarter	409	0.0	25.6	0.00
Weighing edible portion only:				
1 pound of raw meat with skin	585	0.0	36.6	0.00
Without skin:				
Weighed with skin and bones [refuse: bones, approx. 30%; skin, approx. 7%]:				
1 bottom quarter from a 6-lb. 7-oz. ready-to-cook turkey: approx. 1 lb. 11 oz.	534	0.0	19.9	0.00
1 pound of raw bottom quarter	318	0.0	19.9	0.00
Weighing edible portion only:				
1 pound of raw meat without skin (6g/0g/tr/76%/20mg)	503	0.0	31.5	0.00
BOTTOM QUARTER (Drumstick, Thigh, and Back—Dark Meat):				
ROASTED				
Eaten with skin:				
Weighed with skin and bones [refuse: bones, approx. 31%]:				
1 bottom quarter from a 6-lb. 7-oz. ready-to-cook turkey: approx. 1 lb. 3 oz. cooked	680	0.0	35.6	0.00
1 pound of cooked bottom quarter	569	0.0	35.6	0.00
Yield per pound of raw ready-to-cook turkey: approx. 3 oz. cooked	106	0.0	35.6	0.00
Weighing edible portion only:				
1 pound of cooked meat with skin (6g/0g/1g/75%/19mg)	826	0.0	51.6	0.00
Roasted with skin, but skin removed before eating:				
Weighed with skin and bones [refuse: bones, approx. 31%; skin, approx. 10%]:				
1 bottom quarter from a 6-lb. 7-oz. ready-to-cook turkey: approx. 1 lb. 3 oz. cooked	520	0.0	27.1	0.00
1 pound of cooked bottom quarter	434	0.0	27.1	0.00
Yield per pound of raw ready-to-cook turkey: approx. 3 oz. cooked	81	0.0	27.1	0.00
Weighing edible portion only:				
1 pound of cooked meat without skin (8g/0g/1g/66%/23mg)	735	0.0	45.9	0.00
1 cup, chopped or diced (approx. 4.9 oz.)	227	0.0	45.9	0.00
TURKEY PARTS:				
BACK:				
RAW				
Eaten with skin:				
Weighed with skin and bones [refuse: bones, approx. 41%]:				
½ back from a 6-lb. 7-oz. ready-to-cook turkey: approx. 10.9 oz.	275	0.0	25.2	0.00
1 pound of raw backs	403	0.0	25.2	0.00
Weighing edible portion only:				
1 pound of raw meat with skin (6g/0g/2g/72%/17mg)	685	0.0	42.8	0.00
Without skin:				
Weighed with skin and bones [refuse: bones, approx. 41%; skin, approx. 10%]:				
½ back from a 6-lb. 7-oz. ready-to-cook turkey: approx. 10.9 oz.	180	0.0	16.6	0.00
1 pound of raw backs	266	0.0	16.6	0.00

	UNIT Cal.	UNIT Carb.	1 OZ., BY WT. Cal.	1 OZ., BY WT. Carb.
Weighing edible portion only:				
1 pound of raw meat without skin (6g/0g/1g/75%/18mg)	544	0.0	34.0	0.00
ROASTED				
Eaten with skin:				
Weighed with skin and bones [refuse: bones, approx. 41%]:				
½ back from a 6-lb. 7-oz. ready-to-cook turkey: approx. 7.8 oz. cooked	265	0.0	34.1	0.00
1 pound of cooked backs	546	0.0	34.1	0.00
Yield per pound of raw ready-to-cook turkey: approx. 1.2 oz. cooked	41	0.0	34.1	0.00
Weighing edible portion only:				
1 pound of cooked meat with skin (7g/0g/3g/63%/20mg)	925	0.0	57.8	0.00
Roasted with skin, but skin removed before eating:				
Weighed with skin and bones [refuse: bones, approx. 41%; skin, approx. 15%]:				
½ back from a 6-lb. 7-oz. ready-to-cook turkey: approx. 7.8 oz. cooked	164	0.0	21.3	0.00
1 pound of cooked backs	340	0.0	21.3	0.00
Yield per pound of raw ready-to-cook turkey: approx. 1.2 oz. cooked	25	0.0	21.3	0.00
Weighing edible portion only:				
1 pound of cooked meat without skin (8g/0g/2g/66%/21mg)	771	0.0	48.2	0.00
BREAST:				
RAW				
Eaten with skin:				
Weighed with skin and bones [refuse: bones, approx. 12%]:				
½ breast from a 6-lb. 7-oz. ready-to-cook turkey: approx. 1 lb. 1 oz.	543	0.0	31.3	0.00
1 pound of raw breast	500	0.0	31.3	0.00
Weighing edible portion only:				
1 pound of raw meat with skin (7g/0g/1g/73%/14mg)	567	0.0	35.4	0.00
Without skin:				
Weighed with skin and bones [refuse: bones, approx. 12%; skin, approx. 9%]:				
½ breast from a 6-lb. 7-oz. ready-to-cook turkey: approx. 1 lb. 1 oz.	433	0.0	24.8	0.00
1 pound of raw breast	397	0.0	24.8	0.00
Weighing edible portion only:				
1 pound of raw meat without skin (7g/tr/tr/74%/14mg)	504	0.0	31.5	0.00
ROASTED				
Eaten with skin:				
Weighed with skin and bones [refuse: bones, approx. 11%]:				
½ breast from a 6-lb. 7-oz. ready-to-cook turkey: approx. 13.7 oz. cooked	526	0.0	38.6	0.00
1 pound of cooked breast	618	0.0	38.6	0.00
Yield per pound of raw ready-to-cook turkey: approx. 2.1 oz. cooked	82	0.0	38.6	0.00
Weighing edible portion only:				
1 pound of cooked meat with skin (8g/tr/1g/68%/15mg)	694	0.0	43.4	0.00
Roasted with skin, but skin removed before eating:				
Weighed with skin and bones [refuse: bones, approx. 11%; skin, approx. 10%]:				
½ breast from a 6-lb. 7-oz. ready-to-cook turkey: approx. 1 lb. 1 oz. cooked	413	0.0	30.3	0.00
1 pound of cooked breast	484	0.0	30.3	0.00
Yield per pound of raw ready-to-cook turkey: approx. 2.1 oz. cooked	64	0.0	30.3	0.00
Weighing edible portion only:				
1 pound of cooked meat without skin (9g/tr/tr/68%/15mg)	612	0.0	38.3	0.00
LEG (Drumstick and Thigh—Dark Meat):				
RAW				
With skin:				
Weighed with skin and bones [refuse: bones, approx. 23%]:				
1 leg from a 6-lb. 7-oz. ready-to-cook turkey: approx. 1 lb.	412	0.0	25.8	0.00
1 pound of raw leg	413	0.0	25.8	0.00
Weighing edible portion only:				
1 pound of raw meat with skin (6g/0g/1g/76%/20mg)	535	0.0	33.5	0.00
Without skin:				
Weighed with skin and bones [refuse: bones, approx. 23%; skin, approx. 5%]:				
1 leg from a 6-lb. 7-oz. ready-to-cook turkey: approx. 1 lb.	356	0.0	22.1	0.00
1 pound of raw leg	354	0.0	22.1	0.00
Weighing edible portion only:				
1 pound of raw meat without skin (6g/0g/1g/77%/20mg)	490	0.0	30.6	0.00

	UNIT Cal.	UNIT Carb.	1 OZ., BY WT. Cal.	1 OZ., BY WT. Carb.
ROASTED				
Eaten with skin:				
Weighed with skin and bones [refuse: bones, approx. 25%]:				
1 leg from a 6-lb. 7-oz. ready-to-cook turkey: approx. 11.4 oz. cooked	418	0.0	36.3	0.00
1 pound of cooked legs	580	0.0	36.3	0.00
Yield per pound of raw ready-to-cook turkey: approx. 1.8 oz. cooked	65	0.0	36.3	0.00
Weighing edible portion only:				
1 pound of cooked meat with skin (8g/0g/2g/66%/23mg)	771	0.0	48.2	0.00
Roasted with skin, but skin removed before eating:				
Weighed with skin and bones [refuse: bones, approx. 25%; skin, approx. 6%]:				
1 leg from a 6-lb. 7-oz. ready-to-cook turkey: approx. 11.4 oz. cooked	355	0.0	31.1	0.00
1 pound of cooked legs	497	0.0	31.1	0.00
Yield per pound of raw ready-to-cook turkey: approx. 1.8 oz. cooked	55	0.0	31.1	0.00
Weighing edible portion only:				
1 pound of cooked meat without skin (8g/0g/1g/67%/23mg)	721	0.0	45.1	0.00
WING:				
RAW				
With skin:				
Weighed with skin and bones [refuse: bones, approx. 37%]:				
1 wing from a 6-lb. 7-oz. ready-to-cook turkey: approx. 7.2 oz.	203	0.0	28.3	0.00
1 pound of raw wings	453	0.0	28.3	0.00
Weighing edible portion only:				
1 pound of raw meat with skin (6g/2g/tr/71%/16mg)	721	0.0	45.1	0.00
Without skin:				
Weighed with skin and bones [refuse: bones, approx. 37%; skin, approx. 19%]:				
1 wing from a 6-lb. 7-oz. ready-to-cook turkey: approx. 7.2 oz.	96	0.0	13.3	0.00
1 pound of raw wings	212	0.0	13.3	0.00
Weighing edible portion only:				
1 pound of raw meat without skin (6g/tr/tr/76%/19mg)	481	0.0	30.1	0.00
ROASTED				
Eaten with skin:				
Weighed with skin and bones [refuse: bones, approx. 39%]:				
1 wing from a 6-lb. 7-oz. ready-to-cook turkey: approx. 5.2 oz. cooked	186	0.0	35.8	0.00
1 pound of cooked wings	573	0.0	35.8	0.00
Yield per pound of raw ready-to-cook turkey: approx. 0.8 oz. cooked	29	0.0	35.8	0.00
Weighing edible portion only:				
1 pound of cooked meat with skin (8g/0g/3g/62%/21mg)	939	0.0	58.7	0.00
Roasted with skin, but skin removed before eating:				
Weighed with skin and bones [refuse: bones, approx. 39%; skin, approx. 20%]:				
1 wing from a 6-lb. 7-oz. ready-to-cook turkey: approx. 5.2 oz. cooked	98	0.0	18.9	0.00
1 pound of cooked wings	303	0.0	18.9	0.00
Yield per pound of raw ready-to-cook turkey: approx. 0.8 oz. cooked	15	0.0	18.9	0.00
Weighing edible portion only:				
1 pound of cooked meat without skin (9g/0g/1g/66%/23mg)	739	0.0	46.2	0.00
SKIN:				
RAW				
Skin from a 7-lb. turkey: approx. 9.4 oz. (4g/0g/7g/60%/10mg)	754	0.0	80.2	0.00
1 pound of skin	1284	0.0	80.2	0.00
ROASTED				
Skin from a 7-lb. turkey: approx. 8.5 oz. cooked (6g/0g/7g/55%/17mg)	724	0.0	84.8	0.00
1 pound of skin	1356	0.0	84.8	0.00
Young Hen Turkeys				
ENTIRE TURKEY (with neck and giblets):				
RAW				
With skin:				
Weighed with skin and bones [refuse: bones, approx. 22%]:				
1 12-lb. 9-oz. ready-to-cook turkey	7384	4.7	36.6	0.02
1 pound of raw bird, average all parts	586	0.4	36.6	0.02
Weighing edible portion only:				
1 pound of raw meat with skin (6g/0g/2g/70%/18mg)	754	0.5	47.1	0.03

	UNIT Cal.	UNIT Carb.	1 OZ., BY WT. Cal.	1 OZ., BY WT. Carb.
Without skin:				
Weighed with skin and bones [refuse: bones, approx. 22%; skin, approx. 11%]:				
1 12-lb. 9-oz. ready-to-cook turkey	(4709)	(4.7)	(23.4)	(0.02)
1 pound of raw bird, average all parts	(375)	(0.4)	(23.4)	(0.02)
Weighing edible portion only:				
1 pound of raw meat without skin	(568)	(0.5)	(35.5)	(0.03)
ENTIRE TURKEY (with neck and giblets):				
ROASTED				
Eaten with skin:				
Weighed with skin and bones [refuse: bones, approx. 20%]:				
1 12-lb. 9-oz. ready-to-cook turkey: approx. 9 lb. 2 oz. cooked	7094	2.2	48.8	0.02
1 pound of cooked bird, average all parts	780	0.2	48.8	0.02
Yield per pound of raw ready-to-cook turkey: approx. 11.6 oz. cooked	565	0.2	48.8	0.02
Weighing edible portion only:				
1 pound of cooked meat with skin (8g/0g/3g/61%/18mg)	975	0.3	61.0	0.02
Roasted with skin, but skin removed before eating:				
Weighed with skin and bones [refuse: bones, approx. 20%; skin, approx. 9%]:				
1 12-lb. 9-oz. ready-to-cook turkey: approx. 9 lb. 2 oz. cooked	(5204)	(2.2)	(35.6)	(0.02)
1 pound of cooked bird, average all parts	(570)	(0.2)	(35.6)	(0.02)
Yield per pound of raw ready-to-cook turkey: approx. 11.6 oz. cooked	(414)	(0.2)	(35.6)	(0.02)
Weighing edible portion only:				
1 pound of cooked meat without skin	(803)	(0.3)	(50.2)	(0.02)
ENTIRE TURKEY (without neck and giblets):				
RAW				
Eaten with skin:				
Weighed with skin and bones [refuse: bones, approx. 22%]:				
1 11-lb. 9-oz. ready-to-cook turkey	6902	0.0	37.2	0.00
1 pound of raw bird, average all parts	595	0.0	37.2	0.00
Weighing edible portion only:				
1 pound of raw meat with skin (6g/0g/3g/70%/17mg)	762	0.0	47.6	0.00
Without skin:				
Weighed with skin and bones [refuse: bones, approx. 22%; skin, approx. 12%]:				
1 11-lb. 9-oz. ready-to-cook turkey	4210	0.0	22.8	0.00
1 pound of raw bird, average all parts	364	0.0	22.8	0.00
Weighing edible portion only:				
1 pound of raw meat without skin	553	0.0	34.6	0.00
ENTIRE TURKEY (without neck and giblets):				
ROASTED				
Eaten with skin:				
Weighed with skin and bones [refuse: bones, approx. 20%]:				
1 11-lb. 9-oz. ready-to-cook turkey: approx. 8 lb. 7 oz. cooked	6646	0.0	49.4	0.00
1 pound of cooked bird, average all parts	791	0.0	49.4	0.00
Yield per pound of raw ready-to-cook turkey: approx. 11.7 oz. cooked	575	0.0	49.4	0.00
Weighing edible portion only:				
1 pound of cooked meat with skin (8g/0g/3g/61%/18mg)	989	0.0	61.9	0.00
Roasted with skin, but skin removed before eating:				
Weighed with skin and bones [refuse: bones, approx. 20%; skin, approx. 10%]:				
1 11-lb. 9-oz. ready-to-cook turkey: approx. 8 lb. 7 oz. cooked	4661	0.0	34.6	0.00
1 pound of cooked bird, average all parts	554	0.0	34.6	0.00
Yield per pound of raw ready-to-cook turkey: approx. 11.7 oz. cooked	403	0.0	34.6	0.00
Weighing edible portion only:				
1 pound of cooked meat without skin	794	0.0	49.6	0.00
1 cup, chopped or diced (approx. 4.9 oz.)	244	0.0	49.6	0.00
TOP QUARTER (Breast and Wing—Light Meat):				
RAW				
With skin:				
Weighed with skin and bones [refuse: bones, approx. 16%]:				
1 top quarter from an 11-lb. 9-oz. ready-to-cook turkey: approx. 2 lb. 14 oz.	1812	0.0	39.3	0.00
1 pound of raw top quarter	628	0.0	39.3	0.00
Weighing edible portion only:				
1 pound of raw meat with skin	749	0.0	46.8	0.00
Without skin:				
Weighed with skin and bones [refuse: bones, approx. 16%; skin, approx. 14%]:				
1 top quarter from an 11-lb. 9-oz. ready-to-cook turkey: approx. 2 lb. 14 oz.	1066	0.0	23.0	0.00
1 pound of raw top quarter	368	0.0	23.0	0.00

	UNIT Cal.	UNIT Carb.	1 OZ., BY WT. Cal.	1 OZ., BY WT. Carb.
Weighing edible portion only:				
1 pound of raw meat without skin (7g/tr/tr/74%/17mg)	526	0.0	32.9	0.00
ROASTED				
Eaten with skin:				
Weighed with skin and bones [refuse: bones, approx. 14%]:				
1 top quarter from an 11-lb. 9-oz. ready-to-cook turkey: approx. 2 lb. 3 oz. cooked	1778	0.0	50.5	0.00
1 pound of cooked top quarter	808	0.0	50.5	0.00
Yield per pound of raw ready-to-cook turkey: approx. 3 oz. cooked	154	0.0	50.5	0.00
Weighing edible portion only:				
1 pound of cooked meat with skin (8g/0g/3g/62%/17mg)	939	0.0	58.7	0.00
Roasted with skin, but skin removed before eating:				
Weighed with skin and bones [refuse: bones, approx. 14%; skin, approx. 11%]:				
1 top quarter from an 11-lb. 9-oz. ready-to-cook turkey: approx. 2 lb. 3 oz. cooked	1209	0.0	34.3	0.00
1 pound of cooked top quarter	549	0.0	34.3	0.00
Yield per pound of raw ready-to-cook turkey: approx. 3 oz. cooked	105	0.0	34.3	0.00
Weighing edible portion only:				
1 pound of cooked meat without skin (9g/0g/1g/66%/17mg)	730	0.0	45.6	0.00
1 cup, chopped or diced (approx. 4.9 oz.)	226	0.0	45.6	0.00
BOTTOM QUARTER (Drumstick, Thigh, and Back—Dark Meat):				
RAW				
With skin:				
Weighed with skin and bones [refuse: bones, approx. 21%]:				
1 bottom quarter from an 11-lb. 9-oz. ready-to-cook turkey: approx. 2 lb. 14 oz.	1640	0.0	35.6	0.00
1 pound of raw bottom quarter	570	0.0	35.6	0.00
Weighing edible portion only:				
1 pound of raw meat with skin (5g/0g/3g/70%/19mg)	780	0.0	48.8	0.00
Without skin:				
Weighed with skin and bones [refuse: bones, approx. 21%; skin, approx. 11%]:				
1 bottom quarter from an 11-lb. 9-oz. ready-to-cook turkey: approx. 2 lb. 14 oz.	1053	0.0	22.8	0.00
1 pound of raw bottom quarter	365	0.0	22.8	0.00
Weighing edible portion only:				
1 pound of raw meat without skin (6g/0g/1g/74%/21mg)	590	0.0	36.9	0.00
ROASTED				
Eaten with skin:				
Weighed with skin and bones [refuse: bones, approx. 27%]:				
1 bottom quarter from an 11-lb. 9-oz. ready-to-cook turkey: approx. 2 lb. cooked	1544	0.0	48.1	0.00
1 pound of cooked bottom quarter	769	0.0	48.1	0.00
Yield per pound of raw ready-to-cook turkey: approx. 2.8 oz. cooked	134	0.0	48.1	0.00
Weighing edible portion only:				
1 pound of cooked meat with skin (8g/0g/4g/60%/21mg)	1052	0.0	65.8	0.00
Roasted with skin, but skin removed before eating:				
Weighed with skin and bones [refuse: bones, approx. 27%; skin, approx. 9%]:				
1 bottom quarter from an 11-lb. 9-oz. ready-to-cook turkey: approx. 2 lb. cooked	1114	0.0	34.8	0.00
1 pound of cooked bottom quarter	556	0.0	34.8	0.00
Yield per pound of raw ready-to-cook turkey: approx. 2.8 oz. cooked	96	0.0	34.8	0.00
Weighing edible portion only:				
1 pound of cooked meat without skin (8g/0g/2g/63%/22mg)	871	0.0	54.4	0.00
1 cup, chopped or diced (approx. 4.9 oz.)	268	0.0	54.4	0.00
TURKEY PARTS:				
BACK:				
RAW				
With skin:				
Weighed with skin and bones [refuse: bones, approx. 43%]:				
½ back from an 11-lb. 9-oz. ready-to-cook turkey: approx. 1 lb. 2 oz.	651	0.0	35.3	0.00
1 pound of raw back	565	0.0	35.3	0.00
Weighing edible portion only:				
1 pound of raw meat with skin (5g/0g/5g/66%/17mg)	989	0.0	61.8	0.00
ROASTED				
Eaten with skin:				
Weighed with skin and bones [refuse: bones, approx. 41%]:				
½ back from an 11-lb. 9-oz. ready-to-cook turkey: approx. 13.0 oz. cooked	551	0.0	42.4	0.00

	UNIT Cal.	UNIT Carb.	1 OZ., BY WT. Cal.	1 OZ., BY WT. Carb.
1 pound of cooked backs	679	0.0	42.4	0.00
Yield per pound of raw ready-to-cook turkey: approx. 1.1 oz. cooked	48	0.0	42.4	0.00
Weighing edible portion only:				
1 pound of cooked meat with skin (7g/0g/4g/57%/20mg)	1152	0.0	72.0	0.00
Roasted with skin, but skin removed before eating:				
Weighed with skin and bones [refuse: bones, approx. 41%; skin, approx. 13%]:				
½ back from an 11-lb. 9-oz. ready-to-cook turkey: approx. 13.0 oz. cooked	(320)	0.0	(24.6)	0.00
1 pound of cooked backs	(393)	0.0	(24.6)	0.00
Yield per pound of raw ready-to-cook turkey: approx. 1.1 oz. cooked	(28)	0.0	(24.6)	0.00
Weighing edible portion only:				
1 pound of cooked meat without skin	(853)	0.0	(53.3)	0.00
BREAST:				
RAW				
With Skin:				
Weighed with skin and bones [refuse: bones, approx. 11%]:				
½ breast from an 11-lb. 9-oz. ready-to-cook turkey: approx. 2 lb. 3 oz.	1462	0.0	42.2	0.00
1 pound of raw breast	675	0.0	42.2	0.00
Weighing edible portion only:				
1 pound of raw meat with skin (6g/0g/2g/69%/16mg)	758	0.0	47.3	0.00
ROASTED				
Eaten with skin:				
Weighed with skin and bones [refuse: bones, approx. 8%]:				
½ breast from an 11-lb. 9-oz. ready-to-cook turkey: approx. 1 lb. 10 oz. cooked	1330	0.0	50.6	0.00
1 pound of cooked breast	809	0.0	50.6	0.00
Yield per pound of raw ready-to-cook turkey: approx. 2.2 oz. cooked	115	0.0	50.6	0.00
Weighing edible portion only:				
1 pound of cooked meat with skin (8g/0g/2g/63%/16mg)	880	0.0	55.0	0.00
Roasted with skin, but skin removed before eating:				
Weighed with skin and bones [refuse: bone, approx. 8%; skin, approx. 9%]:				
½ breast from an 11-lb. 9-oz. ready-to-cook turkey: approx. 1 lb. 10 oz. cooked	(1007)	0.0	(38.2)	0.00
1 pound of cooked breast	(611)	0.0	(38.2)	0.00
Yield per pound of raw ready-to-cook turkey: approx. 2.2 oz. cooked	(87)	0.0	(38.2)	0.00
Weighing edible portion only:				
1 pound of cooked meat without skin	(736)	0.0	(46.0)	0.00
LEG (Drumstick and Thigh):				
RAW				
With skin:				
Weighed with skin and bones [refuse: bones, approx. 17%]:				
1 leg from 11-lb. 9-oz. ready-to-cook turkey: approx. 1 lb. 12 oz. cooked	989	0.0	35.4	0.00
1 pound of raw leg	567	0.0	35.4	0.00
Weighing edible portion only:				
1 pound of raw meat with skin (6g/0g/2g/72%/20mg)	685	0.0	42.8	0.00
ROASTED				
Eaten with skin:				
Weighed with skin and bones [refuse: bones, approx. 17%]:				
1 leg from an 11-lb. 9-oz. ready-to-cook turkey: approx. 1 lb. 3 oz. cooked	955	0.0	50.1	0.00
1 pound of cooked leg	802	0.0	50.1	0.00
Yield per pound of raw ready-to-cook turkey: approx. 1.6 oz. cooked	83	0.0	50.1	0.00
Weighing edible portion only:				
1 pound of cooked meat with skin (8g/0g/3g/61%/21mg)	966	0.0	60.4	0.00
Roasted with skin, but skin removed before eating:				
Weighed with skin and bones [refuse: bones, approx. 17%; skin, approx. 6%]:				
1 leg from an 11-lb. 9-oz. ready-to-cook turkey: approx. 1 lb. 3 oz. cooked	(820)	0.0	(43.0)	0.00
1 pound of cooked leg	(689)	0.0	(43.0)	0.00
Yield per pound of raw ready-to-cook turkey: approx. 1.6 oz. cooked	(71)	0.0	(43.0)	0.00
Weighing edible portion only:				
1 pound of cooked meat without skin	(895)	0.0	(55.9)	0.00
WING:				
RAW				
With skin:				
Weighed with skin and bones [refuse: bones, approx. 31%]:				
1 wing from an 11-lb. 9-oz. ready-to-cook turkey: approx. 11.5 oz.	471	0.0	41.1	0.00
1 pound of raw wings	658	0.0	41.1	0.00

	UNIT Cal.	UNIT Carb.	1 OZ., BY WT. Cal.	1 OZ., BY WT. Carb.
Weighing edible portion only:				
1 pound of raw meat with skin (6g/0g/4g/65%/15mg)	953	0.0	59.5	0.00
ROASTED				
Eaten with skin:				
Weighed with skin and bones [refuse: bones, approx. 31%]:				
1 wing from an 11-lb. 9-oz. ready-to-cook turkey: approx. 8.9 oz. cooked	414	0.0	46.6	0.00
1 pound of cooked wings	745	0.0	46.6	0.00
Yield per pound of raw ready-to-cook turkey: approx. 0.8 oz. cooked	36	0.0	46.6	0.00
Weighing edible portion only:				
1 pound of cooked meat with skin (8g/0g/4g/59%/16mg)	1080	0.0	67.5	0.00
Roasted with skin, but skin removed before eating:				
Weighed with skin and bones [refuse: bones, approx. 31%; skin, approx. 17%]:				
1 wing from an 11-lb. 9-oz. ready-to-cook turkey: approx. 8.9 oz. cooked	(207)	0.0	(23.2)	0.00
1 pound of cooked wings	(371)	0.0	(23.2)	0.00
Yield per pound of raw ready-to-cook turkey: approx. 0.8 oz. cooked	(18)	0.0	(23.2)	0.00
Weighing edible portion only:				
1 pound of cooked meat without skin	(716)	0.0	(44.7)	0.00
SKIN:				
RAW				
Skin from a 12-lb. 9-oz. turkey: approx. 1 lb. 7 oz. (3g/0g/12g/47%/9mg)	2676	0.0	118.2	0.00
1 pound of raw skin	1892	0.0	118.2	0.00
ROASTED				
Skin from a 12-lb. 9-oz. turkey: approx. 14 oz. cooked (5g/0g/13g/36%/13mg)	1890	0.0	136.7	0.00
1 pound of roasted skin	2187	0.0	136.7	0.00

Young Tom Turkeys

	UNIT Cal.	UNIT Carb.	1 OZ., BY WT. Cal.	1 OZ., BY WT. Carb.
ENTIRE TURKEY (with neck and giblets):				
RAW				
With skin:				
Weighed with skin and bones [refuse: bones, approx. 20%]:				
1 23-lb. 1-oz. ready-to-cook turkey	12,799	7.1	34.6	0.02
1 pound of raw bird, average all parts	553	0.3	34.6	0.02
Weighing edible portion only:				
1 pound of raw meat with skin (6g/tr/2g/71%/20mg)	690	0.4	43.1	0.02
Without skin:				
Weighed with skin and bones [refuse: bones, approx. 20%; skin, approx. 13%]:				
1 23-lb. 1-oz. ready-to-cook turkey	(8439)	(7.1)	(22.9)	(0.02)
1 pound of raw bird, average all parts	(366)	(0.3)	(22.9)	(0.02)
Weighing edible portion only:				
1 pound of raw meat without skin	(413)	(0.4)	(25.8)	(0.02)
ROASTED				
Eaten with skin:				
Weighed with skin and bones [refuse: bones, approx. 21%]:				
1 23-lb. 1-oz. ready-to-cook turkey: approx. 16 lb. 9 oz. cooked	11,873	6.0	44.6	0.02
1 pound of cooked bird, average all parts	714	0.4	44.6	0.02
Yield per pound of raw ready-to-cook turkey: approx. 11.5 oz. cooked	516	0.3	44.6	0.02
Weighing edible portion only:				
1 pound of cooked meat with skin (8g/tr/2g/62%/21mg)	903	0.5	56.4	0.03
Roasted with skin, but skin removed before eating:				
Weighed with skin and bones [refuse: bones, approx. 21%; skin, approx. 10%]:				
1 23-lb. 1-oz. ready-to-cook turkey: approx. 16 lb. 9 oz. cooked	(8717)	(6.0)	(32.8)	(0.02)
1 pound of cooked bird, average all parts	(525)	(0.4)	(32.8)	(0.02)
Yield per pound of raw ready-to-cook turkey: approx. 11.5 oz. cooked	(378)	(0.3)	(32.8)	(0.02)
Weighing edible portion only:				
1 pound of cooked meat without skin	(583)	(0.4)	(36.5)	(0.03)
ENTIRE TURKEY (without neck and giblets):				
RAW				
With skin:				
Weighed with skin and bones [refuse: bones, approx. 19%]:				
1 21-lb. 4-oz. ready-to-cook turkey	12,026	0.0	35.4	0.00
1 pound of raw bird, average all parts	567	0.0	35.4	0.00
Weighing edible portion only:				
1 pound of raw meat with skin (6g/0g/2g/71%/18mg)	699	0.0	43.7	0.00
Without skin:				
Weighed with skin and bones [refuse: bones, approx. 19%; skin, approx. 12%]:				
1 21-lb. 4-oz. ready-to-cook turkey	7734	0.0	22.9	0.00

	UNIT Cal.	UNIT Carb.	1 OZ., BY WT. Cal.	1 OZ., BY WT. Carb.
1 pound of raw bird, average all parts	367	0.0	22.9	0.00
Weighing edible portion only:				
1 pound of raw meat without skin (6g/0g/1g/74%/21mg)	531	0.0	33.2	0.00
ROASTED				
Eaten with skin:				
Weighed with skin and bones [refuse: bones, approx. 20%]:				
1 21-lb. 4-oz. ready-to-cook turkey: approx. 15 lb. 4 oz. cooked	11,090	0.0	45.8	0.00
1 pound of cooked bird, average all parts	732	0.0	45.8	0.00
Yield per pound of raw ready-to-cook turkey: approx. 11.5 oz. cooked	522	0.0	45.8	0.00
Weighing edible portion only:				
1 pound of cooked meat with skin (8g/0g/3g/62%/21mg)	916	0.0	57.3	0.00
Roasted with skin, but skin removed before eating:				
Weighed with skin and bones [refuse: bones, approx. 20%; skin, approx. 11%]:				
1 21-lb. 4-oz. ready-to-cook turkey: approx. 15 lb. 4 oz. cooked	8000	0.0	32.8	0.00
1 pound of cooked bird, average all parts	525	0.0	32.8	0.00
Yield per pound of raw ready-to-cook turkey: approx. 11.5 oz. cooked	376	0.0	32.8	0.00
Weighing edible portion only:				
1 pound of cooked meat without skin	762	0.0	47.6	0.00
1 cup, chopped or diced (approx. 4.9 oz.)	235	0.0	47.6	0.00
TOP QUARTER (Breast and Wing—Light Meat):				
RAW				
With skin:				
Weighed with skin and bones [refuse: bones, approx. 14%]:				
1 top quarter from a 21-lb. 4-oz. ready-to-cook turkey: approx. 5 lb. 8 oz.	3331	0.0	38.0	0.00
1 pound of raw top quarter	608	0.0	38.0	0.00
Weighing edible portion only:				
1 pound of raw meat with skin	708	0.0	44.2	0.00
Without skin:				
Weighed with skin and bones [refuse: bones, approx. 14%; skin, approx. 15%]:				
1 top quarter from a 21-lb. 4-oz. ready-to-cook turkey: approx. 5 lb. 8 oz.	2023	0.0	23.0	0.00
1 pound of raw top quarter	368	0.0	23.0	0.00
Weighing edible portion only:				
1 pound of raw meat without skin (7g/tr/tr/74%/19mg)	517	0.0	32.3	0.00
ROASTED				
Eaten with skin:				
Weighed with skin and bones [refuse: bones, approx. 14%]:				
1 top quarter from a 21-lb. 4-oz. ready-to-cook turkey: approx. 4 lb. cooked	2992	0.0	46.6	0.00
1 pound of cooked top quarter	745	0.0	46.6	0.00
Yield per pound of raw ready-to-cook turkey: approx. 3 oz. cooked	141	0.0	46.6	0.00
Weighing edible portion only:				
1 pound of cooked meat with skin	866	0.0	54.2	0.00
Roasted with skin, but skin removed before eating:				
Weighed with skin and bones [refuse: bones, approx. 14%; skin, approx. 12%]:				
1 top quarter from a 21-lb. 4-oz. ready-to-cook turkey: approx. 4 lb. cooked	2081	0.0	32.3	0.00
1 pound of cooked top quarter	517	0.0	32.3	0.00
Yield per pound of raw ready-to-cook turkey: approx. 3 oz. cooked	98	0.0	32.3	0.00
Weighing edible portion only:				
1 pound of cooked meat without skin (9g/0g/1g/67%/19mg)	699	0.0	43.7	0.00
1 cup, chopped or diced (approx. 4.9 oz.)	215	0.0	43.7	0.00
BOTTOM QUARTER (Drumstick, Thigh, and Back—Dark Meat):				
RAW				
With skin:				
Weighed with skin and bones [refuse: bones, approx. 24%]:				
1 bottom quarter from a 21-lb. 4-oz. ready-to-cook turkey: approx. 5 lb. 2 oz.	2681	0.0	32.9	0.00
1 pound of raw bottom quarter	526	0.0	32.9	0.00
Weighing edible portion only:				
1 pound of raw meat with skin (5g/0g/2g/72%/22mg)	690	0.0	43.1	0.00
Without skin:				
Weighed with skin and bones [refuse: bones, approx. 24%; skin, approx. 10%]:				
1 bottom quarter from a 21-lb. 4-oz. ready-to-cook turkey: approx. 5 lb. 2 oz.	1879	0.0	22.9	0.00
1 pound of raw bottom quarter	367	0.0	22.9	0.00
Weighing edible portion only:				
1 pound of raw meat without skin (6g/0g/1g/75%/23mg)	558	0.0	34.9	0.00

	UNIT Cal.	UNIT Carb.	1 OZ., BY WT. Cal.	1 OZ., BY WT. Carb.
ROASTED				
Eaten with skin:				
Weighed with skin and bones [refuse: bones, approx. 27%]:				
1 bottom quarter from a 21-lb. 4-oz. ready-to-cook turkey: approx. 3 lb. 9 oz. cooked	2553	0.0	44.6	0.00
1 pound of cooked bottom quarter	714	0.0	44.6	0.00
Yield per pound of raw ready-to-cook turkey: approx. 2.7 oz. cooked	120	0.0	44.6	0.00
Weighing edible portion only:				
1 pound of cooked meat with skin (8g/0g/3g/60%/23mg)	980	0.0	61.2	0.00
Roasted with skin, but skin removed before eating:				
Weighed with skin and bones [refuse: bones, approx. 27%; skin, approx. 9%]:				
1 bottom quarter from a 21-lb. 4-oz. ready-to-cook turkey: approx. 3 lb. 9 oz. cooked	1993	0.0	33.6	0.00
1 pound of cooked bottom quarter	538	0.0	33.6	0.00
Yield per pound of raw ready-to-cook turkey: approx. 2.7 oz. cooked	94	0.0	33.6	0.00
Weighing edible portion only:				
1 pound of cooked meat without skin (8g/0g/2g/63%/24mg)	839	0.0	52.5	0.00
1 cup, chopped or diced (approx. 4.9 oz.)	260	0.0	52.5	0.00
TURKEY PARTS:				
BACK:				
RAW				
With skin:				
Weighed with skin and bones [refuse: bones, approx. 38%]:				
½ back from a 21-lb. 4-oz. ready-to-cook turkey: approx. 1 lb. 14 oz.	940	0.0	31.5	0.00
1 pound of raw back	504	0.0	31.5	0.00
Weighing edible portion only:				
1 pound of raw meat with skin (5g/0g/3g/69%/20mg)	812	0.0	50.8	0.00
ROASTED				
Eaten with skin:				
Weighed with skin and bones [refuse: bones, approx. 40%]:				
½ back from a 21-lb. 4-oz. ready-to-cook turkey: approx. 1 lb. 6 oz. cooked	903	0.0	40.4	0.00
1 pound of cooked back	647	0.0	40.4	0.00
Yield per pound of raw ready-to-cook turkey: approx. 1 oz. cooked	42	0.0	40.4	0.00
Weighing edible portion only:				
1 pound of cooked meat with skin (8g/0g/4g/58%/22mg)	1078	0.0	67.5	0.00
Roasted with skin, but skin removed before eating:				
Weighed with skin and bones [refuse: bones, approx. 40%; skin, approx. 13%]:				
½ back from a 21-lb. 4-oz. ready-to-cook turkey: approx. 1 lb. 6 oz. cooked	(506)	0.0	(22.7)	0.00
1 pound of cooked back	(363)	0.0	(22.7)	0.00
Yield per pound of raw ready-to-cook turkey: approx. 1 oz. cooked	(24)	0.0	(22.7)	0.00
Weighing edible portion only:				
1 pound of cooked meat without skin	(771)	0.0	(48.2)	0.00
BREAST:				
RAW				
With skin:				
Weighed with skin and bones [refuse: bones, approx. 9%]:				
½ breast from a 21-lb. 4-oz. ready-to-cook turkey: approx. 4 lb. 5 oz.	2700	0.0	38.9	0.00
1 pound of raw breast	623	0.0	38.9	0.00
Weighing edible portion only:				
1 pound of raw meat with skin (6g/0g/2g/71%/18mg)	685	0.0	42.8	0.00
ROASTED				
Eaten with skin:				
Weighed with skin and bones [refuse: bones, approx. 8%]:				
½ breast from a 21-lb. 4-oz. ready-to-cook turkey: approx. 3 lb. 3 oz. cooked	2510	0.0	49.3	0.00
1 pound of cooked breast	788	0.0	49.3	0.00
Yield per pound of raw ready-to-cook turkey: approx. 2.4 oz. cooked	118	0.0	49.3	0.00
Weighing edible portion only:				
1 pound of cooked meat with skin (8g/0g/2g/63%/19mg)	857	0.0	53.6	0.00
Roasted with skin, but skin removed before eating:				
Weighed with skin and bones [refuse: bones, approx. 8%; skin, approx. 12%]:				
½ breast from a 21-lb. 4-oz. ready-to-cook turkey: approx. 3 lb. 3 oz. cooked	(1951)	0.0	(38.2)	0.00
1 pound of cooked breast	(611)	0.0	(38.2)	0.00
Yield per pound of raw ready-to-cook turkey: approx. 2.4 oz. cooked	(92)	0.0	(38.2)	0.00
Weighing edible portion only:				
1 pound of cooked meat without skin	(764)	0.0	(47.7)	0.00

	UNIT Cal.	UNIT Carb.	1 OZ., BY WT. Cal.	1 OZ., BY WT. Carb.
LEG (Drumstick and Thigh):				
RAW				
With skin:				
Weighed with skin and bones [refuse: bones, approx. 17%]:				
1 leg from a 21-lb. 4-oz. ready-to-cook turkey: approx. 3 lb. 5 oz.	1736	0.0	33.1	0.00
1 pound of raw leg	530	0.0	33.1	0.00
Weighing edible portion only:				
1 pound of raw meat with skin	640	0.0	40.0	0.00
ROASTED				
Eaten with skin:				
Weighed with skin and bones [refuse: bones, approx. 19%]:				
1 leg from a 21-lb. 4-oz. ready-to-cook turkey: approx. 2 lb. 3 oz. cooked	1660	0.0	47.3	0.00
1 pound of cooked leg	757	0.0	47.3	0.00
Yield per pound of raw ready-to-cook turkey: approx. 1.6 oz. cooked	78	0.0	47.3	0.00
Weighing edible portion only:				
1 pound of cooked meat with skin	935	0.0	58.4	0.00
Roasted with skin, but skin removed before eating:				
Weighed with skin and bones [refuse: bones, approx. 19%; skin, approx. 7%]:				
1 leg from a 21-lb. 4-oz. ready-to-cook turkey: approx. 2 lb. 3 oz. cooked	(1323)	0.0	(37.6)	0.00
1 pound of cooked leg	(602)	0.0	(37.6)	0.00
Yield per pound of raw ready-to-cook turkey: approx. 1.6 oz. cooked	(62)	0.0	(37.6)	0.00
Weighing edible portion only:				
1 pound of cooked meat without skin	(813)	0.0	(50.8)	0.00
WING:				
RAW				
With skin:				
Weighed with skin and bones [refuse: bones, approx. 34%]:				
1 wing from a 21-lb. 4-oz. ready-to-cook turkey: approx. 1 lb. 3 oz.	656	0.0	35.3	0.00
1 pound of raw wing	564	0.0	35.3	0.00
Weighing edible portion only:				
1 pound of raw meat with skin	853	0.0	53.3	0.00
ROASTED				
Eaten with skin:				
Weighed with skin and bones [refuse: bones, approx. 37%]:				
1 wing from a 21-lb. 4-oz. ready-to-cook turkey: approx. 13.3 oz. cooked	524	0.0	39.4	0.00
1 pound of cooked wing	631	0.0	39.4	0.00
Yield per pound of raw ready-to-cook turkey: approx. 0.6 oz. cooked	25	0.0	39.4	0.00
Weighing edible portion only:				
1 pound of cooked meat with skin	1003	0.0	62.7	0.00
Roasted with skin, but skin removed before eating:				
Weighed with skin and bones [refuse: bones, approx. 37%; skin, approx. 16%]:				
1 wing from a 21-lb. 4-oz. ready-to-cook turkey: approx. 13.3 oz. cooked	232	0.0	17.4	0.00
1 pound of cooked wing	279	0.0	17.4	0.00
Yield per pound of raw ready-to-cook turkey: approx. 0.6 oz. cooked	11	0.0	17.4	0.00
Weighing edible portion only:				
1 pound of cooked meat without skin	592	0.0	37.0	0.00
SKIN:				
RAW				
Skin from a 23-lb. turkey: approx. 2 lb. 10 oz. (4g/0g/10g/51%/11g)	4360	0.0	104.3	0.00
1 pound of skin	1669	0.0	104.3	0.00
ROASTED				
Skin from a 23-lb. turkey: approx. 1 lb. 10 oz. cooked (6g/0g/11g/42%/17mg)	3110	0.0	119.6	0.00
1 pound of skin	1914	0.0	119.6	0.00
Average, All Classes				
ENTIRE TURKEY (with neck and giblets):				
RAW				
With skin:				
Weighed with skin and bones [refuse: bones, approx. 21%]:				
1 15-lb. 7-oz. ready-to-cook turkey	8738	4.3	35.3	0.02
1 pound of raw bird, average all parts	564	0.3	35.3	0.02
Weighing edible portion only:				
1 pound of raw meat with skin	712	0.4	44.5	0.02

	UNIT Cal.	UNIT Carb.	1 OZ., BY WT. Cal.	1 OZ., BY WT. Carb.
Without skin:				
Weighed with skin and bones [refuse: bones, approx. 21%; skin, approx. 11%]:				
1 15-lb. 7-oz. ready-to-cook turkey	(5702)	(4.3)	(23.1)	(0.02)
1 pound of raw bird, average all parts	(370)	(0.3)	(23.1)	(0.02)
Weighing edible portion only:				
1 pound of raw meat without skin	(543)	(0.4)	(33.9)	(0.02)
ROASTED				
Eaten with skin:				
Weighed with skin and bones [refuse: bones, approx. 21%]:				
1 15-lb. 7-oz. ready-to-cook turkey: approx. 11 lb. 3 oz. cooked	8248	2.9	45.9	0.02
1 pound of cooked bird, average all parts	734	0.3	45.9	0.02
Yield per pound of raw ready-to-cook turkey: approx. 11.6 oz. cooked	534	0.2	45.9	0.02
Weighing edible portion only:				
1 pound of cooked meat with skin	930	0.3	58.1	0.02
Roasted with skin, but skin removed before eating:				
Weighed with skin and bones [refuse: bones, approx. 21%; skin, approx. 9%]:				
1 15-lb. 7-oz. ready-to-cook turkey: approx. 11 lb. 3 oz. cooked	(6056)	(2.9)	(33.8)	(0.02)
1 pound of cooked bird, average all parts	(541)	(0.3)	(33.8)	(0.02)
Yield per pound of raw ready-to-cook turkey: approx. 11.6 oz. cooked	(392)	(0.2)	(33.8)	(0.02)
Weighing edible portion only:				
1 pound of cooked meat without skin	(779)	(0.4)	(48.7)	(0.02)
ENTIRE TURKEY (without neck and giblets):				
RAW				
With skin:				
Weighed with skin and bones [refuse: bones, approx. 21%]:				
1 14-lb. 4-oz. ready-to-cook turkey	8184	0.0	35.8	0.00
1 pound of raw bird, average all parts	572	0.0	35.8	0.00
Weighing edible portion only:				
1 pound of raw meat with skin (5g/0g/2g/71%/20mg)	726	0.0	45.4	0.00
Without skin:				
Weighed with skin and bones [refuse: bones, approx. 21%; skin, approx. 12%]:				
1 14-lb. 4-oz. ready-to-cook turkey	5162	0.0	22.6	0.0
1 pound of raw bird, average all parts	361	0.0	22.6	0.00
Weighing edible portion only:				
1 pound of raw meat without skin	540	0.0	33.7	0.00
ROASTED:				
Eaten with skin:				
Weighed with skin and bones [refuse: bones, approx. 21%]:				
1 14-lb. 4-oz. ready-to-cook turkey: approx. 10 lb. 5 oz. cooked	7714	0.0	46.5	0.00
1 pound of cooked bird, average all parts	744	0.0	46.5	0.00
Yield per pound of raw ready-to-cook turkey: approx. 11.6 oz. cooked	541	0.0	46.5	0.00
Weighing edible portion only:				
1 pound of cooked meat with skin	944	0.0	59.0	0.00
Roasted with skin, but skin removed before eating:				
Weighed with skin and bones [refuse: bones, approx. 21%; skin, approx. 10%]:				
1 14-lb. 4-oz. ready-to-cook turkey: approx. 10 lb. 5 oz. cooked	5488	0.0	33.3	0.00
1 pound of cooked bird, average all parts	532	0.0	33.3	0.00
Yield per pound of raw ready-to-cook turkey: approx. 11.6 oz. cooked	385	0.0	33.3	0.00
Weighing edible portion only:				
1 pound of cooked meat without skin	771	0.0	53.2	0.00
TOP QUARTER (Breast and Wing—Light Meat):				
RAW				
With skin:				
Weighed with skin and bones [refuse: bones, approx. 15%]:				
1 top quarter from a 14-lb. 4-oz. ready-to-cook turkey: approx. 3 lb. 10 oz.	2204	0.0	38.3	0.00
1 pound of raw top quarter	612	0.0	38.3	0.00
Weighing edible portion only:				
1 pound of raw meat with skin	721	0.0	45.1	0.00
Without skin:				
Weighed with skin and bones [refuse: bones, approx. 15%; skin, approx. 14%]:				
1 top quarter from a 14-lb. 4-oz. ready-to-cook turkey: approx. 3 lb. 10 oz.	1326	0.0	23.1	0.00
1 pound of raw top quarter	369	0.0	23.1	0.00
Weighing edible portion only:				
1 pound of raw meat without skin (2g/0g/tr/74%/18mg)	522	0.0	32.6	0.00

	UNIT Cal.	UNIT Carb.	1 OZ., BY WT. Cal.	1 OZ., BY WT. Carb.
ROASTED				
Eaten with skin:				
Weighed with skin and bones [refuse: bones, approx. 14%]:				
1 top quarter from a 14-lb. 4-oz. ready-to-cook turkey: approx. 2 lb. 11 oz. cooked	2069	0.0	48.1	0.00
1 pound of cooked top quarter	769	0.0	48.1	0.00
Yield per pound of raw ready-to-cook turkey: approx. 3 oz. cooked	145	0.0	48.1	0.00
Weighing edible portion only:				
1 pound of cooked meat with skin	894	0.0	55.9	0.00
Roasted with skin, but skin removed before eating:				
Weighed with skin and bones [refuse: bones, approx. 14%; skin, approx. 12%]:				
1 top quarter from a 14-lb. 4-oz. ready-to-cook turkey: approx. 2 lb. 11 oz. cooked	1421	0.0	32.9	0.00
1 pound of cooked top quarter	526	0.0	32.9	0.00
Yield per pound of raw ready-to-cook turkey: approx. 3 oz. cooked	98	0.0	32.9	0.00
Weighing edible portion only:				
1 pound of cooked meat without skin (9g/0g/1g/66%/18mg)	712	0.0	44.5	0.00
1 cup, chopped or diced (approx. 4.9 oz.)	219	0.0	44.5	0.00
BOTTOM QUARTER (Drumstick, Thigh, and Back—Dark Meat):				
RAW				
With skin:				
Weighed with skin and bones [refuse: bones, approx. 26%]:				
1 bottom quarter from a 14-lb. 4-oz. ready-to-cook turkey: approx. 3 lb. 5 oz.	1883	0.0	33.6	0.00
1 pound of raw bottom quarter	538	0.0	33.6	0.00
Weighing edible portion only:				
1 pound of raw meat with skin	726	0.0	45.4	0.00
Without skin:				
Weighed with skin and bones [refuse: bones, approx. 26%; skin, approx. 10%]:				
1 bottom quarter from a 14-lb. 4-oz. ready-to-cook turkey: approx. 3 lb. 5 oz.	1273	0.0	22.7	0.00
1 pound of raw bottom quarter	363	0.0	22.7	0.00
Weighing edible portion only:				
1 pound of raw meat without skin (6g/0g/1g/74%/22mg)	567	0.0	35.4	0.00
ROASTED				
Eaten with skin:				
Weighed with skin and bones [refuse: bones, approx. 27%]:				
1 bottom quarter from a 14-lb. 4-oz. ready-to-cook turkey: approx. 2 lb. 7 oz. cooked	1789	0.0	45.8	0.00
1 pound of cooked bottom quarter	733	0.0	45.8	0.00
Yield per pound of raw ready-to-cook turkey: approx. 2.7 oz. cooked	126	0.0	45.8	0.00
Weighing edible portion only:				
1 pound of cooked meat with skin (8g/0g/3g/60%/22mg)	1003	0.0	62.7	0.00
Roasted with skin, but skin removed before eating:				
Weighed with skin and bones [refuse: bones, approx. 27%; skin, approx. 10%]:				
1 bottom quarter from a 14-lb. 4-oz. ready-to-cook turkey: approx. 2 lb. 7 oz. cooked	1096	0.0	33.4	0.00
1 pound of cooked bottom quarter	535	0.0	33.4	0.00
Yield per pound of raw ready-to-cook turkey: approx. 2.7 oz. cooked	77	0.0	33.4	0.00
Weighing edible portion only:				
1 pound of cooked meat without skin (8g/0g/2g/63%/23mg)	848	0.0	53.0	0.00
1 cup, chopped or diced (approx. 4.9 oz.)	262	0.0	53.0	0.00
TURKEY PARTS:				
BACK:				
RAW				
With skin:				
Weighed with skin and bones [refuse: bones, approx. 40%]:				
½ back from a 14-lb. 4-oz. ready-to-cook turkey: approx. 1 lb. 5 oz.	706	0.0	33.3	0.00
1 pound of raw back	532	0.0	33.3	0.00
Weighing edible portion only:				
1 pound of raw meat with skin (5g/0g/4g/68%/19mg)	889	0.0	55.6	0.00
ROASTED				
Eaten with skin:				
Weighed with skin and bones [refuse: bones, approx. 41%]:				
½ back from a 14-lb. 4-oz. ready-to-cook turkey: approx. 15.6 oz. cooked	637	0.0	40.7	0.00
1 pound of cooked back	651	0.0	40.7	0.00
Yield per pound of raw ready-to-cook turkey: approx. 1.1 oz. cooked	45	0.0	40.7	0.00

	UNIT Cal.	UNIT Carb.	1 OZ., BY WT. Cal.	1 OZ., BY WT. Carb.
Weighing edible portion only:				
1 pound of cooked meat with skin (7g/0g/4g/58%/21mg)	1102	0.0	68.9	0.00
Roasted with skin, but skin removed before eating:				
Weighed with skin and bones [refuse: bones, approx. 41%; skin, approx. 13%]:				
½ back from a 14-lb. 4-oz. ready-to-cook turkey: approx. 15.6 oz. cooked	(381)	0.0	(24.5)	0.00
1 pound of cooked back	(392)	0.0	(24.5)	0.00
Yield per pound of raw ready-to-cook turkey: approx. 1.1 oz. cooked	(27)	0.0	(24.5)	0.00
Weighing edible portion only:				
1 pound of cooked meat without skin	(850)	0.0	(53.1)	0.00
BREAST:				
RAW				
With skin:				
Weighed with skin and bones [refuse: bones, approx. 10%]:				
½ breast from a 14-lb. 4-oz. ready-to-cook turkey: approx. 2 lb. 12 oz.	1775	0.0	40.0	0.00
1 pound of raw breast	640	0.0	40.0	0.00
Weighing edible portion only:				
1 pound of raw meat with skin (6g/0g/2g/70%/17mg)	712	0.0	44.5	0.00
ROASTED				
Eaten with skin:				
Weighed with skin and bones [refuse: bones, approx. 8%]:				
½ breast from a 14-lb. 4-oz. ready-to-cook turkey, approx. 2 lb. 1 oz. cooked	1637	0.0	49.4	0.00
1 pound of cooked breast	791	0.0	49.4	0.00
Yield per pound of raw ready-to-cook turkey: approx. 2.3 oz. cooked	115	0.0	49.4	0.00
Weighing edible portion only:				
1 pound of cooked meat with skin (8g/0g/2g/63%/18mg)	857	0.0	53.6	0.00
Roasted with skin, but skin removed before eating:				
Weighed with skin and bones [refuse: bones, approx. 8%; skin, approx. 11%]:				
½ breast from a 14-lb. 4-oz. ready-to-cook turkey. approx. 2 lb. 1 oz. cooked	(1137)	0.0	(34.2)	0.00
1 pound of cooked breast	(547)	0.0	(34.2)	0.00
Yield per pound of raw ready-to-cook turkey: approx. 2.3 oz. cooked	(80)	0.0	(34.2)	0.00
Weighing edible portion only:				
1 pound of cooked meat without skin	(675)	0.0	(42.2)	0.00
LEG (Drumstick and Thigh):				
RAW				
With skin:				
Weighed with skin and bones [refuse: bones, approx. 17%]:				
1 leg from a 14-lb. 4-oz. ready-to-cook turkey: approx. 2 lb. 3 oz.	1176	0.0	33.9	0.00
1 pound of raw leg	542	0.0	33.9	0.00
Weighing edible portion only:				
1 pound of raw meat with skin (6g/0g/2g/73%/21mg)	653	0.0	40.8	0.00
ROASTED				
Eaten with skin:				
Weighed with skin and bones [refuse: bones; approx. 19%]:				
1 leg from a 14-lb. 4-oz. ready-to-cook turkey: approx. 1 lb. 8 oz. cooked	1133	0.0	47.7	0.00
1 pound of cooked leg	763	0.0	47.7	0.00
Yield per pound of raw ready-to-cook turkey: approx. 1.7 oz. cooked	80	0.0	47.7	0.00
Weighing edible portion only:				
1 pound of cooked meat with skin (8g/0g/3g/61%/22mg)	944	0.0	59.0	0.00
Roasted with skin, but skin removed before eating:				
Weighed with skin and bones [refuse: bones, approx. 19%; skin, approx. 6%]				
1 leg from a 14-lb. 4-oz. ready-to-cook turkey: approx. 1 lb. 8 oz. cooked	(953)	0.0	(39.7)	0.00
1 pound of cooked leg	(635)	0.0	(39.7)	0.00
Yield per pound of raw ready-to-cook turkey: approx. 1.7 oz. cooked	(67)	0.0	(39.7)	0.00
Weighing edible portion only:				
1 pound of cooked meat without skin	(856)	0.0	(53.5)	0.00
WING:				
RAW				
With skin:				
Weighed with skin and bones [refuse: bones, approx. 33%]:				
1 wing from a 14-lb. 4-oz. ready-to-cook turkey: approx. 13.4 oz.	505	0.0	37.5	0.00
1 pound of raw wings	600	0.0	37.5	0.00
Weighing edible portion only:				
1 pound of raw meat with skin (6g/0g/3g/65%/16mg)	894	0.0	55.9	0.00

	UNIT Cal.	UNIT Carb.	1 OZ., BY WT. Cal.	1 OZ., BY WT. Carb.
ROASTED				
Eaten with skin:				
Weighed with skin and bone [refuse: bones approx. 34%]:				
1 wing from a 14-lb. 4-oz. ready-to-cook turkey: approx. 9.9 oz. cooked	426	0.0	42.9	0.00
1 pound of cooked wings	686		42.9	
Yield per pound of raw ready-to-cook turkey: approx. 0.7 oz. cooked	30		42.9	
Weighing edible portion only:				
1 pound of cooked meat with skin (8g/0g/4g/60%/17mg)	1039		64.9	
Roasted with skin, but skin removed before eating:				
Weighed with skin and bone [refuse: bones, approx. 34%; skin, approx. 16%]				
1 wing from a 14-lb. 4-oz. ready-to-cook turkey: approx. 9.9 oz. cooked	(227)	0.0	(27.1)	0.00
1 pound of cooked wings	(434)		(27.1)	
Yield per pound of raw ready-to-cook turkey: approx. 0.7 oz. cooked	(16)		(27.1)	
Weighing edible portion only:				
1 pound of cooked meat without skin	(731)		(45.7)	
GIBLETS (1 each gizzard, heart, and liver):				
RAW				
Giblets from a 15-lb. 8-oz. turkey: approx. 8.6 oz. (5g/1g/1g/73%/25mg)	314	5.1	36.6	0.59
1 pound of giblets	585	9.5	36.6	0.59
SIMMERED				
Giblets from a 15-lb. 8-oz. turkey: approx. 5.6 oz. cooked (7g/1g/1g/65%/17mg)	264	3.3	47.3	0.59
1 pound of giblets	758	9.5	47.3	0.59
GIZZARD:				
RAW				
1 gizzard from a 15-lb. 8-oz. turkey: approx. 4 oz. (5g/tr/1g/76%/23mg)	133	0.7	32.2	0.18
1 pound of gizzards	531	2.8	32.2	0.18
SIMMERED				
1 gizzard from a 15-lb. 8-oz. turkey: approx. 2.4 oz. cooked (8g/tr/1g/65%/15mg)	111	0.4	46.2	0.17
1 pound of gizzards	739	2.7	46.2	0.17
1 cup (approx. 5.1 oz.)	236	0.9	46.2	0.17
HEART:				
RAW				
1 heart from a 15-lb. 8-oz. turkey: approx. 1 oz. (5g/tr/2g/73%/25mg)	41	0.2	40.5	0.18
1 pound of hearts	649	3.0	40.5	0.18
SIMMERED				
1 heart from a 15-lb. 8-oz. turkey: approx. 0.6 oz. cooked (8g/1g/2g/64%/16mg)	30	0.3	50.2	0.58
1 pound of hearts	803	9.3	50.2	0.58
1 cup (approx. 5.1 oz.)	257	3.0	50.2	0.58
LIVER:				
RAW				
1 liver from a 15-lb. 8-oz. turkey: approx. 3.6 oz. cooked (6g/1g/1g/71%/27mg)	140	4.2	38.8	1.17
1 pound of livers	621	18.7	38.8	1.17
SIMMERED				
1 liver from a 15-lb. 8-oz. turkey: approx. 2.6 oz. cooked (7g/1g/2g/66%/18mg)	125	2.5	47.9	0.97
1 pound of livers	767	15.6	47.9	0.97
1 cup (approx. 4.9 oz.)	237	4.8	47.9	0.97
NECK:				
RAW				
Without Skin:				
Weighed with bones [refuse: bones, approx. 42%]				
1 neck from a 14-lb. 4-oz. ready-to-cook turkey: approx. 10.9 oz.	243	0.0	22.2	0.00
1 pound of raw necks	355	0.0	22.2	0.00
Weighing edible portion only:				
1 pound of raw meat without skin	612	0.0	38.3	0.00
SIMMERED				
Simmered with skin, but skin removed before eating:				
Weighed with bones [refuse: bones, approx. 41%]				
1 neck from a 14-lb. 4-oz. ready-to-cook turkey: approx. 9.0 oz. cooked	274	0.0	30.1	0.00
1 pound of cooked necks	482	0.0	30.1	0.00
Yield per pound of raw ready-to-cook turkey: approx. 0.6 oz. cooked	19	0.0	30.1	0.00
Weighing edible portion only:				
1 pound of cooked meat without skin	817	0.0	51.0	0.00
SKIN:				
RAW				
Skin from a 15-lb. 8-oz. turkey: approx. 1 lb. 12 oz. (9g/0g/1g/65%/20mg)	3036	0.0	109.7	0.00
1 pound of skin	1756	0.0	10.7	0.00

	UNIT Cal.	UNIT Carb.	1 OZ., BY WT. Cal.	1 OZ., BY WT. Carb.
ROASTED				
Skin from a 15-lb. 8-oz. turkey: approx. 1 lb. 1 oz. cooked (5g/0g/11g/40%/15mg)	2192	0.0	125.3	0.00
1 pound of skin	2005	0.0	125.3	0.00

Foreign Turkeys, Domesticated Breeds

	UNIT Cal.	UNIT Carb.	1 OZ., BY WT. Cal.	1 OZ., BY WT. Carb.
(Based on data from the Caribbean)				
RAW, dressed, average all parts				
Edible portion, 1 pound	1216	264.5	76.0	16.53
(Based on data from East Asia)				
RAW, average all parts				
As purchased:				
Live, 1 pound [refuse: approx. 39%]	740	177.1	46.2	11.06
Dressed, 1 pound [refuse: approx. 33%]	813	149.8	50.8	9.36
Drawn, 1 pound [refuse: approx. 19%]	990	86.3	61.8	5.39
Edible portion, 1 pound	1216	0.0	76.0	0.00
(Based on data from Far East)				
RAW, average all parts				
As purchased:				
Live, 1 pound [refuse: approx. 39%]	739	0.0	46.2	0.00
Dressed, 1 pound [refuse: approx. 33%]	812	0.0	50.8	0.00
Drawn, 1 pound [refuse: approx. 19%]	989	0.0	61.8	0.00
Edible portion, 1 pound	1216	0.0	76.0	0.00
(Based on data from France)				
RAW				
Edible portion, 1 pound	971	1.8	60.7	0.11
COOKED (method unspecified)				
Edible portion, 1 pound	(1129)	(0.9)	(70.6)	(0.06)
(Based on data from Japan)				
RAW, average all parts				
Edible portion, 1 pound	903	0.0	56.4	0.00
(Based on data from Latin America)				
RAW, medium-fat bird, average all parts				
Edible portion, 1 pound	2116	0.0	56.4	0.00

DUCK

American Domesticated Breeds

	UNIT Cal.	UNIT Carb.	1 OZ., BY WT. Cal.	1 OZ., BY WT. Carb.
ENTIRE DUCK (without neck and giblets):				
RAW				
With skin:				
Weighed with skin and bones [refuse: bones, approx. 28%]:				
1 3-lb. 14-oz. ready-to-cook duck	5122	0.0	82.4	0.00
1 pound of raw bird, average all parts	1318	0.0	82.4	0.00
Weighing edible portion only:				
1 pound of raw meat with skin	1833	0.0	114.5	0.00
Without skin:				
Weighed with skin and bones [refuse: bones, approx. 28%; skin and separable fat, approx. 38%]:				
1 3-lb. 14-oz. ready-to-cook duck:	798	0.0	12.7	0.00
1 pound of raw bird, average all parts	203	0.0	12.7	0.00
Weighing edible portion only:				
1 pound of raw meat without skin	599	0.0	37.4	0.00
ROASTED:				
With skin:				
Weighed with skin and bones [refuse: bones approx. 35%]:				
1 3-lb. 14-oz. ready-to-cook duck: approx. 2 lb. 10 oz. cooked	2574	0.0	62.1	0.00
1 pound of cooked bird, average all parts	993	0.0	62.1	0.00
Yield per pound of raw ready-to-cook duck: approx. 10.8 oz. cooked	664	0.0	62.1	0.00
Weighing edible portion only:				
1 pound of cooked meat with skin	1529	0.0	95.5	0.00
Roasted with skin; but skin removed before eating:				
Weighed with skin and bones [refuse: bones, approx. 35%; skin and separable fat, approx. 27%]:				
1 3-lb. 14-oz. ready-to-cook duck: approx. 2 lb. 10 oz. cooked	890	0.0	21.7	0.00
1 pound of cooked bird, average all parts	347	0.0	21.7	0.00
Yield per pound of raw ready-to-cook duck: approx. 10.8 oz. cooked	230	0.0	21.7	0.00
Weighing edible portion only:				
1 pound of cooked meat without skin	912	0.0	57.0	0.00
LIVER:				
RAW				
1 liver from a 4-lb. 7-oz. duck: approx. 1.6 oz. (5g/1g/1g/72%/na)	60	1.6	38.6	1.00
1 pound of livers	617	16.0	38.6	1.00

	UNIT Cal.	UNIT Carb.	1 OZ., BY WT. Cal.	1 OZ., BY WT. Carb.
Foreign Domesticated Breeds				
(Based on data from Africa)				
RAW, average all parts				
Edible portion, 1 pound	1302	0.0	81.4	0.00
(Based on data from Australia)				
RAW, average all parts				
Edible portion, 1 pound	1583	0.0	95.8	0.00
ROASTED, average all parts				
Edible portion, 1 pound	1449	0.0	90.6	0.00
(Based on data from the Caribbean)				
RAW, average all parts				
Edible portion, 1 pound	1479	0.0	92.4	0.00
(Based on data from East Asia)				
RAW, average all parts				
As purchased:				
Dressed, 1 pound [refuse, approx. 26%: bones, head, feet, inedible viscera]	948	0.0	59.3	0.00
Drawn, 1 pound [refuse: bones approx. 16%]	1243	0.0	77.7	0.00
Edible portion, 1 pound	1479	0.0	92.4	0.00
ROASTED, average all parts				
As purchased, 1 pound [refuse: bones, approx., 32%]	563	2.7	35.2	0.17
Edible portion, 1 pound	830	4.1	51.9	0.26
PICKLED, average all parts				
As purchased, 1 pound [refuse: bones, approx., 30%]	962	14.5	60.1	0.91
Edible portion, 1 pound	1375	20.4	85.9	1.28
SALTED, PRESSED, average all parts				
As purchased, 1 pound [refuse: bones, approx., 30%]	2586	0.0	161.6	0.00
Edible portion, 1 pound	3697	0.0	231.1	0.00
(Based on data from the Far East)				
RAW, average all parts				
As purchased:				
Dressed, 1 pound [refuse: approx. 36%]	948	0.0	59.3	0.00
Drawn, 1 pound [refuse: approx. 16%]	1243	0.0	77.7	0.00
Edible portion, 1 pound	1479	0.0	92.4	0.00
DRIED, SALTED, average all parts				
Edible portion, 1 pound	1874	0.0	117.1	0.00
(Based on data from India)				
RAW, average all parts				
Edible portion, 1 pound	590	0.5	39.9	0.03
(Based on data from Japan)				
RAW, average all parts				
Edible portion, 1 pound	685	0.0	42.8	0.00
(Based on data from Latin America)				
RAW, average all parts				
Edible portion, 1 pound	1479	0.0	92.4	0.00
(Based on data from Singapore)				
RAW, average all parts				
Edible portion, 1 pound	1479	0.0	92.4	0.00
"Canard" (Based on data from France)				
RAW, average all parts				
Edible portion, 1 pound	1030	0.0	64.4	0.00
COOKED (method unspecified)				
Edible portion, 1 pound	(1229)	0.0	(76.8)	0.00
DUCK FEET (Based on data from East Asia):				
RAW				
As purchased, 1 pound [refuse, bones, nails, and tendons, approx. 53%]	290	0.0	18.1	0.00
Edible portion, 1 pound	608	0.0	38.0	0.00
DRIED				
As purchased, 1 pound [refuse: bones, approx. 58%]	762	0.0	47.6	0.00
Edible portion, 1 pound	1819	0.0	113.7	0.00
American Wild Ducks				
ENTIRE DUCK (without neck and giblets):				
RAW				
With skin:				
Weighed with skin and bones [refuse: bones, approx. 38%]:				
1 2-lb. ready-to-cook duck	1142	0.0	36.0	0.00
1 pound of raw bird, average all parts	576	0.0	36.0	0.00
Weighing edible portion only:				
1 pound of raw meat with skin	957	0.0	59.8	0.00

	UNIT Cal.	UNIT Carb.	1 OZ., BY WT. Cal.	1 OZ., BY WT. Carb.
BREAST:				
RAW				
Without skin:				
Weighed with skin and bones [refuse: bones, approx. 15%; skin and separable fat, approx. 31%]				
½ breast from a 2-lb. duck, approx. 10.9 oz.	204	0.0	18.9	0.00
1 pound of raw breasts	302	0.0	18.9	0.00
Weighing edible portion only:				
1 pound of raw meat without skin	558	0.0	34.9	0.00
Foreign Wild Ducks				
(Based on data from Africa)				
RAW, average all parts:				
Edible portion, 1 pound	1302	0.0	81.4	0.00
(Based on data from East Asia)				
RAW, average all parts:				
Edible portion, 1 pound	572	0.0	35.7	0.00
(Based on data from Japan)				
RAW, average all parts:				
Edible portion, 1 pound	572		35.7	
GOOSE				
American Domesticated Breeds				
ENTIRE GOOSE (without neck and giblets):				
RAW				
With skin:				
Weighed with skin and bones [refuse: bones, approx. 19%]:				
1 7-lb. 3-oz. ready-to-cook goose	9786	0.0	85.2	0.00
1 pound of raw bird, average all parts	1363	0.0	85.2	0.00
Weighing edible portion only:				
1 pound of raw meat with skin (4g/0g/10g/50%/21mg)	1683	0.0	105.2	0.00
Without skin:				
Weighed with skin and bones [refuse: bones, approx. 19%; skin and separable fat, approx. 34%]				
1 7-lb. 3-oz. ready-to-cook goose	2474	0.0	21.5	0.00
1 pound of raw bird, average all parts	344	0.0	21.5	0.00
Weighing edible portion only:				
1 pound of raw meat without skin	730	0.0	45.6	0.00
ROASTED				
Eaten with skin:				
Weighed with skin and bones [refuse: bones, approx. 28%]:				
1 7-lb. 3-oz. ready-to-cook goose approx. 4 lb. 12 oz. cooked	4724	0.0	62.3	0.00
1 pound of cooked bird, average all parts	997	0.0	62.3	0.00
Yield per pound of raw ready-to-cook goose: approx. 10.5 oz. cooked	657	0.0	62.3	0.00
Weighing edible portion only:				
1 pound of cooked meat with skin	1384	0.0	86.5	0.00
Roasted with skin, but skin removed before eating:				
Weighed with skin and bones [refuse: bones, approx. 28%; skin and separable fat, approx. 17%]				
1 7-lb. 3-oz. ready-to-cook goose approx. 4 lb. 12 oz. cooked	2812	0.0	37.1	0.00
1 pound of cooked bird, average all parts	594	0.0	37.1	0.00
Yield per pound of raw ready-to-cook goose: approx. 10.5 oz. cooked	391	0.0	37.1	0.00
Weighing edible portion only:				
1 pound of cooked meat without skin	1080	0.0	67.5	0.00
LIVER:				
RAW				
1 liver from a 7-lb. 3-oz. goose: approx. 3.3 oz. (4g/2g/1g/72%/40mg)	125	5.9	37.7	1.79
1 pound of livers	603	28.7	37.7	1.79
Foreign Domesticated Breeds				
(Based on data from the Caribbean)				
RAW, DRESSED, average all parts				
Edible portion, 1 pound	1606	233.2	100.4	14.57
(Based on data from East Asia)				
RAW, average all parts				
As purchased:				
Dressed [refuse: approx. 34%]	499	0.0	31.9	0.00
Edible portion, 1 pound	758	0.0	47.3	0.00
(Based on data from the Far East)				
As purchased:				
Dressed, 1 pound [refuse: approx. 41%]	948	0.0	59.3	0.00

	UNIT Cal.	UNIT Carb.	1 OZ., BY WT. Cal.	1 OZ., BY WT. Carb.
Drawn, 1 pound [refuse: approx. 10%]	1447	0.0	90.4	0.00
Edible portion, 1 pound	1606	0.0	100.4	0.00
(Based on data from France)				
RAW				
Edible portion, 1 pound	1551	0.0	97.0	0.00
COOKED (method unspecified)				
Edible portion, 1 pound	(1801)	0.0	(112.6)	0.00
(Based on data from Latin America)				
Edible portion, 1 pound	1607	0.0	100.4	0.00
LESS FAMILIAR BIRDS				
Dusky Ouzel				
(Based on data from East Asia)				
Edible portion, 1 pound	418	0.0	26.1	0.00
Finch				
RAW, average all parts:				
Edible portion, 1 pound	604		37.7	
Grouse				
(Based on data from the British Isles)				
COOKED (roasted with basting):				
Weighed with bone, 1 pound [refuse: approx. 49%]	517	0.0	32.3	0.00
Edible portion, 1 pound	785	0.0	49.1	0.00
Guinea Fowl				
(Based on data from the British Isles)				
COOKED (roasted with basting):				
Weighed with bone, 1 pound [refuse: approx. 41%]	508	0.0	31.8	0.00
Edible portion, 1 pound	953	0.0	59.5	0.00
Guinea Hen				
ENTIRE GUINEA HEN (without neck and giblets):				
RAW				
With skin:				
Weighed with skin and bones [refuse: bones, approx. 17%]:				
1 1-lb. 13-oz. ready-to-cook guinea hen	1090	0.0	37.2	0.00
1 pound of raw bird, average all parts	595	0.0	37.2	0.00
Weighing edible portion only:				
1 pound of raw meat with skin	717	0.0	44.8	0.00
Without skin:				
Weighed with skin and bones [refuse: bones, approx. 36%; skin, approx. 17%]:				
1 1-lb. 13-oz. ready-to-cook guinea hen	584	0.0	20.1	0.00
1 pound of raw bird, average all parts	321	0.0	20.1	0.00
Weighing edible portion only:				
1 pound of raw meat without skin	499	0.0	31.2	0.00
(Based on data from France)				
COOKED (method unspecified):				
Edible portion, 1 pound	(608)	(2.7)	(38.0)	(0.17)
Partridge				
(Based on data from the British Isles)				
COOKED (roasted with bastings):				
Weighed with bones, 1 pound [refuse: approx. 61%]	576	0.0	36.0	0.00
Edible portion, 1 pound	957	0.0	59.8	0.00
Pheasant				
ENTIRE PHEASANT (without neck and giblets):				
RAW				
With skin:				
Weighed with skin and bones [refuse: bones, approx. 14%]:				
1 2-lb. 1-oz. ready-to-cook pheasant	1446	0.0	44.1	0.00
1 pound of raw bird, average all parts	705	0.0	44.1	0.00
Weighing edible portion only:				
1 pound of raw meat with skin	821	0.0	51.3	0.00
Without skin:				
Weighed with skin and bones [refuse: bones, approx. 14%; skin, approx. 10%]:				
1 2-lb. 1-oz. ready-to-cook pheasant	940	0.0	28.8	0.00
1 pound of raw bird, average all parts	460	0.0	28.8	0.00

	UNIT Cal.	UNIT Carb.	1 OZ., BY WT. Cal.	1 OZ., BY WT. Carb.
Weighing edible portion only:				
1 pound of raw meat without skin	603	0.0	37.7	0.00
BREAST:				
RAW				
Without skin:				
Weighing edible portion only:				
1 breast from a 2-lb. 1-oz. pheasant: approx. 13 oz. (7g/0g/1g/72%/10mg)	486	0.0	37.7	0.00
1 pound of pheasant breast meat	603	0.0	37.7	0.00
LEG:				
RAW				
Without skin:				
Weighing edible portion only:				
1 leg from a 2-lb. 1-oz. pheasant: approx. 3.8 oz. (6g/0g/1g/73%/13mg)	143	0.0	38.0	0.00
1 pound of pheasant leg meat	608	0.0	38.0	0.00
(Based on data from the British Isles)				
COOKED (roasted with bastings):				
Weighed with bone, 1 pound [refuse: approx. 55%]	608	0.0	38.0	0.00
Edible portion, 1 pound	966	0.0	60.4	0.00
(Based on data from East Asia)				
As purchased [refuse: approx. 70%, bones and viscera], 1 pound	191	0.0	11.9	0.00
Edible portion, 1 pound	636	0.0	39.7	0.00
Pigeon (Squab)				
ENTIRE PIGEON (without neck and giblets):				
RAW				
With skin:				
Weighed with skin and bones [refuse: bones, approx. 23%]:				
1 9.1-oz. ready-to-cook squab	584	0.0	64.1	0.00
1 pound of raw bird, average all parts	1025	0.0	64.1	0.00
Weighing edible portion only:				
1 pound of raw meat with skin	1334	0.0	83.4	0.00
Without skin:				
Weighed with skin and bones [refuse: bones, approx. 23%; skin, approx. 14%]:				
1 9.1-oz. ready-to-cook squab	239	0.0	26.3	0.00
1 pound of raw bird, average all parts	420	0.0	26.3	0.00
Weighing edible portion only:				
1 pound of raw meat without skin	644	0.0	40.3	0.00
BREAST:				
RAW				
Weighing edible portion only:				
1 breast from a 9.1-oz. squab, approx. 3.6 oz. (6g/0g/1g/73%/na)	135	0.0	38.0	0.00
1 pound of squab meat	608	0.0	38.0	0.00
(Based on data from Africa)				
RAW, average all parts				
Edible portion, 1 pound	813	1.4	50.8	0.09
(Based on data from the British Isles)				
COOKED (boiled)				
Weighed with bones, 1 pound [refuse: approx. 64%]	435	0.0	27.2	0.00
Edible portion, 1 pound	989	0.0	61.8	0.00
COOKED (ROASTED)				
Weighed with bones, 1 pound [refuse: approx. 72%]	463	0.0	28.9	0.00
Edible portion, 1 pound	1057	0.0	66.1	0.00
(Based on data from East Asia)				
RAW, average all parts				
As purchased: dressed, 1 pound [refuse, approx. 53%: bones, head, feet, inedible viscera]	372	0.0	23.3	0.00
Edible portion, 1 pound	795	0.0	49.6	0.00
(Based on data from the Far East)				
RAW, average all parts				
As purchased: dressed, 1 pound [refuse: approx. 40%]	763	0.0	47.6	0.00
Edible portion, 1 pound	1267	0.0	79.1	0.00
(Based on data from France)				
RAW				
Edible portion, 1 pound	490	2.3	30.6	0.14
COOKED (method unspecified)				
Edible portion, 1 pound	(608)	(2.7)	(38.0)	(0.17)
(Based on data from Latin America)				
RAW, average all parts				
Edible portion, 1 pound	1267	0.0	79.1	0.00

	UNIT Cal.	UNIT Carb.	1 OZ., BY WT. Cal.	1 OZ., BY WT. Carb.
Ptarmigan				
(Based on data from Canada)				
RAW, average all parts				
Edible portion, 1 pound	472	0.0	29.5	0.00
Quail				
(Based on data from East Asia)				
RAW, average all parts				
As purchased: [refuse: bones, approx. 53%]	250	0.0	15.6	0.00
Edible portion, 1 pound	536	0.0	33.5	0.00
(Based on data from Japan)				
RAW, average all parts				
Edible portion, 1 pound	531	0.0	33.2	0.00
(Based on data from Pakistan)				
RAW, average all parts				
Edible portion, 1 pound	522	0.0	32.6	0.00
Quail, Grey				
(Based on data from India)				
RAW, average all parts				
Edible portion, 1 pound	1280	0.0	80.0	0.00
Ruff and Reeve				
(Based on data from India)				
RAW, average all parts:				
Edible portion, 1 pound	562	0.0	35.2	0.00
Sparrow				
(Based on data from East Asia)				
RAW, average all parts				
Edible portion (includes bones), 1 pound	563	0.0	35.2	0.00
(Based on data from Japan)				
RAW, average all parts				
Edible portion (includes bones), 1 pound	562	0.0	35.1	0.00
Squab, see Pigeon				
Swiftlet				
(Based on data from East Asia)				
BIRD'S NEST:				
DRIED				
Edible portion, 1 pound	1565	133.0	97.8	8.31
DRIED, SOAKED, DRAINED				
Edible portion, 1 pound	318	19.0	19.8	1.19
Teal				
(Based on data from East Asia and Japan)				
RAW, average all parts				
Edible portion, 1 pound	604	0.0	37.8	0.00
Turtledove				
(Based on data from Africa and Japan)				
RAW, average all parts				
Edible portion, 1 pound	509	0.0	31.8	0.00
Wild Fowl				
(Based on data from India)				
RAW, average all parts				
Edible portion, 1 pound	1112	0.0	69.5	0.00
Wood Sandpiper				
(Based on data from India)				
RAW, average all parts				
Edible portion, 1 pound	531	6.8	33.2	0.43
PREPACKAGED FRESH POULTRY (TURKEY)				
READY-TO-COOK TURKEY PARTS, based on generic data				
Prebasted, Roasted Turkey (breast meat and skin)				
As purchased [refuse: bones, approx. 8%]				
1 breast, 4 lb. 3 oz. yield: 3 lbs. 13 oz. edible portion	2175	0.0	32.8	0.00
1 pound	525	0.0	32.8	0.00

	UNIT Cal.	UNIT Carb.	1 OZ., BY WT. Cal.	1 OZ., BY WT. Carb.
Edible portion:				
1 pound (6g/tr/1g/71%/113mg)	572	0.0	35.7	0.00
Prebasted, Roasted Turkey (thigh meat and skin)				
As purchased [refuse: bones, approx. 13%]				
1 thigh, 13 oz. [Yield: 11 oz. edible portion]	495	0.0	38.8	0.00
1 pound	621	0.0	38.8	0.00
Edible portion:				
1 pound (5g/tr/3g/71%/125mg)	712	0.0	44.5	0.00
TURKEY PARTS, by brand				
Louis Rich Fresh Turkey Breast Half (package weight varies)				
As purchased, 1 pound (yield: approx. 14.2 oz.)	570	0.0	35.6	0.00
Edible portion, 1 pound	640	0.0	40.0	0.00
Fresh Turkey Boneless Breast Half (package weight varies)				
As purchased, 1 pound, all-edible	640	0.0	40.0	0.00
Fresh Hen Turkey Breast Half (package weight varies)				
As purchased, 1 pound (yield: approx. 14.2 oz.)	570	0.0	35.6	0.00
Edible portion, 1 pound	640	0.0	40.0	0.00
Fresh Turkey Breast Portion (package weight varies)				
As purchased, 1 pound (yield: approx. 14.2 oz.)	570	0.0	35.6	0.00
Edible portion, 1 pound	640	0.0	40.0	0.00
Fresh Turkey Breast Slices (package weight varies)				
As purchased, 1 pound, all-edible	533	0.0	33.3	0.00
Fresh Turkey Breast Tenderloins (package weight varies)				
As purchased, 1 pound, all-edible	533	0.0	33.0	0.00
Fresh Turkey Breast Tenderloin Steaks (package weight varies)				
As purchased, 1 pound, all-edible	533	0.0	33.0	0.00
Fresh Turkey Drumsticks (package weight varies)				
As purchased, 1 pound (yield: approx. 14.2 oz.)	570	0.0	35.6	0.00
Edible portion, 1 pound	640	0.0	40.0	0.00
Fresh Turkey Hindquarter (package weight varies)				
As purchased, 1 pound (yield: approx. 12.0 oz.)	720	0.0	45.0	0.00
Edible portion, 1 pound	960	0.0	60.0	0.00
Fresh Turkey Thigh (package weight varies)				
As purchased, 1 pound (yield: approx. 12.0 oz.)	680	0.0	42.5	0.00
Edible portion, 1 pound	907	0.0	56.7	0.00
Fresh Turkey Wings (package weight varies)				
As purchased, 1 pound (yield: approx. 10.5 oz.)	455	0.0	28.4	0.00
Edible portion, 1 pound	693	0.0	43.3	0.00
Fresh Turkey Wing Drumettes (package weight varies)				
As purchased, 1 pound (yield: approx. 11.0 oz.)	477	0.0	29.8	0.00
Edible portion, 1 pound	694	0.0	43.4	0.00
Prime Young Hen Turkey (package weight varies)				
As purchased, 1 pound (yield: approx. 11.3 oz.)	563	0.0	35.2	0.00
Edible portion, 1 pound	800	0.0	50.0	0.00
Pure Ground Turkey, 1-pound package				
All-edible portion, 1 pound (yield: approx. 13.3 oz. cooked)	840	0.0	52.5	0.00
All edible, cooked, 1 pound	816	0.0	51.0	0.00
FROZEN POULTRY				
FROZEN CHICKEN, by brand				
Barber Foods 2 Boneless Breasts of Chicken Cordon Bleu, 14-oz. box	810	19.0	57.8	1.36
1 breast, approx. 7 oz.	405	9.5	57.8	1.36
2 Boneless Breasts of Chicken Kiev, 14-oz. box	1072	30.1	76.6	2.15
1 breast, approx. 7 oz.	536	15.1	76.6	2.15
4 Breaded Chicken Cutlets, 12-oz. box	868	51.0	72.3	4.25
1 piece, approx. 3 oz.	217	12.8	72.3	4.25
2 Stuffed Boneless Chicken Breasts, 16-oz. (1-lb.) box	980	53.1	61.2	3.32
1 breast, approx. 8 oz.	490	26.6	61.2	3.32
FROZEN TURKEY, Ready-to-Cook, by brand				
Land O'Lakes Whole Young Turkey, 10 lb.	(4800)	0.0	(30.0)	0.00
Buttermoist Boneless Dark Meat Turkey Roast with Gravy, 32-oz. (2-lb.) package	1493	10.7	46.7	0.33
White Meat Turkey Roast with Gravy, 32-oz. (2-lb.) package	1387	10.7	43.3	0.33
Fancy Turkey Breast (with ribs, wing meat, and neck skin), 3-lb. package	1440	0.0	30.0	0.00
6-lb. package	2880	0.0	30.0	0.00
Whole Butter-Knife Tender Self-Basting Young Turkey, 10 lb.	6400	0.0	40.0	0.00
20 lb.	2800	0.0	40.0	0.00
Swift Premium Whole Deep-Basted Butterball Young Turkey, 5–30 lb. (data based on 10-lb. bird)	10,060	0.0	62.9	0.00
Dark meat only, 1 pound	(594)	0.0	(37.1)	0.00
White meat only, 1 pound	(533)	0.0	(33.3)	0.00
Skin only, 1 pound	(1870)	0.0	(117.0)	0.00

	UNIT Cal.	UNIT Carb.	1 OZ., BY WT. Cal.	1 OZ., BY WT. Carb.
Raw, Boneless, Frozen, Seasoned Turkey Roasts (light and dark meat)				
1 box, 2.5 lb. net wt.	1358	72.6	34.0	1.81
1 pound (5g/2g/1g/70%/194mg)	544	29.0	34.0	1.81
Roasted, Boneless, Frozen, Seasoned Turkey Roasts (light and dark meat)				
1 box, 1.7 lb. net wt.	1213	24.0	43.9	0.87
1 pound (6g/1g/2g/68%/194mg)	703	13.9	43.9	0.87
Diced, Light and Dark, Seasoned Turkey				
Edible portion:				
1 pound (5g/tr/2g/72%/243mg)	626	4.5	39.1	0.28

CANNED POULTRY

	UNIT Cal.	UNIT Carb.	1 OZ., BY WT. Cal.	1 OZ., BY WT. Carb.
CANNED CHICKEN, based on generic data				
Canned, Boned Chicken, 5½-oz. can (solid pack)	309	0.0	56.1	0.00
1 cup (approx. 7¼ oz.)	406	0.0	56.1	0.00
1 pound (approx. 2.2 cups)	898	0.0	56.1	0.00
Canned, Boned Chicken with Broth				
Drained solids:				
1 can, 5 oz.	234	0.0	46.8	0.00
1 pound (6g/0g/2g/69%/143mg)	749	0.0	46.8	0.00
CANNED CHICKEN, by brand				
Swanson Boned Chicken With Broth, 5-oz. can	240	0.0	48.0	0.00
Chunk white Chicken, 5-oz. can	220	0.0	44.0	0.00
Tender Chunk Chicken, 6¾-oz. can	259	0.0	38.3	0.00
For comparison: **Worthington** chickenless Soyameat Chicken-like Slices with Sauce, 13-oz. can, approx. 12 slices	798	12.4	61.4	0.95
1 slice, approx. 1.06 oz.	65	1.0	61.4	0.95
CANNED TURKEY, based on generic data				
Canned, Boned Turkey, 5½ oz. can (solid pack)	315	19.5	57.3	3.55
1 cup (approx. 7¼ oz.)	414	25.6	57.3	3.55
1 pound (approx. 2.2 cups)	916	56.7	57.3	3.55
Canned, Boned Turkey with Broth				
Drained solids:				
1 can, 5 oz.	231	0.0	46.2	0.00
1 pound (7g/0g/2g/66%/133mg)	739	0.0	46.2	0.00
CANNED TURKEY, by brand				
Morton House Sliced Turkey and Gravy, 12½-oz. can	280	14.0	22.4	1.12
Swanson Boned Turkey With Broth, 5-oz. can	240	0.0	48.0	0.00
Tender Chunk Turkey, 6¾-oz. can	207	0.0	30.7	0.00
For comparison: **Worthington** turkeyless, Turkey-like flavor, 13-oz. can, approx. 12 slices	877	17.6	67.5	1.35
1 slice, approx. 1.13 oz.	75	1.5	67.5	1.35

6 FISH, SHELLFISH & WATERLIFE •

	UNIT Cal.	UNIT Carb.	1 OZ., BY WT. Cal.	1 OZ., BY WT. Carb.
FRESH FISH AND SHELLFISH				
ABALONE				
RAW:				
Weighed in shell [refuse, approx. 58% shell and viscera], 1 pound as purchased	187	6.5	11.7	0.41
Edible portion, 1 pound (5g/1g/tr/76%/na)	445	15.4	27.8	0.96
Abalone (based on data from Japan)				
RAW:				
Edible portion, 1 pound	485	3.7	30.3	0.23
DRIED:				
All-edible, 1 pound	1166	7.7	72.9	0.48
SEASONED:				
All-edible, 1 pound	603	81.2	37.7	5.06
SALTED:				
All-edible, with viscera, 1 pound	454	4.5	28.4	0.28
BOILED:				
All-edible, 1 pound	458	33.1	28.6	2.07
AGAR, see under SEAWEED				
ALBACORE *(Thunnus alalunga)* (see also TUNA)				
RAW:				
Edible portion, 1 pound	476	0.0	29.8	0.00
ALEWIFE				
RAW:				
Weighed whole [refuse, approx. 51%: head, tail, fins, entrails, scales, bones, and skin], 1 pound as purchased	282	0.0	17.6	0.00
Edible portion, 1 pound (6g/0g/1g/74%/na)	576	0.0	36.0	0.00
ALLIGATOR (based on data from Latin America)				
SEMI-DRIED:				
Edible portion, 1 pound	1052	(0.0)	65.8	(0.00)
AMBERJACK				
Amberjack *(Seriola)*				
RAW:				
Edible portion, 1 pound	435	0.0	27.2	0.00
Redtail Amberjack (*Seriola.* Based on data from East Asia)				
RAW:				
As purchased, 1 pound [refuse, approx. 45%: bones, scales, entrails, and tail]	309	0.0	19.3	0.00
Edible portion, 1 pound	563	0.0	35.2	0.00
Yellowtail Amberjack (*Seriola quinqueradiata.* Based on data from East Asia)				
RAW:				
As purchased, 1 pound [refuse, approx. 33%: bones, scales, and entrails]	390	0.0	24.4	0.00
Edible portion, 1 pound	586	0.0	36.6	0.00
ANCHOVY				
Anchovy *(Engraulidae)*				
RAW:				
Edible portion, 1 pound	422	(0.0)	26.4	(0.00)
Anchovy (based on data from Japan)				
RAW:				
Edible portion, 1 pound	824	2.0	51.4	0.13
DRIED:				
Edible portion, 1 pound	1438	1.4	89.9	0.09
BOILED, DRIED:				
Edible portion, 1 pound	1462	1.4	91.4	0.09
Anchovy, Striped *(Anchoa hepsetus)*				
RAW:				
Edible portion, 1 pound	430		26.9	
Anchovy Larval Fish (based on data from Japan)				
BOILED, DRIED:				
Edible portion, 1 pound	803	1.4	50.2	0.09
ARCTIC CHAR (based on data from Canada)				
RAW:				
Edible portion, 1 pound	594	0.0	3.71	0.00
ARKSHELL (based on data from Japan)				
RAW:				
As purchased, 1 pound [refuse, approx. 83%]	66	2.7	4.1	0.17
Edible portion, 1 pound	386	15.8	24.1	0.99
BAGRE (based on data from Latin America)				
RAW:				
Flesh and skin, 1 pound	617	0.0	38.6	0.00
BAM (*Mastocembelus armatus.* Based on data from India)				
RAW:				
Edible portion, 1 pound	454	31.3	28.4	1.96

	UNIT Cal.	UNIT Carb.	1 OZ., BY WT. Cal.	1 OZ., BY WT. Carb.
BARRACOUTA *(Thyrsiles atun)*				
RAW:				
Edible portion, 1 pound	599	3.2	37.4	0.20
BARRACUDA, PACIFIC				
RAW:				
Edible portion, 1 pound	513	0.0	32.1	0.00
BASS (see also SEA BASS)				
Black Sea Bass				
RAW:				
Edible portion, 1 pound (5g/0g/tr/79%/na)	422	0.0	26.4	0.00
STUFFED, COATED, BAKED:				
Data are based on USDA home recipe with ingredients as follows per pound of fillets: For stuffing, 1.1 oz. bacon, 2 Tbsp. butter, ½ oz. chopped onion, 1⅓ oz. chopped celery. For coating, 1¼ oz. butter or margarine, 1 cup soft breadcrumbs:				
1 pound of fillets, stuffed, coated, baked: yield approx. 15.5 oz. (5g/3g/4g/53%/na)	1114	49.0	71.9	3.16
Baked, stuffed, 1 pound	1150	50.6	71.9	3.16
Smallmouth and Largemouth Bass				
RAW:				
Weighed whole [refuse, approx. 69%: head, fins, entrails, skin, and bones], 1 pound as purchased	146	0.0	9.1	0.00
Edible portion, 1 pound (5g/0g/1g/77%/na)	472	0.0	29.5	0.00
Striped Bass				
RAW:				
Weighed whole [refuse, approx. 57%: head, tail, entrails, scales, bones, and skin], 1 pound as purchased	205	0.0	12.8	0.00
Edible portion, 1 pound (5g/0g/1g/78%/na)	477	0.0	29.8	0.00
COATED, THEN OVEN-FRIED:				
Data are based on USDA home recipe with coating ingredients as follows per pound of fillets: ½ cup milk, 1½ tsp. salt, ½ cup dry breadcrumbs, 2 Tbsp. butter or other fat:				
1 pound of raw striped bass fillets with 7.2 oz. coating (Yield: approx. 16.9 oz.)	941	32.2	55.8	1.90
1 oven-fried striped bass fillet, aprox 8¾" × 4½" × ⅝" (approx. 7.1 oz.) (6g/2g/2g/61%/na)	392	13.4	55.8	1.90
1 pound of oven-fried striped bass fillets	889	30.4	55.8	1.90
White Bass				
RAW:				
Weighed whole [refuse, approx. 61%: head, tail, entrails, fins, scales, bones, and skin], 1 pound as purchased	173	0.0	10.8	0.00
Edible portion, 1 pound (5g/0g/1g/79%/na)	445	0.0	27.8	0.00
BLUEFISH				
RAW:				
Weighed whole [refuse, approx. 49%: head, tail, entrails, fins, bones, and skin], 1 pound as purchased	271	0.0	16.9	0.00
Edible portion, 1 pound (6g/0g/1g/75%/na)	531	0.0	33.2	0.00
BAKED OR BROILED:				
Based on USDA data; cooked with unspecified amount of butter or margarine:				
1 pound of raw bluefish fillets, cooked (yield: approx. 12.9 oz.)	580	0.0	45.1	0.00
1 baked or broiled bluefish fillet, approx. 7⅔" × 3⅞" × ⅜" (approx. 5.5 oz.) (7g/0g/1g/68%/29mg)	246	0.0	45.1	0.00
1 pound of baked or broiled bluefish fillets	721	0.0	45.1	0.00
COATED, THEN FRIED:				
Data are based on USDA home recipe with coating ingredients as follows per pound of fillets: ½ egg, 1½ tsp. milk, ½ cup dry breadcrumbs:				
1 pound of raw bluefish fillets, cooked (yield: approx. 13.6 oz.)	789	18.1	58.1	1.33
1 fried bluefish fillet, approx. 8⅛" × 3¼" × ¼" (6g/1g/3g/61%/41mg)	400	9.2	58.1	1.33
1 pound of fried bluefish fillets	930	21.3	58.1	1.33
BOMBAY DUCK (*Harpodon neherens.* Based on data from India)				
RAW:				
Dried, edible portion, 1 pound	1773	15.2	110.8	0.95

	UNIT Cal.	UNIT Carb.	1 OZ., BY WT. Cal.	1 OZ., BY WT. Carb.
BONITO				
Bonito, from data including Atlantic, Pacific, and Striped				
RAW:				
Weighed whole [refuse, approx. 42%: head, tail, entrails, fins, bones, and skin], 1 pound as purchased	442	0.0	27.6	0.00
Edible portion, 1 pound (7g/0g/2g/68%/na)	763	0.0	47.7	0.00
BONITO EGGS (based on data from Latin America)				
RAW:				
Edible portion, 1 pound	454	0.0	28.4	0.00
BRANCHIOSTEGUS (based on data from Japan)				
RAW:				
Edible portion, 1 pound	467	1.4	29.2	0.09
BREAM				
Bream *(Pagellus)*				
RAW:				
Edible portion, 1 pound (5g/0g/tr/75%/na)	373	0.0	23.3	0.00
Large-eyed Bream *(Montanes grandoculis)*				
RAW:				
Edible portion, 1 pound (5g/tr/tr/78%/na)	411	7.3	25.7	0.45
BRILL, ROUGH SCALED (based on data from East Asia)				
RAW:				
As purchased, 1 pound [refuse, approx. 40%: scales, bones, and entrails]	245	0.0	15.3	0.00
Edible portion, 1 pound	413	0.0	25.8	0.00
BUFFALOFISH				
Buffalofish from unspecified waters				
RAW:				
Weighed whole [refuse, approx. 68%: head, fins, entrails, skin and bones], 1 pound as purchased	164	0.0	10.3	0.00
Edible portion, 1 pound (5g/0g/2g/77%/na)	513	0.0	32.1	0.00
Buffalofish from Great Lakes waters				
RAW:				
Edible portion, 1 pound (5g/0g/1g/78%/na)	481	0.0	30.1	0.00
BULL-FROG (based on data from Japan)				
RAW:				
Edible portion, 1 pound	399	0.0	25.0	0.00
BULLHEAD, BLACK				
RAW:				
Weighed whole [refuse, approx. 81%: head, fins, entrails, and bones], 1 pound as purchased	72	0.0	4.5	0.00
Edible portion, 1 pound (5g/0g/tr/81%/na)	381	0.0	23.8	0.00
BURBOT				
RAW:				
Weighed whole [refuse, approx. 85%: head, tail, fins, entrails, bones, and skin], 1 pound as purchased	56	0.0	3.5	0.00
Edible portion, 1 pound (5g/0g/tr/81%/na)	372	0.0	23.3	0.00
BUTTERFISH				
Butterfish from Northern waters				
RAW:				
Weighed whole [refuse, approx. 49%: head, tail, fins, entrails, bones, and skin], 1 pound as purchased	391	0.0	24.4	0.00
Edible portion, 1 pound (5g/0g/3g/71%/na)	767	0.0	47.9	0.00
Butterfish from Gulf waters				
RAW:				
Weighed whole [refuse, approx. 49%: head, tail, fins, entrails, bones, and skin], 1 pound as purchased	220	0.0	13.8	0.00
Edible portion, 1 pound (5g/0g/1g/78%/na)	431	0.0	26.9	0.00

	UNIT Cal.	UNIT Carb.	1 OZ., BY WT. Cal.	1 OZ., BY WT. Carb.
Butterfish, caught off Block Island, Massachusetts				
Caught in Autumn				
RAW:				
Edible portion, 1 pound (5g/0g/1g/76%/27mg)	535	0.0	33.4	0.00
Caught in Spring				
RAW:				
Edible portion, 1 pound (5g/0g/1g/74%/23mg)	667	0.0	41.7	0.00
CARP				
RAW:				
Weighed whole [refuse, approx. 70%: head, fins, entrails, skin and bones], 1 pound as purchased	156	0.0	9.8	0.00
Edible portion, 1 pound (5g/0g/1g/78%/81mg)	522	0.0	32.6	0.00
Indian Carp (*Labeo*)				
RAW:				
Edible portion, 1 pound (5g/tr/1g/80%/na)	(500)	1.8	(31.2)	0.11
CATFISH (see also MUDFISH)				
Air-Breathing Catfish (*Clariidae*)				
RAW:				
Edible portion, 1 pound (5g/tr/1g/78%/na)	467	0.9	29.2	0.06
Electric Catfish (*Malapterurus electricus*. Based on data from Africa)				
RAW:				
Edible portion, 1 pound	386	0.0	24.1	0.00
Freshwater Catfish				
RAW:				
Edible portion, 1 pound (5g/0g/1g/78%/17mg)	467	0.0	29.2	0.00
Freshwater Catfish (*Clarias batrachus*. Based on data from East Asia)				
RAW:				
As purchased, 1 pound [refuse, approx. 41%: bones and entrails]	259	0.0	16.2	0.00
Edible portion, 1 pound (5g/0g/1g/78%/na)	445	0.0	27.8	0.00
Sea Catfish				
RAW:				
Edible portion, 1 pound (5g/tr/tr/78%/na)	381	2.3	23.9	0.14
Sea Catfish (*Arius*. Based on data from East Asia)				
DRIED, SALTED:				
Edible portion, 1 pound	922	0.0	57.6	0.00
CAVALLI (*Caranx hippos*. Based on data from the Caribbean)				
RAW:				
Edible portion, 1 pound	522	0.0	32.6	0.00
CAVIAR				
RAW:				
Caviar, Sturgeon				
GRANULAR:				
All-edible:				
1 tablespoon (approx. 0.57 oz.)	42	0.5	74.0	0.90
1 cup (approx. 9.1 oz.)	672	8.0	74.0	0.90
1 ounce (approx. 1.8 Tbsp.)	74	0.9	74.0	0.90
1 caviar-pound (a measure used for caviar, it equals 14 oz.)	1036	12.6	74.0	0.90
1 pound (approx. 1¾ cups) (8g/1g/4g/46%/624mg)	1184	14.4	74.0	0.90
PRESSED:				
All-edible:				
1 tablespoon (approx. 0.61 oz.)	54	0.8	90.0	1.34
1 cup (approx. 9.6 oz.)	864	12.8	90.0	1.34
1 ounce (approx. 1.7 Tbsp.)	90	1.3	90.0	1.34
1 caviar-pound (a measure used for caviar, it equals 14 oz.)	1260	18.8	90.0	1.34
1 pound (approx. 1⅔ cups) (10g/1g/5g/36%/na)	1440	21.4	90.0	1.34
German Caviar (based on data from France)				
All-edible, 1 pound	572	12.7	35.7	0.79
Russian Caviar (based on data from France)				
All-edible, 1 pound	1188	20.9	74.3	1.30
CHUB				
Chub from unspecified waters				
RAW:				
Weighed whole [refuse, approx. 67%: head, tail, fins, entrails, scales, bones, and skin], 1 pound as purchased	217	0.0	13.6	0.00
Edible portion, 1 pound (4g/0g/3g/75%/na)	658	0.0	41.1	0.00
Chub from Great Lakes waters				
RAW:				
Edible portion, 1 pound	740	0.0	46.3	0.00
Sea Chub (*Kyphosidae*)				
RAW:				
Edible portion, 1 pound (6g/0g/1g/76%/na)	46.3	(0.0)	28.9	(0.00)
CISCO, LONGJAW (*Coregonus alpenae*) (see also LAKE HERRING)				
RAW:				
Edible portion, 1 pound (5g/0g/1g/80%/na)	(510)	(0.0)	(31.9)	(0.00)
CLAMS				
Clams (*Cardium*. Based on data from East Asia)				
DRIED:				
Edible portion, 1 pound	1594	74.5	99.6	4.66
Bean Clams (*Donax*. Based on data from East Asia)				
RAW:				
As purchased, 1 pound [refuse, approx. 80%: shell and liquid]	64	4.5	4.0	0.28
Edible portion, 1 pound	336	4.5	21.0	1.45
Cherrystone Clams, see Hard Clams				
Chowder Clams, see Hard Clams				
Hard or Round Clams				
RAW:				
As purchased:				
Meat and liquid weighed in shell [refuse: approx. 68%: shell], 1 pound	71	6.1	4.4	0.38
Meat in shell [refuse, approx. 83%: shell and liquid]	62	4.5	3.9	0.28
RAW:				
Edible portion:				
Meat of 1 small clam, approx. 0.26 oz.	6	0.4	22.7	1.67
Meat of 1 medium clam, approx. 0.3 oz.	7	0.5	22.7	1.67
Meat of 1 large clam, approx. 0.4 oz. (3g/2g/tr/80%/58mg)	10	0.7	22.7	1.67
1 cup (approx. 8 oz.; approx. 15 or more little necks, or 11–15 cherrystones, or 7–11 mediums, or 7 or fewer chowders)	184	13.5	22.7	1.67
1 pint (approx. 1 lb., approx. 31 or more little necks, or 22–31 cherrystones, or 14–22 mediums, or 14 or fewer chowders)	(368)	(27.0)	22.7	1.67
1 quart (approx. 2 lb.; approx. 62 or more little necks, or 44–62 cherrystones, or 28–44 mediums, or 28 or fewer chowders)	(736)	(54.0)	22.7	1.67
1 gallon (approx. 8 lb.; approx. 250 or more little necks, or 175–250 cherrystones, 110–175 mediums, or 110 or fewer chowders)	2904	214.2	22.7	1.67
1 pound meat and liquid	222	19.1	13.9	1.19
1 pound meat only	363	26.8	22.7	1.67
Hen Clams (*Mactra*. Based on data from East Asia)				
RAW:				
Meat weighed in shell [refuse, approx. 72%: shell and liquid], 1 pound as purchased	100	2.7	6.2	0.17
Edible portion, 1 pound	377	9.5	23.5	0.60
Little Neck Clams, see Hard Clams				
Razor Clams, Solen (*Solenidae*)				
RAW:				
As purchased, 1 pound [refuse, approx. 49%: shell and liquid]	109	4.5	6.8	0.28
Edible portion, 1 pound	209	8.6	13.0	0.54
Round Clams, see Hard Clams				
Short Neck Clams (*Venerupis semi-decussata*. Based on data from East Asia)				
RAW:				
As purchased, 1 pound [refuse, approx. 76%: shell and liquid]	64	2.7	4.0	0.17
Edible portion, 1 pound	267	11.3	16.7	0.70
Short Neck Clams (based on data from Japan)				
RAW:				
Edible portion, 1 pound	277	11.4	17.3	0.71
PREPARED "TSUKUDANI" STYLE:				
All-edible, 1 pound	1075	132.2	67.2	8.26
Soft Clams				
RAW:				
As purchased:				
Meat and liquid weighed in shell [refuse, approx. 42%: shell], 1 pound	142	5.3	8.9	0.33
Meat in shell [refuse, approx. 65%: shell and liquid]	130	2.1	8.1	0.13

	UNIT Cal.	UNIT Carb.	1 OZ., BY WT. Cal.	1 OZ., BY WT. Carb.
Edible portion:				
Meat of 1 small clam, approx. 0.26 oz. (4g/tr/1g/81%/10mg)	6	0.1	23.3	0.37
Meat of 1 medium clam, approx. 0.3 oz.	7	0.1	23.3	0.37
Meat of 1 large clam, approx. 0.4 oz.	10	0.2	23.3	0.37
1 cup (approx. 8 oz.; 31 small clams, or 27 medium clams, or 19 large clams)	186	3.0	23.3	0.37
1 pint (approx. 1 lb.; approx. 62 or more small clams, or 38–62 medium clams, or 38 or fewer large clams)	(372)	(6.0)	23.3	0.37
1 quart (approx. 2 lb.; approx. 125 or more small clams, or 75 to 125 medium clams, or 75 or fewer large clams)	(744)	(12.0)	23.3	0.37
1 gallon (approx. 8 lb.; approx. 500 or more small clams, or 300 to 500 medium clams, or 300 or fewer large clams)	2977	47.2	23.3	0.37
1 pound meat and liquid (2g/1g/tr/86%/na)	245	9.1	15.3	0.57
1 pound meat only	372	5.9	23.3	0.37
CLIMBING PERCH, see under PERCH				
COCKLES, SAND (*Hemidonax donaciforme.* Based on data from East Asia)				
RAW:				
As purchased, 1 pound [refuse, approx. 88%: shell and liquid]	41	0.0	2.6	0.00
Edible portion, 1 pound	368	0.0	23.0	0.00
COD (see also LINGCOD and TOMCOD)				
RAW:				
Weighed whole [refuse, approx. 69%: head, tail, fins, entrails, scales, bones, and skin], 1 pound as purchased	110	0.0	6.9	0.00
Edible portion, 1 pound (5g/0g/tr/81%/20mg)	354	0.0	22.1	0.00
BROILED:				
Based on USDA data; cooked with unspecified amount of butter or margarine:				
1 cod fillet, raw dimensions: 5″ long (with ends rolled back) × 2½″ wide (at widest point) × ⅞″ thick (at thickest point). (yield: approx. 2.3 oz.)	111	0.0	48.2	0.00
1 cod steak, raw dimensions: 5½″ long (with ends rolled back) × 4″ wide (at widest point) × 1¼″ thick (at thickest point). (yield: approx. 8.3 oz. weighed with bone) [refuse, approx. 12%: bone]	352	0.0	42.4	0.00
1 pound of broiled cod fillet (8g/0g/2g/65%/31mg)	771	0.0	48.2	0.00
DEHYDRATED, LIGHTLY SALTED:				
1 cup, shredded (approx. 1.5 oz.) (23g/0g/1g/12%/2297mg)	158	0.0	106.3	0.00
1 pound (approx. 10.8 cups, shredded)	1701	0.0	106.3	0.00
DRIED, SALTED:				
1 piece, approx. 5½″ long × 1½″ wide (at widest point) × ½″ thick (at thickest point), approx. 2.8 oz.	104	0.0	36.9	0.00
1 pound (8g/0g/tr/52%/na)	590	0.0	36.9	0.00
CONGERS, PIKE (*Muraenespcodae*)				
RAW:				
Edible portion, 1 pound (5g/tr/tr/79%/na)	386	3.6	24.1	0.23
CRABS				
Crabs, from data including Blue, Dungeness, Rock, and King				
STEAMED:				
Weighed and cooked in shell [refuse, approx. 52%: shell], 1 pound	202	1.1	12.6	0.07
Edible portion:				
1 cup, pieces (approx. 5.5 oz.)	144	0.8	26.3	0.14
1 cup, flaked (approx. 4.4 oz.)	116	0.6	26.3	0.14
1 pound (5g/tr/1g/79%/na)	422	2.3	26.3	0.14
Blue Crabs (*Callinectes sapidus*)				
RAW:				
Edible portion, 1 pound (5g/tr/tr/81%/na)	370	5.7	23.1	0.35
Deep Sea Crabs (*Neptunnis*)				
RAW:				
Edible portion, 1 pound (5g/tr/tr/78%/na)	(342)	(1.4)	(21.4)	(0.09)
Dungeness Crabs (*Cancer magister*)				
RAW:				
Edible portion, 1 pound (5g/tr/tr/81%/na)	(386)	na	(24.1)	trace
King Crabs (*Paralithodes camtschatica*)				
RAW:				
Edible portion, 1 pound (5g/tr/tr/81%/na)	(359)	na	(22.4)	trace
Samoan Crabs (*Scylla serrata*)				
RAW:				
Edible portion, 1 pound (4g/tr/1g/80%/na)	(400)	(2.7)	(24.9)	(0.17)

	UNIT Cal.	UNIT Carb.	1 OZ., BY WT. Cal.	1 OZ., BY WT. Carb.
CRAB ROE				
Crab Roe (based on data from Japan)				
SALTED:				
All-edible, 1 pound	1094	65.8	68.4	4.11
Blue Sea Crab Roe (*Neptune; scylla.* Based on data from Africa)				
SALTED:				
All-edible, 1 pound	1112	65.8	69.5	4.11
CRAPPIE, WHITE				
RAW:				
Edible portion, 1 pound	358	0.0	22.4	0.00
CRAWFISH, see CRAYFISH				
CRAYFISH (Crawfish)				
Crayfish, Freshwater (Spiny Lobster)				
RAW:				
In shell [refuse, approx. 88%: shell], 1 pound as purchased	39	0.7	2.4	0.04
Edible portion, 1 pound	327	5.4	20.4	0.34
Crayfish, type unspecified (based on data from Great Britain)				
BOILED:				
Edible portion, 1 pound	403	0.0	25.2	0.00
CROAKER				
Atlantic Croaker				
RAW:				
Whole [refuse, approx. 66%: head, tail, fins, skin, entrails, and bones], 1 pound raw as purchased	148	0.0	9.3	0.00
Edible portion 1 pound	435	0.0	27.2	0.00
White Croaker				
RAW:				
Edible portion, 1 pound	381	0.0	23.8	0.00
Yellowfin Croaker				
RAW:				
Edible portion, 1 pound	404	0.0	25.3	0.00
CROCODILE, Narrow snouted (*Gavialis Gangeticus Gmelin.* Based on data from India)				
RAW:				
Edible portion, 1 pound	395	1.4	24.7	0.09
CUSK				
DRAWN:				
As purchased, 1 pound raw [refuse, approx. 42%: head, tail, fins, skin, and bones]	197	0.0	12.3	0.00
RAW:				
Edible portion, 1 pound	341	0.0	21.3	0.00
COOKED:				
Steamed, 1 pound (7g/0g/tr/74%/21mg)	481	0.0	30.1	0.00
DOGFISH ROE (*Squalus.* Based on data from Africa)				
RAW:				
All-edible, 1 pound	1453	2.3	90.8	0.14
DOGFISH, SPINY (Grayfish)				
RAW:				
Edible portion, 1 pound	708	0.0	44.3	0.00
DOG'S TEETH (*Dentex*)				
RAW:				
As purchased, 1 pound [refuse, approx. 50%: fins, scales, and entrails]	250	0.0	15.6	0.00
Edible portion, 1 pound	504	0.0	31.5	0.00
DOLLY VARDEN TROUT (see also TROUT)				
Dolly Varden from unspecified water				
RAW:				
Edible portion, 1 pound	653	0.0	40.8	0.00

	UNIT Cal.	UNIT Carb.	1 OZ., BY WT. Cal.	1 OZ., BY WT. Carb.
Dolly Varden *(Salvelinas malma)*, caught in Lake Aleknagik, Alaska				
RAW:				
Edible portion, 1 pound	625	0.0	39.1	0.00
DOLPHIN				
Dolphin *(Coryphaena equisetis)*				
RAW:				
Edible portion, 1 pound	428	0.0	26.7	0.00
Dolphin (*Coryphaena hippurus.* Based on data from East Asia)				
RAW;				
Edible portion, 1 pound	400	0.0	25.0	0.00
DORY, see JOHN-DORY				
DOVER SOLE, see under SOLE				
DRUM				
Freshwater Drum				
RAW:				
Weighed whole [refuse, approx. 74%: head, tail, fins, skin, bones, and entrails], 1 pound as purchased	143	0.0	8.9	0.00
Edible portion, 1 pound	549	0.0	34.3	0.00
Red Drum (Redfish)				
RAW:				
Whole [refuse, approx. 59%: head, tail, fins, skin, bones, and entrails], 1 pound as purchased	149	0.0	9.3	0.00
Edible portion, 1 pound	363	0.0	22.7	0.00
EEL				
American Eel				
Edible portion, 1 pound	363	0.0	22.7	0.00
RAW:				
Weighed with head, skin, and entrails removed [refuse: approx. 24%: bones], 1 pound as purchased	803	0.0	50.2	0.00
Edible portion, 1 pound	1057	0.0	66.1	0.00
Conger Eel *(Congridae)*				
RAW:				
Edible portion, 1 pound	501	(0.0)	31.3	(0.00)
Freshwater Eel *(Anguillidae)*				
RAW:				
Edible portion, 1 pound	1116	(0.0)	69.7	(0.00)
Smoked Eel (based on data from Denmark)				
RAW:				
Edible portion, 1 pound	1588	0.0	99.2	0.00
COOKED (method unspecified):				
Edible portion, 1 pound	1361	0.0	85.1	0.00
Snake Eel *(Ophichthidae)*				
RAW:				
Edible portion, 1 pound	369	2.7	23.1	0.17
Swamp Eel (*Synbrachus bengalensis.* Based on data from East Asia)				
RAW:				
As purchased, 1 pound [refuse, approx. 44%: head, entrails, and bones]	218	0.0	13.6	0.00
Edible portion, 1 pound	390	0.0	24.4	0.00
EULACHON (see also SMELT)				
RAW:				
Edible portion, 1 pound	535	0.0	33.4	0.00
FIDDLEFISH, see Sand Shark under SHARK				
FINNAN HADDIE (Smoked Haddock)				
RAW:				
As purchased, 1 pound	468	0.0	29.3	0.00
FISH SAUSAGE, see the SAUSAGES & COLD CUTS chapter				
FLAT FISHES, see under individual names, such as FLOUNDER and SOLE				

	UNIT Cal.	UNIT Carb.	1 OZ., BY WT. Cal.	1 OZ., BY WT. Carb.
FLATHEAD (*Platycephalus indicus.* Based on data from India)				
RAW:				
As purchased, 1 pound [refuse, approx. 46%: bones, fins, scales, and entrails]	237	0.0	14.8	0.00
Edible portion, 1 pound	435	0.0	27.2	0.00
FLOUNDER				
Flounder, type not specified				
RAW:				
Weighed whole [refuse, approx. 67%: head, tail, fins, skin, entrails, and bones], 1 pound as purchased	118	0.0	7.4	0.00
Edible portion, 1 pound	369	0.0	21.1	0.00
BAKED:				
Based on USDA data; cooked with unspecified amount of butter or margarine:				
1 baked flounder fillet dimensions: approx. 6″ long × 2½″ wide (at the widest point) × ¼″ thick (at thickest point), (approx. 2 oz.) (9g/0/2g/58%/67mg)	115	0.0	57.2	0.00
1 baked flounder fillet dimensions: approx. 8¼″ long × 2¾″ wide (at the widest point) × ¼″ thick (at the thickest point), approx. 3.5 oz.)	202	0.0	57.2	0.00
1 pound of baked flounder fillets	916	0.0	57.2	0.00
Blackback Flounder *(Pseudopleuronectes americanus)*, caught in New England waters				
RAW:				
Edible portion, 1 pound	347	0.0	21.7	0.00
Dabs *(Hippoglossoides platessoides)*, caught in New England waters				
Caught in Autumn				
RAW:				
Edible portion, 1 pound	329	0.0	20.6	0.00
Caught in Spring				
RAW:				
Edible portion, 1 pound	333	0.0	20.8	0.00
Greyback Flounder *(Glyptocephalus cynoglossus)*, caught in New England Waters				
RAW:				
Edible portion, 1 pound	296	0.0	18.5	0.00
Winter Flounder *(Pseudopleuronectes americanus)*				
RAW:				
Edible portion, 1 pound	(348)	0.0	(21.8)	0.00
Yellowtail Flounder *(Limanda ferruginea)*, caught in New England waters				
RAW:				
Edible portion, 1 pound	323	0.0	20.2	0.00
FLYING FISH and HALFBEAKS *(Exocoetidae)*				
RAW:				
Edible portion, 1 pound	419	1.8	26.2	0.11
FROG'S LEGS				
RAW:				
As purchased, 1 pound [refuse, approx. 35%: bones]	215	0.0	13.4	0.00
Edible portion, 1 pound	331	0.0	20.7	0.00
Frog's Legs, "Grenouille" or "Cuisses de Grenouille" (based on data from France)				
RAW:				
Edible portion, 1 pound	308	0.0	19.3	0.00
COOKED (method unspecified):				
Edible portion, 1 pound	(308)	0.0	(19.3)	0.00
GIZZARD SHAD, see under SHAD				
GLOBEFISH (*Sphaeroides.* Based on data from East Asia)				
RAW:				
As purchased, 1 pound [refuse, approx. 48%: bones, scales, fins, and entrails]	218	0.0	13.6	0.00
Edible portion, 1 pound	417	0.0	26.1	0.00
GOATFISH				
Goatfish *(Mullidae)*				
RAW:				
Edible portion, 1 pound	482	0.0	30.1	0.00

	UNIT Cal.	UNIT Carb.	1 OZ., BY WT. Cal.	1 OZ., BY WT. Carb.
Dwarf Goatfish *(Upeneus parvus)*				
RAW:				
Edible portion, 1 pound	523	0.0	32.7	0.00
GOBIES *(Gobildae)*				
RAW:				
Edible portion, 1 pound	340	1.4	21.3	0.09
GOLDFISH				
Goldfish (based on data from Africa)				
RAW:				
Edible portion, 1 pound	653	0.0	40.8	0.00
Goldfish (*Carassius auratus.* Based on data from East Asia)				
RAW:				
As purchased, 1 pound [refuse, approx. 60%: bones, scales, head, and entrails]	141	0.0	8.8	0.00
Edible portion, 1 pound	354	0.0	22.1	0.00
GOOSEFISH *(Lophilidae)*				
RAW:				
Edible portion, 1 pound	400	1.4	25.0	0.09
GROUPER				
RAW:				
Weighed whole [refuse, approx. 57%: head, fins, tail, bones, skin, and entrails], 1 pound as purchased	170	0.0	10.6	0.00
Edible portion, 1 pound	395	0.0	24.7	0.00
GRUNTS *(Pomadasyidae)*				
RAW:				
Edible portion, 1 pound	396	10.0	24.8	0.62
HADDOCK				
RAW:				
Whole [refuse, approx. 52%: head, tail, fins, bones, skin, and entrails], 1 pound as purchased	172	0.0	10.8	0.00
Edible portion, 1 pound	359	0.0	22.4	0.00
SMOKED:				
Edible portion, 1 pound (7g/0g/tr/73%/tr)	467	0.0	29.2	0.00
PAN-FRIED OR OVEN-FRIED:				
Based on USDA data; dipped in unspecified quantities of eggs, milk, and breadcrumbs:				
1 pound of raw haddock fillets, cooked (yield: approx. 12.8 oz.) (6g/2g/2g/66%/tr)	597	21.0	46.8	1.65
1 pound of fried haddock fillets	748	26.4	46.8	1.68
HAKE				
Hake from data that include Pacific, Squirrel, and Silver Hake or Whiting				
RAW:				
Whole [refuse, approx. 57%: head, tail, fins, skin, entrails, and bones], 1 pound as purchased	144	0.0	9.0	0.00
Edible portion, 1 pound	336	0.0	21.0	0.00
Squirrel Hake *(Urophyces Chuss)*, caught in New England waters in fall				
RAW:				
Edible portion, 1 pound	326	0.0	20.4	0.00
HALIBUT				
Halibut from data that include Atlantic and Pacific Halibut				
RAW:				
Weighed whole [refuse, approx. 41%: head, tail, fins, entrails, scales, bones, and skin], 1 pound as purchased	268	0.0	16.7	0.00
Edible portion, 1 pound	454	0.0	28.4	0.00
SMOKED:				
Edible portion, 1 pound (6g/0g/4g/49%/na)	1016	0.0	63.6	0.00
BROILED:				
Based on USDA data; cooked with unspecified amount of butter or margarine:				
1 pound of raw halibut fillets, cooked (yield: approx. 12.9 oz.) (7g/0g/2g/67%/tr)	624	0.0	48.5	0.00
1 pound of broiled halibut fillets	776	0.0	48.5	0.00
Atlantic Halibut *(Hippoglossus hippoglossus)*				
RAW:				
Edible portion, 1 pound	572	0.0	35.7	0.00

	UNIT Cal.	UNIT Carb.	1 OZ., BY WT. Cal.	1 OZ., BY WT. Carb.
California Halibut				
RAW:				
Edible portion, 1 pound	440	0.0	27.5	0.00
Greenland Halibut				
RAW:				
Whole [refuse, approx. 48%: head, tail, fins, skin, bones, and entrails], 1 pound as purchased	344	0.0	21.5	0.00
Edible portion, 1 pound	663	0.0	41.4	0.00
Pacific Halibut *(Hippoglossus stenolepis)*				
RAW:				
Edible portion, 1 pound	(428)	0.0	(26.7)	0.00
HAWS, SCARLET				
RAW:				
As purchased, 1 pound [refuse, approx. 20%: core]	316	75.5	19.8	4.72
Edible portion, 1 pound	395	94.4	22.7	5.90
HERRING (see also LAKE HERRING)				
PICKLED (Bismarck type):				
Edible portion, 1 pound	1012	0.0	63.3	0.00
SALTED OR BRINED:				
Edible portion, 1 pound	990	0.0	61.9	0.00
SMOKED:				
Bloaters:				
Edible portion, 1 pound	890	0.0	55.6	0.00
Hard:				
Edible portion, 1 pound	1362	0.0	85.1	0.00
Kippered:				
Edible portion, 1 pound	958	0.0	59.9	0.00
Herring (based on data from Denmark)				
RAW:				
Edible portion, 1 pound	680	0.0	42.5	0.00
PICKLED:				
Edible portion, 1 pound	680	0.0	42.5	0.00
SMOKED:				
Edible portion, 1 pound	862	0.0	53.9	0.00
Herring (based on data from Japan)				
RAW:				
Edible portion, 1 pound	1082	2.2	67.6	0.13
DRIED:				
Edible portion, 1 pound	1736	2.7	108.5	0.17
DRIED, RECONSTITUTED:				
Edible portion, 1 pound	1866	4.5	116.6	0.28
SALTED:				
Edible portion, 1 pound	838	1.1	52.4	0.07
SMOKED:				
Edible portion, 1 pound	1412	4.5	88.3	0.28
Atlantic Herring				
RAW:				
Weighed whole [refuse, approx. 49%: head, tail, fins, entrails, skin, and bones], 1 pound as purchased	407	0.0	25.4	0.00
Edible portion, 1 pound	799	0.0	49.9	0.00
Fimbriated Herring *(Sardinella fimbriata)*				
RAW:				
Edible portion, 1 pound	464	7.7	29.0	0.48
Lake Trout Herring *(Coregonus artedii)* (see also Lake Trout)				
RAW:				
Edible portion, 1 pound	(476)	0.0	(29.7)	0.00
Pacific Herring				
RAW:				
Edible portion, 1 pound	(718)	0.0	(44.9)	0.00
HERRING ROE				
Herring Roe (based on data from East Asia)				
RAW:				
All-edible, 1 pound	663	1.8	41.4	0.11
DRIED:				
All-edible, 1 pound	1752	1.8	109.5	0.11
Herring Roe (based on data from Japan)				
RAW:				
Edible portion, 1 pound	631	1.8	39.4	0.11
DRIED:				
Edible portion, 1 pound	1671	1.8	104.4	0.11

	UNIT Cal.	UNIT Carb.	1 OZ., BY WT. Cal.	1 OZ., BY WT. Carb.
HILSA (*Clupea ilisha.* Based on data from India)				
Edible portion, 1 pound	1239	13.2	77.4	0.82
HORSE MACKEREL (*Caranx melamprgus.* Based on data from India)				
RAW:				
As purchased, 1 pound [refuse, approx. 34%: bones, fins, and entrails]	340	0.0	21.8	0.00
Edible portion, 1 pound	518	0.0	32.4	0.00
JACK MACKEREL (*Trachurus trachurus*)				
RAW:				
Edible portion, 1 pound	(635)	(0.0)	(39.7)	(0.00)
JACKS (*Caranx*)				
RAW:				
Edible portion, 1 pound	(438)	(2.7)	(2.7)	(0.17)
JELLYFISH, MEDUSA (*Rhopilema esculenta.* Based on data from East Asia)				
RAW:				
Edible portion, 1 pound	136	13.2	8.5	0.83
SALTED:				
Edible portion, 1 pound	150	10.0	9.4	0.63
JOHN-DORY				
John-Dory (*Zeidae*)				
RAW:				
Edible portion, 1 pound	363	0.0	22.7	0.00
John-Dory (*Zeus Faber.* Based on data from Africa)				
RAW:				
Edible portion, 1 pound	540	0.0	33.8	0.00
KINGFISH				
Kingfish, Southern, Gulf and Northern (see also WHITING)				
RAW:				
Weighed whole [refuse, approx. 56%: entrails, head, fins, skin, and bones], 1 pound as purchased	210	0.0	13.1	0.00
Edible portion, 1 pound	477	0.0	29.8	0.00
Kingfish (*Scomberomorus commersion.* Based on data from East Asia)				
DRIED:				
As purchased, 1 pound [refuse, approx. 24%: bones]	649	1.4	40.5	0.09
Edible portion, 1 pound	854	1.8	53.3	0.11
LADY FISH (*Megalops cyprinoides.* Based on data from East Asia)				
RAW:				
As purchased, 1 pound [refuse, approx. 52%: bones, entrails, fins, scales]	222	0.0	13.9	0.00
Edible portion, 1 pound	463	0.0	28.9	0.00
LADY VENDI (based on data from India)				
RAW:				
Edible portion, 1 pound	418	15.0	26.1	0.94
LAKE HERRING (Cisco) (see also CISCO; HERRING; and WHITEFISH, LAKE)				
RAW:				
Weighed whole [refuse, approx. 48%: entrails, scales, head, fins, and bones], 1 pound as purchased	226	0.0	14.1	0.00
Edible portion, 1 pound	436	0.0	27.2	0.00
LAKE TROUT (see also WHITEFISH, LAKE)				
Lake Trout (see also HERRING)				
RAW:				
Weighed drawn [refuse, approx. 63%: head, fins, and bones], 1 pound as purchased	282	0.0	17.6	0.00
Edible portion, 1 pound	763	0.0	47.7	0.00

	UNIT Cal.	UNIT Carb.	1 OZ., BY WT. Cal.	1 OZ., BY WT. Carb.
Lake Trout, Siscowet				
Weighing less than 6.5 pounds when caught:				
RAW:				
Weighed whole [refuse, approx. 63%: entrails, head, fins, skin, and bones], 1 pound as purchased	404	0.0	25.3	0.00
Edible portion, 1 pound	1094	0.0	68.4	0.00
Weighing 6.5 pounds and over when caught:				
RAW:				
Weighed whole [refuse, approx. 64%: entrails, head, fins, skin, and bones], 1 pound as purchased	856	0.0	53.5	0.00
Edible portion, 1 pound	2379	0.0	148.7	0.00
LAMPREY (based on data from Japan)				
RAW:				
Edible portion, 1 pound	1149	1.4	71.8	0.09
DRIED:				
Edible portion, 1 pound	1843	2.3	115.2	0.14
LEATHERJACKET				
Leatherjacket (*Scomberoides lysan*)				
RAW:				
Edible portion, 1 pound	(494)	(1.4)	(30.9)	(0.09)
Leatherjacket (*Scomberoides lysan.* Based on data from East Asia)				
RAW:				
As purchased, 1 pound [refuse, approx. 40%: bones, skin, and entrails]	295	0.0	18.4	0.00
Edible portion, 1 pound	490	0.0	30.6	0.00
LINGCOD				
RAW:				
Weighed whole [refuse, approx. 66%: head, tail, fins, entrails, scales, bones, and skin], 1 pound as purchased	130	0.0	8.1	0.00
Edible portion, 1 pound	381	0.0	23.8	0.00
LIZARDFISH				
Lizardfish (*Saurida tumbil*)				
RAW:				
Edible portion, 1 pound	(396)		(24.8)	
Lizardfish (*Saurida undosquamis*)				
RAW:				
Edible portion, 1 pound	(399)	(4.1)	(25.0)	(0.26)
LOBSTER, NORTHERN				
RAW:				
Weighed whole [refuse, approx. 74%: shell], 1 pound raw as purchased	107	0.6	6.7	0.04
Edible portion, 1 pound	412	2.3	25.8	0.14
COOKED (method unspecified):				
Edible portion, 1 pound (5g/tr/tr/77%/59mg)	431	1.4	26.9	0.09
LOBSTER, SPINY, see under CRAYFISH				
LONGJAW CISCO, see CISCO, LONGJAW				
LUNGFISH (*Protopterus.* Based on data from Africa)				
RAW:				
Edible portion, 1 pound	327	0.0	20.4	0.00
SMOKED, DRIED:				
Edible portion, 1 pound	1707	0.0	106.7	0.00
MACKEREL (see also HORSE MACKEREL and JACK MACKEREL)				
SALTED:				
Edible portion, 1 pound (5g/0g/7g/43%/na)	1383	0.0	86.4	0.00
SMOKED:				
Edible portion, 1 pound (7g/0g/4g/59%/na)	994	0.0	62.1	0.00
SMOKED: (based on data from Denmark):				
Edible portion, 1 pound	998	0.0	62.4	0.00
SMOKED: (based on data from France)				
Edible portion, 1 pound	966	0.0	60.4	0.00

Food	UNIT Cal.	UNIT Carb.	1 OZ., BY WT. Cal.	1 OZ., BY WT. Carb.
Atka Mackerel (*Pleurogrammus azonus.* Based on data from East Asia)				
RAW:				
As purchased, 1 pound [refuse, approx. 55%: entrails, scales, fins, and bones]	227	0.0	14.2	0.00
Edible portion, 1 pound	513	0.0	32.1	0.00
Atlantic Mackerel				
RAW:				
Weighed whole [refuse, approx. 46%: head, tail, fins, bones, skin, and entrails], 1 pound as purchased	468	0.0	29.2	0.00
Edible portion, 1 pound (6g/0g/4g/67%/na)	867	0.0	54.2	0.00
Cape Mackerel (*Scomber japonicus.* Based on data from Africa)				
RAW:				
Edible portion, 1 pound	776	0.0	48.5	0.00
Frigate Mackerel (based on data from Japan)				
RAW:				
Edible portion, 1 pound	549	1.4	34.3	0.09
Horse Mackerel, see HORSE				
Indian Mackerel				
RAW:				
Edible portion, 1 pound	443	9.5	27.7	0.60
Jack Mackerel, see JACK				
Rake-Gilled Mackerel (*Rastrelliger.* Based on data from East Asia)				
RAW:				
As purchased, 1 pound [refuse, approx. 43%: bones, fins, and entrails]	254	0.0	15.9	0.00
Edible portion, 1 pound	445	0.0	27.8	0.00
DRIED, SALTED:				
As purchased, 1 pound [refuse, approx. 44%: bones, fins, and entrails]	586	0.0	36.6	0.00
Edible portion, 1 pound	1044	0.0	65.3	0.00
SMOKED:				
As purchased, 1 pound [refuse, approx. 45%: bones, fins, and entrails]	359	0.0	22.4	0.00
Edible portion, 1 pound	658	0.0	41.1	0.00
Spanish Mackerel				
RAW:				
Edible portion, 1 pound (6g/0g/3g/69%/19 mg)	804	0.0	50.2	0.00
Spanish Mackerel (*Scomberomorus commerson.* Based on data from East Asia)				
RAW:				
As purchased, 1 pound [refuse, approx. 35%: bones, scales, fins, and entrails]	304	0.0	19.0	0.00
Edible portion, 1 pound	468	0.0	29.2	0.00
DRIED:				
As purchased, 1 pound [refuse, approx. 24%: bones]	649	1.4	40.5	0.09
Edible portion, 1 pound	854	1.8	53.3	0.11
MARLIN				
Marlin (*Istiophorus.* Based on data from East Asia)				
RAW:				
As purchased, 1 pound [refuse, approx. 35%: bones, fins, scales, and entrails]	381	0.0	23.8	0.00
Edible portion, 1 pound	586	0.0	36.6	0.00
Marlin (based on data from Japan)				
RAW:				
Edible portion, 1 pound	581	1.4	36.3	0.09
MEDUSA, see JELLYFISH				
MILKFISH (*Chanos chanos.* Based on data from Africa)				
RAW:				
As purchased, 1 pound [refuse, approx. 31%: bones, scales, fins, and entrails]	431	0.0	26.9	0.00
Edible portion, 1 pound	627	0.0	39.2	0.00
DRIED, SALTED:				
Edible portion, 1 pound	1444	0.0	90.3	0.00
SMOKED:				
Edible portion, 1 pound	908	0.0	56.8	0.00
MOJARRAS (*Gerreidae*)				
RAW:				
Edible portion, 1 pound	381		23.8	

Food	UNIT Cal.	UNIT Carb.	1 OZ., BY WT. Cal.	1 OZ., BY WT. Carb.
MUDFISH (*Arius.* Based on data from Africa) (see also CATFISH)				
RAW:				
Edible portion, 1 pound	409	0.0	25.5	0.00
DRIED:				
Edible portion, 1 pound	1643	0.0	102.7	0.00
Eaten Whole:				
DRIED:				
1 pound	1471	0.0	91.9	0.00
VERY DRY:				
1 pound	1966	0.0	122.8	0.00
SALTED:				
1 pound	949	0.0	59.3	0.00
SMOKED:				
1 pound	1439	0.0	89.9	0.00
DRIED, SMOKED:				
1 pound	1834	0.0	114.6	0.00
MUDSUCKER (*Labeo.* Based on data from Africa)				
RAW:				
Edible portion, 1 pound	390	0.0	24.4	0.00
DRIED:				
Edible portion, 1 pound	1698	0.0	106.1	0.00
DRIED, SMOKED:				
Edible portion, 1 pound	1594	0.0	99.6	0.00
MULLET				
RAW:				
Edible portion, 1 pound	582	10.0	36.4	0.62
Mullet (*Mugil.* Based on data from Africa)				
RAW:				
Edible portion, 1 pound	522	0.0	32.6	0.00
DRIED, SALTED:				
Edible portion, 1 pound	1276	0.0	79.8	0.00
DRIED, SMOKED:				
Edible portion, 1 pound	1571	0.0	98.2	0.00
BOILED:				
Edible portion, 1 pound	667	0.0	41.7	0.00
Red Mullet (*Mullus barbalus*)				
RAW:				
Edible portion, 1 pound	577	0.0	36.0	0.00
Striped Mullet				
RAW:				
Weighed whole [refuse, approx. 47%: head, tail, fins, bones, skin, and entrails], 1 pound as purchased	351	0.0	22.0	0.00
Edible portion, 1 pound	663	0.0	41.4	0.00
MULLET ROE (based on data from Japan)				
SALTED, SMOKED:				
All-edible, 1 pound	1876	20.9	117.3	1.31
MUSKELLUNGE				
RAW:				
Weighed whole [refuse, approx. 51%: head, tail, fins, skin, bones, and entrails], 1 pound as purchased	242	0.0	15.0	0.00
Edible portion, 1 pound	494	0.0	30.9	0.00
MUSSELS				
Mussels (based on data from France)				
RAW:				
Edible portion, 1 pound	331	10.0	20.7	0.62
COOKED (method unspecified):				
Edible portion, 1 pound	304	5.0	19.0	0.31
Atlantic and Pacific Mussels				
RAW:				
As purchased:				
Meat and liquid weighed in shell [refuse, approx. 49%: shell and beard], 1 pound as purchased	153	7.2	9.6	0.45
Meat weighed in shell [refuse, approx. 71%: shell, beard, and liquid], 1 pound as purchased	125	4.3	7.8	0.27

	UNIT Cal.	UNIT Carb.	1 OZ., BY WT. Cal.	1 OZ., BY WT. Carb.
Edible portion:				
Meat and liquid, edible portion, 1 pound (3g/1g/tr/84%/na)	300	14.1	18.7	0.88
Meat only, edible portion, 1 pound (4g/1g/1g/79%/82 mg)	431	15.0	26.9	0.94
Blue Mussels (*Mytilus viridis.* Based on data from India)				
RAW:				
Edible portion, 1 pound	327	16.3	20.4	1.02
Freshwater Mussels (*Corbicula.* Based on data from East Asia)				
RAW:				
As purchased, 1 pound [refuse, approx. 64%: shell]	132	11.8	8.3	0.74
Edible portion, 1 pound	372	32.7	23.3	2.04
Horse or Sea Mussels (*Mytilus.* Based on data from East Asia)				
RAW:				
Edible portion, 1 pound	227	7.3	14.2	0.45
DRIED:				
Edible portion, 1 pound	1661	62.6	103.8	3.91

MUTI (based on data from India)

	UNIT Cal.	UNIT Carb.	1 OZ., BY WT. Cal.	1 OZ., BY WT. Carb.
DRIED:				
Edible portion, 1 pound	1308	13.6	81.7	0.85

MYSIS (based on data from Japan)

	UNIT Cal.	UNIT Carb.	1 OZ., BY WT. Cal.	1 OZ., BY WT. Carb.
RAW:				
Edible portion, 1 pound	445	4.1	27.8	0.26
DRIED:				
Edible portion, 1 pound	1271	10.0	79.4	0.63
PREPARED "SHIOKARA" STYLE:				
Edible portion, 1 pound	259	1.4	16.2	0.09
PREPARED "TSUKUDANI" STYLE:				
Edible portion, 1 pound	935	104.0	58.4	6.53

NEEDLEFISH

	UNIT Cal.	UNIT Carb.	1 OZ., BY WT. Cal.	1 OZ., BY WT. Carb.
Needlefish *(Belonidae)*				
RAW:				
Edible portion, 1 pound	383	(0.0)	24.0	(0.00)
Needlefish (*Tylosurus crocodilus.* Based on data from East Asia)				
RAW:				
As purchased, 1 pound [refuse, approx. 36%: fins, bones, and entrails]	354	0.0	22.1	0.00
Edible portion, 1 pound	554	0.0	34.6	0.00

OCEAN PERCH, see under PERCH

OCTOPUS

	UNIT Cal.	UNIT Carb.	1 OZ., BY WT. Cal.	1 OZ., BY WT. Carb.
RAW:				
Edible portion, 1 pound	331	0.0	20.7	0.00
Common Octopus (*Octopus vulgaris.* Based on data from East Asia)				
RAW:				
As purchased, 1 pound [refuse, approx. 18%: bone and viscera]	254	0.0	15.9	0.00
Edible portion, 1 pound	309	0.0	19.3	0.00
DRIED:				
Edible portion, 1 pound	1811	0.0	113.2	0.00
Large Octopus (*Octopus.* Based on data from East Asia)				
RAW:				
As purchased, 1 pound [refuse, approx. 12%: bone and viscera]	254	0.0	15.9	0.00
Edible portion, 1 pound	291	0.0	18.2	0.00

OFFAL, see after ZEBRA FISH

OPOSSUM SHRIMP (see also PRAWNS and SHRIMP)

	UNIT Cal.	UNIT Carb.	1 OZ., BY WT. Cal.	1 OZ., BY WT. Carb.
Opossum Shrimp (*Neomysis japonica.* Based on data from East Asia)				
RAW:				
Edible portion, 1 pound	445	4.1	27.8	0.26
DRIED:				
Edible portion, 1 pound	1271	10.0	79.5	0.62
Opossum Shrimp, Processed (based on data from Japan)				
PREPARED "SHIOKARA" STYLE:				
Edible portion, 1 pound	259	1.4	16.2	0.09
PREPARED "TSUKUDANI" STYLE:				
Edible portion, 1 pound	935	104.4	58.4	6.53

OYSTERS

	UNIT Cal.	UNIT Carb.	1 OZ., BY WT. Cal.	1 OZ., BY WT. Carb.
Oysters (*Ostrea.* Based on data from East Asia)				
RAW:				
As purchased, 1 pound [refuse, approx. 82%: shell and liquid]	59	5.0	3.7	0.31
Edible portion, 1 pound	322	26.7	20.1	1.67
DRIED:				
Edible portion, 1 pound	1516	151.6	94.8	9.48
Oysters (based on data from Singapore)				
DRIED:				
Edible portion, 1 pound	1597	107.0	99.8	6.69
Oysters (*Ostrea.* Based on data from Korea)				
SOUSED:				
Edible portion, 1 pound	499	10.9	31.2	0.68
Blue Point Oysters *(Crassostrea virginica)*				
RAW:				
Edible portion, 1 pound	(246)	15.0	(15.4)	0.94
Eastern Oysters				
RAW:				
Weighed in shell [refuse, approx. 90%: shell and liquid], 1 pound as purchased	30	1.5	1.9	0.10
Meat only, edible portion, 1 pound (2g/1g/1g/85%/21 mg)	300	15.4	18.7	0.96
Pacific and Western Oysters *(Olympia)*				
RAW:				
Edible portion, 1 pound (3g/2g/1g/79%/na)	413	29.1	25.8	1.82
FRIED:				
1 Select (medium) oyster, approx. 3" × 1½" (yield: approx. 1¾" × 1", approx. 0.5 oz.) (2g/5g/4g/55%/58 mg)	27	2.1	54.0	4.20

PARROTFISH

	UNIT Cal.	UNIT Carb.	1 OZ., BY WT. Cal.	1 OZ., BY WT. Carb.
Parrotfish *(Scaridae)*				
RAW:				
Edible portion, 1 pound	476	(0.0)	29.8	(0.00)
Parrotfish (*Scarus nuchipunctatus.* Based on data from East Asia)				
RAW:				
As purchased, 1 pound [refuse, approx. 65%: bones, head, scales, fins, and entrails]	136	0.0	8.5	0.00
Edible portion, 1 pound	390	0.0	24.4	0.00

PEJASAPO (based on data from Latin America)

	UNIT Cal.	UNIT Carb.	1 OZ., BY WT. Cal.	1 OZ., BY WT. Carb.
PARBOILED FLESH:				
Edible portion, 1 pound	400	5.9	25.0	0.37

PEJERREY (based on data from Latin America)

	UNIT Cal.	UNIT Carb.	1 OZ., BY WT. Cal.	1 OZ., BY WT. Carb.
RAW:				
Edible portion, 1 pound	395	0.0	24.7	0.00

PELAMID, see BONITO

PERCH

	UNIT Cal.	UNIT Carb.	1 OZ., BY WT. Cal.	1 OZ., BY WT. Carb.
Climbing Perch (*Ctenopoma; Anabas.* Based on data from Africa)				
RAW:				
Edible portion, 1 pound	468	0.0	29.3	0.00
Climbing Perch (*Ctenopoma.* Based on data from East Asia)				
RAW:				
As purchased, 1 pound [refuse, approx. 51%: bones, scales, fins, and entrails]	304	0.0	19.0	0.00
Edible portion, 1 pound	662	0.0	38.9	0.00
Madagascar Perch (*Paratilapia polleni.* Based on data from Africa)				
COOKED (method unspecified):				
Edible portion, 1 pound	350	0.0	21.9	0.00

	UNIT Cal.	UNIT Carb.	1 OZ., BY WT. Cal.	1 OZ., BY WT. Carb.
Nile Perch (*Lates niloxicus*. Based on data from Africa)				
RAW:				
Edible portion, 1 pound	486	0.0	30.4	0.00
DRIED:				
Edible portion, 1 pound	1907	0.0	119.1	0.00
Ocean Perch, Pacific				
RAW:				
Weighed whole [refuse, approx. 73%: head, tail, fins, entrails, scales, bones, and skin], 1 pound as purchased	116	0.0	7.2	0.00
Edible portion, 1 pound	431	0.0	26.9	0.00
Perch, Atlantic Ocean (Redfish)				
RAW:				
Weighed whole [refuse, approx. 69%: head, tail, fins, entrails, scales, and bones], 1 pound as purchased	124	0.0	7.8	0.00
Edible portion, 1 pound	400	0.0	25.0	0.00
FRIED:				
Based on USDA data; dipped in unspecified quantities of egg, milk, and breadcrumbs:				
Edible portion, 1 pound	1030	30.8	64.4	1.93
Sea Perch (*Lates calcarices*. Based on data from East Asia)				
RAW:				
As purchased, 1 pound [refuse, approx. 46%: bones, scales, and entrails]	200	0.0	12.5	0.00
Edible portion, 1 pound	368	0.0	23.0	0.00
White Perch				
RAW:				
Weighed whole [refuse, approx. 64%: head, tail, fins, bones, skin, and entrails], 1 pound as purchased	193	0.0	12.1	0.00
Edible portion, 1 pound (5g/0g/1g/76%/na)	535	0.0	33.4	0.00
Yellow Perch				
RAW:				
Weighed whole [refuse, approx. 61%: head, tail, fins, bones, skin, and entrails], 1 pound as purchased	161	0.0	10.1	0.00
Edible portion, 1 pound (6g/0g/tr/79%/na)	413	0.0	25.8	0.00

PICKEREL, CHAIN

	UNIT Cal.	UNIT Carb.	1 OZ., BY WT. Cal.	1 OZ., BY WT. Carb.
RAW:				
Weighed whole [refuse, approx. 49%: head, tail, fins, skin, entrails, and bones], 1 pound as purchased	194	0.0	12.1	0.00
Edible portion, 1 pound (5g/0g/tr/80%/na)	381	0.0	23.8	0.00

PIKE

	UNIT Cal.	UNIT Carb.	1 OZ., BY WT. Cal.	1 OZ., BY WT. Carb.
Pike (*Hepsetus odoe*. Based on data from Africa)				
RAW:				
Edible portion, 1 pound	390	0.0	24.4	0.00
DRIED:				
Edible portion, 1 pound	1725	0.0	107.8	0.00
Blue Pike				
RAW:				
Weighed whole [refuse, approx. 56%: head, tail, fins, skin, entrails, and bones], 1 pound as purchased	180	0.0	11.3	0.00
Edible portion, 1 pound (5g/0g/tr/79%/na)	408	0.0	25.5	0.00
Northern Pike				
RAW:				
Weighed whole [refuse, approx. 74%: head, tail, fins, skin, entrails, and bones], 1 pound as purchased	104	0.0	6.5	0.00
Edible portion, 1 pound (5g/0g/tr/80%/na)	400	0.0	25.0	0.00
Walleye Pike				
RAW:				
Weighed whole [refuse, approx. 43%: head, tail, fins, entrails and bones], 1 pound as purchased	240	0.0	15.0	0.00
Edible portion, 1 pound (5g/0g/tr/78%/na)	422	0.0	26.4	0.00

PILCHARD *(Sardinops)* (see also SARDINES)

	UNIT Cal.	UNIT Carb.	1 OZ., BY WT. Cal.	1 OZ., BY WT. Carb.
RAW:				
Edible portion, 1 pound	396	0.0	24.8	0.00

PLAICE (based on data from Denmark)

	UNIT Cal.	UNIT Carb.	1 OZ., BY WT. Cal.	1 OZ., BY WT. Carb.
RAW:				
Edible portion, 1 pound	363	0.0	22.7	0.00

POLLOCK

	UNIT Cal.	UNIT Carb.	1 OZ., BY WT. Cal.	1 OZ., BY WT. Carb.
Pollock				
RAW:				
Weighed drawn [refuse, approx. 55%: head, tail, fins, and bones], 1 pound as purchased	194	0.0	12.1	0.00
Edible portion, 1 pound	431	0.0	27.0	0.00
CREAMED:				
Based on USDA data; cooked with unspecified amounts of flour, milk, and shortening:				
1 cup (approx. 8.8 oz.) (4g/1g/2g/75%/31 mg)	320	10.0	36.3	1.14
1 pound (approx. 1.8 cups)	581	18.2	36.3	1.14
Pollock (*Polachius*. Based on data from East Asia)				
DRIED:				
Edible portion, 1 pound	404	0.0	25.3	0.00
Coalfish Pollock (*Pollachius virens*)				
RAW:				
Edible portion, 1 pound	358	0.0	22.4	0.00

POLLOCK INTESTINES (based on data from Korea) (see also under OFFAL, which follows ZEBRA FISH)

	UNIT Cal.	UNIT Carb.	1 OZ., BY WT. Cal.	1 OZ., BY WT. Carb.
SOUSED:				
Edible portion, 1 pound	318	0.9	19.9	0.06

POLLOCK ROE

	UNIT Cal.	UNIT Carb.	1 OZ., BY WT. Cal.	1 OZ., BY WT. Carb.
Pollock Roe (based on data from East Asia)				
RAW:				
All-edible, 1 pound	563	4.5	31.2	0.28
Pollock Roe (based on data from Japan)				
RAW:				
All-edible, 1 pound	531	4.5	33.2	0.28

POMFRET

	UNIT Cal.	UNIT Carb.	1 OZ., BY WT. Cal.	1 OZ., BY WT. Carb.
Pomfret (*Bramidae*)				
RAW:				
Edible portion, 1 pound (5g/1g/tr/77%/na)	423	12.7	26.5	0.79
Black Pomfret (*Stromateus niger*. Based on data from East Asia)				
RAW:				
As purchased, 1 pound [refuse, approx. 42%: bones, scales, fins, entrails]	245	0.0	15.3	0.00
Edible portion, 1 pound	427	0.0	26.7	0.00
White Pomfret (*Pampus argenteus*. Based on data from East Asia)				
RAW:				
As purchased, 1 pound [refuse, approx. 31%: bones, scales, entrails]	372	0.0	23.3	0.00
Edible portion, 1 pound	540	0.0	33.8	0.00

POMPANO *(Trachinotus)*

	UNIT Cal.	UNIT Carb.	1 OZ., BY WT. Cal.	1 OZ., BY WT. Carb.
RAW:				
Edible portion, 1 pound (5g/1g/tr/77%/na)	391	12.7	24.4	0.79

PONDSMELT, see under SMELT

PORGY

	UNIT Cal.	UNIT Carb.	1 OZ., BY WT. Cal.	1 OZ., BY WT. Carb.
RAW:				
Weighed whole [refuse, approx. 59%: head, tail, fins, bones, skin, and entrails], 1 pound as purchased	208	0.0	13.0	0.00
Meat only, edible portion, 1 pound (5g/0g/1g/76%/na)	508	0.0	31.8	0.00
Porgy (*Lethrinus opercularis*. Based on data from East Asia)				
RAW:				
As purchased, 1 pound [refuse, approx. 55%: scales, bones, entrails, fins, and head]	186	0.0	11.6	0.00
Edible portion, 1 pound	413	0.0	25.8	0.00
Big-Eyed Porgy (*Monotaxis grandoculis*. Based on data from East Asia)				
RAW:				
As purchased, 1 pound [refuse, approx. 49%: scales, bones, entrails, and fins]	222	0.0	13.9	0.00
Edible portion, 1 pound	436	0.0	27.3	0.00

	UNIT Cal.	UNIT Carb.	1 OZ., BY WT. Cal.	1 OZ., BY WT. Carb.
PRAWNS (see also SHRIMP)				
Prawns, type not specified				
RAW:				
Edible portion, 1 pound (5g/na/tr/75%/na)	(354)	na	(22.1)	na
Marine Prawns (*Aresteus palaemon.* Based on data from Africa)				
RAW:				
Edible portion, 1 pound	463	21.8	28.9	1.36
DRIED, POWDER *(Parapenaeus):*				
All-edible, 1 pound	1698	20.0	106.1	1.25
SMOKED *(Penaeus):*				
Edible portion, 1 pound	1298	8.2	81.1	0.51
FRIED:				
Edible portion, 1 pound	1049	78.5	65.6	4.91
Marine Prawns (*Penaeus.* Based on data from East Asia)				
RAW:				
Jumbo:				
As purchased, 1 pound [refuse, approx. 43%: shell and head]	222	2.3	13.9	0.14
Edible portion, 1 pound	395	4.1	24.7	0.26
Medium:				
As purchased, 1 pound [refuse, approx. 54%: shell and head]	182	1.8	11.4	1.11
Edible portion, 1 pound	395	4.1	24.7	0.26
DRIED:				
As purchased, 1 pound [refuse, approx. 47%: shell and head]	872	37.7	54.5	2.36
Edible portion, 1 pound	1643	70.8	102.7	4.42
SALTED, FERMENTED:				
Edible portion, 1 pound	300	8.2	18.8	0.51
River Prawns, Common (*Atya.* Based on data from Africa)				
DRIED:				
Edible portion, 1 pound	1494	27.2	93.4	1.70
BOILED:				
Edible portion, 1 pound	486	13.2	30.4	0.83
River Prawns, Common (*Atya.* Based on data from East Asia)				
RAW, SMALL, WHOLE:				
Edible portion, 1 pound	372	1.8	23.3	0.11
DRIED, SALTED:				
Edible portion, 1 pound	1294	3.2	80.9	0.20
Tiger Prawns (based on data from Japan)				
RAW:				
Edible portion, 1 pound	381	6.8	23.8	0.42
PRAWN EGGS (based on data from East Asia)				
All-edible, 1 pound	1362	109.3	85.1	6.83
PRAWN PASTE				
Prawn Paste, Marine, Average (based on data from East Asia)				
All-edible, 1 pound	749	29.5	46.8	1.84
Prawn Paste, River, Average (based on data from East Asia)				
All-edible, 1 pound	513	15.4	32.0	0.96
PUFFER (see also GLOBEFISH)				
Puffer *(Spheroides)*				
RAW:				
Edible portion, 1 pound (7g/0g/tr/74%/na)	(450)	(0.0)	(28.1)	(0.00)
Puffer (*Sphaeroides.* Based on data from East Asia)				
RAW:				
As purchased, 1 pound [refuse, approx. 48%: bones, scales, fins, and entrails]	218	0.0	13.6	0.00
Edible portion, 1 pound	418	0.0	26.1	0.00
Puffer (based on data from Japan)				
RAW:				
Edible portion, 1 pound	400	1.4	25.0	0.09
QUEENFISH (*Chorinemus.* Based on data from Africa)				
RAW:				
Edible portion, 1 pound	436	0.0	27.2	0.00

	UNIT Cal.	UNIT Carb.	1 OZ., BY WT. Cal.	1 OZ., BY WT. Carb.
RABBIT-FISH (*Siganus oramin.* Based on data from Africa)				
RAW:				
Edible portion, 1 pound	386	0.0	24.1	0.00
RAINBOW RUNNER (*Elagatis bipinnulatus.* Based on data from East Asia)				
RAW:				
As purchased, 1 pound [refuse, approx. 56%: bones, entrails, fins, and scales]	177	0.0	11.1	0.00
Edible portion, 1 pound	404	0.0	25.2	0.00
RAJA FISH, see SKATE				
RAY				
Ray (*Pteroplatea.* Based on data from Africa)				
RAW:				
Edible portion, 1 pound	359	0.0	22.4	0.00
Ray (*Raga.* Based on data from Africa)				
RAW:				
Edible portion, 1 pound	463	0.0	28.9	0.00
RAYED SHELL (based on data from East Asia)				
RAW:				
As purchased, 1 pound [refuse: approx. 39%: shell]	136	3.6	8.5	0.23
Edible portion, 1 pound	227	6.4	14.2	0.40
RAZOR CLAMS, see under CLAMS				
RAZOR-FISH (*Papyrocranus afer.* Based on data from Africa)				
RAW:				
Edible portion, 1 pound	400	0.0	25.0	0.00
DRIED, SMOKED:				
Edible portion, 1 pound	1802	0.0	112.6	0.00
REDFISH *(Sebastes marinus)* (see also DRUM and OCEAN PERCH)				
RAW:				
Edible portion, 1 pound (5g/0g/tr/79%/na)	(380)	(0.0)	(23.7)	(0.00)
REDHORSE, SILVER				
RAW:				
Weighed drawn [refuse, approx. 54%: head, tail, fins, bones, and skin], 1 pound as purchased	204	0.0	12.8	0.00
Edible portion, 1 pound (5g/0g/tr/79%/16 mg)	445	0.0	27.8	0.00
RHINO-FISH (*Labeo.* Based on data from Africa)				
RAW:				
Edible portion, 1 pound	390	0.0	24.4	0.00
DRIED:				
Edible portion, 1 pound	1698	0.0	106.1	0.00
DRIED, SMOKED:				
Edible portion, 1 pound	1594	0.0	99.6	0.00
RIBBONFISH (*Tricliurus.* Based on data from East Asia)				
RAW:				
As purchased, 1 pound [refuse, approx. 45%: bones, tail, fins, and entrails]	290	0.0	18.1	0.00
Edible portion, 1 pound	527	0.0	32.9	0.00
SALTED:				
As purchased, 1 pound [refuse, approx. 31%: bones]	527	0.0	32.9	0.00
Edible portion, 1 pound	763	0.0	47.7	0.00
ROACH (based on data from France)				
RAW:				
Edible portion, 1 pound	508	0.0	31.8	0.00

	UNIT Cal.	UNIT Carb.	1 OZ., BY WT. Cal.	1 OZ., BY WT. Carb.
ROBALO (based on data from Latin America)				
RAW:				
Edible portion, 1 pound	427	0.0	26.7	0.00
ROCKFISH				
Rockfish, including Black, Bocaccio, Canary, Rasphead, and Yellowtail (United States)				
RAW:				
Edible portion, 1 pound (5g/0g/1g/79%/17 mg)	440	0.0	27.5	0.00
OVEN-STEAMED (cooked with onion):				
1 pound of raw fillets, cooked (yield: approx. 13 oz.) (5g/1g/1g/75%/19 mg)	396	7.0	30.4	0.54
1 pound of cooked Rockfish	486	8.6	30.4	0.54
Red Rockfish (*Sebastodes matsubarae.* Based on data from East Asia)				
RAW:				
As purchased, 1 pound [refuse, approx. 45%: bones, fins, scales, and entrails]	290	0.0	18.1	0.00
Edible portion, 1 pound	527	0.0	32.9	0.00
ROE				
Roe, average including Carp, Cod, Haddock, Herring, Pike, and Shad				
RAW:				
Edible portion, 1 pound (7g/tr/1g/70%/na)	590	6.8	36.9	0.43
Roe, average including Salmon, Sturgeon, and Turbot				
RAW:				
Edible portion, 1 pound (7g/tr/3g/61%/na)	940	6.4	58.7	0.40
Roe, Average, fish unspecified (based on data from East Asia)				
RAW:				
All-edible, 1 pound	568	11.4	35.5	0.71
Blue Sea Crab Roe (*Neptune; scylla.* Based on data from Africa)				
SALTED:				
All-edible, 1 pound	1112	65.8	69.5	4.11
Bonito Eggs (based on data from Latin America)				
RAW:				
All-edible, 1 pound	454	0.0	28.4	0.00
Crab Roe (based on data from Japan)				
SALTED:				
All-edible, 1 pound	1094	65.8	68.4	4.11
Dogfish Roe (*Squalus.* Based on data from Africa)				
RAW:				
All-edible, 1 pound	1453	2.3	90.8	0.14
Herring Roe (based on data from East Asia)				
RAW:				
All-edible, 1 pound	663	1.8	41.4	0.11
DRIED:				
All-edible, 1 pound	1752	1.8	109.5	0.11
Herring Roe (based on data from Japan)				
RAW:				
All-edible, 1 pound	631	1.8	39.4	0.11
DRIED:				
All-edible, 1 pound	1671	1.8	104.4	0.11
Mullet Roe (based on data from Japan)				
SALTED, SMOKED:				
All-edible, 1 pound	1876	20.9	117.3	1.31
Pollock Roe (based on data from East Asia)				
RAW:				
All-edible, 1 pound	563	4.5	31.2	0.28
Pollock Roe (based on data from Japan)				
RAW:				
All-edible, 1 pound	531	4.5	33.2	0.28
Prawn Eggs (based on data from East Asia)				
RAW:				
All-edible, 1 pound	1362	109.3	85.1	6.84
Salmon Roe				
BAKED OR BROILED:				
Based on USDA data; cooked with unspecified amount of butter or margarine:				
All-edible, 1 pound (7g/1g/3g/61%/na)	576	8.6	35.7	0.53

	UNIT Cal.	UNIT Carb.	1 OZ., BY WT. Cal.	1 OZ., BY WT. Carb.
Salmon Roe (based on data from East Asia)				
SALTED:				
All-edible, 1 pound	1112	3.6	69.5	0.23
Salmon Roe (based on data from Japan)				
SALTED:				
All-edible, 1 pound	1081	3.6	67.5	0.23
Salmon Roe, Red Salmon or Sockeye (United States) (based on data from East Asia)				
SALTED:				
All-edible, 1 pound	1112	3.6	69.5	0.23
Sea Urchin Roe (based on data from Japan)				
RAW:				
All-edible, 1 pound	672	9.1	42.0	0.57
SALTED:				
All-edible, 1 pound	922	23.0	57.6	1.44
Shark Roe (based on data from Japan)				
RAW:				
All-edible, 1 pound	1426	2.3	89.1	0.14
SABLEFISH				
RAW:				
Weighed whole [refuse, approx. 58%: head, tail, fins, entrails, bones, and skin], 1 pound as purchased	362	0.0	22.6	0.00
Edible portion, 1 pound (4g/0g/4g/72%/16mg)	863	0.0	53.9	0.00
SAILFIN (*Polypterus.* Based on data from Africa)				
RAW:				
Edible portion, 1 pound	386	0.0	24.1	0.00
SALMON				
Salmon, type not specified				
SMOKED:				
All-edible, 1 pound	798	0.0	49.9	0.00
Atlantic Salmon				
RAW:				
Weighed whole [refuse, approx. 35%: head, tail, fins, bones, skin, and entrails], 1 pound as purchased	640	0.0	40.0	0.00
Edible portion, 1 pound (6g/0g/3g/64%/na)	985	0.0	61.6	0.00
Cherry or Pink Salmon (*Oncorhynchus masou.* Based on data from East Asia)				
RAW:				
As purchased, 1 pound [refuse, approx. 40%: scales, bones, fins, and entrails]	386	0.0	24.1	0.00
Edible portion, 1 pound	645	0.0	40.3	0.00
Chinook Salmon (King)				
RAW:				
Steak [refuse, approx. 12%: bones], 1 pound as purchased	886	0.0	55.4	0.00
Edible portion, 1 pound (5g/0g/4g/64%/13mg)	1008	0.0	63.0	0.00
Humpback Salmon (Pink)				
RAW:				
Steak [refuse: bones, approx. 12%], 1 pound as purchased	475	0.0	29.7	0.00
Edible portion, 1 pound (6g/0g/1g/76%/18mg)	540	0.0	33.8	0.00
Humpback Salmon (*Oncorhynchus gorbuscha.* Based on data from East Asia)				
RAW:				
As purchased, 1 pound [refuse, approx. 40%: scales, bones, fins, and entrails]	386	0.0	24.1	0.00
Edible portion, 1 pound	645	0.0	40.3	0.00
SALTED:				
As purchased, 1 pound [refuse, approx. 25%: bones]	785	0.0	49.1	0.00
Edible portion, 1 pound	1049	0.0	65.6	0.00
King or Silver Salmon (*Oncorhynchus keta.* Based on data from East Asia)				
RAW:				
As purchased, 1 pound [refuse, approx. 34%: scales, bones, fins, and entrails]	418	0.0	26.1	0.00
Edible portion, 1 pound	636	0.0	39.8	0.00
SLIGHT CURING:				
As purchased, 1 pound [refuse, approx. 30%: bones and skin]	449	0.9	28.1	0.06
Edible portion, 1 pound	645	1.4	40.3	0.09

	UNIT Cal.	UNIT Carb.	1 OZ., BY WT. Cal.	1 OZ., BY WT. Carb.
SALTED:				
As purchased, 1 pound [refuse, approx. 25%: bones]	495	0.9	30.9	0.06
Edible portion, 1 pound	663	1.4	41.4	0.09
SMOKED, SALTED:				
As purchased, 1 pound [refuse, approx. 20%: bones]	881	2.7	55.1	0.17
Edible portion, 1 pound	1099	3.6	68.7	0.22

SALMON ROE

	UNIT Cal.	UNIT Carb.	1 OZ., BY WT. Cal.	1 OZ., BY WT. Carb.
BAKED OR BROILED:				
Based on USDA data; cooked with unspecified amount of butter or margarine:				
All-edible, 1 pound (7g/1g/3g/61%/na)	576	8.6	35.7	0.53
Salmon Roe (based on data from East Asia)				
SALTED:				
All-edible, 1 pound	1112	3.6	69.5	0.23
Salmon Roe (based on data from Japan)				
SALTED:				
All-edible, 1 pound	1081	3.6	67.5	0.23
Sockeye or Red Salmon Roe (based on data from East Asia)				
SALTED:				
All-edible, 1 pound	1112	3.6	69.5	0.23

SARDINELLA (*Sardinella.* Based on data from Africa)

	UNIT Cal.	UNIT Carb.	1 OZ., BY WT. Cal.	1 OZ., BY WT. Carb.
RAW:				
Edible portion, 1 pound	477	0.0	29.8	0.00
SMOKED:				
Edible portion, 1 pound	1330	0.0	83.1	0.00
FRIED IN COCONUT OIL:				
Edible portion, 1 pound	2343	0.0	146.4	0.00

SARDINES

	UNIT Cal.	UNIT Carb.	1 OZ., BY WT. Cal.	1 OZ., BY WT. Carb.
Sardines (*Sardinella eba*)				
RAW:				
Edible portion, 1 pound (5g/0g/1g/77%/na)	(496)	(0.0)	(31.0)	(0.00)
Sardines (based on data from Denmark)				
RAW:				
Edible portion, 1 pound	907	0.0	56.7	0.00
Fimbriated Sardines (*Sardinella fimbriata.* Based on data from East Asia)				
RAW:				
As purchased, 1 pound [refuse, approx. 34%: bones, heads, scales, and entrails]	300	0.0	18.8	0.00
Edible portion, 1 pound	454	0.0	28.4	0.00
Gilt Sardines (*Sardinella aurita*)				
RAW:				
Edible portion, 1 pound (6g/0g/1g/75%/na)	(527)	(0.0)	(32.9)	(0.00)
Indian Sardines (*Sardinella longiceps*)				
RAW:				
Edible portion, 1 pound (5g/tr/1g/76%/na)	467	3.2	29.2	0.20
Pacific Sardines				
RAW:				
Edible portion, 1 pound (5g/0g/2g/71%/na)	726	0.0	45.4	0.00

SAUGER

	UNIT Cal.	UNIT Carb.	1 OZ., BY WT. Cal.	1 OZ., BY WT. Carb.
RAW:				
Weighed whole [refuse, approx. 65%: head, tail, fins, entrails, scales, bones, and skin], 1 pound as purchased	133	0.0	8.3	0.00
Edible portion, 1 pound (5g/0g/tr/81%/na)	381	0.0	23.8	0.00

SCAD (*Decapterus*)

	UNIT Cal.	UNIT Carb.	1 OZ., BY WT. Cal.	1 OZ., BY WT. Carb.
RAW:				
Edible portion, 1 pound (6g/tr/1g/75%/na)	494	5.4	30.9	0.34

SCALLOPS

	UNIT Cal.	UNIT Carb.	1 OZ., BY WT. Cal.	1 OZ., BY WT. Carb.
Scallops (*Pectinidae*)				
RAW:				
Edible portion, 1 pound (5g/tr/tr/79%/na)	(371)	(7.7)	(23.2)	(0.48)
Scallops (based on data from Indonesia)				
DRIED:				
All-edible, 1 pound	1547	54.4	96.7	3.40
Atlantic Bay Scallop (*Pecten irradians*)				
RAW:				
Edible portion, 1 pound (4g/tr/tr/81%/na)	(331)	(7.7)	(20.7)	(0.48)
Bay and Sea Scallop				
RAW:				
Edible portion, 1 pound (4g/1g/tr/80%/na)	368	15.0	23.0	0.94
Calico Scallop				
RAW:				
Edible portion, 1 pound (5g/tr/tr/80%/na)	(344)	(7.7)	(21.5)	(0.48)
Scallops, "Coquille St. Jacques" (based on data from France)				
RAW:				
Edible portion, 1 pound	363	18.1	22.7	1.13
COOKED (method unspecified):				
Edible portion, 1 pound	358	15.9	22.4	0.99

SCORPION FISH (*Scorpaena.* Based on data from Africa)

	UNIT Cal.	UNIT Carb.	1 OZ., BY WT. Cal.	1 OZ., BY WT. Carb.
RAW:				
Edible portion, 1 pound	699	0.0	43.7	0.00

SCUP (*Stenotomus chrysops*)

	UNIT Cal.	UNIT Carb.	1 OZ., BY WT. Cal.	1 OZ., BY WT. Carb.
RAW:				
Edible portion, 1 pound (5g/0g/1g/76%/na)	(492)	(0.0)	(30.8)	(0.00)

SEA BASS (see also BASS)

	UNIT Cal.	UNIT Carb.	1 OZ., BY WT. Cal.	1 OZ., BY WT. Carb.
Sea Bass (based on data from France)				
RAW:				
Edible portion, 1 pound	413	0.0	25.8	0.00
White Sea Bass				
RAW:				
Edible portion, 1 pound (6g/0g/tr/76%/na)	436	0.0	27.2	0.00

SEA BREAM (see also BREAM)

	UNIT Cal.	UNIT Carb.	1 OZ., BY WT. Cal.	1 OZ., BY WT. Carb.
Steenbros Sea Bream (*Pagellus.* Based on data from Africa)				
RAW:				
Edible portion, 1 pound	558	0.0	34.9	0.00
Stumpnose Sea Bream (*Pagellus.* Based on data from Africa)				
RAW:				
Edible portion, 1 pound	440	0.0	27.5	0.00
DRIED:				
Edible portion, 1 pound	1594	0.0	99.6	0.00
DRIED, SALTED:				
Edible portion, 1 pound	1371	0.0	85.7	0.00

SEA CUCUMBER

	UNIT Cal.	UNIT Carb.	1 OZ., BY WT. Cal.	1 OZ., BY WT. Carb.
Sea Cucumber (*Stichopus japonica.* Based on data from East Asia)				
RAW:				
Edible portion (muscle), 1 pound	95	0.9	5.9	0.06
DRIED:				
Edible portion (muscle), 1 pound	1748	21.8	109.3	1.36
DRIED, SOAKED:				
Edible portion (muscle), 1 pound	404	5.0	25.3	0.31
Sea Cucumber (based on data from Japan)				
RAW:				
Edible portion, 1 pound	82	6.8	5.1	0.43
SALTED VISCERA:				
Edible portion, 1 pound	232	2.3	14.5	0.14

SEA PERCH, see under PERCH

SEA TROUT, see WEAKFISH

SEA URCHIN ROE (based on data from Japan)

	UNIT Cal.	UNIT Carb.	1 OZ., BY WT. Cal.	1 OZ., BY WT. Carb.
FRESH:				
All-edible, 1 pound	672	9.1	42.0	0.57
SALTED:				
All-edible, 1 pound	922	23.0	57.6	1.44

SEAWEED (for more extensive information, see the VEGETABLES chapter)

	UNIT Cal.	UNIT Carb.	1 OZ., BY WT. Cal.	1 OZ., BY WT. Carb.
Agar (based on data from East Asia)				
DRIED:				
1 pound	1416	378.7	88.5	23.67

	UNIT Cal.	UNIT Carb.	1 OZ., BY WT. Cal.	1 OZ., BY WT. Carb.
SHAD				
American Shad				
RAW:				
Weighed whole [refuse, approx. 52%: head, tail, fins, bones, skin, and entrails], 1 pound as purchased	370	0.0	23.1	0.00
Edible portion, 1 pound (5g/0g/3g/70%/15mg)	772	0.0	48.2	0.00
BAKED:				
Based on USDA data; prepared with unspecified amounts of butter or margarine and bacon slices:				
1 pound raw fillets, cooked (yield: 12.9 oz.) (7g/0g/3g/64%/22mg)	734	0.0	57.1	0.00
1 pound of baked shad	914	0.0	57.1	0.00
Gizzard Shad				
RAW:				
Weighed whole [refuse, approx. 67%: head, tail, fins, skin, bones, and entrails], 1 pound as purchased	299	0.0	18.7	0.00
Edible portion, 1 pound (5g/0g/4g/68%/na)	908	0.0	56.8	0.00
Gizzard Shad (*Anodontosoma chacunda.* Based on data from East Asia)				
RAW:				
As purchased, 1 pound [refuse, approx. 60%: bones, scales, fins, head, and entrails]	163	0.0	10.2	0.00
Edible portion, 1 pound	409	0.0	25.5	0.00
DRIED, SALTED:				
Edible portion, 1 pound	680	0.0	42.5	0.00
Slender Shad (*Ilisha elongata.* Based on data from East Asia)				
RAW:				
As purchased, 1 pound [refuse, approx. 45%: bones, entrails, and scales]	327	0.0	20.4	0.00
Edible portion, 1 pound	594	0.0	37.1	0.00
West African Shad (based on data from Africa)				
RAW (*Ethmalosa dorsalis*):				
Edible portion, 1 pound	490	0.0	30.6	0.00
DRIED (*Ethmalosa fimbriata*):				
Edible portion, 1 pound	1780	0.0	111.2	0.00
DRIED, SMOKED (*Ethmalosa fimbriata*):				
Edible portion, 1 pound	1448	0.0	90.5	0.00
SHAD ROE, see under ROE				
SHARK				
Shark (average, mixed species)				
RAW:				
Edible portion, 1 pound (6g/0g/tr/76%/na)	458	(0.0)	28.6	(0.00)
Shark (*Carcharias.* Based on data from East Asia)				
RAW:				
As purchased, 1 pound [refuse, approx. 24%: bones]	254	0.0	15.9	0.00
Edible portion, 1 pound	454	0.0	28.4	0.00
DRIED FINS:				
Edible portion, 1 pound	1662	0.0	103.9	0.00
DRIED, SOAKED, AND DRAINED FINS:				
Edible portion, 1 pound	513	0.0	32.1	0.00
DRIED SKIN:				
Edible portion, 1 pound	331	0.0	20.7	0.00
Blue Shark (*Prionace glauca.* Based on data from East Asia)				
RAW:				
As purchased, 1 pound [refuse, approx. 55%: scales, fins, bones, and entrails]	127	0.0	7.9	0.00
Edible portion, 1 pound	286	0.0	17.9	0.00
Great Blue Shark (based on data from Japan)				
RAW:				
Edible portion, 1 pound	291	1.4	18.2	0.09
Sand Shark (*Rhinobatos hynnicephalus.* Based on data from East Asia)				
RAW:				
As purchased, 1 pound [refuse, approx. 56%: bones, fins, and entrails]	254	0.0	15.9	0.00
Edible portion, 1 pound	577	0.0	36.1	0.00
Shark's Fin (based on data from Singapore)				
DRIED FINS:				
As purchased, 1 pound [refuse, approx. 22%]	1362	0.5	85.1	0.03
Edible portion, 1 pound	1743	0.5	108.9	0.03
SHARK ROE (based on data from Japan)				
RAW:				
All-edible, 1 pound	1426	2.3	89.1	0.14

	UNIT Cal.	UNIT Carb.	1 OZ., BY WT. Cal.	1 OZ., BY WT. Carb.
SHEEPSHEAD				
Atlantic Sheepshead				
RAW:				
Weighed whole [refuse, approx. 69%: head, tail, fins, skin, bones, and entrails], 1 pound as purchased	159	0.0	9.9	0.00
Edible portion, 1 pound (6g/0g/1g/76%/29mg)	513	0.0	32.1	0.00
Sheepshead, Fresh Water, see Drum				
SHRIMP (see also PRAWNS)				
RAW:				
Weighed in shell [refuse, approx. 31%: shell], 1 pound as purchased	285	4.7	17.8	0.29
Edible portion, 1 pound (5g/tr/tr/78%/40mg)	413	6.8	25.8	0.43
FRIED:				
Data are based on USDA home recipe with coating ingredients as follows: ½ egg, 1½ tsp. milk, ½ cup dried breadcrumbs:				
1 pound of raw shrimp, coated and French-fried, (yield: approx. 11.8 oz.) (6g/3g/3g/57%/53mg)	(746)	(33.5)	(63.8)	(2.84)
Fried, 1 pound	1021	45.4	63.8	2.84
Shrimp (based on data from Denmark)				
RAW:				
Edible portion, 1 pound	363	0.0	22.7	0.00
Shrimp (based on data from France)				
RAW:				
Edible portion, 1 pound	431	0.0	26.9	0.00
COOKED (method unspecified):				
Edible portion, 1 pound	(435)	0.0	(27.2)	0.00
SISCOWET, see under LAKE TROUT				
SKATE (Raja Fish)				
RAW:				
Edible portion, 1 pound (6g/0g/tr/78%/na)	445	0.0	27.8	0.00
SKIPJACK (*Euthynnus pelamis*)				
RAW:				
Edible portion, 1 pound (7g/0g/1g/70%/na)	(601)	(0.0)	(37.6)	(0.00)
SMELT (see also EULACHON and WHITING)				
Smelt, from data that include Atlantic, Bay, and Jack				
RAW:				
As purchased, 1 pound [refuse, approx. 45%: head, tail, fins, bone, skin, and entrails]	244	0.0	15.3	0.00
Edible portion, 1 pound (5g/0g/1g/79%/na)	445	0.0	27.8	0.00
Pond Smelt (*Hypomesus olidus.* Based on data from East Asia)				
RAW:				
Edible portion, 1 pound	449	0.0	28.1	0.00
Sweet Smelt (*Plecoglossus altivelis.* Based on data from East Asia)				
RAW:				
As purchased, 1 pound [refuse, approx. 25%: bones and entrails]	336	0.0	21.0	0.00
Edible portion, 1 pound	454	0.0	28.4	0.00
Whiting Smelt (*Hypomesus olidus.* Based on data from East Asia)				
RAW:				
As purchased, 1 pound [refuse, approx. 46%: bones and entrails]	236	0.0	14.7	0.00
Edible portion, 1 pound	440	0.0	27.5	0.00
SNAILS				
RAW:				
Edible portion, 1 pound (5g/1g/tr/79%/na)	408	9.1	25.5	0.57
Snails, "Escargot" (based on data from France)				
RAW:				
Edible portion, 1 pound	340	9.1	21.3	0.57
COOKED (method unspecified):				
Edible portion, 1 pound	(318)	(4.5)	(19.8)	(0.28)
African Snails (*Achatina marginata.* Based on data from Africa)				
RAW:				
Edible portion, 1 pound	485	0.0	30.3	0.00

	UNIT Cal.	UNIT Carb.	1 OZ., BY WT. Cal.	1 OZ., BY WT. Carb.
Giant African Snails				
RAW:				
Edible portion, 1 pound (3g/1g/tr/82%/na)	331	20.0	20.7	1.25
Pond Snails (*Viviparuss.* Based on data from East Asia)				
RAW:				
As purchased, 1 pound [refuse, approx. 46%: shell and viscera]	191	11.8	11.9	0.74
Edible portion, 1 pound	349	21.8	21.8	1.36
River Snails (*Viviparuss.* Based on data from East Asia)				
RAW:				
As purchased, 1 pound [refuse, approx. 46%: shell and viscera]	191	11.8	11.9	0.74
Edible portion, 1 pound	349	21.8	21.8	1.36
Sea Snails (*Yetus.* Based on data from Africa)				
BOILED, SUN DRIED:				
Edible portion, 1 pound	844	70.8	52.7	4.42
SNAKEHEAD				
Snakehead (*Parophiocephalus.* Based on data from Africa)				
RAW:				
Edible portion, 1 pound	399	0.0	25.0	0.00
DRY, SMOKED:				
Edible portion, 1 pound	1756	0.0	109.7	0.00
Snakehead (*Ophiocephalus striatus.* Based on data from East Asia)				
RAW:				
As purchased, 1 pound [refuse, approx. 43%: bones, scales, fins, and entrails]	241	0.0	15.1	0.00
Edible portion, 1 pound	422	0.0	26.4	0.00
SNAPPER				
Snapper, from data that include Red and Gray				
RAW:				
Weighed whole [refuse, approx. 48%: head, tail, fins, bones, skin, and entrails], 1 pound as purchased	219	0.0	13.7	0.00
Edible portion, 1 pound (6g/0g/tr/79%/19mg)	422	0.0	26.4	0.00
SNOOKS (*Centropomidae*)				
RAW:				
Edible portion, 1 pound	374	2.7	23.4	0.20
SOLE				
Sole (based on data from France)				
RAW:				
Edible portion, 1 pound	331	0.0	20.7	0.00
COOKED (method unspecified):				
Edible portion, 1 pound	(318)	(0.0)	(19.8)	(0.00)
Sole (*Limanda*)				
RAW:				
Edible portion, 1 pound	(367)	0.0	(23.0)	0.00
Sole (*Soleidae*)				
RAW:				
Edible portion, 1 pound	374	0.0	23.4	0.00
Dover Sole, caught in the Bering Sea				
RAW:				
Edible portion, 1 pound	279	0.0	17.5	0.00
Dover Sole (*Microstomus pacificus*)				
RAW:				
Edible portion, 1 pound (4g/0g/tr/84%/na)	(305)	(0.0)	(19.1)	(0.00)
English Sole, caught in the Bering Sea				
RAW:				
Edible portion, 1 pound	409	0.0	25.6	0.00
English Sole (*Parophys ventulus*)				
RAW:				
Edible portion, 1 pound (5g/0g/tr/81%/na)	367	0.0	23.0	0.00
Flathead Sole, caught in the Bering Sea				
RAW:				
Edible portion, 1 pound	406	0.0	25.4	0.00
Lemon Sole, caught in the Bering Sea				
RAW:				
Edible portion, 1 pound	369	0.0	23.1	0.00

	UNIT Cal.	UNIT Carb.	1 OZ., BY WT. Cal.	1 OZ., BY WT. Carb.
Lemon Sole (based on data from the British Isles)				
STEAMED:				
Weighed with bones and skin [refuse, approx. 38%: head, viscera, fins], 1 pound as purchased	224	0.0	14.0	0.00
Edible portion, 1 pound	384	0.0	24.0	0.00
FRIED:				
Prepared with unspecified amount of batter and breadcrumbs:				
Weighed with bones [refuse, approx. 9%: head, viscera, or fins], 1 pound	1088	20.8	68.0	1.30
Covered with batter, edible portion, 1 pound	1248	24.0	78.0	1.50
Petrole Sole (*Eopsetta jordani*)				
RAW:				
Edible portion, 1 pound (5g/0g/1g/79%/na)	386	0.0	24.1	0.00
Rock Sole (Caught in the Bering Sea)				
RAW:				
Edible portion, 1 pound	401	0.0	25.1	0.00
Yellowfin Sole (Caught in the Bering Sea)				
RAW:				
Edible portion, 1 pound	36	0.0	22.6	0.00
SPANISH MACKEREL, see under MACKEREL				
SPOT				
RAW:				
Edible portion, 1 pound (5g/0g/5g/65%/17mg)	994	0.0	62.1	0.00
BAKED:				
Based on USDA data; cooked with unspecified amount of butter or margarine:				
Edible portion, 1 pound (6g/0g/6g/54%/88mg)	1338	0.0	83.6	0.00
SPRAT (*Clupea sprattus*)				
RAW:				
Edible portion, 1 pound (5g/0g/2g/69%/na)	798	(0.0)	49.9	(0.00)
SQUAWFISH, NORTHERN (*Ptychocheilus oregonensis*)				
RAW:				
Edible portion, 1 pound (5g/0g/1g/79%/na)	(411)	(0.0)	(25.7)	(0.00)
SQUID				
Squid (*Loligo.* Based on data from East Asia)				
RAW:				
As purchased, 1 pound [refuse, approx. 7%: soft bones and viscera]	313	2.7	19.6	0.17
Edible portion, 1 pound	337	2.9	21.1	0.18
DRIED:				
Edible portion, 1 pound	1489	17.7	93.1	1.11
DRIED, SOAKED, DRAINED:				
Edible portion, 1 pound	735	4.5	45.9	0.28
COOKED (method unspecified):				
Edible portion, 1 pound	522	0.9	32.6	0.06
Squid (*Loliginidae*)				
RAW:				
Edible portion, 1 pound (4g/1g/tr/79%/na)	404	13.6	25.2	0.85
Squid (based on data from Japan)				
PREPARED "SURUME" STYLE:				
Edible portion, 1 pound	1535	8.6	95.9	0.54
PREPARED "TSUKUDANI" STYLE, IN STRIPS:				
Edible portion, 1 pound	1309	195.0	81.8	12.19
Squid (based on data from Korea)				
SOUSED:				
Edible portion, 1 pound	1111	79.8	69.5	4.99
Toyama Squid (*Watasemia scintillans.* Based on data from East Asia)				
RAW:				
As purchased, 1 pound [refuse, approx. 10%: soft bones and viscera]	422	2.3	23.4	0.14
Edible portion, 1 pound	472	2.7	29.5	0.17
SQUID VISCERA (based on data from East Asia)				
SALTED:				
Edible portion, 1 pound	463	22.7	28.9	1.42

	UNIT Cal.	UNIT Carb.	1 OZ., BY WT. Cal.	1 OZ., BY WT. Carb.
STINGRAY				
Stingray (*Dasyatis.* Based on data from Africa)				
RAW:				
Edible portion, 1 pound	399	0.0	25.0	0.00
Blue Spotted Stingray (*Dasyatis kuhlii.* Based on data from East Asia)				
RAW:				
As purchased, 1 pound [refuse, approx. 59%: bones, scales, entrails, head, and fins]	145	0.0	9.1	0.00
Edible portion, 1 pound	359	0.0	22.4	0.00
Marbled Stingray (*Dasyatis uarnak.* Based on data from East Asia)				
RAW:				
As purchased, 1 pound [refuse: approx. 60%: bones, scales, entrails, head, and fins]	127	0.0	7.9	0.00
Edible portion, 1 pound	322	0.0	20.1	0.00
STURGEON				
Sturgeon (*Acipenseridae*)				
RAW:				
Sections [refuse, approx. 15%: bones and skin]	362	0.0	22.6	0.00
Edible portion, 1 pound (5g/0g/1g/79%/na)	427	0.0	26.7	0.00
SMOKED:				
Edible portion, 1 pound (9g/0g/1g/64%/na)	676	0.0	42.3	0.00
STEAMED:				
Edible portion, 1 pound (7g/0g/2g/68%/na)	726	0.0	45.4	0.00
Sturgeon (based on data from France)				
RAW:				
Edible portion, 1 pound	567	0.0	35.4	0.00
Sturgeonfish (*Ocan thurus bleekeri.* Based on data from East Asia)				
RAW:				
As purchased, 1 pound [refuse, approx. 51%: bones, scales, entrails, and fins]	186	0.0	11.6	0.00
Edible portion, 1 pound	381	0.0	23.8	0.00
SUCKER				
Sucker, including White and Mullet				
RAW:				
Weighed whole [refuse, approx. 57%: entrails, heads, fins, scales, and bones], 1 pound as purchased	203	0.0	12.7	0.00
Fillets, edible portion, 1 pound (6g/0g/1g/76%/na)	472	0.0	29.5	0.00
Carp Sucker				
RAW:				
Weighed whole [refuse, approx. 61%: head, tail, fins, entrails, bones, and skin], 1 pound as purchased	196	0.0	12.3	0.00
Edible portion, 1 pound (5g/0g/1g/76%/na)	504	0.0	31.5	0.00
SURIMI is listed in the *Frozen Fish and Shellfish* section.				
SUSHI (based on data from Greenwich Village) see the tail end of the Fish Chapter Preface.				
SWAMP EEL, see under EEL				
SWORDFISH				
RAW:				
Edible portion, 1 pound (5g/0g/1g/77%/na)	465	0.0	29.1	0.00
DEHYDRATED:				
All-edible, 1 pound (19g/0g/8g/2%/na)	2379	0.0	148.7	0.00
BROILED (without butter):				
Edible portion, 1 pound (8g/0g/1g/65%/na)	729	0.0	45.6	0.00
Swordfish (*Xiphias gladius.* Based on data from East Asia)				
RAW:				
As purchased, 1 pound [refuse, approx. 35%: bones, entrails, and fins]	340	0.0	21.3	0.00
Edible portion, 1 pound	526	0.0	32.9	0.00
Swordfish (based on data from France)				
RAW:				
Edible portion, 1 pound	531	0.0	33.2	0.00
Swordfish (based on data from Japan)				
RAW:				
Edible portion, 1 pound	581	1.4	36.3	0.09

	UNIT Cal.	UNIT Carb.	1 OZ., BY WT. Cal.	1 OZ., BY WT. Carb.
Broadbill Swordfish (*Xiphias gladius.* Based on data from Africa)				
RAW:				
Edible portion, 1 pound	635	0.0	36.7	0.00
TALAPIA (based on data from Ethiopia)				
RAW:				
Boneless fillet, edible portion, 1 pound	272	0.0	17.0	0.00
TARPON (*Megalops cyprinoides.* Based on data from East Asia)				
RAW:				
As purchased, 1 pound [refuse, approx. 52%: bones, entrails, fins, and scales]	222	0.0	13.9	0.00
Edible portion, 1 pound	463	0.0	28.9	0.00
TAUTOG (Blackfish)				
RAW:				
Weighed whole [refuse, approx. 63%: head, tail, fins, entrails, bones, and skin], 1 pound as purchased	149	0.0	9.3	0.00
Edible portion, 1 pound (5g/0g/tr/79%/na)	404	0.0	25.3	0.00
TENCH (based on data from France)				
RAW:				
Edible portion, 1 pound	345	0.0	21.5	0.00
TEN-POUNDER (based on data from East Asia)				
RAW:				
As purchased, 1 pound [refuse, approx. 44%: bones, entrails, scales, and fins]	277	0.0	17.3	0.00
Edible portion, 1 pound	499	0.0	31.2	0.00
TERRAPIN (Diamondback)				
RAW:				
Weighed in shell [refuse, approx. 79%: shell], 1 pound as purchased	106	0.0	6.6	0.00
Edible portion, 1 pound (5g/0g/1g/77%/na)	503	0.0	31.4	0.00
THREADFIN (based on data from East Asia)				
RAW:				
As purchased, 1 pound [refuse, approx. 59%: bones, scales, head, and entrails]	168	0.0	10.5	0.00
Edible portion, 1 pound	418	0.0	26.1	0.00
DRIED, SALTED:				
Edible portion, 1 pound	853	0.0	53.3	0.00
TIGER FISH (*Hydrocyon.* Based on data from Africa)				
RAW:				
Edible portion, 1 pound	749	0.0	46.8	0.00
DRIED, FLESH ONLY:				
Edible portion, 1 pound	1737	0.0	108.6	0.00
TILAPIA (*Tilipia mossambica.* Based on data from East Asia)				
RAW:				
As purchased, 1 pound [refuse, approx. 34%: bones, entrails, and scales]	182	0.0	11.4	0.00
Edible portion, 1 pound	481	0.0	30.0	0.00
TILE FISH				
RAW:				
Weighed whole [refuse, approx. 49%: head, tail, fins, entrails, bones, and skin], 1 pound as purchased	183	0.0	11.4	0.00
Edible portion, 1 pound (5g/0g/tr/80%/na)	359	0.0	22.4	0.00
BAKED:				
Based on USDA data; cooked with unspecified amount of butter or margarine:				
1 pound (7g/0g/1g/72%/na)	626	0.0	39.1	0.00

	UNIT Cal.	UNIT Carb.	1 OZ., BY WT. Cal.	1 OZ., BY WT. Carb.
Tile Fish (*Branchiostigus*. Based on data from East Asia)				
RAW:				
As purchased, 1 pound [refuse, approx. 34%: bones, entrails, and scales]	295	0.0	18.4	0.00
Edible portion, 1 pound	454	0.0	28.4	0.00
TOMCOD (see also COD)				
Atlantic Tomcod (*Microgadus*)				
RAW:				
Weighed whole [refuse, approx. 61%: head, tail, fins, entrails, bones, and skin], 1 pound as purchased	136	0.0	8.5	0.00
Edible portion, 1 pound (5g/0g/tr/82%/na)	350	0.0	21.8	0.00
TONGUE SOLE				
Tongue Sole (*Cynoglossus*. Based on data from Africa)				
RAW:				
As purchased, 1 pound [refuse, approx. 43%: bones, scales, entrails, and fins]	222	0.0	13.9	0.00
Edible portion, 1 pound	390	0.0	24.4	0.00
Tongue Sole (*Cynoglossus*. Based on data from East Asia)				
RAW:				
As purchased, 1 pound [refuse, approx. 43%: bones, scales, entrails, and fins]	236	0.0	14.7	0.00
Edible portion, 1 pound	408	0.0	25.5	0.00
Tongue Sole (based on data from Japan)				
RAW:				
Edible portion, 1 pound	427	1.4	26.7	0.09
TOP-SHELL (*Turbo cornutus*. Based on data from East Asia)				
RAW:				
As purchased, 1 pound [refuse, approx. 84%: shell and viscera]	77	2.7	4.8	0.17
Edible portion, 1 pound	481	18.1	30.1	1.13
TROUT (see also Dolly Varden Trout, Weakfish [Sea Trout], and Lake Trout)				
Trout (*Salmo*. Based on data from East Asia)				
RAW:				
As purchased, 1 pound [refuse, approx. 30%: bones, entrails, scales, and fins]	485	0.0	30.3	0.00
Edible portion, 1 pound	669	0.0	43.7	0.00
Trout (based on data from France)				
RAW:				
Edible portion, 1 pound	435	0.0	27.2	0.00
Brook Trout				
RAW:				
Weighed whole [refuse, approx. 51%: head, tail, fins, entrails, bones, and skin], 1 pound as purchased	224	0.0	14.0	0.00
Edible portion, 1 pound (5g/0g/1g/78%/na)	459	0.0	28.7	0.00
Rainbow or Steelhead Trout				
RAW:				
Edible portion, 1 pound (6g/0g/3g/66%/na)	885	0.0	55.3	0.00
TUNA				
Big Eye Tuna (*Thunnus obesus*)				
RAW:				
Edible portion, 1 pound (6g/0g/tr/73%/na)	445	(0.0)	27.8	(0.00)
Bluefin Tuna (*Thunnus thynnus*)				
RAW:				
Edible portion, 1 pound (7g/0g/1g/70%/na)	553	(0.0)	34.6	(0.00)
Bluefin Tuna (*Thunnus orientalis*. Based on data from East Asia)				
RAW:				
Lean only:				
Edible portion, 1 pound	549	0.0	34.3	0.00
Fatty portion:				
Edible portion, 1 pound	1438	0.0	89.9	0.00
Bluefin Tuna, Immature (based on data from Japan)				
RAW:				
Edible portion, 1 pound	658	0.0	41.1	0.00
Tunny, Little (*Euthynnus alletteratus*)				
RAW:				
Edible portion, 1 pound (6g/0g/2g/70%/na)	646	(0.0)	40.4	(0.00)

	UNIT Cal.	UNIT Carb.	1 OZ., BY WT. Cal.	1 OZ., BY WT. Carb.
Yellowfin Tuna				
RAW:				
Edible portion, 1 pound (7g/0g/1g/72%/10mg)	604	0.0	37.7	0.00
Yellowfin Tuna (*Thunnus albacares*)				
RAW:				
Edible portion, 1 pound (7g/0g/1g/73%/na)	531	(0.0)	33.2	(0.00)
Yellowfin Tuna (*Thunnus albacares*. Based on data from East Asia)				
RAW:				
As purchased, 1 pound [refuse, approx. 29%: bones and skin]	336	0.0	21.0	0.00
Edible portion, 1 pound	476	0.0	29.8	0.00
Seasoned, all-edible, 1 pound	749	14.5	46.8	0.91
TURBOT				
Turbot (*Thombus maximus*)				
RAW:				
Edible portion, 1 pound (5g/0g/1g/78%/na)	426	(0.0)	26.7	(0.00)
Turbot (*Scophthalmus maximum*. Based on data from Africa)				
RAW:				
Edible portion, 1 pound	608	0.0	38.0	0.00
Turbot (based on data from France)				
RAW:				
Edible portion, 1 pound	535	0.0	33.5	0.00
TURTLE, GREEN				
RAW:				
Weighed in shell [refuse, approx. 76%: shell], 1 pound as purchased	97	0.0	6.1	0.00
Muscle only, edible portion, 1 pound (6g/0g/tr/79%/na)	404	0.0	25.2	0.00
VAJRA (based on data from India)				
RAW:				
Edible portion, 1 pound	422	0.0	26.4	0.00
WALLEYE (*Stizostedion vitreum*)				
RAW:				
Edible portion, 1 pound	411	(0.0)	25.7	(0.00)
WEAKFISH (Sea Trout)				
RAW:				
Weighed whole [refuse, approx. 52%: head, tail, fins, entrails, bones, and skin], 1 pound as purchased	263	0.0	16.4	0.00
Edible portion, 1 pound	549	0.0	34.3	0.00
BROILED				
Based on USDA data; cooked with unspecified amounts of butter or margarine:				
1 pound (7g/0g/3g/61%/159mg)	943	0.0	58.9	0.00
WEEVER (*Trachinus*. Based on data from Africa)				
RAW:				
Edible portion, 1 pound	518	0.0	32.4	0.00
WHALE				
RAW:				
Weighed whole [refuse, approx. 53%: head, tail, fins, entrails, bones, and skin], 1 pound as purchased	329	0.0	20.5	0.00
Weighed drawn [refuse, approx. 49%: head, tail, fins, bones, and skin], 1 pound as purchased	356	0.0	22.3	0.00
Edible portion, 1 pound	708	0.0	44.3	0.00
WHELK				
Whelk (*Buccinum*. Based on data from Africa)				
COOKED, SUN DRIED:				
Edible portion, 1 pound	1448	93.5	90.5	5.84
Whelk (*Eburna japonica*. Based on data from East Asia)				
RAW:				
As purchased, 1 pound [refuse, approx. 56%: shell and viscera]	141	6.8	8.8	0.43
Edible portion, 1 pound	313	15.4	19.6	0.96

	UNIT Cal.	UNIT Carb.	1 OZ., BY WT. Cal.	1 OZ., BY WT. Carb.
WHITEBAIT				
Whitebait (*Stolothrissa tanganical.* Based on data from Africa)				
RAW:				
Edible portion, 1 pound	263	0.0	16.4	0.00
DRIED:				
Edible portion, 1 pound	1370	0.0	85.6	0.00
Whitebait (*Salanx microclon.* Based on data from East Asia)				
RAW:				
Edible portion, 1 pound	440	0.0	27.5	0.00
DRIED, SALTED:				
Edible portion, 1 pound	1660	0.0	103.8	0.00
WHITEFISH, LAKE (see also LAKE TROUT and LAKE HERRING)				
RAW:				
Weighed whole [refuse, approx. 53%: head, tail, fins, entrails, bones, and skin], 1 pound as purchased	330	0.0	20.6	0.00
Weighed drawn [refuse, approx. 49%: head, tail, fins, bones, and skin], 1 pound as purchased	359	0.0	22.4	0.00
Meat only, edible portion, 1 pound (5g/0g/2g/72%/15mg)	703	0.0	43.9	0.00
SMOKED:				
All-edible, 1 pound (6g/0g/2g/68%/na)	518	0.0	32.4	0.00
STUFFED, BAKED:				
Based on USDA data; prepared with unspecified quantities of bacon, butter, or margarine, onion, celery, and breadcrumbs:				
1 pound (4g/2g/4g/63%/55mg)	976	25.6	61.0	1.60
WHITING (see also SMELT)				
Whiting (*Merluccius bilinearis*)				
RAW:				
Edible portion, 1 pound (5g/0g/tr/81%/na)	398	0.0	24.9	0.00
Whiting (based on data from France)				
RAW:				
Edible portion, 1 pound	313	0.0	19.6	0.00
WOLF HERRING (*Chirocentrus dorab.* Based on data from East Asia)				
RAW:				
As purchased, 1 pound [refuse, approx. 26%: bones and entrails]	318	0.0	19.8	0.00
Edible portion, 1 pound	431	0.0	26.9	0.00
WRASSES (*Labrus* and *Crenilabrus.* Based on data from Africa)				
RAW:				
Edible portion, 1 pound	440	0.0	27.5	0.00
WRECKFISH				
RAW:				
Edible portion, 1 pound (5g/0g/1g/77%/na)	518	0.0	32.4	0.00
YELLOWTAIL				
Yellowtail (Pacific Coast)				
RAW:				
Edible portion (fillet), 1 pound (6g/0g/2g/73%/na)	626	0.0	39.1	0.00
Yellowtail, Immature (based on data from Japan)				
RAW:				
Edible portion, 1 pound	740	1.4	46.3	0.09
XENOMYSTUS (based on data from Africa)				
RAW:				
Edible portion, 1 pound	400	0.0	25.0	0.00
ZACCO (*Zacco platypus.* Based on data from East Asia)				
RAW:				
As purchased, 1 pound [refuse, approx. 50%: bones, entrails, scales, and fins]	173	0.0	10.8	0.00
Edible portion, 1 pound	345	0.0	21.6	0.00

	UNIT Cal.	UNIT Carb.	1 OZ., BY WT. Cal.	1 OZ., BY WT. Carb.
ZEBRA FISH (*Diplodus.* Based on data from Africa)				
RAW:				
Edible portion, 1 pound	795	0.0	49.6	0.00
DRIED, SALTED:				
Edible portion, 1 pound	1212	0.0	75.7	0.00
FISH OFFAL (Fish intestines)				
Butterfish, caught in New England waters				
Caught in Autumn				
RAW:				
Edible portion, 1 pound (5g/0g/1g/76%/27mg)	622	0.0	38.9	0.00
Caught in Spring				
RAW:				
Edible portion, 1 pound (5g/0g/3g/74%/23mg)	(797)	0.0	(49.8)	0.00
Dabs				
Caught in Autumn				
RAW:				
Edible portion, 1 pound (5g/0g/tr/81%/24mg)	(402)	0.0	(25.1)	0.00
Caught in Spring				
RAW:				
Edible portion, 1 pound (5g/0g/tr/80%/28mg)	(399)	0.0	(24.9)	0.00
Flounder, caught in New England waters				
Blackback Flounder, caught in Autumn				
RAW:				
Edible portion, 1 pound (5g/0g/tr/80%/23mg)	(437)	0.0	(27.3)	0.00
Greyback Flounder, caught in Autumn				
RAW:				
Edible portion, 1 pound (5g/0g/tr/82%/28mg)	(305)	0.0	(19.1)	0.00
Yellowtail Flounder, caught in Autumn				
RAW:				
Edible portion, 1 pound (5g/0g/tr/81%/22mg)	327	0.0	20.4	0.00
Hake, caught in New England waters				
Silver Hake, caught in Autumn				
RAW:				
Edible portion, 1 pound (5g/0g/tr/81%/26mg)	(341)	0.0	(21.3)	0.00
Silver Hake, caught in Spring				
RAW:				
Edible portion, 1 pound (5g/0g/1g/80%/30mg)	379	0.0	23.7	0.00
Squirrel Hake, caught in Autumn				
RAW:				
Edible portion, 1 pound (5g/0g/tr/82%/26mg)	326	0.0	20.4	0.00
Pollock, caught in New England waters				
Small, caught in Autumn				
RAW:				
Edible portion, 1 pound (5g/0g/tr/78%/24mg)	684	0.0	42.8	0.00
Medium, caught in Spring				
RAW:				
Edible portion, 1 pound (5g/0g/tr/78%/20mg)	630	0.0	39.4	0.00
Large, caught in Autumn				
RAW:				
Edible portion, 1 pound (5g/0g/tr/77%/35mg)	(578)	0.0	(36.1)	0.00
FROZEN FISH AND SHELLFISH				
Catfish, by brand				
Taste O'Sea Ocean Catfish (fillet), 16-oz. (1-lb.) package	400	0.0	25.0	0.00
Clams, by brand				
Matlaw's Clams Oreganata Italian Style, 7-oz. package, 12 clams, weighed without shell	480	36.0	68.6	5.14
Stuffed Clams, 15-oz. package, 6 clams (each approx. 2½ oz.), weighed without shell	720	72.0	48.0	4.80
30-oz. package, 12 clams, weighed without shell	1440	144.0	48.0	4.80
1 clam, approx. 2½ oz., weighed without shell	120	12.0	48.0	4.80
Stuffed Clams Casino Hors d'Oeuvres, 11-oz. box, 12 clams, weighed without shell	480	52.0	43.6	4.73
1 clam, approx. 0.9 oz., weighed without shell	40	4.3	43.6	4.73
Stuffed Clams New England Style, 11-oz. package, 6 clams, weighed without shell	540	54.0	49.1	4.91
1 clam, approx. 1.8 oz., weighed without shell	90	9.0	49.1	4.91
Mrs. Paul's Clam Crêpes, 5½-oz. package, 2 crêpes	280	22.0	50.9	4.00
1 crêpe, approx. 2¾ oz.	140	11.0	50.9	4.00

	UNIT Cal.	UNIT Carb.	1 OZ., BY WT. Cal.	1 OZ., BY WT. Carb.
Fried Clams, 5-oz. package, approx. 80 clams, plus crumbs	540	50.0	108.0	10.00
1 clam, approx. 0.06 oz. (approx. 16 to the oz.)	(7)	(0.6)	108.0	10.00

Cod, by brand

	UNIT Cal.	UNIT Carb.	1 OZ., BY WT. Cal.	1 OZ., BY WT. Carb.
Taste O'Sea 4 Equal Cod Fish Portions, 12-oz. package	240	0.0	20.0	0.00
1 fish portion, approx. 3 oz.	60	0.0	20.0	0.00
Skinless Cod Breaded Fish Portions, 32-oz. (2-lb.) package, 12 portions	960	120.0	30.0	3.75
1 fish portion, approx. 2⅔ oz.	80	10.0	30.0	3.75
16-oz. (1-lb.) package, 8 portions	480	60.0	30.0	3.75
1 fish portion, approx. 2 oz.	60	7.5	30.0	3.75
Skinless Cod fillet, 16-oz. (1-lb.) package	320	0.0	20.0	0.00

Crab, by brand

	UNIT Cal.	UNIT Carb.	1 OZ., BY WT. Cal.	1 OZ., BY WT. Carb.
Mrs. Paul's Crab Crêpes, 5½-oz. package, 2 crêpes	240	24.0	43.6	4.36
1 crêpe, approx. 2¾ oz.	120	12.0	43.6	4.36
Deviled Crabs, 6-oz. package, 2 crab cakes	320	36.0	53.3	6.00
"Family," 15-oz. package, 5 crab cakes	800	90.0	53.3	6.00
1 crab cake, approx. 3 oz.	160	18.0	53.3	6.00
Wakefield Alaska Snow Crabmeat, 6-oz. package	120	2.0	20.0	0.33
Alaska Snow Crabmeat and Shrimp, 6-oz. package	120	2.0	20.0	0.33

Fish Cakes, by brand

	UNIT Cal.	UNIT Carb.	1 OZ., BY WT. Cal.	1 OZ., BY WT. Carb.
A&P 6 Fish Cakes, 12-oz. box	750	87.0	62.5	7.25
1 fish cake, approx. 2 oz.	125	14.5	62.5	7.25
Mrs. Paul's Fish Cakes, 8-oz. package, 4 cakes	420	46.0	52.5	5.75
"Family," 16-oz. (1-lb.) package, 8 cakes	840	92.0	52.5	5.75
1 fish cake, approx. 2 oz.	105	11.5	52.5	5.75
Taste O'Sea 4 Fish Cakes (cod and/or haddock, whiting, hake, pollock), 8-oz. package, 4 cakes	380	46.0	47.5	5.75

Fish Fillets, by brand

	UNIT Cal.	UNIT Carb.	1 OZ., BY WT. Cal.	1 OZ., BY WT. Carb.
Mrs. Paul's Buttered Fish Fillets, 10-oz. package, 4 fillets	775	5.0	77.5	0.50
1 fillet, approx. 2½ oz.	155	1.0	77.5	0.50
Fried Fish Fillets, 8-oz. package, 4 fillets	440	48.0	55.0	6.00
"Family," 14-oz. package, 7 fillets	770	84.0	55.0	6.00
"Party pak," 25-oz. package, 12 fillets	1375	150.0	55.0	6.00
1 fillet, approx. 2 oz.	110	12.0	55.0	6.00
Light Batter Fish Fillets, 9-oz. package, 4 fillets	560	56.0	62.2	6.22
"Family," 16-oz. (1-lb.) package, 7 fillets	995	100.0	62.2	6.22
"Party pak," 27½-oz. package, 12 fillets	1711	171.1	62.2	6.22
1 fillet, approx. 2¼ oz.	140	14.0	62.2	6.22
Supreme Light Batter Fish Fillets, 7¼-oz. package, 2 fillets	437	37.8	60.3	5.21
18¼-oz. package, 5 fillets	1100	95.1	60.3	5.21
1 fillet, approx. 3⅝ oz.	220	19.0	60.3	5.21

Fish Kabobs, by brand

	UNIT Cal.	UNIT Carb.	1 OZ., BY WT. Cal.	1 OZ., BY WT. Carb.
Taste O'Sea Fish Kabobs (Pollock), 16-oz. (1-lb.) package	900	100.0	56.3	6.25

Fish Portions, by brand

	UNIT Cal.	UNIT Carb.	1 OZ., BY WT. Cal.	1 OZ., BY WT. Carb.
A&P 8 Batter Dipped Fish Portions, 24-oz. package	1440	128.0	60.0	5.33
1 fish portion, approx. 3 oz.	180	16.0	60.0	5.33
7 Fish Sandwich Portions, 14-oz. package	910	91.0	65.0	6.50
1 sandwich portion, approx. 2 oz.	130	16.0	65.0	6.50
Taste O'Sea 4 Batter Dipt Fish Portions (Pollock), 12-oz. package	880	60.0	73.3	5.00
1 fish portion, approx. 3 oz.	220	15.0	73.3	5.00

Fish Sticks, based on generic data

	UNIT Cal.	UNIT Carb.	1 OZ., BY WT. Cal.	1 OZ., BY WT. Carb.
Fish Sticks, cooked, 1 container, 8 oz. net wt., approx. 8 fish sticks (5g/2g/3g/66%/na)	400	14.8	50.0	1.85
16 oz. (1 lb.) net wt., approx. 16 fish sticks (each approx. 1 oz.)	798	29.5	50.0	1.85
1 fish stick, approx. 1 oz.	50	1.8	50.0	1.85

Fish Sticks, by brand

	UNIT Cal.	UNIT Carb.	1 OZ., BY WT. Cal.	1 OZ., BY WT. Carb.
A&P Fish Sticks, 8-oz. box	480	48.0	60.0	6.00
1 fish stick, approx. 0.8 oz. (1¼ to the oz.)	48	4.8	60.0	6.00
14 Batter Dipped Fish Sticks, 14-oz. package	880	76.0	62.9	5.43
1 fish stick, approx. 1 oz.	63	5.4	62.9	5.43
Booth Fisheries Fish sticks, 16-oz. (1-lb.) package	880	100.0	55.0	6.25
1 fish stick, approx. 1 oz.	55	6.3	55.0	6.25
Mrs. Paul's Fish Sticks, 9-oz. package, 12 sticks	450	48.0	50.0	5.33
"Family," 14-oz. package, 18 sticks	700	74.6	50.0	5.33
"Party pak," 23-oz. package, 30 sticks	1150	122.6	50.0	5.33
1 fish stick, approx. ¾ oz.	38	4.0	50.0	5.33
16 Fish Sticks (Pollock), 16-oz. (1-lb.) package	1016	92.0	63.5	5.75
1 fish stick, approx. 1 oz.	64	5.8	63.5	5.75
32 Fish Sticks (Pollock), 27-oz. package	1688	168.8	62.5	6.25
1 fish stick, 0.8 oz. (1⅕ to the oz.)	74	7.4	62.5	6.25
8 Batter Dipt Fish Sticks (Pollock), 8-oz. package	620	52.0	77.5	6.50
1 fish stick, approx. 1 oz.	78	6.5	77.5	6.50
Light Batter Fish Sticks, 8¾-oz. package, 10 sticks	575	60.0	65.7	6.86
"Family," 14-oz. package, 16 sticks	920	96.0	65.7	6.86
"Party pak," 21-oz. package, 24 sticks	1380	144.1	65.7	6.86
1 fish stick, approx. ⅞ oz.	58	6.0	65.7	6.86
Taste O'Sea 8 Golden Fried Fish Sticks (Cod), 8-oz. package	508	46.0	63.5	5.75
1 fish stick, approx. 1 oz.	64	5.8	63.5	5.75
16 Golden Fried Fish Sticks (Haddock), 16-oz. (1-lb.) package	880	68.0	55.0	4.25
1 fish stick, approx. 1 oz.	55	4.3	55.0	4.25
8 Golden Fried Fish Sticks (Pollock), 8-oz. package	508	46.0	63.5	5.75
1 fish stick, approx. 1 oz.	64	5.8	63.5	5.75

Fish Thins, by brand

	UNIT Cal.	UNIT Carb.	1 OZ., BY WT. Cal.	1 OZ., BY WT. Carb.
Mrs. Paul's Fish Thins, 10-oz. package, 4 "thins"	640	62.0	64.0	6.20
1 "thin," 2½ oz.	160	15.0	64.0	6.20

Flounder, by brand

	UNIT Cal.	UNIT Carb.	1 OZ., BY WT. Cal.	1 OZ., BY WT. Carb.
Mrs. Paul's Flounder with Lemon Butter, 8½-oz. package	283	143.0	43.3	18.00
Fried Flounder Fillets, 8-oz. package, 4 fillets	440	44.0	55.0	5.50
"Family," 14-oz. package, 7 fillets	770	77.0	55.0	5.50
1 fillet, approx. 2 oz.	110	11.0	55.0	5.50
Taste O'Sea Flounder (fillet), 16-oz. (1-lb.) package	360	0.0	22.5	0.00
8 Flounder Fish Portions, 16-oz. (1-lb.) package	280	36.0	17.5	2.25

Haddock, by brand

	UNIT Cal.	UNIT Carb.	1 OZ., BY WT. Cal.	1 OZ., BY WT. Carb.
Mrs. Paul's Fried Haddock Fillets, 8-oz. package, 4 fillets	460	48.0	57.5	6.00
"Family," 14-oz. package, 7 fillets	805	84.0	57.5	6.00
1 fillet, approx. 2 oz.	115	12.0	57.5	6.00
Taste O'Sea Haddock (fillet), 16-oz. (1-lb.) package	360	0.0	22.5	0.00
4 Equal Haddock Fish Portions, 12-oz. package	280	0.0	23.3	0.00
1 fish portion, approx. 3 oz.	70	0.0	23.3	0.00
4 Batter Dipt Haddock Fish Portions, 12-oz. package	800	56.0	66.7	4.67
1 fish portion, approx. 3 oz.	200	14.0	66.7	4.67
12 Breaded Skinless Haddock Fish Portions, 32-oz. (2-lb.) package	960	120.0	30.0	3.75
1 fish portion, approx. 2⅔ oz.	80	10.0	30.0	3.75
Skinless Haddock (fillet), 16-oz. (1-lb.) package	400	0.0	25.0	0.00

Perch, by brand

	UNIT Cal.	UNIT Carb.	1 OZ., BY WT. Cal.	1 OZ., BY WT. Carb.
Mrs. Paul's Fried Ocean Perch Fillets, 8-oz. package, 4 fillets	500	36.0	62.5	4.50
"Family," 14-oz. package, 7 fillets	875	63.0	62.5	4.50
1 fillet, approx. 2 oz.	125	9.0	62.5	4.50
Taste O'Sea Ocean Perch (fillet), 16-oz. (1-lb.) package	400	0.0	25.0	0.00
12 Breaded Ocean Perch Fish Portions, 32-oz. (2-lb.) package	1200	132.0	37.5	4.13
1 fish portion, approx. 2⅔ oz.	100	11.0	37.5	4.13
4 Equal Ocean Perch Fish Portions, 12-oz. package	400	0.0	33.3	0.00
1 fish portion, approx. 3 oz.	100	0.0	33.3	0.00

Scallops, based on generic data

SEA SCALLOPS

Breaded, Fried, Reheated:

	UNIT Cal.	UNIT Carb.	1 OZ., BY WT. Cal.	1 OZ., BY WT. Carb.
"Random" pack containers (each scallop ranging in weight from 0.2 oz. to 0.7 oz., ranging in size from ⅞" long, ⅞" wide, ⅝" thick to 2¼" long, 1⅝" wide, ⅞" thick) (5g/3g/2g/60%/na)				
7-oz. container (reheated yield: approx. 6⅔ oz., 15 to 20 scallops)	367	19.8	55.0	2.98
12-oz. container (reheated yield: approx. 11⅖ oz., approx. 30 to 35 scallops)	629	34.0	55.0	2.98
1 scallop, approx. 0.4 oz.	19	1.1	55.0	2.98
"Uniform" pack container (packed in counts of 10 to 15, 15 to 20, 20 to 25, 25 to 30, 30 to 35 per pound)				
5-lb. (80-oz.) container (reheated yield: approx. 76⅕ oz.)	4190	226.8	55.0	2.98
1 scallop, 15 to 20 per pound, approx. 0.9 oz.	49	2.6	55.0	2.98
1 scallop, 25 to 30 per pound, approx. 0.5 oz.	29	1.6	55.0	2.98
Random & Uniform packs, 1 pound container (reheated yield: approx. 15¼ oz.)	838	45.4	55.0	2.98
1 pound	880	47.6	55.0	2.98

	UNIT Cal.	UNIT Carb.	1 OZ., BY WT. Cal.	1 OZ., BY WT. Carb.
Scallops, by brand				
A&P Crispy Scallops, 7-oz. box	480	50.0	68.6	7.14
Mrs. Paul's Batter Dipt Scallops, 7-oz. package	380	40.0	54.3	5.70
Fried Scallops, 7-oz. package, approx. 20 scallops	420	48.0	60.0	6.86
1 scallop, approx. 0.4 oz.	(23)	(2.6)	60.0	6.86
"Family," 12-oz. package, approx. 30 scallops	720	81.0	60.0	6.86
1 scallop, approx. 0.4 oz.	(23)	(2.6)	60.0	6.86
Golden Fried Sea Scallops, 8-oz. package	440	36.0	55.0	5.75
Light Batter Scallops, 7-oz. package, approx. 20 scallops	400	42.0	57.1	6.00
1 scallop, approx. 0.4 oz.	(21)	(2.3)	57.1	6.00
Scallops with Butter & Cheese, 7-oz. package	260	11.0	37.1	1.57
Scallop Crêpes, 5½-oz. package, 2 crêpes	220	25.0	40.0	4.55
1 crêpe, approx. 2¾ oz.	110	12.5	40.0	4.55
For comparison: **Worthington** Skallops (vegetarian, scallop-like), 20-oz. can, drained	450	20.0	23.3	1.00
1 cup (approx. 6.0 oz.)	140	6.0	23.3	1.00
1 pound (approx. 2.7 cups)	373	16.0	23.3	1.00
Shrimp, by brand				
A&P Crispy Shrimp, 6-oz. box	460	50.0	76.7	8.33
Gulf Princess Peeled and Deveined Shrimp, 12-oz. bag	212	10.9	17.7	0.91
16-oz. (1-lb.) bag	283	14.6	17.7	0.91
1½-lb. bag	425	21.8	17.7	0.91
3-lb. bag	850	43.7	17.7	0.91
Mrs. Paul's Fried Shrimp, 6-oz. package, approx. 10 pieces	340	34.0	56.7	5.67
1 piece, approx. 0.6 oz.	(34)	(3.4)	56.7	5.67
Shrimp Crêpes, 5½-oz. package, 2 crêpes	250	24.0	45.5	4.36
1 crêpe, approx. 2¾-oz.	125	12.0	45.5	4.36
Taste O'Sea Batter Dipt Shrimp, 6-oz. package	380	38.0	63.3	6.33
Golden Fried Shrimp, 6-oz. package	360	45.0	60.0	7.50
Shrimp Scampi, 7½-oz. package	490	16.0	65.3	2.13
Wakefield Alaska Shrimp, 6-oz. package	132	58.0	22.0	9.67
Alaska Snow Crabmeat and Shrimp, 6-oz. package	120	2.0	20.0	0.33
Sole, by brand				
Mrs. Paul's Sole with Lemon Butter, 8½-oz. package	303	18.9	35.6	2.22
Taste O'Sea 4 Equal Sole Portions, 12-oz. package	280	0.0	23.3	0.00
1 sole portion, approx. 3 oz.	70	0.0	23.3	0.00
Fillet of Sole, 16-oz. (1-lb.) package	360	0.0	22.5	0.00
Sole in lemon butter, 9-oz. package	420	18.0	46.7	2.00
Surimi, based on data provided by the National Food Processors Association, Washington, D.C.				
(There is a discussion of surimi in the FISH Chapter Preface, following "How to Eat Fish")				
Surimi Crab Legs, 1 pound	457	46.4	28.6	2.90
Surimi Scallops, 1 pound	441	48.2	27.6	3.01
Surimi Shrimp, 1 pound	450	41.4	28.1	2.59
Trout, by brand				
Clear Springs Boned Idaho Rainbow Trout, 10-oz. box, 2 trout	250	(0.3)	25.0	(0.03)
1 trout, approx. 5 oz.	125	(0.2)	25.0	(0.03)
Dressed Idaho Rainbow Trout, 10-oz. box, 2 trout	204	(0.2)	20.4	(0.02)
1 trout, approx. 5 oz.	102	(0.1)	20.4	(0.02)
12-oz. box, 2 trout	245	(0.3)	20.4	(0.02)
1 trout, approx. 6 oz.	122	(0.1)	20.4	(0.02)
Thousand Springs Boned Idaho Rainbow Trout, 10-oz. box, 2 trout	250	5.3	25.0	0.53
1 trout, approx. 5 oz.	125	2.6	25.0	0.53
Dressed Idaho Rainbow Trout, 10-oz. box, 2 trout	204	4.3	20.4	0.43
1 trout, approx. 5 oz.	102	2.2	20.4	0.43
16-oz. (1-lb.) tray pack	326	6.9	20.4	0.43
Turbot, by brand				
Taste O'Sea Greenland Turbot (fillet), 16-oz. (1-lb.) package	640	0.0	40.0	0.00
Whiting, by brand				
Taste O'Sea 8 Breaded Whiting Fish Portions, 16-oz. (1-lb.) package	560	64.0	3.50	4.00
1 fish portion, approx. 2 oz.	70	8.0	3.50	4.00
12 Breaded Whiting Fish Portions, 32-oz. (2-lb.) package	1080	120.0	33.8	3.75
1 fish portion, approx. 2⅔ oz.	90	10.0	33.8	3.75
Whiting (fillet), 16-oz. (1-lb.) package	320	0.0	20.0	0.00

CANNED FISH AND SHELLFISH

	UNIT Cal.	UNIT Carb.	1 OZ., BY WT. Cal.	1 OZ., BY WT. Carb.
Abalone, based on generic data				
Solids and liquid, 16-oz. (1-lb.) can (5g/1g/tr/80%/na)	363	10.4	22.7	0.65
Albacore, see Tuna *(Almost all albacore catch is canned as Tuna Fish.)*				
Alewife, solids and liquid, based on generic data				
1 pound (5g/0g/2g/73%/na)	640	0.0	40.0	0.00
Anchovy, based on generic data				
PICKLED, NOT HEAVILY SALTED: *Flat or rolled:*				
Can, solids and liquid, 2 oz. net wt. (10 to 16 anchovies)	(80)	(0.1)	(40.0)	(0.05)
Drained solids (yield: approx. 1.6 oz.) (5g/tr/3g/59%/na)	79	0.1	49.9	0.09
1 anchovy (flat: 4" long, ½" wide, ⅛" thick, or roll: ½"–¾" diameter, ½" thick), approx. 0.14 oz. (approx. 6 to 10 per ounce)	7	0.1	49.9	0.09
Drained solids, 1 pound	798	1.4	49.9	0.09
Bloater (based on data from Great Britain)				
Canned, drained solids, 1 pound	913	0.0	57.1	0.00
Caviar, Sturgeon, based on generic data				
GRANULAR:				
1 jar, 4 oz. net wt.	296	3.6	74.0	0.90
1 tablespoon (approx. 0.57 oz.)	42	0.5	74.0	0.90
1 caviar-pound (a measure used for caviar, it equals 14 oz.)	1036	12.6	74.0	0.90
1 cup (approx. 9.1 oz.)	672	8.0	74.0	0.90
1 pound (approx. 1¾ cups) (8g/1g/4g/46%/624 mg)	1184	14.4	74.0	0.90
PRESSED:				
1 jar, 4 oz. net wt.	360	5.6	90.0	1.34
1 tablespoon (approx. 0.61 oz.)	54	0.8	90.0	1.34
1 caviar-pound (a measure used for caviar, it equals 14 oz.)	1260	18.8	90.0	1.34
1 cup (approx. 9.6 oz.)	864	12.8	90.0	1.34
1 pound (approx. 1⅔ cups) (10g/1g/5g/36%/na)	1440	21.4	90.0	1.34
Clams, based on generic data				
WHOLE:				
Can #8Z Short, 7½–9 oz. net wt. (data based on 7.76 oz.) (2g/1g/tr/86%/na)	(132)	(4.5)	(17.0)	(0.57)
Drained solids (yield: approx. 3.9–4.2 oz.) (data based on 4 oz.) (4g/1g/1g/77%/na)	112	2.2	(27.7)	(0.54)
Liquid ("liquor," "bouillon," or "nectar") approx. 3½ fl. oz. (approx. 3¾ oz. by weight) (1g/1g/tr/94%/na)	(20)	(2.3)	5.4	0.60
Solids, 1 cup (approx. 9 clams)	(157)	(3.0)	(27.7)	(0.54)
1 clam, approx. 0.6 oz.	(17)	(0.3)	(27.7)	(0.54)
CHOPPED OR MINCED:				
Can #8Z Short, 7½–8 oz. net wt. (data based on 7.76 oz.) (2g/1g/tr/86%/na)	(132)	(4.5)	(17.0)	(0.57)
Drained solids (yield: approx. 3.9–4.2 oz.) (data based on 4 oz.) (4g/1g/1g/77%/na)	112	2.2	(27.7)	(0.54)
Liquid ("liquor," "bouillon," or "nectar"), approx. 3½ fl. oz. (approx. 3¾ oz. by weight) (1g/1g/tr/94%/na)	(20)	(2.3)	5.4	0.60
Solids, 1 cup (approx. 5.7 oz.)	(157)	(3.0)	(27.7)	(0.80)
Solids and liquid, 1 pound (2g/1g/tr/86%/na)	(272)	(9.1)	(17.0)	(0.57)
Drained solids, 1 pound (4g/1g/1g/77%/na)	445	8.6	(27.7)	(0.54)
Liquor, Bouillon, or Nectar, 8-fl.-oz. bottle (approx. 1 cup) (1g/1g/tr/94%/na)	46	5.0	5.7	0.63
Can #12Z, 12 fl. oz. (approx. 1½ cups)	68	7.6	5.7	0.63
1 fl. oz. (approx. 1.1 oz. by wt.)	6	0.7	5.7	0.63
Short Neck Clams (based on data from Japan)				
BOILED, CANNED:				
All-edible, 1 pound	431	10.9	26.9	0.68
SEASONED, CANNED:				
All-edible, 1 pound	499	39.9	31.2	2.50
Clams, by brand				
Pacific Pearl Whole Smoked Baby Clams, drained. 3¾-oz. can	293	7.2	78.0	1.93

Cod, based on generic data

	UNIT Cal.	UNIT Carb.	1 OZ., BY WT. Cal.	1 OZ., BY WT. Carb.
Can #1 Picnic, 11 oz. net wt., based on generic data				
Drained Solids (yield: approx. 8½ oz.; 4 pieces, each approx. 3½" long, 2" wide, ⅝" thick)	204	0.0	24.1	0.00
1 piece, approx. 2.1 oz.	51	0.0	24.1	0.00
1 cup, flaked (approx. 4.9 oz.)	(119)	0.0	24.1	0.00
1 pound (approx. 3.3 cups) (5g/0g/tr/79%/na)	386	0.0	24.1	0.00
DRIED, SALTED:				
1 pound (8g/0g/tr/52%/na)	590	0.0	36.9	0.00
1 piece, approx. 2.8 oz. (approx. 5½" long, 1½" wide, ½" thick)	104	0.0	36.9	0.00
DEHYDRATED, LIGHTLY SALTED:				
1 cup, shredded (approx. 1½ oz.)	(158)	0.0	106.0	0.00
1 pound (approx. 10.7 cups) (23g/0g/1g/12%/2297mg)	1696	0.0	106.0	0.00

Cod, by brand

	UNIT Cal.	UNIT Carb.	1 OZ., BY WT. Cal.	1 OZ., BY WT. Carb.
Beardsley Shredded Salt Codfish, 2-oz. box	70	0.0	35.0	0.00
Prepared as package directs for codfish cakes, mixing contents of box with 1½ cups water, 2 cups mashed potatoes, 1 egg, 1 small onion, 1 tsp. pepper, ¼ cup butter. (yield: approx. 31 oz., 4 to 6 fishcakes)	(914)	(54.0)	(29.5)	(1.75)
1 fish cake, approx. 6¼ oz.	(183)	(10.8)	(29.5)	(1.75)
Elf Salted Cod, 16-oz. (1-lb.) package	(1701)	0.0	(106.3)	0.00

Crab, based on generic data

	UNIT Cal.	UNIT Carb.	1 OZ., BY WT. Cal.	1 OZ., BY WT. Carb.
KING CRAB				
Can #½ Flat, 7½ oz. net wt., based on generic data				
Drained solids (yield: approx. 6⅓ oz.; approx. 1⅒ cups, packed) (5g/tr/1g/77%/246 mg)	182	2.0	28.9	0.32
1 cup, drained solids, packed (approx. 5.6 oz.)	(162)	(1.8)	28.9	0.32
BLUE CRAB (claw or white)				
Can #½, 6½ oz. net wt., based on generic data				
Drained solids (yield: approx. 4⅖ oz.) (5g/tr/1g/na/na)	126	1.4	28.6	0.32
1 cup, not packed:				
Claw meat (approx. 4 oz.)	(116)	(1.3)	28.6	0.32
White meat (approx. 4¾ oz.)	(136)	(1.5)	28.6	0.32
1 cup, packed, claw or white meat (approx. 5.6 oz.)	(162)	(1.8)	28.6	0.32
1 pound (approx. 2.9 cups, packed)	458	5.1	28.6	0.32

Crab, by brand

	UNIT Cal.	UNIT Carb.	1 OZ., BY WT. Cal.	1 OZ., BY WT. Carb.
Pacific Pearl Alaska Snow Crab Meat, 6.5-oz. can	138	0.0	21.3	0.00
Wakefield Alaska King Crabmeat, 6-oz. can	120	2.0	20.0	0.33

Crayfish (based on data from Great Britain)

	UNIT Cal.	UNIT Carb.	1 OZ., BY WT. Cal.	1 OZ., BY WT. Carb.
BOILED, DRAINED SOLIDS:				
Sample A, 1 pound	403	0.0	25.2	0.00
Sample B, 1 pound	360	0.0	22.5	0.00

Fish Flakes, based on generic data

	UNIT Cal.	UNIT Carb.	1 OZ., BY WT. Cal.	1 OZ., BY WT. Carb.
Solids and liquids, Can #½, 7 oz. net wt. (approx. 1⅕ cups)	220	0.0	31.4	0.00
1 cup, not packed (approx. 5.8 oz.)	(183)	0.0	31.4	0.00
1 pound (approx. 2¾ cups) (7g/tr/0g/72%/na)	503	0.0	31.4	0.00

Gefilte Fish (and "Whitefish & Pike"), by brand

"Piece" refers to 1 piece of fish and an amount of jelled broth. In a 2-piece can, for example, the jelled broth per "1 piece" would be half the broth in the can. The amount of broth and the size of the piece of fish will vary considerably in varying containers, even for the same manufacturer.

	UNIT Cal.	UNIT Carb.	1 OZ., BY WT. Cal.	1 OZ., BY WT. Carb.
Manischewitz Gefilte Fish, 12-oz. can, 4 pieces	323	12.6	26.9	1.05
1 piece, approx. 3 oz.	81	3.2	26.9	1.05
24-oz. jar, 6 pieces	646	25.2	26.9	1.05
1 piece, approx. 4 oz.	108	4.2	26.9	1.05
27-oz. jar, 8 pieces	726	28.4	26.9	1.05
1 piece approx. 3.3 oz.	90	3.5	26.9	1.05
27-oz. jar, 4 pieces	726	28.4	26.9	1.05
1 piece, approx. 6.7 oz.	179	7.0	26.9	1.05
Gefilte Fish Balls, 12-oz. jar, 8 pieces	323	12.6	26.9	1.05
1 piece, approx. 1½ oz.	40	1.6	26.9	1.05
Gefilte Fish Fishlets, 12-oz. jar, 28 pieces	323	12.6	26.9	1.05
1 piece, approx. 0.4 oz.	12	0.4	26.9	1.05
Whitefish & Pike, 12-oz. can, 4 pieces	162	6.2	23.0	0.88
1 piece, approx. 3 oz.	69	2.6	23.0	0.88
24-oz. jar, 6 pieces	552	21.1	23.0	0.88
1 piece, approx. 4 oz.	92	3.5	23.0	0.88
27-oz. jar, 8 pieces	621	23.8	23.0	0.88
1 piece, approx. 3.3 oz.	78	3.0	23.0	0.88
27-oz. jar, 4 pieces	621	23.8	23.0	0.88
1 piece, approx. 6.7 oz.	153	5.9	23.0	0.88
Whitefish & Pike Fishlets, 12-oz. jar, 28 pieces	276	10.6	23.0	0.88
1 piece approx. 0.4 oz.	10	0.4	23.0	0.88
Mrs. Adler's Gefilte Fish, 16-oz. (1-lb.) jar or can	267	30.3	16.7	1.89
32-oz. (2-lb.) jar	534	60.5	16.7	1.89
64-oz. (4-lb.) can	1069	121.0	16.7	1.89
Rokeach Old Vienna Sweet Recipe Gefilte Fish in Redi-Jelled Broth, 6-oz. jar	112	8.2	18.6	1.37
14-oz. can	260	19.2	18.6	1.37
22-oz. (1-lb. 6-oz.) jar	409	30.1	18.6	1.37
Gefilte Fish in Redi-Jelled Broth, 6-oz. jar	89	2.7	14.9	0.45
24-oz. jar	360	24.0	14.9	0.45
Gefilte Fish, Whitefish-Pike in Redi-Jelled Broth, 24-fl.-oz. (1-lb. 8-oz.) jar	360	24.0	15.0	1.00
Gefilte Fish in Liquid Broth, 16-oz. (1-lb.) jar	221	3.8	13.8	0.24
24-oz. jar	330	5.8	13.8	0.24

Haddock, based on generic data

	UNIT Cal.	UNIT Carb.	1 OZ., BY WT. Cal.	1 OZ., BY WT. Carb.
Smoked Haddock, drained solids, 1 pound	467	0.0	29.2	0.00

Herring, based on generic data

	UNIT Cal.	UNIT Carb.	1 OZ., BY WT. Cal.	1 OZ., BY WT. Carb.
Plain, Can #300, 15 oz. net wt., solids and liquid (drained solids will be approximately 10.6 oz., the drained liquid approximately 4.4 oz. Can will contain approximately 4 pieces, each approximately 3½" long, 2" wide, ¾" thick, weight approximately 2.7 oz.) (6g/0g/4g/63%/na)	884	0.0	58.9	0.00
Solids and liquid, 1 pound	943	0.0	58.9	0.00
In Tomato Sauce, 1 pound (4g/1g/3g/67%/na)	798	16.8	49.9	1.05
1 herring, approx. 4¾" long, 1½" wide, ⅝" thick), and 1 Tbsp. sauce (approx. 0.6 oz.), total weight approx. 1.9 oz.	97	2.0	49.9	1.05
Pickled, 1 pound (6g/0g/4g/59%/na)	1012	0.0	63.3	0.00
1 Bismarck herring, approx. 1¾ oz. (approx. 7" long, 1½" wide, ½" thick)	112	0.0	63.3	0.00
Marinated Pieces, each ranging in weight from 0.1 oz. to 0.8 oz. (ranging in size from ⅝" long, ¾" wide, ¼" thick to 3⅝" long, ¾" wide, ½" thick)				
1 piece, solids and liquid, approx. ½ oz. (approx. 1¾" long, ⅞" wide, ½" thick)	33	0.0	63.3	0.00
Smoked, Kippered, 3¼-oz. can, drained (approx. 2.8 oz.) (contains 2 fillets, each approx. 1.4 oz. or 4 fillets, each approx. 0.7 oz.) (6g/0g/4g/61%/na)	169	0.0	60.4	0.00
1 fillet, drained, approx. 0.7 oz. (approx. 2⅔" long, 1⅜" wide, ¼" thick)	42	0.0	60.4	0.00
1 fillet, drained, approx. 1.4 oz. (approx. 4⅜" long, 1¾" wide, ¼" thick)	84	0.0	60.4	0.00
8-oz. can, drained solids (yield: approx. 6.9 oz.; 3 fillets)	411	0.0	60.4	0.00
1 fillet, approx. 2.3 oz. (approx. 7" long, 2¼" wide, ¼" thick)	137	0.0	60.4	0.00
1 pound, drained	966	0.0	60.4	0.00
Based on data from Great Britain				
Kippers, 1 pound	705	0.0	44.1	0.00

Herring, by brand

	UNIT Cal.	UNIT Carb.	1 OZ., BY WT. Cal.	1 OZ., BY WT. Carb.
A&P Kipper Snacks, fillets of Kippered Herring, salted, solids and liquid, 3¼-oz. can	150	0.0	46.2	0.00
Elf Norwegian, Salted, with Head, drained, 7-lb. pail	(6,923)	0.0	(61.8)	0.00
25-lb. pail	(24,724)	0.0	(61.8)	0.00
38-lb. pail	(37,574)	0.0	(61.8)	0.00
225-lb. barrel	(222,512)	0.0	(61.8)	0.00
Iceland Type, Salted, Headless, drained, 7-lb. pail	(6,923)	0.0	(61.8)	0.00
38-lb. pail	(37,574)	0.0	(61.8)	0.00
225-lb. barrel	(222,512)	0.0	(61.8)	0.00
Lyon Smoked, Boneless, drained, 4½-oz. container	(383)	0.0	(85.1)	0.00
10-lb. box	(13,616)	0.0	(85.1)	0.00
Sea Trader Kipper Snacks, 3¾-oz. can	150	0.0	40.0	0.00

Horse Mackerel (based on data from Japan)

	UNIT Cal.	UNIT Carb.	1 OZ., BY WT. Cal.	1 OZ., BY WT. Carb.
SEASONED:				
All-edible, 1 pound	654	11.4	40.9	0.71

	UNIT Cal.	UNIT Carb.	1 OZ., BY WT. Cal.	1 OZ., BY WT. Carb.
Kippers, see under Herring				
Lobster, based on generic data				
Drained solids, 1 lb. (5g/tr/tr/77%/60mg)	431	1.4	26.9	0.09
Mackerel, based on generic data				
Atlantic Mackerel				
Solids and liquid, 1 pound (5g/0g/3g/66%/na)	830	0.0	51.9	0.00
Pacific Mackerel				
Can #300, 15 oz. net wt., solids and liquid (drained solids will be approximately 12¾ oz., the drained liquid approximately 2¼ oz. Can will contain approximately 2⅔ pieces, each approximately 4" long, 1½" wide, 1" thick, weight approx. 3.4 oz. This will yield approximately 1.9 cups, when flaked.) (6g/0g/3g/66%/na)	765	0.0	51.0	0.00
Solids and liquid, 1 pound	816	0.0	51.0	0.00
1 cup, flaked, solids and liquid (approx. 7.9 oz.)	403	0.0	51.0	0.00
Menhadem, Atlantic, based on generic data				
Solids and liquid, 1 pound (5g/0g/3g/68%/na)	780	0.0	48.8	0.00
Mussels, Pacific, based on generic data				
Drained solids, 1 pound (5g/tr/1g/75%/na)	517	6.8	32.3	0.43
Mussels, by brand				
Pacific Pearl, Smoked Mussels, 3¾-oz. can	271	7.2	72.3	1.93
Ocean Perch, Atlantic, based on generic data				
Frozen, Breaded, Fried, Reheated, 1 pound (5g/5g/5g/43%/na)	1447	74.8	90.4	4.68
Oysters (type not specified), based on generic data				
Solids and liquid, 12-fl.-oz. can (approx. 12.7 oz.)	(273)	(17.6)	(21.5)	(1.39)
1 pound (approx. 1.9 cups)	(344)	(22.2)	(21.5)	(1.39)
Oil added, smoked, 1 pound	1034	48.5	64.6	3.03
Oysters, by brand				
Pacific Pearl Whole Oysters, 8-oz. can, drained wt.	204	14.7	25.5	1.84
Smoked Oysters, 3¾-oz. can, drained wt.	302	15.2	80.5	4.05
Pike, see Gefilte Fish and Whitefish				
Prawns (based on data from Great Britain) (see also Shrimp)				
Canned, drained solids, 1 pound	482	0.0	30.1	0.00
Roe, including Cod, Haddock, and Herring Roe, based on generic data				
Solids and liquid, Can #8Z Tall, Buffet, 8 oz. net wt. (6g/tr/1g/72%/na)	268	0.7	33.5	0.09
Can #300, 15 oz. net wt.	502	1.3	33.5	0.09
1 pound	535	1.4	33.5	0.09
Salmon, based on generic data				
Atlantic Salmon				
Can #½ Flat, solids and liquid, 7¾ oz. net wt.	447	0.0	57.7	0.00
Can #1 Tall, solids and liquid, 16 oz. (1 lb.) net wt.	921	0.0	57.7	0.00
Can, solids and liquid, 64 oz. (4 lb.) net wt.	3682	0.0	57.7	0.00
Solids and liquid, 1 pound (approx. 2 cups) (6g/0g/3g/6470/na)	921	0.0	57.7	0.00
1 cup, not packed (approx. 7¾ oz.)	447	0.0	57.7	0.00
Chinook (King) Salmon				
Can #½ Flat, solids and liquid, 7¾ oz. net wt.	462	0.0	59.6	0.00
Can #1 Tall, solids and liquid, 16 oz. (1 lb.) net wt.	953	0.0	59.6	0.00
Can, solids and liquid, 64 oz. (4 lb.) net wt.	3809	0.0	59.6	0.00
Solids and liquid, 1 pound (approx. 2 cups) (6g/0g/4g/64%/na)	953	0.0	59.6	0.00
1 cup, not packed (approx. 7¾ oz.)	462	0.0	59.6	0.00
Chum Salmon				
Can #½ Flat, solids and liquid, 7¾ oz. net wt.	306	0.0	39.4	0.00

	UNIT Cal.	UNIT Carb.	1 OZ., BY WT. Cal.	1 OZ., BY WT. Carb.
Can #1 Tall, solids and liquid, 16 oz. (1 lb.) net wt.	631	0.0	39.4	0.00
Can, solids and liquid, 64 oz. (4 lb.) net wt.	2521	0.0	39.4	0.00
Solids and liquid, 1 pound (approx. 2 cups) (6g/0g/1g/71%/na)	631	0.0	39.4	0.00
1 cup, not packed (approx. 7¾ oz.)	306	0.0	39.4	0.00
Coho (Silver) Salmon				
Can #½ Flat, solids and liquid, 7¾ oz. net wt.	337	0.0	43.4	0.00
Can #1 Tall, solids and liquid, 16 oz. (1 lb.) net wt.	694	0.0	43.4	0.00
Can, solids and liquid, 64 oz. (4 lb.) net wt.	2775	0.0	43.4	0.00
Solids and liquid, 1 pound (approx. 2 cups) (6g/0g/2g/69%/100mg)	694	0.0	43.4	0.00
1 cup, not packed (approx. 7¾ oz.)	336	0.0	43.4	0.00
Humpback Pink Salmon				
Can #½ Flat, solids and liquid, 7¾ oz. net wt.	310	0.0	40.0	0.00
Can #1 Tall, solids and liquid, 16 oz. (1 lb.) net wt.	640	0.0	40.0	0.00
Can, solids and liquid, 64 oz. (4 lb.) net wt.	2558	0.0	40.0	0.00
Solids and liquid, 1 pound (approx. 2 cups) (6g/0g/2g/71%/110mg)	640	0.0	40.0	0.00
1 cup, not packed (approx. 7¾ oz.)	310	0.0	40.0	0.00
Sockeye (red) Salmon				
Can #½ Flat, solids and liquid, 7¾ oz. net wt.	376	0.0	48.5	0.00
Can #1 Tall, solids and liquid, 16 oz. (1 lb.) net wt.	776	0.0	48.5	0.00
Can, solids and liquid, 64 oz. (4 lb.) net wt.	3102	0.0	48.5	0.00
Solids and liquid, 1 pound (approx. 2 cups) (6g/0g/3g/67%/148mg)	776	0.0	48.5	0.00
1 cup, not packed (approx. 7¾ oz.)	376	0.0	48.5	0.00
Salmon, by brand				
Balanced Salmon, dietetic, without added oil or salt, 3½-oz. can.	(74)	0.0	(21.0)	0.00
7¾-oz. can	(163)	0.0	(21.0)	0.00
Bumble Bee Blueback Salmon, 3¾-oz. can	193	0.0	51.4	0.00
7½-oz. can	386	0.0	51.4	0.00
1 cup, solids and liquid (approx. 7 oz.)	(360)	0.0	51.4	0.00
Pink Salmon, 3¾-oz. can	171	0.0	45.7	0.00
7½-oz. can	343	0.0	45.7	0.00
15½-oz. can	709	0.0	45.7	0.00
1 cup, solids and liquid (approx. 7 oz.)	(320)	0.0	45.7	0.00
Red Salmon, 3¾-oz. can	179	0.0	47.7	0.00
7¾-oz. can	370	0.0	47.7	0.00
15½-oz. can	739	0.0	47.7	0.00
1 cup, solids and liquid (approx. 7 oz.)	(334)	0.0	47.7	0.00
Sardines, based on generic data				
Atlantic Sardines Packed in Oil				
Can #¼ Oil, 3¾ oz. net wt. (6g/tr/7g/51%/145mg)	330	0.6	88.0	0.20
Drained solids (yield: approx. 3¼ oz.) (7g/tr/3g/62%/233mg)	178		57.5	
Liquid, approx. ½-oz. (approx. 1 Tbsp.) (tr/tr/28g/tr/na)	(152)		(250.6)	
1 sardine, from can 3¾ oz. net wt. when packed: 5 per can, each approx. 3½" long, 1½" wide, ⅜" thick (approx. 0.7 oz.)	41		57.5	
8 per can, each approx. 3" long, 1" wide, ½" thick (approx. 0.4 oz.)	24		57.5	
16 to 20 per can, each approx. 2⅔" long, ½" wide, ¼" thick (approx. 0.2 oz.)	10		57.5	
Solids and liquid, 1 pound	1411	2.7	88.0	0.20
Drained solids, 1 pound	921		57.5	
Sardines, by brand				
A&P Norway Brisling Sardines in Olive Oil, solids and liquid, 3¾-oz. can, 16 to 22 sardines	260	1.0	69.3	0.27
Drained solids (yield: approx. 3¼ oz.)	(179)	(1.0)	(55.2)	(0.31)
1 sardine, approx. 0.16 oz.	(9)	trace	(55.2)	(0.31)
Norway Sardines in Norway Sild Sardine Oil, solids and liquid, 3¾-oz. can, 8 to 12 sardines	260	1.0	69.3	0.27
Drained solids (yield: approx. 3¼ oz.)	(179)	(1.0)	(55.2)	(0.31)
1 sardine, approx. 0.33 oz.	(18)	(0.1)	(55.2)	(0.31)
Norway Sardines in Norway Sild Sardine Oil, solids and liquid, 3¾-oz. can, 16 to 24 sardines	260	1.0	69.3	0.27
Drained solids (yield: approx. 3¼ oz.)	(179)	(1.0)	(55.2)	(0.31)
1 sardine, approx. 0.16 oz.	(9)	trace	(55.2)	(0.31)
Norway Sardines in Olive Oil, solids and liquid, 3¾-oz. can, 16 to 24 sardines	260	1.0	69.3	0.27
Drained solids (yield: approx. 3¼ oz.)	(179)	(1.0)	(55.2)	(0.31)
1 sardine, approx. 0.16 oz.	(9)	trace	(55.2)	(0.31)
Betsy Maine Sardines in Soybean Oil, solids and liquid, 4-oz. can, approx. 20 sardines	300	1.0	75.0	0.25
Drained solids (yield: approx. 3½ oz.)	(207)	(1.0)	(59.1)	(0.29)
1 sardine, approx. 0.7 oz.	(10)	(0.1)	(59.1)	(0.29)

	UNIT Cal.	UNIT Carb.	1 OZ., BY WT. Cal.	1 OZ., BY WT. Carb.
Coastal Kitchen Maine Sardines in Mustard Sauce, solids and liquid, 4-oz. can, approx. 9 sardines	170	1.0	42.5	0.25
1 sardine plus ⅑ of the mustard sauce, approx. 0.4 oz.	(19)	(0.1)	42.5	0.25
Maine Sardines in Soybean Oil, solids and liquid, 4-oz. can, approx. 9 sardines	300	1.0	75.0	0.25
Drained solids (yield: approx. 3½ oz.)	(207)	(1.0)	(59.1)	(0.29)
1 sardine, approx. 0.39 oz.	(23)	(0.1)	(59.1)	(0.29)
Sardines in Tomato Sauce, solids and liquid, 4-oz. can, 9 sardines	200	2.0	50.0	0.50
1 sardine plus ⅑ of the tomato sauce, approx. 0.4 oz.	(22)	(0.2)	50.0	0.50
Del Monte Sardines in Tomato Sauce, solids and liquid, 8-oz. can	352	4.3	44.0	0.53
15-oz. can	660	8.0	44.0	0.53
King Oscar Finest Norway Smoked Brisling Sardines in Olive Oil, solids and liquid, 3¾-oz. can, approx. 20 sardines	460	1.0	122.7	0.27
Drained solids (yield: approx. 3 oz.)	260	1.0	(87.8)	(0.34)
1 sardine, approx. 0.15 oz.	(13)	(0.1)	(87.8)	(0.34)
Sardines in Mustard Sauce, solids and liquid 3¾-oz. can, 8 sardines	240	2.0	64.0	0.53
1 sardine plus ⅛ of the mustard sauce, approx. 0.5 oz.	(30)	(0.2)	64.0	0.53
Sardines in Soya Oil, solids and liquid, 3¾-oz. can, approx. 20 sardines	460	1.0	122.7	0.27
Drained solids (yield: approx. 3 oz.)	260	1.0	(87.8)	(0.34)
1 sardine, approx. 0.15 oz.	(13)	(0.1)	(87.8)	(0.34)
Sardines in Tomato Sauce, 3¾-oz. can	240	2.0	64.0	0.53
Norse Girl Norway Sardines in Mustard Sauce, 3¾-oz. can	240	2.0	64.0	0.53
Norway Sardines in Oil, 3¾-oz. can, solids and liquid	460	1.0	122.7	0.27
Drained solids (yield: approx. 3.1 oz.)	260	1.0	85.2	0.33
Norway Sardines in Tomato Sauce, 3¾-oz. can	240	2.0	64.0	0.53
Ocean Delight Maine Sardines in Mustard Sauce, solids and liquid, 4-oz. can, 9 sardines	170	1.0	42.5	0.25
1 sardine plus ⅑ of the mustard sauce, approx. 0.5 oz.	19	0.1	42.5	0.25
Maine Sardines in Tomato Sauce, solids and liquid, 4-oz. can, 9 sardines	200	2.0	50.0	0.50
1 sardine plus ⅑ of the tomato sauce, approx. 0.4 oz.	22	0.2	50.0	0.50
Pacific Pearl Chunk Light Sardines in Water, solids and liquid, 7-oz. can	250	0.0	35.7	0.00
Drained solids, approx. 5.7 oz.	(250)	0.0	(44.1)	0.00
Port Clyde Maine Sardines in Mustard Sauce, solids and liquid, 3¾-oz. can, 8 sardines	160	1.0	42.8	0.27
1 sardine plus ⅛ of the mustard sauce, approx. 0.5 oz.	20	0.1	42.8	0.27
Maine Sardines in Mustard Sauce, solids and liquid, 4-oz. can, 9 sardines	170	1.0	42.8	0.27
1 sardine plus ⅑ of the mustard sauce, approx. 0.5 oz.	19	0.1	42.8	0.27
Maine Sardines in Soybean Oil, solids and liquid, 3¾-oz. can, 8 sardines	280	1.0	74.7	0.27
Drained solids (yield: approx. 3¼ oz.)	187	1.0	57.5	0.31
1 sardine, approx. 0.40 oz.	23	0.1	57.5	0.31
Maine Sardines in Soybean Oil, solids and liquid, 4-oz. can, 9 sardines	300	1.0	75.0	0.25
Drained solids (yield: approx. 3½ oz.)	207	1.0	59.1	0.29
1 sardine, approx. 0.39 oz.	23	0.1	59.1	0.29
Maine Sardines in Soybean Oil, Small, solids and liquid, 4-oz. can, 20 sardines	300	1.0	75.0	0.25
Drained solids (yield: approx. 3½ oz.)	207	1.0	59.1	0.29
1 sardine, approx. 0.17 oz.	10	0.1	59.1	0.29
Maine Sardines in Tomato Sauce, solids and liquid, 3¾-oz. can, 8 sardines	190	2.0	50.7	0.53
1 sardine plus ⅛ of the sauce, approx. 0.5 oz.	24	0.3	50.7	0.53
Maine Sardines in Tomato Sauce, solids and liquid, 4-oz. can, 9 sardines	190	2.0	50.7	0.53
1 sardine plus ⅑ of the sauce, approx. 0.4 oz.	24	0.3	50.7	0.53
Sea Trader Sardines in Oil, 3¾-oz. can, solids and liquid	460	1.0	122.7	0.27
Drained solids (yield: approx. 3.1 oz.)	260	1.0	85.2	0.33
Brisling Sardines in Olive Oil, 3¾-oz. can, solids and liquid	460	1.0	122.7	0.27
Drained solids (yield: approx. 3.05 oz.)	260	1.0	85.2	0.33
Tiny Tots Norway Brisling Sardines in Olive Oil, solids and liquid, 3¾-oz. can	260	1.0	69.3	0.27
Drained solids (yield: approx. 3 oz.)	(179)	(1.0)	(55.2)	(0.34)
Underwood Sardines in Mustard Sauce, solids and liquid, 3¾-oz. can	195	2.3	52.0	0.60
Sardines in Soya Bean Oil, solids and liquid, 3¾-oz. can	233	0.4	62.0	0.10
Sardines in Tomato Sauce, solids and liquid 3¾-oz. can	169	4.5	45.0	1.20

Shrimp, based on generic data (see also Prawns)

	UNIT Cal.	UNIT Carb.	1 OZ., BY WT. Cal.	1 OZ., BY WT. Carb.
Can, 4½ oz. drained wt. (Drained weight is also the declared net weight of can.) (approx. 1 cup, not packed) (7g/tr/tr/70%/na)	148	0.9	32.9	0.20
1 shrimp from can, 4½ oz. declared and drained wt., when shrimp are:				
Large, packed 22 to the can, each approx. 3¼" long when measured along outer curvature (approx. 0.2 oz.)	7	trace	32.9	0.20
Medium, packed 40 to the can, each approx. 2½" long when measured along outer curvature (approx. 0.1 oz.)	4	trace	32.9	0.20
Small, packed 76 to the can, each approx. 2" long when measured along outer curvature (approx. 0.06 oz.)	2	trace	32.9	0.20
1 cup, not packed (approx. 22 large shrimp, 40 medium shrimp, or 76 small shrimp; approximate contents of 4½-oz. can as above)	148	0.9	32.9	0.20
1 pound, drained solids	526	3.2	32.9	0.20

Shrimp, by brand

	UNIT Cal.	UNIT Carb.	1 OZ., BY WT. Cal.	1 OZ., BY WT. Carb.
China Bowl, Dried Miniature Shrimp, 2-oz. container	205	8.8	102.6	4.42
Orleans Jumbo Shrimp, drained, 4¼-oz. can, approx. 12 shrimp	130	0.0	30.6	0.00
1 shrimp, approx. 0.4 oz.	(11)	0.0	30.6	0.00
Jumbo Shrimp, Deveined, drained, 4¼-oz. can, approx. 12 shrimp	130	0.0	30.6	0.00
1 shrimp, approx. 0.4 oz.	(11)	0.0	30.6	0.00
Large Shrimp, drained, 4¼-oz. can, approx. 21 shrimp	130	0.0	30.6	0.00
1 shrimp, approx. 0.2 oz.	(6)	0.0	30.6	0.00
Large Shrimp, Deveined, drained, 4¼-oz. can, approx. 21 shrimp	130	0.0	30.6	0.00
1 shrimp, approx. 0.2 oz.	(6)	0.0	30.6	0.00
Medium Shrimp, drained, 4¼-oz. can, approx. 38 shrimp	130	0.0	30.6	0.00
1 shrimp, approx. 0.1 oz.	(3)	0.0	30.6	0.00
Medium Shrimp, Deveined, drained, 4¼-oz. can, approx. 38 shrimp	130	0.0	30.6	0.00
1 shrimp, approx. 0.1 oz.	(3)	0.0	30.6	0.00
Small Shrimp, drained, 4¼-oz. can, approx. 72 shrimp	130	0.0	30.6	0.00
1 shrimp, approx. 0.06 oz.	(2)	0.0	30.6	0.00
Small Shrimp, Deveined, drained, 4¼-oz. can, approx. 72 shrimp	130	0.0	30.6	0.00
1 shrimp, approx. 0.06 oz.	(2)	0.0	30.6	0.00
Tiny Cocktail Shrimp, drained, 4¼-oz. can, approx. 120 shrimp	130	0.0	30.6	0.00
1 shrimp, approx. 0.04 oz.	(1)	0.0	30.6	0.00
Tiny Cocktail Shrimp, Deveined, drained, 4¼-oz. can, approx. 120 shrimp	130	0.0	30.6	0.00
1 shrimp, approx. 0.04 oz.	(1)	0.0	30.6	0.00
Pacific Pearl Tiny Alaska Shrimp, 4.5-oz. jar	96	0.0	21.3	0.00
Sau-Sea Cooked Shrimp, drained, 8-oz. jar	226	38.0	28.3	4.75
Shrimp Cocktail, solids and liquid, 4-oz. jar, approx. 18 shrimp	113	19.0	28.3	4.75
1 shrimp plus 1/18 sauce, approx. 0.2 oz.	(6)	(1.1)	28.3	4.75
Shrimp Cocktail, Deluxe, solids and liquid, 6-oz. jar, approx. 18 shrimp	170	29.0	28.3	4.83
1 shrimp plus 1/18 sauce, approx. ⅓ oz.	(9)	(1.6)	28.3	4.83
Shrimp Fries, 8-oz. jar	480	44.0	60.0	5.50

Smelt, Atlantic, Jack, and Bay, based on generic data

	UNIT Cal.	UNIT Carb.	1 OZ., BY WT. Cal.	1 OZ., BY WT. Carb.
Solids and liquid, 1 pound (5g/0g/4g/63%/na)	907	0.0	56.7	0.00

Swordfish, based on generic data

	UNIT Cal.	UNIT Carb.	1 OZ., BY WT. Cal.	1 OZ., BY WT. Carb.
Solids and liquid, 1 pound (5g/0g/1g/78%/na)	463	0.0	28.9	0.00

Top-Shell (*Turbo cornutus.* Based on data from East Asia)

	UNIT Cal.	UNIT Carb.	1 OZ., BY WT. Cal.	1 OZ., BY WT. Carb.
SEASONED:				
Edible portion, 1 pound	594	43.5	37.1	2.72

Trout

	UNIT Cal.	UNIT Carb.	1 OZ., BY WT. Cal.	1 OZ., BY WT. Carb.
Trout (*Salmo.* Based on data from East Asia)				
SALTED:				
Edible portion, 1 pound	907	0.0	56.7	0.00
Trout, Rainbow and Steelhead				
Solids and liquid, 1 pound (6g/0g/4g/63%/na)	948	0.0	59.3	0.00

Tuna, based on generic data

	UNIT Cal.	UNIT Carb.	1 OZ., BY WT. Cal.	1 OZ., BY WT. Carb.
TUNA, PACKED IN OIL				
SOLID PACK, Can #½, solids and liquid, 7 oz. net wt. (7g/0g/6g/53%/227mg)	570	0.0	81.6	0.00
Drained solids (yield: approx. 6 oz.; 1.1 cup, not packed) (8g/0g/2g/61%/na)	333	0.0	55.5	0.00
Liquid, approx. 1 oz. (approx. 2 Tbsp.) (tr/tr/28g/tr/na)	(243)	0.0	(243.0)	0.00
Can #1, solids and liquid, 13 oz. net wt.	1063	0.0	81.6	0.00
Drained solids (yield: approx. 11 oz.; 1.8 cups, not packed)	617	0,0	55.5	0.00
Liquid, approx. 2 oz. (approx. 4 Tbsp.)	(446)	0.0	(243.0)	0.00
Can, solids and liquid, 64 oz. (4 lb.) net wt.	5224	0.0	81.6	0.00
Drained solids (yield: approx. 54 oz.; 3 lb. 6 oz.; 9.6 cups, not packed)	3038	0.0	55.5	0.00
Liquid, approx. 10 oz. (approx. 1 cup plus 4 Tbsp.)	2186	0.0	243.0	0.00

	UNIT Cal.	UNIT Carb.	1 OZ., BY WT. Cal.	1 OZ., BY WT. Carb.
CHUNK STYLE, Can #½, solids and liquid, 6½ oz. net wt. (7g/0g/6g/53%/227 mg)	530	0.0	81.6	0.00
Drained solids (yield: approx. 5½ oz.; 1.0 cup, not packed) (8g/0g/2g/61%/na)	309	0.0	55.5	0.00
Liquid, approx. 1 oz. (approx. 2 Tbsp. (tr/tr/28g/tr/na)	(221)	0.0	(221.0)	0.00
"Family" Can, solids and liquid, 9¼ oz. net wt.	755	0.0	81.6	0.00
Drained solids (yield: approx. 7.9 oz., 1.4 cups, not packed)	439	0.0	55.5	0.00
Liquid, approx. 1.4 oz., (approx. 3 tbsp.)	(316)	0.0	(221.0)	0.00
Can, solids and liquid, 60 oz. (3 lb. 12 oz.) net wt.	4899	0.0	81.6	0.00
Drained solids (yield: approx. 51 oz. or 3 lb. 3 oz.; 9 cups, not packed)	2849	0.0	55.5	0.00
Liquid, approx. 9 oz. (approx. 1 cup plus 2 Tbsp.)	2050	0.0	227.8	0.00
TUNA, PACKED IN WATER				
SOLID PACK, Can #¼, solids and liquid, 3½ oz. net wt.	126	0.0	36.0	0.00
Drained solids (yield: approx. 2¾ oz.)	(120)	0.0	(45.6)	0.00
Can #½, solids and liquid, 7 oz. net wt.	251	0.0	36.0	0.00
Drained solids (yield: approx. 5½ oz.)	(251)	0.0	(45.6)	0.00
Can #1, solids and liquid, 13 oz. net wt.	469	0.0	36.0	0.00
Drained solids (yield: approx. 10¼ oz.)	(469)	0.0	(45.6)	0.00
Can, solids and liquid, 66½ oz. (4 lb. 2½ oz.) net wt.	2394	0.0	36.0	0.00
Drained solids (yield: approx. 52.5 oz.)	(2394)	0.0	(45.6)	0.00
Solids and liquid, 1 pound (approx. 1.9 cups) (4g/0g/tr/70%/12mg)	576	0.0	36.0	0.00
Drained solids, 1 pound (approx. 2.7 cups)	(730)	0.0	(45.6)	0.00
TUNA SALAD				
(General figures provided by the USDA for tuna salad prepared with unspecified amounts of mayonnaise-type salad dressing, celery, pickle, onion, and egg.)				
1 cup (approx. 7.2 oz.)	(349)	(7.2)	(48.2)	(0.99)
1 pound (approx. 2.2 cups)	(771)	(15.9)	(48.2)	(0.99)

Tuna, by brand

	UNIT Cal.	UNIT Carb.	1 OZ., BY WT. Cal.	1 OZ., BY WT. Carb.
Balanced Solid White Tuna, no salt added, packed in Water, solids and liquid, 3½-oz. can	120	0.0	34.3	0.00
Drained solids, (yield: approx. 2.8 oz.)	(120)	0.0	(42.9)	0.00
1 cup, not packed:				
Solids and liquid (approx. 5.7 oz.)	(194)	0.0	(34.3)	0.00
Drained solids (yield: approx. 5.6 oz.)	(242)	0.0	(42.9)	0.00
Bumble Bee Chunk Light Tuna, packed in Oil, solids and liquid, 3¼-oz. can	(260)	0.0	(80.0)	0.00
Drained solids (yield: approx. 2¾ oz.)	(153)	0.0	(55.7)	0.00
6½-oz. can	(520)	0.0	(80.0)	0.00
Drained solids (yield: approx. 5½ oz.)	(306)	0.0	(55.7)	0.00
1 cup, not packed:				
Solids and liquid (approx. 8.8 oz.)	(705)	0.0	(80.0)	0.00
Drained solids (yield: approx. 6.0 oz.)	(334)	0.0	(55.7)	0.00
Chunk Light Tuna, packed in Water, solids and liquid, 6½-oz. can	221	0.0	34.0	0.00
Drained solids (yield: approx. 5 oz.)	(221)	0.0	(43.0)	0.00
12½-oz. can	425	0.0	34.0	0.00
Drained solids (yield: approx. 10 oz.)	(425)	0.0	(43.0)	0.00
1 cup, not packed:				
Solids and liquid (approx. 8.8 oz.)	300	0.0	34.0	0.00
Drained solids (yield: approx. 7.0 oz.)	(300)	0.0	(43.0)	0.00
Chunk White Tuna, packed in Oil, solids and liquid, 3¼-oz. can	(260)	0.0	80.0	0.00
Drained solids (yield: approx. 2¾ oz.)	(153)	0.0	53.7	0.00
6½-oz. can	(520)	0.0	(80.0)	0.00
Drained solids (yield: approx. 5½ oz.)	(306)	0.0	55.7	0.00
1 cup, not packed:				
Solids and liquid (approx. 8.8 oz.)	(705)	0.0	80.0	0.00
Drained solids (yield: approx. 6.2 oz.)	334	0.0	53.7	0.00
Chunk White Tuna, packed in Water, solids and liquid, 3¼-oz. can	111	0.0	34.0	0.00
Drained solids (yield: approx. 2.6 oz.)	(111)	0.0	(43.0)	0.00
6½-oz. can	221	0.0	34.0	0.00
Drained solids (yield: approx. 5 oz.)	(221)	0.0	(43.0)	0.00
12½-oz. can	425	0.0	34.0	0.00
Drained solids (yield: approx. 10 oz.)	(425)	0.0	(43.0)	0.00
1 cup, not packed:				
Solids and liquid (approx. 8.0 oz.)	300	0.0	34.0	0.00
Drained solids (yield: approx. 7.0 oz.)	(300)	0.0	(43.0)	0.00
Solid White Tuna, packed in Oil, solids and liquid, 3½-oz. can	(280)	0.0	(80.0)	0.00
Drained solids (yield: approx. 3 oz.)	167	0.0	55.7	0.00
7-oz. can	(560)	0.0	(80.0)	0.00
Drained solids, (yield: approx. 6 oz.)	334	0.0	55.7	0.00
1 cup, not packed:				
Solids and liquid (approx. 8.8 oz.)	(705)	0.0	(80.0)	0.00
Drained solids (approx. 6.0 oz.)	334	0.0	55.7	0.00
Chicken of the Sea Chunk Light Tuna, packed in Oil, solids and liquid, 3¼-oz. can	240	0.0	73.7	0.00
Drained solids (yield: approx. 2.75 oz.)	(127)	0.0	(46.2)	0.00
Solids and liquid, 6½-oz. can	480	0.0	73.7	0.00
Drained solids, (yield: approx. 5½ oz.)	(254)	0.0	(46.2)	0.00
Solids and liquid, 9¼-oz. can	680	0.0	73.7	0.00
Drained solids (yield: approx. 7.8 oz.)	(362)	0.0	(46.2)	0.00
1 cup, not packed:				
Solids and liquid (approx. 8.8 oz.)	(650)	0.0	73.7	0.00
Drained solids (approx. 6.0 oz.)	(277)	0.0	(46.2)	0.00
Chunk White Albacore Tuna, packed in Oil, solids and liquid, 6½-oz. can	530	1.0	81.5	0.15
Drained solids (yield: approx. 5½ oz.)	(316)	(1.0)	(57.5)	(0.18)
1 cup, not packed:				
Solids and liquid (approx. 8.8 oz.)	(717)	(1.0)	81.5	0.15
Drained solids (yield: approx. 6.0 oz.)	(345)	(1.0)	(57.5)	(0.18)
Chunk White Fancy Albacore Tuna, packed in Oil, solids and liquid, 9¼-oz. can	720	1.0	77.8	0.11
Drained solids (yield: approx. 7⅔ oz.)	340	1.0	44.7	0.13
1 cup, not packed:				
Solids and liquid (approx. 8.8 oz.)	(685)	(1.0)	77.8	0.11
Drained solids (approx. 6.0 oz.)	(270)	(0.8)	44.7	0.13
Solid White Albacore Tuna, packed in Oil, solids and liquid, 3½-oz. can	286	0.5	77.1	0.14
Drained solids (yield: approx. 3 oz.)	(167)	(0.5)	(55.7)	(0.17)
Solids and liquid, 7-oz. can	540	1.0	77.1	0.19
Drained solids (yield: approx. 6 oz.)	(334)	(1.0)	(55.7)	(0.17)
1 cup, not packed:				
Solids and liquid (approx. 8.8 oz.)	(680)	(0.5)	77.1	0.14
Drained solids (yield: approx. 6.0 oz.)	(334)	(0.5)	(55.7)	(0.17)
Solid White Fancy Albacore Tuna, packed in Oil, solids and liquid, 10-oz. can	750	1.0	75.0	0.10
Drained solids (yield: approx. 8.5 oz.)	(397)	(1.0)	(47.1)	(0.12)
13-oz. can	970	1.3	75.0	0.10
Drained solids (yield: approx. 11 oz.)	(518)	(1.3)	(47.1)	(0.12)
1 cup, not packed:				
Solids and liquid (approx. 8.8 oz.)	(660)	(0.9)	75.0	0.10
Drained solids (yield: approx. 6.0 oz.)	(283)	(0.7)	(47.1)	(0.12)
Solid White Fancy Albacore Tuna, packed in Water, solid and liquid, 10-oz. can	340	1.0	34.0	1.00
Drained solids, (yield: approx. 7⅔ oz.)	(340)	(1.0)	(44.2)	(0.13)
1 cup, not packed:				
Solids and liquid (approx. 8.8 oz.)	(300)	(1.0)	34.0	1.00
Drained solids (yield: approx. 5.9 oz.)	(261)	(1.0)	(44.2)	(0.13)
Del Monte Light Chunk Tuna, packed in Oil, solids and liquid, 6½-oz. can	450	0.0	69.3	0.00
Drained solids (yield: approx. 5½ oz.)	(220)	0.0	(40.0)	0.00
Solids and liquid, 9½-oz. can	658	0.0	69.3	0.00
Drained solids (yield: approx. 8 oz.)	(322)	0.0	(40.0)	0.00
1 cup, not packed:				
Solids and liquid (approx. 8.8 oz.)	(610)	0.0	69.3	0.00
Drained solids (yield: approx. 5.9 oz.)	(236)	0.0	(40.0)	0.00
Gold Seal Chunk Light Tuna, packed in Oil, solids and liquid, 6-oz. can	(492)	0.0	83.0	0.00
Drained solids (yield: approx. 5 oz.)	(278)	0.0	55.6	0.00
1 cup, not packed:				
Solids and liquid (approx. 8.8 oz.)	(730)	0.0	83.0	0.00
Drained solids (yield: approx. 5.9 oz.)	(328)	0.0	55.6	0.00
Fancy Solid White Tuna, packed in Oil, solids and liquid, 6-oz. can	(510)	0.0	(83.3)	0.00
Drained solids (yield: approx. 5.1 oz.)	290	0.0	56.6	0.00
1 cup, not packed:				
Solids and liquid (approx. 8.8 oz.)	(733)	0.0	(83.3)	0.00
Drained solids (yield: approx. 5.9 oz.)	(333)	0.0	56.6	0.00
Flake White Tuna, packed in Oil, solids and liquid, 6-oz. can	(498)	0.0	83.0	0.00
Drained solids (yield: approx. 5 oz.)	(278)	0.0	55.6	0.00
1 cup, not packed:				
Solids and liquid (approx. 8.8 oz.)	(730)	0.0	83.0	0.00
Drained Solids (yield: approx. 5.9 oz.)	(328)	0.0	55.6	0.00
Halfhill's unspecified cut of Tuna, packed in Oil, solids and liquid, 6½-oz. can	450	0.0	69.2	0.00
Drained solids (yield: approx. 5½ oz.)	(220)	0.0	40.0	0.00
12½-oz. can	882	0.0	69.2	0.00
Drained solids (yield: approx. 10½ oz.)	(422)	0.0	40.0	0.00
1 cup, not packed:				
Solids and liquid (approx. 9.4 oz.)	(650)	0.0	69.2	0.00
Drained solids (yield: approx. 8.5 oz.)	(340)	0.0	40.0	0.00
Chunk Light Tuna, packed in Oil, solids and liquid, 9¼-oz. can	650	0.0	70.3	0.00
Drained solids (yield: approx. 7.9 oz.)	(340)	0.0	(43.0)	0.00
1 cup, not packed:				
Solids and liquid (approx. 8.8 oz.)	(620)	0.0	70.3	0.00
Drained solids (yield: approx. 6.0 oz.)	(260)	0.0	(43.0)	0.00

	UNIT Cal.	UNIT Carb.	1 OZ., BY WT. Cal.	1 OZ., BY WT. Carb.
Chunk Light Tuna, packed in Water, solids and liquid, 6½-oz. can	200	0.0	30.8	0.00
Drained solids (yield: approx. 5⅛ oz.)	200	0.0	39.0	0.00
Solids and liquid, 12½-oz. can	396	0.0	30.8	0.00
Drained solids (yield: approx. 10 oz.)	(396)	0.0	(39.0)	0.00
1 cup, not packed:				
Solids and liquid (approx. 8.8 oz.)	(271)	0.0	30.8	0.00
Drained solids (yield: approx. 5.9 oz.)	(230)	0.0	39.0	0.00
Chunk White Tuna, packed in Water, solids and liquid, 6½-oz. can	240	0.0	36.9	0.00
Drained solids (yield: approx. 5⅛ oz.)	240	0.0	(46.8)	0.00
1 cup, not packed:				
Solids and liquid (approx. 8.8 oz.)	(325)	0.0	36.9	0.00
Drained solids (yield: approx. 5.9 oz.)	(276)	0.0	(46.8)	0.00
Icy Point unspecified cut of Tuna, packed in Oil, solids and liquid, 6-oz. can	(510)	0.0	(83.3)	0.00
Drained solids (yield: approx. 5.1 oz.)	(290)	0.0	56.6	0.00
1 cup, not packed:				
Solids and liquid (approx. 8.8 oz.)	(733)	0.0	(83.3)	0.00
Drained solids (yield: approx. 5.9 oz.)	(334)	0.0	56.6	0.00
Chunk Light Tuna, packed in Oil, solids and liquid, 6-oz. can	(498)	0.0	(83.0)	0.00
Drained solids (yield: approx. 5 oz.)	278	0.0	55.6	0.00
1 cup, not packed:				
Solids and liquid (approx. 8.8 oz.)	(730)	0.0	(83.0)	0.00
Drained solids (yield: approx. 5.9 oz.)	(328)	0.0	55.6	0.00
Fancy Solid White Tuna, packed in Oil, solids and liquid, 6-oz. can	(510)	0.0	(83.3)	0.00
Drained solids (yield: approx. 5.1 oz.)	290	0.0	56.6	0.00
1 cup, not packed:				
Solids and liquid (approx. 8.8 oz.)	(733)	0.0	(83.3)	0.00
Drained solids (yield: approx. 5.9 oz.)	334	0.0	56.6	0.00
Pillar Rock Chunk Light Tuna, packed in Oil, solids and liquid, 6-oz. can	498	0.0	83.0	0.00
Drained solids (yield: approx. 5 oz.)	278	0.0	55.6	0.00
1 cup, not packed:				
Solids and liquid (approx. 8.8 oz.)	(730)	0.0	(83.0)	0.00
Drained solids (yield: approx. 5.9 oz.)	(328)	0.0	55.6	0.00
Fancy Solid Tuna, packed in Oil, solids and liquid, 6-oz. can	510	0.0	83.3	0.00
Drained solids (yield: approx. 5.1 oz.)	290	0.0	56.6	0.00
1 cup, not packed:				
Solids and liquid (approx. 8.8 oz.)	(733)	0.0	83.3	0.00
Drained solids (yield: approx. 6.1 oz.)	(344)	0.0	56.6	0.00
Snow Mist Chunk Light Tuna, packed in Oil, solids and liquid, 6-oz. can	(498)	0.0	(83.0)	0.00
Drained solids (yield: approx. 5 oz.)	278	0.0	55.6	0.00
1 cup, not packed:				
Solids and liquid (approx. 8.8 oz.)	(730)	0.0	(83.0)	0.00
Drained solids (yield: approx. 5.9 oz.)	(328)	0.0	55.6	0.00
Star Kist Chunk Light Tuna, packed in Oil, solids and liquid, 6½-oz. can	450	0.0	69.2	0.00
1 cup, not packed (approx. 8.8 oz.)	609	0.0	69.2	0.00
Chunk Light Tuna, packed in Water, solids and liquid, 6½-oz. can	200	0.0	30.8	0.00
Drained solids (yield: approx. 5 oz.)	(200)	0.0	(40.0)	0.00
1 cup, not packed:				
Solids and liquid (approx. 8.8 oz.)	(271)	0.0	30.8	0.00
Drained solids (yield: approx. 5.9 oz.)	(236)	0.0	(40.0)	0.00
Solid Light Tuna, packed in Spring Water, solids and liquid, 7-oz. can	220	0.0	31.4	0.00
Drained solids (yield: approx. 5.5 oz.)	(220)	0.0	(40.0)	0.00
1 cup, not packed:				
Solids and liquid (approx. 8.8 oz.)	(277)	0.0	31.4	0.00
Drained solids (yield: approx. 5.9 oz.)	(236)	0.0	(40.0)	0.00
Solid White Fancy Albacore Tuna, packed in Oil, solids and liquid, 7-oz. can	520	0.0	74.3	0.00
Drained solids (yield: approx. 6 oz.)	(294)	0.0	(49.0)	0.00
1 cup, not packed:				
Solids and liquid (approx. 8.8 oz.)	(654)	0.0	74.3	0.00
Drained solids (yield: approx. 6.0 oz.)	(294)	0.0	(49.0)	0.00
Solid White Fancy Albacore Tuna, packed in Spring Water, solids and liquid, 7-oz. can	240	0.0	34.3	0.00
Drained solids (yield: approx. 5.5 oz.)	(240)	0.0	(43.6)	0.00
Solids and liquid, 10-oz. can	(340)	0.0	34.0	0.00
Drained solids (yield: approx. 7⅔ oz.)	(340)	0.0	44.2	0.00
1 cup, not packed:				
Solids and liquid (approx. 8.8 oz.)	(302)	0.0	34.0	0.00
Drained solids (yield: approx. 5.9 oz.)	(260)	0.0	(44.0)	0.00

Turtle, Green, based on generic data

	UNIT Cal.	UNIT Carb.	1 OZ., BY WT. Cal.	1 OZ., BY WT. Carb.
Solids and liquid, 1 pound (7g/0g/tr/75%/na)	481	0.0	30.1	0.00

Whitefish, by brand (see also Gefilte Fish)

	UNIT Cal.	UNIT Carb.	1 OZ., BY WT. Cal.	1 OZ., BY WT. Carb.
Elf Smoked Whitefish, 10-lb. tray pack	(7031)	0.0	(43.9)	0.00
1 pound	(702)	0.0	(43.9)	0.00

7 EGGS •

	UNIT		1 OZ., BY WT.		1 CUP	
	Cal.	Carb.	Cal.	Carb.	Cal.	Carb.
CHICKEN EGGS						
(All the data for Chicken Eggs apply equally to white and brown eggs.)						
Raw						
WHOLE, RAW (FRESH OR FROZEN)						
JUMBO, approx. 30 oz. per dozen weighed in shell:						
The dozen	1182	9.0	39.4	0.30		
1 pound:						
Weighed in shell (approx. 6½ Jumbo eggs) [refuse: shell, approx. 10%]	630	4.8	39.4	0.30		
Shelled (approx. 7⅛ Jumbo eggs) (4g/tr/3g/74%/35mg)	717	5.4	44.8	0.34	384	2.9
1 cup (approx. 3⅝ shelled Jumbo eggs)	384	2.9	44.8	0.34	384	2.9
1 egg:						
Approx. 2½ oz. weighed in shell [refuse: shell, approx. 10%]	99	0.8	39.4	0.30		
Approx. 2¼ oz. shelled	99	0.8	44.8	0.34	384	2.9
EXTRA LARGE, 27 oz. per dozen weighed in shell:						
The dozen	1064	8.1	39.4	0.30		
1 pound:						
Weighed in shell (approx. 7¼ Extra Large eggs) [refuse: shell, approx. 10%]	630	4.8	39.4	0.30		
Shelled (approx. 8 Extra Large eggs) (4g/tr/3g/74%/35mg)	717	5.4	44.8	0.34	384	2.9
1 cup (approx. 4¼ shelled Extra Large eggs)	384	2.9	44.8	0.34	384	2.9
1 egg:						
Approx. 2¼ oz. weighed in shell [refuse: shell, approx. 10%]	89	0.7	39.4	0.30		
Approx. 2 oz. shelled	89	0.7	44.8	0.34	384	2.9
LARGE, 24 oz. per dozen weighed in shell:						
The dozen	946	7.2	39.4	0.30		
1 pound:						
Weighed in shell (approx. 9 Large eggs) [refuse: shell, approx. 12%]	630	4.8	39.4	0.30		
Shelled (approx. 9¼ Large eggs) (4g/tr/3g/74%/35mg)	717	5.4	44.8	0.34	384	2.9
1 cup (approx. 4⅞ shelled Large eggs)	384	2.9	44.8	0.34	384	2.9
1 egg:						
Approx. 2 oz. weighed in shell [refuse: shell, approx. 12%]	79	0.6	39.4	0.30		
Approx. 1¾ oz. shelled	79	0.6	44.8	0.34	384	2.9
MEDIUM, approx. 21 oz. per dozen weighed in shell:						
The dozen	827	6.3	39.4	0.30		
1 pound:						
Weighed in shell (approx. 10 Medium eggs) [refuse: shell approx. 12%]	630	4.8	39.4	0.30		

	UNIT		1 OZ., BY WT.		1 CUP	
	Cal.	Carb.	Cal.	Carb.	Cal.	Carb.
Shelled (approx. 11 Medium eggs) (4g/tr/3g/74%/35mg)	717	5.4	44.8	0.34	384	2.9
1 cup (approx. 5½ shelled Medium eggs)	384	2.9	44.8	0.34	384	2.9
1 egg:						
Approx. 1¾ oz. weighed in shell [refuse: shell, approx. 12%]	69	0.5	39.4	0.30		
Approx. 1½ oz. shelled	69	0.5	44.8	0.34	384	2.9
SMALL, approx. 18 oz. per dozen weighed in shell:						
The dozen	709	5.4	39.4	0.30		
1 pound:						
Weighed in shell (approx. 11 Small eggs) [refuse: shell, 12%]	630	4.8	39.4	0.30		
Shelled (approx. 13 Small eggs) (4g/tr/3g/74%/35mg)	717	5.4	44.8	0.34	384	2.9
1 cup (approx. 6⅛ shelled Small eggs)	384	2.9	44.8	0.34	384	2.9
1 egg:						
Approx. 1½ oz. weighed in shell [refuse: shell approx. 13%]	59	0.5	39.4	0.30		
Approx. 1¼ oz. shelled	59	0.5	44.8	0.34	384	2.9
PEEWEE, approx. 15 oz. per dozen weighed in shell:						
The dozen	591	4.5	39.4	0.30		
1 pound:						
Weighed in shell (approx. 12 Peewee eggs) [refuse: shell, approx. 13%]	630	4.8	39.4	0.30		
Shelled (approx. 14½ Peewee eggs) (4g/tr/3g/74%/35mg)	717	5.4	44.8	0.34	384	2.9
1 cup (approx. 6¾ shelled Peewee eggs)	384	2.9	44.8	0.34	384	2.9
1 egg:						
Approx. 1¼ oz. weighed in shell [refuse: shell, approx. 13%]	49	0.4	39.4	0.30		
Approx. 1.1 oz. shelled	49	0.4	44.8	0.34	384	2.9
WHITES ONLY, RAW (FRESH OR FROZEN)						
JUMBO EGGS:						
Whites of 1 dozen eggs (approx. 18 oz.)	239	6.1	13.9	0.35	118	3.0
1 pound egg white (whites of approx. 10⅓ Jumbo eggs) (3g/tr/tr/88%/41mg)	222	5.6	13.9	0.35	118	3.0
1 cup egg white (whites of approx. 5½ Jumbo eggs)	118	3.0	13.9	0.35	118	3.0
White of 1 Jumbo egg (approx. 1½ oz.)	20	0.5	13.9	0.35	118	3.0
EXTRA LARGE EGGS:						
Whites of one dozen Extra Large eggs (approx. 16 oz.)	215	5.5	13.9	0.35	118	3.0
1 pound egg white (whites of approx. 12 Extra Large eggs) (3g/tr/tr/88%/41mg)	222	5.6	13.9	0.35	118	3.0
1 cup egg white (whites of approx. 6½ Extra Large eggs)	118	3.0	13.9	0.35	118	3.0
White of 1 Extra Large egg (approx. 1⅓ oz.)	18	0.5	13.9	0.35	118	3.0

	UNIT Cal.	UNIT Carb.	1 OZ., BY WT. Cal.	1 OZ., BY WT. Carb.	1 CUP Cal.	1 CUP Carb.
LARGE EGGS:						
Whites of 1 dozen Large eggs (approx. 14 oz.)	192	4.9	13.9	0.35	118	3.0
1 pound egg white (whites of approx. 13¾ Large eggs) (3g/tr/tr/88%/41mg)	222	5.6	13.9	0.35	118	3.0
1 cup egg white (whites of approx. 7½ Large eggs)	118	3.0	13.9	0.35	118	3.0
White of 1 Large egg (approx. 1.2 oz.)	16	0.4	13.9	0.35	118	3.0
MEDIUM EGGS:						
Whites of 1 dozen Medium eggs (approx. 12⅓ oz.)	167	4.3	13.9	0.35	118	3.0
1 pound egg white (whites of approx. 17½ Small eggs) (3g/tr/tr/88%/41mg)	222	5.6	13.9	0.35	118	3.0
1 cup egg white (whites of approx. 6½ Medium eggs)	118	3.0	13.9	0.35	118	3.0
White of 1 Medium egg (approx. 1 oz.)	14	0.3	13.9	0.35	118	3.0
SMALL EGGS:						
Whites of 1 dozen Small eggs (approx. 10½ oz.)	144	3.7	13.9	0.35	118	3.0
1 pound egg white (whites of approx. 17½ Small eggs) (3g/tr/tr/88%/41mg)	222	5.6	13.9	0.35	118	3.0
1 cup egg white (whites of approx. 8½ Small eggs)	118	3.0	13.9	0.35	118	3.0
White of 1 Small egg (approx. 0.9 oz.)	12	0.3	13.9	0.35	118	3.0
PEEWEE EGGS:						
Whites of 1 dozen Peewee eggs (approx. 9½ oz.)	120	3.1	13.9	0.35	118	3.0
1 pound egg white (whites of approx. 20 Peewee eggs) (3g/tr/tr/88%/41mg)	222	5.6	13.9	0.35	118	3.0
1 cup egg white (whites of approx. 10½ Peewee eggs)	118	3.0	13.9	0.35	118	3.0
White of 1 Peewee egg (approx. 0.8 oz.)	10	0.3	13.9	0.35	118	3.0
YOLKS, RAW, FRESH						
(The data for whole eggs and egg whites are identical for both fresh and frozen eggs, but the data for fresh and frozen yolks are different. This is because while fresh egg yolks do contain small amounts of egg white, frozen egg yolks contain considerably more.)						
JUMBO EGGS:						
Yolks of 1 dozen Jumbo eggs (approx. 8.8 oz.)	943	0.5	104.6	0.06	897	0.5
1 pound egg yolk (yolks of approx. 21½ Jumbo eggs) (5g/tr/9g/51%/28mg)	1675	1.0	104.6	0.06	897	0.5
1 cup egg yolk (yolks of approx. 11½ Jumbo eggs)	897	0.5	104.6	0.06	897	0.5
Yolk of 1 Jumbo egg (approx. ¾ oz.)	79	trace	104.6	0.06	897	0.5
EXTRA LARGE EGGS:						
Yolks of 1 dozen Extra Large eggs (approx. 8 oz.)	849	0.5	104.6	0.06	897	0.5
1 pound egg yolk (yolks of approx. 23¾ Extra Large eggs) (5g/tr/9g/51%/28mg)	1675	1.0	104.6	0.06	897	0.5
1 cup egg yolk (yolks of approx. 12¾ Extra Large eggs)	897	0.5	104.6	0.06	897	0.5
Yolk of 1 Extra Large egg (approx. 0.7 oz.)	71	trace	104.6	0.06	897	0.5
LARGE EGGS:						
Yolks of 1 dozen Large eggs (approx. 7 oz.)	755	0.4	104.6	0.06	897	0.5
1 pound egg yolk (yolks of approx. 26¾ Large eggs) (5g/tr/9g/51%/28mg)	1675	1.0	104.6	0.06	897	0.5
1 cup egg yolk (yolks of approx. 14⅓ Large eggs)	897	0.5	104.6	0.06	897	0.5
Yolk of 1 Large egg (approx. 0.6 oz.)	63	trace	104.6	0.06	897	0.5
MEDIUM EGGS:						
Yolks of 1 dozen Medium eggs (approx. 6⅓ oz.)	660	0.4	104.6	0.06	897	0.5
1 pound egg yolk (yolks of approx. 30 Medium eggs) (5g/tr/9g/51%/28mg)	1675	1.0	104.6	0.06	897	0.5
1 cup egg yolk (yolks of approx. 16 Medium eggs)	897	0.5	104.6	0.06	897	0.5
Yolk of 1 Medium egg (approx. ½ oz.)	55	trace	104.6	0.06	897	0.5
SMALL EGGS:						
Yolks of 1 dozen Small eggs (approx. 5½ oz.)	565	0.3	104.6	0.06	897	0.5
1 pound egg yolk (yolks of approx. 35 Small eggs) (5g/tr/9g/51%/28mg)	1675	1.0	104.6	0.06	897	0.5
1 cup egg yolk (yolks of approx. 18½ Small eggs)	897	0.5	104.6	0.06	897	0.5
Yolk of 1 Small egg (approx. 0.4 oz.)	47	trace	104.6	0.06	897	0.5
PEEWEE EGGS:						
Yolks of 1 dozen Peewee eggs (approx. 4.6 oz.)	471	0.3	104.6	0.06	897	0.5
1 pound egg yolk (yolks of approx. 41 Peewee eggs) (5g/tr/9g/51%/28mg)	1675	1.0	104.6	0.06	897	0.5
1 cup egg yolk (yolks of approx. 22 Peewee eggs)	897	0.5	104.6	0.06	897	0.5
Yolk of 1 Peewee egg (approx. 0.4 oz.)	39	trace	104.6	0.06	897	0.5

	UNIT Cal.	UNIT Carb.	1 OZ., BY WT. Cal.	1 OZ., BY WT. Carb.	1 CUP Cal.	1 CUP Carb.
YOLKS, RAW, FROZEN						
AVERAGE ALL SIZE EGGS:						
1 pound frozen egg yolks (4g/tr/8g/56%/18mg)	1465	1.6	91.6	0.10		
1 pound frozen egg yolks, sugared (4g/3g/7g/51%/16mg)	1465	43.1	91.6	2.69		
Whole Eggs, Cooked						
BOILED (SOFT, MEDIUM, or HARD):						
1 Jumbo egg:						
Yield: approx. 2½ oz. weighed in shell	99	0.8	39.4	0.30		
approx. 2¼ oz. shelled (4g/tr/3g/73%/35mg)	99	0.8	44.8	0.34	215	1.6
1 Extra Large egg:						
Yield: approx. 2¼ oz. weighed in shell	89	0.7	39.4	0.30		
approx. 2 oz. shelled (4g/tr/3g/73%/35mg)	89	0.7	44.8	0.34	215	1.6
1 Large egg:						
Yield: approx. 2 oz. weighed in shell	79	0.6	39.4	0.30		
approx. 1¾ oz. shelled (4g/tr/3g/73%/35mg)	79	0.6	44.8	0.34	215	1.6
1 Medium egg:						
Yield: approx. 1¾ oz. weighed in shell	69	0.5	39.4	0.30		
approx. 1½ oz. shelled (4g/tr/3g/73%/35mg)	69	0.5	44.8	0.34	215	1.6
1 Small egg:						
Yield: approx. 1½ oz. weighed in shell	59	0.5	39.4	0.30		
approx. 1¼ oz. shelled (4g/tr/3g/73%/35mg)	59	0.5	44.8	0.34	215	1.6
1 Peewee egg:						
Yield: approx. 1¼ oz. weighed in shell	49	0.4	39.4	0.30		
approx. 1 oz. shelled (4g/tr/3g/73%/35mg)	49	0.4	44.8	0.34	215	1.6
FRIED:						
1 Jumbo egg:						
1 Jumbo egg fried in 1 tsp. butter or margarine or 2 tsps. "diet" margarine (yield: approx. 2.0 oz.) (4g/tr/6g/na/na)	(135)	(0.8)	(67.5)	(0.40)	(507)	(3.0)
1 Jumbo egg fried in a 1¼-second application of vegetable cooking spray (yield: approx. 2 oz.)	(101)	(0.8)	(50.5)	(0.40)	(380)	(3.0)
1 Extra Large egg:						
1 Extra Large egg fried in 1 tsp. butter or margarine or 2 tsps. "diet" margarine (yield: approx. 1.9 oz.) (4g/tr/6g/na/na)	(124)	(0.7)	(67.5)	(0.40)	(507)	(3.0)
1 Extra Large egg fried in a 1¼-second application of vegetable cooking spray (yield: approx. 1.9 oz.)	(91)	(0.7)	(50.5)	(0.40)	(380)	(3.0)
1 Large egg:						
1 Large egg fried in 1 tsp. butter or margarine or 2 tsps. "diet" margarine (yield: approx. 1.7 oz.) (4g/tr/6g/na/na)	(113)	(0.6)	(67.5)	(0.40)	(507)	(3.0)
1 Large egg fried in a 1¼-second application of vegetable cooking spray (yield: approx. 1.7 oz.)	(81)	(0.6)	(50.5)	(0.40)	(380)	(3.0)
1 Medium egg:						
1 Medium egg fried in 1 tsp. butter or margarine or 2 tsp. "diet" margarine (yield: approx. 1.5 oz.) (4g/tr/6g/na/na)	(100)	(0.6)	(67.5)	(0.40)	(507)	(3.0)
1 Medium egg fried in a 1¼-second application of vegetable cooking spray (yield: approx. 1.5 oz.)	(71)	(0.6)	(50.5)	(0.40)	(380)	(3.0)
1 Small egg:						
1 Small egg fried in 1 tsp. butter or margarine or 2 tsp. "diet" margarine (yield: approx. 1.3 oz.) (4g/tr/6g/na/na)	(87)	(0.5)	(67.5)	(0.40)	(507)	(3.0)
1 Small egg fried in a 1¼-second application of vegetable cooking spray (yield: approx. 1.3 oz.)	(61)	(0.5)	(50.5)	(0.40)	(380)	(3.0)
1 Peewee egg:						
1 Peewee egg fried in 1 tsp. butter or margarine or 2 tsp. "diet" margarine (yield: approx. 1.1 oz.) (4g/tr/6g/na/na)	(73)	(0.4)	(67.5)	(0.40)	(507)	(3.0)
1 Peewee egg fried in a 1¼-second application of vegetable cooking spray (yield: approx. 1.1 oz.)	(51)	(0.4)	(50.5)	(0.40)	(380)	(3.0)
POACHED:						
1 Jumbo egg (yield: approx. 2.3 oz.) (4g/tr/3g/73%/79mg)	99	0.8	44.5	0.34	(392)	(3.0)
1 Extra Large egg (yield: approx. 2.0 oz.)	89	0.7	44.5	0.34	(392)	(3.0)
1 Large egg (yield: approx. 1.8 oz.)	79	0.6	44.5	0.34	(392)	(3.0)
1 Medium egg (yield: approx. 1.5 oz.)	69	0.5	44.5	0.34	(392)	(3.0)
1 Small egg (yield: approx. 1.4 oz.)	59	0.5	44.5	0.34	(392)	(3.0)
1 Peewee egg (yield: approx. 1.2 oz.)	49	0.4	44.5	0.34	(392)	(3.0)

	UNIT Cal.	UNIT Carb.	1 OZ., BY WT. Cal.	1 OZ., BY WT. Carb.	1 CUP Cal.	1 CUP Carb.
SCRAMBLED OR OMELETS:						
1 Jumbo egg:						
1 Jumbo egg with 1⅓ Tbsp. whole milk, fried in 1 tsp. butter or margarine or 2 tsp. "diet" margarine (yield: approx. 2.9 oz.) (3g/1g/3g/na/na)	(144)	(1.8)	(49.7)	(0.61)	(374)	(4.6)
1 Jumbo egg with 1⅓ Tbsp. skim milk, replacing butter or margarine with a 1¼-second application of vegetable cooking spray (yield: approx. 2.9 oz.) (3g/1g/2g/na/na)	(107)	(1.8)	(36.9)	(0.61)	(278)	(4.6)
1 Extra Large egg:						
1 Extra Large egg with 1⅓ Tbsp. milk cooked in 1 tsp. butter or margarine or 2 tsp. "diet" margarine (yield: approx. 2.7 oz.) (3g/1g/3g/na/na)	(135)	(1.6)	(49.7)	(0.61)	(374)	(4.6)
1 Extra Large egg with 1⅓ Tbsp. skim milk, replacing butter or margarine with a 1¼-second application of vegetable cooking spray (yield: approx. 2.7 oz.) (3g/1g/2g/na/na)	(98)	(1.6)	(36.9)	(0.61)	(278)	(4.6)
1 Large Egg:						
1 Large egg with 1⅓ Tbsp. milk cooked in 1 tsp. butter or margarine or 2 tsp. "diet" margarine. (yield: approx. 2.4 oz.) (3g/1g/3g/na/na)	(125)	(1.4)	(49.7)	(0.61)	(374)	(4.6)
1 Large egg with 1⅓ Tbsp. skim milk, replacing butter or margarine with a 1¼-second application of vegetable cooking spray (yield: approx. 2.4 oz.) (3g/1g/2g/na/na)	(88)	(1.4)	(36.9)	(0.61)	(278)	(4.6)
1 Medium egg:						
1 Medium egg with 1⅓ Tbsp. milk cooked in 1 tsp. butter or margarine (yield: approx. 2.1 oz.) (3g/1g/3g/na/na)	(115)	(1.3)	(49.7)	(0.61)	(374)	(4.6)
1 Medium egg with 1⅓ Tbsp. skim milk, replacing butter or margarine with a 1¼-second application of vegetable cooking spray (yield: approx. 2.1 oz.) (3g/1g/2g/na/na)	(77)	(1.3)	(36.9)	(0.61)	(278)	(4.6)
1 Small egg:						
1 Small egg with 1⅓ Tbsp. milk cooked in 1 tsp. butter or margarine or 2 tsps. "diet" margarine. (yield: approx. 1.8 oz.) (3g/1g/3g/na/na)	(105)	(1.1)	(49.7)	(0.61)	(374)	(4.6)
1 Small egg with 1⅓ Tbsp. skim milk, replacing butter or margarine with a 1¼-second application of vegetable cooking spray (yield approx. 1.8 oz.) (3g/1g/2g/na/na)	(68)	(1.1)	(36.9)	(0.61)	(278)	(4.6)
1 Peewee egg:						
1 Peewee egg with 1⅓ Tbsp. milk cooked in 1 tsp. butter or margarine (yield: approx. 1.5 oz.) (3g/1g/3g/na/na)	(75)	(0.9)	(49.7)	(0.61)	(374)	(4.6)
1 Peewee egg with 1⅓ Tbsp. skim milk, replacing butter or margarine with a 1¼-second application of vegetable cooking spray (3g/1g/2g/na/na)	(58)	(0.9)	(36.9)	(0.61)	(278)	(4.6)

Dried Eggs

	UNIT Cal.	UNIT Carb.	1 OZ., BY WT. Cal.	1 OZ., BY WT. Carb.	1 CUP Cal.	1 CUP Carb.
Whole, 1 pound (13g/1g/12g/4%/121mg)	2697	21.6	168.4	1.35	505	4.1
Whole, stabilized (glucose reduced), 1 pound (14g/1g/12g/2%/126mg)	2791	10.8	174.4	0.67	523	2.0
White:						
Flakes, stabilized (glucose reduced), 1 pound (21g/1g/tr/15%/293mg)	1592	18.9	99.5	1.18		
Powder, stabilized (glucose reduced), 1 pound (23g/1g/tr/9%/313mg)	1706	20.3	106.6	1.27	402	4.8
Yolk, 1 pound (9g/tr/16g/5%/28mg)	3117	1.8	194.8	0.11	460	0.3

CHICKEN EGGS IN OTHER COUNTRIES

	UNIT Cal.	UNIT Carb.	1 OZ., BY WT. Cal.	1 OZ., BY WT. Carb.	1 CUP Cal.	1 CUP Carb.
Based on data from Africa:						
RAW OR BOILED:						
Shelled, 1 pound	636	2.7	39.7	0.17	(340)	(1.5)
Based on data from the Caribbean:						
RAW OR BOILED:						
Shelled, 1 pound	740	4.2	46.2	0.26	(396)	(2.2)
Based on data from East Asia:						
RAW OR BOILED:						
Whole, 1 pound:						
Weighed in shell [refuse: shell, approx. 11%]	658	3.2	41.1	0.20	(397)	(2.0)
Shelled	740	3.6	46.3	0.23	(397)	(2.0)
Whites only:						
1 pound	236	5.0	14.8	0.31	(127)	(2.7)
Yolks only:						
1 pound	1525	4.1	95.3	0.26	(817)	(2.2)
Based on data from China:						
PRESERVED *(known as Black Egg or Pidan Egg)*:						
1 pound	730	9.1	45.6	0.57		
Based on data from Japan:						
RAW OR BOILED:						
Whole, 1 pound:						
Weighed in shell [refuse: shell, approx. 12%]	623		38.9		(380)	
Shelled	708		44.3		(380)	
Whites only:						
1 pound	204		12.8		(110)	
1 cup	(110)		12.8		(110)	
Yolks only:						
1 pound	1648		103.0		(883)	
1 cup	(883)		103.0		(883)	
DRIED:						
Whole, 1 pound	2665		166.6			

EGGS OTHER THAN CHICKEN EGGS

(The primary listing for fish eggs is in the FISH, SHELLFISH & WATERLIFE chapter, under "ROE.")

Caviar, Sturgeon

	UNIT Cal.	UNIT Carb.	1 OZ., BY WT. Cal.	1 OZ., BY WT. Carb.	1 CUP Cal.	1 CUP Carb.
RAW, all-edible:						
GRANULAR:						
1 tablespoon (approx. 0.57 oz.)	42	0.5	74.0	0.90	672	8.0
1 ounce (approx. 1.8 Tbsp.)	74	0.9	74.0	0.90	672	8.0
1 caviar-pound (a measure used for caviar, it equals 14 oz.)	1036	12.6	74.0	0.90	672	8.0
1 pound (approx. 1¾ cups) (8g/1g/4g/46%/624mg)	1184	14.4	74.0	0.90	672	8.0
PRESSED:						
1 tablespoon (approx. 0.61 oz.)	54	0.8	90.0	1.34	864	12.8
1 ounce (approx. 1.7 Tbsp.)	90	1.3	90.0	1.34	864	12.8
1 caviar-pound (a measure used for caviar, it equals 14 oz.)	1260	18.8	90.0	1.34	864	12.8
1 pound (approx. 1⅔ cups) (10g/1g/5g/36%/na)	1440	21.4	90.0	1.34	864	12.8
GERMAN CAVIAR (based on data from France):						
1 pound	572	12.7	35.7	0.79		
RUSSIAN CAVIAR (based on data from France):						
1 pound	1188	20.9	74.3	1.30		

Charapa Eggs (based on data from Latin America)

(Indigenous Peruvian marine reptile—a small tortoise)

	UNIT Cal.	UNIT Carb.	1 OZ., BY WT. Cal.	1 OZ., BY WT. Carb.	1 CUP Cal.	1 CUP Carb.
WHOLE, RAW:						
1 pound weighed without shell	1040	17.7	65.0	1.11		

Duck Eggs

	UNIT Cal.	UNIT Carb.	1 OZ., BY WT. Cal.	1 OZ., BY WT. Carb.	1 CUP Cal.	1 CUP Carb.
WHOLE, RAW:						
LARGE, approx. 40 oz. (2½ pounds) per dozen weighed in shell:						
The dozen	1896	8.4	47.4	0.20	(479)	(2.0)
1 pound:						
Weighed in shell (approx. 4.8 eggs) [refuse: shell, approx. 12%]	758	3.2	47.4	0.20	(479)	(2.0)
Shelled (approx. 5½ eggs) (4g/tr/4g/70%/35mg)	866	3.7	54.1	0.23	(479)	(2.0)
1 cup (approx. 3 shelled eggs)	(479)	(2.0)	54.1	0.23	(479)	(2.0)
1 egg:						
Approx. 3⅓ oz. weighed in shell [refuse: shell, approx. 12%]	158	0.7	47.4	0.20	(479)	(2.0)
Approx. 2.9 oz. shelled	158	0.7	54.1	0.23	(479)	(2.0)
MEDIUM, approx. 33.8 oz. (2.1 pounds) per dozen weighed in shell:						
The dozen	1620	7.2	47.9	0.21	(479)	(2.0)
1 pound:						
Weighed in shell (approx. 5.7 eggs) [refuse: shell, approx. 12%]	766	3.4	47.9	0.21	(479)	(2.0)
Shelled (approx. 6.4 eggs)	866	3.7	54.1	0.23	(479)	(2.0)
1 cup (approx. 3½ shelled eggs)	(479)	(2.0)	54.1	0.23	(479)	(2.0)
1 egg:						
Approx. 2.8 oz. weighed in shell [refuse: shell, approx. 12%]	135	0.6	47.9	0.21	(479)	(2.0)
Approx. 2.5 oz. shelled	135	0.6	54.1	0.23	(479)	(2.0)

	UNIT Cal.	UNIT Carb.	1 OZ., BY WT. Cal.	1 OZ., BY WT. Carb.	1 CUP Cal.	1 CUP Carb.
SMALL, approx. 28.8 oz. (1⅘ pounds) per dozen weighed in shell:						
The dozen	1368	6.0	47.5	0.21	(480)	(2.1)
1 pound:						
Weighed in shell (approx. 6⅔ eggs) [refuse: shell, approx. 12%]	760	3.4	47.5	0.21	(480)	(2.1)
Shelled (approx. 7⅔ eggs)	866	3.7	54.1	0.21	(480)	(2.1)
1 cup (approx. 4¼ shelled eggs)	(480)	(2.1)	54.1	0.21	(480)	(2.1)
1 egg:						
Approx. 2.4 oz. weighed in shell [refuse: shell, approx. 12%]	114	0.5	47.5	0.21	(480)	(2.1)
Approx. 2.1 oz. shelled	114	0.5	54.1	0.21	(480)	(2.1)
WHITES ONLY, RAW:						
Whites of 1 dozen medium duck eggs (approx. 24 oz.)	348	4.8	14.2	0.20	(123)	(1.7)
1 pound egg white (whites of approx. 8 medium duck eggs)	227	3.2	14.2	0.20	(123)	(1.7)
1 cup egg white (whites of approx. 4¼ medium duck eggs)	(123)	(1.7)	14.2	0.20	(123)	(1.7)
White of 1 duck egg (approx. 2 oz.)	29	0.4	14.2	0.20	(123)	(1.7)
YOLKS ONLY, RAW:						
Yolks of 1 dozen medium duck eggs (approx. 14.4 oz.)	1503	2.4	104.4	0.17	(890)	(1.4)
1 pound egg yolk (yolks of approx. 13⅓ medium duck eggs)	1671	2.7	104.4	0.17	(890)	(1.4)
1 cup egg yolk (yolks of approx. 7⅒ medium duck eggs)	(890)	(1.4)	104.4	0.17	(890)	(1.4)
Yolk of 1 duck egg (approx. 1.2 oz.)	125	0.2	104.4	0.17	(890)	(1.4)
WHOLE, PRESERVED, LIMED (Based on data from East Asia):						
Raw, 1 pound:						
Weighed in shell [refuse: shell, approx. 12%]	649	8.2	40.6	0.51		
Shelled	731	9.1	45.7	0.57		
WHOLE, SALTED (Based on data from East Asia):						
Raw, 1 pound:						
Weighed in shell [refuse: shell, approx. 12%]	808	3.2	50.5	0.20		
Shelled	917	3.6	57.3	0.23		
Cooked, 1 pound:						
Weighed in shell [refuse: shell, approx. 12%]	844	14.5	52.8	0.91		
Shelled	963	16.3	60.2	1.02		
EMBRYONATED (Based on data from East Asia):						
1 pound:						
Weighed in shell [refuse: shell, approx. 10%]	767		48.0	trace		
Shelled	853		53.3	trace		
Goose Eggs						
WHOLE, RAW:						
American Goose Eggs, Canadian or Egyptian Species (approx. 3¾ pounds per dozen weighed in shell):						
The dozen	2796	20.4	45.5	0.33	(390)	(2.8)
1 pound:						
Weighed in shell (approx. 3⅛ eggs) [refuse: shell, approx. 13%]	728	5.3	45.5	0.33	(390)	(2.8)
Shelled (approx. 3⅔ eggs) (4g/tr/4g/70%/na)	837	6.1	52.3	0.38	(390)	(2.8)
1 cup (approx. 1⅔ eggs)	(390)	(2.8)	52.3	0.38	(390)	(2.8)
1 egg:						
Approx. 5 oz. weighed in shell [refuse: shell, approx. 13%]	233	1.7	45.5	0.33	(390)	(2.8)
Approx. 4⅓ oz. shelled	233	1.7	52.3	0.38	(390)	(2.8)
American Goose Eggs, African or Emdin Species (approx. 5¼ pounds per dozen weighed in shell):						
The dozen	3816	27.6	45.5	0.33	(390)	(2.8)
1 pound:						
Weighed in shell (approx. 2¼ eggs) [refuse: shell, approx. 13%]	728	5.3	45.5	0.33	(390)	(2.8)
Shelled (approx. 2½ eggs)	837	6.1	52.3	0.38	(390)	(2.8)
1 cup (approx. 1⅕ eggs)	(390)	(2.8)	52.3	0.38	(390)	(2.8)
1 egg:						
Approx. 7 oz. weighed in shell [refuse: shell, approx. 12%]	318	2.3	45.5	0.33	(390)	(2.8)
Approx. 6⅙ oz. shelled	318	2.3	52.3	0.38	(390)	(2.8)
Guinea Hen and Wild Hen Eggs, see Wild Fowl Eggs						

	UNIT Cal.	UNIT Carb.	1 OZ., BY WT. Cal.	1 OZ., BY WT. Carb.	1 CUP Cal.	1 CUP Carb.
Iguana Eggs (based on data from Latin America)						
WHOLE, RAW OR BOILED:						
Shelled, 1 pound	990	19.5	61.9	1.22		
Motelo Eggs (based on data from Latin America)						
WHOLE, RAW:						
Shelled, 1 pound	649	7.3	40.6	0.45		
Pidan (Specially treated Chicken Egg of the Orient, also called Black Egg), see CHICKEN EGGS IN OTHER COUNTRIES						
Pigeon Eggs (based on data from East Asia)						
WHOLE, RAW:						
1 pound:						
Weighed in shell [refuse: shell, approx. 11%]	463	6.4	28.9	0.40	(280)	(3.9)
Shelled	527	7.3	32.9	0.45	(280)	(3.9)
Quail Eggs (based on data from East Asia)						
WHOLE, RAW:						
1 dozen eggs (approx. 4 oz.) [refuse: shell, approx. 8%]	164	9.6	40.6	0.26	(390)	(2.4)
1 pound:						
Weighed in shell (approx. 39⅗ eggs) [refuse: shell, approx. 8%]	649	4.1	40.6	0.26	(390)	(2.4)
Shelled (approx. 53 eggs)	731	4.5	45.7	0.28	(390)	(2.4)
1 cup (approx. 28⅗ shelled eggs)	(390)	(2.4)	45.7	0.28	(390)	(2.4)
1 egg:						
Approx. 0.33 oz. weighed in shell [refuse: shell, approx. 8%]	14	0.1	40.6	0.26	(390)	(2.4)
Approx. 0.30 oz. shelled	14	0.1	45.7	0.28	(390)	(2.4)
Salmon Roe						
BAKED OR BROILED:						
Based on USDA data; cooked with unspecified amount of butter or margarine:						
All-edible, 1 pound (7g/tr/3g/61%/na)	576	8.6	35.7	0.53		
Sea Urchin Roe (based on data from Japan)						
RAW:						
All-edible, 1 pound	672	9.1	42.0	0.57		
SALTED:						
All-edible, 1 pound	922	23.0	57.6	1.44		
Tericaya Eggs (based on data from Latin America)						
Shelled, 1 pound	826	18.2	51.6	1.14	(440)	(9.7)
Turkey Eggs						
WHOLE, RAW:						
LARGE, 44 oz. (2¾ pounds) per dozen weighed in shell:						
The dozen	1884	13.2	42.6	0.28	(416)	(2.9)
1 pound:						
Weighed in shell (approx. 4⅓ Large eggs) [refuse: shell, approx. 12%]	681	4.5	42.6	0.28	(416)	(2.9)
Shelled (approx. 5 Large eggs) (4g/tr/3g/73%/na)	776	5.4	48.5	0.34	(416)	(2.9)
1 cup (approx. 2⅔ shelled Large eggs)	(416)	(2.9)	48.5	0.34	(416)	(2.9)
1 egg:						
Approx. 3⅔ oz. weighed in shell [refuse: shell, approx. 12%]	157	1.1	42.6	0.28	(416)	(2.9)
Approx. 3¼ oz. shelled	157	1.1	48.5	0.34	(416)	(2.9)
MEDIUM, 37.3 oz. (2⅓ pounds) per dozen weighed in shell:						
The dozen	1656	10.8	42.6	0.28	(416)	(2.9)

	UNIT Cal.	UNIT Carb.	1 OZ., BY WT. Cal.	1 OZ., BY WT. Carb.	1 CUP Cal.	1 CUP Carb.
1 pound:						
Weighed in shell (approx. 5 Medium eggs) [refuse: shell, approx. 12%]	682	4.5	42.6	0.28	(416)	(2.9)
Shelled (approx. 5⅔ Medium eggs)	776	5.4	48.5	0.34	(416)	(2.9)
1 cup (approx. 3 Medium eggs)	(416)	(2.9)	48.5	0.34	(416)	(2.9)
1 egg:						
Approx. 3¼ oz. weighed in shell [refuse: shell, approx. 12%]	138	0.9	42.6	0.28	(416)	(2.9)
Approx. 2⅞ oz. shelled	138	0.9	48.5	0.34	(416)	(2.9)
SMALL, 33.6 oz. (2.1 pounds) per dozen weighed in shell:						
1 pound:						
Weighed in shell (approx. 5⅔ Small eggs) [refuse: shell, approx. 12%]	682	4.5	42.6	0.28	(416)	(2.9)
Shelled (approx. 6½ eggs)	776	5.4	48.5	0.34	(416)	(2.9)
1 cup (approx. 3½ eggs)	(416)	(2.9)	48.5	0.34	(416)	(2.9)
1 egg:						
Approx. 2⅞ oz. weighed in shell [refuse: shell, approx. 12%]	119	0.8	42.6	0.28	(416)	(2.9)
Approx. 2½ oz. shelled	119	0.8	48.5	0.34	(416)	(2.9)

Turtle Eggs (based on data from East Asia)

	UNIT Cal.	UNIT Carb.	1 OZ., BY WT. Cal.	1 OZ., BY WT. Carb.	1 CUP Cal.	1 CUP Carb.
WHOLE, RAW:						
1 pound:						
Weighed in shell (approx. 12 to 20 eggs) [refuse: shell, approx. 9%]	613	4.1	38.3	0.26	(360)	(2.4)
Shelled (approx. 13 to 22 eggs)	672	4.5	42.0	0.28	(360)	(2.4)
1 egg:						
Small:						
Approx. 0.76 oz. weighed in shell [refuse: shell, approx. 9%]	29	0.2	38.3	0.26	(360)	(2.4)
Approx. 0.7 oz. shelled	29	0.2	42.0	0.28	(360)	(2.4)
Large:						
Approx. 1.26 oz. weighed in shell [refuse: shell, approx. 9%]	48	0.3	38.3	0.26	(360)	(2.4)
Approx. 1.17 oz. shelled	48	0.3	42.0	0.28	(360)	(2.4)

Wild Fowl Eggs (based on data from Pakistan)

	UNIT Cal.	UNIT Carb.	1 OZ., BY WT. Cal.	1 OZ., BY WT. Carb.	1 CUP Cal.	1 CUP Carb.
Shelled, 1 pound	840	50.0	52.5	3.12	(450)	(26.7)

EGG SUBSTITUTES

EGG SUBSTITUTES, based on generic data

	UNIT Cal.	UNIT Carb.	1 OZ., BY WT. Cal.	1 OZ., BY WT. Carb.	1 CUP Cal.	1 CUP Carb.
Frozen egg substitutes that contain egg white, corn oil, and nonfat dry milk:						
The equivalent of 1 egg:						
¼ cup (approx. 2.1 oz.)	96	1.9	45.4	0.91	384	7.7
The equivalent of 2 eggs:						
½ cup (approx. 4.2 oz.)	192	3.8	45.4	0.91	384	7.7
Liquid egg substitutes that contain egg white, hydrogenated soybean oil, and soy protein:						
The equivalent of 1 egg:						
1 tablespoon (approx. 1.7 oz.)	40	0.3	23.8	0.18	211	1.6
The equivalent of 2 eggs:						
2 tablespoons (approx. 3.4 oz.)	80	0.6	23.8	0.18	211	1.6
Powdered egg substitutes that contain egg white solids, whole egg solids, sweet whey solids, nonfat dry milk, and soy protein:						
The equivalent of 1 egg:						
Approx. 0.35 oz.	44	2.2	125.9	6.18		
The equivalent of 2 eggs:						
Approx. 0.70 oz.	88	4.4	125.9	6.18		

EGG SUBSTITUTES, by brand

	UNIT Cal.	UNIT Carb.	1 OZ., BY WT. Cal.	1 OZ., BY WT. Carb.	1 CUP Cal.	1 CUP Carb.
Breakfast Treat Lucerne Powdered Egg Substitute, 1 package (yield: approx. 8½ oz. prepared)	180	4.0	21.2	0.47	180	4.0
The equivalent of 1 egg: ¼ envelope, prepared with water (yield: approx. 2 tablespoons)	23	0.5	21.2	0.47	180	4.0
The equivalent of 2 eggs: ½ envelope, prepared with water (yield: approx. ¼ cup)	45	1.0	21.2	0.47	180	4.0
Egg Beaters Cholesterol-Free Egg Substitute, 17 oz. package, 2 containers, each 8.5 oz.	320	24.0	18.8	1.41	160	12.0
1 container, 8.5 oz. (equivalent to 4 large eggs)	160	12.0	18.8	1.41	160	12.0
The equivalent of 1 egg:						
¼ cup (approx. 2 oz.)	40	3.0	18.8	1.41	160	12.0
The equivalent of 2 eggs:						
½ cup (approx. 4 oz.)	80	6.0	18.8	1.41	160	12.0
Egg Magic Featherweight, 99.9% Cholesterol Free, Powdered Egg Substitute, 2⅛ oz. package (3 packets)	306	6.0	145.7	2.86		
The equivalent of 1 egg: ½ packet, prepared with water (yield: approx. ⅙ cup)	51	1.0	(30.0)	(0.59)	306	6.0
The equivalent of 2 eggs: 1 packet, prepared with water (yield: approx. ⅓ cup)	102	2.0	(30.0)	(0.59)	306	6.0
Egg Replacer Jolly Joan, Powdered Egg Substitute, 18-oz. box	1800	360.0	100.0	20.00		
The equivalent of 1 egg:						
1 teaspoon (approx. 0.1 oz.)	10	2.0	100.0	20.00	480	96.0
The equivalent of 2 eggs:						
2 teaspoons (approx. 0.2 oz.)	20	4.0	100.0	20.00	480	96.0
Eggstra Tillie Lewis "Tasti Diet" Powdered Egg Substitute						
The equivalent of 1 egg:						
½ envelope (approx. 0.35 oz.)	50	4.0	142.9	11.43	320	25.6
The equivalent of 2 eggs:						
1 envelope (approx. 0.70 oz.)	100	8.0	142.9	11.43	320	25.6

8 CHEESE •

NATURAL CHEESES

Pasteurized Process(ed) Cheese, Cheese Food, Cheese Spread, Cheese Products, are PROCESS(ED) CHEESES and follow the NATURAL CHEESES.

	UNIT Cal.	UNIT Carb.	1 SLICE Cal.	1 SLICE Carb.	1 OZ., BY WT. Cal.	1 OZ., BY WT. Carb.	1 POUND Cal.	1 POUND Carb.
ALEMTEJO Ewe's-Milk Cheese (a rather soft cheese from Portugal), based on generic data (31.5% fat)								
1 pound	(1618)	(9.6)			(101.1)	(0.60)	(1618)	(9.6)
ALOUETTE Cheese, by brand								
Bongrain, 4-oz. tin	422	2.5			105.5	0.62	1688	9.9
APPENZELLER Cheese, by brand								
Zinco, 6-oz. package	(600)				(100.0)		(1600)	
ASIAGO Cheese, based on generic data								
Fresh (28.8% fat) 1 pound	(1606)	(9.6)			(100.4)	(0.60)	(1606)	(9.6)
Old (28.6% fat), 1 pound	(1773)	(9.6)			(110.8)	(0.60)	(1773)	(9.6)
Asiago (25% fat) (Italy), 1 pound	1615	0.0			100.9	0.00	1615	0.0
BABYBEL Cheese, by brand								
Laughing Cow Babybel Cheese, round, red waxed, 8-oz. package	771	0.0			96.4	0.00	1536	0.0
BACKSTEINER Cheese (similar to Limburger), based on generic data (20.5% fat)								
1 pound	(1258)	(9.6)			(78.6)	(0.60)	(1258)	(9.6)

	UNIT Cal.	UNIT Carb.	1 SLICE Cal.	1 SLICE Carb.	1 OZ., BY WT. Cal.	1 OZ., BY WT. Carb.	1 POUND Cal.	1 POUND Carb.
BAKERS' Skim-Milk Cheese (similar to Cottage Cheese and used mostly commercially), based on generic data (0.5% fat)								
1 pound	(581)	(46.4)			(36.3)	(2.90)	(581)	(46.4)
BATTELMATT Cheese (Swiss-type cheese more like Tilsiter than Swiss), based on generic data (25% fat)								
1 pound	(1456)	(9.6)			(91.0)	(0.60)	(1456)	(9.6)
BAUDEN Cheese, see KOPPEN Cheese								
BELLELAY Cheese (similar to Gorgonzola), based on generic data (30% fat)								
1 pound	(1723)	(9.6)			(107.7)	(0.60)	(1723)	(9.6)
BLUE or BLEU Cheese								
Based on generic data:								
1 pound:								
USDA source A (28.74% fat) (8g/1g/6g/42%/396mg)	1600	10.6			100.0	0.66	1600	10.6
USDA source B (30.5% fat) (9g/1g/6g/40%/na)	1669	9.1			104.3	0.60	1669	9.1
1 cubic inch (approx. ⅗ oz.):								
USDA source A	62	0.4			100.0	0.66	1600	10.6
USDA source B	64	0.3			104.4	0.60	1669	9.1
1 cup, crumbled:								
USDA source A:								
Not packed (approx. 4¾ oz.)	477	3.2			100.0	0.66	1600	10.6
Packed (approx. 8.8 oz.)	880	5.8			100.0	0.66	1600	10.6

	UNIT		1 SLICE		1 OZ., BY WT.		1 POUND	
	Cal.	Carb.	Cal.	Carb.	Cal.	Carb.	Cal.	Carb.
USDA source B:								
Not packed (approx. 4¾ oz.)	494	2.9			104.3	0.60	1669	9.1
Packed (approx. 8.8 oz.)	915	5.3			104.3	0.60	1669	9.1
By brand:								
Casino Blue Cheese, 6-oz. chunk	600	6.0			100.0	1.00	1600	16.1
Dorman's Danish Blue Cheese, 5-lb. loaf	8000	52.8			100.0	0.66	1600	10.6
Kraft Cold Pack Blue Cheese, 4-oz. tray	400	4.0			100.0	1.00	1600	16.0
BONBEL Cheese, by brand								
Laughing Cow Bonbel Cheese, wedge, 6-oz. package	578	0.0			96.3	0.00	1541	0.0
Round, yellow waxed, 8-oz. package	771	0.0			96.3	0.00	1541	0.0
BONBINO Cheese, by brand								
Laughing Cow Bonbino Cheese, round, yellow waxed, 8-oz. package	800				101.0	trace	1616	
BONDON Cheese (French Neufchâtel type), based on generic data (23% fat)								
1 pound	(1283)	(9.6)			(80.2)	(0.60)	(1283)	(9.6)
BONDOST Cheese (Swedish farm-type cheese, also made in U.S.), based on generic data (29.7% fat)								
1 pound	(1624)	(9.6)			(101.5)	(0.60)	(1624)	(9.6)
BRÂNDZA DE BRAILA Cheese, see TELEME								
BRICK Cheese								
Based on generic data:								
1 pound:								
USDA source A (29.68% fat) (8g/1g/7g/41%/159mg)	1684	12.7			105.3	0.79	1684	12.7
USDA source B (30.49% fat) (9g/1g/6g/40%/na)	1678	8.6			104.9	0.54	1678	8.6
1 cubic inch (approx. ⅗ oz.):								
USDA source A	64	0.5			105.3	0.79	1684	12.7
USDA source B	63	0.5			104.9	0.54	1678	8.6
1 rectangle, 4½" × 2¾" × 1⅜" (approx. 10 oz.):								
USDA source A	1051	7.9			105.3	0.79	1684	12.7
USDA source B	1051	5.4			104.9	0.54	1678	8.6
1 slice, 7⅛" × 3¾" × 3/32" (approx. 1⅗ oz.):								
USDA source A	168	1.3	168	1.3	105.3	0.79	1684	12.7
USDA source B	167	0.9	167	0.9	104.9	0.54	1678	8.6
1 cup:								
USDA source A:								
Diced, not packed (approx. 4¾ oz.)	500	3.8			105.3	0.79	1684	12.7
Shredded, not packed (approx. 4 oz.)	421	3.2			105.3	0.79	1684	12.7
USDA source B:								
Diced, not packed (approx. 4¾ oz.)	499	2.4			104.9	0.54	1678	8.6
Shredded, not packed (approx. 4 oz.)	420	2.0			104.9	0.54	1678	8.6
By brand:								
Casino Brick Cheese, 8-oz. chunk	880	8.0			110.0	1.00	1760	16.0
12-oz. chunk	1320	12.0			110.0	1.00	1760	16.0
Dorman's Brick Cheese, 6-oz. package, 5 slices	630	4.7			105.0	0.79	1680	12.6
1 slice, approx. 1.2 oz.	126	1.0	126	1.0	105.0	0.79	1680	12.6
Kraft Brick Cheese, 6-oz. package, 8 slices	660	6.0			110.0	1.00	1760	16.0
1 slice, approx. 0.75 oz.	83	0.8	83	0.8	110.0	1.00	1760	16.0
8-oz. package, 11 slices	880	8.0			110.0	1.00	1760	0.0
1 slice, approx. 0.75 oz.	83	0.8	83	0.8	110.0	1.00	1760	0.0
8-oz. package, 9 "Sandwich Size" slices	880	8.0			110.0	1.00	1760	16.0
1 slice, approx. 0.9 oz.	98	0.9	98	0.9	110.0	1.00	1760	16.0
Land O'Lakes Brick Cheese, 7-oz. chunk	770	7.0			110.0	1.00	1760	16.0
11-oz. chunk	1210	11.0			110.0	1.00	1760	16.0
Pure Goat Products (Goat's Milk) Brick Cheese, 8-oz. chunk	846	1.5			106.0	0.19	1696	3.0
5-lb. block	8464	15.4			106.0	0.19	1696	3.0
BRIE Cheese								
Based on generic data (27.68% fat):								
1 pound (8g/tr/6g/48%/178mg)	1516	2.0			94.8	0.13	1516	2.0
By brand:								
Tiny Dane (Imported) Brie Cheese, 5¼-oz. can	525	0.0			100.0	0.00	1600	0.0
BURGUNDY Cheese (soft, white cheese), based on generic data (38.6% fat)								
1 pound	(2110)	(9.6)			(131.9)	(0.60)	(2110)	(9.6)
BUTTER Cheese, based on generic data (28.5% fat)								
1 pound	(1568)	(9.6)			(98.0)	(0.60)	(1568)	(9.6)
CACIOCAVALLO Cheese (a pressed Provolone cheese)								
Based on generic data (24.5% fat):								
1 pound	(1669)	(9.6)			(104.3)	(0.60)	(1669)	(9.6)
Based on data from Italy (29.7% fat):								
1 pound	1755	0.0			109.7	0.00	1755	0.0
CAERPHILLY Cheese								
Based on generic data (30% fat):								
1 pound	(1946)	(9.6)			(121.6)	(0.60)	(1946)	(9.6)
By brand:								
St. Ivel Caerphilly Cheese, 200-gram (7.05-oz.) package	748	trace			106.0	trace	1696	trace
CAMEMBERT Cheese (domestic)								
Based on generic data:								
1 pound:								
USDA source A (24.26% fat) (7g/tr/6g/52%/239mg)	1362	2.1			85.1	0.13	1362	2.1
USDA source B (24.69% fat) (7g/1g/5g/52%/na)	1356	8.2			84.8	0.50	1356	8.2
1 triangle, 2¼" at base, 2⅛" sides, 1⅛" high (approx. 1⅓ oz.):								
USDA source A	113	0.2			85.1	0.13	1362	2.1
USDA source B	114	0.7			84.8	0.51	1356	8.2
1 cubic inch (approx. ⅗ oz.):								
USDA source A	51	0.1			85.1	0.13	1362	2.1
USDA source B	51	0.3			84.8	0.51	1356	8.2
1 cup (approx. 8.6 oz.):								
USDA source A	738	1.1			85.1	0.13	1362	2.1
USDA source B	731	4.3			84.8	0.51	1356	8.2
By brand:								
Borden Camembert Cheese 4-oz. package, 3 wedges	360	3.0			90.0	0.75	1440	12.0
1 wedge, approx. 1⅓ oz.	120	1.0			90.0	0.75	1440	12.0

	UNIT Cal.	UNIT Carb.	1 SLICE Cal.	1 SLICE Carb.	1 OZ., BY WT. Cal.	1 OZ., BY WT. Carb.	1 POUND Cal.	1 POUND Carb.
CANTAL Cheese, based on generic data (31.0% fat)								
1 pound	(1677)	(9.6)			(104.8)	(0.60)	(1677)	(9.6)
CARAWAY Cheese								
Based on generic data (29.3% fat):								
1 pound (8g/1g/7g/39%/196mg)	1707	13.9			106.7	0.87	1707	13.9
By brand:								
Dorman's Endeco Caraway Cheese, 6-oz. package, 5 slices	642	5.2			106.7	0,87	1707	13.9
1 slice, approx. 1.2 oz.	128	1.0	128	1.0	106.7	0.87	1707	13.9
Kraft Caraway Cheese, 8-oz. package, 5 slices	800	8.0			100.0	1.00	1600	16.0
1 slice, approx. 1.6 oz.	160	1.6	160	1.6	100.0	1.00	1600	16.0
CARRÉ DE L'EST Cheese (Camembert-type cheese), based on generic data (22.6% fat)								
1 pound	(1290)	(9.6)			(80.6)	(0.60)	(1290)	(9.6)
CHANTELLE Cheese, based on generic data (26.7% fat)								
1 pound	(1427)	(9.6)			(89.2)	(0.60)	(1427)	(9.6)
CHEDDAR Cheese (domestic)								
Based on generic data:								
1 pound:								
USDA source A (33.14% fat) (9g/tr/7g/37%/176mg)	1830	5.8			114.4	0.36	1830	5.8
USDA source B (32.21% fat) (9g/tr/7g/37%/198mg)	1805	9.5			112.8	0.60	1805	9.5
1 cylindrical piece (Longhorn style), 2⅝″ diameter, 3⅝″ high (approx. 12 oz.):								
USDA source A	1372	4.3			114.4	0.36	1830	5.8
USDA source B	1353	7.1			112.8	0.60	1805	9.5
1 rectangle, 5⅝″ × 1⅝″ × 1¾″ (approx. 10 oz.):								
USDA source A	1144	3.6			114.4	0.36	1830	5.8
USDA source B	1128	6.0			112.8	0.60	1805	9.5
1 slice:								
Round (midget Longhorn style), 3⅓″ diameter × ⅛″ thick (approx. ¾ oz.):								
USDA source A	85	0.3	85	0.3	114.4	0.36	1830	5.8
USDA source B	84	0.4	84	0.4	112.8	0.60	1805	9.5
Semi-circular (Longhorn style), 5⅝″ long, 3½″ wide at center, ⅛″ thick (approx. 1¼ oz.):								
USDA source A	141	0.4	141	0.4	114.4	0.36	1830	5.8
USDA source B	139	0.7	139	0.7	112.8	0.60	1805	9.5
Rectangular, 6⅞″ × 3⅞″ × 3/32″ (approx. 1⅗ oz.):								
USDA source A	182	0.6	182	0.6	114.4	0.36	1830	5.8
USDA source B	179	0.9	179	0.9	112.8	0.60	1805	9.5
1 cubic inch (approx. ⅗ oz.):								
USDA source A	69	0.2			114.4	0.36	1830	5.8
USDA source B	68	0.4			112.8	0.60	1805	9.5
1 cup:								
USDA source A:								
Diced, not packed (approx. 4.6 oz.)	529	1.7			114.4	0.36	1830	5.8
Shredded, medium packed (approx. contents of a 4-oz. package) (approx. 4 oz.)	450	1.4			114.4	0.36	1830	5.8
Shredded, lightly packed (approx. 3½ oz.)	401	1.3			114.4	0.36	1830	5.8
Grated (approx. 4 oz.)	450	1.4			114.4	0.36	1830	5.8

	UNIT Cal.	UNIT Carb.	1 SLICE Cal.	1 SLICE Carb.	1 OZ., BY WT. Cal.	1 OZ., BY WT. Carb.	1 POUND Cal.	1 POUND Carb.
USDA source B:								
Diced, not packed (approx. 4.6 oz.)	520	2.8			112.8	0.60	1805	9.5
Shredded, medium packed (approx. contents of a 4-oz. package) (approx. 4 oz.)	450	2.4			112.8	0.60	1805	9.5
Shredded, lightly packed (approx. 3½ oz.)	396	2.1			112.8	0.60	1805	9.5
Grated (approx. 4 oz.)	450	2.4			112.8	0.60	1805	9.5
1 tablespoon, grated (approx. ¼ oz.):								
USDA source A	29	0.1			114.4	0.36	1830	5.8
USDA source B	28	0.2			112.8	0.60	1805	9.5
By brand:								
Cellu Cheddar Cheese, low sodium ½-lb. package	880	0.0			110.0	0.00	1760	0.0
16-oz. (1-lb.) package	1760	0.0			110.0	0.00	1760	0.0
2½-lb. loaf	4400	0.0			110.0	0.00	1760	0.0
Coon (Kraft) extra sharp Cheddar Cheese, 8-oz. bar	880	8.0			110.0	1.00	1760	0.0
10-oz. package	1100	10.0			110.0	1.00	1760	0.0
Cracker Barrel (Kraft) mellow, mild, sharp, or extra sharp Cheddar Cheese, including Longhorn style, 1¾-oz. wedge	193	1.8			110.0	1.00	1760	16.0
8-oz. wedge	880	8.0			110.0	1.00	1760	16.0
10-oz. stick	1100	10.0			110.0	1.00	1760	16.0
16-oz. (1-lb.) stick	1760	16.0			110.0	1.00	1760	16.0
Harvest Moon (Kraft) mild Cheddar Cheese, 12-oz. chunk	1320	12.0			110.0	1.00	1760	16.0
2-lb. loaf	3520	32.0			110.0	1.00	1760	16.0
Kraft Shredded Cheddar Cheese, 4-oz. package (approx. 1 cup)	440	4.0			110.0	1.00	1760	16.0
Kraft Sliced Cheddar Cheese, 6-oz. package, 8 slices	660	6.0			110.0	1.00	1760	16.0
1 slice, approx. ¾ oz.	83	0.8			110.0	1.00	1760	16.0
Kraft New York extra sharp Cheddar Cheese, 8-oz. chunk	880	8.0			110.0	1.00	1760	16.0
Land O'Lakes mild, medium, or sharp Cheddar Cheese, 7-oz. "half moon"	770	7.0			110.0	1.00	1760	16.0
10-oz. stick	1100	10.0			110.0	1.00	1760	16.0
11-oz. chunk	1210	11.0			110.0	1.00	1760	16.0
16-oz. (1-lb.) midget horn	1760	16.0			110.0	1.00	1760	16.0
Cold Pack, sharp Cheddar Cheese, 8-oz. package	880	8.0			110.0	1.00	1760	16.0
Laughing Cow Cheddar Cheese, round, yellow waxed 8-oz. package	880	trace			110.0	trace	1760	trace
Martin's Rabbit (Kraft) extra sharp Cheddar Cheese, 10-oz. stick	1100	10.0			110.0	1.00	1760	16.0
Pure Goat Products Goat's Milk Cheddar-Type Cheese, 8-oz. chunk	846	1.5			105.8	0.19	1692	3.0
5-lb. block	(8464)	(15.4)			(105.8)	(0.19)	(1692)	(3.0)
Tillamook medium or sharp Cheddar Cheese, 10-oz. stick	1128	6.0			113.0	0.60	1808	9.6
2-lb. loaf	3610	19.0			113.0	0.60	1808	9.6
Sodium Free Cheddar Cheese, 2-lb. loaf	3610	19.0			113.0	0.60	1808	9.6
CHESHIRE Cheese								
Based on generic data (30.6% fat):								
1 pound	1757	21.7			109.8	1.35	1757	21.7
By brand:								
St. Ivel Cheshire Cheese, 200-gram (7.05-oz.) package	762	trace			108.0	trace	1728	trace
COLBY Cheese								
Based on generic data (32.11% fat):								
1 pound	1789	11.7			111.8	0.73	1789	11.7
1 cubic inch (approx. ⅗ oz.)	68	0.4			111.8	0.72	1789	11.7
By brand:								
Cellu low sodium Colby Cheese, 16-oz. (1-lb.) package	1760	0.0			112.0	0.00	1760	0.0
2½-lb. package	4400	0.0			112.0	0.00	1760	0.0
Dorman's Colby Cheese, 6-oz. package, 6 sandwich slices	672	4.4			112.0	0.73	1760	16.0
1 slice, approx. 1 oz.	110	0.0	110	0.0	112.0	0.73	1760	16.0

	UNIT Cal.	UNIT Carb.	1 SLICE Cal.	1 SLICE Carb.	1 OZ., BY WT. Cal.	1 OZ., BY WT. Carb.	1 POUND Cal.	1 POUND Carb.
8-oz. package, 7 slices	880	0.0			112.0	0.73	1760	0.0
1 slice, approx. 1 oz.	126	0.0	126	0.0	112.0	0.73	1760	0.0
Kraft Colby Cheese, mellow, 8-oz. package, 5 slices	880	8.0			110.0	1.00	1760	16.0
1 slice, approx. 1.6 oz.	176	1.6	176	1.6	110.0	1.00	1760	16.0
16-oz. (1-lb.) package, 10 slices	1760	16.0			110.0	1.00	1760	16.0
1 slice, approx. 1.6 oz.	176	1.6	176	1.6	110.0	1.00	1760	16.0
Land O'Lakes Colby Cheese, 7-oz. wedge	770	7.0			110.0	1.00	1760	16.0
10-oz. half moon	1100	10.0			110.0	1.00	1760	16.0
11-oz. sticks	1210	11.0			110.0	1.00	1760	16.0
16-oz. (1-lb.) square	1760	16.0			110.0	1.00	1760	16.0
Pauly (Swift) low sodium Colby Cheese, 8-oz. block	880	8.0			110.0	1.00	1760	16.0
5-lb. block	8800	80.0			110.0	1.00	1760	16.0
COON Cheese (a fully cured, extremely sharp Cheddar cheese)								
Based on generic data (33% fat):								
1 pound	(1853)	(9.6)			(115.8)	(0.60)	(1853)	(9.6)
By brand:								
Coon (Kraft) extra-sharp Cheddar Cheese, 8-oz. bar	880	8.0			110.0	1.00	1760	0.0
10-oz. package	1100	10.0			110.0	1.00	1760	0.0
CORNHUSKER Cheese (similar to, but softer than, Colby and Cheddar cheeses), based on generic data (30% fat)								
1 pound	(1656)	(9.6)			(103.5)	(0.60)	(1656)	(9.6)
COTHERSTONE Cheese (similar to Stilton Cheese), based on generic data (30% fat)								
1 pound	(1675)	(9.6)			(104.7)	(0.60)	(1675)	(9.6)
COTTAGE Cheese								
COTTAGE CHEESE, based on generic data:								
Creamed Cottage Cheese								
USDA source A (4.51% fat), 1 pound (1g/1g/4g/79%/115mg)	468	12.2			29.2	0.76	468	12.2
1 cup:								
Not packed:								
Large curd (approx. 7.9 oz.)	232	6.0			29.2	0.76	468	12.2
Small curd (approx. 7.4 oz.)	216	5.6			29.2	0.76	468	12.2
Packed, large or small curd (approx. 8.6 oz.)	251	6.3			29.2	0.76	468	12.2
1 tablespoon, large or small curd (approx. 0.5 oz.)	15	0.4			29.2	0.76	468	12.2
USDA source B (4.2% fat), 1 pound (1g/1g/4g/78%/65mg)	481	13.2			30.1	0.82	481	13.2
1 cup:								
Not packed:								
Large curd (approx. 7.9 oz.)	239	6.5			30.1	0.82	481	13.1
Small curd (approx. 7.4 oz.)	223	6.1			30.1	0.82	481	13.1
Packed, large or small curd (approx. 8.6 oz.)	260	7.1			30.1	0.82	481	13.1
1 tablespoon (approx. 0.5 oz.)	15	0.4			30.1	0.82	481	13.1
Dry Curd Cottage Cheese								
USDA source A (0.42% fat)								
1 pound (tr/1g/5g/80%/13mg)	384	8.4			24.0	0.52	384	8.4
1 cup:								
Not packed (approx. 5.1 oz.)	123	2.7			24.0	0.52	384	8.4

	UNIT Cal.	UNIT Carb.	1 SLICE Cal.	1 SLICE Carb.	1 OZ., BY WT. Cal.	1 OZ., BY WT. Carb.	1 POUND Cal.	1 POUND Carb.
Packed (approx. 7.1 oz.)	171	3.7			24.0	0.52	384	8.4
1 tablespoon (approx. 0.3 oz.)	8	0.2			24.0	0.52	384	8.4
USDA source B (0.3% fat)								
1 pound (tr/1g/5g/79%/82mg)	390	12.2			24.4	0.76	390	12.2
1 cup, not packed (approx. 5.1 oz.)	124	3.9			24.4	0.76	390	12.2
1 tablespoon (approx. 0.3 oz.)	8	0.2			24.4	0.76	390	12.2
Low-fat (2% fat)								
1 pound:								
USDA source A (1g/1g/4g/79%/115mg)	409	16.5			25.5	1.03	409	16.5
USDA source B	410	5.6			25.6	0.35	410	5.6
1 cup, not packed:								
USDA source A (approx. 8 oz.)	(204)	(8.2)			25.5	1.03	409	16.5
USDA source B (approx. 8 oz.)	205	2.8			25.6	0.35	410	5.6
1 tablespoon:								
USDA source A (approx. 0.5 oz.)	(13)	(0.5)			25.5	1.03	409	16.5
USDA source B (approx. 0.5 oz.)	13	0.2			25.6	0.35	410	5.6
Low-fat (1% fat)								
1 pound:								
USDA source A (tr/1g/4g/82%/115mg)	327	12.3			20.4	0.77	327	12.3
USDA source B	330	3.0			20.6	0.19	330	3.0
1 cup, not packed:								
Source A (approx. 8 oz.)	163	6.1			20.4	0.77	327	12.3
Source B (approx. 8 oz.)	165	1.5			20.6	0.19	330	3.0
1 tablespoon:								
Source A (approx. 0.5 oz.)	10	0.4			20.4	0.77	327	12.3
Source B (approx. 0.5 oz.)	10	0.1			20.6	0.19	330	3.0
COTTAGE CHEESE, by brand								
Whole-milk and skim-milk cottage cheeses are integrated and alphabetized by brand. Flavored cottage cheeses such as Cottage Cheese with Pineapple and Yogurt Cottage Cheese are listed together directly following plain cottage cheese.								
A&P Large Curd Cottage Cheese, 4% fat minimum, 8-oz. container	240	8.0			30.0	1.00	480	16.0
16-oz. (1-lb.) container	480	16.0			30.0	1.00	480	16.0
32-oz. (2-lb.) container	960	32.0			30.0	1.00	480	16.0
1 cup:								
Not packed (approx. 7.9 oz.)	237	7.9			30.0	1.00	480	16.0
Packed (approx. 8.6 oz.)	258	8.6			30.0	1.00	480	16.0
1 tablespoon (approx. 0.5 oz.)	15	0.5			30.0	1.00	480	16.0
Small Curd Cottage Cheese, 4% fat minimum, 8-oz. container	240	8.0			30.0	1.00	480	16.0
16-oz. (1-lb.) container	480	16.0			30.0	1.00	480	16.0
32-oz. (2-lb.) container	960	32.0			30.0	1.00	480	16.0
1 cup:								
Not packed (approx. 7.4 oz.)	222	7.4			30.0	1.00	480	18.0
Packed (approx. 8.6 oz.)	258	8.6			30.0	1.00	480	16.0
1 tablespoon (approx. 0.5 oz.)	14	0.5			30.0	1.00	480	16.0
Axelrod's Low-Fat Cottage Cheese, 1% fat, 8-oz. container	180	8.0			22.5	1.00	360	16.0
16-oz. (1-lb.) container	360	16.0			22.5	1.00	360	16.0
32-oz. (2-lb.) container	720	32.0			22.5	1.00	360	16.0
1 cup:								
Not packed (approx. 8 oz.)	180	8.0			22.5	1.00	360	16.0
1 tablespoon (approx. 0.5 oz.)	11	0.5			22.5	1.00	360	16.0
Cottage Cheese, 4% fat, 8-oz. container	240	8.0			30.0	1.00	480	16.0
16-oz. (1-lb.) container	480	16.0			30.0	1.00	480	16.0
32-oz. (2-lb.) container	960	32.0			30.0	1.00	480	16.0

	UNIT Cal.	UNIT Carb.	1 SLICE Cal.	1 SLICE Carb.	1 OZ., BY WT. Cal.	1 OZ., BY WT. Carb.	1 POUND Cal.	1 POUND Carb.
Breakstone's Dry Curd Cottage Cheese with added skim milk, less than ½% fat, unsalted, 12-oz. container	(400)	(40.0)			(33.0)	(3.34)	(528)	(53.4)
1 cup:								
Not packed (approx. 5.1 oz.)	(168)	(16.8)			(33.0)	(3.34)	(528)	(53.4)
Packed (approx. 7.1 oz.)	(234)	(23.7)			(33.0)	(3.34)	(528)	(53.4)
1 tablespoon (approx. 0.3 oz.)	(11)	(1.1)			(33.0)	(3.34)	(528)	(53.4)
Large Curd Creamed Cottage Cheese, 4% fat minimum, 8-oz. container	240	8.0			30.0	1.00	480	16.0
16-oz. (1-lb.) container	480	16.0			30.0	1.00	480	16.0
24-oz. container	720	24.0			30.0	1.00	480	16.0
1 cup:								
Not packed (approx. 7.9 oz.)	237	7.9			30.0	1.00	480	16.0
Packed (approx. 8.6 oz.)	258	8.6			30.0	1.00	480	16.0
1 tablespoon (approx. 0.5 oz.)	15	0.5			30.0	1.00	480	16.0
Small Curd Creamed Cottage Cheese, 4% fat minimum, 8-oz. container	240	8.0			30.0	1.00	480	16.0
16-oz. (1-lb.) container	480	16.0			30.0	1.00	480	16.0
1 cup:								
Not packed (approx. 7.4 oz.)	222	7.4			30.0	1.00	480	16.0
Packed (approx. 8.6 oz.)	258	8.6			30.0	1.00	480	16.0
1 tablespoon (approx. 0.5 oz.)	14	0.5			30.0	1.00	480	16.0
Tangy Small Curd Cottage Cheese, 4% fat minimum, 8-oz. container	240	8.0			30.0	1.00	480	16.0
16-oz. (1-lb.) container	480	16.0			30.0	1.00	480	16.0
24-oz. container	720	24.0			30.0	1.00	480	16.0
1 cup:								
Not packed (approx. 7.4 oz.)	222	7.4			30.0	1.00	480	16.0
Packed (approx. 8.6 oz.)	258	8.8			30.0	1.00	480	16.0
1 tablespoon (approx. 0.5 oz.)	14	0.5			30.0	1.00	480	16.0
Crowley's No Fat or Salt Added Cottage Cheese, 12-oz. container	240	9.0			20.0	0.75	320	12.0
1 cup, not packed (approx. 8 oz.)	160	6.0			20.0	0.75	320	12.0
1 tablespoon (approx. 0.5 oz.)	10	0.4			20.0	0.75	320	12.0
Foodfair Les-Cal Diet, 12-oz. container	288	12.4			24.0	1.03	384	16.5
Friendship Calorie Meter Cottage Cheese, 2% fat, 12-oz. container	300	12.0			25.0	1.00	400	16.0
Unsalted, 12-oz. container	270	12.0			22.5	1.00	360	16.0
Large Curd Creamed Cottage Cheese, 4% fat minimum, 8-oz. container	240	8.0			30.0	1.00	480	16.0
16-oz. (1-lb.) container	480	16.0			30.0	1.00	480	16.0
32-oz. (2-lb.) container	960	32.0			30.0	1.00	480	16.0
1 cup:								
Not packed (approx. 7.9 oz.)	237	7.9			30.0	1.00	480	16.0
Packed (approx. 8.6 oz.)	258	8.6			30.0	1.00	480	16.0
1 tablespoon (approx. 0.5 oz.)	15	0.5			30.0	1.00	480	16.0
Small Curd Creamed Cottage Cheese, 8-oz. container	240	8.0			30.0	1.00	480	16.0
16-oz. (1-lb.) container	480	16.0			30.0	1.00	480	16.0
32-oz. (2-lb.) container	960	32.0			30.0	1.00	480	16.0
1 cup:								
Not packed (approx. 7.4 oz.)	222	7.4			30.0	1.00	480	16.0
Packed (approx. 8.6 oz.)	258	8.6			30.0	1.00	480	16.0
1 tablespoon (approx. 0.5 oz.)	14	0.5			30.0	1.00	480	16.0
Light n' Lively (Sealtest) 99% Fat-Free Cottage Cheese, 1% fat minimum, 8-oz. container	180	8.0			22.5	1.00	360	16.0
16-oz. (1-lb.) container	360	16.0			22.5	1.00	350	16.0
24-oz. container	540	24.0			22.5	1.00	360	16.0
1 cup:								
Not packed (approx. 7.9 oz.)	178	7.9			22.5	1.00	360	16.0
Packed (approx. 8.5 oz.)	191	8.5			22.5	1.00	360	16.0
1 tablespoon (approx. 0.5 oz.)	11	0.5			22.5	1.00	360	16.0
Small Curd Creamed Cottage Cheese, 4% fat minumum, 16-oz. (1-lb.) container	480	16.0			30.0	1.00	480	16.0
24-oz. container	720	24.0			30.0	1.00	480	16.0
1 cup:								
Not packed (approx. 7.4 oz.)	(222)	(7.4)			30.0	1.00	480	16.0
Packed (approx. 8.6 oz.)	(258)	(8.6)			30.0	1.00	480	16.0
1 tablespoon (approx. 0.5 oz.)	(14)	(0.5)			30.0	1.00	480	16.0
Lucerne (Safeway) Dry Curd Cottage Cheese, 16-oz. (1-lb.) container	320	12.0			20.0	0.75	320	12.0
1 cup:								
Not packed (approx. 5.1 oz.)	102	3.8			20.0	0.75	320	12.0
Packed (approx. 7.1 oz.)	142	5.3			20.0	0.75	320	12.0
1 tablespoon (approx. 0.3 oz.)	6	0.2			20.0	0.75	320	12.0
Low-Fat Cottage Cheese, 2% fat, 16-oz. (1-lb.) container	400	16.0			25.0	1.00	400	16.0
1 cup:								
Not packed (approx. 7.9 oz.)	198	7.9			25.0	1.00	400	16.0
Packed (approx. 8.5 oz.)	215	8.5			25.0	1.00	400	16.0
1 tablespoon (approx. 0.5 oz.)	12	0.5			25.0	1.00	400	16.0
Small Curd Creamed Cottage Cheese, 4% fat minimum, 16-oz. (1-lb.) container	480	16.0			30.0	1.00	480	16.0
1 cup:								
Not packed (approx. 7.4 oz.)	222	7.4			30.0	1.08	480	16.0
Packed (approx. 8.6 oz.)	258	8.6			30.0	1.00	480	16.0
1 tablespoon (approx. 0.5 oz.)	14	0.5			30.0	1.00	480	16.0
Meadow Gold Creamed Cottage Cheese, 4% fat minimum, 16-oz. (1-lb.) container	480	16.0			30.0	1.00	480	16.0
1 cup:								
Not packed (approx. 8 oz.)	240	8.0			30.0	1.00	480	16.0
Packed (approx. 8.6 oz.)	258	8.6			30.0	1.00	480	16.0
1 tablespoon (approx. 0.5 oz.)	15	0.5			30.0	1.00	480	16.0
Sealtest Large Curd Creamed Cottage Cheese, 4% fat minimum, 16-oz. (1-lb.) container	480	16.0			30.0	1.00	480	16.0
24-oz. container	720	24.0			30.0	1.00	480	16.0
1 cup:								
Not packed (approx. 7.9 oz.)	237	7.9			30.0	1.00	480	16.0
Packed (approx. 8.6 oz.)	258	8.6			30.0	1.00	480	16.0
1 tablespoon (approx. 0.5 oz.)	15	0.5			30.0	1.00	480	16.0
Viva Low-Fat Cottage Cheese, 2% fat, 16-oz. (1-lb.) container	400	16.0			25.0	1.00	400	16.0
1 cup:								
Not packed (approx. 8 oz.)	200	8.0			25.0	1.00	400	16.0
Packed (approx. 8.6 oz.)	215	8.6			25.0	1.00	400	16.0
1 tablespoon (approx. 0.5 oz.)	13	0.5			25.0	1.00	400	16.0
Waldbaum Creamed Cottage Cheese, 4% fat, 8-oz. container	260	7.0			33.0	0.88	528	14.1
Weight Watchers Cottage Cheese, 0.9% fat, 16-oz. (1-lb.) container	360	52.0			23.0	3.25	368	52.0
1 cup:								
Not packed (approx. 8 oz.)	(180)	(26.0)			22.5	3.25	360	52.0
Packed (approx. 8.6 oz.)	(194)	(28.0)			22.5	3.25	360	52.0
1 tablespoon (approx. 0.5 oz.)	(11)	(1.6)			22.5	3.25	360	52.0

	UNIT Cal.	UNIT Carb.	1 SLICE Cal.	1 SLICE Carb.	1 OZ., BY WT. Cal.	1 OZ., BY WT. Carb.	1 POUND Cal.	1 POUND Carb.
Zausner Creamed Cottage Cheese, 4% fat minimum, 12-oz. container	390	10.5			33.0	0.88	528	14.1
Sold bulk, 1 pound	528	14.1			33.0	0.88	528	14.1
Sold bulk, 33-lb. supermarket container	17160	464.5			33.0	0.88	528	14.1
Unsalted Creamed Cottage Cheese, sold bulk, 1 pound	528	14.1			33.0	0.88	528	14.1
FLAVORED COTTAGE CHEESE, by flavor								
Cottage Cheese with Chives, **Lucerne (Safeway),** 16-oz. (1-lb.) container	480	16.0			30.0	1.00	480	16.0
Cottage Cheese with Dutch Apple, **Friendship,** 4% fat, 8-oz. container	248	10.0			31.1	1.25	496	20.0
1 cup, not packed (approx. 8 oz.)	248	10.0			31.1	1.25	496	20.0
1 tablespoon (approx. 0.5 oz.)	(16)	(0.6)			31.1	1.25	496	20.0
Cottage Cheese with Fruit Salad, **Axelrod's,** 8-oz. container	280	36.0			35.0	4.50	560	72.0
16-oz. (1-lb.) container	560	72.0			35.0	4.50	560	72.0
1 cup, not packed (approx. 8 oz.)	280	36.0			35.0	4.50	560	72.0
1 tablespoon (approx. 0.5 oz.)	18	2.3			35.0	4.50	560	72.0
Cottage Cheese with Fruit Salad, **Friendship** Calorie Meter, 1.7% fat, 12-oz. container	360	39.0			30.0	3.25	480	52.0
1 tablespoon (approx. 0.5 oz.)	(16)	(0.2)			30.0	3.25	480	52.0
Cottage Cheese with Fruit Salad, **Lucerne (Safeway),** 16-oz. (1-lb.) container	600	60.0			37.5	3.75	600	60.0
1 tablespoon (approx. 0.5 oz.)	(19)	(1.9)			37.5	3.75	600	60.0
Cottage Cheese with Garden Salad, **Axelrod's,** 3.5% fat, 8-oz. container	220	4.0			28.0	0.50	440	8.0
16-oz. (1-lb.) container	440	8.0			28.0	0.50	440	8.0
1 cup, not packed (approx. 8 oz.)	220	4.0			28.0	0.50	440	8.0
1 tablespoon (approx. 0.5 oz.)	14	0.3			28.0	0.50	440	8.0
Garden Salad Cottage Cheese, **Friendship,** 4% fat, 12-oz. container	360	12.0			30.0	1.00	480	16.0
Garden Salad in Low-Fat Cottage Cheese, **Light n' Lively (Sealtest),** 99% Fat Free, 1% fat minimum, 12-oz. container	270	15.0			22.5	1.25	360	20.0
1 cup, not packed (approx. 8 oz.)	180	10.0			22.5	1.25	360	20.0
1 tablespoon (approx. 0.5 oz.)	11	0.6			22.5	1.25	360	20.0
Peach & Pineapple in Low-Fat Cottage Cheese, **Light n' Lively (Sealtest)** 99% Fat Free, 1% fat minimum, 12-oz. container	300	33.0			25.0	2.75	400	44.0
1 cup, not packed (approx. 8 oz.)	200	22.0			25.0	2.75	400	44.0
1 tablespoon (approx. 0.5 oz.)	13	1.4			25.0	2.75	400	44.0
Cottage Cheese with Pineapple, **Axelrod's,** 3.5% fat, 8-oz. container	280	30.0			35.0	3.75	560	60.3
16-oz. (1-lb.) container	560	60.0			35.0	3.75	560	60.3
1 cup, not packed (approx. 8 oz.)	280	30.0			35.0	3.75	560	60.3
1 tablespoon (approx. 0.5 oz.)	18	1.9			35.0	3.75	560	60.3
Cottage Cheese with Pineapple, **Breakstone's,** 4% fat minimum, 16-oz. (1-lb.) container	608	60.0			38.0	3.75	608	60.0
1 cup, not packed (approx. 8 oz.)	304	30.0			38.0	3.75	608	60.0
1 teaspoon (approx. 0.5 oz.)	19	1.9			38.0	3.75	608	60.0
Pineapple Cottage Cheese, **Friendship,** 3.5% fat, 12-oz. container	420	45.0			35.0	3.75	560	60.0
1 cup, not packed (approx. 8 oz.)	280	30.0			35.0	3.75	560	60.0
1 tablespoon (approx. 0.5 oz.)	18	1.9			35.0	3.75	560	60.0
Cottage Cheese with Pineapple, **Lucerne (Safeway)** 16-oz. (1-lb.) container	600	60.0			37.5	3.75	600	60.0
1 cup, not packed (approx. 8 oz.)	300	30.0			37.5	3.75	560	60.0
1 tablespoon (approx. 0.5 oz.)	19	1.9			37.5	3.75	560	60.0
Pineapple Cottage Cheese, **Waldbaum,** 3.5% fat, 12-oz. container	330	21.0			27.5	1.75	440	28.0
1 cup, not packed (approx. 8 oz.)	220	14.0			27.5	1.75	440	28.0
1 tablespoon (approx. 0.5 oz.)	14	0.9			27.5	1.75	440	28.0
Pineapple Cottage Cheese, **Zausner,** 3.5% fat, 12-oz. container	330	21.0			27.5	1.75	440	28.0
1 cup, not packed (approx. 8 oz.)	220	14.0			27.5	1.75	440	28.0
1 tablespoon (approx. 0.5 oz.)	14	0.9			27.5	1.75	440	28.0
Yogurt Cottage Cheese, **Zausner,** 1.4% fat, 12-oz. container	249	9.0			21.0	0.75	336	12.0
Yogurt Cottage Cheese with Blueberry, **Zausner,** 1.4% fat, 12-oz. container	276	21.0			23.0	1.75	368	28.0
Yogurt Cottage Cheese with Pineapple, **Zausner,** 1.4% fat, 12-oz. container	276	21.0			23.0	1.75	368	28.0
Yogurt Cottage Cheese with Raspberry, **Zausner,** 1.4% fat, 12-oz. container	276	21.0			23.0	1.75	368	28.0
Yogurt Cottage Cheese with Strawberry, **Zausner,** 1.4% fat, 12-oz. container	276	21.0			23.0	1.75	368	28.0

COULOMMIERS Cheese (similar to Brie and Camembert, but ripened for a shorter period), based on generic data (23% fat)

	UNIT Cal.	UNIT Carb.	1 SLICE Cal.	1 SLICE Carb.	1 OZ., BY WT. Cal.	1 OZ., BY WT. Carb.	1 POUND Cal.	1 POUND Carb.
1 pound	(1203)	(1.6)			(75.2)	(0.10)	(1203)	(1.6)

COUNTRY CHARM Cheese, by brand

	UNIT Cal.	UNIT Carb.	1 SLICE Cal.	1 SLICE Carb.	1 OZ., BY WT. Cal.	1 OZ., BY WT. Carb.	1 POUND Cal.	1 POUND Carb.
Fisher Longhorn semi-soft part-skim-milk cheese, 14-oz. full moon	1260	trace			90.0	trace	1440	

CREAM Cheese

CREAM CHEESE, based on generic data:

Regular or Whipped. When cream cheese is whipped, it takes up more space. This affects calorie values based on volume, such as cup and tablespoon measures. It does not affect calorie values based on weight. For further discussion of the relationship between weights and volumes, please see ***Methodology,*** *"Weight/Volume relationships."*

	UNIT Cal.	UNIT Carb.	1 SLICE Cal.	1 SLICE Carb.	1 OZ., BY WT. Cal.	1 OZ., BY WT. Carb.	1 POUND Cal.	1 POUND Carb.
Regular, 1 pound:								
USDA source A (34.87% fat), (10g/1g/2g/54%/84mg)	1584	12.1			99.0	0.75	1584	12.1
USDA source B (37.7% fat), (11g/1g/2g/51%/71mg)	1696	9.5			106.0	0.60	1696	9.5
Regular, 1 cubic inch (approx. 0.57 oz.):								
USDA source A	56	0.4			99.0	0.75	1584	12.1
USDA source B	60	0.3			106.0	0.60	1696	9.5
1 cup:								
Regular (approx. 8.2 oz.):								
USDA source A	812	6.2			99.0	0.75	1584	12.1
USDA source B	869	4.9			106.0	0.60	1696	9.5
Whipped (approx. 5.5 oz.):								
USDA source A	545	4.1			99.0	0.75	1584	12.1
USDA source B	583	3.3			106.0	0.60	1696	9.5

	UNIT Cal.	UNIT Carb.	1 SLICE Cal.	1 SLICE Carb.	1 OZ., BY WT. Cal.	1 OZ., BY WT. Carb.	1 POUND Cal.	1 POUND Carb.
1 tablespoon:								
Regular (approx. 0.51 oz.):								
USDA source A	51	0.4			99.0	0.75	1584	12.1
USDA source B	54	0.3			106.0	0.60	1696	9.5
Whipped (approx. 0.34 oz.):								
USDA source A	34	0.3			99.0	0.75	1584	12.1
USDA source B	36	0.2			106.0	0.60	1696	9.5
CREAM CHEESE, by brand								
Regular and whipped are integrated. Flavored cream cheeses, such as "whipped cream cheese with chives," are listed together directly following plain cream cheeses. Imitation cream cheeses are included in the main listing, and appear again in their own listing at the end, alphabetized by brand.								
Acme Whipped Cream Cheese, 8-oz. container	812	3.2			102.0	0.40	1632	6.4
1 cup (approx. 5.5 oz.)	561	2.2			102.0	0.40	1632	6.4
1 tablespoon (approx. 0.3 oz.)	35	0.1			102.0	0.40	1632	6.4
Ann Page (A&P) Cream Cheese, 8-oz. package	800	8.0			100.0	1.00	1600	16.0
1 cup (approx. 8.2 oz.)	820	8.2			100.0	1.00	1600	16.0
1 tablespoon (approx. 0.5 oz.)	51	0.5			100.0	1.00	1600	16.0
Whipped Cream Cheese, 8-oz. container	800	8.0			100.0	1.00	1600	16.0
1 cup (approx. 5.5 oz.)	550	5.5			100.0	1.00	1600	16.0
1 tablespoon (approx. 0.3 oz.)	34	0.3			100.0	1.00	1600	16.0
Breakstone's Cream Cheese, 8-oz. package	800	8.0			100.0	1.00	1600	16.0
1 cup (approx. 8.2 oz.)	820	8.2			100.0	1.00	1600	16.0
1 tablespoon (approx. 0.5 oz.)	51	0.5			100.0	1.00	1600	16.0
Dairygold Cream Cheese, sold bulk, 1 pound	1701	10.1			106.3	0.63	1701	10.1
1 cup (approx. 8.2 oz.)	872	5.2			106.3	0.63	1701	10.1
1 tablespoon (approx. 0.5 oz.)	55	0.3			106.3	0.63	1701	10.1
Dellwood Cream Cheese, sold bulk, 1 pound	1701	10.1			106.3	0.63	1701	10.1
1 cup (approx. 8.2 oz.)	872	5.2			106.3	0.63	1701	10.1
1 tablespoon (approx. 0.5 oz.)	55	0.3			106.3	0.63	1701	10.1
Deutsch Whipped Cream Cheese, 8-oz. container	812	3.2			102.0	0.40	1632	6.4
1 cup (approx. 5.5 oz.)	561	2.2			102.0	0.40	1632	6.4
1 tablespoon (approx. 0.3 oz.)	35	0.1			102.0	0.40	1632	6.4
Fairmont Cream Cheese, sold bulk, 1 pound	1701	10.1			106.3	0.63	1701	10.1
1 cup (approx. 8.2 oz.)	872	5.2			106.3	0.63	1701	10.1
1 tablespoon (approx. 0.5 oz.)	55	0.3			106.3	0.63	1701	10.1
Fanfare Cream Cheese, sold bulk, 1 pound	1859				116.2		1859	
1 cup (approx. 8.2 oz.)	953				116.2		1859	
1 tablespoon (approx. 0.5 oz.)	60				116.2		1859	
Food Town Whipped Cream Cheese, 8-oz. container	812	3.2			101.5	0.40	1624	6.4
1 cup (approx. 5.5 oz.)	558	2.2			101.5	0.40	1624	6.4
1 tablespoon (approx. 0.3 oz.)	35	0.1			101.5	0.40	1624	6.4
Friendship Cream Cheese, sold bulk, 1 pound	1701	10.1			106.3	0.63	1701	10.1
1 cup (approx. 8.2 oz.)	872	5.2			106.3	0.63	1701	10.1
1 tablespoon (approx. 0.5 oz.)	55	0.3			106.3	0.63	1701	10.1
June Dairy Cream Cheese, sold bulk, 1 pound	1701	10.1			106.3	0.63	1701	10.1
1 cup (approx. 8.2 oz.)	872	5.2			106.3	0.63	1701	10.1
1 tablespoon (approx. 0.5 oz.)	55	0.3			106.3	0.63	1701	10.1
Key Food Whipped Cream Cheese, 8-oz. container	812	3.2			101.5	0.40	1624	6.4
1 cup (approx. 5.5 oz.)	558	2.2			101.5	0.40	1624	6.4
1 tablespoon (approx. 0.3 oz.)	35	0.1			101.5	0.40	1624	6.4
King Smoothee Imitation Cream Cheese, 8-oz. package	520	16.0			65.0	2.00	1040	32.0
1 cup (approx. 8.2 oz.)	533	16.4			65.0	2.00	1040	32.0
1 tablespoon (approx. 0.5 oz.)	33	1.0			65.0	2.00	1040	32.0
Kraft American Cheese & Cream Cheese with Jalapeño Peppers, 5-oz. jar	400	5.0			80.0	1.00	1280	16.0
1 tablespoon (approx. 0.5 oz.)	(43)	(0.5)			80.0	1.00	1280	16.0
Lion Cream Cheese, sold bulk, 1 pound	1701	10.1			106.3	0.63	1701	10.1
1 cup (approx. 8.2 oz.)	872	5.2			106.3	0.63	1701	10.1
1 tablespoon (approx. 0.5 oz.)	55	0.3			106.3	0.63	1701	10.1
Lucerne (Safeway) Cream Cheese, 8-oz. package	800	8.0			100.0	1.00	1600	16.0
1 cup (approx. 8.2 oz.)	820	8.2			100.0	1.00	1600	16.0
1 tablespoon (approx. 0.5 oz.)	51	0.5			100.0	1.00	1600	16.0
Whipped Cream Cheese, 8-oz. container	812	3.2			101.5	0.40	1624	6.4
1 cup (approx. 5.5 oz.)	558	2.2			101.5	0.40	1624	6.4
1 tablespoon (approx. 0.3 oz.)	35	0.1			101.5	0.40	1624	6.4
Montrose Cream Cheese, sold bulk, 1 pound	1701	10.1			106.3	0.63	1701	10.1
1 cup (approx. 8.2 oz.)	872	5.2			106.3	0.63	1701	10.1
1 tablespoon (approx. 0.5 oz.)	55	0.3			106.3	0.63	1701	10.1
Penn Maid Cream Cheese, sold bulk, 1 pound	1701	10.1			106.3	0.63	1701	10.1
1 cup (approx. 8.2 oz.)	872	5.2			106.3	0.63	1701	10.1
1 tablespoon (approx. 0.5 oz.)	55	0.3			106.3	0.63	1701	10.1
Philadelphia (Kraft) Cream Cheese, 3-oz. package	300	3.0			100.0	1.00	1600	16.0
8-oz. package	800	8.0			100.0	1.00	1600	16.0
1 cup (approx. 8.2 oz.)	820	8.2			100.0	1.00	1600	16.0
1 tablespoon (approx. 0.5 oz.)	51	0.5			100.0	1.00	1600	16.0
Imitation, reduced calories, Cream Cheese, 8-oz. package	400	16.0			50.0	2.00	800	32.0
1 cup (approx. 8.2 oz.)	410	16.4			50.0	2.00	1600	32.0
1 tablespoon (approx. 0.5 oz.)	26	1.0			50.0	2.00	1600	32.0
"Light," Pasteurized Process Cream Cheese Product, 8-oz. container	480	16.0			60.0	2.00	960	32.0
1 cup (approx. 7.1 oz.)	423	14.1			60.0	2.00	960	32.0
1 tablespoon (approx. 0.4 oz.)	26	0.9			60.0	2.00	960	32.0
Whipped Cream Cheese, 4-oz. container	400	4.0			100.0	1.00	1600	16.0
8-oz. container	800	8.0			100.0	1.00	1600	16.0
1 cup (approx. 5.5 oz.)	550	5.5			100.0	1.00	1600	16.0
1 tablespoon (approx. 0.3 oz.)	34	0.3			100.0	1.00	1600	16.0
Ralph's Whipped Cream Cheese, 8-oz. container	812	3.2			101.5	0.40	1624	6.4
1 cup (approx. 5.5 oz.)	558	2.2			101.5	0.40	1624	6.4
1 tablespoon (approx. 0.3 oz.)	35	0.1			101.5	0.40	1624	6.4
Regent Cream Cheese, sold bulk, 1 pound	1701	10.1			106.3	0.63	1701	10.1
1 cup (approx. 8.2 oz.)	872	5.2			106.3	0.63	1701	10.1
1 tablespoon (approx. 0.5 oz.)	55	0.3			106.3	0.63	1701	10.1
Royal Dairy Whipped Cream Cheese, 8-oz. container	812	3.2			101.5	0.40	1624	6.4
1 cup (approx. 5.5 oz.)	558	2.2			101.5	0.40	1624	6.4
1 tablespoon (approx. 0.3 oz.)	35	0.1			101.5	0.40	1624	6.4
Sanchez Whipped Cream Cheese, 8-oz. container	812	3.2			101.5	0.40	1624	6.4
1 cup (approx. 5.5 oz.)	558	2.2			101.5	0.40	1624	6.4
1 tablespoon (approx. 0.3 oz.)	35	0.1			101.5	0.40	1624	6.4
Shoprite Whipped Cream Cheese, 8-oz. container	812	3.2			101.5	0.40	1624	6.4
1 cup (approx. 5.5 oz.)	558	2.2			101.5	0.40	1624	6.4
1 tablespoon (approx. 0.3 oz.)	35	0.1			101.5	0.40	1624	6.4
Smithfield Cream Cheese, sold bulk, 1 pound	1701	10.1			106.3	0.63	1701	10.1
1 cup (approx. 8.2 oz.)	872	5.2			106.3	0.63	1701	10.1
1 tablespoon (approx. 0.5 oz.)	55	0.3			106.3	0.63	1701	10.1
Sunny Cream Cheese, sold bulk, 1 pound	1701	10.1			106.3	0.63	1701	10.1
1 cup (approx. 8.2 oz.)	872	5.2			106.3	0.63	1701	10.1

	UNIT Cal.	UNIT Carb.	1 SLICE Cal.	1 SLICE Carb.	1 OZ., BY WT. Cal.	1 OZ., BY WT. Carb.	1 POUND Cal.	1 POUND Carb.
1 tablespoon (approx. 0.5 oz.)	55	0.3			106.3	0.63	1701	10.1
Temp Tee Whipped Cream Cheese, 4-oz. container	406	1.6			101.5	0.40	1624	6.4
8-oz. container	812	3.2			101.5	0.40	1624	6.4
1 cup (approx. 5.5 oz.)	558	2.2			101.5	0.40	1624	6.4
1 tablespoon (approx. 0.3 oz.)	35	0.1			101.5	0.40	1624	6.4
Waldbaum Whipped Cream Cheese, 8-oz. container	812	3.2			101.5	0.40	1624	6.4
1 cup (approx. 5.5 oz.)	558	2.2			101.5	0.40	1624	6.4
1 tablespoon (approx. 0.3 oz.)	35	0.1			101.5	0.40	1624	6.4
White Rose Cream Cheese, 8-oz. package	800	16.0			100.0	2.00	1600	32.0
1 cup (approx. 8.2 oz.)	820	16.4			100.0	2.00	1600	32.0
1 tablespoon (approx. 0.5 oz.)	51	1.0			100.0	2.00	1600	32.0
Whipped Cream Cheese, 8-oz. container	880	8.0			110.0	1.00	1760	16.0
1 cup (approx. 5.5 oz.)	605	5.5			110.0	1.00	1760	16.0
1 tablespoon (approx. 0.3 oz.)	38	0.3			110.0	1.00	1760	16.0
Zausner Whipped Cream Cheese, 8-oz. container	812	3.2			101.5	0.40	1624	6.4
1 cup (approx. 5.5 oz.)	558	2.2			101.5	0.40	1624	6.4
1 tablespoon (approx. 0.3 oz.)	35	0.1			101.5	0.40	1624	6.4
FLAVORED CREAM CHEESE, by brand								
Philadelphia (Kraft) Cream Cheese with Bacon & Horseradish, Whipped, 4-oz. container	360	4.0			90.0	1.00	1440	16.0
1 cup (approx. 5.5 oz.)	495	5.5			90.0	1.00	1440	16.0
1 tablespoon (approx. 0.3 oz.)	31	0.3			90.0	1.00	1440	16.0
Cream Cheese and Blue Cheese, Blended, Whipped, 4-oz. container	400	8.0			100.0	2.00	1600	32.0
1 cup (approx. 5.5 oz.)	550	11.0			100.0	2.00	1600	32.0
1 tablespoon (approx. 0.3 oz.)	34	0.7			100.0	2.00	1600	32.0
Cream Cheese with Chives, 3-oz. package	300	3.0			100.0	1.00	1600	16.0
1 cup (approx. 8.2 oz.)	820	8.2			100.0	1.00	1600	16.0
1 tablespoon (approx. 0.5 oz.)	51	0.5			100.0	1.00	1600	16.0
Cream Cheese with Chives, Whipped, 4-oz. container	360	4.0			90.0	1.00	1440	16.0
1 cup (approx. 5.5 oz.)	495	5.5			90.0	1.00	1440	16.0
1 tablespoon (approx. 0.3 oz.)	31	0.3			90.0	1.00	1440	16.0
Cream Cheese with Onions, Whipped, 4-oz. container	360	8.0			90.0	2.00	1440	32.0
8-oz. container	720	16.0			90.0	2.00	1440	32.0
1 cup (approx. 5.5 oz.)	495	11.0			90.0	2.00	1440	32.0
1 tablespoon (approx. 0.3 oz.)	31	0.7			90.0	2.00	1440	32.0
Cream Cheese with Pimentos, 3-oz. package	300	3.0			100.0	1.00	1600	16.0
1 cup (approx. 8.2 oz.)	820	8.2			100.0	1.00	1600	16.0
1 tablespoon (approx. 0.5 oz.)	51	0.5			100.0	1.00	1600	16.0
Cream Cheese with Pimentos, Whipped, 4-oz. container	360	8.0			90.0	2.00	1440	16.0
1 cup (approx. 5.5 oz.)	495	11.0			90.0	2.00	1440	16.0
1 tablespoon (approx. 0.3 oz.)	31	0.7			90.0	2.00	1440	16.0
Cream Cheese with Smoked Salmon, Whipped, 4-oz. container	360	4.0			90.0	1.00	1440	16.0
1 cup (approx. 5.5 oz.)	495	5.5			90.0	1.00	1440	16.0
1 tablespoon (approx. 0.3 oz.)	31	0.3			90.0	1.00	1440	16.0
IMITATION CREAM CHEESE, by brand								
King Smoothee Imitation Cream Cheese, 8-oz. package	520	16.0			65.0	2.00	1040	32.0
1 cup (approx. 8.2 oz.)	533	16.4			65.0	2.00	1040	32.0
1 tablespoon (approx. 0.5 oz.)	33	1.0			65.0	2.00	1040	32.0
Philadelphia (Kraft), Imitation, reduced-calories Cream Cheese, 8-oz. package	400	16.0			50.0	2.00	800	32.0
1 cup (approx. 8.2 oz.)	410	16.4			50.0	2.00	800	32.0
1 tablespoon (approx. 0.5 oz.)	26	1.0			50.0	2.00	800	32.0

	UNIT Cal.	UNIT Carb.	1 SLICE Cal.	1 SLICE Carb.	1 OZ., BY WT. Cal.	1 OZ., BY WT. Carb.	1 POUND Cal.	1 POUND Carb.
DANISH EXPORT Skim-Milk Cheese, based on generic data (16.5% fat)								
1 pound	(1272)				(79.5)		(1272)	
DERBY Cheese (similar to Cheddar cheese)								
Based on generic data (29.3% fat):								
1 pound	(1725)	(9.6)			(107.8)	(0.60)	(1725)	(9.6)
By brand:								
St. Ivel Derby or Sage Derby Cheese, 200-gram (7.05-oz.) package	790				112.0	trace	1792	trace
DOMIATI Cheese (soft, white Egyptian cheese), based on generic data (22.5% fat)								
1 pound	(1240)	(9.6)			(77.5)	(0.60)	(1240)	(9.6)
DORSET Cheese, based on generic data (18.2% fat)								
1 pound	(1379)	(9.6)			(86.2)	(0.60)	(1379)	(9.6)
DOUBLE GLOUCESTER Cheese. by brand								
St. Ivel Double Gloucester Cheese, 200-gram (7.05-oz.) package	790				112.0	trace	1792	trace
DUNLOP Cheese (pressed white Scottish cheese resembling Cheddar), based on generic data (32% fat)								
1 pound	(1794)	(9.6)			(112.1)	(0.60)	(1794)	(9.6)
EDAM Cheese								
Based on generic data (27.8% fat):								
1 pound (8g/tr/7g/42/274mg)	1621	6.5			101.3	0.41	1621	6.5
By brand:								
Dorman's Endeco Edam Cheese, 6-oz. package, 5 slices	606	2.4			101.0	0.40	1616	6.4
1 slice, approx. 1.2 oz.	121	0.5	121	0.5	101.0	0.40	1616	6.4
Fanfare Edam Cheese, with or without cumminseed, 2-lb. (scant) ball	2812				87.9		1406	
5½-lb. loaf	7735				87.9		1406	
Fanfare Edam Cheese, low-sodium with or without cumminseed, 5½-lb. loaf	7735				87.9		1406	
Laughing Cow Edam Cheese, round, red waxed, 8-oz. package	800	trace			100.0	trace	1600	trace
EMILIANO (Parmesan-type) Cheese, based on generic data (32.5% fat)								
1 pound	(1707)	(9.6)			(106.7)	(0.60)	(1707)	(9.6)

	UNIT Cal.	UNIT Carb.	1 SLICE Cal.	1 SLICE Carb.	1 OZ., BY WT. Cal.	1 OZ., BY WT. Carb.	1 POUND Cal.	1 POUND Carb.
EMMENTHAL Cheese, based on data from Italy (30.0% fat)								
1 pound	1751	0.0			109.4	0.00	1751	0.0
ENGADINE Cheese (Swiss whole-milk cheese), based on generic data (11.4% fat)								
1 pound	(1173)	(14.4)			(73.3)	(0.90)	(1173)	(14.4)
FARMER Cheese, by brand								
Friendship Farmer Cheese, 7½-oz. mini-pack	(285)	(5.9)			(38.0)	(0.79)	(608)	(12.7)
16-oz. (1-lb.) package	(608)	(12.7)			(38.0)	(0.79)	(608)	(12.7)
1 cup, crumbled (approx. 4.7 oz.)	(177)	(3.7)			(38.0)	(0.79)	(608)	(12.7)
FETA Cheese (Sheep's Milk), based on generic data (21.28% fat)								
1 pound (6g/1g/4g/55%/316mg)	1199	18.6			74.9	1.16	1199	18.6
1 cup, crumbled (approx. 4.8 oz.)	(357)	(5.5)			74.9	1.16	1199	18.6
1 tablespoon (approx. 0.3 oz.)	(22)	(0.3)			74.9	1.16	1199	18.6
FONTINA Cheese								
Based on generic data (31.14% fat):								
1 pound (9g/tr/7g/38%/na)	1766	7.0			110.4	0.44	1766	7.0
Based on data from Italy (30.4% fat):								
1 pound	1696	0.0			106.0	0.00	1696	0.0
By brand:								
Dorman's Danish Fontina Cheese, 1 pound	1760	7.0			110.0	0.44	1760	7.0
FRIESIAN Cheese, by brand								
Fanfare Friesian Cheese, with cumminseed								
17⅔-lb. wheel	24805				87.8		1404	
Fanfare low-fat Friesian Cheese, with cumminseed, 5½-lb. loaf	5945				67.6		1081	
FRÜHSTÜCK "Breakfast" Cheese (Limburger type), based on generic data (25.5% fat)								
1 pound	(1418)	(9.6)			(88.6)	(0.60)	(1418)	(9.6)
GAMMELOST Skim-Milk Cheese, based on generic data (0.8% fat)								
1 pound	(976)	(14.4)			(61.0)	(0.90)	(976)	(14.4)
GEX Cheese (a Bleu cheese), based on generic data (30% fat)								
1 pound	(1790)	(9.6)			(111.9)	(0.60)	(1790)	(9.6)
GISLEV Cheese (a hard Danish cheese), based on generic data (3% fat)								
1 pound	(941)	(14.4)			(58.5)	(0.90)	(941)	(14.4)
GJETOST Cheese (goat's and cow's milk), based on generic data (29.51% fat)								
1 pound (8g/12g/3g/13%/170mg)	2116	193.6			132.3	12.10	2116	193.6
GLOUCESTER Cheese (similar to Derby cheese), based on generic data (31% fat) (see also DOUBLE GLOUCESTER)								
1 pound	(1790)	(9.6)			(111.9)	(0.60)	(1790)	(9.6)
GORGONZOLA Cheese, based on generic data (32% fat)								
1 pound	(1774)	(9.6)			(110.9)	(0.60)	(1774)	(9.6)
GOUDA Cheese								
Based on generic data (27.44% fat):								
1 pound (8g/1g/7g/42%/232mg)	1616	10.1			101.0	0.63	1616	10.1
By brand:								
Dorman's Holland Gouda cheese, 6-oz. package, 5 slices	606	3.8			101.0	0.63	1616	10.1
1 slice (approx. 1.2 oz.)	121	0.8	121	0.8	101.0	0.63	1616	10.1
Fanfare Gouda cheese, with or without cumminseed, 10.6-oz. loaf	1052				99.0		1584	
14.1-oz. loaf	1399				99.0		1584	
2-lb. (scant) loaf	3150				99.0		1584	
Low-sodium Gouda cheese, with or without cumminseed, 16-oz. (1-lb.) loaf	1577				99.2		1587	
1 slice, approx. 1.2 oz.	121	0.8	121	0.8	101.0	0.63	1616	10.1
Land O'Lakes Gouda cheese, 7-oz. loaf	700	7.0			100.0	1.00	1600	16.0
Laughing Cow Gouda cheese, round, red waxed, 8-oz. package	851	trace			106.0	trace	1696	trace
GRANULAR or Stirred-Curd Cheese (similar to Cheddar and Colby), based on generic data (31.5% fat)								
1 pound	(1850)	(9.6)			(115.6)	(0.60)	(1850)	(9.6)
GRUYERE Cheese								
Based on generic data (33.34% fat):								
1 pound (9g/tr/9g/33%/95mg)	1875	1.6			117.2	0.10	1875	1.6
By brand:								
Dorman's Gruyère Cheese, 16-oz. (1-lb.) package	1872	117.0			117.0	11.00	1872	1.6
Zinco Gruyère Cheese, 6-oz. package	(600)				(100.0)		(1600)	
GRUYERE PROCESS Cheese, see PROCESS(ED) CHEESES								

	UNIT Cal.	UNIT Carb.	1 SLICE Cal.	1 SLICE Carb.	1 OZ., BY WT. Cal.	1 OZ., BY WT. Carb.	1 POUND Cal.	1 POUND Carb.
HARZKÄSE Cheese, based on generic data (2% fat)								
1 pound	(624)	(4.5)			(39.0)	(0.30)	(624)	(4.5)
HERRGÅRDSOST Cheese (medium-hard Swedish cheese with eyes), based on generic data (29% fat)								
1 pound	(1693)	(9.6)			(105.8)	(0.60)	(1693)	(9.6)
ILHA Cheese (hard Portuguese cheese), based on generic data (29.5% fat)								
1 pound	(1723)	(9.6)			(107.7)	(0.60)	(1723)	(9.6)
ISLAND OF ORLEANS Cheese (soft, piquant Canadian cheese), based on generic data (25% fat)								
1 pound	(1379)	(9.6)			(86.2)	(0.60)	(1379)	(9.6)
JARLSBERG Cheese, by brand								
Dorman's Jarlsberg Cheese, 1 pound	1712	0.0			107.0	0.00	1712	0.0
KAJMAK Ewe's-Milk Cream Cheese (also known as Serbian butter), based on generic data (55.79% fat)								
1 pound	(2358)	(9.6)			(147.4)	(0.60)	(2358)	(9.6)
KANTER Cheese, by brand								
Fanfare Kanter Cheese								
17⅔-lb. wheel	24805				87.9		1406	
Lowfat, 5½-lb. loaf	5945				67.0		1072	
KASKAVAL Cheese (Part-Skim ewe's-milk cheese from Rumania), based on generic data (14.1% fat)								
1 pound	(1120)				(70.0)		(1120)	
KATSCHKAWALJ Ewe's-Milk Cheese (like Caciocavallo), based on generic data (31.0% fat)								
1 pound	(1720)	(9.6)			(107.5)	(0.60)	(1720)	(9.6)
KEFIR Cheese, by brand								
Continental Kefir Cheese, 8-oz. package	456	8.0			57.0	1.00	912	16.0
1 cup (approx. 8.2 oz.)	(467)	(8.2)			57.0	1.00	912	16.0
1 tablespoon (approx. 0.5 oz.)	(29)	(0.5)			57.0	1.00	912	16.0

	UNIT Cal.	UNIT Carb.	1 SLICE Cal.	1 SLICE Carb.	1 OZ., BY WT. Cal.	1 OZ., BY WT. Carb.	1 POUND Cal.	1 POUND Carb.
KOPPEN (also called Bauden) Semi-hard Sour Goat's-Milk Cheese, based on generic data (24.5% fat)								
1 pound	(1320)	(9.6)			(82.5)	(0.60)	(1320)	(9.6)
KRUTT (or Kirgischerkäse) (cow's, goat's, ewe's, or camel's milk) Skim-Milk Cheese from Asia, based on generic data								
1 pound	(1518)	(9.6)			(94.9)	(0.60)	(1518)	(9.6)
LAGUIOLE Cheese (hard French cheese similar to Cantal), based on generic data (25.2% fat)								
1 pound	(1576)	(9.6)			(98.5)	(0.60)	(1576)	(9.6)
LANCASHIRE Cheese								
Based on generic data (24.5% fat):								
1 pound	(1494)	(9.6)			(93.4)	(0.60)	(1494)	(9.6)
By brand:								
St. Ivel Lancashire Cheese, 200-gram (7.05-oz.) package	762	trace			108.1	trace	1729	trace
LEICESTER Cheese								
Based on generic data (29.5% fat):								
1 pound	(1771)	(9.6)			(110.7)	(0.60)	(1771)	(9.6)
By brand:								
St. Ivel Leicester Cheese, 200-gram (7.05-oz.) package	776	trace			110.1	trace	1761	trace
LEYDEN Part-Skim Cheese								
Based on generic data (13.5% fat):								
1 pound	(1285)	(9.6)			(80.3)	(0.60)	(1285)	(9.6)
By brand:								
Fanfare Leyden Cheese, with cumminseed, 17⅔-lb. wheel	24805				87.8		1404	
Low-fat Leyden Cheese with cumminseed, 5½-lb. loaf	5504				62.5		1001	
LIEDERKRANZ Cheese								
Based on generic data (28% fat):								
1 pound (8g/1g/6g/45%/na)	(1565)	(10.0)			(97.8)	(0.63)	(1565)	(10.0)
By brand:								
Borden Liederkranz Cheese, 4-oz. package	360	4.0			90.0	1.00	1440	16.0
LIMBURGER Cheese								
Based on generic data:								
1 pound:								
USDA source A (27.25% fat), (8g/tr/6g/48%/227mg)	1485	2.2			92.8	0.14	1485	2.2
USDA source B (28.00% fat), (8g/1g/6g/45%/na)	1565	10.0			97.8	0.63	1565	10.0
1 rectangle, 3⅜" × 1⅞" × 1⅞" (approx. 7 oz.):								
USDA source A	651	1.0			92.8	0.14	1485	2.2
USDA source B	685	4.4			97.8	0.63	1565	10.0
1 slice 1⅞" × ⅞" × ⅛" (approx. ¼ oz.):								
USDA source A	23	trace	23	trace	92.8	0.14	1485	2.2
USDA source B	24	0.2	24	0.2	97.8	0.63	1565	10.0

	UNIT Cal.	UNIT Carb.	1 SLICE Cal.	1 SLICE Carb.	1 OZ., BY WT. Cal.	1 OZ., BY WT. Carb.	1 POUND Cal.	1 POUND Carb.
1 cubic inch (approx. 0.63 oz.):								
USDA source A	58	0.1			92.8	0.14	1485	2.2
USDA source B	62	0.4			97.8	0.63	1565	10.0
By brand:								
Mohawk Valley Limburger cheese **(Kraft)**, 7-oz. bar	700	0.0			100.0	0.00	1600	0.0
LIPTAUER (or Liptoi) Hungarian Ewe's-Milk Cheese, based on generic data (20.8% fat)								
1 pound	(1320)	(9.6)			(82.5)	(0.60)	(1320)	(9.6)
LIVAROT Cheese (Skim-Milk cheese), based on generic data (15% fat)								
1 pound	(1117)				(69.8)		(1117)	
LODIGIANO Cheese (Parmesan-type), based on generic data (20.4% fat)								
1 pound	(1661)	(9.6)			(103.8)	(0.60)	(1661)	(9.6)
LOMBARDO Cheese (Parmesan-type), based on generic data (33% fat)								
1 pound	(1833)				(114.5)		(1833)	
LONGHORN Cheese, see CHEDDAR Cheese								
MAINZER HAND Cheese (Part-Skim cheese), based on generic data (5.55% fat)								
1 pound	(958)				(59.9)		(958)	
MAROLLES Cheese (soft cheese similar to Pont l'Evêque and Livarot), based on generic data (30% fat)								
1 pound	(1597)	(9.6)			(99.8)	(0.60)	(1597)	(9.6)
MILANO (or Stracchino di Milano) Cheese, based on generic data (30% fat)								
1 pound	(1597)	(9.6)			(99.8)	(0.60)	(1597)	(9.6)
MONT D'OR Cheese (similar to Pont l'Evêque cheese), based on generic data (30% fat)								
1 pound	(1597)	(9.6)			(99.8)	(0.60)	(1597)	(9.6)
MONTEREY (or Monterey Jack) Cheese								
Based on generic data (30.28% fat):								
1 pound (9g/tr/7g/41%/152mg)	1693	3.1			105.8	0.19	1693	3.1

	UNIT Cal.	UNIT Carb.	1 SLICE Cal.	1 SLICE Carb.	1 OZ., BY WT. Cal.	1 OZ., BY WT. Carb.	1 POUND Cal.	1 POUND Carb.
By brand:								
Casino (Kraft) Monterey Jack Cheese, 8-oz. chunk	800	8.0			100.0	1.00	1600	16.0
12-oz. chunk	1200	12.0			100.0	1.00	1600	16.0
Dorman's Monterey Jack Cheese, 6-oz. package, 5 slices	636	1.1			106.0	0.19	1696	3.0
1 slice, approx. 1.2 oz.	127	0.2	127	0.2	106.0	0.19	1696	3.0
Kraft Monterey Jack Cheese, 8-oz. chunk	800	8.0			100.0	1.00	1600	16.0
Land O'Lakes Monterey Jack Cheese, 7-oz. chunk	700	7.0			100.0	1.00	1600	16.0
11-oz. chunk	1100	11.0			100.0	1.00	1600	16.0
MOZZARELLA Cheese								
PART SKIM MILK MOZZARELLA Cheese, based on generic data								
Part Skim Milk Mozzarella Cheese (15.92% fat), 1 pound (5g/1g/7g/54%/132mg)	1153	12.6			72.1	0.79	1153	12.6
1 cubic inch (approx. 3/5 oz.)	43	0.5			72.1	0.79	1153	12.6
1 cup:								
Chopped or diced (approx. 3.9 oz.)	281	3.1			72.1	0.79	1153	12.6
Shredded (approx. 4 oz.)	288	3.2			72.1	0.79	1153	12.6
Low Moisture Part Skim Milk Mozzarella Cheese (17.12% fat), 1 pound (5g/1g/8g/49%/150mg)	1271	14.3			79.4	0.89	1271	14.3
1 cup:								
Chopped or diced (approx. 2 oz.)	(160)	(1.8)			79.4	0.89	1271	14.3
Shredded (approx. 2 oz.)	(160)	(1.8)			79.4	0.89	1271	14.3
1 cubic inch (approx. 3/5 oz.)	49	0.5			79.4	0.89	1271	14.3
WHOLE MILK MOZZARELLA Cheese, based on generic data								
Whole Milk Mozzarella Cheese (21.60% fat), 1 pound (6g/1g/6g/54%/106mg)	1276	10.1			79.8	0.63	1276	10.1
Low Moisture Whole Milk Mozzarella Cheese (24.64% fat), 1 pound (7g/1g/6g/48%/118mg)	1444	11.2			90.3	0.70	1444	11.2
1 cubic inch (approx. 3/5 oz.)	54	0.4			90.3	0.70	1444	11.2
1 cup:								
Chopped or diced (approx. 3.9 oz.)	351	2.7			90.3	0.70	1444	11.2
Shredded (approx. 4 oz.)	360	2.8			90.3	0.70	1444	11.2
MOZZARELLA Cheese (based on data from Italy) (22.0% fat)								
1 pound	1207	0.0			75.4	0.00	1207	0.0
PART SKIM MILK MOZZARELLA Cheese, by brand								
Ann Page (A&P) Part Skim Milk Mozzarella Cheese, 6-oz. package	540	6.0			90.0	1.00	1440	16.0
Casino (Kraft) Mozzarella Cheese, 8-oz. chunk	640	8.0			80.0	1.00	1280	16.0
12-oz. chunk	960	12.0			80.0	1.00	1280	16.0
16-oz. (1-lb.) chunk	1040	16.0			80.0	1.00	1280	16.0
Dorman's Endeco Part Skim Milk Mozzarella Cheese, 6-oz. package, 5 slices	432	4.7			72.0	0.78	1152	12.5
1 slice, approx. 1.2 oz.	86	0.9	86	0.9	72.0	0.78	1152	12.5
Dragone Part Skim Milk Mozzarella Cheese, 8-oz. package	506	6.8			63.2	0.85	1012	13.6
12-oz. package	759	10.2			63.2	0.85	1012	13.6
16-oz. (1-lb.) package	1012	13.6			63.2	0.85	1012	13.6
1 slice, approx. 1 oz.	63	0.9	63	0.9	63.2	0.85	1012	13.6
Shredded, 8-oz. package	506	6.8			63.2	0.85	1012	13.6
Kraft Part Skim Milk Mozzarella Cheese, 6-oz. package, 4 slices	480	6.0			80.0	1.00	1280	16.0
1 slice, approx. 1.5 oz.	120	1.5	120	1.5	80.0	1.00	1280	16.0
8-oz. package, 5 slices	640	8.0			80.0	1.00	1280	16.0
1 slice, approx. 1.6 oz.	128	1.6	128	1.6	80.0	1.00	1280	16.0
8-oz. round	640	8.0			80.0	1.00	1280	16.0
12-oz. package, 8 slices	960	12.0			80.0	1.00	1280	16.0
1 slice, approx. 1.5 oz.	120	1.5	120	1.5	80.0	1.00	1280	16.0
12-oz. chunk	960	12.0			80.0	1.00	1280	16.0
16-oz. (1-lb.) package, 10 slices	1280	16.0			80.0	1.00	1280	16.0

	UNIT		1 SLICE		1 OZ., BY WT.		1 POUND	
	Cal.	Carb.	Cal.	Carb.	Cal.	Carb.	Cal.	Carb.
1 slice, approx. 1.6 oz.	128	1.6	128	1.6	80.0	1.00	1280	16.0
16-oz. (1-lb.) chunk	1280	16.0			80.0	1.00	1280	16.0
Shredded, 4-oz. bag (approx. 1 cup)	320	4.0			80.0	1.00	1280	16.0
8-oz. bag (approx. 2 cups)	640	8.0			80.0	1.00	1280	16.0
Land O'Lakes Part Skim Milk Mozzarella Cheese, 7-oz. chunk	560	7.0			80.0	1.00	1280	16.0
11-oz. chunk	880	11.0			80.0	1.00	1280	16.0
Polly-O Part Skim Milk Mozzarella Cheese, 8-oz. package	632	1.6			79.0	0.20	1264	3.2
16-oz. (1-lb.) package	1264	3.2			79.0	0.20	1264	3.2
WHOLE MILK MOZZARELLA Cheese, by brand								
Dragone Whole Milk Mozzarella Cheese, 8-oz. package	590	4.5			73.7	0.57	1179	9.1
12-oz. package	884	6.8			73.7	0.57	1179	9.1
16-oz. (1-lb.) package	1179	9.1			73.7	0.57	1179	9.1
Polly-O Whole Milk Mozzarella Cheese, 8-oz. package	632	1.6			79.0	0.20	1264	3.2
16-oz. (1-lb.) package	1264	3.2			79.0	0.20	1264	3.2
MOZZARELLA CHEESE SUBSTITUTE								
Mozzarella Cheese Substitute **Fisher** "Pizza-Mate" shredded, 8-oz. (approx. 2 cups) pouch	640	trace			80.0	trace	1280	trace

MUENSTER (or MÜNSTER) Cheese

	UNIT		1 SLICE		1 OZ., BY WT.		1 POUND	
	Cal.	Carb.	Cal.	Carb.	Cal.	Carb.	Cal.	Carb.
Based on generic data (30.04% fat):								
1 pound (9g/tr/7g/42%/178mg)	1671	5.1			104.4	0.32	1671	5.1
By brand:								
Ann Page (A&P) natural Muenster Cheese, 6-oz. package, 5 slices	600	6.0			100.0	1.00	1600	16.0
1 slice, approx. 1.2 oz.	120	1.2	120	1.2	100.0	1.00	1600	16.0
8-oz. package	800	8.0			100.0	1.00	1600	16.0
Dorman's Endeco Muenster Cheese, 6-oz. package, 5 slices	624	1.9			104.0	0.32	1664	5.1
1 slice, approx. 1.2 oz.	125	0.4	125	0.4	104.0	0.32	1664	5.1
Sandwich Slices, 6-oz. package, 7 slices	624	1.9			104.0	0.32	1664	5.1
1 slice, approx. 0.86 oz.	89	0.3	89	0.3	104.0	0.32	1664	5.1
5-lb. square or wheel	8320	25.5			104.0	0.32	1664	5.1
Baby Münster Cheese, 10-oz. wheel	1040	3.2			104.0	0.32	1664	5.1
Kraft Muenster Cheese, 8-oz. package, 5 slices	800	8.0			100.0	1.00	1600	16.0
1 slice, approx. 1.6 oz.	160	1.6	160	1.6	100.0	1.00	1600	16.0
Sandwich Slices, 8-oz. package, 8 slices	800	8.0			100.0	1.00	1600	16.0
1 slice, approx. 1 oz.	100	1.0	100	1.0	100.0	1.00	1600	16.0
Kraft Orange Rind Münster Cheese, 8-oz. package, 5 slices	800	8.0			100.0	1.00	1600	16.0
1 slice, approx. 1.6 oz.	160	1.6	160	1.6	100.0	1.00	1600	16.0
Land O'Lakes Muenster Cheese, 7-oz. chunk	700	7.0			100.0	1.00	1600	16.0
11-oz. chunk	1100	11.0			100.0	1.00	1600	16.0

NEUFCHÂTEL Cheese

	UNIT		1 SLICE		1 OZ., BY WT.		1 POUND	
	Cal.	Carb.	Cal.	Carb.	Cal.	Carb.	Cal.	Carb.
Based on generic data (23.43% fat):								
1 pound (7g/1g/3g/62%/113g)	1180	13.3			73.8	0.83	1180	13.3
By brand:								
Borden's "Lite Line" Neufchâtel Cheese, 8-oz. package	640	16.0			80.0	2.00	1280	32.0
Calorie Wise (Kraft) Neufchâtel Cheese, 8-oz. package	560	8.0			70.0	1.00	1120	16.0
New Holland Neufchâtel Cheese, 3-lb. loaf	3840	96.0			80.0	2.00	1280	32.0
Sold bulk, 30-lb. loaf	38400	960.0			80.0	2.00	1280	32.0
Quaker Neufchâtel Cheese, 3-lb. loaf	3840	96.0			80.0	2.00	1280	32.0
Sold bulk, 30-lb. loaf	38400	960.0			80.0	2.00	1280	32.0

OLIVET Cheese, based on generic data (48.2% fat)

	UNIT		1 SLICE		1 OZ., BY WT.		1 POUND	
	Cal.	Carb.	Cal.	Carb.	Cal.	Carb.	Cal.	Carb.
1 pound	(2206)				(137.9)		(2206)	

OLMÜTZER QUARGEL Cheese (with caraway seeds, similar to Mainzer Hand cheese) (5.8% fat), based on generic data:

	UNIT		1 SLICE		1 OZ., BY WT.		1 POUND	
	Cal.	Carb.	Cal.	Carb.	Cal.	Carb.	Cal.	Carb.
1 pound	(1010)				(63.1)		(1010)	

PARMESAN Cheese

Calorie values for Parmesan cheese differ for the cheese that is sold in blocks and cheese that is sold shredded or grated. This difference reflects the difference in moisture content. Block Parmesan cheese is approximately 29.16% water, shredded Parmesan cheese is approximately 25% water, and grated Parmesan cheese is approximately 17.66% water.

	UNIT		1 SLICE		1 OZ., BY WT.		1 POUND	
	Cal.	Carb.	Cal.	Carb.	Cal.	Carb.	Cal.	Carb.
PARMESAN CHEESE, based on generic data:								
Block Parmesan Cheese								
1 pound:								
USDA source A (25.83% fat) (7g/1g/10g/29%/454mg)	1780	14.6			111.3	0.91	1780	14.6
USDA source B (26.10% fat) (7g/1g/10g/30%/208mg)	1783	13.2			111.4	0.80	1783	13.2
1 wedge, 4¼" × 3¼" × 1" high (approx. 5 oz.):								
USDA source A (25.83% fat)	556	4.6			111.2	0.91	1779	14.6
USDA source B (26.10% fat)	557	4.0			111.4	0.80	1783	13.2
Grated Parmesan Cheese								
1 pound (approx. 4½ cups):								
USDA source A (30.02% fat), (9g/1g/12g/18%/93mg)	2068	17.0			129.3	1.06	2068	17.0
USDA source B (27.8% fat)	2118	15.9			132.4	1.00	2118	15.9
1 cup:								
USDA Source A:								
Not packed (approx. 3.5 oz.)	453	3.7			129.3	1.06	2068	17.0
Packed (approx. 4.9 oz.)	634	5.2			129.3	1.06	2068	17.0
USDA source B:								
Not packed (approx. 3.5 oz.)	462	30.5			132.4	8.70	2118	139.7
Packed (approx. 4.9 oz.)	647	42.6			132.4	8.70	2118	139.7
1 tablespoon (approx. 0.18 oz.)	23	0.2			129.3	1.06	2068	17.0
Shredded Parmesan Cheese								
1 pound (approx. 4.6 cups):								
USDA source A (27.36% fat) (9g/1g/13g/25%/100mg)	(1885)	(15.5)			(117.8)	(0.96)	(1885)	(15.5)
USDA source B (27.65% fat)	(1889)	(14.0)			(118.0)	(0.88)	(1889)	(14.0)
1 cup:								
USDA source A:								
Not packed (approx. 2.8 oz.)	(330)	(2.7)			(117.8)	(0.96)	(1885)	(15.5)
Packed (approx. 3.9 oz.)	(460)	(3.7)			(117.8)	(0.96)	(1885)	(15.5)
USDA source B:								
Not packed (approx. 2.8 oz.)	(330)	(2.5)			(118.0)	(0.88)	(1889)	(14.0)
Packed (approx. 3.9 oz.)	(460)	(3.4)			(118.0)	(0.88)	(1889)	(14.0)

	UNIT Cal.	UNIT Carb.	1 SLICE Cal.	1 SLICE Carb.	1 OZ., BY WT. Cal.	1 OZ., BY WT. Carb.	1 POUND Cal.	1 POUND Carb.
1 tablespoon (approx. 0.18 oz.):								
USDA source A	(21)	(0.2)			(117.8)	(0.96)	(1885)	(15.5)
USDA source B	(21)	(0.2)			(118.0)	(0.88)	(1889)	(14.0)
PARMESAN CHEESE, by brand								
Borden Grated Parmesan Cheese, 3-oz. canister (approx. ¾ cups)	420	9.0			140.0	3.00	2240	48.0
8-oz. canister (approx. 2 cups)	1120	24.0			140.0	3.00	2240	48.0
1 tablespoon (approx. ¼ oz.)	(35)	(0.8)			140.0	3.00	2240	48.0
Borden Grated Parmesan & Romano Cheese, 3-oz. canister (approx. ¾ cups)	420	9.0			140.0	3.00	2240	48.0
8-oz. canister (approx. 2 cups)	1120	24.0			140.0	3.00	2240	48.0
16-oz. (1-lb.) canister (approx. 4 cups)	2240	48.0			140.0	3.00	2240	48.0
1 tablespoon (approx. ¼ oz.)	(35)	(0.8)			140.0	3.00	2240	48.0
Dorman's Hard Parmesan Cheese, 13-lb. wheel	23088	189.3			111.0	0.91	1776	14.6
PARMIGIANO Cheese, based on generic data (35% fat)								
1 pound	(1971)	(9.6)			(123.2)	(0.60)	(1971)	(9.6)
PATAGRAS Cheese (hard Cuban cheese similar to Gouda), based on generic data (26% fat)								
1 pound	(1573)	(9.6)			(98.3)	(0.60)	(1573)	(9.6)
PENETELEU Cheese (similar to Caciocavallo cheese), based on generic data (20.1% fat)								
1 pound	(1699)	(9.6)			(106.2)	(0.60)	(1699)	(9.6)
PETIT SUISSE Cheese (similar to Carré cheese), based on generic data (35% fat)								
1 pound	(1550)	(9.6)			(96.9)	(0.60)	(1550)	(9.6)
PINEAPPLE Cheese (named for its shape, not its flavor; originated in Litchfield County, Conn.), based on generic data (39% fat)								
1 pound	(2109)	(9.6)			(131.8)	(0.60)	(2109)	(9.6)
PIORA Cheese (a Swiss cheese similar to Tilsiter), based on generic data (29% fat)								
1 pound	(1595)	(9.6)			(99.7)	(0.60)	(1595)	(9.6)
PONT L'EVÊQUE Cheese, based on generic data (26.7% fat)								
1 pound	(1467)	(9.6)			(91.7)	(0.60)	(1467)	(9.6)

	UNIT Cal.	UNIT Carb.	1 SLICE Cal.	1 SLICE Carb.	1 OZ., BY WT. Cal.	1 OZ., BY WT. Carb.	1 POUND Cal.	1 POUND Carb.
PORT SALUT Cheese								
Based on generic data (28.20% fat):								
1 pound	1598	2.6			99.9	0.16	1598	2.6
By brand:								
Dorman's, 6-oz. package, 6 slices	600	0.9			100.0	0.16	1600	2.6
1 slice, approx. 1 oz.	100	0.2	100	0.2	100.0	0.16	1600	2.6
POT Cheese, by brand								
Friendship Pot Style Cottage Cheese, 12-oz. container	300	12.0			25.0	1.00	400	16.0
1 cup:								
Not packed (approx. 5.1 oz.)	128	5.1			25.0	1.00	400	16.0
Packed (approx. 7.1 oz.)	178	7.1			25.0	1.00	400	16.0
Zausner Pot Cheese, unsalted, sold bulk, 5-lb. container	1704	50.4			21.3	0.63	341	10.1
Sold bulk, 33-lb. supermarket container	11246	332.6			21.3	0.63	341	10.1
PROVATURA Cheese (soft Italian cheese like Caciocavallo), based on generic data (15% fat)								
1 pound	(1019)				(63.7)		(1019)	
PROVOLONE Cheese, based on generic data								
USDA source A (26.62% fat), 1 pound (8g/1g/7g/41%/248mg)	1594	9.7			100.0	0.61	1600	9.8
PROVOLONE DOLCE Cheese, based on data from Italy (29.8% fat)								
1 pound	1742	0.0			108.9	0.00	1742	0.0
PROVOLONE PICCANTE Cheese								
Based on data from Italy (30.3% fat):								
1 pound	1774	0.0			110.8	0.00	1774	0.0
By brand:								
Casino (Kraft) Provolone sharp, 5-oz. wedge	450	5.0			90.0	1.00	1440	16.0
Dorman's Endeco Provolone Cheese, 6-oz. package, 5 slices	600	3.7			100.0	0.61	1600	9.8
1 slice, approx. 1.2 oz.	120	0.7	120	0.7	100.0	0.61	1600	9.8
Kraft Provolone Cheese, 6-oz. package, 4 slices	540	6.0			90.0	1.00	1440	16.0
1 slice, approx. 1.5 oz.	135	1.5	135	1.0	90.0	1.00	1440	16.0
8-oz. package, 5 slices	720	8.0			90.0	1.00	1440	16.0
1 slice, approx. 1.6 oz.	144	1.6	144	1.6	90.0	1.00	1440	16.0
QUARTIROLO Cheese (soft Italian cheese), based on generic data (23.7% fat)								
1 pound	(1346)	(9.6)			(84.1)	(0.60)	(1346)	(9.6)
RABACAL Cheese (ewe's- or goat's-milk cheese from Portugal), based on generic data (37.4% fat)								
1 pound	(2182)	(9.6)			(136.4)	(0.60)	(2182)	(9.6)

	UNIT Cal.	UNIT Carb.	1 SLICE Cal.	1 SLICE Carb.	1 OZ., BY WT. Cal.	1 OZ., BY WT. Carb.	1 POUND Cal.	1 POUND Carb.
RACLETTE Cheese, by brand								
Zinco, 6-oz. package	(600)				(100.0)		(1600)	
REBLOCHON Cheese, based on generic data (20.5% fat)								
1 pound	(1206)	(9.6)			(75.4)	(0.60)	(1206)	(9.6)
REQUEIJÃO Cheese (Brazilian skim cheese), based on generic data (14% fat)								
1 pound	(928)				(58.0)		(928)	
RICOTTA Cheese								
Based on generic data:								
Whole Milk Ricotta Cheese								
USDA source A (12.98% fat):								
1 pound (4g/1g/3g/72%/24mg)	790	13.8			49.4	0.86	790	13.8
1 cup (approx. 8⅔ oz.)	428	76.8			49.4	0.86	790	13.8
Part Skim Milk Ricotta Cheese								
USDA source A (7.91% fat)								
1 pound (2g/1g/3g/74%/35mg)	627	23.3			39.2	1.46	627	23.3
1 cup (approx. 8⅔ oz.)	339	12.6			39.2	1.46	627	23.3
By brand:								
A&P Whole milk Ricotta Cheese, 15-oz. container	638	7.5			42.5	0.50	680	8.0
48-oz (3-lb.) container	2040	24.0			42.5	0.50	680	8.0
Dragone Part skim milk Ricotta Cheese, 15-oz. container	638	22.5			42.5	1.50	680	24.0
16-oz. (1-lb.) container	680	24.0			42.5	1.50	680	24.0
32-oz. (2-lb.) container	1360	48.0			42.5	1.50	680	24.0
Whole milk Ricotta Cheese, 15-oz. container	675	15.0			45.0	1.00	720	16.0
16-oz. (1-lb.) container	720	16.0			45.0	1.00	720	16.0
32-oz. (2-lb.) container	1440	32.0			45.0	1.00	720	16.0
30-lb. container	21600	480.0			45.0	1.00	720	16.0
Polly-O Whole milk Ricotta Cheese, 15-oz. container	750	15.0			50.0	1.00	800	16.0
32-oz. (2-lb.) container	1600	32.0			50.0	1.00	800	16.0
48-oz. (3-lb.) container	2400	48.0			50.0	1.00	800	16.0
Precious Part skim milk Ricotta Cheese, 8-oz. container	340	12.0			42.5	1.50	680	24.0
16-oz. (1-lb.) container	680	24.0			42.5	1.50	680	24.0
ROBBIOLE (ROBIOLO) Cheese (soft Italian cheese)								
Based on generic data (28% fat):								
1 pound	(1514)	(9.6)			(94.8)	(0.60)	(1514)	(9.6)
Based on data from Italy (25.9% fat):								
1 pound	1407	0.0			87.6	0.00	1407	0.0
ROMADUR Cheese (Limburger-type cheese), based on generic data (22.6% fat)								
1 pound	(1322)	(9.6)			(82.6)	(0.60)	(1322)	(9.6)
ROMANO Cheese								
Calorie values for Romano cheese differ for the cheese that is sold in blocks and cheese that is sold shredded or grated. This difference reflects the difference in moisture content. Block Romano cheese is approximately 29.16% water, shredded Romano cheese is approximately 25% water, and grated Romano cheese is approximately 17.66% water.								
Block Romano Cheese, based on generic data (26.9% fat)								
1 pound (8g/1g/9g/29%/340mg)	1754	16.5			109.6	1.03	1754	16.5
1 wedge, 4¼" x 3¼" x 1" high (approx. 5 oz.)	548	5.2			109.6	1.03	1754	16.5
Grated Romano Cheese, based on generic data (31.34% fat):								
1 pound (approx. 5.7 cups) (9g/1g/10g/18%/395mg)	(2040)	(19.2)			(127.5)	(1.20)	(2040)	(19.2)
1 cup:								
Not packed (approx. 2.8 oz.)	(357)	(3.4)			(127.5)	(1.20)	(2040)	(19.2)
Packed (approx. 3.9 oz.)	(497)	(4.7)			(127.5)	(1.20)	(2040)	(19.2)
1 tablespoon not packed (approx. 0.2 oz.)	(26)	(10.2)			(127.5)	(1.20)	(2040)	(19.2)
Shredded Romano Cheese, based on generic data (31.75% fat):								
1 cup:								
Not packed (approx. 2.8 oz.) (8g/1g/9g/25%/358mg)	(325)	(3.1)			(116.1)	(1.09)	(1858)	(17.5)
Packed (approx. 3.9 oz.)	(453)	(4.3)			(116.1)	(1.09)	(1858)	(17.5)
1 tablespoon (approx. 0.2 oz.)	(23)	(0.2)			(116.1)	(1.09)	(1858)	(17.5)
ROMANO CHEESE, by brand								
Borden grated Parmesan and Romano Cheese, 3-oz. canister (approx. ¾ cup)	420	9.0			140.0	3.00	2240	48.0
8-oz. canister (approx. 2 cups)	1120	24.0			140.0	3.00	2240	48.0
16-oz. (1-lb.) canister (approx. 4 cups)	2240	48.0			140.0	3.00	2240	48.0
1 tablespoon (approx. ¼ oz.)	(33)	(0.7)			140.0	3.00	2240	48.0
Carzedda (Dorman's) Romano Cheese Extra Pecorino (made from sheep's milk), 10-lb. wheel	17600	164.8			110.0	1.03	1760	16.5
1 40-lb. case, 4 10-lb. wheels	70400	659.2			110.0	1.03	1760	16.5
Casino (Kraft) Romano Cheese, 5-oz. wedge	550	5.0			110.0	1.03	1760	16.5
Kraft grated Romano Cheese, 3-oz. jar	390	3.0			130.0	1.03	2080	16.5
6-oz. jar	780	6.0			130.0	1.00	2080	16.0
RONDELÉ Semisoft Cheese								
Plain Cheese, 4-oz. package	436	4.0			109.0	1.00	1744	16.0
2½-lb. tub or wheel	4360	40.0			109.0	1.00	1744	16.0
Spiced Cheese with French Onion, 4-oz. package	432	8.0			108.0	2.00	1728	32.0
2½-lb. tub or wheel	4320	80.0			108.0	2.00	1728	32.0
Spiced Cheese with Garlic & Herbs, 4-oz. package	412	4.0			103.0	1.00	1648	16.0
2½-lb. tub or wheel	4120	40.0			103.0	3.00	1648	48.0
Spiced Cheese with Pepper, 4-oz. package	412	4.0			103.0	1.00	1648	16.0
2½-lb. tub or wheel	4120	40.0			103.0	1.00	1648	16.0
ROQUEFORT Cheese (ewe's-milk)								
Based on generic data (30.64% fat):								
1 pound (9g/1g/6g/39%/513mg)	1674	9.1			104.6	0.57	1674	9.1
1 cubic inch (approx. ⅗ oz.)	63	0.3			104.6	0.57	1674	9.1
1 cup, crumbled:								
Not packed (approx. 4¾ oz.)	499	2.7			104.6	0.57	1674	9.1
Packed (approx. 8.8 oz.)	924	5.0			104.6	0.57	1674	9.1
By brand:								
Surchoix (French) Roquefort Cheese, 5-lb. wheel	8400	45.6			105.0	0.57	1680	9.1

	UNIT Cal.	UNIT Carb.	1 SLICE Cal.	1 SLICE Carb.	1 OZ., BY WT. Cal.	1 OZ., BY WT. Carb.	1 POUND Cal.	1 POUND Carb.
1 60-lb. case, 12 5-lb. wheels	100800	547.0			105.0	0.57	1680	9.1
SAGE Cheese, based on generic data								
Whole Milk (30.8% fat), 1 pound	(1746)	(9.6)			(109.1)	(0.60)	(1746)	(9.6)
Part Skim (12.3% fat), 1 pound	(1250)	(9.6)			(78.1)	(0.60)	(1250)	(9.6)
For information by brand, see under DERBY Cheese.								
SALOIO Cheese (soft Portuguese skim cheese), based on generic data (1.8% fat)								
1 pound	(384)	(48.0)			(24.0)	(3.00)	(384)	(48.0)
SAPSAGO Cheese (Skim-Milk cheese), based on generic data (7.2% fat)								
1 pound	(1101)				(68.8)		(1101)	
SCAMORZE Cheese (soft Italian cheese)								
Based on generic data (26% fat):								
1 pound	(1534)	(9.6)			(95.9)	(0.60)	(1534)	(9.6)
By brand:								
Kraft Part skim Scamorze Cheese, 16-oz. (1-lb.) semi-round	1120	16.0			70.0	1.00	1120	16.0
SERBIAN Butter, see KAJMAK Cheese								
SERRA DA ESTRELLA (soft Portuguese cheese), based on generic data (29.5% fat)								
1 pound	(1675)	(9.6)			(104.7)	(0.60)	(1675)	(9.6)
SKANDOR Swedish Cheese, by brand								
Dorman's, 6-oz. package, 5 slices	600	3.9			100.0	0.65	1600	10.4
1 slice, approx. 1.2 oz.	120	0.8	120	0.8	100.0	0.65	1600	10.4
10-oz. chunk	1000	6.5			100.0	0.65	1600	10.4
SKIM MILK Cheese, by brand								
Weight Watchers Natural Semi-Soft Skim Milk Cheese, 8-oz. chunk	640	8.0			80.0	1.00	1280	16.0
For comparison: **Weight Watchers** Pasteurized Process skim milk cheese product, 9% fat, 10-oz. package, 10 slices	500	10.0			50.0	1.00	800	16.0
1 slice, approx. 1 oz.	50	1.0			50.0	1.00	800	16.0
SPALEN Swiss Cheese, based on generic data (33.7% fat)								
1 pound	(1954)	(9.6)			(122.1)	(0.60)	(1954)	(9.6)
STILTON Cheese								
Based on generic data (33% fat):								
1 pound	(1872)	(9.6)			(117.0)	(0.60)	(1872)	(9.6)
By brand:								
St. Ivel Stilton Cheese, 1 pound	2080	trace			130.0	trace	2080	trace

	UNIT Cal.	UNIT Carb.	1 SLICE Cal.	1 SLICE Carb.	1 OZ., BY WT. Cal.	1 OZ., BY WT. Carb.	1 POUND Cal.	1 POUND Carb.
STRACCHINO Cheese, based on generic data (26.4% fat)								
1 pound	(1494)	(9.6)			(93.4)	(0.60)	(1494)	(9.6)
SVECIAOST Cheese (Swedish Gouda-type cheese), based on generic data (26.5% fat)								
1 pound	(1565)	(9.6)			(97.8)	(0.60)	(1565)	(9.6)
SWISS Cheese								
SWISS CHEESE, domestic, based on generic data:								
1 pound:								
USDA source A (27.45% fat) (8g/1g/8g/37%/74mg)	1707	15.3			106.7	0.95	1707	15.3
USDA source B (27.87% fat) (8g/1g/8g/39%/201mg)	1678	7.7			104.9	0.50	1678	7.7
1 rectangle, 6″ × 2″ × 2″ (approx. 12 oz.):								
USDA source A	1284	11.4			106.7	0.95	1707	15.3
USDA source B	1258	5.8			104.8	0.50	1678	7.7
1 slice, 7½″ to 7¾″ × 4″ × 1/16″ (approx. 1¼ oz.):								
USDA source A	134	1.2	134	1.2	106.7	0.95	1707	15.3
USDA source B	130	0.6	130	0.6	104.9	0.50	1678	7.7
1 cubic inch (chunk without holes, approx. 0.53 oz.):								
USDA source A	56	0.5			106.7	0.95	1707	15.3
USDA source B	56	0.3			104.8	0.50	1678	7.7
SWISS CHEESE, imported from Switzerland (30.50% fat), based on generic data:								
1 pound (9g/1g/8g/na/241mg)	1805	15.4			112.8	0.96	1805	15.4
1 rectangle, 6″ × 2″ × 2″ (approx. 12 oz.)	1354	11.5			112.8	0.96	1805	15.4
1 slice, 7½″ to 7¾″ × 4″ × 1/16″ (approx. 1¼ oz.)	141	1.2	141	1.2	112.8	0.96	1805	15.4
1 cubic inch (chunk without holes, approx. 0.53 oz.)	60	0.5			112.8	0.96	1805	15.4
For comparison: Swiss Process Cheese, based on generic data								
1 pound:								
USDA source A (25.01% fat) (7g/1g/6g/44%/440mg)	1516	9.5			94.8	0.60	1516	9.5
USDA source B (26.90% fat) (8g/tr/8g/39%/331mg)	1610	8.0			100.6	0.46	1610	8.0
1 cubic inch (chunk without holes, approx. 0.63 oz.):								
USDA source A	60	0.5			95.0	0.60	1520	9.6
USDA source B	64	0.3			100.6	0.46	1610	7.3
SWISS CHEESE, by brand:								
Ann Page Swiss Cheese, 8-oz. package, 5 slices	800	0.0			100.0	0.00	1600	0.0
1 slice, approx. 1.6 oz.	160	0.0	160	0.0	100.0	0.00	1600	0.0
Dorman's Endeco Domestic Swiss Cheese, 6-oz. package, 5 slices	642	5.8			107.0	0.96	1712	13.4
1 slice, approx. 1.2 oz.	128	1.2	128	1.2	107.0	0.96	1712	15.4
"Sandwich Slices," 6-oz. package, 7 slices	642	5.8			107.0	0.96	1712	15.4
1 slice, approx. 0.86 oz.	92	0.8	92	0.8	107.0	0.96	1712	15.4
Smoked Swiss, 5-oz. cube	(585)	(5.3)			(117.0)	(1.05)	1872	16.8
1 48-lb. case, 4 12-lb. blocks	82176	739.2			107.0	0.96	1712	15.4
1 12-lb. block	20544	184.8			107.0	0.96	1712	15.4
Kraft Domestic Swiss cheese, 6-oz. package, 6 slices	600	0.0			100.0	0.00	1600	0.0
1 slice, approx. 1 oz.	100	0.0	100	0.0	100.0	0.00	1600	0.0
8-oz. package, 5 slices	800	0.0			100.0	0.00	1600	0.0
1 slice, approx. 1.6 oz.	160	0.0	160	0.0	100.0	0.00	1600	0.0
"Sandwich Slices," 8-oz. package, 9 slices	800	0.0			100.0	0.00	1600	0.0
1 slice, approx. 0.89 oz.	89	0.0	89	0.0	100.0	0.00	1600	0.0
12-oz. chunk	1200	0.0			100.0	0.00	1600	0.0
12-oz. package, 10 slices	1200	0.0			100.0	0.00	1600	0.0
1 slice, approx. 1.2 oz.	120	0.0	120	0.0	100.0	0.00	1600	0.0

	UNIT Cal.	UNIT Carb.	1 SLICE Cal.	1 SLICE Carb.	1 OZ., BY WT. Cal.	1 OZ., BY WT. Carb.	1 POUND Cal.	1 POUND Carb.
16-oz. (1-lb.) package, 10 slices	1600	0.0			100.0	0.00	1600	0.0
1 slice, approx. 1.6 oz.	160	0.0	160	0.0	100.0	0.00	1600	0.0
Shredded, 6-oz. package	600	0.0			100.0	0.00	1600	0.0
Kraft Swiss Cheese, Aged, 6-oz. package, 6 slices	600	0.0			100.0	0.00	1600	0.0
1 slice, approx. 1 oz.	100	0.0	100	0.0	100.0	0.00	1600	0.0
8-oz. package, 6 slices	800	0.0			100.0	0.00	1600	0.0
1 slice, approx. 1.33 oz.	133	0.0	133	0.0	100.0	0.00	1600	0.0
"Sandwich Slices," 8-oz. package, 9 slices	800	0.0			100.0	0.00	1600	0.0
1 slice, approx. 0.89 oz.	89	0.0	89	0.0	100.0	0.00	1600	0.0
Swiss Chris Swiss Cheese, reduced cholesterol, no salt added, part skim 10-lb. cut	16,000	0.0			100.0	0.00	1600	0.0
Zinco Swiss Cheese, Imported from Switzerland, 6-oz. package	600	0.0			100.0	0.00	1600	0.0
12-oz. chunk	1200	0.0			100.0	0.00	1600	0.0
TELEME Cheese (also called Brândza de Braila cheese; similar to Feta), based on generic data (37.5% fat)								
1 pound	(2090)	(9.6)			(130.6)	(0.60)	(2090)	(9.6)
TEXEL Cheese (ewe's-milk cheese), based on generic data (18.3% fat)								
1 pound	(1133)	(9.6)			(70.8)	(0.60)	(1133)	(9.6)
THENAY Cheese (Camembert-type cheese), based on generic data (15% fat)								
1 pound	(963)	(14.4)			(60.2)	(0.90)	(963)	(14.4)
TILSITER (TILSIT) Cheese								
Based on generic data:								
Whole milk (25.96% fat), 1 pound	1544	8.5			96.5	0.53	1544	8.5
(17% fat), 1 pound	(1234)	(9.6)			(77.1)	(0.60)	(1234)	(9.6)
By brand:								
Dorman's Danish Tilsiter cheese, 6-oz. package, 5 slices	576	3.6			96.0	0.53	1536	8.5
1 slice, approx. 1.2 oz.	115	0.6	115	0.6	96.0	0.53	1536	8.5
TOPFKÄSE Cheese (cooked-curd cheese), based on generic data (6.5% fat)								
1 pound	(680)				(42.5)		(680)	
TRAPPIST Cheese, based on generic data (26.1% fat)								
1 pound	(1506)	(9.6)			(94.1)	(0.60)	(1506)	(9.6)
VORARLBERG Cheese (sour-milk cheese), based on generic data (17.5% fat)								
1 pound	(1352)	(9.6)			(84.5)	(0.60)	(1352)	(9.6)
WARWICKSHIRE Cheese (similar to Derby cheese), based on generic data (30% fat)								
1 pound	1771	9.6			110.7	0.60	1771	9.6

	UNIT Cal.	UNIT Carb.	1 SLICE Cal.	1 SLICE Carb.	1 OZ., BY WT. Cal.	1 OZ., BY WT. Carb.	1 POUND Cal.	1 POUND Carb.
WENSLEYDALE Cheese								
Based on generic data (32.2% fat):								
1 pound	1824	9.6			114.0	0.60	1824	9.6
By brand:								
St. Ivel Wensleydale Cheese, 200-gram (7.05-oz.) package	754	trace			107.0	trace	1712	trace
WILSTERMARSCH Cheese (similar to Tilsiter cheese), based on generic data								
Whole milk (22% fat), 1 pound	1376	9.6			86.0	0.60	1376	9.6
Skim milk (2.1% fat), 1 pound	762	16.0			47.6	1.00	762	16.0
WILTSHIRE Cheese (similar to Derby cheese), based on generic data (26.9% fat)								
1 pound	1667	9.6			104.2	0.60	1667	9.6
YOGHURT Cheese, based on generic data (30% fat)								
1 pound	1568	9.6			98.0	0.60	1568	9.6
ZIGER Whey Cheese (similar to Ricotta), based on generic data (4% fat)								
1 pound	563	14.4			35.2	0.90	563	14.4

PROCESS(ED) CHEESES

Cheese foods, cheese products, and cheese spreads follow. Other reduced-calorie, imitation, and substitute cheeses are listed last.

PROCESS(ED) CHEESES

	UNIT Cal.	UNIT Carb.	1 SLICE Cal.	1 SLICE Carb.	1 OZ., BY WT. Cal.	1 OZ., BY WT. Carb.	1 POUND Cal.	1 POUND Carb.
Pasteurized Process(ed) AMERICAN Cheese, based on generic data:								
1 pound:								
USDA source A (31.25% fat) (9g/tr/6g/39%/250mg)	1703	7.3			106.4	0.45	1703	7.3
USDA source B (29.98% fat) (9g/1g/8g/40%/322mg)	1680	8.6			105.0	0.54	1680	8.6
1 loaf, 8½" × 2¾" (approx. 2 lbs.)								
USDA source A	3406	14.5			106.4	0.45	1703	7.3
USDA source B	3356	17.2			105.0	0.54	1680	8.6
1 slice, 2½" × 1¾" × ¼" (approx. 1⅓ oz., 1/24 of a 2-lb. loaf)								
USDA source A	142	0.6	142	0.6	106.4	0.45	1703	7.3
USDA source B	140	0.7	140	0.7	105.0	0.54	1680	8.6
Typical sandwich sizes:								
1 slice, 3½" × 3⅜" × ⅛" (approx. 1 oz.)								
USDA source A	106	0.5	106	0.5	106.4	0.45	1703	7.3
USDA source B	105	0.5	105	0.5	105.0	0.54	1680	8.6
1 slice, 3½" × 3⅜" × 3/32" (approx. ¾ oz.)								
USDA source A	80	0.3	80	0.3	106.4	0.45	1703	7.3
USDA source B	79	0.4	79	0.4	105.0	0.54	1680	8.6
Typical cheeseburger sizes:								
1 slice, 3½" × 2¼" × ⅛" (approx. ½ oz.):								
USDA source A	71	0.3	71	0.3	106.4	0.45	1703	7.2
USDA source B	70	0.4	70	0.4	105.0	0.54	1680	8.6

	UNIT		1 SLICE		1 OZ., BY WT.		1 POUND	
	Cal.	Carb.	Cal.	Carb.	Cal.	Carb.	Cal.	Carb.
1 slice, 3½" × 2¼" × 3 3/32" (approx. ¾ oz.):								
USDA source A	79	0.3	79	0.3	106.4	0.45	1703	7.2
USDA source B	78	0.4	78	0.4	105.0	0.54	1680	8.6
1 cubic inch (approx. ⅗ oz.):								
USDA source A	66	0.3			106.4	0.45	1703	7.2
USDA source B	65	0.3			105.0	0.54	1680	8.6
1 cup:								
USDA source A:								
Diced, not packed (approx. 5 oz.)	532	2.3			106.4	0.45	1703	7.2
Shredded, not packed (approx. 4 oz.)	426	1.8			106.4	0.45	1703	7.2
Diced or shredded, packed (approx. 9 oz.)	958	4.1			106.4	0.45	1703	7.2
USDA source B:								
Diced, not packed (approx. 5 oz.)	518	2.7			105.0	0.54	1680	8.6
Shredded, not packed (approx. 4 oz.)	418	2.1			105.0	0.54	1680	8.6
Diced or shredded, packed (approx. 9 oz.)	944	4.8			105.0	0.54	1680	8.6
1 tablespoon, shredded (approx. ¼ oz.):								
USDA source A	27	0.1			106.4	0.45	1703	7.2
USDA source B	27	0.1			105.0	0.54	1680	8.6
Pasteurized Process(ed) AMERICAN Cheese, by brand								
Ann Page (A&P), "Mel-O-Bit," Pasteurized Process(ed) American Cheese, 12-oz. package, 16 slices	1320	12.0			110.0	1.00	1760	16.0
1 slice, approx. ¾ oz.	83	0.8	83	0.8	110.0	1.00	1760	16.0
sharp, 6-oz. package, 8 slices	660	6.0			110.0	1.00	1760	16.0
1 slice, approx. ¾ oz.	83	0.8	83	0.8	110.0	1.00	1760	16.0
Borden Pasteurized Process(ed) American Cheese, yellow or white, 6-oz. package, 8 slices	660	6.0			110.0	1.00	1760	16.0
1 slice, approx. ¾ oz.	83	0.8	83	0.8	110.0	1.00	1760	16.0
12-oz. package, 16 slices	1320	12.0			110.0	1.00	1760	16.0
1 slice, approx. ¾ oz.	83	0.8	83	0.8	110.0	1.00	1760	16.0
16-oz. (1-lb.) package, 24 slices	1760	16.0			110.0	1.00	1760	16.0
1 slice, approx. ¾ oz.	83	0.8	83	0.8	110.0	1.00	1760	16.0
24-oz. package, 32 slices	2460	24.0			110.0	1.00	1760	16.0
1 slice, approx. ¾ oz.	83	0.8	83	0.8	110.0	1.00	1760	16.0
3-lb. package, 24 ribbon slices used in restaurants to make 72 hamburgers into cheeseburgers (each approx. 2 oz., each to top 3 hamburgers)	5280	48.0			110.0	1.00	1760	16.0
Dorman's Endeco Pasteurized Process(ed) American Cheese, yellow or white, 5-lb. box	8480	80.0			106.0	1.00	1696	7.2
Kraft De Luxe Choice Pasteurized Process(ed) American Cheese, yellow or white, 6-oz. package, 8 slices	110	1.0			110.0	1.00	1760	16.0
1 slice, approx. ¾ oz.	83	0.8	83	0.8	110.0	1.00	1760	16.0
8-oz. package, 12 slices	880	8.0			110.0	1.00	1760	16.0
1 slice, approx. ⅔ oz.	73	0.7	73	0.7	110.0	1.00	1760	16.0
12-oz. package, 16 slices	1320	12.0			110.0	1.00	1760	16.0
1 slice, approx. ¾ oz.	83	0.8	83	0.8	110.0	1.00	1760	16.0
24-oz. package, 32 slices	2640	24.0			110.0	1.00	1760	16.0
1 slice, approx. ¾ oz.	83	0.8	83	0.8	110.0	1.00	1760	16.0
48-oz. (3-lb.) package, 64 slices	5280	48.0			110.0	1.00	1760	16.0
1 slice, approx. ¾ oz.	83	0.8	83	0.8	110.0	1.00	1760	16.0
Kraft De Luxe Choice "Old English" sharp Pasteurized Process(ed) American Cheese, 8-oz. package, 8 slices	880	1.0			110.0	1.00	1760	16.0
1 slice, approx. 1 oz.	110	1.0	110	1.0	110.0	1.00	1760	16.0
Land O'Lakes Pasteurized Process(ed) American Cheese, 8-oz. package, 8 slices	880	8.0			110.0	1.00	1760	16.0
1 slice, approx. 1 oz.	110	1.0	110	1.0	110.0	1.00	1760	16.0
32-oz. (2-lb.) loaf	3520	32.0			110.0	1.00	1760	16.0
48-oz. (3-lb.) package, 64 slices	5280	48.0			110.0	1.00	1760	16.0
1 slice, approx. ¾ oz.	83	0.8	83	0.8	110.0	1.00	1760	16.0
96 slices	5280	48.0			110.0	1.00	1760	16.0
1 slice, approx. ½ oz.	55	0.5	55	0.5	110.0	1.00	1760	16.0
Sharp, 48-oz. (3-lb.) package, 96 slices	5280	48.0			110.0	1.00	1760	16.0
1 slice, approx. ½ oz.	55	0.5	55	0.5	110.0	1.00	1760	16.0
Pasteurized Process(ed) AMERICAN/SWISS LOAF, by brand								
Land O'Lakes, 8-oz. package, 8 slices	880	8.0			110.0	1.00	1760	16.0
1 slice approx. 1 oz.	110	1.0	110	1.0	110.0	1.00	1760	16.0
Pasteurized Process(ed) CHEDDAR Cheese, by brand								
Country Store (Borden), sharp or extra sharp 8-oz. bar	880	8.0			110.0	1.00	1760	16.0
For comparison: natural Cheddar Cheese based on generic data (33.14% fat) 1 pound (7g/tr/7g/37%/176mg)	1830	5.8			114.4	0.36	1830	5.8
Process(ed) GRUYERE Cheese, by brand								
Zinco Process(ed) Gruyère Cheese, 6-oz. package	(600)				(100.0)		(1600)	
8-oz. package	(800)				(100.0)		(1600)	
For comparison: natural Gruyère based on generic data (33.34% fat), 1 pound (9g/tr/9g/33%/95mg)	1875	1.6			117.2	0.10	1875	1.6
Pasteurized Process(ed) PIMENTO Cheese, based on generic data:								
1 pound:								
USDA source A (31.20% fat) (9g/tr/6g/39%/405mg)	1703	7.9			106.4	0.49	1703	7.9
USDA source B (30.20% fat) (9g/1g/7g/40%/na)	1683	8.2			105.2	0.51	1683	8.2
1 loaf, 8½" × 2¾" × 2¼" (approx. 2 pounds):								
USDA source A	3406	15.8			106.4	0.49	1703	7.9
USDA source B	3366	16.4			105.2	0.51	1683	8.2
1 slice, 2½" x 1¾" x ¼" (approx. 1⅓ oz., 1/24 of a 2-lb. loaf):								
USDA source A	141	0.7	141	0.7	106.4	0.49	1703	7.9
USDA source B	140	0.7	140	0.7	105.2	0.51	1683	8.2
1 cubic inch (approx. ⅗ oz.):								
USDA source A	66	0.3			106.4	0.49	1703	7.9
USDA source B	65	0.3			105.2	0.50	1683	8.2
1 cup:								
USDA source A:								
Diced, not packed (approx. 5 oz.)	532	2.5			106.4	0.49	1703	7.9
Shredded, not packed (approx. 4 oz.)	426	2.0			106.4	0.49	1703	7.9
Diced or shredded, packed (approx. 9 oz.)	958	4.4			106.4	0.49	1703	7.9
USDA source B:								
Diced, not packed (approx. 5 oz.)	526	2.6			105.2	0.51	1683	8.2
Shredded, not packed (approx. 4 oz.)	421	2.0			105.2	0.51	1683	8.2
Diced or shredded, packed (approx. 9 oz.)	947	4.6			105.2	0.51	1683	8.2
1 tablespoon, shredded (approx. ¼ oz.):								
USDA source A	27	0.1			106.4	0.49	1703	7.9
USDA source B	26	0.1			105.2	0.51	1683	8.2
Typical sandwich sizes:								
1 slice, 3½" × 3⅜" × ⅛" (approx. 1 oz.)								
USDA source A	106	0.5	106	0.5	106.4	0.49	1703	7.9
USDA source B	105	0.5	105	0.5	105.2	0.50	1683	8.2
1 slice, 3½" × 3⅜" × 3/32" (approx. ¾ oz.)								
USDA source A	80	0.4	80	0.4	106.4	0.49	1703	7.9
USDA source B	75	0.4	75	0.4	105.2	0.50	1683	8.2
Pasteurized Process(ed) PIMENTO Cheese, by brand								
Ann Page (A&P) "Mel-O-Bit," Pasteurized Process(ed) Pimento Cheese, 6-oz. package, 8 slices	660	6.0			110.0	1.00	1760	16.0
1 slice, approx. ¾ oz.	83	0.8	83	0.8	110.0	1.00	1760	16.0
Kraft De Luxe Choice Pasteurized Process(ed) Pimento Cheese, 6-oz. package, 8 slices	660	6.0			110.0	1.00	1760	16.0
1 slice, approx. ¾ oz.	83	0.8	83	0.8	110.0	1.00	1760	16.0

	UNIT		1 SLICE		1 OZ., BY WT.		1 POUND	
	Cal.	Carb.	Cal.	Carb.	Cal.	Carb.	Cal.	Carb.
8-oz. package, 12 slices	880	8.0			110.0	1.00	1760	16.0
1 slice, approx. ⅔ oz.	73	0.7	73	0.7	110.0	1.00	1760	16.0
12-oz. package, 16 slices	1320	12.0			110.0	1.00	1760	16.0
1 slice, approx. ¾ oz.	83	0.8	83	0.8	110.0	1.00	1760	16.0
Pasteurized Process(ed) SWISS Cheese, based on generic data:								
1 pound:								
USDA source A (25.01% fat) (7g/1g/6g/44%/440mg)	1516	9.5			94.8	0.60	1516	9.5
USDA source B (26.90% fat) (8g/tr/8g/39%/331mg)	1610	8.0			100.6	0.46	1610	8.0
Typical sandwich sizes:								
1 slice, 3½" × 3⅜" × ⅛" (approx. 1 oz.):								
USDA source A	95	0.6	95	0.6	94.8	0.60	1516	9.5
USDA source B	101	0.5	101	0.5	100.6	0.46	1610	7.3
1 slice, 3½" × 3⅜" × 3/32" (approx. ¾ oz.):								
USDA source A	71	0.5	71	0.5	94.8	0.60	1516	9.5
USDA source B	76	0.3	76	0.3	100.6	0.46	1610	7.3
1 cubic inch (approx. 0.63 oz.):								
USDA source A	60	0.4			94.8	0.60	1516	9.5
USDA source B	63	0.3			100.6	0.46	1610	7.3
1 cup:								
USDA source A:								
Diced, not packed (approx. 4.7 oz.)	446	2.8			94.8	0.60	1516	9.5
Shredded, not packed (approx. 3.7 oz.)	351	2.2			94.8	0.60	1516	9.5
Diced or shredded, packed (approx. 9 oz.)	853	5.4			94.8	0.60	1516	9.5
USDA source B:								
Diced, not packed (approx. 4.7 oz.)	473	2.2			100.6	0.46	1610	7.3
Shredded, not packed (approx. 3.7 oz.)	372	1.7			100.6	0.46	1610	7.3
Diced or shredded, packed (approx. 9 oz.)	905	4.1			100.6	0.46	1610	7.3
1 tablespoon, shredded (approx. 0.23 oz.):								
USDA source A	22	0.1			94.8	0.60	1516	9.5
USDA source B	23	0.1			100.6	0.46	1610	7.3
For comparison: natural domestic Swiss cheese, based on generic data								
1 pound:								
USDA source A (27.45% fat) (8g/1g/8g/37%/74mg)	1707	15.3			106.7	0.95	1707	15.3
USDA source B (27.87% fat) (8g/1g/8g/39%/201mg)	1678	7.7			104.9	0.50	1678	7.7
For comparison: imported Swiss cheese, based on generic data (30.50% fat), 1 pound (9g/1g/8g/na/241mg)	1805	15.4			112.8	0.96	1805	15.4
Pasteurized Process(ed) SWISS Cheese, by brand								
Ann Page (A&P) "Mel-O-Bit," Pasteurized Process(ed) Swiss Cheese, 6-oz. package, 8 slices	600	6.0			100.0	1.00	1600	16.0
1 slice, approx. ¾ oz.	75	0.8	75	0.8	100.0	1.00	1600	16.0
12-oz. package, 16 slices	1200	12.0			100.0	1.00	1600	16.0
1 slice, approx. ¾ oz.	75	0.8	75	0.8	100.0	1.00	1600	16.0
Kraft De Luxe Choice Pasteurized Process(ed) Swiss Cheese, 8-oz. package, 12 slices	720	8.0			90.0	1.00	1440	16.0
1 slice, approx. ⅔ oz.	60	0.7	60	0.7	90.0	1.00	1440	16.0
PASTEURIZED PROCESS(ED) CHEESE FOOD								
Pasteurized Process(ed) AMERICAN Cheese Food, based on generic data:								
1 pound:								
USDA source A (24.44% fat) (7g/2g/6g/43%/274mg)	1504	37.8			94.0	2.36	1504	37.8
USDA source B (23.99% fat) (7g/2g/6g/43%/na)	1465	32.2			92.0	2.00	1465	32.2
Typical sandwich sizes:								
1 slice, 3½" × 3⅜" × ⅛" (approx. 1 oz.)								
USDA source A	94	2.4	94	2.4	94.0	2.36	1504	37.8
USDA source B	92	2.0	92	2.0	92.0	2.00	1465	32.2
1 slice, 3½" × 3⅜" × 3/32" (approx. ¾ oz.)								
USDA source A	71	1.8	71	1.8	94.0	2.36	1504	37.8
USDA source B	68	1.5	68	1.5	92.0	2.00	1465	32.2
1 cubic inch (approx. ⅗ oz.):								
USDA source A	58	1.5			94.0	2.36	1504	32.7
USDA source B	57	1.2			92.0	2.00	1465	32.2
1 cup:								
USDA source A:								
Diced, not packed (approx. 5 oz.)	470	11.8			94.0	2.36	1504	37.7
Shredded, not packed (approx. 4 oz.)	376	9.4			94.0	2.36	1504	37.7
Diced or shredded, packed (approx. 9 oz.)	846	21.2			94.0	2.36	1504	37.7
USDA source B:								
Diced, not packed (approx. 5 oz.)	460	10.0			92.0	2.00	1465	32.2
Shredded, not packed (approx. 4 oz.)	368	8.0			92.0	2.00	1465	32.2
Diced or shredded, packed (approx. 9 oz.)	828	18.0			92.0	2.00	1465	32.2
1 tablespoon (approx. ½ oz.):								
USDA source A	47	1.2			94.0	2.36	1504	37.7
USDA source B	46	1.0			92.0	2.00	1465	32.2
Pasteurized Process(ed) AMERICAN Cheese Food, by brand								
Ann Page (A&P) "Ched-O-Bit," Pasteurized Process(ed) American Cheese Food, yellow or white								
12-oz. package, 16 slices	1080	24.0			90.0	2.00	1440	32.0
1 slice, approx. ¾ oz.	68	1.5	68	1.5	90.0	2.00	1440	32.0
16-oz. (1-lb.) package, 24 slices	1440	32.0			90.0	2.00	1440	32.0
1 slice, approx. ⅔ oz.	60	1.3	60	1.3	90.0	2.00	1440	32.0
Borden Pasteurized Process(ed) American Cheese Food, yellow or white, 8-oz. package, 10 slices	720	16.0			90.0	2.00	1446	32.0
1 slice, approx. ⅘ oz.	72	1.6	72	1.6	90.0	2.00	1440	32.0
12-oz. package, 16 slices	1080	24.0			90.0	2.00	1440	32.0
1 slice, approx. ¾ oz.	68	1.5	68	1.5	90.0	2.00	1440	32.0
16-oz. (1-lb.) package, 24 slices	1440	32.0			90.0	2.00	1440	32.0
1 slice, approx. ¾ oz.	68	1.5	68	1.5	90.0	2.00	1440	32.0
32-oz. (2-lb.) package, 48 slices	2880	64.0			90.0	2.00	1440	32.0
1 slice, approx. ⅔ oz.	60	1.3	60	1.3	90.0	2.00	1440	32.0
Cheez Kisses (Borden) bite-size Pasteurized Process(ed) American Cheese Food, 6-oz. package, approx. 30 kisses	660	6.0			110.0	1.00	1760	16.0
1 kiss, approx. 0.225 oz. (approx. 4½ per ounce)	25	0.2	25	0.2	110.0	1.00	1760	16.0
Kraft "Singles," Pasteurized Process(ed) American Cheese Food, yellow or white, 6-oz. package, 8 slices	540	12.0			90.0	2.00	1440	32.0
1 slice, approx. ¾ oz.	68	1.5	68	1.5	90.0	2.00	1440	32.0
8-oz. package, 12 slices	720	16.0			90.0	2.00	1440	32.0
1 slice, approx. ⅔ oz.	68	1.5	68	1.5	90.0	2.00	1440	32.0
12-oz. package, 16 slices	1080	24.0			90.0	2.00	1440	32.0
1 slice, approx. ¾ oz.	68	1.5	68	1.5	90.0	2.00	1440	32.0
16-oz. (1-lb.) package, 24 slices	1440	32.0			90.0	2.00	1440	32.0
1 slice, approx. ⅔ oz.	68	1.5	68	1.5	90.0	2.00	1440	32.0
48-oz. (3-lb.) package, 64 slices	4320	96.0			90.0	2.00	1440	32.0
1 slice, approx. ¾ oz.	68	1.5	68	1.5	90.0	2.00	1440	32.0
Sharp "Singles," Pasteurized Process(ed) American Cheese Food, 6-oz. package, 8 slices	600	6.0			100.0	1.00	1600	16.0
1 slice, approx. ¾ oz.	75	0.8	75	0.8	100.0	1.00	1600	16.0
Pauly (Swift) Pasteurized Process(ed) American Cheese Food, 12-oz. package, 16 slices	1080	24.0			90.0	2.00	1440	32.0
1 slice, approx. ¾ oz.	68	1.5	68	1.5	90.0	2.00	1440	32.0
Pasteurized Process(ed) PIMENTO Cheese Food, based on generic data (31.18% fat):								
1 pound (9g/tr/na/na/na)	1696	7.8			106.0	0.49	1696	7.8

	UNIT Cal.	UNIT Carb.	1 SLICE Cal.	1 SLICE Carb.	1 OZ., BY WT. Cal.	1 OZ., BY WT. Carb.	1 POUND Cal.	1 POUND Carb.
Typical sandwich sizes:								
1 slice, 3½″ × 3⅜″ × ⅛″ (approx. 1 oz.)	106	0.5	106	0.5	106.0	0.49	1696	7.8
1 slice, 3½″ × 3⅜″ × 3/32″ (approx. ¾ oz.)	80	0.4	80	0.4	106.0	0.49	1696	7.8
1 cubic inch (approx. ⅗ oz.)	64	0.3			106.0	0.49	1696	7.8
1 cup:								
Diced, not packed (approx. 5 oz.)	530	2.5			106.0	0.49	1696	7.8
Shredded, not packed (approx. 4 oz.)	424	2.0			106.0	0.49	1696	7.8
Diced or shredded, packed (approx. 9 oz.)	954	4.4			106.0	0.49	1696	7.8
1 tablespoon (approx. ½ oz.)	53	0.2			106.0	0.49	1696	7.8
Pasteurized Process(ed) PIMENTO Cheese Food, by brand								
Ann Page (A&P) "Ched-O-Bit," Pasteurized Process(ed) Pimento Cheese Food, 8-oz. package, 10 slices	720	16.0			90.0	2.00	1440	32.0
1 slice, approx. ⅘ oz.	72	1.6	72	1.6	90.0	2.00	1440	32.0
Pauly (Swift) Pasteurized Process(ed) Pimento Cheese Food, 8-oz. package, 10 slices	720	8.0			90.0	1.00	1440	16.0
1 slice, approx. ⅘ oz.	72	0.8	72	0.8	90.0	1.00	1440	16.0
Pasteurized Processed SWISS Cheese Food, by brand								
Ann Page (A&P) "Ched-O-Bit," Pasteurized Process(ed) Swiss Cheese Food, 8-oz. package, 10 slices	800	24.0			100.0	3.00	1600	48.0
1 slice, approx. ⅘ oz.	80	2.4	80	2.4	100.0	3.00	1600	48.0
Land O'Lakes Pasteurized Process(ed) Swiss Cheese Food, 7-oz. chunk	700	0.0			100.0	0.00	1600	0.0
6-oz. package, 8 slices	600	0.0			100.0	0.00	1600	0.0
1 slice, approx. ¾ oz.	75	0.0	75	0.0	100.0	0.00	1600	0.0
Pauly (Swift) Pasteurized Process(ed) Swiss Cheese Food, 8-oz. package, 10 slices	720	16.0			90.0	2.00	1440	32.0
1 slice, approx. ⅘ oz.	72	1.6	72	1.6	90.0	2.00	1440	32.0
OTHER Cheese Food, by brand								
Cheez-Ola (Fisher) Pasteurized Process(ed) Filled Cheese Food, 8-oz. chunk	720	trace			90.0	trace	1440	
16-oz. (1-lb.) package	1440	trace			90.0	trace	1440	
32-oz. (2-lb.) package	2880	trace			90.0	trace	1440	
Land O'Lakes Cheese and Salami Process(ed) Cheese Food, 7-oz. chunk	630	14.0			90.0	2.00	1440	32.0
11-oz. chunk	990	22.0			90.0	2.00	1440	32.0
Jalepeño Pepper, Process(ed) Cheese Food, 7-oz. chunk	630	18.0			90.0	2.00	1440	32.0
11-oz. chunk	990	22.0			90.0	2.00	1440	32.0
Ole Smoky Process(ed) Cheese Food, 7-oz. chunk	630	14.0			90.0	2.00	1440	32.0
11-oz. chunk	990	22.0			90.0	2.00	1440	32.0
Pizza Pepperoni Process(ed) Cheese Food, 7-oz. chunk	630	14.0			90.0	2.00	1440	32.0
11-oz. chunk	990	22.0			90.0	2.00	1440	32.0
Tangy Onion Process(ed) Cheese Food, 7-oz. chunk	630	14.0			90.0	2.00	1440	32.0
11-oz. chunk	990	22.0			90.0	2.00	1440	32.0
Munchee (Pauly [Swift]) Sweet Pasteurized Process(ed) Cheese Food, 6-oz. package, 8 slices	600	12.0			100.0	2.00	1600	32.0
1 slice, approx. ¾ oz.	75	1.5	75	1.5	100.0	2.00	1600	32.0
8-oz. chunk	800	16.0			100.0	2.00	1600	32.0

PASTEURIZED PROCESS(ED) CHEESE PRODUCTS

	UNIT Cal.	UNIT Carb.	1 SLICE Cal.	1 SLICE Carb.	1 OZ., BY WT. Cal.	1 OZ., BY WT. Carb.	1 POUND Cal.	1 POUND Carb.
Di-et (Clearfield) Skim Milk, Pasteurized Process(ed) Cheese Product "Singles," 8-oz. package, 12 slices	480	16.0			60.0	2.00	960	32.0
1 slice, approx. ⅔ oz.	40	1.3	40	1.3	60.0	2.00	960	32.0
Light n' Lively (Kraft) American Flavored Pasteurized Cheese product, 12-oz. package, 16 slices	840	24.0			70.0	2.00	1120	32.0
1 slice, approx. ¾ oz.	53	1.5	53	1.5	70.0	2.00	1120	32.0
Lite-Line (Borden) Pasteurized Process(ed) Cheese Product, 8-oz. package, 12 slices	400	8.0			50.0	1.00	800	16.0
1 slice, approx. ⅔ oz.	33	0.7	33	0.7	50.0	1.00	800	16.0
Nuform (Clearfield) Pasteurized Process(ed) Cheese Product, 8-oz. package, 12 slices	400	24.0			50.0	3.00	800	48.0
1 slice, approx. ⅔ oz.	33	2.0	33	2.0	50.0	3.00	800	48.0
Sandwich-Mate (Fisher) 12-oz. package, 16 slices	1080	12.0			90.0	1.00	1440	16.0
1 slice, approx. ¾ oz.	68	0.8	68	0.8	90.0	1.00	1440	16.0
Skim-American (Borden) Pasteurized Process(ed) Cheese Product, 12-oz. package, 16 slices	840	12.0			70.0	1.00	1120	16.0
1 slice, approx. ¾ oz.	53	0.8	53	0.8	70.0	1.00	1120	16.0
Weight Watchers Pasteurized Process(ed) Cheese Product, 10-oz. package, 10 slices	500	10.0			50.0	1.00	800	16.0
1 slice, approx. 1 oz.	50	1.0	50	1.0	50.0	1.00	800	16.0
For comparison: **Kraft** De Luxe Choice, Pasteurized Process(ed) American Cheese, yellow or white, 12-oz. package, 16 slices	1320	12.0			110.0	1.00	1760	16.0
1 slice, approx. ¾ oz.	83	0.8	83	0.8	110.0	1.00	1760	16.0
For comparison: **Kraft** "Singles," Pasteurized Process(ed) American Cheese Food, yellow or white, 12-oz. package, 16 slices	1080	24.0			90.0	2.00	1440	32.0
1 slice, approx. ¾ oz.	68	1.5	68	1.5	90.0	2.00	1440	32.0

PASTEURIZED PROCESS(ED) CHEESE SPREADS

	UNIT Cal.	UNIT Carb.	1 SLICE Cal.	1 SLICE Carb.	1 OZ., BY WT. Cal.	1 OZ., BY WT. Carb.	1 POUND Cal.	1 POUND Carb.
Pasteurized Process(ed) AMERICAN Cheese Spread, based on generic data:								
1 pound:								
USDA source A (21.23% fat) (6g/2g/5g/48%/381mg)	1317	39.6			82.3	2.48	1317	39.6
USDA source B (21.41% fat) (6g/2g/5g/49%/461mg)	1306	37.2			81.6	2.33	1306	37.2
1 Loaf, 8½″ × 2¾″ × 2¼″ [approx. 32 oz. (2 lb.)]:								
USDA source A	2634	79.2			82.3	2.48	1317	39.6
USDA source B	2614	74.4			81.6	2.33	1306	37.2
1 cubic inch (approx. ⅗ oz.):								
USDA source A	51	1.5			82.3	2.48	1317	39.6
USDA source B	50	1.4			81.6	2.31	1306	37.2
1 cup:								
USDA source A:								
Diced, not packed (approx. 5 oz.)	412	12.5			82.3	2.48	1317	39.6
Shredded, not packed (approx. 4 oz.)	329	10.0			82.3	2.48	1317	39.6
Diced or shredded, packed (approx. 9 oz.)	741	22.5			82.3	2.48	1317	39.6
USDA source B:								
Diced, not packed (approx. 5 oz.)	408	11.7			81.6	2.33	1306	37.2
Shredded, not packed (approx. 4 oz.)	326	9.3			81.6	2.33	1306	37.2
Diced or shredded, packed (approx. 9 oz.)	734	21.0			81.6	2.33	1306	37.2
1 tablespoon (approx. ½ oz.):								
USDA source A	41	1.3			82.3	2.48	1317	39.6
USDA source B	40	1.1			81.6	2.33	1306	37.2
Pasteurized Process(ed) Cheese Spreads, by brand								
Cheestix (Birkum) Process(ed) Cheese Snack with Gruyère, 5-stick multipack, 3.3 oz.	290	(1.8)			87.0	(0.54)	1392	(8.6)
1 stick, approx. ⅔ oz.	58	(0.4)			87.0	(0.54)	1392	(8.6)
Process(ed) Cheese Snack with Onion, 5-stick multipack, 3.3 oz.	(270)	(1.8)			81.0	(0.54)	1296	(8.6)
1 stick, approx. ⅔ oz.	54	(0.4)			81.0	(0.54)	1296	(8.6)
Process(ed) Cheese Snack with Pepper, 5-stick multipack, 3.3 oz.	285	(1.8)			85.5	(0.54)	1368	(8.6)
1 stick, approx. ⅔ oz.	57	(0.4)			85.5	(0.54)	1368	(8.6)

	UNIT Cal.	UNIT Carb.	1 SLICE Cal.	1 SLICE Carb.	1 OZ., BY WT. Cal.	1 OZ., BY WT. Carb.	1 POUND Cal.	1 POUND Carb.
Cheez Kisses (Borden) pasteurized process(ed) American Cheese Spread, bite-size, 6-oz. package, approx. 30 kisses	540	18.0			90.0	3.00	1440	48.0
1 kiss, approx. 0.2 oz. (approx. 5 per ounce)	18	0.6			90.0	3.00	1440	48.0
Cheez Whiz (Kraft), 8-oz. jar	600	16.0			75.0	2.00	1200	32.0
16-oz. (1-lb.) jar	1200	32.0			75.0	2.00	1200	32.0
Dorman's process(ed) Gruyère Cheese Spread, 1 pound	1440	16.0			90.0	1.00	1440	16.0
Laughing Cow, 6-oz. package, 6 wedges	434	4.3			72.3	0.71	1157	11.4
1 wedge, approx. 1 oz.	72	0.7			72.3	0.71	1157	11.4
6-oz. package, 8 wedges	434	4.3			72.3	0.71	1157	11.4
1 wedge, approx. ¾ oz.	54	0.5			72.3	0.71	1157	11.4
8-oz. package, 12 wedges	578	5.7			72.3	0.71	1157	11.4
1 wedge, approx. ⅔ oz.	48	0.5			72.3	0.71	1157	11.4
Cheezbits, 4-oz. package, 24 bits	306	2.8			72.3	0.71	1157	11.4
1 bit, approx. 0.18 oz.	13	0.1			72.3	0.71	1157	11.4
Continental Wedges, 6-oz. package, 6 wedges	434	4.3			72.3	0.71	1157	11.4
1 wedge, approx. 1 oz.	72	0.7			72.3	0.71	1157	11.4
Hot Pepper Wedges, 6-oz. package, 8 wedges	434	4.3			72.3	0.71	1157	11.4
1 wedge, approx. ¾ oz.	54	0.5			72.3	0.71	1157	11.4
Reduced Calories Wedges, 6-oz. package, 8 wedges	272	8.0			45.4	1.33	726	21.3
1 wedge, approx. ¾ oz.	32	1.0			45.4	1.33	726	21.3
Neufchâtel (Kraft) Spread with Bacon & Horseradish, 5-oz. jar	350	5.0			70.0	1.00	1120	16.0
1 tablespoon (approx. 0.5 oz.)	(37)	(0.5)			70.0	1.00	1120	16.0
Spread with Blue Cheese, 5-oz. jar	350	10.0			70.0	2.00	1120	32.0
1 tablespoon (approx. 0.5 oz.)	(37)	(1.1)			70.0	2.00	1120	32.0
Spread with Clams, 5-oz. jar	350	10.0			70.0	2.00	1120	32.0
1 tablespoon (approx. 0.5 oz.)	(37)	(1.1)			70.0	2.00	1120	32.0
Spread with Dill Pickles, 5-oz. jar	350	10.0			70.0	2.00	1120	32.0
1 tablespoon (approx. 0.5 oz.)	(37)	(1.1)			70.0	2.00	1120	32.0
Spread with Garlic & Onions, 5-oz. jar	350	10.0			70.0	2.00	1120	32.0
1 tablespoon (approx. 0.5 oz.)	(37)	(1.1)			70.0	2.00	1120	32.0
Spread with Onions, 5-oz. jar	350	15.0			70.0	3.00	1120	48.0
1 tablespoon (approx. 0.5 oz.)	(37)	(1.6)			70.0	3.00	1120	48.0
Spread with Pineapple, 5-oz. jar	350	15.0			70.0	3.00	1120	48.0
1 tablespoon (approx. 0.5 oz.)	(37)	(1.6)			70.0	3.00	1120	48.0
Roka (Kraft) "Blue" Brand, pasteurized cheese spread, 5-oz. jar	400	5.0			80.0	1.00	1280	16.0
Six De Savoie regular, 4-oz. package	363	2.3			90.7	0.57	1451	9.1
Noix, 4-oz. package	336	1.1			83.9	0.28	1342	4.5
Snack Mates (Nabisco) Pasteurized Process(ed) Cheese Spread, American flavor, Nabisco, 4⅝ oz.	370	9.3			80.0	2.00	1280	32.0
Cheddar flavor, 4⅝ oz.	370	9.3			80.0	2.00	1280	32.0
Cheese 'n Bacon flavor, 4⅝ oz.	370	9.3			80.0	2.00	1280	32.0
Chive 'n Green Onion flavor, 4⅝ oz.	370	9.3			80.0	2.00	1280	32.0
Sharp Cheddar flavor, 4⅝ oz.	370	9.3			80.0	2.00	1280	32.0
Squeez-A-Snak (Kraft) Hickory Smoke Flavor pasteurized process(ed) cheese spread, 6-oz. link	540	0.0			90.0	0.00	1440	0.0
Velveeta (Kraft) pasteurized process(ed) cheese spread, 8-oz. loaf	640	16.0			80.0	2.00	1280	32.0
16-oz. (1-lb.) loaf	1280	32.0			80.0	2.00	1280	32.0
32-oz. (2-lb.) loaf	2560	64.0			80.0	2.00	1280	32.0

OTHER REDUCED-CALORIE, IMITATION, AND SUBSTITUTE CHEESES, by brand

	UNIT Cal.	UNIT Carb.	1 SLICE Cal.	1 SLICE Carb.	1 OZ., BY WT. Cal.	1 OZ., BY WT. Carb.	1 POUND Cal.	1 POUND Carb.
Ched-O-Mate (Fisher) Cheddar Cheese Substitute, shredded, 4-oz. bag	360	4.0			90.0	1.00	1440	16.0
8-oz. bag	720	8.0			90.0	1.00	1440	16.0
Chef's Delight Imitation Pasteurized Process(ed) Cheese Spread, 32-oz. (2-lb.) package	2240	128.0			70.0	4.00	1120	64.0
Count Down (Fisher) Imitation Pasteurized Process(ed) Skim Milk Cheese Spread, 32-oz. (2-lb.) box	1280	96.0			40.0	3.00	640	48.0
Laughing Cow Reduced Calories Wedges, 6-oz. package, 8 wedges	272	8.0			45.4	1.33	726	21.3
1 wedge, approx. ¾ oz.	32	1.0			45.4	1.33	726	21.3
Lo-Chol (Dorman's) Imitation Semi-Soft Cheese, 6-oz. package, 4 slices	630	0.0			105.0	0.00	1680	0.0
1 slice, approx. 1.5 oz.	158	0.0	158	0.0	105.0	0.00	1680	0.0
Pizza-Mate (Fisher) Mozzarella Cheese Substitute, 8-oz. chunk	640	trace			80.0	trace	1280	trace
16-oz. (1-lb.) chunk	1280	trace			80.0	trace	1280	trace
shredded, 4-oz. bag	320	trace			80.0	trace	1280	trace
8-oz. bag	640	trace			80.0	trace	1280	trace
12-oz. bag	960	trace			80.0	trace	1280	trace
Sandwich-Mate (Fisher) American Cheese Substitute, 12-oz. package, 16 slices	1080	12.0			90.0	1.00	1440	16.0
1 slice, approx. ¾ oz.	90	1.0	90	1.0	90.0	1.00	1440	16.0

9 PASTA •

MACARONI And SPAGHETTI

	ENTIRE BOX		1 OZ., BY WT. DRY		1 OZ., BY WT. BOILED		1 CUP	
	Cal.	Carb.	Cal.	Carb.	Cal.	Carb.	Cal.	Carb.
PASTA ALIMENTORE (based on data from Italy), 1 pound	1678	375.6	104.9	23.48				
Cooked medium [yield: approx. 46 oz. (2.9 lb.)]	1678	375.6			36.8	8.28		
"Al dente" [yield: approx. 40 oz. (2.5 lb.)]	1678	375.6			42.0	9.39		
"Tender" [yield: approx. 52 oz. (3.3 lb.)]	1678	375.6			31.5	7.18		
By brand:								
ACINI DI PEPE #44								
La Rosa, 1-lb. box	1674	341.1	104.6	21.32			(624)	(127.1)
Cooked medium [yield: approx. 46 oz. (2.9 lb.), 7.2 cups]	1674	341.1			36.7	7.52	(231)	(47.4)
"Al dente" [yield: approx. 40 oz. (2.5 lb.)]	1674	341.1			41.9	8.53		
"Tender" [yield: approx. 52 oz. (3.3 lb.)]	1674	341.1			31.4	6.52		
ALPHABET #51								
La Rosa Alphabet #51, 1-lb. box	1674	341.1	104.6	21.32				
Cooked medium [yield: approx. 46 oz. (2.9 lb.)]	1674	341.1			36.7	7.52		
BUCATINE #7								
Ronzoni Bucatine #7, 1-lb. box	1674	341.1	104.6	21.32				
Cooked medium [yield: approx. 46 oz. (2.9 lb.)]	1674	341.1			36.7	7.52		
CANNELLONI #82 (Tufoli)								
La Rosa Cannelloni #82, 1-lb. box	1674	341.1	104.6	21.32				
Cooked medium [yield: approx. 46 oz. (2.9 lb.)]	1674	341.1			36.7	7.52		
"Al dente" [yield: approx. 40 oz. (2.5 lb.)]	1674	341.1			41.9	8.53		
"Tender" [yield: approx. 52 oz. (3.3 lb.)]	1674	341.1			31.4	6.52		
Ronzoni Cannelloni #82, 12-oz. box	1255	255.8	104.6	21.32				
Cooked medium [yield: approx. 35 oz. (2.2 lb.)]	1255	255.8			36.7	7.52		
CAPELLINI #11								
La Rosa Capellini #11, 1-lb. box	1674	341.1	104.6	21.32				
Cooked medium [yield: approx. 46 oz. (2.9 lb.), 7.5 cups]	1674	341.1			36.7	7.52	(223)	(45.8)
CAVATTI #120								
Ronzoni Cavatti #120, 1-lb. box	1674	341.1	104.6	21.32				
Cooked medium [yield: approx. 46 oz. (2.9 lb.)]	1674	341.1			36.7	7.52		
CONCHIGLIE (for Stuffing)								
Mennucci Conchiglie, 14-oz. box	1465	298.5	104.6	21.32				
Cooked medium [yield: approx. 40 oz. (2.5 lb.)]	1465	298.5			36.7	7.52		
DITALI #39								
La Rosa Ditali #39, 1-lb. box	1674	341.1	104.6	21.32				
Cooked medium [yield: approx. 46 oz. (2.9 lb.)]	1674	341.1			36.7	7.52		
Ronzoni Ditali #39, 1-lb. box	1674	341.1	104.6	21.32				
Cooked medium [yield: approx. 46 oz. (2.9 lb.)]	1674	341.1			36.7	7.52		
DITALINI #40								
La Rosa Ditalini #40, 1-lb. box	1674	341.1	104.6	21.32			(365)	(74.4)
Cooked medium [yield: approx. 46 oz. (2.9 lb.), 10.5 cups]	1674	341.1			36.7	7.52	(160)	(32.8)
Ronzoni Ditalini #40, 1-lb. box	1674	341.1	104.6	21.32			(365)	(74.4)
Cooked medium [yield: approx. 46 oz. (2.9 lb.), 10.5 cups]	1674	341.1			36.7	7.52	(160)	(32.8)
ELBOWS								
Ann Page (A&P) Elbows #20, 1-lb. box	1674	341.1	104.6	21.32			(446)	(90.9)
Cooked medium [yield: approx. 46 oz. (2.9 lb.), 10 cups]	1674	341.1			36.7	7.52	(168)	(34.4)
48-oz. (3-lb.) box	5021	1023.4	104.6	21.32			(446)	(90.9)
Cooked medium [yield: approx. 138 oz. (8.6 lb.), 29.9 cups]	5021	1023.4			36.7	7.52	(168)	(34.4)
Buitoni Pasta Romana Elbows, 1-lb. box	1674	341.1	104.6	21.32				
Cooked medium [yield: approx. 46 oz. (2.9 lb.)]	1674	341.1			36.7	7.52		
La Rosa Elbows #35, 1-lb. box	1674	341.1	104.6	21.32			(485)	(98.9)
Cooked medium [yield: approx. 46 oz. (2.9 lb.), 9.1 cups]	1674	341.1			36.7	7.52	(183)	(37.4)
Mueller Elbows, 1-lb. box	1674	341.1	104.6	21.32			(485)	(98.9)
Cooked medium [yield: approx. 46 oz. (2.9 lb.), 9.9 cups]	1674	341.1			36.7	7.52	(169)	(34.6)
8-oz. box	837	170.6	104.6	21.32			(485)	(98.9)

	ENTIRE BOX		1 OZ., BY WT. DRY		1 OZ., BY WT. BOILED		1 CUP	
	Cal.	Carb.	Cal.	Carb.	Cal.	Carb.	Cal.	Carb.
Cooked medium [yield: approx. 23 oz. (1.4 lb.), 5 cups]	837	170.6			36.7	7.52	(169)	(34.6)
Progresso Elbows #34, 1-lb. box	1674	341.1	104.6	21.32				
Cooked medium [yield: approx. 46 oz. (2.9 lb.)]	1674	341.1			36.7	7.52		
Ronzoni Elbows, 1-lb. box	1674	341.1	104.6	21.32				
Cooked medium [yield: approx. 46 oz. (2.9 lb.)]	1674	341.1			36.7	7.52		
"Al dente" [yield: approx. 40 oz. (2.5 lb.)]	1674	341.1			41.9	8.53		
"Tender" [yield: approx. 52 oz. (3.3 lb.)]	1674	341.1			31.4	6.52		
ELBOW TWISTS								
Ronzoni Elbow Twists #36, 1-lb. box	1674	341.1	104.6	21.32			(283)	(57.7)
Cooked medium [yield: approx. 46 oz. (2.9 lb.) 13.2 cups]	1674	341.1			36.7	7.52	(127)	(25.8)
FIDEOS								
La Rosa Fideos #79, 6-oz. cello bag	628	127.9	104.6	21.32				
Cooked medium [yield: approx. 17½ oz. (1 lb. 1.5 oz.)]	628	127.9			36.7	7.52		
12-oz. cello bag	1255	255.8	104.6	21.32				
Cooked medium [yield: approx. 35 oz. (2.2 lb.)]	1255	255.8			36.7	7.52		
La Rosa Fideos #80, 6-oz. cello bag	628	127.9	104.6	21.32				
Cooked medium [yield: approx. 17½ oz. (1 lb. 1.5 oz.), 3⅔ cups]	628	127.9			36.7	7.52		
12-oz. cello bag	1255	255.8	104.6	21.32				
Cooked medium [yield: approx. 35 oz. (2.2 lb.)]	1255	255.8			36.7	7.52		
Ronzoni Fideos #166, 6-oz. box	628	127.9	104.6	21.32				
Cooked medium [yield: approx. 17½ oz. (1 lb. 1.5 oz.), 4 cups]	628	127.9			36.7	7.52	(156)	(31.5)
12-oz. box	1255	255.8	104.6	21.32				
Cooked medium [yield: approx. 35 oz. (2.2 lb.), 8.1 cups]	1255	255.8			36.7	7.52	(156)	(31.5)
Ronzoni Fideos #168, 12-oz. box	1255	255.8	104.6	21.32				
Cooked medium [yield: approx. 35 oz. (2.2 lb.)]	1255	255.8			36.7	7.52		
FUSILLI #115								
Ronzoni Fusilli #115, 1-lb. box	1674	341.1	104.6	21.32				
Cooked medium [yield: approx. 46 oz. (2.9 lb.), 13.5 cups]	1674	341.1			36.7	7.52	(124)	(25.5)
LASAGNA								
Ann Page (A&P) Lasagna #80, 1-lb. box	1674	341.1	104.6	21.32				
Cooked medium [yield: approx. 46 oz. (2.9 lb.), 13.8 cups]	1674	341.1			36.7	7.52	(120)	(24.7)
"Al dente" [yield: approx. 40 oz. (2.5 lb.)]	1674	341.1			41.9	8.53		
"Tender" [yield: approx. 52 oz. (3.3 lb.)]	1674	341.1			31.4	6.52		
Filli de Cecco Di Filippo Lasagna (Large Doppia Riccia), 1-lb. box	1674	341.1	104.6	21.32				
Cooked medium [yield: approx. 46 oz. (2.9 lb.)]	1674	341.1			36.7	7.52		
La Rosa Lasagna #123 (Ribbed), 1-lb. box	1674	341.1	104.6	21.32				
Cooked medium [yield: approx. 46 oz. (2.9 lb.)]	1674	341.1			36.7	7.52		
Mueller's Lasagna, 1-lb. box	1674	341.1	104.6	21.32				
Cooked medium [yield: approx. 46 oz. (2.9 lb.)]	1674	341.1			36.7	7.52		
8-oz. box	837	170.6	104.6	21.32				
Cooked medium [yield: approx. 23 oz. (1.4 lb.)]	837	170.6			36.7	7.52		
Progresso Lasagna #71 (Ricci), 1-lb. box	1674	341.1	104.6	21.32				
Cooked medium [yield: approx. 46 oz. (2.9 lb.)]	1674	341.1			36.7	7.52		
Ronzoni Lasagna #80 (Curly Edge), 1-lb. box	1674	341.1	104.6	21.32				
Cooked medium [yield: approx. 46 oz. (2.9 lb.), 13.8 cups]	1674	341.1			36.7	7.52	(120)	(24.7)
Ronzoni Lasagna #123, 1-lb. box	1674	341.1	104.6	21.32				
Cooked medium [yield: approx. 46 oz. (2.9 lb.)]	1674	341.1			36.7	7.52		
San Giorgio Lasagna (Rippled Edge), 1-lb. box	1674	341.1	104.6	21.32				
Cooked medium [yield: approx. 46 oz. (2.9 lb.)]	1674	341.1			36.7	7.52		
LINGUINE								
Ann Page (A&P) Linguine #12, 1-lb. box	1674	341.1	104.6	21.32				
Cooked medium [yield: approx. 46 oz. (2.9 lb.)]	1674	341.1			36.7	7.52		
Buitoni High Protein Linguine #8, 8-oz. box	840	148.0	105.0	18.50				
Cooked medium [yield: approx. 23 oz. (1.4 lb.), 6.8 cups]	840	148.0			36.7	6.43	(124)	(21.8)
Buitoni Pasta Romana (Linguine #17), 1-lb. box	1674	341.1	104.6	21.32				
Cooked medium [yield: approx. 46 oz. (2.9 lb), 9.7 cups]	1674	341.1			36.7	7.52	(172)	(35.3)
La Rosa Linguine #17, 1-lb. box	1674	341.1	104.6	21.32				
Cooked medium [yield: approx. 46 oz. (2.9 lb.), 9.7 cups]	1674	341.1			36.7	7.52	(172)	(35.3)
Ronzoni Linguine #17, 1-lb. box	1674	341.1	104.6	21.32				
Cooked medium [yield: approx. 46 oz. (2.9 lb.), 9.7 cups]	1674	341.1			36.7	7.52	(172)	(35.3)
Ronzoni Linguine Fine, #18, 1-lb. box	1674	341.1	104.6	21.32				
Cooked medium [yield: approx. 46 oz. (2.9 lb.), 10.2 cups]	1674	341.1			36.7	7.52	(164)	(33.6)
MACAROLI								
Mueller Macaroli, 12-oz. bag	1255	255.8	104.6	21.32				
Cooked medium [yield: approx. 35 oz. (2.2 lb.)]	1255	255.8			36.7	7.52		
MACARONI								
Buitoni High Protein Macaroni Moon Buggies, 8-oz. box	840	148.0	105.0	18.50				
Cooked medium [yield: approx. 23 oz. (1.4 lb.)]	840	148.0			36.7	6.43		
"Al dente" [yield: approx. 20 oz. (1.3 lb.)]	840	148.0			41.9	8.53		
"Tender" [yield: approx. 26 oz. (1.6 lb.)]	840	148.0			31.4	6.52		
Cooked medium: 1 Moon Buggie, approx. 0.13 oz., 8 to the oz.	(5)	(0.8)			36.7	6.43		
Buitoni High Protein Macaroni Space Robots, 8-oz. box	840	148.0	105.0	18.50				
Cooked medium [yield: approx. 23 oz. (1.4 lb.)]	840	148.0			36.7	6.43		
Cooked medium 1 Space Robot, approx. 0.17 oz.; 6 to the oz.	(6)	(1.1)			36.7	6.43		
Buitoni High Protein Macaroni Spacemen, 8-oz. box	840	148.0	105.0	18.50				
Cooked medium [yield: approx. 23 oz. (1.4 lb.)]	840	148.0			36.7	6.43		
Cooked medium: 1 Spaceman, approx. 0.19 oz.; 5.4 to the oz.	(7)	(1.2)			36.7	6.43		
La Rosa Macaroni #4 (Long) (Perciatelli-Bucatini), 1-lb. box	1674	341.1	104.6	21.32				
Cooked medium [yield: approx. 46 oz. (2.9 lb.)]	1674	341.1			36.7	7.52		
La Rosa Macaroni #5, 1-lb. box	1674	341.1	104.6	21.32				
Cooked medium [yield: approx. 46 oz. (2.9 lb.)]	1674	341.1			36.7	7.52		
Ronzoni Macaroni #5 (cut Maccaroncelli), 1-lb. box	1674	341.1	104.6	21.32				
Cooked medium [yield: approx. 46 oz. (2.9 lb.)]	1674	341.1			36.7	7.52		
"Al dente" [yield: approx. 40 oz. (2.5 lb.)]	1674	341.1			41.9	8.53		
"Tender" [yield: approx. 52 oz. (3.3 lb.)]	1674	341.1			31.4	6.52		
MANICOTTI								
La Rosa Manicotti #126 (Ribbed), 5-oz. box	523	106.6	104.6	21.32				

	ENTIRE BOX		1 OZ., BY WT. DRY		1 OZ., BY WT. BOILED		1 CUP	
	Cal.	Carb.	Cal.	Carb.	Cal.	Carb.	Cal.	Carb.
Cooked medium [yield: approx. 14.3 oz.]	523	106.6			36.7	7.52		
Mennucci Manicotti, 8-oz. box	837	170.6	104.6	21.32				
Cooked medium [yield: approx. 23 oz. (1.4 lb.)]	837	170.6			36.7	7.52		
"Al dente" [yield: approx. 40 oz. (2.5 lb.)]	1674	341.1			41.9	8.53		
"Tender" [yield: approx. 52 oz. (3.3 lb.)]	1674	341.1			31.4	6.52		
Cooked medium: 1 manicotti, 12 to the box, approx. ⅔ oz. dry (1.9 oz. cooked)	(24)	5.0			36.7	7.52		
Ronzoni Manicotti #90, 8-oz. box	837	170.6	104.6	21.32				
Cooked medium [yield: approx. 23 oz. (1.4 lb.)]	837	170.6			36.7	7.52		
MARGHERITE								
Ronzoni Margherite #114, 1-lb. box	1674	341.1	104.6	21.32				
Cooked medium [yield: approx. 46 oz. (2.9 lb.)]	1674	341.1			36.7	7.52		
MARUZELLE, see SHELLS #21 and SHELLS #22								
MEZZANI								
Ann Page (A&P) Mezzani #26, 1-lb. box	1674	341.1	104.6	21.32				
Cooked medium [yield: approx. 46 oz. (2.9 lb.)]	1674	341.1			36.7	7.52		
Ann Page (A&P) Mezzani Rigati #81, 1-lb. box	1674	341.1	104.6	21.32				
Cooked medium [yield: approx. 46 oz. (2.9 lb.)]	1674	341.1			36.7	7.52		
La Rosa Mezzani #3, 1-lb. box	1674	341.1	104.6	21.32			(309)	(63.0)
Cooked medium [yield: approx. 46 oz. (2.9 lb.), 10.7 cups]	1674	341.1			36.7	7.52	(156)	(32.0)
Ronzoni Mezzani #3, 1-lb. box	1674	341.1	104.6	21.32			(309)	(63.0)
Cooked medium [yield: approx. 46 oz. (2.9 lb.), 10.7 cups]	1674	341.1			36.7	7.52	(156)	(32.0)
"Al dente" [yield: approx. 40 oz. (2.5 lb.)]	1674	341.1			41.9	8.53		
"Tender" [yield: approx. 52 oz. (3.3 lb.)]	1674	341.1			31.4	6.52		
Ronzoni Mezzani Rigati #4, 1-lb. box	1674	341.1	104.6	21.32			(314)	(63.9)
Cooked medium [yield: approx. 46 oz. (2.9 lb.), 13.4 cups]	1674	341.1			36.7	7.52	(125)	(25.6)
MOSTACCIOLI								
La Rosa Mostaccioli #84, 1-lb. box	1674	341.1	104.6	21.32				
Cooked medium [yield: approx. 46 oz. (2.9 lb.), 9¾ cups]	1674	341.1			36.7	7.52		
La Rosa Mostaccioli Rigati #86, 1-lb. box	1674	341.1	104.6	21.32			(223)	(45.5)
Cooked medium [yield: approx. 46 oz. (2.9 lb.), 10.7 cups]	1674	341.1			36.7	7.52	(157)	(32.1)
Ronzoni Mostaccioli #86, 1-lb. box	1674	341.1	104.6	21.32			(223)	(45.5)
Cooked medium [yield: approx. 46 oz. (2.9 lb.), 10.7 cups]	1674	341.1			36.7	7.52	(157)	(32.1)
NOODLES								
La Rosa Fine Noodles, 6-oz. box or bag	628	127.9	104.6	21.32				
Cooked medium [yield: approx. 17½ oz. (1 lb. 1.5 oz.)]	628	127.9			36.7	7.52		
12-oz. box or bag	1255	255.8	104.6	21.32				
Cooked medium [yield: approx. 35 oz. (2.2 lb.)]	1255	255.8			36.7	7.52		
"Al dente" [yield: approx. 30 oz. (1.9 lb.)]	1255	255.8			41.9	8.53		
"Tender" [yield: approx. 39 oz. (2.4 lb.)]	1255	255.8			31.4	6.52		
Medium Noodles, 6-oz. box or bag	628	127.9	104.6	21.32				
Cooked medium [yield: approx. 17½ oz. (1 lb. 1.5 oz.)]	628	127.9			36.7	7.52		
12-oz. box or bag	1255	255.8	104.6	21.32				
Cooked medium [yield: approx. 35 oz. (2.2 lb.)]	1255	255.8			36.7	7.52		

	ENTIRE BOX		1 OZ., BY WT. DRY		1 OZ., BY WT. BOILED		1 CUP	
	Cal.	Carb.	Cal.	Carb.	Cal.	Carb.	Cal.	Carb.
"Al dente" [yield: approx. 30 oz. (1.9 lb.)]	1255	255.8			41.9	8.53		
"Tender" [yield: approx. 39 oz. (2.4 lb.)]	1255	255.8			31.4	6.52		
Wide noodles, 6-oz. box or bag	628	127.9	104.6	21.32				
Cooked medium [yield: approx. 17½ oz. (1 lb. 1.5 oz.)]	628	127.9			36.7	7.52		
"Al dente" [yield: approx. 30 oz. (1.9 lb.)]	628	127.9			41.9	8.53		
"Tender" [yield: approx. 39 oz. (2.4 lb.)]	628	127.9			31.4	6.52		
12-oz. box or bag	1255	255.8	104.6	21.32				
Cooked medium [yield: approx. 35 oz. (2.2 lb.)]	1255	255.8			36.7	7.52		
OCCHIO DI LUPO #26								
La Rosa Occhio Di Lupo #26, 1-lb. box	1674	341.1	104.6	21.32				
Cooked medium [yield: approx. 46 oz. (2.9 lb.)]	1674	341.1			36.7	7.52		
Ronzoni Occhio Di Lupo #26, 1-lb. box	1674	341.1	104.6	21.32				
Cooked medium [yield: approx. 46 oz. (2.9 lb.)]	1674	341.1			36.7	7.52		
ORZO #47								
La Rosa Orzo #47, 1-lb. box	1674	341.1	104.6	21.32			(637)	(129.9)
Cooked medium [yield: approx. 46 oz. (2.9 lb.), 8.4 cups]	1674	341.1			36.7	7.52	(200)	(41.0)
Ronzoni Orzo #47, 1-lb. box	1674	341.1	104.6	21.32			(637)	(129.9)
Cooked medium [yield: approx. 46 oz. (2.9 lb.), 8.4 cups]	1674	341.1			36.7	7.52	(200)	(41.0)
PERCIATELLI #6								
Ronzoni Perciatelli #6, 1-lb. box	1674	341.1	104.6	21.32				
Cooked medium [yield: approx. 46 oz. (2.9 lb.), 9.7 cups]	1674	341.1			36.7	7.52	(172)	(35.1)
RIGATONI								
Ann Page (A&P) Rigatoni #28, 1-lb. box	1674	341.1	104.6	21.32				
Cooked medium [yield: approx. 46 oz. (2.9 lb.)]	1674	341.1			36.7	7.52		
Buitoni Pasta Romana Rigatoni #131, 1-lb. box	1674	341.1	104.6	21.32				
Cooked medium [yield: approx. 46 oz. (2.9 lb.)]	1674	341.1			36.7	7.52		
La Rosa Rigatoni #27, 1-lb. box	1674	341.1	104.6	21.32			(233)	(47.6)
Cooked medium [yield: approx. 46 oz. (2.9 lb.), 9.9 cups]	1674	341.1			36.7	7.52	(169)	(34.6)
Mueller Rigatoni, 1-lb. box	1674	341.1	104.6	21.32				
Cooked medium [yield: approx. 46 oz. (2.9 lb.)]	1674	341.1			36.7	7.52		
Progresso Rigatoni #57, 1-lb. box	1674	341.1	104.6	21.32				
Cooked medium [yield: approx. 46 oz. (2.9 lb.)]	1674	341.1			36.7	7.52		
"Al dente" [yield: approx. 40 oz. (2.5 lb.)]	1674	341.1			41.9	8.53		
"Tender" [yield: approx. 52 oz. (3.3 lb.)]	1674	341.1			31.4	6.52		
Ronzoni Rigatoni #27, 1-lb. box	1674	341.1	104.6	21.32			(233)	(47.6)
Cooked medium [yield: approx. 46 oz. (2.9 lb.), 9.9 cups]	1674	341.1			36.7	7.52	(169)	(34.6)
RIGOLETTI #88 (TWISTS)								
La Rosa Rigoletti #88, 1-lb. box	1674	341.1	104.6	21.32				
Cooked medium [yield: approx. 46 oz. (2.9 lb.)]	1674	341.1			36.7	7.52		
ROTELLE #124								
La Rosa Rotelle #124, 1-lb. box	1674	341.1	104.6	21.32			(260)	(53.0)
Cooked medium [yield: approx. 46 oz. (2.9 lb.), 11.3 cups]	1674	341.1			36.7	7.52	(148)	(30.4)
ROTINI								
San Giorgio Rotini, 1-lb. box	1674	341.1	104.6	21.32				
Cooked medium [yield: approx. 46 oz. (2.9 lb.)]	1674	341.1			36.7	7.52		
SHELLS								
Ann Page (A&P) Maruzelle Shells #21, 1-lb. box	1674	341.1	104.6	21.32			(248)	(50.6)

	ENTIRE BOX		1 OZ., BY WT. DRY		1 OZ., BY WT. BOILED		1 CUP	
	Cal.	Carb.	Cal.	Carb.	Cal.	Carb.	Cal.	Carb.
Cooked medium [yield: approx. 46 oz. (2.9 lb.), 11.3 cups]	1674	341.1			36.7	7.52	(148)	(30.4)
Buitoni Pasta Romana, Maruzelle Shells #22, 1-lb. box	1674	341.1	104.6	21.32			(284)	(57.9)
Cooked medium [yield: approx. 46 oz. (2.9 lb.), 9.1 cups]	1674	341.1			36.7	7.52	(184)	(37.8)
La Rosa Jumbo Shells #20, 5-oz. package	523	106.6	104.6	21.32				
Cooked medium [yield: approx. 14⅓ oz.]	523	106.6			36.7	7.52		
"Al dente" [yield: approx. 12½ oz.]	523	106.6			41.9	8.53		
"Tender" [yield: approx. 16 oz. (1 lb.)]	523	106.6			31.4	6.52		
La Rosa Large Shells #21, 5-oz. package	523	106.6	104.6	21.32			(248)	(50.6)
Cooked medium [yield: approx. 14⅓ oz., 3.5 cups]	523	106.6			36.7	7.52	(148)	(30.4)
La Rosa Small Shells #23, 5-oz. package	523	106.6	104.6	21.32				
Cooked medium [yield: approx. 14⅓ oz.]	523	106.6			36.7	7.52		
Mueller Sea Shells, 1-lb. box	1674	341.1	104.6	21.32			(260)	(53.0)
Cooked medium [yield: approx. 46 oz. (2.9 lb.), 12.8 cups]	1674	341.1			36.7	7.52	(131)	(26.8)
8-oz. box	837	170.6	104.6	21.32			(130)	(26.5)
Cooked medium [yield: approx. 23 oz. (1.4 lb.), 6.4 cups]	837	170.6			36.7	7.52	(131)	(26.8)
"Al dente" [yield: approx. 20 oz. (1.3 lb.)]	837	170.6			41.9	8.53		
"Tender" [yield: approx. 26 oz. (1.6 lb.)]	837	170.6			31.4	6.52		
Ronzoni Jumbo Shells #95 (for filling), 12-oz. box	1255	255.8	104.6	21.32			(173)	(35.3)
Cooked medium [yield: approx. 35 oz. (2.2 lb.), 9.6 cups]	1255	255.8			36.7	7.52	(131)	(26.8)
Ronzoni Large Shells #21, 1-lb. box	1674	341.1	104.6	21.32			(248)	(50.6)
Cooked medium [yield: approx. 46 oz. (2.9 lb.), 11.3 cups]	1674	341.1			36.7	7.52	(148)	(30.4)
San Giorgio Shell Macaroni (Maruzelli) #51, 1-lb. box	1674	341.1	104.6	21.32			(305)	(62.2)
Cooked medium [yield: approx. 46 oz. (2.9 lb.), 10 cups]	1674	341.1			36.7	7.52	(167)	(34.3)
SPAGHETTI								
Ann Page (A&P) Spaghetti #6, 1-lb. box	1674	341.1	104.6	21.32				
Cooked medium [yield: approx. 46 oz. (2.9 lb.)]	1674	341.1			36.7	7.52		
48-oz. (3-lb.) box	5021	1023.4	104.6	21.32				
Cooked medium [yield: approx. 138 oz. (8.6 lb.)]	5021	1023.4			36.7	7.52		
Ann Page (A&P) Spaghetti #9 ("Thin"), 1-lb. box	1674	341.1	104.6	21.32				
Cooked medium [yield: approx. 46 oz. (2.9 lb.), 9 cups]	1674	341.1			36.7	7.52	(185)	(37.9)
48-oz. (3-lb.) box	5021	1023.4	104.6	21.32				
Cooked medium [yield: 138 oz. (8.6 lb.), 27.1 cups]	5021	1023.4			36.7	7.52	(185)	(37.9)
Buitoni Spaghetti #2 ("Very Thin"), 8-oz. box	840	148.0	104.6	21.32				
Cooked medium [yield: approx. 23 oz. (1.4 lb.)]	840	148.0			36.7	7.52		
Buitoni Spaghetti #3 ("Thin"), 8-oz. box	840	148.0	104.6	21.32				
Cooked medium [yield: approx. 23 oz. (1.4 lb.)]	840	148.0			36.7	7.52		
Buitoni Pasta Romana, Spaghetti #8, 1-lb. box	1674	341.1	104.6	21.32				
Cooked medium [yield: approx. 46 oz. (2.9 lb.), 9¾ cups]	1674	341.1			36.7	7.52	(155)	(31.7)
Buitoni Pasta Romana, Spaghetti #9, 1-lb. box	1674	341.1	104.6	21.32				
Cooked medium [yield: approx. 46 oz. (2.9 lb.), 10.8 cups]	1674	341.1			36.7	7.52	(185)	(37.9)
La Rosa Spaghetti #8, 1-lb. box	1674	341.1	104.6	21.32				

	ENTIRE BOX		1 OZ., BY WT. DRY		1 OZ., BY WT. BOILED		1 CUP	
	Cal.	Carb.	Cal.	Carb.	Cal.	Carb.	Cal.	Carb.
Cooked medium [yield: approx. 46 oz. (2.9 lb.), 9 cups]	1674	341.1			36.7	7.52	(155)	(31.7)
La Rosa #9 ("Thin"), Spaghettini, 1-lb. box	1674	341.1	104.6	21.32				
Cooked medium [yield: approx. 46 oz. (2.9 lb.), 10.8 cups]	1674	341.1			36.7	7.52	(185)	(37.9)
La Rosa #115, Slip Pruf Spaghetti Fusilli, 1-lb. box	1674	341.1	104.6	21.32				
Cooked medium [yield: approx. 46 oz. (2.9 lb.)]	1674	341.1			36.7	7.52		
Mueller Spaghetti #1 ("X-Thin"), 1-lb. cello bag	1674	341.1	104.6	21.32				
Cooked medium [yield: approx. 46 oz. (2.9 lb.)]	1674	341.1			36.7	7.52		
"Al dente" [yield: approx. 40 oz. (2.5 lb.)]	1674	341.1			41.9	8.53		
"Tender" [yield: approx. 52 oz. (3.3 lb.)]	1674	341.1			31.4	6.52		
Mueller Spaghetti #9, 1-lb. box	1674	341.1	104.6	21.32				
Cooked medium [yield: approx. 46 oz. (2.9 lb.), 10.8 cups]	1674	341.1			36.7	7.52	(185)	(37.9)
Progresso Spaghetti #8, 1-lb. box	1674	341.1	104.6	21.32				
Cooked medium [yield: approx. 46 oz. (2.9 lb.), 9 cups]	1674	341.1			36.7	7.52	(155)	(31.7)
"Al dente" [yield: approx. 40 oz. (2.5 lb.)]	1674	341.1			41.9	8.53		
"Tender" [yield: approx. 52 oz. (3.3 lb.)]	1674	341.1			31.4	6.52		
Ronzoni Spaghetti #8, 1-lb. box	1674	341.1	104.6	21.32				
Cooked medium [yield: approx. 46 oz. (2.9 lb.), 10.8 cups]	1674	341.1			36.7	7.52	(155)	(31.7)
Ronzoni Spaghetti #9, 1-lb. box	1674	341.1	104.6	21.32				
Cooked medium [yield: approx. 46 oz. (2.9 lb.), 9 cups]	1674	341.1			36.7	7.52	(185)	(37.9)
San Giorgio Spaghetti #9 ("Thin"), 1-lb. box	1674	341.1	104.6	21.32				
Cooked medium [yield: approx. 46 oz. (2.9 lb.), 9 cups]	1674	341.1			36.7	7.52	(185)	(37.9)
SPAGHETTI TWISTS								
Buitoni High Protein Spaghetti Twists #37, 8-oz. box	840	148.0	105.0	18.50			(269)	(47.3)
Cooked medium [yield: approx. 23 oz. (1.4 lb.), 7.9 cups]	840	148.0			36.7	6.43	(106)	(18.6)
"Al dente" [yield: approx. 20 oz. (1.3 lb.)]	840	148.0			41.9	8.53		
"Tender" [yield: approx. 26 oz. (1.6 lb.)]	840	148.0			31.4	6.52		
Ronzoni Spaghetti Twists #126, 1-lb. box	1674	341.1	104.6	21.32				
Cooked medium [yield: approx. 46 oz. (2.9 lb.)]	1674	341.1			36.7	7.52		
SPIEDINI #144								
La Rosa Spiedini #144, 1-lb. box	1674	341.1	104.6	21.32				
Cooked medium [yield: approx. 46 oz. (2.9 lb.)]	1674	341.1			36.7	7.52		
SPIRELLE #47								
Ann Page (A&P) Spirelle #47, 1-lb. box	1647	341.1	104.6	21.32				
Cooked medium [yield: approx. 46 oz. (2.9 lb.)]	1674	341.1			36.7	7.52		
STELLETTE								
Filli de Cecco Di Filippo Stellette, 1-lb. box	1674	341.1	104.6	21.32				
Cooked medium [yield: approx. 46 oz. (2.9 lb.)]	1674	341.1			36.7	7.52		
TUBETTI #41								
La Rosa Tubetti #41, 1-lb. box	1674	341.1	104.6	21.32			(559)	(113.9)
Cooked medium [yield: approx. 46 oz. (2.9 lb.), 9.4 cups]	1674	341.1			36.7	7.52	(179)	(36.6)
Ronzoni Tubetti #41, 1-lb. box	1674	341.1	104.6	21.32			(559)	(113.9)
Cooked medium [yield: approx. 46 oz. (2.9 lb.), 9.4 cups]	1674	341.1			36.7	7.52	(179)	(36.6)

	ENTIRE BOX		1 OZ., BY WT. DRY		1 OZ., BY WT. BOILED		1 CUP	
	Cal.	Carb.	Cal.	Carb.	Cal.	Carb.	Cal.	Carb.
TUBETTINI #42								
La Rosa Tubettini #42, 1-lb. box	1674	341.1	104.6	21.32			(552)	(112.4)
Cooked medium [yield: approx. 46 oz. (2.9 lb.), 8.8 cups]	1674	341.1			36.7	7.52	(190)	(38.9)
Ronzoni Tubettini #42, 1-lb. box	1674	341.1	104.6	21.32			(552)	(112.4)
Cooked medium [yield: approx. 46 oz. (2.9 lb.), 8.8 cups]	1674	341.1			36.7	7.52	(190)	(38.9)
TWISTS								
Mueller, 1-lb. box	1674	341.1	104.6	21.32			(234)	(47.7)
Cooked medium [yield: approx. 46 oz. (2.9 lb.), 10.8 cups]	1674	341.1			36.7	7.52	(155)	(31.7)
8-oz. box	837	170.6	104.6	21.32			(234)	(47.7)
Cooked medium [yield: approx. 23 oz. (1.4 lb.), 5.4 cups]	837	170.6			36.7	7.52	(155)	(31.7)
VERMICELLI								
Ann Page (A&P) Vermicelli #8, 1-lb. box	1674	341.1	104.6	21.32				
Cooked medium [yield: approx. 46 oz. (2.9 lb.)]	1674	341.1			36.7	7.52		
Buitoni Pasta Romana, Vermicelli #10, 1-lb. box	1674	341.1	104.6	21.32				
Cooked medium [yield: approx. 46 oz. (2.9 lb.), 9.1 cups]	1674	341.1			36.7	7.52	(183)	(37.5)
"Al dente" [yield: approx. 40 oz. (2.5 lb.)]	1674	341.1			41.9	8.53		
"Tender" [yield: approx. 52 oz. (3.3 lb.)]	1674	341.1			31.4	6.52		
ZITI								
Buitoni High Protein Ziti #29, 8-oz. box	840	148.0	105.0	18.50			(303)	(53.3)
Cooked medium [yield: approx. 23 oz. (1.4 lb.), 5.4 cups]	840	148.0			36.7	6.43	(155)	(27.2)
Buitoni Pasta Romana, (Cut Ziti), 1-lb. box	1674	341.1	104.6	21.32				
Cooked medium [yield: approx. 46 oz. (2.9 lb.)]	1674	341.1			36.7	7.52		
La Rosa Ziti #2, 1-lb. box	1674	341.1	104.6	21.32			(324)	(66.0)
Cooked medium [yield: approx. 46 oz. (2.9 lb.), 12.5 cups]	1674	341.1			36.7	7.52	(134)	(27.5)
La Rosa Ziti Rigati #32, 1-lb. box	1674	341.1	104.6	21.32				
Cooked medium [yield: approx. 46 oz. (2.9 lb.)]	1674	341.1			36.7	7.52		
"Al dente" [yield: approx. 40 oz. (2.5 lb.)]	1674	341.1			41.9	8.53		
"Tender" [yield: approx. 52 oz. (3.3 lb.)]	1674	341.1			31.4	6.52		
Ronzoni Ziti, 1-lb. box	1674	341.1	104.6	21.32				
Cooked medium [yield: approx. 46 oz. (2.9 lb.)]	1674	341.1			36.7	7.52		
San Giorgio Ziti #28 (Magliette Lisce), 1-lb. box	1674	341.1	104.6	21.32				
Cooked medium [yield: approx. 46 oz. (2.9 lb.)]	1674	341.1			36.7	7.52		

Frozen Macaroni and Spaghetti

	ENTIRE BOX		1 OZ., BY WT. DRY		1 OZ., BY WT. BOILED		1 CUP	
	Cal.	Carb.	Cal.	Carb.	Cal.	Carb.	Cal.	Carb.
Reames, 8-oz. package	288	48.4			(36.0)	(6.05)		
Silverstar Fresh Frozen Cavatelli, 16-oz. (1-lb.) box	1350	293.4	84.4	18.34				

EGG NOODLES

	ENTIRE BOX		1 OZ., BY WT. DRY		1 OZ., BY WT. BOILED		1 CUP	
	Cal.	Carb.	Cal.	Carb.	Cal.	Carb.	Cal.	Carb.
ALPHABET EGG								
Pennsylvania Dutch, 8-oz. bag	840	160.0	105.0	20.00				
Cooked medium [yield: approx. 25 oz. (1.6 lb.)]	840	160.0			(33.8)	(6.48)		
BARLEY SHAPE, TOASTED								
Goodman's, 8-oz. box	880	160.0	110.0	20.00			(751)	(136.5)
Cooked medium [yield: approx. 25 oz. (1.6 lb.), 4 cups]	880	160.0			(34.5)	(6.48)	(222)	(41.7)
BOTT BOI								
Pennsylvania Dutch, 12-oz. bag	1260	240.0	105.0	20.00				
Cooked medium [yield: approx. 37 oz. (2.3 lb.)]	1260	240.0			(33.8)	(6.48)		
COUNTRY KITCHEN								
Ronzoni, 1-lb. box	1760	320.0	110.0	20.00				
Cooked medium [yield: approx. 50 oz. (3.1 lb.)]	1760	320.0			(35.4)	(6.48)		
12-oz. box	1320	240.0	110.0	20.00				
Cooked medium [yield: approx. 37 oz. (2.3 lb.)]	1320	240.0			(35.4)	(6.48)		
"Al dente" [yield: approx. 22 oz. (1.4 lb.)]	840	160.0			38.6	7.35		
"Tender" [yield: approx. 29 oz. (1.8 lb.)]	840	160.0			28.9	5.62		
EGG BOWS								
Goodman's Egg Bows, 8-oz. box	880	160.0	110.0	20.00			(263)	(47.8)
Cooked medium [yield: approx. 25 oz. (1.6 lb.), 7.8 cups]	880	160.0			(35.4)	(6.48)	(113)	(20.7)
La Rosa Egg Bows #66 (Farfalle), 8-oz. box	880	164.0	110.0	20.41				
Cooked medium [yield: approx. 25 oz. (1.6 lb.)]	880	164.0			35.4	6.61		
Pennsylvania Dutch Egg Bows, 12-oz. bag	1260	240.0	105.0	20.00			(187)	(35.6)
Cooked medium [yield: approx. 37 oz. (2.3 lb.), 11.7 cups]	1260	240.0			(33.8)	(6.48)	(107)	(20.6)
EGG PASTINA								
La Rosa Egg Pastina #119, 12-oz. box	1320	244.9	110.0	20.41				
Cooked medium [yield: approx. 37 oz. (2.3 lb.)]	1320	244.9			35.4	6.61		
"Al dente" [yield: approx. 30 oz. (1.9 lb.)]	1320	244.9			44.0	8.16		
"Tender" [yield: approx. 44 oz. (2.8 lb.)]	1320	244.9			30.0	5.57		
Ronzoni Egg Pastina #150, 6-oz. box	660	120.0	110.0	20.00				
Cooked medium [yield: approx. 19 oz. (1 lb. 3 oz.)]	660	120.0			35.4	6.45		
Ronzoni Egg Pastina #155, 12-oz. box	1320	144.0	110.0	20.00			(617)	(112.2)
Cooked medium [yield: approx. 37 oz. (2.3 lb.)]	1320	144.0			35.4	6.45	(287)	(52.3)
FETTUCCINE, EXTRA LONG								
La Rosa Fettuccine #135, 10-oz. box	1100	204.1	110.0	20.41				
Cooked medium [yield: approx. 31 oz. (1 lb. 15 oz.)]	1100	204.1			35.4	6.61		
Ronzoni Fettuccine #134, 12-oz. box	1320	240.0	110.0	20.00			(424)	(77.0)
Cooked medium [yield: approx. 37 oz. (2.3 lb.), 10.5 cups]	1320	240.0			35.4	6.45	(126)	(23.0)
"Al dente" [yield: approx. 30 oz. (1.9 lb.)]	1320	240.0			44.0	8.00		
"Tender" [yield: approx. 44 oz. (2.8 lb.)]	1320	240.0			30.0	5.45		
FLAKES								
Goodman's, 8-oz. box	880	160.0	110.0	20.00			(651)	(118.3)
Cooked medium [yield: approx. 25 oz. (1.6 lb.), 5.2 cups]	880	160.0			35.4	6.40	(168)	(30.4)
GOLDEN MEDIUM								
Mueller, 10-oz. bag	1100	204.1	110.0	20.41				
Cooked medium [yield: approx. 31 oz. (1 lb. 15 oz.)]	1100	204.1			35.4	6.61		
GOLDEN WIDE								
Mueller, 10-oz. bag	1100	204.1	110.0	20.41				
Cooked medium [yield: approx. 31 oz. (1 lb. 15 oz.)]	1100	204.1			35.4	6.61		
HEARTY								
Mueller, 1-lb. bag	1760	326.6	110.0	20.41			(169)	(31.3)
Cooked medium [yield: approx. 50 oz. (3.1 lb.), 18 cups]	1760	326.6			35.4	6.61	(98)	(18.3)
KLOPS								
Mueller, 8-oz. bag	880	163.3	110.0	20.41			(178)	(33.0)
Cooked medium [yield: approx. 25 oz. (1.6 lb.), 6.8 cups]	880	163.3			35.4	6.61	(130)	(24.2)
KLUSKI								
Mueller, 8-oz. bag	880	163.3	110.0	20.41				
Cooked medium [yield: approx. 25 oz. (1.6 lb.)]	880	163.3			35.4	6.61		
Pennsylvania Dutch, 8-oz. bag	840	160.0	105.0	20.00				
Cooked medium [yield: approx. 25 oz. (1.6 lb.)]	840	160.0			(34.0)	(6.48)		

	ENTIRE BOX		1 OZ., BY WT. DRY		1 OZ., BY WT. BOILED		1 CUP	
	Cal.	Carb.	Cal.	Carb.	Cal.	Carb.	Cal.	Carb.
MUNCHEN								
Mueller, 8-oz. bag	880	163.3	110.0	20.41				
Cooked medium [yield: approx. 25 oz. (1.6 lb.)]	880	163.3			35.4	6.61		
NOODLE LOOPS								
Ronzoni, 8-oz. box	880	160.0	110.0	20.00			(178)	(32.4)
Cooked medium [yield: approx. 25 oz. (1.6 lb.), 6.8 cups]	880	160.0			35.4	6.45	(130)	(120.0)
OLD FASHIONED								
Goodman's, 1-lb. box	1760	320.0	110.0	20.00			(242)	(27.6)
Cooked medium [yield: approx. 50 oz. (3.1 lb.), 9.6 cups]	1760	320.0			35.4	6.45	(184)	(33.6)
8-oz. box	880	160.0	110.0	20.00			(242)	(27.6)
Cooked medium [yield: approx. 25 oz. (1.6 lb.), 4.8 cups]	880	160.0			35.4	6.45	(184)	(33.6)
"Al dente" [yield: approx. 20 oz. (1.3 lb.)]	880	160.0			44.0	8.00		
"Tender" [yield: approx. 29 oz. (1.6 lb.)]	880	160.0			30.0	5.45		
OLD FASHIONED FINE								
Mueller, 1-lb. bag	1760	326.6	110.0	20.41				
Cooked medium [yield: approx. 50 oz. (3.1 lb.)]	1760	326.6			35.4	6.61		
8-oz. bag	880	163.3	110.0	20.41				
Cooked medium [yield: approx. 25 oz. (1.6 lb.)]	880	163.3			35.4	6.61		
OLD FASHIONED WIDE								
Mueller, 1-lb. bag	1760	326.6	110.0	20.41			(375)	(69.7)
Cooked medium [yield: approx. 50 oz. (3.1 lb.), 12.2 cups]	1760	326.6			35.4	6.61	(144)	(26.8)
8-oz. bag	880	163.3	110.0	20.41			(375)	(69.7)
Cooked medium [yield: approx. 25 oz. (1.6 lb.), 6.1 cups]	880	163.3			35.4	6.61	(144)	(26.8)
REGULAR FINE								
Mueller, 8-oz. bag	880	163.3	110.0	20.41				
Cooked medium [yield: approx. 25 oz. (1.6 lb.)]	880	163.3			35.4	6.61		
12-oz. bag	1320	244.9	110.0	20.41				
Cooked medium [yield: approx. 37 oz. (2.3 lb.)]	1320	244.9			35.4	6.61		
REGULAR MEDIUM								
Mueller, 8-oz. bag	880	163.3	110.0	20.41				
Cooked medium [yield: approx. 25 oz. (1.6 lb.)]	880	163.3			35.4	6.61		
12-oz. bag	1320	244.9	110.0	20.41				
Cooked medium [yield: approx. 37 oz. (2.3 lb.)]	1320	244.9			35.4	6.61		
REGULAR WIDE								
Mueller, 8-oz. bag	880	163.3	110.0	20.41				
Cooked medium [yield: approx. 25 oz. (1.6 lb.)]	880	163.3			35.4	6.61		
12-oz. bag	1320	244.9	110.0	20.41				
Cooked medium [yield: approx. 37 oz. (2.3 lb.)]	1320	244.9			35.4	6.61		
RUFFLES								
Pennsylvania Dutch Ruffles, 8-oz. bag	840	160.0	105.0	20.00				
Cooked medium [yield: approx. 25 oz. (1.6 lb.)]	840	160.0			(34.0)	(6.48)		
STROGANOFF								
Pennsylvania Dutch Stroganoff Noodles, 8-oz. bag	840	160.0	105.0	20.00			(169)	(32.1)
Cooked medium [yield: approx. 25 oz. (1.6 lb.), 5.2 cups]	840	160.0			(34.0)	(6.48)	(161)	(30.7)
ORIENTAL NOODLES								
China Bowl Cellophane Noodles, 3¾-oz. package	(362)	(88.1)	(96.4)	(23.48)				
Chinese Noodles, 10-oz. package	(1012)	(212.6)	(101.2)	(21.26)				
China Bowl Glutinous Rice Noodles, 8-oz. package	(814)	(171.0)	(101.8)	(21.38)			(204)	(42.8)
Rice Noodle Sticks, 7-oz. package	(715)	(162.3)	(102.1)	(23.19)				
HARD NOODLES (CRISP CHOW MEIN NOODLES)								
Chun King, 3-oz. can	385	na	128.3	na			(251)	na
La Choy, 16-oz. (1-lb.) can	2454	252.6	153.4	15.79			306	31.6
Wide, 7-oz. can	1047	111.8	149.5	15.98			298	32.0

	ENTIRE BOX		1 OZ., BY WT. DRY		1 OZ., BY WT. BOILED		1 CUP	
	Cal.	Carb.	Cal.	Carb.	Cal.	Carb.	Cal.	Carb.
SPINACH NOODLES								
SPINACH EGG NOODLES #156								
La Rosa Spinach Egg Noodles #156, 12-oz. box	1320	244.9	110.0	20.41				
Cooked medium [yield: approx. 37 oz. (2.3 lb.)]	1320	244.9			35.4	6.61		
Ronzoni Spinach Egg Noodles #156, 8-oz. box	880	160.0	110.0	20.00				
Cooked medium [yield: approx. 25 oz. (1.6 lb.)]	880	160.0			35.4	6.45		
"Al dente" [yield: approx. 20 oz. (1.3 lb.)]	880	160.0			44.0	8.00		
"Tender" [yield: approx. 29 oz. (1.6 lb.)]	880	160.0			30.0	5.45		
SPINACH LASAGNA								
Mannucci Spinach Lasagna, 14-oz. box	1464	298.5	104.6	21.32				
Cooked medium [yield: approx. 40 oz. (2.5 lb.)]	1464	298.5			(36.7)	(7.52)		
SPINACH MACARONI #15								
Buitoni High Protein Spinach Macaroni #115, 8-oz. box	840	148.0	104.6	18.50				
Cooked medium [yield: approx. 25 oz. (1.6 lb.)]	840	148.0			(36.7)	(6.43)		
WHOLE WHEAT And OTHER GRAIN PASTAS, by brand								
A Proten:								
Anellini Lo-Protein Imitation Vermicelli, 7.1-oz. package	431	105.6	60.7	14.87				
Cooked medium [yield: approx. 17.1 oz. (1.1 lb.), 2.2 cups]	431	105.6			25.2	6.18	196	48.0
Ditalini Lo-Protein Imitation Macaroni, 8.8-oz. package	456	112.0	51.8	12.73				
Cooked medium [yield: approx. 13.7 oz. (0.9 lb.), 4 cups]	456	112.0			33.1	8.14	114	28.0
Rigatini Lo-Protein Imitation Macaroni, 8.8-oz. package	456	112.0	51.8	12.73				
Cooked medium [yield: approx. 13.7 oz. (0.9 lb.), 4 cups]	456	112.0			33.1	8.14	114	28.0
Spaghettini Lo-Protein Imitation Noodles, 8.8-oz. package	713	176.7	81.0	20.08				
Cooked medium [yield: approx. 27.9 oz. (1.7 lb.), 3⅓ cups]	713	176.7			25.6	6.33	214	53.0
Tagliatelle Lo-Protein Imitation Noodles, 8.8-oz. package	800	176.7	90.9	20.08				
Cooked medium [yield: approx. 28.2 oz. (1.8 lb.), 3⅓ cups]	800	176.7			28.4	6.26	240	53.0
Alimento:								
Whole Wheat Lasagna, 1-lb. box	1674	341.1	104.6	21.32				
Cooked medium [yield: approx. 50 oz. (3.1 lb.)]	1674	341.1			36.7	7.52		
"Al dente" [yield: approx. 40 oz. (2.5 lb.)]	1674	341.1			41.9	8.53		
"Tender" [yield: approx. 52 oz. (3.3 lb.)]	1674	341.1			31.4	6.52		
Whole Wheat Ribbons, 12-oz. box	1255	255.8	104.6	21.32				
Cooked medium [yield: approx. 37 oz. (2.3 lb.)]	1255	255.8			36.7	7.52		
Whole Wheat Shells, 1-lb. box	1674	341.1	104.6	21.32				
Cooked medium [yield: approx. 50 oz. (3.1 lb.)]	1674	341.1			36.7	7.52		
Golden Harvest:								
Curly Macaroni (Wheat Soy Spaghetti made with Wheat Gluten), 12-oz. box	1260	216.0	105.0	18.00				
Cooked medium [yield: approx. 37 oz. (2.3 lb.)]	1260	216.0			36.7	6.17		
"Al dente" [yield: approx. 30 oz. (1.9 lb.)]	1260	216.0			41.9	8.53		
"Tender" [yield: approx. 40 oz. (2.5 lb.)]	1260	216.0			31.4	6.52		

	ENTIRE BOX Cal.	ENTIRE BOX Carb.	1 OZ., BY WT. DRY Cal.	1 OZ., BY WT. DRY Carb.	1 OZ., BY WT. BOILED Cal.	1 OZ., BY WT. BOILED Carb.	1 CUP Cal.	1 CUP Carb.
"Thin" Spaghetti (Wheat Soy Spaghetti made with Wheat Gluten), 1-lb. box	1680	288.0	105.0	18.00				
Cooked medium [yield: approx. 46 oz. (2.9 lb.)]	1680	288.0			36.7	6.17		
Wheat Free Pasta Corn Ribbons, 10-oz. package	1050	220.0	105.0	22.00				
Wheat Free Pasta Elbows, 12-oz. package	1260	264.0	105.0	22.00				
Wheat Free Pasta Medium Shells, 12-oz. package	1260	264.0	105.0	22.00				
Wheat Free Pasta Spaghetti Substitute, 12-oz. package	1260	264.0	105.0	22.00				
Whole Wheat Egg Noodles, 12-oz. package	1380	288.0	115.0	24.00				
Cooked medium [yield: approx. 39.3 oz. (2½ lb.)]	1380	288.0			(35.1)	(7.33)		
Whole Wheat Elbow Macaroni, 12-oz. package	1380	288.0	115.0	24.00				
Cooked medium [yield: approx. 39.3 oz. (2½ lb.)]	1380	288.0			(35.1)	(7.33)		
Whole Wheat Lasagna, 10-oz. package	1150	240.0	115.0	24.00				
Cooked medium [yield: approx. 32.8 oz. (2 lb.)]	1150	240.0			(35.1)	(7.33)		
Whole Wheat Shell Macaroni, 8-oz. package	920	192.0	115.0	24.00				
Cooked medium [yield: approx. 26.2 oz. (1.6 lb.)]	920	192.0			(35.1)	(7.33)		
Whole Wheat Thin Spaghetti, 1-lb. package	1840	384.0	115.0	24.00				
Cooked medium [yield: approx. 52.4 oz. (3.3 lb.)]	1840	384.0			(35.1)	(7.33)		
Whole Wheat Ziti Macaroni, 8-oz. package	920	192.0	115.0	24.00				
Cooked medium [yield: approx. 26.6 oz. (1.6 lb.)]	920	192.0			(35.1)	(7.33)		

SPAGHETTI SAUCE (see also the BASIC BAKING & COOKING INGREDIENTS chapter)

	ENTIRE CONTAINER Cal.	ENTIRE CONTAINER Carb.	1 OZ., BY WT. Cal.	1 OZ., BY WT. Carb.	1 CUP Cal.	1 CUP Carb.	1 TABLE-SPOON Cal.	1 TABLE-SPOON Carb.
Ann Page (A & P) Flavored With Meat Spaghetti Sauce, 32-oz. (2-lb.) jar	640	96.0	20.0	3.00	(175)	(26.2)	(11)	(1.6)
Marinara Spaghetti Sauce, 32-oz. (2-lb.) jar	560	104.0	17.5	3.25	(153)	(28.4)	(10)	(1.8)
Meatless, No Mushrooms, "Plain" Spaghetti Sauce, 32-oz. (2-lb.) jar	560	104.0	17.5	3.25	(153)	(28.4)	(10)	(1.8)
Meatless, With Mushrooms, Spaghetti Sauce, 32-oz. (2-lb.) jar	560	104.0	17.5	3.25	(153)	(28.4)	(10)	(1.8)
Buitoni Marinara Sauce, 10¼-oz. can	174	20.3	17.0	1.98	(149)	(17.3)	(9)	(1.1)
15-oz. jar	255	29.7	17.0	1.98	(149)	(17.3)	(9)	(1.1)
29-oz. jar	493	57.4	17.0	1.98	(149)	(17.3)	(9)	(1.1)
Meatless Sauce, 10¼-oz. can	195	24.4	19.0	2.38	(166)	(20.8)	(10)	(1.3)
15-oz. jar	285	35.7	19.0	2.38	(166)	(20.8)	(10)	(1.3)
29-oz. jar	551	69.0	19.0	2.38	(166)	(20.8)	(10)	(1.3)
Mushroom Sauce, 10¼-oz. can	174	19.5	17.0	1.90	(149)	(16.6)	(9)	(1.0)
15-oz. jar	255	28.5	17.0	1.90	(149)	(16.6)	(9)	(1.0)
29-oz. jar	493	55.1	17.0	1.90	(149)	(16.6)	(9)	(1.0)
Red Clam Sauce, 10¼-oz. can	267	3.5	26.0	0.34	(227)	(3.0)	(14)	(0.2)
White Clam Sauce, 10¼-oz. can	359	5.5	35.0	0.54	(306)	(4.7)	(19)	(0.3)
Contadina Tomato Sauce, 8-oz. jar	82	17.4	10.3	2.17	90	19.0	6	1.2
15-oz. jar	155	32.6	10.3	2.17	90	19.0	6	1.2
Del Monte Tomato Sauce, 8-oz. can	80	17.0	10.0	2.13	80	17.0	5	1.1
15-oz. can	150	31.9	10.0	2.13	80	17.0	5	1.1
Tomato Sauce With Mushrooms, 8-oz. can	100	22.0	12.5	2.75	100	22.0	6	1.4
Tomato Sauce With Onion, 8-oz. can	100	23.0	12.5	2.88	100	23.0	6	1.4
Tomato Sauce With Tidbits, 15-oz. can	150	35.6	10.0	2.38	80	19.0	5	1.2
Durkee Mushroom Spaghetti Sauce Mix, 1¼-oz. envelope	69	16.0	55.2	12.80				
Prepared as package directs, add 6 oz. tomato paste and 2 cups water (yield: approx. 2⅔ cups)	208	48.0	(9.0)	(2.10)	78	18.0	5	1.1
Spaghetti Sauce Mix, 1½-oz. envelope	85	20.0	56.7	13.30				
Prepared as package directs, add 6 oz. tomato paste and 1¾ cups water (yield: approx. 2½ cups)	224	52.0	(10.7)	(2.50)	90	20.8	6	1.3
Featherweight low-sodium Spaghetti Sauce, 14½-oz. jar	232	29.0	16.0	2.00	(140)	(17.5)	(9)	(1.1)
French's Italian Style Spaghetti Sauce Mix, 1½-oz. envelope	120	20.0	80.0	13.33				
Prepared as package directs, add 6 oz. tomato paste, 2 tablespoons cooking oil, 1¾ cups water (yield: approx. 2½ cups)	400	52.0	(17.8)	(2.31)	160	20.8	10	1.3
Spaghetti Sauce With Mushrooms Mix, 1¼-oz. envelope	120	20.0	96.0	16.00				
Prepared as package directs, add 6 oz. tomato paste, 2 tablespoons cooking oil, 1¾ cups water (yield: approx. 2½ cups)	400	52.0	(17.8)	(2.31)	160	20.8	10	1.3
Ragu Chunky Gardenstyle Spaghetti Sauce, Extra Tomatoes, Garlic, and Onions, 15½-oz. jar	310	54.3	20.0	3.50	172	30.1	11	1.9
32-oz. (2-lb.) jar	640	112.0	20.0	3.50	172	30.1	11	1.9
48-oz. (3-lb.) jar	960	168.0	20.0	3.50	172	30.1	11	1.9
Chunky Gardenstyle Spaghetti Sauce, Green Pepper and Mushrooms, 15½-oz. jar	310	54.3	20.0	3.50	172	30.1	11	1.9
32-oz. (2-lb.) jar	640	112.0	20.0	3.50	172	30.1	11	1.9
48-oz. (3-lb.) jar	960	168.0	20.0	3.50	172	30.1	11	1.9
Chunky Gardenstyle Spaghetti Sauce, Italian Garden Combo, 15½-oz. jar	310	54.3	20.0	3.50	172	30.1	11	1.9
32-oz. (2-lb.) jar	640	112.0	20.0	3.50	172	30.1	11	1.9
48-oz. (3-lb.) jar	960	168.0	20.0	3.50	172	30.1	11	1.9
Chunky Gardenstyle Spaghetti Sauce, Mushrooms and Onions, 15½-oz. jar	310	54.3	20.0	3.50	172	30.1	11	1.9
32-oz. (2-lb.) jar	640	112.0	20.0	3.50	172	30.1	11	1.9
48-oz. (3-lb.) jar	960	168.0	20.0	3.50	172	30.1	11	1.9
Chunky Gardenstyle Spaghetti Sauce, Sweet Green and Red Peppers, 15½-oz. jar	310	54.3	20.0	3.50	172	30.1	11	1.9
32-oz. (2-lb.) jar	640	112.0	20.0	3.50	172	30.1	11	1.9
48-oz. (3-lb.) jar	960	168.0	20.0	3.50	172	30.1	11	1.9
Extra Thick and Zesty Spaghetti Sauce, Plain, 15½-oz. jar	388	58.1	25.0	3.75	235	35.3	15	2.2
32-oz. (2-lb.) jar	800	120.0	25.0	3.75	235	35.3	15	2.2
48-oz. (3-lb.) jar	1200	180.0	25.0	3.75	235	35.3	15	2.2
Extra Thick and Zesty Spaghetti Sauce, Meat, 15½-oz. jar	388	54.3	25.0	3.50	235	33.0	15	2.1
32-oz. (2-lb.) jar	800	112.0	25.0	3.50	235	33.0	15	2.1
48-oz. (3-lb.) jar	1200	168.0	25.0	3.50	235	33.0	15	2.1
Extra Thick and Zesty Spaghetti Sauce, Mushroom, 15½-oz. jar	426	50.4	27.5	3.25	259	30.6	16	1.9
32-oz. (2-lb.) jar	880	104.0	27.5	3.25	259	30.6	16	1.9
48-oz. (3-lb.) jar	1320	156.0	27.5	3.25	259	30.6	16	1.9
Homestyle Spaghetti Sauce, Plain, 15½-oz. jar	271	46.5	17.5	3.00	148	26.2	9	1.6
32-oz. (2-lb.) jar	560	96.0	17.5	3.00	148	26.2	9	1.6
48-oz. (3-lb.) jar	840	144.0	17.5	3.00	148	26.2	9	1.6
Homestyle Spaghetti Sauce, Meat, 15½-oz. jar	310	46.5	20.0	3.00	169	25.4	11	1.6
32-oz. (2-lb.) jar	640	96.0	20.0	3.00	169	25.4	11	1.6
48-oz. (3-lb.) jar	960	144.0	20.0	3.00	169	25.4	11	1.6
Homestyle Spaghetti Sauce, Mushroom, 15½-oz. jar	271	46.5	17.5	3.00	148	25.4	9	1.6
32-oz. (2-lb.) jar	560	96.0	17.5	3.00	148	25.4	9	1.6
48-oz. (3-lb.) jar	840	144.0	17.5	3.00	148	25.4	9	1.6
Old World Style Spaghetti Sauce, Plain, 15½-oz. jar	310	42.6	20.0	2.75	169	23.2	11	1.5
32-oz. (2-lb.) jar	640	88.0	20.0	2.75	169	23.2	11	1.5
48-oz. (3-lb.) jar	960	132.0	20.0	2.75	169	23.2	11	1.5

	ENTIRE CONTAINER		1 OZ., BY WT.		1 CUP		1 TABLE-SPOON	
	Cal.	Carb.	Cal.	Carb.	Cal.	Carb.	Cal.	Carb.
Old World Style Spaghetti Sauce, Extra Cheese, 15½-oz. jar	310	42.6	20.0	2.75	169	23.2	11	1.5
32-oz. (2-lb.) jar	640	88.0	20.0	2.75	169	23.2	11	1.5
48-oz. (3-lb.) jar	960	132.0	20.0	2.75	169	23.2	11	1.5
Old World Style Spaghetti Sauce, Extra Garlic, 15½-oz. jar	310	42.6	20.0	2.75	169	23.2	11	1.5
32-oz. (2-lb.) jar	640	88.0	20.0	2.75	169	23.2	11	1.5
48-oz. (3-lb.) jar	960	132.0	20.0	2.75	169	23.2	11	1.5
Old World Style Spaghetti Sauce, Marinara, 15½-oz. jar	349	46.5	22.5	3.00	190	26.2	12	1.6
32-oz. (2-lb.) jar	720	96.0	22.5	3.00	190	26.2	12	1.6
48-oz. (3-lb.) jar	1080	144.0	22.5	3.00	190	26.2	12	1.6
Old World Style Spaghetti Sauce, Meat, 15½-oz. jar	310	42.6	20.0	2.75	169	23.2	11	1.6
32-oz. (2-lb.) jar	640	88.0	20.0	2.75	169	23.2	11	1.6
48-oz. (3-lb.) jar	960	132.0	20.0	2.75	169	23.2	11	1.6

	ENTIRE CONTAINER		1 OZ., BY WT.		1 CUP		1 TABLE-SPOON	
	Cal.	Carb.	Cal.	Carb.	Cal.	Carb.	Cal.	Carb.
Old World Style Spaghetti Sauce, Mushroom, 15½-oz. jar	349	34.9	22.5	2.25	190	20.3	12	1.3
32-oz. (2-lb.) jar	720	72.0	22.5	2.25	190	20.3	12	1.3
48-oz. (3-lb.) jar	1080	108.0	22.5	2.25	190	20.3	12	1.3
Ronzoni All-Purpose Meatless Sauce, 15-oz. jar	169	26.3	11.3	1.75	(98)	(15.3)	(6)	(1.0)
Lite 'n' Natural, Spaghetti Sauce Flavored With Italian Sausage, 15-oz. jar	188	26.3	12.5	1.75	(109)	(15.3)	(7)	(1.0)
Marinara Sauce, 15-oz. jar	169	26.3	11.3	1.75	(98)	(15.3)	(6)	(1.0)
Spaghetti Sauce Flavored With Meat, 15-oz. jar	188	26.3	12.5	1.75	(109)	(15.3)	(7)	(1.0)
Stokely Tomato Sauce, 8-oz. can	65	12.0	8.1	1.50	70	13.0	4	0.8
15-oz. can	122	22.5	8.1	1.50	70	13.0	4	0.8

10 COMBINATION MAIN DISHES •

FROZEN DINNERS AND ENTREES

	UNIT Cal.	UNIT Carb.	1 OZ., BY WT. Cal.	1 OZ., BY WT. Carb.
A&P				
Batter-Dipped Fish & Chips, 16-oz. (1-lb.) package	750	81.0	46.9	5.06
8 Batter-Dipped Fish Portions, 24-oz. package	1440	128.0	60.0	5.33
1 fish portion, approx. 3 oz.	180	16.0	60.0	5.33
14 Batter-Dipped Fish Sticks, 14-oz. package	880	76.0	62.9	5.43
1 fish stick, approx. 1 oz.	63	5.4	62.9	5.43
Crispy Scallops, 7-oz. box	480	50.0	68.6	7.14
Crispy Shrimp, 6-oz. box	460	50.0	76.7	8.33
6 Fish Cakes, 12-oz. box	750	87.0	62.5	7.25
1 fish cake, approx. 2 oz.	125	14.5	62.5	7.25
7 Fish Sandwich Portions, 14-oz. package	910	91.0	65.0	6.50
1 sandwich portion, approx. 2 oz.	130	16.0	65.0	6.50
10 Fish Sticks, 8-oz. box	480	48.0	60.0	6.00
1 fish stick, approx. 0.8 oz.	48	4.8	60.0	6.00
BANQUET DINNERS, including Cookin' Bags, and Man-Pleaser Dinners				
BBQ Sauce with Sliced Beef Cookin' Bag (barbecue sauce, sliced beef), 5-oz. bag	126	12.5	25.2	2.50
Beans & Frankfurters Dinner (beans, frankfurters, sauce, carrots and peas, corn bread), 10¾-oz. tray	591	63.1	55.0	5.87
Beef Chop Suey Buffet Supper, 32-oz. (2-lb.) package	418	39.1	13.1	1.22
Beef Chop Suey Cookin' Bag (beef chop suey, no rice), 7-oz. bag	73	9.5	10.4	1.36
Beef Chop Suey Dinner (beef chop suey, rice), 12-oz. tray	282	38.8	23.5	3.23
Beef Dinner (beef, gravy, mashed potatoes, carrots), 11-oz. tray	312	24.9	28.4	1.90
Beef Enchilada with Cheese and Chili Gravy Buffet Dinner, 32-oz. (2-lb.) package	1118	118.2	34.9	3.69
Beef Enchilada Dinner (beef enchiladas, chili gravy, refried beans, rice), 12-oz. tray	479	63.6	39.9	5.30
2 Beef Enchiladas with Sauce Cookin' Bag (beef enchiladas, sauce), 6-oz. bag	207	28.9	34.5	4.82
Beef Stew Buffet Supper, 32-oz. (2-lb.) package	700	90.9	21.9	2.84
Cheese Enchilada Dinner (cheese enchiladas, chili gravy, refried beans, rice), 12-oz. tray	459	58.8	38.3	4.90
Chicken à la King Cookin' Bag, 5-oz. bag	138	10.4	27.6	2.08
Chicken Chow Mein Buffet Supper, 32-oz. (2-lb.) package	345	36.4	10.8	1.14
Chicken Chow Mein Cookin' Bag (chicken chow mein, no noodles), 7-oz. bag	89	9.7	12.7	1.39
Chicken Chow Mein Dinner (chicken chow mein, rice, no noodles), 12-oz. tray	282	38.8	23.5	3.23
Chicken and Dumplings Buffet Supper, 32-oz. (2-lb.) package	1209	128.2	37.8	4.01
Chicken Man-Pleaser Dinner (chicken, mashed potatoes, carrots and peas, apple cobbler), 17-oz. tray	1026	89.2	60.4	5.25
Chicken and Noodles Buffet Supper, 32-oz. (2-lb.) package	764	79.1	23.9	2.47
Chopped Beef Dinner (chopped beef, gravy, mashed potatoes, carrots), 11-oz. tray	443	32.8	40.3	2.98
Corned Beef Hash Dinner (corned beef hash, carrots and peas, corn bread), 10-oz. tray	372	42.6	37.2	4.26
Creamed Chipped Beef Cookin' Bag (creamed chipped beef), 5-oz. bag	124	10.5	24.8	2.10
Fish Dinner [breaded fried fish (pollock), carrots and peas, potato puffs], 8¾-oz. tray	382	43.6	43.7	4.98
Fried Chicken Dinner (chicken, mashed potatoes, carrots), 11-oz. tray	530	48.4	48.2	4.40
Gravy and Sliced Beef Cookin' Bag (gravy, sliced beef), 5-oz. bag	116	4.8	23.2	0.96
Haddock Dinner (Haddock, potato puffs, carrots and peas), 8¾-oz. tray	419	45.4	47.9	5.19
Ham Dinner (ham, barbecue sauce, candied yams, carrots and peas, corn bread), 10-oz. tray	369	47.7	36.9	4.77
Italian Style Dinner (mostaccioli, meatballs, sauce, garlic bread), 11-oz. tray	446	44.6	40.5	4.05
Macaroni and Beef Buffet Supper, 32-oz. (2-lb.) container	1000	106.4	31.3	3.31
Macaroni and Beef Dinner, 12-oz. tray	394	55.1	32.8	4.59
Macaroni and Cheese Buffet Supper, 32-oz. (2-lb.) container	1027	110.1	32.1	3.44
Macaroni and Cheese Cookin' Bag, 8-oz. package	261	28.6	32.6	3.58
Macaroni and Cheese Dinner (macaroni, cheese), 12-oz. tray	326	45.6	27.2	3.80
Macaroni and Cheese Entrée (macaroni, cheese), 8-oz. tray	279	36.9	34.9	4.61
Meat Loaf Buffet Supper, 32-oz. (2-lb.) package	1445	464.0	45.2	14.50
Meat Loaf Cookin' Bag (meat loaf, tomato sauce), 5-oz. bag	224	13.6	44.8	2.72
Meat Loaf Dinner (meat loaf, tomato sauce, mashed potatoes, carrots and peas), 11-oz. tray	412	29.0	37.5	2.64
Meat Loaf Man-Pleaser Dinner (meat loaf, tomato sauce, mashed potatoes, carrots and peas, apple strudel), 18-oz. tray	916	63.6	50.9	3.53
Mexican Style Combination Dinner (beef enchiladas, chili gravy, refried beans, beef tacos), 12-oz. tray	571	72.1	47.6	6.01
Mexican Style Dinner (tamale, beef enchilada, chili gravy, refried beans, rice), 16-oz. (1-lb.) tray	608	73.5	38.0	4.59
Noodles and Beef Buffet Dinner, 32-oz. (2-lb.) package	754	83.6	23.6	2.61
Salisbury Steak Dinner (Salisbury steak, gravy, mashed potatoes, carrots and peas), 11-oz. tray	390	24.0	35.5	2.18
Salisbury Steak and Gravy Buffet Supper, 32-oz. (2-lb.) package	1454	48.2	45.4	1.51
Salisbury Steak and Gravy Cookin' Bag (Salisbury steak, gravy), 5-oz. bag	246	7.8	49.2	1.56
Salisbury Steak Man-Pleaser Dinner (Salisbury steak, mashed potatoes, carrots and peas, apple cobbler), 19-oz. tray	873	17.7	45.9	0.93
Sliced Beef and Gravy, 32-oz. (2-lb.) package	782	34.5	24.4	1.08
Sliced Turkey and Giblet Gravy, Cookin' Bag (giblet gravy, sliced turkey), 5-oz. bag	98	5.3	19.6	1.06

	UNIT Cal.	UNIT Carb.	1 OZ., BY WT. Cal.	1 OZ., BY WT. Carb.
Spaghetti and Meatballs, 11½-oz. tray	405	46.4	35.2	4.03
32-oz. (2-lb.) container	1127	129.1	35.2	4.03
Spaghetti and Meatballs Dinner, 11½-oz. tray	450	62.9	39.1	5.47
Spaghetti with Meat Sauce Entrée (spaghetti, meat sauce), 8-oz. tray	311	31.3	38.9	3.91
Turkey Dinner (turkey, gravy, dressing, mashed potatoes, carrots), 11-oz. tray	293	27.8	26.6	2.53
Turkey and Giblet Gravy Buffet Supper, 32-oz. (2-lb.) package	564	28.2	17.6	0.88
Turkey Man-Pleaser Dinner (turkey, gravy, dressing, mashed potatoes, carrots and peas, cherry strudel), 19-oz. tray	620	73.8	34.4	3.88
Veal Parmesan Cookin' Bag (breaded veal parmesan), 5-oz. bag	287	19.5	57.4	4.88
Veal Parmesan Dinner [breaded veal (beef added) patty, tomato sauce, mashed potatoes, peas], 11-oz. tray	421	42.1	38.3	3.83
Veal Parmesan with Tomato Sauce Buffet Supper, 32-oz. (2-lb.) package	1563	119.1	48.8	3.72
Western Dinner (gravy, beef patty, beans, chili sauce, fried potatoes), 11-oz. tray	417	32.4	37.9	2.95
BOIL-IN-BAG ENTREES And TOAST TOPPERS), see GREEN GIANT				
BOOTH FISHERIES				
Fishsticks, 16-oz. (1-lb.) package, 16 fishsticks	880	100.0	55.0	6.25
1 fishstick, approx. 1 oz.	55	6.3	55.0	6.25
BUITONI				
Cheese Ravioli, 11-oz. tray, 12 ravioli	747	83.1	67.9	7.56
1 ravioli, approx. 0.9 oz.	62	6.9	67.9	7.56
15-oz. tray, 40 ravioli	1194	181.4	79.6	12.09
1 ravioli, approx. 0.38 oz.	30	4.5	79.6	12.09
Cheese Ravioli Parmesan, 12-oz. tray	456	70.2	38.0	5.85
Eggplant Parmesan, 12-oz. tray	624	57.7	52.0	4.81
Lasagne with Meat Sauce Casserole, 14-oz. tray	596	74.6	42.6	5.33
Manicotti filled with Ricotta Cheese, without sauce, 17-oz. package	839	91.8	49.3	5.40
Manicotti in Sauce, 14-oz. tray	616	70.1	44.0	5.01
Meat Ravioli, 15-oz. tray, 40 ravioli	1281	182.2	85.4	12.15
1 ravioli, approx. 0.38 oz.	32	4.6	85.4	12.15
Meat Ravioli Parmesan, 12-oz. tray	576	61.6	48.0	5.13
Sausage and Peppers with Mostaccioli Rigati, 19-oz. tray	784	56.4	41.3	2.97
Shells in Sauce, 12-oz. tray	408	74.4	34.0	6.20
Shrimp Marinara with Shells, 17-oz. tray	486	80.5	28.6	4.73
Veal Parmesan with Spaghetti Twists, 19-oz. tray	767	77.8	40.4	4.09
Ziti in Sauce, Baked, 12-oz. tray	408	77.2	34.0	6.43
CELANTANO				
Eggplant Parmigiana, 12-oz. box	660	38.0	55.0	6.33
26-oz. box	1400	80.0	53.8	12.31
Lasagna, 26-oz. box	1120	104.0	43.1	4.00
Manicotti, 18-oz. box, 5 manicotti	970	70.0	53.9	3.89
1 manicotti, approx. 3.6 oz.	194	14.0	53.9	3.89
Ravioli, 13-oz. box, 12 ravioli	820	80.0	63.1	6.15
1 ravioli, approx. 1.1 oz.	68	6.7	63.1	6.15
Ricotta Cavatelli, 15-oz. box	1290	249.0	86.0	16.60
Stuffed Shells (Conconi Stufati), 9-oz. box, 6 shells	892	76.0	99.1	8.44
1 shell, approx. 1.5 oz.	149	12.7	99.1	8.44
COOKIN' BAG, see BANQUET				
COUNTRY TABLE DINNERS And ENTREES, see MORTON				
GOLDEN				
Cheese Blintzes, 15-oz. box, 6 blintzes	1278	23.2	85.2	1.55
1 blintz, approx. 2.5 oz.	213	3.9	85.2	1.55
GREEN GIANT, including Boil-in-Bags and Toast Toppers				
Beef Stew and Biscuits Oven Bake Entrée, 14-oz. package	365	83.4	26.1	5.95
Chicken à la King Boil-in-Bag Toast Topper, 5-oz. pouch	170	80.0	34.0	1.60
Chicken and Biscuits Oven Bake Entrée, 14-oz. package	389	37.3	27.8	2.67
Chicken Chow Mein without Noodles Dinner, Boil-in-Bag Entrée, 9-oz. pouch	130	15.0	14.4	1.67
Chicken and Noodles, Boil-in-Bag Entrée, 9-oz. pouch	250	24.0	27.8	2.67
Creamed Tuna with Peas, Boil-in-Bag Toast Topper, 5-oz. pouch	140	11.0	28.0	2.20
Gravy and Sliced Beef, Boil-in-Bag Toast Topper, 5-oz. pouch	130	7.0	26.0	1.40
Gravy and Sliced Turkey, Boil-in-Bag Toast Topper, 5-oz. pouch	100	70.0	20.0	1.40
Lasagna with Meat and Sauce, 14-oz. container	588	55.6	42.0	3.97
Macaroni and Beef with Tomato Sauce, Boil-in-Bag Entrée, 9-oz. pouch	240	31.0	26.7	3.44
Macaroni and Cheese, Boil-in-Bag Entrée, 9-oz. pouch	330	36.0	36.7	4.00
Macaroni and Cheese Oven Bake Entrée, 16-oz. (1-lb.) container	571	145.1	35.7	9.07
Salisbury Steak with Gravy Oven Bake Entrée, 14-oz. package	547	55.6	39.1	3.97
Salisbury Steaks with Tomato Sauce, Boil-in-Bag Entrée, 9-oz. pouch	390	22.0	43.3	2.44
Sloppy Joe Seasoned with Tomato Sauce and Beef, Boil-in-Bag Toast Topper, 5-oz. pouch	160	15.0	32.0	3.00
Spaghetti and Meatballs with Tomato Sauce, Boil-in-Bag Entrée, 9-oz. pouch	280	30.0	31.1	3.33
Stuffed Cabbage Rolls with Beef in Tomato Sauce, 14-oz. package	417	32.9	29.8	2.35
Stuffed Green Peppers with Beef in Creole Sauce, 14-oz. package	400	36.1	28.6	2.58
Veal Parmigiana, Breaded, made with Veal Patties, 14-oz. container	619	36.5	44.2	2.61
Welsh Rarebit Seasoned with Cheddar and Swiss Cheese, Boil-in-Bag Toast Topper, 5-oz. pouch	220	12.0	44.0	2.40
HUNGRY MAN DINNERS And ENTREES), see SWANSON				
LA CHOY Dinners and Entrees				
Beef Chow Mein Dinner (chow mein, sweet and sour pork, rice, egg rolls, apple dessert rolls), 11-oz. tray	342	55.6	31.1	5.05
Beef Chow Mein Entrée (chow mein), 16-oz. (1-lb.) tray	194	23.2	12.1	1.43
Chicken Chow Mein Dinner (chow mein, sweet and sour pork, rice, egg rolls, apple dessert rolls), 11-oz. tray	354	7.6	32.2	0.69
Chicken Chow Mein Entrée (chow mein), 16-oz. (1-lb.) tray	215	18.2	13.4	1.14
Fried Rice and Pork Entrée (fried rice and pork), 12-oz. tray	490	77.6	40.9	6.47
Pepper Oriental Dinner (vegetables, sauce, beef, sweet and sour pork, rice, egg rolls, apple dessert rolls), 11-oz. tray	349	7.3	31.7	0.66
Pepper Oriental Entrée (pepper oriental), 15-oz. tray	207	23.0	13.8	1.53
Shrimp Chow Mein Dinner (chow mein, sweet and sour pork, fried rice, egg rolls, apple dessert rolls), 11-oz. tray	325	5.6	29.5	0.51
Shrimp Chow Mein Entrée (chow mein), 16-oz. (1-lb.) tray	147	21.8	9.2	1.36
Sweet & Sour Pork Entrée (sweet and sour pork), 15-oz. tray	460	90.7	30.6	6.04
LAND O' LAKES				
Breaded Turkey Breast Fillets with Cheese, 10-oz. package (approx. 2 fillets)	270	9.0	27.0	0.90
1 fillet, approx. 5 oz.	135	4.5	27.0	0.90
Breaded Turkey Patties, 13.5-oz. package, approx. 6 patties	1080	60.0	80.0	4.40
1 patty, approx. 2¼ oz.	180	9.9	80.0	4.40
Turkey Sticks, 10-oz. package, approx. 10 sticks	800	45.0	80.0	4.50
1 stick, approx. 1 oz.	80	4.5	80.0	4.50
LEAN CUISINE, see STOUFFER'S LEAN CUISINE				
LE MENU DINNERS, see SWANSON				
MAN-PLEASER DINNERS, see BANQUET				
MORTON, including Steak House Dinners and Country Table Dinners and Entrées				
Beans and Beef Franks Dinner (beans, frankfurters, tomato sauce, sliced apples, cornbread), 10¾-oz. tray	530	79.0	49.3	7.25
Beef Dinner (sliced beef, gravy, mashed potatoes, seasoned carrots), 10-oz. tray	260	20.0	26.0	2.00
Beef Enchilada Dinner (enchiladas, chili gravy, cheese, beans, rice), 12-oz. tray	350	47.0	29.2	3.92
Beef Tenderloin Steak, Steak House Dinner (filet mignon, fried tater bites, fried onion rings), 9½-oz. tray	890	43.0	93.7	4.53
Boneless Chicken Dinner (chicken, dressing, gravy, mashed potatoes, seasoned carrots and peas), 10-oz. tray	230	24.0	23.0	2.40
Chicken 'N Dumplings Dinner (chicken, dumplings, gravy, mashed potatoes, seasoned carrots and peas), 11-oz. tray	280	30.0	25.5	2.73
Chicken 'N Noodles Dinner (chicken, noodles, sliced apples, seasoned carrots and peas), 10¼-oz. tray	260	40.0	25.4	3.90
Chopped Sirloin Steak, Steak House Dinner (steak, fried steak house potatoes, fried diced onion rings), 9½-oz. tray	760	43.0	80.0	4.53
Fish Dinner (breaded fish, whipped potatoes, seasoned carrots and peas), 9-oz. tray	260	22.0	28.9	2.44
Fried Chicken Country Table Dinner (fried chicken, whipped potatoes, seasoned carrots and peas, cornbread, apple/cranberry treat), 15-oz. tray	710	96.0	47.3	6.40
Fried Chicken Country Table Entrée (fried chicken and whipped potatoes), 12-oz. tray	600	26.0	50.0	2.17
Fried Chicken Dinner (fried chicken, mashed potatoes, seasoned carrots), 11-oz. tray	460	49.0	41.8	4.45
Ham Dinner (sliced ham, sauce, sliced apples, seasoned carrots and peas, sweet potatoes), 10-oz. tray	440	57.0	44.0	5.70
Macaroni and Beef Dinner (macaroni, meat sauce, sliced apples, carrots and peas), 10-oz. tray	260	46.0	26.0	4.60
Macaroni and Cheese Dinner (macaroni, cheese, sliced apples, seasoned carrots), 11-oz. tray	320	54.0	29.1	4.91
Meat Loaf Country Table Dinner (meat loaf, tomato sauce, whipped potatoes, seasoned carrots and peas, spaghetti, apple cobbler), 15-oz. tray	480	59.0	32.0	3.93
Meat Loaf Dinner (meat loaf, tomato sauce, mashed potatoes, seasoned carrots and peas), 11-oz. tray	340	28.0	30.9	2.55
Mexican Style Dinner (tamale, beef enchilada, chili gravy, cheese, beans, rice), 12-oz. tray	410	50.0	34.2	4.17

	UNIT Cal.	UNIT Carb.	1 OZ., BY WT. Cal.	1 OZ., BY WT. Carb.
Rib Eye Steak, Steak House Dinner (steak, fried crinkle cut potatoes, fried diced onion rings), 9-oz. tray	820	38.0	91.1	4.22
Salisbury Steak Country Table Dinner (Salisbury steak, gravy, whipped potatoes, seasoned carrots and peas, macaroni and cheese, peach cobbler), 15-oz. tray	500	62.0	33.3	4.13
Salisbury Steak Country Table Entrée (Salisbury steak, gravy, tater bites), 10¼-oz. tray	500	36.0	48.8	3.51
Salisbury Steak Dinner (Salisbury steak, gravy, mashed potatoes, seasoned carrots), 11-oz. tray	290	25.0	26.4	2.27
Sirloin Strip Steak Dinner (steak, fried tater rounds, fried diced onion rings), 9½-oz. tray	760	43.0	80.0	4.53
Sliced Beef Country Table Dinner (beef, gravy, whipped potatoes, seasoned carrots and peas, macaroni and cheese, brownie), 14-oz. tray	510	57.0	36.4	4.07
Sliced Turkey Country Table Dinner (turkey, gravy, dressing, whipped potatoes, seasoned carrots and peas, brownie, apple-cranberry treat), 15-oz. tray	550	80.0	36.7	5.33
Sliced Turkey Country Table Entrée (turkey, gravy, dressing, whipped potatoes), 12¼-oz. tray	370	34.0	30.2	2.78
Spaghetti and Meatballs Dinner (spaghetti, meatballs, tomato sauce, sliced apples, garlic bread), 11-oz. tray	360	61.0	32.7	5.55
Turkey Dinner (turkey, gravy, dressing, mashed potatoes, seasoned carrots), 11-oz. tray	340	35.0	30.9	3.18
Veal Parmesan Dinner [breaded veal (beef added) patty, seasoned peas, mashed potatoes], 11-oz. tray	250	27.0	22.7	2.45
Western Style Dinner (grilled beef patty, gravy, beans, chili sauce, mashed potatoes), 11¾-oz. tray	400	32.0	34.0	2.72
MRS. PAUL'S				
Clam Crêpes, 5½-oz. package, approx. 2 clam crêpes	280	22.0	50.9	4.00
1 clam crêpe, approx. 2¾ oz.	140	11.0	50.9	4.00
Clams, Fried, 5-oz. package, approx. 80 clams, plus crumbs	540	50.0	108.0	10.0
1 clam, approx. 0.06 oz. (approx. 19 to the oz.)	(7)	(0.6)	108.0	10.00
Combination Seafood Platter, 9-oz. package	510	57.0	56.7	6.33
Crab Crêpes, 5½-oz. package, 2 crab crêpes	240	24.0	43.6	4.36
1 crab crêpe, approx. 2¾ oz.	120	12.0	43.6	4.36
Deviled Crabs, 6-oz. package, 2 crab cakes	320	36.0	53.3	6.00
"Family," 15-oz. package, 5 crab cakes	800	90.0	53.3	6.00
1 crab cake, approx. 3 oz.	160	18.0	53.3	6.00
Deviled Crab Miniatures, 7-oz. package	440	52.0	62.9	7.43
Eggplant Parmesan Casserole, 11-oz. tray	500	42.0	45.5	3.82
Fish au Gratin, 10-oz. tray	500	46.0	50.0	4.60
Fish Cakes, 8-oz. package, 4 fish cakes	420	46.0	52.5	5.75
"Family," 16-oz. (1-lb.) package, 8 fish cakes	840	92.0	52.5	5.75
1 fish cake, approx. 2 oz.	105	11.5	52.5	5.75
Fish Fillets, Buttered, 10-oz. package, 4 fillets	775	5.0	77.5	0.50
1 fillet, approx. 2½ oz.	155	1.0	77.5	0.50
Fish Fillets, Fried, 8-oz. package, 4 fillets	440	48.0	55.0	6.00
"Family," 14-oz. package, 7 fillets	770	84.0	55.0	6.00
"Party pak," 25-oz. package, 12 fillets	1375	150.0	55.0	6.00
1 fillet, approx. 2 oz.	110	12.0	55.0	6.00
Fish Fillets, Light Batter, 9-oz. package, 4 fillets	560	56.0	62.2	6.22
"Family," 16-oz. (1-lb.) package, 7 fillets	995	100.0	62.2	6.22
"Party pak," 27½-oz. package, 12 fillets	1711	171.1	62.2	6.22
1 fillet, approx. 2¼ oz.	140	14.0	62.2	6.22
Fish Fillets, Supreme Light Batter, 7¼-oz. package, 2 fillets	437	37.8	60.3	5.21
18¼-oz. package, 5 fillets	1100	95.1	60.3	5.21
1 fillet, approx. 3⅝ oz.	220	19.0	60.3	5.21
Fish Miniatures, Light Batter, 9-oz. package	450	45.0	50.0	5.00
Fish 'N Chips, Light Batter, 14-oz. package	740	90.0	52.9	6.43
Fish Parmesan, 10-oz. tray	440	40.0	44.0	4.00
16-oz. (1-lb.) tray	704	64.0	44.0	4.00
Fish Sticks, 9-oz. package, 12 fish sticks	450	48.0	50.0	5.33
"Family," 14-oz. package, 18 fish sticks	700	74.6	50.0	5.33
"Party pak," 23-oz. package, 30 fish sticks	1150	122.6	50.0	5.33
1 stick, approx. ¾ oz.	38	4.0	50.0	5.33
Fish Sticks, Light Batter, 8¾-oz. package, 10 fish sticks	575	60.0	65.7	6.86
"Family," 14-oz. package, 16 fish sticks	920	96.0	65.7	6.86
"Party pak," 21-oz. package, 24 fish sticks	1380	144.1	65.7	6.86
1 fish stick, approx. ⅞ oz.	58	6.0	65.7	6.86
Fish Thins, 10-oz. package, 4 fish "thins"	640	62.0	64.0	6.20
1 fish "thin," approx. 2½ oz.	160	15.0	64.0	6.20
Flounder Fillets, Fried, 8-oz. package, 4 fillets	440	44.0	55.0	5.50
"Family," 14-oz. package, 7 fillets	770	77.0	55.0	5.50
1 fillet, approx. 2 oz.	110	11.0	55.0	5.50
Flounder with Lemon Butter, 8½-oz. package	283	143.0	43.3	18.00
Haddock Fillets, Fried, 8-oz. package, 4 fillets	460	48.0	57.5	6.00
"Family," 14-oz. package, 7 fillets	805	84.0	57.5	6.00
1 fillet, approx. 2 oz.	115	12.0	57.5	6.00
Ocean Perch Fillets, Fried, 8-oz. package, 4 fillets	500	36.0	62.5	4.50
"Family," 14-oz. package, 7 fillets	875	63.0	62.5	4.50
1 fillet, approx. 2 oz.	125	9.0	62.5	4.50
Scallops with Butter and Cheese, 7-oz. package	260	11.0	37.1	1.57

	UNIT Cal.	UNIT Carb.	1 OZ., BY WT. Cal.	1 OZ., BY WT. Carb.
Scallop Crêpes, 5½-oz. package, 2 scallop crêpes	220	25.0	40.0	4.55
1 scallop crêpe, approx. 2¾ oz.	110	12.5	40.0	4.55
Scallops, Fried, 7-oz. package, approx. 20 scallops	420	48.0	60.0	6.86
"Family," 12-oz. package, approx. 30 scallops	720	81.0	60.0	6.86
1 scallop, approx. 0.4 oz.	(23)	(2.6)	60.0	6.86
Scallops, Light Batter, 7-oz. package, approx. 20 scallops	400	42.0	57.1	6.00
1 scallop, approx. 0.4 oz.	(21)	(2.3)	57.1	6.00
Shrimp Crêpes, 5½-oz. package, 2 crêpes	250	24.0	45.5	4.36
1 crêpe, approx. 2¾ oz.	125	12.0	45.5	4.36
Shrimp, Fried, 6-oz. package, approx. 10 pieces	340	34.0	56.7	5.67
Sole with Lemon Butter, 8½-oz. package	303	18.9	35.6	2.22
REAMES				
Flat Dumplins, 12-oz. tray	432	72.6	36.0	6.05
Mini Dumplins, 12-oz. tray	432	72.6	36.0	6.05
RONZONI				
Fettuccine Alfredo, 8-oz. package	430	37.0	53.7	4.63
Fettuccine Alfredo with butter and cheese, 16-oz. (1-lb.) package	760	60.0	47.5	3.75
Lasagna with Fresh Ricotta Cheese, 23-oz. package	800	110.0	34.8	4.78
Linguine with White Clam Sauce, 16-oz. (1-lb.) package	480	64.0	30.0	4.00
Macaroni and Eggplant Casserole, 8-oz. package	260	34.0	32.5	4.25
Manicotti with Fresh Ricotta Cheese, 15-oz. package, 5 manicotti	700	90.0	46.7	6.00
1 manicotti, approx. 3 oz.	140	18.0	46.7	6.00
Rotelle alla Romana, 15-oz. package	480	64.0	32.0	4.27
Stuffed Shells with Fresh Ricotta Cheese, 15-oz. package, 3 shells	750	81.0	50.0	5.40
1 shell, approx. 5 oz.	250	27.0	50.0	5.40
Ziti, Baked, 8-oz. package	250	37.0	31.2	4.63
Ziti, Baked, with Fresh Ricotta Cheese, 18-oz. package	520	76.0	28.9	4.22
ROSETTO FOODS				
Cooked Pierogis with Potato and Cheese Filling, 30-oz. bag, 50 pierogis	1430	268.0	47.7	8.93
1 pierogi, approx. 0.6 oz.	29	5.4	47.7	8.93
Cooked Ravioli with Beef Filling, 30-oz. bag, 50 ravioli	1680	290.3	56.0	9.68
1 ravioli, approx. 0.6 oz.	34	5.5	56.0	9.68
Cooked Ravioli with Chicken, 30-oz. bag, 50 ravioli	1550	246.8	51.7	8.23
1 ravioli, approx. 0.6 oz.	31	4.9	51.7	8.23
Cooked Ravioli with Italian Sausage Filling, 30-oz. bag, 50 ravioli	1940	298.4	64;7	9.95
1 ravioli, approx. 0.6 oz.	39	6.0	64.7	9.95
Cooked Ravioli with Ricotta Cheese, 30-oz. bag, 50 ravioli	1520	291.4	50.7	9.71
1 ravioli, approx. 0.6 oz.	30	5.8	50.7	9.71
SILVER STAR				
Cheese-filled Manicotti, 14-oz. box, 6 manicotti	1020	60.0	72.9	4.29
1 manicotti, approx. 2⅓ oz.	170	10.0	72.9	4.29
Cheese Ravioli, 16-oz. (1-lb.) box, 50 ravioli	1250	203.0	78.1	12.69
1 ravioli, approx. 0.3 oz.	25	4.1	78.1	12.69
Cheese Ravioli, Round, 12-oz. box, 12 ravioli	930	92.7	77.5	7.73
1 ravioli, approx. 1 oz.	78	7.7	77.5	7.73
Jumbo Stuffed Shells, 18-oz. box, 9 shells	960	87.0	53.3	4.83
1 shell, approx. 2 oz.	107	9.7	53.3	4.83
Meat Ravioli, 19-oz. box, 50 ravioli	1450	219.0	76.3	11.53
1 ravioli, approx. 0.38 oz.	29	4.3	76.3	11.53
STEAK HOUSE DINNERS, see MORTON				
STOUFFER'S				
Baked Breast of Chicken, 16-oz. package	770	10.0	48.1	0.63
Beef Burgundy Crêpes, 6¼-oz. package	335	24.0	53.6	3.84
Beef Chop Suey with Rice, 12-oz. package	355	48.0	29.6	4.00
Beef and Spinach Stuffed Pasta Shells with Tomato Sauce, 9-oz. package	290	28.0	32.2	3.11
Beef Stew, 10-oz. package	310	16.0	31.0	1.60
Beef Stroganoff with Parsley and Noodles, 9¾-oz. package, 2 pouches	390	31.0	40.0	3.18
1 pouch, 4.88 oz.	195	15.5	40.0	3.18
Beef Teriyaki with Rice and Vegetables, 10-oz. package	365	41.0	36.5	4.10
Cheese Soufflé, 12-oz. package	710	28.0	59.2	2.33
Cheese Stuffed Pasta Shells with Meat Sauce, 9-oz. package	320	30.0	35.6	3.33
Chicken à la King with Rice, 9½-oz. package, 2 pouches	330	38.0	34.7	4.00
1 pouch, approx. 4¾ oz.	165	19.0	34.7	4.00
Chicken Cacciatore with Spaghetti, 11¼-oz. package	310	29.0	27.6	2.58
Chicken Chow Mein without Noodles, 8-oz. package	145	10.0	18.1	1.25
Chicken Crêpes in Mushroom Sauce, 8¼-oz. package	390	19.0	47.3	2.30
Chicken Divan (chicken, broccoli in sauce), 8½-oz. tray	335	14.0	39.4	1.65
Chicken Paprikash with Egg Noodles, 10½-oz. package	385	32.0	36.7	3.05
Chicken Stuffed Pasta Shells with Cheese Sauce, 9-oz. package	400	24.0	44.4	2.67
Chili Con Carne with Beans, 8¾-oz. package	270	26.0	30.9	2.97
Creamed Chicken, 6½-oz. single serving pouch	300	6.0	46.2	0.92

	UNIT Cal.	UNIT Carb.	1 OZ., BY WT. Cal.	1 OZ., BY WT. Carb.
Creamed Chipped Beef, 11-oz. package, 2 pouches	470	20.0	42.7	1.82
1 pouch, approx. 5½ oz.	235	10.0	42.7	1.82
Escalloped Chicken and Noodles, 11½-oz. tray	500	32.0	43.5	2.78
Fettuccine Alfredo, 10-oz. package	540	38.0	54.0	3.80
Green Pepper Steak, Chinese Style with Rice, 10½-oz. package, 2 pouches	350	35.0	33.3	3.33
1 pouch, approx. 5¼ oz.	175	17.5	33.3	3.33
Ham and Asparagus Crêpes, 6¼-oz. package	325	21.0	52.0	3.36
Ham and Swiss Cheese Crêpes, 7½-oz. package	410	23.0	54.7	3.07
Italian Meatball Sandwich, 7¾-oz. package	410	44.0	52.9	5.68
Italian Mild Sausage Sandwich, 8¼-oz. package	470	40.0	57.0	4.85
Lasagna, 21-oz. package	770	72.0	36.7	3.43
10½-oz. package	385	36.0	36.7	3.43
Linguini with Clam Sauce, 10½-oz. package	285	36.0	27.1	3.43
Lobster Newburg, 6½-oz. package	350	9.0	53.8	1.38
Macaroni and Beef with Tomatoes, 11½-oz. package	380	40.0	33.0	3.48
Macaroni and Cheese, 12-oz. package	520	48.0	32.5	3.00
Mushroom Crêpes, 6¼-oz. package	255	27.0	40.8	4.32
Noodles Romanoff, 8-oz. package	340	32.0	42.5	4.00
12-oz. package	510	48.0	42.5	4.00
Salisbury Steak with Onion Gravy, 12-oz. tray	500	10.0	41.7	0.83
Short Ribs of Beef, Boneless, with Vegetable Gravy, 11½-oz. package	700	4.0	60.9	0.35
Shrimp Newburg, 6½-oz. package	350	2.0	53.8	0.31
Shrimp and Scallops Mariner with Rice, 10¼-oz. package, 2 pouches	400	40.0	39.0	3.90
Spaghetti with Meat Sauce, 14-oz. tray	445	62.0	31.8	4.43
Spinach Crêpes, 9½-oz. package	415	30.0	43.7	3.16
Stuffed Green Peppers with Beef in Tomato Sauce, 15½-oz. package	550	36.0	35.5	2.32
Stuffed Peppers, 15½-oz. package	450	36.0	29.0	2.32
Swedish Meatballs with Parsley Noodles, 11-oz. package	475	33.0	43.2	3.00
Sweet and Sour Chicken Crêpes with Sweet and Sour Sauce, 8½-oz. package	280	35.0	32.9	4.12
Swiss Cheese Crêpes with Mustard Sauce, 8⅜-oz. package	570	43.0	68.1	5.13
Tuna Noodle Casserole, 11½-oz. tray	400	36.0	34.8	3.13
Turkey Casserole with Gravy and Dressing, 9¾-oz. package	370	29.0	37.9	2.97
Turkey Tetrazzini, 12-oz. tray	480	34.0	40.0	2.83
Welsh Rarebit, 10-oz. package	710	34.0	71.0	3.40
STOUFFER'S LEAN CUISINE				
Beef and Pork Canneloni with Mornay Sauce, 9⅝-oz. tray	240	22.0	24.9	2.29
Chicken Chow Mein with Rice, 11¼-oz. tray	240	36.0	21.3	3.20
Chicken and Vegetables with Vermicelli, 12¾-oz. tray	260	28.0	20.4	2.20
Filet of Fish Divan, 12⅜-oz. tray	240	23.0	19.4	1.86
Filet of Fish Florentine, 9-oz. tray	200	11.0	22.2	1.22
Glazed Chicken with Vegetable Rice, 8½-oz. tray	270	23.0	31.8	2.70
Meatball Stew, 10-oz. tray	240	19.0	24.0	1.90
Oriental Beef with Vegetables & Rice, 8⅝-oz. tray	280	30.0	34.0	3.94
Oriental Scallops and Vegetables with Rice, 11-oz. tray	230	32.0	20.9	2.91
Salisbury Steak with Italian Style Sauce and Vegetables, 9½-oz. tray	260	27.4	27.4	1.58
Spaghetti with Beef and Mushroom Sauce, 11½-oz. tray	280	38.0	24.3	3.30
Zucchini Lasagna, 11-oz. tray	260	34.0	23.6	3.09
SWANSON, including TV Dinners and Entrées, Hungry-Man Dinners and Entrées, 3-Course Dinners, and Le Menu Dinners				
Barbecue Flavored Fried Chicken Hungry-Man Dinner (barbecue flavored fried chicken, whipped potatoes, mixed vegetables in seasoned sauce, apple cake cobbler), 16½-oz. tray	760	72.0	46.1	4.36
Barbecue Flavored Fried Chicken Hungry-Man Entrée, 12-oz. tray	620	37.0	51.7	3.08
Barbecue Flavored Fried Chicken TV Dinner (2 pieces fried breaded chicken, whipped potatoes, corn in seasoned sauce, apple cake cobbler), 11¼-oz. tray	530	47.0	47.1	4.18
Beans and Beef Patties TV Dinner, 11-oz. tray	500	73.0	45.5	6.64
Beans and Franks TV Dinner (beans, frankfurters, tomato sauce, apple slices, chocolate cake), 11¼-oz. tray	550	75.0	48.9	6.67
Beef Enchiladas TV Dinner (enchiladas, chili sauce, refried beans, Mexican rice, hot pepper sauce), 15-oz. tray	570	72.0	38.0	4.80
Beef Sirloin Tips Le Menu Dinner (beef sirloin tips, mushroom gravy, O'Brien potatoes, broccoli with cheddar cheese sauce), 11½-oz. tray	390	24.0	33.9	2.09
Beef 3-Course Dinner (beef, gravy, hashed brown potatoes, corn in seasoned sauce, Campbell's cream of tomato soup, apple cake cobbler), 15-oz. tray	490	58.0	32.7	3.87
Beef TV Dinner (sliced beef, gravy, whipped potatoes, peas and carrots in seasoned sauce, apple cake cobbler), 11½-oz. tray	370	34.0	32.2	2.96
Boneless Chicken Hungry-Man Dinner (chicken, gravy, dressing, whipped potatoes, peas in seasoned sauce, peach cake cobbler), 19-oz. tray	730	74.0	38.4	3.89
Breast of Chicken Parmigiana Le Menu Dinner (breast of chicken parmigiana, fettuccine alfredo, Italian beans), 11½-oz. tray	410	26.0	35.7	2.26

	UNIT Cal.	UNIT Carb.	1 OZ., BY WT. Cal.	1 OZ., BY WT. Carb.
Chicken à la King Le Menu Dinner (chicken à la king, seasoned rice, green beans almondine), 10½-oz. tray	320	26.0	30.5	2.48
Chicken Nibbles with French Fries TV Entrée (4 pieces fried breaded chicken wings, french fries), 6-oz. tray	370	31.0	61.7	5.17
Chopped Beefsteak Hungry-Man Dinner (beefsteak patties, gravy, whipped potatoes, mixed vegetables with seasoned sauce, apple-blueberry cake cobbler), 18-oz. tray	730	70.0	40.6	3.89
Chopped Sirloin Beef TV Dinner (beef, brown gravy, peas and carrots in seasoned sauce, french fried potatoes, blueberry muffin), 10-oz. tray	460	37.0	46.0	3.70
Chopped Sirloin Beef with Mushroom Gravy Le Menu Dinner (chopped sirloin beef, mushroom gravy, potatoes au gratin, green beans), 12¼-oz. tray	440	22.0	35.9	1.80
Crisp Fried Chicken TV Dinner (fried breaded chicken, peas and carrots in butter sauce, hash brown potato nuggets, apple cake cobbler), 10-oz. tray	650	51.0	65.0	5.10
English Style, Batter Dipped Fish 'N Chips TV Entrée (fried breaded fish, french fries), 5-oz. tray	290	25.0	58.0	5.00
Fish 'N Chips Hungry-Man Dinner, 15¾-oz. tray	760	68.0	48.3	4.32
Fish 'N Chips TV Dinner (batter-dipped fried ocean perch, corn in seasoned sauce, crinkle cut potatoes, stewed tomatoes), 10¼-oz. tray	450	40.0	43.9	3.90
French Toast with Sausages TV Entrée (french toast, sausages with soy protein concentrate added), 4½-oz. tray	300	22.0	66.7	4.89
Fried Chicken Hungry-Man Dinner (4 pieces fried breaded chicken, crinkle cut fried potatoes, corn in seasoned sauce, apple-raisin cake cobbler), 15¾-oz. tray	910	78.0	57.8	4.95
Fried Chicken Hungry-Man Entrée (4 pieces fried breaded chicken, whipped potatoes), 12-oz. tray	620	37.0	51.7	3.08
Fried Chicken 3-Course Dinner (Campbell's vegetable soup, fried breaded chicken, whipped potatoes, corn in seasoned sauce, apple cake cobbler), 15-oz. tray	630	64.0	42.0	4.27
Fried Chicken TV Dinner (fried breaded chicken, whipped potatoes, mixed vegetables in seasoned sauce, apple cake cobbler), 11½-oz. tray	570	48.0	49.6	4.17
Fried Chicken with Whipped Potatoes TV Entrée, 7-oz. tray	360	25.0	51.4	3.47
German Style Dinner TV Dinner (sliced beef, sauerbraten gravy, German style whipped potatoes, applesauce cake), 11¾-oz. tray	430	40.0	36.6	3.40
Gravy and Sliced Beef with Whipped Potatoes TV Entrée (beef, gravy, whipped potatoes), 8-oz. tray	190	23.0	23.8	2.88
Ham TV Dinner (seasoned and formed ham, sauce, sweet potato, peas and carrots in seasoned sauce, corn muffin), 10¼-oz. tray	380	47.0	37.1	4.59
Italian Style TV Dinner, 13-oz. tray	420	55.0	32.3	4.23
Lasagna Hungry-Man Entrée, 12¾-oz. tray	540	51.0	42.4	4.00
Lasagna with Meat Hungry-Man Dinner (lasagna with meat, tomato sauce, bean salad, pudding cake, garlic roll), 17¾-oz. tray	740	86.0	41.7	4.85
Loin of Pork TV Dinner (loin of pork, brown gravy, whipped potatoes, mixed vegetables in seasoned sauce, apple compote), 11¼-oz. tray	470	48.0	41.8	4.27
Macaroni and Beef TV Dinner (macaroni and beef in tomato sauce, corn in seasoned sauce, chocolate pudding), 12-oz. tray	400	56.0	33.3	4.67
Macaroni and Cheese TV Dinner (macaroni and cheese, apple slices, peas and carrots in seasoned sauce), 12½-oz. tray	390	55.0	31.2	4.40
Meatballs with Brown Gravy and Whipped Potatoes TV Entrée (meatballs, brown gravy, whipped potatoes), 9¼-oz. tray	330	26.0	35.7	2.81
Meatballs TV Dinner, 11¾-oz. tray	400	35.0	34.0	2.98
Meat Loaf TV Dinner (meat loaf, tomato sauce, green beans in seasoned sauce, hash brown potato nuggets, chocolate nut brownie), 10¾-oz. tray	530	48.0	49.3	4.47
Meat Loaf TV Entrée (meat loaf, tomato sauce, whipped potatoes), 9-oz. tray	330	27.0	36.7	3.00
Mexican Style Combination TV Dinner (beef tamales, beef enchilada, chili with meat, refried beans, Mexican rice, hot pepper sauce), 16-oz. (1-lb.) tray	600	72.0	37.5	4.50
Noodles and Chicken TV Dinner (noodles, chicken, chicken gravy, corn in seasoned sauce, chocolate cake), 10¼-oz. tray	390	53.0	38.0	5.17
Pancakes and Sausages TV Dinner [pancakes with sausages (soy protein concentrate added to sausages)], 6-oz. tray	500	50.0	83.3	8.33
Peppersteak Le Menu Dinner (peppersteak, oriental vegetables, long grain rice), 11½-oz. tray	350	28	30.4	2.43
Polynesian Style TV Dinner (sweet and sour chicken with vegetables, vegetable chow mein, oriental style rice, orange tea cake), 13-oz. tray	490	65.0	37.7	5.00
Salisbury Steak with Crinkle Cut Potatoes TV Entrée (steak, crinkle cut potatoes), 5½-oz. tray	370	28.0	67.3	5.09
Salisbury Steak Hungry-Man Dinner (steak, brown onion gravy, hash brown potato nuggets, peas and carrots in seasoned sauce, apple cake cobbler), 17-oz. tray	870	65.0	51.2	3.82
Salisbury Steak Hungry-Man Entrée (steak, brown onion gravy, crinkle cut potatoes), 12½-oz. tray	640	39.0	51.2	3.12
Salisbury Steak 3-Course Dinner, 16-oz. (1-lb.) tray	490	48.0	30.6	3.00

	UNIT Cal.	UNIT Carb.	1 OZ., BY WT. Cal.	1 OZ., BY WT. Carb.
Salisbury Steak TV Dinner (steak, gravy, potatoes, corn in seasoned sauce, chocolate cake), 11½-oz. tray	500	40.0	43.5	3.48
Sliced Beef Hungry-Man Entrée (beef, gravy, whipped potatoes), 12¼-oz. tray	330	23.0	26.9	1.88
Sliced Turkey Breast with Mushroom Gravy Le Menu Dinner (sliced turkey breast, mushroom gravy, long grain wild rice, garden vegetable medley), 11¼-oz. tray	460	34.0	40.9	3.02
Spaghetti and Meatballs Hungry-Man Dinner, 18½-oz. tray	660	83.0	35.7	4.49
Spaghetti and Meatballs TV Dinner (spaghetti, meatballs, tomato sauce, peas in seasoned sauce, vanilla pudding), 12½-oz. tray	410	57.0	32.8	4.56
Spaghetti in Tomato Sauce with Breaded Veal TV Entrée, 8¼-oz. package	290	24.0	35.2	2.91
Sweet & Sour Chicken Le Menu Dinner (sweet & sour chicken, seasoned rice, green beans, oriental vegetables), 11¼-oz. tray	470	41.0	41.8	3.64
Swiss Steak TV Dinner (steak, tomato-beef gravy, mixed vegetables in seasoned sauce, hash brown potato nuggets, apple cake cobbler), 10-oz. package	350	40.0	35.0	4.00
Turkey, Gravy, Dressing with Whipped Potatoes TV Entrée (turkey, gravy, dressing, whipped potatoes), 8¾-oz. tray	260	27.0	29.7	3.09
Turkey Hungry-Man Dinner, ("mostly white meat" turkey, gravy, dressing, whipped potatoes, peas in seasoned sauce, apple-cranberry cake cobbler), 19-oz. tray	740	80.0	38.9	4.21
Turkey Hungry-Man Entrée ("mostly white meat" turkey, gravy, dressing, whipped potatoes), 15¼-oz. tray	438	40.3	28.7	2.64
Turkey 3-Course Dinner ("mostly white meat" turkey, gravy, dressing, whipped potatoes, peas and carrots in seasoned sauce, apple-cranberry cake cobbler), 16-oz. (1-lb.) tray	520	60.0	32.5	3.75
Turkey TV Entrée ("mostly white meat" turkey, gravy, dressing, whipped potatoes, peas and carrots in seasoned sauce, apple-cranberry cake cobbler), 11½-oz. tray	360	45.0	31.3	3.91
Veal Parmesan Hungry-Man Dinner (breaded chopped veal, tomato sauce, macaroni and cheese, green beans in seasoned sauce, peach cake cobbler), 20½-oz. tray	910	70.0	44.4	3.41
Veal Parmesan TV Dinner (breaded chopped veal, tomato sauce, apple slices, peas in seasoned sauce, lemon muffin), 12¼-oz. tray	520	47.0	42.4	3.84
Western Style Hungry-Man Dinner (broiled chopped beef steaks, gravy, beans in sauce, corn in seasoned sauce, chocolate cake), 17¾-oz. tray	890	77.0	50.1	4.34
Western Style TV Dinner (chopped beef steak, gravy, beans and sauce, corn in seasoned sauce, apple cake cobbler), 11¾-oz. tray	460	41.0	39.1	3.49
Yankee Pot Roast Le Menu Dinner (yankee pot roast, mushroom gravy, browned potatoes, carrots with pearl onions), 11-oz. tray	360	28.0	32.7	2.55
TASTE O'SEA				
Batter Dipt Cod Dinner (fried breaded cod, potato puffs), 8¾-oz. tray	500	48.0	57.1	5.49
Batter Dipt Fish and Chips, English Style (potatoes, fried breaded pollock), 16-oz. (1-lb.) tray	1000	92.0	62.5	5.75
Batter Dipt Scrod Dinner (fried breaded scrod, potato puffs), 8¾-oz. package	500	48.0	57.1	5.49
Cod fillet, skinless, 16-oz. (1-lb.) package	320	0.0	20.0	0.00
Fish Cakes (cod and/or haddock, whiting, hake, pollock), 8-oz. package, 4 cakes	380	46.0	47.5	5.75
Fish Cake Dinner (fried breaded codfish or other fish, peas, potato puffs), 8-oz. tray	380	46.0	47.5	5.75
Fish Dinner (fried breaded pollock, peas, potato puffs), 9-oz. tray	390	39.0	43.3	4.33
Fish Kabobs (Pollock), 16-oz. (1-lb.) package	900	100.0	56.3	6.25
Fish Portions (Cod), 12-oz. package, 4 equal fish portions	240	0.0	20.0	0.00
1 fish portion, approx. 3 oz.	60	0.0	20.0	0.00
Fish Portions (skinless Cod), Breaded, 32-oz. (2-lb.) package, 12 fish portions	960	120.0	30.0	3.75
1 fish portion, approx. 2⅔ oz.	80	10.0	30.0	3.75
16-oz. (1-lb.) package, 8 fish portions	480	60.0	30.0	3.75
1 fish portion, approx. 2 oz.	60	7.5	30.0	3.75
Fish Portions (Flounder), 16-oz. (1-lb.) package, 8 fish portions	280	36.0	17.5	2.25
Fish Portions (Haddock), 12-oz. package, 4 equal fish portions	280	0.0	23.3	0.00
1 fish portion, approx. 3 oz.	70	0.0	23.3	0.00
Fish Portions (Haddock), Batter Dipt, 12-oz. package, 4 fish portions	800	56.0	66.7	4.67
1 fish portion, approx. 3 oz.	200	14.0	66.7	4.67
Fish Portions (Haddock), Breaded skinless, 32-oz. (2-lb.) package, 12 fish portions	960	120.0	30.0	3.75
1 fish portion, approx. 2⅔ oz.	80	10.0	30.0	3.75
Fish Portions (Ocean Perch), 12-oz. package, 4 equal fish portions	400	0.0	33.3	0.00
1 fish portion, approx. 3 oz.	100	0.0	33.3	0.00
Fish Portions (Ocean Perch), Breaded, 32-oz. (2-lb.) package, 12 fish portions	1200	132.0	37.5	4.13
1 fish portion, approx. 2⅔ oz.	100	11.0	37.5	4.13
Fish Portions (Pollock), Batter Dipt, 12-oz. package, 4 fish portions	880	60.0	73.3	5.00
1 fish portion, approx. 3 oz.	220	15.0	73.3	5.00
Fish Portions (Sole), 12-oz. package, 4 equal portions	280	0.0	23.3	0.00
1 sole portion, approx. 3 oz.	70	0.0	23.3	0.00
Fish Portions (Whiting), Breaded, 32-oz. (2-lb.) package, 12 fish portions	1080	120.0	33.8	3.75
1 fish portion, approx. 2⅔ oz.	90	10.0	33.8	3.75
16-oz. (1-lb.) package, 8 fish portions	560	64.0	35.0	4.00
1 fish portion, approx. 2 oz.	70	0.0	35.0	4.00
Fish Sticks (Cod), Golden Fried, 8-oz. package, 8 fish sticks	508	46.0	63.5	5.75
1 fish stick, approx. 1 oz.	64	5.8	63.5	5.75
Fish Sticks (Haddock), Golden Fried, 16-oz. (1-lb.) package, 16 fish sticks	880	68.0	55.0	4.25
1 stick, approx. 1 oz.	55	4.3	55.0	4.25
Fish Sticks (Pollock), 27-oz. package, 32 fish sticks	1688	168.8	62.5	6.25
1 fish stick, approx. 0.8 oz.	53	5.3	62.5	6.25
16-oz. (1-lb.) package	1016	92.0	63.5	5.75
1 fish stick, approx. 1 oz.	64	5.8	63.5	5.75
Fish Sticks (Pollock), Batter Dipt, 8-oz. package, 8 fish sticks	620	52.0	77.5	6.50
1 fish stick, approx. 1 oz.	78	6.5	77.5	6.50
Fish Sticks (Pollock), Golden Fried, 8-oz. package, 8 fish sticks	508	46.0	63.5	5.75
1 fish stick, approx. 1 oz.	64	5.8	63.5	5.75
Flounder (fillet), 16-oz. (1-lb.) package	360	0.0	22.5	0.00
Flounder Dinner (fried breaded flounder, peas, potato puffs), 9-oz. tray	350	35.0	38.9	3.89
Greenland Turbot (fillet), 16-oz. (1-lb.) package	640	0.0	40.0	0.00
Haddock (fillet), 16-oz. (1-lb.) package	360	0.0	22.5	0.00
Haddock, skinless (fillet), 16-oz. (1-lb.) package	400	0.0	25.0	0.00
Haddock Dinner (fried breaded haddock, peas, potato puffs), 9-oz. tray	380	36.0	42.2	4.00
Moby Dick Dinner, 9-oz. tray	430	44.0	47.8	4.89
New England Clam Platter (fried breaded clams, potato puffs), 6½-oz. tray	540	55.0	83.1	8.46
Ocean Catfish (fillet), 16-oz. (1-lb.) package	400	0.0	25.0	0.00
Ocean Perch (fillet), 16-oz. (1-lb.) package	400	0.0	25.0	0.00
Scallops, Batter Dipt, 7-oz. package	380	40.0	54.3	5.70
Scallop Dinner (sea scallops, peas, potato puffs), 8-oz. tray	380	45.0	47.5	5.63
Sea Scallops, Golden Fried, 8-oz. package	440	46.0	55.0	5.80
Seafood Platter (potato puffs, cod and/or haddock, whiting, hake, pollock), 9-oz. package	520	57.0	57.8	6.33
Shrimp, Batter Dipt, 6-oz. package	380	38.0	63.3	6.33
Shrimp Dinner (fried breaded shrimp, peas, potato puffs), 7-oz. tray	350	45.0	50.0	6.43
Shrimp, Golden Fried, 6-oz. package	360	45.0	60.0	7.50
Shrimp Patty Dinner (fried breaded shrimp, peas, potato puffs), 8-oz. tray	390	48.0	48.8	6.00
Shrimp Scampi, 7½-oz. package	490	16.0	65.3	2.13
Sole (fillet), 16-oz. (1-lb.) package	360	0.0	22.5	0.00
Sole Dinner (fried breaded sole, peas, potato puffs), 9-oz. tray	330	28.0	36.7	3.11
Sole in Lemon Butter, 9-oz. package	420	18.0	46.7	2.00
Whiting (fillet), 16-oz. (1-lb.) package	320	0.0	20.0	0.00
TOAST TOPPERS, see GREEN GIANT				
TREE TAVERN				
Eggplant Parmigiana, 10-oz. box	370	25.0	37.0	2.50
TV DINNERS And ENTRÉES, see SWANSON				
WEAVER				
Chicken Croquettes, 24-oz. package (approx. 8 croquettes)	1176	158.6	49.0	6.61
1 croquette, approx. 3 oz.	147	19.8	49.0	6.61
Chicken Turnovers, 16-oz. (1-lb.) package (approx. 4 turnovers)	1289	120.3	80.6	7.52
1 turnover, approx. 4 oz.	322	30.1	80.6	7.52
WEIGHT WATCHERS				
Beef Steak (chopped and formed) in Green Pepper and Mushroom Sauce, Crinkle Cut Carrots, 9¾-oz. tray	340	12.0	34.9	1.23
Beef Steak and Mushrooms Dinner (chopped beef steak, carrots, green peppers, mushroom sauce), 10-oz. tray	390	11.0	39.0	1.10
Beef Steak and Peppers Luncheon, 10-oz. tray	321	6.0	32.1	0.60
Canneloni Florentine Dinner (pasta, veal, spinach, cheese, sauce), 13-oz. tray	450	46.0	34.6	3.54
Cheese Pizza Pie, 6-oz. tray	370	31.0	61.7	5.17
Cheese and Tomato Pies, 12-oz. tray, 2 pies	760	74.0	63.3	6.17
1 pie, approx. 6 oz.	380	37.0	63.3	6.17
Chicken à la King, 10-oz. tray	240	17.0	24.0	1.70
Chicken Creole Lunch Casserole, 13-oz. tray	250	12.0	19.3	0.92
Chicken Livers and Onions Luncheon (livers, onions, broccoli, soy sauce), 10½-oz. tray	220	11.0	21.0	1.05

	UNIT Cal.	UNIT Carb.	1 OZ., BY WT. Cal.	1 OZ., BY WT. Carb.
Chicken Parmigiana, Italian Cut Beans, 7¾-oz. tray	220	11.0	28.4	1.42
Chili Con Carne with Beans, 10-oz. tray	290	33.0	29.0	3.30
Eggplant Parmigiana, 13-oz. tray	290	25.0	22.3	1.92
Flounder Dinner (flounder, broccoli, carrots and peas, lobster sauce), 16-oz. (1-lb.) tray	260	14.0	16.3	0.88
Flounder with Lemon Flavored Bread Crumbs, Vegetable Medley, 6½-oz. tray	140	12.0	21.5	1.85
Flounder Luncheon (flounder, broccoli, cauliflower, red pepper, bread crumbs), 8½-oz. tray	162	13.0	19.1	1.53
Haddock Dinner, 16-oz. (1-lb.) tray	270	18.0	16.9	1.13
Haddock Luncheon, 8¾-oz. tray	172	10.0	19.7	1.14
Lasagna with Veal, Tomato Sauce, and Cheese, 12¾-oz. tray	380	40.0	29.8	3.14
Perch Dinner, 16-oz. (1-lb.) tray	311	17.0	19.4	1.06
Perch Luncheon, 8½-oz. tray	202	13.0	23.8	1.53
Sausage, Cheese, and Tomato Pies, 14-oz. tray, 2 pies	780	70.0	55.7	5.00
1 pie, approx. 7 oz.	390	35.0	55.7	5.00
Sirloin of Beef Dinner, 16-oz. (1-lb.) tray	510	10.0	31.9	0.63
Sirloin of Beef (chopped and formed) in Mushroom Sauce, Cut Green Beans, Cauliflower, 13-oz. tray	410	16.0	31.5	1.23
Sliced Breast of Turkey Dinner (turkey, stuffing, gravy, broccoli, carrots), 19-oz. tray	380	21.0	20.0	11.11
Sliced Chicken Luncheon (chicken, peas, onions), 9-oz. tray	245	24.0	27.2	2.67
Sliced Turkey with Gravy and Stuffing, Carrots, Broccoli, 15¼-oz. tray	390	37.0	25.6	2.46
Sole Dinner (sole, peas and mushrooms, lobster sauce), 9½-oz. tray	210	14.0	22.1	1.54
Sole in Lemon Sauce, Peas and Onions, 9¼-oz. tray	200	17.0	21.6	1.84
Sole Luncheon, 9½-oz. tray	234	8.0	24.6	0.84
Turbot Dinner, 16-oz. (1-lb.) tray	416	14.1	26.0	0.88
Turbot Luncheon, 8-oz. tray	234	8.0	29.3	1.00
Turkey Tetrazzini with Cheese, Mushrooms, and Red Peppers, 13-oz. tray	400	37.0	30.7	2.85
Ziti Macaroni with Veal, Tomato Sauce, and Cheese, 12½-oz. tray	340	41.0	27.2	3.28

FROZEN HEAT-AND-SERVE PIZZA

	UNIT Cal.	UNIT Carb.	1 OZ., BY WT. Cal.	1 OZ., BY WT. Carb.
APPIAN WAY				
Cheese Pizza, 13½-oz. pie	1100	142.0	66.7	10.52
Pizza, Regular, 12½-oz. pie	800	144.0	64.0	11.52
CELANTANO				
Elegante Pizza, 15-oz. pie	960	156.0	64.0	10.40
Mini Pizza, 14-oz. pie, 8 slices	840	116.0	60.0	8.29
1 slice, approx. 1¾ oz.	105	14.5	60.0	8.29
Pizza, not presliced, 11-oz. pie	840	93.0	76.5	8.47
CELESTE				
Cheese Pizza, 19-oz. pie, 4 slices	1280	145.0	67.4	7.63
1 slice, approx. 4.75 oz.	320	36.2	67.4	7.63
7-oz. pie, 2 slices	490	63.3	70.0	9.04
1 slice, approx. 3.5 oz.	245	31.7	70.0	9.04
Cheese Pizza, Sicilian Style, 20-oz. pie, 4 slices	1316	170.2	65.8	8.51
1 slice, approx. 5 oz.	329	42.5	65.8	8.51
Cheese Mushroom Pizza, 21-oz. pie, 4 slices	1190	121.2	56.8	5.77
1 slice, approx. 5¼ oz.	298	30.3	56.8	5.77
8-oz. pie, 2 slices	454	64.0	56.8	8.00
1 slice, approx. 4 oz.	227	32.0	56.8	8.00
DeLuxe Pizza, 23.5-oz. pie, 4 slices	1468	135.7	62.5	5.77
1 slice, approx. 5.9 oz.	367	33.9	62.5	5.77
9-oz. pie, 2 slices	596	55.4	66.2	6.16
1 slice, approx. 4.5 oz.	298	27.7	66.2	6.16
Pepperoni Pizza, 20-oz. pie, 4 slices	1424	126.7	71.2	6.33
1 slice, approx. 5 oz.	356	31.7	71.2	6.33
7¼-oz. pie, 2 slices	528	51.7	72.8	7.14
1 slice, approx. 3.6 oz.	264	25.9	72.8	7.14
Pizza, 9-oz. pie, 2 slices	570	58.0	63.3	6.44
1 slice, approx. 4.5 oz.	285	29.0	63.3	6.44
Sausage Pizza, 22-oz. pie, 4 slices	1500	135.7	68.1	6.17
1 slice, approx. 5.5 oz.	375	33.9	68.1	6.17
8-oz. pie, 2 slices	562	51.6	70.3	6.45
1 slice, approx. 4 oz.	281	25.8	70.3	6.45
Sausage and Mushroom Pizza, 24-oz. pie, 4 slices	1516	137.3	63.2	5.72
1 slice, approx. 6 oz.	379	34.3	63.2	5.72
JENO'S				
Cheese Pizza, 13-oz. pie, 6 slices	840	108.0	64.6	8.31
1 slice, approx. 2.2 oz.	140	18.0	64.6	8.31
Cheese Pizza, Deluxe, 20.1-oz. pie, 6 slices	1470	171.0	73.1	8.51
1 slice, approx. 3.3 oz.	245	28.5	73.1	8.51
Combination Pizza, 23.1-oz. pie, 6 slices	1680	165.0	72.7	7.14
1 slice, approx. 3.9 oz.	280	27.5	72.7	7.14

	UNIT Cal.	UNIT Carb.	1 OZ., BY WT. Cal.	1 OZ., BY WT. Carb.
Hamburger Pizza, 13.5 oz. pie, 6 slices	880	114.0	65.2	8.44
1 slice, approx. 2.3 oz.	147	19.0	65.2	8.44
Pepperoni Pizza, 13-oz. pie, 6 slices	900	114.0	69.2	8.77
1 slice, approx. 2.2 oz.	150	19.0	69.2	8.77
Sausage Pizza, 13.5-oz. pie, 6 slices	900	114.0	66.7	8.44
1 slice, approx. 2.3 oz.	150	19.0	66.7	8.44
Sausage Pizza, Deluxe, 21-oz. pie, 6 slices	1500	159.0	71.4	7.57
1 slice, approx. 3.5 oz.	250	26.5	71.4	7.57
LA PIZZERIA				
Cheese Pizza, not presliced, 20-oz. pie	1160	132.0	58.0	6.60
Cheese Pizza, Thick Crust, not presliced, 18.5-oz. pie	1230	138.0	66.5	7.46
Combination Pizza, not presliced, 13.5-oz. pie	840	86.0	62.1	6.37
Pepperoni Pizza, not presliced, 21-oz. pie	1320	168.0	62.9	8.00
Sausage Pizza, not presliced, 13-oz. pie	860	82.0	66.1	6.31
LIGHTSTYLE				
Incredible Frozen Pizza, 26-oz. pie, 12 slices	1776	204.0	68.3	7.85
1 slice, approx. 2.2 oz.	148	17.0	68.3	7.85
ORE-IDA				
Sausage Pizza, 23-oz. pie	1520	164.0	66.1	7.13
STOUFFER'S				
Cheese Pizza, 10¼-oz. pie	660	86.0	64.4	8.39
Deluxe Pizza, 12.38-oz. pie	800	92.0	64.6	7.43
Mushroom Pizza, 12-oz. pie	680	86.0	56.7	7.17
Pepperoni Pizza, 11.25-oz. pie	800	84.0	71.1	7.47
Stouffer's French Bread Pizzas:				
Hamburger Pizza, 12¼-oz. package	800	78.0	65.3	6.37
Sausage Pizza, 12-oz. package	840	88.0	70.0	7.33
Sausage and Mushroom Pizza, 12½-oz. package	790	80.0	63.2	6.40
TOTINO'S				
Canadian Bacon Pizza	700	94.0		
1 slice, ¼ of the pie	175	23.5		
Cheese Pizza	880	106.0		
1 slice, ¼ of the pie	220	26.5		
Combination Pizza, Classic	1680	153.0		
Combination Pizza, Deep Crust	1860	198.0		
Hamburger Pizza	920	102.0		
Pepperoni Pizza	920	104.0		
Pepperoni Pizza, Deep Crust	1800	204.0		
Pepperoni and Mushroom Pizza, Classic	1500	153.0		
Sausage Pizza	940	108.0		
Sausage Pizza, Deep Crust	1800	198.0		
Sausage and Mushroom Pizza, Classic	1680	141.0		
TREE TAVERN				
Cheese Pizza, 16-oz. (1-lb.) pie, 6 slices	960	128.0	60.0	8.00
1 slice, approx. 2.7 oz.	160	21.3	60.0	8.00
Pizza, 16-oz. (1-lb.) pie, 4 slices	960	128.0	60.0	8.00
1 slice, approx. 4 oz.	240	32.0	60.0	8.00
WEIGHT WATCHERS				
Cheese Pizza Pie, 6-oz. tray	370	31.0	61.7	5.17
2 Cheese and Tomato Pies, 12-oz. tray	760	63.3	63.3	6.17
2 Sausage, Cheese, and Tomato Pies, 14-oz. tray	780	70.0	55.7	5.00

PIZZA NOVELTIES

	UNIT Cal.	UNIT Carb.	1 OZ., BY WT. Cal.	1 OZ., BY WT. Carb.
JENO'S				
Cheeseburger Pizza Rolls, 6-oz. package, 12 rolls	540	54.0	90.0	9.00
1 roll, approx. ½ oz.	45	4.5	90.0	9.00
Pepperoni and Cheese Pizza Rolls, 6-oz. package, 12 rolls	520	50.0	86.7	8.33
1 roll, approx. ½ oz.	43	4.2	86.7	8.33
Sausage and Cheese Pizza Rolls, 6-oz. package, 12 rolls	520	50.0	86.7	8.33
1 roll, approx. ½ oz.	43	4.2	86.7	8.33
Shrimp and Cheese Pizza Rolls, 6-oz. package, 12 rolls	440	46.0	73.3	7.67
1 roll, approx. ½ oz.	37	3.8	73.3	7.67
LENDER'S				
Cheese Pizza Bagels, 12-oz. package, 6 bagels	840	102.0	70.0	8.50
1 bagel, approx. 2 oz.	140	17.0	70.0	8.50
Mushroom Pizza Bagels, 13½-oz. package, 6 bagels	900	108.0	66.7	8.00
1 bagel, approx. 2¼ oz.	150	18.0	66.7	8.00
Onion Pizza Bagels, 13½-oz. package, 6 bagels	840	114.0	62.2	8.44
1 bagel, approx. 2¼ oz.	140	19.0	62.2	8.44
"The Works," Onions, Peppers, and Mushrooms Pizza Bagels, 16½-oz. package, 6 bagels	1020	137.9	61.8	8.36
1 bagel, approx. 2¾ oz.	170	23.0	61.8	8.36

FROZEN POT PIES

	UNIT Cal.	UNIT Carb.	1 OZ., BY WT. Cal.	1 OZ., BY WT. Carb.
BANQUET				
Beef Pot Pie, 8-oz. pie	409	40.9	51.1	5.11

	UNIT Cal.	UNIT Carb.	1 OZ., BY WT. Cal.	1 OZ., BY WT. Carb.
Chicken Pot Pie, 8-oz. pie	427	39.0	53.4	4.88
Tuna Pot Pie, 8-oz. pie	434	42.7	54.3	5.34
Turkey Pot Pie, 8-oz. pie	415	40.6	51.9	5.08
MORTON				
Beef Pot Pie, 8-oz. pie	320	31.0	40.0	3.88
Chicken Pot Pie, 8-oz. pie	350	30.0	43.8	3.75
Tuna Pot Pie, 8-oz. pie	370	36.0	46.3	4.50
Turkey Pot Pie, 8-oz. pie	320	31.0	40.0	3.88
STOUFFER'S				
Beef Pot Pie, 10-oz. pie	550	38.0	55.0	3.80
Chicken Pot Pie, 10-oz. pie	500	40.0	50.0	4.00
Turkey Pot Pie, 10-oz. pie	460	35.0	46.0	3.50
SWANSON				
Beef Pot Pie, 8-oz. pie	430	43.0	53.8	5.38
Beef Pot Pie, Hungry-Man, 16-oz. (1-lb.) pie	770	65.0	48.1	4.06
Chicken Pot Pie, 8-oz. pie	450	44.0	56.3	5.50
Chicken Pot Pie, Hungry-Man, 16-oz. (1-lb.) pie	780	66.0	48.8	4.13
Macaroni and Cheese Pot Pie, 7-oz. pie	230	26.0	32.9	3.71
Sirloin Burger Pot Pie, Hungry-Man, 16-oz. (1-lb.) pie	800	55.0	50.0	3.44
Turkey Pot Pie, 8-oz. pie	450	40.0	56.3	5.00
Turkey Pot Pie, Hungry-Man, 16-oz. (1-lb.) pie	790	60.0	49.4	3.75
WORTHINGTON				
Vegetarian Beef-Like Pot Pie (all vegetable), 8-oz. pie	470	51.0	58.8	6.38
Vegetarian Chicken-Like Pot Pie (all vegetable), 8-oz. pie	450	42.0	56.3	5.25

COMBINATION MAIN DISHES IN CANS OR JARS, based on generic data

	UNIT Cal.	UNIT Carb.	1 OZ., BY WT. Cal.	1 OZ., BY WT. Carb.
BEEF AND VEGETABLE STEW:				
15-oz. can	336	30.2	22.4	2.01
24-oz. (1½-lb.) can	537	48.3	22.4	2.01
50-oz. (3-lb. 2-oz.) can	1120	100.7	22.4	2.01
1 cup (approx. 8.6 oz.)	194	17.4	22.4	2.01
1 pound (approx. 1.9 cups)	358	32.2	22.4	2.01
CHICKEN CHOW MEIN (WITHOUT NOODLES):				
1 can, 16 oz. (1 lb.)	172	32.2	10.8	2.01
1 cup (approx. 8.8 oz.)	95	17.8	10.8	2.01
1 pound (approx. 1.8 cups)	172	32.2	10.8	2.01
For comparison:				
Chicken Chow Mein (without noodles), based on a USDA home recipe with ingredients as follows: ¾ cup boned, canned chicken, ½ tsp. cornstarch, 1 cup mung bean sprouts, ½ cup diced celery, 3 Tbsp. chopped onion, 2 Tbsp. canned mushrooms, ½ cup broth, ½ Tbsp. water, 2 tsp. soy sauce, ½ Tbsp. cooking oil, 1 tsp. sugar, dash of salt. (Loss of 12% has been applied for evaporation in cooking.) (Yield: approx. 2 cups, or 17 oz.)	278	10.9	15.9	0.63
1 cup, prepared (approx. 8.8 oz.)	139	5.5	15.9	0.63
CHILI CON CARNE WITH BEANS:				
15-oz. can	566	51.9	37.7	3.46
108-oz. (6-lb. 12-oz.) can	4072	373.6	37.7	3.46
1 cup (approx. 9 oz.)	339	31.1	37.7	3.46
1 pound (approx. 1.8 cups)	603	55.3	37.7	3.46
CHILI CON CARNE WITHOUT BEANS: *(contains at least 60 percent meat and no more than 8 percent cereals and seasonings)*				
15-oz. can	851	24.6	56.7	1.64
1 pound	907	26.2	56.7	1.64
CORNED BEEF HASH MADE WITH POTATO:				
15½-oz. can	795	47.0	51.3	3.03
24-oz. (1½-lb.) can	1231	72.8	51.3	3.03
1 cup (approx. 7¾ oz.)	398	23.5	51.3	3.03
1 pound (approx. 2.1 cups)	821	48.5	51.3	3.03
MACARONI AND CHEESE:				
15¼-oz. can	409	46.0	26.9	3.03
50-oz. (3-lb. 2-oz.) can	1347	151.7	26.9	3.03
1 cup (approx. 8.5 oz.)	228	25.7	26.9	3.03
SPAGHETTI IN TOMATO SAUCE WITH CHEESE:				
15¼-oz. can	328	66.5	21.6	4.37
26-oz. (1-lb. 10-oz.) can	565	114.6	21.6	4.37
51-oz. (3-lb. 3-oz.) can	1099	222.7	21.6	4.37
1 cup (approx. 8.8 oz.)	190	38.5	21.6	4.37
SPAGHETTI IN TOMATO SAUCE WITH MEATBALLS:				
15-oz. can	438	48.5	29.2	3.23
1 cup (approx. 8.8 oz.)	258	28.5	29.2	3.23

COMBINATION MAIN DISHES IN CANS OR JARS, by brand

	UNIT Cal.	UNIT Carb.	1 OZ., BY WT. Cal.	1 OZ., BY WT. Carb.
ARMOUR				
Beef Stew, 24-oz. can	630	39.1	26.3	1.63
Beef Tamales, 15½-oz. can (approx. 7 tamales)	800	68.0	51.9	4.15
Beef Tamales, 13½-oz. jar (approx. 6 tamales)	700	56.0	51.9	4.15
1 tamale, approx. 2¼ oz.	117	9.3	51.9	4.15
Chili with Beans, 15½-oz. can	740	56.0	47.7	3.61
Chili without Beans, 15-oz. can	860	32.0	57.3	2.13
Corned Beef Hash, 15¼-oz. can	800	38.0	52.4	2.49
Pork Brains in Milk Gravy, 5½-oz. can	200	0.0	36.4	0.00
Sloppy Joe, Beef, 15½-oz. can	673	53.0	43.4	3.42
Sloppy Joe, Pork, 15½-oz. can	653	40.8	42.1	2.63
Texas Chili with beans, 15½-oz. can	680	54.0	43.9	3.48
Texas Chili without beans, 15-oz. can	860	28.0	57.3	1.87
CHEF BOY-AR-DEE				
Beef Ravioli in Tomato Sauce, 7½-oz. can	230	36.0	30.7	4.80
Mini Ravioli, 15-oz. can	440	64.0	29.3	4.27
CHUN KING				
Stir-Fry Pepper Steak, 28-oz. can with 1¾-oz. sauce mix	2300	430.2	77.3	14.46
DERBY				
Beef Tamales, with Sauce, 13½-oz. jar (approx. 6 tamales, 2.2 oz. each)	736	39.9	54.5	2.95
1 tamale, approx. 2.2 oz.	120	6.5	54.5	2.95
DINTY MOORE				
Beef Stew, 40-oz. (2½-lb.) can	960	74.8	24.0	1.87
15-oz. can	360	28.0	24.0	1.87
7½-oz. can	180	14.0	24.0	1.87
Vegetable Stew, 7.5-oz. can	160	20.0	21.3	2.67
24-oz. can	512	64.0	21.3	2.67
FRANCO AMERICAN				
Macaroni and Cheese, 14¾-oz. can	366	46.8	24.8	3.17
GEBHARDT				
Chili Plain, 15-oz. can	924	89.3	61.6	1.45
Refried Beans, 15-oz. can	428	69.8	28.5	4.65
Tamales, 7½-oz. can	401	38.3	53.4	5.10
HORMEL				
Beef Tamales, 15-oz. can (approx. 15 tamales, each approx. 1 oz.)	560	36.0	37.3	2.40
1 tamale, approx. 1 oz.	37	2.4	37.3	2.40
Chili with Beans, 15-oz. can	640	48.0	42.6	3.20
7.5-oz. can	320	24.0	42.6	3.20
Chili without Beans, 10.5-oz. can	476	12.6	45.3	1.20
7.5-oz. can	340	9.0	45.3	1.20
Pork Chow Mein, "Short Orders," 7½-oz. can	140	13.0	18.7	1.73
LA CHOY				
Chop Suey Vegetables, 16-oz. (1-lb.) can, prepared as directed	105	20.0	6.6	1.25
For comparison:				
Chop Suey With Meat (without noodles), based on a USDA home recipe with ingredients as follows: 4½ oz. of cooked lean beef (trimmed of separable fat), 3½ oz. cooked lean pork (trimmed of separable fat), 2 Tbsp. flour, 1 medium green pepper, chopped (or ½ cup), ½ cup chopped onion, 1 cup diced celery, 1 cup mung bean sprouts, ½ cup canned mushrooms, ¼ cup broth, 3 Tbsp. table fat and 2 Tbsp. soy sauce. (Loss of 10% has been applied for evaporation in cooking.) (Yield: approx. 3½ cups, or 30 oz.)	562	24.0	18.8	0.80
Beef Chow Mein, 14-oz. can	126	9.9	9.0	0.71
Beef Chow Mein, 42-oz. bipack, prepared as package directs (yield, drained: approx. 28.5 oz.)	296	36.2	10.4	1.28
1 cup (approx. 8.0 oz.)	83	10.3	10.4	1.28
Chicken Chow Mein, 14-oz. can	118	9.1	8.4	0.65
Chicken Chow Mein, 42-oz. bipack; prepared as package directs (yield, drained: approx. 28.5 oz.)	359	33.1	12.6	1.16
1 cup (approx. 8.0 oz.)	101	9.5	12.6	1.16
Meatless Chow Mein, 16-oz. (1-lb.) can	93	11.8	5.8	0.74
1 cup (approx. 8.0 oz.)	47	5.9	5.8	0.74
Mushroom Chow Mein, 42-oz. bipack, prepared as package directs (yield, drained: approx. 28½ oz.)	302	38.0	10.6	1.33
1 cup (approx. 8.0 oz.)	85	10.6	10.6	1.33
Pepper Oriental Chow Mein, 16-oz. (1-lb.) can	178	20.5	11.1	1.28
Pepper Oriental Chow Mein, 42-oz. bipack, prepared as package directs (yield, drained: approx. 28½ oz.)	316	39.6	11.1	1.39
1 cup (approx. 8.0 oz.)	89	11.1	11.1	1.39
Pork Chow Mein, 42-oz. bipack (yield, drained: approx. 28½ oz.)	428	37.8	15.0	1.33
1 cup (approx. 8.0 oz.)	120	10.6	15.0	1.33
Shrimp Chow Mein, 14-oz. can	107	9.9	7.6	0.71
Shrimp Chow Mein, 42-oz. bipack, prepared as package directs (yield, drained: approx. 28½ oz.)	(392)	(34.8)	13.8	1.22
1 cup (approx. 8.0 oz.)	(110)	(9.7)	13.8	1.22
Sweet and Sour Vegetables with Chicken, 17-oz. can	680	142.4	40.0	8.38
1 cup (approx. 10.7 oz.)	427	89.3	40.0	8.38

	UNIT Cal.	UNIT Carb.	1 OZ., BY WT. Cal.	1 OZ., BY WT. Carb.
Sweet and Sour Vegetables with Pork, 17-oz. can	723	138.1	42.5	8.13
1 cup (approx. 10.7 oz.)	453	86.7	42.5	8.13
LIBBY'S				
Sloppy Joe, Pork, 15¼-oz. can	642	40.1	42.1	2.63
MARY KITCHEN				
Corned Beef Hash, 15-oz. can	800	40.0	53.3	2.67
7.5-oz. can	400	20.0	53.3	2.67
Roast Beef Hash, 15-oz. can	780	34.0	52.0	2.27
7.5-oz. can	390	17.0	52.0	2.27
MORTON HOUSE				
Beef Stew, 24-oz. can	720	51.0	30.0	2.13
Chili, 22½-oz. can	1020	81.0	45.3	3.60
15-oz. can	680	54.0	45.3	3.60
Chili without Beans, 15-oz. can	680	28.0	45.3	1.87
Meatball Stew, 24-oz. can	870	54.0	36.3	2.25
Pork and Gravy, sliced, 12½-oz. can	380	18.0	30.4	1.44
Salisbury Steak and Mushroom Gravy, 12½-oz. can	480	21.0	38.4	1.68
Sliced Beef and Gravy, 12½-oz. can	380	16.0	30.4	1.28
Sloppy Joe, Beef, with Barbecue Sauce, 15-oz. can	720	57.0	48.0	3.80
Turkey and Gravy, sliced, 12½-oz. can	280	14.0	22.4	1.12
SWANSON				
Chicken à la King, 10½-oz. can	380	18.0	36.2	1.71
Chicken and Dumplings, 15-oz. can	460	36.0	30.7	2.40
Chili con Carne, 15½-oz. can	620	56.0	40.0	3.61
WORTHINGTON (For other Worthington main dishes, see the VEGETARIAN FOODS Chapter)				
Meatless Chili, 20-oz. can	770	81.0	38.5	4.05

COMBINATION MAIN DISHES IN BOXES, by brand

	UNIT Cal.	UNIT Carb.	1 OZ., BY WT. Cal.	1 OZ., BY WT. Carb.
ANN PAGE (A&P)				
Macaroni and Cheese Dinner, 7¼-oz. box	760	148.0	104.8	20.41
Prepared as package directs (yield: approx. 21.2 oz., or 3 cups)	1160	148.0	54.7	6.98
1 cup (approx. 7.1 oz.)	387	49.3	54.7	6.98
BETTY CROCKER CASSEROLE AND SIDE DISHES				
Macaroni and Cheese Casserole, 7¼-oz. package	800	148.0	110.3	20.41
Prepared as package directs, adding 1 Tbsp. of butter and 1 Tbsp. of milk (yield: approx. 40.0 oz., or 5 cups)	1240	152.0	31.0	3.80
1 cup (approx. 8.0 oz.)	248	30.4	31.0	3.80
Noodles Almondine, 5½-oz. package	760	100.0	138.1	18.18
Prepared as package directs, adding ½ Tbsp. of butter and ⅙ cup of milk (yield: approx. 19 oz., or 2⅔ cups)	1040	108.0	54.7	5.68
1 cup (approx. 7.1 oz.)	386	40.0	54.7	5.68
Noodles Stroganoff, 5¼-oz. package	600	96.0	114.3	18.29
Prepared as package directs, adding ½ Tbsp. of butter and ⅙ cup of milk (yield: approx. 19 oz., or 2⅔ cups)	677	98.0	35.6	5.16
1 cup (approx. 7.1 oz.)	251	36.3	35.6	5.16
BETTY CROCKER SIDE QUICKS				
Egg Noodles and Cheese Sauce, 4.3-oz. box prepared as package directs (yield: approx. 14 oz., or 2 cups)	480	76.0	34.3	5.43
1 cup (approx. 7.0 oz.)	240	38.0	34.3	5.43
Egg Noodles and Chicken Sauce, 4.2-oz. box prepared as package directs (yield: approx. 14 oz., or 2 cups)	480	76.0	34.2	5.43
1 cup (approx. 7.0 oz.)	240	38.0	34.2	5.43
FEARN				
Bean Barley Stew, 3.5-oz. box	328	66.0	93.7	18.90
1 package, prepared as package directs, with 2 cups of water and 1 Tbsp. of oil (yield: approx. 19.8 oz.)	(448)	(66.0)	(22.6)	(3.33)
1 cup (approx. 9.9 oz.)	(224)	(33.0)	(22.6)	(3.33)
Blackbean Creole, 3.75-oz. box	260	50.0	69.3	13.33
1 package, prepared as package directs, with 2 cups of water and 1 Tbsp. of oil (yield: approx. 19.8 oz.)	(380)	(50.0)	(19.2)	(2.53)
1 cup (approx. 9.9 oz.)	(190)	(25.0)	(19.2)	(2.53)
Tri-Bean Casserole, 3.75-oz. box	358	54.0	95.5	14.40
1 package, prepared as package directs, with 2 cups of water and 1 Tbsp. of oil (yield: approx. 19.8 oz.)	(478)	(54.0)	(24.2)	(2.75)
1 cup (approx. 9.9 oz.)	(239)	(27.0)	(24.2)	(2.75)
GOLDEN GRAIN				
Macaroni and Cheddar, 7¼-oz. box	806	153.1	111.2	21.12
Prepared as package directs (yield: approx. 19 oz., or 2.8 cups)	806	153.1	40.6	7.70
1 cup (approx. 7.0 oz.)	286	54.3	40.6	7.70
HAMBURGER HELPER				
Hash Dinner, 6-oz. package	650	120.0	108.3	20.00
Prepared as package directs (yield: approx. 18½ oz.)	1500	120.0	81.1	6.49
KRAFT				
Egg Noodles with Chicken, 7-oz. box	760	120.0	108.6	17.14
Prepared as package directs (yield: approx. 3 cups, or 28.2 oz.)	960	120.0	34.0	4.25
1 cup (approx. 9.4 oz.)	320	40.0	34.0	4.25
Macaroni and Cheese Dinner, 7¼-oz. box	760	140.0	104.8	19.31
Prepared as package directs (yield: approx. 3 cups, or 22.2 oz.)	1200	144.0	54.5	6.55
1 cup (approx. 7.3 oz.)	400	48.0	54.5	6.55
Deluxe Dinner, 14-oz. box	1250	170.0	89.3	12.14
Prepared as package directs (yield: approx. 6 cups, or 44 oz.)	1250	170.0	28.4	3.86
1 cup (approx. 7.3 oz.)	208	28.3	28.4	3.86
Spaghetti Dinner, American Style, 8-oz. box	800	152.0	100.0	19.00
Prepared as package directs (yield: approx. 4 cups, or 34 oz.)	1080	176.0	31.8	5.10
1 cup (approx. 8.5 oz.)	270	44.0	31.8	5.10
Spaghetti with Meat Sauce, 1-lb. 3½-oz. box	920	124.0	47.2	6.40
Prepared as package directs (yield: approx. 3 cups, or 24 oz.)	1000	124.0	41.7	5.17
1 cup (approx. 8.0 oz.)	333	41.3	41.7	5.17
Tangy Style Spaghetti Dinner, 8-oz. box	780	148.0	97.5	18.50
Prepared as package directs (yield: approx. 4 cups, or 34.1 oz.)	1040	156.0	30.5	4.60
1 cup (approx. 8.5 oz.)	260	39.0	30.5	4.60
NEAR EAST				
Precooked Medium Grain Couscous, 16-oz. (1-lb.) box	1600	672.0	100.0	42.00
1 package, prepared as package directs (not including butter) (approx. 6.8 oz.)	1600	672.0	(23.5)	(9.88)
1 cup (approx. 8.5 oz.)	200	84.0	(23.5)	(9.88)
Tabouleh Wheat Salad Mix, 7-oz. box	690	192.0	91.4	28.43
Prepared as package directs (not including butter), 1 cup (approx. 8.5 oz.)	160	48.0	(18.8)	(5.65)
NOODLE RONI				
Parmesano, 6-oz. package	650	115.0	108.3	19.17
Prepared as package directs (yield: approx. 2½ cups, or 24 oz.)	1129	121.0	47.0	5.09
1 cup (approx. 9.6 oz.)	452	48.4	47.0	5.09
ORTEGA				
Taco Shell, approx. 0.4 oz.	50	6.0	128.9	15.46
Prepared according to label directions, filled with 2 Tbsp. meat filling, and 1 Tbsp. each of cheese, lettuce, tomato and taco sauce, approx. 1.8 oz.	200	13.0	(113.6)	(7.40)
P & Q (A&P)				
Macaroni and Cheese, 7¼-oz. net box	760	148.0	104.8	20.41
1 box, prepared as package directs (yield: approx. 21.2 oz., or 3 cups)	800	152.0	37.8	7.18
1 cup (approx. 7.1 oz.)	267	50.7	37.8	7.18
PENNSYLVANIA DUTCH				
Macaroni and Cheese, 5¼-oz. package	640	100.0	121.9	19.05
Prepared as package directs (yield: approx. 2 cups, or approx. 12.0 oz.)	640	100.0	(53.3)	(8.33)
1 cup (approx. 6.0 oz.)	320	50.0	(53.3)	(8.33)
Noodles Plus Butter, 4¾-oz. package	600	92.0	126.3	19.37
Prepared as package directs (yield: approx. 2 cups, or 12 oz.)	600	92.0	(50.0)	(7.67)
1 cup (approx. 6.0 oz.)	300	46.0	(50.0)	(7.67)
Noodles Plus Cheese, 4¾-oz. package	600	96.0	126.3	20.21
Prepared as package directs (yield: approx. 2 cups, or 12 oz.)	600	96.0	50.0	8.00
1 cup (approx. 6.0 oz.)	300	48.0	50.0	8.00
Noodles Plus Chicken, 4¾-oz. package	600	100.0	126.3	21.05
Prepared as package directs (yield: approx. 2 cups, or 12 oz.)	600	100.0	(50.0)	(8.33)
1 cup (approx. 6.0 oz.)	300	50.0	(50.0)	(8.33)
Noodles Plus Sauce, Beef, 4½-oz. package	520	96.0	115.6	21.33
Prepared as package directs (yield: approx. 2 cups, or 12 oz.)	520	96.0	(43.3)	(8.00)
1 cup (approx. 6.0 oz.)	260	48.0	(43.3)	(8.00)
STIR-N-SERV				
Lasagna Dinner (noodles and Italian sauce mix), 7.5-oz. box	750	139.3	100.0	18.57

11 SOUPS •

	UNIT		1 OZ., BY WT.		1 FLUID OZ.		1 CUP	
	Cal.	Carb.	Cal.	Carb.	Cal.	Carb.	Cal.	Carb.
CONDENSED AND READY-TO-SERVE SOUPS, based on generic data								
Asparagus, Cream of, condensed, 10¾-oz. can	210	26.0	19.6	2.42				
Prepared with an equal amount of whole milk (yield: approx. 19.5 fl. oz.)	392	39.8	18.4	1.87	20.1	2.05	161	16.4
Prepared with an equal amount of water (yield: approx. 19.3 fl. oz.)	210	26.0	9.9	1.24	10.9	1.34	87	10.7
Bean with Bacon, condensed, 11½-oz. can	420	55.3	36.6	4.81				
Prepared with an equal amount of water (yield: approx. 19.4 fl. oz.)	420	55.3	19.3	2.55	21.6	2.85	173	22.8
Bean with Frankfurters, condensed, 11¼-oz. can	454	53.4	40.3	4.75				
Prepared with an equal amount of water (yield: approx. 19.4 fl. oz.)	454	53.4	21.3	2.50	23.4	2.75	187	22.0
Bean with Ham, Chunky, ready to serve 19¼-oz. can	519	60.9	26.9	3.16	28.9	3.39	231	27.1
Beef Broth or Bouillon, ready to serve, 14-oz. can	27	0.2	2.0	0.01	2.0	0.01	16	0.1
Beef, Chunky, ready to serve, 19-oz. can	383	43.9	20.1	2.31	21.4	2.45	171	19.6
Beef Noodle, condensed, 10¾-oz. can	204	21.8	19.0	2.03				
Prepared with an equal amount of water (yield: approx. 19.4 fl. oz.)	204	21.8	9.6	1.04	10.5	1.12	84	9.0
Black Bean, condensed, 11-oz. can	285	48.1	25.8	4.37				
Prepared with an equal amount of water (yield: approx. 19.4 fl. oz.)	285	48.1	13.3	2.27	14.5	2.48	116	19.8
Celery, Cream of, condensed, 10¾-oz. can	219	21.5	20.4	1.99				
Prepared with an equal amount of whole milk (yield: approx. 19.4 fl. oz.)	400	35.3	18.7	1.66	20.6	1.82	165	14.5
Prepared with an equal amount of water (yield: approx. 19.4 fl. oz.)	219	21.5	10.5	1.03	11.3	1.10	90	8.8
Cheese, condensed, 11-oz. can	377	25.6	34.3	2.32				
Prepared with an equal amount of whole milk (yield: approx. 19.4 fl. oz.)	558	39.4	26.1	1.83	28.8	2.03	230	16.2
Prepared with an equal amount of water (yield: approx. 19.4 fl. oz.)	377	25.6	17.9	1.21	19.4	1.32	155	10.5
Chicken Broth, condensed, 10¾-oz. can	94	2.3	8.7	0.21				
Prepared with an equal amount of water (yield: approx. 19.4 fl. oz.)	94	2.3	4.5	0.11	4.9	0.12	39	0.9
Chicken, Chunky, ready to serve, 10¾-oz. can	216	21.0	20.1	1.95	22.3	2.16	178	17.3
Chicken, Cream of, condensed, 10¾-oz. can	283	22.5	26.4	2.09				
Prepared with an equal amount of whole milk (yield: approx. 19.4 fl. oz.)	464	36.3	21.8	1.71	23.9	1.87	191	15.0
Prepared with an equal amount of water (yield: approx. 19.5 fl. oz.)	283	22.5	13.6	1.08	14.5	1.16	116	9.3
Chicken and Dumplings, condensed, 10½-oz. can	236	14.7	22.5	1.40				
Prepared with an equal amount of water (yield: approx. 19.5 fl. oz.)	236	14.7	11.3	0.71	12.1	0.76	97	6.0
Chicken Gumbo, condensed, 10¾-oz. can	137	20.3	12.8	1.89				
Prepared with an equal amount of water (yield: approx. 19.6 fl. oz.)	137	20.3	6.5	0.97	7.0	1.05	56	8.4
Chicken Noodle, condensed, 10½-oz. can	182	22.7	17.3	2.16				
Prepared with an equal amount of water (yield: approx. 19.4 fl. oz.)	182	22.7	8.8	1.10	9.4	1.17	75	9.4
Chicken Noodle with Meatballs, ready to serve, 20-oz. can	227	19.1	11.3	1.00	12.4	1.05	99	8.4
Chicken Rice, condensed, 10½-oz. can	146	17.4	14.0	1.66				
Prepared with an equal amount of water (yield: approx. 19.5 fl. oz.)	146	17.4	7.1	0.84	7.5	0.89	60	7.2
Chicken Rice, Chunky, ready to serve, 19-oz. can	286	29.2	15.0	1.53	15.9	1.62	127	13.0
Chicken Vegetable, condensed, 10½-oz. can	181	20.9	17.3	1.99				
Prepared with an equal amount of water (yield: approx. 19.5 fl. oz.)	181	20.9	8.8	1.01	9.3	2.43	74	8.6
Chicken Vegetable, Chunky, ready to serve, 19-oz. can	374	42.4	19.6	2.23	20.9	2.36	167	18.9
Chili Beef, condensed, 11¼-oz. can	411	52.1	36.6	4.63				
Prepared with an equal amount of water (yield: approx. 19.5 fl. oz.)	411	52.1	19.3	2.43	21.1	2.68	169	21.5

	UNIT		1 OZ., BY WT.		1 FLUID OZ.		1 CUP	
	Cal.	Carb.	Cal.	Carb.	Cal.	Carb.	Cal.	Carb.
Clam Chowder, Manhattan, condensed, 10¾-oz. can	187	29.7	17.3	2.76				
Prepared with an equal amount of water (yield: approx. 19.4 fl. oz.)	190	29.7	9.1	0.43	9.8	1.53	78	12.2
Clam Chowder, Chunky Manhattan, ready to serve, 19-oz. can	299	42.3	15.9	2.22	16.6	2.35	133	18.8
Clam Chowder, New England, condensed, 10¾-oz. can	214	26.5	19.8	2.46				
Prepared with an equal amount of whole milk (yield: approx. 19.4 fl. oz.)	396	40.3	18.7	2.00	20.4	2.08	163	16.6
Prepared with an equal amount of water (yield: approx. 19.4 fl. oz.)	214	26.5	10.2	1.27	11.0	1.36	88	10.9
Consommé with Gelatin, condensed, 10½-oz. can	71	4.3	6.8	0.41				
Prepared with an equal amount of water (yield: approx. 19.7 fl. oz.)	71	4.3	3.4	0.21	3.6	0.22	29	1.8
Crab, ready to serve, 13-oz. can	114	15.6	8.8	1.20	9.5	1.29	76	10.3
Escarole, ready to serve, 20-oz. can	61	4.0	3.1	0.20	3.4	0.22	27	1.8
Gazpacho, ready to serve, 13-oz. can	87	1.2	6.5	0.09	7.1	0.10	57	0.8
Groundnut (Peanut) (based on data from Ghana), 16-oz. (1-lb.) can	667	0.9	41.7	0.06				
Lentil, (based on data from Middle East), 16-oz. (1-lb.) can	327	(42.6)	20.4	(2.67)				
Lentil with Ham, ready to serve, 20-oz. can	320	46.3	16.0	2.32	17.5	2.53	140	20.2
Minestrone, condensed, 10½-oz. can	202	27.3	19.3	2.60				
Prepared with an equal amount of water (yield: approx. 19.4 fl. oz.)	202	27.3	9.6	1.32	10.4	1.41	83	11.2
Minestrone, Chunky, ready to serve, 19-oz. can	285	46.6	15.0	2.45	15.9	2.59	127	20.7
Mushroom, Cream of, condensed, 10¾-oz. can	313	22.6	29.2	2.10				
Prepared with an equal amount of whole milk (yield: approx. 19.4 fl. oz.)	494	36.4	23.2	1.72	25.4	1.88	203	15.0
Prepared with an equal amount of water (yield: approx. 19.5 fl. oz.)	313	22.6	15.0	1.08	16.1	1.16	129	9.3
Mushroom with Beef Stock, condensed, 10¾-oz. can	208	22.6	19.3	2.10				
Prepared with an equal amount of water (yield: approx. 19.6 fl. oz.)	208	22.6	9.9	1.08	10.6	1.16	85	9.3
Onion, condensed, 10½-oz. can	138	19.9	13.0	1.89				
Prepared with an equal amount of water (yield: approx. 19.4 fl. oz.)	138	19.9	6.8	0.96	7.1	1.02	57	8.2
Oyster Stew, condensed, 10½-oz. can	144	9.9	13.6	0.94				
Prepared with an equal amount of whole milk (yield: approx. 19.3 fl. oz.)	325	23.7	15.6	1.13	16.8	1.22	134	9.9
Prepared with an equal amount of water (yield: approx. 19.5 fl. oz.)	144	9.9	6.8	0.47	7.4	0.51	59	4.1
Pea, Green, condensed, 11¼-oz. can	398	64.4	35.4	5.72				
Prepared with an equal amount of whole milk (yield: approx. 19.4 fl. oz.)	579	78.6	26.7	3.60	29.9	4.03	239	32.2
Prepared with an equal amount of water (yield: approx. 19.4 fl. oz.)	398	64.4	18.7	3.01	20.5	3.31	164	26.5
Pea, Split, with Ham, condensed, 11½-oz. can	459	67.8	40.0	5.90				
Prepared with an equal amount of water (yield: approx. 19.4 fl. oz.)	459	67.8	21.3	3.13	23.6	3.49	189	28.0
Pea, Split, with Ham, Chunky, ready to serve, 19-oz. can	413	60.2	21.8	3.17	23.0	3.35	184	26.8
Pepperpot. condensed, 10½-oz. can	251	22.8	23.8	2.17				
Prepared with an equal amount of water (yield: approx. 19.5 fl. oz.)	251	22.8	12.2	1.10	12.9	1.17	103	9.4
Potato, Cream of, condensed, 10¾-oz. can	178	27.9	16.7	2.59				

	UNIT		1 OZ., BY WT.		1 FLUID OZ.		1 CUP	
	Cal.	Carb.	Cal.	Carb.	Cal.	Carb.	Cal.	Carb.
Prepared with an equal amount of whole milk (yield: approx. 19.5 fl. oz.)	360	41.7	17.0	1.96	18.5	2.15	148	17.2
Prepared with an equal amount of water (yield: approx. 19.6 fl. oz.)	178	27.9	8.5	1.33	9.1	1.43	73	11.5
Scotch Broth, condensed, 10½-oz. can	195	23.0	18.7	2.19				
Prepared with an equal amount of water (yield: approx. 19.5 fl. oz.)	195	23.0	9.4	1.11	10.0	1.18	80	9.5
Shrimp, Cream of, condensed, 10¾-oz. can	219	19.9	20.4	1.85				
Prepared with an equal amount of whole milk (yield: approx. 19.4 fl. oz.)	400	33.8	18.7	1.59	20.6	1.74	165	13.9
Prepared with an equal amount of water (yield: approx. 19.4 fl. oz.)	219	19.9	10.5	0.95	11.3	1.02	90	8.2
Stockpot, condensed, 11-oz. can	242	27.9	22.1	2.54				
Prepared with an equal amount of water (yield: approx. 19.4 fl. oz.)	242	27.9	11.3	1.32	12.5	1.44	100	11.5
Tomato, condensed, 10¾-oz. can	208	40.3	19.3	3.75				
Prepared with an equal amount of whole milk (yield: approx. 19.5 fl. oz.)	389	54.1	18.4	2.55	20.0	2.79	160	22.3
Prepared with an equal amount of water (yield: approx. 19.3 fl. oz.)	208	40.3	9.9	1.93	10.8	2.07	86	16.6
Tomato Beef with Noodle, condensed, 10¾-oz. can	341	51.4	31.8	4.78				
Prepared with an equal amount of water (yield: approx. 19.5 fl. oz.)	341	51.4	16.2	2.46	17.5	2.65	140	21.2
Tomato Bisque, condensed, 11-oz. can	300	57.6	27.2	5.24				
Prepared with an equal amount of whole milk (yield: approx. 19.4 fl. oz.)	481	71.4	22.4	3.33	24.8	3.68	198	29.4
Prepared with an equal amount of water (yield: approx. 19.5 fl. oz.)	300	57.6	14.2	2.72	15.4	2.97	123	23.7
Tomato Rice, condensed, 11-oz. can	291	53.3	26.4	4.84				
Prepared with an equal amount of water (yield: approx. 19.4 fl. oz.)	291	53.3	13.6	2.52	15.0	2.74	120	21.9
Turkey, Chunky, ready to serve, 18¾-oz. can	306	31.7	16.2	1.69	17.0	1.76	136	14.1
Turkey Noodle, condensed, 10¾-oz. can	168	21.0	15.6	1.95				
Prepared with an equal amount of water (yield: approx. 19.5 fl. oz.)	168	21.0	7.9	1.00	8.6	1.08	69	8.6
Turkey Vegetable, condensed, 10½-oz. can	179	21.0	17.0	2.00				
Prepared with an equal amount of water (yield: approx. 19.2 fl. oz.)	179	21.0	8.5	1.02	9.3	1.08	74	8.6
Vegetable (based on data from France), 16-oz. (1-lb.) can	113	24.5	7.0	1.53				
Vegetable with Beef, condensed, 10¾-oz. can	192	24.7	17.9	2.30				
Prepared with an equal amount of water (yield: approx. 19.4 fl. oz.)	192	24.7	9.1	1.18	9.9	1.27	79	10.2
Vegetable with Beef Broth, condensed, 10½-oz. can	197	31.9	18.7	3.03				
Prepared with an equal amount of water (yield: approx. 19.5 fl. oz.)	197	31.9	9.6	1.54	10.1	1.64	81	13.1
Vegetable, Chunky, ready to serve, 19-oz. can	274	42.7	14.5	2.25	15.3	2.38	122	19.0
Vegetable, Vegetarian, condensed, 10½-oz. can	176	29.1	16.7	2.77				
Prepared with an equal amount of water (yield: approx. 19.5 fl. oz.)	176	29.1	8.5	1.41	9.0	1.50	72	12.0
DEHYDRATED SOUPS, based on generic data								
Asparagus, Cream of, 2¼-oz. package	234	35.6	103.8	15.81				
Prepared with 4½ cups of water (yield: approx. 36 fl. oz.)	265	40.3	6.5	1.01	7.4	1.12	59	9.0

	UNIT Cal.	UNIT Carb.	1 OZ., BY WT. Cal.	1 OZ., BY WT. Carb.	1 FLUID OZ. Cal.	1 FLUID OZ. Carb.	1 CUP Cal.	1 CUP Carb.
Bean with Bacon, 1-oz. package	105	16.4	104.9	16.37				
Prepared with 1 cup of water (yield: approx. 8 fl. oz.)	105	16.4	11.3	1.75	13.1	2.05	105	16.4
Beef Bouillon or Broth, 0.2-oz. packet	14	1.4	67.5	6.71				
Prepared with ¾ cup of water (yield: approx. 6 fl. oz.)	14	1.4	2.3	0.23	2.4	0.24	19	1.9
Beef Broth, cubed, 0.12-oz. cube	6	0.6	48.2	4.56				
Prepared with ¾ cup of water (yield: approx. 6 fl. oz.)	6	0.6	0.9	0.09	1.0	0.10	8	0.8
Beef Noodle, 0.3-oz. package	30	6.9	93.6	13.79				
Prepared with 1 cup of water (yield: approx. 8 fl. oz.)	30	6.9	4.5	0.68	5.1	0.75	30	4.5
Cauliflower, 0.7-oz. package	68	10.7	102.1	16.04				
Prepared with 1 cup of water (yield: approx. 8 fl. oz.)	68	10.7	7.7	1.19	8.5	1.34	68	10.7
Celery, Cream of, 0.6-oz. package	62	9.7	101.5	15.85				
Prepared with 1 cup of water (yield: approx. 8 fl. oz.)	62	9.7	7.1	1.09	7.9	1.22	62	9.7
Chicken Bouillon or Broth, 0.21-oz. package	16	1.1	75.7	5.11				
Prepared with ¾ cup of water (yield: approx. 6 fl. oz.)	16	1.1	2.6	0.17	2.6	0.18	21	1.4
Chicken Broth, cubed, 0.17-oz. package	9	1.1	56.1	6.66				
Prepared with ¾ cup of water (yield: approx. 6 fl. oz.	9	1.1	1.4	0.18	1.6	0.19	13	1.5
Chicken, Cream of, 0.6-oz. package	80	9.9	123.6	15.41				
Prepared with ¾ cup water (yield: approx. 6 fl. oz.)	80	9.9	11.6	1.45	13.4	1.67	107	13.4
Chicken Noodle, 2.6-oz. package	257	36.0	97.8	13.72				
Prepared with 5 cups of water (yield: approx. 39 fl. oz.)	257	36.0	6.0	0.83	6.6	0.93	53	7.4
Chicken Rice, 0.6-oz. package	60	9.3	104.6	16.20				
Prepared with 1 cup of water (yield: approx. 8 fl. oz.)	60	9.3	6.8	1.04	7.5	1.16	60	9.3
Chicken Vegetable, 0.4-oz. package	37	5.8	98.1	15.60				
Prepared with ¾ cup of water (yield: approx. 6 fl. oz.)	37	5.8	5.7	0.88	6.1	1.00	49	7.8
Clam Chowder, Manhattan, 0.7-oz. package	65	10.9	97.8	16.29				
Prepared with 1 cup of water (yield: approx. 8 fl. oz.)	65	10.9	7.2	1.21	8.1	1.36	65	10.9
Consommé, with Gelatin Added, 2-oz. package	77	9.3	38.8	4.62				
Prepared with 4½ cups of water (yield: approx. 37 fl. oz.)	77	9.3	2.0	0.24	2.1	0.26	17	2.1
Leek, 2.75-oz. package	294	47.4	106.9	17.23				
Prepared with 4 cups of water (yield: approx. 33 fl. oz.)	294	47.4	7.9	1.28	8.9	1.43	71	11.4
Minestrone, 2.75-oz. package	279	41.8	101.5	15.20				
Prepared with 3½ cups of water (yield: approx. 28 fl. oz.)	279	41.8	8.8	1.32	9.9	1.49	79	11.9
Mushroom, 2.6-oz. package	328	38.1	125.0	14.51				
Prepared with 4½ cups of water (yield: approx. 27 fl. oz.)	328	38.1	10.8	1.25	12.0	1.39	74	8.5
Onion, 1.4-oz. package	115	20.9	83.4	15.17				
Prepared with 4 cups of water (yield: approx. 33 fl. oz.)	115	20.9	3.1	0.58	3.5	0.63	28	5.1
Oxtail, 2.6-oz. package	280	35.6	106.9	13.58				
Prepared with 4 cups of water (yield: approx. 32 fl. oz.)	280	35.6	7.9	1.00	8.9	1.12	71	9.0
Pea, Green or Split, 4-oz. package	402	68.6	100.9	17.20				
Prepared with 3 cups of water (yield: approx. 24 fl. oz.)	402	68.6	13.9	2.37	16.7	2.84	133	22.7
Tomato, 0.75-oz. package	77	14.6	102.1	19.36				
Prepared with ¾ cup of water (yield: approx. 6 fl. oz.)	77	14.6	11.1	2.08	12.8	2.43	102	19.4
Tomato Vegetable, 1.4-oz. package	125	23.1	92.1	16.98				
Prepared with 2¼ cups of water (yield: approx. 18 fl. oz.)	125	23.1	6.2	1.15	6.9	1.28	55	10.2
Vegetable Beef, 2.6-oz. package	256	38.5	97.5	14.67				
Prepared with 5 cups of water (yield: approx. 39 fl. oz.)	256	38.5	6.0	0.09	6.6	1.00	53	8.0
Vegetable, Cream of, 0.6-oz. package	79	9.2	126.5	14.77				
Prepared with ¾ cup of water (yield: approx. 6 fl. oz.)	79	9.2	11.6	1.34	13.1	1.54	105	12.3

SOUPS, by brand

BALANCED

	UNIT Cal.	UNIT Carb.	1 OZ., BY WT. Cal.	1 OZ., BY WT. Carb.	1 FLUID OZ. Cal.	1 FLUID OZ. Carb.	1 CUP Cal.	1 CUP Carb.
Condensed Soups:								
Dietetic Pea, 8-oz. can	195	38.1	26.0	5.08			(220)	(42.8)
Prepared with an equal amount of water (yield: approx. 16 fl. oz.)	195	38.1	(12.2)	(2.38)	(12.2)	(2.38)	(104)	(20.3)
Dietetic Tomato, 8-oz. can	146	29.3	19.5	3.99			(160)	(32.2)
Prepared with an equal amount of water (yield: approx. 16 fl. oz.)	146	29.3	(9.1)	(1.83)	(9.1)	(1.83)	(78)	(15.7)

CAMPBELL'S

	UNIT Cal.	UNIT Carb.	1 OZ., BY WT. Cal.	1 OZ., BY WT. Carb.	1 FLUID OZ. Cal.	1 FLUID OZ. Carb.	1 CUP Cal.	1 CUP Carb.
Condensed, Semi-Condensed, and Ready To Serve Soups:								
Asparagus, Cream of, condensed, 10¾-oz. can	200	24.0	18.6	2.23			160	19.2
Prepared with an equal amount of water (yield: approx. 20 fl. oz.)	200	24.0	9.5	1.13	10.0	1.20	80	9.6
Prepared with ½ can water and ½ can whole milk (yield: approx. 20 fl. oz.)	314	33.3	9.5	1.13	15.7	1.67	126	13.3
Bean with Bacon, condensed, 11½-oz. can	380	52.0	33.0	4.52			304	41.6
Prepared with an equal amount of water (yield: approx. 20 fl. oz.)	380	52.0	17.4	2.37	19.0	2.60	152	20.8
Bean, Old Fashioned, semi-condensed, "Soup For One," 7¾-oz. can	210	28.0	27.1	3.61			252	33.6
Prepared with ½ can of water (yield: approx. 11⅝ oz.)	210	28.0	14.3	1.91	18.1	2.41	168	22.4
Black Bean, condensed, 11-oz. can	260	44.0	23.6	4.00			208	35.2
Prepared with an equal amount of water (yield: approx. 20 fl. oz.)	260	44.0	12.2	2.06	13.0	2.20	104	17.6
Beef, condensed, 11-oz. can	200	28.0	18.2	2.55			160	22.4
Prepared with an equal amount of water (yield: approx. 20 fl. oz.)	200	28.0	9.4	1.31	10.0	1.40	80	11.2
Beef Broth (Bouillon), condensed, 10½-oz. can	70	6.0	6.7	0.57			56	4.8
Prepared with an equal amount of water (yield: approx. 20 fl. oz.)	70	6.0			3.5	0.30	28	2.4
Beef Noodle, condensed, 10¾-oz. can	180	20.0	16.7	1.88			144	16.0
Prepared with an equal amount of water (yield: approx. 20 fl. oz.)	180	20.0	8.6	0.96	9.0	1.00	72	8.0
Celery, Cream of, condensed, 10¾-oz. can	220	20.0	20.5	1.86			176	16.0
Prepared with an equal amount of water (yield: approx. 20 fl. oz.)	220	20.0	(10.4)	(0.95)	11.0	1.00	88	8.0
Prepared with ½ can of water and ½ can of whole milk (yield: approx. 20 fl. oz.)	(319)	(27.5)	(15.1)	(1.30)	16.0	1.38	128	11.0

	UNIT		1 OZ., BY WT.		1 FLUID OZ.		1 CUP	
	Cal.	Carb.	Cal.	Carb.	Cal.	Carb.	Cal.	Carb.
Cheddar Cheese, condensed, 11-oz. can	360	24.0	32.7	2.18			288	19.2
Prepared with an equal amount of water (yield: approx. 20 fl. oz.)	360	24.0	(16.8)	(1.12)	18.0	1.20	144	9.6
Prepared with ½ can of water and ½ can of whole milk (yield: approx. 20 fl. oz.)	459	31.5	(21.5)	(1.47)	23.0	1.58	184	12.6
Chicken Alphabet, condensed, 10¾-oz. can	220	30.0	20.5	2.79			(176)	(24.0)
Prepared with an equal amount of water (yield: approx. 20 fl. oz.)	220	30.0	(10.4)	(1.42)	11.0	1.50	88	12.0
Chicken Broth, condensed, 10¾-oz. can	100	6.0	9.3	0.56			80	4.8
Prepared with an equal amount of water (yield: approx. 20 fl. oz.)	100	6.0			5.0	0.30	40	2.4
Chicken, Cream of, condensed, 10¾-oz. can	280	20.0	26.0	1.86			224	16.0
Prepared with an equal amount of water (yield: approx. 20 fl. oz.)	280	20.0	(13.2)	(0.95)	14.0	1.00	112	8.0
Prepared with ½ can of water and ½ can of whole milk (yield: approx. 20 fl. oz.	(379)	(27.5)	(17.9)	(1.30)	19.0	1.38	152	11.0
Chicken 'n Dumplings, condensed, 10½-oz. can	240	14.0	22.9	1.33			192	11.2
Prepared with an equal amount of water (yield: approx. 20 fl. oz.)	240	14.0	(11.5)	(0.67)	12.0	0.70	96	5.6
Chicken Gumbo, condensed, 10¾-oz. can	140	20.0	13.0	1.86			112	16.0
Prepared with an equal amount of water (yield: approx. 20 fl. oz.)	140	20.0	(6.6)	(0.95)	7.0	1.00	56	8.0
Chicken Noodle, condensed, 10¾-oz. can	180	22.0	16.7	2.05			144	17.6
Prepared with an equal amount of water (yield: approx. 20 fl. oz.)	180	22.0	(8.5)	(1.04)	9.0	1.10	72	8.8
Chicken & Noodles, Golden, semi-condensed, "Soup For One," 7¾-oz. can	120	14.0	15.5	1.81			144	16.8
Prepared with ½ can of water (yield: approx. 11⅝ oz.)	120	14.0	(8.2)	(0.96)	10.3	1.20	96	11.2
Chicken Noodle-o's, condensed, 10¼-oz. can	180	24.0	17.6	2.34			144	19.2
Prepared with an equal amount of water (yield: approx. 20 fl. oz.)	180	24.0	(8.7)	(1.16)	9.0	1.20	72	9.6
Chicken with Rice, condensed, 10½-oz. can	160	18.0	15.2	1.71			128	14.4
Prepared with an equal amount of water (yield: approx. 20 fl. oz.)	160	18.0	(7.7)	(0.86)	8.0	0.90	64	7.2
Chicken 'N Stars, condensed, 10½-oz. can	160	18.0	15.2	1.71			128	14.4
Prepared with an equal amount of water (yield: approx. 20 fl. oz.)	160	18.0	(7.7)	(0.86)	8.0	0.90	64	7.2
Chicken Vegetable, condensed, 10½-oz. can	180	20.0	17.1	1.90			144	16.0
Prepared with an equal amount of water (yield: approx. 20 fl. oz.)	180	20.0	(8.6)	(0.96)	9.0	1.00	72	8.0
Chicken Vegetable, "Full Flavor," semi-condensed, "Soup For One," 7¾-oz. can	130	14.0					156	16.8
Prepared with ½ can of water (yield: approx. 11⅝ oz.)	130	14.0	(11.2)	(1.20)	13.0	1.40	104	11.2
Chili Beef, condensed, 11¼-oz. can	380	48.0	33.8	4.27			304	38.4
Prepared with an equal amount of water (yield: approx. 20 fl. oz.)	380	48.0	(17.6)	(2.22)	19.0	2.40	152	19.2
Clam Chowder, Manhattan Style, condensed, 10¾-oz. can	200	30.0	18.6	2.79			160	24.0
Prepared with an equal amount of water (yield: approx. 20 fl. oz.)	200	30.0	(9.5)	(1.42)	10.0	1.50	80	12.0
Clam Chowder, New England, condensed, 10¾-oz. can	200	13.0	18.6	1.21			160	10.4
Prepared with ½ can of water and ½ can of whole milk (yield: approx. 20 fl. oz.)	(299)	(20.5)	(14.1)	(0.97)	15.0	1.03	120	8.2
Prepared with an equal amount of whole milk (yield: approx. 20 fl. oz.)	399	28.0	(18.9)	(1.32)	20.0	1.40	160	11.2
Clam Chowder, New England, semi-condensed, "Soup For One," 7¾-oz. can	125	16.0	16.1	2.06			129	16.5
Prepared with ½ can of water (yield: approx. 11⅝ oz.)	125	16.0	(8.5)	(1.09)	10.8	1.38	88	11.0
Prepared with ½ can of whole milk (yield: approx. 11⅝ oz.)	200	21.0	(13.7)	(1.43)	17.2	1.81	138	14.5
Consommé, Beef (Gelatin Added), condensed, 10½-oz. can	90	8.0	8.6	0.76			72	6.4
Prepared with an equal amount of water (yield: approx. 20 fl. oz.)	90	8.0			4.5	0.40	36	3.2
Golden Soups, see Individual flavors								
Hotdog Bean, condensed, 11¼-oz. can	420	50.0	37.3	4.44			336	40.0
Prepared with an equal amount of water (yield: approx. 20 fl. oz.)	430	50.0	(19.9)	(2.31)	21.0	2.50	168	20.0
Meatball Alphabet, condensed, 10¾-oz. can	280	32.0	26.0	2.98			224	25.6
Prepared with an equal amount of water (yield: approx. 20 fl. oz.)	280	32.0	(13.2)	(1.51)	14.0	1.60	112	12.8
Minestrone, condensed, 10½-oz. can	220	30.0	21.0	2.88			176	24.0
Prepared with an equal amount of water (yield: approx. 20 fl. oz.)	220	3.00	(10.5)	(1.44)	11.0	1.50	88	12.0
Mushroom, Cream of, condensed, 10¾-oz. can	300	22.0	27.9	2.05			240	17.6
Prepared with an equal amount of water (yield: approx. 20 fl. oz.)	300	22.0	(14.2)	(1.04)	15.0	1.10	120	8.8
Prepared with ½ can of water and ½ can of whole milk (yield: approx. 20 fl. oz.)	399	29.5	(18.9)	(1.39)	20.0	1.48	160	11.8
Mushroom, Cream of, low sodium, ready to serve, 7¼-oz. can	140	10.0	19.3	1.38	20.7	1.48	166	11.9
Mushroom, Golden, condensed, 10¾-oz. can	220	22.0	20.5	2.05			176	17.6
Prepared with an equal amount of water (yield: approx. 20 fl. oz.)	220	22.0	(10.4)	(1.04)	11.0	1.10	88	8.8
Mushroom, Savory Cream of, with Wine, semi-condensed, "Soup For One," 7½-oz. can	160	12.0	21.3	1.60			171	12.9
Prepared with ½ can of water (yield: approx. 10.5 fl. oz.)	160	12.0	(11.1)	(0.83)	15.2	1.14	114	8.6
Prepared with ½ can of whole milk (yield: approx. 10.5 fl. oz.)	237	17.4	(16.5)	(1.21)	22.6	1.66	181	13.3
Noodles & Beef Broth, condensed, 10¾-oz. can	160	20.0	14.9	1.86			128	16.0
Prepared with an equal amount of water (yield: approx. 20 fl. oz.)	160	20.0	(7.6)	(0.95)	8.0	1.00	64	8.0
Noodles & Chicken Broth, condensed, 10¾-oz. can	160	20.0	14.9	1.86			128	16.0
Prepared with an equal amount of water (yield: approx. 20 fl. oz.)	160	20.0	(7.6)	(0.95)	8.0	1.00	64	8.0
(Curly) Noodle with Chicken, condensed, 10¾-oz. can	200	24.0	18.6	2.23			160	19.2
Prepared with an equal amount of water (yield: approx. 20 fl. oz.)	200	24.0	(9.5)	(1.13)	10.0	1.20	80	9.6
Noodles & Ground Beef, condensed, 10¾-oz. can	220	28.0	20.5	2.60			176	22.4
Prepared with an equal amount of water (yield: approx. 20 fl. oz.)	220	28.0	(10.4)	(1.32)	11.0	1.40	88	11.2
Onion, condensed, 10½ oz. can	160	18.0	15.2	1.71			128	14.4
Prepared with an equal amount of water (yield: approx. 20 fl. oz.)	160	18.0	(7.7)	(0.86)	8.0	0.90	64	7.2
Onion, Cream of, condensed, 10¾-oz. can	160	18.0	14.9	1.67			128	14.4
Prepared with an equal amount of water (yield: approx. 20 fl. oz.)	160	18.0	(7.6)	(0.86)	8.0	0.90	64	7.2

	UNIT		1 OZ., BY WT.		1 FLUID OZ.		1 CUP	
	Cal.	Carb.	Cal.	Carb.	Cal.	Carb.	Cal.	Carb.
Prepared with ½ can of water and ½ can of whole milk (yield: approx. 20 fl. oz.)	259	25.5	(12.3)	(1.21)	13.0	1.28	104	10.2
Oyster Stew, condensed, 10½-oz.	140	10.0	13.3	0.95			112	8.0
Prepared with an equal amount of water (yield: approx. 20 fl. oz.)	140	10.0	(6.7)	(0.48)	7.0	0.50	56	4.0
Prepared with ½ can of water and ½ can of whole milk (yield: approx. 20 fl. oz.)	239	17.5	(11.4)	(0.84)	12.0	0.88	96	7.0
Pea, Green, condensed, 11¾-oz. can	360	56.0	32.0	4.98			288	44.8
Prepared with an equal amount of water (yield: approx. 20 fl. oz.)	360	56.0	(16.6)	(2.59)	18.0	2.80	144	22.4
Prepared with ½ can of water and ½ can of whole milk (yield: approx. 20 fl. oz.)	459	63.5	(21.2)	(2.93)	23.0	3.18	184	25.4
Pea, Green, low sodium, ready to serve, 7½-oz. can	150	24.0	20.0	3.20	22.5	3.60	180	28.8
Pea, Split with Ham & Bacon, condensed, 11½-oz. can	420	60.0	36.5	5.22			336	48.0
Prepared with an equal amount of water (yield: approx. 20 fl. oz.)	420	60.0	(19.2)	(2.74)	21.0	3.00	168	24.0
Prepared with ½ can of water and ½ can of whole milk (yield: approx. 20 fl. oz.)	519	67.5	(23.7)	(3.08)	26.0	3.38	208	27.0
Pepper Pot, condensed, 10½-oz. can	260	24.0	24.8	2.29			208	19.2
Prepared with an equal amount of water (yield: approx. 20 fl. oz.)	260	24.0	(12.4)	(1.15)	13.0	1.20	104	9.6
Potato, Cream of, condensed, 10¾-oz. can	180	28.0	16.7	2.60			144	22.4
Prepared with an equal amount of water (yield: approx. 20 fl. oz.)	180	28.0	(8.5)	(1.32)	9.0	1.40	72	11.2
Prepared with ½ can of water and ½ can of whole milk (yield: approx. 20 fl. oz.)	(279)	(35.5)	(13.2)	(1.68)	14.0	1.78	112	14.2
Scotch Broth, condensed, 10½-oz. can	200	22.0	19.0	2.10			160	17.6
Prepared with an equal amount of water (yield: approx. 20 fl. oz.)	200	22.0			10.0	1.10	80	8.8
Shrimp, Cream of, condensed, 10¾-oz. can	220	20.0	20.5	1.86			176	16.0
Prepared with an equal amount of water (yield: approx. 20 fl. oz.)	220	20.0	(10.4)	(0.95)	11.0	1.00	88	8.0
Prepared with ½ can of water and ½ can of whole milk (yield: approx. 20 fl. oz.)	319	27.7	(15.1)	(1.31)	16.0	1.39	128	11.1
Stock Pot, Vegetables & Beef, condensed, 11-oz. can	240	26.0	21.8	2.36			192	20.8
Prepared with an equal amount of water (yield: approx. 20 fl. oz.)	240	26.0	(11.2)	(1.21)	12.0	1.30	96	10.4
Tomato, condensed, 10¾-oz. can	220	40.0	20.5	3.72			176	32.0
Prepared with an equal amount of water (yield: approx. 20 fl. oz.)	220	40.0	(10.4)	(1.89)	11.0	2.00	88	16.0
Prepared with ½ can of water and ½ can of whole milk (yield: approx. 20 fl. oz.)	319	47.5	(15.1)	(2.25)	16.0	2.38	128	15.0
Tomato, low sodium, ready to serve, 7¼-oz. can	130	22.0	17.9	3.03	19.2	3.25	154	26.0
Tomato-Beef Noodle-o's, condensed, 10¾-oz. can	320	48.0	29.8	4.47			256	38.4
Prepared with an equal amount of water (yield: approx. 20 fl. oz.)	320	48.0	(15.1)	(2.27)	16.0	2.40	128	19.2
Tomato Bisque, condensed, 11-oz. can	280	54.0	25.5	4.91			224	43.2
Prepared with an equal amount of water (yield: approx. 20 fl. oz.)	280	54.0	(13.1)	(2.52)	14.0	2.70	112	21.6
Prepared with ½ can of water and ½ can of whole milk (yield: approx. 20 fl. oz.)	379	61.5	(17.7)	(2.87)	19.0	3.08	152	24.5
Tomato Rice, Old Fashioned, condensed, 11-oz. can	260	52.0	23.6	4.73			208	41.8
Prepared with an equal amount of water (yield: approx. 20 fl. oz.)	260	52.0	(12.2)	(2.43)	13.0	2.60	104	20.8
Tomato Royale, semi-condensed, "Soup For One," 7¾-oz. can	180	33.0	23.2	4.26				
Prepared with ½ can of water (yield: approx. 10.5 fl. oz.)	180	33.0	(15.5)	(2.83)	17.1	3.14	133	25.1
Prepared with ½ can of whole milk (yield: approx. 10.5 fl. oz.)	(250)	(43.6)	(21.1)	(3.67)	23.8	4.15	170	29.4
Turkey Noodle, condensed, 10¾-oz. can	160	20.0	14.9	1.86			128	16.0
Prepared with an equal amount of water (yield: approx. 20 fl. oz.)	160	20.0	(7.6)	(0.95)	8.0	1.00	64	8.0
Turkey Noodle, low sodium, ready to serve, 7¼-oz. can	60	7.0	8.3	0.97	8.9	1.04	71	8.3
Turkey Vegetable, condensed, 10½-oz. can	180	20.0	17.1	1.90			144	16.0
Prepared with an equal amount of water (yield: approx. 20 fl. oz.)	180	20.0	(8.6)	(0.96)	9.0	1.00	72	8.0
Vegetable, condensed, 10½-oz. can	200	34.0	19.0	3.24			160	27.2
Prepared with an equal amount of water (yield: approx. 20 fl. oz.)	200	34.0	(9.6)	(1.63)	10.0	1.70	80	13.6
Vegetable, low sodium, ready to serve, 7½-oz. can	90	15.0	12.0	2.00	13.0	2.10	104	16.8
Vegetable Beef, condensed, 10½-oz. can	180	20.0	17.1	1.90			144	16.0
Prepared with an equal amount of water (yield: approx. 20 fl. oz.)	180	20.0	(8.6)	(0.96)	9.0	1.00	72	8.0
Vegetable Beef, low sodium, ready to serve, 7¼-oz. can	80	8.0	11.0	1.10	11.5	1.16	92	9.2
Vegetable Noodle-o's, Golden, condensed, 10½-oz. can	180	26.0	17.1	2.48			144	20.8
Prepared with an equal amount of water (yield: approx. 20 fl. oz.)	180	26.0	(8.6)	(1.24)	9.0	1.30	72	10.4
Vegetable, Old Fashioned, condensed, 10½-oz. can	180	22.0	17.1	2.10			144	17.6
Prepared with an equal amount of water (yield: approx. 20 fl. oz.)	180	22.0	(8.6)	(1.05)	9.0	1.10	72	8.8
Vegetable, Old World, semi-condensed, "Soup For One," 7¾-oz. can	125	18.0	16.1	2.32			139	19.5
Prepared with ½ can of water (yield: approx. 11⅝ oz.)	125	18.0	(8.5)	(1.23)	11.3	1.63	90	13.0
Vegetarian Vegetable Soup, Condensed, 10½-oz. can	180	28.0	17.1	2.67			144	22.4
Prepared with an equal amount of water (yield: approx. 20 fl. oz.)	180	28.0	8.6	1.33	9.0	1.40	72	11.2
CAMPBELL'S CHUNKY								
Ready-to-Serve Soups:								
Chunky Beef, 10¾-oz. can	(215)	(22.6)	20.0	2.11	21.1	2.22	169	17.8
19-oz. can	380	40.0	20.0	2.11	21.1	2.22	169	17.8
Chunky Chicken, 10¾-oz. can	215	23.1	20.0	2.15	21.1	2.34	169	18.7
19-oz. can	380	42.0	20.0	2.15	21.1	2.34	169	18.7
Chunky Chicken with Rice, 19-oz. can	320	32.0	16.8	1.68	17.8	1.78	142	14.2
Chunky Chicken Vegetable, 19-oz. can	380	42.0	20.0	2.50	21.1	2.34	169	18.7
Chunky Chili Beef, 11-oz. can	(293)	37.0	26.7	3.36	28.9	3.55	231	28.4
19½-oz. can	520	(65.6)	26.7	3.36	28.9	3.55	231	28.4
Chunky Manhattan Style Clam Chowder, 19-oz. can	320	46.0	16.8	2.42	17.8	2.55	142	20.4
Chunky Minestrone, 19-oz. can	320	50.0	16.8	2.63	17.8	2.78	142	22.2
Chunky Old Fashioned Bean with Ham, 11-oz. can	(301)	(35.9)	27.4	3.26	28.9	3.44	231	27.6
19-oz. can	520	62.0	27.4	3.26	28.9	3.44	231	27.6
Chunky Old Fashioned Vegetable Beef, 19-oz. can	320	38.0	16.8	1.95	17.8	1.11	142	8.9
Chunky Sirloin Burger, 10¾-oz. can	(238)	(23.8)	22.1	2.21	23.4	2.34	187	18.7
19-oz. can	420	42.0	22.1	2.21	23.4	2.34	187	18.7

	UNIT		1 OZ., BY WT.		1 FLUID OZ.		1 CUP	
	Cal.	Carb.	Cal.	Carb.	Cal.	Carb.	Cal.	Carb.
Chunky Split Pea with Ham, 19-oz. can	440	60.0	23.2	3.16	24.5	1.66	196	13.3
Chunky Steak & Potato, 19-oz. can	380	46.0	20.0	2.42	21.1	2.55	169	20.4
Chunky Turkey, 18½-oz. can	320	34.0	17.5	1.84	17.8	1.89	142	15.1
Chunky Vegetable, 10¾-oz. can	(158)	(24.9)	14.7	2.32	15.5	2.45	124	19.6
19-oz. can	280	44.0	14.7	2.32	15.5	2.45	124	19.6
CARMEL KOSHER								
Dry Soup Mixes:								
Mushroom, instant, 5-oz. jar	336	56.0	67.2	11.20				
Prepared with 6 fl. oz. of water and 1 teaspoon mix (yield: approx. 6 fl. oz.)	12	2.0	1.9	0.31	2.0	0.33	16	2.7
Onion, instant, 5-oz. jar	336	67.2	67.2	13.44				
Prepared with 6 fl. oz. of water and 1 teaspoon mix (yield: approx. 6 fl. oz.)	12	2.4	1.9	0.37	2.0	0.40	16	3.2
Parve Soup Mix, "Tastes Like Beef Soup," 5-oz. jar	336	50.4	67.2	10.08				
Prepared with 6 fl. oz. of water and 1 teaspoon mix (yield: approx. 6 fl. oz.)	12	1.8	1.9	0.28	2.0	0.30	16	2.4
Parve Soup Mix, "Tastes Like Chicken Soup," 5-oz. jar	336	50.4	67.2	10.08				
Prepared with 6 fl. oz. of water and 1 teaspoon mix (yield: approx. 6 fl. oz.)	12	1.8	1.9	0.28	2.0	0.30	16	2.4
CROSSE & BLACKWELL								
Ready-to-Serve Soups:								
Black Bean with Sherry, 13-oz. can	160	36.0	12.3	2.77	(13.5)	(3.05)	(108)	(24.4)
Clam Chowder, Manhattan Style, 13-oz. can	100	18.0	7.7	1.35	(8.3)	(1.50)	(66)	(12.0)
Clam Chowder, New England, 13-oz. can	180	28.0	13.9	2.15	(15.0)	(2.31)	(120)	(18.5)
Consommé Madrilene, Clear, 13-oz. can	50	0.0	3.9	0.00	(4.1)	0.00	(33)	0.0
Consommé Madrilene, Red, 13-oz. can	60	0.0	4.6	0.00	(4.9)	0.00	(39)	0.0
Crab à la Maryland, 13-oz. can	100	16.0	7.7	1.23	(8.1)	(1.31)	(65)	(10.5)
Gazpacho, 13-oz. can	60	2.0	4.6	0.15	(4.9)	(0.15)	(39)	(1.2)
Lentil with Ham, 13-oz. can	160	26.0	12.3	2.00	(13.3)	(2.15)	(106)	(17.2)
Minestrone, 13-oz. can	180	36.0	13.9	2.77	(15.0)	(2.98)	(120)	(23.8)
Mushroom Bisque, Cream of, 13-oz. can	180	16.0	13.1	1.23	(14.8)	(1.31)	(118)	(10.5)
Shrimp, Cream of, 13-oz. can	180	14.0	13.9	1.08	(14.8)	(1.15)	(118)	(9.2)
Vichyssoise, Cream of, 13-oz. can	140	10.0	10.8	0.78	(11.5)	(0.83)	(92)	(6.6)
CUP O'NOODLES								
Dry Soup Mixes:								
Beef, 1.2-oz. package	151	18.2	126.2	15.17				
Filled to brim with water (yield: approx. 6 fl. oz.)	151	18.2	20.3	2.45	25.2	3.03	173	20.8
2.5-oz. package	343	39.2	137.2	15.70				
Filled to brim with water (yield: approx. 12 fl. oz.)	343	39.2	22.9	2.62	28.6	3.27	229	26.1
Chicken, 1.2-oz. package	155	18.6	129.0	15.50				
Filled to brim with water (yield: approx. 6 fl. oz.)	155	18.6	20.8	2.50	25.8	3.10	177	24.8
2.5-oz. package	343	40.0	137.0	15.98				
Filled to brim with water (yield: approx. 12 fl. oz.)	343	40.0	22.9	2.67	28.6	3.33	229	26.6
Shrimp, 2.5-oz. package	335	39.0	134.0	15.60				
Filled to brim with water (yield: approx. 12 fl. oz.)	335	39.0	22.4	2.60	27.9	3.25	223	26.0
DIA-MEL								
Condensed Soups:								
Beef Noodle, condensed, 8-oz. can	140	10.0	17.5	1.25			140	10.0
Prepared with an equal amount of water (yield: approx. 16 fl. oz.)	140	10.0	8.6	0.61	8.8	0.63	70	5.0
Chicken Broth, condensed, 8-oz. can	36	2.0	4.5	0.25			36	2.0
Prepared with an equal amount of water (yield: approx. 16 fl. oz.)	36	2.0	2.2	0.12	2.3	0.13	18	1.0
Chicken Noodle, condensed, 8-oz. can	100	14.0	12.5	1.75			100	14.0
Prepared with an equal amount of water (yield: approx. 16 fl. oz.)	100	14.0	6.1	0.86	6.3	0.88	50	7.0

	UNIT		1 OZ., BY WT.		1 FLUID OZ.		1 CUP	
	Cal.	Carb.	Cal.	Carb.	Cal.	Carb.	Cal.	Carb.
Green Pea, condensed, 8-oz. can	220	36.0	27.5	4.50			220	36.0
Prepared with an equal amount of water (yield: approx. 16 fl. oz.)	220	36.0	13.5	2.21	13.8	2.25	110	18.0
Mushroom, Cream of, condensed, 8-oz. can	90	18.0	11.3	2.5			90	18.0
Prepared with an equal amount of water (yield: approx. 16 fl. oz.)	90	18.0	5.5	1.10	5.6	1.13	45	9.0
Tomato, condensed, 8-oz. can	100	22.0	12.5	2.75			100	22.0
Prepared with an equal amount of water (yield: approx. 16 fl. oz.)	100	22.0	6.1	1.35	6.3	1.38	50	11.0
Vegetable, condensed, 8-oz. can	120	24.0	15.0	3.00			120	24.0
Prepared with an equal amount of water (yield: approx. 16 fl. oz.)	120	24.0	7.4	1.47	7.5	1.50	60	12.0
Vegetable Beef, condensed, 8-oz. can	160	22.0	20.0	2.75			160	22.0
Prepared with an equal amount of water (yield: approx. 16 fl. oz.)	160	22.0	9.8	1.35	10.0	1.38	80	11.0
DOXSEE								
Condensed Soups:								
New England Clam Chowder, condensed, 10½-oz. can	150	26.7	15.0	2.67				
Prepared with an equal amount of water (yield: approx. 20 fl. oz.)	150	26.7	7.2	1.28	7.5	1.33	60	10.6
15-oz. can	225	40.0	15.0	2.67				
Prepared with an equal amount of water (yield: approx. 30 fl. oz.)	225	40.0	7.2	1.28	7.5	1.33	60	10.6
24-oz. can	360	64.1	15.0	2.67				
Prepared with an equal amount of water (yield: approx. 48 fl. oz.)	360	64.1	7.2	1.28	7.5	1.33	60	10.6
51-oz. (institutional) can	765	136.2	15.0	2.67				
Prepared with an equal amount of water (yield: approx. 102 fl. oz.)	765	136.2	7.2	1.28	7.5	1.33	60	10.6
FEARN								
Dry Soup Mix:								
Lentil Minestrone, 3.75-oz. box	316	66.0	84.3	17.60				
Prepared with 2 cups of water and 1 tablespoon oil (yield: approx. 16 fl. oz.)	436	66.0	20.9	3.17	27.0	4.10	218	33.0
FEATHERWEIGHT								
Condensed Soups:								
Chicken Noodle, low sodium, condensed, 8-oz. can	240	32.0	30.0	4.00			240	32.0
Prepared with an equal amount of water (yield: approx. 16 fl. oz.)	240	32.0	14.7	1.96	15.0	2.00	120	16.0
Green Pea, low sodium, condensed, 8-oz. can	360	64.0	45.0	8.00			360	64.0
Prepared with an equal amount of water (yield: approx. 16 fl. oz.)	360	64.0	22.1	3.93	22.5	4.00	180	32.0
Mushroom, Cream of, low sodium, condensed, 8-oz. can	240	36.0	30.0	4.50			240	36.0
Prepared with an equal amount of water (yield: approx. 16 fl. oz.)	240	36.0	14.7	2.21	15.0	2.25	120	18.0
Tomato, low sodium, condensed, 8-oz. can	240	60.0	30.0	7.50			240	60.0
Prepared with an equal amount of water (yield: approx. 16 fl. oz.)	240	60.0	14.7	3.68	15.0	3.75	120	30.0
Vegetable Beef, low sodium, condensed, 8-oz. can	360	56.0	45.0	7.33			360	56.0
Prepared with an equal amount of water (yield: approx. 16 fl. oz.)	360	56.0	22.1	3.44	22.5	3.50	180	28.0
FRENCH'S								
Dry Stock Bases:								
Beef Flavor Stock Base, 2⅝-oz. jar	161	40.2	61.3	15.32				
1 teaspoon (approx. 0.13 oz.)	8	2.0	61.3	15.32	48.0	12.00	384	96.0

	UNIT		1 OZ., BY WT.		1 FLUID OZ.		1 CUP	
	Cal.	Carb.	Cal.	Carb.	Cal.	Carb.	Cal.	Carb.
Chicken Flavor Stock Base, 2½-oz. jar	177	22.1	70.9	8.86				
1 teaspoon (approx. 0.13 oz.)	8	1.0	70.9	8.86	48.0	12.00	384	48.0
HAIN								
Dry Soup Mixes:								
Creamy Chicken, 1.9-oz. package, prepared (yield: approx. 3 cups)	672	42.0	24.9	1.56	28.0	1.73	224	14.0
Mushroom, Cream of, 2-oz. package, prepared (yield: approx. 3 cups)	825	51.0	29.5	1.82	34.4	2.13	275	17.0
Onion, Zesty, 2.75-oz. package, prepared (yield: approx. 3 cups)	771	51.0	26.6	1.76	32.1	2.13	257	17.0
Savory Split Pea, 3-2-oz. package, prepared (yield: approx. 3 cups)	780	66.0	26.9	2.28	32.5	2.75	260	22.0
Tangy Tomato, 3.45-oz. package, prepared (yield: approx. 3 cups)	1080	78.0	37.2	2.69	45.4	3.25	363	26.0
Vegetable, Hearty, 2.6-oz. package, prepared (yield: approx. 3 cups)	453	45.0	16.2	1.61	18.9	1.89	151	15.0
HERB-OX								
Dry Soup Mixes and Bouillon Cubes:								
Beef Flavored Bouillon Cubes, 0.7-oz. package, 5 cubes	30	5.0	46.0	7.66				
1.6-oz. container, 12 cubes	72	12.0	46.0	7.66				
3.3-oz. package, 25 cubes	150	25.0	46.0	7.66				
1 cube, approx. 0.13 oz., prepared with 1 cup of water (yield: approx. 8 fl. oz.)	6	1.0	0.7	0.12	0.8	0.13	6	1.0
Beef Flavored Instant Broth and Seasoning, 1.25-oz. box, 8 envelopes	64	8.0	50.6	6.33				
1 envelope, approx. 0.16 oz., prepared with 6 oz. of water (yield: approx. 6 fl. oz.)	8	1.0	1.3	0.16	1.3	0.17	11	1.3
Chicken Flavored Bouillon Cubes, 0.7-oz. package, 5 cubes	30	5.0	44.8	7.46				
1.6-oz. box, 12 cubes	72	12.0	44.8	7.46				
3.4-oz. box, 25 cubes	150	25.0	44.8	7.46				
1 cube, approx. 0.13 oz., prepared with 1 cup of water (yield: approx. 8 fl. oz.)	6	1.0	0.7	0.12	0.8	0.13	6	1.0
Chicken Packets, 1.5-oz. package, 8 envelopes	96	16.0	64.2	10.70				
1 envelope, approx. 0.19 oz., prepared with 6 oz. of water (yield: approx. 6 fl. oz.)	12	2.0	1.9	0.31	2.0	0.33	16	2.7
Onion Cubes, 1.5-oz. package, 12 cubes	120	12.0	78.9	7.88				
1 cube, approx. 0.13 oz., prepared with 6 oz. of water (yield: approx. 6 fl. oz.)	10	1.0	1.6	0.16	1.6	0.16	13	1.3
Onion Packets, 1.5-oz. package, 8 envelopes	112	16.0	74.9	10.70				
1 envelope, approx. 0.19 oz., prepared with 6 oz. of water (yield: approx. 6 fl. oz.)	14	2.0	2.2	0.31	2.3	0.33	18	2.7
Vegetarian Style Bouillon Cubes, 0.7-oz. package, 5 cubes	30	5.0	44.8	7.46				
3.4-oz. package, 12 cubes	72	12.0	44.8	7.46				
3.4-oz. package, 25 cubes	150	25.0	44.8	7.46				
1 cup, approx. 0.13 oz., prepared with one cup of water (yield: approx. 8 fl. oz.)	6	1.0	0.7	0.12	0.8	0.13	6	1.0
Vegetarian Packets, 1.4-oz. package, 8 envelopes	96	16.0	68.1	11.43				
1 envelope, 0.18 oz., prepared with 6 oz. of water (yield: approx. 6 fl. oz.)	12	2.0	1.9	0.31	2.0	0.33	16	2.7
HUGLI								
Dry Soup Mixes:								
Mushroom, Cream of, Mix, 2¾-oz. package	360	42.0	130.9	15.27				
Prepared with 4½ cups of water (yield: 36 fl. oz.)	360	42.0	9.0	1.05	10.0	1.17	80	9.4

	UNIT		1 OZ., BY WT.		1 FLUID OZ.		1 CUP	
	Cal.	Carb.	Cal.	Carb.	Cal.	Carb.	Cal.	Carb.
Tomato, Cream of, Mix, 3-oz. package	420	60.0	140.0	20.00				
Prepared with 4½ cups of water (yield: 36 fl. oz.)	420	60.0	10.4	1.49	11.7	1.67	94	13.4
Vegetable, Cream of, Mix, 2¾-oz. package	360	48.0	130.9	17.45				
Prepared with 4½ cups of water (yield: 36 fl. oz.)	360	48.0	9.0	1.20	10.0	1.33	80	10.7
LIPTON								
Dry Soup Mixes:								
Beef Mushroom, 2.5-oz. package, 2 envelopes	270	42.0	108.0	16.80				
1 envelope, prepared with 3 cups of water (yield: approx. 24 fl. oz.)	135	21.0	5.2	0.80	5.6	0.88	45	7.0
Beefy Onion, 2.25-oz. package, 2 envelopes	240	32.0	106.7	14.22				
1 envelope, prepared with 4 cups of water (yield: approx. 32 fl. oz.)	120	16.0	3.5	0.47	3.8	0.50	30	4.0
Chicken Noodle With Chicken Meat, 3.2-oz. package, 2 envelopes	420	54.0	120.0	15.43				
1 envelope, prepared with 3 cups of water (yield: approx. 24 fl. oz.)	210	27.0	7.9	1.02	8.8	1.13	70	9.0
Chicken Rice, 3.0-oz. package, 2 envelopes	360	48.0	120.0	16.00				
1 envelope, prepared with 3 cups of water (yield: approx. 24 fl. oz.)	180	24.0	6.8	0.91	7.5	1.00	60	8.0
Chicken Ripple Noodle, 2.5-oz. package, 2 envelopes	320	48.0	128.0	19.20				
1 envelope, prepared with 2 cups of water (yield: approx. 16 fl. oz.)	160	24.0	9.0	1.34	10.0	1.50	80	12.0
Giggle Noodle, 4-oz. package, 2 envelopes	480	72.0	120.0	18.00				
1 envelope, prepared with 3 cups of water (yield: approx. 24 fl. oz.)	240	36.0	8.9	1.34	10.0	1.50	80	12.0
Noodle with Chicken Broth, 4-oz. package, 2 envelopes	480	64.0	120.0	16.00				
1 envelope, prepared with 4 cups of water (yield: approx. 32 fl. oz.)	240	32.0	6.8	0.91	7.5	1.00	60	8.0
Onion, 2.75-oz. package, 2 envelopes	280	48.0	101.8	17.45				
1 envelope, prepared with 4 cups of water (yield: approx. 32 fl. oz.)	140	24.0	4.1	0.69	4.4	0.75	35	6.0
Onion Mushroom, 2-oz. package, 2 envelopes	200	30.0	100.0	15.00				
1 envelope, prepared with 2½ cups of water (yield: approx. 20 fl. oz.)	100	15.0	4.6	0.69	5.0	0.75	40	6.0
Ring-O-Noodle, 4.25-oz. package, 2 envelopes	480	72.0	94.1	16.94				
1 envelope, prepared with 4 cups of water (yield: approx. 32 fl. oz.)	240	36.0	6.8	1.02	7.5	1.13	60	9.0
Vegetable Beef, 3.5-oz. package, 2 envelopes	360	54.0	102.9	15.43				
1 envelope, prepared with 3 cups of water (yield: approx. 24 fl. oz.)	180	26.0	6.8	0.98	7.5	1.13	60	9.0
Vegetable Beef with Shells, 3.5-oz. package, 2 envelopes	400	72.0	114.3	20.57				
1 envelope, prepared with 2 cups of water (yield: approx. 16 fl. oz.)	200	36.0	10.9	1.96	12.5	2.25	100	18.0
Vegetable, Country, 4-oz. package, 2 envelopes	480	84.0	120.0	21.00				
1 envelope, prepared with 3 cups of water (yield: approx. 24 fl. oz.)	240	42.0	8.9	1.56	10.0	1.75	80	14.0
LIPTON CUP-A-BROTH								
Dry Soup Mixes:								
Chicken Flavored, 1.6-oz. package, 8 envelopes	200	24.0	125.0	15.00				
1 envelope, prepared with 6 fl. oz. of water (yield: approx. 6 fl. oz.)	25	3.0	3.9	0.47	4.2	0.50	33	4.0
LIPTON CUP-A-SOUP								
Dry Soup Mixes:								
Alphabet Vegetable, 1.5-oz. package, 4 envelopes	160	24.0	106.7	16.00				
1 envelope, prepared with 6 fl. oz. of water (yield: approx. 6 fl. oz.)	40	6.0	6.1	0.91	6.7	1.00	53	8.0

	UNIT		1 OZ., BY WT.		1 FLUID OZ.		1 CUP	
	Cal.	Carb.	Cal.	Carb.	Cal.	Carb.	Cal.	Carb.
Beef Flavor Noodle, 1.3-oz. package, 4 envelopes	140	24.0	107.7	18.46				
1 envelope, prepared with 6 fl. oz. of water (yield: approx. 6 fl. oz.)	35	6.0	5.3	0.92	5.8	1.00	46	8.0
Chicken, Cream of, 2.4-oz. package, 4 envelopes	320	40.0	133.3	16.67				
1 envelope, prepared with 6 fl. oz. of water (yield: approx. 6 fl. oz.)	80	10.0	11.7	1.46	13.4	1.63	107	13.0
Chicken, Hearty, 1.2-oz. package, 2 envelopes	140	11.0	116.7	9.17				
1 envelope, prepared with 6 fl. oz. of water (yield: approx. 6 fl. oz.)	70	5.5	10.2	0.80	11.7	0.92	93	7.3
Chicken Noodle with Meat, 1.5-oz. package, 4 envelopes	180	24.0	120.0	16.00				
1 envelope, prepared with 6 fl. oz. of water (yield: approx. 6 fl. oz.)	45	6.0	6.8	0.91	7.5	1.00	60	8.0
Chicken Supreme, 1.3-oz. package, 2 envelopes	180	22.0	138.5	16.92				
1 envelope, prepared with 6 fl. oz. of water (yield: approx. 6 fl. oz.)	90	11.0	13.1	1.60	15.0	1.83	120	14.7
Chicken Vegetable, 1.5-oz. package, 4 envelopes	160	28.0	106.7	18.67				
1 envelope, prepared with 6 fl. oz. of water (yield: approx. 6 fl. oz.)	40	7.0	6.1	1.06	6.7	1.17	53	9.3
Giggle Noodle, 1.5-oz. package, 4 envelopes	160	32.0	106.7	21.33				
1 envelope, prepared with 6 fl. oz. of water (yield: approx. 6 fl. oz.)	40	8.0	6.1	1.21	6.6	1.33	53	10.7
Green Pea, 4-oz. package, 4 envelopes	480	80.0	120.0	20.00				
1 envelope, prepared with 6 fl. oz. of water (yield: approx. 6 fl. oz.)	120	20.0	16.6	2.77	20.0	3.33	160	26.7
Harvest Vegetable, 1.7-oz. package, 2 envelopes	200	40.0	117.6	23.53				
1 envelope, prepared with 6 fl. oz. of water (yield: approx. 6 fl. oz.)	100	20.0	14.1	2.82	16.7	3.33	133	26.7
Mushroom, Cream of, 2.3-oz. package, 4 envelopes	320	44.0	139.1	19.13				
1 envelope, prepared with 6 fl. oz. of water (yield: approx. 6 fl. oz.)	80	11.0	11.8	1.62	13.3	1.84	106	14.7
Onion, 1-oz. package, 4 envelopes	120	20.0	120.0	20.00				
1 envelope, prepared with 6 fl. oz. of water (yield: approx. 6 fl. oz.)	30	5.0	4.6	0.77	5.0	0.83	40	6.6
Ring Noodle, 1.8-oz. package, 4 envelopes	160	32.0	88.9	17.78				
1 envelope, prepared with 6 fl. oz. of water (yield: approx. 6 fl. oz.)	40	8.0	6.0	1.20	6.6	1.33	53	10.7
Spring Vegetable, 1.7-oz. package, 4 envelopes	180	28.0	105.9	16.47				
1 envelope, prepared with 6 fl. oz. of water (yield: approx. 6 fl. oz.)	45	7.0	6.8	1.05	7.5	1.17	60	9.3
Tomato, 3-oz. package, 4 envelopes	280	52.0	93.3	17.30				
1 envelope, prepared with 6 fl. oz. of water (yield: approx. 6 fl. oz.)	70	13.0	10.0	1.86	11.7	3.16	93	25.3
Vegetable Beef, 2-oz. package, 4 envelopes	240	36.0	120.0	18.00				
1 envelope, prepared with 6 fl. oz. of water (yield: approx. 6 fl. oz.)	60	9.0	8.9	1.34	10.0	1.50	80	12.0
Virginia Pea, 2.1-oz., 2 envelopes	280	36.0	133.3	17.14				
1 envelope, prepared with 6 fl. oz. of water (yield: approx. 6 fl. oz.)	140	18.0	19.1	2.45	23.3	3.00	187	24.0
MAGGI								
Bouillon:								
Beef bouillon, 1.5-oz. box, 12 cubes	72	0.0	48.6	0.00				
1 cube, approx. 0.12 oz., prepared with 6 fl. oz. of water (yield: approx. 6 fl. oz.)	6	0.0	0.9	0.00	1.0	0.00	8	0.0
Chicken bouillon, 1.56-oz. box, 12 cubes	84	12.0	53.9	7.70				

	UNIT		1 OZ., BY WT.		1 FLUID OZ.		1 CUP	
	Cal.	Carb.	Cal.	Carb.	Cal.	Carb.	Cal.	Carb.
1 cube, approx. 0.13 oz. prepared with 6 fl. oz. of water (yield: approx. 6 fl. oz.)	7	1.0	1.1	0.16	1.2	0.17	9	1.3
MANISCHEWITZ								
Condensed and Ready-to-Serve Soups, and Dry Soup Mix:								
Beef Cabbage, condensed, 10½-oz. can	166	23.9	15.6	2.28				
Prepared with an equal amount of water (yield: approx. 20 fl. oz.)	166	23.9	7.9	1.14	8.1	1.20	64	9.2
Borscht, ready to serve, 32-fl. oz. (1 quart) jar	288	70.1	9.0	2.19	9.0	2.19	72	17.5
Borscht, low calorie, ready to serve, 32-fl. oz. (1 quart) jar	100	19.8	3.1	0.62	3.1	0.62	25	5.0
Chicken Barley, condensed, 10½-oz. can	220	32.7	10.4	3.11				
Prepared with an equal amount of water (yield: approx. 20 fl. oz)	220	32.7	10.5	1.56	11.0	1.64	88	13.1
Chicken Noodle, condensed, 10½-oz. can	119	10.8	11.3	1.03				
Prepared with an equal amount of water (yield: approx. 20 fl. oz.)	119	10.8	5.7	0.51	6.0	0.54	48	10.8
Chicken Rice, condensed, 10½-oz. can	125	14.2	11.9	1.36				
Prepared with an equal amount of water (yield: approx. 20 fl. oz.)	125	14.2	6.0	0.68	6.3	0.71	50	5.7
Chicken Vegetable, condensed, 10½-oz. can	143	20.2	13.6	1.92				
Prepared with an equal amount of water (yield: approx. 20 fl. oz.)	143	20.2	6.8	0.96	7.2	1.01	57	8.1
Mushroom Barley, condensed, 10½-oz. can	190	32.3	18.1	3.07				
Prepared with an equal amount of water (yield: approx. 21 fl. oz.)	190	32.3	9.0	1.54	9.5	1.62	76	12.9
Schav, ready to serve, 25-fl. oz. jar	34	6.6	1.4	0.26	1.4	0.26	11	2.1
Split Pea, dry mix, 6-oz. package	531	90.2						
Prepared with 4 cups of water (yield: approx. 4 cups)	531	90.2	16.6	2.82	17.9	3.04	143	24.3
Tomato, condensed, 10½-oz. can	158	9.0	15.1	0.86				
Prepared with an equal amount of water (yield: approx. 20 fl. oz.)	158	9.0	7.6	0.43	7.9	0.45	63	3.6
Vegetable, condensed, 10½-oz. can	166	26.5	15.8	2.52				
Prepared with an equal amount of water (yield: approx. 20 fl. oz.)	166	26.5	8.0	1.27	8.3	1.33	66	10.6
MARX BROTHERS								
Duck Soup	0	0.0	0.0	0.00	0.0	0.00	0	0.0
MBT								
Instant Broth:								
Beef Flavored, 1.55-oz. box, 8 envelopes	112	16.0	72.3	10.32				
1 envelope, approx. 0.19 oz., prepared with 6 oz. of water (yield: approx. 6 fl. oz.)	14	2.0	2.2	0.31	2.3	0.33	19	2.7
Chicken Flavored, 1.55-oz. box, 8 envelopes	96	16.0	61.9	10.32				
1 envelope, approx. 0.19 oz., prepared with 6 oz. of water (yield: approx. 6 fl. oz.)	12	2.0	1.9	0.31	2.0	0.33	16	2.7
Onion Broth and Dip Mix, 1.7-oz. box, 8 envelopes	128	16.0	75.3	9.41				
1 envelope, approx. 0.21 oz., prepared with 6 oz. of water (yield: approx. 6 fl. oz.)	16	2.0	2.5	0.31	2.7	0.33	21	2.7
Vegetable Broth, 1.55-oz. box, 8 envelopes	96	16.0	61.9	10.30				
1 envelope, approx. 0.19 oz., prepared with 6 oz. of water (yield: approx. 6 fl. oz.)	12	2.0	1.9	0.31	2.0	0.33	16	2.7
NESTLÊ SOUPTIME "10 SECOND SOUP"								
Dry Mixes:								
Beef Noodle, 1.3-oz. box, 4 envelopes	120	16.0	92.3	12.31				

	UNIT Cal.	UNIT Carb.	1 OZ., BY WT. Cal.	1 OZ., BY WT. Carb.	1 FLUID OZ. Cal.	1 FLUID OZ. Carb.	1 CUP Cal.	1 CUP Carb.
1 envelope, approx. ⅓ oz., add 6 oz. of water (yield: approx. 6 fl. oz.)	30	4.0	4.6	0.61	5.0	0.67	40	5.3
Chicken, Cream of, 2.7-oz. box, 4 envelopes	400	32.0	148.1	11.90				
1 envelope, approx. 0.7 oz., add 6 oz. of water (yield: approx. 6 fl. oz.)	100	8.0	14.5	1.16	16.7	1.33	133	10.7
Chicken Noodle, 1.4-oz. box, 4 envelopes	120	16.0	85.7	11.43				
1 envelope, approx. ⅓ oz., add 6 oz. of water (yield: approx. 6 fl. oz.)	30	4.0	4.6	0.61	5.0	0.67	40	0.7
French Style Onion, 1.0-oz. box, 4 envelopes	80	16.0	80.0	16.00				
1 envelope, approx. ¼ oz., add 6 oz. of water (yield: approx. 6 fl. oz.)	20	4.0	3.1	0.62	3.3	0.67	27	5.3
Garden Vegetable, Cream of, 2.5-oz. box, 4 envelopes	320	36.0	128.0	14.40				
1 envelope, approx. ⅔ oz., add 6 oz. of water (yield: approx. 6 fl. oz.)	80	9.0	11.6	1.31	13.3	1.50	106	12.0
Green Pea, 3.2-oz. box, 4 envelopes	280	56.0	87.5	17.50				
1 envelope, approx. 0.8 oz., add 6 oz. of water (yield: approx. 6 fl. oz.)	70	14.0	10.0	1.99	11.7	2.33	94	18.7
Tomato, 2.7-oz. box, 4 envelopes	280	52.0	103.7	19.30				
1 envelope, approx. 0.7 oz., add 6 oz. of water (yield: approx. 6 fl. oz.)	70	13.0	0.1	1.88	11.7	2.17	93	17.4
PEPPERIDGE FARM								
Semi-Condensed and Ready-to-Serve Soups:								
Bacon, Lettuce and Tomato Soup, semi-condensed, 10¾-oz. can	160	12.5	14.9	0.70			128	10.0
Prepared with ½ can of whole milk (yield: approx. 15 fl. oz.)	260	20.0	16.3	1.25	17.3	1.33	138	10.6
Borscht, semi-condensed, 11-oz. can	180	40.0	16.4	3.64			144	32.0
Prepared with ½ can of water (yield: approx. 15 fl. oz.)	180	40.0	11.1	2.47	12.0	2.67	96	21.4
Chicken Curry, semi-condensed, 11-oz. can	360	30.0	32.7	2.73			288	21.8
Prepared with ½ can of water (yield: approx. 15 fl. oz.)	360	30.0	22.2	1.85	24.0	2.00	192	16.0
Chicken with Wild Rice, semi-condensed, 10¾-oz. can	180	16.0	16.7	1.49			144	12.8
Prepared with ½ can of water (yield: approx. 15 fl. oz.)	180	16.0	11.3	1.00	12.0	1.07	96	8.5
Clam Chowder, New England, semi-condensed, 10½-oz. can	160	11.4	15.8	1.08			128	9.1
Prepared with ½ can of whole milk (yield: approx. 15 fl. oz.)	280	20.0	17.8	1.27	18.7	1.33	150	10.7
Prepared with ½ can of light cream (yield: approx. 15 fl. oz.)	500	18.2	31.8	1.16	33.3	1.21	267	9.7
Consommé Madrilene, ready to serve or semi-condensed, 10¾-oz. can	90	10.0	8.4	0.93			72	8.0
When prepared with ½ can of water (yield: approx. 15 fl. oz.)	90	10.0	5.6	0.63	6.0	0.67	48	5.3
Consommé Printanier, ready to serve or semi-condensed, 10½-oz. can	100	12.0	9.5	1.14			80	9.6
When prepared with ½ can of water (yield: approx. 15 fl. oz.)	100	12.0	6.4	0.76	6.7	0.80	53	6.4
Corn Chowder, semi-condensed, 11-oz. can	171	15.7	15.5	1.43			137	12.6
Prepared with ½ can of whole milk (yield: approx. 15 fl. oz.)	280	24.0	17.3	1.48	18.7	1.60	150	12.8
Prepared with ½ can of light cream (yield: approx. 15 fl. oz.)	519	22.8	32.0	1.41	34.6	1.52	277	12.2
Crab, semi-condensed, 11-oz. can	160	24.0	14.6	2.18			128	19.2
Prepared with ½ can of water (yield: approx. 15 fl. oz.)	160	24.0	9.9	1.48	10.7	1.60	86	12.8

	UNIT Cal.	UNIT Carb.	1 OZ., BY WT. Cal.	1 OZ., BY WT. Carb.	1 FLUID OZ. Cal.	1 FLUID OZ. Carb.	1 CUP Cal.	1 CUP Carb.
French Onion, semi-condensed, 10¾-oz. can	220	40.0	20.5	3.72			176	32.0
Prepared with ½ can of water (yield: approx. 15 fl. oz.)	220	40.0	13.8	2.51	14.7	2.67	118	21.4
Gazpacho, semi-condensed, 11-oz. can	120	18.0	10.9	1.64			96	14.4
Prepared with ½ can of water (yield: approx. 15 fl. oz.)	120	18.0	7.4	1.11	8.0	1.20	64	9.6
Hunter's, semi-condensed, 10¾-oz. can	220	16.0	20.5	1.49			176	12.8
Prepared with ½ can of water (yield: approx. 15 fl. oz.)	220	16.0	13.8	1.00	14.7	1.07	118	8.6
Lobster Bisque with White Wine, semi-condensed, 10¾-oz. can	340	20.0	31.6	1.86			272	10.6
Prepared with ½ can of water (yield: approx. 15 fl. oz.)	340	20.0	21.3	1.25	22.7	1.33	182	10.6
Prepared with ½ can of whole milk (yield: approx. 15 fl. oz.)	447	28.1	28.0	1.76	29.8	1.87	238	15.0
Mushroom Consommé, ready to serve or semi-condensed, 10½-oz. can	70	4.0	6.7	0.38			56	3.2
When prepared with ½ can of water (yield: approx. 15 fl. oz.)	70	4.0	4.5	0.25	4.7	0.27	38	2.2
Mushroom, Shitake, semi-condensed, 10¾-oz. can	140	16.0	13.0	1.45			112	12.8
Prepared with ½ can of water (yield: approx. 15 fl. oz.)	140	16.0	8.9	1.02	9.3	1.06	75	8.5
Orange with Apricot, ready to serve, 11-oz. can	240	56.0	21.8	5.09	24.0	5.60	192	44.8
Oyster Stew, semi-condensed, 10¾-oz. can	113	11.9	10.5	1.11			90	9.5
Prepared with ½ can of whole milk (yield: approx. 15 fl. oz.)	220	20.0	13.8	1.25	14.7	1.33	118	10.6
Prepared with ½ can of light cream (yield: approx. 15 fl. oz.)	455	18.8	28.5	1.18	30.3	1.25	242	10.0
Peach Apple, ready to serve, 10¾-oz. can	240	54.0	22.3	5.02	24.0	5.40	192	43.2
Strawberry with Sauterne, ready to serve, 10¾-oz. can	300	72.0	27.9	6.70	30.0	7.20	240	57.6
Watercress, semi-condensed, 10¾-oz. can	53	10.9	4.9	0.92			42	0.7
Prepared with ½ can of whole milk (yield: approx. 15 fl. oz.)	160	18.0	10.0	1.13	10.7	11.20	86	9.6
Prepared with ½ can of light cream (yield: approx. 15 fl. oz.)	395	16.8	24.8	1.05	26.3	1.12	210	9.0
PROGRESSO								
Ready-to-Serve Soups:								
Chicarina, 20-oz. can	250	20.0	12.5	1.00	(13.3)	(1.06)	(106)	(8.5)
Clam Chowder, Manhattan, 20-oz. can	250	40.0	12.5	2.00	(13.5)	(2.15)	(108)	(17.2)
Escarole in Chicken Broth, 20-oz. can	62	2.6	3.1	0.13	(3.1)	(0.13)	(25)	(1.0)
Lentil, 20-oz. can	376	55.0	18.8	2.75	(20.3)	(2.98)	(162)	(23.7)
Tomato, 20-oz. can	276	57.6	13.8	2.85	(14.9)	(3.10)	(119)	(24.8)
RICHTER BROS.								
Bouillon Cubes:								
Instant Bouillon Cubes with Sea Salt, 30-oz. package, 40 cubes	2400	17.2	80.0	0.57				
1 cube, approx. 0.75 oz., prepared with 6 fl. oz. of water (yield: 6 fl. oz.)	60	0.4	8.6	0.06	10.0	0.07	80	0.5
Instant Bouillon Cubes without Salt, 30-oz. package, 40 cubes	4040	136.0	134.7	4.53				
1 cube, approx. 0.75 oz., prepared with 6 fl. oz. of water (yield: 6 fl. oz.)	101	3.4	14.5	0.49	16.8	0.57	135	4.5
ROKEACH								
Condensed and Ready-to-Serve Soups:								
Borscht, ready to serve, 32-fl. oz. (1-quart) jar	(361)	(85.8)	9.9	2.35	(11.3)	(2.68)	(90)	(21.5)
Vegetable, condensed 10¾-oz. can	194	32.3	19.4	3.23				
Prepared with 1 can of water (yield: approx. 20 fl. oz.)	194	32.3	9.2	1.53	9.7	1.62	78	13.0

	UNIT		1 OZ., BY WT.		1 FLUID OZ.		1 CUP	
	Cal.	Carb.	Cal.	Carb.	Cal.	Carb.	Cal.	Carb.
SMITHERS								
Beef Tea, 4.5-oz. bottle, 18 servings	54	3.6	12.0	0.80				
1 serving, prepared with 6 fl. oz. water (yield: 6 fl. oz.)	3	0.2	0.5	0.03	0.5	0.03	4	trace
STEERO								
Bouillon Cubes and Powder:								
Bouillon Cubes, 4.13-oz. jar	(120)	27.3	(29.1)	6.63				
1 cube, approx. 0.14 oz., prepared with 8 fl. oz. of water (yield: approx. 8 fl. oz.)	(4)	0.9	(0.5)	(0.11)	(0.5)	0.11	(4)	0.9
Instant Powdered Bouillon, 5¾-oz. jar	(180)	41.0	(31.3)	6.63				
1 teaspoon, approx. 0.14 oz., prepared with 8 fl. oz. of water (yield: approx. 8 fl. oz.)	(4)	0.9	(0.5)	0.11	(0.5)	0.11	(4)	0.9
TABATCHNICK								
Frozen Soups:								
Barley and Mushroom, "Boil in Bag," 15-oz. box, 2 pouches	184	32.0	12.3	2.13	11.5	2.00	92	16.0
1 pouch, approx. 7½ oz.	92	16.0	12.3	2.13	11.5	2.00	92	16.0
1 pouch, approx. 7½ oz.	63	22.0	8.4	2.93	7.9	2.75	63	22.0
Bean and Barley, "Boil in Bag," 15-oz. box, 2 pouches	126	44.0	8.4	2.91	7.9	2.75	63	22.0
1 pouch, approx. 7½ oz.	63	22.0	8.4	2.93	7.9	2.75	63	22.0
Lentil, "Boil in Bag," 15-oz. box, 2 pouches	346	54.0	23.1	3.60	21.6	3.38	173	27.0
1 pouch, approx. 7½ oz.	173	27.0	23.1	3.60	21.6	3.38	173	27.0
Minestrone, "Boil in Bag," 15-oz. box, 2 pouches	294	48.0	19.6	3.20	18.4	3.00	147	24.0
1 pouch, approx. 74 oz.	147	24.0	19.6	3.20	18.4	3.00	147	24.0
Northern Bean, "Boil in Bag," 15-oz. box, 2 pouches	160	58.0	10.6	3.87	10.0	3.63	80	29.0
1 pouch, approx. 7½ oz.	80	29.0	10.6	3.87	10.0	3.63	80	29.0
Pea, "Boil in Bag," 15-oz. box, 2 pouches	372	62.0	24.8	4.13	23.3	3.88	186	31.0
1 pouch, approx. 7½ oz.	186	31.0	24.8	4.13	23.3	3.88	186	31.0
Potato, "Boil in Bag," 15-oz. box, 2 pouches	190	38.0	12.6	2.53	11.9	2.38	95	19.0
1 pouch, approx. 7½ oz.	95	19.0	12.6	2.53	11.9	2.38	95	19.0
Vegetable, "Boil in Bag," 15-oz. box, 2 pouches	208	38.0	13.8	2.53	13.0	2.37	104	19.0
1 pouch, approx. 7½ oz.	103	19.0	13.8	2.53	13.0	2.37	104	19.0
TOWN HOUSE								
Condensed Soups:								
Celery, Cream of, condensed, 10¾-oz. can	220	24.0	20.5	2.23			176	19.2
Prepared with an equal amount of water (yield: approx. 20 fl. oz.)	220	24.0	10.4	1.14	11.0	1.20	88	9.6
Prepared with an equal amount of whole milk (yield: approx. 20 fl. oz.)	440	40.0	20.8	1.89	22.0	2.00	176	16.0

	UNIT		1 OZ., BY WT.		1 FLUID OZ.		1 CUP	
	Cal.	Carb.	Cal.	Carb.	Cal.	Carb.	Cal.	Carb.
Mushroom, Cream of, condensed, 10¾-oz. can	320	28.0	29.8	2.60			256	22.4
Prepared with an equal amount of water (yield: approx. 20 fl. oz.)	320	28.0	15.1	1.33	16.0	1.40	128	11.2
Prepared with an equal amount of whole milk (yield: approx. 20 fl. oz.)	540	44.0	25.6	2.08	27.0	2.20	216	17.6
Potato, Cream of, condensed, 10¾-oz. can	200	32.0	18.6	2.98			160	25.6
Prepared with an equal amount of water (yield: approx. 20 fl. oz.)	200	32.0	9.5	1.51	10.0	1.60	80	12.8
Tomato, condensed, 10¾-oz. can	200	46.0	18.6	4.28			160	36.3
Prepared with an equal amount of water (yield: approx. 20 fl. oz.)	200	46.0	9.5	2.18	10.0	2.30	80	18.4
Prepared with an equal amount of whole milk (yield: approx. 20 fl. oz.)	420	62.0	19.9	2.93	21.0	3.10	168	24.8
Tomato with Rice, condensed, 11-oz. can	300	23.0	27.3	2.09			240	18.4
Prepared with an equal amount of water (yield: approx. 20 fl. oz.)	300	23.0	14.0	1.08	15.0	1.15	120	9.2
WASHINGTON'S								
Rich Brown Seasoning and Broth, 1.1-oz. box, 8 envelopes	48	8.0	43.5	7.27				
1 envelope, approx. 0.14 oz. prepared with 6 fl. oz. of water (yield: approx. 6 fl. oz.)	6	1.0	0.9	0.16	1.0	0.17	8	1.3
WEIGHT WATCHERS								
Dry Broth Mixes:								
Beef Flavored Broth and Seasoning, 1¼-oz. box, 8 envelopes	80	13.6	64.0	10.88				
1 envelope, approx. 0.16 oz., prepared with 6 fl. oz. of water (yield: approx. 6 fl. oz.)	10	2.0	1.6	0.31	1.7	0.33	13	2.7
Chicken Flavored Broth and Seasoning, 1¼-oz. box, 8 envelopes	72	7.2	57.6	5.76				
1 envelope, approx. 0.16 oz., prepared with 6 fl. oz. of water (yield: approx. 6 fl. oz.)	9	0.9	1.4	0.14	1.5	0.15	23	2.3
Onion Flavored Broth and Seasoning, 1¼-oz. box, 8 envelopes	80	13.6	64.0	10.88				
1 envelope, approx. 0.16 oz., prepared with 6 fl. oz. of water (yield: approx. 6 fl. oz.)	10	2.0	1.6	0.31	1.7	0.33	13	2.7

12 BEVERAGES •

VEGETABLE JUICES

	UNIT		1 FLUID OZ.		1 CUP		1 TABLESPOON	
	Cal.	Carb.	Cal.	Carb.	Cal.	Carb.	Cal.	Carb.
BEETROOT JUICE								
Biotta, 17-fl.-oz. bottle	(202)	(43.4)	(11.9)	(2.55)	(95)	(20.4)	(5.9)	(1.28)
CARROT JUICE								
Balanced, 12-fl-oz. can	144	(30.0)	12.0	(2.50)	96	(20.0)	6.0	(1.25)
Biotta, 17-fl-oz. bottle	(174)	(37.8)	(10.2)	(2.22)	(82)	(17.8)	(5.1)	(1.11)
Eveready, 12-fl-oz. can	140	32.0	11.7	2.67	94	21.3	5.9	1.33
Hain, 12 fl. oz.	126	28.0	10.5	2.33	84	18.7	5.3	1.17
Hollywood, 12-fl.-oz. can	126	28.0	10.5	2.33	84	18.7	5.3	1.17
CELERY JUICE								
Balanced, 12-fl-oz. can	(60)	(10.2)	(5.0)	(0.85)	(40)	(6.8)	(2.5)	(0.43)
Biotta, 17-fl.-oz. bottle	(182)	(35.5)	(10.7)	(2.09)	(86)	(16.7)	(5.4)	(1.05)
CLAM AND TOMATO JUICE								
Mott's Clamato, 5½-fl.-oz. can	73	17.4	13.3	3.17	106	25.4	6.7	1.59
16-fl.-oz. (1-pint) can	213	50.7	13.3	3.17	106	25.4	6.7	1.59
32-fl-oz. (1-quart) bottle	426	101.4	13.3	3.17	106	25.4	6.7	1.59
46-fl-oz. can	612	145.8	13.3	3.17	106	25.4	6.7	1.59
SAUERKRAUT JUICE								
Biotta, 17-fl.-oz. bottle	(58)	(10.7)	(3.4)	(0.63)	(27)	(5.0)	(1.7)	(0.32)
Libby's, 5½-fl.-oz. can	18	3.7	3.3	0.67	26	5.4	1.6	0.34
TOMATO JUICE								
Balanced, 18-fl.-oz. can	(99)	(23.4)	(5.5)	(1.30)	(44)	(10.4)	(2.8)	(0.65)
Biotta, 17-fl.-oz. bottle	(81)	(15.6)	(4.7)	(0.92)	(38)	(7.4)	(2.4)	(0.46)
Campbell's, 6-fl.-oz. can	35	8.0	5.8	1.33	46	10.7	2.9	0.67
Del Monte, 6-fl.-oz. can	35	8.0	5.8	1.33	47	10.7	2.9	0.67
32-fl.-oz. (1-quart) can	181	42.7	5.8	1.33	47	10.7	2.9	0.67
Diet Delight, 12-fl.-oz. can	70	14.0	5.8	1.17	47	9.3	2.9	0.58
low sodium, 12-fl.-oz. can	70	14.0	5.8	1.17	47	9.4	2.9	0.58
Featherweight, no salt/no sugar, 12-fl.-oz. can	70	14.0	5.8	1.17	47	9.4	2.9	0.58
18-fl.-oz. can	104	21.1	5.8	1.17	47	9.4	2.9	0.58
salt-free, 12-fl.-oz. can	70	16.0	5.8	1.35	47	10.8	2.9	0.68
18-fl.-oz. can	105	24.0	5.8	1.35	47	10.8	2.9	0.68
Golden Harvest, 12-fl.-oz. can	70	16.0	5.8	1.33	46	10.6	2.9	0.67
Libby's, 5½-fl.-oz. can	32	7.3	5.8	1.33	47	10.7	2.9	0.67
18-fl.-oz. can	105	24.0	5.8	1.33	47	10.7	2.9	0.67
Pet, Inc., 46-fl.-oz. can	230	53.8	5.0	1.17	40	9.4	2.5	0.59
Sacramento, 5½-fl.-oz. can	35	7.0	6.4	1.27	51	10.2	3.2	0.64
7-fl.-oz. can	45	8.9	6.4	1.27	51	10.2	3.2	0.64
12-fl.-oz. can	77	15.2	6.4	1.27	51	10.2	3.2	0.64
46-fl.-oz. can	294	58.4	6.4	1.27	51	10.2	3.2	0.64
Snap-E-Tom, 6-fl.-oz. can	38	6.8	6.3	1.13	51	9.1	3.2	0.57
10-fl.-oz. can	63	11.3	6.3	1.13	51	9.1	3.2	0.57
32-fl.-oz. (1-quart) bottle	203	36.3	6.3	1.13	51	9.1	3.2	0.57

	UNIT		1 FLUID OZ.		1 CUP		1 TABLESPOON	
	Cal.	Carb.	Cal.	Carb.	Cal.	Carb.	Cal.	Carb.
Stokely, 5½-fl.-oz. can	28	6.2	5.0	1.13	40	9.0	2.5	0.56
46-fl.-oz. can	230	52.0	5.0	1.13	40	9.0	2.5	0.56
S & W Nutradiet, 12-fl.-oz. can	70	16.0	5.8	1.33	47	10.7	2.9	0.67
Tillie Lewis "Tasti Diet," 12-fl.-oz. can	70	16.0	5.8	1.33	46	10.7	2.9	0.67
Town House Fancy, 18-fl.-oz. can	105	24.0	5.8	1.33	47	10.6	2.9	0.67
Welch's, 32-fl.-oz. (1-quart) bottle	187	37.3	5.8	1.17	47	9.3	2.9	0.58
48-fl.-oz. (3-pint) bottle	280	56.0	5.8	1.17	47	9.3	2.9	0.58
Welch's (with vitamin C), 32-fl.-oz. (1-quart) bottle	200	40.0	6.3	1.25	50	10.0	3.1	0.63
TOMATO JUICE COCKTAIL								
Mott's Nutrimato, Tomato Flavor Cocktail with Beef Broth, 32 fl. oz. (1 quart)	374	90.6	11.7	2.83	94	22.6	5.9	1.42
Ocean Spray Firehouse Jubilee, Tomato Cocktail, 32-fl.-oz. (1-quart) bottle	240	48.0	7.5	1.50	60	12.0	3.8	0.75
TOMATO PLUS VEGETABLE COCKTAIL								
Sacramento, 5½-fl.-oz. can	35	7.0	6.4	1.27	51	10.2	3.2	0.64
VEGETABLE COCKTAIL								
Campbell's V-8 Vegetable Juice Cocktail, 6-fl.-oz. can	35	8.0	5.8	1.33	46	10.7	2.9	0.67
Campbell's V-8 Spicy Hot Vegetable Juice Cocktail, 6-fl.-oz. can	35	8.0	5.8	1.33	46	10.7	2.9	0.67
Seneca, 46-fl.-oz. bottle	230	53.7	5.0	1.17	40	9.4	2.5	0.59
Town House, 46-fl.-oz. can	268	61.3	5.8	1.33	47	10.7	2.9	0.67
VEGETABLE JUICE								
Biotta, 17-fl.-oz. bottle	(134)	(27.4)	(7.9)	(1.61)	(63)	(12.9)	(4.0)	(0.81)

FRUIT JUICES AND DRINKS

(Fruit-flavored drinks sold as dry mixes are in a separate list that follows the canned and bottled fruit juices.)

	UNIT		1 FLUID OZ.		1 CUP		1 TABLESPOON	
	Cal.	Carb.	Cal.	Carb.	Cal.	Carb.	Cal.	Carb.
ACEROLA JUICE, based on generic data								
1 pint	102	23.2	6.4	1.45	51	11.6	3.2	0.73
1 pound (approx. 1.9 cups) (tr/1g/tr/94%/1mg)	95	21.8	6.4	1.45	51	11.6	3.2	0.73
1 quart (approx. 34.2 oz. by wt.)	204	46.5	6.4	1.45	51	11.6	3.2	0.73
"A.M." FRUIT DRINK								
Mott's, 5½-fl.-oz. can	83	20.2	15.0	3.67	120	29.4	7.5	1.84
6-pack (six 5½-fl.-oz. cans, 33 fl. oz.)	495	121.2	15.0	3.67	120	29.4	7.5	1.84

	UNIT		1 FLUID OZ.		1 CUP		1 TABLE-SPOON	
	Cal.	Carb.	Cal.	Carb.	Cal.	Carb.	Cal.	Carb.
APPLE DELIGHT DRINK								
Golden Harvest, 32-fl.-oz. (1-quart) bottle	400	104.0	12.5	3.25	100	26.0	6.3	1.63
APPLE DRINK								
Capri Sun natural 10% juice, 6.75-fl.-oz. can	90	22.7	13.3	3.36	107	26.9	7.0	1.70
APPLE JUICE, based on generic data								
CANNED OR BOTTLED (Based on USDA data that do not specify "sweetened" or "unsweetened."):								
1 pint	232	57.9	14.5	3.62	116	29.0	7.3	1.81
1 pound (approx. 1.8 cups) (tr/3g/tr/88%/1mg)	213	53.0	14.5	3.62	116	29.0	7.3	1.81
1 quart (approx. 34.8 oz. by wt.)	464	115.8	14.5	3.62	116	29.0	7.3	1.81
FROZEN:								
Concentrated:								
1 pint	932	230.7	58.3	14.42	466	115.4	29.1	7.21
1 pound (approx. 1.6 cups) (tr/12g/tr/57%/7mg)	754	11.6	58.3	14.42	466	115.4	29.1	7.21
1 quart (approx. 39.6 oz. by wt.)	1864	461.4	58.3	14.42	466	115.4	29.1	7.21
Diluted with 3 parts water by volume:								
1 pint	222	55.2	13.9	3.45	111	27.6	6.9	1.72
1 pound (approx. 1.9 cups) (tr/3g/tr/88%/2mg)	195	51.3	13.9	3.45	111	27.6	6.9	1.72
1 quart (approx. 36.4 oz. by wt.)	444	110.3	13.9	3.45	111	27.6	6.9	1.72
APPLE JUICE, by brand								
A&P, 32-fl.-oz. (1-quart) bottle	480	117.3	15.0	3.67	120	29.4	7.5	1.84
40-fl.-oz. bottle	600	146.8	15.0	3.67	120	29.4	7.5	1.84
Ann Page (A&P), 64-fl.-oz. (2-quart) bottle	960	243.9	15.0	3.67	120	29.4	7.5	1.84
Hansen's, 6-fl.-oz. can	99	24.5	16.5	4.08	132	32.6	8.3	2.04
6-pack (six 6-fl.-oz. cans, 36 fl. oz.)	594	147.0	16.5	4.08	132	32.6	8.3	2.04
33.8-fl.-oz. (1-liter) bottle	549	135.8	16.5	4.08	132	32.6	8.3	2.04
128-fl.-oz. (1-gallon) bottle	2112	522.3	16.5	4.08	132	32.6	8.3	2.04
Lehr, 23-fl.-oz. bottle	286	69.5	12.4	3.02	99	24.2	6.2	1.51
Lucky Leaf, 46-fl.-oz. can	690	161.0	15.0	3.50	120	28.0	7.5	1.75
Mott's, 5½-fl.-oz. can	73	17.4	13.3	3.17	106	25.4	6.7	1.59
12-fl.-oz. can	160	38.0	13.3	3.17	106	25.4	6.7	1.59
32-fl.-oz. (1-quart) bottle	426	101.4	13.3	3.17	106	25.4	6.7	1.59
40-fl.-oz. bottle	532	126.8	13.3	3.17	106	25.4	6.7	1.59
64-fl.-oz. (2-quart) bottle	851	202.9	13.3	3.17	106	25.4	6.7	1.59
Musselman, 5½-fl.-oz. can	73	19.3	13.3	3.50	106	28.0	6.6	1.75
32-fl.-oz. (1-quart) bottle	426	112.0	13.3	3.50	106	28.0	6.6	1.75
46-fl.-oz. can	612	161.0	13.3	3.50	106	28.0	6.6	1.75
Red Cheek, 5½-fl.-oz. can	76	19.3	13.9	3.51	111	28.1	6.9	1.76
32-fl.-oz. (1-quart) bottle	444	112.4	13.9	3.51	111	28.1	6.9	1.76
40-fl.-oz. bottle	555	141.6	13.9	3.51	111	28.1	6.9	1.76
64-fl.-oz. (2-quart) bottle	888	22.6	13.9	3.51	111	28.1	6.9	1.76
128-fl. oz. (1-gallon) bottle	1776	449.6	13.9	3.51	111	28.1	6.9	1.76
Seneca, 32-fl.-oz. (1-quart) bottle	480	117.3	15.0	3.67	120	29.3	7.5	1.83
48-fl.-oz. (3-pint) bottle	720	176.0	15.0	3.67	120	29.3	7.5	1.83
64-fl.-oz. (2-quart) bottle	960	234.7	15.0	3.67	120	29.3	7.5	1.83
Concentrated, 6-fl.-oz. can	360	88.0	60.0	14.67	480	117.3	30.0	7.33
Prepared as label directs, adding 3 cans (18 fl. oz.) water (yield: 24 fl. oz.)	360	88.0	15.0	3.67	120	29.3	7.5	1.83
12-fl.-oz. can	960	176.0	60.0	14.67	480	117.3	30.0	7.33
Prepared as label directs, adding 3 cans (36 fl. oz.) water [yield: approx. 48 fl. oz. (3 pints)]	720	176.0	15.0	3.67	120	29.3	7.5	1.83
16-fl.-oz. (1-pint) can	960	234.7	60.0	14.67	480	117.3	30.0	7.33
Prepared as label directs, adding 3 cans (48 fl. oz.) water [yield: approx. 64 fl. oz. (2 quarts)]	960	234.7	15.0	3.67	120	29.3	7.5	1.83
Natural Style, 48-fl.-oz. (3-pint) bottle	720	176.0	15.0	3.67	120	29.3	7.5	1.83
64-fl.-oz. (2-quart) bottle	960	234.7	15.0	3.67	120	29.3	7.5	1.83
Concentrated Natural Style, 12-fl.-oz. can	672	176.0	56.0	14.67	448	117.3	28.0	7.33
Prepared as label directs, adding 3 cans (36 fl. oz.) water [yield: approx. 48 fl. oz. (3 pints)]	672	176.0	14.0	3.67	112	29.3	7.5	1.83

	UNIT		1 FLUID OZ.		1 CUP		1 TABLE-SPOON	
	Cal.	Carb.	Cal.	Carb.	Cal.	Carb.	Cal.	Carb.
Tropicana, 5½-fl.-oz. container	80	19.5	14.5	3.54	116	28.3	7.3	1.77
32-fl.-oz. (1-quart) bottle	464	113.3	14.5	3.54	116	28.3	7.3	1.77
APPLE BLACKBERRY JUICE								
Hansen's, 12-fl.-oz. bottle	213	51.8	17.8	4.32	142	34.6	8.9	2.16
32-fl.-oz. (1-quart) bottle	570	138.2	17.8	4.32	142	34.6	8.9	2.16
APPLE GRAPE JUICE								
Red Cheek, 32-fl.-oz. (1-quart) bottle	475	120.8	14.8	3.78	119	30.2	7.0	1.90
64-fl.-oz. (2-quart) bottle	950	241.7	14.8	3.78	119	30.2	7.0	1.90
APPLE PEACH JUICE								
Hansen's, 8-fl.-oz. bottle	130	31.9	16.3	3.99	130	31.9	8.1	1.99
12-fl.-oz. can	195	47.9	16.3	3.99	130	31.9	8.1	1.99
33.8-fl.-oz. (1-liter) bottle	542	132.8	16.3	3.99	130	31.9	8.1	1.99
APPLE STRAWBERRY JUICE								
Hansen's, 6-fl.-oz. can	106	25.9	17.7	4.32	142	34.6	8.9	2.16
8-fl.-oz. bottle	142	34.6	17.7	4.32	142	34.6	8.9	2.16
12-fl.-oz. can	212	51.8	17.7	4.32	142	34.6	8.9	2.16
64-fl.-oz. (2-quart) bottle	1133	276.5	17.7	4.32	142	34.6	8.9	2.16
APRICOT NECTAR, canned, based on generic data								
1 pint	282	72.2	17.6	4.51	141	36.1	8.8	2.26
1 pound (approx. 1.8 cups) (tr/4g/tr/85%/1mg)	254	65.3	17.6	4.51	141	36.1	8.8	2.26
1 quart (approx. 35.5 oz. by wt.)	564	144.4	17.6	4.51	141	36.1	8.8	2.26
APRICOT NECTAR, by brand								
Del Monte, 6-fl.-oz. can	100	26.0	16.7	4.33	133	34.7	8.3	2.17
46-fl.-oz. can	767	199.3	16.7	4.33	133	34.7	8.3	2.17
Heart's Delight, 6⅔-fl.-oz. can	111	28.9	16.7	4.33	133	34.7	8.3	2.17
Libby's, 5½-fl.-oz. can	101	24.8	18.3	4.50	146	36.0	9.1	2.25
12-fl.-oz. can	220	54.0	18.3	4.50	146	36.0	9.1	2.25
Town House, 12 fl. oz.	220	56.0	18.3	4.67	147	37.3	9.1	2.33
BANANA ORANGE JUICE								
Biotta, 12-fl.-oz. can	258		15.2		122		7.6	
CHERRY DRINK								
Ann Page (A&P) 10% fruit, 46-fl.-oz. can	690	178.3	15.0	3.88	120	31.0	7.5	1.94
Donaukrone Sour Cherry Beverage, 23-fl.-oz. bottle	260	62.6	11.3	2.72	90	21.8	5.7	1.36
Scotch Buy, 46-fl.-oz. can	690	166.8	15.0	3.63	120	29.0	7.5	1.82
CITRUS COOLER DRINK								
Scotch Buy, 46-fl.-oz. can	690	166.8	15.0	3.68	120	29.0	7.5	1.82
COCONUT CREAM								
Coco Lopez Cream of Coconut, 15½-fl.-oz. can	924	35.7	59.6	2.30	477	18.4	29.8	1.15
COCONUT MILK, based on generic data								
Coconut milk, 1 cup (8 fl. oz.)	605	12.5	75.6	1.56	605	12.5	37.8	0.78
COCONUT WATER, based on generic data								
Coconut water, 1 cup (8 fl. oz.)	53	11.3	6.6	1.41	53	11.3	3.3	0.71
CRANBERRY APPLE DRINK								
Ocean Spray Cranapple, 5½-fl.-oz. can	119	29.3	21.7	5.33	173	42.7	10.8	2.67
32-fl.-oz. (1-quart) bottle	694	170.6	21.7	5.33	173	42.7	10.8	2.67
46-fl.-oz. can	998	245.3	21.7	5.33	173	42.7	10.8	2.67
128-fl.-oz. (1-gallon) bottle	2778	682.2	21.7	5.33	173	42.7	10.8	2.67
CRANBERRY APPLE JUICE COCKTAIL								
Veryfine, 32-fl.-oz. (1-quart) bottle	533	133.3	16.7	4.17	133	33.3	8.3	2.08
Welch's concentrated, 12-fl.-oz. can	880	216.0	73.3	18.00	587	144.0	37.0	9.00
Prepared as label directs, adding 3 cans (36 fl. oz.) water [yield: 48 fl. oz. (3 pints)]	880	216.0	18.3	4.50	146	36.0	9.0	2.30
CRANBERRY APRICOT JUICE DRINK								
Ocean Spray Cranicot, 32-fl.-oz. (1-quart) bottle	640	160.0	20.0	5.00	160	40.0	10.0	2.50
CRANBERRY GRAPE DRINK								
Ocean Spray Crangrape, 32-fl.-oz. (1-quart) bottle	586	144.0	18.3	4.50	147	36.0	9.2	2.25
48-fl.-oz. (3-pint) bottle	880	208.0	18.3	4.50	147	36.0	9.2	2.25

	UNIT		1 FLUID OZ.		1 CUP		1 TABLE-SPOON	
	Cal.	Carb.	Cal.	Carb.	Cal.	Carb.	Cal.	Carb.
CRANBERRY GRAPE JUICE COCKTAIL								
Welch's concentrated, 12-fl.-oz. can	880	216.0	73.3	18.00	587	144.0	37.0	9.00
Prepared as label directs, adding 3 cans (36 fl. oz.) water [yield: 48 fl. oz. (3 pints)]	880	216.0	18.3	4.50	146	36.0	9.0	2.30
CRANBERRY JUICE COCKTAIL, bottled, based on generic data								
1 pint	294	75.3	18.4	4.71	294	75.3	9.2	2.35
1 pound (approx. 1.8 cups) (tr/4g/tr/85%/1mg)	263	67.6	18.4	4.71	294	75.3	9.2	2.35
1 quart (approx. 35.8 oz. by wt.)	588	150.6	18.4	4.71	294	75.3	9.2	2.35
CRANBERRY JUICE COCKTAIL, by brand								
A&P, 32-fl.-oz. (1-quart) bottle	640	16.0	20.0	5.00	160	40.0	10.0	2.50
Ocean Spray, 5½-fl.-oz. can	100	23.8	18.3	4.33	147	34.7	9.2	2.17
32-fl.-oz. (1 quart) bottle	586	138.7	18.3	4.33	147	34.7	9.2	2.17
46-fl.-oz. can	842	199.3	18.3	4.33	147	34.7	9.2	2.17
128-fl.-oz. (1-gallon) bottle	2342	554.7	18.3	4.33	147	34.7	9.2	2.17
Frozen concentrate, 6-fl.-oz. can	440	112.0	73.3	18.67	587	149.3	37.0	9.30
Prepared as label directs, adding 3 cans (18 fl. oz.) water (yield: approx. 24 fl. oz.)	440	112.0	18.3	4.67	146	37.4	9.0	2.30
Low calorie (sweetened with saccharin), 32-fl.-oz. (1-quart) bottle	186	48.0	5.8	1.50	47	12.0	2.9	0.75
128-fl.-oz. (1-gallon) bottle	742	192.0	5.8	1.50	47	12.0	2.9	0.75
P&Q (A&P), 64-fl.-oz. (2-quart) bottle	1280	320.0	20.0	5.00	160	40.0	10.0	2.50
Town House, 32-fl.-oz. (1-quart) can	587	144.0	18.3	4.50	147	36.0	9.2	2.25
48-fl.-oz. (3-pint) can	1120	272.0	23.3	5.67	187	45.3	11.7	2.83
Welch's, 40-fl.-oz. bottle	700	190.0	17.5	4.75	140	38.0	8.8	2.38
Concentrated, 6-fl.-oz. can	480	120.0	80.0	20.00	640	160.0	40.0	10.00
Prepared as label directs, adding 3 cans (18 fl. oz.) water (yield: approx. 24 fl. oz.)	480	120.0	20.0	5.00	160	40.0	10.0	2.50
12-fl.-oz. can	960	240.0	80.0	20.00	640	160.0	40.0	10.00
Prepared as label directs, adding 3 cans (36 fl. oz.) water [yield: 48 fl. oz. (3 pints)]	960	240.0	20.0	5.00	160	40.0	10.0	2.50
Low calorie (sweetened with saccharin) 32-fl.-oz. (1-quart) bottle	160	37.4	5.0	1.17	40	9.4	2.5	0.59
CRANBERRY PRUNE JUICE DRINK								
Ocean Spray Cranprune, 32-fl.-oz. (1-quart) bottle	640	154.6	20.0	4.83	160	38.7	10.0	2.42
CURRANT JUICE, based on data from France (also see RED CURRANT BEVERAGE)								
Currant Juice, Black, 1-liter (33.8-fl.-oz.) container	608	146.7	18.0	4.34	144	34.7	9.0	2.17
Currant Juice, White, 1-liter (33.8-fl.-oz.) container	524	125.7	15.5	3.72	124	29.8	7.8	1.86
CURRANT JUICE, by brand								
Currant Juice, Black, **Lehr's,** 23-fl.-oz. bottle	381	91.3	16.6	3.97	133	31.7	8.3	1.98
FRUIT PUNCH DRINK								
P&Q (A&P), 46-fl.-oz. can	676	168.8	14.7	3.67	118	29.3	7.4	1.83
Tropi-Cal Lo, low cal, 64-fl.-oz. (2-quart) bottle	294	64.0	4.6	1.00	37	8.0	2.3	0.50
Tropicana, 10-fl.-oz. bottle	187	(47.1)	18.7	(4.71)	150	(31.7)	9.4	(2.36)
GATORADE, see ORANGE DRINK								
GRANADILLA JUICE, see PASSION FRUIT JUICE								
GRAPE DRINK								
A&P 10% grape juice, 32-fl.-oz. (1-quart) bottle	480	124.2	15.0	3.88	120	31.0	7.5	1.94
Ann Page (A&P), 46-fl.-oz. can	690	178.5	15.0	3.88	120	31.0	7.5	1.94
Golden Harvest Delight, 32-fl.-oz. (1-quart) bottle	400	104.0	12.5	3.25	100	26.0	6.3	1.63
P&Q (A&P), 46-fl.-oz. container	676	168.8	14.7	3.67	118	29.3	7.4	1.83
Artificially Flavored, 64-fl.-oz. (2-quart) container	960	248.0	15.0	3.88	120	31.0	7.5	1.94

	UNIT		1 FLUID OZ.		1 CUP		1 TABLE-SPOON	
	Cal.	Carb.	Cal.	Carb.	Cal.	Carb.	Cal.	Carb.
Romeo, 46-fl.-oz. can	690	172.5	15.0	3.75	120	30.0	7.5	1.88
Scotch Buy Artificially Flavored, 46-fl.-oz. can	690	166.8	15.0	3.63	120	29.0	7.5	1.82
Tropi-Cal-Lo reduced calorie, 64-fl.-oz. (2-quart) bottle	294	64.0	4.6	1.00	37	8.0	2.3	0.50
Tropicana, 10-fl.-oz. bottle	188	(48.2)	18.8	(4.82)	150	(38.6)	9.4	(2.41)
Wagner 10% grape juice, 32-fl. oz. (1-quart) bottle	534	133.4	16.7	4.17	134	33.4	8.4	2.09
Diet, 32-fl.-oz. (1-quart) bottle	128	32.0	4.0	1.00	32	8.0	2.0	0.50
Welch's Welchade, 5.5-fl.-oz. can	83	21.1	15.0	3.84	120	30.7	7.5	1.92
12-fl.-oz. can	180	46.1	15.0	3.84	120	30.7	7.5	1.92
46-fl.-oz. can	690	176.6	15.0	3.84	120	30.7	7.5	1.92
Concentrated, 12-fl.-oz. can	720	184.0	60.0	15.33	480	122.7	30.0	7.70
Prepared as label directs, adding 3 cans (36 fl. oz.) water [yield: approx. 48 fl. oz. (3 pints)]	720	184.0	15.0	3.83	120	30.7	8.0	1.90
GRAPE JUICE, canned or bottled, based on generic data								
1 pint	310	75.7	19.4	4.73	155	37.9	9.7	2.37
1 pound (approx. 1.8 cups) (tr/4g/tr/84%/1mg)	277	67.9	19.4	4.73	155	37.9	9.7	2.37
1 quart (approx. 35.8 oz. by wt.)	620	151.4	19.4	4.73	155	37.9	9.7	2.37
GRAPE JUICE, canned or bottled, by brand								
Balanced Concord, 24-fl.-oz. can	511	(122.4)	21.3	(5.10)	170	(40.8)	10.6	(2.55)
Hansen's Concord, 6-fl.-oz. can	119	27.9	19.8	4.65	158	37.2	9.9	2.33
12-fl.-oz. can	238	55.8	19.8	4.65	158	37.2	9.9	2.33
46-fl.-oz. can	911	213.9	19.8	4.65	158	37.2	9.9	2.33
Lehr's Red, 23-fl.-oz. bottle	463	103.6	20.1	4.50	161	36.0	10.1	2.25
White, 23-fl.-oz. bottle	470	114.0	20.4	4.96	163	39.6	10.2	2.48
White, Sparkling, 23-fl.-oz. bottle	449	(101.0)	19.5	(4.39)	156	(35.1)	9.8	(2.20)
Meier's Catawba, 25.4-fl.-oz. (750-ml.) bottle	(533)	(131.9)	(21.0)	(5.20)	(168)	(41.6)	(11.0)	(2.60)
50.7-fl.-oz. bottle (1.5-liter)	(1066)	(263.9)	(21.0)	(5.20)	(168)	(41.6)	(11.0)	(2.60)
Catawba, Pink, 25.4-fl.-oz. (750-ml.) bottle	(533)	(131.9)	(21.0)	(5.20)	(168)	(41.6)	(11.0)	(2.60)
50.7-fl.-oz. (1.5-liter) bottle	(1066)	(263.9)	(21.0)	(5.20)	(168)	(41.6)	(11.0)	(2.60)
Catawba, Sparkling, 25.4-fl.-oz. (750-ml.) bottle	(533)	(131.9)	(21.0)	(5.20)	(168)	(41.6)	(11.0)	(2.60)
50.7-fl.-oz. (1.5-liter) bottle	(1066)	(263.9)	(21.0)	(5.20)	(168)	(41.6)	(11.0)	(2.60)
Catawba, Pink Sparkling, 25.4-fl.-oz. (750-ml.) bottle	(533)	(131.9)	(21.0)	(5.20)	(168)	(41.6)	(11.0)	(2.60)
50.7-fl.-oz. (1.5 liter) bottle	(1066)	(263.9)	(21.0)	(5.20)	(168)	(41.6)	(11.0)	(2.60)
Cold Duck, 25.4-fl.-oz. (750-ml.) bottle	(533)	(131.9)	(21.0)	(5.20)	(168)	(41.6)	(11.0)	(2.60)
50.7-fl.-oz. (1.5-liter) bottle	(1066)	(263.9)	(21.0)	(5.20)	(168)	(41.6)	(11.0)	(2.60)
Seneca, 32-fl.-oz. (1-quart) bottle	640	160.0	20.0	5.00	160	40.0	10.0	2.50
48-fl.-oz. (3-pint) bottle	960	240.0	20.0	5.00	160	40.0	10.0	2.50
80-fl.-oz. (5-pint) bottle	1600	400.0	20.0	5.00	160	40.0	10.0	2.50
Welch's Purple, 4-fl.-oz. bottle	80	20.0	20.0	5.00	160	40.0	10.0	2.50
12-fl.-oz. bottle	240	60.0	20.0	5.00	160	40.0	10.0	2.50
24-fl.-oz. bottle	480	120.0	20.0	5.00	160	40.0	10.0	2.50
40-fl.-oz. bottle	800	200.0	20.0	5.00	160	40.0	10.0	2.50
Red, 24-fl.-oz. bottle	480	120.0	20.0	5.00	160	40.0	10.0	2.50
Red, Sparkling, 25.4-fl.-oz. bottle	508	127.0	20.0	5.00	160	40.0	10.0	2.50
White, 24-fl.-oz. bottle	480	120.0	20.0	5.00	160	40.0	10.0	2.50
White, Sparkling, 25.4-fl.-oz. bottle	508	127.0	20.0	5.00	160	40.0	10.0	2.50
GRAPE JUICE, frozen concentrate, sweetened, based on generic data								
Concentrated:								
1 pint	1029	255.5	64.3	15.97	515	127.7	32.2	7.98
1 pound (approx. 1.6 cups) (tr/13g/tr/54%/2mg)	813	201.4	64.3	15.97	515	127.7	32.2	7.98
1 quart (approx. 40.5 oz. by wt.)	2059	511.0	64.3	15.97	515	127.7	32.2	7.98
Diluted with 3 parts water by volume:								
1 pint	256	63.7	16.0	3.98	128	31.9	8.0	1.99
1 pound (approx. 1.8 cups) (tr/4g/tr/87%/1mg)	232	57.9	16.0	3.98	128	31.9	8.0	1.99
1 quart (approx. 35.4 oz. by wt.)	512	127.5	16.0	3.98	128	31.9	8.0	1.99

	UNIT		1 FLUID OZ.		1 CUP		1 TABLESPOON	
	Cal.	Carb.	Cal.	Carb.	Cal.	Carb.	Cal.	Carb.
GRAPE JUICE, frozen concentrate, by brand								
Minute Maid Sweetened, 6-fl.-oz. can	396	100.1	66.0	16.70	528	133.5	33.0	8.33
Prepared as label directs, adding 3 cans (18 fl. oz.) water (yield: approx. 24 fl. oz.)	396	100.1	16.5	4.17	132	33.3	8.3	2.08
Welch's, 6-fl.-oz. can	400	100.0	66.7	16.67	533	133.3	33.0	8.00
Prepared as label directs, adding 3 cans (18 fl. oz.) water (yield: approx. 24 fl. oz.)	400	100.0	16.7	4.17	133	33.3	8.00	2.10
12-fl.-oz. can	800	200.0	66.7	16.67	533	133.3	33.0	8.30
Prepared as label directs, adding 3 cans (36 fl. oz.) water [yield: 48 fl. oz. (3 pints)]	800	200.0	16.7	4.17	133	33.3	8.0	2.10
16-fl.-oz. (1-pint) can	1067	266.7	66.7	16.67	533	133.3	33.0	8.30
Prepared as label directs, adding 3 cans (48 fl. oz.) water [yield: approx. 64 fl. oz. (2 quarts)]	1067	266.7	16.7	4.17	133	33.3	8.0	2.10
GRAPE JUICE DRINK								
Welch's, 32-fl.-oz. (1-quart) bottle	586	144.0	18.3	4.50	147	36.0	9.2	2.25
48-fl.-oz. (3-pint) bottle	880	216.0	18.3	4.50	147	36.0	9.2	2.25
64-fl.-oz. (2-quart) bottle	1171	288.0	18.3	4.50	147	36.0	9.2	2.25
GRAPEFRUIT DRINK								
Tropicana, 10-fl.-oz. bottle	166	(42.1)	16.6	(4.21)	133	(33.6)	8.3	(2.10)
Wagner, 12 fl. oz.	180	45.9	15.0	3.83	120	30.6	7.5	1.91
Diet, 12 fl. oz.	36	8.0	3.0	0.67	24	5.3	1.5	0.33
GRAPEFRUIT JUICE, fresh or canned, based on generic data								
FRESH:								
For more information on fresh grapefruit juice, see the FRUITS chapter								
1 pint	192	45.4	12.0	2.84	96	22.6	6.0	1.42
1 pound (approx. 1.9 cups) (tr/3g/tr/90%/tr)	176	41.6	12.0	2.84	96	22.6	6.0	1.42
1 quart (approx. 34.7 oz. by wt.)	384	90.8	12.0	2.84	96	22.6	6.0	1.42
CANNED:								
Unsweetened:								
1 pint	186	44.2	11.6	2.76	93	22.1	5.8	1.38
1 pound (approx. 1.9 cups) (tr/3g/tr/90%/tr)	173	40.7	11.6	2.76	93	22.1	5.8	1.38
1 quart (approx. 34.5 oz. by wt.)	372	88.2	11.6	2.76	93	22.1	5.8	1.38
Sweetened:								
1 pint	232	55.7	14.5	3.48	116	27.8	7.3	1.74
1 pound (approx. 1.8 cups) (tr/3g/tr/87%/1mg)	209	50.5	14.5	3.48	116	27.8	7.3	1.74
1 quart (approx. 35.5 oz. by wt.)	464	111.4	14.5	3.48	116	27.8	7.3	1.74
GRAPEFRUIT JUICE, canned or bottled, by brand								
Del Monte Sweetened, 6-fl.-oz. can	80	21.0	13.3	3.50	107	28.0	6.7	1.75
46-fl.-oz. can	613	161.0	13.3	3.50	107	28.0	6.7	1.75
Unsweetened, 6-fl.-oz. can	70	17.0	11.7	2.83	93	22.7	5.8	1.42
46-fl.-oz. can	537	130.3	11.7	2.83	93	22.7	5.8	1.42
Featherweight Unsweetened, 12-fl.-oz. can	130	27.0	10.8	2.25	86	18.0	5.4	0.56
32-fl.-oz. (1-quart) bottle	342	73.5	10.7	2.30	86	18.4	5.4	1.15
Hansen's Natural Delight, 6-fl.-oz. bottle	64	14.4	10.7	2.30	86	18.4	5.4	1.15
12-fl.-oz. bottle	128	28.7	10.7	2.30	86	18.4	5.4	1.15
Libby's Sweetened, 6-fl.-oz. can	100	24.0	16.7	4.00	134	32.0	8.4	2.00
18-fl.-oz. can	300	72.0	16.7	4.00	134	32.0	8.4	2.00
Unsweetened, 6-fl.-oz. can	75	18.0	12.5	3.00	100	24.0	6.3	1.50
18-fl.-oz. can	225	54.0	12.5	3.00	100	24.0	6.3	1.50
Ocean Spray, 32-fl.-oz. (1-quart) bottle	320	80.0	10.0	2.50	80	20.0	5.0	1.30
48-fl.-oz. (3-pint) bottle	480	120.0	10.0	2.50	80	20.0	5.0	1.30
64-fl.-oz. (2-quart) bottle	640	160.0	10.0	2.50	80	20.0	5.0	1.30
Royal Sun, 32-fl.-oz. (1-quart) bottle	403	(98.3)	12.6	(3.07)	101	(24.6)	6.3	(1.54)
Tropicana, 5½-fl.-oz. bottle	69	(16.8)	12.6	(3.06)	101	(24.5)	6.3	(1.53)
7-fl.-oz. bottle	88	(21.4)	12.6	(3.06)	101	(24.5)	6.3	(1.53)
32-fl.-oz. (1-quart) bottle	403	(97.9)	12.6	(3.06)	101	(24.5)	6.3	(1.53)
64-fl.-oz. (2-quart) bottle	806	(192.8)	12.6	(3.06)	101	(24.5)	6.3	(1.53)

	UNIT		1 FLUID OZ.		1 CUP		1 TABLESPOON	
	Cal.	Carb.	Cal.	Carb.	Cal.	Carb.	Cal.	Carb.
GRAPEFRUIT JUICE, frozen concentrate, based on generic data								
Concentrated:								
1 pint	808	191.2	50.5	11.95	404	95.6	25.3	5.98
1 pound (approx. 1.7 cups) (1g/10g/tr/62%/1mg)	663	156.9	50.5	11.95	404	95.6	25.3	5.98
1 quart (approx. 39 oz. by wt.)	1616	382.5	50.5	11.95	404	95.6	25.3	5.98
Diluted with 3 parts water by volume:								
1 pint	204	48.1	12.8	3.01	102	24.0	6.4	1.50
1 pound (approx. 1.9 cups) (tr/3g/tr/89%/tr)	186	44.2	12.8	3.01	102	24.0	6.4	1.50
1 quart (approx. 35.1 oz. by wt.)	408	96.2	12.8	3.01	102	24.0	6.4	1.50
GRAPEFRUIT JUICE, frozen concentrate, by brand								
Minute Maid, 6-fl.-oz. can	300	39.0	50.0	6.50	400	52.0	25.0	3.25
Prepared as label directs, adding 3 cans (18 fl. oz.) water (yield: approx. 24 fl. oz.)	300	39.0	12.5	1.63	100	13.0	6.3	0.82
12-fl.-oz. can	600	78.0	50.0	6.50	400	52.0	25.0	3.25
Prepared as label directs, adding 3 cans (36 fl. oz.) water [yield: 48 fl. oz. (3 pints)]	600	78.0	12.5	1.63	100	13.0	6.3	0.82
Tropicana, 6-fl.-oz. can	302	(73.7)	50.4	(12.30)	403	(98.4)	25.2	(6.15)
Prepared as label directs, adding 3 cans (18 fl. oz.) water (yield: approx. 24 fl. oz.)	302	(73.7)	12.6	(3.07)	101	(24.6)	6.3	(1.54)
12-fl.-oz. can	605	(147.6)	50.4	(12.30)	403	(98.4)	25.2	(6.15)
Prepared as label directs, adding 3 cans (36 fl. oz.) water [yield: approx. 48 fl. oz. (3 pints)]	605	(147.6)	12.6	(3.07)	101	(24.6)	6.3	(1.54)
GRAPEFRUIT JUICE COCKTAIL, by brand								
Ocean Spray Pink Grapefruit Juice Cocktail, 48-fl.-oz. (3-pint) bottle	640	160.0	13.3	3.33	107	26.7	7.0	1.67
GUAVA DRINK								
Dole, 46-fl.-oz. can	690	176.3	15.0	3.83	120	30.6	7.5	1.90
HAWAIIAN PUNCH								
Hawaiian Punch Apple-Red, 10% fruit juice Fruit Punch, 46-fl.-oz. can	690	168.4	15.0	3.66	120	29.3	7.5	1.83
Cherry Fruit Punch, 46-fl.-oz. can	690	168.4	15.0	3.66	120	29.3	7.5	1.83
Fruit Juicy Red Fruit Punch, 46-fl.-oz. can	690	168.4	15.0	3.66	120	29.3	7.5	1.83
Grape Fruit Punch, 46-fl.-oz. can	690	168.4	15.0	3.66	120	29.3	7.5	1.83
Low Sugar Fruit Punch, reduced calorie, 46-fl.-oz. can	230	61.2	5.0	1.33	40	10.7	2.5	0.67
Orange Fruit Punch, 46-fl.-oz. can	690	168.4	15.0	3.66	120	29.3	7.5	1.83
Very Berry Fruit Punch, 46-fl.-oz. can	690	168.4	15.0	3.66	120	29.3	7.5	1.83
HI-C								
Hi-C Apple Drink, 10% fruit juice, 46-fl.-oz. can	705	176.3	15.3	3.83	123	30.7	7.7	1.92
64-fl-oz. (2-quart) bottle	979	245.1	15.3	3.83	123	30.7	7.7	1.92
Cherry Drink, 10% fruit juice, 12-fl.-oz. can	186	46.0	15.5	3.83	124	30.7	7.7	1.92
46-fl.-oz. can	713	176.3	15.5	3.83	124	30.7	7.7	1.92
Citrus Cooler Drink, 10% fruit juice, 46-fl.-oz. can	713	176.3	15.5	3.83	124	30.7	7.7	1.92
Grape Drink, 10% fruit juice, 12-fl.-oz. can	178	44.0	14.8	3.67	119	29.3	7.4	1.84
46-fl.-oz. can	682	168.7	14.8	3.67	119	29.3	7.4	1.84
67.6-fl.-oz. (2-liter) bottle	870	219.7	12.9	3.25	103	26.0	6.4	1.63
Grape Soft Drink, no fruit juice, 12-fl.-oz. can	160	40.0	13.3	3.33	106	26.6	6.7	1.67
67.6-fl.-oz. (2-liter) bottle	899	225.3	13.3	3.33	106	26.6	6.7	1.67
Lemonade, 67.6-fl.-oz. (2-liter) bottle	820	202.8	12.1	3.00	97	24.0	6.1	1.50
Lemonade Soft Drink, no fruit juice, 12-fl.-oz. can	160	40.0	13.3	3.33	106	26.6	6.7	1.67
67.6-fl.-oz. (2-liter) bottle	899	225.3	13.3	3.33	106	26.6	6.7	1.67
Orange Drink, 67.6-fl.-oz. (2-liter) bottle	862	219.7	12.8	3.25	102	26.0	6.4	1.63
Orange Drink, 10% fruit juice, 12-fl.-oz. can	184	46.0	15.3	3.83	123	30.7	7.7	1.92

	UNIT		1 FLUID OZ.		1 CUP		1 TABLE-SPOON	
	Cal.	Carb.	Cal.	Carb.	Cal.	Carb.	Cal.	Carb.
46-fl.-oz. can	705	176.3	15.3	3.83	123	30.7	7.7	1.92
64-fl.-oz. (2-quart) bottle	979	245.1	15.3	3.83	123	30.7	7.7	1.92
Orange Soft Drink, no fruit juice, 12-fl.-oz. can	160	40.0	13.3	3.33	106	26.6	6.7	1.67
67.6-fl. oz. (2-liter) bottle	899	225.3	13.3	3.33	106	26.6	6.7	1.67
Orange-Pineapple Drink, 10% fruit juice, 46-fl.-oz. can	721	176.3	15.7	3.83	125	30.7	7.9	1.92
Peach Drink, 10% fruit juice, 12-fl.-oz. can	180	46.0	15.0	3.83	120	30.7	7.5	1.92
46-fl.-oz. can	690	176.3	15.0	3.83	120	30.7	7.5	1.92
Red Punch, 67.6-fl.-oz. (2-liter) bottle	870	219.7	12.9	3.25	103	26.0	6.4	1.63
Strawberry Drink, 10% fruit juice, 46-fl.-oz. can	680	168.7	14.8	3.67	119	29.3	7.4	1.84
Tangerine Drink, 10% fruit juice, 46-fl.-oz. can	692	176.3	15.0	3.83	120	30.7	7.5	1.92
Wild Berry Drink, 10% fruit juice, 46-fl.-oz. can	675	168.7	14.7	3.67	117	29.3	7.4	1.84
LEMONADE								
Ann Page (A&P) frozen concentrate, 6-fl.-oz. can	400	104.0	66.7	17.33	533	138.7	33.4	8.67
Prepared as label directs, adding 4⅓ cans water [yield: approx. 32 fl. oz. (1 quart)]	400	104.0	12.5	3.25	100	26.0	6.3	1.63
Pink, 6-fl.-oz. can	400	104.0	66.7	17.33	533	138.7	33.4	8.67
Prepared as label directs, adding 4⅓ cans water [yield: approx. 32 fl. oz. (1 quart)]	400	104.0	12.5	3.25	100	26.0	6.3	1.63
Capri Sun Natural Lemonade Drink, 6¾-fl.-oz. container	63	23.3	9.3	3.45	74	27.6	4.7	1.70
Minute Maid frozen concentrate, 6-fl.-oz. can	395	104.5	65.8	17.42	526	139.4	32.9	8.71
Prepared as label directs, adding 4⅓ cans water [yield: approx. 32 fl. oz. (1 quart)]	395	104.5	12.3	3.27	99	26.1	6.2	1.64
12-fl.-oz. can	790	209.0	65.8	17.42	526	139.4	32.9	8.71
Prepared as label directs, adding 4⅓ cans water [yield: approx. 64 fl. oz. (2 quarts)]	790	209.0	12.3	3.27	99	26.1	6.2	1.64
Sunkist frozen concentrate, 6-fl.-oz. can	324	80.1	54.0	13.35	432	106.8	27.0	6.68
Prepared as label directs, adding 3 cans (18 fl. oz.) water (yield: approx. 24 fl. oz.)	324	80.1	13.5	3.34	108	26.7	6.8	1.67
12-fl.-oz. can	648	160.2	54.0	13.35	432	106.8	27.0	6.68
Prepared as label directs, adding 3 cans (36 fl. oz.) water [yield: approx. 48 fl. oz. (3 pints)]	648	16.2	13.5	3.34	108	26.7	6.8	1.67
LEMONADE FLAVOR DRINK								
Lemon Tree, 8-fl.-oz. container	90	23.0	11.3	2.88	90	23.0	5.6	1.44
12-fl.-oz. container	136	34.6	11.3	2.88	90	23.0	5.6	1.44
Sugar Free, 8-fl.-oz. container	40	10.0	5.0	1.25	40	10.0	2.5	0.63
12-fl.-oz. container	60	15.0	5.0	1.25	40	10.0	2.5	0.63
LEMON JUICE, based on generic data								
FRESH:								
For more information on fresh lemon juice, see the FRUITS chapter								
1 pint	122	39.0	7.6	2.44	61	19.5	3.8	1.22
1 pound (approx. 1.9 cups) (tr/2g/tr/91%/tr)	114	36.3	7.6	2.44	61	19.5	3.8	1.22
1 quart (approx. 33.8 oz. by wt.)	244	78.1	7.6	2.44	61	19.5	3.8	1.22
Juice of 1 medium lemon (approx. 3 tablespoons, approx. 1.7 oz.)	(12)	(3.8)	7.6	2.44	61	19.5	3.8	1.22
(based on data from France), 33.8 fl. oz. (1 liter)	379	83.8	11.2	2.48	89	19.9	5.6	1.24
CANNED OR BOTTLED:								
1 pint	104	31.6	6.5	1.98	52	15.8	3.3	0.98
1 pound (approx. 1.9 cups) (tr/2g/tr/92%/6mg)	95	29.4	6.5	1.98	52	15.8	3.3	0.98
1 quart (approx. 34.9 oz. by wt.)	208	63.3	6.5	1.98	52	15.8	3.3	0.98
FROZEN, single strength:								
1 pint	106	31.7	6.6	1.98	53	15.9	3.3	0.99
1 pound (approx. 1.9 cups) (tr/2g/tr/92%/tr)	100	29.5	6.6	1.98	53	15.9	3.3	0.99
1 quart (approx. 34.0 oz. by wt.)	212	63.4	6.6	1.98	53	15.9	3.3	0.99

	UNIT		1 FLUID OZ.		1 CUP		1 TABLE-SPOON	
	Cal.	Carb.	Cal.	Carb.	Cal.	Carb.	Cal.	Carb.
LEMON JUICE, by brand								
Minute Maid Lemon Juice, reconstituted, 7½-fl.-oz. can	50	16.5	6.7	2.20	53	17.6	3.3	1.10
P&Q (A&P), 1-quart container	192	64.0	6.0	2.00	48	16.0	3.0	1.00
RealLemon, reconstituted, 8-fl.-oz. bottle	48	16.0	6.0	2.00	48	16.0	3.0	1.00
16-fl.-oz. (1-pint) bottle	96	32.0	6.0	2.00	48	16.0	3.0	1.00
32-fl.-oz. (1-quart) bottle	192	64.0	6.0	2.00	48	16.0	3.0	1.00
Town House, 24-fl.-oz. bottle	144	48.0	6.0	2.00	48	16.0	3.0	1.00
LEMON/LIME FLAVORED DRINK								
Stokely Gatorade, 32-fl.-oz. (1-quart) bottle	202	56.0	6.3	1.75	50	14.0	3.2	0.88
LEMON-LIMEADE								
Minute Maid frozen concentrate, 6-fl.-oz. can	400	104.5	66.7	17.42	534	139.4	33.4	8.71
Prepared as label directs, adding 4⅓ cans water [yield: approx. 32 fl. oz. (1 quart)]	400	104.5	12.5	3.27	100	26.1	6.3	1.64
12-fl.-oz. can	800	209.0	66.7	17.42	534	139.4	33.4	6.21
Prepared as label directs, adding 4⅓ cans water [yield: approx. 64 fl. oz. (2 quarts)]	800	209.0	12.5	3.27	100	26.1	6.3	1.64
LIMEADE								
Minute Maid frozen concentrate, 6-fl.-oz. can	400	107.2	66.7	17.87	534	143.0	33.4	8.94
Prepared as label directs, adding 4⅓ cans water [approx. 32 fl. oz. (1 quart)]	400	107.2	12.5	3.35	100	26.8	6.3	1.68
12-fl.-oz. can	800	214.4	66.7	17.87	534	143.0	33.4	8.94
Prepared as label directs, adding 4⅓ cans water [yield: approx. 64 fl. oz. (2 quarts)]	800	214.4	12.5	3.35	100	26.8	6.3	1.68
LIME JUICE, based on generic data								
FRESH:								
1 pint	132	44.3	8.3	2.77	66	22.2	4.1	1.39
1 pound (approx. 1.9 cups) (tr/3g/tr/90%/tr)	123	40.9	8.3	2.77	66	22.2	4.1	1.39
1 quart (approx. 34.5 oz. by wt.)	264	88.6	8.3	2.77	66	22.2	4.1	1.39
CANNED OR BOTTLED:								
1 pint	102	32.9	6.4	2.06	51	16.5	3.2	1.03
1 pound (approx. 1.9 cups) (tr/2g/tr/93%/5mg)	95	30.4	6.4	2.06	51	16.5	3.2	1.03
1 quart (approx. 34.2 oz. by wt.)	204	65.8	6.4	2.06	51	16.5	3.2	1.03
LIME JUICE, by brand								
ReaLime, reconstituted, 8-fl.-oz. bottle	32	8.0	4.0	1.00	32	8.0	2.0	0.50
MULBERRY JUICE, based on data from East Asia								
32 fl. oz. (1 quart)	476	118.1	14.9	3.69	119	29.5	7.4	1.84
ORANGEADE								
Minute Maid frozen concentrate, 6-fl.-oz. can	501	121.1	83.5	20.18	668	161.4	41.8	10.09
Prepared as label directs, adding 4⅓ cans water [yield: approx. 32 fl. oz. (1 quart)]	501	121.1	15.7	3.78	125	30.3	7.9	1.89
12-fl.-oz. can	1002	242.2	83.5	20.18	668	161.4	41.8	10.09
Prepared as label directs, adding 4⅓ cans water [yield: approx. 64 fl. oz. (2 quarts)]	1002	242.2	15.7	3.78	125	30.3	7.9	1.89
ORANGE APRICOT DRINK								
Ann Page (A&P), 64-fl.-oz. (2-quart) can	960	248.3	15.0	3.88	120	31.0	7.5	1.94
ORANGE DRINK								
A&P, 10% orange juice, 32-fl.-oz. (1-quart) bottle	480	120.0	15.0	3.75	120	30.0	7.5	1.88
Ann Page (A&P) 10% fruit, 46-fl.-oz. can	690	172.5	15.0	3.75	120	30.0	7.5	1.88
Capri Sun Natural, 6¾-fl.-oz. container	103	26.1	15.3	3.87	122	30.9	7.7	1.90
Dole Passion, 46-fl.-oz. can	690	184.0	15.0	4.00	120	32.0	7.5	2.00
Gatorade Orange Flavored Drink, 32-fl.-oz. (1-quart) bottle	202	56.0	6.3	1.75	50	14.0	3.2	0.88
P&Q (A&P), 46-fl.-oz. container	676	168.8	14.7	3.67	118	29.3	7.4	1.83
Romeo, 46-fl.-oz. can	690	172.5	15.0	3.75	120	30.0	7.5	1.88
Scotch Buy, 46-fl.-oz. can	690	166.8	15.0	3.68	120	29.0	7.5	1.82

	UNIT		1 FLUID OZ.		1 CUP		1 TABLE-SPOON	
	Cal.	Carb.	Cal.	Carb.	Cal.	Carb.	Cal.	Carb.
Tropi-Cal Lo, 64-fl.-oz. (2-quart) bottle	294	64.0	4.6	1.00	37	8.0	2.3	0.50
Tropicana, 10-fl.-oz. bottle	179	(45.6)	17.9	(4.56)	143	(36.4)	9.0	(2.28)
Wagner, 12 fl. oz.	180	42.0	15.0	3.50	120	28.0	7.5	1.75
Diet, 12 fl. oz.	30	6.0	2.5	0.50	20	4.0	1.3	0.25
ORANGE GRAPEFRUIT JUICE, canned, based on generic data								
1 pint	214	50.8	13.4	3.18	107	25.4	6.7	1.59
1 pound (approx. 1.9 cups) (tr/3g/tr/89%/1mg)	195	46.7	13.4	3.18	107	25.4	6.7	1.59
1 quart (approx. 35.1 oz. by wt.)	428	101.6	13.4	3.18	107	25.4	6.7	1.59
ORANGE GRAPEFRUIT DRINK, by brand								
Del Monte Sweetened, Orange & Grapefruit Drink, 46-fl.-oz. can	613	153.3	13.3	3.33	107	26.7	6.7	1.67
Unsweetened, 46-fl.-oz. can	613	145.7	13.3	3.17	107	25.4	6.7	1.58
ORANGE GRAPEFRUIT JUICE, by brand								
Libby's Unsweetened Orange & Grapefruit Juice, 46-fl.-oz. can	612	145.8	13.3	3.17	107	25.4	6.7	1.58
Minute Maid Orange Grapefruit Blend, frozen concentrate, 6-fl.-oz. can	305	76.3	50.8	12.72	406	101.8	25.4	6.40
Prepared as label directs, adding 3 cans (18 fl. oz.) water (yield: approx. 24 fl. oz.)	305	76.3	12.7	3.18	101	25.5	6.3	1.59
12-fl.-oz. can	610	152.6	50.8	12.72	406	101.8	25.4	6.40
Prepared as label directs, adding 3 cans (36 fl. oz.) water [yield: approx. 48 fl. oz. (3 pints)]	610	152.6	12.7	3.18	101	25.5	6.3	1.59
ORANGE JUICE, fresh or canned, based on generic data								
FRESH:								
For more information on fresh orange juice, see the FRUITS chapter								
1 pint	224	51.6	13.9	3.22	112	25.8	6.9	1.61
1 pound (approx. 1.8 cups) (tr/3g/tr/88%/tr)	205	47.5	13.9	3.22	112	25.8	6.9	1.61
1 quart (approx. 34.8 oz. by wt.)	448	103.2	13.9	3.22	112	25.8	6.9	1.61
CANNED (Based on USDA data that do not specify "sweetened" or "unsweetened."):								
1 pint	208	49.0	13.0	3.06	104	24.5	6.5	1.53
1 pound (approx. 1.8 cups) (tr/3g/tr/89%/1mg)	191	44.7	13.0	3.06	104	24.5	6.5	1.53
1 quart (approx. 34.9 oz. by wt.)	416	98.0	13.0	3.06	104	24.5	6.5	1.53
ORANGE JUICE, canned or bottled, by brand								
Del Monte Sweetened, 46-fl.-oz. can	537	138.0	11.7	3.00	93	24.0	7.7	1.50
Unsweetened, 6-fl.-oz. can	80	19.0	13.3	3.17	107	25.3	6.7	1.58
46-fl.-oz. can	613	145.7	13.3	3.17	107	25.3	6.7	1.58
Gold-N-Pure, 64-fl.-oz. (2-quart) carton	864		13.5		90		5.6	
Grove Queen, 32-fl.-oz. (1-quart) bottle	432	(102.9)	13.5	(3.21)	108	(25.7)	6.8	(1.61)
64-fl.-oz. (2-quart) bottle	864	(205.4)	13.5	(3.21)	108	(25.7)	6.8	(1.61)
Hansen's, 6-fl.-oz. can	78	18.1	13.0	3.02	104	24.2	6.5	1.51
12-fl.-oz. can	156	36.3	13.0	3.02	104	24.2	6.5	1.51
33.3-fl.-oz. (1-liter) bottle	433	100.5	13.0	3.02	104	24.2	6.5	1.51
64-fl.-oz. (2-quart) bottle	832	193.3	13.0	3.02	104	24.2	6.5	1.51
Libby's Sweetened, 6-fl.-oz. can	100	23.0	16.7	3.83	133	30.7	8.3	1.92
18-fl.-oz. can	300	69.0	16.7	3.83	133	30.7	8.3	1.92
Unsweetened, 6-fl.-oz. can	90	20.0	15.0	3.33	120	26.7	5.6	1.67
18-fl.-oz. can	270	60.0	15.0	3.33	120	26.7	5.6	1.67
Minute Maid from concentrate, 32-fl.-oz. (1-quart) carton	442	105.0	13.8	3.28	111	26.3	6.9	1.64
64-fl.-oz. (2-quart) carton	884	210.0	13.8	3.28	111	26.3	6.9	1.64
Royal Sun, 32-fl.-oz. (1-quart) bottle	432	(102.9)	13.5	(3.21)	108	(25.7)	6.8	(1.61)
64-fl.-oz. (2-quart) bottle	864	(205.4)	13.5	(3.21)	108	(25.7)	6.8	(1.61)
Tropicana, 5½-fl.-oz. container	74	(17.6)	13.5	(3.20)	108	(25.6)	6.8	(1.60)
7-fl.-oz. bottle	95	(22.4)	13.5	(3.20)	108	(25.6)	6.8	(1.60)
16-fl.-oz. container	216	(51.2)	13.5	(3.20)	108	(25.6)	6.8	(1.60)

	UNIT		1 FLUID OZ.		1 CUP		1 TABLE-SPOON	
	Cal.	Carb.	Cal.	Carb.	Cal.	Carb.	Cal.	Carb.
32-fl.-oz. (1-quart) container	432	(102.4)	13.5	(3.20)	108	(25.6)	6.8	(1.60)
64-fl.-oz. (2-quart) container	864	(204.8)	13.5	(3.20)	108	(25.6)	6.8	(1.60)
ORANGE JUICE, frozen concentrate, based on generic data								
Concentrated:								
1 pint	908	217.3	56.8	13.58	454	108.7	28.4	6.79
1 pound (approx. 1.6 cups) (1g/11g/tr/58%/1mg)	722	173.3	56.8	13.58	454	108.7	28.4	6.79
1 quart (approx. 40.3 oz. by wt.)	1816	434.6	56.8	13.58	454	108.7	28.4	6.79
Diluted with 3 parts water by volume:								
1 pint	224	53.7	14.0	3.35	112	26.8	7.0	1.68
1 pound (approx. 1.8 cups) (tr/3g/tr/88%/tr)	204	48.9	14.0	3.35	112	26.8	7.0	1.68
1 quart (approx. 35.1 oz. by wt.)	448	107.3	14.0	3.35	112	26.8	7.0	1.68
ORANGE JUICE, frozen concentrate, by brand								
Minute Maid, 6-fl.-oz. can	360	85.7	60.0	14.28	480	114.3	30.0	7.14
Prepared as label directs, adding 3 cans (18 fl. oz.) water (yield: approx. 24 fl. oz.)	360	85.7	15.0	3.57	120	28.5	7.5	1.78
12-fl.-oz. can	720	171.4	60.0	14.28	480	114.3	30.0	7.14
Prepared as label directs, adding 3 cans (36 fl. oz.) water [yield: approx. 48 fl. oz. (3 pints)]	720	171.4	15.0	3.57	120	28.5	7.5	1.78
24-fl.-oz. can	1440	342.8	60.0	14.28	480	114.3	30.0	7.14
Prepared as label directs, adding 3 cans (72 fl. oz.) water [yield: approx. 96 fl. oz. (3 quarts)]	1440	342.8	15.0	3.57	120	28.5	7.5	1.78
Snow Crop, 6-fl.-oz. can	360	85.7	60.0	14.28	480	114.2	30.0	7.14
Prepared as label directs, adding 3 cans (18 fl. oz.) water (yield: approx. 24 fl. oz.)	360	85.7	15.0	3.57	120	28.5	7.5	1.78
12-fl.-oz. can	720	171.4	60.0	14.28	480	114.2	30.0	7.14
Prepared as label directs, adding 3 cans (36 fl. oz.) water [yield: approx. 48 fl. oz. (3 pints)]	720	171.4	15.0	3.57	120	28.5	7.5	1.78
24-fl.-oz. can	1440	342.8	60.0	14.28	480	114.2	30.0	7.14
Prepared as label directs, adding 3 cans (72 fl. oz.) water [yield: approx. 96 fl. oz. (3 quarts)]	1440	342.8	15.0	3.57	120	28.5	7.5	1.78
Sunkist, 6-fl.-oz. can	321	80.1	53.5	13.35	428	106.8	26.8	6.68
Prepared as label directs, adding 3 cans (18 fl. oz.) water (yield: approx. 24 fl. oz.)	321	80.1	13.4	3.34	107	26.7	6.7	1.67
12-fl.-oz. can	642	160.2	53.5	13.35	428	106.8	26.8	6.68
Prepared as label directs, adding 3 cans (36 fl. oz.) water [yield: approx. 48 fl. oz. (3 pints)]	642	160.2	13.4	3.34	107	26.7	6.7	1.67
Tropicana, 6-fl.-oz. can	324	(77.1)	54.0	(12.86)	432	(102.9)	27.0	(6.43)
Prepared as label directs, adding 3 cans (18 fl. oz.) water (yield: approx. 24 fl. oz.)	324	(77.1)	13.5	(3.20)	108	(25.6)	6.8	(1.60)
16-fl.-oz. can	864	(205.7)	54.0	(12.86)	432	(102.9)	27.0	(6.43)
Prepared as label directs, adding 3 cans (48 fl. oz.) water [yield: approx. 64 fl. oz. (2 quarts)]	864	(205.7)	13.5	(3.20)	108	(25.6)	6.8	(1.60)
ORANGE JUICE, imitation, frozen concentrate								
Birds Eye Awake, 12-fl.-oz. can	720	168.0	60.0	14.00	480	112.0	30.0	7.00
Prepared as label directs, adding 3 cans (36 fl. oz.) water [yield: 48 fl. oz. (3 pints)]	720	168.0	15.0	3.50	120	28.0	7.5	1.75
Minute Maid Bright & Early, 6-fl.-oz. can	360	85.7	60.0	14.28	480	114.2	30.0	7.14
Prepared as label directs, adding 3 cans (18 fl. oz.) water (yield: approx. 24 fl. oz.)	360	85.7	15.0	3.60	120	28.8	7.5	1.80
12-fl.-oz. can	720	171.4	60.0	14.28	480	114.2	30.0	7.14
Prepared as label directs, adding 3 cans (36 fl. oz.) water [yield: approx. 48 fl. oz. (3 pints)]	720	171.4	15.0	3.60	120	28.8	7.5	1.80

	UNIT		1 FLUID OZ.		1 CUP		1 TABLE-SPOON	
	Cal.	Carb.	Cal.	Carb.	Cal.	Carb.	Cal.	Carb.
24-fl.-oz. can	1440	342.8	60.0	14.28	480	114.2	30.0	7.14
Prepared as label directs, adding 3 cans (72 fl. oz.) water [yield: approx. 96 fl. oz. (3 quarts)]	1440	342.8	15.0	3.60	120	28.8	7.5	1.80
Orange Plus frozen concentrate, 12-fl.-oz. can	800	192.0	66.7	16.00	534	128.0	33.4	8.00
Prepared as label directs, adding 3 cans (36 fl. oz.) water [yield: approx. 48 fl. oz. (3 pints)]	800	192.0	16.7	4.00	133	32.0	8.3	2.00
ORANGE PINEAPPLE DRINK								
Ann Page (A&P), 46-fl.-oz. can	690	178.3	15.0	3.88	120	31.0	7.5	1.94
Tropicana, 10-fl.-oz. bottle	173	(43.6)	17.3	(4.36)	138	(34.9)	8.7	(2.18)
Wagner, 12-fl.-oz. container	160	42.0	13.3	3.50	106	28.0	6.6	1.75
"P.M." FRUIT DRINK								
Mott's, 5½-fl.-oz. can	83	20.2	15.1	3.67	120	29.4	7.5	1.84
6-pack (six 5½-fl.-oz. cans, 33 fl. oz.)	495	121.2	15.1	3.67	120	29.4	7.5	1.84
PAPAYA CONCENTRATE								
Golden Harvest, 32-fl.-oz. (1-quart) bottle	1440	352.0	45.0	11.00	360	88.0	22.5	5.60
Prepared as label directs, adding 3 bottles (96 fl. oz.) water [yield: approx. 128 fl. oz. (4 quarts)]	1440	352.0	11.3	2.25	90	22.0	5.7	1.38
Prepared as label directs, adding 5 bottles (160 fl. oz.) water [yield: approx. 192 fl. oz. (6 quarts)]	1440	352.0	7.5	1.83	60	14.7	3.8	0.92
PAPAYA JUICE, based on data from East Asia								
33.8 fl. oz. (1 liter)	723	174.1	21.4	5.15	171	41.2	10.7	2.57
Canned, 33.8 fl. oz. (1 liter)	713	181.2	21.1	5.36	169	42.9	10.5	2.68
PAPAYA NECTAR, canned, based on generic data								
1 pint	284	72.6	17.8	4.54	142	36.3	8.9	2.27
1 pound (approx. 1.8 cups) (tr/4g/tr/85%/1mg)	259	65.8	17.8	4.54	142	36.3	8.9	2.27
1 quart (approx. 35.1 oz. by wt.)	568	145.1	17.8	4.54	142	36.3	8.9	2.27
PAPAYA NECTAR, by brand								
Golden Harvest, 32-oz. (1-quart) bottle	400	104.0	12.5	3.25	100	26.0	6.3	1.63
PASSION FRUIT JUICE (Granadilla Juice), based on generic data								
Purple Passion Fruit Juice (based on data from Hawaii), 32 fl. oz. (1 quart)	504	134.4	15.8	4.20	126	33.6	7.9	2.10
Yellow Passion Fruit Juice (based on data from East Asia), canned sweetened, 33.8 fl. oz. (1 liter)	1835	461.0	54.3	13.64	434	109.1	27.1	6.82
Yellow Passion Fruit Juice (based on data from Hawaii), 32 fl. oz. (1 quart)	524	135.6	16.4	4.24	131	33.9	8.2	2.12
PEACH JUICE, based on data from France								
33.8 fl. oz. (1 liter)	554	136.2	16.4	4.03	131	32.2	8.2	2.02
PEACH NECTAR, canned, based on generic data								
1 pint	268	69.3	16.8	4.33	134	34.7	8.4	2.17
1 pound (approx. 1.8 cups) (tr/4g/tr/86%/2mg)	245	63.2	16.8	4.33	134	34.7	8.4	2.17
1 quart (approx. 35.0 oz. by wt.)	536	138.7	16.8	4.33	134	34.7	8.4	2.17
PEACH NECTAR, by brand								
Del Monte, 12-fl.-oz. can	200	54.0	16.7	4.50	133	36.0	8.3	2.55
Heart's Delight, 12-fl.-oz. can	200	50.0	16.7	4.17	133	33.4	8.3	2.09
Libby's, 5½-fl.-oz. can	83	21.1	15.0	3.83	120	30.6	7.5	1.91
PEAR NECTAR, canned, based on generic data								
1 pint	298	78.8	18.6	4.93	149	39.4	9.3	2.46
1 pound (approx. 1.8 cups) (tr/4g/tr/84%/2mg)	272	71.6	18.6	4.93	149	39.4	9.3	2.46
1 quart (approx. 35.0 oz. by wt.)	596	157.6	18.6	4.93	149	39.4	9.3	2.46
PEAR NECTAR, by brand								
Del Monte, 12-fl.-oz. can	220	60.0	18.3	5.00	147	40.0	9.2	2.50
Heart's Delight, 12-fl.-oz. can	200	52.0	16.7	4.33	133	34.6	8.3	2.17

	UNIT		1 FLUID OZ.		1 CUP		1 TABLE-SPOON	
	Cal.	Carb.	Cal.	Carb.	Cal.	Carb.	Cal.	Carb.
Libby's, 5½-fl.-oz. can	92	22.9	16.7	4.17	133	33.3	8.3	2.08
12-fl.-oz. can	200	50.0	16.7	4.17	133	33.3	8.3	2.08
PINEAPPLE COCONUT JUICE								
Hansen's, 6-fl.-oz. can	131	30.0	21.9	5.00	175	40.0	10.9	2.50
8-fl.-oz. bottle	175	40.0	21.9	5.00	175	40.0	10.9	2.50
12-fl.-oz. can	263	60.0	21.9	5.00	175	40.0	10.9	2.50
128-fl.-oz. (1-gallon) bottle	2803	640.0	21.9	5.00	175	40.0	10.9	2.50
PINEAPPLE GRAPEFRUIT JUICE DRINK								
Pineapple Grapefruit Drink, **Romeo,** 46-fl.-oz. can	748	178.3	16.3	3.88	130	31.0	8.2	1.94
Pineapple-Grapefruit Juice, **Dole,** 46-fl.-oz. can	767	199.3	16.7	4.33	133	34.6	8.0	2.20
Pineapple Pink Grapefruit Juice, **Del Monte,** 6-fl.-oz. can	90	24.0	15.0	4.00	120	32.0	7.5	2.00
46-fl.-oz. can	690	184.0	15.0	4.00	120	32.0	7.5	2.00
Dole, 6-fl.-oz. can	91	23.0	15.2	3.83	121	30.7	7.6	1.92
46-fl.-oz. can	698	176.3	15.2	3.83	121	30.7	7.6	1.92
Town House, 46-fl.-oz. can	690	184.0	15.0	4.00	120	32.0	7.5	2.00
Pineapple Pink Grapefruit Juice Drink, **Del Monte,** 46-fl.-oz. can	690	184.0	15.0	4.00	120	32.0	7.5	2.00
PINEAPPLE JUICE, canned, based on generic data								
1 pint	278	68.9	17.4	4.31	139	34.4	8.7	2.15
1 pound (approx. 1.8 cups) (tr/4g/tr/86%/tr)	254	62.6	17.4	4.31	139	34.4	8.7	2.15
1 quart (approx. 35.0 oz. by wt.)	556	137.8	17.4	4.31	139	34.4	8.7	2.15
PINEAPPLE JUICE, canned, by brand								
A&P Unsweetened, 46-fl.-oz. can	768	191.7	16.7	4.17	133	33.3	8.3	2.08
Balanced Dietetic, Hawaiian (no salt or sugar added), 18-fl.-oz. can	256	(61.2)	14.2	(3.40)	114	(27.2)	7.1	(1.70)
Del Monte, 6-fl.-oz. can	100	25.0	16.7	4.17	133	33.3	8.3	2.08
46-fl.-oz. can	767	191.7	16.7	4.17	133	33.3	8.3	2.08
Dole, 6-fl.-oz. can	93	22.8	15.5	3.80	124	30.4	7.8	1.90
Hawaiian Punch, 46-fl.-oz. can	787	193.7	17.1	4.21	137	33.7	8.6	2.11
Town House Unsweetened Hawaiian, 46-fl.-oz. can	767	191.7	16.7	4.17	133	33.3	8.3	2.08
PINEAPPLE JUICE, frozen concentrate, based on generic data								
Concentrated:								
1 pint	1032	255.2	64.5	15.95	516	127.6	32.3	7.97
1 pound (approx. 1.6 cups) (tr/13g/tr/53%/1mg)	813	201.1	64.5	15.95	516	127.6	32.3	7.97
1 quart (approx. 40.6 oz. by wt.)	2064	510.3	64.5	15.95	516	127.6	32.3	7.97
Diluted with 3 parts water by volume:								
1 pint	258	63.9	16.1	3.99	129	31.9	8.1	2.00
1 pound (approx. 1.8 cups) (tr/4g/tr/87%/tr)	236	58.0	16.1	3.99	129	31.9	8.1	2.00
1 quart (approx. 35.0 oz. by wt.)	516	127.7	16.1	3.99	129	31.9	8.1	2.00
PINEAPPLE JUICE, frozen concentrate, by brand								
Minute Maid, 6-fl.-oz. can	367	90.7	61.2	15.12	490	121.0	30.6	7.56
Prepared as label directs, adding 3 cans (18 fl. oz.) water (yield: approx. 24 fl. oz.)	367	90.7	15.3	3.78	123	30.3	7.7	1.89
12-fl.-oz. can	734	181.4	61.2	15.12	490	121.0	30.6	7.56
Prepared as label directs, adding 3 cans (36 fl. oz.) water [yield: approx. 48 fl. oz. (3 pints)]	734	181.4	15.3	3.78	123	30.3	7.7	1.89
PINEAPPLE ORANGE DRINK								
Minute Maid Pineapple Orange frozen concentrate, 6-fl.-oz. can	377	91.9	62.8	15.32	502	122.6	31.4	7.66
Prepared as label directs, adding 3 cans (18 fl. oz.) water (yield: approx. 24 fl. oz.)	377	91.9	15.7	3.83	125	30.7	7.8	1.92
12-fl.-oz. can	754	183.8	62.8	15.32	502	122.6	31.4	7.66
Prepared as label directs, adding 3 cans (36 fl. oz.) water [yield: approx. 48 fl. oz. (3 pints)]	754	183.8	15.7	3.83	125	30.7	7.8	1.92
Scotch Buy, 46-fl.-oz. can	690	166.8	15.0	3.68	120	29.0	7.5	1.82

	UNIT		1 FLUID OZ.		1 CUP		1 TABLE-SPOON	
	Cal.	Carb.	Cal.	Carb.	Cal.	Carb.	Cal.	Carb.
PINEAPPLE ORANGE GRAPEFRUIT JUICE								
Dole, 6-fl.-oz. can	90	23.0	15.0	3.83	120	30.7	7.5	1.92
46-fl.-oz. can	690	176.3	15.0	3.83	120	30.7	7.5	1.92
POMEGRANATE JUICE, based on data from Pakistan								
Red Pomegranate Juice, 33.8 fl. oz. (1 liter)	649	148.7	19.2	4.40	154	35.2	9.6	2.20
PRUNE JUICE, canned, based on generic data								
1 pint	362	89.3	22.6	5.58	181	44.7	11.3	2.79
1 pound (approx. 1.8 cups) (tr/5g/tr/81%/1mg)	322	79.2	22.6	5.58	181	44.7	11.3	2.79
1 quart (approx. 35.9 oz. by wt.)	724	178.6	22.6	5.58	181	44.7	11.3	2.79
PRUNE JUICE, by brand								
A&P, 32-fl.-oz. (1-quart) bottle	747	181.3	23.3	5.67	187	45.3	11.7	2.83
40-fl.-oz. bottle	933	226.7	23.3	5.67	187	45.3	11.7	2.83
Del Monte, 32-fl.-oz. (1-quart) bottle	640	176.0	20.0	5.50	160	44.0	10.0	2.75
40-fl.-oz. bottle	800	220.0	20.0	5.50	160	44.0	10.0	2.75
Mott's, 32-fl.-oz. (1-quart) bottle	746	181.4	23.3	5.67	187	45.3	11.7	2.83
40-fl.-oz. bottle	932	226.8	23.3	5.67	187	45.3	11.7	2.83
48-fl.-oz. (3-pint) bottle	1118	272.2	23.3	5.67	187	45.3	11.7	2.83
Mott's blended with Prune Pulp, 32-fl.-oz. (1-quart) bottle	640	160.0	20.0	5.00	160	40.0	10.0	2.50
40-fl.-oz. bottle	800	200	20.0	5.00	160	40.0	10.0	2.50
48-fl.-oz. (3-pint) bottle	960	240.0	20.0	5.00	160	40.0	10.0	2.50
Sunsweet, 4-fl.-oz. bottle	80	22.0	20.0	5.50	160	44.0	10.0	2.75
5½-fl.-oz. can	110	30.3	20.0	5.50	160	44.0	10.0	2.75
12-fl.-oz. can	240	66.0	20.0	5.50	160	44.0	10.0	2.75
32-fl.-oz. (1-quart) bottle	640	176.0	20.0	5.50	160	44.0	10.0	2.75
40-fl.-oz. bottle	800	220.0	20.0	5.50	160	44.0	10.0	2.75
46-fl.-oz. can	920	253.0	20.0	5.50	16	440	10.0	2.75
48-fl.-oz. (3-pint) bottle	960	264.0	20.0	5.50	160	44.0	10.0	2.75
Super Mott's Unsweetened, 32-fl.-oz. (1-quart) bottle	746	181.4	23.3	5.67	187	45.3	11.7	2.83
Town House, 32 fl. oz. (1-quart)	747	186.7	23.3	5.83	187	46.7	11.7	2.92
Welch's, 46-fl.-oz. bottle	1150	276.0	25.0	6.00	200	48.0	12.5	3.00
PRUNE NECTAR								
Mott's, 32-fl.-oz. (1-quart) bottle	534	133.4	16.7	4.17	134	33.4	8.4	2.09
PUNCH, see HAWAIIAN PUNCH and TROPICAL PUNCH								
RASPBERRY JUICE, based on data from France								
33.8 fl. oz. (1 liter)	470	115.3	13.9	3.41	112	27.3	7.0	1.70
RED CURRANT BEVERAGE (see also CURRANT JUICE)								
Donaukrone, Red Currant Beverage, 23-fl.-oz. bottle	345	81.4	15.0	3.54	120	28.3	7.5	1.77
SOURSOP JUICE, based on data from Hawaii								
32 fl. oz. (1 quart)	(789)	(202.3)	(24.7)	(6.32)	(197)	(50.6)	(12.3)	(3.16)
TANGELO JUICE, see the FRUITS chapter								
TANGERINE JUICE, based on generic data								
FRESH:								
1 pint	212	49.9	13.3	3.12	106	25.0	6.6	1.56
1 pound (approx. 1.9 cups) (tr/3g/tr/89%/tr)	195	45.9	13.3	3.12	106	25.0	6.6	1.56
1 quart (approx. 34.8 oz. by wt.)	424	99.8	13.3	3.12	106	25.0	6.6	1.56
CANNED, SWEETENED:								
1 pint	250	59.8	15.6	3.74	125	30.0	7.8	1.87
1 pound (approx. 1.8 cups) (tr/3g/tr/87%/tr)	227	54.5	15.6	3.74	125	30.0	7.8	1.87
1 quart (approx. 35.2 oz. by wt.)	500	119.5	15.6	3.74	125	30.0	7.8	1.87
FROZEN, SWEETENED:								
Concentrated:								
1 pint	917	886.8	57.3	13.86	459	443.4	28.7	27.71
1 pound (approx. 1.6 cups) (tr/11g/tr/58%/1mg)	731	176.4	57.3	13.86	459	443.4	28.7	27.71
1 quart (approx. 40.2 oz. by wt.)	1835	1773.7	57.3	13.86	459	444.3	28.7	27.71
Diluted with 3 parts water by volume:								
1 pint	220	53.3	13.8	3.33	110	26.7	6.9	1.67
1 pound (approx. 1.8 cups) (tr/3g/tr/88%/tr)	209	50.2	13.8	3.33	110	26.7	6.9	1.67
1 quart (approx. 33.7 oz. by wt.)	440	106.6	13.8	3.33	110	26.7	6.9	1.67
(Based on data from France)								
32 fl. oz. (1 quart)	427	91.3	13.3	2.85	107	22.8	6.7	1.43
TANGERINE JUICE, frozen concentrate, by brand								
Minute Maid Sweetened, 6-fl.-oz. can	341	83.3	56.8	13.89	454	111.1	28.4	6.95
Prepared as label directs, adding 3 cans (18 fl. oz.) water (yield: approx. 24 fl. oz.)	341	83.3	14.2	3.47	113	27.7	7.1	1.73
12-fl.-oz. can	682	166.6	56.8	13.89	454	111.1	28.4	6.95
Prepared as label directs, adding 3 cans (36 fl. oz.) water [yield: approx. 48 fl. oz. (3 pints)]	682	166.6	14.2	3.47	113	27.7	7.1	1.73
TROPICAL PUNCH								
A&P 10% fruit juice, 32-fl.-oz. (1-quart) bottle	480	120.0	15.0	3.75	120	30.0	7.5	1.88
Ann Page (A&P) 10% fruit juice, 46-fl.-oz. can	690	172.5	15.0	3.75	120	30.0	7.5	1.88
Romeo, 46-fl.-oz. can	690	172.5	15.0	3.75	120	20.0	7.5	1.88
Scotch Buy, 46-fl.-oz. can	690	166.8	15.0	3.63	120	29.0	7.5	1.82
Wagner, 32-fl.-oz. (1-quart) bottle	480	117.4	15.0	3.67	120	29.3	7.5	1.83
WILD BERRY								
Scotch Buy, Artificially Flavored Drink, 46-fl.-oz. can	690	166.8	15.0	3.63	120	29.0	7.5	1.82

FRUIT-FLAVORED DRINK MIXES (alphabetized by brand)

	UNIT		1 FLUID OZ.		1 CUP		1 TABLE-SPOON	
	Cal.	Carb.	Cal.	Carb.	Cal.	Carb.	Cal.	Carb.
Elam's dry mix:								
Natural Lemonade Flavor with Fructose, 36¾-oz. package	4160	(1041.0)						
Prepared as label directs, adding 2 gallons of water (yield: 256 fl. oz., or 2 gallons)	4160	(1041.0)	16.3	(4.13)	130	(33.0)	81.1	2.06
Hawaiian Punch dry mixes:								
Cherry Punch, sugar sweetened, 28½-oz. can	3200	800.0						
Prepared as label directs, adding approx. 2 gallons water [yield: 2 gallons (32 cups)]	3200	800.0	12.5	3.13	100	25.0	6.3	1.56
1 "scoop," approx. ¼ cup (2 "suggested" servings)	200	50.0						
Prepared as label directs, adding 2 cups (1 pint) water [yield: approx. 1 pint (2 cups)]	200	50.0	12.5	3.13	100	25.0	6.3	1.56
Grape Punch, not presweetened, 0.22-oz. packet	16	0						
Prepared as label directs, adding 2 quarts water and 1 cup sugar [yield: approx. 2 quarts (8 cups)]	800	200.0	12.5	3.13	100	25.0	6.3	1.56
sugar sweetened, 28½-oz. can	3200	800.0						
Prepared as label directs, adding 2 gallons water [yield: approx. 2 gallons, 256 fl. oz. (32 cups)]	3200	800.0	12.5	3.13	100	25.0	6.3	1.56
1 "scoop," approx. ¼ cup (2 "suggested" servings)	200	50.0						
Prepared as label directs, adding 2 cups (1 pint) water [yield: approx. 1 pint (2 cups)]	200	50.0	12.5	3.13	100	25.0	6.3	1.56
Lemonade Punch, not presweetened, 0.36-oz. packet	26	0.0						
Prepared as label directs, adding 2 quarts water and 1 cup sugar [yield: approx. 2 quarts (8 cups)]	800	200.0	12.5	3.13	100	25.0	6.3	1.56
Orange Punch, not presweetened, 0.28-oz. packet	16	0.0						
Prepared as label directs, adding 2 quarts water and 1 cup sugar [yield: approx. 2 quarts (8 cups)]	800	200.0	12.5	3.13	100	25.0	6.3	1.56

	UNIT		1 FLUID OZ.		1 CUP		1 TABLE-SPOON	
	Cal.	Carb.	Cal.	Carb.	Cal.	Carb.	Cal.	Carb.
sugar sweetened, 27½-oz. can	3200	800.0	(100.0)	(25.00)	(800)	(200.0)	(50.0)	(12.50)
Prepared as label directs, adding approx. 2 gallons water [yield: 2 gallons (32 cups)]	3200	800.0	12.5	3.13	100	25.0	6.3	1.56
1 "scoop," approx. ¼ cup (2 "suggested" servings)	200	50.0	(100.0)	(25.00)	(800)	(200.0)	(50.0)	(12.50)
Prepared as label directs, adding 2 cups (1 pint) water [yield: approx. 1 pint (2 cups)]	200	50.0	12.5	3.13	100	25.0	6.3	1.56
Raspberry Punch, not presweetened, 0.19-oz. packet	16	0.0						
Prepared as label directs, adding 2 quarts water and 1 cup sugar [yield: approx. 2 quarts (8 cups)]	800	200.0	12.5	3.13	100	25.0	6.3	1.56
Red Punch, not presweetened, 0.24-oz. packet	16	0.0						
Prepared as label directs, adding 2 quarts water and 1 cup sugar [yield: approx. 2 quarts (8 cups)]	800	200.0	12.5	3.13	100	25.0	6.3	1.56
sugar sweetened, 7¼-oz. can	800	200.0	(100.0)	(25.09)	(800)	(100.0)	(50.0)	(6.25)
Prepared as label directs, adding 2 quarts water [yield: approx. 2 quarts (8 cups)]	800	200.0	12.5	3.13	100	25.0	6.3	1.56
Strawberry Punch, not presweetened, 0.24-oz. packet	16	0.0						
Prepared as label directs, adding 2 quarts water and 1 cup sugar [yield: approx. 2 quarts (8 cups)]	800	200.0	12.5	3.13	100	25.0	6.3	1.56
Hi-C dry mixes:								
Cherry, sugar sweetened, 29.2-oz. container	3243	810.7						
Prepared as label directs, adding 8 quarts water [yield: approx. 8 quarts (32 cups)]	3243	810.7	12.7	3.17	101	25.4	6.3	1.59
43.8-oz. container	4865	1216.1						
Prepared as label directs, adding 12 quarts water [yield: approx. 12 quarts (48 cups)]	4865	1216.1	12.7	3.17	101	25.4	6.3	1.59
1 "scoop" (2 "suggested" servings)	203	50.7						
Prepared as label directs, adding 1 pint water [yield: approx. 1 pint (2 cups)]	203	50.7	12.7	3.17	101	25.4	6.3	1.59
Grape, sugar sweetened, 29.2-oz. container	3243	810.7						
Prepared as label directs, adding 8 quarts water [yield: approx. 8 quarts (32 cups)]	3243	810.7	12.7	3.17	101	25.4	6.3	1.59
43.8-oz. container	4865	116.1						
Prepared as label directs, adding 12 quarts water [yield: approx. 12 quarts (48 cups)]	4865	1216.1	12.7	3.17	101	25.4	6.3	1.59
1 "scoop" (2 "suggested" servings)	203	50.7						
Prepared as label directs, adding 1 pint water [yield: approx. 1 pint (2 cups)]	203	50.7	12.7	3.17	101	25.4	6.3	1.59
Lemonade, sugar sweetened, 29.2-oz. container	3243	810.7						
Prepared as label directs, adding 8 quarts water [yield: approx. 8 quarts (32 cups)]	3243	810.7	12.7	3.17	101	25.4	6.3	1.59
43.8-oz. container	4865	1216.1						
Prepared as label directs, adding 12 quarts water [yield: approx. 12 quarts (48 cups)]	4865	1216.1	12.7	3.17	101	25.4	6.3	1.59
1 "scoop" (2 "suggested" servings)	203	50.7						
Prepared as label directs, adding 1 pint water [yield: approx. 1 pint (2 cups)]	203	50.7	12.7	3.17	101	25.4	6.3	1.59
Orange, sugar sweetened, 29.2-oz. container	3243	810.7						
Prepared as label directs, adding 8 quarts water [yield: approx. 8 quarts (32 cups)]	3423	810.7	12.7	3.17	101	25.4	6.3	1.59
43.8-oz. container	4865	1216.7						
Prepared as label directs, adding 12 quarts water [yield: approx. 12 quarts (48 cups)]	4865	1216.7	12.7	3.17	101	25.4	6.3	1.59
1 "scoop" (2 "suggested" servings)	203	50.7						
Prepared as label directs, adding 1 pint water [yield: approx. 1 pint (2 cups)]	203	50.7	12.7	3.17	101	25.4	6.3	1.59
Peach, sugar sweetened, 29.2-oz. container	3243	810.7						
Prepared as label directs, adding 8 quarts water [yield: approx. 8 quarts (32 cups)]	3243	810.7	12.7	3.17	101	25.4	6.3	1.59
43.8-oz. container	4865	1216.1						
Prepared as label directs, adding 12 quarts water [yield: approx. 12 quarts (48 cups)]	4865	1216.1	12.7	3.17	101	25.4	6.3	1.59
1 "scoop" (2 "suggested" servings)	203	50.7						
Prepared as label directs, adding 1 pint water [yield: approx. 1 pint (2 cups)]	203	50.7	12.7	3.17	101	25.4	6.3	1.59
Punch, sugar sweetened, 29.2-oz. container	3242	810.7						
Prepared as label directs, adding 8 quarts water [yield: approx. 8 quarts (32 cups)]	3242	810.7	12.7	3.17	101	25.4	6.3	1.59
43.8-oz. container	4865	1216.7						
Prepared as label directs, adding 12 quarts water [yield: approx. 12 quarts (48 cups)]	4865	1216.7	12.7	3.17	101	25.4	6.3	1.59
1 "scoop" (2 "suggested" servings)	203	50.7						
Prepared as label directs, adding 1 pint water [yield: approx. 1 pint (2 cups)]	203	50.7	12.7	3.17	101	25.4	6.3	1.59
Strawberry, sugar sweetened, 29.2-oz. container	3242	810.7						
Prepared as label directs, adding 8 quarts water [yield: approx. 8 quarts (32 cups)]	3242	810.7	12.7	3.17	101	25.4	6.3	1.59
43.8-oz. container	4865	1216.7						
Prepared as label directs, adding 12 quarts water [yield: approx. 12 quarts (48 cups)]	4865	1216.7	12.7	3.17	101	25.4	6.3	1.59
1 "scoop" (2 "suggested" servings)	203	50.7						
Prepared as label directs, adding 1 pint water [yield: approx. 1 pint (2 cups)]	203	50.7	12.7	3.17	101	25.4	6.3	1.59
Kool Aid dry mixes:								
Black Cherry, not presweetened, 0.23-oz. packet	16	0.0						
Prepared as label directs, adding 2 quarts water and 1 cup sugar [yield: approx. 2 quarts (8 cups)]	800	200.3	12.5	3.13	100	25.0	6.3	1.56
Cherry, not presweetened, 0.24-oz. packet	16	0.0						
Prepared as label directs, adding 2 quarts water and 1 cup sugar [yield: approx. 2 quarts (8 cups)]	800	200.3	12.5	3.13	100	25.0	6.3	1.56
sugar sweetened, 7.2-oz. packet	720	184.0						
Prepared as label directs, adding 2 quarts water [yield: approx. 2 quarts (8 cups)]	720	184.0	11.3	2.89	90	23.0	5.6	1.44
Grape, not presweetened, 0.23-oz. packet	16	0.0						
Prepared as label directs, adding 2 quarts water and 1 cup sugar [yield: approx. 2 quarts (8 cups)]	800	200.3	12.5	3.13	100	25.0	6.3	1.56

	UNIT		1 FLUID OZ.		1 CUP		1 TABLE-SPOON	
	Cal.	Carb.	Cal.	Carb.	Cal.	Carb.	Cal.	Carb.
sugar sweetened, 6.6-oz. packet	720	184.0						
Prepared as label directs, adding 2 quarts water [yield: approx. 2 quarts (8 cups)]	720	184.0	11.3	2.89	90	23.0	5.6	1.44
Lemonade, not presweetened, 0.46-oz. packet	16	0.0						
Prepared as label directs, adding 2 quarts water and 1 cup sugar [yield: approx. 2 quarts (8 cups)]	800	200.3	12.5	3.13	100	25.0	6.3	1.56
sugar sweetened, 6.7-oz. packet	720	184.0						
Prepared as label directs, adding 2 quarts water [yield: approx. 2 quarts (8 cups)]	720	184.0	11.3	2.89	90	23.0	5.6	1.44
Lemonade Flavor, not presweetened, 0.64-oz. packet	16	0.0						
Prepared as label directs, adding 2 quarts water and 1 cup sugar [yield: approx. 2 quarts (8 cups)]	800	200.3	12.5	3.13	100	25.0	6.3	1.56
Lemon-Lime, not presweetened, 0.23-oz. packet	16	0.0						
Prepared as label directs, adding 2 quarts water and 1 cup sugar [yield: approx. 2 quarts (8 cups)]	800	200.3	12.5	3.13	100	25.0	6.3	1.56
Orange Flavor, not presweetened, 0.16-oz. packet	16	0.0						
Prepared as label directs, adding 2 quarts water and 1 cup sugar [yield: approx. 2 quarts (8 cups)]	800	200.3	12.5	3.13	100	25.0	6.3	1.56
sugar sweetened, 6.8-oz. packet	720	184.0						
Prepared as label directs, adding 2 quarts water [yield: approx. 2 quarts (8 cups)]	720	184.0	11.3	2.89	90	23.0	5.6	1.44
Punch, not presweetened, 0.26-oz. packet	16	0.0						
Prepared as label directs, adding 2 quarts water and 1 cup sugar [yield: approx. 2 quarts (8 cups)]	800	200.3	12.5	3.13	100	25.0	6.3	1.56
Raspberry Flavor, not presweetened, 0.24-oz. packet	16	0.0						
Prepared as label directs, adding 2 quarts water and 1 cup sugar [yield: approx. 2 quarts (8 cups)]	800	200.3	12.5	3.13	100	25.0	6.3	1.56
sugar sweetened, 6.7-oz. packet	720	184.0						
Prepared as label directs, adding 2 quarts water [yield: approx. 2 quarts (8 cups)]	720	184.0	11.3	2.89	90	23.0	5.6	1.44
Strawberry Flavor, not presweetened, 0.23-oz. packet	16	0.0						
Prepared as label directs, adding 2 quarts water and 1 cup sugar [yield: approx. 2 quarts (8 cups)]	800	200.3	12.5	3.13	100	25.0	6.3	1.56
sugar sweetened, 6.7-oz. packet	720	184.0						
Prepared as label directs, adding 2 quarts water [yield: approx. 2 quarts (8 cups)]	720	184.0	11.3	2.89	90	23.0	5.6	1.44
Tropical Punch, sugar sweetened, 7.2-oz. packet	720	184.0						
Prepared as label directs, adding 2 quarts water [yield: approx. 2 quarts (8 cups)]	720	184.0	11.3	2.89	90	23.0	5.6	1.44
Lemon Tree dry mixes:								
Lemonade, 3.2-oz. package	360	(90.6)						
Prepared as label directs, adding 4 cups water [yield: approx. 1 quart (4 cups)]	360	(90.6)	11.3	(2.88)	90	(23.0)	5.6	(1.44)

	UNIT		1 FLUID OZ.		1 CUP		1 TABLE-SPOON	
	Cal.	Carb.	Cal.	Carb.	Cal.	Carb.	Cal.	Carb.
Low Calorie Lemonade, prepared as label directs, adding 4 cups water [yield: approx. 1 quart (4 cups)]	32	8.0	1.0	0.25	8	2.0	0.5	0.13
Pink Lemonade, 32-oz. (2-lb.) package	3600	(905.6)						
Prepared as label directs, adding 10 quarts water [yield: approx. 10 quarts (40 cups)]	3600	(905.6)	11.3	(2.83)	90	(22.6)	5.6	(1.41)
Unsweetened Lemonade, prepared as label directs, adding 10 quarts water [yield: approx. 10 quarts (40 cups)]	240	80.0	0.8	0.25	6	2.0	0.4	0.13
Minute Maid dry mixes:								
LEMONADE CRYSTALS, 30.7-oz. container	3405	853.3						
Prepared as label directs, adding 8 quarts water [yield: approx. 8 quarts (32 cups)]	3405	853.3	13.3	3.30	106	26.7	6.6	1.67
46.1-oz. container	5120	1280.0						
Prepared as label directs, adding 12 quarts water [yield: approx. 12 quarts (48 cups)]	5120	1280.0	13.3	3.30	106	26.7	6.6	1.67
Pink Lemonade Crystals, 30.7-oz. container	3405	853.3						
Prepared as label directs, adding 8 quarts water [yield: approx. 8 quarts (32 cups)]	3405	853.3	13.3	3.30	106	26.7	6.6	1.67
46.1-oz. container	5120	1280.0						
Prepared as label directs, adding 12 quarts water [yield: approx. 12 quarts (48 cups)]	5120	1280.0	13.3	3.30	106	26.7	6.6	1.67
P & Q (A&P) dry mix:								
Lemonade, 31-oz. package	3200	840.0						
Prepared as label directs, adding 10 quarts water [yield: approx. 10 quarts (40 cups)]	3200	840.0	10.0	2.63	80	21.0	5.0	1.31
Start dry mix:								
Instant Breakfast Drink, 4⅝-oz. jar	480	112.0	(87.6)	(20.31)	(701)	(162.5)	(43.8)	(10.16)
Sweet 'N Low dry mixes:								
Cherry Flavor, 17-oz. canister	1600	360.0						
Prepared as label directs, adding 10 quarts water [yield: approx. 10 quarts (40 cups)]	1600	360.0	5.0	1.13	40	9.0	2.5	0.56
Cranberry Apple Natural Flavor, 19-oz. canister	2240	504.0						
Prepared as label directs, adding 7 quarts water [yield: approx. 7 quarts (28 cups)]	2240	504.0	10.0	2.25	80	18.0	5.0	1.13
Fruit Punch Flavor, 17-oz. canister	1600	360.0						
Prepared as label directs, adding 10 quarts water [yield: approx. 10 quarts (40 cups)]	1600	360.0	5.0	1.13	40	9.0	2.5	0.56
Grape Flavor, 17-oz. canister	1600	360.0						
Prepared as label directs, adding 10 quarts water [yield: approx. 10 quarts (40 cups)]	1600	360.0	5.0	1.13	40	9.4	2.5	0.59
Lemonade Flavor, 17-oz. canister	1600	360.0						
Prepared as label directs, adding 10 quarts water [yield: approx. 10 quarts (40 cups)]	1600	360.0	5.0	1.13	40	9.0	2.5	0.56
Orange Flavor, 19-oz. canister	2240	504.0						
Prepared as label directs, adding 7 quarts water [yield: approx. 7 quarts (28 cups)]	2240	504.0	10.0	2.25	80	18.0	5.0	1.13
Tang Instant Breakfast Drinks:								
Grape Flavored, 18-oz. jar	1920	480.0	(90.0)	(22.50)	(720)	(180.0)	(45.0)	(11.25)
Prepared as label directs, adding 4 quarts water [yield: approx. 4 quarts (16 cups)]	1920	480.0	15.0	3.75	120	30.0	7.5	1.88
"Suggested" serving, 2 rounded teaspoons mix (approx. ⅕ oz.) to ½ cup water [yield: approx. 4 fl. oz. (½ cup)]	60	15.0	15.0	3.75	120	30.0	7.5	1.88

	UNIT		1 FLUID OZ.		1 CUP		1 TABLE-SPOON	
	Cal.	Carb.	Cal.	Carb.	Cal.	Carb.	Cal.	Carb.
Grapefruit Flavored, 18-oz. jar	1600	416.0	(75.0)	(19.50)	(600)	(156.0)	(37.5)	(9.75)
Prepared as label directs, adding 4 quarts water [yield: approx. 4 quarts (16 cups)]	1600	416.0	12.5	3.25	100	26.0	6.3	1.63
"Suggested" serving, 2 rounded teaspoons mix (approx. ⅕ oz.) to ½ cup water [yield: approx. 4 fl. oz. (½ cup)]	50	13.0	12.5	3.25	100	26.0	6.3	1.63
Orange Flavored, 18-oz. jar	1920	448.0	(90.0)	(21.00)	(720)	(168.0)	(45.0)	(10.50)
Prepared as label directs, adding 4 quarts water [yield: approx. 4 quarts (16 cups)]	1920	448.0	15.0	3.50	120	28.0	7.5	1.75
"Suggested" serving, 2 rounded teaspoons mix (approx. ⅕ oz.) to ½ cup water [yield: approx. 4 fl. oz. (½ cup)]	60	14.0	15.0	3.50	120	28.0	7.5	1.75
White Rose dry mix:								
Cherry Drink, presweetened, 24-oz. container	2560	672.0						
Prepared as label directs, adding ¾ oz. mix to 8 fl. oz. water [yield: approx. 8 oz. (1 cup)]	2560	672.0	10.0	2.63	80	21.0	5.0	1.31
Wylers dry mix:								
Lemonade Flavor, unsweetened, 0.5-oz. package	48	(16.0)						
Prepared as label directs, adding 1 cup sugar and 2 quarts water [yield: approx. 2 quarts (8 cups)]	880	216.0	13.8	3.38	110	27.0	6.9	1.69

SODA (Carbonated Soft Drinks)

Soda, based on generic data

	Cal.	Carb.	Cal.	Carb.	Cal.	Carb.	Cal.	Carb.
Carbonated waters, sweetened (quinine or tonic sodas), 12-fl.-oz. bottle	113	29.3	9.4	2.44	75	19.5	4.7	1.22
Club soda, 12-fl.-oz. bottle	0	0.0	0.0	0.00	0	0.0	0.0	0.00
Cola type, 12-fl.-oz. bottle	144	36.9	12.0	3.08	96	24.8	6.0	1.55
Cream soda, 12-fl.-oz. bottle	160	40.8	13.3	3.40	106	27.2	6.6	1.70
Fruit flavored sodas (citrus, cherry, grape, strawberry, Tom Collins mixer, other, 10–13% sugar), 12-fl.-oz. bottle	171	44.6	14.8	3.71	118	29.7	7.4	1.86
Ginger ale, pale dry and golden, 12-fl.-oz. bottle	113	29.3	9.4	2.44	75	19.5	4.7	1.22
Root beer, 12-fl.-oz. bottle	152	38.9	12.7	3.24	102	25.9	6.4	1.62
Special dietary drinks with artificial sweetener (less than 1 calorie per ounce), 12-fl.-oz. bottle			trace	trace			trace	trace

Soda, by brand

	Cal.	Carb.	Cal.	Carb.	Cal.	Carb.	Cal.	Carb.
APPLE								
Shasta Red Apple Soda, 12-fl.-oz. can	168	42.5	14.0	3.54	112	28.3	7.0	1.77
Diet, 12-fl.-oz. bottle	2	0.5	0.2	0.05	1	0.4	0.1	0.03
Slice, diet, with 10% fruit juices, 12-fl.-oz. can	20	4.0	1.7	0.33	13	2.7	0.8	0.17
BIRCH BEER (see also ROOT BEER)								
Canada Dry, 12-fl.-oz. can	165	42.0	13.8	3.50	110	28.0	6.9	1.75
16-fl.-oz. (1-pint) bottle	220	56.0	13.8	3.50	110	28.0	6.9	1.75
BITTER LEMON								
Canada Dry, 7-fl.-oz. bottle	88	22.8	12.5	3.25	100	26.0	6.3	1.63
32-fl.-oz. (1-quart) bottle	400	104.0	12.5	3.25	100	26.0	6.3	1.63
Hoffman, 10-fl.-oz. bottle	143	35.8	14.3	3.58	114	28.6	7.1	1.79
12-fl.-oz. can	172	43.0	14.3	3.58	114	28.6	7.1	1.79
Schweppes, 10-fl.-oz. bottle	140	33.8	14.0	3.38	112	27.0	7.0	1.69
BLACK CHERRY								
Canada Dry diet, 12-fl.-oz. can	3	0.5	0.3	0.04	2	0.3	0.1	0.02
16-fl.-oz. (1-pint) bottle	4	0.6	0.3	0.04	2	0.3	0.1	0.02
32-fl.-oz. (1-quart) bottle	8	1.2	0.3	0.04	2	0.3	0.1	0.02
Cragmont diet, 28-fl.-oz. bottle	2	0.6	0.1	0.02	1	0.2	0.1	0.01
Kirsch, 12-fl.-oz. can	175	43.8	14.6	3.65	117	29.2	7.3	1.83
16-fl.-oz. (1-pint) bottle	234	58.4	14.6	3.65	117	29.2	7.3	1.84

	UNIT		1 FLUID OZ.		1 CUP		1 TABLE-SPOON	
	Cal.	Carb.	Cal.	Carb.	Cal.	Carb.	Cal.	Carb.
No-Cal diet, 16-fl.-oz. (1-pint) bottle	0	0.0	0.0	0.00	0	0.0	0.0	0.00
28-fl.-oz. bottle	0	0.0	0.0	0.00	0	0.0	0.0	0.00
Shasta, 12-fl.-oz. can	168	42.5	14.0	3.54	112	42.5	7.0	2.66
diet, 12-fl.-oz. bottle	0	0.0	0.0	0.00	0	0.0	0.0	0.00
Tab diet, 12-fl.-oz.	3	0.5	0.3	0.04	2	0.3	0.1	0.02
Weight Watchers diet, 12-fl.-oz. can	(4)	(1.0)	(0.3)	(0.08)	(3)	(0.7)	(0.2)	(0.04)
White Rock, 12-fl.-oz. can	178	45.0	14.8	3.75	118	30.0	7.4	1.88
67.6-fl.-oz. (2-liter) bottle	1000	253.5	14.8	3.75	118	30.0	7.4	1.88
BLACK RASPBERRY, see RASPBERRY								
CACTUS COOLER								
Canada Dry, 12-fl.-oz. can	180	43.5	15.0	3.63	120	29.0	7.5	1.81
16-fl.-oz. (1-pint) bottle	240	58.0	15.0	3.63	120	29.0	7.5	1.81
32-fl.-oz. (1-quart) bottle	480	116.0	15.0	3.63	120	29.0	7.5	1.81
CEL-RAY								
Dr. Brown's, 10-fl.-oz. bottle	(108)	(26.9)	(10.8)	(2.69)	(86)	(21.5)	(5.4)	(1.34)
12-fl.-oz. can	(130)	(32.3)	(10.8)	(2.69)	(86)	(21.5)	(5.4)	(1.34)
28-fl.-oz. bottle	(302)	(75.3)	(10.8)	(2.69)	(86)	(21.5)	(5.4)	(1.34)
diet, 10-fl.-oz. bottle	2	0.5	0.2	0.05	2	0.4	0.1	0.03
CHERRI BERRI								
Hoffman diet, 12-fl.-oz. can	4	0.8	0.3	0.07	2	0.6	0.1	0.04
16-fl.-oz. (1-pint) bottle	5	1.1	0.3	0.07	2	0.6	0.1	0.04
CHERRY								
Canada Dry Wild Cherry, 12-fl.-oz. can	195	48.0	16.3	4.00	130	32.0	8.1	2.00
16-fl.-oz. (1-pint) bottle	260	64.0	16.3	4.00	130	32.0	8.1	2.00
32-fl.-oz. (1-quart) bottle	520	128.0	16.3	4.00	130	32.0	8.1	2.00
Cragmont diet, 28-fl.-oz. bottle	2	0.6	0.1	0.02	1	0.2	0.1	0.01
Dr. Brown's, 10-fl.-oz. bottle	147	36.8	14.7	3.68	118	29.4	7.4	1.84
12-fl.-oz. can	176	44.2	14.7	3.68	118	29.4	7.4	1.84
28-fl.-oz. bottle	412	103.0	14.7	3.68	118	29.4	7.4	1.84
Hoffman, 10-fl.-oz. bottle	147	36.8	14.7	3.68	118	29.4	7.4	1.84
12-fl.-oz. can	176	44.2	14.7	3.68	118	29.4	7.4	1.84
diet, 12-fl.-oz. can	9	2.2	0.7	0.18	6	1.4	0.4	0.09
16-fl.-oz. (1-pint) bottle	11	2.9	0.7	0.18	6	1.4	0.4	0.09
CHERRY COLA								
Canfield's diet, Cherry Ola Cola, 12-fl.-oz. can	8	0.0	0.7	0.00	5	0.0	0.3	0.00
Coke diet, 12-fl.-oz. can	0	trace	0.0	0.00	0	trace	0.0	0.00
Shasta, 12-fl.-oz. can	136	37.0	11.3	3.08	90	24.7	5.6	1.54
diet, 12-fl.-oz. bottle	0	0.0	0.0	0.00	0	0.0	0.0	0.00
Slice diet, with 10% fruit juices, 12-fl.-oz. can	20	6.0	1.7	0.50	13	4.0	0.8	0.25
Weight Watchers diet, 12-fl.-oz. can	(4)	(1.0)	(0.3)	(0.08)	(3)	(0.7)	(0.2)	(0.04)
CHOCOLATE								
Canada Dry diet, 12-fl.-oz. can	3	1.5	0.3	0.13	2	1.0	0.1	0.12
16-fl.-oz. (1-pint) bottle	4	2.0	0.3	0.13	2	1.0	0.1	0.12
32-fl.-oz. (1-quart) bottle	8	4.0	0.3	0.13	2	1.0	0.1	0.12
Canfield's diet, Chocolate Fudge, 12-fl.-oz. can	4	0.0	0.3	0.00	2	0.0	0.1	0.00
Hoffman diet, 12-fl.-oz. can	1	0.4	0.1	0.03	1	0.2	0.1	0.01
16-fl.-oz. (1-pint) bottle	2	0.5	0.1	0.03	1	0.2	0.1	0.01
No-Cal diet, 16-fl.-oz. (1-pint) bottle	4	0.1	0.3	0.01	2	0.1	0.1	0.12
Shasta diet, 12-fl.-oz. bottle	0	0.0	0.0	0.00	0	0.0	0.0	0.00
Weight Watchers diet, 12-fl.-oz. can	(4)	(1.0)	(0.3)	(0.08)	(3)	(0.7)	(0.2)	(0.04)
For Comparison: **Yoo-hoo,** diet, Chocolate Fudge, 12-fl.-oz. can	4	0.0	0.3	0.00	2	0.0	0.1	0.00
CHOCOLATE CREAM								
Hoffman, 10-fl.-oz. bottle	144	35.9	14.4	3.59	115	28.7	7.2	1.79
12-fl.-oz. can	172	43.1	14.4	3.59	115	28.7	7.2	1.79
CITRUS								
No-Cal "TNT" Tart & Tingly, 16-fl.-oz. (1-pint) bottle	0	0.0	0.0	0.00	0	0.0	0.0	0.00
CLUB								
Canada Dry, 16-fl.-oz. (1-pint) bottle	0	0.0	0.0	0.00	0	0.0	0.0	0.00
32-fl.-oz. (1-quart) bottle	0	0.0	0.0	0.00	0	0.0	0.0	0.00
Dr. Brown's, 10-fl.-oz. bottle	0	0.0	0.0	0.00	0	0.0	0.0	0.00
12-fl.-oz. can	0	0.0	0.0	0.00	0	0.0	0.0	0.00
28-fl.-oz. bottle	0	0.0	0.0	0.00	0	0.0	0.0	0.00
Hoffman, 10-fl.-oz. bottle	0	0.0	0.0	0.00	0	0.0	0.0	0.00
12-fl.-oz. can	0	0.0	0.0	0.00	0	0.0	0.0	0.00
low sodium, 12-fl.-oz. can	0	0.0	0.0	0.00	0	0.0	0.0	0.00
16-fl.-oz. (1-pint) bottle	0	0.0	0.0	0.00	0	0.0	0.0	0.00

	UNIT		1 FLUID OZ.		1 CUP		1 TABLE-SPOON	
	Cal.	Carb.	Cal.	Carb.	Cal.	Carb.	Cal.	Carb.
No-Cal low sodium, 16-fl.-oz. bottle	0	0.0	0.0	0.00	0	0.0	0.0	0.00
28-fl.-oz. bottle	0	0.0	0.0	0.00	0	0.0	0.0	0.00
Schweppes, 10-fl.-oz. bottle	0	0.0	0.0	0.00	0	0.0	0.0	0.00
COFFEE								
Hoffman, 10-fl.-oz. bottle	117	29.2	11.7	2.92	94	23.4	5.9	1.46
12-fl.-oz. can	140	35.0	11.7	2.92	94	23.4	5.9	1.46
diet, 12-fl.-oz. can	0	0.1	0.0	0.01	0	0.1	0.0	0.01
16-fl.-oz. (1-pint) bottle	0	0.2	0.0	0.01	0	0.1	0.0	0.01
No-Cal diet, 16-fl.-oz. (1-pint) bottle	5	0.8	0.3	0.05	2	0.4	0.1	0.03
COLA								
Canada Dry Jamaica, 12-fl.-oz. can	165	40.5	13.8	3.38	110	27.0	6.9	1.69
16-fl.-oz. (1-pint) bottle	220	54.0	13.8	3.38	110	27.0	6.9	1.69
32-fl.-oz. (1-quart) bottle	440	108.0	13.8	3.38	110	27.0	6.9	1.69
diet, 12-fl.-oz. can	3	1.2	0.3	0.10	2	0.8	0.1	0.05
16-fl.-oz. (1-pint) bottle	4	1.6	0.3	0.10	2	0.8	0.1	0.05
32-fl.-oz. (1-quart) bottle	8	3.2	0.3	0.10	2	0.8	0.1	0.05
Canfield's, diet, 12-fl.-oz. can	0	0.0	0.0	0.00	0	0.0	0.0	0.00
Coca-Cola, 6½-fl.-oz. bottle	78	19.5	12.0	3.00	96	24.0	6.0	1.50
7-fl.-oz. bottle	84	21.0	12.0	3.00	96	24.0	6.0	1.50
10-fl.-oz. bottle	120	30.0	12.0	3.00	96	24.0	6.0	1.50
12-fl.-oz. can	144	36.0	12.0	3.00	96	24.0	6.0	1.50
16-fl.-oz. (1-pint) bottle	192	48.0	12.0	3.00	96	24.0	6.0	1.50
16.9-fl.-oz. (½-liter) bottle	202	50.7	12.0	3.00	96	24.0	6.0	1.50
32-fl.-oz. (1-quart) bottle	384	96.0	12.0	3.00	96	24.0	6.0	1.50
33.8-fl.-oz. (1-liter) bottle	405	101.4	12.0	3.00	96	24.0	6.0	1.50
67.6-fl.-oz. (2-liter) bottle	811	202.8	12.0	3.00	96	24.0	6.0	1.50
Cragmont diet, 28-fl.-oz. bottle	2	0.6	0.1	0.02	1	0.2	0.1	0.01
Diet Rite, 12-fl.-oz. can	1	0.1	0.1	0.01	1	0.1	0.1	0.01
16-fl.-oz. (1-pint) bottle	1	0.2	0.1	0.01	1	0.1	0.1	0.01
Dr. Brown's, 10-fl.-oz. bottle	132	33.0	13.2	3.30	106	26.4	6.6	1.65
12-fl.-oz. can	159	39.6	13.2	3.30	106	26.4	6.6	1.65
28-fl.-oz. bottle	370	92.4	13.2	3.30	106	26.4	6.6	1.65
Hoffman, 10-fl.-oz. bottle	132	33.0	13.2	3.30	106	26.4	6.6	1.65
12-fl.-oz. can	159	39.6	13.2	3.30	106	26.4	6.6	1.65
diet, 12-fl.-oz. can	1	0.1	trace	0.01	trace	0.1	trace	0.01
16-fl.-oz. (1-pint) bottle	1	0.2	trace	0.01	trace	0.1	trace	0.01
Kirsch, 12-fl.-oz. can	162	40.3	13.5	3.36	108	26.9	6.8	1.68
16-fl.-oz. (1-pint) bottle	216	53.8	13.5	3.36	108	26.9	6.8	1.68
No-Cal diet, 16-fl.-oz (1-pint) bottle	0	0.0	0.0	0.00	0	0.0	0.0	0.00
Pepsi-Cola, 10-fl.-oz. bottle	131	3.3	13.1	3.30	105	26.4	6.6	1.65
12-fl.-oz. can	157	39.6	13.1	3.30	105	26.4	6.6	1.65
16-fl.-oz (1-pint) bottle	210	52.8	13.1	3.30	105	26.4	6.6	1.65
32-fl.-oz. (1-quart) bottle	419	105.6	13.1	3.30	105	26.4	6.6	1.65
33.8-fl.-oz. (1-liter) bottle	443	111.5	13.1	3.30	105	26.4	6.6	1.65
67.6-fl.-oz. (2-liter) bottle	886	223.1	13.1	3.30	105	26.4	6.6	1.65
Pepsi Light, 12-fl.-oz. can	(0)	(0.0)	(0.0)	(0.00)	(0)	(0.0)	(0.0)	(0.00)
67.6-fl.-oz. (2-liter) bottle	(0)	(0.0)	(0.0)	(0.00)	(0)	(0.0)	(0.0)	(0.00)
Pepsi diet, 12-fl.-oz. can	(0)	(0.0)	(0.0)	(0.00)	(0)	(0.0)	(0.0)	(0.00)
32-fl.-oz. (1-quart) bottle	(0)	(0.0)	(0.0)	(0.00)	(0)	(0.0)	(0.0)	(0.00)
67.6-fl.-oz. (2-liter) bottle	(0)	(0.0)	(0.0)	(0.00)	(0)	(0.0)	(0.0)	(0.00)
Royal Crown, 10-fl.-oz. bottle	130	32.4	13.0	3.24	104	25.9	6.5	1.62
12-fl.-oz. can	156	38.9	13.0	3.24	104	25.9	6.5	1.62
16-fl.-oz. (1-pint) bottle	208	51.8	13.0	3.24	104	25.9	6.5	1.62
32-fl.-oz. (1-quart) bottle	416	103.7	13.0	3.24	104	25.9	6.5	1.62
33.8-fl.-oz (1-liter) bottle	439	109.5	13.0	3.24	104	25.9	6.5	1.62
64-fl.-oz. (2-quart) bottle	832	207.4	13.0	3.24	104	25.9	6.5	1.62
67.6-fl.-oz (2-liter) bottle	879	219.0	13.0	3.24	104	25.9	6.5	1.62
RC 100 diet cola, 12-fl.-oz. can	1	0.1	0.1	0.01	trace	0.1	trace	0.01
16-fl.-oz. (1-pint) bottle	1	0.2	0.1	0.01	trace	0.1	trace	0.01
67.6-fl.-oz (2-liter) bottle	3	0.7	0.1	0.01	trace	0.1	trace	0.01
Shasta, 8-fl.-oz. can	95	26.0	11.9	3.25	95	26.0	5.9	1.63
12-fl.-oz. can	143	39.0	11.9	3.25	95	26.0	5.9	1.63
diet, 8-fl.-oz. can	0	0.0	0.0	0.00	0	0.0	0.0	0.00
12-fl.-oz. can	0	0.0	0.0	0.00	0	0.0	0.0	0.00
Tab, 12-fl.-oz. can	5	0.0	0.4	0.00	3	0.0	(0.2)	(0.04)
Weight Watchers diet, 12-fl.-oz. can	(4)	(1.0)	(0.3)	(0.08)	(3)	(0.7)	(0.2)	(0.04)
White Rock, 12-fl.-oz. can	168	44.4	14.0	3.70	112	29.6	7.0	1.85
16-fl.-oz. (1-pint) bottle	224	59.2	14.0	3.70	112	29.6	7.0	1.85
67.6-fl.-oz. (2-liter) bottle	946	250.1	14.0	3.70	112	29.6	7.0	1.85
CREAM (or CREME)								
Cragmont diet, 28-fl.-oz. bottle	2	trace	0.1	trace	1	trace	0.1	trace

	UNIT		1 FLUID OZ.		1 CUP		1 TABLE-SPOON	
	Cal.	Carb.	Cal.	Carb.	Cal.	Carb.	Cal.	Carb.
Dr. Brown's, 10-fl.-oz. bottle	146	36.5	14.6	3.65	117	29.2	7.3	1.83
12-fl.-oz. can	175	43.8	14.6	3.65	117	29.2	7.3	1.83
28-fl.-oz. bottle	409	102.2	14.6	3.65	117	29.2	7.3	1.83
Hoffman, 10-fl.-oz. bottle	146	32.5	14.6	3.65	117	29.2	7.3	1.83
12-fl.-oz. can	175	43.8	14.6	3.65	117	29.2	7.3	1.83
diet, 12-fl.-oz. can	3	0.7	0.3	0.06	2	0.5	0.1	0.03
16-fl.-oz. (1-pint) bottle	4	1.0	0.3	0.06	2	0.5	0.1	0.03
No-Cal diet, 16-fl.-oz. (1-pint) bottle	0	0.0	0.0	0.00	0	0.0	0.0	0.00
28-fl.-oz. bottle	0	0.0	0.0	0.00	0	0.0	0.0	0.00
Shasta, 12-fl.-oz. can	150	41.0	12.5	3.42	100	27.3	6.3	1.71
diet, 12-fl.-oz. bottle	0	0.0	0.0	0.00	0	0.0	0.0	0.00
Weight Watchers diet, 12-fl.-oz. can	(4)	(1.0)	(0.3)	(0.08)	(3)	(0.7)	(0.2)	(0.04)
White Rock, 12-fl.-oz. can	178	45.0	14.8	3.75	118	30.0	7.4	1.88
28-fl.-oz. bottle	414	105.0	14.8	3.75	118	30.0	7.4	1.88
67.6-fl.-oz. (2-liter) bottle	1000	253.5	14.8	3.75	118	30.0	7.4	1.88
DR PEPPER								
Dr Pepper, 12-fl.-oz. can	150	39.7	12.5	3.31	100	26.5	6.1	1.53
64-fl.-oz. (½-gallon) bottle	802	211.8	12.5	3.31	100	26.5	6.1	1.53
diet, 12-fl.-oz. can	3	0.8	0.3	0.06	2	0.5	0.1	0.03
64-fl.-oz (½-gallon) bottle	16	4.0	0.3	0.06	2	0.5	0.1	0.03
FRESCA								
Fresca, 12-fl.-oz. can	3	0.0	0.3	0.00	2	0.0	0.1	0.03
FROSTA								
Weight Watchers, 12-fl.-oz. can	(4)	(1.0)	(0.3)	(0.08)	(3)	(0.7)	(0.2)	(0.04)
FRUIT PUNCH								
Nehi, 12-fl.-oz. bottle	182	45.6	15.2	3.80	122	30.4	7.6	1.90
Shasta, 12-fl.-oz. can	168	46.0	14.0	3.83	112	30.6	7.6	1.90
GINGER ALE								
Canada Dry, 12-fl.-oz. can	135	31.5	11.3	2.63	90	21.0	5.6	1.31
16-fl.-oz. (1-pint) bottle	180	42.0	11.3	2.63	90	21.0	5.6	1.31
Golden, 12-fl.-oz. can	150	36.0	12.5	3.00	100	24.0	6.3	1.50
16-fl.-oz. (1-pint) bottle	200	48.0	12.5	3.00	100	24.0	6.3	1.50
32-fl.-oz. (1-quart) bottle	400	96.0	12.5	3.00	100	24.0	6.3	1.50
diet, 12-fl.-oz. can	3	0.0	0.3	0.00	2	0.0	0.1	0.00
16-fl.-oz. (1-pint) bottle	4	0.0	0.3	0.00	2	0.0	0.1	0.00
32-fl.-oz. (1-quart) bottle	8	0.0	0.3	0.00	2	0.0	0.1	0.00
Canfield's, diet, 12-fl.-oz. can	4	0.0	0.3	0.00	2	0.0	0.1	0.00
Cragmont diet, 28-fl.-oz. bottle	2	trace	0.1	trace	1	trace	0.1	trace
Dr. Brown's, 10-fl.-oz. bottle	100	25.0	10.0	2.50	80	20.0	5.0	1.25
12-fl.-oz. can	120	30.0	10.0	2.50	80	20.0	5.0	1.25
28-fl.-oz. bottle	280	70.0	10.0	2.50	80	20.0	5.0	1.25
Fanta, 12-fl.-oz. can	126	31.5	10.5	2.63	84	21.0	5.3	1.31
Hoffman, 10-fl.-oz. bottle	100	25.0	10.0	2.50	80	20.0	5.0	1.25
12-fl.-oz. can	120	30.0	10.0	2.50	80	20.0	5.0	1.25
diet, 12-fl.-oz. can	3	0.7	0.3	0.06	2	0.5	0.1	0.03
16-fl.-oz. (1-pint) bottle	4	1.0	0.3	0.06	2	0.5	0.1	0.03
Kirsch, 12-fl.-oz. can	119	29.5	9.9	2.46	79	19.7	4.9	1.23
16-fl.-oz. (1-pint) bottle	158	39.4	9.9	2.46	79	19.7	4.9	1.23
Nehi, 12-fl.-oz. bottle	137	33.1	11.4	2.76	91	22.1	5.7	1.38
No-Cal diet, 16-fl.-oz. (1-pint) bottle	0	0.0	0.0	0.00	0	0.0	0.0	0.00
28-fl.-oz. bottle	0	0.0	0.0	0.00	0	0.0	0.0	0.00
Royal Crown, 12-fl.-oz. can	137	33.1	11.4	2.76	91	22.1	5.7	1.38
16-fl.-oz. (1-pint) bottle	183	44.2	11.4	2.76	91	22.1	5.7	1.38
Schweppes, 10-fl.-oz. bottle	110	27.1	11.0	2.71	88	21.7	5.5	1.36
12-fl.-oz. can	132	32.5	11.0	2.71	88	21.7	5.5	1.36
28-fl.-oz. bottle	308	75.9	11.0	2.71	88	21.7	5.5	1.36
32-oz. (1-quart) bottle	352	86.7	11.0	2.71	88	21.7	5.5	1.36
Sugar Free, 6-fl.-oz. can	2	0.0	0.3	0.00	3	0.0	0.2	0.00
12-fl.-oz. bottle	4	0.0	0.3	0.00	3	0.0	0.2	0.00
28-fl.-oz. bottle	9	0.0	0.3	0.00	3	0.0	0.2	0.00
32-fl.-oz. (1-quart) bottle	11	0.0	0.3	0.00	3	0.0	0.2	0.00
Shasta, 12-fl.-oz. can	117	32.0	9.8	2.67	78	21.3	4.9	1.33
diet, 8-fl.-oz. can	0	0.0	0.0	0.00	0	0.0	0.0	0.00
12-fl.-oz. can	0	0.0	0.0	0.00	0	0.0	0.0	0.00
Weight Watchers diet, 12-fl.-oz. can	(4)	(1.0)	(0.3)	(0.08)	(3)	(0.7)	(0.2)	(0.04)
White Rock Pale Dry, 12-fl.-oz. can	124	30.0	10.3	2.50	82	20.0	5.2	1.25
28-fl.-oz. bottle	288	70.0	10.3	2.50	82	20.0	5.2	1.25
67.6-fl.-oz. (2-liter) bottle	696	169.0	10.3	2.50	82	20.0	5.2	1.25
GINGER BEER								
Schweppes, 10-fl.-oz. bottle	120	28.0	12.0	2.80	96	22.4	6.0	1.40
12-fl.-oz. can	144	33.6	12.0	2.80	96	22.4	6.0	1.40
28-fl.-oz. bottle	336	78.4	12.0	2.80	96	22.4	6.0	1.40
32-fl.-oz. (1-quart) bottle	384	89.6	12.0	2.80	96	22.4	6.0	1.40

	UNIT		1 FLUID OZ.		1 CUP		1 TABLE-SPOON	
	Cal.	Carb.	Cal.	Carb.	Cal.	Carb.	Cal.	Carb.
GRAPE								
Canada Dry, 12-fl.-oz. can	195	48.0	16.3	4.00	130	32.0	8.1	2.00
16-fl.-oz. (1-pint) bottle	260	64.0	16.3	4.00	130	32.0	8.1	2.00
diet, 12-fl.-oz. can	3	0.0	0.3	0.00	2	0.0	0.1	0.00
16-fl.-oz (1-pint) bottle	4	0.0	0.3	0.00	2	0.0	0.1	0.00
Dr. Brown's, 10-fl.-oz. bottle	149	37.3	14.9	3.73	119	29.8	7.4	1.86
12-fl.-oz. can	179	44.8	14.9	3.73	119	29.8	7.4	1.86
Fanta, 12-fl.-oz. can	171	43.5	14.3	3.63	114	29.0	7.1	1.81
Hoffman, 10-fl.-oz. bottle	149	37.3	14.9	3.73	119	29.8	7.4	1.86
12-fl.-oz. can	179	44.8	14.9	3.73	119	29.8	7.4	1.86
diet, 10-fl.-oz. bottle	1	0.2	0.1	0.02	1	0.2	0.1	0.01
12-fl.-oz. can	2	0.3	0.1	0.02	1	0.2	0.1	0.01
Nehi, 12-fl.-oz. bottle	174	43.6	14.5	3.63	116	29.0	7.3	1.81
No-Cal, 16-fl.-oz. (1-pint) bottle	0	0.0	0.0	0.00	0	0.0	0.0	0.00
Patio, 12-fl.-oz. can	(192)	(48.0)	(16.0)	(4.00)	(128)	(32.0)	(8.0)	(2.00)
16-fl.-oz. (1-pint) bottle	(256)	(64.0)	(16.0)	(4.00)	(128)	(32.0)	(8.0)	(2.00)
Royal Crown, 12-fl.-oz. can	175	43.6	14.6	3.63	117	29.0	7.3	1.81
16-fl.-oz. (1-pint) bottle	233	58.1	14.6	3.63	117	29.0	7.3	1.81
Schweppes, 10-fl.-oz. bottle	161	39.6	16.1	3.96	129	31.7	8.1	1.98
Shasta, 12-fl.-oz. can	172	47.0	14.3	3.92	115	31.4	7.2	1.96
diet, 12-fl.-oz. bottle	1	trace	0.1	trace	1	trace	0.1	trace
Weight Watchers diet, 12-fl.-oz. can	(4)	(1.0)	(0.3)	(0.08)	(3)	(0.7)	(0.2)	(0.04)
White Rock, 12-fl.-oz. can	178	45.0	14.8	3.75	118	30.0	7.4	1.88
16-fl.-oz. (1-pint) bottle	237	60.0	14.8	3.75	118	30.0	7.4	1.88
67.6-fl.-oz (2-liter) bottle	1000	253.5	14.8	3.75	118	30.0	7.4	1.88
GRAPEFRUIT								
Hoffman, 10-fl.-oz. bottle	141	35.3	14.1	3.53	113	28.2	7.1	1.76
12-fl.-oz. can	169	42.4	14.1	3.53	113	28.2	7.1	1.76
diet, 12-fl.-oz. can	9	2.3	0.8	0.19	6	1.5	0.4	0.09
16-fl.-oz. (1-pint) bottle	13	3.0	0.8	0.19	6	1.5	0.4	0.09
Shasta, 12-fl.-oz. can	158	43.0	13.2	3.58	106	28.7	6.6	1.79
diet, 10-fl.-oz. bottle	2	0.5	0.2	0.04	1	0.3	0.1	0.02
HALF & HALF								
Canada Dry, 7-fl.-oz. bottle	96	22.8	13.8	3.25	110	26.0	6.9	1.63
16-fl.-oz (1-pint) bottle	220	52.0	13.8	3.25	110	26.0	6.9	1.63
Hoffman, 10-fl.-oz. bottle	132	33.0	13.2	3.30	106	26.4	6.6	1.65
12-fl.-oz. can	158	39.6	13.2	3.30	106	26.4	6.6	1.65
diet, 12-fl.-oz. can	5	1.3	0.4	0.11	3	0.9	0.2	0.06
16-fl.-oz. (1-pint) bottle	7	1.8	0.4	0.11	3	0.9	0.2	0.06
HI SPOT								
Canada Dry, 12-fl.-oz. can	150	37.5	12.5	3.13	100	25.0	6.3	1.56
16-fl.-oz. (1-pint) bottle	200	50.0	12.5	3.13	100	25.0	6.3	1.56
32-fl.-oz. (1-quart) bottle	400	100.0	12.5	3.13	100	25.0	6.3	1.56
KICK								
Nehi, 12-fl.-oz. bottle	178	44.3	14.8	3.69	118	29.5	7.4	1.84
LEMON								
Canada Dry diet, 12-fl.-oz. can	3	0.0	0.3	0.00	2	0.0	0.1	0.00
16-fl.-oz. (1-pint) bottle	4	0.0	0.3	0.00	2	0.0	0.1	0.00
32-fl.-oz. (1-quart) bottle	8	0.0	0.3	0.00	0	0.0	0.0	0.00
Hoffman diet, 12-fl.-oz. can	4	1.1	0.4	0.09	3	0.7	0.2	0.04
16-fl.-oz. (1-pint) bottle	6	1.4	0.4	0.09	3	0.7	0.2	0.04
LEMONADE								
Shasta, 12-fl.-oz. can	142	38.0	11.8	3.17	94	25.3	5.9	1.58
BITTER LEMON								
Canada Dry, 7-fl.-oz. bottle	88	22.8	12.5	3.25	100	26.0	6.3	1.63
32-fl.-oz. (1-quart) bottle	400	104.0	12.5	3.25	100	26.0	6.3	1.63
Hoffman, 10-fl.-oz. bottle	143	35.8	14.3	3.58	114	28.6	7.1	1.79
12-fl.-oz. can	172	43.0	14.3	3.58	114	28.6	7.1	1.79
Schweppes, 10-fl.-oz. bottle	140	33.8	14.0	3.38	112	27.0	7.0	1.69
LEMON-LIME								
Hoffman, 10-fl.-oz. bottle	125	31.2	12.5	3.12	100	25.0	6.3	1.56
12-fl.-oz. can	150	37.0	12.5	3.12	100	25.0	6.3	1.56
No-Cal Shape-Up, 16-fl.-oz. (1-pint) bottle	0	0.0	0.0	0.00	0	0.0	0.0	0.00
28-fl.-oz. bottle	0	0.0	0.0	0.00	0	0.0	0.0	0.00
Shasta, 12-fl.-oz. can	139	38.0	11.6	3.17	93	25.3	5.8	1.58
diet, 12-fl.-oz. bottle	0	0.0	0.0	0.00	0	0.0	0.0	0.00
Slice diet, with 10% fruit juices, 12-fl.-oz. can	28	6.0	2.3	0.50	18	4.0	1.2	0.25
Weight Watchers diet, 12-fl.-oz. can	(4)	(1.0)	(0.3)	(0.08)	(3)	(0.7)	(0.2)	(0.04)
LIME								
Canada Dry, 12-fl.-oz. can	195	49.5	16.3	4.13	130	33.0	8.1	2.06
16-fl.-oz. (1-pint) bottle	260	66.0	16.3	4.13	130	33.0	8.1	2.06
32-fl.-oz. (1-quart) bottle	520	132.0	16.3	4.13	130	33.0	8.1	2.06
MANDARIN ORANGE								
Slice diet, with 10% fruit juices, 12-fl.-oz. can	20	4.0	1.7	0.33	13	2.7	0.8	0.17

	UNIT		1 FLUID OZ.		1 CUP		1 TABLE-SPOON	
	Cal.	Carb.	Cal.	Carb.	Cal.	Carb.	Cal.	Carb.
MELLO YELLO								
Mello Yello, 12-fl.-oz. can	175	45.0	14.5	3.75	116	30.0	7.3	1.88
MINERAL WATER								
Perrier, 23-fl.-oz. bottle	0	0.0	0.0	0.00	0	0.0	0.0	0.00
With a twist of lemon, 23-fl.-oz. bottle	0	0.0	0.0	0.00	0	0.0	0.0	0.00
With a twist of lime, 23-fl.-oz. bottle	0	0.0	0.0	0.00	0	0.0	0.0	0.00
With a twist of orange, 23-fl.-oz. bottle	0	0.0	0.0	0.00	0	0.0	0.0	0.00
Schweppes, 12-fl.-oz. can	0	0.0	0.0	0.00	0	0.0	0.0	0.00
MOUNTAIN DEW								
Mountain Dew, 12-fl.-oz. can	176	43.9	14.7	3.66	117	29.3	7.3	1.83
67.6-fl.-oz (2-liter) bottle	990	247.5	14.7	3.66	117	29.3	7.3	1.83
MR. PIBB								
Mr. Pibb, 12-fl.-oz. can	140	37.5	11.6	3.13	93	25.0	5.8	1.56
diet, 12-fl.-oz. can	2	0.4	0.1	0.02	1	0.2	0.1	0.01
NEAR BEER								
Birell, 12-fl.-oz. bottle	75	15.6	6.3	1.30	50	10.4	3.1	0.65
Kingsbury Brew, 12-fl.-oz. can	63		5.3		42		2.6	
For comparison: Beer, **Miller High Life,** 12-fl.-oz. bottle or can	150	14.0	12.5	1.17	100	9.3	6.3	0.58
For comparison: **Miller Lite,** 12-fl.-oz. bottle or can	96	2.8	8.0	0.23	64	1.8	4.0	0.11
NEHI								
Nehi, 12-fl.-oz. bottle	147	36.6	12.2	3.05	98	24.4	6.1	1.53
NU GRAPE								
Nu Grape, 12-fl.-oz. can	0	0.0	0.0	0.00	0	0.0	0.0	0.00
ORANGE								
Canada Dry, Sunripe, 12-fl.-oz. can	195	49.5	16.3	4.13	130	33.0	8.1	2.06
16-fl.-oz. (1-pint) bottle	260	66.0	16.3	4.13	130	33.0	8.1	2.06
32-fl.-oz. (1-quart) bottle	520	132.0	16.3	4.13	130	33.0	8.1	2.06
Cragmont diet, 12-fl.-oz. can	1	0.3	0.1	0.02	1	0.2	0.1	0.01
16-fl.-oz. (1-pint) bottle	1	0.4	0.1	0.02	1	0.2	0.1	0.01
28-fl.-oz. bottle	2	0.6	0.1	0.02	1	0.2	0.1	0.01
32-fl.-oz. (1-quart) bottle	3	0.8	0.1	0.02	1	0.2	0.1	0.01
Crush diet, with 10% real juice, 12-fl.-oz. can	24	6.0	2.0	0.50	16	4.0	1.0	0.25
Dr. Brown's, 10-fl.-oz. bottle	152	38.1	15.2	3.81	122	30.5	7.6	1.91
12-fl.-oz. can	183	45.7	15.2	3.81	122	30.5	7.6	1.91
28-fl.-oz. bottle	426	106.7	15.2	3.81	122	30.5	7.6	1.91
Fanta, 12-fl.-oz. can	176	45.0	14.6	3.75	117	30.0	7.3	1.88
Hoffman, 10-fl.-oz. bottle	152	38.1	15.2	3.81	122	30.5	7.6	1.91
12-fl.-oz. can	183	45.7	15.2	3.81	122	30.5	7.6	1.91
diet, 12-fl.-oz. can	3	0.7	0.2	0.06	2	0.5	0.1	0.03
16-fl.-oz. (1-pint) bottle	4	1.0	0.2	0.06	2	0.5	0.1	0.03
Nehi, 12-fl.-oz. bottle	190	47.5	15.8	3.96	127	31.7	7.9	1.98
Pepsico, 12-fl.-oz. can	210	52.4	17.5	4.37	140	35.0	8.8	2.19
16-fl.-oz. (1-pint) bottle	280	69.9	17.5	4.37	140	35.0	8.8	2.19
Royal Crown, 12-fl.-oz. can	188	46.9	15.6	3.91	125	31.3	7.8	1.96
16-fl.-oz. (1-pint) bottle	250	62.6	15.6	3.91	125	31.3	7.8	1.96
Schweppes Sparkling, 12-fl.-oz. can	178	44.0	14.8	3.67	118	29.4	7.4	1.84
Shasta, 12-fl.-oz. can	172	47.0	14.3	3.92	114	31.3	7.1	1.96
diet, 12-fl.-oz. bottle	0	0.0	0.0	0.00	0	0.0	0.0	0.00
Sunkist diet, with 10% real fruit juices, 12-fl.-oz. can	24	6.0	2.0	0.50	16	4.0	1.0	0.25
Weight Watchers diet, 12-fl.-oz. can	(4)	(1.0)	(0.3)	(0.08)	(3)	(0.7)	(0.2)	(0.04)
White Rock, 12-fl.-oz. can	180	45.6	15.0	3.80	120	30.4	7.5	1.90
16-fl.-oz. (1-pint) bottle	240	60.8	15.0	3.80	120	30.4	7.5	1.90
67.6-fl.-oz. (2-liter) bottle	1014	256.9	15.0	3.80	120	30.4	7.5	1.90
ORANGE JAFFA								
White Rock, 12-fl.-oz. can	166	42.0	13.8	3.50	110	28.0	6.9	1.75
64-fl.-oz. (2-quart) bottle	885	224.0	13.8	3.50	110	28.0	6.9	1.75
PEACH								
Nehi, 12-fl.-oz. bottle	184	46.1	15.4	3.84	123	30.7	7.7	1.92
PINEAPPLE								
Canada Dry, 12-fl.-oz. can	165	39.0	13.8	3.25	110	26.0	6.9	1.63
16-fl.-oz. (1-pint) bottle	220	52.0	13.8	3.25	110	26.0	6.9	1.63
32-fl.-oz. (1-quart) bottle	440	104.0	13.8	3.25	110	26.0	6.9	1.63
Hoffman, 10-fl.-oz. bottle	151	37.6	15.1	3.77	120	30.1	7.5	1.88
12-fl.-oz. can	181	45.1	15.1	3.77	120	30.1	7.5	1.88
diet, 12-fl.-oz. can	1	1.2	0.1	0.10	1	0.8	0.1	0.05
16-fl.-oz. (1-pint) bottle	1	1.6	0.1	0.10	1	1.1	0.1	0.07
PUNCH & FRUITS								
White Rock, 12-fl.-oz. can	166	40.0	13.8	3.33	110	26.7	6.9	1.67
64-fl.-oz. (2-quart) bottle	885	213.1	13.8	3.33	110	26.7	6.9	1.67

	UNIT		1 FLUID OZ.		1 CUP		1 TABLE-SPOON	
	Cal.	Carb.	Cal.	Carb.	Cal.	Carb.	Cal.	Carb.
PURPLE PASSION								
Canada Dry, 12-fl.-oz. can	180	45.0	15.0	3.75	120	30.0	7.5	1.88
16-fl.-oz. (1-pint) bottle	240	60.0	15.0	3.75	120	30.0	7.5	1.88
32-fl.-oz. (2-pint) bottle	480	120.0	15.0	3.75	120	30.0	7.5	1.88
QUININE								
Hoffman, 10-fl.-oz. bottle	108	26.9	10.8	2.69	86	21.5	5.4	1.34
12-fl.-oz. can	129	32.3	10.8	2.69	86	21.5	5.4	1.34
RASPBERRY								
Canada Dry, 12-fl.-oz. can	3	0.0	0.3	0.00	2	0.0	0.1	0.00
16-fl.-oz. (1-pint) bottle	4	0.0	0.3	0.00	2	0.0	0.1	0.00
32-fl.-oz. (1-quart) bottle	8	0.0	0.3	0.00	2	0.0	0.1	0.00
Hoffman, 10-fl.-oz. bottle	152	37.9	15.2	3.79	121	30.3	7.6	1.89
12-fl.-oz. can	182	45.5	15.2	3.79	121	30.3	7.6	1.89
diet, 12-fl.-oz. can	2	0.6	0.2	0.05	2	0.4	0.1	0.03
16-fl.-oz. (1-pint) bottle	3	0.8	0.2	0.05	2	0.4	0.1	0.03
No-Cal Black Raspberry, 16-fl.-oz. (1-pint) bottle	4	0.8	0.3	0.05	2	0.4	0.1	0.03
Shasta Wild Raspberry, 12-fl.-oz. can	168	42.5	14.0	3.54	112	28.3	7.0	1.77
diet, 12-fl.-oz. bottle	0	0.0	0.0	0.00	0	0.0	0.0	0.00
RASPBERRY CREME								
Weight Watchers diet, 12-fl.-oz. can	(4)	(1.0)	(0.3)	(0.08)	(3)	(0.7)	(0.2)	(0.04)
RED CREME								
Schweppes, 12-fl.-oz. can	173	42.6	14.4	3.55	115	28.4	7.2	1.78
RED POP								
Canfield's diet, strawberry-cherry, 12-fl.-oz. can	4	0.0	0.3	0.00	2	0.0	0.1	0.00
No-Cal diet, 16-fl.-oz. (1-pint) bottle	0	0.0	0.0	0.00	0	0.0	0.0	0.00
RONDO								
Schweppes, 12-fl.-oz. can	153	39.1	12.8	3.26	102	26.1	6.4	1.63
Sugar-free, 12-fl.-oz. can	0	0.0	0.0	0.00	0	0.0	0.0	0.00
ROOT BEER								
A&W, 10-fl.-oz. bottle	140	35.0	14.0	3.50	112	28.0	7.0	1.75
67.6-fl.-oz. (2-liter) bottle	947	236.8	14.0	3.50	112	28.0	7.0	1.75
diet, 10-fl.-oz. bottle	1		0.1	trace	1		0.1	
32-fl.-oz. (1-quart) bottle	5		0.1	trace	1		0.1	
Barrelhead, 12-fl.-oz. can	165	39.0	13.8	3.25	110	26.0	6.9	1.63
16-fl.-oz. (1-pint) bottle	220	52.0	13.8	3.25	110	26.0	6.9	1.63
32-fl.-oz. (1-quart) bottle	440	104.0	13.8	3.25	110	26.0	6.9	1.63
diet, 12-fl.-oz. can	3	1.5	0.3	0.13	2	1.0	0.1	0.06
16-fl.-oz. (1-pint) bottle	4	2.0	0.3	0.13	2	1.0	0.1	0.06
32-fl.-oz. (1-quart) bottle	8	4.0	0.3	0.13	2	1.0	0.1	0.06
Canada Dry Rooti, 12-fl.-oz. can	165	39.0	13.8	3.25	110	26.0	6.9	1.63
16-fl.-oz. (1-pint) bottle	220	52.0	13.8	3.25	110	26.0	6.9	1.63
32-fl.-oz. (1-quart) bottle	440	104.0	13.8	3.25	110	26.0	6.9	1.63
diet, 12-fl.-oz. can	3	1.5	0.3	0.13	2	1.0	0.1	0.06
16-fl.-oz. (1-pint) bottle	4	2.0	0.3	0.13	2	1.0	0.1	0.06
32-fl.-oz. (1-quart) bottle	8	4.0	0.3	0.13	2	1.0	0.1	0.06
Cragmont diet, 28-fl.-oz. bottle	2	0.6	0.1	0.02	1	0.2	0.1	0.01
Sugar-free, 12-fl.-oz. can	1	0.4	0.1	0.04	1	0.3	0.1	0.02
Dr. Brown's, 12-fl.-oz. can	156	39.1	13.0	3.26	104	26.1	6.5	1.63
28-fl.-oz. bottle	364	91.3	13.0	3.26	104	26.1	6.5	1.63
Fanta, 12-fl.-oz. can	155	40.5	12.9	3.28	103	27.0	6.4	1.69
Hoffman, 10-fl.-oz. bottle	130	32.6	13.0	3.26	104	26.1	6.5	1.63
12-fl.-oz. can	156	39.1	13.0	3.26	104	26.1	6.5	1.63
diet, 12-fl.-oz. can	trace	0.1	trace	0.01	trace	0.1	trace	0.01
16-fl.-oz. (1-pint) bottle	(1)	0.2	trace	0.01	trace	0.1	trace	0.01
Nehi, 12-fl.-oz. bottle	175	43.7	14.6	3.64	117	29.1	7.3	1.82
No-Cal Draft Style, 16-fl.-oz. (1-pint) bottle	0	0.1	0.0	0.01	0	0.1	0.0	0.01
28-fl.-oz. bottle	0	0.2	0.0	0.01	0	0.1	0.0	0.01
Pepsico, 12-fl.-oz. can	180	45.1	15.0	3.76	120	30.1	7.5	1.88
16-fl.-oz. (1-pint) bottle	240	60.2	15.0	3.76	120	30.1	7.5	1.88
Ramblin' 12-fl.-oz. can	177	46.5	14.8	3.88	118	31.0	7.4	1.94
Royal Crown, 12-fl.-oz. can	175	43.7	14.6	3.64	117	29.1	7.3	1.82
16-fl.-oz. (1-pint) bottle	233	58.2	14.6	3.64	117	29.1	7.3	1.82
Schweppes, 12-fl.-oz. can	157	38.6	13.1	3.22	105	25.8	6.6	1.61
Shasta Draft, 12-fl.-oz. can	150	41.0	12.5	3.42	100	27.3	6.3	1.71
diet, 8-fl.-oz. can	trace	trace	trace	trace	trace	trace	trace	trace
12-fl.-oz. can	1	trace	0.1	trace	trace	trace	trace	trace
Weight Watchers diet, 12-fl.-oz. can	(4)	(1.0)	(0.3)	(0.08)	(3)	(0.7)	(0.2)	(0.04)
White Rock, 12-fl.-oz. can	162	40.8	13.5	3.40	108	27.2	6.8	1.70
28-fl.-oz. bottle	378	95.2	13.5	3.40	108	27.2	6.8	1.70
67.6-fl.-oz. (2-liter) bottle	913	230	13.5	3.40	108	27.2	6.8	1.70
SARSAPARILLA								
Hoffman, 10-fl.-oz. bottle	136	34.0	13.6	3.40	109	27.2	6.8	1.70
12-fl.-oz. can	163	40.8	13.6	3.40	109	27.2	6.8	1.70
White Rock, 12-fl.-oz. can	178	45.0	14.8	3.75	118	30.0	7.4	1.89
28-fl.-oz. bottle	414	105.0	14.8	3.75	118	30.0	7.4	1.89
SELTZER WATER								
Old Original, no salt added, Vintage, 28-fl.-oz. bottle	0	0.0	0.0	0.00	0	0.0	0.0	0.00
7-UP								
Seven-Up, 12-fl.-oz. can	144	36.3	12.0	3.02	96	24.1	6.0	1.51
diet, 12-fl.-oz. can	4	1.0	0.3	0.08	3	0.6	0.2	0.04
SPRING WATER								
Poland Springs, 28-fl.-oz. bottle	0	0.0	0.0	0.00	0	0.0	0.0	0.00
Cherry Essence, 28-fl.-oz. bottle	0	0.0	0.0	0.00	0	0.0	0.0	0.00
Cherry Berry Cola Essence, 28-fl.-oz. bottle	0	0.0	0.0	0.00	0	0.0	0.0	0.00
Lime Essence, 28-fl.-oz. bottle	0	0.0	0.0	0.00	0	0.0	0.0	0.00
Orange Essence, 28-fl.-oz. bottle	0	0.0	0.0	0.00	0	0.0	0.0	0.00
SPRITE								
Sprite, 12-fl.-oz. can	143	36.0	11.9	3.00	95	24.0	5.9	1.50
67.6-fl.-oz. (2-liter) bottle	804	202.8	11.9	3.00	95	24.0	5.9	1.50
diet, 12-fl.-oz. can	5	0.0	0.4	0.00	3	0.0	0.2	0.00
67.6-fl.-oz. (2-liter) bottle	27	0.0	0.4	0.00	3	0.0	0.2	0.00
STRAWBERRY								
Canada Dry, 12-fl.-oz. can	180	45.0	15.0	3.75	120	30.0	7.5	1.88
16-fl.-oz. (1-pint) bottle	240	60.0	15.0	3.75	120	30.0	7.5	1.88
32-fl.-oz. (1-quart) bottle	480	120.0	15.0	3.75	120	30.0	7.5	1.88
diet, 12-fl.-oz. can	3	0.0	0.3	0.00	2	0.0	0.1	0.00
16-fl.-oz. (1-pint) bottle	4	0.0	0.3	0.00	2	0.0	0.1	0.00
32-fl.-oz. (1-quart) bottle	8	0.0	0.3	0.00	2	0.0	0.1	0.00
Hoffman, 10-fl.-oz. bottle	150	37.4	15.0	3.74	120	29.9	7.5	1.87
12-fl.-oz. can	180	44.9	15.0	3.74	120	29.9	7.5	1.87
diet, 12-fl.-oz. can	2	0.4	0.1	0.03	1	0.2	0.1	0.01
16-fl.-oz. (1-pint) bottle	2	0.5	0.1	0.03	1	0.2	0.1	0.01
Nehi, 12-fl.-oz. bottle	175	43.7	14.6	3.64	117	29.1	7.3	1.82
Royal Crown, 12-fl.-oz. can	174	43.6	14.5	3.63	116	29.0	7.3	1.81
16-fl.-oz. (1-pint) bottle	232	58.1	14.5	3.63	116	29.0	7.3	1.81
Shasta, 12-fl.-oz. can	143	39.0	11.9	3.25	95	26.0	5.9	1.63
diet, 12-fl.-oz. bottle	trace	trace	trace	trace	trace	trace	trace	trace
Weight Watchers diet, 12-fl.-oz. can	(4)	(1.0)	(0.3)	(0.08)	(3)	(0.7)	(0.2)	(0.04)
TAB								
Tab, 12-fl.-oz. can	1	0.1	0.1	0.01	1	0.1	0.1	0.01
TAHITIAN TREAT								
Canada Dry, 12-fl.-oz. can	195	48.0	16.3	4.00	130	32.0	8.1	2.00
16-fl.-oz. (1-pint) bottle	260	64.0	16.3	4.00	130	32.0	8.1	2.00
32-fl.-oz. (1-quart) bottle	520	128.0	16.3	4.00	130	32.0	8.1	2.00
TEEM								
Teem, 12-fl.-oz. can	(139)	(26.3)	(11.6)	(2.19)	(93)	(17.5)	(5.8)	(1.09)
16-fl.-oz. (1-pint) bottle	(186)	(35.0)	(11.6)	(2.19)	(93)	(17.5)	(5.8)	(1.09)
TIKI								
Shasta, 12-fl.-oz. can	160	40.6	13.3	3.38	106	27.1	6.6	1.69
TIME OUT								
White Rock, 12-fl.-oz. can	144	38.4	12.0	3.20	96	25.6	6.0	1.60
28-fl.-oz. bottle	336	89.6	12.0	3.20	96	25.6	6.0	1.60
67.6-fl.-oz. (2-liter) bottle	811	216.3	12.0	3.20	96	25.6	6.0	160
TONIC WATER								
Canada Dry, 7-fl.-oz. bottle	79	19.3	11.3	2.75	90	22.0	5.6	1.38
16-fl.-oz. (1-pint) bottle	180	44.0	11.3	2.75	90	22.0	5.6	1.38
diet, 12-fl.-oz. can	3	0.0	0.3	0.00	2	0.0	0.1	0.00
16-fl.-oz. (1-pint) bottle	4	0.0	0.3	0.00	2	0.0	0.1	0.00
32-fl.-oz. (1-quart) bottle	8	0.0	0.3	0.00	2	0.0	0.1	0.00
No-Cal diet, 16-fl.-oz. (1-pint) bottle	0	0.0	0.0	0.00	0	0.0	0.0	0.00
Schweppes, 10-oz. bottle	110	27.5	11.0	2.75	88	22.0	5.5	1.38
12-oz. can	132	33.0	11.0	2.75	88	22.0	5.5	1.38
28-oz. bottle	308	77.0	11.0	2.75	88	22.0	5.5	1.38
32-oz. (1-quart) bottle	352	88.0	11.0	2.75	88	22.0	5.5	1.38
Sugar Free, 6-oz. bottle	1	0.0	0.2	0.00	1	0.0	0.1	0.00
12-oz. can	2	0.0	0.2	0.00	1	0.0	0.1	0.00
28-oz. bottle	5	0.0	0.2	0.00	1	0.0	0.1	0.00
32-oz. (1-quart) bottle	5	0.0	0.2	0.00	1	0.0	0.1	0.00
Shasta, 12-fl.-oz. can	114	28.8	9.5	2.40	76	19.2	4.8	1.20
White Rock, 7-fl.-oz. bottle	72	17.5	10.3	2.50	84	20.0	5.3	1.25
12-fl.-oz. can	124	30.0	10.3	2.50	84	20.0	5.3	1.25
UPPER 10								
Royal Crown, 12-fl.-oz. can	152	38.4	12.7	3.20	102	25.6	6.4	1.60
16-fl.-oz. (1-pint) bottle	202	51.2	12.7	3.20	102	25.6	6.4	1.60

	UNIT		1 FLUID OZ.		1 CUP		1 TABLESPOON	
	Cal.	Carb.	Cal.	Carb.	Cal.	Carb.	Cal.	Carb.
VANILLA CREAM								
Canada Dry, 12-fl.-oz. can	195	48.0	16.3	4.00	130	32.0	8.1	2.00
16-fl.-oz. (1-pint) bottle	260	64.0	16.3	4.00	130	32.0	8.1	2.00
32-fl.-oz. (1-quart) bottle	520	128.0	16.3	4.00	130	32.0	8.1	2.00
diet, 12-fl.-oz. can	3	0.5	0.3	0.04	2	0.3	0.1	0.02
16-fl.-oz. (1-pint) bottle	4	0.6	0.3	0.04	2	0.3	0.1	0.02
32-fl.-oz. (1-quart) bottle	8	1.3	0.3	0.04	2	0.3	0.1	0.02
VICHY WATER								
Schweppes, 12-fl.-oz. can	0	0.0	0.0	0.00	0	0.0	0.0	0.00
WATER, see MINERAL WATER, SELTZER WATER, SPRING WATER, TONIC WATER, and VICHY WATER								
WILD CHERRY, see CHERRY								
WILD RASPBERRY, see RASPBERRY								
WINK								
Canada Dry, 7-fl.-oz. bottle	105	26.3	15.0	3.75	120	30.0	7.5	1.88
32-fl.-oz. (1-quart) bottle	480	120.0	15.0	3.75	120	30.0	7.5	1.88
diet, 12-fl.-oz. can	3	0.0	0.3	0.00	2	0.0	0.1	0.00
16-fl.-oz. (1-pint) bottle	4	0.0	0.3	0.00	2	0.0	0.1	0.00
32-fl.-oz. (1-quart) bottle	8	0.0	0.3	0.00	2	0.0	0.1	0.00

MILK

This section is for milk from cows. Milk from other animals follows.
Cream, including half and half, has its own listing farther on in this chapter, following MILK DRINKS AND MIXES, by brand.

	UNIT		1 FLUID OZ.		1 CUP		1 TABLESPOON	
	Cal.	Carb.	Cal.	Carb.	Cal.	Carb.	Cal.	Carb.
BUTTERMILK								
Buttermilk, cultured, based on generic data (0.9% fat), 1 quart (1g/1g/tr/90%/30mg)	396	46.9	12.4	1.47	99	11.7	6.2	0.73
Axelrod Buttermilk, 1 quart	440	48.0	13.8	1.50	110	12.0	6.9	0.75
CONDENSED MILK, canned								
Sweetened Condensed Milk, based on generic data (8.7% fat), 1 quart (2g/15g/2g/27%/36mg)	3929	665.9	122.8	20.80	982	166.5	61.4	10.41
Borden Eagle Brand, Sweetened Condensed Milk, 14-oz. can	1680	259.0	120.0	18.50	960	156.0	60.0	9.75
DRY MILK								
Whole Dry Milk, based on generic data (26.71% fat), 1 cup dry (7g/11g/8g/2%/105mg)	635	49.2	79.4	6.15	635	49.2	39.7	3.08
Prepared with 1 quart water [yield: approx. 1 quart (4 cups)]	635	49.2	19.8	1.54	159	12.3	9.9	0.77
Non-fat Dry Milk, based on generic data (0.77% fat), 1 cup dry (10g/15g/tr/3%/152mg)	435	62.4	54.4	7.80	435	62.4	27.2	3.90
Prepared with 1 quart water [yield: approx. 1 quart (4 cups)]	435	62.4	13.6	1.95	109	15.6	6.8	0.97
Instantized Non-fat Dry Milk, based on generic data (0.72% fat), 1⅓ cup dry (10g/15g/tr/4%/156mg)	326	47.5	30.5	4.44	244	35.5	15.3	2.22
Prepared with 1 quart water [yield: approx. 1 quart (4 cups)]	326	47.5	10.2	1.48	82	11.9	5.1	0.74
Fearn Non-fat Dry Milk, 3-lb. package	4950	715.0						
Prepared as label directs, adding 13¾ quarts water (yield: approx. 55 cups)	4950	715.0	11.3	1.63	90	13.0	5.6	0.81
EVAPORATED MILK								
Evaporated Skim Milk, canned, based on generic data (0.20% fat), 1 quart (2g/3g/tr/79%/33mg)	794	28.9	24.8	3.62	198	28.9	12.4	1.81
Evaporated Whole Milk, canned, based on generic data (7.56% fat), 1 quart (2g/3g/2g/74%/30mg)	1344	25.3	42.0	3.16	338	25.3	21.1	1.58
Carnation Evaporated Milk, 13-fl.-oz. can	491	35.1	37.8	2.70	302	21.6	18.9	1.35
Dairymate Evaporated "Filled" Milk, 13-fl.-oz. can	487	39.0	37.5	3.00	300	24.0	18.8	1.50
P&Q (A&P) Evaporated Milk, 13-fl.-oz. can	553	39.0	42.5	3.00	340	24.0	21.3	1.50

	UNIT		1 FLUID OZ.		1 CUP		1 TABLESPOON	
	Cal.	Carb.	Cal.	Carb.	Cal.	Carb.	Cal.	Carb.
Pet Evaporated Milk, 5.33-fl.-oz. can	231	16.6	43.4	3.11	340	24.0	21.3	1.50
13-fl.-oz. can	564	40.4	43.4	3.11	340	24.0	21.3	1.50
Evaporated Skimmed Milk, 13-fl.-oz. can	299	41.9	23.0	3.23	184	25.8	11.5	1.62
KEFIR (Cultured Milk)								
Alta Dena Dairy Plain Kefir, 8-fl.-oz. container	200	24.0	25.0	3.00	200	24.0	12.5	1.50
Apple Kefir, 8-fl.-oz. container	200	24.0	25.0	3.00	200	24.0	12.5	1.50
Black Cherry Kefir, 8-fl.-oz. container	200	24.0	25.0	3.00	200	24.0	12.5	1.50
Boysenberry Kefir, 8-fl.-oz. container	200	24.0	25.0	3.00	200	24.0	12.5	1.50
Lemon Kefir, 8-fl.-oz. container	200	24.0	25.0	3.00	200	24.0	12.5	1.50
Peach Kefir, 8-fl.-oz. container	200	24.0	25.0	3.00	200	24.0	12.5	1.50
Pineapple Kefir, 8-fl.-oz. container	200	24.0	25.0	3.00	200	24.0	12.5	1.50
Red Raspberry Kefir, 8-fl.-oz. container	200	24.0	25.0	3.00	200	24.0	12.5	1.50
Strawberry Kefir, 8-fl.-oz. container	200	24.0	25.0	3.00	200	24.0	12.5	1.50
MILK, arranged in ascending order of fat content, based on generic data								
(Values apply equally to pasteurized and raw milk.)								
Skim Milk (0.18% fat), 1 quart (1g/2g/tr/91%/15mg)	343	47.5	10.7	1.49	86	11.9	5.4	0.74
Skim Milk (0.25% fat) with non-fat milk solids added, 1 quart (1g/1g/tr/90%/17mg)	361	49.2	11.3	1.54	90	12.3	5.6	0.77
Skim Milk, Protein-fortified, (0.25% fat), 1 quart (1g/2g/tr/89%/15mg)	400	54.7	12.6	1.71	100	13.7	6.3	0.86
Low-fat Milk (1% fat) 1 quart (1g/1g/tr/90%/44mg)	410	46.7	12.8	1.46	102	11.7	6.4	0.73
Low-fat Milk (1% fat) with non-fat milk solids added, 1 quart (1g/1g/tr/90%/15mg)	418	48.7	13.0	1.52	104	12.2	6.5	0.80
Low-fat Milk, Protein fortified, (1% fat) 1 quart (1g/2g/tr/89%/16mg)	477	54.3	14.9	1.68	119	13.4	7.4	0.84
Low-fat Milk (2% fat), 1 quart (1g/1g/1g/89%/14mg)	485	46.9	15.3	1.46	121	11.7	7.6	0.73
Low-fat Milk (2% fat) with non-fat milk solids added, 1 quart (1g/1g/1g/89%/15mg)	500	48.5	15.6	1.52	125	12.2	7.8	0.76
Low-fat Milk, Protein fortified, (2% fat), 1 quart (1g/2g/1g/88%/17mg)	546	54.0	17.2	1.69	137	13.5	8.6	0.84
Whole Milk (3.3% fat), 1 quart (1g/1g/1g/88%/14mg)	600	45.5	18.8	1.42	150	11.4	9.4	0.71
Whole milk (3.5% fat) (Based on USDA data published in 1975. This analysis seems popular among manufacturers. Many manufacturers used the number "160 calories," a rounded version of the USDA's "159," in reporting calories for products that require whole milk to be added by the consumer.) 1 quart (1g/1g/1g/88%/14mg)	634	47.8	19.8	1.49	159	12.0	9.9	0.75
Whole Milk, low sodium (3.5% fat), 1 quart (1g/1g/1g/88%/1mg)	595	43.5	18.6	1.36	149	10.9	9.3	0.68
Whole milk, producer, (3.7% fat), 1 quart (1g/1g/1g/88%/14mg)	625	45.4	19.5	1.42	157	11.4	9.8	0.71
MILK, by brand								
Within each brand, whole milk is listed first, followed by low-fat, and then skim or non-fat milk.								
A&P Whole Homogenized Vitamin D Milk, 1 quart	600	44.0	18.8	1.38	150	11.0	9.4	0.69
Look-Fit Low-fat (1% fat) Protein Fortified Vitamin A & D Milk, 1 quart	440	56.0	13.8	1.75	110	14.0	6.9	0.88
Low-fat (2% fat) Vitamin A & D Milk, 1 quart	480	44.0	150	1.38	120	11.0	7.5	0.69
Skim (0.5% fat) Vitamin A & D Milk, 1 quart	400	56.0	12.5	1.75	100	14.0	6.3	0.88
Brisk 'N Bouncy Lowfat (1% fat) "99% Fat Free" Vitamin A & D Milk, 1 quart	400	44.0	12.5	1.38	100	11.0	6.3	0.69

	UNIT		1 FLUID OZ.		1 CUP		1 TABLE-SPOON	
	Cal.	Carb.	Cal.	Carb.	Cal.	Carb.	Cal.	Carb.
Caldwell Farms Whole Homogenized Vitamin D Milk, 1 quart	600	44.0	18.8	1.38	150	11.0	9.4	0.69
Dairylea Whole Homogenized Vitamin D Milk, 1 quart	600	44.0	18.8	1.38	150	11.0	9.4	0.69
Skim (0.5% fat) Protein Fortified Vitamin A & D Milk, 1 quart	360	44.0	11.3	1.38	90	11.0	5.7	0.69
Daitch Whole Homogenized Vitamin D "Country Packaged" Milk, 1 quart	600	44.0	18.8	1.38	150	11.0	9.4	0.69
Skim Protein Fortified Vitamin A & D Milk, 1 quart	400	52.0	12.5	1.63	100	13.0	6.3	0.81
Dari-Lean Low-fat (1% fat) Protein Fortified Vitamin A & D Milk, 1 quart	480	44.0	15.0	1.38	120	11.0	7.5	0.69
Dellwood Whole Homogenized Vitamin D Milk, 1 quart	600	44.0	18.8	1.38	150	11.0	9.4	0.69
Low-fat (1% fat) Protein Fortified Vitamin A & D Milk, 1 quart	440	56.0	13.8	1.75	110	14.0	6.9	0.88
Skim (0.5% fat) Vitamin A & D Milk, 1 quart	400	56.0	12.5	1.75	100	14.0	6.3	0.88
Elmhurst Dairy Whole Homogenized Vitamin D Milk, 1 quart	600	44.0	18.8	1.38	150	11.0	9.4	0.69
Low-fat (1% fat) Vitamin A & D "Skinny" Milk, 1 quart	400	44.0	12.5	1.38	100	11.0	6.3	0.69
Family Friend Low-fat (2% fat) "98% Fat Free" Vitamin A & D Milk, 1 quart	480	44.0	15.0	1.38	120	11.0	7.5	0.69
Farmland Low-fat (1% fat) Vitamin A & D "Slender" Milk, 1 quart	400	44.0	12.5	1.38	100	11.0	6.3	0.69
Hood Nuform Fortified Low-fat (1% fat) Milk, 1 quart	440	52.0	13.8	1.63	110	13.0	6.9	0.81
Whole Milk (3.5% fat), 1 quart	600	44.0	18.8	1.38	150	11.0	9.4	0.69
Kings Whole Vitamin D Milk, 1 quart	600	44.0	18.8	1.38	150	11.0	9.4	0.69
Knudsen Whole (3.5%) Vitamin D Milk, 1 quart	600	48.0	18.8	1.50	150	12.0	9.4	0.75
Vitamin A & D Non-fat (0% fat) Milk, 1 quart	360	48.0	11.3	1.50	90	12.0	5.6	0.75
LSM low sodium Whole, Sterilized, "Ready-to-Drink" Milk, 1-quart can	675	46.0	21.1	1.44	169	11.5	10.6	0.72
Low sodium Low-fat (1% fat) Protein Fortified Vitamin A & D "Ready-to-Drink" Milk, 8-fl.-oz. cans	110	13.0	13.8	1.63	110	13.0	6.9	0.81
1 quart	440	52.0	13.8	1.63	110	13.0	6.9	0.81
Meadow Gold Whole Homogenized Vitamin D Milk, 1 quart	557	40.6	17.4	1.27	139	10.2	8.7	0.64
Skim (0.1% fat) Vitamin A & D Milk, 1 quart	333	40.6	10.4	1.27	83	10.2	5.2	0.64
Queens Farms Whole Homogenized Vitamin D Milk, 1 quart	600	44.0	18.8	1.38	150	11.0	9.4	0.69
Skim Protein Fortified Vitamin A & D Milk, 1 quart	400	52.0	12.5	1.63	100	13.0	6.3	0.81
Russell Farms Low-fat (2% fat) Lactobacillus Acidophilus Culture-added Vitamin A & D "Selected Sweet" Milk, 1 quart	480	44.0	15.0	1.38	120	11.0	7.5	0.69
Safeway Lucerne, Extra Rich Vitamin D Milk, 1 quart	680	44.0	21.3	1.38	170	11.0	10.7	0.69
Whole (3.5% fat) Vitamin D Milk, 1 quart	600	44.0	18.8	1.38	150	11.0	9.4	0.69
Whole Concentrated Vitamin D Milk, reconstituted, 1 quart	600	44.0	18.8	1.38	150	11.0	9.4	0.69
Low-fat (2% fat) Lactobacillus Acidophilus Culture-added Milk, 1 quart	560	52.0	17.5	1.63	140	13.0	8.8	0.81
Low-fat (2% fat) Protein Fortified Vitamin A & D "Two Ten" Milk, 1 quart	560	52.0	17.5	1.63	140	13.0	8.8	0.81
Non-fat (0% fat) Vitamin A & D Milk, 1 quart	360	48.0	11.3	1.50	90	12.0	5.7	0.75
Trim N' Tasty Low-fat (1% fat) Protein Fortified "99% Fat-Free" Vitamin A & D Milk, 1 quart	440	52.0	13.8	1.63	110	13.0	6.9	0.81
Viva Low-fat (2% fat) Vitamin A & D Milk, 1 quart	480	33.3	15.0	1.04	120	16.6	7.5	1.04
WHEY, based on generic data								
fluid, 1 cup	246	12.5	30.8	1.56	246	12.5	15.4	0.78

	UNIT		1 FLUID OZ.		1 CUP		1 TABLE-SPOON	
	Cal.	Carb.	Cal.	Carb.	Cal.	Carb.	Cal.	Carb.
dried, 1 pound (4g/21g/tr/3%/306mg)	1583	333.4	98.9	20.84				
MILK FROM OTHER ANIMALS								
GOAT MILK								
Whole, 4.14% fat, 1 quart, based on generic data	673	43.4	21.0	1.35	168	10.9	10.5	0.88
Pure Goat Products, Pasteurized Whole Milk, 1 quart	680	46.0	21.3	1.44	170	11.5	10.6	0.72
Pasteurized Buttermilk, 1 quart	680	46.0	21.3	1.44	170	11.5	10.6	0.72
HUMAN MILK								
Africa, 3.1% fat, 1 quart	(660)	(89.7)	(20.6)	(2.80)	(165)	(22.4)	(10.3)	(1.40)
Canada (percentage of fat unavailable), 1 quart	(710)	(73.0)	(22.1)	(2.28)	(178)	(18.2)	(11.1)	(1.14)
East Asia, 3.2% fat, 1 quart	(611)	(69.1)	(19.1)	(2.16)	(153)	(17.3)	(9.5)	(1.08)
France, 5.0% fat, 1 quart	(749)	(64.0)	(23.4)	(2.00)	(187)	(16.0)	(11.7)	(1.00)
United States, 4.38% fat, 1 quart	684	67.8	21.4	2.11	171	17.0	10.7	1.06
INDIAN BUFFALO MILK								
Whole, 6.9% fat, 1 quart	947	50.6	29.6	1.58	237	12.6	14.8	0.79
REINDEER MILK								
Whole, 19.6% fat, 1 quart	2320	40.8	72.5	1.28	580	10.2	36.3	0.64
SHEEP MILK								
Whole, 7% fat, 1 quart	1058	52.5	33.1	1.64	265	13.1	16.6	0.82
VEGETABLE-DERIVED MILK								
COCONUT MILK, based on generic data								
(Liquid expressed from mixture of grated coconut meat and coconut water)								
1 cup (approx. 8 oz.)	(605)	(12.5)	75.6	1.56	(605)	(12.5)	(37.8)	(0.78)
PEANUT MILK, based on data from East Asia								
1 quart	(282)	(11.7)	(8.8)	(0.37)	(71)	(2.9)	(4.4)	(0.18)
SOY MILK, by brand:								
Soy Moo Soy Milk, 30-fl.-oz. carton	484	37.5	16.1	1.25	129	10.0	8.1	0.63
Soy Moo Carob Soy Milk, 30-fl.-oz. carton	484	60.0	16.1	2.00	129	16.0	8.1	1.00
FLAVORED MILK DRINKS AND MILK-DRINK MIXES								
CHOCOLATE- and CAROB-FLAVORED MILK, by brand								
Dairylea Chocolate Milk, 1 quart	720	96.0	22.5	3.00	180	24.0	11.3	1.50
Gilbert H. Brockmeyer's Natural Caroby Carob Milk, 1 quart	880	104.0	27.5	3.25	220	26.0	13.8	6.50
Knudsen Chocolate Low-fat (1% fat) Milk, 1 quart	800	124.2	25.0	3.88	200	31.0	12.5	1.94
CHOCOLATE-FLAVORED SYRUPS FOR MILK, by brand								
There are other chocolate-flavored syrups in the SUGARS, SWEETENERS & TOPPINGS chapter.								
Hershey's Chocolate Flavored Syrup, 24-oz. bottle	2160	528.0	(90.0)	(22.00)	(720)	(176.0)	(45.0)	(11.00)
Louis Sherry (Dia-Mel) reduced calorie, Choco-Syrup, Chocolate Syrup and Topping, 8-oz. jar	225	45.0	30.0	6.00	240	48.0	15.0	3.00
1 serving, 1 tablespoon	15	3.0	30.0	6.00	240	48.0	15.0	3.00
Prepared as label directs, mixing 1 serving with 1 cup (8 fl. oz.) milk (yield: approx. 8 fl. oz.)								
Made with whole milk (3.5% fat)	187	17.6	23.4	2.20	187	17.6	11.7	1.10
Made with skim milk (0.1% fat)	116	18.3	14.5	2.29	116	18.3	7.3	1.14
Milk-Mate Chocolate Flavor Syrup, 20-oz. bottle	1500	360.6						
36-oz. bottle	2700	649.1						

	UNIT		1 FLUID OZ.		1 CUP		1 TABLE-SPOON	
	Cal.	Carb.	Cal.	Carb.	Cal.	Carb.	Cal.	Carb.
1 serving, 1½ tablespoons	75	18.3						
Prepared as label directs, mixing 1 serving with 1 cup (8 fl. oz.) milk (yield: approx. 8 fl. oz.)								
Made with whole milk (3.5% fat)	(234)	(30.0)	29.3	3.75	(234)	(30.0)	(14.6)	(1.88)
Made with skim milk (0.1% fat)	163	30.5	20.4	3.82	163	30.5	10.2	1.91
COCOA DRINKS, by brand, are listed below in the MILK DRINKS AND MIXES section								
COCOA POWDER, see the BASIC BAKING & COOKING INGREDIENTS chapter								
EGGNOG, based on generic data								
7.48% fat, 32 fl. oz. (1 quart) (approx. 35.8 oz.)	1368	137.6	42.8	4.30	342	34.4	21.4	2.15
1 cup	342	34.4	42.8	4.30	342	34.4	21.4	2.15
1 tablespoon (approx. 0.5 oz.)	21	2.2	42.8	4.30	342	34.4	21.4	2.15
EGGNOG DRINKS, by brand, are listed in the MILK DRINKS AND MIXES section								
MALTED MILK, based on USDA home recipe								
Natural Flavor, ¾ oz. (by weight), or approx. 2 to 3 heaping teaspoons	86	15.2	(120.0)	(20.25)				
Prepared by adding ¾ oz. powder to 1 cup (8 fl. oz.) milk (yield: approx. 8 fl. oz.):								
Made with whole milk (3.5% fat)	(245)	(27.2)	(30.6)	(3.40)	(245)	(27.2)	(15.3)	(1.70)
Made with skim milk (0.1% fat)	(175)	(27.7)	(21.9)	(3.46)	(175)	(27.7)	(10.9)	(1.73)
Chocolate Flavor, ¾ oz. (by weight), or approx. 2 to 3 heaping teaspoons	83	17.8	(110.0)	(23.75)				
Prepared by adding ¾ oz. powder to 1 cup (8 fl. oz.) milk (yield: approx. 8 fl. oz.):								
Made with whole milk (3.5% fat)	(242)	(29.8)	(30.3)	(3.73)	(242)	(29.8)	(15.1)	(1.86)
Made with skim milk (0.1% fat)	(172)	(30.3)	(21.5)	(3.79)	(172)	(30.3)	(10.8)	(1.89)
MILK DRINKS AND MIXES, by brand								
A&P Instant Chocolate Flavor Mix, 32-oz. (2-lb.) box	3420	836.0	(90.0)	(22.00)				
1 serving, 2 level tablespoons	90	220	(90.0)	(22.00)				
Prepared as package directs, mixing 1 serving with 1 cup (8 fl. oz.) milk (yield: approx. 8 fl. oz.):								
Made with whole milk (3.5% fat)	249	34.0	31.1	4.25	249	34.0	15.6	2.13
Made with skim milk (0.1% fat)	179	34.5	22.4	4.31	179	34.5	11.2	2.16
Alba '66 Hot Cocoa Mix, 6.8-oz. box, 10 envelopes	600	100.0	(35.0)	(5.82)				
1 envelope, approx. 0.68 oz.	60	10.0	(35.0)	(5.82)				
Prepared as package directs, mixing 1 envelope with 6 fl. oz. water (yield: approx. 6 fl. oz.)	60	10.0	10.0	1.66	80	13.3	5.0	0.83
12.15-oz. box	1080	120.0	(35.0)	(5.82)				
1 scoop, approx. 0.33 oz.	60	10.0	(35.0)	(5.82)				
Prepared as package directs, mixing 1 level scoop with 6-oz. water (yield: approx. 6 fl. oz.)	60	10.0	10.0	1.67	80	13.3	5.0	0.83
Chocolate Marshmallow Flavor, 6.8-oz. box. 10 envelopes	600	100.0	(32.6)	(5.44)				
1 envelope, approx. 0.68 oz.	60	10.0	(32.6)	(5.44)				
Prepared as package directs, mixing 1 envelope with 6 fl. oz. water (yield: approx. 6 fl. oz.)	60	10.0	10.0	1.66	80	13.3	5.0	0.83
Alba '77 Fit 'N Frosty, Chocolate Flavor, 7.5-oz. box, 10 envelopes	700	110.0	(33.2)	(5.68)				

	UNIT		1 FLUID OZ.		1 CUP		1 TABLE-SPOON	
	Cal.	Carb.	Cal.	Carb.	Cal.	Carb.	Cal.	Carb.
1 envelope, approx. 0.75 oz.	70	11.0	(33.3)	(5.68)				
Prepared as package directs, mixing 1 envelope with 4 fl. oz. cold water and 3 ice cubes or ⅓ cup crushed ice (2 fl. oz. when melted) (yield: approx. 6 fl. oz.)	70	11.0	11.7	1.83	93	14.7	5.8	0.92
Chocolate and artificial Marshmallow Flavor, 7.5-oz. box	700	110.0						
1 envelope, approx. 0.75 oz.	70	11.0						
Prepared as package directs, mixing 1 envelope with 4 oz. cold water (yield: approx. 6 fl. oz.)	70	11.0	(11.7)	(1.83)	(93)	(14.7)	5.8	0.92
Strawberry Flavor, 7.5-oz. box, 10 envelopes	700	120.0	(36.6)	(6.26)				
1 envelope, approx. 0.75 oz.	70	12.0	(36.6)	(6.26)				
Prepared as package directs, mixing 1 envelope with 4 fl. oz. cold water and 3 ice cubes or ⅓ cup crushed ice (2 fl. oz. when melted) (yield: approx. 6 fl. oz.)	70	12.0	(11.7)	(1.83)	(93)	14.7	5.8	0.92
Vanilla Flavor, 7.5-oz. box, 10 envelopes	700	110.0	(34.3)	(5.86)				
1 envelope, approx. 0.75 oz.	70	11.0	(34.3)	(5.86)				
Prepared as package directs, mixing 1 envelope with 4 fl. oz. cold water and 3 ice cubes or ⅓ cup crushed ice (2 fl. oz. when melted) (yield: approx. 6 fl. oz.)	70	11.0	(11.7)	(1.83)	(93)	14.7	5.8	0.92
Borden Eggnog, 32-fl. oz. (1-quart) can	1283	128.0	40.0	4.00	320	32.0	20.0	2.00
"Frosted," Chocolate Flavored Shake, 7½-fl. oz. can	270	37.0	36.0	4.93	288	39.4	18.0	2.46
Chocolate Fudge Flavored Shake, 7½-fl.-oz. can	270	37.0	36.0	4.93	288	39.4	18.0	2.46
Coffee Flavored Shake, 7½-fl.-oz. can	270	36.0	36.0	4.80	288	38.4	18.0	2.46
Strawberry Flavored Shake, 7½-fl.-oz. can	270	36.0	36.0	4.80	288	38.4	18.0	2.46
Vanilla Flavored Shake, 7½-fl.-oz. can	270	36.0	36.0	4.80	288	38.4	18.0	2.46
Carnation Instant Breakfast Mix, Chocolate, 7.56-oz. box, 6 envelopes	780	138.0	(65.0)	(12.50)				
1 envelope, approx. 1.26 oz.	130	23.0	(65.0)	(12.50)				
Prepared as package directs, mixing 1 envelope with 1 cup (8 fl. oz.) milk (yield: approx. 8 fl. oz.):								
Made with whole milk (3.5% fat)	289	35.0	36.1	4.38	289	35.0	18.1	2.19
Made with skim milk (0.1% fat)	218	35.5	27.3	4.44	218	35.5	13.6	2.22
Instant Breakfast Mix, Chocolate Malt, 7.26-oz. box, 6 envelopes	780	132.0	(66.3)	(12.50)				
1 envelope, approx. 1.21 oz.	130	22.0	(66.3)	(12.50)				
Prepared as package directs, mixing 1 envelope with 1 cup (8 fl. oz.) milk (yield: approx. 8 fl. oz.):								
Made with whole milk (3.5% fat)	289	34.0	36.1	4.25	289	34.0	18.1	2.13
Made with skim milk (0.1% fat)	218	34.5	27.3	4.31	218	34.5	13.6	2.16
Instant Breakfast Mix, Coffee, 7.56-oz. box, 6 envelopes	780	144.0	(65.0)	(12.50)				
1 envelope, approx. 1.26 oz.	130	24.0	(65.0)	(12.50)				
Prepared as package directs, mixing 1 envelope with 1 cup (8 fl. oz.) milk (yield: approx. 8 fl. oz.):								
Made with whole milk (3.5% fat)	289	36.0	36.1	4.50	289	36.0	18.1	2.25

	UNIT		1 FLUID OZ.		1 CUP		1 TABLESPOON	
	Cal.	Carb.	Cal.	Carb.	Cal.	Carb.	Cal.	Carb.
Made with skim milk (0.1% fat)	218	36.5	27.3	4.56	218	36.5	13.6	2.28
Instant Breakfast Mix, Eggnog, 7.26-oz. box, 6 envelopes	780	138.0	(66.3)	(12.50)				
1 envelope, approx. 1.21 oz.	130	23.0	(66.3)	(12.50)				
Prepared as package directs, mixing 1 envelope with 1 cup (8 fl. oz.) milk (yield: approx. 8 fl. oz.):								
Made with whole milk (3.5% fat)	289	35.0	36.1	4.38	289	35.0	18.1	2.19
Made with skim milk (0.1% fat)	218	35.5	27.3	4.44	218	35.5	13.6	2.22
Instant Chocolate Malted Milk, 15-oz. jar	1711	372.8	(68.8)	(12.50)				
1 serving, 3 heaping tablespoons	84	18.4	(68.8)	(12.50)				
Prepared as package directs, mixing 1 serving with 1 cup (8 fl. oz.) milk (yield: approx. 8 fl. oz.):								
Made with whole milk (3.5% fat)	243	30.4	30.4	3.80	243	30.4	15.2	1.90
Made with skim milk (0.1% fat)	172	30.9	21.5	3.86	172	30.9	10.8	1.93
Instant Hot Cocoa Mix, Chocolate & Artificial Marshmallow Flavor, 12-oz. box, 12 envelopes	1344	264.0	(68.8)	(12.50)				
1 envelope, approx. 1 oz.	112	22.0	(68.8)	(12.50)				
Prepared as package directs, mixing 1 envelope with 6 fl. oz. water (yield: approx. 6 fl. oz.)	112	22.0	18.7	3.67	149	29.3	9.3	1.83
12-oz. can	1344	264.0	(68.8)	(12.50)				
1 serving, 2 heaping teaspoons (approx. 1 oz.)	112	22.0	(68.8)	(12.50)				
Prepared as package directs, mixing 1 serving with 6 fl. oz. water (yield: approx. 6 fl. oz.)	112	22.0	18.7	3.67	149	29.3	9.3	1.83
20-oz. jar	2226	437.0	(68.8)	(12.50)				
Instant Hot Cocoa Mix, Cocoa Supreme Flavor, 9-oz. box, 8 envelopes	1040	184.0	(68.8)	(12.50)				
1 envelope, approx. 1⅛ oz.	130	23.0	(68.8)	(12.50)				
Prepared as package directs, mixing 1 envelope with 6 fl. oz. water (yield: approx. 6 fl. oz.)	130	23.0	21.7	3.83	173	30.7	10.8	1.92
Instant Hot Cocoa Mix, Rich Chocolate Flavor, 12-oz. box, 12 envelopes	1344	264.0	(68.8)	(12.50)				
1 envelope, approx. 1 oz.	112	22.0	(68.8)	(12.50)				
Prepared as package directs, mixing 1 envelope with 6 fl. oz. water (yield: approx. 6 fl. oz.)	112	22.0	18.7	3.67	149	29.3	9.3	1.83
20-oz. jar	2226	437.0	(68.8)	(12.50)				
Instant Natural Malted Milk, 15-oz. jar	1868	315.4	(78.8)	(12.50)				
1 serving, 3 heaping tablespoons	90	15.6	(78.8)	(12.50)				
Prepared as package directs, mixing 1 serving with 1 cup (8 fl. oz.) milk (yield: approx. 8 fl. oz.):								
Made with whole milk (3.5% fat)	249	27.6	31.1	3.45	249	27.6	15.6	1.73
Made with skim milk (0.1% fat)	178	28.1	22.3	3.51	178	27.6	11.1	1.73
Slender, Butterscotch, 10-fl.-oz. can	225	34.0	22.5	3.40	180	27.2	11.3	1.70
Slender, Chocolate, 4.08-oz. box, 4 envelopes	440	80.0	(68.8)	(12.50)				
1 envelope, approx. 1.02 oz.	110	20.0	(68.8)	(12.50)				
Prepared as package directs, mixing 1 envelope with 1 cup (8 fl. oz.) milk (yield: approx. 8 fl. oz.):								
Made with whole milk (3.5% fat)	(309)	(35.0)	(30.9)	(3.50)	(247)	(28.0)	15.4	1.75
Made with skim milk (0.1% fat)	(220)	(35.6)	(22.0)	(3.56)	(176)	(28.5)	(11.0)	(1.78)
10-fl.-oz. can	225	34.0	22.5	3.40	180	27.2	11.3	1.70
Slender, Chocolate Fudge, 10-fl.-oz. can	225	34.0	22.5	3.40	180	27.2	11.3	1.70
Slender, Chocolate Malt, 3.96-oz. box, 4 envelopes	440	80.0	(68.8)	(12.50)				
1 envelope, approx. 0.99 oz.	110	20.0	(68.8)	(12.50)				
Prepared as package directs, mixing 1 envelope with 1 cup (8 fl. oz.) milk (yield: approx. 8 fl. oz.):								
Made with whole milk (3.5% fat)	(309)	(35.9)	(30.9)	(3.59)	(247)	(28.7)	(15.4)	(1.79)
Made with skim milk (0.1% fat)	(220)	(36.5)	(22.0)	(3.65)	(176)	(29.2)	(11.0)	(1.83)
10-fl.-oz. can	225	34.0	22.5	3.40	180	27.2	11.3	1.70
Slender, Chocolate Marshmallow, 10-fl.-oz. can	225	34.0	22.5	3.40	180	27.2	11.3	1.70
Slender, Coffee, 4-oz. box, 4 envelopes	440	84.0	(68.8)	(12.50)				
1 envelope, approx. 1 oz.	110	21.0	(68.8)	(12.50)				
Prepared as package directs, mixing 1 envelope with 1 cup (8 fl. oz.) milk (yield: approx. 8 fl. oz.):								
Made with whole milk (3.5% fat)	(309)	(36.9)	(30.9)	(3.69)	(247)	(29.5)	(15.4)	(1.84)
Made with skim milk (0.1% fat)	(220)	(37.5)	(22.0)	(3.75)	(176)	(30.0)	(11.0)	(1.88)
10-fl.-oz. can	225	34.0	22.5	3.40	180	27.2	11.3	1.70
Slender, Dutch Chocolate, 4.08-oz. box, 4 envelopes	440	80.0	(68.8)	(12.50)				
1 envelope, approx. 1.02 oz.	110	20.0	(68.8)	(12.50)				
Prepared as package directs, mixing 1 envelope with 1 cup (8 fl. oz.) milk (yield: approx. 8 fl. oz.):								
Made with whole milk (3.5% fat)	(309)	(35.9)	(30.9)	(3.59)	(247)	(28.7)	(15.4)	(1.79)
Made with skim milk (0.1% fat)	(220)	(36.5)	(22.0)	(3.65)	(176)	(29.2)	(11.0)	(1.83)
Slender, Eggnog, 10-fl.-oz. can	225	34.0	22.5	3.40	180	27.2	11.3	1.70
Slender, French Vanilla, 4-oz. box, 4 envelopes	440	84.0	(68.8)	(12.50)				
1 envelope, approx. 1 oz.	110	21.0	(68.8)	(12.50)				
Prepared as package directs, mixing 1 envelope with 1 cup (8 fl. oz.) milk (yield: approx. 8 fl. oz.):								
Made with whole milk (3.5% fat)	(309)	(37.5)	(30.9)	(3.75)	(247)	(30.0)	(15.4)	(1.88)
Made with skim milk (0.1% fat)	(220)	(38.1)	(22.0)	(3.81)	(176)	(30.5)	(11.0)	(1.91)
Slender, Milk Chocolate, 10-fl.-oz. can	225	34.0	22.5	3.40	180	27.2	11.3	1.70
Slender, Vanilla, 10-fl.-oz. can	225	34.0	22.5	3.40	180	27.2	11.3	1.70
Slender, Wild Strawberry, 4-oz. box, 4 envelopes	440	84.0	(68.8)	(12.50)				
1 envelope, approx. 1 oz.	110	21.0	(68.8)	(12.50)				
Prepared as package directs, mixing 1 envelope with 1 cup (8 fl. oz.) milk (yield: approx. 8 fl. oz.):								
Made with whole milk (3.5% fat)	(309)	(36.9)	(30.9)	(3.69)	(247)	(29.5)	(15.4)	(1.84)
Made with skim milk (0.1% fat)	(220)	(37.5)	(22.0)	(3.75)	(176)	(30.0)	(11.0)	(1.88)
Chocolate Cow High Protein Chocolate Flavored Dairy Drink, 6-pack, 66 fl. oz.	1020	216.0	15.5	3.27	124	26.2	7.8	1.64
1 can, approx. 11 fl. oz.	170	36.0	15.5	3.27	124	26.2	7.8	1.64
Chocolate Time, 11½-fl.-oz. can	196	47.2	17.0	4.10	136	32.8	8.5	2.05
Fearn Shake Mix, Natural Carob Flavor, 12-oz. can	1263	126.3						
1 pouch, ⅓ cup (approx. 1.0 oz.)	(100)	(10.0)						
Prepared as package directs, mixing ⅓ cup with 1 cup (8 fl. oz.) whole milk (yield: approx. 8 fl. oz.)	(250)	(22.0)	(32.5)	(2.75)	(250)	(22.0)	(15.6)	(1.38)
Natural Chocolate Flavor, 12-oz. can	1263	113.6						

	UNIT		1 FLUID OZ.		1 CUP		1 TABLE-SPOON	
	Cal.	Carb.	Cal.	Carb.	Cal.	Carb.	Cal.	Carb.
1 pouch, ⅓ cup (approx. 1.0 oz.)	100	9.0						
Prepared as package directs, mixing ⅓ cup with 1 cup (8 fl. oz.) whole milk (yield: approx. 8 fl. oz.)	(260)	(21.0)	(32.5)	(2.65)	(260)	(21.0)	(16.3)	(1.31)
Natural Vanilla Flavor, 12-oz. can	1263	126.3						
1 pouch, ⅓ cup (approx. 1.0 oz.)	(100)	(10.0)						
Prepared as package directs, mixing ⅓ cup with 1 cup (8 fl. oz.) whole milk (yield: approx. 8 fl. oz.)	(250)	(22.0)	(32.5)	(2.75)	(250)	(22.0)	(15.6)	(1.38)
Featherweight Rich Tasting Hot Cocoa Mix, 4.5 oz. box, 10 envelopes	500	80.0						
1 envelope, approx. 0.45 oz.	50	8.0						
Prepared as package directs, mixing 0.45 oz. with 6 fl. oz. hot water (yield: approx. 6 fl. oz.)	50	8.0	8.3	1.33	67	10.7	4.2	0.67
Golden Harvest Instant Carob Drink Mix, 20-oz. package	2350	470.0						
1 serving, 2 heaping teaspoons, approx. 0.4 oz.	50	10.0						
Prepared as package directs, mixing 2 heaping teaspoons with 1 cup (8 fl. oz.) whole milk (yield: approx. 8 fl. oz.)	200	22.0	25.0	2.75	200	22.0	12.5	1.38
Hershey's Cocoa Mix, 8-oz. can	960	112.0			(360)	(42.0)		
1 serving, approx. 5 tablespoons (⅓ cup)	120	14.0			(360)	(42.0)		
Prepared as package directs, mixing 1 serving with 2 teaspoons sugar, dash salt, and 1 cup (8 fl. oz.) milk (yield: approx. 8 fl. oz.):								
Made with whole milk (3.5% fat)	(297)	(40.4)	(37.1)	(5.05)	(297)	(40.4)	(18.6)	(2.53)
Made with skim milk (0.1% fat)	(226)	(40.9)	(28.2)	(5.11)	(226)	(40.9)	(14.1)	(2.56)
16-oz. (1-lb.) can	1920	224.0	(83.0)	(9.60)				
1 serving, 1 heaping teaspoon	120	14.0	(83.0)	(9.60)				
Prepared as package directs, mixing 1 serving with 2 teaspoons sugar, dash salt, and 1 cup (8 fl. oz.) milk (yield: approx. 8 fl. oz.):								
Made with whole milk (3.5% fat)	(297)	(40.4)	(37.0)	(5.10)	(297)	(40.4)	(18.6)	(2.53)
Made with skim milk (0.1% fat)	(226)	(40.9)	(28.0)	(5.10)	(226)	(40.9)	(14.1)	(2.56)
Hot Cocoa Mix, 16-oz. (1-lb.) can	1920	336.0						
1 serving, 3 heaping teaspoons	120	21.0						
Prepared as package directs, mixing 1 serving with 6 fl. oz. liquid (yield: approx. 6 fl. oz.):								
Made with whole milk (3.5% fat)	(239)	(30.0)	(39.3)	(5.00)	(314)	(40.0)	(19.6)	(2.50)
Made with skim milk (0.1% fat)	(187)	(30.4)	(31.2)	(5.07)	(250)	(40.5)	(15.6)	(2.53)
Made with water	120	21.0	20.0	3.50	160	28.0	10.0	1.75
12-oz. box (12 envelopes)	1440	252.0						
Prepared as package directs, mixing 1 envelope with 8 fl. oz. water (yield: approx. 8 fl. oz.)	120	21.0	20.0	3.50	160	28.0	10.0	1.75
Instant Chocolate Mix, 16-oz. (1-lb.) can	1680	357.0	(60.0)	(12.75)				
Prepared Cold:								
1 serving, 2 heaping teaspoons	80	17.0	(60.0)	(12.75)				
Prepared as package directs, mixing 1 serving with 1 tall glass (8 fl. oz.) liquid (yield: approx. 8 fl. oz.):								
Made with whole milk (3.5% fat)	240	29.0	30.0	3.63	240	29.0	15.0	1.81
Made with skim milk (0.1% fat)	168	29.5	21.0	3.69	168	29.5	10.5	1.84
Made with water	80	17.0	10.0	2.13	80	17.0	5.0	1.06
Prepared Hot:								
1 serving, 2 heaping teaspoons	80	17.0	(60.0)	(12.75)				
Prepared as package directs, mixing 1 serving with 6 fl. oz. liquid (yield: approx. 6 fl. oz.):								
Made with whole milk (3.5% fat)	(193)	(26.0)	(32.2)	(4.33)	(258)	(34.6)	(16.1)	(2.16)
Made with skim milk (0.1% fat)	(148)	(26.7)	(24.6)	(4.40)	(197)	(35.2)	(12.3)	(2.20)
Made with water	(80)	(17.0)	(13.3)	(2.83)	(106)	(22.7)	(6.6)	(1.42)
Kraft Instantized Malted Milk, Chocolate Flavor, 13½-oz. jar	1800	360.0	(50.0)	(10.00)				
1 serving, 3 heaping teaspoons	90	18.0	(50.0)	(10.00)				
Prepared as package directs, mixing 1 serving with 1 cup (8 fl. oz.) milk (yield: approx. 8 fl. oz.):								
Made with whole milk (3.5% fat)	240	30.0	30.0	3.80	240	30.0	15.0	1.88
Made with skim milk (0.1% fat)	(179)	(30.5)	(22.4)	(3.81)	(179)	(30.5)	(11.2)	1.91
Lucerne Instant Chocolate Flavored Mix, 32-oz. (2-lb.) can	3420	798.0						
1 serving, 2 teaspoons, approx. 0.8 oz.	90	21.0						
Prepared as package directs, mixing 2 teaspoonsful with 6 fl. oz. whole milk (yield: approx. 6 fl. oz.)	215	27.0	35.4	4.50	287	36.0	17.9	2.25
Nestlé Hot Cocoa Mix, 14-oz. canister	1540	308.0						
24-oz. canister	2640	528.0						
1 serving, 4 heaping teaspoons	110	22.0						
Prepared as package directs, mixing 1 serving with 6 fl. oz. water (yield: approx. 6 fl. oz.)	110	22.0	18.3	3.67	147	29.3	9.2	1.83
Quik, Chocolate Flavor, 8-oz. can	756	205.2						
1 serving, 2 heaping teaspoons	70	19.0						
Prepared as package directs, mixing 1 serving with 1 cup (8 fl. oz.) milk (yield: approx. 8 fl. oz.):								
Made with whole milk (3.5% fat)	(253)	(37.7)	(31.7)	(4.71)	(254)	(37.7)	(15.9)	(2.36)
Made with skim milk (0.1% fat)	(182)	(38.2)	(22.8)	(4.77)	(182)	(38.2)	(11.2)	(2.39)
16-oz. (1-lb.) can	1512	410.4						
32-oz. (2-lb.) can	3024	820.8						
1 serving, 2 heaping teaspoons	70	19.0						
Prepared as package directs, mixing 1 serving with 1 cup (8 fl. oz.) milk (yield: approx. 8 fl. oz.):								
Made with whole milk (3.5% fat)	(253)	(37.7)	(31.7)	(4.71)	(254)	(37.7)	(15.9)	(2.36)
Made with skim milk (0.1% fat)	(182)	(38.2)	(22.8)	(4.77)	(182)	(38.2)	(11.2)	(2.39)
Quik, Strawberry Flavor, 16-oz. (1-lb.) can	1728	453.6						
32-oz. (2-lb.) can	3456	907.2						
1 serving, 2 heaping teaspoons	80	21.0						
Prepared as package directs, mixing 1 serving with 1 cup (8 fl. oz.) milk (yield: approx. 8 fl. oz.):								
Made with whole milk (3.5% fat)	267	40.4	33.4	5.04	267	40.4	16.7	2.53
Made with skim milk (0.1% fat)	(196)	(40.9)	(24.5)	(5.11)	(196)	(40.9)	(12.3)	(2.56)
Ovaltine Chocolate Flavor, 4.5-oz. jar	480	96.0						
9-oz. jar	960	204.0						
1 serving, ¾ oz.	80	16.0						

	UNIT Cal.	UNIT Carb.	1 FLUID OZ. Cal.	1 FLUID OZ. Carb.	1 CUP Cal.	1 CUP Carb.	1 TABLESPOON Cal.	1 TABLESPOON Carb.
Prepared as package directs, mixing 1 serving with 1 cup (8 fl. oz.) milk (yield: approx. 8 fl. oz.):								
Made with whole milk (3.5% fat)	239	28.0	29.9	3.50	239	28.0	14.9	1.75
Made with skim milk (0.1% fat)	169	28.5	21.1	3.56	169	28.0	10.6	1.75
Chocolate Malt Flavor, 4.5-oz. jar	480	102.0						
9-oz. jar	960	204.0						
1 serving, ¾ oz.	80	17.0						
Prepared as package directs, mixing 1 serving with 1 cup (8 fl. oz.) milk (yield: approx. 8 fl. oz.):								
Made with whole milk (3.5% fat)	239	29.0	29.9	3.63	239	29.0	14.9	1.81
Made with skim milk (0.1% fat)	169	29.5	21.1	3.69	169	29.5	10.6	1.81
Reduced calorie Hot Cocoa Mix, 6.9-oz. box, 10 envelopes	800	150.0						
1 envelope, approx. 0.69 oz.	80	15.0						
Prepared as package directs, mixing 1 envelope with 6 fl. oz. water (yield: approx. 6 fl. oz.)	80	15.0	13.3	2.50	106	20.0	6.6	1.25
Pillsbury Instant Breakfast Mix, Chocolate Flavor, 7.75-oz. box, 6 pouches	780	156.0						
1 pouch, approx. 1.3 oz.	130	26.0						
Prepared as package directs, mixing 1 pouch with 1 cup (8 fl. oz.) milk (yield: approx. 8 fl. oz.):								
Made with whole milk (3.5% fat)	290	38.0	36.3	4.75	290	38.0	18.1	2.38
Made with skim milk (0.1% fat)	218	38.5	27.3	4.81	218	38.0	13.6	2.38
Instant Breakfast Mix, Chocolate Malt Flavor, 7.5-oz. box, 6 pouches	780	156.0						
1 pouch, approx. 1.25 oz.	130	26.0						
Prepared as package directs, mixing 1 pouch with 1 cup (8 fl. oz.) milk (yield: approx. 8 fl. oz.):								
Made with whole milk (3.5% fat)	290	38.0	36.3	4.75	290	38.0	18.1	2.38
Made with skim milk (0.1% fat)	218	38.5	27.3	4.81	218	38.5	13.6	2.41
13-oz. box, 10 pouches	1300	260.0						
1 envelope, approx. 1.3 oz.	130	26.0						
Prepared as package directs, mixing 1 envelope with 1 cup (8 fl. oz.) milk (yield: approx. 8 fl. oz.):								
Made with whole milk (3.5% fat)	289	36.0	36.1	4.50	289	36.0	18.1	2.25
Made with skim milk (0.1% fat)	218	36.5	27.3	4.56	218	36.5	13.6	2.28
Instant Breakfast Mix, Strawberry Flavor, 7.5-oz. box, 6 pouches	780	156.0						
1 pouch, approx. 1.25 oz.	130	27.0						
Prepared as package directs, mixing 1 pouch with 1 cup (8 fl. oz.) milk (yield: approx. 8 fl. oz.):								
Made with whole milk (3.5% fat)	290	39.0	36.3	4.88	290	39.0	18.1	2.44
Made with skim milk (0.1% fat)	218	39.5	36.3	4.94	218	39.5	18.1	2.47
13-oz. box, 10 pouches	1300	260.0						
1 envelope, approx. 1.3 oz.	130	26.0						
Prepared as package directs, mixing 1 envelope with 1 cup (8 fl. oz.) milk (yield: approx. 8 fl. oz.):								
Made with whole milk (3.5% fat)	289	36.0	36.1	4.50	289	36.0	18.1	2.25
Made with skim milk (0.1% fat)	218	36.5	27.3	4.58	218	36.5	13.6	2.28
Instant Breakfast Mix, Vanilla Flavor, 7.75-oz. box, 6 pouches	780	156.0						
1 pouch, approx. 1.3 oz.	130	27.0						
Prepared as package directs, mixing 1 pouch with 1 cup (8 fl. oz.) milk (yield: approx. 8 fl. oz.):								
Made with whole milk (3.5% fat)	290	39.0	36.3	4.88	290	39.0	18.1	2.44
Made with skim milk (0.1% fat)	218	39.5	27.3	4.94	218	39.5	13.6	2.47
Swiss Miss Hot Cocoa Mix, 12-oz. box, 12 envelopes	1344	252.0						
1 envelope, approx. 1 oz.	112	21.0						
Prepared as package directs, mixing 1 envelope with 6 fl. oz. water (yield: approx. 6 fl. oz.)	112	21.0	18.7	3.50	150	28.0	9.4	1.75
14-oz. can	1568	294.0						
1 serving, prepared as package directs, mixing 1 envelope with 6 fl. oz. water (yield: approx. 6 fl. oz.)	112	21.0	18.7	3.50	150	28.0	9.4	1.75
Hot Cocoa Mix, Double Rich								
1 envelope, approx. 1.6 oz.	120	20.0						
Prepared as package directs, mixing 1 envelope to 6 fl. oz. water (yield: approx. 6 fl. oz.)	120	20.0	20.0	3.33	160	26.7	10.0	1.67
14-oz. can	1680	280.0						
1 serving, 1 oz.	120	20.0						
Prepared as package directs, mixing 1 serving with 6 fl. oz. water (yield: approx. 6 fl. oz.)	120	20.0	20.0	3.33	160	26.7	10.0	1.67
Hot Cocoa Mix, Lite, 9-oz. box, 12 envelopes	840	204.0						
1 envelope, ¾ oz.	70	17.0						
Prepared as package directs, mixing 1 envelope with 6 fl. oz. water (yield: 6 fl. oz.)	70	17.0	11.7	2.83	93	22.7	5.8	1.42
Town House Instant Breakfast Drink, 27-oz. can	2880	768.0						
1 serving, 2 heaping teaspoons, approx. 0.6 oz.	60	16.0						
Prepared as package directs, mixing 2 heaping teaspoons with 4 fl. oz. whole milk (yield: approx. 4 fl. oz.)	120	22.0	30.0	5.50	240	44.0	15.0	2.75
Prepared with skim milk (yield: approx. 4 fl. oz.)	105	22.3	26.3	5.56	210	44.5	13.1	2.78
Yoo-hoo Chocolate Flavored Drink, 9½-fl.-oz. bottle	180	40.0	18.9	4.21	151	33.7	9.4	2.12
diet Chocolate Fudge, 12-fl.-oz. can	4	0.0	0.3	0.00	2	0.0	0.1	0.00
Coconut Flavored Shake, 9½-fl.-oz. bottle	140	29.0	14.7	3.10	117	24.4	7.3	1.53
Strawberry Flavored Shake, 9½-fl.-oz. bottle	150	33.0	15.8	3.48	127	27.8	7.9	1.74
Vanilla Flavored Shake, 9½-fl.-oz. bottle	150	33.0	15.8	3.48	127	27.8	7.9	1.74

CREAM

	UNIT Cal.	UNIT Carb.	1 FLUID OZ. Cal.	1 FLUID OZ. Carb.	1 CUP Cal.	1 CUP Carb.	1 TABLESPOON Cal.	1 TABLESPOON Carb.
CREAM, arranged in ascending order of fat content, based on generic data								
Half-and-Half (milk and cream) Cream, 11.5% fat, 1 quart	1296	44.4	40.0	1.40	324	11.1	20.3	0.69
Light Coffee or Table Cream, 19.31% fat, 1 quart	2024	41.2	64.0	1.20	506	10.3	31.6	0.64
Medium Cream, 25% fat, 1 quart	2332	33.3	74.0	1.04	583	8.3	36.4	0.52
Light Whipping Cream, 30.9% fat, 1 quart	2796	28.3	88.0	0.88	699	7.1	43.7	0.44
Whipped, 30.9% fat, 1 quart	1398	14.2	44.0	0.44	350	3.6	21.9	0.23
Heavy Whipping Cream, 37% fat, 1 quart	3284	26.6	104.0	0.84	821	6.6	51.3	0.41
Whipped, 37% fat, 1 quart	1642	13.3	52.0	0.42	411	3.3	25.7	0.21
CREAM, by brand								
Dellwood Half-and-Half (11% fat), 16 fl. oz. (1 pint)	576	32.0	36.0	2.00	288	16.0	18.0	1.00
1 quart	1152	64.0	36.0	2.00	288	16.0	18.0	1.00

	UNIT		1 FLUID OZ.		1 CUP		1 TABLE-SPOON	
	Cal.	Carb.	Cal.	Carb.	Cal.	Carb.	Cal.	Carb.
Heavy Whipping Cream (36% fat), 8 fl. oz.	800	8.0	100.0	1.00	800	8.0	50.0	0.50
1 quart	3200	32.0	100.0	1.00	800	8.0	50.0	0.50
Hood "All Purpose" Cream, 16 fl. oz. (1 pint)	1400	14.0	87.5	0.88	700	7.0	43.8	0.44
Heavy Cream, 8 fl. oz.	820	7.0	102.5	0.88	820	7.0	51.3	0.44
COFFEE WHITENERS (Non-Dairy)								
COFFEE WHITENERS, based on generic data								
Liquid (frozen) containing hydrogenated vegetable oil and soy protein								
1 cup (approx. 8.5 oz.)	326	27.3	40.8	3.41	326	27.3	20.4	1.71
1 tablespoon (approx. 0.5 oz.)	20	1.7	40.8	3.41	326	27.3	20.4	1.71
1 teaspoon (approx. 0.2 oz.)	7	0.6	40.8	3.41	326	27.3	20.4	1.71
Liquid (frozen) containing Lauric Acid Oil and Sodium Caseinate (Lauric oils include modified coconut oil, hydrogenated coconut oil and/or palm kernel oil.)								
1 cup (approx. 8.5 oz.)	328	23.9	41.0	2.99	328	23.9	20.5	1.49
1 tablespoon (approx. 0.5 oz.)	21	1.5	41.0	2.99	328	23.9	20.5	1.49
1 teaspoon (approx. 0.2 oz.)	7	0.5	41.0	2.99	328	23.9	20.5	1.49
Powdered containing Lauric Acid Oil and Sodium Caseinate								
1 cup (approx. 3.3 oz.)	514	51.6	155.8	15.64	514	51.6	32.2	3.23
1 tablespoon (approx. 0.2 oz.)	32	3.2	155.8	15.64	514	51.6	32.2	3.23
1 teaspoon (approx. 0.1 oz.)	11	1.1	155.8	15.64	514	51.6	32.2	3.23
COFFEE WHITENERS, by brand								
Lucerne Cereal Blend non-dairy creamer, 32-fl.-oz. (1-quart) container	1280	64.0	40.0	2.00	320	16.0	20.0	1.00
1 cup	320	16.0	40.0	2.00	320	16.0	20.0	1.00
1 tablespoon	20	1.0	40.0	2.00	320	16.0	20.0	1.00
1 teaspoon	7	0.3	40.0	2.00	320	16.0	20.0	1.00
P&Q (A&P) Non-Dairy Creamer, 22-oz. container	1584	132.0	72.0	6.00	576	48.0	36.0	3.00
1 cup (approx. 3.4 oz.)	576	48.0	72.0	6.00	576	48.0	36.0	3.00
1 tablespoon (approx. 0.5 oz.)	36	3.0	72.0	6.00	576	48.0	36.0	3.00
1 teaspoon (approx. 0.17 oz.)	12	1.0	72.0	6.00	576	48.0	36.0	3.00
Rich Products Coffee Rich, 16-oz. (1-lb.) package	640	64.0	(44.0)	(4.40)	(352)	(35.2)	(22.0)	(2.20)
1 cup	(352)	(35.2)	(44.0)	(4.40)	(352)	(35.2)	(22.0)	(2.20)
1 tablespoon (approx. 0.6 oz.)	(22)	(2.2)	(44.0)	(4.40)	(352)	(35.2)	(22.0)	(2.20)
1 teaspoon (approx. 0.2 oz.)	(7)	(0.7)	(44.0)	(4.40)	(352)	(35.2)	(22.0)	(2.20)
Poly Rich, 16-oz. (1-lb.) package	640	64.0	(44.0)	(4.40)	(352)	(35.2)	(22.0)	(2.20)
1 cup	(352)	(35.2)	(44.0)	(4.40)	(352)	(35.2)	(22.0)	(2.20)
1 tablespoon (approx. 0.6 oz.)	(22)	(2.2)	(44.0)	(4.40)	(352)	(35.2)	(22.0)	(2.20)
1 teaspoon (approx. 0.2 oz.)	(7)	(0.7)	(44.0)	(4.40)	(352)	(35.2)	(22.0)	(2.20)
COFFEE, by brand								
1 level tablespoon of most ground coffees equals just a fraction less than 1/5 oz. by weight. A teaspoon of coffee weighs about 1/16 oz.								
GROUND COFFEE								
Chase & Sanborn Ground Coffee, 16-oz. (1-lb.) can (yield: approx. 64 servings)	128	trace	(0.3)	trace	(2)	trace	(0.1)	trace
Institutional, 3-lb. can (yield: 192 servings)	384	trace	(0.3)	trace	(2)	trace	(0.1)	trace
Hills Bros. Ground Coffee, 16-oz. (1-lb.) can (yield: approx. 384 fl. oz., 64 servings)	128	trace	(0.3)	trace	(2)	trace	(0.1)	trace
"Suggested" serving, rounded tablespoon, dry (yield: approx. 6 fl. oz.)	(2)	trace	(0.3)	trace	(2)	trace	(0.1)	trace

	UNIT		1 FLUID OZ.		1 CUP		1 TABLE-SPOON	
	Cal.	Carb.	Cal.	Carb.	Cal.	Carb.	Cal.	Carb.
High Yield Coffee, 13-oz. can (yield: approx. 384 fl. oz., 64 servings)	128	trace	(0.3)	trace	(2)	trace	(0.1)	trace
"Suggested" serving, 1 rounded tablespoon, dry (yield: approx. 6 fl. oz.)	(2)	trace	(0.3)	trace	(2)	trace	(0.1)	trace
Maxwell House Regular Coffee, 16-oz. (1-lb.) can (yield: approx. 468 fl. oz., 78 servings)	99	0.9	0.2	trace	2	trace	0.1	trace
"Suggested" serving, 1 level tablespoon, dry (yield: approx. 6 fl. oz.)	1	trace	0.2	trace	2	trace	0.1	trace
Drip Coffee, 16-oz. (1-lb.) can (yield: approx. 468 fl. oz., 78 servings)	99	0.9	0.2	trace	2	trace	0.1	trace
"Suggested" serving, 1 level tablespoon, dry (yield: approx. 6 fl. oz.)	1	trace	0.2	trace	2	trace	0.1	trace
Electra-Perk Coffee, 16-oz. (1-lb.) can (yield: approx. 468 fl. oz., 78 servings)	99	0.9	0.2	trace	2	trace	0.1	trace
"Suggested" serving, 1 level tablespoon, dry (yield: approx. 6 fl. oz.)	1	trace	0.2	trace	2	trace	0.1	trace
Fine Grind Coffee, 16-oz. (1-lb.) can (yield: approx. 468 fl. oz., 78 servings)	99	0.9	0.2	trace	2	trace	0.1	trace
"Suggested" serving, 1 level tablespoon, dry (yield: approx. 6 fl. oz.)	1	trace	0.2	trace	2	trace	0.1	trace
Max-Pax, Ground Coffee Filter Rings, 24-oz. container, 20 rings (yield: approx. 660 fl. oz., 120 servings)	149	2.0	0.2	trace	2	trace	0.1	trace
1 filter ring (yield: approx. six 5½-oz. servings)	8	0.1	0.2	trace	2	trace	0.1	trace
"Suggested" serving, ⅙ ring (yield: approx. 5½ fl. oz.)	1	trace	0.2	trace	2	trace	0.1	trace
Yuban Regular Coffee, 16-oz. (1-lb.) can (yield: approx. 468 fl. oz., 78 servings)	99	0.9	0.2	trace	2	trace	0.1	trace
"Suggested" serving, 1 level tablespoon, dry (yield: approx. 6 fl. oz.)	1	trace	0.2	trace	2	trace	0.1	trace
Drip Coffee, 16-oz. (1-lb.) can (yield: approx. 468 fl. oz., 78 servings)	99	0.9	0.2	trace	2	trace	0.1	trace
"Suggested" serving, 1 level tablespoon, dry (yield: approx. 6 fl. oz.)	1	trace	0.2	trace	2	trace	0.1	trace
GROUND DECAFFEINATED								
Brim Decaffeinated Coffee, Regular Grind, 16-oz. (1-lb.) package (yield: approx. 78 servings)	99	0.9	0.2	trace	2	trace	0.1	trace
"Suggested" serving, 1 level tablespoon, dry (yield: approx. 6 fl. oz.)	1	trace	0.2	trace	2	trace	0.1	trace
Drip Grind, 16-oz. (1-lb.) package (yield: approx. 468 fl. oz., 78 servings)	99	0.9	0.2	trace	2	trace	0.1	trace
"Suggested" serving, 1 level tablespoon, dry (yield: approx. 6 fl. oz.)	1	trace	0.2	trace	2	trace	0.1	trace
Electric-Perk, 16-oz. (1-lb.) package (yield: approx. 468 fl. oz., 78 servings)	99	0.9	0.2	trace	2	trace	0.1	trace
"Suggested" serving, 1 level tablespoon, dry (yield: approx. 6 fl. oz.)	1	trace	0.2	trace	2	trace	0.1	trace
Sanka 97% Caffeine Free Regular Grind Coffee, 16-oz. (1-lb.) can (yield: approx. 468 fl. oz., 78 servings)	99	0.9	0.2	trace	2	trace	0.1	trace
"Suggested" serving, 1 level tablespoon, dry (yield: approx. 6 fl. oz.)	1	trace	0.2	trace	2	trace	0.1	trace
Drip Grind Coffee, 16-oz. (1-lb.) can (yield: approx. 468 fl. oz., 78 servings)	99	0.9	0.2	trace	2	trace	0.1	trace
"Suggested" serving, 1 level tablespoon, dry (yield: approx. 6 fl. oz.)	1	trace	0.2	trace	2	trace	0.1	trace
INSTANT COFFEE								
Hills Bros. 10-oz. jar (yield: approx. 900 oz., approx. 150 servings)	27		0.3	trace	3	trace	0.2	trace
"Suggested" serving, 1 rounded teaspoon, dry (yield: approx. 6 fl. oz.)	2	trace	0.3	trace	3	trace	0.2	trace

	UNIT		1 FLUID OZ.		1 CUP		1 TABLE-SPOON	
	Cal.	Carb.	Cal.	Carb.	Cal.	Carb.	Cal.	Carb.
Maxim 100% Freeze-Dried Coffee, 4-oz. jar (yield: approx. 63 servings)	190	47.7	0.5	0.13	4	trace	0.3	trace
"Suggested" serving, 1 level teaspoon, dry (yield: approx. 6 fl. oz.)	3	0.8	0.5	0.13	4	1.0	0.3	0.06
Maxwell House 6-oz. jar (yield: approx. 570 fl. oz., 95 servings)	297	74.5	0.5	0.13	4	1.0	0.3	0.06
"Suggested" serving, 1 level teaspoon, dry (yield: approx. 6 fl. oz.)	3	0.8	0.5	0.13	4	1.0	0.3	0.06
Nescafé 2-oz. jar (yield: approx. 180 fl. oz., 30 servings)	120	30.0	0.7	0.17	5	1.0	0.3	0.06
6-oz. jar (yield: approx. 540 fl. oz., 90 servings)	360	90.0	0.7	0.17	5	1.0	0.3	0.06
10-oz. jar (yield: approx. 900 fl. oz., 150 servings)	600	150.0	0.7	0.17	5	1.0	0.3	0.06
"Suggested" serving, 1 level teaspoon, dry (yield: approx. 6 fl. oz.)	4	1.0	0.7	0.17	5	1.0	0.3	0.06
Taster's Choice Freeze-Dried, 2-oz. jar (yield: approx. 180 fl. oz., 30 servings)	120	30.0	0.7	0.17	5	1.0	0.3	0.06
4-oz. jar (yield: approx. 360 fl. oz., 60 servings)	240	60.0	0.7	0.17	5	1.0	0.3	0.06
8-oz. jar (yield: approx. 720 fl. oz., 120 servings)	480	120.0	0.7	0.17	5	1.0	0.3	0.06
"Suggested" serving, 1 level teaspoon, dry (yield: approx. 6 fl. oz.)	4	1.0	0.7	0.17	5	1.0	0.3	0.06
Yuban 2-oz. jar (yield: approx. 180 fl. oz., 30 servings)	103	23.9	0.6	0.13	5	1.0	0.3	0.06
"Suggested" serving, 1 level teaspoon, dry (yield: approx. 6 fl. oz.)	3	0.8	0.6	0.13	5	1.0	0.3	0.06
DECAFFEINATED INSTANT								
Brim Freeze-Dried 4-oz. jar (yield: approx. 378 fl. oz., 63 servings)	208	52.2	0.6	0.14	4	1.1	0.3	0.07
"Suggested" serving, 1 level teaspoon, dry (yield: approx. 6 fl. oz.)	3	0.8	0.6	0.14	4	1.1	0.3	0.07
Decaf Instant Coffee, 2-oz. jar (yield: approx. 180 fl. oz., 30 servings)	120	30.0	0.7	0.17	5	1.3	0.3	0.08
4-oz. jar (yield: approx. 360 fl. oz., 60 servings)	240	60.0	0.7	0.17	5	1.3	0.3	0.08
8-oz. jar (yield: approx. 720 fl. oz., 120 servings)	480	120.0	0.7	0.17	5	1.3	0.3	0.08
"Suggested" serving, 1 level teaspoon, dry (yield: approx. 6 fl. oz.)	4	1.0	0.7	0.17	5	1.3	0.3	0.08
Nescafé Decaffeinated Freeze-dried Coffee, 2-oz. jar (yield: approx. 180 fl. oz., 30 servings)	120	30.0	0.7	0.17	6	1.3	0.4	0.08
4-oz. jar (yield: approx. 360 fl. oz., 60 servings)	240	60.0	0.7	0.17	6	1.3	0.4	0.08
8-oz. jar (yield: approx. 720 fl. oz., 120 servings)	480	120.0	0.7	0.17	6	1.3	0.4	0.08
"Suggested" serving, 1 level teaspoon, dry (yield: approx. 6 fl. oz.)	4	1.0	0.7	0.17	6	1.3	0.4	0.08
Sanka Freeze-dried 97% Caffeine Free Coffee, 4-oz. jar (yield: approx. 378 fl. oz., 63 servings)	227	52.2	0.6	0.14	5	1.1	0.3	0.07
"Suggested" serving, 1 level teaspoon, dry (yield: approx. 6 fl. oz.)	3	0.8	0.6	0.14	5	1.1	0.3	0.07
Instant 97% Caffeine Free Coffee, 2-oz. jar (yield: approx. 192 fl. oz., 32 servings)	103	23.6	0.5	0.12	4	1.0	0.3	0.06
"Suggested" serving, 1 level teaspoon, dry (yield: approx. 6 fl. oz.)	3	0.7	0.5	0.12	4	1.0	0.3	0.06
Taster's Choice Decaffeinated Freeze-dried Coffee, 2-oz. jar (yield: approx. 180 fl. oz., 30 servings)	120	30.0	0.7	0.17	6	1.3	0.4	0.08
4-oz. jar (yield: approx. 360 fl. oz., 60 servings)	240	60.0	0.7	0.17	6	1.3	0.4	0.08
8-oz. jar (yield: approx. 720 fl. oz., 120 servings)	480	120.0	0.7	0.17	6	1.3	0.4	0.08
"Suggested" serving, 1 level teaspoon, dry (yield: approx. 6 fl. oz.)	4	1.0	0.7	0.17	6	1.3	0.4	0.08

	UNIT		1 FLUID OZ.		1 CUP		1 TABLE-SPOON	
	Cal.	Carb.	Cal.	Carb.	Cal.	Carb.	Cal.	Carb.
FLAVORED COFFEES								
Almond Mocha Coffee, **Hills Bros.,** 8-oz. can (yield: approx. 96 fl. oz., 16 servings)	960	176.0	10.0	1.83	80	14.7	5.0	0.92
"Suggested" serving, 2 rounded teaspoons, dry (yield: approx. 6 fl. oz.)	60	11.0	10.0	1.83	80	14.7	5.0	0.92
Bavarian Mint Coffee, **Hills Bros.,** 8-oz. can (yield: approx. 96 fl. oz., 16 servings)	928	192.0	9.7	2.00	77	16.0	4.8	1.00
"Suggested" serving, 2 rounded teaspoons, dry (yield: approx. 6 fl. oz.)	58	12.0	9.7	2.00	77	16.0	4.8	1.00
Café Français Coffee, **General Foods International Coffees,** 8-oz. tin (yield: approx. 138 fl. oz., 23 servings)	(1380)	(234.6)	10.0	1.70	80	13.6	5.0	0.85
"Suggested" serving, 2 heaping teaspoons (1.1 tablespoons), dry (yield: approx. 6 fl. oz.)	60	10.2	10.0	1.70	80	13.6	5.0	0.85
Café Mocha Coffee, **Hills Bros.,** 8-oz. can (yield: approx. 96 fl. oz., 16 servings)	928	192.0	9.7	2.00	78	16.0	4.9	1.00
"Suggested" serving, 2 rounded teaspoons, dry (yield: approx. 6 fl. oz.)	58	12.0	9.7	2.00	78	16.0	4.9	1.00
Café Vienna Coffee, **General Foods International Coffees,** 10-oz. tin (yield: approx. 174 fl. oz., 29 servings)	(1750)	(315.0)	10.0	1.83	80	14.7	5.0	0.92
"Suggested" serving, 2 heaping teaspoons (1.1 tablespoons), dry (yield: approx. 6 fl. oz.)	60	11.0	10.0	1.83	80	14.7	5.0	0.92
Suisse Mocha Coffee, **General Foods International Coffees,** 8-oz. tin (yield: approx. 156 fl. oz., 26 servings)	(1380)	(160.0)	10.0	1.17	80	9.3	5.0	0.58
"Suggested" serving, 2 heaping teaspoons (1.1 tablespoons), dry (yield: approx. 6 fl. oz.)	60	7.0	10.0	1.17	80	9.3	5.0	0.58
Toffee Mocha Coffee, **Hills Bros.,** 8-oz. can (yield: approx. 96 fl. oz., 16 servings)	800	208.0	8.3	2.17	66	17.3	4.1	1.08
"Suggested" serving, 2 rounded teaspoons, dry (yield: approx. 6 fl. oz.)	50	13.0	8.3	2.17	66	17.3	4.1	1.08
COFFEE SUBSTITUTES and CEREAL BEVERAGES								
Cafix no caffeine Instant Natural Cereal Beverage, 1¾-oz. tin (yield: approx. 198 fl. oz., 33 servings)	(231)	(24.4)	0.9	0.09	7	0.7	0.4	0.04
7-oz. tin (yield: approx. 798 fl. oz., 133 servings)	(931)	(98.4)	0.9	0.09	7	0.7	0.4	0.04
"Suggested" serving, 1 level teaspoon, dry (yield: approx. 6 fl. oz.)	7	0.7	0.9	0.09	7	0.7	0.4	0.04
Coffisub Coffee Substitute, 4-oz. box. 32 bags [yield: approx. 6 quarts (24 cups)]	179	trace	0.9	trace	8	trace	trace	trace
1 bag, prepared as label directs, adding 6 fl. oz. water (yield: approx. 6 fl. oz.)	6	trace	0.9	trace	8	trace	trace	trace
Kathreiner's Malzkaffee Ready Beverage Cereal Beverage, 8.8-oz. box								
1 serving, prepared as label directs, adding 6 fl. oz. water (yield: approx. 6 fl. oz.)	7	1.6	1.1	0.26	9	2.0	0.6	0.13
Mellow Roast Brewed Ground Coffee & Grain (Wheat) Beverage, 16-oz. (1-lb.) can (yield: approx. 384 fl. oz., 64 servings)	424	95.5	1.1	0.25	9	2.2	0.6	0.14
"Suggested" serving, 1 tablespoon (¼ oz.), dry (yield: approx. 6 fl. oz.)	7	1.5	1.1	0.25	9	2.2	0.6	0.14
Instant Coffee & Grain (Wheat & Molasses) Beverage, 8-oz. jar (yield: approx. 504 fl. oz., 84 servings)	669	145.6	1.3	0.29	8	2.3	0.5	0.14
"Suggested" serving, 1 rounded teaspoon, dry (yield: approx. 6 fl. oz.)	8	1.7	1.3	0.29	8	2.3	0.5	0.14

	UNIT		1 FLUID OZ.		1 CUP		1 TABLESPOON	
	Cal.	Carb.	Cal.	Carb.	Cal.	Carb.	Cal.	Carb.
Pero Instant Cereal Beverage, 1¾-oz. tin (yield: approx. 186 fl. oz., 31 servings)	188	43.2	(0.8)	(0.18)	(6)	(1.4)	(0.4)	(0.08)
3½-oz. tin (yield: approx. 378 fl. oz., 63 servings)	377	86.3	(0.8)	(0.18)	(6)	(1.4)	(0.4)	(0.08)
7-oz. tin (yield: approx. 756 fl. oz., 126 servings)	754	172.7	(0.8)	(0.18)	(6)	(1.4)	(0.4)	(0.08)
"Suggested" serving, 1 level teaspoon, dry (yield: approx. 6 fl. oz.)	(6)	1.4	(0.8)	(0.18)	(6)	(1.4)	(0.4)	(0.08)
Postum Instant Cereal Beverage, 4-oz. package, 50 envelopes, 300 oz.	500	100.0	1.7	0.33	13	2.6	0.8	0.16
1 envelope, prepared as label directs, adding 6 fl. oz. water (yield: approx. 6 fl. oz.)	10	2.0	1.7	0.33	13	2.6	0.8	0.16
TEA								
Lipton Tea Bags, 16-bag box	(32)	(8.0)	(0.3)	(0.08)	(2)	(0.5)	(0.1)	(0.03)
48-bag box	(96)	(24.0)	(0.3)	(0.08)	(2)	(0.5)	(0.1)	(0.03)
100-bag box	(200)	(50.0)	(0.3)	(0.08)	(2)	(0.5)	(0.1)	(0.03)
Instant Tea, 4-oz. jar (yield: approx. 8 fl. oz.)	(0)	(0.0)	(0.0)	(0.00)	(0)	(0.0)	(0.0)	(0.00)
Nestea Instant Tea, 1-oz. jar	(0)	(0.0)	(0.0)	(0.00)	(0)	(0.0)	(0.0)	(0.00)
Tender Leaf Tea, 16-bag package	(16)	(0.0)	(0.1)	(0.00)	(1)	(0.0)	(0.1)	(0.00)
FLAVORED TEAS								
Almond Pleasure Tea, **Lipton Herbal Tea,** 16-bag box	(96)	(16.0)	(0.8)	(0.13)	(6)	(1.0)	(0.4)	(0.06)
Apricot Flavored Tea, **Rose,** 4-oz. tin	(0)	(0.0)	(0.0)	(0.00)	(0)	(0.0)	(0.0)	(0.00)
Assam Tea, **Twinings,** 227- and 113-gram tins	(0)	(0.0)	(0.0)	(0.00)	(0)	(0.0)	(0.0)	(0.00)
Black Tea, **Brooke Bond,** 1 tea bag	2	trace	0.3	trace	2	trace	0.1	trace
Black Currant Flavor Tea, **Rose,** 4-oz. tin	(0)	(0.0)	(0.0)	(0.00)	(0)	(0.0)	(0.0)	(0.00)
Black Rum Tea, **Lipton Flavored Tea,** 16-bag box	(32)	(8.0)	(0.3)	(0.06)	(2)	(0.5)	(0.1)	(0.03)
Ceylon Afternoon Tea, **Olde London,** 125-gram tin (4.4 oz.)	(0)	(0.0)	(0.0)	(0.00)	(0)	(0.0)	(0.0)	(0.00)
Ceylon Breakfast Tea, **Twinings,** 227- and 113-gram tins	(0)	(0.0)	(0.0)	(0.00)	(0)	(0.0)	(0.0)	(0.00)
Chamomile Tea, **Hunza,** 20-bag box	(0)	(0.0)	(0.0)	(0.00)	(0)	(0.0)	(0.0)	(0.00)
(Quietly) Chamomile Tea, **Lipton Herbal Tea,** 16-bag box	(32)	(8.0)	(0.3)	(0.06)	(2)	(0.5)	(0.1)	(0.03)
China Black Tea, **Twinings,** 227- and 113-gram tins	(0)	(0.0)	(0.0)	(0.00)	(0)	(0.0)	(0.0)	(0.00)
Cinnamon Tea, **Lipton Flavored Tea,** 16-bag box	(32)	(8.0)	(0.3)	(0.06)	(2)	(0.5)	(0.1)	(0.03)
Darjeeling Tea, **Olde London,** 125-gram tin (4.4 oz.)	(0)	(0.0)	(0.0)	(0.00)	(0)	(0.0)	(0.0)	(0.00)
Twinings, 227- and 113-gram tins	(0)	(0.0)	(0.0)	(0.00)	(0)	(0.0)	(0.0)	(0.00)
(Vintage) Darjeeling Tea, **Twinings,** 227- and 113-gram tins	(0)	(0.0)	(0.0)	(0.00)	(0)	(0.0)	(0.0)	(0.00)
Dinner Tea, **China Bowl,** 16-bag package (1.25 oz.)	(0)	(0.0)	(0.0)	(0.00)	(0)	(0.0)	(0.0)	(0.00)
Earl Grey Tea, **Olde London,** 125-gram tin (4.4 oz.)	(0)	(0.0)	(0.0)	(0.00)	(0)	(0.0)	(0.0)	(0.00)
Rose, 4-oz. tin	(0)	(0.0)	(0.0)	(0.00)	(0)	(0.0)	(0.0)	(0.00)
Twinings, 227- and 113-gram tins	(0)	(0.0)	(0.0)	(0.00)	(0)	(0.0)	(0.0)	(0.00)
English Breakfast Tea, **Olde London,** 125-gram tin (4.4 oz.)	(0)	(0.0)	(0.0)	(0.00)	(0)	(0.0)	(0.0)	(0.00)
Twinings, 227- and 113-gram tins	(0)	(0.0)	(0.0)	(0.00)	(0)	(0.0)	(0.0)	(0.00)
Formosa Oolong Tea, **Twinings,** 227- and 113-gram tins	(0)	(0.0)	(0.0)	(0.00)	(0)	(0.0)	(0.0)	(0.00)
Fruit, **Tisa,** Instant Tea Beverage Cubes, 2-oz. box	(216)	(56.7)	(3.4)	(0.89)	(27)	(7.1)	(1.7)	(0.44)
Green Gunpowder Tea, **Twinings,** 227- and 113-gram tins	(0)	(0.0)	(0.0)	(0.00)	(0)	(0.0)	(0.0)	(0.00)
Gunpowder Green Tea, **Rose,** 4-oz. tin	(0)	(0.0)	(0.0)	(0.00)	(0)	(0.0)	(0.0)	(0.00)
Hibiscus Red Tea, **Lipton Herbal Tea,** 16-bag box	32	(8.0)	0.3	(0.06)	2	(0.5)	0.1	(0.03)

	UNIT		1 FLUID OZ.		1 CUP		1 TABLESPOON	
	Cal.	Carb.	Cal.	Carb.	Cal.	Carb.	Cal.	Carb.
Irish Breakfast Tea, **Twining's,** 8-oz. tin (yield: approx. 100 cups)	(0)	(0.0)	(0.0)	(0.00)	(0)	(0.0)	(0.0)	(0.00)
Jasmine Tea, **Rose,** 4-oz. tin	(0)	(0.0)	(0.0)	(0.00)	(0)	(0.0)	(0.0)	(0.00)
Twining's, 8-oz. tin (yield: approx. 100 cups)	(0)	(0.0)	(0.0)	(0.00)	(0)	(0.0)	(0.0)	(0.00)
Keemun China Tea, **Olde London,** 125-gram tin (4.4 oz.)	(0)	(0.0)	(0.0)	(0.00)	(0)	(0.0)	(0.0)	(0.00)
Lapsang Souchong Tea, **Rose,** 4-oz. tin	(0)	(0.0)	(0.0)	(0.00)	(0)	(0.0)	(0.0)	(0.00)
Twining's, 8-oz. tin (yield: approx. 100 cups)	(0)	(0.0)	(0.0)	(0.00)	(0)	(0.0)	(0.0)	(0.00)
Lemon Tea, **Olde London,** 125-gram tin	(0)	(0.0)	(0.0)	(0.00)	(0)	(0.0)	(0.0)	(0.00)
Twining's, 8-oz. tin (yield: approx. 100 cups)	(0)	(0.0)	(0.0)	(0.00)	(0)	(0.0)	(0.0)	(0.00)
Lemon Flavor Tea, **Nestea,** 2-oz. container (yield: approx. 65 6-oz. servings)	(130)	(9.8)	(0.3)	(0.03)	(3)	(0.2)	(0.2)	(0.01)
4-oz. container (yield: approx. 130 6-oz. servings)	(260)	(19.5)	(0.3)	(0.03)	(3)	(0.2)	(0.2)	(0.01)
0.9 grams (yield: approx. 6 fl. oz.)	(2)	(0.2)	(0.3)	(0.03)	(3)	(0.2)	(0.2)	(0.01)
Lemon Rose Tea, **Rose,** 4-oz. tin	(0)	(0.0)	(0.0)	(0.00)	(0)	(0.0)	(0.0)	(0.00)
Lemon Scented Tea, **Rose,** 4-oz. tin	(0)	(0.0)	(0.0)	(0.00)	(0)	(0.0)	(0.0)	(0.00)
Lemon & Spice Tea, **Lipton Flavored Tea,** 16-bag box	32	(8.0)	0.3	(0.06)	2	(0.5)	0.1	(0.03)
Lime Scented Tea, **Rose,** 4-oz. tin	(0)	(0.0)	(0.0)	(0.00)	(0)	(0.0)	(0.0)	(0.00)
Mint Tea, **Lipton Tea,** 16-bag box	32	(8.0)	0.3	(0.06)	2	(0.5)	0.1	(0.03)
Rose, 4-oz. tin	(0)	(0.0)	(0.0)	(0.00)	(0)	(0.0)	(0.0)	(0.00)
(Dessert) Mint Tea, **Lipton Herbal Tea,** 16-bag box	32	(8.0)	0.3	(0.06)	2	(0.5)	0.1	(0.03)
Orange Blossom Scented Tea, **Rose,** 4-oz. tin	(0)	(0.0)	(0.0)	(0.00)	(0)	(0.0)	(0.0)	(0.00)
(Gentle) Orange Tea, **Lipton Herbal Tea,** 16-bag box	32	(8.0)	0.3	(0.06)	2	(0.5)	0.1	(0.03)
Orange Pekoe Tea, **Twining's,** 8-oz. tin (yield: approx. 100 cups)	(0)	(0.0)	(0.0)	(0.00)	(0)	(0.0)	(0.0)	(0.00)
Orange Scented Tea, **Rose,** 4-oz. tin	(0)	(0.0)	(0.0)	(0.00)	(0)	(0.0)	(0.0)	(0.00)
Orange & Spice Tea, **Lipton Flavored Tea,** 16-bag box	32	(8.0)	0.3	(0.06)	2	(0.5)	0.1	(0.03)
Peach Flavored Tea, **Rose,** 4-oz. tin	(0)	(0.0)	(0.0)	(0.00)	(0)	(0.0)	(0.0)	(0.00)
Peppermint Tea, **Hain,** 20-bag box	(0)	(0.0)	(0.0)	(0.00)	(0)	(0.0)	(0.0)	(0.00)
Tisa, Instant Beverage cubes, 2-oz. box (yield: approx. 8 cups)	(224)	(56.7)	(3.5)	(0.89)	(28)	(7.1)	(1.8)	(0.44)
0.25-oz. cube (yield: approx. 1 cup)	(28)	(7.1)	(3.5)	(0.89)	(28)	(7.1)	(1.8)	(0.44)
Prince of Wales Tea, **Twining's,** 8-oz. tin (yield: approx. 100 cups)	(0)	(0.0)	(0.0)	(0.00)	(0)	(0.0)	(0.0)	(0.00)
Queen Mary Tea, **Twining's,** 8-oz. tin (yield: approx. 100 cups)	(0)	(0.0)	(0.0)	(0.00)	(0)	(0.0)	(0.0)	(0.00)
Rose Hips, **Hunza,** 20-bag box	(0)	(0.0)	(0.0)	(0.00)	(0)	(0.0)	(0.0)	(0.00)
Tisa, Instant Tea Beverage Cubes, 2-oz. box (yield: approx. 8 cups)	(208)	(56.7)	(3.3)	(0.89)	(26)	(7.1)	(1.6)	(0.44)
0.25 cube (yield: approx. 1 cup)	(26)	(7.1)	(3.3)	(0.89)	(26)	(7.1)	(1.6)	(0.44)
Royal Rose Tea, **Rose,** 4-oz. tin	(0)	(0.0)	(0.0)	(0.00)	(0)	(0.0)	(0.0)	(0.00)
Russian Tea, **Rose,** 4-oz. tin	(0)	(0.0)	(0.0)	(0.00)	(0)	(0.0)	(0.0)	(0.00)
Russian Caravan Tea, **Twining's,** 8-oz. tin (yield: approx. 100 cups)	(0)	(0.0)	(0.0)	(0.00)	(0)	(0.0)	(0.0)	(0.00)
Spearmint Tea, **Hunza,** 20-bag box	(0)	(0.0)	(0.0)	(0.00)	(0)	(0.0)	(0.0)	(0.00)
(Toasty) Spice Tea, **Lipton Herbal Tea,** 16-bag box	32	(8.0)	0.3	(0.04)	2	(0.5)	0.1	(0.03)
Spiced Tea, **Rose,** 4-oz. tin	(0)	(0.0)	(0.0)	(0.00)	(0)	(0.0)	(0.0)	(0.00)
Twining's, 8-oz. tin (yield: approx. 100 cups)	(0)	(0.0)	(0.0)	(0.00)	(0)	(0.0)	(0.0)	(0.00)
ICED TEA, Ready-to-Serve								
Lipton Lemon Flavored Iced Tea, 12-fl.-oz. can	135	33.0	11.3	2.75	90	22.0	5.6	1.38
16-fl.-oz. (1-pint) bottle	(173)	(42.7)	(10.8)	(2.67)	(87)	(2.7)	(5.4)	(0.17)
Sugar-free, 10-fl.-oz. can	(2)	(0.0)	(0.2)	(0.00)	(1)	(0.0)	(0.1)	(0.00)

	UNIT		1 FLUID OZ.		1 CUP		1 TABLESPOON	
	Cal.	Carb.	Cal.	Carb.	Cal.	Carb.	Cal.	Carb.
Shasta Iced Tea, 12-fl.-oz. can	121	33.0	10.1	2.75	81	22.0	5.1	1.38
Diet Iced Tea, 12-fl.-oz. can	0	0.0	0.0	0.00	0	0.0	0.0	0.00
Weight Watchers diet Iced Tea, 12-fl.-oz. can	(4)	(1.0)	(0.3)	(0.08)	(3)	(0.7)	(0.2)	(0.04)
ICED TEA MIXES								
Lipton, Lemon Flavored Instant Tea (40 to 80 servings per container) 4 fl. oz. [yield: approx. 20 quarts (80 cups)]	(320)	(80.0)	(0.5)	(0.13)	(4)	(1.0)	(0.3)	(0.06)
1 cup, prepared	(4)	(1.0)	(0.5)	(0.13)	(4)	(1.0)	(0.3)	(0.06)
Nestea Lemon Flavored Iced Tea, 4-oz. container (yield: approx. 90 8-oz. servings)	(180)	(18.9)	(0.3)	(0.03)	(2)	(0.2)	(0.1)	(0.01)
2-oz. container (yield: approx. 45 8-oz. servings)	(90)	(9.5)	(0.3)	(0.03)	(2)	(0.2)	(0.1)	(0.01)
1 cup, prepared	(2)	(0.2)	(0.3)	(0.03)	(2)	(0.2)	(0.1)	(0.01)
Lemon & Sugar Iced Tea Mix, 3.2-oz. envelope (yield: approx. five 6-oz. servings)	(350)	(85.0)	(11.7)	(2.83)	(94)	(22.7)	(5.9)	(1.42)
1.6 oz. (10-envelope box)	(1750)	(425.0)	(11.7)	(2.83)	(94)	(22.7)	(5.9)	(1.42)
1.6-oz. envelope (yield: approx. 2½ 6-oz. servings)	(175)	(42.5)	(11.7)	(2.83)	(94)	(22.7)	(5.9)	(1.42)
Salada, 32-oz. (2-lb.) canister	1802	(436.2)						
Prepared as label directs, adding 10 quarts water [yield: approx. 10 quarts (40 cups)]	1802	(436.2)	5.6	(1.36)	45	(10.9)	2.8	0.68
24-oz. canister	1351	(327.1)						
Prepared as label directs, adding 7½ quarts water [yield: approx. 7½ quarts (30 cups)]	1351	(327.1)	5.6	(1.36)	45	(10.9)	2.8	0.68
Mint, 24-oz. canister	1351	(327.1)						
Prepared as label directs, adding 7½ quarts water [yield: approx. 7½ quarts (30 cups)]	1351	(327.1)	5.6	(1.36)	45	(10.9)	2.8	0.68
32-oz. (2-lb.) canister	1802	(436.2)						
Prepared as label directs, adding 10 quarts water [yield: approx. 10 quarts (40 cups)]	1802	(436.2)	5.6	(1.36)	45	(10.9)	2.8	0.68

13 FATS & OILS •

TABLE FATS

	UNIT Cal.	UNIT Carb.	1 OZ., BY WT. Cal.	1 OZ., BY WT. Carb.	1 CUP Cal.	1 CUP Carb.	1 TABLESPOON Cal.	1 TABLESPOON Carb.
BUTTER, based on generic data								
NOT WHIPPED:								
1 stick, 4 oz. net wt. (approx. ½ cup)	812	0.5	203.0	0.11	1625	0.9	102	0.1
1 cup (approx. 8 oz. net wt., 2 of the sticks)	1625	0.9	203.0	0.11	1625	0.9	102	0.1
1 pound (approx. 2 cups) (0g/0g/23g/16%/280mg)	3248	1.8	203.0	0.11	1625	0.9	102	0.1
1 teaspoon (approx. ⅙ oz., 1/24 of the stick)	34	trace	203.0	0.11	1625	0.9	102	0.1
1 tablespoon (approx. ½ oz., ⅛ of the stick)	102	0.1	203.0	0.11	1625	0.9	102	0.1
1 "pat," 1" × 1" × ⅓" high (approx. 0.18 oz., 90 pats per pound)	36	trace	203.0	0.11	1625	0.9	102	0.1
1 cubic inch (approx. ½ oz.)	105	0.1	203.0	0.11	1625	0.9	102	0.1
WHIPPED:								
1 stick, 2⅔ oz. net wt. (approx. ½ cup)	541	0.3	203.0	0.11	1081	0.6	67	trace
1 cup (approx. 2 of the sticks, or ⅔ of an 8-oz. container)	1081	0.6	203.0	0.11	1081	0.6	67	trace
1 pound (approx. 3 cups) (0g/0g/23g/16%/280mg)	3248	1.8	203.0	0.11	1081	0.6	67	trace
1 teaspoon (approx. ⅑ oz., 1/24 of the stick)	23	trace	203.0	0.11	1081	0.6	67	trace
1 tablespoon (approx. ⅓ oz., ⅛ of the stick)	67	trace	203.0	0.11	1081	0.6	67	trace
1 "pat," 1¼" × 1¼" × ⅓" high (approx. 0.13 oz., 120 pats per pound)	27	trace	203.0	0.11	1081	0.6	67	trace
For comparison: Mayonnaise, 1 pound (approx. 2.1 cups)	3258	9.9	203.6	0.62	1580	4.8	101	0.3
For comparison: Peanut butter, 1 pound (approx. 1¾ cups)	2672	85.3	167.0	5.33	1520	48.5	95	3.0
BUTTER, by brand								
Including regular and whipped butters.								
Land O'Lakes Lightly Salted, Sweet Cream Butter, 16-oz. (1-lb.) carton (4 sticks)	3240	0.0	202.5	0.00	1600	0.0	100	0.0
4-oz. stick	810	0.0	202.5	0.00	1600	0.0	100	0.0
Unsalted Sweet Butter, 16-oz. (1-lb.) carton (4 sticks)	3240	0.0	202.5	0.00	1600	0.0	100	0.0
4-oz. stick	810	0.0	202.5	0.00	1600	0.0	100	0.0
Whipped Sweet Cream Butter, 16-oz. (1-lb.) package (2 8-oz. tubs)	3240	0.0	202.5	0.00	960	0.0	60	0.0
8-oz. tub	1620	0.0	202.5	0.00	960	0.0	60	0.0
Whipped Unsalted Sweet Cream Butter, 16-oz. (1-lb.) package (2 8-oz. tubs)	3240	0.0	202.5	0.00	960	0.0	60	0.0
8-oz. tub	1620	0.0	202.5	0.00	960	0.0	60	0.0
Meadow Gold Butter, 16-oz. (1-lb.) carton	3150	0.0	196.9	0.00	1680	0.0	105	0.0
Pantry Pride Lightly Salted Butter, 16-oz. (1-lb.) carton	3375	0.0	210.9	0.00	1800	0.0	113	0.0
MARGARINE, based on generic data								
REGULAR OR SOFT, BUT NOT WHIPPED:								
1 stick, [approx. 4 oz. net wt. (approx. ½ cup)]	816	0.5	204.1	0.11	1634	0.9	102	0.1
1 cup (approx. 8 oz. net wt., 2 sticks)	1634	0.9	204.1	0.11	1634	0.9	102	0.1
1 pound (approx. 2 cups) (0g/0g/23g/16%/280mg)	3266	1.8	204.1	0.11	1634	0.9	102	0.1
1 teaspoon (approx. ⅙ oz., 1/24 of the stick)	34	trace	204.1	0.11	1634	0.9	102	0.1
1 tablespoon (approx. ½ oz., ⅛ of the stick)	102	0.1	204.1	0.11	1634	0.9	102	0.1
1 "pat," 1" × 1" × ⅓" high (approx. 0.18 oz., approx. 90 pats per pound)	36	trace	204.1	0.11	1634	0.9	102	0.1
1 cubic inch (approx. ½ oz.)	106	0.1	204.1	0.11	1634	0.9	102	0.1
WHIPPED:								
1 stick [approx. 2⅔ oz. net wt. (approx. ½ cup)]	544	0.3	204.1	0.11	1087	0.6	68	trace
1 cup (approx. 2 sticks)	1087	0.6	204.1	0.11	1087	0.6	68	trace
1 pound [6 sticks (approx. 3 cups)] (0g/0g/23g/16%/280mg)	3266	1.8	204.1	0.11	1087	0.6	68	trace
1 teaspoon (approx. ⅑ oz., 1/24 of the stick)	23	trace	204.1	0.11	1087	0.6	68	trace
1 tablespoon (approx. ⅓ oz., ⅛ of the stick)	68	trace	204.1	0.11	1087	0.6	68	trace
1 "pat," 1¼" × 1¼" × ⅓" high (approx. 13% of 1 oz., approx. 120 pats per pound)	27	trace	204.1	0.11	1087	0.6	68	trace
MARGARINE, by brand								
Including regular and whipped margarines, and diet margarines and spreads.								
Allsweet Margarine, 16-oz. (1-lb.) carton (4 sticks)	3200	0.0	200.0	0.00	1600	0.0	100	0.0
4-oz. stick	800	0.0	200.0	0.00	1600	0.0	100	0.0

	UNIT		1 OZ., BY WT.		1 CUP		1 TABLESPOON	
	Cal.	Carb.	Cal.	Carb.	Cal.	Carb.	Cal.	Carb.
A&P Corn Oil Table Spread Margarine, 16-oz. (1-lb.) carton (4 sticks)	3200	0.0	200.0	0.00	1600	0.0	100	0.0
4-oz. stick	800	0.0	200.0	0.00	1600	0.0	100	0.0
Premium Margarine, 16-oz. (1-lb.) carton (4 sticks)	3200	0.0	200.0	0.00	1600	0.0	100	0.0
4-oz. stick	800	0.0	200.0	0.00	1600	0.0	100	0.0
Ann Page (A&P) Margarine, 16-oz. (1-lb.) carton (4 sticks)	3200	0.0	200.0	0.00	1600	0.0	100	0.0
4-oz. stick	800	0.0	200.0	0.00	1600	0.0	100	0.0
Autumn Margarine, 16-oz. (1-lb.) carton (2 8-oz. tubs)	3200	0.0	200.0	0.00	1600	0.0	100	0.0
8-oz. tub	1600	0.0	200.0	0.00	1600	0.0	100	0.0
Blue Bonnet Diet Margarine, 16-oz. (1-lb.) carton	1600	0.0	100.0	0.00	800	0.0	50	0.0
Margarine, 16-oz. (1-lb.) carton (4 sticks)	3200	0.0	200.0	0.00	1600	0.0	100	0.0
4-oz. stick	800	0.0	200.0	0.00	1600	0.0	100	0.0
Soft Margarine, 16-oz. (1-lb.) carton (2 8-oz. tubs)	3200	0.0	200.0	0.00	1600	0.0	100	0.0
8-oz. tub	1600	0.0	200.0	0.00	1600	0.0	100	0.0
Spread, 16-oz. (1-lb.) carton	2560	0.0	160.0	0.00	1280	0.0	80	0.0
Stick margarine, 16-oz. (1-lb.) carton	3200	0.0	200.0	0.00	1600	0.0	100	0.0
"25% less fat and calories" Light Tasty Spread, 32-oz. (2-lb.) tub	5120	0.0	160.0	0.00	1280	0.0	80	0.0
Whipped Soft Margarine, 16-oz. (1-lb.) carton	3360	0.0	210.0	0.00	1120	0.0	70	0.0
Whipped Stick Margarine, 16-oz. (1-lb.) carton	3360	0.0	210.0	0.00	1120	0.0	70	0.0
Chiffon "Lite" Spread, 16-oz. (1-lb.) carton	2442	0.0	153.0	0.00	1120	0.0	70	0.0
Regular Soft Margarine, 16-oz. (1-lb.) carton	3200	0.0	200.0	0.00	1600	0.0	100	0.0
Stick margarine, 16-oz. (1-lb.) carton	3200	0.0	200.0	0.00	1600	0.0	100	0.0
Sweet Unsalted Margarine, 16-oz. (1-lb.) carton	3200	0.0	200.0	0.00	1600	0.0	100	0.0
Whipped Soft Margarine, 16-oz. (1-lb.) carton	3175	0.0	198.0	0.00	1120	0.0	70	0.0
Coldbrook Soft Spread Margarine, 16-oz. (1-lb.) carton	2560	0.0	160.0	0.00	1280	0.0	80	0.0
Dalewood Margarine, 16-oz. (1-lb.) carton	3200	0.0	200.0	0.00	1600	0.0	100	0.0
Empress Corn Oil Margarine, 16-oz. (1-lb.) carton	3200	0.0	200.0	0.00	1600	0.0	100	0.0
Soft Corn Oil Margarine, 16-oz. (1-lb.) carton	3200	0.0	200.0	0.00	1600	0.0	100	0.0
Vegetable Oil Margarine, 16-oz. (1-lb.) carton	3200	0.0	200.0	0.00	1600	0.0	100	0.0
Fleischmann's Diet Margarine, 16-oz. (1-lb.) carton (2 8-oz. tubs)	1600	0.0	100.0	0.00	800	0.0	50	0.0
8-oz. tub	800	0.0	100.0	0.00	800	0.0	50	0.0
100% Corn Oil Margarine, 16-oz. (1-lb.) carton	3200	0.0	200.0	0.00	1600	0.0	100	0.0
Soft Corn Oil Margarine, 16-oz. (1-lb.) carton	3200	0.0	200.0	0.00	1600	0.0	100	0.0
Spread, 32-oz. (2-lb.) carton	5120	0.0	160.0	0.00	1280	0.0	80	0.0
Stick Margarine, 16-oz. (1-lb.) carton	3200	0.0	200.0	0.00	1600	0.0	100	0.0
Unsalted Stick Margarine, 16-oz. (1-lb.) carton	3200	0.0	200.0	0.00	1600	0.0	100	0.0
Hain Safflower Oil Margarine, 16-oz. (1-lb.) carton	3200	0.0	200.0	0.00	1600	0.0	100	0.0
Holiday Margarine, 16-oz. (1-lb.) carton	3200	0.0	200.0	0.00	1600	0.0	100	0.0
Hollywood Safflower Oil Margarine, 16-oz. (1-lb.) carton	3200	0.0	200.0	0.00	1600	0.0	100	0.0
Imperial Margarine, 16-oz. (1-lb.) carton	3200	0.0	200.0	0.00	1600	0.0	100	0.0
Soft Diet Margarine, 16-oz. (1-lb.) carton	1595	0.6	99.7	0.04	798	0.3	50	trace
Soft Spread Margarine, 16-oz. (1-lb.) carton	3259	2.7	203.7	0.17	1630	1.4	102	0.1
Soft Whipped Margarine, 16-oz. (1-lb.) carton	3259	2.7	203.7	0.17	1040	0.9	65	0.1
Stick Margarine, 16-oz. (1-lb.) carton	3200	0.0	200.0	0.00	1600	0.0	100	0.0
Keller's Margarine, 16-oz. (1-lb.) carton	3200	0.0	200.0	0.00	1600	0.0	100	0.0
Kingston Soft Margarine, 16-oz. (1-lb.) carton	3200	0.0	200.0	0.00	1600	0.0	100	0.0
Land O'Lakes Corn Oil Margarine, 16-oz. (1-lb.) carton (4 sticks)	3200	0.0	200.0	0.00	1600	0.0	100	0.0
4-oz. stick	800	0.0	200.0	0.00	1600	0.0	100	0.0
Mazola Diet Imitation Margarine, 16-oz. (1-lb.) carton	1600	0.0	100.0	0.00	800	0.0	50	0.0
Margarine with Corn Oil, 16-oz. (1-lb.) carton	3200	0.0	200.0	0.00	1600	0.0	100	0.0
No Stick Margarine, 16-oz. (1-lb.) carton	3200	0.0	200.0	0.00	1600	0.0	100	0.0
Unsalted Sweet Margarine, 16-oz. (1-lb.) carton	3200	0.0	200.0	0.00	1600	0.0	100	0.0
Monarch Margarine, 16-oz. (1-lb.) carton (4 sticks)	3712	0.4	232.0	0.00	1856	0.0	116	0.0
4-oz. stick	928	0.1	232.0	0.00	1856	0.0	116	0.0
Mother's Margarine, 16-oz. (1-lb.) carton (4 sticks)	3200	0.0	200.0	0.00	1600	0.0	100	0.0
4-oz. stick	800	0.0	200.0	0.00	1600	0.0	100	0.0
Mrs. Filbert's Golden Quarters Margarine, 16-oz. (1-lb.) carton	3200	0.0	200.0	0.00	1600	0.0	100	0.0
100% Corn Oil Margarine, 16-oz. (1-lb.) carton	3200	0.0	200.0	0.00	1600	0.0	100	0.0
4-oz. stick	800	0.0	200.0	0.00	1600	0.0	100	0.0
Soft Golden Margarine, 16-oz. (1-lb.) carton	3200	0.0	200.0	0.00	1600	0.0	100	0.0
Parkay Light Spread Margarine, 16-oz. (1-lb.) carton	2275	0.0	142.2	0.00	1120	0.0	70	0.0
Margarine, 16-oz. (1-lb.) carton (4 sticks)	3200	0.0	200.0	0.00	1600	0.0	100	0.0
4-oz. stick	800	0.0	200.0	0.00	1600	0.0	100	0.0
Soft Margarine, 16-oz. (1-lb.) carton	3200	0.0	200.0	0.00	1600	0.0	100	0.0
Squeeze Margarine, 16-oz. (1-lb.) carton	3200	0.0	200.0	0.00	1600	0.0	100	0.0
Whipped Margarine, 16-oz. (1-lb.) carton	3200	0.0	200.0	0.00	960	0.0	60	0.0
Promise Stick Margarine, 16-oz. (1-lb.) carton	3200	0.0	200.0	0.00	1600	0.0	100	0.0
Sunflower Oil Margarine, 16-oz. (1-lb.) carton (4 sticks)	3200	0.0	200.0	0.00	1600	0.0	100	0.0
4-oz. stick	800	0.0	200.0	0.00	1600	0.0	100	0.0
Sunflower Oil Soft Margarine, 16-oz. (1-lb.) carton	3200	0.0	200.0	0.00	1600	0.0	100	0.0
Ralph's Soft Corn Oil Margarine, 16-oz. (1-lb.) carton	3200	0.0	200.0	0.00	1600	0.0	100	0.0
Saffola Cube Margarine, 16-oz. (1-lb.) carton	3200	0.0	200.0	0.00	1600	0.0	100	0.0
Soft Margarine, 16-oz. (1-lb.) carton	3200	0.0	200.0	0.00	1600	0.0	100	0.0
Scotch Buy Soft Margarine, 16-oz. (1-lb.) tub	3200	0.0	200.0	0.00	1600	0.0	100	0.0
Vegetable Oil Margarine, 16-oz. (1-lb.) carton (2 8-oz. patties)	3200	0.0	200.0	0.00	1600	0.0	100	0.0
8-oz. patty	1600	0.0	200.0	0.00	1600	0.0	200	0.0
Shedd's Reduced Fat Content Vegetable Oil Table Spread, 32-oz. (2-lb.) tub	5120	0.0	160.0	0.00	1280	0.0	80	0.0
Whipped Margarine, 8-oz. tub	1600	0.0	200.0	0.00	1120	0.0	70	0.0
Weight Watchers Imitation Margarine, 16-oz. (1-lb.) carton	1512	0.0	94.5	0.00	800	0.0	50	0.0
Willow Run Soybean Margarine, 16-oz. (1-lb.) carton (4 sticks)	3200	0.0	200.0	0.00	1600	0.0	100	0.0
4-oz. stick	800	0.0	200.0	0.00	1600	0.0	100	0.0

SALAD AND COOKING OILS

SALAD AND COOKING OILS, based on generic data

	UNIT		1 OZ., BY WT.		1 CUP		1 TABLESPOON	
	Cal.	Carb.	Cal.	Carb.	Cal.	Carb.	Cal.	Carb.
Apricot Kernel Oil, 1 quart (approx. 30.8 oz. net wt.) (0g/0g/28g/0%/0mg)	7708	0.0	250.6	0.00	1927	0.0	120	0.0
Cocoa (cacao) butter, 1 quart (approx. 30.8 oz. net wt.) (0g/0g/28g/0%/0mg)	7708	0.0	250.6	0.00	1927	0.0	120	0.0
Coconut Oil (based on data from East Asia), 1 pound	4005	0.0	250.3	0.00				
Corn Oil, 1 quart (approx. 30.9 oz. net wt.) (0g/0g/28g/0%/0mg)	7708	0.0	250.6	0.00	1927	0.0	120	0.0
Cottonseed Oil, 1 quart (approx. 30.9 oz. net wt.) (0g/0g/28g/0%/0mg)	7708	0.0	250.6	0.00	1927	0.0	120	0.0

	UNIT		1 OZ., BY WT.		1 CUP		1 TABLESPOON	
	Cal.	Carb.	Cal.	Carb.	Cal.	Carb.	Cal.	Carb.
Fish Liver Oil (based on data from India), 1 pound	4082	0.0	255.2	0.00				
Grapeseed Oil, 1 quart (approx. 30.9 oz. net wt.) (0g/0g/28g/0%/0mg)	7708	0.0	250.6	0.00	1927	0.0	120	0.0
Hazelnut Oil, 1 quart (approx. 30.9 oz. net wt.) (0g/0g/28g/0%/0mg)	7708	0.0	250.6	0.00	1927	0.0	120	0.0
Linseed Oil, 1 quart (approx. 30.9 oz. net wt.) (0g/0g/28g/0%/0mg)	7708	0.0	250.6	0.00	1927	0.0	120	0.0
Nutmeg Butter, 1 quart (approx. 30.9 oz. net wt.) (0g/0g/28g/0%/0mg)	7708	0.0	250.6	0.00	1927	0.0	120	0.0
Olive Oil, 1 quart (approx. 30.5 oz. net wt.) (0g/0g/28g/0%/0mg)	7638	0.0	250.6	0.00	1910	0.0	119	0.0
Olive Oil (based on data from Italy), 1 pound	4082	0.0	255.2	0.00				
Palm Kernel Oil, 1 quart (approx. 30.9 oz. net wt.) (0g/0g/28g/0%/0mg)	7708	0.0	250.6	0.00	1927	0.0	120	0.0
Peanut Oil, 1 quart (approx. 30.5 oz. net wt.) (0g/0g/28g/0%/0mg)	7638	0.0	250.6	0.00	1910	0.0	119	0.0
Safflower Oil, 1 quart (approx. 30.9 oz. net wt.) (0g/0g/28g/0%/0mg)	7708	0.0	250.6	0.00	1927	0.0	120	0.0
Sesame Oil, 1 quart (approx. 30.9 oz. net wt.) (0g/0g/28g/0%/0mg)	7708	0.0	250.6	0.00	1927	0.0	120	0.0
Soybean Oil, 1 quart (approx. 30.9 oz. net wt.) (0g/0g/28g/0%/0mg)	7708	0.0	250.6	0.00	1927	0.0	120	0.0
Soybean-Cottonseed Oil Blend, 1 quart (approx. 30.9 oz. net wt.) (0g/0g/28g/0%/0mg)	7708	0.0	250.6	0.00	1927	0.0	120	0.0
SALAD AND COOKING OILS, by brand								
ALMOND OIL:								
Hain Pure Cold Pressed, 16-fl.-oz. (1-pint) bottle	3840	0.0	(250.0)	0.00	1920	0.0	120	0.0
CORN OIL:								
Arrowhead Mills, 16-fl.-oz. (1-pint) bottle	3840	0.0	(250.0)	0.00	1920	0.0	120	0.0
Deaf Smith Unrefined, 16-fl.-oz. (1-pint) bottle	3840	0.0	(250.0)	0.00	1920	0.0	120	0.0
Golden Harvest Pure, 32-fl.-oz. (1-quart) bottle	(7708)	0.0	(250.6)	0.00	(1927)	0.0	(120)	0.0
Hain Pure Cold Pressed, 16-fl.-oz. (1-pint) bottle	3840	0.0	(250.0)	0.00	1920	0.0	120	0.0
Hollywood, 32-fl.-oz. (1-quart) bottle	7680	0.0	(250.0)	0.00	1920	0.0	120	0.0
Hunza, 16-fl.-oz. (1-pint) bottle	3840	0.0	(250.0)	0.00	1920	0.0	120	0.0
Mazola, 16-fl.-oz. (1-pint) bottle	3840	0.0	(250.0)	0.00	1920	0.0	120	0.0
Nu Made, 16-fl.-oz. (1-pint) bottle	3840	0.0	(250.0)	0.00	1920	0.0	120	0.0
24-fl.-oz. bottle	5760	0.0	(250.0)	0.00	1920	0.0	120	0.0
32-fl.-oz. (1-quart) bottle	7680	0.0	(250.0)	0.00	1920	0.0	120	0.0
48-fl.-oz. bottle	11520	0.0	(250.0)	0.00	1920	0.0	120	0.0
OLIVE OIL:								
Arrowhead Mills, 16-fl.-oz. (1-pint) bottle	3840	0.0	(250.0)	0.00	1920	0.0	120	0.0
Avallo Blended 10%, 128-fl.-oz. (1-gallon) tin	(30720)	0.0	(250.0)	0.00	(1920)	0.0	(120)	0.0
Blended 20%, 128-fl.-oz. (1-gallon) tin	(30720)	0.0	(250.0)	0.00	(1920)	0.0	(120)	0.0
Hain Pure Cold Pressed (California Virgin), 6-fl.-oz. bottle	1440	0.0	(240.0)	0.00	1920	0.0	120	0.0
16-fl.-oz. (1-pint) bottle	3840	0.0	(240.0)	0.00	1920	0.0	120	0.0
Laco, 32-fl.-oz. (1-quart) tin	7638	0.0	(248.0)	0.00	1910	0.0	119	0.0
128-fl.-oz. (1-gallon) tin	30552	0.0	(248.0)	0.00	1910	0.0	119	0.0
Pompeian, 2-fl.-oz. bottle	477	0.0	(248.0)	0.00	1910	0.0	119	0.0
4-fl.-oz. bottle	955	0.0	(248.0)	0.00	1910	0.0	119	0.0
8-fl.-oz. bottle	1910	0.0	(248.0)	0.00	1910	0.0	119	0.0
16-fl.-oz. (1-pint) bottle	3819	0.0	(248.0)	0.00	1910	0.0	119	0.0
32-fl.-oz. (1-quart) tin	7638	0.0	(248.0)	0.00	1910	0.0	119	0.0
128-fl.-oz. (1-gallon) tin	30552	0.0	(248.0)	0.00	1910	0.0	119	0.0
Romanza, 128-fl.-oz. (1-gallon) tin	30552	0.0	(248.0)	0.00	1910	0.0	119	0.0
PEANUT OIL:								
Arrowhead Mills, 16-fl.-oz. (1-pint) bottle	3840	0.0	(250.0)	0.00	1920	0.0	120	0.0
Hain Pure Cold Pressed, 5-fl.-oz. bottle	1200	0.0	(250.0)	0.00	1920	0.0	120	0.0

	UNIT		1 OZ., BY WT.		1 CUP		1 TABLESPOON	
	Cal.	Carb.	Cal.	Carb.	Cal.	Carb.	Cal.	Carb.
Hollywood, 32-fl.-oz. (1-quart) bottle	7680	0.0	(250.0)	0.00	1920	0.0	120	0.0
Hunza, 16-fl.-oz. (1-pint) bottle	3840	0.0	(250.0)	0.00	1920	0.0	120	0.0
Planters, 24-fl.-oz. bottle	(6240)	0.0	(260.0)	0.00	(2080)	0.0	(130)	0.0
SAFFLOWER OIL:								
Arrowhead Mills, 16-fl.-oz. (1-pint) bottle	3840	0.0	(250.0)	0.00	1920	0.0	120	0.0
Deaf Smith Unrefined, 16-fl.-oz. (1-pint) bottle	3840	0.0	(250.0)	0.00	1920	0.0	120	0.0
Golden Harvest Pure Cold Pressed, 32-fl.-oz. (1-quart) bottle	(8320)	0.0	(250.6)	0.00	(2080)	0.0	(130)	0.0
Hain Cold Pressed SupEr E, 16-fl.-oz. (1-pint) bottle	3840	0.0	(250.0)	0.00	1920	0.0	120	0.0
Hollywood, 32-fl.-oz. (1-quart) bottle	7680	0.0	(250.0)	0.00	1920	0.0	120	0.0
Hunza, 16-fl.-oz. (1-pint) bottle	3840	0.0	(250.0)	0.00	1920	0.0	120	0.0
32-fl.-oz. (1-quart) bottle	7680	0.0	(250.0)	0.00	1920	0.0	120	0.0
Nu Made, 24-fl.-oz. bottle	5760	0.0	(250.0)	0.00	1920	0.0	120	0.0
SESAME OIL:								
Arrowhead Mills, 16-fl.-oz. (1-pint) bottle	3840	0.0	(250.0)	0.00	1920	0.0	120	0.0
China Bowl, 5-fl.-oz. bottle	1250	0.0	(250.0)	0.03	1920	0.0	120	trace
Hain Pure Cold Pressed, 6-fl.-oz. bottle	1440	0.0	(250.0)	0.00	1920	0.0	120	0.0
Hunza, 16-fl.-oz. (1-pint) bottle	3840	0.0	(250.0)	0.00	1920	0.0	120	0.0
SOYBEAN OIL:								
Arrowhead Mills, 16-fl.-oz. (1-pint) bottle	3840	0.0	(250.0)	0.00	1920	0.0	120	0.0
Hain Pure Cold Pressed Soy Oil, 16-fl.-oz. (1-pint) bottle	3840	0.0	(250.0)	0.00	1920	0.0	120	0.0
Hollywood Soy Salad Oil, 32-fl.-oz. (1-quart) bottle	7680	0.0	(250.0)	0.00	1920	0.0	120	0.0
Hunza Soy Oil, 16-fl.-oz. (1-pint) bottle	3840	0.0	(250.0)	0.00	1920	0.0	120	0.0
32-fl.-oz. (1-quart) bottle	7680	0.0	(250.0)	0.00	1920	0.0	120	0.0
Jewel, 16-fl.-oz. (1-pint) bottle	3840	0.0	(250.0)	0.00	1920	0.0	120	0.0
Sterling, 420-lb. industrial drum	1,612,-800	0.0	(250.0)	0.00	1920	0.0	120	0.0
SUNFLOWER OIL:								
Arrowhead Mills, 16-fl.-oz. (1-pint) bottle	3840	0.0	(250.0)	0.00	1920	0.0	120	0.0
Golden Harvest, 32-fl.-oz. (1-quart) bottle	(7708)	0.0	(250.6)	0.00	(1927)	0.0	(120)	0.0
Hain Pure Cold Pressed, 6-fl.-oz. bottle	1440	0.0	(250.0)	0.00	1920	0.0	120	0.0
Hollywood, 32-fl.-oz. (1-quart) bottle	7680	0.0	(250.0)	0.00	1920	0.0	120	0.0
Hunza, 16-fl.-oz. (1-pint) bottle	3840	0.0	(250.0)	0.00	1920	0.0	120	0.0
Sunlite, 32-fl.-oz. (1-quart) bottle	7680	0.0	(250.0)	0.00	1920	0.0	120	0.0
VEGETABLE OIL:								
Nu Made, 16-fl.-oz. (1-pint) bottle	3840	0.0	(250.0)	0.00	1920	0.0	120	0.0
24-fl.-oz. bottle	5760	0.0	(250.0)	0.00	1920	0.0	120	0.0
38-fl.-oz. bottle	9120	0.0	(250.0)	0.00	1920	0.0	120	0.0
48-fl.-oz. (3-pint) bottle	11520	0.0	(250.0)	0.00	1920	0.0	120	0.0
128-fl.-oz. (1-gallon) bottle	30720	0.0	(250.0)	0.00	1920	0.0	120	0.0
Puritan 100% Pure, 16-fl.-oz. (1-pint) bottle	3840	0.0	(250.0)	0.00	1920	0.0	120	0.0
WALNUT OIL:								
Hain Cold Pressed, 16-fl.-oz. (1-pint) bottle	3840	0.0	(250.0)	0.00	1920	0.0	120	0.0
WHEAT GERM OIL:								
Arrowhead Mills, 16-fl.-oz. (1-pint) bottle	3840	0.0	(250.0)	0.00	1920	0.0	120	0.0
Hain Pure Cold Pressed, 16-fl.-oz. (1-pint) bottle	3840	0.0	(250.0)	0.00	1920	0.0	120	0.0
BLENDED OILS:								
Arrowhead Mills Blended Oil, 16-fl.-oz. (1-pint) bottle	3840	0.0	(250.0)	0.00	1920	0.0	120	0.0
Crisco Soybean, Vegetable Oil, 12-fl.-oz. bottle	2880	0.0	(250.0)	0.00	1920	0.0	120	0.0
16-fl.-oz. (1-pint) bottle	3840	0.0	(250.0)	0.00	1920	0.0	120	0.0
24-fl.-oz. bottle	5760	0.0	(250.0)	0.00	1920	0.0	120	0.0
38-fl.-oz. bottle	9120	0.0	(250.0)	0.00	1920	0.0	120	0.0
48-fl.-oz. (3-pint) bottle	11520	0.0	(250.0)	0.00	1920	0.0	120	0.0
Hain Pure Cold Pressed (soy, walnut, peanut, and safflower oils), 64-fl.-oz. (2-quart) bottle	15360	0.0	(250.0)	0.00	1920	0.0	120	0.0
Hunza, 16-fl.-oz. (1-pint) bottle	3840	0.0	(250.0)	0.00	1920	0.0	120	0.0

	UNIT Cal.	UNIT Carb.	1 OZ., BY WT. Cal.	1 OZ., BY WT. Carb.	1 CUP Cal.	1 CUP Carb.	1 TABLESPOON Cal.	1 TABLESPOON Carb.
Saffola Salad Oil, 24-fl.-oz. bottle	5865	0.0	(253.8)	0.00	1955	0.0	122	0.0
SupEr E (soy, peanut, walnut, and safflower oils), 16-fl.-oz. (1-pint) bottle	3840	0.0	(250.0)	0.00	1920	0.0	120	0.0
OTHER OILS:								
China Bowl Hot Oil, 5-oz. bottle	1252	0.0	250.4	0.00	1920	0.0	120	0.0
Planters Popcorn Oil (oil *for,* not *from,* popcorn), 12-fl.-oz. bottle	(3120)	0.0	(260.0)	0.00	(2080)	0.0	(130)	0.0

COOKING AND BAKING FATS

	UNIT Cal.	UNIT Carb.	1 OZ., BY WT. Cal.	1 OZ., BY WT. Carb.	1 CUP Cal.	1 CUP Carb.	1 TABLESPOON Cal.	1 TABLESPOON Carb.
FATS, based on generic data								
Bacon Fat, 1 pound (tr/0g/28g/0%/tr)	4073	0.0	254.4	0.00				
Beef Drippings (based on data from Great Britain), 1 pound	4178	0.0	261.1	0.00				
Chicken Fat, 1 pound (approx. 2.2 cups) (0g/0g/28g/tr%/0mg)	2853	0.0	178.3	0.00	(1297)	0.0	(81)	0.0
Coconut Butter (based on data from the Middle East), 1 quart (approx. 30.9 oz. net wt.)	7762	0.0	251.2	0.00	1941	0.0	121	0.0
Duck Fat, 1 pound (0g/0g/28g/tr%/0mg)	4084	0.0	255.3	0.00	1846	0.0	115	0.0
Ghee (Butter Oil) (based on data from India), 1 pound	4082	0.0	255.2	0.00				
Goose Fat, 1 pound (0g/0g/28g/tr%/0mg)	4084	0.0	255.3	0.00	1846	0.0	115	0.0
Kidney Fat (tallow, suet) (based on data from the Caribbean), 1 pound	3874	0.0	242.1	0.00				
Lard, 1 pound (approx. 2.2 cups) (0g/0g/28g/0%/0mg)	4091	0.0	255.7	0.00	1849	0.0	117	0.0
Mutton Tallow, 1 pound (0g/0g/28g/0%/0mg)	4091	0.0	255.7	0.00	1849	0.0	115	0.0
Salt Pork (based on data from the Far East) as purchased, 1 pound (yield: approx. 14.9 oz.)	3016	0.0	188.5	0.00				
Edible portion, 14.9 oz. (yield from 1 lb. as purchased)	3227	0.0	201.7	0.00				
Suet (Beef) (based on data from France) 1 pound (1g/0g/28g/0%/4mg)	3701	0.0	231.3	0.00				
Turkey Fat, 1 pound (0g/0g/28g/0%/0mg)	4084	0.0	255.3	0.00	1846	0.0	115	0.0
SHORTENING, based on generic data								
1 cup (approx. 7¼ oz.)	1845	0.0	255.2	0.00	1845	0.0	115	0.0
1 pound (approx. 2.2 cups) (0g/0g/28g/0%/0mg)	4082	0.0	255.2	0.00	1845	0.0	115	0.0
1 tablespoon (approx. 0.45 oz.)	115	0.0	255.2	0.00	1845	0.0	115	0.0
1 teaspoon (approx. 0.15 oz.)	38	0.0	255.2	0.00	1845	0.0	115	0.0
1 container, 48-oz. (3-lbs.)	5535	0.0	255.2	0.00	1845	0.0	115	0.0
SHORTENING, by brand								
Crisco, 16-oz. (1-lb.) container	4180	0.0	261.3	0.00	1760	0.0	110	0.0
3-lb. container	12540	0.0	261.3	0.00	1760	0.0	110	0.0
6-lb. container	25080	0.0	261.3	0.00	1760	0.0	110	0.0
Fluffo, 3-lb. container	12430	0.0	259.0	0.00	1760	0.0	110	0.0
Light Spry, 2-lb. 10-oz. container	10608	0.0	252.6	0.00	1414	0.0	88	0.0

COOKING SPRAYS, by brand

	UNIT Cal.	UNIT Carb.	1 OZ., BY WT. Cal.	1 OZ., BY WT. Carb.	1 CUP Cal.	1 CUP Carb.	1 TABLESPOON Cal.	1 TABLESPOON Carb.
Mazola 2-Second Spray, 2.3 oz. container, 82 "sprays" per container	(600)	0.0	(260.0)	0.00				
"Suggested" spray, 2 seconds, approx. 0.8 grams	(8)	0.0	(260.0)	0.00				
Pam Vegetable Cooking Spray, 4.2-oz. container, 150 "sprays"	1050	0.0	248.1	0.00				
"Suggested" spray, 1¼ seconds, approx. 0.8 grams	(7)	0.0	248.1	0.00				

14 SUGARS, SWEETENERS & TOPPINGS •

	UNIT		1 OZ., BY WT.		1 CUP		1 TABLE-SPOON	
	Cal.	Carb.	Cal.	Carb.	Cal.	Carb.	Cal.	Carb.
SOLID SUGARS								
BROWN SUGAR, based on generic data								
1 tablespoon (not packed, 0.32 oz.)	34	8.7	105.8	27.33	541	139.8	34	8.7
1 cup:								
Not packed (approx. 5.1 oz.)	541	139.8	105.8	27.33	541	139.8	34	8.7
Packed (approx. 7¾ oz.)	821	212.1	105.8	27.33	821	212.1	51	13.3
1 pound (approx. 3 1/10 cups not packed; 2 cups packed) (0g/28g/0g/2%/9mg)	1692	437.3	105.8	27.33				
CINNAMON SUGAR								
French's, 3-oz. jar	317	79.1	105.5	25.37	768	192.0	48	12.0
1 teaspoon, approx. 0.15 oz.	16	4.0	105.5	25.37	768	192.0	48	12.0
For comparison: Cinnamon, 1 pound (1g/23g/1g/10%/7mg)	1184	361.8	74.0	22.61	288	86.9	18	5.4
CONFECTIONERS' SUGAR (10X OR POWDERED), based on generic data								
Unsifted:								
1 tablespoon (approx. 0.26 oz.)	29	7.5	109.1	28.21	462	119.4	29	7.5
1 cup (approx. 4¼ oz.)	462	119.4	109.1	28.21	462	119.4	29	7.5
1 pound (approx. 3¾ cups) (0g/28g/0g/1%/tr)	1746	451.3	109.1	28.21	462	119.4	29	7.5
Sifted:								
1 cup (approx. 3½ oz.)	385	99.5	109.1	28.21	385	99.5	24	6.2
1 pound (approx. 4½ cups)	1746	451.3	109.1	28.21	385	99.5	24	6.2
DEXTROSE								
Richter, Assorted Flavor Dextrose Cubes, 36-oz. box, 48 cubes	3827	1019.5	106.3	28.32				
1 cube, ¾ oz.	80	21.2	106.3	28.32				
FRUCTOSE								
Golden Harvest, 48-oz. package	5760	1360.8	120.0	28.35				
5-oz. box, 50 packets	600	141.8	120.0	28.35				
1 packet, 0.1 oz.	12	2.8	120.0	28.35				
MAPLE SUGAR, based on generic data								
1 piece, 1¾" × 1¼" × ½" (approx. 1 oz.)	99	25.5	99.0	25.50				
1 pound (0g/26g/0g/8%/na)	1584	408.0	99.0	25.50	(497)	(128.0)	(31)	(8.0)
TURBINADO SUGAR								
Hollywood, 24-oz. box	(2619)	(677.0)	(109.1)	(28.21)	(736)	(190.4)	(46)	(11.9)
3-lb. box	(5238)	(1354.1)	(109.1)	(28.21)	(736)	(190.4)	(46)	(11.9)
Sugar-in-the-Raw, 32-oz. (2-lb.) box	(3492)	(902.7)	(109.1)	(28.21)				
UNREFINED CANE SUGAR								
Sugar-in-the-Raw, 16-oz. (1-lb.) box	(1746)	(451.4)	(109.1)	(28.21)				
WHITE SUGAR (GRANULATED SUGAR), based on generic data								
1 tablespoon (approx. 0.44 oz.)	46	11.9	109.1	28.21	770	199.0	46	11.9
1 teaspoon (approx. 0.14 oz.)	15	4.0	109.1	28.21	770	199.0	46	11.9
1 lump, 1⅛" × ¾" × 5/16" (approx. 0.14 oz.)	15	3.9	109.1	28.21				
1 cube, ½" (approx. 0.08 oz.)	9	2.3	109.1	28.21				
1 restaurant-type packet (0.24 oz., approx. 1/33 cup)	26	6.7	109.1	28.21				
1 cup (approx. 7.1 oz.)	770	199.0	109.1	28.21	770	199.0	46	11.9
1 pound (approx. 2¼ cups) (0g/28g/0g/1%/tr)	1746	451.3	109.1	28.21	770	199.0	46	11.9
SUGAR SUBSTITUTES, by brand								
Dia-Mel Sweet 'n It "No Calorie," 5-oz. jar	0	0.0	0.0	0.00	0	0.0	0	0.0
Equal Low-Calorie Sweetener, 1.75 oz. box, 50 packets	200	(45.5)	114.3	(25.97)				
1 packet, 0.04 oz. (equivalent sweetness of 2 teaspoons sugar)	4	(0.9)	114.3	(25.97)				
Featherweight Liquid Sweetening, 8-oz. package	0	0.0	0.0	0.00	0	0.0	0	0.0
Saccharin, .28 package, 500 tablets	0	0.0	0.0	0.00	0	0.0	0	0.0
¼-grain tablet (approx. 16.2 mg.)	0	0.0	0.0	0.00	0	0.0	0	0.0
Milani Sugar Twin Brown Bulk, 1.7-oz. box	181	45.8	106.3	26.93	528	135.3	33	8.5
1 teaspoon (approx. 0.10 oz.)	11	0.4	106.3	26.93	528	135.3	33	8.5
White Bulk, 7.13-oz. box	758	192.0	106.3	26.93	528	135.3	33	8.5
1 teaspoon (approx. 0.10 oz.)	11	0.4	106.3	26.93	528	135.3	33	8.5
White Sugar Twin packets, 28.2-oz. box, 1,000 packets	3000	760.0	106.3	26.93	528	135.3	33	8.5
1 packet, 0.03 oz. (equivalent sweetness of 2 teaspoons sugar)	3	0.8	106.3	26.93	528	135.3	33	8.5
Pillsbury Sprinkle Sweet, 4½-oz. package	464	116.0	103.1	25.78	96	24.0	6	1.5
Equivalent sweetness of 1 teaspoon sugar, 0.02 oz.	2	0.5	103.1	25.78	96	24.0	6	1.5
Sweet-10, 12-fl.-oz. container	0	0.0	0.0	0.00	0	0.0	0	0.0

	UNIT		1 OZ., BY WT.		1 CUP		1 TABLE-SPOON	
	Cal.	Carb.	Cal.	Carb.	Cal.	Carb.	Cal.	Carb.
Slim-ette Liquid Sugarless Sweetener, 6-fl.-oz. bottle	0	0.0	0.0	0.00	0	0.0	0	0.0
Sweet 'n Low Brown or White, 8-oz. box	794	204.2	99.2	25.52				
3.6-oz. box, 100 packets	357	81.7	99.2	25.52				
1.8-oz. box, 50 packets	179	45.0	99.2	25.52				
1 packet, 0.035 oz.	4	0.9	99.2	25.52				
Sweet Magic Sugar Substitute, 3.2-oz. box	0	0.0	0.0	0.00	0	0.0	0	0.0
2.12-oz. box, 100 packets	0	0.0	0.0	0.00	0	0.0	0	0.0
1 packet, 0.02 oz.	0	0.0	0.0	0.00	0	0.0	0	0.0
Weight Watchers Granulated Sweet'ner, 1¾-oz. box, 50 packets	200	45.0	114.3	25.71				
3.5-oz. box, 100 packets	400	90.0	114.3	25.71				
4.2-oz. box, 120 packets	480	108.0	114.3	25.71				
1 packet, 0.04 oz.	4	0.9	114.3	25.71				
Zero-Cal Liquid Sweetener, 8-fl.-oz. bottle	0	0.0	0.0	0.00	0	0.0	0	0.0
SYRUPS, based on generic data								
CANE JUICE, concentrated								
1 teaspoon (approx. ¼ oz.)	17	4.5	73.8	19.01	832	214.4	52	13.4
1 cup (approx. 11¼ oz.)	832	214.4	73.8	19.01	832	214.4	52	13.4
1 pound (approx. 1.4 cups)	1180	304.2	73.8	19.01	832	214.4	52	13.4
For comparison: Cane Juice for drinking (based on data from the Far East), 1 cup (approx. 11¼ oz.)	(179)	(47.8)	15.9	4.25	(179)	(47.8)	(11)	(3.0)
For comparison: Sugar Cane Stalks, Peeled (based on data from the Far East), 1 pound	304	79.8	19.0	4.99				
CANE SYRUP								
1 teaspoon (approx. ¼ oz.)	19	4.8	80.6	20.60	909	232.3	57	14.5
1 cup (approx. 11¼ oz.)	909	232.3	80.6	20.60	909	232.3	57	14.5
1 pound (approx. 1.4 cups)	1289	329.7	80.6	20.60	909	232.3	57	14.5
(Based on data from the Far East) 1 cup (approx. 11¼ oz.)	(826)	(213.8)	73.4	(19.00)	(826)	(213.8)	(52)	(13.4)
CORN SYRUP, light or dark								
1 tablespoon (approx. 0.72 oz.)	59	15.4	82.2	21.26	951	246.0	59	15.4
1 cup (approx. 11½ oz.)	951	246.0	82.2	21.26	951	246.0	59	15.4
1 pound (approx. 1.4 cups) (0/21g/0/24%/19mg)	1315	340.2	82.2	21.26	951	246.0	59	15.4
1 16-fl.-oz. (1-pint) bottle	1905	492.8	82.2	21.26	951	246.0	59	15.4
HONEY, strained or extracted								
1 tablespoon (approx. 0.74 oz.)	64	17.4	86.2	23.33	1031	279.0	64	17.4
1 cup (approx. 11.9 oz.)	1031	279.0	86.2	23.33	1031	279.0	64	17.4
1 pound (approx. 1⅓ cups) (tr/23g/0g/17%/1mg)	1379	373.3	86.2	23.33	1031	279.0	64	17.4
1 16-oz. (1-lb.) jar	1379	373.3	86.2	23.33	1031	279.0	64	17.4
(Based on data from Africa) 1 pound (approx. 1⅓ cups)	1411	363.4	88.2	22.71	(1050)	(270.2)	(66)	(16.9)
(Based on data from the Caribbean), 1 pound (approx. 1⅓ cups)	1315	358.3	82.2	22.40	(978)	(266.6)	(61)	(16.7)
(Based on data from Great Britain), 1 pound (approx. 1⅓ cups)	1387	346.6	86.7	21.66	(1032)	(257.8)	(65)	(16.1)
(Based on data from Japan), 1 pound (approx. 1⅓ cups)	1393	359.3	87.0	22.46	(1035)	(267.3)	(65)	(16.7)
(Based on data from Latin America), 1 pound (approx. 1⅓ cups)	1388	353.8	86.3	22.11	(1033)	(263.1)	(65)	(16.4)
MAPLE SYRUP								
1 tablespoon (approx. 0.70 oz.)	50	12.8	71.4	18.43	794	204.8	50	12.8
1 cup (approx. 11.1 oz.)	794	204.8	71.4	18.43	794	204.8	50	12.8
1 pound (approx. 1.44 cups) (na/18g/na/33%/3mg)	1142	294.9	71.4	18.43	794	204.8	50	12.8
1 12-fl.-oz. bottle	1189	306.9	71.4	18.43	794	204.8	50	12.8
MOLASSES, CANE								
BARBADOS MOLASSES:								
1 tablespoon (approx. 0.73 oz.)	56	14.4	76.8	19.84	889	229.6	56	14.4
1 cup (approx. 11½ oz.)	889	229.6	76.8	19.84	889	229.6	56	14.4
1 pound (approx. 1⅖ cups) (na/20g/na/24%/na)	1229	317.4	76.8	19.84	889	229.6	56	14.4
1 12-fl.-oz. bottle	1332	344.4	76.8	19.84	889	229.6	56	14.4

	UNIT		1 OZ., BY WT.		1 CUP		1 TABLE-SPOON	
	Cal.	Carb.	Cal.	Carb.	Cal.	Carb.	Cal.	Carb.
LIGHT MOLASSES, First extraction:								
1 tablespoon (approx. 0.73 oz.)	52	13.3	71.4	18.43	827	213.2	52	13.3
1 cup (approx. 11½ oz.)	827	213.2	71.4	18.43	827	213.2	52	13.3
1 pound (approx. 1⅖ cups) (na/18g/na/24%/4mg)	1142	294.9	71.4	18.43	827	213.2	52	13.3
1 12-fl.-oz. bottle	1242	320.5	71.4	18.43	827	213.2	52	13.3
MEDIUM MOLASSES, Second extraction:								
1 tablespoon (approx. 0.73 oz.)	48	12.3	65.8	17.01	761	196.8	48	12.3
1 cup (approx. 11½ oz.)	761	196.8	65.8	17.01	761	196.8	48	12.3
1 pound (approx. 1⅖ cups) (na/17g/na/24%/10mg)	1053	272.2	65.8	17.01	761	196.8	48	12.3
1 12-fl.-oz. bottle	1144	295.8	65.8	17.01	761	196.8	48	12.3
BLACKSTRAP MOLASSES, Third extraction:								
1 tablespoon (approx. 0.73 oz.)	44	11.3	60.4	15.60	699	180.4	44	11.3
1 cup (approx. 11½ oz.)	699	180.4	60.4	15.60	699	180.4	44	11.3
1 pound (approx. 1⅖ cups) (na/16g/na/24%/27mg)	966	249.6	60.4	15.60	699	180.4	44	11.3
1 12-fl.-oz. bottle	1050	271.2	60.4	15.60	699	180.4	44	11.3
SORGHUM								
1 tablespoon (approx. 0.73 oz.)	53	14.0	72.9	19.28	848	224.4	53	14.0
1 cup (approx. 11.6 oz.)	848	224.4	72.9	19.28	848	224.4	53	14.0
1 pound (approx. 1.4 cups) (na/19g/na/23%/na)	1166	308.4	72.9	19.28	848	224.4	53	14.0
1 12-fl.-oz. bottle	1272	336.6	72.9	19.28	848	224.4	53	14.0
TABLE BLENDS								
CHIEFLY CORN SYRUP:								
1 tablespoon (approx. 0.72 oz.)	59	15.4	82.2	21.26	951	246.0	59	15.4
1 cup (approx. 11½ oz.)	951	246.0	82.2	21.26	951	246.0	59	15.4
1 pound (approx. 1.4 cups) (0/21g/0/24%/19mg)	1315	340.2	82.2	21.26	951	246.0	59	15.4
1 12-fl.-oz. bottle	1427	369.0	82.2	21.26	951	246.0	59	15.4
CANE AND MAPLE MIXTURE:								
1 tablespoon (approx. 0.70 oz.)	50	12.8	71.4	18.43	794	204.8	50	12.8
1 cup (approx. 11.1 oz.)	794	204.8	71.4	18.43	794	204.8	50	12.8
1 pound (approx. 1.4 cups) (0g/18g/0g/33%/tr)	1142	294.9	71.4	18.43	794	204.8	50	12.8
1 12-fl.-oz. bottle	1189	306.8	71.4	18.43	784	204.8	50	12.8
SYRUPS AND TOPPINGS, based on generic data								
"THIN" SYRUP, CHOCOLATE FLAVORED								
1 can, 12 fl. oz. (approx. 1 lb.) (1g/18g/1g/32%/17mg)	1111	284.4	69.4	17.78	735	188.1	46	11.8
1 cup (approx. 10.6 oz.)	735	188.1	69.4	17.78	735	188.1	46	11.8
1 fl. oz. (approx. 1.3 oz.)	92	23.5	69.4	17.78	735	188.1	46	11.8
"THICK," FUDGE TYPE, CHOCOLATE FLAVORED								
1 can, 12 fl. oz. (approx. 1 lb.) (2g/15g/5g/25%/30mg)	1497	244.9	93.6	15.31	990	162.0	62	10.1
1 cup (approx. 10.6 oz.)	990	162.0	93.6	15.31	990	162.0	62	10.1
1 fl. oz. (approx. 1.3 oz.)	124	20.3	93.6	15.31	990	162.0	62	10.1
SYRUPS AND TOPPINGS, by brand								
Apricot syrup, **Smucker's,** 12-fl.-oz. jar	1200	312.0	74.6	19.40	800	208.0	50	13.0
Blackberry syrup, **Smucker's,** 12-fl.-oz. jar	1200	312.0	74.6	19.40	800	208.0	50	13.0
Blueberry syrup, reduced calorie, **Featherweight,** 7¾-fl.-oz. bottle	217	46.5	(19.7)	(4.23)	224	48.0	14	3.0
Blueberry syrup, **Smucker's,** 12-fl.-oz. jar	1200	312.0	74.6	19.40	800	208.0	50	13.0
Boysenberry syrup, **Smucker's,** 12-fl.-oz. jar	1200	312.0	74.6	19.40	800	208.0	50	13.0
Butterscotch artificially flavored topping, **Kraft,** 12-oz. jar	1047	209.4	87.3	17.45	960	192.0	60	12.0
Butterscotch flavored topping, **Smucker's,** 6-fl.-oz. jar	560	132.1	93.3	22.02	1120	264.0	70	16.5
18.5-fl.-oz. jar	1727	407.1	93.3	22.02	1120	264.0	70	16.5
Caramel topping, **Kraft,** 12-oz. jar	872	209.4	72.7	17.45	800	192.0	50	12.0

	UNIT		1 OZ., BY WT.		1 CUP		1 TABLESPOON	
	Cal.	Carb.	Cal.	Carb.	Cal.	Carb.	Cal.	Carb.
Caramel topping, chocolate flavored, **Kraft,** 12-oz. jar	872	209.4	72.7	17.45	800	192.0	50	12.0
Caramel flavored topping, **Smucker's,** 6-fl.-oz. jar	560	132.0	93.3	22.02	1120	264.0	70	16.5
18.5-fl.-oz. jar	1680	396.0	93.3	22.02	1120	264.0	70	16.5
Cherry topping, **Smucker's,** 6-fl.-oz. jar	520	128.1	88.5	21.35	1040	256.0	65	16.0
Chocolate flavored syrup, **Bosco,** 11-oz. jar	750	195.0	68.2	17.73	800	208.0	50	13.0
Chocolate flavored syrup, **Hershey's,** 5½-oz. can	495	121.0	90.0	22.00	(720)	(176.0)	(45)	(11.0)
24-oz. bottle	2160	528.0	90.0	22.00	(720)	(176.0)	(45)	(11.0)
Chocolate flavored topping, **Kraft,** 12-oz. jar	872	209.4	72.7	17.45	800	192.0	50	12.0
Chocolate flavored syrup, **Milk-Mate,** 20-oz. bottle	1500	360.6	75.0	18.03	(795)	(191.1)	(50)	(11.9)
36-oz. bottle	2700	649.1	75.0	18.03	(795)	(191.1)	(50)	(11.9)
Chocolate flavored syrup topping, **Smucker's,** 11.75-fl.-oz. jar	1040	216.0	88.5	18.38	1040	216.0	65	13.5
17.75-fl.-oz. jar	1560	326.2	88.5	18.38	1040	216.0	65	13.5
Chocolate flavored topping, low calorie, **Tillie Lewis** "Tasti-Diet," 8-oz. jar	128	32.0	16.0	4.00	128	32.0	8	2.0
Chocolate Fudge topping, **Hershey's,** 16-oz. (1-lb.) can	1440	160.0	90.0	10.00	(720)	(80.0)	(45)	(5.0)
Chocolate Fudge topping, **Smucker's,** 6-fl.-oz. jar	520	124.1	86.7	20.68	1040	248.0	65	15.5
18-fl.-oz. jar	1561	324.2	86.7	20.68	1040	248.0	65	15.5
Chocolate Fudge topping, Swiss Milk, **Smucker's,** 12-fl.-oz. jar	1121	248.1	93.4	20.68	1121	248.0	70	15.5
Chocolate-Mint Fudge Topping, **Smucker's,** 12-fl.-oz. jar	1121	248.1	93.4	20.68	1120	248.0	70	15.5
Choco-Syp and topping, low calorie, **Dia-Mel,** 8-oz. jar	225	45.0	28.1	5.63	240	48.0	15	3.0
Corn syrup, dark, **Karo,** 16-fl.-oz. (1-pint) bottle	1920	480.0	(82.8)	(20.71)	960	240.0	60	15.0
Corn syrup, light, **Karo,** 16-fl.-oz. (1-pint) bottle	1920	480.0	(82.8)	(20.71)	960	240.0	60	15.0
Maple syrup, imitation, **Karo,** 24-fl.-oz. bottle	2820	720.0	(82.8)	(20.71)	960	240.0	60	15.0
Maple syrup, imitation, **Log Cabin,** 24-fl.-oz. bottle	2400	624.0	(74.6)	(19.40)	800	208.0	50	13.0
Maple syrup, imitation, "buttered," **Log Cabin,** 24-fl.-oz. bottle	2400	624.0	(74.6)	(19.40)	800	208.0	50	13.0
Maple flavored syrup, 100% natural, **Staley,** 1.5-fl.-oz. pack	170	42.0	78.3	19.40	906	224.0	57	14.0
Maple Honey flavor syrup, imitation, **Log Cabin,** 24-fl.-oz. bottle	2400	672.0	(74.6)	(20.89)	800	224.0	50	14.0
Marshmallow topping, **Kraft,** 7-oz. jar	569	146.4	81.3	20.91	560	144.0	35	9.0
41-oz. jar	895	230.1	81.3	20.91	560	144.0	35	9.0
Molasses, **Brer Rabbit** "Green Label," 12-fl.-oz. bottle	804	260.8	(46.2)	(15.00)	536	173.9	34	10.9
Pancake syrup, reduced calorie, **Diet Delight,** 12-fl.-oz. bottle	329	94.0	(19.3)	(5.52)	219	62.6	14	4.0
Pancake syrup, reduced calorie, **Featherweight,** 7¾-fl.-oz. bottle	248	62.0	(22.5)	(5.64)	256	64.0	16	4.0
Pancake syrup, **Golden Griddle,** 16-fl.-oz. (1-pint) bottle	1600	448.0	(74.6)	(20.89)	800	224.0	50	14.0
Pancake & Waffle syrup, **Karo,** 16-fl.-oz. (1-pint) bottle	1920	480.0	(82.8)	(20.71)	960	240.0	60	15.0
Pancake syrup, **Mrs. Butterworth's,** 24-fl.-oz. bottle	2560	624.0	(76.8)	(18.72)	853	208.0	53	13.0
36-fl.-oz. bottle	3840	936.0	(76.8)	(18.72)	853	208.0	53	13.0
Pancake & Waffle topping, reduced calorie, **Tillie Lewis** "Tasti-Diet," 12-fl.-oz. bottle	100	25.0	(5.9)	(1.47)	67	16.7	4	1.0
Pancake or Table Syrup, **Winston,** (commonly served in restaurants), 1½-fl.-oz. container	(174)	(42.0)			(928)	(224.0)	(58)	(14.0)
Papaya Concentrate, **Golden Harvest,** 32-fl.-oz. (1-quart) bottle	1440	352.0			360	88.0	23	5.6
Peanut Butter Caramel topping, **Smucker's,** 11.5-fl.-oz. jar	1226	237.0	106.6	20.61	1226	237.0	75	14.5
Pecans in syrup topping, **Smucker's,** 4-fl.-oz. jar	418	90.0	104.5	22.50	1040	224.0	65	14.0
Pineapple topping, **Kraft,** 12-oz. jar	872	226.8	72.7	18.90	800	208.0	50	13.0
Pineapple topping, **Smucker's,** 6-fl.-oz. jar	520	128.1	86.7	21.34	1040	256.0	65	16.0
18-fl.-oz. jar	1561	384.2	86.7	21.34	1040	256.0	65	16.0
Red Raspberry syrup, **Smucker's,** 12-fl.-oz. jar	1200	312.0	74.6	19.40	800	208.0	50	13.0
Rice syrup, **Yinnies,** 16-oz. (1-lb.) jar	1371	347.4	85.7	21.71	(997)	(252.7)	(62)	(15.8)
Strawberry syrup, **Smucker's,** 12-fl.-oz. jar	1200	312.0	74.6	19.40	800	208.0	50	13.0
Strawberry topping, **Kraft,** 12-oz. jar	872	226.8	72.7	18.90	800	208.0	50	13.0
Strawberry topping, **Smucker's,** 6-fl.-oz. jar	480	120.1	80.0	20.02	960	240.0	60	15.0
11.75-fl.-oz. jar	940	235.1	80.0	20.02	960	240.0	60	15.0
Table syrup, reduced calorie, **Dia-Mel,** 8-fl.-oz. jar	240	60.0	(21.4)	(5.36)	240	60.0	15	3.8
Table syrup, reduced calorie, **E. D. Smith,** 8-fl.-oz. jar	307	67.2	(27.4)	(6.00)	307	67.2	19	4.2
Walnut topping, **Kraft,** 5-oz. jar	654	72.7	130.8	14.54	1440	160.0	90	10.0
Walnuts in syrup topping, **Smucker's,** 5-fl.-oz. jar	523	108.6	104.6	21.72	1040	216.0	65	13.5

WHIPPED TOPPINGS, based on generic data

	UNIT		1 OZ., BY WT.		1 CUP		1 TABLESPOON	
	Cal.	Carb.	Cal.	Carb.	Cal.	Carb.	Cal.	Carb.
DAIRY *(arranged in ascending order of fat content)*								
Sweetened Condensed Milk, canned, 8.7% fat, 1 cup	982	166.5	91.0	15.42	982	166.5	61	10.4
Half-and-Half (milk and cream) Cream, 11.5% fat, 1 cup (approx. 8.8 oz.)	324	11.1	36.9	1.22	324	11.1	20	0.7
Light Whipping Cream, 30.9% fat, 1 cup (approx. 8.4 oz.)	699	7.1	82.8	0.84	699	7.1	44	0.4
whipped, 1 cup (approx. 4.2 oz.)	350	3.6	82.8	0.84	350	3.6	22	0.2
Heavy Whipping Cream, 37% fat, 1 cup (approx. 8.4 oz.)	821	6.6	97.8	0.79	821	6.6	51	0.4
whipped, 1 cup (approx. 4.2 oz.)	411	3.3	97.8	0.79	411	3.3	26	0.2
NONDAIRY								
Powdered Topping containing Lauric Acid Oil and Sodium Caseinate (Lauric oils include modified coconut oil, hydrogenated coconut oil and/or palm kernel oil.):								
Unprepared: 1.5 oz. (common amount used for mixing) 11g/4g/1g/1%/35mg)	245	22.3	163.4	14.88				
Prepared: Mix 1.5 oz. powdered dessert topping with ½ cup whole milk (yield: approx. 2 cups, 5.6 oz.) (4g/5g/1g/67%/66mg)	302	26.4	53.9	4.69	151	13.2	8	0.7
1 tablespoon (approx. 0.18 oz.)	8	0.7	53.9	4.69	151	13.2	8	0.7
1 cup (approx. 2.8 oz.)	151	13.2	53.9	4.69	151	13.2	8	0.7
PRESSURIZED TOPPING:								
1 tablespoon (approx. 0.14 oz.)	11	0.6	74.5	4.58	184	11.3	12	0.7
1 cup (approx. 2.5 oz.)	184	11.3	74.5	4.58	184	11.3	12	0.7
SEMISOLID (FROZEN) TOPPING:								
1 tablespoon (approx. 0.14 oz.)	15	1.1	90.3	6.54	239	17.3	15	1.1
1 cup (approx. 2.6 oz.)	239	17.3	90.3	6.54	239	17.3	15	1.1

WHIPPED TOPPINGS (NONDAIRY), by brand

	UNIT		1 OZ., BY WT.		1 CUP		1 TABLESPOON	
	Cal.	Carb.	Cal.	Carb.	Cal.	Carb.	Cal.	Carb.
Dieter's Gourmet Whipped Topping Mix, 1.6-oz. package	256	0.0	160.0	0.00	128	0.0	8	0.0
Dream Whip Whipped Topping Mix, 6 oz.	512	64.0	85.3	10.67				
Prepared with milk	640	64.0	20.0	2.00	160	16.0	10	1.0
Featherweight Whipped Topping, 2.5-oz. package	(30)	(5.0)	(12.0)	(2.00)	48	8.0	3	0.5

	UNIT		1 OZ., BY WT.		1 CUP		1 TABLE-SPOON	
	Cal.	Carb.	Cal.	Carb.	Cal.	Carb.	Cal.	Carb.
Heller's Whirl Whip Frozen Dessert Topping, 10-oz. carton	800	40.0	80.0	4.00	160	8.0	10	0.5
Lucky Whip Aerosol Dessert Topping, 9-oz. can, net wt.	699	27.6	77.7	3.06	192	8.0	12	0.5
Powdered Topping Mix, 4-oz. box	662	59.6	165.6	14.90				
6-oz. box	994	89.4	165.6	14.90				
Prepared as directed			64.3	5.95	160	3.2	10	0.2
Monarch Whip Aerosol Whipped Topping, 7.05-oz. canister	568	42.0	80.5	5.95	(200)	(14.8)	(13)	(0.9)
Quick Whip Powdered Topping Mix, 2-oz. box	331	29.8	165.6	14.90				
Prepared as directed			64.3	5.95	(160)	(3.2)	(10)	(0.2)
Rich 'N Whipped Spoon 'n Serve Topping, 5-oz. tub	486	33.9	97.2	6.78	256	17.6	16	1.1
9-oz. tub	875	61.0	97.2	6.78	256	17.6	16	1.1
Rich's Aerosol Whip Topping, 9-oz. can	720	36.0	80.0	4.00	(197)	(9.9)	(12)	(0.6)
12-oz. can	960	48.0	80.0	4.00	(197)	(9.9)	(12)	(0.6)
Richwhip Whipped Topping, 8-oz. container	640	320.0	80.0	4.00	160	8.0	10	0.5

MISCELLANEOUS TOPPINGS, based on generic data

	UNIT		1 OZ., BY WT.		1 CUP		1 TABLE-SPOON	
	Cal.	Carb.	Cal.	Carb.	Cal.	Carb.	Cal.	Carb.
Cherry, Maraschino, 1 med., (approx. 0.2 oz.)	(6)	(1.4)	32.9	8.34	352	89.2	22	5.6
Coconut, dried, sweetened, shredded, 1 teaspoon (approx. 0.06 oz.)	(11)	(1.1)	155.4	15.08	(528)	(51.3)	(33)	(3.2)
Walnuts, English or Persian, chopped, 1 teaspoon (approx. 0.09 oz.)	17	0.4	184.5	4.48	781	19.0	52	1.3

15 SALTS & SPICES •

	UNIT		1 PINCH		1 OZ., BY WT.		1 TEASPOON	
	Cal.	Carb.	Cal.	Carb.	Cal.	Carb.	Cal.	Carb.
SALTS								
Table Salt								
Based on USDA data, 1 pound	0	0.0	0.0	0.00	0.0	0.00	0	0.0
Diamond Crystal Plain, 16-oz. (1-lb.) canister	0	0.0	0.0	0.00	0.0	0.00	0	0.0
Iodized, 16-oz. (1-lb.) canister	1	0.2	0.0	0.00	0.1	0.01	trace	trace
Morton Plain, 26-oz. canister	0	0.0	0.0	0.00	0.0	0.00	0	0.0
Iodized, 16-oz. (1-lb.) canister	1	0.2	0.0	0.00	trace	0.01	trace	trace
26-oz. canister	1	0.3	0.0	0.00	trace	0.01	trace	trace
Other Salts								
Butter Flavor Salt (Imitation), **French's,** 2½-oz. jar	158	0.0		0.00	63.0	0.00	8	0.0
Celery Salt, **French's,** 3¼-oz. jar	40	na	0.0	0.00	12.3	na	6	trace
Garlic Salt, **French's,** 4-oz. jar	80	19.9	0.0	0.00	19.9	4.97	4	1.0
6⅜-oz. jar	127	31.7	0.0	0.00	19.9	4.97	4	1.0
Garlic Salt, Parslied, **French's,** 2⅞-oz. jar	119	19.9	0.0	0.00	41.5	6.91	6	1.0
Hickory Smoked Salt, **French's,** 3-oz. jar	40	na	0.0	0.00	13.2	na	2	trace
Lite Salt (Iodized Salt and Potassium Chloride Mixture), **Morton,** 11-oz. canister	1	0.1	0.0	0.00	0.1	0.01	trace	trace
Onion Salt, **French's,** 3¾-oz. jar	120	20.1	0.0	0.00	32.1	5.35	6	1.0
Sea Salt, "Plain," **Hollywood,** 16-oz. (1-lb.) canister	0	0.0	0.0	0.00	0.0	0.00	0	0.0
Sea Salt, **Salin Du Midi,** 26-oz. canister	0	0.0	0.0	0.00	0.0	0.00	0	0.0
Seasoning Salt, **Salin Du Midi,** 3-oz. jar	40	19.8	trace	trace	13.2	6.59	2	1.0
Vegetable Salt, **Salin Du Midi,** 16-oz. (1-lb.) canister	0	0.0	0.0	0.00	0.0	0.00	0	0.0
SALT SUBSTITUTES								
Featherweight Salt Substitute, 3-oz. container	0	0.0	0.0	0.00	0.0	0.00	0	0.0
Garlic Salt Substitute, 3-oz. container	0	0.0	0.0	0.00	0.0	0.00	0	0.0
Seasoned Salt Substitute, 3-oz. container	0	0.0	0.0	0.00	0.0	0.00	0	0.0
Nu-Salt Salt Substitute, 3-oz. box	53	14.2			17.6	4.72		
1 packet, 0.04 oz.	1	0.2			17.6	4.72		

	UNIT		1 PINCH		1 OZ., BY WT.		1 TEASPOON	
	Cal.	Carb.	Cal.	Carb.	Cal.	Carb.	Cal.	Carb.
Salt It Salt Substitute, 3-oz. container	0	0.0	0.0	0.00	0.0	0.00	0	0.0
SPICES								
Accent, see Monosodium Glutamate								
Allspice, ground								
Based on USDA data, 1 pound	1194	327.2	(0.5)	(0.12)	74.6	20.45	5	1.4
1 teaspoon (approx. 0.07 oz.)	5	1.4	(0.5)	(0.12)	74.6	20.45	5	1.4
1 tablespoon (approx. 0.21 oz.)	16	4.3	(0.5)	(0.12)	74.6	20.45	5	1.4
American Spice Trade Association data, 1 pound	1723	337.4			107.7	21.09	7	1.3
Durkee, 1¾-oz. tin	188	36.9	(0.7)	(0.13)	107.7	21.09	7	1.3
Ehlers, 1½-oz. bottle	162	31.6	(0.7)	(0.13)	107.7	21.09	7	1.3
McCormick, 1¼-oz. bottle	188	36.9	(0.7)	(0.13)	107.7	21.09	7	1.3
Spice Islands, 1.7-oz. bottle	183	35.9	(0.7)	(0.13)	107.7	21.09	7	1.3
Anise seed, ground								
Based on USDA data, 1 pound	1528	226.9			95.5	14.18	7	1.1
1 teaspoon (approx. 0.07 oz.)	7	1.1			95.5	14.18	7	1.1
1 tablespoon (approx. 0.24 oz.)	23	3.4			95.5	14.18	7	1.1
China Bowl, 1-oz. bottle	118	12.8			117.7	12.84		
Ehlers, 1½-oz. bottle	177	19.3			117.7	12.84	7	1.1
Basil, ground								
Based on USDA data, 1 pound	1139	276.5			71.2	17.28	4	0.9
1 teaspoon (approx. 0.05 oz.)	4	0.9			71.2	17.28	4	0.9
1 tablespoon (approx. 0.16 oz.)	11	2.7			71.2	17.28	4	0.9
American Spice Trade Association data, 1 pound	1476	280.1			92.1	17.49	4	0.7
Durkee, ½-oz. glass jar	46	8.8	(0.6)	(0.11)	92.1	17.49	4	0.7
Ehlers, ⅜-oz. tin	29	6.6			77.3	17.50	3	0.7
McCormick, ½-oz. bottle	46	8.8	(0.6)	(0.11)	92.1	17.49	4	0.7
Spice Islands, 0.49-oz. bottle	45	8.6	(0.6)	(0.11)	92.1	17.49	4	0.7

	UNIT Cal.	UNIT Carb.	1 PINCH Cal.	1 PINCH Carb.	1 OZ., BY WT. Cal.	1 OZ., BY WT. Carb.	1 TEASPOON Cal.	1 TEASPOON Carb.
Bay Leaves, crumbled								
Based on USDA data, 1 pound	1419	340.0			88.7	21.25	2	0.5
1 teaspoon (approx. 0.02 oz.)	2	0.5			88.7	21.25	2	0.5
1 tablespoon (approx. 0.24 oz.)	6	1.4			88.7	21.25	2	0.5
American Spice Trade Association data, 1 pound	1861	342.3			116.2	21.38	5	1.0
Ehlers, ¼-oz. tin	27	5.3			109.0	21.40	5	1.0
Bay Leaves, whole								
McCormick, ¼-oz. bottle	29	5.3			116.2	21.38	5	1.0
Spice Islands, ¾-oz. bottle	87	16.0			116.2	21.38	5	1.0
Buttery Seasoning								
Jolly Time Instant, 7⅞-oz. jar	2				0.2			
Caraway Seed								
Based on USDA data, 1 pound	1510	226.4	(1.3)	(0.19)	94.4	14.15	7	1.1
1 teaspoon (approx. 0.07 oz.)	7	1.1	(1.3)	(0.19)	94.4	14.15	7	1.1
1 tablespoon (approx. 0.24 oz.)	22	3.3	(1.3)	(0.19)	94.4	14.15	7	1.1
American Spice Trade Association data, 1 pound	2109	167.3	(1.8)	(0.17)	131.8	12.33	8	0.8
Durkee, 1¾-oz. carton	231	21.6	(1.8)	(0.17)	131.8	12.33	8	0.8
Ehlers, 1¾-oz. bottle	231	21.6	(1.8)	(0.17)	131.8	12.33	8	0.8
McCormick, 1¾-oz. bottle	231	21.6			131.8	12.33	8	0.8
Spice Islands, 2.1-oz. bottle	277	25.9	(1.8)	(0.17)	131.8	12.33	8	0.8
Cardamom Seed, ground								
Based on USDA data, 1 pound	1411	310.6			88.2	19.41	6	1.4
1 teaspoon (approx. 0.07 oz.)	6	1.4			88.2	19.41	6	1.4
1 tablespoon (approx. 0.20 oz.)	18	4.0			88.2	19.41	6	1.4
American Spice Trade Association data, 1 pound	1634	336.7			102.1	21.04	7	1.3
Durkee, 1⅝-oz. carton	166	34.2			102.2	21.05	7	1.3
Ehlers, 1-oz. bottle	102	21.1			102.2	21.05	7	1.3
McCormick, ½-oz. bottle	51	10.2			102.2	21.04	7	1.3
Spice Islands, 1.9-oz. bottle	164	40.0			102.2	21.05	7	1.3
Cassia, see Cinnamon								
Cayenne, see Pepper								
Celery Seed, ground								
Based on USDA data, 1 pound	1776	187.5	(1.1)	(0.12)	111.0	11.72	8	0.8
1 teaspoon (approx. 0.07 oz.)	8	0.8	(1.1)	(0.12)	111.0	11.72	8	0.8
1 tablespoon (approx. 0.23 oz.)	25	2.7	(1.1)	(0.12)	111.0	11.72	8	0.8
American Spice Trade Association data, 1 pound	2042	168.7	(1.3)	(0.12)	127.6	12.42	7	1.1
McCormick, 1⅝-oz. bottle	207	20.2	(1.3)	(0.12)	127.6	12.42	7	1.1
Spice Islands, 1.8-oz. bottle	230	22.3	(1.3)	(0.12)	127.6	12.42	7	1.1
Celery Seed, whole								
Ehlers, 2-oz. tin	260	24.8			129.9	12.41	11	1.1
Chervil, dried								
Based on USDA data, 1 pound	1075	222.7			67.2	13.92	1	0.3
1 teaspoon (approx. 0.02 oz.)	1	0.3			67.2	13.92	1	0.3
1 tablespoon (approx. 0.07 oz.)	4	0.9			67.2	13.92	1	0.3

	UNIT Cal.	UNIT Carb.	1 PINCH Cal.	1 PINCH Carb.	1 OZ., BY WT. Cal.	1 OZ., BY WT. Carb.	1 TEASPOON Cal.	1 TEASPOON Carb.
Chervil, fresh, see the VEGETABLES chapter								
Chili Powder								
(83% Red Pepper, 9% Cumin, 4% Oregano, 2.5% Salt, 1.5% Garlic Powder)								
Based on USDA data, 1 pound	1424	248.0			89.0	15.50	8	1.4
1 teaspoon (approx. 0.09 oz.)	8	1.4			89.0	15.50	8	1.4
1 tablespoon (approx. 0.26 oz.)	24	4.1			89.0	15.50	8	1.4
Chives, freeze dried								
Armanino Farms, 2-oz. package	187	38.7			93.6	19.36		
Chives, fresh, see the VEGETABLES chapter								
Cinnamon, ground								
Based on USDA data, 1 pound	1184	361.8	(0.3)	(0.10)	74.0	22.61	6	1.8
1 teaspoon (approx. 0.08 oz.)	6	1.8	(0.3)	(0.10)	74.0	22.61	6	1.8
1 tablespoon (approx. 0.24 oz.)	18	5.4	(0.3)	(0.10)	74.0	22.61	6	1.8
American Spice Trade Association data, 1 pound	1610	361.9	(0.4)	(0.10)	100.6	22.62	6	1.4
Durkee, 1-oz. tin	101	22.6	(0.4)	(0.10)	100.6	22.62	6	1.4
Ehlers, 1-oz. bottle	101	22.6	(0.4)	(0.10)	100.6	22.62	6	1.4
McCormick, 1¾-oz. bottle	176	39.6	(0.4)	(0.10)	100.6	22.62	6	1.4
Spice Islands, 1.9-oz. bottle	161	43.0	(0.4)	(0.10)	100.6	22.62	6	1.4
Cloves, ground								
Based on USDA data, 1 pound	1466	277.8	(0.2)	(0.05)	91.6	17.36	7	1.3
1 teaspoon (approx. 0.07 oz.)	7	1.3	(0.2)	(0.05)	91.6	17.36	7	1.3
1 tablespoon (approx. 0.23 oz.)	21	4.0	(0.2)	(0.05)	91.6	17.36	7	1.3
American Spice Trade Association data, 1 pound	1650	312.0	(0.3)	(0.05)	121.9	19.50	7	1.2
Durkee, 1⅞-oz. tin	229	36.6	(0.3)	(0.05)	121.9	19.50		
Ehlers, 1⅛-oz. bottle	137	21.9	(0.3)	(0.05)	121.9	19.50	7	1.2
McCormick, 1¼-oz. bottle	153	24.4	(0.3)	(0.05)	121.9	19.50	7	1.2
Spice Islands, 1.9-oz. bottle	232	37.1	(0.3)	(0.05)	121.9	19.50	7	1.2
Coriander Leaf, dried								
Based on USDA data, 1 pound	1266	236.3			79.1	14.77	2	0.3
1 teaspoon (approx. 0.02 oz.)	2	0.3			79.1	14.77	2	0.3
1 tablespoon (approx. 0.06 oz.)	5	0.9			79.1	14.77	2	0.3
Coriander Seed, ground								
American Spice Trade Association data, 1 pound	2042	256.3	(1.2)	(0.50)	127.6	16.02	6	0.8
McCormick, 1⅛-oz. bottle	144	18.0	(1.2)	(0.50)	127.6	16.02	6	0.8
Spice Islands, 1.6-oz. bottle	204	25.6	(1.2)	(0.50)	127.6	16.02	6	0.8
Coriander Seed, whole								
Based on USDA data, 1 pound	1352	249.4			84.5	15.59	5	1.0
1 teaspoon (approx. 0.06 oz.)	5	1.0			84.5	15.59	5	1.0
1 tablespoon (approx. 0.18 oz.)	15	2.8			84.5	15.59	5	1.0

	UNIT		1 PINCH		1 OZ., BY WT.		1 TEASPOON	
	Cal.	Carb.	Cal.	Carb.	Cal.	Carb.	Cal.	Carb.
Cumin Seed, ground								
Based on USDA data, 1 pound	1701	200.6	(1.0)	(0.12)	106.3	12.54	8	0.9
1 teaspoon (approx. 0.07 oz.)	8	0.9	(1.0)	(0.12)	106.3	12.54	8	0.9
1 tablespoon (approx. 0.21 oz.)	22	2.7	(1.0)	(0.12)	106.3	12.54	8	0.9
American Spice Trade Association data, 1 pound	2086	202.2	(1.2)	(0.12)	130.4	12.64	7	0.7
Durkee, 1¾-oz. tin	228	22.1	(1.2)	(0.12)	130.4	12.64	7	0.7
Ehlers, 1¼-oz. bottle	163	15.8	(1.2)	(0.12)	130.4	12.64	7	0.7
McCormick, 1½-oz. bottle	196	19.0	(1.2)	(0.12)	130.4	12.64	7	0.7
Spice Islands, 1.8-oz. bottle	235	22.8	(1.2)	(0.12)	130.4	12.64	7	0.7
Curry Powder								
(36% Coriander Seed, 28% Turmeric, 10% Cumin, 10% Fenugreek Seed, 5% White Pepper, 4% Allspice, 3% Yellow Mustard, 2% Red Pepper, 2% Ginger)								
Based on USDA data, 1 pound	1474	263.8			92.1	16.49	6	1.2
1 teaspoon (approx. 0.07 oz.)	6	1.2			92.1	16.49	6	1.2
1 tablespoon (approx. 0.22 oz.)	20	3.7			92.1	16.49	6	1.2
Dill Seed, ground								
American Spice Trade Association data, 1 pound	1973	255.8			123.3	15.99	9	1.2
McCormick, 1½-oz. bottle	185	24.0			123.3	15.99	9	1.2
Spice Islands, 2-oz. bottle	247	32.0			123.3	15.99	9	1.2
Dill Seed, whole								
Based on USDA data, 1 pound	1384	250.2			86.5	15.64	6	1.2
1 teaspoon (approx. 0.07 oz.)	6	1.2			86.5	15.64	6	1.2
1 tablespoon (approx. 0.23 oz.)	20	3.6			86.5	15.64	6	1.2
Durkee, 1⅝-oz. carton	200	26.0			123.3	15.99	9	1.1
Ehlers, 1¾-oz. bottle	216	28.0			123.3	15.99	9	1.1
Dill Weed, dried								
Based on USDA data, 1 pound	1147	253.3			71.7	15.83	3	0.6
1 teaspoon (approx. 0.04 oz.)	3	0.6			71.7	15.83	3	0.6
1 tablespoon (approx. 0.11 oz.)	8	1.7			71.7	15.83	3	0.6
Fennel Seed, ground								
American Spice Trade Association data, 1 pound	1678	275.8			104.9	17.24	8	1.3
McCormick, 1½-oz. bottle	157	25.9			104.9	17.24	8	1.3
Spice Islands, 1.8-oz. bottle	189	31.0			104.9	17.24	8	1.3
Fennel Seed, whole								
Based on USDA data, 1 pound	1147	253.3			97.8	14.83	7	1.1
1 teaspoon (approx. 0.07 oz.)	7	1.1			97.8	14.83	7	1.1
1 tablespoon (approx. 0.20 oz.)	20	3.0			97.8	14.83	7	1.1
Ehlers, 1½-oz. tin	162	25.9			108.0	17.20	8	1.3
Fenugreek Seed, whole								
Based on USDA data, 1 pound	1466	264.6			91.6	16.54	12	2.2
1 teaspoon (approx. 0.13 oz.)	12	2.2			91.6	16.54	12	2.2
1 tablespoon (approx. 0.32 oz.)	36	6.5			91.6	16.54	12	2.2
Garlic Cloves, see the VEGETABLES chapter								

	UNIT		1 PINCH		1 OZ., BY WT.		1 TEASPOON	
	Cal.	Carb.	Cal.	Carb.	Cal.	Carb.	Cal.	Carb.
Garlic Powder								
Based on USDA data, 1 pound	1506	329.9	(0.5)	(0.10)	94.1	20.62	9	2.0
1 teaspoon (approx. 0.10 oz.)	9	2.0	(0.5)	(0.10)	94.1	20.62	9	2.0
1 tablespoon (approx. 0.30 oz.)	28	6.1	(0.5)	(0.10)	94.1	20.62	9	2.0
American Spice Trade Association data, 1 pound	1656	332.5	(0.5)	(0.10)	103.5	20.78	5	1.1
Durkee, 2-oz. glass jar	207	41.6	(0.5)	(0.10)	103.5	20.78	5	1.1
McCormick, 2⅜-oz. bottle	246	49.4	(0.5)	(0.10)	103.5	20.78	5	1.1
Spice Islands, 2.6-oz. bottle	269	54.0	(0.5)	(0.10)	103.5	20.78	5	1.1
Ginger, ground								
Based on USDA data, 1 pound	1574	321.1	(0.5)	(0.10)	98.4	20.07	6	1.3
1 teaspoon (approx. 0.06 oz.)	6	1.3	(0.5)	(0.10)	98.4	20.07	6	1.3
1 tablespoon (approx. 0.19 oz.)	19	3.8	(0.5)	(0.10)	98.4	20.07	6	1.3
American Spice Trade Association data, 1 pound	1723	328.0	(0.6)	(0.11)	107.7	20.50	6	1.2
Durkee, 1¾-oz. tin	188	35.9	(0.6)	(0.11)	107.7	20.50	6	1.2
Ehlers, 1-oz. bottle	108	20.5	(0.6)	(0.11)	107.7	20.50	6	1.2
McCormick, 2-oz. bottle	216	41.1	(0.6)	(0.11)	107.7	20.50	6	1.2
Spice Islands, 1.9-oz. bottle	205	39.0	(0.6)	(0.11)	107.7	20.50	6	1.2
Lemon Flavor Crystals								
Single Serv, 0.03-oz. packet (equivalent to juice of ¼ lemon)	3	0.7			100.0	25.47		
Mace, ground								
Based on USDA data, 1 pound	2155	229.1			134.7	14.32	8	0.9
1 teaspoon (approx. 0.06 oz.)	8	0.9			134.7	14.32	8	0.9
1 tablespoon (approx. 0.19 oz.)	25	2.7			134.7	14.32	8	0.9
American Spice Trade Association data, 1 pound	3562	209.3			160.1	13.08	10	0.8
Durkee, 17-oz. tin	300	11.4			160.1	13.08	10	0.8
Ehlers, 1⅛-oz. bottle	180	14.7			160.1	13.08	10	0.8
McCormick, 1⅞-oz. bottle	301	24.5			160.1	13.08	10	0.8
Spice Islands, 1.7-oz. bottle	272	22.2			160.1	13.08	10	0.8
Marjoram, ground								
Based on USDA data, 1 pound	1229	274.7	(0.3)	(0.07)	76.8	17.17	2	0.4
1 teaspoon (approx. 0.02 oz.)	2	0.4	(0.3)	(0.07)	76.8	17.17	2	0.4
1 tablespoon (approx. 0.06 oz.)	5	1.0	(0.3)	(0.07)	76.8	17.17	2	0.4
American Spice Trade Association data, 1 pound	1656	292.2	(0.4)	(0.08)	103.5	18.26	4	0.8
Durkee, 1⅛-oz. tin	116	20.5	(0.4)	(0.08)	103.5	18.26	4	0.8
McCormick, 1½-oz. bottle	155	27.4	(0.4)	(0.08)	103.5	18.26	4	0.8
Spice Islands, ½-oz. bottle	51	8.9	(0.4)	(0.08)	103.6	18.26	4	0.8
Mint, fresh, see the VEGETABLES chapter								
Monosodium Glutamate								
Accent Flavor Enhancer, 2-oz. canister	163				81.6	trace	9	trace
4½-oz. canister	367				81.6	trace	9	trace
10-oz. canister	816				81.6	trace	9	trace
Mustard Powder								
American Spice Trade Association data, 1 pound	2630	83.8	(0.8)	(0.03)	164.4	5.24	9	0.3
China Bowl, 2⅜-oz. bottle	316	19.0	(0.6)	(0.05)	133.0	8.00	7	0.4
Ehlers, 1⅛-oz. bottle	185	5.9	(0.8)	(0.03)	164.4	5.24	9	0.3
McCormick, 1¾-oz. bottle	288	9.9	(0.8)	(0.03)	164.6	5.25	9	0.3
Spice Islands, 1.8 -oz. bottle	296	9.5	(0.8)	(0.03)	164.6	5.25	9	0.3

	UNIT		1 PINCH		1 OZ., BY WT.		1 TEASPOON	
	Cal.	Carb.	Cal.	Carb.	Cal.	Carb.	Cal.	Carb.
Mustard, Prepared, see the CONDIMENTS chapter								
Mustard Seed, yellow								
Based on USDA data, 1 pound	2128	158.6			133.0	9.91	15	1.2
1 teaspoon (approx. 0.12 oz.)	15	1.2			133.0	9.91	15	1.2
1 tablespoon (approx. 0.40 oz.)	53	3.9			133.0	9.91	15	1.2
Ehlers, 3-oz. bottle	(2131)	(158.6)			(133.2)	(9.91)	(15)	(1.2)
Nutmeg, ground								
Based on USDA data, 1 pound	2382	223.7	(1.0)	(0.10)	148.9	13.98	12	1.1
1 teaspoon (approx. 0.08 oz.)	12	1.1	(1.0)	(0.10)	148.9	13.98	12	1.1
1 tablespoon (approx. 0.25 oz.)	37	3.5	(1.0)	(0.10)	148.9	13.98	12	1.1
American Spice Trade Association data, 1 pound	2563	214.6	(1.1)	(0.09)	160.2	13.41	11	0.9
Durkee, 1⅛-oz. tin	180	15.1	(1.1)	(0.09)	160.2	13.41	11	0.9
Ehlers, 1⅛-oz. tin	185	15.1	(1.1)	(0.09)	164.1	13.41	11	0.9
McCormick, 2¼-oz. bottle	361	30.2	(1.1)	(0.09)	160.2	13.41	11	0.9
Spice Islands, 2.1-oz. bottle	336	28.2	(1.1)	(0.09)	160.2	13.41	11	0.9
Onion Flakes, dehydrated								
Based on USDA data, 1 pound	1588	372.4			99.2	23.28	7	1.7
1 teaspoon (approx. 0.07 oz.)	7	1.7			99.2	23.28	7	1.7
1 tablespoon (approx. 0.22 oz.)	22	5.1			99.2	23.28	7	1.7
Onion Powder								
Based on USDA data, 1 pound	1574	365.9	(0.7)	(0.15)	98.4	22.87	7	1.7
1 teaspoon (approx. 0.07 oz.)	7	1.7	(0.7)	(0.15)	98.4	22.87	7	1.7
1 tablespoon (approx. 0.23 oz.)	23	5.2	(0.7)	(0.15)	98.4	22.87	7	1.7
American Spice Trade Association data, 1 pound	1678	362.1	(0.7)	(0.16)	104.9	22.82	8	1.7
Durkee, 1½-oz. glass jar	157	34.2	(0.7)	(0.16)	104.9	22.82	8	1.7
Ehlers, 1¼-oz. bottle	131	28.5	(0.7)	(0.16)	104.9	22.82	8	1.7
2-oz. bottle	210	45.6	(0.7)	(0.16)	104.9	22.82	8	1.7
5-oz. bottle	525	114.1	(0.7)	(0.16)	104.9	22.82	8	1.7
McCormick, 1¾-oz. bottle	184	40.0	(0.7)	(0.16)	104.9	22.82	8	1.7
Spice Islands, 1.9-oz. bottle	199	43.4	(0.7)	(0.16)	104.9	22.82	8	1.7
Oregano, ground								
Based on USDA data, 1 pound	1389	292.3	(0.7)	(0.14)	86.8	18.27	5	1.0
1 teaspoon (approx. 0.05 oz.)	5	1.0	(0.7)	(0.14)	86.8	18.27	5	1.0
1 tablespoon (approx. 0.16 oz.)	14	2.9	(0.7)	(0.14)	86.8	18.27	5	1.0
American Spice Trade Association data, 1 pound	1634	294.6	(0.8)	(0.14)	102.1	18.39	6	1.0
Durkee, 1¼-oz. glass jar	128	23.0	(0.8)	(0.14)	102.1	18.39	6	1.0
McCormick, 1¾-oz. jar	179	32.2	(0.8)	(0.14)	102.1	18.39	6	1.0
Spice Islands, 0.49-oz. jar	50	9.0	(0.8)	(0.14)	102.1	18.39	6	1.0
Oregano Leaves, whole								
Ehlers, ½-oz. tin	53	9.2			106.3	18.39	6	1.0
Paprika, domestic								
Based on USDA data, 1 pound	1310	252.8	(0.4)	(0.07)	81.9	15.80	6	1.2
1 teaspoon (approx. 0.07 oz.)	6	1.2	(0.4)	(0.07)	81.9	15.80	6	1.2
1 tablespoon (approx. 0.24 oz.)	20	3.9	(0.4)	(0.07)	81.9	15.80	6	1.2

	UNIT		1 PINCH		1 OZ., BY WT.		1 TEASPOON	
	Cal.	Carb.	Cal.	Carb.	Cal.	Carb.	Cal.	Carb.
Durkee, 1¼-oz. tin	138	21.4	(0.5)	(0.07)	110.6	17.10	7	1.2
McCormick, 2⅛-oz. tin	235	36.3	(0.5)	(0.07)	110.6	17.10	7	1.2
Spice Islands, 2.3-oz. bottle	254	36.3	(0.5)	(0.07)	110.6	17.10	7	1.2
Paprika, imported								
Durkee, 2-oz. jar	218	32.9			109.2	16.45	7	1.1
McCormick, 1¾-oz. bottle	191	28.8			109.2	16.45	7	1.1
Spice Islands, 2.3-oz. bottle	251	37.9			109.2	16.46	7	1.1
Parsley Flakes								
Based on USDA data, 1 pound	1253	234.4	(0.3)	(0.06)	78.3	14.65	1	0.2
1 teaspoon (approx. 0.01 oz.)	1	0.2	(0.3)	(0.06)	78.3	14.65	1	0.2
1 tablespoon (approx. 0.04 oz.)	4	0.7	(0.3)	(0.06)	78.3	14.65	1	0.2
American Spice Trade Association data, 1 pound	1611	246.4	(0.4)	(0.07)	100.7	15.40	7	0.6
Durkee, ¼-oz. tin	25	3.9	(0.4)	(0.07)	100.7	15.40	7	0.6
Ehlers, 1⅛-oz. bottle	113	17.3	(0.4)	(0.07)	100.7	15.40	7	0.6
¼-oz. bottle	25	3.9	(0.4)	(0.07)	100.7	15.40	7	0.6
McCormick, ⅝-oz. bottle	63	9.0	(0.4)	(0.07)	100.7	15.40	7	0.6
Spice Islands, 0.39-oz. bottle	39	6.0	(0.4)	(0.07)	100.7	15.40	7	0.6
Parsley, fresh, see the VEGETABLES chapter								
Pepper, Black, ground								
American Spice Trade Association data, 1 pound	1814	301.6	(0.7)	(0.12)	113.4	18.85	9	1.5
Durkee, 1-oz. tin	113	18.9	(0.7)	(0.12)	113.4	18.85	9	1.5
Ehlers, 1⅜-oz. tin	153	25.9	(0.7)	(0.12)	110.9	18.85	9	1.5
McCormick, 1¾-oz. bottle	199	33.0	(0.7)	(0.12)	113.4	18.87	9	1.5
Spice Islands, 2.1-oz. bottle	238	39.6	(0.7)	(0.12)	113.4	18.87	9	1.5
Pepper, Black, whole								
Based on USDA data, 1 pound	1157	294.1			72.3	18.38	5	1.4
1 teaspoon (approx. 0.07 oz.)	5	1.4			72.3	18.38	5	1.4
1 tablespoon (approx. 0.23 oz.)	16	4.2			72.3	18.38	5	1.4
Pepper, Chili, ground								
American Spice Trade Association data, 1 pound	1893	264.0	(0.7)	(0.12)	117.7	16.50	9	1.2
McCormick, 1¾-oz. bottle	206	28.9	(0.7)	(0.12)	117.7	16.50	9	1.2
Pepper, Red or Cayenne								
Based on USDA data, 1 pound	1443	257.0	(0.6)	(0.10)	90.2	16.06	6	1.0
1 teaspoon (approx. 0.06 oz.)	6	1.0	(0.6)	(0.10)	90.2	16.06	6	1.0
1 tablespoon (approx. 0.19 oz.)	17	3.0	(0.6)	(0.10)	90.2	16.06	6	1.0
American Spice Trade Association data, 1 pound	1902	246.2	(0.8)	(0.10)	119.1	15.39	9	1.1
Durkee, 1⅞-oz. tin	223	28.9	(0.8)	(0.10)	119.1	15.39	9	1.1
Ehlers, 1-oz. bottle	119	15.4	(0.8)	(0.10)	119.1	15.39	9	1.1
McCormick, 1⅞-oz. bottle	223	28.9	(0.8)	(0.10)	119.1	15.39	9	1.1
Spice Islands, 1.8-oz. bottle	215	27.7	(0.8)	(0.10)	119.1	15.39	9	1.1
Pepper, Seasoned								
French's, 2-oz. tin	156	19.6			78.2	9.78	8	1.0
Pepper, White								
Based on USDA data, 1 pound	1342	311.7	(0.3)	(0.07)	83.9	19.48	7	1.7
1 teaspoon (approx. 0.08 oz.)	7	1.7	(0.3)	(0.07)	83.9	19.48	7	1.7
1 tablespoon (approx. 0.25 oz.)	21	4.9	(0.3)	(0.07)	83.9	19.48	7	1.7

	UNIT		1 PINCH		1 OZ., BY WT.		1 TEASPOON	
	Cal.	Carb.	Cal.	Carb.	Cal.	Carb.	Cal.	Carb.
American Spice Trade Association data, 1 pound	1792	313.0	(0.4)	(0.07)	112.0	19.56	9	1.5
Durkee, 1-oz. tin	112	19.6	(0.4)	(0.07)	112.0	19.56	9	1.5
Ehlers, 1⅛-oz. tin	130	22.0	(0.4)	(0.07)	116.0	19.56	9	1.5
McCormick, 1¾-oz. bottle	196	34.3	(0.4)	(0.07)	112.0	19.56	9	1.5
Spice Islands, 2½-oz. bottle	280	48.8	(0.4)	(0.07)	112.0	19.56	9	1.5
Pizza Sprinkles								
Scotch Buy, 8-oz. package	720	8.0			90.0	1.00		
Poppy Seed								
Based on USDA data, 1 pound	2418	107.5			151.1	6.72	15	0.7
1 teaspoon (approx. 0.10 oz.)	15	0.7			151.1	6.72	15	0.7
1 tablespoon (approx. 0.31 oz.)	47	2.1			151.1	6.72	15	0.7
American Spice Trade Association data, 1 pound	2405	137.0			150.3	8.56	13	0.8
Durkee, 2¼-oz. tin	338	19.3			150.3	8.56	13	0.8
Ehlers, 2½-oz. bottle	376	21.4			150.3	8.56	13	0.8
McCormick, 2⅛-oz. bottle	320	18.2			150.3	8.56	13	0.8
Spice Islands, 2.7-oz. bottle	406	23.1			150.3	8.56	13	0.8
Poultry Seasoning								
(35% White Pepper, 15% Sage, 10% Thyme, 10% Marjoram, 10% Savory, 10% Ginger, 5% Allspice, 5% Nutmeg)								
Based on USDA data, 1 pound	1392	297.6			87.0	18.60	5	1.0
1 teaspoon (approx. 0.05 oz.)	5	1.0			87.0	18.60	5	1.0
1 tablespoon (approx. 0.13 oz.)	11	2.4			87.0	18.60	5	1.0
Pumpkin Pie Spice								
(40% Cinnamon, 20% Ginger, 20% Nutmeg, 10% Allspice, 10% Cloves)								
Based on USDA data, 1 pound	1552	314.2			97.0	19.64	6	1.2
1 teaspoon (approx. 0.06 oz.)	6	1.2			97.0	19.64	6	1.2
1 tablespoon (approx. 0.20 oz.)	19	1.9			97.0	19.64	6	1.2
Rosemary, dried								
Based on USDA data, 1 pound	1501	290.6			93.8	18.16	4	0.8
1 teaspoon (approx. 0.04 oz.)	4	0.8			93.8	18.16	4	0.8
1 tablespoon (approx. 0.12 oz.)	11	2.1			93.8	18.16	4	0.8
Ehlers, ¾-oz. tin	89	13.8			118.1	18.36	5	0.8
Rosemary, ground								
American Spice Trade Association data, 1 pound	1995	301.1			124.7	18.82	5	0.8
McCormick, ⅝-oz. bottle	78	11.8			124.7	18.82	5	0.8
Spice Islands, ¾-oz. bottle	94	14.1			124.7	18.82	3	0.8
Saffron								
Based on USDA data, 1 pound	1406	296.5			87.9	18.53	2	0.5
1 teaspoon (approx. 0.02 oz.)	2	0.5			87.9	18.53	2	0.5
1 tablespoon (approx. 0.07 oz.)	7	1.4			87.9	18.53	2	0.5
Sage, ground								
Based on USDA data, 1 pound	89	17.2	(0.3)	(0.06)	89.3	17.22	2	0.4
1 teaspoon (approx. 0.02 oz.)	2	0.4	(0.3)	(0.06)	89.3	17.22	2	0.4
1 tablespoon (approx. 0.07 oz.)	6	1.2	(0.3)	(0.06)	89.3	17.22	2	0.4
American Spice Trade Association data, 1 pound	1883	282.7	(0.04)	(0.05)	117.7	17.66	4	0.6

	UNIT		1 PINCH		1 OZ., BY WT.		1 TEASPOON	
	Cal.	Carb.	Cal.	Carb.	Cal.	Carb.	Cal.	Carb.
Durkee, ½-oz. tin	59	8.8	(0.4)	(0.05)	117.7	17.65	4	0.6
Ehlers, ⅝-oz. bottle	74	11.0	(0.4)	(0.05)	117.7	17.66	4	0.6
McCormick, ⅞-oz. bottle	103	12.2	(0.4)	(0.05)	117.7	17.66	4	0.6
Spice Islands, ¾-oz. bottle	88	13.2	(0.4)	(0.05)	117.7	17.66	4	0.6
Savory, ground								
Based on USDA data, 1 pound	1234	311.8	(0.4)	(0.10)	77.1	19.49	4	1.0
1 teaspoon (approx. 0.05 oz.)	4	1.0	(0.4)	(0.10)	77.1	19.49	4	1.0
1 tablespoon (approx. 0.16 oz.)	12	3.0	(0.4)	(0.10)	77.1	19.49	4	1.0
American Spice Trade Association data, 1 pound	1610	317.1	(0.5)	(0.10)	100.6	19.82	5	1.0
McCormick, 1½-oz. bottle	151	69.8	(0.5)	(0.10)	100.6	19.82	5	1.0
Spice Islands, ¾-oz. bottle	75	14.9	(0.5)	(0.10)	100.6	19.83	5	1.0
Sesame Seed, decorticated (skinned)								
Based on USDA data, 1 pound	2667	42.6	(0.9)	(0.01)	166.7	2.66	16	0.3
1 teaspoon (approx. 0.10 oz.)	16	0.3	(0.9)	(0.01)	166.7	2.66	16	0.3
1 tablespoon (approx. 0.28 oz.)	47	0.8	(0.9)	(0.01)	166.7	2.66	16	0.3
American Spice Trade Association data, 1 pound	2178	213.6	(0.7)	(0.07)	136.1	13.35	9	0.9
Durkee, 2⅜-oz. carton	187	18.4	(0.7)	(0.07)	136.2	13.36	9	0.9
Ehlers, 2½-oz. bottle	341	33.4	(0.7)	(0.07)	136.2	13.36	9	0.9
McCormick, 2⅛-oz. bottle	289	28.4	(0.7)	(0.07)	136.2	13.36	9	0.9
Spice Islands, 2.6-oz. bottle	354	34.7	(0.7)	(0.07)	136.2	13.36	9	0.9
Sesame Seed, whole, see the NUTS & SEEDS chapter								
Soup Greens								
Durkee, 2½-oz. jar	216	43.0			86.4	17.20	12	2.4
Tarragon, ground								
Based on USDA data, 1 pound	1338	227.8	(0.4)	(0.07)	83.6	14.24	5	0.8
1 teaspoon (approx. 0.06 oz.)	5	0.8	(0.4)	(0.07)	83.6	14.24	5	0.8
1 tablespoon (approx. 0.17 oz.)	14	2.4	(0.4)	(0.07)	83.6	14.24	5	0.8
American Spice Trade Association data, 1 pound	1656	233.6	(0.5)	(0.07)	103.5	14.60	5	0.7
McCormick, ⅜-oz. bottle	39	5.5	(0.5)	(0.07)	103.5	14.60	5	0.7
Spice Islands, 0.49-oz. bottle	65	9.1	(0.5)	(0.07)	103.5	14.60	5	0.7
Tarragon, whole leaves								
Ehlers, ⅜-oz. tin	38	5.5			101.3	14.60	5	0.7
Thyme, ground								
Based on USDA data, 1 pound	1253	290.1	(0.3)	(0.08)	78.3	18.13	4	0.9
1 teaspoon (approx. 0.05 oz.)	4	0.9	(0.3)	(0.08)	78.3	18.13	4	0.9
1 tablespoon (approx. 0.15 oz.)	12	2.8	(0.3)	(0.08)	78.3	18.13	4	0.9
American Spice Trade Association data, 1 pound	1542	309.8	(0.4)	(0.07)	96.4	19.36	5	1.0
Durkee, ⅝-oz. tin	157	31.5	(0.4)	(0.07)	96.4	19.36	5	1.0
Ehlers, ⅞-oz. bottle	84	13.4	(0.4)	(0.07)	96.4	19.36	5	1.0
McCormick, 1¼-oz. bottle	121	24.2	(0.4)	(0.07)	96.4	19.36	5	1.0
Spice Islands, ¾-oz. bottle	76	14.5	(0.4)	(0.07)	96.4	19.36	5	1.0
Turmeric, ground								
Based on USDA data, 1 pound	1606	294.6	(0.7)	(0.13)	100.4	18.41	8	1.4
1 teaspoon (approx. 0.8 oz.)	8	1.4	(0.7)	(0.13)	100.4	18.41	8	1.4
1 tablespoon (approx. 0.24 oz.)	24	4.4	(0.7)	(0.13)	100.4	18.41	8	1.4

	UNIT Cal.	UNIT Carb.	1 PINCH Cal.	1 PINCH Carb.	1 OZ., BY WT. Cal.	1 OZ., BY WT. Carb.	1 TEASPOON Cal.	1 TEASPOON Carb.
American Spice Trade Association data, 1 pound	1770	317.1	(0.8)	(0.14)	110.6	19.83	7	1.3
Durkee, 2-oz. tin	221	39.7	(0.8)	(0.14)	110.6	19.83	7	1.3
Ehlers, 1¼-oz. tin	131	24.8	(0.7)	(0.14)	104.4	19.83	7	1.3
McCormick, 2-oz. bottle	221	39.7	(0.8)	(0.14)	110.6	19.83	7	1.3
Spice Islands, 2.3-oz. bottle	254	45.6	(0.8)	(0.14)	110.6	19.83	7	1.3

Vegetable Flakes, dehydrated

	UNIT Cal.	UNIT Carb.	1 PINCH Cal.	1 PINCH Carb.	1 OZ., BY WT. Cal.	1 OZ., BY WT. Carb.	1 TEASPOON Cal.	1 TEASPOON Carb.
French's, 1-oz. bottle	95	23.8			95.0	23.80	4	1.0
1 tablespoon (approx. 0.13 oz.)	12	3.0			95.0	23.80	4	1.0

16 NUTS & SEEDS •

	UNIT		1 OZ., BY WT.		1 POUND		Fiber per oz. (GMS.)
	Cal.	Carb.	Cal.	Carb.	Cal.	Carb.	
ACORNS (based on data from the Middle East)							
Edible portion, 1 pound	1216	239.5	76.0	14.97	1216	239.5	
ALFALFA SEEDS							
Natural Brand, 3-oz. package	294	30.0	98.0	10.00	1568	160.0	
9-oz. package	882	90.0	98.0	10.00	1568	160.0	
ALMONDS							
DRIED:							
As purchased in shell [refuse: shells, skin, approx. 60%]:							
1 medium almond (approx. 0.08 oz., 13 per ounce)	6	0.2	67.8	2.21	1085	35.4	
1 cup (approx. 2¾ oz., 34 medium almonds)	187	6.1	67.8	2.21	1085	35.4	
1 pound (approx. 5.8 cups, 200 medium almonds)	1085	35.4	67.8	2.21	1085	35.4	
Shelled:							
Whole:							
1 medium almond (approx. 0.04 oz., 28 per ounce)	6	0.2	169.8	5.54	2717	88.6	0.74
1 cup (approx. 5 oz., 142 medium almonds)	849	27.7	169.8	5.54	2717	88.6	0.74
1 pound (approx. 3¼ cups, 453 medium almonds [yield from approx. 2.5 lb. almonds in the shell) (5g/6g/15g/5%/1mg])	2717	88.6	169.8	5.54	2717	88.6	0.74
Chopped:							
1 tablespoon (approx. 0.3 oz.)	49	1.6	169.8	5.54	2717	88.6	0.74
1 cup (approx. 4.6 oz.)	777	25.4	169.8	5.54	2717	88.6	0.74
Slivered (split in half, then sliced to 3/16" wide):							
1 cup:							
Packed (approx. 4¾ oz.)	807	26.3	169.8	5.54	2717	88.6	0.74
Not packed (approx. 4 oz.)	688	22.4	169.8	5.54	2717	88.6	0.74
Sliced:							
1 cup (approx. 3⅓ oz.)	568	18.5	169.8	5.54	2717	88.6	0.74
ROASTED IN OIL, SALTED:							
Whole:							
1 almond (approx. 0.05 oz., 22 per ounce)	8	0.3	177.8	5.53	2844	88.5	0.74
1 cup (approx. 5½ oz., approx. 120 nuts)	984	30.6	177.8	5.53	2844	88.5	0.74
1 pound (approx. 2.9 cups, 350 nuts) (5g/6g/16g/1%/56mg)	2844	88.5	177.8	5.53	2844	88.5	0.74
CHOCOLATE-COATED:							
1 chocolate-coated almond (approx. 0.14 oz., 7 per ounce)	23	1.6	161.3	11.23	2581	179.6	0.43
1 cup (approx. 5.8 oz., 40–46 almonds that are not clustered)	939	65.3	161.3	11.23	2581	179.6	0.43
1 pound (approx. 2¾ cups, 96–128 almonds) (3g/11g/12g/2%/17mg)	2581	179.6	161.3	11.23	2581	179.6	0.43
SUGAR-COATED:							
1 sugar-coated almond (approx. 0.13 oz., 8 per ounce)	(17)	(2.6)	129.3	19.90	2068	318.4	0.26
1 cup (approx. 6.8 oz., 55 almonds)	889	136.7	129.3	19.90	2068	318.4	0.26
1 pound (approx. 2⅓ cups, 128 almonds) (2g/20g/5g/8%/6mg)	2068	318.4	129.3	19.90	2068	318.4	0.26
For comparison: Butter Almond Ice Cream, **Breyer's,** 1 cup (approx. 4.9 oz.)	340	30.0	68.8	6.07	1101	97.1	
ALMONDS, by brand							
Fisher Dried, Shelled Almonds, 7½-oz. jar	1275	31.3	170.0	5.50	2720	88.0	
1 cup (approx. 5.0 oz.)	(851)	(27.5)	170.0	5.50	2720	88.0	
Golden Harvest Barbecue Roasted Almonds, 6-oz. can	1080	24.0	180.0	4.00	2880	64.0	
1 cup (approx. 5.0 oz.)	(901)	(20.0)	180.0	4.00	2880	64.0	
Hickory Smoked Almonds, 6-oz. can	1080	24.0	180.0	4.00	2880	64.0	
1 cup (approx. 5.0 oz.)	(901)	(20.0)	180.0	4.00	2880	64.0	
100% Natural: Raw, Uncooked, Unbleached Almonds, 6-oz. bag	1080	36.0	180.0	6.00	2880	96.0	
1 cup (approx. 5.0 oz.)	(908)	(30.3)	180.0	6.00	2880	96.0	
Onion & Garlic Flavor Almonds, 6-oz. package	1080	24.0	180.0	4.00	2880	64.0	
1 cup (approx. 5.0 oz.)	(901)	(20.0)	180.0	4.00	2880	64.0	
Granny Goose Almonds, 1-oz. package	155	7.5	155.0	7.50	2480	120.0	
3-oz. package	465	22.6	155.0	7.50	2480	120.0	
1 cup (approx. 5.0 oz.)	(776)	(37.6)	155.0	7.50	2480	120.0	
Laura Scudder's Dry Roasted Smoke Flavored Almonds, 7½-oz. jar	1358	32.3	181.0	4.30	2896	68.8	
1 cup (approx. 5.0 oz.)	(914)	(21.7)	181.0	4.30	2896	68.8	
Planters Almonds, 7¼-oz. can	1233	43.5	170.0	6.00	2720	96.0	
1 cup (approx. 5.0 oz.)	(851)	(30.1)	170.0	6.00	2720	96.0	
Sun Giant Blanched Almonds, Slivered, 6-oz. pouch	(1020)	(33.0)	(170.0)	(5.50)	(2720)	(88.0)	
1 cup (approx. 4.0 oz.)	(688)	(22.4)	(170.0)	(5.50)	(2720)	(88.0)	
Blanched Almonds, Whole, 6-oz. pouch	(407)	(13.3)	(67.8)	(2.21)	(1085)	(35.4)	
1 cup (approx. 2.8 oz.)	(187)	(6.1)	(67.8)	(2.21)	(1085)	(35.4)	
Dry Roasted, Hickory Smoke Flavored Almonds, 4-oz. can	720	24.0	180.0	6.00	2880	96.0	
8-oz. jar	1440	48.0	180.0	6.00	2880	96.0	
1 cup (approx. 5.3 oz.)	(997)	(33.2)	180.0	6.00	2880	96.0	
Natural Almonds, Diced, 6-oz. pouch	(1020)	(33.0)	(170.0)	(5.50)	(2720)	(88.0)	
1 cup (approx. 4.6 oz.)	(777)	(25.4)	(170.0)	(5.50)	(2720)	(88.0)	

	UNIT Cal.	UNIT Carb.	1 OZ., BY WT. Cal.	1 OZ., BY WT. Carb.	1 POUND Cal.	1 POUND Carb.	Fiber per oz. (GMS.)
Natural Almonds, Whole, 4-oz. can	(271)	(8.9)	(67.8)	(2.21)	(1085)	(35.4)	
6-oz. pouch	(407)	(13.3)	(67.8)	(2.21)	(1085)	(35.4)	
8-oz. can	(542)	(17.7)	(67.8)	(2.21)	(1085)	(35.4)	
Salted Almonds, 4-oz. can	720	24.0	180.0	6.00	2880	96.0	
8-oz. jar	1440	48.0	180.0	6.00	2880	96.0	
1 cup (approx. 5.1 oz.)	(909)	(30.3)	180.0	6.00	2880	96.0	
Taco Flavored Almonds, 4-oz. can	720	24.0	180.0	6.00	2880	96.0	
8-oz. jar	1440	48.0	180.0	6.00	2880	96.0	
1 cup (approx. 5.1 oz.)	(909)	(30.3)	180.0	6.00	2880	96.0	
Almond Products							
ALMOND BUTTER							
Hain unsalted raw blanched Almond Butter, 11-oz. jar	1851	29.2	168.3	2.66	2693	42.6	
1 cup (approx. 9.1 oz.)	1520	24.0	168.3	2.66	2693	42.6	
ALMOND CANDY							
Schrafft's Almond Cluster, 5½-oz. box	902	61.6	164.0	11.20	2624	179.2	
Rainbow Jordan Almonds, 4½-oz. box	683	61.4	151.9	13.64	2430	218.2	
ALMOND MEAL							
Balanced All Natural Fancy Grade, 10-oz. can	(1166)	(82.4)	(116.6)	(8.24)	(1866)	(131.8)	
1 cup (approx. 8.0 oz.)	933	65.9	(116.6)	(8.24)	(1866)	(131.8)	
ALMOND OIL							
Hain Pure Cold Pressed Almond Oil, 16-fl.-oz. (1-pint) bottle	3840	0.0	(250.0)	0.00	(4000)	0.0	
1 cup (approx. 7.7 oz.)	1920	0.0	(250.0)	0.00	(4000)	0.0	
ALMOND PASTE							
1 pound (based on data from France) (2g/18g/5g/na/1mg)	2046	291.7	127.9	18.23	2046	291.7	
APRICOT KERNELS (based on data from East Asia)							
DRIED:							
Edible portion, 1 pound (8g/4g/13g/8%/na)	2490	58.5	155.6	3.66	2490	58.6	0.85
BEECHNUTS							
RAW:							
As purchased in shell [refuse: shells, approx. 39%]							
1 pound	1572	56.2	98.3	3.51	1572	56.2	
Shelled, 1 pound (5g/6g/14g/7%/na)	2576	92.1	161.1	5.76	2576	92.2	
BRAZIL NUTS							
RAW, WHOLE:							
As purchased in shell [refuse: shells, approx. 52%]:							
1 nut:							
1 medium nut (approx. 0.9" diameter, 0.28 oz., 3½ per ounce)	25	0.4	89.1	1.48	1426	23.7	
1 large Brazil Nut (approx. 1.1" diameter, 0.32 oz., 3 per ounce)	30	0.5	89.1	1.48	1426	23.7	
1 extra large nut (approx. 1.2" diameter, 0.36 oz., 2¾ per ounce)	32	0.5	89.1	1.48	1426	23.7	
1 cup (approx. 4.3 oz., 15 medium Brazil Nuts)	383	6.4	89.1	1.48	1424	23.7	
1 pound (approx. 3¾ cups, 45 extra large nuts, 50 large nuts, or 57 medium nuts)	1424	23.7	89.1	1.48	1424	23.7	
Shelled:							
1 nut:							
1 medium Brazil Nut (approx. 0.12 oz., 8¼ per ounce)	25	0.4	185.4	3.09	2966	49.4	0.88
1 large Brazil Nut (approx. 0.16 oz.)	30	0.5	185.4	3.09	2966	49.4	0.88
1 extra large Brazil Nut (approx. 0.17 oz., 6 per ounce)	32	0.5	185.4	3.09	2966	49.4	0.88
1 cup (approx. 4.9 oz., 32 large Brazil Nuts)	916	15.3	185.4	3.09	2966	49.4	0.88
1 pound (approx. 3¼ cups, 94 extra large, 103 large, 133 medium nuts [yield from approx. 2.1 lbs. of Brazil Nuts in the shell]) (4g/3g/19g/5%/tr)	2967	49.4	185.4	3.09	2966	49.4	0.88
BRAZIL NUTS, by brand							
Fisher Brazil Nuts, Shelled, 1-lb. package	2960	49.6	185.0	3.10	2960	49.6	
1 cup (approx. 4.6 oz.)	(855)	(14.3)	185.0	3.10	2960	49.6	

	UNIT Cal.	UNIT Carb.	1 OZ., BY WT. Cal.	1 OZ., BY WT. Carb.	1 POUND Cal.	1 POUND Carb.	Fiber per oz. (GMS.)
BUTTERNUTS							
RAW:							
As purchased in shell [refuse: shells, approx. 86%]:							
1 pound	399	5.3	24.9	0.33	399	5.3	
Shelled:							
1 butternut (approx. 0.12 oz., 8⅓ per ounce)	21	0.3	178.3	2.38	2853	38.1	
1 pound (approx. 136 butternuts) (7g/2g/17g/4%/tr)	2853	38.1	178.3	2.38	2853	38.1	
CASHEW NUTS							
ROASTED IN OIL:							
Shelled:							
Whole:							
1 nut:							
1 small cashew (approx. 0.04 oz., 26 per ounce)	6	0.3	159.0	8.30	2545	132.9	0.40
1 medium cashew (approx. 0.06 oz., 18 per ounce)	9	0.5	159.0	8.30	2545	132.9	0.40
1 large cashew (approx. 0.07 oz., 14 per ounce)	12	0.6	159.0	8.30	2545	132.9	0.40
1 cup (approx. 4.9 oz., 88 medium cashews)	785	41.0	159.0	8.30	2545	132.9	0.40
1 pound (approx. 3¼ cups, 200–240 large, 260–320 medium, or 350–500 small cashews (5g/8g/13g/5%/17mg)	2545	132.9	159.0	8.30	2545	132.9	0.40
CASHEW NUTS, by brand							
Ann Page (A&P) Dry Roasted Cashews, 7-oz. jar	1190	56.0	170.0	8.00	2720	128.0	
1 cup (approx. 4.8 oz.)	(816)	(38.4)	170.0	8.00	2720	128.0	
Fancy Salted Cashews, 6½ oz.	1125	50.0	180.0	8.00	2880	128.0	
1 cup (approx. 4.8 oz.)	(863)	(38.4)	180.0	8.00	2880	128.0	
Fisher Cashews, Roasted In Oil, 6½-oz. package	1034	54.0	159.0	8.30	2544	132.8	
12-oz. package	1908	99.6	159.0	8.30	2544	132.8	
1 cup (approx. 4.8 oz.)	(755)	(39.4)	159.0	8.30	2544	132.8	
Frito-Lay Cashews, ⅝-oz. bag	105	5.4	168.1	8.65	2690	138.4	
1¾-oz. bag	294	15.1	168.1	8.65	2690	138.4	
1 cup (approx. 4.8 oz.)	(806)	(41.5)	168.1	8.65	2690	138.4	
Golden Harvest Roasted Cashews, with Sea Salt, 2½-oz. bag	440	15.0	176.0	6.00	2816	96.0	
1 cup (approx. 4.8 oz.)	(845)	(28.8)	176.0	6.00	2816	96.0	
Granny Goose Cashews, 1-oz. package	169	7.0	169.0	7.00	2704	112.0	
2-oz. package	338	14.1	169.0	7.00	2704	112.0	
3-oz. package	507	21.2	169.0	7.00	2704	112.0	
3.3-oz. package	596	24.9	169.0	7.00	2704	112.0	
4-oz. package	676	28.2	169.0	7.00	2704	112.0	
1 cup (approx. 4.8 oz.)	(811)	(33.6)	169.0	7.00	2704	112.0	
Laura Scudder's Cashews, Roasted in Oil, ¾-oz. bag	119	6.2	159.0	8.30	2544	132.8	
1½-oz. bag	239	12.5	159.0	8.30	2544	132.8	
6-oz. can	954	49.8	159.0	8.30	2544	132.8	
12-oz. can	1908	99.6	159.0	8.30	2544	132.8	
1 cup (approx. 4.8 oz.)	(763)	(39.8)	159.0	8.30	2544	132.8	
Dry Roasted Cashews, 7-oz. jar	1190	54.6	170.0	7.80	2720	124.8	
1 cup (approx. 4.8 oz.)	(816)	(37.4)	170.0	7.80	2720	124.8	
Planters Cashews, Roasted in Oil, Salted, 7-oz. can	1190	56.0	170.0	8.00	2720	128.0	
1 cup (approx. 4.8 oz.)	(813)	(38.2)	170.0	8.00	2720	128.0	
Dry Roasted Cashews, Salted, 7-oz. can	1120	63.0	160.0	9.00	2560	144.0	
1 cup (approx. 4.8 oz.)	(765)	(43.0)	160.0	9.00	2560	144.0	
Dry Roasted Cashews, Unsalted, 7½-oz. can	1200	67.5	160.0	9.00	2560	144.0	
1 cup (approx. 4.8 oz.)	(765)	(43.0)	160.0	9.00	2560	144.0	
Skippy Dry Roasted Cashews, 7-oz. jar	1155	56.0	165.0	8.00	2640	128.0	
1 cup (approx. 4.8 oz.)	(789)	(38.2)	165.0	8.00	2640	128.0	
Cashew Products							
CASHEW BUTTER							
Hain Unsalted Raw Cashew Butter, 11-oz. jar	1851	78.0	168.3	7.10	2693	113.4	
1 cup (approx. 9.1 oz.)	1520	64.0	168.3	7.10	2693	113.4	

	UNIT Cal.	UNIT Carb.	1 OZ., BY WT. Cal.	1 OZ., BY WT. Carb.	1 POUND Cal.	1 POUND Carb.	Fiber per oz. (GMS.)
CHESTNUTS							
RAW:							
As purchased in shell [refuse: shells, approx. 19%]:							
1 small chestnut (approx. 0.18 oz., 5½ per ounce)	8	1.8	44.6	9.67	713	154.7	
1 large chestnut (approx. 1½" diameter, ⅓ oz., 3 per ounce)	15	3.2	44.6	9.67	713	154.7	
1 cup (approx. 4¼ oz., 13 large or 24 small chestnuts)	189	40.9	44.6	9.67	713	154.7	
1 pound (approx. 3¾ cups, 50 large or 89 small chestnuts)	713	154.7	44.6	9.67	713	154.7	
Shelled:							
1 cup (approx. 5.6 oz.)	310	67.0	55.0	11.94	880	191.0	0.31
1 pound (approx. 2.8 cups) (1g/12g/tr/53%/2mg)	880	191.0	55.0	11.94	880	191.0	0.31
DRIED:							
As purchased in shell [refuse: shells, approx. 18%]:							
1 pound	377	78.6	23.6	4.91	377	78.6	
Shelled:							
1 cup (approx. 5.6 oz.)	310	67.0	55.0	11.94	880	191.0	0.71
1 pound (2g/22g/1g/8%/3mg)	880	191.0	55.0	11.94	880	191.0	0.71
Chestnut Products							
CHESTNUT FLOUR							
1 pound	1642	345.6	102.6	21.60	1642	345.6	
CHESTNUT PASTE (based on data from France)							
1 pound	481	103.4	30.1	6.46	481	103.4	
COCONUTS							
RAW:							
As purchased:							
1 medium coconut (approx. 4⅝" diameter, 4⅞" high, 1⅔ lb.) [refuse: shell, brown skin, water, approx. 48%]	1373	37.3	51.5	1.40	824	22.4	
Edible portion:							
1 medium coconut (approx. 14 oz.)	1373	37.3	98.1	2.66	1569	42.6	1.14
1 piece (approx. 2" × 2" × ½", 1.6 oz.) (1g/3g/10g/51%/7mg)	156	4.2	98.1	2.66	1569	42.6	1.14
1 pound (1g/3g/10g/51%/7mg)	1569	42.6	98.1	2.66	1569	42.6	1.14
Shredded or grated:							
1 cup:							
Not packed (approx. 2.8 oz.)	277	7.5	98.1	2.66	1569	42.6	1.14
Packed (approx. 4.6 oz.)	450	12.2	98.1	2.66	1569	42.6	1.14
1 pound (approx. 5.7 cups not packed, or 3.5 cups packed)	1569	42.6	98.1	2.66	1569	42.6	1.14
(for shredded coconut by brand, see the BASIC BAKING & COOKING INGREDIENTS chapter)							
DRIED:							
Unsweetened, shredded:							
1 cup (approx. 3.2 oz.)	(596)	(20.7)	187.7	6.52	3003	104.3	1.11
1 pound (approx. 5 cups) (2g/7g/18g/4%/na)	3003	104.3	187.7	6.52	3003	104.3	1.11
Sweetened, shredded:							
1 cup (approx. 3.4 oz.)	528	51.3	155.4	15.08	2486	241.3	1.16
1 pound (approx. 4.71 cups) (1g/15g/11g/3%/na)	2486	241.3	155.4	15.08	2486	241.3	1.16
Coconut Products							
COCONUT BUTTER (based on data from France):							
1 pound	4019	0.0	251.2	0.00	4019	0.0	
COCONUT CREAM (liquid expressed from grated coconut meat)							
1 cup (approx. 8.5 oz.)	(802)	(19.9)	94.4	2.34	1510	37.4	
1 pound (approx. 1.9 cups) (1g/2g/9g/54%/1mg)	1510	37.4	94.4	2.34	1510	37.4	
1 tablespoon (approx. 0.5 oz.)	50	1.2	94.4	2.34	1510	37.4	
COCONUT MILK (liquid expressed from mixture of grated coconut meat and coconut water)							
1 cup (approx. 8.5 oz.) (1g/1g/7g/66%/na)	605	12.5	71.2	1.47	1132	23.5	

	UNIT Cal.	UNIT Carb.	1 OZ., BY WT. Cal.	1 OZ., BY WT. Carb.	1 POUND Cal.	1 POUND Carb.	Fiber per oz. (GMS.)
COCONUT OIL (based on data from East Asia), 1 pound	4005	0.0	250.3	0.00	4005	0.0	
COCONUT WATER (liquid from coconuts)							
1 cup (approx. 8.5 oz.) (tr/1g/tr/94%/na)	53	11.3	6.2	1.34	100	21.3	
FILBERTS (Hazelnuts)							
RAW:							
As purchased in shell [refuse: shells, approx. 54%]							
1 filbert (approx. ⅕ oz., 5 per ounce)	18	0.5	82.7	2.18	1323	34.9	
1 cup (approx. 8.9 oz., 45 filberts)	735	19.4	82.7	2.18	1323	34.9	
1 pound (1¾ cups, 80 filberts)	1323	34.9	82.7	2.18	1323	34.9	
Shelled:							
Whole:							
1 filbert (approx. 1/20 oz., 20 per ounce)	9	0.2	179.9	4.73	2879	75.7	0.85
1 cup (approx. 4¾ oz., 95 filberts)	856	22.5	179.9	4.73	2879	75.7	
1 pound (approx. 3.4 cups, 320 filberts) (4g/5g/18g/6%/tr)	2879	75.7	179.9	4.73	2879	75.7	0.85
Chopped:							
1 cup (approx. 4.1 oz.)	729	19.2	179.9	4.74	2879	75.8	0.85
1 tablespoon (approx. ¼ oz.)	46	1.2	179.9	4.74	2879	75.8	0.85
Ground:							
1 cup (approx. 2.6 oz.)	476	12.5	179.9	4.74	2879	75.8	0.85
FILBERTS (Hazelnuts), by brand							
Fisher Shelled Filberts, 2-oz. bag	360	9.4	180.0	4.70	2880	75.2	0.85
1 cup (approx. 4.7 oz.)	(851)	(22.2)	180.0	4.70	2880	75.2	
GOOBERS, see PEANUTS							
GROUNDNUTS, see PEANUTS							
HAZELNUTS, see FILBERTS							
HICKORY NUTS							
RAW:							
As purchased in shell [refuse: shells, approx. 65%]:							
1 pound	1068	20.3	66.8	1.27	1068	20.3	
Shelled:							
1 small hickory nut (approx. 0.04 oz., 25 per ounce)	6	0.1	190.8	3.63	3053	58.1	0.54
1 pound (approx. 400 small hickory nuts) (4g/4g/19g/3%/tr)	3053	58.1	190.8	3.63	3053	58.1	0.54
MACADAMIA NUTS							
RAW:							
As purchased in shell [refuse: shells, approx. 69%]:							
1 pound	972	22.4	60.8	1.40	972	22.4	
Shelled:							
1 cup:							
Whole (approx. 4.7 oz. [yield from 1 pound of macadamia nuts in the shell])	(926)	(21.3)	195.9	4.51	3134	72.1	0.71
Chopped (approx. 4.1 oz., yield from ¼ pound of macadamia nuts)	(795)	(18.3)	195.9	4.51	3134	72.1	0.71
1 pound (approx. 3.4 cups) (2g/5g/20g/3%/tr)	3134	72.1	195.9	4.51	3134	72.1	0.71
ROASTED IN OIL:							
1 nut:							
1 small Macadamia nut (approx. ⅝" × ⅝", 0.07 oz., 14 per ounce)	15	0.2	208.3	2.83	3333	45.3	0.71
1 medium Macadamia nut (approx. ⅝ × ⅞", 0.14 oz., 7 per ounce)	29	0.4	208.3	2.83	3333	45.3	0.71
1 large Macadamia nut (approx. ¾" × 1", 0.21 oz., 4¾ per ounce)	44	0.6	208.3	2.83	3333	45.3	0.71
1 cup (approx. 4.7 oz., 34 medium macadamia nuts)	974	13.4	208.3	2.83	3300	45.3	0.71

	UNIT Cal.	UNIT Carb.	1 OZ., BY WT. Cal.	1 OZ., BY WT. Carb.	1 POUND Cal.	1 POUND Carb.	Fiber per oz. (GMS.)
1 pound (approx. 3¼ cups, 112 medium macadamia nuts)	3300	45.3	208.3	2.83	3300	45.3	0.71

PEANUTS

	UNIT Cal.	UNIT Carb.	1 OZ., BY WT. Cal.	1 OZ., BY WT. Carb.	1 POUND Cal.	1 POUND Carb.	Fiber per oz. (GMS.)
RAW:							
As purchased in shell [refuse: shells, approx. 27%]:							
1 pound	1868	61.6	116.8	3.85	1868	61.6	
Shelled:							
1 pound (14g/5g/7g/5%/1mg)	2558	84.4	159.9	5.28	2558	84.5	0.68
BOILED:							
1 cup (approx. 5.1 oz.)	(542)	(20.5)	106.7	4.11	1707	65.8	
1 pound (approx. 5 cups) (4g/4g/9g/36%/1mg)	1707	65.8	106.7	4.11	1707	65.8	0.51
ROASTED IN SHELL:							
As purchased in shell [refuse: shells, approx. 33%]:							
1 jumbo peanut (approx. 0.1 oz., 10 per ounce)	11	0.4	110.6	3.91	1769	62.6	
1 pound (approx. 160 jumbo peanuts)	1769	62.6	110.6	3.91	1769	62.6	
Shelled:							
Whole:							
1 pound (approx. 3.1 cups [yield from approx. 1½ lbs. nuts in shell]) (7g/6g/14g/2%/1mg)	2640	93.4	165.1	5.85	2640	93.4	0.77
1 peanut:							
Spanish (approx. 0.02 oz., 60 per ounce)	3	0.1	165.1	5.85	2640	93.4	0.77
Virginia (approx. 0.04 oz., 30 per ounce)	6	0.2	165.1	5.85	2640	93.4	0.77
Chopped:							
1 tablespoon (approx. ⅓ oz.)	52	1.9	165.1	5.85	2640	93.4	0.77
1 cup (approx. 5.1 oz., 140 Virginia or 280 Spanish peanuts)	838	29.7	165.1	5.85	2640	93.4	0.77
ROASTED, SALTED (Spanish and Virginia types):							
Shelled:							
Whole:							
1 pound (approx. 3.1 cups, 500 Virginia or 1000 Spanish Peanuts) (7g/6g/14g/2%/118mg)	2654	85.3	165.9	5.33	2654	85.3	0.68
1 peanut:							
Spanish (approx. 0.02 oz., 60 per ounce)	3	0.1	165.9	5.33	2654	85.9	0.68
Virginia (approx. 0.04 oz., 30 per ounce)	6	0.2	165.9	5.33	2654	85.9	0.68
Chopped:							
1 tablespoon (approx. ⅓ oz.)	53	1.7	165.9	5.33	2654	85.9	0.68
1 cup (approx. 5.1 oz., 159 Virginia or 319 Spanish Peanuts)	842	27.1	165.9	5.33	2654	85.9	0.68
BASED ON DATA FROM AFRICA							
Roasted, 1 pound	2704	98.4	169.0	6.15	2704	98.4	0.90
PEANUTS, by brand							
Ann Page (A&P) Dry Roasted Peanuts, Salted, 8-oz. jar	1440	48.0	180.0	6.00	2880	96.0	
12-oz. jar	2160	72.0	180.0	6.00	2880	96.0	
1 cup (approx. 5.1 oz.)	(918)	(30.6)	180.0	6.00	2880	96.0	
Salted "Party" Peanuts, Roasted in Oil, 12-oz. tin	2160	60.0	180.0	5.00	2880	80.0	
2-lb., 8 oz. tin	7200	200.0	180.0	5.00	2880	80.0	
1 cup (approx. 5.1 oz.)	(918)	(25.5)	180.0	5.00	2880	80.0	
Salted Spanish Peanuts, 6½-oz. tin	1170	32.5	180.0	5.00	2880	80.0	
12-oz. tin	2160	60.0	180.0	5.00	2880	80.0	
1 cup (approx. 5.1 oz.)	(918)	(25.5)	180.0	5.00	2880	80.0	
Balanced Dry Roasted Peanuts, Unsalted, 16-oz. (1-lb.) tin	3120	100.3	195.0	6.27	3120	100.3	
1 cup (approx. 5.1 oz.)	(995)	(32.0)	195.0	6.27	3120	100.3	
Fine Food Distributors Reduced Calorie Peanuts, "50% less calories," partially defatted peanuts, 7-oz. tin	950	na	135.7	na	2171	na	
1 cup (approx. 5.1 oz.)	(692)	na	135.7	na	2171	na	
Fisher Peanuts Roasted in Shell With Skins, 12-oz. package	1260	44.4	105.0	3.70	1680	59.2	
1 cup (approx. 5.1 oz.)	(563)	(19.8)	105.0	3.70	1680	59.2	
Spanish Peanuts, Roasted, Salted, 12-oz. package	1992	63.6	166.0	5.30	2656	84.8	
1 cup (approx. 5.1 oz.)	(843)	(20.9)	166.0	5.30	2656	84.8	
Virginia Peanuts, 12-oz. package	1992	63.6	166.0	5.30	2656	84.8	
1 cup (approx. 5.1 oz.)	(843)	(26.9)	166.0	5.30	2656	84.8	
Frito-Lay Salted-In-The-Shell Peanuts, 5¼-oz. bag	633	22.2	120.6	4.22	1930	67.5	
Salted Peanuts, Shelled, 1⅜-oz. bag	237	8.6	172.1	6.24	2754	99.8	
5-oz. bag	860	31.0	172.1	6.24	2754	99.8	
1 cup (approx. 5.4 oz.)	(922)	(33.4)	172.1	6.24	2754	99.8	
Golden Harvest Raw Spanish Peanuts, 12-oz. package	2040	60.0	170.0	5.00	2720	80.0	
Granny Goose Goobers, 1-oz. package	166	4.9	166.0	4.90	2656	78.4	
2-oz. package	332	9.8	166.0	4.90	2656	78.4	
3-oz. package	499	14.6	166.0	4.90	2656	78.4	
3.3-oz. package	586	17.2	166.0	4.90	2656	78.4	
4-oz. package	664	19.5	166.0	4.90	2656	78.4	
1 "Goober," 0.06 oz. (15 to 16 per ounce)	11	0.3	166.0	4.90	2656	78.4	
1 cup (approx. 5.4 oz.)	(890)	(26.3)	166.0	4.90	2656	78.4	
Spanish Peanuts, 1-oz. package	168	4.0	168.0	4.00	2688	64.0	
2-oz. package	337	8.0	168.0	4.00	2688	64.0	
3-oz. package	505	12.1	168.0	4.00	2688	64.0	
3.3-oz. package	594	14.2	168.0	4.00	2688	64.0	
4-oz. package	674	16.1	168.0	4.00	2688	64.0	
1 cup (approx. 5.1 oz.)	(853)	(20.3)	168.0	4.00	2688	64.0	
Virginia Peanuts, 1-oz. package	166	4.6	166.0	4.60	2656	73.6	
2-oz. package	333	9.2	166.0	4.60	2656	73.6	
3-oz. package	500	13.8	166.0	4.60	2656	73.6	
3.3-oz. package	587	(16.2)	166.0	4.60	2656	73.6	
4-oz. package	666	18.4	166.0	4.60	2656	73.6	
1 cup (approx. 5.1 oz.)	(843)	(23.4)	166.0	4.60	2656	73.6	
Laura Scudder's Goobers, Roasted in Shell [refuse: approx. 33%], 1¾ oz. bag	194	6.8	111.0	3.90	1776	62.4	
4-oz. bag	444	15.6	111.0	3.90	1776	62.4	
7-oz. bag	777	27.3	111.0	3.90	1776	62.4	
2-lb. bag	3552	124.8	111.0	3.90	1776	62.4	
Dry Roasted Snackin' Peanuts, 8-oz. jar	1400	31.2	175.0	3.90	2800	62.4	
12-oz. jar	2100	46.8	175.0	3.90	2800	62.4	
1 cup (approx. 5.1 oz.)	(893)	(19.9)	175.0	3.90	2800	62.4	
Spanish Peanuts, Roasted in Oil, shelled, salted, 5-oz. bag	905	17.0	181.0	3.40	2896	54.4	
6-oz. can	1086	20.4	181.0	3.40	2896	54.4	
12-oz. can or bag	2172	40.8	181.0	3.40	2896	54.4	
1 cup (approx. 5.1 oz.)	(923)	(17.3)	181.0	3.40	2896	54.4	
Virginia Peanuts, Roasted in Oil, shelled, salted, 1¼-oz. bag	228	4.0	182.0	3.20	2912	51.2	
4-oz. bag	728	12.8	182.0	3.20	2912	51.2	
10-oz. bag	1820	32.0	182.0	3.20	2912	51.2	
1-lb. bag	2912	51.2	182.0	3.20	2912	51.2	
1 cup (approx. 5.1 oz.)	(928)	(16.3)	182.0	3.20	2912	51.2	
Party Pride Dry Roasted Peanuts, unsalted, 8¼-oz. tin	1403	41.3	170.0	5.00	2720	80.0	
1 cup (approx. 5.1 oz.)	(864)	(25.4)	170.0	5.00	2720	80.0	
Planters Cocktail Peanuts, Roasted in Oil, 16-oz. (1-lb.) jar	2720	80.0	170.0	5.00	2720	80.0	
1 cup (approx. 5.1 oz.)	(867)	(25.5)	170.0	5.00	2720	80.0	
Dry Roasted Peanuts, salted, 8-oz. jar	1280	48.0	160.0	6.00	2560	96.0	
24-oz. jar	3840	144.0	160.0	6.00	2560	96.0	
1 cup (approx. 5.0 oz.)	(800)	(30.0)	160.0	6.00	2560	96.0	
Unsalted, 8¼-oz. jar	1403	41.3	170.0	5.00	2720	80.0	
16-oz. (1-lb.) jar	2720	80.0	170.0	5.00	2720	80.0	
Vending machine size, ½-oz. cello-pack	85	2.5	170.0	5.00	2720	80.0	
1 cup (approx. 5.4 oz.)	(911)	(26.8)	170.0	5.00	2720	80.0	
Old Fashioned Peanuts, Roasted in Oil, 16-oz. (1-lb.) jar	2720	80.0	170.0	5.00	2720	80.0	
1 cup (approx. 5.4 oz.)	(911)	(26.8)	170.0	5.00	2720	80.0	
Vending machine size, ½-oz. foil pack	85	2.5	170.0	5.00	2720	80.0	
1 cup (approx. 5.4 oz.)	(911)	(26.8)	170.0	5.00	2720	80.0	
Peanuts, Roasted in Oil, 16-oz. (1-lb.) jar	2720	96.0	170.0	6.00	2720	96.0	
1 cup (approx. 5.1 oz.)	(864)	(30.5)	170.0	6.00	2720	96.0	
Redskin Virginia Peanuts, 16-oz. (1-lb.) jar	2720	80.0	170.0	5.00	2720	80.0	
Spanish Peanuts, Dry Roasted, 16-oz. (1-lb.) jar	2560	96.0	160.0	6.00	2560	96.0	
1 cup (approx. 5.1 oz.)	(813)	(30.5)	160.0	6.00	2560	96.0	

Peanut Products

	UNIT Cal.	UNIT Carb.	1 OZ., BY WT. Cal.	1 OZ., BY WT. Carb.	1 POUND Cal.	1 POUND Carb.	Fiber per oz. (GMS.)
PEANUT BUTTER							
Planters Creamy Peanut Butter, 16-oz. (1-lb.) jar	2693	85.1	168.3	5.32	2693	85.1	
1 cup (approx. 9 oz.)	1520	48.0	168.3	5.32	2693	85.1	

	UNIT Cal.	UNIT Carb.	1 OZ., BY WT. Cal.	1 OZ., BY WT. Carb.	1 POUND Cal.	1 POUND Carb.	Fiber per oz. (GMS.)
Skippy Super Chunk Peanut Butter, 18-oz. jar	3029	63.7	168.3	3.54	2693	56.6	
PEANUT CANDY							
CaraCoa (El Molino) Carob Coated Peanuts, 1-oz. package	160	12.0	160.0	12.00	2560	192.0	
Cracker Jack, 1-oz. box	120	22.0	120.0	22.00	1920	352.0	
Goldenberg's Peanut Chews, 2-oz. bar	278	35.0	138.7	17.69	2219	283.0	
Planters Old Fashioned Peanut Candy Bar, 1.6-oz. bar	224	24.0	140.0	15.00	2240	240.0	
Ward Goobers, 1-oz. box	153	12.0	153.0	12.00	2448	192.0	
PEANUT FLOUR, defatted, based on generic data							
1 cup (approx. 2.1 oz.)	223	18.9	105.2	8.92	1683	142.6	
1 pound (approx. 7.5 cups) (14g/9g/3g/7%/3mg)	1683	142.6	105.2	8.92	1683	142.6	
PEANUT MILK, based on data from East Asia							
1 quart (approx. 34.4 oz.)	(282)	(11.7)	8.2	0.34	132	5.4	
PEANUT OIL, based on generic data							
1 cup (approx. 7.6 oz.)	1910	0.0	250.6	0.00	4010	0.0	
1 quart (approx. 30.5 oz.) (0g/0g/28g/0%/0mg)	7638	0.0	250.6	0.00	4010	0.0	

PECANS

	UNIT Cal.	UNIT Carb.	1 OZ., BY WT. Cal.	1 OZ., BY WT. Carb.	1 POUND Cal.	1 POUND Carb.	Fiber per oz. (GMS.)
RAW:							
As purchased in shell [refuse: shells, approx. 47%]:							
1 nut:							
1 Large pecan (approx. 0.2 oz., 64–77 per pound)	24	0.5	103.3	2.19	1652	35.1	
1 Extra large pecan (approx. 0.27 oz., 56–63 per pound)	28	0.6	103.3	2.19	1652	35.1	
1 Oversize pecan (approx. 0.29 oz. each, no more than 55 per pound)	30	0.6	103.3	2.19	1652	35.1	
1 cup (approx. 7.1 oz., 30 large pecans)	(734)	(15.6)	103.3	2.19	1652	35.1	
1 pound (approx. 2¼ cups, 68 large pecans)	1652	35.1	103.3	2.19	1652	35.1	
Shelled, halves:							
Whole:							
1 Extra large pecan (approx. 0.14 oz.)	(28)	(0.6)	194.8	4.14	3116	66.2	
1 cup (approx. 3.8 oz., 26 pecans)	(739)	(16.7)	194.8	4.14	3116	66.2	
1 pound (approx. 4.2 cups, 111 pecans [yield from approx. 1.9 lb. pecans in the shell]) (3g/4g/20g/3%/tr)	3116	66.2	194.8	4.14	3116	66.2	
Chopped:							
1 tablespoon (approx. ¼ oz.)	52	1.1	194.8	4.14	3116	66.2	
1 cup (approx. 4.1 oz., 28 pecans)	811	17.2	194.8	4.14	3116	66.2	
Ground:							
1 cup (approx. 3⅓ oz.)	653	13.9	194.8	4.14	3116	66.2	
For comparison: Butter Pecan Ice Cream, **Breyer's,** 1 cup (approx. 4.9 oz.)	360	30.0	72.9	6.07	1166	97.1	
For comparison: Caramel Pecan Frozen Yogurt, **Johnston's,** 1 cup (approx. 6.0 oz.)	200	37.0	(33.3)	(6.17)	(533)	(98.7)	
PECANS, by brand							
Diamond Sunsweet Shelled Pecans, 4-oz. can	(780)	(16.4)	(195.0)	(4.10)	(3120)	(65.6)	
5-oz. bag	(975)	(20.5)	(195.0)	(4.10)	(3120)	(65.6)	
8-oz. can	(1560)	(32.8)	(195.0)	(4.10)	(3120)	(65.6)	
1 cup (approx. 3.8 oz.)	(743)	(15.6)	(195.0)	(4.10)	(3120)	(65.6)	
Fisher Pecans, Shelled, 6-oz. package	1170	24.6	195.0	4.10	3120	65.6	
1 cup (approx. 3.8 oz.)	(743)	(15.6)	195.0	4.10	3120	65.6	
Granny Goose Shelled Pecans, 1-oz. package	203	3.1	203.0	3.10	3248	49.6	
2-oz. package	406	6.3	203.0	3.10	3248	49.6	
3-oz. package	609	9.4	203.0	3.10	3248	49.6	
3.3-oz. package	(716)	(11.1)	203.0	3.10	3248	49.6	
4-oz. package	812	12.4	203.0	3.10	3248	49.6	
1 cup (approx. 3.8 oz.)	(773)	(11.8)	203.0	3.10	3248	49.6	
Planters "Southern Belle" Pecan Pieces, 3-oz. bag	570	15.0	190.0	5.00	3040	80.0	
1 cup (approx. 3.8 oz.)	(732)	(19.0)	190.0	5.00	3040	80.0	
Southland's Natural Pecans, 12-oz. bag	2338	49.7	194.8	4.14	3117	66.2	
16-oz. (1-lb.) bag or carton	3117	66.2	194.8	4.14	3117	66.2	
5-lb. carton	15584	331.2	194.8	4.14	3117	66.2	
1 cup (approx. 3.8 oz.)	(742)	(15.8)	194.8	4.14	3117	66.2	

PILINUTS

	UNIT Cal.	UNIT Carb.	1 OZ., BY WT. Cal.	1 OZ., BY WT. Carb.	1 POUND Cal.	1 POUND Carb.	Fiber per oz. (GMS.)
RAW:							
As purchased in shell [refuse: shells, approx. 82%]:							
1 pound	546	6.9	34.1	0.43	546	6.9	
Shelled:							
1 pound (3g/2g/20g/6%/1mg)	3037	38.1	189.8	2.38	3037	38.1	0.77

PINENUTS

	UNIT Cal.	UNIT Carb.	1 OZ., BY WT. Cal.	1 OZ., BY WT. Carb.	1 POUND Cal.	1 POUND Carb.	Fiber per oz. (GMS.)
Pignolis							
RAW:							
Shelled:							
1 pound (9g/3g/13g/6%/na)	2496	52.8	156.0	3.30	2496	52.8	0.31
Piñons							
RAW:							
As purchased in shell [refuse: shells, approx. 42%]:							
1 pound	1671	53.9	104.4	3.37	1671	53.9	
Shelled:							
1 pound (4g/6g/17g/3%/na)	2880	97.8	180.0	5.80	2880	97.8	

PISTACHIO NUTS

	UNIT Cal.	UNIT Carb.	1 OZ., BY WT. Cal.	1 OZ., BY WT. Carb.	1 POUND Cal.	1 POUND Carb.	Fiber per oz. (GMS.)
RAW:							
As purchased in shell [refuse: shells, approx. 50%]:							
1 pistachio nut (approx. 0.02 oz., 42 per ounce)	2	0.1	84.2	2.69	1347	43.1	
1 cup (approx. 4.7 oz., 198 pistachio nuts)	(395)	(12.6)	84.2	2.69	1347	43.1	
1 pound (approx. 3⅓ cups, 674 pistachio nuts)	1347	43.1	84.2	2.69	1347	43.1	
Shelled:							
1 cup (approx. 4.4 oz.)	(745)	(23.8)	169.0	5.40	2704	86.4	
1 pound (approx. 3.6 cups [yield from approx. 2 lbs. nuts in the shell] (5g/5g/15g/5%/na)	2704	86.4	169.0	5.40	2704	86.4	0.54
PISTACHIO NUTS, by brand							
Fisher Pistachios, Shelled, Whole, 7-oz. package	1183	37.8	169.0	5.40	2704	86.4	
1 cup (approx. 4.4 oz.)	(745)	(23.8)	169.0	5.40	2704	86.4	
Frito-Lay Pistachios In-The-Shell, 1¾-oz. bag	165	5.5	94.5	3.13	1512	50.1	
1 cup (approx. 4.7 oz.)	(443)	(14.7)	94.5	3.13	1512	50.1	
Shelled Pistachios, 1¾-oz. bag	300	10.2	175.0	5.80	2800	92.8	
1 cup (approx. 4.4 oz.)	(772)	(25.6)	175.0	5.80	2800	92.8	
Fruit Pac, 8-oz. package	(1347)	(43.1)	(168.4)	(5.39)	(2694)	(86.2)	
1 cup (approx. 4.4 oz.)	(743)	(23.8)	(168.4)	(5.39)	(2694)	(86.2)	
Granny Goose Shelled Pistachios, 1-oz. package	172	5.0	172.0	5.00	2752	80.0	
2-oz. package	344	9.9	172.0	5.00	2752	80.0	
3-oz. package	516	14.9	172.0	5.00	2752	80.0	
3.3-oz. package	(607)	(17.5)	172.0	5.00	2752	80.0	
4-oz. package	732	21.1	172.0	5.00	2752	80.0	
1 cup (approx. 4.4 oz.)	(758)	(22.0)	172.0	5.00	2752	80.0	
Laura Scudder's Pistachios, Roasted-In-Shell [refuse: shells, approx. 50%], 7-oz. jar	(589)	(18.8)	(84.2)	(2.69)	(1347)	(43.0)	
1 cup (approx. 4.7 oz.)	(807)	(12.6)	(84.2)	(2.69)	(1347)	(43.0)	
Planters Natural Pistachios, 7-oz. jar	1190	42.0	170.0	6.00	2720	96.0	
1 cup (approx. 4.4 oz.)	(750)	(26.5)	170.0	6.00	2720	96.0	
"Southern Belle" Pistachios, Salted In Shell, 1-oz. package	170	6.0	170.0	6.00	2720	96.0	
1 cup (approx. 4.4 oz.)	(750)	(26.5)	170.0	6.00	2720	96.0	
Sonoma Pistachios, 10-oz. package	(1684)	(53.9)	(168.4)	(5.39)	(2694)	(86.2)	
1 cup (approx. 4.4 oz.)	(743)	(23.8)	(168.4)	(5.39)	(2694)	(86.2)	
Sun Giant "Colossal" Pistachios, Roasted, Salted, In Shell, 6½-oz. jar	585	19.5	90.0	3.00	1440	48.0	
1 cup (approx. 4.7 oz.)	(422)	(14.1)	90.0	3.00	1440	48.0	
Natural Roasted or Red Dyed Pistachios, 3½-oz. can	(295)	(9.4)	(84.2)	(2.69)	(1347)	(43.0)	
4½-oz. pouch	(379)	(12.1)	(84.2)	(2.69)	(1347)	(43.0)	
6½-oz. jar	(547)	(17.5)	(84.2)	(2.69)	(1347)	(43.0)	
1 cup (approx. 4.7 oz.)	(395)	(12.6)	(84.2)	(2.69)	(1347)	(43.0)	
Timber Crest, 5-lb. package	(13472)	(431.2)	(168.4)	(5.39)	(2694)	(86.2)	
1 cup (approx. 4.4 oz.)	(743)	(23.8)	(168.4)	(5.39)	(2694)	(86.2)	

	UNIT Cal.	UNIT Carb.	1 OZ., BY WT. Cal.	1 OZ., BY WT. Carb.	1 POUND Cal.	1 POUND Carb.	Fiber per oz. (GMS.)
PUMPKIN SEEDS (and Squash Seeds)							
DRY:							
As purchased in hull [refuse: hulls, approx. 26%]:							
1 pound	1856	50.4	116.0	3.15	1856	50.4	
Hulled:							
1 pound (approx. 3¼ cups [yield from approx. 1⅓ lbs. seeds in the shell] (8g/4g/13g/4%/na)	2508	68.0	156.8	4.25	2508	68.0	0.54
1 cup (approx. 4.9 oz.)	774	21.0	156.8	4.25	2508	68.0	0.51
PUMPKIN SEEDS, by brand							
Golden Harvest raw, hulled Pumpkin Seeds, 8-oz. bag	1280	32.0	160.0	4.00	2560	64.0	
16-oz. (1-lb.) bag	2560	64.0	160.0	4.00	2560	64.0	
Pumpkin Seed Products							
PUMPKIN SEED MEAL							
David's Pumpkin Seeds, 1-oz. package	120	1.0	120.0	1.00	1920	16.0	
Natural Brand Pumpkin Seed Meal, 16-oz. (1-lb.) jar	2560	na	160.0	na	2560	na	1.00
1 cup (approx. 7.8 oz.)	(1248)	na	160.0	na	2560	na	1.00
SAFFLOWER SEEDS							
DRY:							
As purchased in hull [refuse: hulls, approx. 49%]:							
1 pound	1424	28.7	89.0	1.80	1424	28.7	
Hulled:							
1 pound [yield from approx. 2 lbs. seeds in hull] (5g/3g/17g/5%/16mg)	2792	56.3	174.5	3.52	2792	56.3	
Safflower Seed Products							
SAFFLOWER OIL							
1 cup (approx. 7.7 oz.)	1927	0.0	250.6	0.00	4010	0.0	
1 quart (approx. 30.9 oz. net wt.) (0g/0g/28g/0%/0mg)	7708	0.0	250.6	0.00	4010	0.0	
SESAME SEEDS							
DRY:							
All-edible:							
Whole:							
1 pound (5g/7g/14g/5%/3mg)	2598	106.4	162.4	6.65	2598	106.4	
Decorticated (skinned):							
1 tablespoon (approx. 0.28 oz.)	47	0.8	166.7	2.66	2667	42.6	0.68
1 cup (approx. 5.3 oz.)	884	14.1	166.7	2.66	2667	42.6	0.68
1 pound (approx. 3 cups) (7g/3g/16g/5%/11mg)	2667	42.6	166.7	2.66	2667	42.6	0.68
SESAME SEEDS, by brand							
David's Raw Hulled Sesame Seeds, 1-oz. package	120	1.0	120.0	1.00	1920	16.0	
Golden Harvest Toasted Sesame Seeds, 16-oz. (1-lb.) package	2720	96.0	170.0	6.00	2720	96.0	
1 cup (approx. 5.3 oz.)	(901)	(31.8)	170.0	6.00	2720	96.0	
Sesame Products							
HALVAH							
Based on data from the Middle East, 1 pound	2341	257.6	146.3	16.10	2341	257.6	
Joyva Marble Halvah, 0.8-oz. bar	128	9.6	160.0	12.00	2560	192.0	
Marble Halvah With Assorted Nuts, 1-lb. block	2560	192.0	160.0	12.00	2560	192.0	
SESAME BUTTER (TAHINI)							
Based on data from the Middle East, 1 pound	3139	46.3	196.2	2.89	3139	46.3	
Hain Raw, Unsalted Sesame Butter, 11-oz. jar	1755	68.2	159.5	6.20	2552	99.2	
1 cup (approx. 9.0 oz.)	1440	56.0	159.5	6.20	2552	99.2	
Joyva Tahini, 17-oz. can	3230	51.0	190.0	3.00	3040	48.0	
1 cup (approx. 9.0 oz.)	(1710)	(27.0)	190.0	3.00	3040	48.0	
SESAME CANDY							
Joyva Sesame Bar, 1⅛-oz. bar	200	28.1	178.0	25.00	2848	400.0	
Sesamettes, 11-oz. can	1958	275.0	178.0	25.00	2848	400.0	
SESAME OIL							
Arrowhead Mills Sesame Oil, 16 fl. oz. (1 pint)	3840	0.0	(250.0)	0.00	(4000)	0.0	0.00
1 cup (approx. 7.7 oz.)	1920	0.0	(250.0)	0.00	(4000)	0.0	0.00

	UNIT Cal.	UNIT Carb.	1 OZ., BY WT. Cal.	1 OZ., BY WT. Carb.	1 POUND Cal.	1 POUND Carb.	Fiber per oz. (GMS.)
SESAME SEED MEAL							
Balanced Raw Sesame Meal, 10-oz. can	(1608)	(61.6)	(160.8)	(6.16)	(2573)	(98.6)	
1 cup (approx. 8.0 oz.)	(1286)	(49.3)	(160.8)	(6.16)	(2573)	(98.6)	
SOYBEANS							
MATURE SEEDS, RAW, DRIED:							
1 cup (approx. 7.4 oz.)	846	70.3	114.3	9.50	1828	152.0	
1 pound (approx. 2.2 cups) (10g/9g/5g/10%/1mg)	1828	152.0	114.3	9.50	1828	152.0	
SOYBEANS, by brand							
Balanced Dry Roasted Soybeans, Unsalted or With Sea Salt, 8-oz. can	1040	48.0	130.0	6.00	2080	96.0	
1 cup (approx. 6.3 oz.)	(825)	(38.1)	130.0	6.00	2080	96.0	
El Molino Carob Coated Soy Beans, 1-oz. package	145	12.0	145.0	12.00	(885)	(73.2)	
4½-oz. package	653	54.0	145.0	12.00	(885)	(73.2)	
Golden Harvest Barbecue-Flavored Soybeans, 12-oz. bag	1680	108.0	140.0	9.00	2240	144.0	
1 cup (approx. 6.1 oz.)	(854)	(54.9)	140.0	9.00	2240	144.0	
Garlic-Flavored Soybeans, 12-oz. bag	1680	108.0	140.0	9.00	2240	144.0	
1 cup (approx. 6.1 oz.)	(854)	(54.9)	140.0	9.00	2240	144.0	
Onion-Flavored Soybeans, 12-oz. bag	1680	108.0	140.0	9.00	2240	144.0	
1 cup (approx. 6.1 oz.)	(854)	(54.9)	140.0	9.00	2240	144.0	
Toasted Soybeans, Unsalted or With Sea Salt, ¾-oz. bag	110	7.0	140.0	9.00	2240	144.0	
2½-oz. bag	350	22.5	140.0	9.00	2240	144.0	
12-oz. bag	1680	108.0	140.0	9.00	2240	144.0	
1 cup (approx. 6.1 oz.)	(854)	(54.9)	140.0	9.00	2240	144.0	
Whole Yellow Soybeans, ¾-oz. package	83	5.3	110.0	7.00	1760	112.0	
1 cup (approx. 7.4 oz.)	(814)	(51.8)	110.0	7.00	1760	112.0	
Soy Ahoy Dry Roasted Soybeans, 8-oz. jar	1040	48.0	130.0	6.00	2080	96.0	
1 cup (approx. 6.3 oz.)	(825)	(38.1)	130.0	6.00	2080	96.0	
Roasted In Oil, 8-oz. jar	1120	40.0	140.0	5.00	2240	80.0	
1 cup (approx. 6.4 oz.)	(889)	(31.7)	140.0	5.00	2240	80.0	
Soy Town Roasted Soybeans, 8-oz. package	1120	40.0	140.0	5.00	2240	80.0	
1 cup (approx. 8 oz.)	(1036)	(111.0)	140.0	5.00	2240	80.0	
Taste of Nature Dry Roasted Barbecue Soybeans			130.0	5.00	1760	80.0	
SQUASH SEEDS, see PUMPKIN SEEDS							
SUNFLOWER SEEDS							
DRY:							
As purchased in hull [refuse: hulls, approx. 46%]:							
1 cup	257	9.1	85.7	3.04	1371	48.7	
1 pound	1371	48.7	85.7	3.04	1371	48.7	
Hulled:							
1 pound (approx. 3.1 cups [yield from approx. 1.9 lbs. seeds in the hull]) (7g/6g/13g/5%/9mg)	2540	90.2	158.8	5.64	2540	90.2	1.08
1 cup (approx. 5.1 oz.)	812	28.9	158.8	5.64	2541	90.2	1.08
SUNFLOWER SEEDS, by brand							
David's Sunflower Kernels, 1-oz. package	180	4.0	180.0	4.00	2880	64.0	
Sunflower Seeds, roasted and salted in the shell, 1-oz. package	90	2.0	90.0	2.00	1440	32.0	
Fisher Sunflower Kernels, Dry, in Hull, 4½-oz. bag	386	13.5	85.7	3.00	1371	48.0	
1 cup (approx. 4.4 oz.)	(377)	(13.2)	85.7	3.00	1371	48.0	
Dry, Hulled, 4½-oz. bag	716	25.2	159.0	5.60	2544	89.6	
1 cup (approx. 5.1 oz.)	(811)	(28.6)	159.0	5.60	2544	89.6	
Frito-Lay Sunflower Kernels, Salted in Shell, 1⅞-oz. package	166	4.3	88.7	2.30	1419	36.8	
1 cup (approx. 4.4 oz.)	(390)	(10.1)	88.7	2.30	1419	36.8	
Sunflower Kernels, Shelled, 1-oz. package	181	4.7	181.0	4.70	2896	75.2	
1 cup (approx. 5.1 oz.)	(923)	(24.0)	181.0	4.70	2896	75.2	
Golden Harvest Sunflower Kernels, Raw, Hulled, 14-oz. package	2240	98.0	160.0	7.00	2560	112.0	
1 cup (approx. 5.1 oz.)	(816)	(35.7)	160.0	7.00	2560	112.0	
BBQ Flavored Sunflower Kernels, 10-oz. bag	1770	90.0	177.0	9.00	2832	144.0	
1 cup (approx. 5.1 oz.)	(903)	(45.9)	177.0	9.00	2832	144.0	
Onion & Garlic Flavored Sunflower Kernels, 10-oz. bag	1800	50.0	180.0	5.00	2880	80.0	
1 cup (approx. 5.1 oz.)	(918)	(25.5)	180.0	5.00	2880	80.0	

	UNIT Cal.	UNIT Carb.	1 OZ., BY WT. Cal.	1 OZ., BY WT. Carb.	1 POUND Cal.	1 POUND Carb.	Fiber per oz. (GMS.)
Roasted Sunflower Kernels, Salted, 14-oz. tin	2520	70.0	180.0	5.00	2880	80.0	
1 cup (approx. 5.1 oz.)	(918)	(25.5)	180.0	5.00	2880	80.0	
Toasted Sunflower Kernels, Salted or Unsalted, 14-oz. tin	2520	70.0	180.0	5.00	2880	80.0	
1 cup (approx. 5.1 oz.)	(918)	(25.5)	180.0	5.00	2880	80.0	
"Zesty" Sunflower Kernels, Cleaned, Hulled, Toasted in Soybean Oil, 9-oz. package	1620	45.0	180.0	5.00	2880	80.0	
1 cup (approx. 5.1 oz.)	(918)	(25.5)	180.0	5.00	2880	80.0	
Granny Goose Sunflower Kernels, Whole, 1-oz. package	159	4.2	159.0	4.20	2544	67.2	
2-oz. package	369	8.4	159.0	4.20	2544	67.2	
3-oz. package	476	12.7	159.0	4.20	2544	67.2	
3.3-oz. package	(561)	(14.9)	159.0	4.20	2544	67.2	
4-oz. package	636	16.9	159.0	4.20	2544	67.2	
1 cup (approx. 5.1 oz.)	(811)	(21.4)	159.0	4.20	2544	67.2	
Sunflower Seeds, Shelled, 1-oz. package	174	3.7	174.0	3.68	2784	58.9	
2-oz. package	347	7.4	174.0	3.68	2784	58.9	
3-oz. package	521	11.1	174.0	3.68	2784	58.9	
3.3-oz. package	(612)	(13.0)	174.0	3.68	2784	58.9	
4-oz. package	694	14.7	174.0	3.68	2784	58.9	
1 cup (approx. 5.1 oz.)	(887)	(18.8)	174.0	3.68	2784	58.9	
Laura Scudder's Dry Roasted Sunflower Nuts, 7¼-oz. bag	1044	81.2	144.0	11.20	2304	179.2	
Sunflower Nuts, Roasted in Shell [refuse: approx. 46%], 4-oz. bag	344	12.0	86.0	3.00	1376	48.0	
1 cup (approx. 4.4 oz.)	(378)	(13.2)	86.0	3.00	1376	48.0	
Sunflower Nuts, Shelled, Roasted in Oil, Salted, 3-oz. bag	570	8.4	190.0	2.80	3040	44.8	
1 cup (approx. 5.1 oz.)	(969)	(14.3)	190.0	2.80	3040	44.8	
Planters Sunflower Nuts, Dry Roasted, Shelled, Salted, 7¼-oz. package	1160	36.3	160.0	5.00	2560	80.0	
1 cup (approx. 5.1 oz.)	(816)	(25.5)	160.0	5.00	2560	80.0	
Unsalted, 7¼-oz. package	1233	36.3	170.0	5.00	2720	80.0	
1 cup (approx. 5.1 oz.)	(867)	(25.5)	170.0	5.00	2720	50.0	
Sunflower Seed Products							
SUNFLOWER OIL							
Arrowhead Mills, 16-fl.-oz. (1-pint) bottle	3840	0.0	(250.0)	0.00	(4000)	0.0	
SUNFLOWER SEED MEAL							
Natural Brand, 16-oz. (1-lb.) jar	2560	112.0	160.0	7.00	2560	112.0	
1 cup (approx. 7.8 oz.)	(1248)	(54.6)	160.0	7.00	2560	112.0	
WALNUTS							
Black Walnuts							
As purchased in shell [refuse: shells, approx. 78%]: 1 pound	627	14.8	39.2	0.93	627	14.8	
Shelled: Whole: 1 walnut (approx. 1⁄10 oz., 10 per ounce)	18	0.4	178.1	4.19	2849	67.1	0.48
1 cup (approx. 4.4 oz., 43 walnuts)	785	18.5	178.1	4.19	2849	67.1	0.48
1 pound (approx. 3⅔ cups, 158 walnuts [yield from approx. 4½ pounds of walnuts in the shell]) (6g/4g/17g/3%/1mg)	2849	67.1	178.1	4.19	2849	67.1	0.48
Chopped or broken kernels: 1 tablespoon (approx. 0.3 oz.)	50	1.2	178.1	4.19	2849	67.0	0.48
1 cup (approx. 4.4 oz.)	785	18.5	178.1	4.19	2849	67.0	0.48
Ground: 1 cup (approx. 2.8 oz.)	502	11.8	178.1	4.19	2849	67.0	0.48
For comparison: Black Walnut Ice Cream, **Meadow Gold,** 1 cup (approx. 4.7 oz.)	320	32.0	68.3	6.83	1093	109.3	
English or Persian Walnuts							
As purchased in shell [refuse: shells, approx. 55%]: 1 walnut (approx. 1⅝" diameter, 0.4 oz., 2½ per ounce)	32	0.8	83.1	2.01	1329	32.2	
1 pound	1329	32.2	83.1	2.01	1329	32.2	
Shelled: Whole: 1 walnut (approx. 0.14 oz., 7 per ounce)	32	0.8	184.6	4.48	2954	71.7	0.60
1 pound (approx. 3¾ cups, 92 walnuts, chopped [yield from 2¼ lbs. walnuts in the shell]) (4g/4g/18g/4%/1mg)	2953	71.7	184.6	4.48	2954	71.7	0.60

	UNIT Cal.	UNIT Carb.	1 OZ., BY WT. Cal.	1 OZ., BY WT. Carb.	1 POUND Cal.	1 POUND Carb.	Fiber per oz. (GMS.)
Halves: 1 cup (approx. 3½ oz., 50 halves)	646	15.7	184.6	4.48	2954	71.7	0.60
Chopped: 1 tablespoon (approx. 0.3 oz.)	52	1.3	184.6	4.48	2952	71.8	0.60
1 cup (approx. 4¼ oz., 30 nuts)	781	19.0	184.6	4.48	2952	71.8	0.60
WALNUTS, by brand							
Diamond/Sunsweet California Walnuts, Shelled, 3-oz. bag	578	10.9	192.5	3.63	3080	58.1	
4-oz. bag	770	14.5	192.5	3.63	3080	58.1	
10-oz. bag	1925	36.3	192.5	3.63	3080	58.1	
1-lb. bag or can	3080	58.1	192.5	3.63	3080	58.1	
2-lb. bag	6160	116.2	192.5	3.63	3080	58.1	
30-lb. box	92400	1742.4	192.5	3.63	3080	58.1	
1 cup (approx. 4.0 oz.)	(770)	(14.5)	192.5	3.63	3080	58.1	
In Shell, 1-lb. bag	(647)	(12.2)	(40.4)	(0.76)	(647)	(12.2)	
2-lb. bag	(1294)	(24.4)	(40.4)	(0.76)	(647)	(12.2)	
Fisher Black, Shelled, 8-oz. package	1424	33.6	178.0	4.20	2848	67.2	
1 cup (approx. 4 oz.)	(712)	(16.8)	178.0	4.20	2848	67.2	
Persian or English, Shelled, 8-oz. package	1480	36.0	185.0	4.50	2960	72.0	
1 cup (approx. 4.0 oz.)	(740)	(18.0)	185.0	4.50	2960	72.0	
Granny Goose Shelled, 1-oz. package	189	3.6	189.0	3.60	3024	57.6	
2-oz. package	378	7.3	189.0	3.60	3024	57.6	
3-oz. package	568	11.0	189.0	3.60	3024	57.6	
3.3-oz. package	(667)	(12.9)	189.0	3.60	3024	57.6	
4-oz. package	756	14.6	189.0	3.60	3024	57.6	
1 cup (approx. 4.0 oz.)	(756)	(14.6)	189.0	3.60	3024	57.6	
Walnut Products							
WALNUT OIL							
Hain Cold Pressed, 16-fl.-oz. (1-pint) bottle	3840	0.0	(250.0)	0.00	(4000)	0.0	
1 cup (approx. 7.7 oz.)	1920	0.0	(250.0)	0.00	(4000)	0.0	
WALNUT TOPPING							
Kraft, 5-oz. jar	654	72.7	130.8	14.54	2093	232.6	
WATERMELON SEEDS (based on data from Africa)							
WHOLE, DRIED: As purchased, 1 pound	2350	145.2	146.9	9.07	2350	145.2	6.36
Without shell, 1 pound	2572	68.5	160.7	4.28	2572	68.5	6.55
Roasted, 1 pound	2635	73.9	164.7	4.62	2635	73.9	1.42
Fermented Seed-Cake (popular African recipe), 1 pound	1583	28.6	98.9	1.79	1583	28.6	1.79
WHEAT SNACK PRODUCTS (Nut-like products made from wheat)							
David's Snack 'n Wheat, Cheese Flavored, 1-oz. package	150	15.0	150.0	15.00	2400	240.0	
Pillsbury Wheat Nuts, 1-oz. bag	200	5.0	200.0	5.00	3200	80.0	
10½-oz. jar	2100	52.5	200.0	5.00	3200	80.0	
MIXED NUTS							
Ann Page (A&P) Salted Mixed Nuts (peanuts, cashews, unblanched almonds, filberts, pecans) 7-oz. jar	1260	49.0	180.0	7.00	2880	112.0	
Roasted in Oil, Salted, "less than 50% peanuts," 12-oz. tin	2280	60.0	190.0	5.00	3040	80.0	
Golden Harvest Roasted in Oil, Sea Salted or Unsalted Mixed Nuts (peanuts, almonds, filberts, brazils, cashews), 6-oz. package	960	60.0	160.0	10.00	2560	160.0	
Granny Goose Mixed Nuts, 1-oz. package	168	5.7	168.0	5.70	2688	91.2	
2-oz. package	336	11.4	168.0	5.70	2688	91.2	
3-oz. package	504	17.2	168.0	5.70	2688	91.2	
Planters Dry Roasted, Salted Mixed Nuts, 16-oz. (1-lb.) tin	2560	112.0	160.0	7.00	2560	112.0	
Dry Roasted, Unsalted Mixed Nuts, 16-oz. (1-lb.) tin	2720	112.0	170.0	7.00	2720	112.0	
Mixed Nuts with Peanuts, Roasted in Oil, Salted, 16-oz. (1-lb.) tin	2880	96.0	180.0	6.00	2880	96.0	
Mixed Nuts without Peanuts, Roasted in Oil, Salted, 16-oz. (1-lb.) tin	2880	96.0	180.0	6.00	2880	96.0	

	UNIT Cal.	UNIT Carb.	1 OZ., BY WT. Cal.	1 OZ., BY WT. Carb.	1 POUND Cal.	1 POUND Carb.	Fiber per oz. (GMS.)
Skippy Dry Roasted, 16-oz. (1-lb.) jar	2722	86.6	170.0	5.40	2722	86.6	

MIXTURES OF NUTS, SEEDS, AND DRIED FRUITS

	UNIT Cal.	UNIT Carb.	1 OZ., BY WT. Cal.	1 OZ., BY WT. Carb.	1 POUND Cal.	1 POUND Carb.	Fiber per oz. (GMS.)
Golden Harvest Alpine Pack 'n Snack (raisins, sunflower seeds, dry roasted peanuts, cashews, almonds, soybean oil, sea salt) raw, 6-oz. bag	780	54.0	130.0	9.00	2080	144.0	
Roasted, 6-oz. bag	840	30.0	140.0	5.00	2240	80.0	
Nature's Energy Mix (sunflower seeds, raisins, almonds, cashews, dates), 6-oz. bag	780	60.0	130.0	10.00	2080	160.0	
Party Mix (Virginia peanuts, soybeans, hulled sunflower kernels, raisins, almonds, cashews, soybean oil, sea salt), salted or unsalted, 9-oz. bag	1440	54.0	160.0	6.00	2560	96.0	
Wilderness Pack (peanuts, raisins, sunflower seeds, dates, dried apricots, filberts, whole cashews, almonds, coconut, soybean oil), 4-oz. bag	560	52.0	140.0	13.00	2240	208.0	

17 CONFITURES & NUT BUTTERS •

	UNIT		1 OZ., BY WT.		1 CUP		1 TABLESPOON	
	Cal.	Carb.	Cal.	Carb.	Cal.	Carb.	Cal.	Carb.
CONFITURES								
Fruit Butters, by brand								
Apple Butter, **Empress,** 10-oz. jar	525	126.0	52.5	12.60	600	144.0	38	9.0
Apple Butter, Chunky, **Polaner,** 16-oz. (1-lb.) jar	760	193.8	47.5	12.11	480	122.4	30	7.7
Apple Butter, Smooth, **Polaner,** 16-oz. (1-lb.) jar	760	193.8	47.5	12.11	480	122.4	30	7.7
Apple Butter, **Tap 'N Apple,** 18-oz. jar	976	237.8	54.2	13.21	(539)	(131.4)	(34)	(8.2)
Apricot Butter, **Max Ams,** 17-oz. jar	1110	277.5	65.3	16.32	720	180.0	45	11.3
Apricot Butter, **Polaner,** 17-oz. jar	1110	277.5	65.3	16.32	720	180.0	45	11.3
Prune Butter, **Max Ams,** 17-oz. jar	1073	266.4	63.1	15.67	696	172.8	44	10.8
Prune Butter, **Polaner,** 17-oz. jar	1073	266.4	63.1	15.67	696	172.8	44	10.8
Fruit Spreads, by brand								
Apple Spread, Chunky, **Polaner,** 15-oz. jar	532	136.8	35.5	9.12	336	86.4	21	5.4
Apple Spread, Smooth, **Polaner,** 15-oz. jar	532	136.8	35.5	9.12	336	86.4	21	5.4
Apple Spread, low sugar, **Smucker's,** 8.5-oz. jar	336	84.0	39.5	9.88	384	96.0	24	6.0
Apricot Spread, low sugar, **Smucker's,** 8.5-oz. jar	336	84.0	39.5	9.88	384	96.0	24	6.0
Blackberry Spread, low sugar, **Smucker's,** 8.5-oz. jar	336	84.0	39.5	9.88	384	96.0	24	6.0
Boysenberry Spread, low sugar, **Smucker's,** 8.5-oz. jar	336	84.0	39.5	9.88	384	96.0	24	6.0
Cherry Spread, low sugar, **Smucker's,** 8.5-oz. jar	336	84.0	39.5	9.88	384	96.0	24	6.0
Grape Spread, low sugar, **Smucker's,** 8.5-oz. jar	336	84.0	39.5	9.88	384	96.0	24	6.0
Grape Spread, lite, **Welch's,** 18-oz. jar	851	212.6	47.3	11.81	480	120.0	30	7.5
29.25-oz. jar	1384	345.4	47.3	11.81	480	120.0	30	7.5
Orange Marmalade Spread, low sugar, **Smucker's,** 8.5-oz. jar	336	84.0	39.5	9.88	384	96.0	24	6.0
Red Raspberry Spread, low sugar, **Smucker's,** 8.5-oz. jar	336	84.0	39.5	9.88	384	96.0	24	6.0
Strawberry Spread, low sugar, **Smucker's,** 8.5-oz. jar	336	84.0	39.5	9.88	384	96.0	24	6.0

	UNIT		1 OZ., BY WT.		1 CUP		1 TABLESPOON	
	Cal.	Carb.	Cal.	Carb.	Cal.	Carb.	Cal.	Carb.
Strawberry Spread, lite, **Welch's,** 18-oz. jar	851	212.6	47.3	11.81	480	120.0	30	7.5
29.25-oz. jar	1384	345.4	47.3	11.81	480	120.0	30	7.5
Jams								
JAMS, all flavors, based on generic data								
1 jar, 10 oz. net wt.	772	198.8	77.2	19.88	864	224.0	54	14.1
1 jar, 32 oz. (2 lb.) net wt.	2467	634.9	77.2	19.88	864	224.0	54	14.1
1 cup (approx. 11.2 oz.)	864	224.0	77.2	19.88	864	224.0	54	14.1
1 pound (approx. 1.4 cups) (tr/20g/tr/29%/3mg)	1235	224.0	77.2	19.88	864	224.0	54	14.1
JAMS, by brand								
Apricot Jam, low calorie, imitation, **Slenderella,** 8½-oz. jar	288	72.0	33.9	8.47	384	96.0	24	6.0
Blackberry Jam, **Smucker's,** 12-oz. jar	933	240.0	77.7	20.00	840	216.0	53	6.0
Black Raspberry Jam, **Smucker's,** 12-oz. jar	933	240.0	77.7	20.00	840	216.0	53	13.5
Boysenberry Jam, low calorie, imitation, **Slenderella,** 8½-oz. jar	288	72.0	34.0	8.50	384	96.0	24	6.0
Boysenberry Jam, **Smucker's,** 12-oz. jar	933	240.0	77.7	20.00	840	216.0	53	13.5
Dutch Apple Jam, Chunky, **Polaner,** 12-oz. jar	(930)	(240.6)	(77.5)	(20.05)	(819)	(211.8)	(51)	(13.2)
Grape Jam, **Empress,** 10-oz. jar	735	189.0	73.5	18.90	840	216.0	53	13.0
Grape Jam, **Kraft,** 10-oz. jar	698	174.5	69.8	17.45	768	192.0	48	12.0
18-oz. jar	1256	314.1	69.8	17.45	768	192.0	48	12.0
32-oz. (2-lb.) jar	2233	558.4	69.8	17.45	768	192.0	48	12.0
Grape Jam, **Polaner,** 12-oz. jar	(933)	(240.6)	(77.5)	(20.05)	(819)	(211.8)	(49)	(12.7)
Grape Jam, **Smucker's,** 12-oz. jar	933	240.0	77.7	20.00	840	216.0	53	13.5
Grape Jam, **Welch's,** 10-oz. jar	735	189.0	73.5	18.90	840	216.0	53	13.5
18-oz. jar	1343	345.2	74.6	19.18	840	216.0	53	13.5
32-oz. (2-lb.) jar	2387	613.8	74.6	19.18	840	216.0	53	13.5
48-oz. (3-lb.) jar	3581	920.6	74.6	19.18	840	216.0	53	13.5
Red Raspberry Jam, **Smucker's,** 12-oz. jar	933	240.0	77.7	20.00	840	216.0	53	13.5
Strawberry Jam, **Kraft,** 32-oz. (2-lb.) jar	2233	558.4	69.8	17.45	768	192.0	48	12.0
Strawberry Jam, low calorie, imitation, **Slenderella,** 8½-oz. jar	288	72.0	34.0	8.50	367	91.8	24	6.0
Strawberry Jam, **Smucker's,** 12-oz. jar	933	240.0	77.7	20.00	840	216.0	53	13.5

	UNIT		1 OZ., BY WT.		1 CUP		1 TABLE-SPOON	
	Cal.	Carb.	Cal.	Carb.	Cal.	Carb.	Cal.	Carb.
Strawberry Jam, artificially sweetened, **Smucker's,** 7½-oz. jar	32	32.0	4.3	4.27	48	48.0	3	3.0
Strawberry Jam, **Welch's,** 32-oz. (2-lb.) jar	2352	604.8	73.5	18.90	840	216	53	13.5
Jellies								
JELLIES, all flavors, based on generic data								
1 jar, 10 oz. net wt.	775	200.5	77.5	20.05	819	211.8	51	13.2
1 jar, 32 oz. (2 lb.) net wt.	2476	640.3	77.5	20.05	819	211.8	51	13.2
1 cup (approx. 10.5 oz.)	819	211.8	77.5	20.05	819	211.8	51	13.2
1 pound (approx. 1.5 cups) (tr/20g/tr/29%/5mg)	1240	320.8	77.5	20.05	819	211.8	51	13.2
JELLIES, by brand								
Apple Jelly, Mint Flavored, **Crosse & Blackwell,** 12-oz. jar	900	234.0	75.0	19.50	800	207.8	50	13.0
Apple Jelly, **Empress,** 10-oz. jar	735	189.0	73.5	18.90	840	216.0	53	13.5
Apple Jelly, fructose sweetened, **Featherweight,** 8-oz. jar	252	56.0	31.5	7.00	288	64.0	18	4.0
Apple Jelly, no sugar, artificially sweetened, **Featherweight,** 8-oz. jar	224	42.0	28.0	5.25	256	48.0	16	3.0
Apple Jelly, **Kraft,** 10-oz. jar	698	174.5	69.8	17.45	768	192.0	48	12.0
18-oz. jar	1256	314.0	69.8	17.45	768	192.0	48	12.0
32-oz. (2-lb.) jar	2233	558.4	69.8	17.45	768	192.0	48	12.0
Apple Jelly, Mint Flavored, **Kraft,** 10-oz. jar	698	174.5	69.8	17.45	768	192.0	48	12.0
Apple Jelly, Homestyle, **Polaner,** 10-oz. jar	(933)	(240.6)	(77.5)	(20.05)	(819)	(211.8)	(49)	(12.7)
Apple Jelly, **Shopwell,** 10-oz. jar	752	188.0	75.2	18.80	768	192.0	48	12.0
Apple Jelly, low calorie, imitation, **Slenderella,** 8½-oz. jar	288	72.0	34.0	8.50	384	96.0	24	6.0
Apple Jelly, **Smucker's,** 10-oz. jar	778	200.0	77.7	20.00	840	216.0	53	13.5
Apple Jelly, Cinnamon Flavor, **Smucker's,** 10-oz. jar	778	200.0	77.7	20.00	840	216.0	53	13.5
Apple Jelly, Mint Flavor, **Smucker's,** 10-oz. jar	778	200.0	77.7	20.00	840	216.0	53	13.5
Apple Jelly, no sugar added, artificially sweetened, **Tillie Lewis** "Tasti Diet," 8-oz. jar	188	47.0	23.5	5.87	192	48.0	12	3.0
Apple-Blackberry Jelly, **Dutch Girl,** 18-oz. jar	1398	360.0	77.7	20.00	840	216.0	53	13.5
Apple-Blackberry Jelly, **Kraft,** 18-oz. jar	1256	314.1	69.8	17.45	768	192.0	48	12.0
Apple-Grape Jelly, **Dutch Girl,** 18-oz. jar	1398	360.0	77.7	20.00	840	216.0	53	13.5
Apple-Grape Jelly, **Kraft,** 8-oz. jar	698	174.5	69.8	17.45	768	192.0	48	12.0
32-oz. (2-lb.) jar	2233	558.4	69.8	17.45	768	192.0	48	12.0
Apple Mint Jelly, **Gristede's,** 10-oz. jar	752	188.0	75.2	18.80	768	192.0	48	12.0
Apple Mint Jelly, **Shopwell,** 10-oz. jar	752	188.0	75.2	18.80	768	192.0	48	12.0
Apple-Plum Jelly, **Kraft,** 18-oz. jar	1256	314.1	69.8	17.45	768	192.0	48	12.0
Apple-Strawberry Jelly, **Dutch Girl,** 18-oz. jar	1398	360.0	77.7	20.00	840	216.0	53	13.5
Apple Strawberry Jelly, **Kraft,** 18-oz. jar	1256	314.1	69.8	17.45	768	192.0	48	12.0
Blackberry Jelly, **Empress,** 10-oz. jar	735	189.0	73.5	18.90	840	216.0	53	13.5
Blackberry Jelly, fructose sweetened, **Featherweight,** 8-oz. jar	224	56.0	28.0	7.00	256	63.8	16	4.0
Blackberry Jelly, **Kraft,** 10-oz. jar	698	174.5	69.8	17.45	768	192.0	48	12.0
18-oz. jar	1256	314.1	69.8	17.45	768	192.0	48	12.0
Blackberry Jelly, **Polaner,** 10-oz. jar	(775)	(200.5)	(77.5)	(20.05)	(819)	(211.9)	(51)	(13.2)
Blackberry Jelly, **Shopwell,** 10-oz. jar	752	188.0	75.2	18.80	768	192.0	48	12.0
Blackberry Jelly, low calorie, imitation, **Slenderella,** 8½-oz. jar	288	72.0	34.0	8.50	384	96.0	24	6.0
Blackberry Jelly, **Smucker's,** 10-oz. jar	778	200.0	77.7	20.00	840	216.0	53	13.5
Blackberry Jelly, imitation, artificially sweetened, **Smucker's,** ⅜-oz. jar	4	1.0	10.7	2.67	116	28.8	21	5.7
Black Raspberry Jelly, **Crosse & Blackwell,** 12-oz. jar	900	234.0	75.0	19.50	800	207.8	50	13.0

	UNIT		1 OZ., BY WT.		1 CUP		1 TABLE-SPOON	
	Cal.	Carb.	Cal.	Carb.	Cal.	Carb.	Cal.	Carb.
Black Raspberry Jelly, **Shopwell,** 10-oz. jar	752	188.0	75.2	18.80	768	192.0	48	12.0
Black Raspberry Jelly, **Smucker's,** 10-oz. jar	778	200.0	77.7	20.00	840	216.0	53	13.5
Boysenberry Jelly, **Smucker's,** 10-oz. jar	778	200.0	77.7	20.00	840	216.0	53	13.5
Cherry Jelly, **Crosse & Blackwell,** 12-oz. jar	900	234.0	75.0	19.50	800	207.8	50	13.0
Cherry Jelly, imitation, low calorie, **Slenderella,** 8½-oz. jar	288	72.0	34.0	8.50	384	96.0	24	13.0
Cherry Jelly, **Smucker's,** 10-oz. jar	778	200.0	77.7	20.00	840	216.0	53	13.5
Cherry Jelly, imitation, artificially sweetened, **Smucker's,** ⅜-oz. jar	4	1.0	10.7	2.67	116	28.8	22	5.7
Crab Apple Jelly, **Crosse & Blackwell,** 12-oz. jar	900	234.0	75.0	19.50	800	207.8	50	13.0
Crab Apple Jelly, **Gristede's,** 10-oz. jar	752	188.0	75.2	18.80	768	192.0	48	12.0
Crab Apple Jelly, Homestyle, **Polaner,** 10-oz. jar	(775)	(200.5)	(77.5)	(20.05)	(819)	(211.8)	(51)	(13.2)
Crab Apple Jelly, **Shopwell,** 10-oz. jar	752	188.0	75.2	18.80	768	192.0	48	12.0
Crab Apple Jelly, **Smucker's,** 10-oz. jar	778	200.0	77.7	20.00	840	216.0	53	13.5
Currant Jelly, **Gristede's,** 10-oz. jar	752	188.0	75.2	18.80	768	192.0	48	12.0
Currant Jelly, **Shopwell,** 10-oz. jar	752	188.0	75.2	18.80	768	192.0	48	12.0
Currant Jelly, **Smucker's,** 10-oz. jar	778	200.0	77.7	20.00	840	216.0	53	13.5
Damson Plum Jelly, **Crosse & Blackwell,** 12-oz. jar	900	234.0	75.0	19.50	800	207.8	50	13.0
Damson Plum Jelly, **Kraft,** 10-oz. jar	698	174.5	69.8	17.45	768	192.0	48	12.0
Elderberry Jelly, **Kraft,** 10-oz. jar	698	174.5	69.8	17.45	768	192.0	48	12.0
18-oz. jar	1256	314.1	69.8	17.45	768	192.0	48	12.0
Elderberry Jelly, **Polaner,** 10-oz. jar	(775)	(200.5)	(77.5)	(20.05)	(819)	(211.8)	(51)	(13.2)
Elderberry Jelly, **Smucker's,** 10-oz. jar	778	200.0	77.7	20.00	840	216.0	53	13.5
Goober Grape (peanut butter with grape jelly), **Smucker's,** 12-oz. jar	1500	168.0	125.0	14.40	1226	137.4	77	8.6
Grape Jelly, **Crosse & Blackwell,** 12-oz. jar	900	234.0	75.0	19.50	800	207.8	50	13.0
Grape Jelly, imitation Concord, no sugar added, artificially sweetened, **Dia-Mel,** 8-oz. jar	80	(0.0)	10.0	(0.00)	96	(0.0)	6	(0.0)
Grape Jelly, fructose sweetened, **Featherweight,** 8-oz. jar	224	56.0	28.0	7.00	256	63.8	16	4.0
Grape Jelly, no sugar, artificially sweetened, **Featherweight,** 8-oz. jar	84	14.0	10.4	1.75	96	16.0	6	0.9
Grape Jelly, imitation, no sugar added, artificially sweetened, **Featherweight,** 14-oz. jar	146	24.5	10.4	1.75	96	16.0	6	0.9
Grape Jelly, pure, **Home Brands,** 10-oz. jar	700	180.0	70.0	18.00	840	216.0	53	13.5
12-oz. jar	840	216.0	70.0	18.00	840	216.0	53	13.5
18-oz. jar	1260	324.0	70.0	18.00	840	216.0	53	13.5
32-oz. (2-lb.) jar	2240	576.0	70.0	18.00	840	216.0	53	13.5
Grape Jelly, **Kraft,** 10-oz. jar	698	174.5	69.8	17.45	768	192.0	48	12.0
½-oz. restaurant package size	35	8.7	69.8	17.45	768	192.0	48	12.0
Grape Jelly, Concord, **Kraft,** 10-oz. jar	698	174.5	69.8	17.45	768	192.0	48	12.0
Grape Jelly, low calorie, imitation, **Kraft,** 8½-oz. jar	258	(64.5)	30.4	(7.60)	288	(72.0)	18	(4.5)
Grape Jelly, pure, **Old Virginia,** 16-oz. (1-lb.) jar	1224	340.0	76.5	21.25	864	24.0	54	15.0
Grape Jelly, Concord, **Polaner,** 18-oz. jar	(1395)	(360.9)	(77.5)	(20.05)	(819)	(211.8)	(51)	(13.2)
Grape Jelly, imitation, no sugar added, artificially sweetened, **Polaner,** 7½-oz. jar	(105)	(23.4)	(14.0)	(3.12)	(148.1)	(33.0)	(28)	(6.2)
Grape Jelly, **Shop-Mor,** 32-oz. (2-lb.) jar	2418	604.0	75.5	18.88	768	192.0	48	12.0
Grape Jelly, **Shopwell,** 10-oz. jar	752	188.0	75.2	18.80	768	192.0	48	12.0
18-oz. jar	1354	338.4	75.2	18.80	768	192.0	48	12.0
32-oz. (2-lb.) jar	2406	601.6	75.2	18.80	768	192.0	48	12.0
Grape Jelly, low calorie, imitation, **Slenderella,** 8½-oz. jar	288	72.0	34.0	8.50	384	96.0	24	6.0

	UNIT		1 OZ., BY WT.		1 CUP		1 TABLE-SPOON	
	Cal.	Carb.	Cal.	Carb.	Cal.	Carb.	Cal.	Carb.
Grape Jelly, **Smucker's,** 10-oz. jar	778	200.0	77.7	20.00	840	216.0	53	13.5
Grape Jelly, artificially sweetened, **Smucker's,** 7½-oz. jar	80	20.0	10.7	2.67	116	28.8	22	5.7
Grape Jelly, imitation, artificially sweetened, **Smucker's,** ⅜-oz. package	4	1.0	10.7	2.67	116	28.8	22	5.7
Grape Jelly, no sugar added, artificially sweetened, **Tillie Lewis** "Tasti Diet," 8-oz. jar	188	47.0	23.5	5.87	192	48.0	12	3.0
Grape Jelly, **Welch's,** 10-oz. jar	735	189.0	73.5	18.90	840	216.0	53	13.8
Grape Jelly, Red, **Welch's,** 20-oz. jar	1470	378.0	73.5	18.90	840	216.0	53	13.8
Grape Jelly, **White Rose,** 18-oz. jar	1354	338.4	75.2	18.80	768	192.0	48	12.0
Guava Jelly, **Crosse & Blackwell,** 12-oz. jar	900	234.0	75.0	19.50	800	207.8	50	13.0
Guava Jelly, **Empress,** 10-oz. jar	735	189.0	73.5	18.90	840	216.0	53	13.5
Guava Jelly, **Kraft,** 10-oz. jar	698	174.5	69.8	17.45	768	192.0	48	12.0
18-oz. jar	1256	314.1	69.8	17.45	768	192.0	48	12.0
Guava Jelly, Tropical, **Polaner,** 10-oz. jar	(775)	(200.5)	(77.5)	(20.05)	(819)	(211.8)	(51)	(13.2)
Guava Jelly, **Smucker's,** 10-oz. jar	778	200.0	77.7	20.00	840	216.0	53	13.5
Mint Jelly, real, **Polaner,** 10-oz. jar	(775)	(200.5)	(77.5)	(20.05)	(819)	(211.8)	(51)	(13.2)
Mixed Fruit Jelly, **Smucker's,** 10-oz. jar.	778	200.0	77.7	20.00	840	216.0	53	13.5
Plum Jelly, **Empress,** 10-oz. jar	735	189.0	73.5	18.90	840	216.0	53	13.5
Plum Jelly, fructose sweetened, **Featherweight,** 8-oz. jar	224	56.0	28.0	7.00	256	63.8	16	4.0
Plum Jelly, **Smucker's,** 10-oz. jar	778	200.0	77.7	20.00	840	216.0	53	13.5
Quince Jelly, **Crosse & Blackwell,** 12-oz. jar	900	234.0	75.0	19.50	800	207.8	50	13.0
Quince Jelly, **Smucker's,** 10-oz. jar	778	200.0	77.7	20.00	840	216.0	53	13.5
Red Currant Jelly, **Crosse & Blackwell,** 12-oz. jar	900	234.0	75.0	19.50	800	207.8	50	13.0
Red Currant Jelly, **Kraft,** 10-oz. jar	698	174.5	69.8	17.45	768	192.0	48	12.0
Red Currant Jelly, **Polaner,** 10-oz. jar	(775)	(200.5)	(77.5)	(20.05)	(819)	(211.8)	(51)	(13.2)
Red Raspberry Jelly, **Polaner,** 10-oz. jar	(775)	(200.5)	(77.5)	(20.05)	(819)	(211.8)	(51)	(13.2)
Red Raspberry Jelly, **Shopwell,** 10-oz. jar	752	188.0	75.2	18.80	768	192.0	48	12.0
Red Raspberry Jelly, **Smucker's,** 10-oz. jar	778	200.0	77.7	20.00	840	216.0	53	13.5
Strawberry Jelly, fructose sweetened, **Featherweight,** 8-oz. jar	224	56.0	28.0	7.00	256	63.8	16	4.0
Strawberry Jelly, **Kraft,** 10-oz. jar	698	174.5	69.8	17.45	768	192.0	48	12.0
Strawberry Jelly, **Polaner,** 10-oz. jar	(775)	(200.5)	(77.5)	(20.05)	(819)	(211.8)	(51)	(13.2)
Strawberry Jelly, **Shopwell,** 10-oz. jar	752	188.0	75.2	18.80	768	192.0	48	12.0
Strawberry Jelly, **Smucker's,** 10-oz. jar	778	200.0	77.7	20.00	840	216.0	53	13.5

Marmalades

	UNIT		1 OZ., BY WT.		1 CUP		1 TABLE-SPOON	
	Cal.	Carb.	Cal.	Carb.	Cal.	Carb.	Cal.	Carb.
MARMALADES, based on generic data								
1 jar, 12 oz. net wt.	874	238.3	72.8	19.86	816	224.0	51	14.1
1 cup (approx. 11.2 oz.)	816	224.0	72.8	19.86	816	224.0	51	14.1
1 pound (approx. 1.4 cups) (tr/20g/tr/29%/4mg)	1165	317.8	72.8	19.86	816	224.0	51	14.1
MARMALADES, by brand								
Grapefruit Marmalade, **Keiller,** 16-oz. (1-lb.) crock	1174	313.0	73.4	19.56	882	235.0	55	14.7
Lemon Marmalade, Rough Cut, **Keiller,** 16-oz. (1-lb.) crock	1174	313.0	73.4	19.56	882	235.0	55	14.7
Orange Marmalade, pure Seville, **Crosse & Blackwell,** 16-oz. (1-lb.) jar	1278	319.4	79.9	19.96	960	240.0	60	15.0
Orange Marmalade, Sweet, **Crosse & Blackwell,** 12-oz. jar	959	239.6	79.9	19.96	960	240.0	60	15.0
Orange Marmalade, imitation, artificially sweetened, **Dia-Mel,** 8-oz. jar	80	(0.0)	10.0	(0.00)	96	(0.0)	60	(0.0)
Orange Marmalade, California style, **Empress,** 10-oz. jar	735	189.0	73.5	18.90	840	216.0	53	13.5
Orange Marmalade, English style, **Empress,** 10-oz. jar	735	189.0	73.5	18.90	840	216.0	53	13.5
Orange Marmalade, fructose sweetened, **Featherweight,** 8-oz. jar	(194)	(48.3)	(24.2)	(6.04)	256	64.0	16	4.0
Orange Marmalade, **Gristede's,** 10-oz. jar	752	188.0	75.2	18.80	768	192.0	48	12.0
Orange Marmalade, Seville, **Keiller,** 16-oz. (1-lb.) jar	1174	313.0	73.4	19.56	882	235.0	55	14.5
Orange Marmalade, **Kraft,** 10-oz. jar	698	174.5	69.8	17.45	768	192.0	48	12.0
18-oz. jar	1256	314.1	69.8	17.45	768	192.0	48	12.0
½-oz. restaurant package size	35	8.7	69.8	17.45	768	192.0	48	12.0
Orange Marmalade, Honeyberry, sweetened with honey, **Louis Sherry,** 8½-oz. jar	120	24.0	14.1	2.82	144	28.8	9	1.8
Orange Marmalade, imitation, no sugar added, artificially sweetened, **Louis Sherry,** 8-oz. jar	80	(0.0)	10.0	(0.00)	96	(0.0)	6	(0.0)
Orange Marmalade, Bitter, English style, **Polaner,** 12-oz. jar	(933)	(240.6)	(77.5)	(20.05)	(819)	(211.8)	(51)	(13.2)
Orange Marmalade, Sweet, "California Navel," **Polaner,** 12-oz. jar	(933)	(240.6)	(77.5)	(20.05)	(819)	(211.8)	(51)	(13.2)
Orange Marmalade, **Shopwell,** 12-oz. jar	902	225.6	75.2	18.80	768	192.0	48	12.0
18-oz. jar	1354	338.4	75.2	18.80	768	192.0	48	12.0
Orange Marmalade, low calorie, imitation, **Slenderella,** 8½-oz. jar	288	72.0	34.0	8.50	367	91.8	24	6.0
Orange Marmalade, **Smucker's,** 12-oz. jar	933	240.0	77.7	20.00	840	216.0	53	13.5
Orange Marmalade, reduced calorie, low sugar, **Smucker's,** 8½-oz. jar	336	84.0	39.5	9.88	384	96.0	24	6.0
Orange Marmalade Substitute, no sugar added, artificially flavored, **Tillie Lewis** "Tasti Diet," 8-oz. jar	188	47.0	23.5	5.87	192	48.0	12	3.0
Orange Marmalade, **Welch's,** 10-oz. jar	735	189.0	73.5	18.90	840	216.0	53	13.5
Orange Marmalade, **White Rose,** 18-oz. jar	1360	340.0	75.6	18.90	768	192.0	48	13.5
Three Fruits Marmalade, (Lemon, Orange, Grapefruit), **Crosse & Blackwell,** 16-oz. (1-lb.) jar	1278	319.4	79.9	19.96	960	240.0	60	15.0
Three Fruits Marmalade, (Lemon, Orange, Grapefruit), **Keiller,** 16-oz. (1-lb.) jar	1174	313.0	73.4	19.56	(882)	(235.0)	(55)	(14.7)

Preserves

	UNIT		1 OZ., BY WT.		1 CUP		1 TABLE-SPOON	
	Cal.	Carb.	Cal.	Carb.	Cal.	Carb.	Cal.	Carb.
PRESERVES, all flavors, based on generic data								
1 jar, 10 oz. net wt.	772	198.8	77.2	19.88	864	224.0	54	14.1
1 jar, 32 oz. (2 lb.) net wt.	2467	634.9	77.2	19.88	864	224.0	54	14.1
1 cup (approx. 11.2 oz.)	864	224.0	77.2	19.88	864	224.0	54	14.1
1 pound (approx. 1.4 cups) (tr/20g/tr/29%/3mg)	1235	318.1	77.2	19.88	864	224.0	54	14.1
PRESERVES, by brand								
Apricot Preserves, **Crosse & Blackwell,** 12-oz. jar	959	239.6	79.9	19.96	960	240.0	60	15.0
Apricot Preserves, **Empress,** 10-oz. jar	735	189.0	73.5	18.90	840	216.0	53	13.5
Apricot Preserves, fructose sweetened, **Featherweight,** 8-oz. jar	(194)	(48.3)	(24.2)	(6.04)	256	64.0	16	4.0
Apricot Preserves, **Kraft,** 10-oz. jar	698	174.5	69.8	17.45	768	192.0	48	12.0
Apricot Preserves, imitation, artificially sweetened, **Louis Sherry,** 8-oz. jar	80	(0.0)	10.0	(0.00)	96	(0.0)	6	(0.0)
Apricot Preserves, **Polaner,** 10-oz. jar	(775)	(200.5)	(77.5)	(20.05)	(819)	(211.8)	(51)	(13.2)
Apricot Preserves, Chunky, **Polaner,** 18-oz. jar	(1395)	(360.9)	(77.5)	(20.05)	(819)	(211.8)	(51)	(13.2)
Apricot Preserves, **Shopwell,** 12-oz. jar	912	228.0	76.0	19.00	768	192.0	48	12.0
18-oz. jar	1368	342.0	76.0	19.00	768	192.0	48	12.0
Apricot Preserves, **Smucker's,** 12-oz. jar	933	240.0	77.7	20.00	840	216.0	53	13.5
Apricot-Pineapple Preserves, **Empress,** 10-oz. jar	735	189.0	73.5	18.90	840	216.0	53	13.5

	UNIT		1 OZ., BY WT.		1 CUP		1 TABLE-SPOON	
	Cal.	Carb.	Cal.	Carb.	Cal.	Carb.	Cal.	Carb.
Apricot-Pineapple Preserves, no sugar, artificially sweetened, **Featherweight,** 8-oz. jar	(73)	(12.1)	(9.1)	(1.51)	96	16.0	6	1.0
Apricot-Pineapple Preserves, Chunky, **Polaner,** 12-oz. jar	(930)	(240.6)	(77.5)	(20.05)	(819)	(211.8)	(51)	(13.2)
Apricot-Pineapple Preserves, **Smucker's,** 12-oz. jar	933	240.0	77.7	20.00	840	216.0	53	13.5
Apricot-Pineapple Preserve Substitute, no sugar added, **Tillie Lewis** "Tasti Diet," 8-oz. jar	188	47.0	23.5	5.87	192	48.0	12	3.0
Blackberry Preserves, **Crosse & Blackwell,** 12-oz. jar	959	239.6	79.9	19.96	960	240.0	6	15.0
Blackberry Preserves, seedless, **Empress,** 10-oz. jar	735	189.0	73.5	18.90	840	216.0	53	13.5
Blackberry Preserves, fructose sweetened, **Featherweight,** 8-oz. jar	224	56.0	28.0	7.00	256	63.8	16	4.0
Blackberry Preserves, **Kraft,** 10-oz. jar	698	174.5	69.8	17.45	768	192.0	48	12.0
18-oz. jar	1256	314.1	69.8	17.45	768	192.0	48	12.0
Blackberry Preserves, seedless, **Kraft,** 10-oz. jar	698	174.5	69.8	17.45	768	192.0	48	12.0
18-oz. jar	1256	314.1	69.8	17.45	768	192.0	48	12.0
Blackberry Preserves, **Polaner,** 10-oz. jar	(775)	(200.5)	(77.5)	(20.05)	(819)	(211.8)	(51)	(13.2)
Blackberry Preserves, **Shopwell,** 12-oz. jar	912	228.0	76.0	9.00	768	192.0	48	12.0
Black Cherry Preserves, **Empress,** 10-oz. jar	735	189.0	73.5	18.90	840	216.0	52	13.5
Black Raspberry Preserves, artificially sweetened, imitation, seedless, **Dia-Mel,** 8-oz. jar	80	(0.0)	10.0	(0.00)	96	(0.0)	6	(0.0)
Black Raspberry Preserves, seedless, **Empress,** 10-oz. jar	735	189.0	73.5	18.90	840	216.0	53	13.5
Black Raspberry Preserves, seedless, **Gristede's,** 10-oz. jar	760	190.0	76.0	19.00	768	192.0	48	12.0
Black Raspberry Preserves, imitation, seedless, no sugar added, artificially sweetened, **Louis Sherry,** 8-oz. jar	80	(0.0)	10.0	(0.00)	96	(0.0)	6	(0.0)
Black Raspberry Preserves, seedless, **Polaner,** 10-oz. jar	(775)	(200.5)	(77.5)	(20.05)	(819)	(211.8)	(51)	(13.2)
Black Raspberry Preserves, **Shopwell,** 12-oz. jar	912	228.0	76.0	19.00	768	192.0	48	12.0
Blueberry Preserves, **Crosse & Blackwell,** 12-oz. jar	959	239.6	79.9	19.96	960	240.0	60	15.0
Blueberry Preserves, imitation, no sugar added, artificially sweetened, **Dia-Mel,** 8-oz. jar	80	(0.0)	10.0	(0.00)	96	(0.0)	6	(0.0)
Blueberry Preserves, fructose sweetened, **Featherweight,** 8-oz. jar	(194)	(48.3)	(24.2)	(6.04)	256	64.0	16	4.0
Blueberry Preserves, **Kraft,** 10-oz. jar	698	174.5	69.8	17.45	768	192.0	48	12.0
Blueberry Preserves, **Polaner,** 12-oz. jar	(930)	(240.6)	(77.5)	(20.05)	(819)	(211.8)	(51)	(13.2)
Blueberry Preserves, **Shopwell,** 12-oz. jar	912	228.0	76.0	9.00	768	192.0	48	12.0
Blueberry Preserves, **Smucker's,** 12-oz. jar	933	240.0	77.7	20.00	840	216.0	53	13.5
Boysenberry Preserves, **Empress,** 10-oz. jar	735	189.0	73.5	18.90	840	216.0	53	13.5
Boysenberry Preserves, **Smucker's,** 12-oz. jar	933	240.0	77.7	20.00	840	216.0	53	13.5
Cherry Preserves, imitation, no sugar added, artificially sweetened, **Dia-Mel,** 8-oz. jar	80	(0.0)	10.0	(0.00)	96	(0.0)	6	(0.0)
Cherry Preserves, fructose sweetened, **Featherweight,** 8-oz. jar	(194)	(48.3)	(24.2)	(6.04)	256	64.0	16	4.0
Cherry Preserves, **Gristede's,** 10-oz. jar	760	190.0	76.0	19.00	768	192.0	48	12.0
Cherry Preserves, **Kraft,** 10-oz. jar	698	174.5	69.8	17.45	768	192.0	48	12.0
18-oz. jar	1256	314.1	69.8	17.45	768	192.0	48	12.0
Cherry Preserves, **Shopwell,** 12-oz. jar	912	228.0	76.0	19.00	768	192.0	48	12.0
Cherry Preserves, **Smucker's,** 12-oz. jar	933	239.7	77.7	20.00	840	216.0	53	13.5
Damson Plum Preserves, **Crosse & Blackwell,** 12-oz. jar	959	239.6	79.9	19.96	960	240.0	53	13.5
Damson Plum Preserves, Chunky, **Polaner,** 12-oz. jar	(930)	(240.6)	(77.5)	(20.05)	(819)	(211.8)	(51)	(13.2)
Four Fruit Preserves (Cherry, Peach, Pineapple, Strawberry), **Smucker's,** 12-oz. jar	933	239.7	77.7	20.00	840	216.0	53	13.5

	UNIT		1 OZ., BY WT.		1 CUP		1 TABLE-SPOON	
	Cal.	Carb.	Cal.	Carb.	Cal.	Carb.	Cal.	Carb.
Grape Preserves Whole, **Kraft,** 10-oz. jar	698	174.5	69.8	17.45	768	192.0	48	12.0
18-oz. jar	1256	314.1	69.8	17.45	768	192.0	48	12.0
Grape Preserves, **Shopwell,** 12-oz. jar	912	228.0	76.0	19.00	768	192.0	48	12.0
18-oz. jar	1368	342.0	76.0	19.00	768	192.0	48	12.0
Grape Preserves, **Welch's,** 10-oz. jar	735	189.0	73.5	18.90	840	216.0	53	13.5
Peach Preserves, imitation, no sugar added, artificially sweetened, **Dia-Mel,** 8-oz. jar	80	(0.0)	10.0	(0.00)	96	(0.0)	6	(0.0)
Peach Preserves, **Empress,** 10-oz. jar	735	189.0	73.5	18.90	840	216.0	53	13.5
Peach Preserves, fructose sweetened, **Featherweight,** 8-oz. jar	(194)	(48.3)	(24.2)	(6.04)	256	64.0	16	4.0
Peach Preserves, no sugar, artificially sweetened, **Featherweight,** 8-oz. jar	73	12.1	9.1	1.51	96	16.0	6	0.9
Peach Preserves, **Gristede's,** 10-oz. jar	760	190.0	76.0	19.00	768	192.0	48	12.0
Peach Preserves, **Kraft,** 10-oz. jar	698	174.5	69.8	17.45	768	192.0	48	12.0
18-oz. jar	1256	314.1	69.8	17.45	768	192.0	48	12.0
Peach Preserves, imitation, artificially sweetened, **Louis Sherry,** 8-oz. jar	80	(0.0)	10.0	(0.00)	96	(0.0)	6	(0.0)
Peach Preserves, Elberta Freestone, **Polaner,** 12-oz. jar	(930)	(240.6)	(77.5)	(20.05)	(819)	(211.8)	(51)	(13.2)
Peach Preserves, **Shopwell,** 12-oz. jar	912	228.0	76.0	19.00	768	192.0	48	12.0
Peach Preserves, **Smucker's,** 12-oz. jar	933	240.0	77.7	20.00	840	216.0	53	13.5
Peach Preserve Substitute, Elberta, no sugar added, artificially flavored, **Tillie Lewis** "Tasti Diet," 8-oz. jar	188	47.0	23.5	5.87	192	48.0	12	3.0
Peach-Pineapple Preserves, **Empress,** 10-oz. jar	735	189.0	73.5	18.90	840	216.0	53	13.5
Pineapple Preserves, fructose sweetened, **Featherweight,** 8-oz. jar	(194)	(48.3)	(24.2)	(6.04)	256	64.0	16	4.0
Pineapple Preserves, **Kraft,** 10-oz. jar	698	174.5	69.8	17.45	768	192.0	48	12.0
18-oz. jar	1256	314.1	69.8	17.45	768	192.0	48	12.0
Pineapple Preserves, Chunky, **Polaner,** 12-oz. jar	(930)	(240.6)	(77.5)	(20.05)	(819)	(211.8)	(51)	(13.2)
Pineapple Preserves, **Shopwell,** 12-oz. jar	912	228.0	76.0	19.00	768	192.0	48	12.0
Pineapple Preserves, **Smucker's,** 12-oz. jar	933	240.0	77.7	20.00	840	216.0	53	13.5
Plum Preserves, **Empress,** 10-oz. jar	735	189.0	73.5	18.90	840	216.0	53	13.5
Plum Preserves, **Shopwell,** 12-oz. jar	912	228.0	76.0	19.00	768	192.0	48	12.0
Plum Preserves, **Smucker's,** 12-oz. jar	933	240.0	77.7	20.00	840	216.0	53	13.5
Raspberry Preserves, **Crosse & Blackwell,** 12-oz. jar	959	239.6	79.9	19.96	960	240.0	60	15.0
Red Cherry Preserves, **Empress,** 10-oz. jar	735	189.0	73.5	18.90	840	216.0	53	13.5
Red Cherry Preserves, **Polaner,** 12-oz. jar	(930)	(240.6)	(77.5)	(20.05)	(819)	(211.8)	(51)	(13.2)
Red Plum Preserves, **Kraft,** 10-oz. jar	698	174.5	69.8	17.45	768	192.0	48	12.0
18-oz. jar	1256	314.1	69.8	17.45	768	192.0	48	12.0
Red Raspberry Preserves, **Empress,** 10-oz. jar	735	189.0	73.5	18.90	840	216.0	53	13.5
Red Raspberry Preserves, fructose sweetened, **Featherweight,** 8-oz. jar	(194)	(48.3)	(24.2)	(6.04)	256	64.0	16	4.0
Red Raspberry Preserves, seedless, **Gristede's,** 10-oz. jar	760	190.0	76.0	19.00	768	192.0	48	12.0
Red Raspberry Preserves, **Kraft,** 10-oz. jar	698	174.5	69.8	17.45	768	192.0	48	12.0
18-oz. jar	1256	174.5	69.8	17.45	768	192.0	48	12.0
Red Raspberry Preserves, imitation, artificially sweetened, **Louis Sherry,** 8-oz. jar	80	(0.0)	10.0	(0.00)	96	(0.0)	6	(0.0)
Red Raspberry Preserves, seedless, **Polaner,** 18-oz. jar	(1395)	(360.9)	(77.5)	(20.05)	(819)	(211.8)	(51)	(13.2)
Red Raspberry Preserves, **Shopwell,** 12-oz. jar	912	228.0	76.0	19.00	768	192.0	48	12.0
Red Raspberry Preserves, **Smucker's,** 12-oz. jar	933	240.0	77.7	20.00	840	216.0	53	13.5
Strawberry Preserves, **Crosse & Blackwell,** 12-oz. jar	959	239.6	79.9	19.96	960	240.0	60	15.0

	UNIT		1 OZ., BY WT.		1 CUP		1 TABLESPOON	
	Cal.	Carb.	Cal.	Carb.	Cal.	Carb.	Cal.	Carb.
Strawberry Preserves, imitation, no sugar added, artificially sweetened, **Dia-Mel,** 14-oz. jar	80	(0.0)	10.0	(0.00)	96	(0.0)	6	(0.0)
Strawberry Preserves, **Empress,** 10-oz. jar	735	189.0	73.5	18.90	840	216.0	53	13.5
Strawberry Preserves, fructose sweetened, **Featherweight,** 8-oz. jar	(194)	(48.3)	(24.2)	(6.04)	256	64.0	16	4.0
16-oz. (1-lb.) jar	(387)	(96.6)	(24.2)	(6.04)	256	64.0	16	4.0
Strawberry Preserves, pure, **Home Brands,** 10-oz. jar	700	180.0	70.0	18.00	840	216.0	53	13.5
12-oz. jar	840	216.0	70.0	18.00	840	216.0	53	13.5
18-oz. jar	1260	324.0	70.0	18.00	840	216.0	53	13.5
32-oz. (2-lb.) jar	2240	576.0	70.0	18.00	840	216.0	53	13.5
Strawberry Preserves, **Kern's,** 10-oz. jar	756	210.0	75.6	21.00	864	240.0	60	15.0
Strawberry Preserves, imitation, low calorie, **Kraft,** 8½-oz. jar	258	86.1	30.4	10.13	288	96.0	18	6.0
Strawberry Preserves, **Polaner,** 12-oz. jar	(930)	(240.6)	(77.5)	(20.05)	(819)	(211.8)	(51)	(13.2)
Strawberry Preserves, **Shop-Mor,** 32-oz. (2-lb.) jar	2418	604.0	75.5	18.88	768	192.0	48	12.0
Strawberry Preserves, **Shopwell,** 12-oz. jar	912	228.0	76.0	19.00	768	192.0	48	12.0
18-oz. jar	1368	342.0	76.0	19.00	768	192.0	48	12.0
32-oz. (2-lb.) jar	2432	608.0	76.0	19.00	768	192.0	48	12.0
Strawberry Preserves, **Smucker's,** 12-oz. jar	933	240.0	77.7	20.00	840	216.0	53	13.5
Strawberry Preserve Substitute, no sugar added, artificially flavored, **Tillie Lewis** "Tasti Diet," 8-oz. jar	188	47.0	23.5	5.87	192	48.0	12	3.0
Strawberry Preserves, **Welch's,** 10-oz. jar	735	189.0	73.5	18.90	840	216.0	53	13.5
18-oz. jar	1323	340.2	73.3	18.90	840	216.0	53	13.5
Strawberry Preserves, **White Rose,** 18-oz. jar	1360	340.0	75.6	18.89	768	192.0	48	12.0
Strawberry Rhubarb Preserves, Chunky, **Polaner,** 12-oz. jar	(930)	(240.6)	(77.5)	(20.05)	(819)	(211.8)	(51)	(13.2)
Tomato Preserves, **Smucker's,** 12-oz. jar	933	240.0	77.7	20.00	840	216.0	53	13.5
Wild Strawberry Preserves, imitation, no sugar added, artificially sweetened, **Louis Sherry,** 14-oz. jar	140	(0.0)	10.0	(0.00)	96	(0.0)	6	(0.0)
Wild Strawberry Preserves, **Polaner,** 10-oz. jar	(775)	(200.5)	(77.5)	(20.05)	(819)	(211.8)	(51)	(13.2)
NUT AND SEED BUTTERS								
ALMOND BUTTER, by brand								
Golden Harvest Unsalted Almond Butter, 12-oz. jar	2160	36.0	180.0	3.00	(1626)	(27.1)	(102)	(1.7)
1 teaspoon (approx. ⅙ oz.)	(34)	(0.6)	180.0	3.00	(1626)	(27.1)	(102)	(1.7)
Hain Unsalted, Raw, Blanched Almond Butter, 11-oz. jar	1851	29.2	168.3	2.66	1520	24.0	95	1.5
1 teaspoon (approx. ⅙ oz.)	32	0.5	168.3	2.66	1520	24.0	95	1.5
CASHEW BUTTER, by brand								
Golden Harvest Unsalted Cashew Butter, 12-oz. jar	2160	72.0	180.0	6.00	(1626)	(54.2)	102	3.4
1 teaspoon (approx. ⅙ oz.)	34	1.1	180.0	6.00	(1626)	(54.2)	102	3.4
Hain Unsalted Raw Cashew Butter, 11-oz. jar	1851	78.0	168.3	7.10	1520	64.0	95	4.0
1 teaspoon (approx. ⅙ oz.)	32	1.3	168.3	7.10	1520	64.0	95	4.0
Hollywood Roasted Cashew Butter, 11-oz. jar	1851	78.0	168.3	7.10	1520	64.0	95	4.0
1 teaspoon (approx. ⅙ oz.)	32	1.3	168.3	7.10	1520	64.0	94	4.0
PEANUT BUTTER, based on generic data								
"Creamy" or "Chunky," made with moderate amounts of added fat, sugar, and salt:								
1 #10 can, 110 oz. net wt. (6 lb. 14 oz.)	18365	586.2	167.0	5.33	1520	48.5	95	3.0
Sold in glass jars, 1 jar, 12 oz. net wt.	2003	63.9	167.0	5.33	1520	48.5	95	3.0
1 jar, 18 oz. net wt. (1 lb. 2 oz.)	3004	95.9	167.0	5.33	1520	48.5	95	3.0
1 jar, 28 oz. net wt. (1 lb. 12 oz.)	4677	149.3	167.0	5.33	1520	48.5	95	3.0
1 pound (approx. 1¾ cups) (7g/6g/14g/2%/172mg)	2672	85.3	167.0	5.33	1520	48.5	95	3.0
1 cup (approx. 9.1 oz.)	1520	48.5	167.0	5.33	1520	48.5	95	3.0
1 tablespoon (approx. ½ oz.)	94	3.0	167.0	5.33	1520	48.5	95	3.0
1 teaspoon (approx. ⅙ oz.)	31	1.0	167.0	5.33	1520	48.5	95	3.0
"Creamy" or "Chunky," made with small amounts of added fat, sugar, and salt:								
1 pound (approx. 1¾ cups) (7g/5g/14g/2%/172mg)	2640	88.5	165.0	5.53	(1502)	(50.3)	(94)	(3.1)
1 teaspoon (approx. ⅙ oz.)	(31)	(16.8)	165.0	5.53	(1502)	(50.3)	(94)	(3.1)
PEANUT BUTTER, by brand								
Arrowhead Mills Peanut Butter, 18-oz. jar	2970	104.4	165.0	5.80	1584	55.7	99	3.5
28-oz. jar	4620	162.4	165.0	5.80	1584	55.7	99	3.5
1 teaspoon (approx. ⅙ oz.)	33	1.2	165.0	5.80	1584	55.7	99	3.5
Cellu Low Sodium Peanut Butter, 6-oz. jar	1080	24.0	180.0	4.00	1638	36.4	102	2.3
12-oz. container	2160	48.0	180.0	4.00	1638	36.4	102	2.3
1 teaspoon (approx. ⅙ oz.)	34	0.8	180.0	4.00	1638	36.8	102	2.3
Country Pure Chunky Peanut Butter, 38-oz. jar	6080	192.0	168.3	5.32	1520	48.0	95	3.0
Creamy Peanut Butter, 40-oz. jar	6460	204.0	168.3	5.32	1520	48.0	95	3.0
1 teaspoon (approx. ⅙ oz.)	32	1.0	168.3	5.32	1520	48.0	95	3.0
Deaf Smith Creamy Old Fashioned Peanut Butter, 16-oz. (1-lb.) jar	2640	92.8	165.0	5.80	1502	52.8	94	3.3
18-oz. jar	2970	104.4	165.0	5.80	1502	52.8	94	3.3
28-oz. jar	4620	162.4	165.0	5.80	1502	52.8	94	3.3
1 teaspoon (approx. ⅙ oz.)	33	1.0	165.0	5.80	1502	52.8	94	3.3
Crunchy Peanut Butter, 18-oz. jar	2970	104.4	165.0	5.80	1502	52.8	94	3.3
28-oz. jar	4620	162.4	165.0	5.80	1502	52.8	94	3.3
1 teaspoon (approx. ⅙ oz.)	31	1.1	165.0	5.80	1502	52.8	94	3.3
Golden Harvest Salted Old Fashioned Peanut Butter, 12-oz. jar	2040	72.0	170.0	6.00	1547	54.6	97	3.4
1 teaspoon (approx. ⅙ oz.)	32	1.1	170.0	6.00	1547	54.6	97	3.4
Unsalted Natural Peanut Butter With Embryo Wheat Germ, 12-oz. jar	2040	48.0	170.0	4.00	1547	36.4	97	2.3
1 teaspoon (approx. ⅙ oz.)	32	0.8	170.0	4.00	1547	36.4	97	2.3
Unsalted 100% Pure Old Fashioned Peanut Butter, 26-oz. jar	4420	156.0	170.0	6.00	1547	54.6	97	3.4
1 teaspoon (approx. ⅙ oz.)	32	1.1	170.0	6.00	1547	54.6	97	3.4
Golden State Homogenized Peanut Butter, 48-oz. (3-lb.) jar	8386	239.5	174.7	5.00	1576	44.8	98	2.8
1 teaspoon (approx. ⅙ oz.)	33	0.9	174.7	5.00	1576	44.8	98	2.8
Home Brands Natural Peanut Butter, 18-oz. jar	3040	96.0	168.9	5.33	1520	48.0	95	3.0
1 teaspoon (approx. ⅙ oz.)	32	2.5	168.9	5.33	1520	48.0	95	3.0
Real Peanut Butter, 16-oz. (1-lb.) jar	2844	56.9	177.8	3.56	1600	32.0	100	2.0
1 teaspoon (approx. ⅙ oz.)	33	1.0	177.8	3.56	1600	32.0	100	2.0
Jif Peanut Butter, 12-oz. jar	2027	52.8	168.9	4.40	1520	40.0	95	2.5
18-oz. jar	3040	80.0	168.9	4.40	1520	40.0	95	2.5
28-oz. jar	4729	123.2	168.9	4.40	1520	40.0	95	2.5
40-oz. jar	6756	476.0	168.9	4.40	1520	40.0	95	2.5
1 teaspoon (approx. ⅙ oz.)	32	0.8	168.9	4.40	1520	40.0	95	2.5
Kitchen King Creamy Peanut Butter, 12-oz. jar	2021	85.1	168.3	7.10	1520	64.0	95	4.0
28-oz. jar	4714	198.5	168.3	7.10	1520	64.0	95	4.0
1 teaspoon (approx. ⅙ oz.)	32	1.3	168.3	7.10	1520	64.0	95	4.0
Crunchy Peanut Butter, 12-oz. jar	2021	85.1	168.3	7.10	1520	64.0	95	4.0
28-oz. jar	4714	198.5	168.3	7.10	1520	64.0	95	4.0
1 teaspoon (approx. ⅙ oz.)	32	1.3	168.3	7.10	1520	64.0	95	4.0
Laura Scudder's Old Fashioned Peanut Butter, 16-oz. (1-lb.) jar	2678	49.0	179.2	3.10	1616	28.0	101	1.7
32-oz. (2-lb.) jar	5734	99.2	179.2	3.10	1616	28.0	101	1.7
1 teaspoon (approx. ⅙ oz.)	167.3	3.0	179.2	3.10	1616	28.0	101	1.7
Nu Made Chunky Peanut Butter, 12-oz. jar	2017	53.0	168.1	4.42	1520	40.0	95	2.5
18-oz. jar	3026	79.6	168.1	4.42	1520	40.0	95	2.5
28-oz. jar	4707	(132.8)	168.1	4.42	1520	40.0	95	2.5
1 teaspoon (approx. ⅙ oz.)	32	0.8	168.1	4.42	1520	40.0	95	2.5

	UNIT		1 OZ., BY WT.		1 CUP		1 TABLE-SPOON	
	Cal.	Carb.	Cal.	Carb.	Cal.	Carb.	Cal.	Carb.
Creamy Peanut Butter, 12-oz. jar	(2017)	(53.0)	(168.1)	(4.42)	1520	40.0	95	2.5
18-oz. jar	(3026)	(79.6)	(168.1)	(4.42)	1520	40.0	95	2.5
28-oz. jar	(4707)	(123.8)	(168.1)	(4.42)	1520	40.0	95	2.5
1 teaspoon (approx. ⅙ oz.)	32	0.8	(168.1)	(4.42)	1520	40.0	95	2.5
Extra Chunky Peanut Butter, 28-oz. jar	(4707)	(123.8)	(168.1)	(4.42)	1520	40.0	95	2.5
1 teaspoon (approx. ⅙ oz.)	32	0.8	(168.1)	(4.42)	1520	40.0	95	2.5
Smooth 'n Creamy Peanut Butter, 28-oz. jar	(4707)	(123.8)	(168.1)	(4.42)	1520	40.0	95	2.5
1 teaspoon (approx. ⅙ oz.)	32	2.5	(168.1)	(4.42)	1520	40.0	95	2.5
P & Q (A&P) Peanut Butter, 18-oz. jar	3200	112.0	177.8	6.22	1600	56.0	100	3.5
1 teaspoon (approx. ⅙ oz.)	33	1.2	177.8	6.22	1600	56.0	100	3.5
Peter Pan Crunchy Peanut Butter, 6-oz. jar	1010	31.9	168.3	5.30	1520	48.0	95	3.0
48-oz. (3-lb.) jar	8080	255.3	168.3	5.30	1520	48.0	95	3.0
1 teaspoon (approx. ⅙ oz.)	32	1.0	168.3	5.30	1520	48.0	95	3.0
Low Sodium Peanut Butter, 8-oz. jar	1347	35.4	168.3	4.40	1520	40.0	95	2.5
1 teaspoon (approx. ⅙ oz.)	32	0.8	168.3	4.40	1520	40.0	95	2.5
Smooth Peanut Butter, 6-oz. jar	1010	31.9	168.3	5.30	1520	48.0	95	3.0
48-oz. (3-lb.) jar	8080	255.3	168.3	5.30	1520	48.0	95	3.0
1 teaspoon (approx. ⅙ oz.)	32	1.0	168.3	5.30	1520	48.0	95	3.0
Planters Creamy Peanut Butter, 12-oz. jar	2020	63.8	168.3	5.32	1520	48.0	95	3.0
18-oz. jar	3029	95.8	168.3	5.32	1520	48.0	95	3.0
1 teaspoon (approx. ⅙ oz.)	32	1.0	168.3	5.32	1520	48.0	95	3.0
Crunchy Peanut Butter, 12-oz. jar	2020	63.8	168.3	5.32	1520	48.0	95	3.0
18-oz. jar	3029	95.8	168.3	5.32	1520	48.0	95	3.0
1 teaspoon (approx. ⅙ oz.)	32	1.0	168.3	5.32	1520	48.0	95	3.0
Skippy Old Fashioned Creamy Peanut Butter, 16-oz. (1-lb.) jar	2693	56.7	168.3	3.54	1520	32.0	95	2.0
1 teaspoon (approx. ⅙ oz.)	32	0.7	168.3	3.54	1520	32.0	95	2.0
Old Fashioned Super Chunk Peanut Butter, 16-oz. (1-lb.) jar	2693	56.7	168.3	3.54	1520	32.0	95	2.0
1 teaspoon (approx. ⅙ oz.)	32	0.7	168.3	3.54	1520	32.0	95	2.0
Super Chunk Peanut Butter, 18-oz. jar	3029	63.7	168.3	3.54	1520	32.0	95	2.0
1 teaspoon (approx. ⅙ oz.)	32	0.7	168.3	3.54	1520	32.0	95	2.0
Smucker's Chunky Natural Peanut Butter, 18-oz. jar	2126	63.8	177.2	5.32	1600	48.0	100	3.0
1 teaspoon (approx. ⅙ oz.)	33	1.0	177.2	5.32	1600	48.0	100	3.0
Creamy Peanut Butter, 12-oz. jar	2021	85.1	168.3	7.10	1520	64.0	95	4.0
18-oz. jar	3029	127.8	168.3	7.10	1520	64.0	95	4.0
28-oz. jar	4714	198.5	168.3	7.10	1520	64.0	95	4.0
1 teaspoon (approx. ⅙ oz.)	32	1.3	168.3	7.10	1520	64.0	95	4.0

	UNIT		1 OZ., BY WT.		1 CUP		1 TABLE-SPOON	
	Cal.	Carb.	Cal.	Carb.	Cal.	Carb.	Cal.	Carb.
Crunchy Peanut Butter, 12-oz. jar	2021	85.1	168.3	7.10	1520	64.0	95	4.0
18-oz. jar	3029	127.8	168.3	7.10	1520	64.0	95	4.0
28-oz. jar	4714	198.5	168.3	7.10	1520	64.0	95	4.0
1 teaspoon (approx. ⅙ oz.)	32	1.3	168.3	7.10	1520	64.0	95	4.0
Goober Grape Peanut Butter with Grape Jelly, 12-oz. jar	1500	168.0	125.0	14.00	1226	137.4	77	8.6
18-oz. jar	2250	252.0	125.0	14.00	1226	137.4	77	8.6
1 teaspoon (approx. ⅙ oz.)	26	2.9	125.0	14.00	1226	137.4	77	8.6
Natural Peanut Butter, 12-oz. jar	2126	63.8	177.0	5.30	1600	48.0	100	3.0
18-oz. jar	3189	95.8	177.0	5.30	1600	48.0	100	3.0
1 teaspoon (approx. ⅙ oz.)	33	1.0	177.0	5.30	1600	48.0	100	3.0
Spred-Lite Creamy Old Fashioned Peanut Butter, 16-oz. (1-lb.) jar	2800	56.0	175.0	3.50	1549	31.0	97	2.0
1 teaspoon (approx. ⅙ oz.)	32	0.7	175.0	3.50	1549	31.0	97	2.0
Crunchy Old Fashioned Peanut Butter, 16-oz. (1-lb.) jar	2800	56.0	175.0	3.50	1549	31.0	97	2.0
1 teaspoon (approx. ⅙ oz.)	32	0.7	175.0	3.50	1549	31.0	97	2.0
PEANUT BUTTER CANDIES (For more peanut butter candies, see the SWEET LITTLE NOTHINGS chapter)								
Carob Coated Peanut Butter Bar, **Hi-Protein,** 2-oz. bar	270	33.0	135.0	16.50				
Peanut Butter Bar, **Frito-Lay,** 1¾-oz. bar	274	27.4	156.6	15.66				
Peanut Butter Cups, **Reese's,** 1.2-oz. package	190	18.0	158.3	15.00				
SESAME BUTTER (TAHINI)								
Golden Harvest No Salt Added Sesame Butter, 12-oz. jar	2280	36.0	190.0	3.00	1710	27.0	107	1.7
1 teaspoon (approx. ⅙ oz.)	36	0.6	190.0	3.00	1710	27.0	107	1.7
Hain Unsalted Raw Sesame Butter, 11-oz. jar	1755	68.2	159.5	6.20	1440	56.0	90	3.5
1 teaspoon (approx. ⅙ oz.)	30	1.2	159.5	6.20	1440	56.0	90	3.5
Joyva Sesame Tahini, 17-oz. can	3230	51.0	190.0	3.00	(1710)	(27.0)	(107)	(1.7)
1 teaspoon (approx. ⅙ oz.)	(36)	(0.6)	190.0	3.00	(1710)	(27.0)	(107)	(1.7)
Protein Aide 100% pure Sesame Tahini, 12-oz. jar	2160	48.0	180.0	4.00	1620	36.0	101	2.3
1 teaspoon (approx. ⅙ oz.)	34	0.8	180.0	4.00	1620	36.0	101	2.3
SESAME CANDIES (For more sesame candies, see the SWEET LITTLE NOTHINGS chapter)								
Sesame Crunch Bar, dry roasted, **Sahadi,** ¾-oz. bar	113	8.1	150.0	10.83				

18 BASIC BAKING & COOKING INGREDIENTS •

	UNIT		1 OZ., BY WT.		1 CUP		1 TABLE-SPOON	
	Cal.	Carb.	Cal.	Carb.	Cal.	Carb.	Cal.	Carb.
GRAIN AND ITS IMMEDIATE PRODUCTS								
Unprocessed Grains, as Harvested								
MILLET, based on generic data								
Millet, Proso (Broomcorn, Hogmillet), 1 pound (3g/21g/1g/12%/na)	1484	331.0	92.8	20.69	(371)	(82.8)	(23)	(5.2)
MILLET, by brand								
Millet, whole, **Golden Harvest,** 16-oz. (1-lb.) package	1600	304.0	100.0	19.00	(400)	(76.0)	(25)	(4.8)
1 cup (approx. 4 oz.)	(400)	(76.0)	100.0	19.00	(400)	(76.0)	(25)	(4.8)
RYE, based on generic data								
Rye, 1 pound (3g/21g/tr/11%/tr)	1516	333.0	94.8	20.83				
SORGHUM GRAIN, based on generic data								
Sorghum Grain (all types), 1 pound (3g/21g/1g/11%/na)	1507	331.4	94.2	20.71				
WHEAT, WHOLE GRAIN, based on generic data								
Values are adjusted to a 12% moisture content. This is the moisture content of wheat as it reaches the mill prior to tempering.								
Durum, 1 pound (4g/20g/1g/13%/1mg)	1507	318.3	94.2	19.89	(415)	(87.7)	(26)	(5.5)
Hard Red Spring, 1 pound (4g/20g/1g/13%/1mg)	1498	313.7	93.5	19.60	(412)	(86.4)	(26)	(5.4)
Hard Red Winter, 1 pound (3g/20g/1g/13%/1mg)	1498	325.5	93.6	20.34	(413)	(89.7)	(26)	(5.6)
Soft Red Winter, 1 pound (3g/20g/1g/14%/1mg)	1480	327.3	92.5	20.46	(408)	(90.2)	(26)	(5.6)
White, 1 pound (3g/21g/1g/12%/1mg)	1521	342.3	95.1	21.39	(419)	(94.3)	(26)	(5.9)
Meal								
ALMOND MEAL, based on generic data								
Almond Meal, partially defatted								
1 cup (approx. 8 oz.)	(928)	(65.2)	116.0	8.20	(928)	(65.2)	(58)	(4.1)
1 pound (approx. 2 cups)	1856	132.2	116.0	8.20	(928)	(65.2)	(58)	(4.1)

	UNIT		1 OZ., BY WT.		1 CUP		1 TABLE-SPOON	
	Cal.	Carb.	Cal.	Carb.	Cal.	Carb.	Cal.	Carb.
ALMOND MEAL, by brand								
Almond Meal, raw, **Balanced,** 10-oz. can	(1166)	(82.4)	(116.6)	(8.24)	933	65.9	58	4.1
1 cup (approx. 8 oz.)	933	65.9	(116.6)	(8.24)	933	65.9	58	4.1
1 pound (approx. 2 cups)	(1866)	(131.8)	(116.6)	(8.24)	933	65.9	58	4.1
CORN MEAL								
Corn Meal, White, **Albers,** 20-oz. box	2000	440.0	100.0	22.00	600	132.0	37	8.3
Corn Meal, Yellow, **Albers,** 20-oz. box	2000	440.0	100.0	22.00	600	132.0	37	8.3
1 cup (approx. 6 oz.)	600	132.0	100.0	22.00	600	132.0	37	8.3
1 pound (approx. 2.7 cups)	1600	352.0	100.0	22.00	600	132.0	37	8.3
Corn Meal, White, enriched, **Aunt Jemima,** 1½-lb. box	2448	532.8	102.0	22.20	541	117.6	34	7.4
32-oz. (2-lb.) box	3264	710.4	102.0	22.20	541	117.6	34	7.4
1 cup (approx. 5.3 oz.)	541	117.6	102.0	22.20	541	117.6	34	7.4
1 pound (approx. 3 cups)	1632	355.2	102.0	22.20	541	117.6	34	7.4
Corn Meal, Yellow, enriched, **Aunt Jemima,** 1½-lb. box	2448	532.8	102.0	22.20	541	117.6	34	7.4
32-oz. (2-lb.) box	3264	710.4	102.0	22.20	541	117.6	34	7.4
1 cup (approx. 5.3 oz.)	541	117.6	102.0	22.20	541	117.6	34	7.4
1 pound (approx. 3 cups)	1632	355.2	102.0	22.20	541	117.6	34	7.4
Corn Meal, White, Self-Rising, **Aunt Jemima,** 32-oz. (2-lb.) box	3136	675.2	98.0	21.20	588	126.6	37	7.9
5-lb. box	7840	1688.0	98.0	21.10	588	126.6	37	7.9
1 cup (approx. 6 oz.)	588	126.6	98.0	21.10	588	126.6	37	7.9
1 pound (approx. 2.7 cups)	1568	337.6	98.0	21.10	588	126.6	37	7.9
Corn Meal, White, Self-Rising, bolted, **Aunt Jemima,** 32-oz. (2-lb.) box	3168	652.8	99.0	20.40	594	122.4	37	7.6
5-lb. box	7920	1632.0	99.0	20.40	594	122.4	37	7.6
1 cup (approx. 6 oz.)	594	122.4	99.0	20.40	594	122.4	37	7.6
1 pound (approx. 2.7 cups)	1584	326.4	99.0	20.40	594	122.4	37	7.6
Corn Meal, Yellow, 100% Whole, stone ground, **Elam's,** 32-oz. (2-lb.) package	3366	662.0	105.2	20.70	(490)	(96.4)	(31)	(6.0)
1 cup (approx. 4.7 oz.)	(490)	(96.4)	105.2	20.70	(490)	(96.4)	(31)	(6.0)
1 pound (approx. 3.4 cups)	1683	331.0	105.2	20.70	(490)	(96.4)	(31)	(6.0)
Corn Meal, White, enriched, stone ground, **Indian Head,** 32-oz. (2-lb.) bag	3200	672.0	100.0	21.00	400	84.0	25	5.3
1 cup (approx. 4 oz.)	400	84.0	100.0	21.00	400	84.0	25	5.3
1 pound (approx. 4 cups)	1600	336.0	100.0	21.00	400	84.0	25	5.3
Corn Meal, Yellow, enriched, old fashioned stone ground, **Indian Head,** 32-oz. (2-lb.) bag	3200	672.0	100.0	21.00	400	84.0	25	5.3
1 cup (approx. 4 oz.)	400	84.0	100.0	21.00	400	84.0	25	5.3
1 pound (approx. 4 cups)	1600	336.0	100.0	21.00	400	84.0	25	5.3

	UNIT		1 OZ., BY WT.		1 CUP		1 TABLESPOON	
	Cal.	Carb.	Cal.	Carb.	Cal.	Carb.	Cal.	Carb.
Corn Meal, White, enriched, **Quaker,** 1½-lb. box	2448	532.8	102.0	22.20	541	117.6	34	7.4
2-lb. box	3264	710.0	102.0	22.20	541	117.6	34	7.4
1 cup (approx. 5.3 oz.)	541	117.6	102.0	22.20	541	117.6	34	7.4
1 pound (approx. 3 cups)	1632	355.2	102.0	22.20	541	117.6	34	7.4
Corn Meal, Yellow, enriched, **Quaker,** 1½-lb. box	2448	532.8	102.0	22.20	541	117.6	34	7.4
2-lb. box	3264	710.0	102.0	22.20	541	117.6	34	7.4
1 cup (approx. 5.3 oz.)	541	117.6	102.0	22.20	541	117.6	34	7.4
1 pound (approx. 3 cups)	1632	355.2	102.0	22.20	541	117.6	34	7.4
CORN MEAL MIX								
Corn Meal Mix, White, bolted, **Aunt Jemima,** 32-oz. (2-lb.) box	3168	665.6	99.0	20.80	594	124.8	37	7.8
5-lb. box	7920	1664.0	99.0	20.80	594	124.8	37	7.8
1 cup (approx. 6 oz.)	594	124.8	99.0	20.80	594	124.8	37	7.8
1 pound (approx. 2.7 cups)	1584	332.8	99.0	20.80	594	124.8	37	7.8
COTTONSEED MEAL (based on data from the Caribbean)								
1 pound	1806	166.5	112.8	10.41				
CRACKER MEAL								
Cracker Meal, **Nabisco,** 9½-oz. box	1045	225.6	110.0	23.75	440	95.0	28	5.9
FLAX SEED MEAL								
Flax Seed Meal, ground, **Natural Brand,** 16-oz. (1-lb.) package	2240	64.0	140.0	4.00				
OATMEAL, see the BREAKFAST CEREALS & BREAKFAST BREADS chapter								
MASA HARINA								
Masa Harina, **Quaker,** 32-oz. (2-lb.) box	3373	675.0	105.4	21.08	411	82.2	26	5.1
5-lb. box	8432	1686.4	105.4	21.08	411	82.2	26	5.1
1 cup (approx. 3.9 oz.)	411	82.2	105.4	21.08	411	82.2	26	5.1
1 pound (approx. 4.1 cups)	1686	337.3	105.4	21.08	411	82.2	26	5.1
MATZO MEAL								
Matzo Meal, **Manischewitz,** 10-oz. box	1069	235.0	106.9	23.50	438	96.3	27	6.0
1 cup (approx. 4.1 oz.)	438	96.3	106.9	23.50	438	96.3	27	6.0
1 pound (approx. 3.9 cups)	1710	376.0	106.9	23.50	438	96.3	27	6.0
MILLET MEAL								
Millet Meal, **Natural Brand,** 3-lb. package	4800	912.0	100.0	19.00				
PUMPKIN SEED MEAL								
Pumpkin Seed Meal, **Natural Brand,** 16-oz. (1-lb.) package	2560	na	160.0	na	(1248)	na	(78)	na
1 cup (approx. 7.8 oz.)	(1248)	na	160.0	na	(1248)	na	(78)	na
SAFFLOWER SEED MEAL								
Safflower Seed Meal, partially defatted, based on generic data:								
1 pound	1612	165.7	100.7	10.36				
SESAME SEED MEAL								
Sesame Seed Meal, raw, **Balanced,** 10-oz. can	(1608)	(61.6)	(160.8)	(6.16)	1286	49.3	80	3.1
1 cup (approx. 8 oz.)	1286	49.3	(160.8)	(6.16)	1286	49.3	80	3.1
1 pound (approx. 2 cups)	(2573)	(98.6)	(160.8)	(6.16)	1286	49.3	80	3.1
SUNFLOWER SEED MEAL								
Sunflower Seed Meal, **Natural Brand,** 16-oz. (1-lb.) jar	2560	112.0	160.0	7.00	(1248)	(54.6)	(78)	(3.4)
1 cup (approx. 7.8 oz.)	(1248)	(54.6)	160.0	7.00	(1248)	(54.6)	(78)	(3.4)

Bran

	UNIT		1 OZ., BY WT.		1 CUP		1 TABLESPOON	
	Cal.	Carb.	Cal.	Carb.	Cal.	Carb.	Cal.	Carb.
BRAN, based on generic data								
Additional brans are listed as cold cereals in the Breakfast Cereals & Breakfast Breads chapter.								
Crude commercially milled Wheat Bran								
1 cup (approx. 2.1 oz.)	128	37.2	60.4	17.56	128	37.2	8	2.3
1 pound (approx. 7.5 cups) (5g/18g/1g/12%/3mg)	967	281.0	60.4	17.56	128	37.2	8	2.3
BRAN, by brand								
Miller's Bran, **Elam's,** 13-oz. package	1133	178.7	87.2	13.75	(185)	(29.1)	(12)	(1.8)
1 cup (approx. 2.1 oz.)	(185)	(29.1)	87.2	13.75	(185)	(29.1)	(12)	(1.8)
1 pound (approx. 7.5 cups)	1395	220.0	87.2	13.75	(185)	(29.1)	(12)	(1.8)
Rice Bran, gluten free, **Elam's,** 8-oz. package	650	121.6	81.2	15.20	203	38.0	13	2.4
1 cup (approx. 2.5 oz.)	203	38.0	81.2	15.20	203	38.0	13	2.4
1 pound (approx. 6.4 cups)	1299	243.2	81.2	15.20	203	38.0	13	2.4
Wheat Bran, pure natural, **Jolly Joan,** 8-oz. package	800	144.0	100.0	18.00	200	36.0	13	2.3
1 cup (approx. 2 oz.)	200	36.0	100.0	18.00	200	36.0	13	2.3
1 pound (approx. 8 cups)	1600	288.0	100.0	18.00	200	36.0	13	2.3

Germ

	UNIT		1 OZ., BY WT.		1 CUP		1 TABLESPOON	
	Cal.	Carb.	Cal.	Carb.	Cal.	Carb.	Cal.	Carb.
CORN GERM								
Corn Germ, toasted, **Naturfresh (Fearn),** 10-oz. pouch	1660	120.0	166.0	12.00	664	48.0	42	3.0
WHEAT GERM								
Wheat Germ with Brown Sugar & Honey, **Kretchmer,** 10-oz. jar	1100	170.0	110.0	17.00	440	68.0	28	4.3
1 cup (approx. 4 oz.)	440	68.0	110.0	17.00	440	68.0	28	4.3
1 pound (approx. 4 cups)	1760	272.0	110.0	17.00	440	68.0	28	4.3
Wheat Germ, natural, not toasted, **Fisher From Krustez,** 12-oz. package	1236	168.0	103.0	14.00	412	56.0	26	3.5
1 cup (approx. 4 oz.)	412	56.0	103.0	14.00	412	56.0	26	3.5
1 pound (approx. 4 cups)	1648	224.0	103.0	14.00	412	56.0	26	3.5
Wheat Germ, raw, **Golden Harvest,** 16-oz. (1-lb.) jar	1600	240.0	100.0	15.00	300	45.0	19	2.8
Wheat Germ, raw, **Naturfresh (Fearn)** 10-oz. pouch	1100	130.0	110.0	13.00	440	52.0	28	3.3
Wheat Germ, regular, **Kretchmer,** 12-oz. jar	1320	156.0	110.0	13.00	440	52.0	28	3.5
1 cup (approx. 4 oz.)	440	52.0	110.0	13.00	440	52.0	28	3.5
1 pound (approx. 4 cups)	1760	208.0	110.0	13.00	440	52.0	28	3.5

Grains Before Fine Milling

	UNIT		1 OZ., BY WT.		1 CUP		1 TABLESPOON	
	Cal.	Carb.	Cal.	Carb.	Cal.	Carb.	Cal.	Carb.
BARLEY, PEARLED, based on generic data								
Light, 1 pound (2g/22g/tr/11%/na)	1584	357.6	99.0	22.35	698	157.6	44	9.9
Pot or Scotch, 1 pound (3g/22g/tr/11%/na)	1584	350.4	99.0	21.90	698	154.4	44	9.9
BARLEY, PEARLED, by brand								
Pearled Barley, **Golden Harvest,** 32-oz. (2-lb.) package	3200	672.0	100.0	21.00	680	142.8	43	8.9
1 cup (approx. 6.8 oz.)	680	142.8	100.0	21.00	680	142.8	43	8.9
Pearled Barley, Regular, "Scotch" Brand, **Quaker,** 16-oz. (1-lb.) box	1619	341.6	101.2	21.35	688	145.2	43	9.1
1 cup (approx. 6.8 oz.)	688	145.2	101.2	21.35	688	145.2	43	9.1
1 serving, prepared as package directs (yield: approx. 1 cup, 8.5 oz.)	(172)	(36.3)	(20.2)	(4.27)	(172)	(36.3)	(11)	(2.3)
Quick, 11-oz. box	1113	234.9	101.2	21.35	688	145.2	43	9.1
1 cup (approx. 6.8 oz.)	688	145.2	101.2	21.35	688	145.2	43	9.1
1 serving, prepared as package directs (yield: approx. ¾ cup, 7.2 oz.)	(172)	(36.3)	(23.9)	(5.04)	(226)	(47.8)	(14)	(3.0)
BULGHUR (Cracked Wheat), based on generic data								
Dry, commercial:								
Made from Club Wheat:								
1 cup (approx. 6.2 oz.)	628	139.1	101.3	22.44	628	139.1	39	8.7
1 pound (approx. 2.6 cups) (2g/22g/tr/9%/na)	1621	359.0	101.3	22.44	628	139.1	39	8.7
Made from Hard Red Winter Wheat:								
1 cup (approx. 6 oz.)	602	128.7	100.3	21.45	602	128.7	38	8.0
1 pound (approx. 2⅔ cups) (3g/21g/tr/10%/na)	1605	343.4	100.3	21.45	602	128.7	38	8.0
Made from White Wheat:								
1 cup (approx. 5.5 oz.)	553	121.8	100.5	22.14	553	121.8	35	7.6
1 pound (approx. 2.9 cups) (3g/22g/tr/9%/na)	1608	354.3	100.5	22.14	553	121.8	35	7.6
BULGHUR, by brand								
Bulghur Wheat, **Jolly Joan,** 1½-lb. box	2400	528.0	100.0	22.00	600	132.0	38	8.2
1 cup (approx. 6 oz.)	600	132.0	100.0	22.00	600	132.0	38	8.2
1 pound (approx. 2.7 cups)	1600	352.0	100.0	22.00	600	132.0	38	8.2

	UNIT		1 OZ., BY WT.		1 CUP		1 TABLE-SPOON	
	Cal.	Carb.	Cal.	Carb.	Cal.	Carb.	Cal.	Carb.
CORN GRITS, see the BREAKFAST CEREALS & BREAKFAST BREADS chapter								
FLOUR								
Flours Not Made From Wheat								
ARROWROOT FLOUR (based on data from the Caribbean)								
1 cup (approx. 4½ oz.)	(436)	(108.9)	96.4	24.10	(436)	(108.9)	(27)	(6.8)
1 pound (approx. 3½ cups)	1542	385.6	96.4	24.10	(436)	(108.9)	(27)	(6.8)
BANANA FLOUR (based on data from Africa)								
1 pound	1542	361.1	96.4	22.57				
BARLEY FLOUR								
Barley Flour, **Featherweight,** 32-oz. (2-lb.) bag	3120	672.0	97.5	21.00	390	84.0	24	5.3
Unsifted, spooned into cup:								
1 cup (approx. 3.6 oz.)	(351)	(75.6)	97.5	21.00	(351)	(75.6)	(22)	(4.7)
1 pound (approx. 4½ cups)	1560	336.0	97.5	21.00	(351)	(75.6)	(22)	(4.7)
BEAN FLOUR, see SOY BEAN FLOUR, LIMA BEAN FLOUR, PEA FLOUR, and PEANUT FLOUR								
BUCKWHEAT FLOUR								
Buckwheat Flour, **Elam's,** 32-oz. (2-lb.) package	3213	694.1	100.4	21.69	(347)	(75.0)	(22)	(4.7)
1 cup (approx. 3½ oz.)	(347)	(75.0)	100.4	21.69	(347)	(75.0)	(22)	(4.7)
1 pound (approx. 4½ cups)	1606	347.0	100.4	21.69	(347)	(75.0)	(22)	(4.7)
Buckwheat Flour, **Larrowe's,** 2½-lb. sack	4320	850.4	108.0	21.26	(373)	(73.5)	(23)	(4.6)
5-pound sack	8640	1700.8	108.0	21.26	(373)	(73.5)	(23)	(4.6)
1 cup (approx. 3½ oz.)	(373)	(73.5)	108.0	21.26	(373)	(73.5)	(23)	(4.6)
1 pound (approx. 4½ cups)	1728	340.2	108.0	21.26	(373)	(73.5)	(23)	(4.6)
CHESTNUT FLOUR, based on generic data								
1 pound (2g/22g/1g/11%/3mg)	1642	345.6	102.6	21.60				
CORN FLOUR, based on generic data								
Unsifted, spooned into cup:								
1 cup (approx. 4.2 oz.)	431	89.9	104.3	21.78	431	89.9	27	5.6
1 pound (approx. 3.9 cups) (2g/22g/1g/12%/tr)	1669	348.4	104.3	21.78	431	89.9	27	5.6
CORN FLOUR, by brand								
Corn Flour, **Featherweight,** 32-oz. (2-lb.) bag	3280	720.0	102.5	22.50	410	90.0	26	5.6
CORNSTARCH, based on generic data								
1 cup (approx. 4½ oz.)	463	112.1	102.5	24.83	463	112.1	29	7.0
1 pound (approx. 3½ cups)	1640	397.3	102.5	24.83	463	112.1	29	7.0
COTTONSEED FLOUR, based on generic data								
1 pound (14g/9g/2g/6%/na)	1615	149.7	100.9	9.36				
GRASSHOPPER FLOUR (based on data from Africa)								
1 pound	1905	71.7	119.1	4.48				
LIMA BEAN FLOUR, based on generic data								
Sifted, spooned into cup:								
1 cup (approx. 4.4 oz.)	432	79.4	97.3	17.86	432	79.4	27	5.0
1 pound (approx. 3.6 cups) (6g/18g/tr/11%/na)	1556	285.8	97.3	17.86	432	79.4	27	5.0
OAT FLOUR								
Oat Flour, **Featherweight** 32-oz. (2-lb.) bag	3440	584.0	107.5	18.25	430	73.0	27	4.6
PEA FLOUR (based on data from Africa)								
1 pound	1556	282.6	97.2	17.66				
PEANUT FLOUR, defatted, based on generic data								
1 cup (approx. 2.1 oz.)	223	18.9	105.2	8.92	223	18.9	14	1.2
1 pound (approx. 7.5 cups) (14g/9g/3g/7%/3mg)	1683	142.6	105.2	8.92	223	18.9	14	1.2
PEANUT FLOUR (based on data from Africa)								
1 pound	1756	174.2	109.7	10.89				
POTATO FLOUR, based on generic data								
Unsifted, spooned into cup:								
1 cup (approx. 6⅓ oz.)	629	143.1	99.6	22.67	629	143.1	39	8.9
1 pound (approx. 2½ cups) (2g/23g/tr/8%/10mg)	1594	362.7	99.6	22.67	629	143.1	39	8.9
RICE FLOUR, based on generic data								
1 cup (approx. 4.8 oz.)	(498)	(109.4)	(103.8)	(22.80)	(498)	(109.4)	(31)	(6.8)
1 pound (approx. 3⅓ cups) (3g/23g/tr/4%/1mg)	(1661)	(364.7)	(103.8)	(22.80)	(498)	(109.4)	(31)	(6.8)
RICE FLOUR, by brand								
Rice Flour, **Fearn,** 3-lb. package	(4980)	(1094.1)	(103.8)	(22.80)	(498)	(109.4)	(31)	(6.8)
Rice Flour, **Featherweight,** 32-oz. (2-lb.) bag	3200	723.2	100.0	22.60	500	113.0	31	7.1
Rice Flour, **Jolly Joan,** 1½-lb. box	2150	490.0	89.6	20.42	430	98.0	27	6.1
RYE FLOUR, based on generic data								
Dark Rye Flour, sifted, spooned into cup:								
1 cup (approx. 4.5 oz.)	419	87.2	92.9	19.33	419	87.2	26	5.5
1 pound (approx. 3½ cups) (5g/19g/1g/11%/tr)	1486	309.3	92.9	19.33	419	87.2	26	5.5
Light Rye Flour, sifted, spooned into cup:								
1 cup (approx. 3.1 oz.)	314	68.6	101.3	22.12	314	68.6	20	4.3
1 pound (approx. 5⅕ cups) (3g/22g/tr/11%/tr)	1620	353.9	101.3	22.12	314	68.6	20	4.3
Light Rye Flour, unsifted, spooned into cup:								
1 cup (approx. 3.6 oz.)	364	79.5	101.3	22.12	364	79.5	23	5.0
1 pound (approx. 4½ cups) (3g/22g/tr/11%/tr)	1620	353.9	101.3	22.12	364	79.5	23	5.0
Medium Rye Flour, sifted, spooned into cup:								
1 cup (approx. 3.1 oz.)	308	65.8	99.3	21.22	308	65.8	19	4.1
1 pound (approx. 5⅕ cups) (3g/21g/tr/11%/tr)	1589	339.5	99.3	21.22	308	65.8	19	4.1
RYE FLOUR, by brand								
Rye Flour, Stone Ground Whole, **Elam's,** 5-lb. package	8096	1612.8	101.2	20.16	(293)	(58.3)	(18)	(3.6)
Rye Flour, Medium, **Pillsbury,** 5-lb. package	8400	1780.0	105.0	22.25	420	89.0	26	5.6
Rye and enriched Wheat Flour, Bohemian Style, **Pillsbury,** 5-lb. package	8000	1720.0	100.0	21.50	400	86.0	25	5.4
SOYBEAN FLOUR, based on generic data								
Defatted Soybean Flour:								
Stirred:								
1 cup (approx. 3.5 oz.)	326	38.1	92.4	10.80	326	38.1	20	2.4
1 pound (approx. 4½ cups) (13g/11g/tr/8%/tr)	1479	172.8	92.4	10.80	326	38.1	20	2.4
Full Fat Soybean Flour:								
1 cup:								
Not stirred (approx. 3 oz.)	358	25.8	119.3	8.62	358	25.8	22	1.6
Stirred (approx. 2.5 oz.)	295	21.3	119.3	8.62	295	21.3	18	1.3
1 pound (approx. 5⅓ cups not stirred and approx. 6½ cups stirred) (10g/9g/6g/8%/tr)	1910	137.9	119.3	8.62				
Low Fat Soybean Flour:								
Stirred:								
1 cup (approx. 3.1 oz.)	313	32.2	100.9	10.38	313	32.2	20	2.0
1 pound (approx. 5⅕ cups) (12g/10g/2g/8%/tr)	1615	166.0	100.9	10.38	313	32.2	20	2.0
SOYBEAN FLOUR, by brand								
Soybean Flour, **Deaf Smith Farms,** 1½-lb. package	3000	216.0	125.0	9.00	(500)	(36.0)	(31)	(2.3)
Soybean Flour, **Featherweight,** 32-oz. (2-lb.) bag	3674	90.9	114.8	2.84	405	10.0	25	0.6
SUNFLOWER SEED FLOUR, partially defatted, based on generic data								
1 pound (13g/11g/1g/7%/16mg)	1539	171.2	96.2	10.70				
SWEET POTATO FLOUR (based on data from Africa)								
1 pound	1520	362.9	95.0	22.68				
TAPIOCA FLOUR, based on generic data								
Unsifted, spooned into cup:								
1 cup (approx. 4¼ oz.)	424	104.0	99.8	24.50	424	104.0	27	6.5

	UNIT		1 OZ., BY WT.		1 CUP		1 TABLESPOON	
	Cal.	Carb.	Cal.	Carb.	Cal.	Carb.	Cal.	Carb.
1 pound (approx. 3¾ cups) (tr/25g/tr/13%/3mg)	1597	392.0	99.8	24.50	424	104.0	27	6.5
TAPIOCA STARCH FLOUR								
Featherweight, 2-lb. bag	3120	800.0	97.5	25.00	390	100.0	24	6.3
YAM FLOUR (based on data from Africa)								
1 pound	1520	362.9	95.0	22.68				

Wheat Flours

	UNIT		1 OZ., BY WT.		1 CUP		1 TABLESPOON	
	Cal.	Carb.	Cal.	Carb.	Cal.	Carb.	Cal.	Carb.
WHEAT FLOUR, based on generic data								
"80% extraction" flour (from hard wheats), 1 pound (3g/21g/tr/12%/1mg)	1656	336.2	103.5	21.01				
Straight flour, hard wheats, 1 pound (3g/21g/tr/12%/1mg)	1656	337.9	103.5	21.12				
Straight flour, soft wheats, 1 pound (3g/22g/tr/12%/1mg)	1651	348.9	103.2	21.80				
ALL PURPOSE or FAMILY FLOUR, enriched or unenriched, based on generic data								
Unsifted, standard granulation:								
Dipped with cup:								
1 cup (approx. 4.8 oz.)	499	104.3	103.3	21.59	499	104.3	31	6.5
1 pound (approx. 3⅓ cups) (3g/22g/tr/12%/1mg)	1654	345.4	103.3	21.59	499	104.3	31	6.5
Spooned into cup:								
1 cup (approx. 4.4 oz.)	419	87.5	103.3	21.59	419	87.5	26	5.5
1 pound (approx. 3⅔ cups)	1654	345.4	103.3	21.59	419	87.5	26	5.5
Unsifted, instant blending:								
Spooned into cup:								
1 cup (approx. 4.5 oz.)	470	98.2	103.3	21.59	470	98.2	29	6.1
1 pound (approx. 3½ cups)	1654	345.4	103.3	21.59	470	98.2	29	6.1
Sifted, standard granulation:								
1 cup (approx. 4 oz.)	419	87.5	103.3	21.59	419	87.5	26	5.5
1 pound (approx. 3.9 cups)	1654	345.4	103.3	21.59	419	87.5	26	5.5
ALL PURPOSE FLOUR, by brand								
All Purpose Flour, enriched, bleached, **Ann Page (A&P),** 32-oz. (2-lb.) bag (approx. 8 cups)	3200	696.0	100.0	21.80	400	87.0	25	5.4
5-lb. bag (approx. 20 cups)	8000	1740.0	100.0	21.80	400	87.0	25	5.4
1 cup (approx. 4 oz.)	400	87.0	100.0	21.80	400	87.0	25	5.4
1 pound (approx. 4 cups)	1600	348.0	100.0	21.80	400	87.0	25	5.4
All Purpose Flour, plain, enriched, **Ballard,** 32-oz. (2-lb.) bag (approx. 8 cups)	3200	696.0	100.0	21.80	400	87.0	25	5.4
1 cup (approx. 4 oz.)	400	87.0	100.0	21.80	400	87.0	25	5.4
1 pound (approx. 4 cups)	1600	348.0	100.0	21.80	400	87.0	25	5.4
All Purpose unbleached Flour, **Ceresota,** 5-lb. bag	7800	1650.0	97.5	20.63	390	82.5	24	5.2
1 cup (approx. 4.0 oz.)	390	82.5	97.5	20.63	390	82.5	24	5.2
1 pound (approx. 4 cups)	1560	330.0	97.5	20.63	390	82.5	24	5.2
All Purpose White Flour, **Heckers,** 32-oz. (2-lb.) bag (approx. 8 cups)	3120	660.0	97.5	20.60	390	82.5	24	5.2
1 cup (approx. 4 oz.)	390	82.5	97.5	20.60	390	82.5	24	5.2
1 pound (approx. 4 cups)	1560	330.0	97.5	20.60	390	82.5	24	5.2
All Purpose Flour, unbleached, enriched, sifted, **Pillsbury,** 5-lb. bag (approx. 20 cups)	8000	1720.0	100.0	21.50	400	86.0	25	5.4
10-lb. bag (approx. 40 cups)	16000	3440.0	100.0	21.50	400	86.0	25	5.4
1 cup (approx. 4 oz.)	400	86.0	100.0	21.50	400	86.0	25	5.4
1 pound (approx. 4 cups)	1600	344.0	100.0	21.50	400	86.0	25	5.4
All Purpose Flour, enriched, bleached, **Pillsbury's Best XXXX,** 2-lb. package (approx. 8 cups)	3200	696.0	100.0	21.80	400	87.0	25	5.4
5-lb. package (approx. 20 cups)	8000	1740.0	100.0	21.80	400	87.0	25	5.4
10-lb. package (approx. 40 cups)	16000	3480.0	100.0	21.80	400	87.0	25	5.4
25-lb. package (approx. 100 cups)	40000	8700.0	100.0	21.80	400	87.0	25	5.4
50-lb. package (approx. 200 cups)	80000	1740.0	100.0	21.80	400	87.0	25	5.4
1 cup (approx. 4 oz.)	400	87.0	100.0	21.00	400	87.0	25	5.4
1 pound (approx. 4 cups)	1600	348.0	100.0	21.80	400	87.0	25	5.4

	UNIT		1 OZ., BY WT.		1 CUP		1 TABLESPOON	
	Cal.	Carb.	Cal.	Carb.	Cal.	Carb.	Cal.	Carb.
BREAD FLOUR, enriched or unenriched, standard granulation, based on generic data								
Unsifted, dipped with cup:								
1 cup (approx. 4.8 oz.)	500	102.3	103.6	21.19	500	102.3	31	6.4
1 pound (approx. 3⅓ cups) (3g/21g/tr/12%/1mg)	1658	339.1	103.6	21.19	500	102.3	31	6.4
Sifted, spooned into cup:								
1 cup (approx. 4 oz.)	420	85.9	103.6	21.19	420	85.9	26	5.4
1 pound (approx. 3.9 cups)	1658	339.1	103.6	21.19	420	85.9	26	5.4
CAKE or PASTRY FLOUR, based on generic data								
Unsifted:								
Dipped with cup:								
1 cup (approx. 4.2 oz.)	430	93.7	103.2	22.50	430	93.7	27	5.9
1 pound (approx. 3.8 cups) (2g/23g/tr/12%/1mg)	1650	360.4	103.2	22.50	430	93.7	27	5.9
Spooned into cup:								
1 cup (approx. 3.8 oz.)	397	86.5	103.2	22.50	397	86.5	25	5.4
1 pound (approx. 4.2 cups)	1650	360.4	103.2	22.50	397	86.5	25	5.4
Sifted, spooned into cup:								
1 cup (approx. 3.4 oz.)	349	76.2	103.2	22.50	349	76.2	22	4.8
1 pound (approx. 4¼ cups)	1650	360.4	103.2	22.50	349	76.2	22	4.8
CAKE FLOUR, by brand								
Cake Flour, **Swans Down,** 32-oz. (2-lb.) bag (approx. 7.8 cups)	3129	711.2	97.8	22.20	400	88.0	25	5.5
1 cup (approx. 4.1 oz.)	400	88.0	97.8	22.20	400	88.0	25	5.5
1 pound (approx. 3.9 cups)	1565	355.6	97.8	22.20	400	88.0	25	5.5
ENRICHED FLOUR, by brand								
Enriched Flour, High Altitude, Hungarian, **Peavey Family Flour,** 32-oz. (2-lb.) bag	3200	696.0	100.0	21.75	400	87.0	25	5.4
1 cup (approx. 4.0 oz.)	400	87.0	100.0	21.75	400	87.0	25	5.4
1 pound (approx. 4 cups)	1600	348.0	100.0	21.75	400	87.0	25	5.4
Enriched Flour, King Midas, **Peavey Family Flour,** 32-oz. (2-lb.) bag	3200	696.0	100.0	21.75	400	87.0	25	5.4
1 cup (approx. 4.0 oz.)	400	87.0	100.0	21.75	400	87.0	25	5.4
1 pound (approx. 4 cups)	1600	348.0	100.0	21.75	400	87.0	25	5.4
Enriched Flour, Occident, **Peavey Family Flour,** 32-oz. (2-lb.) bag	3200	696.0	100.0	21.75	400	87.0	25	5.4
1 cup (approx. 4.0 oz.)	400	87.0	100.0	21.75	400	87.0	25	5.4
1 pound (approx. 4 cups)	1600	348.0	100.0	21.75	400	87.0	25	5.4
GLUTEN FLOUR (45% gluten, 55% patent white flour), based on generic data								
Unsifted, dipped with cup:								
1 cup (approx. 4.9 oz.)	529	66.1	107.2	13.39	529	66.1	33	4.1
1 pound (approx. 3¼ cups) (12g/13g/1g/9%/1mg)	1715	214.2	107.2	13.39	529	66.1	33	4.1
Unsifted or sifted, spooned into cup:								
1 cup (approx. 4¾ oz.)	510	63.7	107.2	13.39	510	63.7	32	4.0
1 pound (approx. 3⅓ cups)	1715	214.2	107.2	13.39	510	63.7	32	4.0
GLUTEN FLOUR, by brand								
Featherweight, 2-lb. bag	(3430)	(428.5)	(107.2)	(13.39)	420	55.0	26	3.4
GRAHAM FLOUR, see WHOLE WHEAT FLOUR								
SAUCE & GRAVY FLOUR								
Sauce & Gravy Flour, **Pillsbury,** 13.5-oz. container (approx. 27 teaspoons)	1350	297.0	100.0	22.00	400	88.0	25	5.5
1 cup (approx. 4 oz.)	400	88.0	100.0	22.00	400	88.0	25	5.5
1 pound (approx. 4 cups)	1600	352.0	100.0	22.00	400	88.0	25	5.5
SELF-RISING FLOUR (anhydrous monocalcium phosphate used as a baking acid), based on generic data								
Unsifted, spooned into cup:								
1 cup (approx. 4.4 oz.)	440	92.8	99.9	21.05	440	92.8	28	5.8
1 pound (approx. 3⅔ cups) (3g/21g/tr/12%/306mg)	1598	336.7	99.9	21.05	440	92.8	28	5.8
Sifted, spooned into cup:								
1 cup (approx. 4 oz.)	405	85.3	99.9	21.05	405	85.3	25	5.3
1 pound (approx. 3.9 cups)	1599	336.7	99.9	21.05	405	85.3	25	5.3
SELF-RISING FLOUR, by brand								
Self-Rising Flour, **Aunt Jemima,** 32-oz. (2-lb.) box (approx. 8 cups)	3488	755.2	109.0	23.60	436	94.4	27	5.9

	UNIT		1 OZ., BY WT.		1 CUP		1 TABLE-SPOON	
	Cal.	Carb.	Cal.	Carb.	Cal.	Carb.	Cal.	Carb.
1 cup (approx. 4 oz.)	436	94.4	109.0	23.60	436	94.4	27	5.9
1 pound (approx. 4 cups)	1744	377.6	109.0	23.60	436	94.4	27	5.9
Self-Rising Flour, **Ballard,** 32-oz. (2-lb.) bag (approx. 8 cups)	3040	672.0	95.0	21.00	380	84.0	24	5.3
5-lb. bag (approx. 20 cups)	7600	1680.0	95.0	21.00	380	84.0	24	5.3
10-lb. bag (approx. 40 cups)	15200	3360.0	95.0	21.00	380	84.0	24	5.3
25-lb. bag (approx. 100 cups)	38000	8400.0	95.0	21.00	380	84.0	24	5.3
1 cup (approx. 4 oz.)	380	84.0	95.0	21.00	380	84.0	24	5.3
1 pound (approx. 4 cups)	1520	335.0	95.0	21.00	380	84.0	24	5.3
Self-Rising Flour, **Pillsbury's Best XXX,** 32-oz. (2-lb.) bag (approx. 8 cups)	3040	672.0	95.0	21.00	380	84.0	24	5.3
5-lb. bag (approx. 20 cups)	7600	1680.0	95.0	21.00	380	84.0	24	5.3
10-lb. bag (approx. 40 cups)	15200	3360.0	95.0	21.00	380	84.0	24	5.3
25-lb. bag (approx. 100 cups)	38000	8400.0	95.0	21.00	380	84.0	24	5.3
1 cup (approx. 4 oz.)	380	84.0	95.0	21.00	380	84.0	24	5.3
1 pound (approx. 4 cups)	1520	335.0	95.0	21.00	380	84.0	24	5.3
Self-Rising Cake Flour, **Presto,** 16-oz. (1-lb.) box (approx. 4 cups)	1634	350.7	102.4	21.90	400	86.6	25	5.4
32-oz. (2-lb.) box (approx. 8 cups)	3267	701.4	102.4	21.90	400	86.6	25	5.4
1 cup (approx. 3.9 oz.)	400	86.6	102.4	21.90	400	86.6	25	5.4
1 pound (approx. 4.1 cups)	1634	350.7	102.4	21.90	400	86.6	25	5.4
SEMOLINA FLOUR								
Aproten, 5-lb. package	7680	1936.0	96.0	24.20	(910)	(228.0)	(57)	(14.3)
WHOLE WHEAT FLOUR (from hard wheats), based on generic data								
Stirred, spooned into cup:								
1 cup (approx. 4¼ oz.)	400	85.2	94.6	20.14	400	85.2	25	5.3
1 pound (approx. 3.8 cups) (4g/20g/1g/12%/3mg)	1513	322.2	94.6	20.14	400	85.2	25	5.3
WHOLE WHEAT FLOUR, by brand								
Whole Wheat Flour, **Ceresota,** 32-oz. (2-lb.) bag	3200	640.0	100.0	20.00	(400)	(80.0)	(25)	(5.0)
1 cup (approx. 4.0 oz.)	(400)	(80.0)	100.0	20.00	(400)	(80.0)	(25)	(5.0)
1 pound (approx. 4 cups)	1600	320.0	100.0	20.00	(400)	(80.0)	(25)	(5.0)
Whole Wheat Flour, Stone Ground, **Deaf Smith Farms,** 32-oz. (2-lb.) package	3200	640.0	100.0	20.00	(423)	(84.7)	(26)	(5.3)
1 cup (approx. 4.2 oz.)	(423)	(84.7)	100.0	20.00	(423)	(84.7)	(26)	(5.3)
1 pound (approx. 3.8 oz.)	1600	320.0	100.0	20.00	(423)	(84.7)	(26)	(5.3)
Whole Wheat Graham Flour, **Pillsbury's Best XXXX,** 5-lb. bag	8000	1600.0	100.0	20.00	400	80.0	25	5.0
1 cup (approx. 4 oz.)	400	80.0	100.0	20.00	400	80.0	25	5.0
1 pound (approx. 4 cups)	1600	320.0	100.0	20.00	400	80.0	25	5.0
EXTENDERS								
Hamburger Helper, **Betty Crocker:**								
For Beef Noodle, Egg Noodles & Sauce Mix, 6½-oz. box	700	130.0	107.7	20.00				
Prepared as package directs, adding 1 pound of hamburger meat to mix (yield: approx. 5 cups, 43 oz.)	1600	130.0	(37.2)	(3.02)	320	26.0	20	1.6
For comparison: 1 pound of hamburger alone	(800)	0.0	(50.0)	0.00				
For Cheesburger Macaroni, Macaroni and Cheese Sauce Mix, 8-oz. box	900	140.0	112.5	17.50				
Prepared as package directs, adding 1 pound of hamburger meat to mix (yield: approx. 5 cups, 43 oz.)	1800	140.0	(41.9)	(3.26)	360	28.0	23	1.8
For Chili Tomato, Macaroni, Tomato Sauce Mix With Chili Seasoning, 7¼-oz. box	700	145.0	96.6	20.00				
Prepared as package directs, adding 1 pound of hamburger meat to mix (yield: approx. 5 cups, 43 oz.)	1600	145.0	(37.2)	(3.37)	320	29.0	20	1.8
For Hamburger Pizza Dish, 8½-oz. box	800	165.0	94.1	19.41				

	UNIT		1 OZ., BY WT.		1 CUP		1 TABLE-SPOON	
	Cal.	Carb.	Cal.	Carb.	Cal.	Carb.	Cal.	Carb.
Prepared as package directs, adding 1 pound of hamburger meat to mix (yield: approx. 2½ cups, 21 oz.)	1700	165.0	(81.0)	(7.86)	680	62.8	43	3.9
For Hamburger Stew, 5½-oz. box	550	115.0	100.0	20.91				
Prepared as package directs, adding 1 pound of hamburger meat to mix (yield: approx. 2½ cups, 18 oz.)	1450	115.0	(80.6)	(6.39)	580	46.0	36	2.9
For Lasagne, Lasagne Macaroni & Italian Style Sauce Mix, 7¾-oz. box	750	160.0	96.8	20.70				
Prepared as package directs, adding 1 pound of hamburger meat to mix (yield: approx. 5 cups, 43 oz.)	1650	160.0	(38.4)	(3.72)	330	32.0	21	2.0
For Potatoes Stroganoff, 7-oz. box	750	145.0	107.1	20.71				
Prepared as package directs, adding 1 pound of hamburger meat to mix (yield: approx. 2½ cups, 19 oz.)	1650	145.0	86.8	7.63	660	58.0	41	3.6
For Rice Oriental, Long Grain Rice and Soy Sauce Mix, 8-oz. box	800	175.0	100.0	21.90				
Prepared as package directs, adding 1 pound of hamburger meat to mix (yield: approx. 5 cups, 43 oz.)	1700	175.0	(39.5)	(4.07)	340	35.0	21	2.2
For Spaghetti, Spaghetti & Tomato Sauce Mix, 7½-oz. box	750	155.0	100.0	20.70				
Prepared as package directs, adding 1 pound of hamburger meat to mix (yield: approx. 5 cups, 43 oz.)	1650	155.0	(38.4)	(3.60)	330	31.0	21	1.9
Sesame Burger Mix, **Fearn,** 10-oz. box	1276	63.8	127.6	6.38	464	23.2	29	1.5
Prepared as package directs	1485	64.9						
Soya Granules, **Fearn,** 16-oz. (1-lb.) box	1560	144.0	97.5	9.00	520	48.0	33	3.0
3-lb. bag	4680	432.0	97.5	9.00	520	48.0	33	3.0
1 cup, dry (approx. 5.4 oz.)	520	48.0	97.5	9.00	520	48.0	33	3.0
Soya Powder, **Fearn,** 11-oz. box	1800	108.0	163.6	9.82	400	24.0	25	1.5
36-oz. bag	5890	353.5	163.6	9.82	400	24.0	25	1.5
1 cup, dry (approx. 2.4 oz.)	400	24.0	163.6	9.82	400	24.0	25	1.5
Soya Protein, **Fearn,** 10-oz. container	975	na	97.5	trace	200	na	13	trace
40-oz. container	3900	na	97.5	trace	200	na	13	trace
1 cup, dry (approx. 2.1 oz.)	200	na	97.5	trace	200	na	13	trace
Tuna Helper, **Betty Crocker**								
For Country Dumplings Noodles 'n Tuna, 8-oz. box	850	155.0	106.3	19.38				
Prepared as package directs, adding drained contents of one 6½-oz. can of tuna packed in oil (yield: approx. 5 cups, 40 oz.)	1150	155.6	(28.8)	(3.89)	230	31.1	14	1.9
For comparison: drained contents of one 6½-oz. can of chunk-style tuna packed in oil, alone (approx. 5½ oz.)	(309)	(0.0)	(55.5	(0.00)	309	0.0	19	0.0
For Creamy Noodles 'N Tuna, 8¾-oz. box	1100	150.0	125.7	17.10				
Prepared as package directs, adding drained contents of one 6½-oz. can of tuna (yield: approx. 5 cups, 40 oz.)	1400	150.0	35.0	3.75	(280)	(30.0)	(18)	(1.9)
For Noodles, Cheese Sauce 'N Tuna, 7¾-oz. box	850	140.0	109.7	18.10				
Prepared as package directs, adding drained contents of one 6½-oz. can of tuna (yield: approx. 5 cups, 40 oz.)	1150	140.0	28.8	3.50	(230)	(28.0)	(14)	(1.8)

CRUMBS, COATINGS, CROUTONS, and STUFFINGS

	UNIT		1 OZ., BY WT.		1 CUP		1 TABLE-SPOON	
	Cal.	Carb.	Cal.	Carb.	Cal.	Carb.	Cal.	Carb.
BREADCRUMBS AND OTHER CRUMBS (The BREADS chapter has a column for breadcrumbs. See Prepackaged Bread, by brand)								
Breadcrumbs, dry, grated, based on generic data, 1 pound (approx. 2 cups) (4g/21g/1g/7%/209mg)	1778	332.9	111.1	20.81	(444)	(83.2)	(28)	(5.3)
Breadcrumbs, Seasoned, **Contadina,** 9-oz. container	909	176.8	101.0	19.64	(411)	(79.9)	(26)	(5.0)
Corn Flake Crumbs, **Kellogg's,** 21-oz. box	2310	504.0	110.0	24.00	(440)	(96.0)	(28)	(6.0)
Graham Cracker Crumbs, **Nabisco,** 13½-oz. box	1540	264.0	114.1	19.56	(420)	(84.0)	(26)	(5.3)
Graham Cracker Crumbs, **Sunshine,** 13½-oz. bag	1610	298.4	119.3	22.10	(358)	(66.3)	(22)	(4.1)
COATING MIXES								
Shake 'N Bake For Chicken, 2⅜-oz. box	279	42.4	117.5	17.85				
For Chicken, Barbecue Style, 3.75-oz. box	366	83.0	97.6	22.13				
For Chicken, Crispy Country, 2⅜-oz. box	318	41.9	133.9	17.64				
For Chicken, Italian Flavor, 2⅜-oz. box	286	41.3	120.4	17.39				
For Fish, 2-oz. box	226	33.8	113.0	16.90				
For Hamburger, 2-oz. box	163	33.2	81.5	16.60				
For Pork, 2⅜-oz. box	260	47.0	109.5	19.79				
For Pork and Ribs, Barbecue Style, 2⅞-oz. box	290	60.5	100.9	21.04				
CROUTONS								
Artificial Bacon Croutons, **Bel Air,** 2¾-oz. box	320	48.0	116.4	17.45	(160)	(24.0)		
Buttery Toasted Croutons, **Brownberry,** 6-oz. box	793	109.0	132.2	18.16	(331)	(45.5)		
Caesar Seasoned Croutons, **Brownberry,** 6-oz. box	800	95.5	133.4	15.92	(334)	(39.8)		
Cheddar Cheese Croutons, **Brownberry,** 6-oz. box	827	97.2	137.9	16.20	(345)	(40.5)		
Cheddar Cheese Croutons, **Pepperidge Farm,** 6½-oz. package	845	123.5	130.0	19.00	(193)	(28.1)		
Cheese & Garlic Croutons, **Bel Air,** 3-oz. box	400	48.0	133.3	16.00	(200)	(24.0)		
Cheese-Garlic Croutons, **Pepperidge Farm,** 6-oz. package	840	102.0	140.0	17.00	(207)	(25.2)		
Croutettes, Herb Seasoned Croutons, **Kellogg's,** 7-oz. box	700	150.0	100.0	21.43	(141)	(30.2)		
French Style Garlic Croutons, **Arnold,** 6-oz. box	792	109.6	132.0	18.26	(165)	(22.8)		
Garlic Croutons, **Bel Air,** 2¾-oz. box	320	48.0	116.4	17.45	(160)	(24.0)		
Italian Cheese Croutons, **Bel Air,** 3-oz. box	400	48.0	133.3	16.00	(200)	(24.0)		
Italian Style Seasoned Croutons, **Arnold,** 6-oz. box	786	108.4	131.0	18.07	(164)	(22.6)		
Onion & Garlic Croutons, **Brownberry,** 6-oz. box	797	101.1	132.8	16.85	(332)	(42.1)		
Onion-Garlic Croutons, **Pepperidge Farm,** 6-oz. package	840	114.0	140.0	19.00	(207)	(28.1)		
Plain Croutons, **Bel Air,** 2½-oz. box	240	56.0	96.0	22.40	(120)	(28.0)		
Plain Croutons, **Pepperidge Farm,** 6½-oz. package	910	130.0	140.0	20.00	(207)	(29.6)		
Seasoned Croutons, **Bel Air,** 2¾-oz. box	360	48.0	130.9	17.45	(180)	(24.0)		
Seasoned Croutons, **Brownberry,** 6-oz. box	788	107.8	131.4	17.96	(329)	(44.9)		
Seasoned Croutons, **Pepperidge Farm,** 6-oz. package	840	114.0	140.0	19.00	(207)	(28.1)		
"Something Better Than Croutons," **NSB,** 3.6-oz. package	320	16.0	88.9	4.44	(111)	(5.8)		
Sour Cream & Chives Croutons, **Pepperidge Farm,** 6-oz. package	840	102.0	140.0	17.00	(207)	(25.2)		
Sourdough Croutons, no sugar, no oils, **Pioneer,** 8-oz. box	560	112.0	70.0	14.00	(103)	(20.8)		

	UNIT		1 OZ., BY WT.		1 CUP		1 TABLE-SPOON	
	Cal.	Carb.	Cal.	Carb.	Cal.	Carb.	Cal.	Carb.
STUFFINGS								
All Purpose Seasoned Stuffing, **Arnold,** 7-oz. bag	833	140.8	119.0	20.12	(149)	(25.2)	(9)	(1.6)
Prepared as package directs, adding ½ cup butter and 1 cup water (yield: approx. 19.4 oz.)	(1633)	(140.8)	(84.2)	(7.26)				
Chicken Flavor Bread Stuffing Mix, **Uncle Ben's Stuff 'N Such,** 6-oz. box	613	123.6	102.1	20.53	(256)	(51.4)	(16)	(3.2)
Chicken & Herb Pan Style Stuffing, **Pepperidge Farm,** 6-oz. package	660	120.0	110.0	20.00	(275)	(50.1)	(17)	(3.1)
Cornbread Stuffing, **Arnold,** 7-oz. bag	816	153.4	116.6	21.92	(146)	(27.4)	(9)	(1.7)
Prepared as package directs, adding ½ cup butter and 1 cup water (yield: approx. 19.4 oz.)	(1616)	(153.4)	(83.3)	(7.91)				
Corn Bread Stuffing, **Pepperidge Farm,** 8-oz. package	880	168.0	110.0	21.00	(275)	(52.6)	(17)	(3.3)
16-oz. (1-lb.) package	1760	336.0	110.0	21.00	(275)	(52.6)	(17)	(3.3)
Cornbread Stuffing Mix, **Uncle Ben's Stuff 'N Such,** 6-oz. box	613	127.6	102.1	21.26	(256)	(51.4)	(16)	(3.2)
Croutettes, Herb Seasoned Croutons, **Kellogg's,** 7-oz. box	700	150.0	100.0	21.43	(141)	(30.2)		
Prepared for stuffing as package directs, mixing 7 oz. croutettes with 4 oz. margarine or butter (yield: approx. 11 oz.)	1500	150.0	136.4	13.63	300	30.0	19	1.9
Cube Stuffing, **Pepperidge Farm,** 7-oz. package	770	147.0	110.0	21.00	(275)	(52.6)	(17)	(3.3)
Herb Seasoned Stuffing, **Brownberry,** 8-oz. box	870	162.7	108.7	20.34	(272)	(50.9)	(17)	(3.2)
Herb Stuffing, **Pepperidge Farm,** 8-oz. package	880	184.0	110.0	23.00	(275)	(57.6)	(17)	(3.6)
16-oz. (1-lb.) package	1760	368.0	110.0	23.00	(275)	(57.6)	(17)	(3.6)
Ready Mixed Stuffing, **Bell's,** 6-oz. box	650	120.0	108.3	20.00	260	48.0	16	3.0
Prepared as package directs, adding ¼ cup butter (yield: approx. 2.4 cups, 6 oz.)	1100	125.0	183.3	20.83	440	50.0	28	3.1
Sage Bread Stuffing Mix, **Uncle Ben's Stuff 'N Such,** 6-oz. box	613	123.0	102.1	20.50	(256)	(51.4)	(16)	(3.2)
Seasoned, Pan Style Stuffing, **Pepperidge Farm,** 6-oz. package	660	12.6	110.0	21.00	(275)	(52.6)	(17)	(3.2)
LEAVENINGS								
AIR, see the chapter, THREE FRUGAL REPASTS								
BAKING POWDER, based on generic data								
For home use:								
Sodium aluminum sulfate:								
With monocalcium phosphate monohydrate, 1 teaspoon (approx. 0.1 oz.) (tr/9g/tr/2%/3105mg)	4	0.9	36.1	8.76	224	54.4	14	3.4
With monocalcium phosphate monohydrate and calcium carbonate, 1 teaspoon (approx. 0.1 oz.) (tr/5g/tr/1%/3294mg)	2	0.6	23.2	5.41	144	33.6	9	2.1
With monocalcium phosphate monohydrate and calcium sulfate, 1 teaspoon (approx. 0.1 oz.) (tr/7g/tr/1%/2835mg)	3	0.7	29.7	7.02	176	41.6	11	2.6
Straight phosphate:								
1 teaspoon (approx. 0.13 oz.) (tr/8g/tr/2%/2331mg)	5	1.1	34.0	8.39	240	59.2	15	3.7
Tartrate, Cream of Tartar with tartaric acid:								
1 teaspoon (approx. 0.09 oz.) (tr/5g/tr/1%/2070mg)	2	0.5	20.9	5.37	112	28.8	7	1.8
Special low-sodium preparations:								
Commercial powder, 1 teaspoon (approx. 0.15 oz.) (tr/12g/tr/2%/2mg)	7	1.8	48.3	11.80	368	89.6	23	5.6

	UNIT		1 OZ., BY WT.		1 CUP		1 TABLESPOON	
	Cal.	Carb.	Cal.	Carb.	Cal.	Carb.	Cal.	Carb.
Noncommercial formula (potassium bitartrate [cream of tartar] 42.7%, potassium bicarbonate 30.3%, cornstarch 21.3%, tartaric acid 5.7%), 1 teaspoon (approx. 0.1 oz.) (tr/6g/tr/1%/na)	2	0.6	(18.9)	(5.67)	96	28.8	6	1.8
For commercial use:								
Pyrophosphate:								
No additional leavening acid, 1 oz. (tr/8g/tr/1%/4764mg)	31	7.5	30.9	7.51	(192)	(46.6)	(12)	(2.9)
With monocalcium phosphate monohydrate, 1 oz. (tr/7g/tr/1%/4596mg)	30	7.2	29.8	7.23	(185)	(44.9)	(12)	(2.8)
With monocalcium phosphate monohydrate and calcium lactate, 1 oz. (tr/7g/tr/1%/4521mg)	29	7.1	29.2	7.09	(181)	(44.0)	(11)	(2.7)
BAKING POWDER, by brand								
Baking Powder, **Davis,** 8-oz. can	(250)	0.0	(31.4)	0.00	240	0.0	15	0.0
BAKING SODA, by brand								
Baking Soda, **Arm & Hammer,** 8-oz. box	0	0.0	0.0	0.00	0	0.0	0	0.0
16-oz. (1-lb.) box	0	0.0	0.0	0.00	0	0.0	0	0.0
32-oz. (2-lb.) box	0	0.0	0.0	0.00	0	0.0	0	0.0
CREAM OF TARTAR, based on generic data								
1 teaspoon (approx. 0.1 oz.) (tr/5g/tr/1%/2070mg)	2	0.5	20.9	5.37	112	28.8	7	1.8
YEAST, based on generic data								
For nutritional yeast, see the Weight Loss, Weight Gain, Supplements & Boosters chapter.								
Baker's Compressed yeast, 0.6-oz. package (one piece, approx. 1¼" square, ¾" high) (3g/3g/tr/71%/5mg)	15	2.0	23.6	3.15				
Dry yeast, ¼-oz. package (approx. 1 scant Tbsp.) (10g/11g/tr/5%/15mg)	20	2.7	81.0	10.94	(368)	(49.7)	(23)	(3.1)
YEAST, by brand								
Fleischmann's Active Dry Yeast, 4-oz. jar	320	(48.0)	80.0	12.00	(401)	(49.7)	(25)	(3.1)
Fresh, Active Yeast, 0.6-oz. package	15	2.0	25.0	3.33				
Household Yeast, 2-oz. package	60	8.0	30.0	4.00				
Golden Harvest Patent Yeast, 16-oz. (1-lb.) package	1960	224.0	122.5	14.00	(752)	(85.2)	(47)	(5.3)
Red Star Active Dry Yeast, 0.75-oz. package, 3 envelopes	60	(7.4)	80.0	(9.92)	(401)	(49.7)	(25)	(3.1)
1 envelope, approx. ¼ oz.	20	(2.5)	80.0	(9.92)	(401)	(49.7)	(25)	(3.1)
Consumer Compressed Yeast, ⅝-oz. foil pack	19	(2.2)	30.0	(3.54)				
1-oz. wax pack	30	(3.5)	30.0	(3.54)				
8-oz. wax pack	240	(28.3)	30.0	(3.54)				

EXTRACTS

	UNIT		1 FLUID OZ.		1 CUP		1 TABLESPOON	
	Cal.	Carb.	Cal.	Carb.	Cal.	Carb.	Cal.	Carb.
ALMOND								
Pure Almond Extract, **Durkee,** 1-fl.-oz. bottle	78		78.0		624		39	
1 teaspoon	13		78.0		624		39	
Pure Almond Extract, **Ehlers,** 1-fl.-oz. bottle	72		72.0		576		36	
1 teaspoon	12		72.0		576		36	
Pure Almond Extract, **French's,** 1-fl.-oz. bottle	60		60.0		480		30	
1 teaspoon	10		60.0		480		30	
ANISE								
Imitation Anise Extract, **Durkee,** 1-fl.-oz. bottle	96		96.0		768		48	
1 teaspoon	16		96.0		768		48	
Pure Anise Extract, **Ehlers,** 1-fl.-oz. bottle	158		158.0		1248		79	
1 teaspoon	26		158.0		1248		79	
Pure Anise Extract, **French's,** 1-fl.-oz. bottle	150		150.0		1200		75	
1 teaspoon	25		150.0		1200		75	
BANANA								
Imitation Banana Extract, **Durkee,** 1-fl.-oz. bottle	90		90.0		720		45	
1 teaspoon	15		90.0		720		45	
Imitation Banana Extract, **Ehlers,** 1-fl.-oz. bottle	120		120.0		960		60	
1 teaspoon	20		120.0		960		60	
Imitation Banana Extract, **French's,** 1-fl.-oz. bottle	120		120.0		1200		60	
1 teaspoon	20		120.0		1200		60	
BLACK WALNUT								
Imitation Black Walnut Flavor, **Durkee,** 1-fl.-oz. bottle	24		24.0		192		12	
1 teaspoon	4		24.0		192		12	
Imitation Black Walnut Flavor, **French's,** 1-fl.-oz. bottle	60		60.0		480		30	
1 teaspoon	10		60.0		480		30	
BRANDY								
Imitation Brandy Extract, **Durkee,** 1-fl.-oz. bottle	90		90.0		720		45	
1 teaspoon	15		90.0		720		45	
Pure Brandy Extract, **Ehlers,** 1-fl.-oz. bottle	96		96.0		768		48	
1 teaspoon	16		96.0		768		48	
Pure Brandy Extract, **French's,** 1-fl.-oz. bottle	90		90.0		720		45	
1 teaspoon	15		90.0		720		45	
BUTTER								
Imitation Butter Extract, **Ehlers,** 1-fl.-oz. bottle	48		48.0		384		24	
1 teaspoon	8		48.0		384		24	
Imitation Butter Flavor, **Durkee,** 1-fl.-oz. bottle	18		18.0		144		9	
1 teaspoon	3		18.0		144		9	
Imitation Butter Flavor, **French's,** 1-fl.-oz. bottle	60		60.0		480		30	
1 teaspoon	10		60.0		480		30	
CHERRY								
Imitation Cherry Extract, **Ehlers,** 1-fl.-oz. bottle	96		96.0		768		48	
1 teaspoon	16		96.0		768		48	
Imitation Cherry Extract, **French's,** 1-fl.-oz. bottle	90		90.0		720		45	
1 teaspoon	15		90.0		720		45	
CHOCOLATE								
Imitation Chocolate Extract, **Durkee,** 1-fl.-oz. bottle	42		42.0		336		21	
1 teaspoon	7		42.0		336		21	
Imitation Chocolate Extract, **Ehlers,** 1-fl.-oz. bottle	60		60.0		480		30	
1 teaspoon	10		60.0		480		30	
Imitation Chocolate Flavoring, **French's,** 2-fl.-oz. bottle	120		60.0		480		30	
1 teaspoon	10		60.0		480		30	
COCONUT								
Imitation Coconut Extract, **Ehlers,** 1-fl.-oz. bottle	102		102.0		816		51	
1 teaspoon	17		102.0		816		51	
Imitation Coconut Flavor, **Durkee,** 1-fl.-oz. bottle	48		48.0		384		24	
1 teaspoon	8		48.0		384		24	
Imitation Coconut Flavor, **French's,** 1-fl.-oz. bottle	90		90.0		720		45	
1 teaspoon	15		90.0		720		45	
LEMON								
Imitation Lemon Extract, **Durkee,** 1-fl.-oz. bottle	36		36.0		288		18	
1 teaspoon	6		36.0		288		18	
Pure Lemon Extract, **Ehlers,** 1-fl.-oz. bottle	180		180.0		1440		90	
2-fl.-oz. bottle	360		180.0		1440		90	
1 teaspoon	30		180.0		1440		90	
Pure Lemon Extract, **French's,** 1-fl.-oz. bottle	180		180.0		1440		90	
1 teaspoon	30		180.0		1440		90	
MAPLE								
Imitation Maple Extract, **Durkee,** 1-fl.-oz. bottle	82		82.0		656		41	
1 teaspoon	14		82.0		656		41	
Imitation Maple Extract, **Ehlers,** 1-fl.-oz. bottle	54		54.0		432		27	
1 teaspoon	9		54.0		432		27	
Imitation Maple Flavor, **French's,** 1-fl.-oz. bottle	60		60.0		480		30	
1 teaspoon	10		60.0		480		30	

	UNIT		1 FLUID OZ.		1 CUP		1 TABLE-SPOON	
	Cal.	Carb.	Cal.	Carb.	Cal.	Carb.	Cal.	Carb.
ORANGE								
Imitation Orange Extract, **Durkee,** 1-fl.-oz. bottle	84		84.0		672		42	
1 teaspoon	14		84.0		672		42	
Pure Orange Extract, **Ehlers,** 1-fl.-oz. bottle	180		180.0		1440		90	
1 teaspoon	30		180.0		1440		90	
Pure Orange Extract, **French's,** 1-fl.-oz. bottle	180		180.0		1440		90	
1 teaspoon	30		180.0		1440		90	
PEACH								
Imitation Peach Extract, **French's,** 1-fl.-oz. bottle	150		150.0		1200		75	
1 teaspoon	25		150.0		1200		75	
PEPPERMINT								
Imitation Peppermint Extract, **Durkee,** 1-fl.-oz. bottle	90		90.0		720		45	
1 teaspoon	15		90.0		720		45	
Pure Peppermint Extract, **Ehlers,** 1-fl.-oz. bottle	144		144.0		1152		72	
1 teaspoon	24		144.0		1152		72	
Pure Peppermint Extract, **French's,** 1-fl.-oz. bottle	150		150.0		1200		75	
1 teaspoon	25		150.0		1200		75	
PINEAPPLE								
Imitation Pineapple Extract, **Durkee,** 1-fl.-oz. bottle	36		36.0		288		18	
1 teaspoon	6		36.0		288		18	
Imitation Pineapple Extract, **Ehlers,** 1-fl.-oz. bottle	84		84.0		672		42	
1 teaspoon	14		84.0		672		42	
Imitation Pineapple Extract, **French's,** 1-fl.-oz. bottle	90		90.0		720		45	
1 teaspoon	15		90.0		720		45	
PISTACHIO								
Imitation Pistachio Flavor, **French's,** 1-fl.-oz. bottle	90		90.0		720		45	
1 teaspoon	15		90.0		720		45	
RASPBERRY								
Imitation Raspberry Extract, **Ehlers,** 1-fl.-oz. bottle	84		84.0		672		42	
1 teaspoon	14		84.0		672		42	
Imitation Raspberry Extract, **French's,** 1-fl.-oz. bottle	90		90.0		720		45	
1 teaspoon	15		90.0		720		45	
RUM								
Imitation Rum Extract, **Durkee,** 1-fl.-oz. bottle	84		84.0		672		42	
1 teaspoon	14		84.0		672		42	
Pure Rum Extract, **Ehlers,** 1-fl.-oz. bottle	114		114.0		912		57	
1 teaspoon	19		114.0		912		57	
Pure Rum Flavor, **French's,** 1-fl.-oz. bottle	120		120.0		960		60	
1 teaspoon	20		120.0		960		60	
SHERRY								
Pure Sherry Flavor, **French's,** 1-fl.-oz. bottle	90		90.0		720		45	
1 teaspoon	15		90.0		720		45	
STRAWBERRY								
Imitation Strawberry Extract, **Durkee,** 1-fl.-oz. bottle	72		72.0		576		36	
1 teaspoon	12		72.0		576		36	
Imitation Strawberry Extract, **Ehlers,** 1-fl.-oz. bottle	96		96.0		768		48	
1 teaspoon	16		96.0		768		48	
Imitation Strawberry Extract, **French's,** 1-fl.-oz. bottle	90		90.0		720		45	
1 teaspoon	15		90.0		720		45	
VANILLA								
Imitation Vanilla Extract, **Durkee,** 1-fl.-oz. bottle	18		18.0		144		9	
1 teaspoon	3		18.0		144		9	
Imitation Vanilla, clear, **French's,** 2-fl.-oz. bottle	180		90.0		720		45	
1 teaspoon	15		90.0		720		45	
Pure Vanilla Extract, **Durkee,** 1-fl.-oz. bottle	48		48.0		384		24	
1 teaspoon	8		48.0		384		24	
Pure Vanilla Extract, **Ehlers,** 1-fl.-oz. bottle	78		78.0		624		39	
2-fl.-oz. bottle	156		78.0		624		39	
4-fl.-oz. bottle	312		78.0		624		39	
1 teaspoon	13		78.0		624		39	

	UNIT		1 FLUID OZ.		1 CUP		1 TABLE-SPOON	
	Cal.	Carb.	Cal.	Carb.	Cal.	Carb.	Cal.	Carb.
Pure Vanilla Extract, **French's,** 1-fl.-oz. bottle	60		60.0		480		30	
1 teaspoon	10		60.0		480		30	
WINTERGREEN								
Pure Wintergreen Extract, **French's,** 1-fl.-oz. bottle	150		150.0		1200		75	
2-fl.-oz. bottle	300		150.0		1200		75	
4-fl.-oz. bottle	600		150.0		1200		75	
1 teaspoon	25		150.0		1200		75	

BAKING AND CANDY-MAKING CHOCOLATE

	UNIT		1 OZ., BY WT.		1 CUP		1 TABLE-SPOON	
	Cal.	Carb.	Cal.	Carb.	Cal.	Carb.	Cal.	Carb.
BAKING OR BITTER CHOCOLATE, based on generic data								
1 pound (approx. 3.4 cups grated) (3g/8g/15g/2%/1mg)	2288	131.2	143.0	8.20	667	38.1	42	2.4
Grated, 1 cup (approx. 4.7 oz.)	667	38.1	143.0	8.20	667	38.1	42	2.4
1 tablespoon (approx. 0.3 oz.)	42	2.4	143.0	8.20	667	38.1	42	2.4
BAKING CHOCOLATE, by brand								
Baker's Unsweetened Chocolate, 8-oz. box, 8 squares	1086	68.3	135.8	8.53				
1 pound (approx. 3.4 cups grated, 54.4 Tbsp.)	2173	136.5	135.8	8.53	(632)	(39.7)	(40)	(2.5)
1 square, approx. 1 oz.	136	8.5	135.8	8.53				
Grated, 1 cup (approx. 4.7 oz.)	(632)	(39.7)	135.8	8.53	(632)	(39.7)	(40)	(2.5)
1 tablespoon (approx. 0.3 oz.)	(40)	(2.5)	135.8	8.53	(632)	(39.7)	(40)	(2.5)
Semi-Sweet Chocolate, 8-oz. box, 8 squares	1055	133.1	131.8	16.64				
1 pound (approx. 3.4 cups grated, 54.4 Tbsp.)	2109	266.2	131.8	16.64	(613)	(77.4)	(38)	(4.8)
1 square, approx. 1 oz.	132	16.6	131.8	16.64				
Grated, 1 cup (approx. 4.7 oz.)	(613)	(77.4)	131.8	16.64	(613)	(77.4)	(38)	(4.8)
1 tablespoon (approx. 0.3 oz.)	(38)	(4.8)	131.8	16.64	(613)	(77.4)	(38)	(4.8)
Sweet Chocolate, German's, 4-oz. bar	563	68.7	140.9	17.18				
1 pound (approx. 3.4 cups grated, 54.4 Tbsp.)	2254	274.9	140.9	17.18	(655)	(79.9)	(41)	(5.0)
Grated, 1 cup (approx. 4.7 oz.)	(655)	(79.9)	140.9	17.18	(655)	(79.9)	(41)	(5.0)
1 tablespoon (approx. 0.3 oz.)	(41)	(5.0)	140.9	17.18	(655)	(79.9)	(41)	(5.0)
Hershey's Baking Chocolate, 8-oz. package, 8 blocks	1520	56.0	190.0	7.00				
1 pound, 16 blocks	3040	112.0	190.0	7.00				
1 block, approx. 1 oz.	190	7.0	190.0	7.00				
Nestlé Choco-Bake Pre-Melted Chocolate Flavored Liquid For Baking, 8-oz. box, 8 packets	1360	96.0	170.0	12.00				
1 pound, 16 packets	2720	192.0	170.0	12.00				
1 packet, approx. 1 oz.	170	12.0	170.0	12.00				
CHOCOLATE CHIPS and MORSELS, based on generic data								
Semi-Sweet, 6-oz. package (approx. 360 small pieces)	862	96.9	144.0	16.16	862	96.9	(54)	(6.1)
1 pound (approx. 2.7 cups, 960 pieces)	2304	258.6	144.0	16.16	862	96.9	(54)	(6.1)
1 cup (approx. 6 oz., 360 small pieces)	862	96.9	144.0	16.16	862	96.9	(54)	(6.1)
1 chip or morsel, approx. 0.02 oz.	(2)	0.3	144.0	16.16	862	96.9	(54)	(6.1)
CHOCOLATE CHIPS and MORSELS, by brand								
Baker's Chocolate Flavored Baking Chips, 12-oz. package (approx. 720 chips)	1510	228.2	125.9	19.02	(806)	(121.7)	(50)	(7.6)
1 pound (approx. 2.5 cups, 960 chips)	2014	304.3	125.9	19.02	(806)	(121.7)	(50)	(7.6)
1 cup (approx. 6.4 oz., 380 chips)	(806)	(121.7)	125.9	19.02	(806)	(121.7)	(50)	(7.6)
1 chip (approx. 0.02 oz.)	(2)	(0.3)	125.9	19.02	(806)	(121.7)	(50)	(7.6)

	UNIT		1 OZ., BY WT.		1 CUP		1 TABLE-SPOON	
	Cal.	Carb.	Cal.	Carb.	Cal.	Carb.	Cal.	Carb.
Hershey's Milk Chocolate Chips, 11½-oz. bag (approx. 690 chips)	1725	195.5	150.0	17.00	(900)	(102.0)	(56)	(6.4)
1 pound (approx. 2.7 cups, 960 chips)	2400	272.0	150.0	17.00	(900)	(102.0)	(56)	(6.4)
1 cup (approx. 6 oz., 360 chips)	(900)	(102.0)	150.0	17.00	(900)	(102.0)	(56)	(6.4)
1 chip (approx. 0.02 oz.)	(3)	(0.3)	150.0	17.00	(900)	(102.0)	(56)	(6.4)
Semi-Sweet Chocolate Chips, 6-oz. package	880	104.0	146.5	17.32	880	104.0	(55)	(6.5)
12-oz. package	1758	207.8	146.5	17.32	880	104.0	(55)	(6.5)
1 pound (approx. 2.7 cups)	2344	277.1	146.5	17.32	880	104.0	(55)	(6.5)
1 cup (approx. 6 oz.)	880	104.0	146.5	17.32	880	104.0	(55)	(6.5)
Semi-Sweet Chocolate Mini Chips, 12-oz. package	1758	207.8	146.5	17.32	880	104.0	(55)	(6.5)
1 pound (approx. 2.7 cups)	2344	277.1	146.5	17.32	880	104.0	(55)	(6.5)
1 cup (approx. 6 oz.)	880	104.0	146.5	17.32	880	104.0	(55)	(6.5)
Nestlé "Tollhouse" Semi-Sweet Chocolate Morsels, 6-oz. bag (approx. 360 morsels)	900	108.0	150.0	18.00	(900)	(108.0)	(56)	(6.8)
1 pound (approx. 2.7 cups, 960 morsels)	2400	288.0	150.0	18.00	(900)	(108.0)	(56)	(6.8)
12-oz. bag (approx. 720 morsels)	1800	216.0	150.0	18.00	(900)	(108.0)	(56)	(6.8)
1 cup (approx. 6 oz., 360 morsels)	(900)	(108.0)	150.0	18.00	(900)	(108.0)	(56)	(6.8)
1 morsel (approx. 0.02 oz.)	(3)	(0.3)	150.0	18.00	(900)	(108.0)	(56)	(6.8)
Semi-Sweet Chocolate Morsels with Milk Chocolate Morsels, 11½-oz. bag (approx. 690 morsels)	1725	201.3	150.0	17.50	(900)	(105.0)	(56)	(6.5)
1 pound (approx. 2.7 cups, 960 morsels)	2400	280.0	150.0	17.50	(900)	(105.0)	(56)	(6.5)
1 cup (approx. 6 oz., 360 morsels)	(900)	(105.0)	150.0	17.50	(900)	(105.0)	(56)	(6.5)
1 morsel (approx. 0.02 oz.)	(3)	(0.3)	150.0	17.50	(900)	(105.0)	(56)	(6.5)

BAKING CHIPS and MORSELS OTHER THAN CHOCOLATE

	Cal.	Carb.	Cal.	Carb.	Cal.	Carb.	Cal.	Carb.
Bits O'Peppermint, **Heath,** 1 pound	1996	358.4	124.8	22.40	998	179.2	(62)	(11.2)
Butterscotch Flavored Morsels, **Nestlé,** 6-oz. bag (approx. 360 morsels)	900	114.0	150.0	19.00	900	114.0	(56)	(7.1)
1 pound (approx. 2.7 cups, 960 morsels)	2400	304.0	150.0	19.00	900	114.0	(56)	(7.1)
12-oz. bag (approx. 720 morsels)	1800	228.0	150.0	19.00	900	114.0	(56)	(7.1)
1 cup (approx. 6 oz., 360 morsels)	900	114.9	150.0	19.00	900	114.0	(56)	(7.1)
1 morsel (approx. 0.02 oz.)	(3)	(0.3)	150.0	19.00	900	114.0	(56)	(7.1)
Caramel, **Kraft,** 14-oz. bag (approx. 48 caramels)	1715	294.0	122.5	21.00	980	168.0	(61)	(10.5)
1 pound (approx. 2.7 cups, 55 caramels)	1960	336.0	122.5	21.00	980	168.0	(61)	(10.5)
30-oz. bag (approx. 103 caramels)	3675	630.0	122.5	21.00	980	168.0	(61)	(10.5)
1 cup (approx. 6 oz., 21 caramels)	980	168.0	122.5	21.00	980	168.0	(61)	(10.5)
1 caramel (approx. 0.29 oz.)	36	6.1	122.5	21.00	980	168.0	(61)	(10.5)
Carob Coated Caramels, **Caracoa (El Molino),** sold bulk, 1 pound (approx. 2.9 cups, 73 caramels)	1760	336.0	110.0	21.00	(605)	(155.5)	(38)	(7.2)
1 cup (approx. 5½ oz., 25 caramels)	(605)	(115.5)	110.0	21.00	(605)	(115.5)	(38)	(7.2)
1 caramel (approx. 0.22 oz.)	24	4.6	110.0	21.00	(605)	(115.5)	(38)	(7.2)
Carob Nuggets, **Caracoa (El Molino),** 6-oz. bag	840	120.0	140.0	20.00	882	126.0	(55)	(7.9)
1 pound (approx. 2.5 cups)	2240	320.0	140.0	20.00	882	126.0	(55)	(7.9)
1 cup (approx. 6.3 oz.)	882	126.0	140.0	20.00	882	126.0	(55)	(7.9)
Peanut Butter Flavored Chips, **Reese's,** 12-oz. package	1840	152.0	153.3	12.67	920	76.0	(58)	(4.8)
16-oz. (1-lb.) package (approx. 2.7 cups)	2453	202.7	153.3	12.67	920	76.0	(58)	(4.8)
1 cup (approx. 6 oz.)	920	76.0	153.3	12.67	920	76.0	(58)	(4.8)

COCOA POWDER, based on generic data

See the BEVERAGES chapter for cocoa drinks by brand.

	UNIT		1 OZ., BY WT.		1 CUP		1 TABLE-SPOON	
	Cal.	Carb.	Cal.	Carb.	Cal.	Carb.	Cal.	Carb.
High-Fat or Breakfast Cocoa (23.7% fat)								
Plain:								
1 cup (approx. 3 oz.)	257	41.5	84.8	13.69	257	41.5	16	2.6
1 pound (approx. 5.3 cups) (5g/14g/7g/3%/2mg)	1357	219.0	84.8	13.69	257	41.5	16	2.6
1 tablespoon (approx. 0.2 oz.)	16	2.6	84.8	13.69	257	41.5	16	2.6
Processed with alkali:								
1 cup (approx. 3 oz.)	224	39.0	83.6	12.87	224	39.0	16	2.4
1 pound (approx. 5.3 cups) (5g/13g/7g/3%/203mg)	1338	205.9	83.6	12.87	224	39.0	16	2.4
1 tablespoon (approx. 0.2 oz.)	16	2.4	83.6	12.87	224	39.0	16	2.4
High–Medium-Fat Cocoa (19% fat)								
Plain:								
1 cup (approx. 3 oz.)	228	44.3	75.0	14.60	228	44.3	14	2.8
1 pound (approx. 5.3 cups) (5g/15g/5g/4%/2mg)	1200	233.6	75.0	14.60	228	44.3	14	2.8
1 tablespoon (approx. 0.2 oz.)	14	2.8	75.0	14.60	228	44.3	14	2.8
Processed with alkali:								
1 cup (approx. 3 oz.)	224	41.7	74.0	13.70	224	41.7	14	2.6
1 pound (approx. 5.3 cups) (5g/14g/5g/4%/203mg)	1184	219.2	74.0	13.70	224	41.7	14	2.6
1 tablespoon (approx. 0.2 oz.)	14	2.6	74.0	13.70	224	41.7	14	2.6
Low–Medium-Fat Cocoa (12.7% fat)								
Plain:								
1 cup (approx. 3 oz.)	189	46.3	62.0	15.30	189	46.3	12	2.9
1 pound (approx. 5.3 cups) (5g/15g/4g/5%/2mg)	992	91.8	62.0	15.30	189	46.3	12	2.9
1 tablespoon (approx. 0.2 oz.)	12	2.9	62.0	15.30	189	46.3	12	2.9
Processed with alkali:								
1 cup (approx. 3 oz.)	185	43.2	61.0	14.20	185	43.2	12	2.7
1 pound (approx. 5.3 cups) (5g/14g/4g/5%/203mg)	976	227.2	61.0	14.20	185	43.2	12	2.7
1 tablespoon (approx. 0.2 oz.)	12	2.7	61.0	14.20	185	43.2	12	2.7
Low-Fat Cocoa (7.9% fat)								
1 cup (approx. 5.3 oz.)	160	49.9	53.0	16.44	160	49.9	51	10.5
1 pound (approx. 5.3 cups) (6g/16g/2g/4%/2mg)	848	263.1	53.0	16.44	160	49.9	51	10.5
1 tablespoon (approx. 0.2 oz.)	51	10.5	53.0	16.44	160	49.9	51	10.5

CHOCOLATE-FLAVORED SYRUPS AND TOPPINGS, based on generic data

See the SUGARS, SWEETENERS & TOPPINGS chapters for listings by brand.

	Cal.	Carb.	Cal.	Carb.	Cal.	Carb.	Cal.	Carb.
"THIN" SYRUP, CHOCOLATE FLAVORED								
1 can, 12 fl. oz. (approx. 1 lb.) (1g/18g/1g/32%/17mg)	1111	284.4	69.4	17.78	735	188.1	46	11.8
1 cup (approx. 10.6 oz.)	735	188.1	69.4	17.78	735	188.1	46	11.8
1 fl. oz. (approx. 1.3 oz.)	92	23.5	69.4	17.78	735	188.1	46	11.8
"THICK," FUDGE TYPE								
1 can, 12 fl. oz. (approx. 1 lb.) (2g/15g/5g/25%/30mg)	1497	244.9	93.6	15.31	990	162.0	62	10.1
1 cup (approx. 10.6 oz.)	990	162.0	93.6	15.31	990	162.0	62	10.1
1 fl. oz. (approx. 1.3 oz.)	124	20.3	93.6	15.31	990	162.0	62	10.1

COOKING WINES

Other alcoholic beverages used in cooking, such as rum, brandy, etc., can be found in the ALCOHOLIC BEVERAGES chapter.

	Cal.	Carb.	Cal.	Carb.	Cal.	Carb.	Cal.	Carb.
Cooking Burgundy, **Regina,** 12-fl.-oz. bottle (figures apply to wine after the alcohol evaporates in cooking)	12	2.7	(1.0)	(0.22)	8	1.8	1	0.1

	UNIT		1 OZ., BY WT.		1 CUP		1 TABLESPOON	
	Cal.	Carb.	Cal.	Carb.	Cal.	Carb.	Cal.	Carb.
Cooking Sherry, **Regina,** 12-fl.-oz. bottle (figures apply to wine after the alcohol evaporates in cooking)	114	28.3	(9.5)	(2.36)	76	18.9	5	1.2
Cooking Wine, **China Bowl,** 10-fl.-oz. bottle	320	9.1	(30.8)	(0.87)	256	7.3	16	0.5
Sauterne Cooking Wine, **Regina,** 12-fl.-oz. bottle (figures apply to wine after the alcohol evaporates in cooking)	12	2.7	(1.0)	(0.22)	8	1.8	1	0.1
Vermouth Cooking Wine, **Holland House,** 16-fl.-oz. (1-pint) bottle	488	19.2	(27.0)	(1.16)	224	9.6	14	0.6
¾ liter (25 fl. oz.)	717	30.7	(27.0)	(1.16)	224	9.6	14	0.6

MARINADES and TENDERIZERS

	UNIT		1 OZ., BY WT.		1 CUP		1 TABLESPOON	
	Cal.	Carb.	Cal.	Carb.	Cal.	Carb.	Cal.	Carb.
Marinade for Chicken, **Adolph's,** 0.8-oz. package	51	10.8	64.2	13.51	485	102.1	26	5.5
Marinade for Meat, **Adolph's,** 0.8-oz. package	32	7.3	40.5	9.07	376	84.2	24	5.3
Marinade for Meat, Dry Mix. **Durkee,** 1-oz. package	47	9.0	47.0	9.00				
Prepared with ¼ cup water and 2 Tbsp. vinegar, yield: approx. ½ cup (approx. 4 oz.)	51	9.0	12.8	2.25	102	18.0	6	1.1
Marinade Mix for Meat, **French's,** 1-oz. package	80	16.0	80.0	1.00				
Meat Tenderizer, Unseasoned, **Adolph's,** 3½-oz. package	37	8.8	10.6	2.51	88	20.9	5	1.2
Meat Tenderizer, Seasoned, **Adolph's,** 3½-oz. package	14	2.9	4.1	0.84	32	6.5	2	0.4
Meat Tenderizer, **French's,** 3½-oz. jar	40	trace	11.3	trace	96	trace	6	trace
6¼-oz. jar	71	trace	11.3	trace	96	trace	6	trace
Meat Tenderizer, Seasoned, **French's,** 3½-oz. jar	40	trace	11.3	trace	96	trace	6	trace

SEASONING MIXES

Values are given for seasonings as they are packaged. Calculations do not include the meat, chicken, etc. to which the seasonings are added.

	UNIT		1 OZ., BY WT.		1 CUP		1 TABLESPOON	
	Cal.	Carb.	Cal.	Carb.	Cal.	Carb.	Cal.	Carb.
Barbecue Seasoning, **French's,** 1¾-oz. jar	119	19.9	68.0	11.34				
Beef Stew Seasoning Mix, **Durkee,** 1¾-oz. package	99	22.0	56.6	12.57				
Beef Stew Seasoning Mix, **French's,** 1⅞-oz. package	150	30.0	80.0	16.00				
Chili Con Carne Seasoning Mix, **Durkee,** 1¾-oz. package	148	33.0	84.6	18.86				
Chili-O Mexican Seasoning Mix, **French's,** 1¾-oz. package	150	30.0	85.7	17.14				
Chop Suey Seasoning Mix, **Durkee,** 1½-oz. package	128	19.5	85.3	12.67				
Egg Seasoning Mixes, **Durkee** *(these dry seasoned egg mixes are dehydrated eggs with seasoning that the consumer reconstitutes with water. They have a rehydration yield of 2 eggs.*								
Scrambled Egg, 0.83-oz. package	124	4.0	148.9	4.80				
Scrambled Egg with Bacon, **Durkee,** 1¼-oz. package	181	6.0	144.8	4.80				
Western Omelet, 1¼-oz. package	170	9.0	136.0	7.20				
Enchilada Sauce Seasoning Mix, **Durkee,** 1.1-oz. package	89	18.0	79.1	16.00				
Enchilada Seasoning Mexican Seasoning Mix, **French's,** 1⅜-oz. package	120	20.0	87.3	14.55				
Ground Beef Seasoning Mix, **Durkee,** 1.1-oz. package	91	18.0	80.9	16.00				
Ground Beef with Onion Seasoning Mix, **Durkee,** 1.1-oz. package	102	13.0	90.9	11.59				
Ground Beef Seasoning with Onion Mix, **French's,** 1⅛-oz, package	100	24.0	88.9	21.34				
Hamburger Seasoning Mix, **Durkee,** 1-oz. package	110	15.0	110.0	15.00				
Hamburger Seasoning Mix, **French's,** 1-oz. package	100	20.0	100.0	20.00				
Italian Meatball Seasoning Mix, **Durkee,** 1-oz. package	22	9.0	22.0	9.00				
Italian Meatball With Cheese Seasoning Mix, **Durkee,** 1-oz. package	85	9.0	85.0	9.00				
Lemon & Pepper Seasoning, **French's,** 2½-oz. jar	118	19.7	47.3	7.88				
Meatball Seasoning Mix, **French's,** 1½-oz. package	140	28.0	93.3	18.67				
Meatloaf Seasoning Mix, **French's,** 1½-oz. package	160	40.0	106.7	26.67				
Omelet Seasoning Mixes, **Durkee** *(these do not contain dehydrated egg, but are meant to be added to fresh eggs in order to make seasoned omelets):*								
Bacon Seasoned Omelet Mix, 1¼-oz. package	128	18.0	102.4	14.40				
Cheese Seasoned Omelet Mix, 1¼-oz. package	125	12.0	100.0	9.60				
Puffy Seasoned Omelet Mix, 1¼-oz. package	112	19.0	89.6	15.20				
Western Seasoned Omelet Mix, 1¼-oz. package	110	20.0	88.0	16.00				
Pizza Seasoning, **French's,** 2½-oz. jar	79	19.7	31.5	7.88				
Pizza Sprinkles, **Scotch Buy,** 8-oz. package	720	8.0	90.0	1.00				
Seafood Seasoning, **French's,** 3½-oz. jar	40		11.3					
Seasoning for Sloppy Hot Dogs, **French's,** 1½-oz. package	160	28.0	106.7	18.67				
Sloppy Joe Seasoning Mix, **French's,** 1½-oz. package	128	32.0	85.3	21.33				
Taco Seasoning Mexican Seasoning Mix, **French's,** 1¼-oz. package	120	24.0	96.0	19.20				

SAUCES and GRAVIES

Many other SAUCES can be found in the CONDIMENTS chapter.

	UNIT		1 OZ., BY WT.		1 CUP		1 TABLESPOON	
	Cal.	Carb.	Cal.	Carb.	Cal.	Carb.	Cal.	Carb.
SAUCES AND GRAVIES, Ready-to-Serve, based on generic data								
Au Jus Gravy, 10½ oz. can	48	7.5	4.5	0.71	38	6.0	2	0.4
Barbecue Sauce, 16-fl.-oz. (1-pint) bottle	341	58.1	21.3	3.63	188	32.0	12	2.0
Beef Gravy, 10¼-oz. can	155	14.0	15.0	1.36	124	11.2	8	0.7
Chicken Gravy, 10½ oz. can	236	16.2	22.4	1.54	189	13.0	12	0.8
Chili Sauce, 1 cup (approx. 8.7 oz.) (tr/1g/tr/94%/na)	50	12.4	5.7	1.42	50	12.4	3	0.8
Mushroom Gravy, 10½-oz. can	150	16.3	14.2	1.55	120	13.0	8	0.8
Soy Sauce, 1 cup, 10.2 oz. (2g/3g/tr/63%/2077mg)	197	27.6	19.3	2.69	197	27.6	12	1.7
Spaghetti Sauce, made-from-scratch, 1 cup, 8.7 oz., based on USDA home recipe (4g/2g/1g/87%/416mg)	(155)	(14.3)	(17.7)	(1.64)	(155)	(14.3)	(10)	(0.9)
Tehineh (Tahini) (based on data from Middle East), 1 pound (6g/3g/18g/3%/na)	3139	46.3	196.2	2.89				
Teriyaki Sauce, 1 cup	(240)	(45.9)	23.8	4.52	(240)	(45.9)	(15)	(2.9)
Turkey Gravy, 10½ oz. can	152	15.2	14.5	1.45	122	12.2	8	0.8
White Sauce, made-from-scratch, based on USDA home recipes:								
Thin: with ingredients as follows: 1 cup whole milk, 1 Tbsp. flour, 1 Tbsp. table fat, ¼ tsp. salt (yield: approx. 1 cup, approx. 8.8 oz.) (1g/2g/2g/79%/100mg)	303	18.0	34.3	2.04	303	18.0	19	1.1
Medium: with ingredients as follows: 1 cup whole milk, 2 Tbsp. flour, 2 Tbsp. table fat, ¼ tsp. salt (yield: approx. 1 cup, approx. 8.8 oz.) (1g/2g/4g/73%/107mg)	405	22.0	46.0	2.50	405	22.0	25	1.4
Thick: with ingredients as follows: 1 cup whole milk, 3½ Tbsp. flour, 3 Tbsp. table fat, ¼ tsp. salt (yield: approx. 1 cup, approx. 8.8 oz.) (1g/3g/4g/68%/113mg)	495	27.5	56.3	3.13	495	27.5	31	1.7

	UNIT		1 OZ., BY WT.		1 CUP		1 TABLESPOON	
	Cal.	Carb.	Cal.	Carb.	Cal.	Carb.	Cal.	Carb.
SAUCES AND GRAVIES, Ready-to-Serve, by brand								
Barbeque Sauce, **Chris & Pitts,** 14-fl.-oz. bottle	330	88.0	23.6	6.29	240	64.0	15	4.0
Barbeque Sauce, **French's,** 18-fl.-oz. bottle	419	90.0	23.3	5.00	224	48.0	14	3.0
Barbecue Sauce, **Kraft,** 18-fl.-oz. bottle	696	139.2	38.7	7.73	368	72.0	23	4.5
28-fl.-oz. bottle	1082	216.5	38.7	7.73	368	72.0	23	4.5
Barbeque Sauce, Hickory Smoke Flavor, **Open Pit,** 18-fl.-oz. bottle	474	109.7	26.4	6.10	256	64.0	16	4.0
Barbeque Sauce, Hot, **French's,** 18-fl.-oz. bottle	419	90.0	23.3	5.00	224	48.0	14	3.0
Barbeque Sauce, "Liquid Smoke For Barbeque," **Liquid Smoke,** 4-fl.-oz. bottle	38	28.3	(9.6)	(7.07)	77	56.6	5	3.5
Barbeque Sauce, Original Flavor, **Open Pit,** 18-fl.-oz. bottle	464	107.6	25.8	5.98	256	64.0	16	4.0
Barbeque Sauce, Original Flavor with Onions, **Open Pit,** 18-fl.-oz. bottle	489	113.2	27.2	6.29	288	64.0	18	4.0
Beef Gravy, **Franco-American,** 10¼-oz. can	154	15.4	15.0	1.50	(123)	(12.3)	(8)	(0.8)
Beef Microwave Browning Sauce, **Holland House,** 7.5-oz. can	423	89.3	56.4	11.91				
Brown Gravy, **La Choy,** 5-oz. can	416	101.2	83.1	20.23	(727)	(177.1)	(45)	(11.1)
Brown Gravy with Mushroom Broth, **Dawn Fresh,** 5¾-oz. can	51	9.1	8.8	1.58	80	16.0	5	1.0
Brown Gravy with Onion, **Franco-American,** 10½-oz. can	131	21.0	12.5	2.00	(105)	(16.8)	(7)	(1.1)
Chicken Gravy, **Franco-American,** 10½-oz. can	263	15.8	25.0	1.50	(210)	(12.6)	(13)	(0.8)
Chicken, Gravy Mix for, **Weaver,** prepared as package directs (yield: 1 cup approx. 9¼ oz.)	(120)	(12.2)	(13.0)	(1.32)	(120)	(12.2)	(8)	(0.8)
Chicken Microwave Browning Sauce, **Holland House,** 7.5-fl.-oz. jar	443	95.7	63.3	12.76				
Clam Juice, **Doxsee,** 8-fl.-oz. bottle	20	4.0	(2.5)	(0.50)	20	4.0	1	0.3
1 teaspoon (approx. 0.2 oz.)	trace	trace	(2.5)	(0.50)	20	4.0	1	0.3
Clam Sauce, Red, **Buitoni,** 10¼-oz. can	267	3.5	26.0	0.34	(227)	(3.0)	(14)	(0.2)
Clam Sauce, White, **Buitoni,** 10¼-oz. can	359	5.5	35.0	0.54	(306)	(4.7)	(19)	(0.3)
Famous Sauce, **Durkee,** 6½-oz. bottle	828	26.4	127.4	4.06	1104	35.2	69	2.2
Fish Sauce, **China Bowl,** 6-oz. bottle	87	1.9	14.5	0.31	(120)	(2.6)	(8)	(0.2)
Gravy Master Seasoning and Browning Sauce, **Gravy Master,** 2-fl.-oz. bottle	111	21.8	55.3	10.88	588	115.2	37	7.2
5-fl.-oz. bottle	277	54.4	55.3	10.88	588	115.2	37	7.2
Green Chile Salsa, **Ortega,** 7-oz. can	42	7.0	6.0	1.00	(5.8)	(9.6)	(4)	(0.6)
12-oz. jar	42	7.0	6.0	1.00	(5.8)	(9.6)	(4)	(0.6)
28-oz. can	42	7.0	6.0	1.00	(5.8)	(9.6)	(4)	(0.6)
Italian Cooking Sauce, **Contadina,** 15-oz. can (13.5-fl. oz.)	291	49.8	19.4	3.32	172	29.5	11	1.8
Italian Cooking Sauce, Delicate Wine, **Ragu,** 16-oz. (1-lb.) jar	308	76.7	19.3	4.98	173	44.8	11	2.8
21-oz. jar	404	104.6	19.3	4.98	173	44.8	11	2.8
Italian Cooking Sauce, Mild Herbs, **Ragu,** 16-oz. (1-lb.) jar	238	81.4	14.9	5.09	134	46.0	8	2.9
21-oz. jar	312	106.7	14.9	5.09	134	46.0	8	2.9
Italian Cooking Sauce, Savory Peppers, **Ragu,** 16-oz. (1-lb.) jar	205	54.2	12.8	3.39	114	30.1	7	1.9
21-oz. jar	270	71.2	12.8	3.39	114	30.1	7	1.9
Italian Cooking Sauce, Traditional, **Ragu,** 16-oz. (1-lb.) jar	192	76.2	12.0	4.76	104	41.4	7	2.6
21-oz. jar	251	100.0	12.0	4.76	104	41.4	7	2.6
Marinara Sauce, **Buitoni,** 10¼-oz. can	174	20.3	17.0	1.98	(149)	(17.3)	(9)	(1.1)
15-oz. jar	255	29.7	17.0	1.98	(149)	(17.3)	(9)	(1.1)
29-oz. jar	493	57.4	17.0	1.98	(149)	(17.3)	(9)	(1.1)
Marinara Sauce, Lite 'n' Natural, **Ronzoni,** 15-oz. jar	169	26.3	11.3	1.75	(98)	(15.3)	(6)	(1.0)
Meatless Sauce, **Buitoni,** 10¼-oz. can	195	24.4	19.0	2.38	(166)	(20.8)	(10)	(1.3)
15-oz. jar	285	35.7	19.0	2.38	(166)	(20.8)	(10)	(1.3)
29-oz. jar	551	69.0	19.0	2.38	(166)	(20.8)	(10)	(1.3)
Meatless Sauce, All-Purpose, Lite 'n' Natural, **Ronzoni,** 15-oz. jar	169	26.3	11.3	1.75	(98)	(15.3)	(6)	(1.0)
Mushroom Gravy, **Franco-American,** 10½-oz. can	184	21.0	17.5	2.00	(147)	(16.8)	(9)	(1.1)
Mushroom Sauce, **Buitoni,** 10¼-oz. can	174	19.5	17.0	1.90	(149)	(16.6)	(9)	(1.0)
15-oz. jar	255	28.5	17.0	1.90	(149)	(16.6)	(9)	(1.0)
29-oz. jar	493	55.1	17.0	1.90	(149)	(16.6)	(9)	(1.0)
Mushroom Steak Sauce, **Dawn Fresh,** 5¾-oz. can	51	10.1	8.8	1.76	72	16.0	5	1.0
10½-oz. can	92	18.5	8.8	1.76	72	16.0	5	1.0
Oyster Sauce, **China Bowl,** 10-oz. bottle	256	39.7	32.0	4.96	(256)	(39.7)	(16)	(2.5)
Picante Sauce, **Picante,** 16-oz. (1-lb.) jar	180	30.0	11.3	1.88	96	16.0	6	1.0
Pizza Sauce, **Buitoni,** 10¼-oz. jar	195	25.6	19.0	2.50	(166)	(21.9)	(10)	(1.4)
15-oz. jar	285	37.5	19.0	2.50	(166)	(21.9)	(10)	(1.4)
Pizza Sauce, **Contadina,** 8-oz. jar	140	23.0	17.5	2.88	(153)	(25.2)	(10)	(1.6)
15-oz. jar	263	43.2	17.5	2.88	(153)	(25.2)	(10)	(1.6)
Pizza Topping, Appian Way **Armour,** 6-oz.	100	11.0	16.7	1.83	(146)	(16.0)	(9)	(1.0)
Pork Microwave Browning Sauce, **Holland House,** 7.5 oz. jar	504	117.0	67.2	15.59				
Soy Sauce, **La Choy,** 5-oz. bottle	83	9.1	16.6	1.81	(170)	(18.5)	(11)	(1.2)
10-oz. bottle	166	18.1	16.6	1.81	(170)	(18.5)	(11)	(1.2)
16-oz. (1-lb.) bottle	266	29.0	16.6	1.81	(170)	(18.5)	(11)	(1.2)
Soy Sauce, Dark, **China Bowl,** 5-oz. bottle	122	21.4	24.4	4.28	(249)	(43.8)	(16)	(2.7)
12-oz. bottle	293	51.4	24.4	4.28	(249)	(43.8)	(16)	(2.7)
Soy Sauce, Light, **China Bowl,** 5-oz. bottle	78	11.5	15.6	2.30	(160)	(23.5)	(10)	(1.5)
12-oz. bottle	187	27.6	15.6	2.30	(160)	(23.5)	(10)	(1.5)
Soy Sauce, Tamari, **Arrowhead Mills,** 16-fl.-oz. (1-pint) bottle	480	64.0	(30.0)	(4.00)	240	32.0	15	2.0
Spaghetti Sauce, **Town House,** 32-oz. (2-lb.) jar	520	104.0	16.3	3.25	141	28.2	9	1.8
Spaghetti Sauce, Extra Cheese, Old World Style, **Ragu,** 15½-oz.	310	42.6	20.0	2.75	169	23.2	11	1.5
32-oz. (2-lb.) jar	640	88.0	20.0	2.75	169	23.2	11	1.5
48-oz. (3-lb.) jar	960	132.0	20.0	2.75	169	23.2	11	1.5
Spaghetti Sauce, Extra Garlic, Old World Style, **Ragu,** 15½-oz. jar	310	42.6	20.0	2.75	169	23.2	11	1.5
32-oz. (2-lb.) jar	640	88.0	20.0	2.75	169	23.2	11	1.5
48-oz. (3-lb.) jar	960	132.0	20.0	2.75	169	23.2	11	1.5
Spaghetti Sauce, Extra Tomatoes, Garlic, and Onions, Chunky Gardenstyle, **Ragu,** 15½-oz. jar	310	54.3	20.0	3.50	172	30.1	11	1.9
32-oz. (2-lb.) jar	640	112.0	20.0	3.50	172	30.1	11	1.9
48-oz. (3-lb.) jar	960	168.0	20.0	3.50	172	30.1	11	1.9
Spaghetti Sauce, Green Pepper and Mushrooms, Chunky Gardenstyle, **Ragu,** 15½-oz. jar	310	54.3	20.0	3.50	172	30.1	11	1.9
32-oz. (2-lb.) jar	640	112.0	20.0	3.50	172	30.1	11	1.9
48-oz. (3-lb.) jar	960	168.0	20.0	3.50	172	30.1	11	1.9
Spaghetti Sauce, Italian Garden Combo, Chunky Gardenstyle, **Ragu,** 15½-oz. jar	310	54.3	20.0	3.50	172	30.1	11	1.9
32-oz. (2-lb.) jar	640	112.0	20.0	3.50	172	30.1	11	1.9
48-oz. (3-lb.) jar	960	168.0	20.0	3.50	172	30.1	11	1.9
Spaghetti Sauce flavored with Italian Sausage, Lite 'n' Natural, **Ronzoni,** 15-oz. jar	188	26.3	12.5	1.75	(109)	(15.3)	(7)	(1.0)
Spaghetti Sauce, Low Sodium, **Featherweight,** 14½-oz. jar	232	29.0	16.0	2.00	(140)	(17.5)	(9)	(1.1)
Spaghetti Sauce, Marinara, **Ann Page (A&P)** 32-oz. (2-lb.) jar	560	104.0	17.5	3.25	(153)	(28.4)	(10)	(1.8)
Spaghetti Sauce, Marinara, Old World Style, **Ragu,** 15½-oz. jar	349	46.5	22.5	3.00	190	26.2	12	1.6
32-oz. (2-lb.) jar	720	96.0	22.5	3.00	190	26.2	12	1.6
48-oz. (3-lb.) jar	1080	144.0	22.5	3.00	190	26.2	12	1.6
Spaghetti Sauce flavored with Meat, **Ann Page (A&P),** 32-oz. (2-lb.) jar	640	96.0	20.0	3.00	(175)	(26.2)	(11)	(1.6)

	UNIT		1 OZ., BY WT.		1 CUP		1 TABLESPOON	
	Cal.	Carb.	Cal.	Carb.	Cal.	Carb.	Cal.	Carb.
Spaghetti Sauce, Meat, Extra Thick and Zesty, **Ragu,** 15½-oz. jar	388	54.3	25.0	3.50	235	33.0	15	2.1
32-oz. (2-lb.) jar	800	112.0	25.0	3.50	235	33.0	15	2.1
48-oz. (3-lb.) jar	1200	168.0	25.0	3.50	235	33.0	15	2.1
Spaghetti Sauce, Meat, Homestyle, **Ragu,** 15½-oz. jar	310	46.5	20.0	3.00	169	25.4	11	1.6
32-oz. (2-lb.) jar	640	96.0	20.0	3.00	169	25.4	11	1.6
48-oz. (3-lb.) jar	960	144.0	20.0	3.00	169	25.4	11	1.6
Spaghetti Sauce, Meat, Old World Style, **Ragu,** 15½-oz. jar	310	42.6	20.0	2.75	169	23.2	11	1.6
32-oz. (2-lb.) jar	640	88.0	20.0	2.75	169	23.2	11	1.6
48-oz. (3-lb.) jar	960	132.0	20.0	2.75	169	23.2	11	1.6
Spaghetti Sauce flavored with Meat, Lite 'n' Natural, **Ronzoni,** 15-oz. jar	188	26.3	12.5	1.75	(109)	(15.3)	(7)	(1.0)
Spaghetti Sauce, Meat Flavored, **Town House,** 32-oz. (2-lb.) jar	590	103.3	18.4	3.23	160	28.0	10	1.8
Spaghetti Sauce, Meatless, No Mushrooms, "Plain" Spaghetti Sauce, **Ann Page (A&P),** 32-oz. (2-lb.) jar	560	104.0	17.5	3.25	(153)	(28.4)	(10)	(1.8)
Spaghetti Sauce, Meatless, with Mushrooms, **Ann Page (A&P),** 32-oz. (2-lb.) jar	560	104.0	17.5	3.25	(153)	(28.4)	(10)	(1.8)
Spaghetti Sauce, Mushroom, Extra Thick and Zesty, **Ragu,** 15½-oz. jar	426	50.4	27.5	3.25	258	30.6	16	1.9
32-oz. (2-lb.) jar	880	104.0	27.5	3.25	258	30.6	16	1.9
48-oz. (3-lb.) jar	1320	156.0	27.5	3.25	258	30.6	16	1.9
Spaghetti Sauce, Mushroom, Homestyle **Ragu,** 15½-oz. jar	271	46.5	17.5	3.00	148	25.4	9	1.6
32-oz. (2-lb.) jar	560	96.0	17.5	3.00	148	25.4	9	1.6
48-oz. (3-lb.) jar	840	144.0	17.5	3.00	148	25.4	9	1.6
Spaghetti Sauce, Mushroom, Old World Style, **Ragu,** 15½-oz. jar	349	34.9	22.5	2.25	190	20.3	12	1.3
32-oz. (2-lb.) jar	720	72.0	22.5	2.25	190	20.3	12	1.3
48-oz. (3-lb.) jar	1080	108.0	22.5	2.25	190	20.3	12	1.3
Spaghetti Sauce with Mushrooms, **Town House,** 32-oz. (2-lb.) jar	590	103.3	18.4	3.23	160	28.0	10	1.8
Spaghetti Sauce, Mushrooms and Onions, Chunky Gardenstyle, **Ragu,** 15½-oz. jar	310	54.3	20.0	3.50	172	30.1	11	1.9
32-oz. (2-lb.) jar	640	112.0	20.0	3.50	172	30.1	11	1.9
48-oz. (3-lb.) jar	960	168.0	20.0	3.50	172	30.1	11	1.9
Spaghetti Sauce, Plain, Extra Thick and Zesty, **Ragu,** 15½-oz. jar	388	58.1	25.0	3.75	235	35.3	15	2.2
32-oz. (2-lb.) jar	800	120.0	25.0	3.75	235	35.3	15	2.2
48-oz. (3-lb.) jar	1200	180.0	25.0	3.75	235	35.3	15	2.2
Spaghetti Sauce, Plain, Homestyle, **Ragu,** 15½-oz. jar	271	46.5	17.5	3.00	148	26.2	9	1.6
32-oz. (2-lb.) jar	560	96.0	17.5	3.00	148	26.2	9	1.6
48-oz. (3-lb.) jar	840	144.0	17.5	3.00	148	26.2	9	1.6
Spaghetti Sauce, Plain, Old World Style, **Ragu,** 15½-oz. jar	310	42.6	20.0	2.75	169	23.2	11	1.5
32-oz. (2-lb.) jar	640	88.0	20.0	2.75	169	23.2	11	1.5
48-oz. (3-lb.) jar	960	132.0	20.0	2.75	169	23.2	11	1.5
Spaghetti Sauce, Sweet Green and Red Peppers, Chunky Gardenstyle, **Ragu,** 15½-oz. jar	310	54.3	20.0	3.50	172	30.1	11	1.9
32-oz. (2-lb.) jar	640	112.0	20.0	3.50	172	30.1	11	1.9
48-oz. (3-lb.) jar	960	168.0	20.0	3.50	172	30.1	11	1.9
Sweet and Sour Sauce, **La Choy,** 10-oz. can	514	125.7	51.4	12.57	(450)	(110.0)	(28)	(6.9)
Sweet 'N Sour Cookbook Sauce, **Contadina,** 16-oz. (1-lb.) can	545	111.1	34.1	6.95	316	64.4	20	4.0
Swiss Steak Cookbook Sauce, **Contadina,** 15-oz. can	(180)	(37.5)	(11.2)	(2.33)	96	20.0	6	1.3
Tabasco Pepper Sauce, **Tabasco,** 2-fl.-oz. bottle	7	0.7	3.1	0.31	26	2.7	2	0.2
12-fl.-oz. bottle	40	4.0	3.1	0.31	26	2.7	2	0.2
Taco Sauce, Hot, **Ortega,** 8-fl.-oz. bottle	352	80.0	36.7	8.34	352	80.0	22	5.0
Taco Sauce, Regular, **Ortega,** 8-fl.-oz. bottle	352	80.0	36.7	8.34	352	80.0	22	5.0
Tomato Paste, Fancy California, **Town House,** 6-oz. can	150	35.0	25.0	5.83	225	52.5	14	3.3

	UNIT		1 OZ., BY WT.		1 CUP		1 TABLESPOON	
	Cal.	Carb.	Cal.	Carb.	Cal.	Carb.	Cal.	Carb.
Tomato Sauce, **Contadina,** 8-oz. jar	82	17.4	10.3	2.17	90	19.0	6	1.2
15-oz. jar	155	32.6	10.3	2.17	90	19.0	6	1.2
Tomato Sauce, **Del Monte,** 8-oz. can	80	17.0	10.0	2.13	80	17.0	5	1.1
15-oz. can	150	31.9	10.0	2.13	80	17.0	5	1.1
Tomato Sauce, **Stokely,** 8-oz. can	65	12.0	8.1	1.50	70	13.0	4	0.8
15-oz. can	122	22.5	8.1	1.50	70	13.0	4	0.8
Tomato Sauce with Mushrooms, **Del Monte,** 8-oz. can	100	22.0	12.5	2.75	100	22.0	6	1.4
Tomato Sauce with Onion, **Del Monte,** 8-oz. can	100	23.0	12.5	2.88	100	23.0	6	1.4
Tomato Sauce, Spanish Style, **Ann Page (A&P),** 8-oz. can	74	16.8	9.3	2.10	80	18.0	5	1.1
15-oz. can	140	31.5	9.3	2.10	80	18.0	5	1.1
Tomato Sauce, Spanish Style, **Town House,** 8-oz. can	80	18.0	10.0	2.25	(84)	(18.8)	(5)	(1.2)
Tomato Sauce with Tidbits, **Del Monte,** 15-oz. can	150	35.6	10.0	2.38	80	19.0	5	1.2
Welsh Rare-Bit Cheese Sauce, **Snow's,** 10½-oz. jar	450	40.0	42.9	3.81	360	32.0	23	2.0
Worcestershire Sauce, Regular, **French's,** 5-oz. bottle	89	17.7	17.7	3.54	160	32.0	10	2.0
Worcestershire Sauce, Smoky, **French's,** 5-oz. bottle	89	17.7	17.7	3.54	160	32.0	10	2.0
SAUCES AND GRAVIES, DEHYDRATED, based on generic data								
Au Jus Gravy, 0.8-oz. package	79	9.9	94.1	11.79				
Prepared with 2½ cups water (yield: approx. 2½ cups)	48	6.0	2.3	0.28	19	2.0	1	0.1
Bearnaise Sauce, 0.9-oz. package	90	14.8	102.6	16.94				
Prepared with 1½ cups milk and butter (yield: approx. 1½ cups)	1052	26.3	78.0	1.95	701	17.5	44	1.1
Brown Gravy, 0.9-oz. package	85	14.8	97.0	16.92				
Prepared with 9½ cups water (yield: approx. 9½ cups)	85	14.8	0.9	0.16	9	1.5	1	0.1
Cheese Sauce, 1.25-oz. package	158	11.9	127.0	9.54				
Prepared with 1 cup milk (yield: approx. 1 cup)	307	23.2	31.2	2.36	307	23.2	19	1.5
Chicken Gravy, 0.8-oz. package	83	14.3	102.4	17.60				
Prepared with 1 cup water (yield: approx. 1 cup)	83	14.3	9.1	1.57	83	14.3	5	0.9
Curry Sauce, 1.25-oz. package	151	17.9	121.1	14.35				
Prepared with 1¼ cups milk (yield: approx. 1¼ cups)	337	32.2	28.1	2.68	270	25.7	17	1.6
Hollandaise Sauce with Butterfat, 1.2-oz. package	187	10.8	157.1	9.10				
Prepared with ¾ cups water (yield: approx. ¾ cup)	187	10.8	26.1	1.51	237	13.8	15	0.9
Hollandaise Sauce with Vegetable Oil, 0.9-oz. package	93	15.5	106.0	17.71				
Prepared with 1½ cups milk & butter (yield: approx. 1½ cups)	1055	26.9	78.3	2.00	703	18.0	44	1.1
Mushroom Gravy, 0.75-oz. package	70	13.8	93.0	18.33				
Prepared with 1 cup water (yield: approx. 1 cup)	70	13.8	7.7	1.51	70	13.8	8	1.7
Mushroom Sauce, 1-oz. package	99	15.5	99.0	15.51				
Prepared with 1¼ cups milk (yield: approx. 1¼ cups)	285	29.7	24.1	2.53	228	23.8	14	1.5
Onion Gravy, 0.85-oz. package	80	16.8	91.3	19.18				
Prepared with 1 cup water (yield: approx. 1.2 cup)	80	16.8	8.8	1.82	80	16.8	10	2.0
Pork Gravy, 0.75-oz. package	76	13.4	101.5	17.86				
Prepared with 1 cup water (yield: approx. 1.2 cup)	76	13.4	8.5	1.47	76	13.4	9	1.6
Sour Cream Sauce, 1.25-oz. package	180	17.0	145.2	13.70				
Prepared with ½ cup milk (yield: approx. ½ cup)	255	22.7	45.9	4.09	509	45.4	32	2.8
Spaghetti Sauce, 1.5-oz. package	118	27.0	79.7	18.22				
Spaghetti Sauce with Mushrooms, 1.4-oz. package	118	19.1	86.2	13.89				
Stroganoff Sauce, 1.6-oz. package	161	26.5	99.5	16.35				

	UNIT		1 OZ., BY WT.		1 CUP		1 TABLE-SPOON	
	Cal.	Carb.	Cal.	Carb.	Cal.	Carb.	Cal.	Carb.
Prepared with 1 cup milk and water (yield: approx. 1.1 cups)	292	36.5	26.1	3.25	271	33.9	17	2.1
Sweet & Sour Sauce, 2.0-oz. package	220	54.5	110.3	27.26				
Prepared with ¾ cup water (yield: approx. ¾ cup)	220	54.5	26.7	6.57	294	72.1	18	4.5
Teriyaki Sauce, 1.6-oz. package	130	27.6	80.3	17.01				
Prepared with 1 cup water (yield: approx. 1 cup)	130	27.6	13.0	2.77	130	27.6	8	1.7
Turkey Gravy, 0.88-oz. package	87	15.1	99.2	17.22				
Prepared with 1 cup water (yield: approx. 1 cup)	87	15.1	9.4	1.63	87	15.1	10	1.8
White Sauce, 1.75-oz. package	230	25.1	131.3	14.34				
Prepared with 2½ cups milk (yield: approx. 2½ cups)	602	53.5	25.8	2.30	241	21.4	15	1.3
SAUCE AND GRAVY MIXES, DEHYDRATED, by brand								
DRY MIXES								
A La King Sauce Mix, **Durkee,** 1.1-oz. package	133	14.0	118.2	12.44				
Prepared as package directs (excluding chicken or turkey), add 1 cup water (yield: approx. 1 cup)	133	14.0	14.6	1.53	133	14.0	8	0.9
Au Jus Gravy Mix and Roastin' Bag, **Durkee,** 1-oz. package	62	13.0	62.0	13.00				
Prepared as package directs (excluding beef), add 1 cup water (yield: approx. 1 cup)	62	13.0	3.7	0.76	31	6.5	2	0.4
Au Jus Gravy Mix, **French's,** ¾-oz. package	64	16.0	85.3	21.30				
Prepared as package directs, add 2 cups water (yield: approx. 2 cups)	64	16.0	3.8	0.96	32	8.0	2	0.5
Brown Gravy Mix, **Durkee,** ¾-oz. package	59	10.0	78.5	13.31				
Prepared as package directs, add 1 cup water (yield: approx. 1 cup)	59	10.0	6.7	1.14	59	10.0	4	0.6
Brown Gravy Mix, **Ehlers,** ⅞ oz. package	87	14.0	99.4	16.00				
Prepared as package directs, add 1 cup water (yield: approx. 1 cup)	87	14.0	(9.4)	(1.51)	87	14.0	5	0.9
Brown Gravy Mix, **French's,** ¾-oz. package	80	12.0	106.7	16.00				
Prepared as package directs, add 1 cup water (yield: approx. 1 cup)	80	12.0	9.1	1.37	80	12.0	5	0.8
Brown Gravy Mix, **Pillsbury**	60	12.0						
Prepared as package directs (yield: approx. 1 cup)	60	12.0	(7.5)	(1.50)	60	12.0	4	0.8
Brown Gravy Mix, **Weight Watchers,** 0.44-oz. envelope	27	3.4	61.5	7.69				
Prepared as package directs, add 1 cup water (yield: approx. 1 cup)	27	3.4	(3.1)	(0.38)	27	3.4	2	0.2
Brown Gravy Mix with Mushrooms, **Durkee,** ¾-oz. package	59	11.0	78.9	14.71				
Prepared as package directs, add 1 cup water (yield: approx. 1 cup)	59	11.0	6.7	1.26	59	11.0	4	0.7
Brown Gravy Mix with Mushrooms, **Weight Watchers,** 0.5-oz. envelope	31	3.9	61.5	7.69				
Prepared as package directs, add 1 cup water (yield: approx. 1 cup)	31	3.9	(3.5)	(0.44)	31	3.9	2	0.2
Brown Gravy Mix with Onions, **Durkee,** ⅘-oz. package	66	13.0	82.8	16.31				
Prepared as package directs, add 1 cup water (yield: approx. 1 cup)	66	13.0	7.5	1.48	66	13.0	4	0.8
Brown Gravy Mix with Onions, **Weight Watchers,** 0.51-oz. envelope	31	3.9	61.5	30.15				
Prepared as package directs, add 1 cup water (yield: approx. 1 cup)	31	3.9	(3.6)	(0.44)	31	3.9	2	0.3
Brown Gravy Quik, **Loma Linda,** 0.88-oz. package	87	13.7	98.7	15.62				
Prepared with 1 cup water (yield: approx. 1 cup)	87	13.7	(9.4)	(1.48)	87	13.7	5	0.8

	UNIT		1 OZ., BY WT.		1 CUP		1 TABLE-SPOON	
	Cal.	Carb.	Cal.	Carb.	Cal.	Carb.	Cal.	Carb.
Cheese Sauce Mix, **Durkee,** 1.1-oz. package	175	7.0	155.6	6.22				
Prepared as package directs, add 1 cup milk (yield: approx. 1 cup)	337	19.0	36.9	2.08	337	19.0	21	1.2
Cheese Sauce Mix, **French's,** 1¼-oz. package	160	16.0	128.0	12.80				
Prepared as package directs, add 1 cup milk (yield: approx. 1 cup)	320	28.0	33.7	2.95	320	28.0	20	1.8
Chicken-Flavored Gravy Mix, **Weight Watchers,** 0.5-oz. envelope	36	4.6	72.7	9.09				
Prepared as package directs, add 1 cup water (yield: approx. 1 cup)	36	4.6	(4.1)	(0.51)	36	4.6	2	0.3
Chicken Gravy Mix, **Durkee,** 1-oz. package	87	14.0	87.0	14.00				
Prepared as package directs, add 1 cup water (yield: approx. 1 cup)	87	14.0	9.7	1.56	87	14.0	5	0.9
Chicken Gravy Mix and Roastin' Bag, **Durkee,** 1½-oz. package	122	24.0	81.3	16.00				
Prepared as package directs (excluding chicken), add 1 cup water (yield: approx. 1 cup)	122	24.0	12.8	2.53	122	24.0	8	1.5
Chicken Gravy Mix, **Ehlers,** ⅞-oz. package	84	16.0	96.0	18.29				
Prepared as package directs, add 1 cup water (yield: approx. 1 cup)	84	16.0	(9.1)	(1.73)	84	16.0	5	1.0
Chicken, Gravy Mix for, **French's,** ⅞-oz. package	100	16.0	114.3	18.30				
Prepared as package directs, add 1 cup water (yield: approx. 1 cup)	100	16.0	11.3	1.80	100	16.0	6	1.0
Chicken Gravy Mix, **Pillsbury,** ⅝-oz. package	100	16.0	160.0	25.60				
Prepared as package directs, add 1 cup water (yield: approx. 1 cup)	100	16.0	(12.5)	(2.00)	100	16.0	6	1.0
Chicken Gravy Mix, Creamy Style, **Durkee,** 1⅕-oz. package	156	14.0	128.2	11.50				
Prepared as package directs, add 1 cup water (yield: approx. 1 cup)	156	14.0	17.3	1.56	156	14.0	10	0.9
Chicken Gravy Mix, Creamy Style, and Roastin' Bag, **Durkee,** 2-oz. package	242	22.0	121.0	11.00	242	22.0	15	1.4
Prepared as package directs (excluding chicken), add 1 cup water (yield: approx. 1 cup)	242	22.0	24.2	2.20				
Chicken Italian Style Gravy Mix and Roastin' Bag, **Durkee,** 1½-oz. package	144	31.0	96.1	20.68				
Prepared as package directs (excluding chicken), add 1 cup water (yield: approx. 1 cup)	144	31.0	15.2	3.26	144	31.0	9	1.9
Country Gravy Quik, **Loma Linda,** 0.88-oz. package	88	14.4	99.8	16.36				
Prepared with 1 cup milk (yield: approx. 1 cup)	(247)	(26.4)	(26.3)	(2.81)	(247)	(26.4)	(15)	(1.7)
Hollandaise Sauce Mix, **Durkee,** 1-oz. package	173	11.0	173.0	11.00				
Prepared as package directs, add ⅔ cup water (yield: approx. ¾ cup)	173	11.0	27.3	1.74	231	14.7	14	0.9
Hollandaise Sauce Mix, **French's,** 1⅛-oz. package	180	8.0	160.0	7.11				
Prepared as package directs, add 1 cup water (yield: approx. 1 cup)	180	8.0	25.7	1.14	240	10.7	15	0.7
Homestyle Gravy Mix, **Durkee,** ¾-oz. package	70	11.0	93.3	14.67				
Prepared as package directs, add 1 cup water (yield: approx. 1 cup)	70	11.0	8.0	1.26	70	11.0	4	0.7
Homestyle Gravy Mix, **French's,** ⅞-oz. package	100	16.0	114.3	18.30				
Prepared as package directs, add 1 cup water (yield: approx. 1 cup)	100	16.0	11.3	1.80	100	16.0	6	1.0
Home Style Gravy Mix, **Pillsbury,** ⅝-oz. package	60	12.0	96.0	19.20				
Prepared as package directs (yield: approx. 1 cup)	60	12.0	(7.5)	(1.50)	60	12.0	4	0.8

	UNIT		1 OZ., BY WT.		1 CUP		1 TABLE-SPOON	
	Cal.	Carb.	Cal.	Carb.	Cal.	Carb.	Cal.	Carb.
Lemon Butter-Flavored Sauce Mix, **Weight Watchers,** 0.41-oz. envelope	15	3.7	36.4	9.09				
Prepared as package directs, add 1 cup water (yield: approx. 1 cup)	15	3.7	(1.6)	(0.43)	15	3.7	1	0.2
Meatloaf Gravy Mix and Roastin' Bag, **Durkee,** 1½-oz. package	129	18.0	86.1	12.00				
Mushroom Gravy Mix, **Durkee,** ¾-oz. package	60	11.0	80.0	14.67				
Prepared as package directs, add 1 cup water (yield: approx. 1 cup)	60	11.0	6.9	1.26	60	11.0	4	0.7
Mushroom Gravy Mix, **French's,** ¾-oz. package	80	12.0	106.7	16.00				
Prepared as package directs, add 1 cup water (yield: approx. 1 cup)	80	12.0	9.1	1.37	80	12.0	5	0.8
Mushroom Gravy Quik, **Loma Linda,** 0.88-oz. package	87	14.4	99.0	16.36				
Prepared with 1 cup water (yield: approx. 1 cup)	87	14.4	(9.4)	(1.55)	87	14.4	5	0.9
Onion Gravy Mix, **Durkee,** 1-oz. package	84	15.0	84.0	15.00				
Prepared as package directs, add 1 cup water (yield: approx. 1 cup)	84	15.0	9.3	1.67	84	15.0	5	0.9
Onion Gravy Mix, **French's,** ⅞-oz. package	100	16.0	114.3	18.30				
Prepared as package directs, add 1 cup water (yield: approx. 1 cup)	100	16.0	11.3	1.80	100	16.0	6	1.0
Onion Gravy Quik, **Loma Linda,** 0.88-oz. package	90	16.0	102.6	18.15				
Prepared with 1 cup water (yield: approx. 1 cup)	90	16.0	(9.7)	(1.72)	90	16.0	6	1.0
Onion Pot Roast Gravy Mix and Roastin' Bag, **Durkee,** 1½-oz. package	124	24.0	82.7	16.01				
Prepared as package directs (excluding pot roast), add ¾ cup water (yield: approx. 1 cup)	124	24.0	13.1	2.53	124	24.0	8	1.5
Pork Gravy Mix, **Durkee,** 1-oz. package	70	14.0	70.0	14.00				
Prepared as package directs, add 1 cup water (yield: approx. 1 cup)	70	14.0	7.8	1.56	70	14.0	4	0.9
Pork Gravy Mix and Roastin' Bag, **Durkee,** 1½-oz. package	130	26.0	86.7	17.34				
Prepared as package directs (excluding pork chops), add 1 cup water (yield: approx. 1 cup)	130	26.0	13.7	27.40	130	26.0	8	1.6
Pork, Gravy Mix for, **French's,** ¾-oz. package	80	12.0	106.7	16.00				
Prepared as package directs, add 1 cup water (yield: approx. 1 cup)	80	12.0	9.1	1.37	80	12.0	5	0.8
Pot Roast and Stew Gravy Mix and Roastin' Bag, **Durkee,** 1½-oz. package	125	25.0	83.4	16.78				
Prepared as package directs (excluding meat), add 1 cup water (yield: approx. 1 cup)	125	25.0	13.2	2.63	125	25.0	8	1.6
Smoky Bits Gravy Quik, **Loma Linda,** 0.88-oz. package	85	11.9	96.1	13.47				
Prepared with 1 cup milk (yield: approx. 9 oz.)	(244)	(23.9)	(26.0)	(2.54)	(244)	(23.9)	(15)	(1.5)
Sour Cream Sauce Mix, **Durkee,** 1-oz. package	135	9.0	135.0	9.00				
Prepared as package directs, add ½ cup water (yield: approx. ⅔ cup)	214	15.0	42.8	3.00	321	22.5	20	1.4
Sour Cream Sauce Mix, **French's,** 1¼-oz. package	160	16.0	128.0	12.80				
Prepared as package directs, add ½ cup milk (yield: approx. ½ cup)	240	20.0	68.0	5.67	480	40.0	24	2.0
Spaghetti Sauce Mix, **Durkee,** 1½-oz. package	85	20.0	56.7	13.30				
Prepared as package directs, add 6 oz. tomato paste and 1¾ cups water (yield: approx. 2½ cups)	224	52.0	(10.7)	(2.50)	90	20.8	6	1.3
Spaghetti Sauce Mix, Italian Style, **French's,** 1½-oz. package	120	20.0	80.0	13.33				
Prepared as package directs, add 6 oz. tomato paste, 2 Tbsp. cooking oil, 1¾ cups water (yield: approx. 2½ cups)	400	52.0	(17.8)	(2.31)	160	20.8	10	1.3
Spaghetti Sauce Mix, Mushroom, **Durkee,** 1¼-oz. package	69	16.0	55.2	12.80				
Prepared as package directs, add 6 oz. tomato paste and 2 cups water (yield: approx. 2⅔ cups)	208	48.0	(9.0)	(2.10)	78	18.0	5	1.1
Spaghetti Sauce With Mushrooms Mix, **French's,** 1¼-oz. package	120	20.0	96.0	16.00				
Prepared as package directs, add 6 oz. tomato paste, 2 Tbsp. cooking oil, 1¾ cups water (yield: approx. 2½ cups)	400	52.0	(17.8)	(2.31)	160	20.8	10	1.3
Sparerib Sauce Gravy Mix and Roastin' Bag, **Durkee,** 1.9-oz. package	162	37.0	86.7	19.79				
Prepared as package directs (excluding spare ribs), add 8 oz. tomato sauce (yield: approx. 1 cup)	(250)	(57.2)	(25.3)	(5.78)	(250)	(57.2)	(16)	(3.6)
Stroganoff Sauce Mix, **Durkee,** 1¼-oz. package	90	18.0	72.0	14.40				
Prepared as package directs, add 1½ lbs. beef, 2 Tbsp. oil, 1 cup sour cream (yield: approx. 4 cups)	3280	26.0	102.5	0.81	820	6.5	51	0.4
Stroganoff Sauce Mix, **French's,** 1¾-oz. package	220	28.0	125.7	16.00				
Prepared as package directs, add 1⅓ cups milk (yield: approx. 1⅓ cup)	440	44.0	41.2	4.12	330	33.0	21	2.1
Sweet & Sour Sauce Mix, **Durkee,** 2-oz. package	230	45.0	115.0	22.50				
Prepared as package directs, add 1 cup water (yield: approx. 1 cup)	230	45.0	(22.1)	(4.33)	230	45.0	14	2.8
Sweet N Sour Sauce Mix, **French's,** 2-oz. package	220	56.0	110.0	28.00				
Prepared as package directs, add ½ cup water plus ¼ cup vinegar (yield: approx. ¾ cup)	220	56.0	27.5	7.00	293	74.7	18	4.7
Swiss Steak Gravy Mix, **Durkee,** 1-oz. package	68	16.0	68.0	16.00				
Prepared as package directs, add 1½ cups water (yield: approx. 1½ cups)	68	16.0	5.2	1.23	45	10.7	3	0.7
Swiss Steak Gravy Mix and Roastin' Bag, **Durkee,** 1½-oz. package	115	28.0	76.7	18.68				
Prepared as package directs (excluding meat), add 1½ cups water (yield: approx. 1½ cups)	115	28.0	8.5	2.07	77	18.7	5	1.2
Teriyaki Sauce Mix, **French's,** 1⅝-oz. package	140	28.0	86.2	17.20				
Prepared as package directs, add ½ cup water (yield: approx. ½ cup)	140	28.0	24.9	4.98	280	56.0	18	3.5
Turkey Gravy Mix, **Durkee,** 1-oz. package	93	14.0	93.0	14.00				
Prepared as package directs, add 1 cup water (yield: approx. 1 cup)	93	14.0	10.3	1.56	93	14.0	6	0.9
Turkey, Gravy Mix for, **French's,** ⅞-oz. package	100	16.0	114.3	18.29				
Prepared as package directs, add 1 cup water (yield: approx. 1 cup)	100	16.0	11.3	1.80	100	16.0	6	1.0
White Sauce Mix, **Durkee,** 1-oz. package	158	35.0	158.0	35.00				
Prepared as package directs, add 1 cup milk (yield: approx. 1 cup)	238	41.0	26.4	4.56	238	41.0	15	2.6
GRAVY CONCENTRATES, by brand								
Au Jus "Pan Rich" Concentrate for Gravy, **French's,** 1 5/16-oz. bar	240	8.0	182.9	6.10				
Prepared as package directs, add 2 cups water (yield: approx. 2 cups)	240	8.0	(13.3)	(0.44)	120	4.0	8	0.3
Brown "Pan Rich" Concentrate for Gravy, **French's,** 1 5/16-oz. bar	240	16.0	(182.9)	(12.19)				

	UNIT		1 OZ., BY WT.		1 CUP		1 TABLESPOON	
	Cal.	Carb.	Cal.	Carb.	Cal.	Carb.	Cal.	Carb.
Prepared as package directs, add 1 cup water (yield: approx. 1 cup)	240	16.0	(24.7)	(1.65)	240	16.0	15	1.0
Chicken "Pan Rich" Concentrate for Gravy, **French's**, 1 9/16-oz. bar	240	16.0	(153.6)	(10.24)				
Prepared as package directs, add 1 cup water (yield: approx. 1 cup)	240	16.0	(24.7)	(1.65)	240	16.0	15	1.0
Onion "Pan Rich" Concentrate for Gravy, **French's**, 1 5/16-oz. bar	200	16.0	(152.4)	(12.19)				
Prepared as package directs, add 1 cup water (yield: approx. 1 cup)	200	16.0	(20.6)	(1.65)	200	16.0	13	1.0

A POTPOURRI OF BAKING AND COOKING INGREDIENTS BORROWED FROM OTHER CHAPTERS

Eggs

For a more complete listing, see the EGGS chapter.

	UNIT		1 OZ., BY WT.		1 CUP		1 TABLESPOON	
	Cal.	Carb.	Cal.	Carb.	Cal.	Carb.	Cal.	Carb.
RAW:								
1 large whole chicken egg, (approx. 1¾ oz.)	79	0.6	44.8	0.34	384	2.9	24	0.2
1 cup (approx. 8.6 oz.)	384	2.9	44.8	0.34	384	2.9	24	0.2
White from 1 large egg (approx. 1.2 oz.)	16	0.4	13.9	0.35	118	3.0	7	0.2
1 cup (approx. 8.5 oz.)	118	3.0	13.9	0.35	118	3.0	7	0.2
Yolk from 1 large egg (approx. 0.6 oz.)	63	trace	104.6	0.06	897	0.5	56	trace
1 cup (approx. 8.6 oz.)	897	0.5	104.6	0.06	897	0.5	56	trace

Milk and Cream

For a more complete listing, see the BEVERAGES chapter.

	UNIT		1 OZ., BY WT.		1 CUP		1 TABLESPOON	
	Cal.	Carb.	Cal.	Carb.	Cal.	Carb.	Cal.	Carb.
MILK, based on generic data								
Buttermilk, cultured, 0.9% fat, 1 cup	99	11.7	11.3	1.36	99	11.7	6	0.7
Condensed Milk, Sweetened (canned), 8.7% fat, 1 cup	982	166.5	91.0	15.40	982	166.5	61	10.4
Dry Milk, Whole, 27.61% fat, 1 cup dry	635	49.2	140.6	10.89	635	49.2	40	3.1
Evaporated Milk, Skim (canned), 0.2% fat, 1 cup	198	28.9	22.1	3.22	198	28.9	12	1.8
Evaporated Milk, Whole (canned), 7.56% fat, 1 cup	338	25.3	38.0	2.85	338	25.3	21	1.6
Low-fat Milk, 1% fat, 1 cup	102	11.7	11.9	1.36	102	11.7	6	0.7
Low-fat Milk, 1% fat with nonfat milk solids added, 1 cup	104	12.2	12.2	1.41	104	12.2	7	0.8
Low-fat Milk, protein fortified, 1% fat, 1 cup	119	13.4	13.6	1.57	119	13.4	7	0.8
Low-fat Milk, 2% fat, 1 cup	121	11.7	14.2	1.36	121	11.7	8	0.7
Low-fat Milk, 2% fat, with nonfat milk solids added, 1 cup	125	12.2	14.5	1.41	125	12.2	8	0.8
Low-fat Milk, protein fortified, 2% fat, 1 cup	137	13.5	15.9	1.56	137	13.5	9	0.8
Skim Milk, 0.18% fat, 1 cup	86	11.9	9.9	1.38	86	11.9	5	0.7
Skim Milk, 0.25% fat, with nonfat milk solids added, 1 cup	90	12.3	10.5	1.42	90	12.3	6	0.8
Skim Milk, protein fortified, 0.25% fat, 1 cup	100	13.7	11.6	1.58	100	13.7	6	0.9
Whole Milk, 3.3% fat, 1 cup	150	11.4	17.3	1.32	150	11.4	9	0.7
Whole milk (3.5% fat) (based on USDA data published in 1975. This analysis seems popular among manufacturers. Many manufacturers used the number "160 calories," a rounded version of the USDA's "159," in reporting calories for products that require whole milk to be added by the consumer.), 1 quart (1g/1g/1g/88%/14mg)	634	47.8	19.8	1.49	159	12.0	9.9	0.75
Whole Milk, Low Sodium, 3.5% fat, 1 cup	149	10.9	17.3	1.26	149	10.9	9	0.7
Whole Milk, 3.7% fat, 1 cup	157	11.4	18.2	1.32	157	11.4	10	0.7

	UNIT		1 OZ., BY WT.		1 CUP		1 TABLESPOON	
	Cal.	Carb.	Cal.	Carb.	Cal.	Carb.	Cal.	Carb.
CREAM, based on generic data								
Heavy Whipping Cream, 37% fat, 1 cup	821	6.6	97.8	0.79	821	6.6	51	0.4
Light Cream, 30.9% fat, 1 cup	699	7.1	82.8	0.84	699	7.1	44	0.4
WHIPPED CREAM, by brand								
Ralph's real Whipped Cream (with decorator tip), 6½-oz. container (yield: approx. 3½ cups, whipped)	420	14.0	64.6	0.88	120	4.0	8	0.3

Cheese, Sour Cream, and Yogurt

For more complete listings, see the CHEESE, CONDIMENTS, and YOGURT chapters, respectively.

	UNIT		1 OZ., BY WT.		1 CUP		1 TABLESPOON	
	Cal.	Carb.	Cal.	Carb.	Cal.	Carb.	Cal.	Carb.
CHEESE, based on generic data								
Cottage Cheese, creamed, small curd, 4.51% fat, 1 cup (approx. 7.4 oz.)	216	5.6	29.2	0.76	216	5.6	14	0.4
Cottage Cheese, dry curd, 0.42% fat, 1 cup not packed (approx. 5.1 oz.)	123	2.7	24.0	0.52	123	2.7	8	0.2
Cream Cheese, 37.7% fat, 1 cup (approx. 8.2 oz.)	869	4.9	106.0	0.60	869	4.9	54	0.3
Mozzarella Cheese, whole milk, 1 cup, shredded (approx. 4 oz.)	360	2.8	90.3	0.70	360	2.8	22	0.2
Parmesan Cheese, 1 cup, grated, not packed, (approx. 3.5 oz.)	453	3.7	129.3	1.06	453	3.7	23	0.2
Ricotta Cheese, whole milk, 1 cup (approx. 8.7 oz.)	428	76.8	49.4	0.86	428	76.8	27	4.8
SOUR CREAM, based on generic data								
Half and Half Sour Cream (12% fat)								
1 cup (approx. 8.5 oz.)	320	28.8	38.3	3.40	320	28.8	20	1.8
1 pound (approx. 1.9 cups)	613	54.4	38.3	3.40	320	28.8	20	1.8
1 teaspoon (approx. 0.2 oz.)	7	0.6	38.3	3.40	320	28.8	20	1.8
Sour Cream (20.96% fat)								
1 cup (approx. 8.1 oz.)	492	9.2	60.7	1.21	492	9.2	31	0.6
1 pound (approx. 2 cups)	971	19.4	60.7	1.21	492	9.2	31	0.6
1 teaspoon (approx. 0.2 oz.)	10	0.2	60.7	1.21	492	9.2	31	0.6
Imitation Sour Cream Nondairy (19.5% fat)								
1 cup (approx. 8.1 oz.)	479	15.3	59.0	1.88	479	15.3	30	1.0
1 pound (approx. 2 cups)	946	30.1	59.0	1.88	479	15.3	30	1.0
1 teaspoon (approx. 0.2 oz.)	10	0.3	59.0	1.88	479	15.3	30	1.0
YOGURT, based on generic data								
Skim Milk Yogurt, 0.18% fat, 1 8-oz. container	127	17.4	15.9	2.18	(139)	(19.1)	(9)	(1.2)
Low-fat Yogurt, 1.55% fat, 1 8-oz. container	144	16.0	17.9	2.00	(158)	(17.5)	(10)	(1.1)
Whole Milk Yogurt, 3.25% fat, 1 8-oz. container	139	10.6	17.3	1.32	(150)	(11.4)	(9)	(0.7)

Fats and Oils

For a more complete listing, see the FATS & OILS chapter.

	UNIT		1 OZ., BY WT.		1 CUP		1 TABLESPOON	
	Cal.	Carb.	Cal.	Carb.	Cal.	Carb.	Cal.	Carb.
BUTTER (not whipped), based on generic data								
1 stick, 4 oz. net wt. (approx. ½ cup)	812	0.5	203.0	0.11	1625	0.9	102	0.1
1 cup (approx. 8 oz. net wt. (2 sticks as above)	1625	0.9	203.0	0.11	1625	0.9	102	0.1
1 pound (approx. 2 cups)	3248	1.8	203.0	0.11	1625	0.9	102	0.1
1 teaspoon (approx. ⅙ oz. (1/24 of stick as above)	34	trace	203.0	0.11	1625	0.9	102	0.1
MARGARINE, Regular or Soft (not whipped), based on generic data								
1 stick, 4 oz. net wt. (approx. ½ cup)	816	0.5	204.1	0.11	1634	0.9	102	0.1
1 cup (approx. 8 oz. net wt., 2 sticks as above)	1634	0.9	204.1	0.11	1634	0.9	102	0.1
1 pound (approx. 2 cups)	3266	1.8	204.1	0.11	1634	0.9	102	0.1
1 teaspoon (approx. ⅙ oz., 1/24 of stick as above)	34	trace	204.1	0.11	1634	0.9	102	0.1

	UNIT		1 OZ., BY WT.		1 CUP		1 TABLESPOON	
	Cal.	Carb.	Cal.	Carb.	Cal.	Carb.	Cal.	Carb.
OIL, based on generic data								
Corn Oil, 1 quart (approx. 30.9 oz. net wt.)	7708	0.0	250.6	0.00	1927	0.0	120	0.0
Safflower Oil, 1 quart (approx. 30.9 oz. net wt.)	7708	0.0	250.6	0.00	1927	0.0	120	0.0
SHORTENING, based on generic data								
1 cup (approx. 7¼ oz.)	1845	0.0	255.2	0.00	1845	0.0	115	0.0
1 pound (approx. 2.2 cups)	4082	0.0	255.2	0.00	1845	0.0	115	0.0
1 tablespoon (approx. 0.44 oz.)	115	0.0	255.2	0.00	1845	0.0	115	0.0
1 teaspoon (approx. 0.15 oz.)	38	0.0	255.2	0.00	1845	0.0	115	0.0
1 container, 48 oz. (3 lbs.)	12250	0.0	255.2	0.00	1845	0.0	115	0.0

Nuts and Nut Products

For a more complete listing, see the NUTS & SEEDS chapter.

	UNIT		1 OZ., BY WT.		1 CUP		1 TABLESPOON	
	Cal.	Carb.	Cal.	Carb.	Cal.	Carb.	Cal.	Carb.
ALMOND PASTE (based on data from France)								
1 pound	2046	291.7	127.9	18.23				
ALMONDS, based on generic data								
Dried, Shelled:								
Chopped:								
1 cup (approx. 4.6 oz.)	777	25.4	169.8	5.54	777	25.4	49	1.6
1 tablespoon (approx. 0.3 oz.)	49	1.6	169.8	5.54	777	25.4	49	1.6
Slivered (split in half, then sliced to 3/16" wide):								
1 cup:								
Packed (approx. 4¾ oz.)	807	26.3	169.8	5.54	807	26.3	50	1.6
Not packed (approx. 4.0 oz.)	688	22.4	169.8	5.54	688	22.4	43	1.4
Sliced:								
1 cup (approx. 3⅓ oz.)	568	18.5	169.8	5.54	568	18.5	36	1.2
CHESTNUT PASTE (based on data from France)								
1 pound	481	103.4	30.1	6.46				
COCONUT, based on generic data								
Dried, Unsweetened, Shredded:								
1 cup (approx. 3.2 oz.)	596	20.7	187.7	6.52	596	20.7	37	1.3
1 pound (approx. 5 cups)	3003	104.3	187.7	6.52	596	20.7	37	1.3
Sweetened, Shredded:								
1 cup (approx. 3.4 oz.)	528	51.3	155.4	15.08	528	51.3	33	3.2
1 pound (approx. 4.71 cups)	2486	241.3	155.4	15.08	528	51.3	33	3.2
COCONUT, by brand								
Baker's Angel Flake sweetened flaked Coconut, 3½-oz. can	448	39.0	128.0	11.20	360	32.0	23	2.0
7-oz. bag	896	78.0	128.0	11.20	360	32.0	23	2.0
1 cup (approx. 2.7 oz.)	360	32.0	128.0	11.20	360	32.0	23	2.0
1 tablespoon (approx. 0.2 oz.)	23	2.0	128.0	11.20	360	32.0	23	2.0
Cookie Coconut, 7-oz. bag	982	85.1	140.3	12.20	560	48.0	35	3.0
1 cup (approx. 4 oz.)	560	48.0	140.3	12.20	560	48.0	35	3.0
1 tablespoon (approx. ¼ oz.)	35	3.0	140.3	12.20	560	48.0	35	3.0
Premium Shred shredded sweetened Coconut, 4-oz. bag	558	48.4	139.5	12.10	412	36.0	26	2.3
8-oz. bag	1116	96.8	139.5	12.10	412	36.0	26	2.3
16-oz. (1-lb.) bag	2232	193.6	139.5	12.10	412	36.0	26	2.3
1 cup (approx. 2.9 oz.)	412	36.0	139.5	12.10	412	36.0	26	2.3
1 tablespoon (approx. 0.2 oz.)	26	2.3	139.5	12.10	412	36.0	26	2.3
Southern Style Premium Shred shredded sweetened Coconut, 4-oz. can	508	44.5	127.0	11.11	376	32.9	24	2.1
1 cup (approx. 2.9 oz.)	376	32.9	127.0	11.11	376	32.9	24	2.1
1 tablespoon (approx. 0.2 oz.)	24	2.1	127.0	11.11	376	32.9	24	2.1
Durkee Shredded Coconut, 8-oz. package	277	8.0	34.6	1.00				
Townhouse Sweetened Fancy Shred Coconut, 16-oz. (1-lb.) package	2646	243.1	165.4	15.20	579	53.2	36	3.3
1 cup (approx. 3.5 oz.)	579	53.2	165.4	15.20	579	53.2	36	3.3
1 tablespoon (approx. 0.2 oz.)	36	3.3	165.4	15.20	579	53.2	36	3.3
Sweetened Flaked Coconut, 14-oz. package	2316	212.8	165.4	15.20	579	53.2	36	3.3
1 cup (approx. 3.5 oz.)	579	53.2	165.4	15.20	579	53.2	36	3.3
1 tablespoon (approx. 0.2 oz.)	36	3.3	165.4	15.20	579	53.2	36	3.3
PECANS, based on generic data								
Chopped:								
1 cup (approx. 4.1 oz.)	811	17.2	194.8	4.14	811	17.2	52	1.1
1 tablespoon (approx. ¼ oz.)	52	1.1	194.8	4.14	811	17.2	52	1.1
Ground:								
1 cup (approx. 3⅓ oz.)	653	13.9	194.8	4.14	653	13.9	41	0.9
WALNUTS, based on generic data								
Shelled:								
Black Walnuts:								
Chopped:								
1 tablespoon (approx. 0.3 oz.)	50	1.2	178.1	4.19	785	18.5	50	1.2
1 cup (approx. 4.4 oz.)	785	18.5	178.1	4.19	785	18.5	50	1.2
Ground:								
1 cup (approx. 2.8 oz.)	502	11.8	178.1	4.19	502	11.8	31	0.7
English or Persian Walnuts:								
Chopped:								
1 tablespoon (approx. 0.3 oz.)	52	1.3	184.6	4.48	781	19.0	52	1.3
1 cup (approx. 4¼ oz., 30 nuts)	781	19.0	184.6	4.48	781	19.0	52	1.3

Marshmallows

There are more marshmallows in the SWEET LITTLE NOTHINGS chapter.

	UNIT		1 OZ., BY WT.		1 CUP		1 TABLESPOON	
	Cal.	Carb.	Cal.	Carb.	Cal.	Carb.	Cal.	Carb.
Kraft miniature Marshmallows, 6¼-oz. bag, approx. 300 marshmallows (each approx. 0.02 oz.)	591	147.7	94.5	23.63	(756)	(188.8)	(47)	(11.8)
10½-oz. bag, approx. 500 marshmallows (each approx. 0.02 oz.)	992	248.1	94.5	23.63	(756)	(188.8)	(47)	(11.8)
1 marshmallow (approx. 0.02 oz.)	2	0.5	94.5	23.63	(756)	(188.8)	(47)	(11.8)

Fruits

For fresh fruits and dried fruits, see the FRUITS chapter.

	UNIT		1 OZ., BY WT.		1 CUP		1 TABLESPOON	
	Cal.	Carb.	Cal.	Carb.	Cal.	Carb.	Cal.	Carb.
Candied Fruits, based on generic data								
(See also Fruit Peels, following.)								
Apricots, 1 pound	1549	395.4	96.8	24.71	(514)	(131.2)	(32)	(8.2)
Cherries, 4-oz. container (approx. ¾ cup)	383	98.0	96.0	24.60	511	130.7	32	8.2
1 cup (approx. 5.3 oz.)	511	130.7	96.0	24.60	511	130.7	32	8.2
1 pound (approx. 130 cherries)	1536	393.6	96.0	24.60	511	130.7	32	8.2
1 cherry (approx. 0.12 oz.)	12	3.0	96.0	24.60	511	130.7	32	8.2
Citron, 4-oz. container	356	90.8	89.0	22.70	525	133.9	33	8.4
1 pound	1424	363.2	89.0	22.70	525	133.9	33	8.4
Ginger Root, crystallized, 1 pound	1542	395.1	96.4	24.69	771	197.6	48	12.4
Pear, 1 pound	1374	344.3	85.9	21.52	(456)	(114.3)	(29)	(7.1)
Pineapple, 4-oz. container (2 slices or approx. ½ cup of chunks, approx. 27 chunks)	357	90.4	89.6	22.68	714	180.8	45	11.4
8-oz. container (4 slices or approx. 1 cup of chunks packed, or 1⅛ cups not packed (approx. 55 chunks)	717	181.6	89.6	22.68	714	180.8	45	11.4
1 slice, approx. 2 oz.	179	45.2	89.6	22.68	7.14	180.8	45	11.4
Pineapple Chunks:								
1 chunk, approx. 0.15 oz.	14	3.4	90.0	22.70				
1 cup, not packed (approx. 7.1 oz.)	(639)	(161.2)	90.0	22.70	(639)	(161.2)	(40)	(10.1)
1 cup, packed (approx. 8 oz.)	(717)	(181.6)	90.0	22.70	(717)	(181.6)	(45)	(11.4)
1 pound (approx. 8 slices or 110 chunks)	1440	363.2	90.0	22.70				
Fruit Peels, based on generic data								
Grapefruit Peel, candied, 1 pound	1440	366.4	90.0	22.96	720	183.2	45	11.5
Lemon Peel:								
Raw, medium grated, 1 pound (approx. 75⅔ Tbsp.)	(362)	72.6	(22.6)	4.54	(77)	15.5	(5)	1.0

	UNIT		1 OZ., BY WT.		1 CUP		1 TABLE-SPOON	
	Cal.	Carb.	Cal.	Carb.	Cal.	Carb.	Cal.	Carb.
1 tablespoon (approx. 0.2 oz.)	(5)	1.0	(22.6)	4.54	(77)	15.5	(5)	1.0
1 teaspoon (approx. 0.1 oz.)	(2)	0.3	(22.6)	4.54	(77)	15.5	(5)	1.0
Candied, 1 pound	1440	366.4	90.0	22.90	720	183.2	45	11.5
Orange Peel:								
Raw, medium grated, 1 pound (approx. 75⅔ Tbsp.)	(538)	113.4	(33.6)	7.09	(113)	23.8	(7)	1.5
1 tablespoon (approx. 0.2 oz.)	(7)	1.5	(33.6)	7.09	(113)	23.8	(7)	1.5
1 teaspoon (approx. 0.1 oz.)	(2)	0.5	(33.6)	7.09	(113)	23.8	(7)	1.5
Candied, 1 pound	1433	365.6	89.6	22.85	720	183.2	45	11.5

Sweeteners, based on generic data

For a more complete listing, see the SUGARS, SWEETENERS & TOPPINGS chapter.

	UNIT		1 OZ., BY WT.		1 CUP		1 TABLE-SPOON	
	Cal.	Carb.	Cal.	Carb.	Cal.	Carb.	Cal.	Carb.
Corn Syrup, light or dark, 1 cup (approx. 11.5 oz.)	951	246.0	82.2	21.26	951	246.0	59	15.4
Honey, strained or extracted, 1 cup (approx. 11.9 oz.)	1031	279.0	86.2	23.31	1031	279.0	64	17.4
Maple Syrup, 1 cup (approx. 11.1 oz.)	794	204.8	71.4	18.43	794	204.8	50	12.8
Molasses, light, 1 cup (approx. 11.5 oz.)	827	213.2	71.4	18.43	827	213.2	52	13.3
medium, 1 cup (approx. 11.5 oz.)	761	196.8	65.8	17.01	761	196.8	48	12.3
blackstrap, 1 cup (approx. 11.5 oz.)	699	180.4	60.4	15.60	699	180.4	44	11.3
Sugar:								
brown, 1 cup, not packed (approx. 5.1 oz.)	541	139.8	105.8	27.33	541	139.8	34	8.7
packed (approx. 7.75 oz.)	821	212.1	105.8	27.33	821	212.1	51	13.3
white, granulated, 1 cup (approx. 7 oz.)	736	190.4	109.1	28.14	736	190.4	46	11.9
powdered (10X or confectioners), unsifted, 1 cup (approx. 4.25 oz.)	462	119.4	109.1	28.21	462	119.4	29	7.5
sifted, 1 cup (approx. 3.5 oz.)	385	99.5	109.1	28.21	385	99.5	24	6.2
ARTIFICIAL SWEETENER, by brand								
Granulated Sweet'ner, **Weight Watchers,** 1 packet, 0.04 oz.	4	0.9	114.3	25.71				

. . . And Not So Sweeteners

	UNIT		1 OZ., BY WT.		1 CUP		1 TABLE-SPOON	
	Cal.	Carb.	Cal.	Carb.	Cal.	Carb.	Cal.	Carb.
LEMON JUICE								
Lemon Juice, fresh, based on generic data								
Juice of 1 medium lemon (approx. 3 Tbsp., approx. 1.7 oz.)	(12)	(3.8)	7.6	2.44	61	19.5	4	1.2
1 teaspoon (approx. 0.17 oz.)	1	0.4	7.6	2.44	61	19.5	4	1.2
1 tablespoon (approx. 0.5 oz.)	4	1.2	7.6	2.44	61	19.5	4	1.2
1 cup (approx. 8.6 oz.)	61	19.5	7.6	2.44	61	19.5	4	1.2
Lemon Juice, reconstituted, **ReaLemon,** 8-fl.-oz.-bottle	48	16.0	(5.6)	(1.86)	48	16.0	3.0	1.00
Lemon Flavor Crystals, **Single Serv,** 0.03-oz. packet (equivalent to juice of ¼ lemon)	3	0.7	100.0	25.47				
LIME JUICE								
Lime Juice, reconstituted, **ReaLime,** 8-fl.-oz. bottle	32	8.0	(3.7)	(0.92)	32	8.0	2.0	0.50
VINEGAR								
Vinegar, cider, 1 cup (approx. 8.5 oz.)	34	14.2	4.0	1.77	34	14.2	2	0.8
Vinegar, distilled, 1 cup (approx. 8.5 oz.)	29	12.0	3.4	1.40	29	12.0	2	0.8

19 BREADS •

BREADS MADE FROM SCRATCH, based on USDA home recipes

	UNIT		1 BISCUIT, ROLL, OR MUFFIN		1 OZ., BY WT.	
	Cal.	Carb.	Cal.	Carb.	Cal.	Carb.
BISCUITS						
BAKING POWDER BISCUITS made with enriched or unenriched flour:						
Made from 2 cups flour, ¾ cup fluid skim milk, 5¾ Tbsp. cooking fat, 3 tsp. baking powder, ½ tsp. salt [yield: approx. 16 oz. (1 lb.), prepared] (2g/13g/5g/27%/177mg)	(1670)	(207.6)			104.6	12.98
1 biscuit as above, approx. 0.98 oz.			103	12.8	104.6	12.98
1 pound (approx. 16¼ biscuits)	1674	207.7			104.6	12.98
BAKING POWDER BISCUITS made with self-rising flour:						
Made from 2 cups flour, ⅔ cup fluid skim milk, 5 Tbsp. cooking fat (yield: approx. 15 oz., prepared) (2g/13g/5g/27%/177mg)	(1582)	(195.6)			105.4	13.04
1 biscuit as above, approx. 0.99 oz.			104	12.9	105.4	13.04
1 pound (approx. 16¼ biscuits)	1687	208.7			105.4	13.04
CORN BREAD						
CORN PONE made with white and whole-ground corn meal:						
Made from 1⅓ cups water, 1⅓ Tbsp. cooking fat, 2 cups unbolted corn meal, 2 tsp. baking powder, ½ tsp. salt (yield: approx. 17.1 oz., prepared)	989	175.9			57.8	10.28
1 slice as above, approx. 2.1 oz.	122	21.7	122	21.7	57.8	10.28
1 pound (approx. 7.6 slices) (1g/10g/2g/52%/112mg)	925	164.5			57.8	10.28
SOUTHERN-STYLE CORN BREAD made with degermed corn meal:						
Made from 2 cups buttermilk, 2⅓ Tbsp. cooking fat, 2 large eggs, 2 cups unbolted corn meal, ½ tsp. baking soda, 2 tsp. baking powder, 1 tsp. salt (yield: approx. 26.3 oz., prepared) (2g/10g/2g/50%/168mg)	1673	259.2			63.5	9.84
1 slice as above, approx. 2.9 oz.			186	28.8	63.5	9.84
1 pound (approx. 5½ pieces)	1016	157.4			63.5	9.84
SOUTHERN-STYLE CORN BREAD made with whole-ground corn meal:						
Made from 2 cups buttermilk, 2⅓ Tbsp. cooking fat, 2 large eggs, 2 cups unbolted corn meal, ½ tsp. baking soda, 2 tsp. baking powder, 1 tsp. salt (yield: approx. 24.8 oz., prepared) (2g/8g/2g/54%/77mg)	1455	204.6			58.7	8.25
1 slice as above, approx. 2¾ oz.			161	22.7	58.7	8.25
1 pound (approx. 6 pieces)	939	132.0			58.7	8.25

	UNIT		1 BISCUIT, ROLL, OR MUFFIN		1 OZ., BY WT.	
	Cal.	Carb.	Cal.	Carb.	Cal.	Carb.
SPOONBREAD made with white, whole-ground corn meal:						
Made from ¾ cup water, 1½ cup milk, 3 Tbsp. cooking fat, 3 large eggs, 1 cup unbolted corn meal, 1 tsp. baking soda, 1 tsp. salt (yield: approx. 2⅔ cups, prepared; approx. 22.8 oz.)	1258	109.0			55.3	4.79
1 cup (approx. 8.5 oz.)	468	40.6	468	40.6	55.3	4.79
1 pound (approx. 1.9 cups) (2g/5g/3g/63%/137mg)	885	76.7			55.3	4.79
MUFFINS						
PLAIN MUFFINS						
Made from 2 cups flour, 1 cup fluid skim milk, 3½ Tbsp. cooking fat, 1 large egg, 2 Tbsp. sugar, 2 tsp. baking powder, ½ tsp. salt (yield: approx. 17 oz.), 12 muffins (each 1½" high, with 3" diameter at top and 2" diameter at bottom)	1426	205.2			83.4	11.99
1 muffin as above, approx. 1.4 oz. (yield from approx. 3 Tbsp. batter)			118	16.9	83.4	11.99
1 pound (approx. 11⅓ muffins, as above) (2g/12g/3g/38%/125mg)	1134	191.9			83.4	11.99
BLUEBERRY MUFFINS						
Made from 1⅛ cups flour, ½ cup whole milk, 1½ Tbsp. cooking fat, 1 large egg, 2½ Tbsp. sugar, 1 tsp. baking powder, ⅔ tsp. salt, ¼ cup unsweetened frozen blueberries (yield: approx. 11 1/10 oz.), 8 muffins (each 1½" high, 2⅜" at top, 2" diameter at bottom)	885	132.0			79.7	11.88
1 muffin as above, approx. 1.4 oz. (yield from approx. 3 Tbsp. batter)			112	16.8	79.7	11.88
1 pound (approx. 11⅓ muffins as above) (2g/12g/3g/39%/179mg)	1275	190.1			79.7	11.88
BRAN MUFFINS						
Made from ½ cup flour, ½ cup milk, 4 tsp. cooking fat, 1 large egg, 2½ Tbsp. molasses, 1½ tsp. baking powder, ¼ tsp. salt, 1 cup bran (yield: approx. 10.4 oz.), 7½ muffins (each 1⅜" high, 2⅝" diameter at top, 2" diameter at bottom)	770	127.1			74.0	12.21
1 muffin as above, approx. 1.4 oz. (yield from approx. ¼ cup batter)			104	17.2	74.0	12.21
1 pound (approx. 11⅓ muffins as above) (2g/12g/3g/35%/127mg)	1184	195.5			74.0	12.21
DEGERMED CORNMEAL CORN MUFFINS						
Made from ⅔ cup flour, 1 cup whole milk, 3 Tbsp. cooking fat, 1 large egg, 2 Tbsp. sugar, 3 tsp. baking powder, ½ tsp. salt, 1⅓ cups degermed yellow cornmeal (yield: approx. 18⅓ oz.), 13 muffins (each 1½" high, with 2⅜" diameter at top, 2" diameter at bottom)	1633	250.1			89.0	13.64
1 muffin as above, approx. 1.4 oz. (yield from approx. ¼ cup batter)			126	19.2	89.0	13.64

	UNIT Cal.	UNIT Carb.	1 BISCUIT, ROLL, OR MUFFIN Cal.	1 BISCUIT, ROLL, OR MUFFIN Carb.	1 OZ., BY WT. Cal.	1 OZ., BY WT. Carb.
1 pound (approx. 11⅓ muffins as above) (2g/14g/3g/33%/136mg)	1424	218.2			89.0	13.64
WHOLE-GROUND CORNMEAL CORN MUFFINS						
Made from ⅔ cup flour, 1 cup milk, 3 Tbsp. cooking fat, 1 large egg, 2 Tbsp. sugar, 3 tsp. baking powder, ½ tsp. salt (yield: approx. 17⅔ oz.), 12½ muffins (each 1½" high, with 2⅜" diameter at top, 2" diameter at bottom)	1440	212.5			81.6	12.05
1 muffin as above, 1.4 oz. (yield from approx. ¼ cup batter)			115	17.0	81.6	12.05
1 pound (approx. 11⅓ muffins as above) (2g/12g/3g/38%/140mg)	1306	192.8			81.6	12.05
POPOVERS						
Made from 1 cup flour, 1 cup milk, 1 Tbsp. cooking fat, 2 large eggs, ¼ tsp. salt (yield: approx. 7 popovers, approx. 9.7 oz.)	(621)	(71.0)			63.8	7.30
1 popover as above, approx. 1.4 oz.			90	10.3	63.8	7.30
1 pound (approx. 11⅓ popovers)	1021	116.8			63.8	7.30
ROLLS OR BUNS made with milk and enriched flour:						
Made from 5 cups plus 1 Tbsp. flour, ¼ cup water, 1 cup milk, 5 Tbsp. cooking fat, 1 large egg, ¼ cup sugar, ⅓ tsp. dry yeast, ½ tsp. salt (yield: approx. 28 rolls or buns, approx. 38.4 oz.)	(3344)	(553.7)			96.1	15.91
1 roll or bun as above, approx. 1¼ oz.			119	19.6	96.1	15.91
1 pound (approx. 13 rolls or buns)	1538	254.5			96.1	15.91

BREADS MADE FROM MIXES, by brand

	UNIT Cal.	UNIT Carb.	1 SLICE OR ROLL Cal.	1 SLICE OR ROLL Carb.	1 OZ., BY WT. Cal.	1 OZ., BY WT. Carb.
Applesauce Spice Bread Mix, **Pillsbury** "Quick Bread," 15-oz. box	1760	336.0			117.3	22.40
As prepared (yield: 1 loaf, approx. 23 oz.)	(1920)	(336.0)			(83.5)	(14.61)
Apricot Nut Bread Mix, **Pillsbury** "Quick Bread," 15.7-oz. box	1760	352.0			112.1	22.42
As prepared (yield: 1 loaf, approx. 23 oz.)	(1760)	(352.0)			(76.5)	(15.30)
Banana Bread Mix, **Pillsbury** "Quick Bread," 15-oz. box	1920	336.0			128.0	22.40
As prepared (yield: 1 loaf, approx. 23 oz.)	(1920)	(336.0)			(83.5)	(14.61)
Barley Mix, Wheat Free, **Jolly Joan,** 20-oz. box	1850	405.0			92.5	20.25
As prepared (yield: 2 loaves, approx. 36 oz.)	(2733)	(459.0)			(85.4)	(14.34)
1 loaf, approx. 16 oz. (1 lb.)	(1367)	(229.5)			(85.4)	(14.34)
Blueberry Nut Bread Mix, **Pillsbury** "Quick Bread," 14.5-oz. box	1760	336.0			121.4	23.17
As prepared (yield: 1 loaf, approx. 22 oz.)	(1760)	(336.0)			(80.0)	(15.27)
Cherry Nut Bread Mix, **Pillsbury** "Quick Bread," 16.6-oz. box	1920	352.0			115.7	21.20
As prepared (yield: 1 loaf, approx. 24 oz.)	(2080)	(352.0)			(86.7)	(14.67)
Corn Bread:						
Corn Bread Mix, **Aunt Jemima** "Easy Mix," 10-oz. box	1206	199.4			120.6	19.94
As prepared (weight of yield is not available)	(1326)	(205.4)			120.6	19.94
Corn Bread Mix, **Ballard,** 19-oz. box	1920	384.0			101.1	20.21
As prepared (yield: 2 loaves, approx. 35 oz.)	(2560)	(416.0)			(73.1)	(11.89)
1 loaf, approx. 17½ oz.	(1280)	(208.0)			(73.1)	(11.89)
Corn Bread Mix, **Dromedary,** 15-oz. box	1760	288.0			117.3	19.20
As prepared (yield: 1 loaf, approx. 23 oz.)	(2080)	(304.0)			(90.4)	(13.22)
Corn Bread Mix, **Elam's,** 32-oz. (2-lb.) box	3312	612.5			103.5	19.14
As prepared (yield: 1 loaf, approx. 40 oz.)	(3840)	(656.0)			96.0	16.40
Corn Bread Mix, **Fearn Soy/O,** 16-oz. (1-lb.) package	1120	224.0			70.0	14.00
As prepared for bread or muffins (yield: 16 muffins or 1⅓ loaf, approx. 26.4 oz.)	2160	240.0			(81.6)	(9.07)
1 muffin, approx. 1.7 oz.	(135)	(15.0)			(81.6)	(9.07)
Corn Bread Mix, wheat free, gluten free, **Jolly Joan,** 20-oz. box	1911	426.7			95.6	21.33
As prepared (yield: 4½ loaves, approx. 44.4 oz.)	(3751)	(491.6)			(84.4)	(11.06)
1 loaf, approx. 10 oz.	(844)	(110.6)			(84.4)	(11.06)
Country Style Corn Bread & Muffin Mix, **Vermont General Store & Grist Mill,** 17.2-oz. bag	1680	360.0			97.7	20.93
Multi Grain Corn Bread Mix, **Arrowhead Mills,** 32-oz. (2-lb.) bag	3680	608.0			115.0	19.00
As prepared (yield: 2 8" square pans, approx. 49 oz.)	(3680)	(608.0)			(75.1)	(12.40)
1 pan, approx. 24½ oz.	1840	304.0			(75.1)	(12.40)
As prepared (yield: 1 loaf, approx. 25 oz.)	(2520)	(372.0)			(100.8)	(14.88)
Multigrain Corn Bread Mix, **Deaf Smith Farms,** 32-oz. (2-lb.) package	3200	608.0			100.0	19.00
As prepared (yield: 4 loaves, approx. 69 oz.)	(5120)	(608.0)			(73.8)	(8.76)
1 loaf, approx. 17.6 oz.	(1280)	(152.0)			(73.8)	(8.76)
Cranberry Bread Mix, **Pillsbury** "Quick Bread," 16-oz. (1-lb.) box	1760	352.0			110.0	22.00
As prepared (yield: 1 loaf, approx. 23 oz.)	(1920)	(252.0)			(83.5)	(15.30)
Date Bread Mix, **Pillsbury** "Quick Bread," 17-oz. box	1920	400.0			112.9	23.53
As prepared (yield: 1 loaf, approx. 24 oz.)	(2080)	(400.0)			(86.7)	(16.67)
Grainless Bread Mix, **Featherweight,** 32-oz. (2-lb.) package	3760	496.0			117.5	15.50
3 cups mix, prepared as directed (yield: 1 loaf, approx. 22.0 oz.)	(1781)	(226.7)			(81.7)	(10.40)
Low Gluten Bread Mix, **Featherweight,** 32-oz. (2-lb.) package	3000	690.0			93.8	21.56
As prepared for bread (yield: 3 loaves, approx. 51.0 oz.)	3300	690.0			64.7	13.53
1 loaf, approx. 17 oz.	(1100)	(230.0)			64.7	13.53
As prepared for muffins (yield: 58 muffins, approx. 82 oz.)	(5233)	(754.0)			(63.8)	(9.20)
1 muffin, approx. 1.4 oz.	(89)	(12.9)			(63.8)	(9.20)
Low Protein Baking Mix, **Paygel,** 64-oz. (4-lb.) package	7040	1536.0			110.0	24.00
As prepared (yield: 1 loaf, approx. 29.0 oz.)	(1965)	(425.0)			(67.8)	(14.66)
Low Protein Bread Mix, **Jolly Joan,** 20-oz. package	2000	480.0			100.0	24.00
As prepared [yield: 2 loaves, approx. 32 oz. (2 lb.)]	(2059)	(481.6)			64.3	15.05
1 loaf, approx. 16 oz. (1 lb.)	(1030)	(240.8)			64.3	15.05
Masa Trigo Instant Wheat Flour Tortilla Mix, **Quaker,** 64-oz. (4-lb.) box	5610	929.9			87.7	14.53
8-lb. box	11,219	1859.8			87.7	14.53
Nut Bread Mix, **Pillsbury** "Quick Bread," 16.1-oz. box	1920	320.0			119.3	19.88
As prepared (yield: 1 loaf, approx. 24 oz.)	(1920)	(320.0)			(81.7)	(13.62)
Oatmeal Raisin Mix, **Pillsbury** "Quick Bread," 16½-oz. box	1760	352.0			106.7	21.33
As prepared (yield: 1 loaf, approx. 24 oz.)	(1920)	(352.0)			(80.0)	(14.67)
Oat Mix, wheat free, **Jolly Joan,** 20-oz. box	2000	370.0			100.0	18.50
As prepared [yield: 2 loaves, approx. 32 oz. (2 lb.)]	(3535)	(523.5)			(110.5)	(16.36)
1 loaf, approx. 16 oz. (1 lb.)	(1768)	(261.8)			(110.5)	(16.36)
Potato Mix, wheat free, gluten free, **Jolly Joan,** 24-oz. box	2200	544.0			91.7	22.67
As prepared (yield: 2 loaves, approx. 36 oz.)	(3580)	(602.0)			(99.4)	(16.72)
1 loaf, approx. 18 oz.	(1790)	(301.0)			(99.4)	(16.72)
Rice Mix, wheat free, gluten free, low sodium, **Jolly Joan,** 24-oz. box	2500	545.0			104.2	22.71
Prepared as yeast bread [yield: 2 loaves, approx. 32 oz. (2 lbs.)]	(3200)	(580.0)			(100.0)	(18.13)
1 loaf, approx. 16 oz. (1 lb.)	(1600)	(290.0)			(100.0)	(18.13)
Prepared as quick bread (yield: 2.4 loaves, approx. 38.4 oz.)	(3852)	(622.8)			(100.3)	(16.22)
1 loaf, approx. 16 oz. (1 lb.)	(1605)	(259.5)			(100.3)	(16.22)
Rice Mix, wheat free, gluten free, **Jolly Joan,** 24-oz. box	2352	514.0			98.0	21.40
Prepared as yeast bread (yield: 2 loaves, approx. 42 oz.)	(3232)	(580.7)			(77.0)	(13.83)
1 loaf, approx. 21 oz.	(1616)	(290.4)			(77.0)	(13.83)
Prepared as quick bread (yield: 2½ loaves, approx. 47.5 oz.)	(4100)	(607.5)			(86.3)	(12.79)
1 loaf, approx. 19 oz.	(1640)	(243.0)			(86.3)	(12.79)
Rice 'N Rye Bread Mix, wheat free, **Jolly Joan,** 20-oz. box	1950	430.0			97.5	21.50
As prepared [yield: 2 loaves, approx. 32 oz. (2-lb.)]	(3330)	(521.0)			(104.1)	(16.28)
1 loaf, approx. 16 oz. (1 lb.)	(1665)	(260.5)			(104.1)	(16.28)
Rye Bread Mix, **Elam's,** 32-oz. (2-lb.) box	3283	633.3			102.6	19.79
As prepared (yield: 2 loaves, approx. 31½ oz.)	(2310)	(441.0)			(73.3)	(14.00)
1 loaf, approx. 15¾ oz.	(1155)	(221.1)			(73.3)	(14.00)
Wheatless Mix, **Featherweight,** 32-oz. (2-lb.) package	3600	608.0			112.5	19.00
White Bread Mix, **Elam's,** 32-oz. (2-lb.) box	3258	694.1			10.2	21.69
As prepared (yield: 2 loaves, approx. 31⅓ oz.)	(2310)	(441.1)			(73.3)	(14.00)
1 loaf, approx. 15¾ oz.	(1155)	(220.5)			(73.3)	(14.00)

	UNIT Cal.	UNIT Carb.	1 SLICE OR ROLL Cal.	1 SLICE OR ROLL Carb.	1 OZ., BY WT. Cal.	1 OZ., BY WT. Carb.
Whole Wheat Bread Mix, Stone Ground, **Deaf Smith Farms,** 32-oz. (2-lb.) package	3200	624.0			100.0	19.50
As prepared [yield: 2 loaves, approx. 48 oz. (3 lb.)]	3600	648.0			75.0	13.50
1 loaf, approx. 24 oz.	(1800)	(324.0)			75.0	13.50

BISCUIT, MUFFIN, and ROLL MIXES, by brand

BISCUITS

	UNIT Cal.	UNIT Carb.	1 SLICE OR ROLL Cal.	1 SLICE OR ROLL Carb.	1 OZ., BY WT. Cal.	1 OZ., BY WT. Carb.
Baking (Biscuit) Mix, **Jiffy,** 40-oz. box	4640	760.0			116.0	19.00
Buttermilk Biscuit Mix, **Jiffy,** 8-oz. box	920	149.6			115.0	18.70
Whole Grain Biscuit Mix, **Arrowhead Mills,** 32-oz. (2-lb.) bag	3200	608.0			100.0	19.00
As prepared (yield: 32 biscuits, approx. 54 oz.)	(3840)	(608.0)			(71.3)	(11.28)
1 biscuit, approx. 1.7 oz.			(120)	(19.0)	(71.3)	(11.28)

MUFFINS

	UNIT Cal.	UNIT Carb.	1 SLICE OR ROLL Cal.	1 SLICE OR ROLL Carb.	1 OZ., BY WT. Cal.	1 OZ., BY WT. Carb.
Apple Cinnamon Muffin Mix, **Jiffy,** 7-oz. box	872	136.8			124.6	19.54
As prepared (yield: 8 muffins, approx. 9.3 oz.)	1024	137.6			110.3	14.83
1 muffin, approx. 1.16 oz.			128	17.2	110.3	14.83
Barley Mix, wheat free, **Jolly Joan,** 20-oz. box	1850	405.0			92.5	20.25
As prepared (yield: 30 small muffins, approx. 42 oz.)	(3150)	(467.5)			(74.4)	(11.00)
1 muffin, approx. 1.4 oz.			(105)	(15.6)	(74.4)	(11.00)
Blueberry Muffin Mix, **Jiffy,** 7-oz. box	880	139.2			(125.7)	(19.89)
As prepared (yield: 8 muffins, approx. 9.3 oz.)	1000	139.2			(107.5)	(14.96)
1 muffin, approx. 1.16 oz.			125	17.4	(107.5)	(14.96)
(Wild) Blueberry Muffin Mix, **Betty Crocker,** 13½-oz. box	1200	216.0			88.9	16.00
As prepared (yield: 12 muffins, approx. 16.5 oz.)	1400	228.0			(84.7)	(13.41)
1 muffin, approx. 1.4 oz.			120	19.0	(84.7)	(13.41)
(Wild) Blueberry Muffin Mix, **Duncan Hines,** 13-oz. box	1200	204.0			92.3	15.69
As prepared (yield: 12 muffins, approx. 17 oz.)	1320	204.0			(77.6)	(12.00)
1 muffin, approx. 1.4 oz.			110	17.0	(77.6)	(12.00)
Bran Muffin Mix, Whole Grain, **Arrowhead Mills,** 32-oz. (2-lb.) bag						
As prepared (yield: 40 muffins, approx. 56 oz.)	5400	860.0			(96.4)	(15.36)
1 muffin, approx. 1.4 oz.			135	21.6	(96.4)	(15.36)
Bran Muffin Mix, Whole Grain, **Deaf Smith Farms,** 32-oz. (2-lb.) package	3200	576.0			100.0	18.00
As prepared (yield: 40 muffins, approx. 68 oz.)	5400	860.0			(80.1)	(12.75)
1 muffin, approx. 1.7 oz.			135	21.5	(80.1)	(12.75)
Bran Muffin Mix, **Fearn Soy/O,** 12-oz. box	1080	252.0			90.0	21.00
As prepared (yield: 12 muffins, approx. 17 oz.)	1680	270.0			(98.8)	(15.88)
1 muffin, approx. 1.44 oz.			140	22.5	(98.8)	(15.88)
Bran Muffin Mix, **Golden Harvest,** 18-oz. bag	1610	345.0			89.4	19.17
As prepared (yield: 23 muffins, approx. 26 oz.)	2070	368.0			(79.7)	(14.15)
1 muffin, approx. 1.1 oz.			90	16.0	(79.7)	(14.15)
Bran Muffin Mix, (Stone Ground Whole Grain), **Vermont General Store & Grist Mill,** 20.3-oz. bag	1920	360.0			94.6	17.73
As prepared (yield: 24 muffins, approx. 42 oz.)	2640	384.0			62.9	9.14
1 muffin, approx. 1.4 oz. (based on 30 muffins per bag)			88	12.8	62.9	9.14
Bran with Dates Muffin Mix, **Jiffy,** 7-oz. box	872	136.8			124.6	19.54
As prepared (yield: 8 muffins, approx. 9.3 oz.)	1024	137.6			110.1	14.80
1 muffin, approx. 1.16 oz.			128	17.2	110.1	14.80
Cinnamon Nut Muffin Mix, **Betty Crocker,** 13.5-oz. box	1560	240.0			115.6	17.78
As prepared (yield: 12 muffins, approx. 17.3 oz.)	1800	252.0			(104.0)	(14.37)
1 muffin, approx. 1.44 oz.			150	21.0	(104.0)	(14.37)
Corn Bread & Muffin Mix (Country Style), **Vermont General Store & Grist Mill,** 17.2-oz. bag	1680	360.0			97.7	20.93
As prepared (yield: 12 muffins, approx. 24 oz.)	2520	372.0			105.0	15.50
1 muffin, approx. 2 oz.			210	31.0	105.0	15.50
Corn Meal & Rye Muffin Mix, **Golden Harvest,** 18-oz. box	2400	480.0			133.3	26.67
As prepared (yield: 40 muffins, approx. 31.5 oz.)	2800	520.0			(88.9)	(16.51)
1 muffin, approx. 0.8 oz.			70	13.0	(88.9)	(16.51)
Corn Mix, wheat free, gluten free, **Jolly Joan,** 20-oz. box	1911	426.7			95.6	21.33
As prepared (yield: 35½ muffins, approx. 44.4 oz.)	(3751)	(491.6)			(84.4)	(11.06)
1 muffin, approx. 1.25 oz.			(106)	(13.8)	(84.4)	(11.06)
Corn Muffin Mix, **Betty Crocker,** 14-oz. box	1680	288.0			120.0	20.57
As prepared (yield: 12 muffins, approx. 21.0 oz.)	1920	300.0			(91.4)	(14.29)
1 muffin, approx. 1.8 oz.			160	25.0	(91.4)	(14.29)
Corn Muffin Mix, **Dromedary,** 8-oz. box	1040	160.0			120.0	20.00
As prepared (yield: 8 muffins, approx. 11.4 oz.)	1040	160.0			(91.2)	(14.04)
1 muffin, approx. 1.4 oz.			130	20.0	(91.2)	(14.04)
Corn Muffin Mix, **Flako,** 12-oz. box	1392	234.0			116.0	19.50
As prepared (yield: 12 muffins, approx. 17.1 oz.)	1499	244.6			(87.7)	(14.30)
1 muffin, approx. 1.4 oz.			125	20.4	(87.7)	(14.30)
Corn Muffin Mix, **Jiffy,** 8½-oz. box	1016	173.6			119.5	20.42
As prepared (yield: 8 muffins, approx. 11 oz.)	1128	170.4			(102.5)	(15.49)
1 muffin, approx. 1.37 oz.			141	21.3	(102.5)	(15.49)
Corn Muffin Mix, **Pillsbury**	780	120.0				
As prepared (yield: 6 muffins)	780	120.0				
1 muffin			130	20.0		
Grainless Muffin Mix, **Featherweight,** 32-oz. (2-lb.) package	3760	496.0			117.5	15.50
As prepared (yield: 48 muffins, approx. 67 oz.)	(5368)	(596.0)			(78.9)	(8.76)
1 muffin, approx. 1.4 oz.			(112)	(12.4)	(78.9)	(8.76)
Honey Date Muffin Mix, **Jiffy,** 7-oz. box	824	144.8			117.7	20.69
As prepared (yield: 8 muffins, approx. 9⅓ oz.)	960	145.6			102.6	15.55
1 muffin, approx. 1.17 oz.			120	18.2	102.6	15.55
Multi-grain Muffin Mix, **Ell Liberty Natural Mixes,** 8-oz. package	840	144.0			105.0	18.00
As prepared (yield: 12 muffins, approx. 18.5 oz.)	1440	163.2			(77.8)	(8.82)
1 muffin, approx. 1.5 oz.			120	13.6	(77.8)	(8.82)
Oat Mix, wheat free, **Jolly Joan,** 20-oz. box	2000	370.0			100.0	18.50
As prepared for muffins (yield: 27 muffins, approx. 38.6 oz.)	(2378)	(406.7)			(62.9)	(10.76)
1 muffin, approx. 1.4 oz.			(90)	(15.3)	(62.9)	(10.76)
Popover Mix, **Flako,** 6-oz. box	612	117.6			102.0	19.60
Prepared as package directs (yield: 6 popovers)	946	133.6				
1 popover			158	22.3		
Potato Mix, wheat free, gluten free, **Jolly Joan,** 24-oz. box	2200	544.0			91.7	22.67
As prepared for muffins (yield: 30 muffins, approx. 43 oz.)	(6120)	(1064.7)			(143.9)	(24.76)
1 muffin, approx. 1.4 oz.			204	35.1	(143.9)	(24.76)
Rice Mix, low sodium, **Jolly Joan,** 24-oz. box	2500	545.0			104.2	22.71
As prepared for muffins (yield: 30 muffins, approx. 43 oz.)	(3813)	(600.0)			(88.7)	(13.95)
1 muffin, approx. 1.4 oz.			(127)	(20.0)	(88.7)	(13.95)
Rice Mix, wheat free, gluten free, **Jolly Joan,** 24-oz. box	2352	514.0			98.0	21.40
As prepared for muffins (yield: 30 muffins, approx. 43 oz.)	(3838)	(597.5)			(90.3)	(14.06)
1 muffin, approx. 1.4 oz.			(128)	(19.9)	(90.3)	(14.06)
Rice 'N Rye Bread Mix, wheat free, **Jolly Joan,** 20-oz. box	1950	430.0			97.5	21.50
As prepared for muffins (yield: 30 muffins, approx. 43 oz.)	(3263)	(107.5)			(76.8)	(12.06)
1 muffin, approx. 1.4 oz.			(109)	(17.1)	(76.8)	(12.06)
Whole Wheat Muffin Mix, **Elam's** 3-in-1, 32-oz. (2-lb.) package	3203	637.8			100.1	19.93
As prepared (yield: approx. 75.5 oz., 47 muffins)	(5035)	(821.7)			(66.7)	(10.88)
1 muffin, approx. 1.6 oz.			(107)	(17.5)	(66.7)	(10.88)

ROLLS

	UNIT Cal.	UNIT Carb.	1 SLICE OR ROLL Cal.	1 SLICE OR ROLL Carb.	1 OZ., BY WT. Cal.	1 OZ., BY WT. Carb.
Hot Roll Mix, **Pillsbury,** 13¾-oz. box	1440	248.0			104.7	18.04
As prepared (yield: approx. 19½ oz., 16 rolls)	1520	248.0			(78.5)	(12.81)
1 roll, approx. 1.2 oz.			95	15.5	(78.5)	(12.81)

PREPACKAGED BREADS AND ROLLS, based on generic data

	UNIT Cal.	UNIT Carb.	1 SLICE OR ROLL Cal.	1 SLICE OR ROLL Carb.	1 OZ., BY WT. Cal.	1 OZ., BY WT. Carb.	Fiber per oz. (GMS.)
CRACKED WHEAT BREAD							
1 loaf, 16 oz. (1 lb.) (2g/15g/1g/35%/147mg)	1193	236.3			74.6	14.77	0.14
Toasted (yield: approx. 13.4 oz.) (3g/18g/1g/23%/179mg)	1193	236.3			88.8	17.58	0.17
1 slice, approx. 1/18 of loaf, approx. 4" wide, 4½" high, 9/16" thick (approx. 0.9 oz.)			66	13.0	74.6	14.77	0.14
Toasted (yield: approx. ¾ oz.)			66	13.0	88.8	17.58	0.17
1 pound of toasted cracked wheat bread	1420	281.3			88.8	17.58	0.17
FRENCH BREAD AND ROLLS							
1 loaf, 16 oz. (1 lb.) (3g/16g/1g/31%/164mg)	1315	251.4			82.2	15.71	0.06
1 slice:							
Approx. 1/30 of loaf, 2½" wide, 2" high, ½" thick (approx. 0.5 oz.)			44	8.3	82.2	15.71	0.06
Approx. 1/13 of loaf, 5" wide, 2½" high, 1" thick (approx. 1.2 oz.)			102	19.3	82.2	15.71	0.06
1 roll, hoagie or submarine, 11½" long, 3" wide, 2½" thick (approx. 4.8 oz.)	392	74.8			82.2	15.71	0.06
1 pound of toasted French bread (3g/17g/1g/19%/191mg)	1445	276.2			90.3	17.26	0.07
ITALIAN BREAD							
1 loaf, 16 oz. (1 lb.) (3g/16g/tr/32%/585mg)	1252	255.8			78.3	15.99	0.06
1 slice:							
Approx. 1/46 of loaf, 3¼" wide, 2½" high, ½" thick (approx. 0.4 oz.)			27	5.6	78.3	15.99	0.06
Approx. 1/15 of loaf, 4½" wide, 3¼" high, ¾" thick (approx. 1.1 oz.)			86	17.6	78.3	15.99	0.06
PUMPERNICKEL BREAD							
1 loaf, 16 oz. (1 lb.) (3g/15g/tr/34%/101mg)	1116	240.9			69.8	15.06	0.31
1 slice, approx. 1/14 of loaf, 5" wide, 4" high, ⅜" thick (approx. 1.1 oz.)			79	17.0	69.8	15.06	0.31
1 slice, from "snack-sized" loaf, approx. 1/32 of an 8-oz. (½-lb.) loaf, approx. 1½" wide, 2" high, ¼" thick (approx. ¼ oz.)			17	3.8	69.8	15.06	0.31
RAISIN BREAD							
1 loaf, 16 oz. (1 lb.) (2g/15g/1g/35%/103mg)	1188	243.1			74.3	15.19	0.26
Toasted (yield: approx. 13.26 oz.) (2g/18g/1g/22%/125mg)	1188	243.1			89.6	18.33	0.31
1 slice, approx. 1/18 of loaf, 3¾" wide, 3⅝" high, ½" thick (approx. 0.9 oz.)			66	13.4	74.3	15.19	0.26
Toasted (yield: approx. ¾ oz.)			66	13.4	89.6	18.33	0.31
1 pound of toasted raisin bread	1433	293.3			89.6	18.35	0.31
RYE BREAD (made from ⅔ clear flour, ⅓ rye flour)							
1 loaf, 16 oz. (1 lb.) (3g/15g/tr/36%/158mg)	1102	236.3			68.9	14.77	0.11
Toasted (yield: approx. 13.8 oz.) (3g/17g/tr/25%/na)	1102	236.3			79.9	17.15	0.14
1 slice, approx. 1/18 of loaf, 4¾" wide, 3¾" high, 7/16" thick, approx. 0.9 oz.			66	13.0	68.9	14.77	0.11
Toasted (yield: approx. 0.76 oz.)			66	13.0	79.9	17.15	0.14
1 slice, from "snack-sized" loaf, approx. 1/32 of an 8-oz. (½-lb.) loaf, 1½" wide, 2" high, ¼" thick (approx. ¼ oz.)			17	3.6	68.9	14.77	
Toasted (yield: approx. 0.2 oz.)			17	3.6	79.9	17.15	0.14
1 pound of toasted rye bread	1279	274.4			79.9	17.15	0.14
SALT-RISING BREAD							
1 loaf, 16 oz. (1 lb.) (2g/15g/1g/37%/75mg)	1211	236.8			75.7	14.80	0.28
Toasted (yield: approx. 14.4 oz.) (2g/16g/1g/29%/83mg)	1211	236.8			84.1	16.44	0.28
1 slice, approx. 1/19 of loaf, 4⅛" wide, 4½" high, 7/16" thick, (approx. 0.9 oz.)			64	12.6	75.7	14.80	0.28
Toasted (yield: approx. 0.8 oz.)			66	12.8	84.1	16.44	0.28
1 pound of toasted salt-rising bread	1346	236.8			84.1	16.44	0.28

	UNIT Cal.	UNIT Carb.	1 SLICE OR ROLL Cal.	1 SLICE OR ROLL Carb.	1 OZ., BY WT. Cal.	1 OZ., BY WT. Carb.	Fiber per oz. (GMS.)
VIENNA BREAD and ROLLS							
1 loaf, 16 oz. (1 lb.) (3g/16g/1g/31%/164mg)	1315	251.4			82.2	15.71	0.06
1 slice, approx. 1/18 of loaf, 4¾" wide, 4" high, ½" thick (approx. 0.9 oz.)			73	13.9	82.2	15.71	0.06
1 roll, hoagie or submarine, 11½" long, 3" wide, 2½" thick, (approx. 4.8 oz.)	392	74.8			82.2	15.71	0.06
1 pound of toasted Vienna bread (3g/17g/1g/19%/191mg)	1445	276.2			90.3	17.26	
WHITE BREAD, soft-crumb type (made by continuous mix or conventional method)							
1 loaf, 16 oz. (1 lb.) (2g/14g/1g/36%/144mg)	1225	229.1			76.6	14.32	0.06
Toasted (yield: approx. 13.75 oz. (3g/17g/1g/25%/167mg)	1225	229.1			89.0	16.66	0.07
1 slice, approx. 1/18 of loaf, 4" wide, 4¼" high, 9/16" thick (approx. 0.88 oz.)			68	12.6	76.6	14.32	0.06
Toasted (yield: approx. 0.77 oz.)			68	12.6	89.0	16.66	0.07
"Thin slice," 1/22 of loaf, 4" wide, 4" high, 7/16" thick (approx. 0.7 oz.)			54	10.1	76.6	14.32	0.06
Toasted, yield: approx. 0.6 oz.			54	10.1	89.0	16.66	0.07
1 loaf, 24 oz.	1836	343.4			76.6	14.32	0.06
Toasted (yield: approx. 20.63 oz.)	1836	343.4			89.0	16.66	0.06
1 slice, approx. 1/24 of loaf, 4⅜" wide, 4" high, 9/16" thick (approx. 1 oz.)			76	14.3	76.6	14.32	0.06
Toasted (yield: approx. 0.85 oz.)			76	14.3	89.0	16.66	0.07
"Thin slice," 1/28 of loaf, 4" wide, 3⅞" high, ½" thick (approx. 0.85 oz.)			65	12.1	76.6	14.32	0.06
Toasted (yield: approx. 0.74 oz.)			65	12.1	89.0	16.66	0.07
WHITE BREAD, firm-crumb type (made by conventional method)							
1 loaf, 16 oz. (1 lb.) (3g/14g/1g/35%/140mg)	1247	227.7			77.9	14.23	0.06
Toasted (yield: approx. 13¾ oz. (3g/17g/2g/24%/163mg)	1247	227.7			90.6	16.55	0.07
1 slice:							
Approx. 1/20 of loaf, 3¾" wide, 4" high, 7/16" thick (approx. 0.81 oz.)			63	11.5	77.9	14.23	0.06
Toasted (yield: approx. 0.7 oz.)			63	16.5	90.7	16.55	0.07
Approx. 1/30 of loaf, 3¾" wide, 4" high, ¼" thick (approx. 0.53 oz.)			41	7.5	77.9	14.23	0.06
Toasted (yield: approx. 0.45 oz.)			41	7.5	90.7	16.55	0.07
1 loaf, 32 oz. (2 lbs.)	2494	455.3			77.9	14.23	0.06
Toasted (yield: approx. 27½ oz.)	2494	455.3			90.7	16.55	0.07
1 slice, approx. 1/34 of loaf, 3⅝" wide, 4¼" high, 7/16" thick (approx. 0.95 oz.)			74	13.6	77.9	14.23	0.06
Toasted (yield: approx. 0.81 oz.)			74	13.6	90.7	16.55	0.07
WHOLE WHEAT BREAD, firm-crumb type							
1 loaf, 16 oz. (1 lb.) (3g/14g/1g/36%/149mg)	1102	216.4			68.9	13.53	0.45
Toasted (yield: approx. 13.44 oz. (4g/16g/1g/24%/178mg)	1102	216.4			82.2	16.15	0.54
1 slice, approx. 1/20 of loaf, 3⅞" wide, 3⅝" high, 7/16" thick (approx. 0.81 oz.)			56	11.0	68.9	13.53	0.45
Toasted (yield: approx. 0.67 oz.)			56	11.0	82.2	16.15	0.54
1 slice, approx. 1/18 of loaf, rounded top, 4" wide, 4" high, 7/16" thick (approx. 0.88 oz.)			66	11.9	68.9	13.53	0.45
Toasted (yield: approx. 0.74 oz.)			66	11.9	82.2	16.15	0.54
1 pound of toasted firm-crumb whole wheat bread	1311	257.2			82.2	16.15	0.54
WHOLE WHEAT BREAD, soft-crumb type							
1 loaf, 16 oz. (1 lb.) (3g/14g/1g/36%/150mg)	1093	223.6			68.3	13.98	0.45
Toasted (yield: approx. 13.44 oz. (3g/17g/1g/24%/179mg)	1093	223.6			81.6	16.69	0.54
1 slice, 1/16 of loaf, 4⅛" wide, 3⅝" high, 9/16" thick (approx. 1 oz.)			67	13.8	68.3	13.98	0.45
Toasted (yield: approx. 0.85 oz.)			67	13.8	81.6	16.69	0.54
1 pound of toasted soft-crumb whole wheat bread	1302	226.3			81.6	16.69	0.54

PREPACKAGED BREAD, by brand

	ENTIRE LOAF Cal.	ENTIRE LOAF Carb.	1 SLICE Cal.	1 SLICE Carb.	1 OZ., BY WT. Cal.	1 OZ., BY WT. Carb.	1 CUP CRUMBS FINE, DRY Cal.	1 CUP CRUMBS FINE, DRY Carb.
AMERICAN GRANARY								
American Granary Bread, **Arnold,** 16-oz. (1-lb.) loaf (approx. 18 slices)	1260	225.0			78.8	14.06	(297)	(53.0)
1 slice, approx. 0.89 oz.			70	12.5	78.8	14.06	(297)	(53.0)
BAGELS are listed toward the end of this chapter under Specialty Breads And Rolls.								
BAGUETTE and BATARD, see FRENCH BREAD								
BLACK BREAD								
Old World Style Black Bread, **Mrs. Wright's,** 16-oz. (1-lb.) loaf (approx. 20 slices)	1106	210.2			69.1	13.14	(261)	(49.5)
1 slice, approx. 0.72 oz.			50	9.5	69.1	13.14	(261)	(49.5)
Russian Black Bread, **Old Stone Mill,** 16-oz. (1-lb.) loaf (approx. 16 slices)	1280	240.0			80.0	15.00	(302)	(56.6)
1 slice, approx. 1 oz.			80	15.0	80.0	15.00	(302)	(56.6)
BRAN								
Bran For Life Bread, **Bran For Life,** 24-oz. loaf (approx. 20 slices)	1500	280.0			62.5	11.67	(236)	(44.1)
1 slice, approx. 1.2 oz.			75	14.0	62.5	11.67	(236)	(44.1)
BRAN PITA, see Pita Bread toward the end of this chapter under Specialty Breads And Rolls								
Bran'Nola, Original, **Arnold** 24-oz. loaf (approx. 20 slices)	1800	324.0			75.0	13.50	(283)	(50.9)
1 slice, approx. 1.2 oz.			100	18.0	75.0	18.50	(283)	(50.9)
Grain Belt Granola Bran Bread, **Mrs. Wright's,** 24-oz. loaf (approx. 20 slices)	1790	313.4			74.6	13.06	(281)	(49.2)
1 slice, approx. 1.2 oz.			100	17.5	74.6	13.06	(281)	(49.2)
Whole Bran Bread, **Branberry,** 16-oz. (1-lb.) loaf (approx. 16 slices)	1200	240.0			75.0	15.00	(283)	(56.6)
1 slice, approx. 1 oz.			75	15.0	75.0	15.00	(283)	(56.6)
Whole Bran & Honey Bread, **Hearth Farms,** 24-oz. loaf (approx. 18 slices)	1740	336.0			72.5	14.00	(274)	(528)
1 slice, approx. 1⅓ oz.			97	18.7	72.5	14.00	(274)	(528)
BROWN BREAD								
Brown Bread, **Underwood,** 16-oz. (1-lb.) can (not presliced)	832	182.4			52.0	11.40	(196)	(43.0)
Brown Bread with Raisins, **Underwood,** 16-oz. (1-lb.) can (not presliced)	832	177.6			52.0	11.10	(196)	(41.8)
BUCKWHEAT								
Buckwheat Bread, **Butternut,** 20-oz. loaf (approx. 20 slices)	1500	250.0			75.0	12.50	(284)	(47.3)
1 slice, approx. 1 oz.			75	12.5	75.0	12.50	(284)	(47.3)
Buckwheat Bread, **Millbrook,** 24-oz. loaf (approx. 24 slices)	1800	300.0			75.0	12.50	(284)	(47.3)
1 slice, approx. 1 oz.			75	12.5	75.0	12.50	(284)	(47.3)
BUNS are listed toward the end of this chapter under Prepackaged Buns And Rolls.								
BUTTER & EGG								
Butter & Egg Bread, **Mrs. Wright's,** 16-oz. loaf (approx. 16 slices) (1-lb.)	1200	200.0			75.0	12.50	(283)	(47.1)
1 slice, approx. 1 oz.			75	12.5	75.0	12.50	(283)	(47.1)
BUTTER TOP								
Butter Top Bread, **Home Pride,** 20-oz. loaf (approx. 20 slices)	1500	260.0			75.0	13.00	(283)	(49.0)
1 slice, approx. 1 oz.			75	13.0	75.0	13.00	(283)	(49.0)
Homestyle Butter Top Wheat Bread, **Mrs. Wright's,** 24-oz. loaf (approx. 20 slices)	1866	329.2			77.7	13.72	(293)	(51.7)
1 slice, approx. 1.09 oz.			85	15.0	77.7	13.72	(293)	(51.7)
BUTTERMILK								
Buttermilk Bread, **Butternut,** 20-oz. loaf (approx. 20 slices)	1600	270.0			80.0	13.50	(302)	(51.0)
1 slice, approx. 1 oz.			80	13.5	80.0	13.50	(302)	(51.0)
Buttermilk Bread, **Eddy's,** 24-oz. loaf (approx. 24 slices)	1800	324.0			75.0	13.50	(284)	(51.0)
1 slice, approx. 1 oz.			75	13.5	75.0	13.50	(284)	(51.0)
Buttermilk Bread, **Millbrook,** 24-oz. loaf (approx. 24 slices)	1800	324.0			75.0	13.50	(284)	(51.0)
1 slice, approx. 1 oz.			75	13.5	75.0	13.50	(284)	(51.0)
Buttermilk Bread, **Mrs. Karl's,** 24-oz. loaf (approx. 24 slices)	1920	324.0			80.0	13.50	(302)	(51.0)
1 slice, approx. 1 oz.			80	13.5	80.0	13.50	(302)	(51.0)
Buttermilk Bread, **Sweetheart,** 24-oz. loaf (approx. 24 slices)	1800	324.0			75.0	13.50	(284)	(51.0)
1 slice, approx. 1 oz.			75	13.5	75.0	13.50	(284)	(51.0)
CEREAL GRAIN								
Cereal Grain Bread, **Mrs. Wright's,** 24-oz. loaf (approx. 16 slices)	1791	313.3			74.6	13.06	(281)	(49.2)
1 slice, approx. 1.34 oz.			100	17.5	74.6	13.06	(281)	(49.2)
CHALLAH BREAD								
Enriched Challah Bread, **Jane Parker (A&P),** 16-oz. (1-lb.) loaf (approx. 16 slices)	1200	208.0			75.0	13.00	(283)	(49.0)
1 slice, approx. 1 oz.			75	13.0	75.0	13.00	(283)	(49.0)
CHAPATI BREAD								
Chapati Bread, Unleavened, **Garden of Eatin',** 8-oz. (approx. 6 slices)	672	126.2			84.0	15.77	(317)	(59.5)
1 slice, approx. 1.33 oz.			112	21.0	84.0	15.77	(317)	(59.5)
CHEESE ONION								
Cheese Onion Bread, **Mrs. Wright's,** 24-oz. loaf (approx. 16 slices)	1790	313.3			74.6	13.06	(281)	(49.2)
1 slice, approx. 1.34 oz.			112	21.0	74.6	13.06	(281)	(49.2)
CINNAMON								
Cinnamon Bread, **Pepperidge Farm,** 16-oz. (1-lb.) loaf (approx. 16 slices)	1280	200.0			80.0	12.50	(604)	(94.4)
1 slice, approx. 1 oz.			80	12.5	80.0	12.50	(604)	(94.4)
Cinnamon Raisin Loaf, **Thomas',** 12-oz. loaf (approx. 16 slices)	935	174.8			78.0	14.57	(294)	(55.0)
1 slice, approx. 0.78 oz.			60	11.5	78.0	14.57	(294)	(55.0)
CORN								
Corn Bread, **Brownberry,** 16-oz. (1-lb.) loaf (approx. 16 slices)	1200	248.0			75.0	15.50	(283)	(58.4)
1 slice, approx. 1 oz.			75	15.5	75.0	15.50	(283)	(58.4)
Corn & Molasses Bread, **Pepperidge Farm,** 16-oz. (1-lb.) loaf (approx. 18 slices)	1260	243.0			78.8	15.19	(297)	(57.3)
1 slice, approx. 0.89 oz.			70	13.5	78.8	15.19	(297)	(57.3)
Indian Corn Bread, **Balanced,** 16-oz. (1-lb.) loaf (approx. 16 slices)	1280	256.0			80.0	16.00	(302)	(60.3)
1 slice, approx. 1 oz.			80	16.0	80.0	16.00	(302)	(60.3)
CORNTILLAS								
Corntillas, **Garden of Eatin',** 12-oz. package, (approx. 12 slices)	768	136.2			64.0	11.35		
1 slice, approx. 1 oz.			64	11.3	64.0	11.35		
COUNTRY OAT								
Country Oat, **Bran-nola,** 24-oz. loaf (approx. 18 slices)	1980	342.0			82.5	14.25	(311)	(53.7)
1 slice, approx. 1.3 oz.			110	19.0	82.5	14.25	(311)	(53.7)
CRACKED WHEAT								
Cracked Wheat Bread, **Pepperidge Farm,** 16-oz. (1-lb.) loaf (approx. 18 slices)	1260	264.0			78.8	14.63	(297)	(55.2)
1 slice, approx. 0.89 oz.			70	13.0	78.8	14.63	(297)	(55.2)
Cracked Wheat Bread, **Wonder,** 16-oz. (1-lb.) loaf (approx. 16 slices)	1200	216.0			75.0	13.50	(283)	(50.9)
1 slice, approx. 1 oz.			75	13.5	75.0	13.50	(283)	(50.9)
CROISSANTS are listed toward the end of this chapter under Specialty Breads And Rolls.								
CRUSHED WHEAT								
Crushed Wheat Bread, **Mrs. Wright's,** 16-oz. (1-lb.) loaf (approx. 16 slices)	1362	254.0			85.1	15.88	(321)	(59.9)
1 slice, approx. 1 oz.			85	15.9	85.1	15.88	(321)	(59.9)
24-oz. loaf (approx. 20 slices)	1866	362.1			77.7	15.09	(293)	(56.9)
1 slice, approx. 1.09 oz.			85	16.5	77.7	15.09	(293)	(56.9)

	ENTIRE LOAF Cal.	ENTIRE LOAF Carb.	1 SLICE Cal.	1 SLICE Carb.	1 OZ., BY WT. Cal.	1 OZ., BY WT. Carb.	1 CUP CRUMBS FINE, DRY Cal.	1 CUP CRUMBS FINE, DRY Carb.
Crushed Wheat Sandwich Bread, **Mrs. Wright's,** 24-oz. loaf (approx. 26 slices)	1805	361.0			75.2	15.04	(284)	(56.7)
1 slice, approx. 0.86 oz.			65	13.0	75.2	15.04	(284)	(56.7)
DARK BREAD								
Dark Bread, **Hollywood,** 16-oz. (1-lb.) loaf (approx. 16 slices)	1120	200.0			70.0	12.50	(264)	(47.1)
1 slice, approx. 1 oz.			70	12.5	70.0	12.50	(264)	(47.1)
Dark Bread, **Profile,** 16-oz. (1-lb.) loaf (approx. 16 slices)	1200	200.0			75.0	12.50	(283)	(47.1)
1 slice, approx. 1 oz.			75	12.5	75.0	12.50	(283)	(47.1)
Dark Style Bread, **Mrs. Wright's,** 16-oz. (1-lb.) loaf (approx. 20 slices)	1106	199.1			69.1	12.45	(261)	(46.9)
1 slice, approx. 0.8 oz.			50	9.0	69.1	12.45	(261)	(46.9)
Dark Wheat Bread, **Bran'nola** (Arnold), 24-oz. loaf (approx. 18 slices)	1800	324.0			75.0	13.50	(283)	(50.9)
1 slice, approx. 1⅓ oz.			100	18.0	75.0	13.50	(283)	(50.9)
Sandwich Dark Bread, **Branberry,** 24-oz. loaf (approx. 24 slices)	1680	348.0			70.0	14.50	(264)	(54.7)
1 slice, approx. 1 oz.			70	14.5	70.0	14.50	(264)	(54.7)
DATE NUT								
Date Nut Loaf, **Shiloh Farms,** 24-oz. loaf (approx. 10 slices)	2120	380.0			88.3	15.83	(333)	(59.7)
1 slice, approx. 2.4 oz.			212	38.0	88.3	15.83	(333)	(59.7)
Date Walnut Bread, **Pepperidge Farm,** 16-oz. (1-lb.) loaf (approx. 16 slices)	1200	200.0			75.0	11.50	(566)	(43.4)
1 slice, approx. 1 oz.			75	11.5	75.0	11.50	(566)	(43.4)
EGG								
Egg Twist, **Millbrook,** 24-oz. loaf (approx. 24 slices)	1800	336.0			75.0	14.00	(284)	(52.9)
1 slice, approx. 1 oz.			75	14.0	75.0	14.00	(284)	(52.9)
ENGLISH MUFFINS are listed toward the end of this chapter under Specialty Breads And Rolls.								
English Muffin Style Enriched Bread, **Mrs. Wright's,** 16-oz. (1-lb.) loaf (approx. 18 slices)	1210	231.8			75.6	14.49	(285)	(54.6)
1 slice, approx. 0.79 oz.			60	11.5	75.6	14.49	(285)	(54.6)
English Muffin Toasting Bread, **Northridge,** 16-oz. (1-lb.) loaf (approx. 14 slices)	1120	210.0			70.0	13.13	(264)	(49.5)
1 slice, approx. 1.14 oz.			80	15.0	70.0	13.13	(264)	(49.5)
ENRICHED *(There are many enriched breads throughout the chapter, but the following are breads named, simply, "Enriched.")*								
Enriched Bread, **Heavenly,** 20-oz. loaf (approx. 20 slices)	1500	290.0			75.0	14.50	(284)	(54.8)
1 slice, approx. 1 oz.			75	14.5	75.0	14.50	(284)	(54.8)
Enriched Bread, **Homestyle,** 24-oz. loaf (approx. 24 slices)	1646	307.3			68.6	12.80	(259)	(48.3)
1 slice, approx. 1.1 oz.			75	14.0	68.6	12.80	(259)	(48.3)
Enriched Bread, **Mrs. Wright's,** 24-oz. loaf (approx. 20 slices)	1757	329.2			73.2	13.72	(276)	(51.7)
1 slice, approx. 1.09 oz.			80	15.0	73.2	13.72	(276)	(51.7)
Enriched Bread, **Safeway,** 24-oz. loaf (approx. 20 slices)	1866	362.1			77.7	15.09	(293)	(56.9)
1 slice, approx. 1.09 oz.			85	16.5	77.7	15.00	(293)	(56.9)
Enriched Bread, **Sloan's,** 22-oz. loaf (approx. 22 slices)	1650	297.0			75.0	13.50	(284)	(51.0)
1 slice, approx. 1 oz.			75	13.5	75.0	13.50	(284)	(51.0)
Enriched Bread made with Buttermilk, **A&P,** 22-oz. loaf (approx. 22 slices)	1650	286.0			75.0	13.00	(284)	(49.1)
1 slice, approx. 1 oz.			75	13.0	75.0	13.00	(284)	(49.1)
Enriched Thin Bread, **Millbrook,** 24-oz. loaf (approx. 24 slices)	1800	324.0			75.0	13.50	(284)	(51.0)
1 slice, approx. 1 oz.			75	13.5	75.0	13.50	(284)	(51.0)
14 GRAIN								
14 Grain Bread, Stone Ground, **Foods for Life Bakery,** 16-oz. (1-lb.) loaf, approx. 16 slices)	1280	232.0			80.0	14.50	(302)	(54.7)
1 slice, approx. 1 oz.			80	14.5	80.0	14.50	(302)	(54.7)
FRENCH BREAD								
Baguette (sugar-free French bread), **Country French, Cie,** 8-oz. loaf (not presliced)	560	136.0			70.0	17.00	(264)	(64.1)

	ENTIRE LOAF Cal.	ENTIRE LOAF Carb.	1 SLICE Cal.	1 SLICE Carb.	1 OZ., BY WT. Cal.	1 OZ., BY WT. Carb.	1 CUP CRUMBS FINE, DRY Cal.	1 CUP CRUMBS FINE, DRY Carb.
Barbecue French Style Bread, **Mrs. Wright's,** 16-oz. (1-lb.) loaf (approx. 18 slices)	1179	217.7			73.7	13.61	(278)	(51.3)
1 slice, approx. 0.89 oz.			65	12.0	73.7	13.61	(278)	(51.3)
Batard (sugar-free French bread), **Country French, Cie,** 16-oz. (1-lb.) loaf (not presliced)	1120	272.0			70.0	17.00	(264)	(64.1)
Brown & Serve French Bread, **Pepperidge Farm,** 16-oz. (1-lb.) loaf (approx. 16 slices)	1200	216.0			75.0	13.50	(264)	(50.9)
1 slice, approx. 1 oz.			75	13.5	75.0	13.50	(264)	(50.9)
Enriched French Bread, **Eddy's,** 16-oz. (1-lb.) loaf (approx. 16 slices)	1200	232.0			75.0	14.50	(284)	(54.8)
1 slice, approx. 1 oz.			75	14.5	75.0	14.50	(284)	(54.8)
Extra Sour Dark Crusty French Bread, **Parisian,** 16-oz. (1-lb.) loaf, (approx. 16 slices)	1088	216.0			68.0	13.50	(256)	(50.9)
1 slice, approx. 1 oz.			68	13.5	68.0	13.50	(256)	(50.9)
French Bread, **Eddy's,** 16-oz. (1-lb.) loaf (approx. 16 slices)	1200	232.0			75.0	14.50	(284)	(54.8)
1 slice, approx. 1 oz.			75	14.5	75.0	14.50	(284)	(54.8)
French Bread, **Pepperidge Farm,** 16-oz. (1-lb.) loaf (approx. 16 slices)	1200	224.0			75.0	14.00	(283)	(52.8)
1 slice, approx. 1 oz.			75	14.0	75.0	14.00	(283)	(52.8)
French Bread, **Pioneer,** 16-oz. (1-lb.) loaf (approx. 16 slices)	1200	240.0			75.0	15.00	(283)	(56.6)
1 slice, approx. 1 oz.			75	15.0	75.0	15.00	(283)	(56.6)
French Bread, **Wonder,** 16-oz. (1-lb.) loaf (approx. 16 slices)	1200	216.0			75.0	13.50	(264)	(50.9)
1 slice, approx. 1 oz.			75	13.5	75.0	13.50	(264)	(50.9)
French Sour Dough Bread, **Millbrook,** 16-oz. (1-lb.) loaf (approx. 16 slices)	1200	248.0			75.0	15.50	(284)	(58.6)
1 slice, approx. 1 oz.			75	15.5	75.0	15.50	(284)	(58.6)
French Style Bread, **Mrs. Wright's,** 16-oz. (1-lb.) loaf (approx. 18 slices)	1179	217.7			73.7	13.61	(278)	(51.3)
1 slice, approx. 0.88 oz.			65	12.0	73.7	13.61	(278)	(51.3)
French Style Enriched Bread, **Butternut,** 16-oz. (1-lb.) loaf (approx. 16 slices)	1200	304.0			75.0	19.00	(284)	(71.8)
1 slice, approx. 1 oz.			75	19.0	75.0	19.00	(284)	(71.8)
French Style Enriched Bread, **Dutch Hearth,** 16-oz. (1-lb.) loaf (approx. 16 slices)	1120	232.0			70.0	14.50	(265)	(54.8)
1 slice, approx. 16 oz.			70	14.5	70.0	14.50	(265)	(54.8)
French Style Enriched Bread, **Holsum,** 16-oz. (1-lb.) loaf (approx. 16 slices)	1200	232.0			75.0	14.50	(284)	(54.8)
1 slice, approx. 1 oz.			75	14.5	75.0	14.50	(284)	(54.8)
Old Country Type, Extra Sour French Bread, **Toscana's,** 16-oz. (1-lb.) loaf (approx. 16 slices)	1120	240.0			70.0	15.00	(264)	(56.6)
1 slice, approx. 1 oz.			70	15.0	70.0	15.00	(264)	(56.6)
Old Country Type, Sweet French Bread, **Toscana's,** 16-oz. (1-lb.) loaf (approx. 16 slices)	1120	224.0			70.0	14.00	(264)	(52.8)
1 slice, approx. 1 oz.			70	14.0	70.0	14.00	(264)	(52.8)
San Francisco Fisherman's Wharf Style, Extra Sour French Bread, **Toscana's,** 16-oz. (1-lb.) loaf (approx. 16 slices)	1200	264.0			75.0	16.50	(283)	(62.2)
1 slice, approx. 1 oz.			75	16.5	75.0	16.50	(283)	(62.2)
Sour Dough French Bread, **Hearth Farms,** 24-oz. loaf (approx. 18 slices)	1680	348.0			70.0	14.50	(264)	(54.7)
1 slice, approx. 1⅓ oz.			93	19.3	70.0	14.50	(264)	(54.7)
Sour Dough French Bread, **Weber's,** 16-oz. (1-lb.) loaf (approx. 16 slices)	1200	248.0			75.0	15.50	(284)	(58.6)
1 slice, approx. 1 oz.			75	15.5	75.0	15.50	(284)	(58.6)
Sour French Bread, **Parisian,** 16-oz. (1-lb.) loaf (approx. 16 slices)	1088	216.0			68.0	13.50	(256)	(50.9)
1 slice, approx. 1 oz.			68	13.5	68.0	13.50	(256)	(50.9)
Sweet French Bread, **Parisian,** 16-oz. (1-lb.) loaf (approx. 16 slices)	1088	216.0			68.0	13.50	(256)	(50.9)
1 slice, approx. 1 oz.			68	13.5	68.0	13.50	(256)	(50.9)

	ENTIRE LOAF		1 SLICE		1 OZ., BY WT.		1 CUP CRUMBS FINE, DRY	
	Cal.	Carb.	Cal.	Carb.	Cal.	Carb.	Cal.	Carb.
Sweet French Bread, low cholesterol, **Parisian,** 16-oz. (1-lb.) loaf (approx. 16 slices)	1224	424.0			76.5	26.50	(288)	(99.9)
1 slice, approx. 1 oz.			77	26.5	76.5	26.50	(288)	(99.9)
Sweet French Bread, **Toscana's,** 16-oz. (1-lb.) loaf (approx. 16 slices)	1200	248.0			75.0	15.50	(283)	(58.4)
1 slice, approx. 1 oz.			75	15.5	75.0	15.50	(283)	(58.4)
GARLIC BREAD								
Garlic Bread, **Bellacicco,** 8-oz. loaf (not presliced)	656	104.0			82.0	13.00	(309)	(49.0)
Garlic Bread, **Stouffer's,** 10-oz. loaf (approx. 16 slices)	1280	144.0			128.0	14.40	(483)	(54.3)
1 slice, approx. 0.63 oz.			80	9.0	128.0	14.40	(483)	(54.3)
Jewish Garlic Bread, **Empire,** 8 oz. package, 2 loaves (not presliced)	656	96.0			82.0	12.00	(309)	(45.2)
"Suggested" slice, 2 oz. (approx. 4" slice)			164	24.0	82.0	12.00	(309)	(45.2)
GLUTEN BREAD								
Gluten Bread, **Thomas'** "Glutogen," 8-oz. loaf (approx. 19 slices)	570	100.5			70.9	12.56	(268)	(47.4)
1 slice, approx. 0.42 oz.			30	6.0	70.9	12.56	(268)	(47.4)
GRAHAM								
Graham Bread, **Mrs. Wright's,** 24-oz. loaf (approx. 16 slices)	1790	304.3			74.6	12.68	(281)	(47.8)
1 slice, approx. 1.34 oz.			100	17.0	74.6	12.68	(281)	(47.8)
GRAIN BELT								
Grain Belt Bread, **Mrs. Wright's,** 24-oz. loaf (approx. 20 slices)	1982	330.3			82.6	13.76	(311)	(51.9)
1 slice, approx. 1.2 oz.			99	16.5	82.6	13.76	(311)	(51.9)
Grain Belt Granola Bran Bread, **Mrs. Wright's,** 24-oz. loaf (approx. 16 slices)	1790	313.4			74.6	13.06	(281)	(49.2)
1 slice, approx. 1.34 oz.			100	17.5	74.6	13.06	(281)	(49.2)
Grain Belt Yogurt-Oatmeal Bread, **Mrs. Wright's,** 24-oz. loaf (approx. 16 slices)	1790	313.4			74.6	13.06	(281)	(49.2)
1 slice, approx. 1.5 oz.			112	19.6	74.6	13.06	(281)	(49.2)
GRANOLA								
Granola Brown Bread, **Mrs. Wright's,** 24-oz. loaf (approx. 20 slices)	1866	318.3			77.7	13.26	(293)	(49.0)
1 slice, approx. 1.2 oz.			93	15.9	77.7	13.26	(293)	(49.0)
GRECIAN STYLE								
Grecian Style Enriched Bread with sesame seeds, **Mrs. Wright's,** 16-oz. (1-lb.) loaf (approx. 10 slices)	1134	209.0			70.9	13.06	(267)	(49.2)
1 slice, approx. 1.6 oz.			113	20.9	70.9	13.06	(267)	(49.2)
HAMBURGER BUNS AND ROLLS are listed toward the end of this chapter under Prepackaged Buns And Rolls.								
HEALTH NUT								
Health Nut Bread, **Brownberry,** 16-oz. (1-lb.) loaf (approx. 16 slices)	1360	240.0			85.0	15.00	(320)	(56.6)
1 slice, approx. 1 oz.			85	15.0	85.0	15.00	(320)	(56.6)
HILLBILLY								
Hillbilly Bread, **Hillbilly,** 20-oz. loaf (approx. 20 slices)	1400	250.0			70.0	12.50	(264)	(47.1)
1 slice, approx. 1 oz.			70	12.5	70.0	12.50	(264)	(47.1)
HONEY								
Honey Bran Bread, **Mrs. Wright's,** 24-oz. loaf (approx. 18 slices)	1901	320.0			79.2	13.30	(299)	(50.1)
1 slice, approx. 1.3 oz.			95	16.0	79.2	13.30	(299)	(50.1)
Honey Bran Bread, **Pepperidge Farm,** 24-oz. loaf (approx. 20 slices)	1800	360.0			75.0	15.00	(283)	(56.6)
1 slice, approx. 1.2 oz.			90	18.0	75.0	15.00	(283)	(56.6)
Honey 'n Egg Bread, **Northridge Oroweat,** 16-oz. (1-lb.) loaf (approx. 16 slices)	1120	216.0			70.0	13.50	(264)	(50.9)
1 slice, approx. 1 oz.			70	13.5	70.0	13.50	(264)	(50.9)
Honey Wheat Berry Bread, **Arnold,** 24-oz. loaf (approx. 20 slices)	1800	320.0			75.0	13.33	(283)	(50.3)
1 slice, approx. 1.2 oz.			90	16.0	75.0	13.33	(283)	(50.3)
Honey Wheat Berry Bread, **Oroweat,** 24-oz. loaf (approx. 20 slices)	1700	320.0			70.8	13.33	(267)	(50.3)
1 slice, approx. 1.2 oz.			85	16.0	70.8	13.33	(267)	(50.3)
Honey Wheat Berry Bread, **Pepperidge Farm,** 16-oz. (1-lb.) loaf (approx. 18 slices)	1080	207.0			67.5	12.94	(255)	(48.8)
1 slice, approx. 0.89 oz.			60	11.5	67.5	12.94	(255)	(48.8)
HOT DOG BUNS AND ROLLS are listed toward the end of this chapter under Prepackaged Buns And Rolls.								
HUNTERS GRAIN								
Hunters Grain Bread, **Hearth Farms** (Thomas'), 24-oz. loaf (18 slices)	1800	336.0			75.0	14.00	(283)	(52.7)
1 slice, approx. 1.34 oz.			100	18.7	75.0	14.00	(283)	(52.7)
ITALIAN BREAD								
Brown & Serve Italian Bread, **Pepperidge Farm,** 16-oz. (1-lb.) loaf (approx. 16 slices)	1200	216.0			75.0	13.50	(283)	(50.9)
1 slice, approx. 1 oz.			75	13.5	75.0	13.50	(283)	(50.9)
Italian Bread, sliced, **A&P,** 16-oz. (1-lb.) loaf (approx. 16 slices)	1120	224.0			70.0	14.00	(112)	(22.4)
1 slice, approx. 1 oz.			70	14.0	70.0	14.00	(112)	(22.4)
Italian Bread, **Bel Pane** (Wonder), 16-oz. (1-lb.) loaf (approx. 16 slices)	1040	200.0			65.0	12.50	(245)	(47.1)
1 slice, approx. 1 oz.			65	12.5	65.0	12.50	(245)	(47.1)
Italian Bread, **Pepperidge Farm,** 16-oz. (1-lb.) loaf (not presliced)	1200	224.0			75.0	14.00	(283)	(52.8)
Italian Enriched Bread, **Millbrook,** 18-oz. loaf (approx. 18 slices)	1350	243.0			75.0	13.50	(284)	(51.0)
1 slice, approx. 1 oz.			75	13.5	75.0	13.50	(284)	(51.0)
Italian Style Enriched Bread, **Holsum,** 24-oz. loaf (approx. 24 slices)	1800	348.0			75.0	14.50	(284)	(54.8)
1 slice, approx. 1 oz.			75	14.5	75.0	14.50	(284)	(54.8)
Italiano Bien, **D'Agostino's (Taystee),** 16-oz. (1-lb.) loaf (approx. 16 slices)	1200	216.0			75.0	13.50	(283)	(50.9)
1 slice, approx. 1 oz.			75	13.5	75.0	13.50	(283)	(50.9)
Old Fashioned Italian Bread, **Mrs. Wright's,** 20-oz. loaf (approx. 16 slices)	1418	268.6			70.9	13.43	(113)	(21.4)
1 slice, approx. 1¼ oz.			89	16.7	70.9	13.43	(113)	(21.4)
Old Fashioned Italian Enriched Bread, **Mrs. Wright's,** 24-oz. loaf (approx. 18 slices)	1701	322.3			70.9	13.43	(267)	(50.6)
1 slice, approx. 1.34 oz.			95	18.0	70.9	13.43	(267)	(50.6)
Real Italian Bread, **D'Italiano,** 16-oz. loaf (approx. 16 slices)	1200	216.0			75.0	13.50	(283)	(50.9)
1 slice, approx. 1 oz.			75	13.5	75.0	13.50	(283)	(50.9)
KOMMISBROT								
Kommisbrot Country Bread, **Rubschlager,** 16-oz. (1-lb.) loaf (approx. 27 slices)	1280	208.0			80.0	13.00	(302)	(49.0)
1 slice, approx. 0.6 oz.			40	6.5	80.0	13.00	(302)	(49.0)
LESS								
Less, "The Reduced Calorie Bread," **Stroehmann,** 16-oz. (1-lb.) loaf (approx. 20 slices)	800	140.0			50.0	8.75	(189)	(33.1)
1 slice, approx. 0.8 oz.			40	7.0	50.0	8.75	(189)	(33.1)
Less, "The Reduced Calorie Wheat Bread," **Stroehmann,** 16-oz. (1-lb.) loaf (approx. 20 slices)	800	140.0			50.0	8.75	(189)	(33.1)
1 slice, approx. 0.8 oz.			40	7.0	50.0	8.75	(189)	(33.1)
LIGHT BREAD								
Light Bread, **Hollywood,** 16-oz. (1-lb.) loaf (approx. 16 slices)	1120	216.0			70.0	13.50	(265)	(51.0)
1 slice, approx. 1 oz.			70	13.5	70.0	13.50	(265)	(51.0)
Light Bread, **Profile,** 16-oz. (1-lb.) loaf (approx. 16 slices)	1200	208.0			75.0	13.00	(283)	(49.0)
1 slice, approx. 1 oz.			75	13.0	75.0	13.00	(283)	(49.0)
Light Bread, Wheat, **Wonder,** 16-oz. (1-lb.) loaf (approx. 20 slices)	800	140.0			50.0	8.75	(189)	(33.3)
1 slice, approx. 0.8 oz.			40	7.0	50.0	8.75	(189)	(33.1)
Light Bread, White, **Wonder,** 16-oz. (1-lb.) loaf (approx. 20 slices)	800	140.0			50.0	8.75	(189)	(33.1)
1 slice, approx. 0.8 oz.			40	7.0	50.0	8.75	(189)	(33.1)

	ENTIRE LOAF Cal.	Carb.	1 SLICE Cal.	Carb.	1 OZ., BY WT. Cal.	Carb.	1 CUP CRUMBS FINE, DRY Cal.	Carb.
Special Formula Light Style Bread, **Mrs. Wright's,** 16-oz. (1-lb.) loaf (approx. 20 slices)	1106	199.1			69.1	12.45	(261)	(46.9)
1 slice, approx. 0.72 oz.			50	9.0	69.1	12.45	(261)	(46.9)
LOW SODIUM								
Low Sodium Bread, no salt added, **Mrs. Wright's,** 16-oz. (1-lb.) loaf (approx. 20 slices)	1106	221.3			69.1	13.83	(261)	(52.1)
1 slice, approx. 0.72 oz.			50	10.0	69.1	13.83	(261)	(52.1)
Low Sodium Bread, **Wonder,** 16-oz. (1-lb.) loaf (approx. 16 slices)	1120	216.0			70.0	13.50	(264)	(50.9)
1 slice, approx. 1 oz.			70	13.5	70.0	13.50	(264)	(50.9)
MATZOS are listed toward the end of this chapter under Specialty Breads And Rolls.								
MOUNTAIN OAT								
Mountain Oat Bread, **Hearth Farms,** 24-oz. loaf (approx. 18 slices)	1800	348.0			75.0	14.50	(283)	(54.6)
1 slice, approx. 1⅓ oz.			100	19.3	75.0	14.50	(283)	(54.6)
MUFFINS are listed toward the end of this chapter under Specialty Breads And Rolls.								
MULTI-GRAIN								
Multi Grain Bread, Very Thin, **Pepperidge Farm,** 16-oz. loaf (approx. 28 slices)	1120	196.0			70.0	12.25	(265)	(46.4)
1 slice, approx. 0.57 oz.			40	7.0	70.0	12.25	(265)	(46.4)
MULTI-MEAL								
Multi-Meal Bread, **Mrs. Wright's,** 16-oz. (1-lb.) loaf (approx. 16 slices)	1269	217.7			79.3	13.61	(299)	(51.3)
1 slice, approx. 0.88 oz.			70	12.0	79.3	13.61	(299)	(51.3)
24-oz. loaf (approx. 20 slices)	1866	328.2			77.7	13.72	(293)	(51.7)
1 slice, approx. 1.09 oz.			85	15.0	77.7	13.72	(293)	(51.7)
Multi-Meal Sandwich Bread, **Mrs. Wright's,** 24-oz. loaf (approx. 26 slices)	1805	333.3			75.2	13.89	(284)	(52.4)
1 slice, approx. 0.86 oz.			65	12.0	75.2	13.89	(284)	(52.4)
NATURAL								
Natural Bread, **Arnold,** 16-oz. (1-lb.) loaf (approx. 18 slices)	1260	189.0			78.8	11.81	(297)	(44.5)
1 slice, approx. 0.89 oz.			70	10.5	78.8	11.81	(297)	(44.5)
Natural Grains Bread, **Arnold,** 16-oz. loaf (approx. 20 slices)	1200	230.0			75.0	14.38	(283)	(54.2)
1 slice, approx. 0.8 oz.			60	11.5	75.0	14.38	(283)	(54.2)
Natural Health Loaf, **Arnold,** 16-oz. (1-lb.) loaf (approx. 18 slices)	1260	189.0			78.8	11.81	(297)	(44.5)
1 slice, approx. 0.89 oz.			70	10.5	78.8	11.81	(297)	(44.5)
OATMEAL								
Oatmeal Bread, **Brownberry,** 16-oz. (1-lb.) loaf (approx. 16 slices)	1280	240.0			80.0	15.00	(302)	(56.6)
1 slice, approx. 1 oz.			80	15.0	80.0	15.00	(302)	(56.6)
Oatmeal Bread, **Mrs. Wright's,** 24-oz. loaf (approx. 20 slices)	1431	363.3			59.6	15.14	(225)	(57.1)
1 slice, approx. 1.09 oz.			65	16.5	59.6	15.14	(225)	(57.1)
Oatmeal Bread, **Northridge,** 16-oz. (1-lb.) loaf (approx. 16 slices)	1120	208.0			70.0	13.00	(264)	(49.0)
1 slice, approx. 1 oz.			70	13.0	70.0	13.00	(264)	(49.0)
Oatmeal Bread, **Pepperidge Farm,** 16-oz. (1-lb.) loaf (approx. 18 slices)	1170	216.0			73.1	13.50	(275)	(50.9)
1 slice, approx. 0.89 oz.			65	12.0	73.1	13.50	(275)	(50.9)
OLD FASHION(ED)								
Old Fashion Bread, **Hillbilly,** 24-oz. loaf (approx. 24 slices)	1680	300.0			70.0	12.50	(265)	(47.3)
1 slice, approx. 1 oz.			70	12.5	70.0	12.50	(265)	(47.3)
Old Fashioned Enriched Bread, **Millbrook,** 24-oz. loaf (approx. 24 slices)	1680	348.0			70.0	14.50	(265)	(54.8)
1 slice, approx. 1 oz.			70	14.5	70.0	14.50	(265)	(54.8)
OLD STYLE								
Old Style Bread, **Roman Meal,** 24-oz. loaf (approx. 24 slices)	1680	324.0			70.0	13.50	(264)	(50.9)
1 slice, approx. 1 oz.			70	13.5	70.0	13.50	(264)	(50.9)

	ENTIRE LOAF Cal.	Carb.	1 SLICE Cal.	Carb.	1 OZ., BY WT. Cal.	Carb.	1 CUP CRUMBS FINE, DRY Cal.	Carb.
OLYMPIC MEAL								
Olympic Meal Bread, **Eddy's,** 24-oz. loaf (approx. 24 slices)	1800	300.0			75.0	12.50	(284)	(47.3)
1 slice, approx. 1 oz.			75	12.5	75.0	12.50	(284)	(47.3)
Olympic Meal Bread, **Hart's,** 24-oz. loaf (approx. 24 slices)	1800	300.0			75.0	12.50	(284)	(47.3)
1 slice, approx. 1 oz.			75	12.5	75.0	12.50	(284)	(47.3)
Olympic Meal Bread, **Holsum,** 24-oz. loaf (approx. 24 slices)	1800	300.0			75.0	12.50	(284)	(47.3)
1 slice, approx. 1 oz.			75	12.5	75.0	12.50	(284)	(47.3)
Olympic Meal Bread, **Millbrook,** 24-oz. loaf (approx. 24 slices)	1800	300.0			75.0	12.50	(284)	(47.3)
1 slice, approx. 1 oz.			75	12.5	75.0	12.50	(284)	(47.3)
ONION RYE								
Onion Rye Bread, **Jane Parker (A&P),** 16-oz. (1-lb.) loaf (approx. 26 slices)	1170	234.0			73.1	14.63	(275)	(55.1)
1 slice, approx. 0.62 oz.			90	18.0	73.1	14.63	(275)	(55.1)
PITA BREAD and POCKET BREAD are both listed toward the end of this chapter under Specialty Breads And Rolls.								
POPPY SEED								
Poppy Seed Vienna Style Bread, **Mrs. Wright's,** 16-oz. (1-lb.) loaf (approx. 18 slices)	1109	221.8			69.3	13.86	(261)	(52.3)
1 slice, approx. 0.79 oz.			55	11.0	69.3	13.86	(261)	(52.3)
POTATO BREAD								
Potato Bread, **Mrs. Wright's,** 24-oz. loaf (approx. 20 slices)	1866	351.2			77.7	14.63	(293)	(55.2)
1 slice, approx. 1.09 oz.			85	16.0	77.7	14.63	(293)	(55.2)
PROTEIN BREAD								
Protein Bread, **Thomas'** Protogen, 13-oz. loaf (approx. 18 slices)	830	151.3			63.8	11.62	(241)	(43.9)
1 slice, approx. 0.71 oz.			45	8.2	63.8	11.62	(241)	(43.9)
PUMPERNICKEL								
Cocktail Pumpernickel, **Rubschlager,** 16-oz. (1-lb.) loaf (approx. 22 slices)	1210	209.0			75.6	13.06	(283)	(49.2)
1 slice, approx. 0.38 oz.			29	5.0	75.6	13.06	(283)	(49.2)
Danish Pumpernickel, **Rubschlager,** 16-oz. (1-lb.) loaf (approx. 15 slices)	1125	215.5			70.3	13.59	(264)	(51.2)
1 slice, approx. 1.1 oz.			75	14.5	70.3	13.59	(264)	(51.2)
Old Style German Pumpernickel, **Rubschlager,** 24-oz. loaf (approx. 18 slices)	1710	315.0			71.3	13.13	(269)	(49.5)
1 slice, approx. 1.33 oz.			95	17.5	71.3	13.13	(269)	(49.5)
Party Pumpernickel, **Pepperidge Farm,** 8-oz. loaf (approx. 38 slices)	855	133.0			106.9	16.60	(403)	(62.6)
1 slice, approx. 0.21 oz.			23	3.5	106.9	16.60	(403)	(62.6)
Pumpernickel, **Arnold,** 14-oz. loaf (approx. 14 slices)	1050	196.0			75.0	14.00	(283)	(52.8)
1 slice, approx. 1 oz.			75	14.0	75.0	14.00	(283)	(52.8)
Pumpernickel, **Pepperidge Farm,** 16-oz. (1-lb.) loaf (approx. 14 slices)	1200	224.0			75.0	14.00	(283)	(52.8)
1 slice, approx. 1.14 oz.			86	16.0	75.0	14.00	(283)	(52.8)
Real Pumpernickel, **Levy's,** 16-oz. (1-lb.) loaf (approx. 16 slices)	1200	232.0			75.0	14.50	(283)	(54.7)
1 slice, approx. 1 oz.			75	14.5	75.0	14.50	(283)	(54.7)
Traditional Pumpernickel, **Jane Parker (A&P),** 16-oz. (1-lb.) loaf (approx. 16 slices)	1120	216.0			70.0	13.50	(264)	(50.9)
1 slice, approx. 1 oz.			70	13.5	70.0	13.50	(264)	(50.9)
Westphalian Pumpernickel, **Rubschlager,** 16-oz. (1-lb.) loaf (approx. 15 slices)	1125	215.5			70.3	13.59	(264)	(51.2)
1 slice, approx. 1.1 oz.			75	14.5	70.3	13.59	(264)	(51.2)
RAISIN BREAD								
Cinnamon Raisin Loaf, **Thomas',** 12-oz. loaf (approx. 16 slices)	935	174.8			78.0	14.57	(294)	(55.0)
1 slice, approx. 0.78 oz.			60	11.5	78.0	14.57	(294)	(55.0)
Enriched Raisin Bread, **A&P,** 16-oz. (1-lb.) loaf (approx. 16 slices)	1280	232.0	80	14.5	80.0	14.50	(300)	(54.7)
1 slice, approx. 1 oz.					80.0	14.50	(300)	(54.7)
Raisin Bread, **Butternut,** 16-oz. (1-lb.) loaf (approx. 16 slices)	1280	208.0			80.0	13.00	(302)	(49.1)
1 slice, approx. 1 oz.			80	13.0	80.0	13.00	(302)	(49.1)

	ENTIRE LOAF		1 SLICE		1 OZ., BY WT.		1 CUP CRUMBS FINE, DRY	
	Cal.	Carb.	Cal.	Carb.	Cal.	Carb.	Cal.	Carb.
Raisin Bread, **Mrs. Wright's,** 16-oz. (1-lb.) loaf (approx. 16 slices)	1200	24.0			75.0	15.00	(283)	(56.6)
1 slice, approx. 1 oz.			75	15.0	75.0	15.00	(283)	(56.6)
Raisin Bread, **Pepperidge Farm,** 16-oz. (1-lb.) loaf (approx. 18 slices)	1350	234.0			84.4	14.63	(318)	(55.2)
1 slice, approx. 0.89 oz.			75	13.0	84.4	14.63	(318)	(55.2)
Raisin Bread Cinnamon Swirl, **Sun-Maid,** 16-oz. (1-lb.) loaf (approx. 16 slices)	1200	208.0			75.0	13.00	(282)	(49.0)
1 slice, approx. 1 oz.			75	13.0	75.0	13.00	(282)	(49.0)
Raisin Cinnamon Bread, **Brownberry,** 16-oz. (1-lb.) loaf (approx. 16 slices)	1360	264.0			85.0	16.50	(320)	(62.2)
1 slice, approx. 1 oz.			85	16.5	85.0	16.50	(320)	(62.2)
Raisin Date Honey Loaf, **Holland Honey Co.,** 13-oz. loaf (not presliced)	1120	266.1			86.2	20.47	(325)	(77.2)
"Suggested" slice, 0.93 oz. (approx. ½" slice)			80	19.0	86.2	20.47	(325)	(77.2)
Raisin Nut Bread, **Brownberry,** 16-oz. (1-lb.) loaf (approx. 16 slices)	1520	232.0			95.0	14.50	(358)	(54.7)
1 slice, approx. 1 oz.			95	14.5	95.0	14.50	(358)	(54.7)
Raisin Whole Wheat Bread, no sugar added, **Balanced,** 14-oz. loaf (approx. 14 slices)	1120	196.0			80.0	14.00	(302)	(52.8)
1 slice, approx. 1 oz.			80	14.0	80.0	14.00	(302)	(52.8)
Raisin Whole Wheat Bread, **Shiloh Farms,** 16-oz. (1-lb.) loaf (approx. 12 slices)	1202	226.1			75.8	14.25	(286)	(53.7)
1 slice, approx. 1.3 oz.			101	19.0	75.8	14.25	(286)	(53.7)
Stonehedge Farm Raisin Bread, **Mrs. Wright's,** 16-oz. (1-lb.) loaf, (approx. 16 slices)	1200	224.0			75.0	14.00	(283)	(52.8)
1 slice, approx. 1 oz.			75	14.0	75.0	14.00	(283)	(52.8)
Thin Sliced Raisin Tea Loaf, **Arnold,** 16-oz. (1-lb.) loaf (approx. 18 slices)	1260	216.0			78.8	13.59	(297)	(50.9)
1 slice, approx. 0.89 oz.			70	12.0	78.8	13.59	(297)	(50.9)
ROLLS are listed toward the end of this chapter under Prepackaged Buns And Rolls.								
ROMAN MEAL								
Roman Meal Bread, **Butternut,** 24-oz. loaf (approx. 24 slices)	1680	324.0			70.0	13.50	(265)	(51.0)
1 slice, approx. 1 oz.			70	13.5	70.0	13.50	(265)	(51.0)
Roman Meal Bread, **Holsum,** 24-oz. loaf (approx. 24 slices)	1680	324.0			70.0	13.50	(265)	(51.0)
1 slice, approx. 1 oz.			70	13.5	70.0	13.50	(265)	(51.0)
Roman Meal Bread, **Millbrook,** 24-oz. loaf (approx. 24 slices)	1680	342.0			70.0	13.50	(265)	(51.0)
1 slice, approx. 1 oz.			70	13.5	70.0	13.50	(265)	(51.0)
Roman Meal Bread, **Mrs. Karl's,** 24-oz. loaf (approx. 24 slices)	1680	324.0			70.0	13.50	(265)	(51.0)
1 slice, approx. 1 oz.			70	13.5	70.0	13.50	(265)	(51.0)
Roman Meal Bread, **Roman Meal (Taystee),** 16-oz. (1-lb.) loaf (approx. 16 slices)	1120	216.0			70.0	13.50	(264)	(50.9)
1 slice, approx. 1 oz.			70	13.5	70.0	13.50	(264)	(50.9)
"Small Family Size" 12-oz. loaf (approx. 12 slices)	840	162.0			70.0	13.50	(264)	(50.9)
1 slice, approx. 1 oz.			70	13.5	70.0	13.50	(264)	(50.9)
Roman Meal Bread, **Sweetheart,** 24-oz. loaf (approx. 24 slices)	1680	324.0			70.0	13.50	(265)	(51.0)
1 slice, approx. 1 oz.			70	13.5	70.0	13.50	(265)	(51.0)
Roman Meal Bread, **Weber's,** 24-oz. loaf (approx. 24 slices)	1680	324.0			70.0	13.50	(265)	(51.0)
1 slice, approx. 1 oz.			70	13.5	70.0	13.50	(265)	(51.0)
Roman Meal Round Top Bread, **Roman Meal (Taystee),** 20-oz. loaf (approx. 20 slices)	1400	270.0			70.0	13.50	(264)	(50.9)
1 slice, approx. 1 oz.			70	13.5	70.0	13.50	(264)	(50.9)
ROUND LOAF								
Round Loaf, sliced, **Raviolo,** 12-oz. package (approx. 14 slices)	980	147			80.0	12.00	(303)	(45.2)
1 slice, approx. 1 oz.			80	12.0	80.0	12.00	(303)	(45.2)
RYE								
Cocktail Rye Bread, **Rubschlager,** 16-oz. (1-lb.) loaf (approx. 44 slices)	1100	198.0			68.8	12.38	(259)	(46.7)
1 slice, approx. 0.38 oz. (approx. 2⅔ slices per ounce)			25	4.5	68.8	12.38	(259)	(46.7)
Country Club Rye Bread without Seeds, **Grossinger's,** 16-oz. (1-lb.) loaf, (approx. 16 slices)	1120	216.0			70.0	13.50	(265)	(51.0)
1 slice, approx. 1 oz.			70	13.5	70.0	13.50	(265)	(51.0)
Deli Rye, **Hearth Farms,** 24-oz. loaf (approx. 18 slices)	1800	348.0			75.0	14.50	(283)	(54.6)
1 slice, approx. 1⅓ oz.			100	19.3	75.0	14.50	(283)	(54.6)
Dill Rye Bread, **Mrs. Wright's,** 24-oz. loaf (approx. 16 slices)	1702	313.4			70.9	13.06	(267)	(49.2)
1 slice, approx. 1.34 oz.			95	17.5	70.9	13.06	(267)	(49.2)
Family Rye Bread, **Pepperidge Farm,** 16-oz. (1-lb.) loaf (approx. 14 slices)	1120	203.0			70.0	12.69	(264)	(47.8)
1 slice, approx. 1.14 oz.			80	14.5	70.0	12.69	(264)	(47.8)
German Rye Bread, **Rubschlager,** 24-oz. loaf (approx. 27 slices and ends)	1755	297.0			73.1	12.38	(276)	(46.7)
1 slice, approx. 0.9 oz.			65	11.0	73.1	12.38	(276)	(46.7)
Giant Jewish Rye Bread, **Rubschlager,** 16-oz. (1-lb.) loaf (approx. 16 slices)	1200	208.0			75.0	13.00		
1 slice, approx. 1 oz.			75	13.0	75.0	13.00		
Jewish Deli Rye Bread, **Rubschlager,** 16-oz. (1-lb.) (approx. 16 slices)	1200	208.0			75.0	13.00		
1 slice, approx. 1 oz.			75	13.0	75.0	13.00		
Jewish Rye Bread, **Pepperidge Farm,** 16-oz. (1-lb.) loaf (approx. 14 slices)	1190	224.0			74.4	14.00	(280)	(52.8)
1 slice, approx. 1.14 oz.			85	16.0	74.4	14.00	(280)	(52.8)
Jewish Rye Bread, **Rubschlager,** 18-oz. loaf, unsliced	1350	234.0			75.0	13.00		
Jewish Rye Bread without Seeds, **Arnold,** 16-oz. (1-lb.) loaf (approx. 14 slices)	1050	175.0			65.6	10.94	(247)	(41.2)
1 slice, approx. 1.14 oz.			75	12.5	65.6	10.94	(247)	(41.2)
Jewish Rye Bread without Seeds, **Jane Parker (A&P),** 16-oz. (1-lb.) loaf (approx. 16 slices)	1120	216.0			70.0	13.50	(264)	(50.9)
1 slice, approx. 1 oz.			70	13.5	70.0	13.50	(264)	(50.9)
Jewish Rye Bread with Seeds, **Mrs. Wright's,** 16-oz. (1-lb.) loaf (approx. 14 slices)	1200	232.0			75.0	14.50	(283)	(54.7)
1 slice, approx. 1 oz.			75	14.5	75.0	14.50	(283)	(54.7)
Melba Thin Rye Bread with Caraway Seeds, thin sliced, **Arnold,** 16-oz. (1-lb.) loaf (approx. 22 slices)	1100	209.0			68.8	13.06	(259)	(49.2)
1 slice, approx. 0.73 oz.			50	9.5	68.8	13.06	(259)	(49.2)
Onion Rye Bread, **Jane Parker (A&P),** 16-oz. (1-lb.) loaf (approx. 26 slices)	1170	234.0			73.1	14.63	(275)	(55.1)
1 slice, approx. 0.62 oz.			90	18.0	73.1	14.63	(275)	(55.1)
Party Rye Bread, **Pepperidge Farm,** 8-oz. loaf (approx. 38 slices)	665	114.0			83.1	14.25	(313)	(53.7)
1 slice, approx. 0.21 oz.			18	3.0	83.1	14.25	(313)	(53.7)
Real Jewish Rye Bread with Caraway Seeds, **Levy's,** 16-oz. (1-lb.) loaf (approx. 16 slices)	1120	216.0			70.0	13.50	(264)	(50.9)
1 slice, approx. 1 oz.			70	13.5	70.0	13.50	(264)	(50.9)
Real Jewish Rye Bread without Seeds, **Levy's,** 16-oz. (1-lb.) loaf, 16 slices	1120	216.0			70.0	13.50	(264)	(50.9)
1 slice, approx. 1 oz.			70	13.5	70.0	13.50	(264)	(50.9)
Rye Bread, **Wonder,** 16-oz. (1-lb.) loaf (approx. 16 slices)	1200	216.0			75.0	13.50	(283)	(50.9)
1 slice, approx. 1 oz.			75	13.5	75.0	13.50	(283)	(50.9)
Rye Bread with Seeds, **Mrs. Wright's,** 16-oz. (1-lb.) loaf (approx. 20 slices)	1106	210.2			69.1	13.14	(261)	(49.5)
1 slice, approx. 0.72 oz.			50	9.5	69.1	13.14	(261)	(49.5)
Rye Sandwich Pockets, see Pocket Bread toward the end of this chapter under Specialty Breads And Rolls								
Seeded Dill Rye Bread, **Arnold,** 16-oz. (1-lb.) loaf (approx. 16 slices)	1200	215.0			75.0	13.50	(283)	(50.9)
1 slice, approx. 1 oz.			75	13.5	75.0	13.50	(283)	(50.9)

	ENTIRE LOAF Cal.	ENTIRE LOAF Carb.	1 SLICE Cal.	1 SLICE Carb.	1 OZ., BY WT. Cal.	1 OZ., BY WT. Carb.	1 CUP CRUMBS FINE, DRY Cal.	1 CUP CRUMBS FINE, DRY Carb.
Soft Rye Bread, **Arnold,** 16-oz. (1-lb.) loaf (approx. 14 slices)	1050	210.0			65.6	13.13	(236)	(49.5)
1 slice, approx. 1.14 oz.			75	15.0	65.6	13.13	(236)	(49.5)
Swedish Limpa Rye Bread, **Rubschlager,** 16-oz. (1-lb.) loaf (approx. 18 slices)	1170	20.0			73.1	12.94		
1 slice, approx. 0.89 oz.			65	11.5	73.1	12.94		
Thin Jewish Rye Bread with Caraway Seeds, **Arnold,** 16-oz. (1-lb.) loaf (approx. 14 slices)	1050	196.0			65.6	12.25	(247)	(46.2)
1 slice, approx. 1.14 oz.			75	14.0	65.6	12.25	(247)	(46.2)
SANDWICH BREAD								
Crushed Wheat Sandwich Bread, **Mrs. Wright's,** 24-oz. loaf (approx. 26 slices)	1805	361.0			75.2	15.04	(284)	(56.7)
1 slice, approx. 0.86 oz.			65	13.0	75.2	15.04	(284)	(56.7)
Extra Thin Sliced White Sandwich Bread, **Northridge,** 16-oz. (1-lb.) loaf (approx. 24 slices)	1080	204.0			67.5	12.75	(254)	(48.1)
1 slice, approx. 0.66 oz.			45	8.5	67.5	12.75	(254)	(48.1)
Sandwich Bread, **Butternut,** 24-oz. loaf (approx. 24 slices)	1800	336.0			75.0	14.00	(284)	(52.9)
1 slice, approx. 1 oz.			75	14.0	75.0	14.00	(284)	(52.9)
Sandwich Bread, **Eddy's,** 24-oz. loaf (approx. 24 slices)	1800	336.0			75.0	14.00	(284)	(52.9)
1 slice, approx. 1 oz.			75	14.0	75.0	14.00	(284)	(52.9)
Sandwich Bread, **Mrs. Karl's,** 24-oz. loaf (approx. 24 slices)	1800	336.0			75.0	14.00	(284)	(52.9)
1 slice, approx. 1 oz.			75	14.0	75.0	14.00	(284)	(52.9)
Sandwich Bread, **Roman Meal,** 24-oz. loaf (approx. 24 slices)	1680	324.0			70.0	13.50	(264)	(50.9)
1 slice, approx. 1 oz.			70	13.5	70.0	13.50	(264)	(50.9)
Sandwich Bread, **Sweetheart,** 24-oz. loaf (approx. 24 slices)	1800	336.0			75.0	14.00	(284)	(52.9)
1 slice, approx. 1 oz.			75	14.0	75.0	14.00	(284)	(52.9)
Sandwich Bread, made with Buttermilk, **Mrs. Wright's,** 24-oz. loaf (approx. 26 slices)	1805	319.4			75.2	13.31	(284)	(50.2)
1 slice, approx. 0.86 oz.			65	11.5	75.2	13.31	(284)	(50.2)
Sandwich White Enriched Brand, **The Food Emporium,** 22-oz. loaf (approx. 22 slices)	1540	297.0			70.0	13.50	(263)	(50.9)
1 slice, approx. 1 oz.			70	13.5	70.0	13.50	(263)	(50.9)
Super Soft Sandwich Bread, **Mrs. Wright's,** 24-oz. loaf (approx. 30 slices)	1899	363.9			79.1	15.16	(298)	(57.2)
1 slice, approx. 0.76 oz.			60	11.5	79.1	15.16	(298)	(57.2)
16-oz. (1-lb.) loaf (approx. 20 slices)	1217	243.4			76.1	15.21	(287)	(57.3)
1 slice, approx. 0.72 oz.			55	11.0	76.1	15.21	(287)	(57.3)
Thin Sandwich Bread, **Hart's,** 24-oz. loaf (approx. 24 slices)	1800	336.0			75.0	14.00	(284)	(52.9)
1 slice, approx. 1 oz.			75	14.0	75.0	14.00	(284)	(52.9)
Thin Sandwich Bread, **Holsum,** 24-oz. loaf (approx. 24 slices)	1800	348.0			75.0	14.50	(284)	(54.8)
1 slice, approx. 1 oz.			75	14.5	75.0	14.50	(284)	(54.8)
Thin Sliced Sandwich Bread, **Eddy's,** 24-oz. loaf (approx. 24 slices)	1800	336.0			75.0	14.00	(284)	(52.9)
1 slice, approx. 1 oz.			75	14.0	75.0	14.00	(284)	(52.9)
Thin Sliced Sandwich Bread, **Ovenjoy,** 24-oz. loaf (approx. 24 slices)	1560	276.0			65.0	11.50	(246)	(43.4)
1 slice, approx. 1 oz.			65	11.5	65.0	11.50	(246)	(43.4)
Thin Sliced Sandwich Bread, **Weber's,** 24-oz. loaf (approx. 24 slices)	1800	336.0			75.0	14.00	(284)	(52.9)
1 slice, approx. 1 oz.			75	14.0	75.0	14.00	(284)	(52.9)
Very Thin Sandwich Bread, **Dutch Hearth,** 16-oz. (1-lb.) loaf (approx. 32 slices)	1120	224.0			70.0	14.00	(265)	(52.9)
1 slice, approx. 0.5 oz.			35	7.0	70.0	14.00	(265)	(52.9)
White Enriched Sandwich Bread, **Ovenjoy,** 22-oz. loaf	1663	318.8			75.6	14.49	(283)	(54.7)
1 slice, approx. 0.8 oz.			60	11.5	75.6	14.49	(283)	(54.7)
White Sandwich Bread, **Brownberry,** 24-oz. loaf (24 slices)	1800	372.0			75.0	15.50	(283)	(58.4)
1 slice, approx. 1 oz.			75	15.5	75.0	15.50	(283)	(58.4)

	ENTIRE LOAF Cal.	ENTIRE LOAF Carb.	1 SLICE Cal.	1 SLICE Carb.	1 OZ., BY WT. Cal.	1 OZ., BY WT. Carb.	1 CUP CRUMBS FINE, DRY Cal.	1 CUP CRUMBS FINE, DRY Carb.
White Sandwich Bread, **Pepperidge Farm,** 16-oz. (1-lb.) loaf (approx. 20 slices)	1300	240.0			81.3	15.00	(307)	(56.6)
1 slice, approx. 0.8 oz.			65	12.0	81.3	15.00	(307)	(56.6)
White Sandwich Pockets, see Pocket Bread toward the end of this chapter under Specialty Breads And Rolls								
SESAME								
Sesame Pita, see Pita Bread toward the end of this chapter under Specialty Breads And Rolls								
Sesame Seed Buns, **Pepperidge Farm,** 8¼-oz. bag (6 buns)	720	114.0			87.3	13.81		
1 bun, approx. 1.38 oz.			120	19.0	87.3	13.81		
SEVEN GRAIN								
Seven Grain Bread, **Better Way,** 24-oz. loaf (approx. 24 slices)	1680	276.0			70.0	11.50	(265)	(43.5)
1 slice, approx. 1 oz.			70	11.5	70.0	11.50	(265)	(43.5)
Seven Grain Bread, **Mrs. Wright's,** 24-oz. loaf (approx. 16 slices)	1790	313.4			74.6	13.06	(281)	(49.2)
1 slice, approx. 1.34 oz.			100	17.5	74.6	13.06	(281)	(49.2)
7 Whole Grain Bread, **Hearth Farms** (Arnold), 24-oz. loaf (approx. 18 slices)	2220	456.0			92.5	19.0	(348)	(71.9)
1 slice, approx. 1⅓ oz.			123	25.3	92.5	19.0	(348)	(71.9)
SOURDOUGH BREAD								
Sour Dough Bread, **DiCarlo,** 16-oz. (1-lb.) loaf (approx. 16 slices)	1120	216.0			70.0	13.50	(264)	(50.9)
1 slice, approx. 1 oz.			70	13.5	70.0	13.50	(264)	(50.9)
Sourdough Bread, **Mrs. Wright's,** 24-oz. loaf (approx. 20 slices)	1756	329.2			73.2	13.72	(276)	(51.7)
1 slice, approx. 1.2 oz.			88	16.5	73.2	13.72	(276)	(51.7)
Sourdough Bread, no sugar, **Pioneer,** 24-oz. loaf (approx. 12 slices)	1680	360.0			70.0	15.00	(264)	(56.6)
1 slice, approx. 2 oz.			140	30.0	70.0	15.00	(264)	(56.6)
Sourdough Bread, sugar-free, **Pioneer,** 16-oz. (1-lb.) loaf, unsliced	1120	240.0			70.0	15.00	(264)	(56.6)
Sour Dough French Bread, **Hearth Farms,** 24-oz. loaf (approx. 18 slices)	1680	348.0			70.0	14.50	(264)	(54.7)
1 slice, approx. 1⅓ oz.			93	19.3	70.0	14.50	(264)	(54.7)
SPLIT TOP								
Split Top Bread, **Roman Meal,** 20-oz. loaf (approx. 20 slices)	1400	270.0			70.0	13.50	(264)	(50.9)
1 slice, approx. 1 oz.			70	13.5	70.0	13.50	(264)	(50.9)
Split Top White Bread, **Mrs. Wright's,** 24-oz. loaf (approx. 20 slices)	1600	300.0			66.7	12.50	(251)	(47.1)
1 slice, approx. 1.1 oz.			80	15.5	66.7	12.50	(251)	(47.1)
SPROUTED WHEAT								
Sprouted Stone Ground Wheat Bread, **Pepperidge Farm,** 24-oz. loaf (approx. 20 slices)	1800	340.0			75.0	14.17	(283)	(53.4)
1 slice, approx. 1.2 oz.			90	17.0	75.0	14.17	(283)	(53.4)
Sprouted Wheat Bread, **Arnold,** 16-oz. (1-lb.) loaf (approx. 13 slices)	1170	216.0			73.1	13.50	(276)	(50.1)
1 slice, approx. 0.89 oz.			65	12.0	73.1	13.50	(276)	(50.1)
Sprouted Wheat Bread, **Pepperidge Farm,** 16-oz. (1-lb.) loaf (approx. 18 slices)	1170	207.0			73.1	12.94	(276)	(48.8)
1 slice, approx. 0.89 oz.			65	11.5	73.1	12.94	(276)	(48.8)
Stone Ground Sprouted Wheat Bread, **Oroweat,** 16-oz. (1-lb.) loaf (approx. 16 slices)	1040	160.0			65.0	10.00	(245)	(37.7)
1 slice, approx. 1 oz.			65	10.0	65.0	10.00	(245)	(37.7)
STUFFING BREAD								
Stuffing Enriched Bread, **Mrs. Wright's,** 24-oz. (not presliced)	1905	367.4			79.4	15.31	(299)	(57.7)
1 "Suggested" slice, approx. 0.88 oz.			70	13.5	79.4	15.31	(299)	(57.7)
TACO SHELLS, TORTILLAS, and TOSTADA SHELLS are listed toward the end of this chapter under Specialty Breads And Rolls.								

	ENTIRE LOAF		1 SLICE		1 OZ., BY WT.		1 CUP CRUMBS FINE, DRY	
	Cal.	Carb.	Cal.	Carb.	Cal.	Carb.	Cal.	Carb.
UPSIDE DOWN								
Upside Down Enriched Bread, **Butternut,** 16-oz. (1-lb.) loaf (approx. 16 slices)	1200	216.0			75.0	13.50	(284)	(51.0)
1 slice, approx. 1 oz.			75	13.5	75.0	13.50	(284)	(51.0)
VIENNA								
Vienna Enriched Bread, **Butternut,** 16-oz. (1-lb.) loaf (approx. 16 slices)	1200	224.0			75.0	14.00	(284)	(52.9)
1 slice, approx. 1 oz.			75	14.0	75.0	14.00	(284)	(52.9)
WESTERN FARM								
Western Farm Bread, **Mrs. Wright's,** 24-oz. loaf (approx. 20 slices)	1756	329.2			73.2	13.72	(276)	(51.7)
1 slice, approx. 1.2 oz.			88	16.5	73.2	13.72	(276)	(51.7)
WHEAT BREAD (see also Whole Wheat Bread)								
Bran'Nola Dark Wheat Natural Bread with Bran, **Arnold,** 24-oz. loaf (approx. 18 slices)	1800	324.0			75.0	13.50	(282)	(50.0)
1 slice, approx. 1.34 oz.			100	18.0	75.0	13.50	(282)	(50.0)
Country Wheat, **Arnold,** 24-oz. loaf (approx. 18 slices)	1800	288.0			75.0	12.00	(282)	(45.1)
1 slice, approx. 1.34 oz.			100	16.0	75.0	12.00	(282)	(45.1)
Family Wheat Bread, **Pepperidge Farm,** 32-oz. (2-lb.) loaf (approx. 34 slices)	2380	425.0			74.4	13.28	(280)	(50.1)
1 slice, approx. 0.94 oz.			70	12.5	74.4	13.28	(280)	(50.1)
Hearty Wheat Natural Bread with Bran, **Bran'nola,** 24-oz. loaf (approx. 18 slices)	1890	315.0			78.0	13.13	(297)	(49.5)
1 slice, approx. 1.3 oz.			105	17.5	78.8	13.13	(297)	(49.5)
Home Style Butter Top Wheat Bread, **Mrs. Wright's,** 24-oz. loaf (20 slices)	1866	329.2			77.7	13.72	(293)	(51.7)
1 slice, approx. 1.09 oz.			85	15.0	77.7	13.72	(293)	(51.7)
Less, "The Reduced Calorie Wheat Bread," **Stroehmann,** 16-oz. (1-lb.) loaf, (approx. 20 slices)	800	140.0			50.0	8.75	(189)	(33.1)
1 slice, approx. 0.8 oz.			40	7.0	50.0	8.75	(189)	(33.1)
Light Wheat Bread, **Butternut,** 16-oz. (1-lb.) loaf (approx. 16 slices)	880	168.0			55.0	10.50	(208)	(39.7)
1 slice, approx. 1 oz.			55	10.5	55.0	10.50	(208)	(39.7)
Light Wheat Bread, **Hart's,** 16-oz. (1-lb.) loaf (approx. 16 slices)	880	168.0			55.0	10.50	(208)	(39.7)
1 slice, approx. 1 oz.			55	10.5	55.0	10.50	(208)	(39.7)
Light Wheat Bread, **Holsum,** 16-oz. (1-lb.) loaf (approx. 16 slices)	880	168.0			55.0	10.50	(208)	(39.7)
1 slice, approx. 1 oz.			55	10.5	55.0	10.50	(208)	(39.7)
Light Wheat Bread, **Millbrook,** 16-oz. (1-lb.) loaf (approx. 16 slices)	880	168.0			55.0	10.50	(208)	(39.7)
1 slice, approx. 1 oz.			55	10.5	55.0	10.50	(208)	(39.7)
Light Wheat Bread, **Mrs. Karl's,** 16-oz. (1-lb.) loaf (approx. 16 slices)	880	168.0			55.0	10.50	(208)	(39.7)
1 slice, approx. 1 oz.			55	10.5	55.0	10.50	(208)	(39.7)
Natural Wheat Bread, **Brownberry,** 24-oz. loaf (approx. 20 slices)	1700	360.0			70.8	15.00	(267)	(56.6)
1 slice, 1.2 oz.			85	18.0	70.8	15.00	(267)	(56.6)
Proclaim Wheat Bread, **Wonder,** 16-oz. (1-lb.) loaf (approx. 16 slices)	1120	176.0			70.0	11.00	(264)	(41.5)
1 slice, approx. 1 oz.			70	11.0	70.0	11.00	(264)	(41.5)
Thin Sliced Wheat Germ Bread, **Pepperidge Farm,** 16-oz. (1-lb.) loaf (approx. 18 slices)	1170	225.0			65.0	12.50	(245)	(47.1)
1 slice, approx. 0.89 oz.			65	12.5	65.0	12.50	(245)	(47.1)
Wheat Bread, **Fresh Horizons,** 16-oz. (1-lb.) loaf (approx. 16 slices)	800	136.0			50.0	8.50	(189)	(32.1)
1 slice, approx. 1 oz.			50	8.5	50.0	8.50	(189)	(32.1)
Wheat Bread, **Home Pride,** 20-oz. loaf (approx. 20 slices)	1500	260.0			75.0	13.00	(283)	(49.0)
1 slice, approx. 1 oz.			75	13.0	75.0	13.00	(283)	(49.0)
Wheat Bread, **Pepperidge Farm,** 24-oz. loaf (approx. 20 slices)	1900	340.0			79.2	14.17	(298)	(52.5)
1 slice, approx. 1.2 oz.			95	17.0	79.2	14.17	(298)	(52.5)
Wheat Bread, sliced, **Weber's,** 24-oz. (1-lb. 8-oz.) loaf (approx. 24 slices)	1680	324.0			70.0	13.50	(265)	(51.0)
1 slice, approx. 1 oz.			70	13.5	70.0	13.50	(265)	(51.0)

	ENTIRE LOAF		1 SLICE		1 OZ., BY WT.		1 CUP CRUMBS FINE, DRY	
	Cal.	Carb.	Cal.	Carb.	Cal.	Carb.	Cal.	Carb.
Wheat Nugget Bread, **Better Way,** 24-oz. loaf (approx. 24 slices)	1680	276.0			70.0	11.50	(265)	(43.5)
1 slice, approx. 1 oz.			70	11.5	70.0	11.50	(265)	(43.5)
Wheatberry Bread, **Home Pride,** 24-oz. loaf (approx. 24 slices)	1680	300.0			70.0	12.50	(264)	(47.1)
1 slice, approx. 1 oz.			70	12.5	70.0	12.50	(264)	(47.1)
WHITE BREAD								
Brick Oven White Bread, **Arnold,** 16-oz. (1-lb.) loaf (approx. 20 slices)	1300	200.0			81.3	12.50	(307)	(47.1)
1 slice, approx. 0.8 oz.			65	10.0	81.3	12.50	(307)	(47.1)
Buttercrust White Enriched Bread, **A&P,** 20-oz. loaf (approx. 20 slices)	1500	260.0			75.0	13.00	(283)	(49.0)
1 slice, approx. 1 oz.			75	13.0	75.0	13.00	(283)	(49.0)
Country White Bread, **Arnold,** 24-oz. loaf (approx. 20 slices)	1900	330.0			79.2	13.75	(299)	(51.8)
1 slice, approx. 1.2 oz.			95	16.5	79.2	13.75	(299)	(51.8)
Extra Thin Sliced Sandwich White Bread, **Northridge,** 16-oz. (1-lb.) loaf (approx. 24 slices)	1080	204.0			67.5	12.75	(254)	(48.1)
1 slice, approx. 0.7 oz.			45	8.5	67.5	12.75	(254)	(48.1)
Family White Bread, **Pepperidge Farm,** 32-oz. (2-lb.) loaf (approx. 34 slices)	2550	459.0			79.7	14.34	(300)	(54.1)
1 slice, approx. 0.9 oz.			75	13.5	79.7	14.34	(300)	(54.1)
Family White Bread, Round, **Bellacicco,** 13-oz. loaf (approx. 14 slices)	910	189.0			70.0	14.54	(264)	(54.8)
1 slice, approx. 0.93 oz.			65	13.5	70.0	14.54	(264)	(54.8)
Golden Circles White Bread, **Taystee,** 16-oz. (1-lb.) loaf (approx. 16 slices)	1280	208.0			80.0	13.00	(302)	(49.0)
1 slice, approx. 1 oz.			80	13.0	80.0	13.00	(302)	(49.0)
Golden Split Top White Bread, **Taystee,** 20-oz. loaf (approx. 20 slices)	1500	270.0			75.0	13.50	(283)	(50.9)
1 slice, approx. 1 oz.			75	13.5	75.0	13.50	(283)	(50.9)
Hearthstone Country White Bread, **Arnold,** 16-oz. (1-lb.) loaf (approx. 18 slices)	1350	234.0			84.4	14.63	(318)	(55.2)
1 slice, approx. 0.89 oz.			75	13.0	84.4	14.63	(318)	(55.2)
Hearthstone White Bread, **Arnold,** 32-oz. (2-lb.) loaf (approx. 30 slices)	2550	450.0			76.7	14.06	(289)	(53.0)
1 slice, approx. 1.07 oz.			85	15.0	76.7	14.06	(289)	(53.0)
Home Style White Bread, **Mrs. Wright's,** 24-oz. loaf (approx. 16 slices)	1440	272.0			60.0	11.33	(226)	(42.7)
1 slice, approx. 1.5 oz.			90	17.0	60.0	11.33	(226)	(42.7)
Home Style White Bread, Unsliced, **Pepperidge Farm,** 16-oz. (1-lb.) loaf (approx. 16 slices)	1200	208.0			75.0	13.00	(283)	(49.0)
1 slice, approx. 1 oz.			75	13.0	75.0	13.00	(283)	(49.0)
Light White Bread, **Butternut,** 16-oz. (1-lb.) loaf (approx. 16 slices)	880	176.0			55.0	11.00	(208)	(41.6)
1 slice, approx. 1 oz.			55	11.0	55.0	11.00	(208)	(41.6)
Light White Bread, **Holsum,** 16-oz. (1-lb.) loaf (approx. 16 slices)	880	176.0			55.0	11.00	(208)	(41.6)
1 slice, approx. 1 oz.			55	11.0	55.0	11.00	(208)	(41.6)
Light White Bread, **Millbrook,** 16-oz. (1-lb.) loaf (approx. 16 slices)	880	176.0			55.0	11.00	(208)	(41.6)
1 slice, approx. 1 oz.			55	11.0	55.0	11.00	(208)	(41.6)
Light White Bread, **Mrs. Karl's,** 16-oz. (1-lb.) loaf (approx. 16 slices)	880	176.0			55.0	11.00	(208)	(41.6)
1 slice, approx. 1 oz.			55	11.0	55.0	11.00	(208)	(41.6)
Measure Up White Bread, **Arnold,** 16-oz. (1-lb.) loaf (approx. 30 slices)	1200	210.0			75.0	13.13	(283)	(49.5)
1 slice, approx. 0.53 oz.			40	0.7	75.0	13.13	(283)	(49.5)
Old Fashioned White Bread, **Weight Watchers,** 16-oz. (1-lb.) loaf (approx. 28 slices)	1120	210.0			70.0	13.13	(264)	(49.5)
1 slice, approx. 0.57 oz.			40	7.5	70.0	13.13	(264)	(49.5)
Old Style White Bread, **Bran'nola,** 24-oz. loaf (approx. 18 slices)	1890	342.0			78.8	14.25	(297)	(53.7)
1 slice, approx. 1.3 oz.			105	19.0	78.8	14.25	(297)	(53.7)

	ENTIRE LOAF		1 SLICE		1 OZ., BY WT.		1 CUP CRUMBS FINE, DRY	
	Cal.	Carb.	Cal.	Carb.	Cal.	Carb.	Cal.	Carb.
Premium White Bread, **Safeway,** 24-oz. loaf (approx. 20 slices)	1600	300.0			66.7	12.50	(251)	(47.1)
1 slice, approx. 1.2 oz.			80	15.0	66.7	12.50	(251)	(47.1)
Premium White Enriched Bread, **Safeway,** 16-oz. (1-lb.) loaf (approx. 16 slices)	1270	235.9			79.4	14.74	(299)	(55.6)
1 slice, approx. 0.88 oz.			70	13.0	79.4	14.74	(299)	(55.6)
24-oz. loaf (approx. 20 slices)	1866	351.2			77.7	14.63	(293)	(55.2)
1 slice, approx. 1.09 oz.			85	16.0	77.7	14.63	(293)	(55.2)
Proclaim White Bread, **Wonder,** 16-oz. (1-lb.) loaf (approx. 16 slices)	1120	176.0			70.0	11.00	(264)	(41.5)
1 slice, approx. 1 oz.			70	11.0	70.0	11.00	(264)	(41.5)
Round Top White Bread, **Shopwell,** 22-oz. loaf (approx. 22 slices)	1650	297.0			75.0	13.50	(283)	(50.9)
1 slice, approx. 1 oz.			58	10.4	75.0	13.50	(283)	(50.9)
Sandwich White Bread, **Brownberry,** 24-oz. loaf (approx. 24 slices)	1800	372.0			75.0	15.50	(283)	(58.4)
1 slice, approx. 1 oz.			75	15.5	75.0	15.50	(283)	(58.4)
Sandwich White Bread, **Pepperidge Farm,** 16-oz. (1-lb.) loaf (approx. 20 slices)	1300	240.0			81.3	15.00	(307)	(56.6)
1 slice, approx. 0.8 oz.			65	12.0	81.3	15.00	(307)	(56.6)
Split Top White Bread, **Mrs. Wright's,** 24-oz. loaf (approx. 20 slices)	1600	300.0			66.7	12.50	(251)	(47.1)
1 slice, approx. 1.2 oz.			80	15.0	66.7	12.50	(251)	(47.1)
Split Top White Enriched Bread, **Mrs. Wright's,** 24-oz. (1-lb. 8-oz.) loaf (approx. 20 slices)	1756	329.2			73.2	13.72	(276)	(51.7)
1 slice, approx. 1.09 oz.			80	15.0	73.2	13.72	(276)	(51.7)
Sourdough White Bread, **Mrs. Wright's,** 24-oz. loaf (approx. 20 slices)	1600	300.0			66.7	12.50	(251)	(47.1)
1 slice, approx. 1.2 oz.			80	15.0	66.7	12.50	(251)	(47.1)
Super Soft Enriched White Bread, **Mrs. Wright's,** 16-oz. (1-lb.) loaf (approx. 20 slices)	1217	243.4			76.1	15.21	(287)	(57.3)
1 slice, approx. 0.72 oz.			55	11.0	76.1	15.21	(287)	(57.3)
24-oz. (1-lb. 8-oz.) loaf (approx. 30 slices)	1899	348.1			79.1	14.50	(298)	(54.7)
1 slice, approx. 0.8 oz.			63	11.6	79.1	14.50	(298)	(54.7)
Super Soft Sandwich White Bread, **Mrs. Wright's,** 24-oz. loaf (approx. 30 slices)	1800	315.0			75.0	13.13	(283)	(49.5)
1 slice, approx. 0.8 oz.			60	10.5	75.0	13.13	(283)	(49.5)
Super Soft White Bread, **Mrs. Wright's,** 24-oz. loaf (approx. 30 slices)	1650	315.0			68.8	13.13	(259)	(49.5)
1 slice, approx. 0.77 oz.			55	10.5	68.8	13.13	(259)	(49.5)
16-oz. (1-lb.) loaf (approx. 20 slices)	1200	210.0			75.0	13.13	(283)	(49.5)
1 slice, approx. 0.8 oz.			60	10.5	75.0	13.13	(283)	(49.5)
Thin Sliced Premium White Bread, **Safeway,** 24-oz. loaf (approx. 26 slices)	1690	299.0			70.4	12.46	(265)	(47.0)
1 slice, approx. 0.92 oz.			65	11.5	70.4	12.46	(265)	(47.0)
Thin Sliced White Bread, **Mrs. Wright's** Stonehedge Farm, 16-oz. (1-lb.) loaf (approx. 14 slices)	1050	189.0			65.6	11.81	(247)	(44.5)
1 slice, approx. 1.14 oz.			75	13.5	65.6	11.81	(247)	(44.5)
Thin Sliced White Bread, **Pepperidge Farm,** 16-oz. (1-lb.) loaf (approx. 18 slices)	1350	234.0			84.4	14.63	(318)	(55.2)
1 slice, approx. 0.9 oz.			75	13.0	84.4	14.63	(318)	(55.2)
Thin Sliced White Bread, **Safeway,** 16-oz. (1-lb.) loaf (approx. 18 slices)	1311	241.9			81.9	15.12	(309)	(57.0)
1 slice, approx. 0.79 oz.			65	12.0	81.9	15.12	(309)	(57.0)
24-oz. loaf (approx. 26 slices)	1805	347.1			75.2	14.46	(284)	(54.5)
1 slice, approx. 0.86 oz.			65	12.5	75.2	14.46	(284)	(54.5)
Toasting White Bread, **Pepperidge Farm,** 16-oz. (1-lb.) loaf (approx. 14 slices)	1190	224.0			74.4	14.00	(280)	(52.8)
1 slice, approx. 1.1 oz.			85	16.0	74.4	14.00	(280)	(52.8)
Very Thin Sliced White Bread, **Pepperidge Farm,** 16-oz. (1-lb.) loaf (approx. 18 slices)	1120	224.0			70.0	14.00	(264)	(52.8)
1 slice, approx. 0.89 oz.			62	12.5	70.0	14.00	(264)	(52.8)

	ENTIRE LOAF		1 SLICE		1 OZ., BY WT.		1 CUP CRUMBS FINE, DRY	
	Cal.	Carb.	Cal.	Carb.	Cal.	Carb.	Cal.	Carb.
White Bread, **Brownberry,** 16-oz. (1-lb.) loaf (approx. 16 slices)	1200	248.0			75.0	15.50	(283)	(58.4)
1 slice, approx. 1 oz.			75	15.5	75.0	15.50	(283)	(58.4)
White Bread, **E&B,** 22-oz. loaf (approx. 22 slices)	1650	148.5			75.0	13.50	(283)	(50.9)
1 slice, approx. 1 oz.			75	13.5	75.0	13.50	(283)	(50.9)
White Bread, **Fresh Horizons,** 16-oz. (1-lb.) loaf (approx. 16 slices)	800	136.0			50.0	8.50	(189)	(32.0)
1 slice, approx. 1 oz.			50	8.5	50.0	8.50	(189)	(32.0)
White Bread, **Kilpatrick's,** 24-oz. loaf (approx. 24 slices)	1800	336.0			75.0	14.00	(283)	(52.8)
1 slice, approx. 1 oz.			75	14.0	75.0	14.00	(283)	(52.8)
White Bread, **Levy's,** 16-oz.(1-lb.) loaf (approx. 16 slices)	1280	240.0			80.0	15.00	(302)	(56.6)
1 slice, approx. 1 oz.			80	15.0	80.0	15.00	(302)	(56.6)
White Bread, no salt added, **Levy's,** 14-oz. loaf (approx. 14 slices)	1280	224.0			80.0	14.00	(302)	(52.8)
1 slice, approx. 1 oz.			80	14.0	80.0	14.00	(302)	(52.8)
White Bread, **Marvel (A&P)** 20-oz. loaf (approx. 20 slices)	1500	270.0			75.0	13.50	(283)	(50.9)
1 slice, approx. 1 oz.			75	13.5	75.0	13.50	(283)	(50.9)
White Bread, **Millbrook,** 24-oz. loaf (approx. 24 slices)	1800	336.0			75.0	14.00	(284)	(52.9)
1 slice, approx. 1 oz.			75	14.0	75.0	14.00	(284)	(52.9)
White Bread, **Northridge,** 16-oz. (1-lb.) loaf (approx. 16 slices)	1120	208.0			70.0	13.00	(264)	(49.0)
1 slice, approx. 1 oz.			70	13.0	70.0	13.00	(264)	(49.0)
White Bread, low sodium, **Orowheat,** 16-oz. (1-lb.) loaf (approx. 18 slices)	1260	225.0			78.8	14.06	(297)	(53.0)
1 slice, approx. 0.9 oz.			70	12.5	78.8	14.06	(297)	(53.0)
White Bread, **Pepperidge Farm,** 8-oz. loaf (approx. 8 slices)	675	117.0			84.4	14.63	(251)	(55.1)
1 slice, approx. 1 oz.			84	14.6	84.4	14.63	(251)	(55.1)
16-oz. (1-lb.) loaf (approx. 18 slices)	1350	234.0			84.4	14.63	(318)	(55.2)
1 slice, approx. 0.9 oz.			75	13.0	84.4	14.63	(318)	(55.2)
32-oz. (2-lb.) loaf (approx. 34 slices)	2550	459.0			75.0	13.50	(283)	(50.9)
1 slice, approx. 0.9 oz.			75	13.5	75.0	13.50	(283)	(50.9)
White Bread, **Safeway,** 16-oz. (1-lb.) loaf (approx. 16 slices)	1040	192.0			65.0	12.00	(245)	(45.2)
White Bread, **Sweetheart,** 24-oz. loaf (approx. 24 slices)	1800	336.0			75.0	14.00	(284)	(52.9)
1 slice, approx. 1 oz.			75	14.0	75.0	14.00	(284)	(52.9)
White Bread, **Tip Top,** 22-oz. loaf (approx. 22 slices)	1650	308.0			75.0	14.00	(283)	(52.8)
1 slice, approx. 1 oz.			75	14.0	75.0	14.00	(283)	(52.8)
White Bread, **Wonder,** 22½-oz. loaf (approx. 22½ slices)	1688	303.8			75.0	13.50	(283)	(50.9)
1 slice, approx. 1 oz.			75	13.5	75.0	13.50	(283)	(50.9)
White Bread made with Buttermilk, **Millbrook,** 20-oz. loaf (approx. 20 slices)	1600	270.0			80.0	13.50	(302)	(51.2)
1 slice, approx. 1 oz.			80	13.5	80.0	13.50	(302)	(51.2)
White Bread, made with Buttermilk, **Mrs. Wright's,** 24-oz. loaf (approx. 20 slices)	1600	300.0			66.7	12.50	(251)	(47.1)
1 slice, approx. 1.2 oz.			80	15.0	66.7	12.50	(251)	(47.1)
White Bread with Buttermilk, **Wonder,** 16-oz. (1-lb.) loaf (approx. 16 slices)	1200	216.0			75.0	13.50	(283)	(50.9)
1 slice, approx. 1 oz.			75	13.5	75.0	13.50	(283)	(50.9)
White Enriched Bread, **Monks' Bread,** 16-oz. (1-lb.) loaf (approx. 16 slices)	960	160.0			60.0	10.00	(227)	(37.8)
1 slice, approx. 1 oz.			60	10.0	60.0	10.00	(227)	(37.8)
White Enriched Bread, **Scotch Buy,** 16-oz. (1-lb.) loaf (approx. 16 slices)	1270	244.9			79.4	15.31	(299)	(57.7)
1 slice, approx.0.88 oz.			70	13.5	79.4	15.31	(299)	(57.7)
22-oz. loaf (approx. 20 slices)	1760	330.0			80.0	15.00	(302)	(56.6)
1 slice, approx. 1 oz.			80	15.0	80.0	15.00	(302)	(56.6)
White Enriched Bread, Large, **The Food Emporium,** 22-oz. loaf (approx. 22 slices)	1540	297.0			70.0	13.50	(263)	(50.9)
1 slice, approx. 1 oz.			70	13.5	70.0	13.50	(263)	(50.9)

	ENTIRE LOAF Cal.	Carb.	1 SLICE Cal.	Carb.	1 OZ., BY WT. Cal.	Carb.	1 CUP CRUMBS FINE, DRY Cal.	Carb.
White Enriched Sandwich Bread, **Scotch Buy,** 22-oz. loaf (approx. 26 slices)	1143	332.6			75.6	15.12	(285)	(57.0)
1 slice, approx. 0.79 oz.			60	12.0	75.6	15.12	(285)	(57.0)
24-oz. loaf (approx. 26 slices)	1805	347.1			75.2	14.46	(284)	(54.6)
1 slice, approx. 0.86 oz.			65	12.5	75.2	14.46	(284)	(54.6)
White Sandwich Pockets, see Pocket Bread toward the end of this chapter under Specialty Breads And Rolls								
WHOLE GRAIN								
European Style Whole Grain Bread, **Rubschlager,** 16-oz. (1-lb.) loaf (approx. 15 slices)	1050	180.0			65.6	11.25	(247)	(42.4)
1 slice, approx. 1.1 oz.			70	12.0	65.6	11.25	(247)	(42.4)
Whole Grain Bread, **Rubschlager,** 16-oz. (1-lb.) loaf (approx. 15 slices)	1050	180.0			65.6	11.25		
1 slice, approx. 1.1 oz.			70	11.9	65.6	11.25		
WHOLE WHEAT								
Brick Oven 100% Whole Wheat Bread, **Arnold,** 16-oz. (1-lb.) loaf (approx. 20 slices)	1200	190.0			75.0	11.88	(283)	(44.8)
1 slice, approx. 0.8 oz.			60	9.5	75.0	11.88	(283)	(44.8)
32-oz. (2-lb.) loaf (approx. 40 slices)	2400	380.0			75.0	11.88	(283)	(44.8)
1 slice, approx. 0.8 oz.			60	9.5	75.0	11.88	(283)	(44.8)
Brick Oven 100% Whole Wheat Bread, **Arnold,** Small Family 8-oz. loaf (approx. 10 slices)	600	95.0			75.0	11.88	(283)	(44.8)
1 slice, approx. 0.8 oz.			60	9.5	75.0	11.88	(283)	(44.8)
Measure Up Whole Wheat Bread, **Arnold,** 16-oz. (1-lb.) loaf (approx. 30 slices)	1200	210.0			75.0	13.13	(283)	(49.5)
1 slice, approx. 0.53 oz.			40	7.0	75.0	13.13	(283)	(49.5)
100% Stone Ground Whole Wheat Bread, **Hearth Farms,** 24-oz. loaf (approx. 24 slices)	1800	336.0			75.0	14.0	(284)	(53.0)
1 slice, approx. 1 oz.			75	14.0	75.0	14.0	(284)	53.0)
100% Stone-Ground Whole Wheat Bread, **Rubschlager,** 16-oz. (1-lb.) loaf (approx. 18 slices)	1170	198.0			73.1	12.38		
1 slice, approx. 0.88 oz.			65	11.0	73.1	12.38		
100% Whole Wheat Bread, **A&P,** 16-oz. (1-lb.) loaf (approx. 16 slices)	1120	200.0			70.0	12.50	(264)	(47.1)
1 slice, approx. 1 oz.			70	12.5	70.0	12.50	(264)	(47.1)
100% Whole Wheat Bread, **Thomas',** 16-oz. (1-lb.) loaf (approx. 21 slices)	1045	198.0			65.2	12.36	(246)	(46.6)
1 slice, approx. 0.77 oz.			50	10.1	65.2	12.36	(246)	(46.6)
100% Whole Wheat Sandwich Bread, **Northridge,** 16-oz. (1-lb.) loaf (approx. 24 slices)	1080	216.0			67.5	13.50	(254)	(50.0)
1 slice, approx. 0.67 oz.			45	9.0	67.5	13.50	(254)	(50.0)
Raisin Whole Wheat Bread, no sugar added, **Balanced,** 14-oz. loaf, (approx. 14 slices)	1120	196.0			80.0	14.00	(302)	(52.8)
1 slice, approx. 1 oz.			80	14.0	80.0	14.00	(302)	(52.8)
Raisin Whole Wheat, **Shiloh Farms,** 16-oz. (1-lb.) loaf (approx. 12 slices)	1202	226.1			75.8	14.25	(286)	(53.7)
1 slice, approx. 1.3 oz.			101	19.0	75.8	14.25	(286)	(53.7)
Stone Ground 100% Whole Wheat Bread, **Northridge,** 16-oz. (1-lb.) loaf (approx. 16 slices)	1120	216.0			70.0	13.50	(264)	(50.9)
1 slice, approx. 1 oz.			70	13.5	70.0	13.50	(264)	(50.9)
Stone Ground Whole Wheat Bread, **Nathan Pritikin,** 16-oz. (1-lb.) loaf (approx. 16 slices)	1040	200.0			65.0	12.50	(245)	(47.1)
1 slice, approx. 1 oz.			65	12.5	65.0	12.50	(245)	(47.1)
Thin Sliced Whole Wheat Bread, **Pepperidge Farm,** 16-oz. (1-lb.) loaf (approx. 28 slices)	1120	196.0			70.0	12.25	(264)	(46.2)
1 slice, approx. 0.57 oz.			40	7.0	70.0	12.25	(264)	(46.2)
Whole Wheat & Bran Matzo, see Matzos toward the end of this chapter under Specialty Breads And Rolls								
Whole Wheat Bread, **Balanced,** 16-oz. (1-lb.) loaf (approx. 16 slices)	1120	205.3			70.0	12.83	(264)	(48.4)
1 slice, approx. 1 oz.			70	12.8	70.0	12.83	(264)	(48.4)

	ENTIRE LOAF Cal.	Carb.	1 SLICE Cal.	Carb.	1 OZ., BY WT. Cal.	Carb.	1 CUP CRUMBS FINE, DRY Cal.	Carb.
Whole Wheat Bread, salt free, **Balanced,** 16-oz. (1-lb.) loaf (approx. 16 slices)	1120	205.3			70.0	12.83	(263)	(48.4)
1 slice, approx. 1 oz.			70	12.8	70.0	12.83	(263)	(48.4)
Whole Wheat Bread, **Pepperidge Farm,** 16-oz. (1-lb.) loaf (approx. 18 slices)	1260	216.0			78.8	12.30	(297)	(46.4)
1 slice, approx. 0.89 oz.			70	12.0	78.8	12.30	(297)	(46.4)
Whole Wheat Bread, no salt added, **Shiloh Farms,** 16-oz. (1-lb.) loaf (approx. 16 slices)	1200	224.0			75.0	14.00	(283)	(52.8)
1 slice, approx. 1 oz.			75	14.0	75.0	14.00	(283)	(52.8)
Whole Wheat Matzos, see Matzos toward the end of this chapter under Specialty Breads And Rolls								
Whole Wheat Pita Bread, see Pita Bread toward the end of this chapter under Specialty Breads And Rolls								
100% Whole Wheat Pita Bread, see Pita Bread toward the end of this chapter under Specialty Breads And Rolls								
100% Whole Wheat Pocket Bread, see Pocket Bread toward the end of this chapter under Specialty Breads And Rolls								

PREPACKAGED BUNS AND ROLLS, by brand

	ENTIRE PACKAGE Cal.	Carb.	1 BUN OR ROLL Cal.	Carb.	1 OZ., BY WT. Cal.	Carb.
BAGELS are listed toward the end of this chapter under Specialty Breads And Rolls.						
Bake 'n Serve Rolls, **Jane Parker (A&P),** 11-oz. bag (12 twin rolls)	990	180.0			90.0	16.36
1 roll, approx. 0.92 oz.			83	15.0	90.0	16.36
Big Marty's Large Rolls, **Martin's,** 18-oz. package (8 rolls)	1376	256.0			76.4	14.20
1 roll, approx. 2.25 oz.			172	32.0	76.4	14.20
BOULE						
Boule, sugar free, **Country French,** 16-oz. (1-lb.) bag (16 rolls)	1120	272.0			70.0	17.0
1 roll, approx. 1 oz.			70	17.0	70.0	17.0
Petite Boule, **Country French,** 12-oz. bag (10 rolls)	700	170.0			58.3	14.17
1 roll, approx. 1.2 oz.			70	17.0	58.3	14.17
BRAN ROLLS						
Parti Pak Bran Rolls, **Bellacicco,** 16-oz. (1-lb.) bag (12 rolls)	1104	223.6			69.0	13.97
1 roll, approx. 1.33 oz.			92	18.6	69.0	13.97
BROWN 'N' SERVE ROLLS						
Brown 'n' Serve Rolls, **Butternut,** 12-oz. bag (12 rolls)	1020	132.0			85.0	11.00
1 roll, approx. 1 oz.			85	11.0	85.0	11.00
14-oz. bag (12 rolls)	960	144.0			68.6	12.00
1 roll, approx. 1.2 oz.			80	14.4	68.6	12.00
Brown 'n' Serve Rolls, **Dutch Hearth,** 12-oz. bag (12 rolls)	1020	174.0			85.0	14.50
1 roll, approx. 1 oz.			85	14.5	85.0	14.50
Brown 'n' Serve Rolls, **Eddy's,** 11-oz. bag (12 rolls)	1020	132.0			92.7	12.00
1 roll, approx. 0.92 oz.			85	11.4	92.7	12.00
Brown 'n' Serve Rolls, **Hart's,** 12-oz. bag (12 rolls)	1020	138.0			85.0	11.50
1 roll, approx. 1 oz.			85	11.5	85.0	11.50
Brown 'n' Serve Rolls, **Millbrook,** 12-oz. bag (12 rolls)	1020	132.0			85.0	11.00
1 roll, approx. 1 oz.			85	11.0	85.0	11.00
Brown 'n' Serve Rolls, **Mrs. Karl's,** 12-oz. bag (12 rolls)	960	144.0			80.0	12.00
1 roll, approx. 1 oz.			80	12.0	80.0	12.00
Brown 'n' Serve enriched rolls with Buttermilk, **Mrs. Wright's,** 11½-oz. bag (12 rolls)	1200	168.0			104.3	14.60
1 roll, approx. 0.96 oz.			100	14.0	104.3	14.60
Brown 'n' Serve Buttermilk Rolls, **Wonder,** 12-oz. package (12 rolls)	1020	156.0			85.0	13.00
1 roll, approx. 1 oz.			85	13.0	85.0	13.00
Brown 'n' Serve Chef Rolls, Enriched, **Lovenbest,** 12-oz. package (12 rolls)	960	144.0			80.0	12.00
1 roll, approx. 1 oz.			80	12.0	80.0	12.00

	ENTIRE PACKAGE Cal.	Carb.	1 BUN OR ROLL Cal.	Carb.	1 OZ., BY WT. Cal.	Carb.
Brown 'n' Serve Chef Rolls, **Millbrook,** 12-oz. bag (12 rolls)	1020	132.0			85.0	11.00
1 roll, approx. 1 oz.			85	11.0	85.0	11.00
Brown 'n' Serve Cloverleaf Rolls, **Mrs. Wright's,** 11½-oz. bag (12 rolls)	1200	168.0			104.3	14.60
1 roll, approx. 0.96 oz			100	14.0	104.3	14.60
Brown 'n' Serve Club Rolls, **Pepperidge Farm,** 8-oz. package (6 rolls)	720	138.0			90.0	17.25
1 roll, approx. 1.33 oz.			120	23.0	90.0	17.25
Brown 'n' Serve Crown Rolls, **Millbrook,** 12-oz. bag (12 rolls)	960	144.0			80.0	12.00
1 roll, approx. 1 oz.			80	12.0	80.0	12.00
Brown 'n' Serve Enriched Rolls, **Wonder,** 12-oz. package (12 rolls)	1020	156.0			85.0	13.00
1 roll, approx. 1 oz.			85	13.0	85.0	13.00
Brown 'n' Serve Flaky Rolls, **A&P,** 11-oz. package (12 rolls)	1140	156.0			103.6	14.18
1 roll, approx. 0.92 oz.			95	13.0	103.6	14.18
Brown 'n' Serve Flaky Gem Rolls, **Mrs. Wright's,** 11½-oz. bag (12 rolls)	1200	168.0			104.3	14.60
1 roll, approx. 0.96 oz.			100	14.0	104.3	14.60
Brown 'n' Serve French Rolls, **Millbrook,** 12-oz. bag (12 rolls)	960	144.0			80.0	12.00
1 roll, approx. 1 oz.			80	12.0	80.0	12.00
Brown 'n' Serve French Rolls, **Wonder,** 12-oz. package (12 rolls)	1020	162.0			85.0	13.50
1 roll, approx. 1 oz.			85	13.5	85.0	13.50
Brown 'n' Serve Gem Style Rolls, **Wonder,** 12-oz. package (12 rolls)	1020	162.0			85.0	13.50
1 roll, approx. 1 oz.			85	13.5	85.0	13.50
Brown 'n' Serve Half & Half Rolls, **Wonder,** 12-oz. package (12 rolls)	1020	156.0			85.0	13.00
1 roll, approx. 1 oz.			85	13.0	85.0	13.00
Brown 'n' Serve Home Bake Rolls, **Wonder,** 15-oz. package (15 rolls)	1275	195.0			85.0	13.00
1 roll, approx. 1 oz.			85	13.0	85.0	13.00
Brown 'n' Serve Poppyseed Rolls, **Mrs. Wright's,** 10½-oz. package (10 rolls)	821	154.0			78.2	14.66
1 roll, approx. 1.05 oz.			80	15.0	78.2	14.66
Brown 'n' Serve Sour French Rolls, **Parisian Fisherman's Wharf,** 14-oz. package (8 rolls)	960	192.0			68.6	13.71
1 roll, approx. 1.7 oz.			120	24.0	68.6	13.71
Brown 'n' Serve Sour French Rolls, **Roman Meal,** 10-oz. package (12 rolls)	900	138.0			90.0	13.80
1 roll, approx. 0.83 oz.			75	11.5	90.0	13.80
Brown 'n' Serve Sour French Rolls, **Sweetheart,** 12-oz. bag (12 rolls)	1020	132.0			85.0	11.00
1 roll, approx. 1 oz.			85	11.0	85.0	11.00
Brown 'n' Serve Sour French Rolls, **Taystee,** 11-oz. bag (12 rolls)	990	180.0			90.0	16.36
1 roll, approx. 0.92 oz.			83	15.0	90.0	16.36
Brown 'n' Serve Sour French Rolls, **Weber's,** 12-oz. bag (12 rolls)	1020	132.0			85.0	11.00
1 roll, approx. 1 oz.			85	11.0	85.0	11.00
Brown 'n' Serve Twin Rolls, **Mrs. Wright's,** 11½-oz. bag (12 rolls)	1200	168.0			104.3	14.60
1 roll, approx. 0.96 oz.			100	14.0	104.3	14.60
BUTTER CRESCENT ROLLS						
Butter Crescent Rolls, **Pepperidge Farm,** 6½-oz. package (6 rolls)	780	90.0			120.0	13.85
1 roll, approx. 1.08 oz.			130	15.0	120.0	13.85
CHALLAH ROLLS						
Enriched Challah Rolls, **Mighty Good,** 12-oz. package (6 rolls)	900	312.0			75.0	13.00
1 roll, approx. 2 oz.			150	26.0	75.0	13.00
CROISSANTS are listed toward the end of this chapter under Specialty Breads And Rolls.						
DINNER ROLLS						
Dinner Rolls, **Butternut,** 12-oz. bag (12 rolls)	1020	132.0			85.0	11.00
1 roll, approx. 1 oz.			85	11.0	85.0	11.00
Dinner Rolls, **Home Pride,** 8-oz. package (10 rolls)	720	108.0			90.0	13.50
1 roll, approx. 0.8 oz.			72	10.8	90.0	13.50
Dinner Rolls, **Millbrook,** 12-oz. bag (12 rolls)	1020	132.0			85.0	11.00
1 roll, approx. 1 oz.			85	11.0	85.0	11.00
Dinner Rolls, **Mrs. Karl's,** 12-oz. bag (12 rolls)	960	144.0			80.0	12.00
1 roll, approx. 1 oz.			80	12.0	80.0	12.00
Dinner Rolls, **Pepperidge Farm,** 8-oz. package (12 rolls)	780	120.0			97.5	15.00
1 roll, approx. 1.67 oz.			65	10.0	97.5	15.00
Dinner Rolls, **Weber's,** 11-oz. bag (12 rolls)	1020	132.0			92.7	12.00
1 roll, approx. 0.917 oz.			85	11.0	92.7	12.00

	ENTIRE PACKAGE Cal.	Carb.	1 BUN OR ROLL Cal.	Carb.	1 OZ., BY WT. Cal.	Carb.
Dinner Rolls, **Wonder,** 12-oz. package (12 rolls)	1008	163.2			84.0	13.60
1 roll, approx. 1 oz.			84	13.6	84.0	13.60
EGG						
Egg Twist Dinner Rolls, **Wenner's,** 20-oz. package (12 rolls)	1680	264.0			84.0	13.20
1 roll, approx. 1¾ oz.			140	22.0	84.0	13.20
Enriched Egg Buns, **Millbrook,** 11½-oz. bag (8 buns)	960	144.0			83.5	12.52
1 bun, approx. 1.44 oz.			12	18.3	83.5	12.52
ENRICHED BUNS *(There are many enriched buns throughout the chapter, but the following are buns named, simply, "Enriched.")*						
Enriched Buns, **Eddy's,** 12-oz. bag (8 buns)	880	168.0			73.3	14.00
1 bun, approx. 1.5 oz.			110	21.0	73.3	14.00
Enriched Buns, **Hart's,** 12-oz. bag (8 buns)	880	168.0			73.3	13.30
1 bun, approx. 1.5 oz.			110	20.0	73.3	13.30
Enriched Buns, **Holsum,** 13-oz. bag (8 buns)	1360	240.0			104.6	18.40
1 bun, approx. 1.63 oz.			171	30.0	104.6	18.40
Enriched Buns, **Millbrook,** 11½-oz. bag (8 buns)	880	168.0			76.5	14.60
1 bun, approx. 1.44 oz.			110	21.4	76.5	14.60
Enriched Buns, **Sweetheart,** 12-oz. bag (8 buns)	880	168.0			73.3	14.00
1 bun, approx. 1.5 oz.			110	21.0	73.3	14.00
FINGER ROLLS						
Finger Rolls with Poppy Seeds, **Pepperidge Farm,** 7½-oz. package (12 rolls)	600	108.0			80.0	14.40
1 roll, approx. 0.6 oz.			50	9.0	80.0	14.40
Sesame Finger Rolls, **Pepperidge Farm,** 7½-oz. package (12 rolls)	720	108.0			96.0	14.40
1 roll, approx. 0.63 oz.			60	9.0	96.0	14.40
FRANKFURTER ROLLS, see Hot Dog and Frankfurter Buns and Rolls						
FRENCH ROLLS						
French Rolls, **Old Country,** 14-oz. bag (12 rolls)	1200	216.0			85.7	15.40
1 roll, approx. 1.17 oz.			100	18.0	85.7	15.40
French Rolls, **Weber's,** 14-oz. bag (12 rolls)	960	144.0			68.6	10.30
1 roll, approx. 1.17 oz.			80	12.2	68.6	10.30
French Rolls, Brown 'n' Serve, **Wonder,** 12-oz. package (12 rolls)	1020	162.0			85.0	13.50
1 roll, approx. 1 oz.			85	13.5	85.0	13.50
French Style Rolls, **Pepperidge Farm,** 12-oz. bag (9 rolls)	990	171.0			82.5	14.33
1 roll, approx. 1.3 oz.			110	19.0	82.5	14.33
Large French Rolls, **Pepperidge Farm,** 10-oz. package (2 rolls)	760	154.0			76.0	15.40
1 roll, approx. 5 oz.			380	76.0	76.0	15.40
Small French Rolls, **Pepperidge Farm,** 10-oz. package (3 rolls)	780	150.0			78.0	15.00
1 roll, approx. 3.3 oz.			260	50.0	78.0	15.00
Sour French Rolls, **Pepperidge Farm,** 12-oz. package (9 rolls)	900	153.0			75.0	12.75
1 roll, approx. 1.3 oz.			100	17.0	75.0	12.75
Sour French Rolls, **Toscana's,** 15-oz. package (6 rolls)	1140	246.0			76.0	16.40
1 roll, approx. 2.5 oz.			190	41.0	76.0	16.40
10½-oz. package (8 rolls)	807	169.6			76.9	16.15
1 roll, approx. 1.3 oz.			100	21.0	76.9	16.15
Sour French Rolls, Brown 'n' Serve, **Parisian,** 14-oz. package (8 rolls)	960	192.0			68.6	13.71
1 roll, approx. 1.7 oz.			120	24.0	68.6	13.71
Sourdough French Style Enriched Rolls, Fransico **Arnold,** 11-oz. bag (10 rolls)	1000	190.0			90.9	17.27
1 roll, approx. 1.2 oz.			100	19.0	90.9	17.27
Sweet French Rolls, **Toscana's,** 12½-oz. package (6 rolls)	960	192.0			76.8	15.36
1 roll, approx. 2.1 oz.			160	32.0	76.8	15.36
FUN BUNS						
Fun Buns, **Butternut,** 12-oz. bag (8 buns)	880	168.0			73.3	14.00
1 bun, approx. 1.5 oz.			110	21.0	73.3	14.00
Fun Buns, **Millbrook,** 12-oz. bag (8 buns)	880	168.0			73.3	14.00
1 bun, approx. 1.5 oz.			110	21.0	73.3	14.00
Fun Buns, **Mrs. Karl's,** 12-oz. bag (8 buns)	880	168.0			73.3	14.00
1 bun, approx. 1.5 oz.			110	21.0	73.3	14.00
Fun Buns, **Weber's,** 12-oz. bag (8 buns)	960	176.0			80.0	14.67
1 bun, approx. 1.5 oz.			120	22.0	80.0	14.67
GOLDEN TWIST ROLLS						
Golden Twist Rolls, **Pepperidge Farm,** 6¼-oz. package (6 rolls)	720	90.0			115.2	14.40
1 roll, approx. 1.04 oz.			120	15.0	115.2	14.40

	ENTIRE PACKAGE		1 BUN OR ROLL		1 OZ., BY WT.	
	Cal.	Carb.	Cal.	Carb.	Cal.	Carb.
HALF & HALF ROLLS						
Half & Half Rolls, Brown 'n' Serve, **Wonder,** 12-oz. package (12 rolls)	1020	156.0			85.0	13.00
1 roll, approx. 1 oz.			85	13.0	85.0	13.00
HAMBURGER BUNS AND ROLLS						
8 Enriched Hamburger Rolls, sliced, **A&P,** 10-oz. package (8 rolls)	720	136.0			72.0	13.60
1 roll, approx. 1.25 oz.			90	17.0	72.0	13.60
8 Enriched Hamburger Rolls, sliced, **P&Q (A&P),** 10-oz. package (8 rolls)	720	136.0			72.0	13.60
1 roll, approx. 1.25 oz.			90	17.0	72.0	13.60
8 Enriched Rolls, **The Food Emporium,** 12-oz. bag (8 rolls)	880	160.0			73.3	13.33
1 roll, approx. 1.5 oz.			110	20.0	73.3	13.33
Giant Hamburger Buns, **Mrs. Wright's,** 14-oz. bag (6 buns)	1200	204.0			85.7	14.50
1 bun, approx. 2.33 oz.			200	34.0	85.7	14.50
Hamburger Buns, **Arnold,** 11-oz. bag (8 buns)	1040	176.0			95.5	16.00
1 bun, approx. 1.38 oz.			130	22.0	95.5	16.00
Hamburger Buns, **Millbrook,** 12-oz. bag (8 buns)	880	160.0			73.3	13.30
1 bun, approx. 1.5 oz.			110	20.0	73.3	13.30
Hamburger Buns, **Mrs. Wright's,** 12-oz. bag (8 buns)	1040	192.0			86.7	16.00
1 bun, approx. 1.52 oz.			130	24.0	86.7	16.00
13-oz. bag (8 buns)	1120	208.0			86.2	16.00
1 bun, approx. 1.62 oz.			140	26.0	86.2	16.00
Hamburger Buns, **Sloan's,** 10-oz. bag (8 buns)	1040	192.0			104.0	19.20
1 bun, approx. 1.25 oz.			130	24.0	104.0	19.20
Hamburger Buns, **Wonder,** 12.5-oz. bag (10 buns)	1000	181.3			80.0	14.50
1 bun, approx. 1.25 oz.			100	18.1	80.0	14.50
Hamburger Rolls, **Jane Parker (A&P),** 12-oz. bag (8 rolls)	960	176.0			80.0	14.67
1 roll, approx. 1.5 oz.			120	22.0	80.0	14.67
Hamburger Rolls, **Pepperidge Farm,** 8-oz. bag (6 rolls)	660	120.0			82.5	15.00
1 roll, approx. 1.33 oz.			110	20.0	82.5	15.00
Kaiser-Hoagie Buns, **Kaiser-Hoagie,** 21-oz. bag (4 rolls)	1610	287.0			76.7	13.67
1 bun, approx. 5.25 oz.			403	71.8	76.7	13.67
Multi-Meal Hamburger Buns, **Mrs. Wright's,** 13-oz. bag (8 buns)	1040	192.0			80.0	14.70
1 bun, approx. 1.62 oz.			130	24.0	80.0	14.70
Natural Hamburger Buns, **Roman Meal,** 12-oz. bag (8 buns)	1120	200.0			93.3	16.67
1 bun, approx. 1.5 oz.			140	25.0	93.3	16.67
Roman Meal Hamburger Buns, **Butternut,** 12-oz. bag (8 buns)	960	152.0			80.0	12.65
1 bun, approx. 1.5 oz.			120	19.0	80.0	12.65
Roman Meal Hamburger Buns, **Mrs. Karl's,** 12-oz. bag (8 buns)	960	152.0			80.0	12.65
1 bun, approx. 1.5 oz.			120	19.0	80.0	12.65
Roman Meal Hamburger Buns, **Weber's,** 12-oz. bag (8 buns)	1440	228.0			120.0	19.00
1 bun, approx. 1.5 oz.			180	28.5	120.0	19.00
Sesame Hamburger Buns, **Mrs. Wright's,** 12½-oz. bag (8 buns)	1120	192.0			89.6	15.30
1 bun, approx. 1.56 oz.			140	24.0	89.6	15.30
13½-oz. bag (8 buns)	1200	208.0			88.9	15.40
1 bun, approx. 1.69 oz.			150	26.0	88.9	15.40
Sesame Seed Buns, **Pepperidge Farm,** 8¼-oz. bag (6 buns)	720	114.0			87.3	13.81
1 bun, approx. 1.38 oz.			120	19.0	87.3	13.81
Sliced Hamburger Buns, **Mrs. Wright's,** 16½-oz. bag (12 buns)	1320	240.0			80.0	14.50
1 bun, approx. 1.38 oz.			110	20.0	80.0	14.50
Taystee Eights, **Taystee,** 10-oz. bag (8 "eights")	880	160.0			88.0	16.00
1 "eight," approx. 1.25 oz.			110	20.0	88.0	16.00
HARD ROLLS						
Hard Rolls, 12 Enriched, **West Side Bakery,** 20-oz. package (12 rolls)	1920	336.0			96.0	16.80
1 roll, approx. 1.7 oz.			160	28.0	96.0	16.80
HAWAIIAN SWEET ROLLS						
Hawaiian Sweet Rolls, **International,** 16-oz. package (6 rolls)	1546	230.1			96.6	14.38
1 roll, approx. 2.4 oz.			235	35.0	96.6	14.38
HEARTH ROLLS						
Hearth Rolls, **Pepperidge Farm,** 8½-oz. package (12 rolls)	720	138.0			84.7	16.24
1 roll, approx. 0.71 oz.			60	11.5	84.7	16.24

	ENTIRE PACKAGE		1 BUN OR ROLL		1 OZ., BY WT.	
	Cal.	Carb.	Cal.	Carb.	Cal.	Carb.
HOME BAKE ROLLS						
Home Bake Rolls, Brown 'n' Serve, **Wonder,** 15-oz. package (15 rolls)	1275	195.0			85.0	13.00
1 roll, approx. 1 oz.			85	13.0	85.0	13.00
HOT DOG AND FRANKFURTER BUNS AND ROLLS						
Buns made with Honey 'n' Egg, **Taystee,** 10-oz. bag (8 buns)	1080	176.0			108.0	17.60
1 bun, approx. 1.25 oz.			135	22.0	108.0	17.60
8 Enriched Hot Dog Rolls, sliced, **A&P,** 10-oz. package (8 rolls)	720	136.0			72.0	13.60
1 roll, approx. 1.25 oz.			90	17.0	72.0	13.60
8 Enriched Hot Dog Rolls, sliced, **P&Q (A&P),** 10-oz. package (8 rolls)	720	136.0			72.0	13.60
1 roll, approx. 1.25 oz.			90	17.0	72.0	13.60
8 Enriched Rolls, **The Food Emporium,** 12-oz. bag (8 rolls)	880	160.0			73.3	13.33
1 roll, approx. 1.5 oz.			110	20.0	73.3	13.33
Enriched Frankfurter Rolls, side sliced, **Pepperidge Farm,** 14-oz. package (8 rolls)	960	176.0			68.6	12.57
1 roll, approx. 1.75 oz.			120	22.0	68.6	12.57
Frankfurter Rolls, **Pepperidge Farm,** 8-oz. bag (6 rolls)	720	120.0			90.0	15.00
1 roll, approx. 1.33 oz.			120	20.0	90.0	15.00
Hot Dog Buns, **Millbrook,** 12-oz. bag (8 buns)	880	160.0			73.3	13.30
1 bun, approx. 1.5 oz.			110	20.0	73.3	13.30
Hot Dog Buns, **Mrs. Wright's,** 11-oz. bag (8 buns)	960	176.0			87.3	16.00
1 bun, approx. 1.38 oz.			120	22.0	87.3	16.00
Hot Dog Buns, **Sloan's,** 10-oz. bag (8 buns)	1040	192.0			104.0	19.20
1 bun, approx. 1.25 oz.			130	24.0	104.0	19.20
Hot Dog Buns, **Wonder,** 12½-oz. bag (10 buns)	1000	181.3			80.0	14.50
1 bun, approx. 1.25 oz.			100	18.1	80.0	14.50
Hot Dog Buns, sliced, **Mrs. Wright's,** 13½-oz. bag (10 buns)	1100	190.0			81.5	14.70
1 bun, approx. 1.34 oz.			110	19.0	81.5	14.70
Hot Dog Rolls, **Jane Parker (A&P),** 10-oz. bag (8 rolls)	880	160.0			88.0	16.00
1 roll, approx. 1.25 oz.			110	20.0	88.0	16.00
Multi-Meal B'n'S Hot Dog Buns, **Mrs. Wright's,** 12-oz. bag (12 buns)	1200	180.0			100.0	15.00
1 bun, approx. 1 oz.			100	15.0		
Natural Whole Grain Hot Dog Buns, **Roman Meal,** 12½-oz. bag (8 buns)	1121	200.4			89.7	16.03
1 bun, approx. 1.56 oz.			140	25.0	89.7	16.03
Roman Meal Hot Dog Buns, **Butternut,** 12-oz. bag (8 buns)	960	152.0			80.0	12.60
1 bun, approx. 1.5 oz.			120	19.0	80.0	12.60
Roman Meal Hot Dog Buns, **Weber's,** 12½-oz. bag (8 buns)	960	152.0			80.0	12.65
1 bun, approx. 1.6 oz.			120	20.2	80.0	12.65
U-Shaped Hot Dog & Sandwich Rolls, **Caddies,** 10-oz. bag (8 rolls)	1040	160.0			104.0	16.00
1 roll, approx. 1.25 oz.			130	20.0	104.0	16.00
KAISER ROLLS						
Kaiser Rolls, **Jane Parker (A&P),** 10-oz. bag, (6 rolls)	1440	276.0			144.0	27.60
1 roll, approx. 0.83 oz.			120	23.0	144.0	27.60
Kaiser Rolls, Enriched, **Jane Parker (A&P),** 12-oz. package (6 rolls)	900	168.0			75.0	14.00
1 roll, approx. 2 oz.			150	28.0	75.0	14.00
OLD FASHIONED ROLLS						
Old Fashioned Rolls, **Pepperidge Farm,** 7-oz. package (12 rolls)	440	64.0			62.9	9.14
1 roll, approx. 0.58 oz.			37	5.3	62.9	9.14
Old Fashioned Style Pull Apart Pan Rolls, **Taystee,** 10-oz. package (24 rolls)	900	156.0			90.0	15.60
1 roll, approx. 0.42 oz.			38	6.5	90.0	15.60
ONION ROLLS						
Onion Rolls, **Levy's,** 12-oz. package (6 rolls)	1020	180.0			85.0	15.00
1 roll, approx. 2 oz.			170	30.0	85.0	15.00
PARKERHOUSE ROLLS						
Parkerhouse Dinner Party Rolls, **Arnold,** 8-oz. package (12 rolls)	780	126.0			97.5	15.75
1 roll, approx. 0.67 oz.			65	10.5	97.5	15.75
Parker House Rolls, **Pepperidge Farm,** 7½-oz. package (12 rolls)	720	116.0			96.0	15.47
1 roll, approx. 0.63 oz.			60	9.7	96.0	15.47
Parkerhouse Rolls, **Sara Lee,** 7-oz. package (9 rolls)	661	92.9			94.4	13.27
1 roll, approx. 0.78 oz.			73	10.3	94.4	13.27
Parkerhouse Style Rolls, **Bridgeford,** 25-oz. package (24 rolls)	2250	375.0			90.0	15.00
1 roll, approx. 1.04 oz.			94	15.6	90.0	15.00

	ENTIRE PACKAGE Cal.	Carb.	1 BUN OR ROLL Cal.	Carb.	1 OZ., BY WT. Cal.	Carb.
PARTI PAK ROLLS						
Parti Pak Rolls, **Bellacicco,** 16-oz. (1-lb.) package (12 rolls)	810	150.0			50.6	9.38
1 roll, approx. 1.33 oz.			68	12.5	50.6	9.38
Parti Pak Bran Rolls, **Bellacicco,** 16-oz. (1-lb.) package (12 rolls)	1104	223.6			69.0	13.97
1 roll, approx. 1.33 oz.			92	18.6	69.0	13.97
PARTY ROLLS						
Party Pan Rolls, **Pepperidge Farm,** 7½-oz. package (20 rolls)	700	110.0			93.3	14.67
1 roll, approx. 0.38 oz.			35	5.5	93.3	14.67
Party Rolls, **Sara Lee,** 7-oz. package (12 rolls)	661	92.9			94.4	13.27
1 roll, approx. 0.58 oz.			55	7.7	94.4	13.27
PETITE LISA ROLLS						
Petite Lisa Rolls, **Country French,** 12-oz. bag (10 rolls)	700	170.0			58.3	14.70
1 roll, approx. 1.2 oz.			70	17.0	58.3	14.17
POTATO ROLLS						
Potato Rolls, **Martin's,** sliced, 15-oz. package (12 rolls)	1080	216.0			72.0	14.40
1 roll, approx. 1.25 oz.			90	18.0	72.0	14.40
Potato Sandwich Rolls, **Martin's,** 15-oz. package (8 rolls)	1168	224.0			96.0	16.80
1 roll, approx. 1.87 oz.			146	28.0	96.0	16.80
ROLLS						
Rolls, **Levy's,** 12-oz. package (9 rolls)	1017	180.0			84.7	15.00
1 roll, approx. 1.33 oz.			113	20.0	84.7	15.00
SANDWICH BUNS AND ROLLS						
Dutch Egg Sandwich Buns, with Sesame Seeds, **Arnold,** 12½-oz. bag (8 buns)	1200	176.0			96.0	14.08
1 bun, approx. 1.56 oz.			150	22.0	96.0	14.08
Enriched Sandwich Buns with Poppy Seeds, **Pepperidge Farm,** 13-oz. package (8 rolls)	880	160.0			67.7	12.31
1 roll, approx. 1.63 oz.			110	20.0	67.7	12.31
Enriched Sandwich Buns with Sesame Seeds, **Pepperidge Farm,** 13-oz. package (8 rolls)	640	104.0			49.2	8.00
1 roll, approx. 1.63 oz.			80	13.0	49.2	8.00
Onion Sandwich Buns, **Arnold,** 13-oz. package (8 rolls)	1040	176.0			80.0	13.54
1 roll, approx. 1.63 oz.			130	22.0	80.0	13.54
Onion Sandwich Buns with Poppy Seeds, **Pepperidge Farm,** 15-oz. package (8 rolls)	1200	208.0			80.0	13.87
1 roll, approx. 1.88 oz.			150	26.0	80.0	13.87
Potato Sandwich Rolls, **Martin's,** 15-oz. package (8 rolls)	1168	224.0			96.0	16.80
1 roll, approx. 1.87 oz.			146	28.0	96.0	16.80
San'wich Rolls, **Toscana's,** 14-oz. package (6 rolls)	1022	216.3			73.0	15.45
1 roll, approx. 2.33 oz.			170	36.0	73.0	15.45
Soft Sandwich Rolls, **Arnold,** 16-oz. (1-lb.) package (12 rolls)	1320	216.0			82.5	13.50
1 roll, approx. 1.33 oz.			110	18.0	82.5	13.50
SESAME ROLLS						
Sesame Crisp Rolls, **Pepperidge Farm,** 7-oz. package (9 rolls)	630	110.0			90.0	15.86
1 roll, approx. 0.78 oz.			70	12.3	90.0	15.86
Sesame Rolls, **Mrs. Wright's,** 14-oz. package (12 rolls)	1200	192.0			85.7	13.71
1 roll, approx. 1.2 oz.			100	16.0	85.7	13.71
Sesame Seed Rolls, **Sara Lee,** 7-oz. package (12 rolls)	661	92.9			94.4	13.27
1 roll, approx. 0.58 oz.			55	7.7	94.4	13.27
SOFT ROLLS						
Soft Family Rolls, **Pepperidge Farm,** 12¼-oz. bag (10 rolls)	900	150.0			73.5	12.24
1 roll, approx. 1.2 oz.			90	15.0	73.5	12.24
SOURDOUGH (see also Brown 'n' Serve and French Rolls)						
Fisherman's Wharf Sour Rolls, **Parisian,** 16-oz. (1-lb.) package (6 rolls)	1272	252.0			79.5	15.75
1 roll, approx. 2.7 oz.			212	42.0	79.5	15.75
Natural Sourdough Rolls, **Pioneer,** 13-oz. bag (3 rolls)	930	198.0			71.5	15.20
1 roll, approx. 4.3 oz.			310	66.0	71.5	15.20
Sourdough Flute Rolls, **Pioneer,** 16-oz. (1-lb.) bag (2 rolls)	1120	240.0			70.0	15.00
1 roll, approx. 8 oz.			560	120.0	70.0	15.00
STEAK ROLLS						
Steak Rolls, **Jane Parker (A&P),** 16-oz. (1-lb.) package (6 rolls)	1260	210.0			84.0	14.00
1 roll, approx. 2.5 oz.			210	35.0	84.0	14.00
Steak-Umm Rolls, **Table Treats,** 12-oz. package (6 rolls)	930	192.0			77.5	16.00
1 roll, approx. 2 oz.			155	32.0	77.5	16.00
SWEET ROLLS						
Fisherman's Wharf Sweet Rolls, **Parisian,** 16-oz. (1-lb.) package (6 rolls)	1254	252.0			78.4	15.75
1 roll, approx. 2.7 oz.			209	42.0	78.4	15.75
Sweet Farm Style Rolls, **Mrs. Wright's,** 12-oz. package (12 rolls)	1200	204.0			100.0	17.00
1 roll, approx. 1 oz.			100	17.0	100.0	17.00

SPECIALTY BREADS AND ROLLS

Bagels

	ENTIRE PACKAGE Cal.	Carb.	1 BAGEL Cal.	Carb.	1 OZ., BY WT. Cal.	Carb.
Bagelettes (Baby Bagels), **Lender's,** 11-oz. bag (12 bagels)	960	180.0			87.3	16.36
1 bagel, approx. 0.92 oz.			80	15.0	87.3	16.36
Bagels, **International,** 15-oz. bag (6 bagels)	1164	230.3			77.6	15.35
1 bagel, approx. 2.46 oz.			190	37.6	77.6	15.35
Bagels, **Lender's,** 12-oz. bag (6 bagels)	960	186.0			80.0	15.50
1 bagel, approx. 2 oz.			160	31.0	80.0	15.50
Egg Bagels, **International,** 15-oz. package (6 bagels)	1167	233.4			77.8	15.56
1 bagel, approx. 2.31 oz.			179	35.8	77.8	15.56
Egg Flavored Bagels, **Lender's,** 12-oz. bag (6 bagels)	960	186.0			80.0	15.50
1 bagel, approx. 2 oz.			160	31.0	80.0	15.50
Garlic Bagels, **Lender's,** 12-oz. bag (6 bagels)	961	192.0			80.0	16.00
1 bagel, approx. 2 oz.			160	32.0	80.0	16.00
Onion Bagels, **International,** 15-oz. package (6 bagels)	1250	246.0			83.3	16.40
1 bagel, approx. 2.31 oz.			193	38.0	83.3	16.40
Onion Bagels, **Lender's,** 12-oz. bag (6 bagels)	960	192.0			80.0	16.00
1 bagel, approx. 2 oz.			160	32.0	80.0	16.00
Pizza Bagels:						
Cheese Pizza Bagels, **Lender's,** 12-oz. package (6 bagels)	840	102.0			70.0	8.50
1 cheese pizza bagel, approx. 2 oz.			140	17.0	70.0	8.50
Mushroom Pizza Bagels, **Lender's,** 13½-oz. package (6 bagels)	900	108.0			66.7	8.00
1 mushroom pizza bagel, approx. 2.25 oz.			150	18.0	66.7	8.00
Onion Pizza Bagels, **Lender's,** 13½-oz. package (6 bagels)	840	114.0			62.2	8.44
1 onion pizza bagel, approx. 2.25 oz.			140	19.0	62.2	8.44
"The Works," Onions, Peppers & Mushrooms Pizza Bagels, **Lender's,** 16½-oz. package (6 bagels)	1020	137.9			61.8	8.36
1 combination pizza bagel, approx. 2.75 oz.			170	23.0	61.8	8.36
Pumpernickel Bagels, **Lender's,** 12-oz. bag (6 bagels)	960	186.0			80.0	15.50
1 bagel, approx. 2 oz.			160	31.0	80.0	15.50
Raisin 'n Honey Bagels, **Lender's,** 15-oz. bag (6 bagels)	1200	240.0			80.0	16.00
1 bagel, approx. 2.46 oz.			200	40.0	80.0	16.00
Raisin 'n Honey Cinnamon Bagels, **Lender's,** 15-oz. bag (6 bagels)	1200	240.0			80.0	16.00
1 bagel, approx. 2.46 oz.			200	40.0	80.0	16.00
Rye Bagels, **Lender's,** 12-oz. bag (6 bagels)	960	186.0			80.0	15.50
1 bagel, approx. 2 oz.			160	31.0	80.0	15.50
"Sesame Rings of the Middle East," **Toufayan's,** 11-oz. package (5 sesame rings)	800	130.0			72.7	11.82
1 ring, approx. 2.2 oz.			160	26.0	72.7	11.82
Sesame Seed Bagels, **Lender's,** 12-oz. bag (6 bagels)	960	192.0			80.0	16.00
1 bagel, approx. 2 oz.			160	32.0	80.0	16.00
Wheat 'n Honey Hi-Fiber Bagels, **Lender's,** 15-oz. package (6 bagels)	1200	228.0			80.0	15.20
1 bagel, approx. 2.46 oz.			200	38.0	80.0	15.20

Bagel Chips

	ENTIRE PACKAGE Cal.	ENTIRE PACKAGE Carb.	1 BAGEL CHIP Cal.	1 BAGEL CHIP Carb.	1 OZ., BY WT. Cal.	1 OZ., BY WT. Carb.
(So what's a bagel chip? See "How To Eat Bread" in the BREADS chapter preface)						
Bagel Chips, Poppy Seed, **Balducci's,** 1 package, approx. 16 oz. (1 lb.) (approx. 20 slices, each of different weight)	(1280)	(24.8)			(80.0)	(15.50)
1 slice, approx. 0.8 oz. (including ⅛ tsp. of seeds)			(64)	(12.4)	(80.0)	(15.50)
Bagel Chips, Sesame Seed, **Balducci's,** 1 package, approx. 18¼ oz., (approx. 20 slices, each of different weight)	(1460)	(282.9)			(80.0)	(15.50)
1 slice, approx. 0.9 oz. (including ⅛ tsp. of seeds)			(68)	(13.2)	(80.0)	(15.50)
Bagel Chips, Unseeded Plain or Rye, **Balducci's,** 1 package, approx. 15.7 oz. (approx. 20 slices, each of different weight)	(1256)	(243.4)			(80.0)	(15.50)
1 slice, approx. 0.8 oz.			(62)	(12.1)	(80.0)	(15.50)
Bagel Chips, Whole Wheat, unseeded, **Balducci's,** 1 package, approx. 12.3 oz. (approx. 18–20 slices, each of different weight)	(986)	(187.3)			(80.0)	(15.20)
1 slice, approx. 0.7 oz.			(52)	(9.9)	(80.0)	(15.20)

Croissants

	ENTIRE PACKAGE Cal.	ENTIRE PACKAGE Carb.	1 CROISSANT Cal.	1 CROISSANT Carb.	1 OZ., BY WT. Cal.	1 OZ., BY WT. Carb.
Croissants (based on generic data from France), 1 pound	1171	213.3			73.2	13.33
All Butter Croissants, **Pepperidge Farm,** 4-oz. package (2 croissants)	400	38.0			100.0	9.50
1 croissant, approx. 2 oz.			200	19.0	100.0	9.50
All Butter Croissants, **Sara Lee,** 6-oz. package (4 croissants)	680	76.0			113.0	12.67
1 croissant, approx. 1.5 oz.			170	19.0	113.0	12.67
Almond Croissants, **Pepperidge Farm,** 4-oz. package (2 croissants)	420	42.0			105.0	10.50
1 croissant, approx. 2 oz.			210	21.0	105.0	10.50
Cheese Croissants, **Sara Lee,** 6-oz. package (4 croissants)	680	76.0			113.0	12.67
1 croissant, approx. 1.5 oz.			170	19.0	113.0	12.67
Cinnamon Croissants, **Pepperidge Farm,** 4-oz. package (2 croissants)	400	46.0			100.0	11.50
1 croissant, approx. 2 oz.			200	23.0	100.0	11.50
Raisin Croissants, **Pepperidge Farm,** 4-oz. package (2 croissants)	400	48.0			100.0	12.00
1 croissant, approx. 2 oz.			200	24.0	100.0	12.00
Wheat 'n' Honey Croissants, **Sara Lee,** 6-oz. package (4 croissants)	680	72.0			113.0	12.00
1 croissant, approx. 1.5 oz.			170	18.0	113.0	12.00

English Muffins

	ENTIRE PACKAGE Cal.	ENTIRE PACKAGE Carb.	1 MUFFIN Cal.	1 MUFFIN Carb.	1 OZ., BY WT. Cal.	1 OZ., BY WT. Carb.
Bran'nola Natural Muffins with Bran, **Bran'nola,** 14-oz. bag (6 muffins)	960	180.0			68.6	12.86
1 muffin, approx. 2.33 oz.			160	30.0	68.6	12.86
English Muffins, plain, **Jane Parker (A&P),** 12-oz. package (6 muffins)	780	150.0			65.0	12.50
1 muffin, approx. 2 oz.			130	25.0	65.0	12.50
English Muffins, plain, **Morton,** 11-oz. package (6 muffins)	720	132.0			65.5	12.00
1 muffin, approx. 1.75 oz.			120	22.0	65.5	12.00
English Muffins, plain, **Newly Weds,** 10-oz. package (4 muffins)	612	117.2			61.1	11.70
15-oz. package (6 muffins)	918	175.8			61.1	11.70
7.8-lb. package (50 muffins)	7650	1460.2			61.1	11.70
1 muffin, approx. 2.5 oz.			153	29.3	61.1	11.70
English Muffins, plain, **Pepperidge Farm,** 12-oz. package (6 muffins)	840	162.0			70.0	13.50
1 muffin, approx. 2 oz.			140	27.0	70.0	13.50
English Muffins, plain, **Super-Value,** 12-oz. package (6 muffins)	780	147.6			65.0	12.30
1 muffin, approx. 2 oz.			130	25.0	65.0	12.30
English Muffins, plain, **Thomas',** 7.75-oz. package (4 muffins)	540	104.0			64.7	12.93
12-oz. package (6 muffins)	776	155.2			64.7	12.93
24-oz. package (12 muffins)	1553	310.3			64.7	12.93
1 muffin, approx. 2 oz.			130	26.0	64.7	12.93
English Muffins, plain, **Wonder,** 12-oz. package (6 muffins)	780	156.0			65.0	13.00
1 muffin, approx. 2 oz.			130	26.0	65.0	13.00
Extra Crisp Muffins, **Arnold,** 14-oz. (6 muffins)	900	180.0			64.3	12.80
1 muffin, approx. 2.33 oz.			150	30.0	64.3	12.80
28-oz. package (12 muffins)	1800	360.0			64.3	12.80
1 muffin, approx. 2.33 oz.			150	30.0	64.3	12.80
Honey Wheat English Muffins, **Thomas',** 12-oz. package (6 muffins)	780	162.0			65.0	13.50
1 muffin, approx. 2 oz.			130	27.0	65.0	13.50
Raisin English Muffins, **Thomas',** 13-oz. package (6 muffins)	900	174.0			69.2	13.38
1 muffin, approx. 2.16 oz.			150	29.0	69.2	13.38
7-Grain Sprouted Wheat Honey English Muffins, **Natural Food Mill Bakery,** 16-oz. (1-lb.) package (6 muffins)	840	174.0			52.5	10.88
1 muffin, approx. 2.67 oz.			140	29.0	52.5	10.88
Seven Grain Wheat English Muffins, **Ralph's,** 13-oz. package (6 muffins)	900	168.0			69.2	12.90
1 muffin, approx. 2.17 oz.			150	28.0	69.2	12.90

Matzos

	ENTIRE PACKAGE Cal.	ENTIRE PACKAGE Carb.	1 MATZO Cal.	1 MATZO Carb.	1 OZ., BY WT. Cal.	1 OZ., BY WT. Carb.	1 CUP CRUMBS FINE, DRY Cal.	1 CUP CRUMBS FINE, DRY Carb.
(For matzo crackers, see the COOKIES & CRACKERS chapter.)								
Daily Matzo Thins, **Manischewitz,** 10-oz. box (approx. 12 pieces)	1094	236.6			109.4	23.66	(412)	(89.1)
1 matzo, approx. 0.8 oz.			90	19.7	109.4	23.66	(412)	(89.1)
Daily Thin Tea Matzos, **Manischewitz,** 10-oz. box (approx. 10 pieces)	1092	238.5			109.2	23.85	(412)	(89.1)
1 matzo, approx. 1.0 oz.			110	24.8	109.2	23.85	(412)	(89.1)
Dietetic Matzo Snax, **Streit's,** 10-oz. box (approx. 11 matzos)	1200	230.0			120.0	23.00	(452)	(86.7)
1 matzo, approx. 1 oz.			120	23.0	120.0	23.00	(452)	(86.7)
Dietetic Matzos for sodium-restricted diets, **Goodman's,** 10-oz. box (approx. 12 matzos)	1080	240.0			108.0	24.00	(406)	(90.4)
1 matzo, approx. 0.83 oz.			90	20.0	108.0	24.00	(406)	(90.4)
Dietetic Matzo-Thins, **Manischewitz,** 10-oz. box (approx. 12 matzos)	1080	240.0			108.4	24.10	(408)	(90.8)
1 matzo, approx. 0.83 oz.			90	20.0	108.4	24.10	(408)	(90.8)
Egg Matzo, **Manischewitz,** 12-oz. box (approx. 10 matzos)	1320	266.0			110.0	22.17	(415)	(83.5)
1 matzo, approx. 1.20 oz.			132	26.6	110.0	22.17	(415)	(83.5)
Egg n' Onion Matzo, **Manischewitz,** 10-oz. box (approx. 10 matzos)	1100	235.5			110.0	23.55	(415)	(88.7)
1 matzo, approx. 1 oz.			110	23.6	110.0	23.55	(415)	(88.7)
"Plain" ("Daily") Matzo, **Goodman's,** 10-oz. box (approx. 10 matzos)	1200	240.0			120.0	24.00	(452)	(90.5)
1 matzo, approx. 1 oz.			120	24.0	120.0	24.00	(452)	(90.5)
Matzo, "Regular," **Manischewitz,** 10-oz. box (approx. 10 matzos)	1019	263.4			101.9	26.34	(384)	(99.2)
1 matzo, approx. 1.0 oz.			102	26.3	101.9	26.34	(384)	(99.2)
Unsalted Matzo, **Goodman's,** 11-oz. box, (approx. 11 matzos)	1430	286.0			130.0	26.00	(490)	(98.0)
1 matzo, approx. 1 oz.			130	26.0	130.0	26.00	(490)	(98.0)
Whole Wheat Matzo, **Manischewitz,** 10-oz. box (approx. 10 matzos)	1100	220.0			110.0	22.00	(415)	(82.9)
1 matzo, approx. 1 oz.			110	22.0	110.0	22.00	(415)	(82.9)
Whole Wheat & Bran Matzo, **Goodman's,** 10-oz. box (approx. 10 matzos)	1000	200.0			100.0	20.00	(377)	(75.4)
1 matzo, approx. 1 oz.			100	20.0	100.0	20.00	(377)	(75.4)

Muffins (see also English Muffins)

	ENTIRE PACKAGE		1 MUFFIN		1 OZ., BY WT.	
	Cal.	Carb.	Cal.	Carb.	Cal.	Carb.
Blueberry Muffins, **Morton** "Donut Shop," 9½-oz. package (6 muffins)	722	138.3			75.9	14.56
1 muffin, approx. 1.58 oz.			120	23.0	75.9	14.56
Blueberry Muffin Rounds, toaster-ready, **Morton** "Donut Shop," 9-oz. package (6 muffins)	660	126.0			73.3	14.00
1 muffin, approx. 1.5 oz.			110	21.0	73.3	14.00
Bran with Honey Muffins, **Pepperidge Farm,** 12-oz. package (6 muffins)	660	132.0			55.0	11.00
1 muffin, approx. 2 oz.			110	22.0	55.0	11.00
Bran'nola, **Orowheat,** with bran, honey & molasses, 14-oz. package (6 muffins)	1020	192.0			72.9	13.71
1 muffin, approx. 2.33 oz.			170	32.0	72.9	13.71
Cinnamon Apple Muffins, **Pepperidge Farm,** 12-oz. package (6 muffins)	720	132.0			60.0	11.00
1 muffin, approx. 2 oz.			120	22.0	60.0	11.00
Corn Muffins, **Morton** "Donut Shop," 10-oz. package (6 muffins)	783	120.5			78.3	12.05
1 muffin, approx. 1.66 oz.			130	20.0	78.3	12.05
Corn Muffin Rounds, toaster-ready, **Morton** "Donut Shop," 9-oz. package (6 muffins)	780	126.0			86.7	14.00
1 muffin, approx. 1.5 oz.			130	21.0	86.7	14.00
Corn Muffins, **Thomas'** 8-oz. package (4 muffins)	770	105.3			96.2	13.20
1 muffin, approx. 2 oz.			190	26.0	96.2	13.20
Granola Bran Muffins, **Mrs. Wright's,** 12-oz. package (6 muffins)	960	180.0			68.6	12.80
1 muffin, approx. 2.33 oz.			160	30.0	68.6	12.80
Orange with Honey Muffins, **Pepperidge Farm,** 12-oz. package (6 muffins)	720	150.0			60.0	12.50
1 muffin, approx. 2 oz.			120	25.0	60.0	12.50
Raisin Muffins, **Arnold,** 15-oz. package (6 muffins)	1020	210.0			68.0	14.00
1 muffin, approx. 2.5 oz.			170	35.0	68.0	14.00
Seven Grain Sprouted Wheat Raisin Muffins, **Foods for Life Bakery,** 16-oz. (1-lb.) package (6 muffins)	1120	224.0			70.0	14.00
1 muffin, approx. 2.7 oz.			187	37.4	70.0	14.00

Pita Bread (see also Pocket Bread)

	ENTIRE PACKAGE		1 PITA		1 OZ., BY WT.	
	Cal.	Carb.	Cal.	Carb.	Cal.	Carb.
Bible Bread, Pita, **Garden of Eatin',** 12-oz. package (6 pitas)	1026	173.2			85.5	14.43
1 pita, approx. 2 oz.			171	28.9	85.5	14.43
Bran Pita Bread, **International,** 10-oz. bag (6 pitas)	822	148.2			82.2	14.82
1 pita, approx. 1.76 oz.			137	24.7	82.2	14.82
100% Whole Wheat Pita Bread, **Old Stone Mill,** 12-oz. bag (6 pitas)	960	156.0			80.0	13.00
1 pita, approx. 2 oz.			160	26.0	80.0	13.00
100% Whole Wheat Mini-Size Pitas, **Sahara (Thomas'),** 8-oz. bag (8 pitas)	560	112.0			70.0	14.00
1 pita, approx. 1 oz.			70	14.0	70.0	14.00
100% Whole Wheat Pita, **Toufayan's,** 12-oz. bag (6 pitas)	960	156.0			80.0	13.00
1 pita, approx. 2 oz.			160	26.0	80.0	13.00
100% Whole Wheat Pita "1-ounce" Pitettes, **Toufayan's,** 8-oz. bag (8 pitettes)	560	104.0			70.0	13.00
1 pitette, approx. 1 oz.			70	13.0	70.0	13.00
Onion Pita "The Pocket Bialy," **Toufayan's,** 12-oz. package (6 pitas)	960	192.0			80.0	16.00
1 pita, approx. 2 oz.			160	32.0	80.0	16.00
Pita Bread, **Beirut Bakers,** 10-oz. bag (6 pitas)	800	150.0			80.0	15.00
1 pita, approx. 1.67 oz.			134	25.1	80.0	15.00
Pita Bread, **Sabra Breads,** 12-oz. bag (6 pitas)	912	192.0			76.0	16.00
1 pita, approx. 2 oz.			152	32.0	76.0	16.00
Pita Bread, **Toufayan's,** 12-oz. bag (6 pitas)	960	180.0			80.0	15.00
1 pita, approx. 2 oz.			160	30.0	80.0	15.00
Pitettes, **Toufayan's,** 8-oz. bag (8 pitettes)	560	120.0			70.0	15.00
1 pitette, approx. 1 oz.			70	15.0	70.0	15.00
Sahara Minisize Pitas, **Sahara (Thomas'),** 8-oz. bag (8 pitas)	640	128.0			80.0	16.00
1 pita, approx. 1 oz.			80	16.0	80.0	16.00
Sahara Pita Bread, **Sahara (Thomas')** 12-oz. bag (6 pitas)	960	192.0			80.0	16.00
1 pita, approx. 2 oz.			160.0	32.0	80.0	16.00
Sesame Pita Bread, **Damascus,** 12-oz. bag (6 pitas)	1200	192.0			100.0	16.00
1 pita, approx. 2 oz.			200	32.0	100.0	16.00
Sesame Pita Bread, **International,** 10-oz. bag (6 pitas)	840	162.0			84.0	16.20
1 pita, approx. 1.69 oz.			140	27.0	84.0	16.20
Toaster Size Pita Bread, **Aladdin,** 8-oz. bag (8 pitas)	640	104.0			80.0	13.00
1 pita, approx. 1 oz.			80	13.0	80.0	13.00
Toaster Size Sesame Pita Bread, **Aladdin,** 9-oz. bag (6 pitas)	720	117.0			80.0	13.00
1 pita, approx. 1.5 oz.			120	19.5	80.0	13.00
Whole Wheat Pita Bread, **Beirut Bakers,** 10-oz. bag (6 pitas)	800	150.0			80.0	15.00
1 pita, approx. 1.67 oz.			134	25.1	80.0	15.00
Whole Wheat Pita Bread, **Sabra Breads,** 12-oz. bag (6 pitas)	870	168.0			72.5	14.00
1 pita, approx. 2 oz.			145	28.0	72.5	14.00
Whole Wheat Pitas, **Damascus,** 12-oz. bag (6 pitas)	870	168.0			72.5	14.00
1 pita, approx. 2 oz.			145	28.0	72.5	14.00
Whole Wheat Sesame Pita Bread, **International,** 10-oz. package (6 pitas)	840	144.0			84.0	14.40
1 pita, approx. 1.67 oz.			140	24.0	84.0	14.40

Pocket Bread (see also Pita Bread)

	ENTIRE PACKAGE		1 POCKET		1 OZ., BY WT.	
	Cal.	Carb.	Cal.	Carb.	Cal.	Carb.
Mideast Pocket Bread, **Sahara,** 12-oz. bag (4 pockets)	920	184.0			76.7	15.33
1 pocket, approx. 3 oz.			230	46.0	76.7	15.33
8-oz. bag (8 "mini-size" pockets)	640	120.0			80.0	15.00
1 pocket, approx. 1 oz.			80	15.0	80.0	15.00
10-oz. bag (10 "mini-size" pockets)	800	150.0			80.0	15.00
1 pocket, approx. 1 oz.			80	15.0	80.0	15.00
100% Whole Wheat Pocket Bread, **Sahara,** 8-oz. bag (8 mini-size pockets)	560	112.0			70.0	14.00
1 pocket, approx. 1 oz.			70	14.0	70.0	14.00
Pita Pocket Bread, **International,** 20-oz. package (12 pitas)	1740	360.0			87.0	18.00
1 pita, approx. 1.67 oz.			145	30.0	87.0	18.00
Rye Sandwich Pockets, **Pepperidge Farm,** 8-oz. bag (8 pockets)	640	128.0			80.0	16.00
1 pocket, approx. 1 oz.			80	16.0	80.0	16.00
White Sandwich Pockets, **Pepperidge Farm,** 8-oz. bag (8 pockets)	640	120.0			80.0	15.00
1 pocket, approx. 1 oz.			80	15.0	80.0	15.00

Taco Shells, Tortillas, and Tostada Shells

	ENTIRE PACKAGE		1 PIECE		1 OZ., BY WT.	
	Cal.	Carb.	Cal.	Carb.	Cal.	Carb.
Ortega Taco Shells, 3.9-oz. package (10 shells)	500	60.0			128.9	15.46
4.7-oz. package (12 shells)	600	72.0			128.9	15.46
6.2-oz. package (16 shells)	800	96.0			128.9	15.46
1 shell, approx. 0.39 oz.			50	6.0	128.9	15.46
Ortega Tostada Shells, 3.1-oz. package (8 shells)	400	48.0			128.9	15.46
3.9-oz. package (10 shells)	500	60.0			128.9	15.46
1 shell, approx. 0.39 oz.			50	6.0	128.9	15.46
Thin, Round Enriched Flour Tortillas, **Mariachi,** 13-oz. package (10 tortillas)	1120	200.0			86.2	15.38
1 tortilla, approx. 1.3 oz. (7¼" diameter)			112	20.0	86.2	15.38
Whole Grain Stoneground Corn Tortillas, **Mariachi,** 12-oz. package (12 tortillas)	600	120.0			50.0	10.00
1 tortilla, approx. 1 oz. (6" diameter)			50	10.0	50.0	10.00

Miscellaneous Breads

	ENTIRE PACKAGE Cal.	ENTIRE PACKAGE Carb.	1 PIECE Cal.	1 PIECE Carb.	1 OZ., BY WT. Cal.	1 OZ., BY WT. Carb.
Cheese Blintzes, **Golden,** 15-oz. box (6 blintzes)	(1278)	(23.2)			(85.2)	(1.55)
1 blintz, 2.5 oz.			(213)	(3.9)	(85.2)	(1.55)
Crêpe Mix, Low Cholesterol & Sugar Restricted, **Sweet 'n Low,** 8-oz. carton	1120	192.0			140.0	24.00
As prepared (yield: approx. 16 7″ crêpes)	1120	192.0				
1 7″ crêpe			70	12.0		
Frozen Prepackaged Homestyle Roll Dough, **Rich's,** 25-oz. package	1920	336.0			76.8	13.44
1 roll, baked, approx. 1.9 oz.			80	14.0	84.2	14.73
Potato Pancakes, **Golden,** 12-oz. box (8 pancakes)	(680)	(58.4)			(56.7)	(4.87)
1 pancake, approx. 1.5 oz.			(85)	(7.3)	(56.7)	(4.87)
Rusks, Low Protein Toasted Bread, **Aproten,** 8.5-oz. package (24 slices)	1032	192.0			121.4	22.59
1 slice, approx. 0.4 oz.			43	8.0	121.4	22.59
White Bread Dough, Frozen Prepackaged, **Rich's,** 1 package (2 1-pound loaves)	2040	391.0			63.8	12.22
As prepared (yield: 2 loaves, approx. 29.4 oz.)	2040	391.0			(69.3)	(13.28)
1 loaf, approx. 14.7 oz.			1020	195.5	(69.3)	(13.28)

20 BREAKFAST CEREALS & BREAKFAST BREADS •

	UNIT		1 OZ., BY WT. UN-PREPARED		1 OZ., BY WT. PREPARED		1 CUP	
	Cal.	Carb.	Cal.	Carb.	Cal.	Carb.	Cal.	Carb.
HOT BREAKFAST CEREALS								
(Alphabetized under the grain that is their main ingredient. See under Buckwheat [Kasha], Corn Grits [Hominy Grits], Millet, Oats, Rice, Rye, and Wheat.)								
BUCKWHEAT (KASHA)								
Wolfe's Buckwheat Groats, white, 16-oz. (1-lb.) box	1688	344.8					(560)	(114.9)
1 serving prepared as directed, ¼ cups groats to 1 cup water (yield: approx. 1 cup, 5 oz.)	(140)	(28.7)			(28.0)	(5.74)	(140)	(28.7)
Roasted, brown, 16-oz. (1-lb.) box	1792	376.5	112.0	23.53			(597)	(122.5)
1 serving prepared as directed, ¼ cup groats to 1 cup water (yield: approx. 1 cup, 5 oz.)	(119)	(24.5)			(23.9)	(4.90)	(119)	(24.5)
CORN GRITS (HOMINY GRITS)								
Degermed, based on generic data:								
(Unenriched or enriched. Enriching corn grits does not affect the calorie or carbohydrate content. Data apply to "regular" or "quick-cooking.")								
DRY:								
1 cup (approx. 5.6 oz. (tr/22g/2g/12%/tr)	579	125.0	103.4	22.32			579	125.0
1 pound (approx. 2.8 cups)	1642	354.3	103.4	22.32			579	125.0
COOKED:								
1 cup (approx. 8.6 oz.) (tr/3g/tr/87%/58mg)	125	27.0			14.5	3.14	125	27.0
1 pound (approx. 1.9 cups)	231	49.9			14.5	3.14	125	27.0
By brand:								
Instant Grits Product, **Quaker,** 8-oz. box, 10 packets	790	177.0	98.8	22.10			237	53.1
18-oz. box, 22 packets	1778	397.3	98.8	22.13			237	53.1
36-oz. box, 45 packets	3555	796.7	98.8	22.13			237	53.1
1 packet (approx. 0.8 oz.) prepared as directed, add ¾ cup water (yield: approx. 5.8 oz.)	79	17.7			(13.7)	(3.07)	(118)	(26.4)
With Artificial Cheese Flavor, 8-oz. box, 8 packets	832	172.8	104.0	21.60			832	172.8
1 packet (approx. 1 oz.) prepared as directed, add ¾ cup water (yield: approx. 7.7 oz.)	104	21.6			(14.4)	(3.00)	(124)	(23.8)
With Imitation Bacon Bits, 8-oz. box, 8 packets	808	172.8	101.0	21.60			(808)	(172.8)
1 packet (approx. 1 oz.) prepared as directed, add ¾ cup water (yield: approx. 7.2 oz.)	101	21.6			(14.0)	(3.00)	(120)	(25.8)
With Imitation Ham Bits, 8-oz. box, 8 packets	792	170.4	99.0	21.30			(792)	(170.4)
1 packet (approx. 1 oz.) prepared as directed, add ¾ cup water (yield: approx. 7.2 oz.)	99	21.3			(13.8)	(2.96)	(119)	(25.5)
Quick Hominy Grits, **Albers,** 20-oz. box	2000	440.0	100.0	22.00			600	132.0
1 cup (approx. 6 oz.)	600	132.0	100.0	22.00			600	132.0
1 serving, prepared as directed (yield: approx. 10.7 oz.)	150	33.0			(14.0)	(3.09)	(120)	(26.5)
Quick Hominy Grits, **Aunt Jemima,** 16-oz. (1-lb.) box	1616	358.0	101.0	22.40			539	119.5
24-oz. box	2424	537.6	101.0	22.40			539	119.5
32-oz. (2-lb.) box	3232	716.8	101.0	22.40			539	119.5
40-oz. box	4040	896.0	101.0	22.40			539	119.5
80-oz. (5-lb.) box	8080	1792.0	101.0	22.40			539	119.5
1 serving prepared as directed, 3 tablespoons uncooked cereal to 1 cup water (yield: approx. 7.2 oz.)	101	22.0			(14.0)	(3.30)	(120)	(28.4)
Quick Hominy Grits, **Quaker,** 16-oz. (1-lb.) box	1616	358.4	101.0	22.40			539	119.5
24-oz. box	2424	537.6	101.0	22.40			539	119.5
32-oz. (2-lb.) box	3232	716.8	101.0	22.40			539	119.5
40-oz. box	4040	896.0	101.0	22.40			539	119.5
80-oz. (5-lb.) box	8080	1792.0	101.0	22.40			539	119.5
1 serving prepared as directed, 3 tablespoons uncooked cereal to 1 cup water (yield: approx. 7.2 oz.)	101	22.0			(14.0)	(3.30)	(120)	(28.4)
White Hominy Grits, enriched, **Aunt Jemima,** Regular, 16-oz. (1-lb.) box	1616	358.4	101.0	22.40			539	119.5
24-oz. box	2424	537.6	101.0	22.40			539	119.5
32-oz. (2-lb.) box	3232	716.8	101.0	22.40			539	119.5
40-oz. box	4040	896.0	101.0	22.40			539	119.5
80-oz. (5-lb.) box	8030	1792.0	101.0	22.40			539	119.5

	UNIT		1 OZ., BY WT. UN-PREPARED		1 OZ., BY WT. PREPARED		1 CUP	
	Cal.	Carb.	Cal.	Carb.	Cal.	Carb.	Cal.	Carb.
1 serving prepared as directed, 3 tablespoons uncooked cereal to 1 cup water (yield: approx. 7.2 oz.)	101	22.4			(14.0)	(3.30)	(120)	(28.4)
White Hominy Grits, enriched, **Quaker,** Regular, 16-oz. (1-lb.) box	1616	358.4	101.0	22.40			539	119.5
24-oz. box	2424	537.6	101.0	22.40			539	119.5
32-oz. (2-lb.) box	3232	716.8	101.0	22.40			539	119.5
40-oz. box	4040	896.0	101.0	22.40			539	119.5
80-oz. (5-lb.) box	8080	1792.0	101.0	22.40			539	119.5
1 serving prepared as directed, 3 tablespoons uncooked cereal to 1 cup water (yield: approx. 7.2 oz.)	101	22.4			(14.0)	(3.30)	(120)	(28.4)
KASHA, see BUCKWHEAT								
MILLET								
Golden Harvest Whole Millet, 16-oz. (1-lb.) package	1600	304.0	100.0	19.00			(400)	(76.0)
1 serving prepared as directed, ¼ cup uncooked cereal to ⅔ cups water (yield: approx. ⅔ cup)	100	19.0			(20.0)	(3.80)	(174)	(33.0)
OATS								
Instant Oatmeal								
Instant Oatmeal, **H-O,** Regular, 10-oz. box, 10 packets	1100	180.0	107.5	17.60			260	44.0
1 packet prepared as directed, 1 oz. uncooked cereal to ⅔ cup water (yield: approx. ¾ cup)	(100)	(18.0)			(17.4)	(3.12)	150	27.0
16-oz. (1-lb.) box	1690	286.0	108.4	183.40			260	44.0
1 serving prepared as directed, ½ cup uncooked cereal to ⅔ cup water (yield: approx. ¾ cup)	(130)	(22.0)			(17.6)	(2.97)	173	29.3
Instant Oatmeal, Regular, **Quaker,** 10-oz. box, 10 packets	(1050)	(181.0)	105.0	18.10			(336)	(57.9)
1 packet prepared as directed, 1 oz. uncooked cereal to ¾ cup water (yield: approx. ¾ cup)	105	18.1			(14.4)	(2.48)	(140)	(24.1)
Apple & Cinnamon and Artificial Apple Flavor, **H-O,** 10-oz. box, 8 packets	1040	208.0	104.0	20.80			(250)	(49.9)
1 packet prepared as directed, 1¼ oz. uncooked cereal to ½ cup water (yield: approx. ½ cup)	130	26.0			(23.9)	(4.77)	(260)	(52.0)
Apples & Cinnamon, **Quaker,** 10-oz. box, 8 packets	(1072)	(208.0)	(107.2)	(20.80)			(343)	(66.6)
1 packet prepared as directed, 1½ oz. uncooked cereal to ¾ cup water (yield: approx. ¾ cup)	134	26.0			(20.6)	(4.00)	179	34.7
Bran & Raisin, **H-O,** 12-oz. box, 8 packets	1200	232.0	100.0	19.33			(240)	(46.4)
1 packet prepared as directed, 1½ oz. uncooked cereal to ¾ cup water (yield: approx. ⅔ cup)	150	29.0			(21.1)	(4.08)	(225)	(43.5)
Bran & Raisins, **Quaker,** 12-oz. box, 8 packets	(1260)	(233.6)	(105.0)	(19.47)			(392)	(74.8)
1 packet, prepared as directed, 1½ oz. uncooked cereal to ¾ cup water (yield: approx. ¾ cup)	153	29.2			(19.6)	(3.74)	(204)	(38.9)
Cinnamon & Spice, **Quaker,** 13-oz. box, 8 packets	1440	280.0	110.8	21.54			(355)	(68.9)
1 packet prepared as directed, 1⅝ oz. uncooked cereal to ¾ cup water (yield: approx. ¾ cup)	180	35.0			(22.7)	(4.41)	(240)	(46.7)
Country Apple Brown Sugar, **H-O,** 9-oz. box, 8 packets	960	184.0	106.7	20.40			(256)	(48.9)
1 packet prepared as directed, 1⅛ oz. uncooked cereal to ⅔ cup water (yield: approx. ⅔ cup)	120	23.0			(18.2)	(3.45)	(182)	(34.5)
Flavor Variety, **Quaker,** Regular (2 1-oz. packets), Cinnamon & Spice (2 1⅝-oz. packets), Artificial Maple & Brown Sugar (2 1½-oz. packets), Apples & Cinnamon (2 1½-oz. packets)	1180	222.0	118.0	22.20				
Maple & Brown Sugar Flavors, **H-O,** 12-oz. box, 8 packets	1280	256.0	105.5	21.20			(253)	(50.6)
1 packet prepared as directed, 1½ oz. uncooked cereal to ½ cup water (yield: approx. ⅔ cup)	160	32.0			(28.1)	(5.61)	240	48.0
Maple & Brown Sugar, **Quaker,** 12-oz. box, 8 packets	(1304)	(255.2)	(108.7)	(21.27)			(417)	(81.7)
1 packet prepared as directed, 1½ oz. uncooked cereal to ¾ cup water (yield: approx. ¾ cup)	163	31.9			(26.3)	(5.15)	(217)	(42.5)
Maple Flavor, Artificial, "30-Second Oatmeal," **Maypo,** 14-oz. box	1722	266.0	123.0	19.00			492	76.0
1 serving prepared as directed, ¼ cup uncooked cereal to ½ cup water (yield: approx. ½ cup)	123	19.0			(24.6)	(3.80)	(246)	(38.0)
Raisins & Spice, **H-O,** 12-oz. box, 8 packets	1360	264.0	107.1	20.79			(257)	(49.9)
1 packet prepared as directed, 1½ oz. uncooked cereal to ½ cup water (yield: approx. ½ cup)	170	33.0			(29.8)	(5.79)	(340)	(66.0)
Raisins & Spice, **Quaker,** 12-oz. box, 8 packets	(1272)	(251.2)	(106.0)	(20.93)			(407)	(80.4)
1 packet prepared as directed, 1½ oz. uncooked cereal to ¾ cup water (yield: approx. ¾ cup)	159	31.4			(20.4)	(4.03)	(212)	(41.9)
Sweet & Mellow, **H-O,** 11⅓-oz. box, 8 packets	1200	232.0	106.3	20.55			300	58.0
1 packet prepared as directed, 1⅓ oz. uncooked cereal to ½ cup water (yield: approx. ½ cup)	150	29.0			(27.1)	(5.24)	(300)	(29.0)
Vermont Style "30-Second Oatmeal," **Maypo,** 19-oz. box	2090	380.0	110.0	20.00			440	4.0
1 serving prepared as directed, ¼ cup uncooked cereal to ¾ cup water (yield: approx. ¾ cup)	110	20.0			(17.8)	(3.23)	(147)	(26.7)
Other Oatmeals								
Old Fashioned Oats, **H-O,** 16-oz. (1-lb.) box	1680	288.0	107.3	18.39			280	48.0
18-oz. box	1931	338.1	107.3	18.39			280	48.0
42-oz. box	4507	772.3	107.3	18.39			280	48.0
1 serving prepared as directed, ½ cup uncooked cereal to ¾ cup water (yield: approx. ¾ cup)	140	24.0			(18.7)	(3.20)	187	32.0
Old Fashioned Oats, **Quaker,** 18-oz. package	(1962)	(331.2)	(109.0)	(18.40)			(327)	(55.2)
42-oz. package	(4578)	(772.8)	(109.0)	(18.40)			(327)	(55.2)
1 serving prepared as package directs, ⅓ cup uncooked cereal to ¾ cup water (yield: approx. ¾ cup)	(109)	(18.4)			(20.2)	(3.41)	(163)	(27.6)
Quick Oats, **A&P,** 18-oz. box	1980	342.0	110.0	19.00			220	19.0
1 serving prepared as directed, ⅓ cup uncooked cereal to ⅔ cup water (yield: approx. ⅔ cup)	110	19.0			(20.4)	(3.52)	(165)	(28.5)
Quick Oats, **H-O,** 16-oz. (1-lb.) box	1685	298.0	105.3	18.63			260	46.0
32-oz. (2-lb.) box	3370	596.0	105.3	18.63			260	46.0
1 serving prepared as directed, ½ cup uncooked cereal to ¾ cup water (yield: approx. ¾ cup)	130	23.0			(17.6)	(3.11)	173	30.7
Quick Oats, **Quaker,** 18-oz. package	(1962)	(331.2)	(109.0)	(18.40)			(327)	(55.2)
1 serving prepared as package directs, ⅓ cup uncooked cereal to ⅔ cup water (yield: approx. ⅔ cup)	(109)	(18.4)			(20.2)	(3.41)	(163)	(27.6)
Quick Oats, **Ralston,** 18-oz. (1 lb. 2 oz.) box	1980	342.0	110.0	19.00			330	57.6
1 serving prepared as directed, ⅓ cup uncooked cereal to ¾ cup water (yield: approx. ¾ cup)	(110)	(19.0)			(17.8)	(3.08)	(147)	(25.3)
Quick Oats, **Safeway,** 42-oz. box	4620	798.0	110.0	19.00			330	57.0
1 serving prepared as directed, ⅓ cup uncooked cereal to ¾ cup water (yield: approx. ¾ cup)	110	19.0			(17.7)	(3.06)	(142)	(24.5)

	UNIT		1 OZ., BY WT. UN-PREPARED		1 OZ., BY WT. PREPARED		1 CUP	
	Cal.	Carb.	Cal.	Carb.	Cal.	Carb.	Cal.	Carb.
Regular Oats, **Ralston,** 18-oz. box	1980	342.0	110.0	19.00			333	57.6
1 serving prepared as directed, 1/3 cup uncooked cereal to 3/4 cup water (yield: approx. 3/4 cup)	110	19.0			(17.8)	(3.07)	(147)	(25.3)
Rolled Oats, **Golden Harvest,** 24-oz. box	2640	432.0	110.0	18.00			(308)	(50.4)
1 serving prepared as directed, 1/2 cup uncooked cereal to 1 cup water (yield: approx. 1 cup)	(154)	(25.2)			(18.1)	(2.96)	(154)	(25.2)
100% Rolled Oats, **Golden Harvest,** 16-oz. (1-lb.) box	1760	288.0	110.0	18.00			220	36.0
1 serving prepared as directed, 1/2 cup uncooked cereal to 3/4 cup water (yield: approx. 3/4 cup)	110	18.0			(17.7)	(2.90)	(147)	(24.0)
Scotch Style Oatmeal, **Elam's,** 28-oz. package	3016	517.7	107.7	18.49			(285)	(48.9)
1 serving prepared as directed, 1/3 cup uncooked cereal to 1 cup water (yield: approx. 1 cup)	(95)	(16.3)			(11.7)	(2.01)	(95)	(16.3)
Steel Cut Oatmeal, **Elam's,** 28-oz. package	3063	532.0	109.4	19.00			(289)	(50.3)
1 serving prepared as directed, 1/4 cup uncooked cereal to 3/4 cup water (yield: approx. 3/4 cup)	(48)	(8.4)			(11.8)	(2.03)	(97)	(16.8)
Steel Cut Oatmeal, **Golden Harvest,** 32-oz. (2-lb.) bag	3520	576.0	110.0	18.00			(220)	(36.0)
1 serving prepared as directed, 1/2 cup uncooked cereal to 1 1/4 cup water (yield: approx. 1 cup)	(110)	(18.0)			(14.3)	(2.34)	110	18.0
RICE								
Cream of Rice, **Nabisco,** 16-oz. (1-lb.) box	1920	416.0	120.0	26.00			(720)	(156.0)
1 serving prepared as directed, 1/6 cup uncooked cereal to 3/4 cups water (yield: approx. 3/4 cup)	120	26.0			(18.4)	(3.99)	160	34.7
Cream of Rice, **Grocery Store Products Co.,** 21 1/2-oz. box	2040	442.0	95.0	20.60				
1 serving prepared as directed, 3 Tbsp. uncooked cereal to 3/4 cup water (yield: approx. 3/4 cup)	120	26.0			(18.4)	(3.99)	(160)	(34.7)
Pure Rice Bran, **Jolly Joan,** 8-oz. box	421	116.6	52.6	14.57			130	36.0
1 serving prepared as directed, 1 cup uncooked cereal to 1 cup water (yield: approx. 1 cup)	130	38.0			(15.1)	(4.41)	130	36.0
RYE								
Cream of Rye, **ConAgra,** 10-oz. box	900	190.0	90.0	19.00			720	152.0
1 serving prepared as directed, 1/4 cup uncooked cereal to 3/4 cup water (yield: approx. 3/4 cup)	90	19.0			(14.1)	(2.98)	(120)	(25.4)
100% Rolled Rye, **Golden Harvest,** 16-oz. (1-lb.) box	1600	352.0	100.0	22.00			300	66.0
1 serving prepared as directed, 1/3 cup uncooked cereal to 3/4 cup water (yield: approx. 3/4 cup)	100	22.0			(16.1)	(3.55)	(133)	(29.3)
WHEAT								
Bear Mush, **Arrowhead Mills,** 24-oz. bag	2400	484.0	100.0	21.00			800	168.0
1 serving prepared as directed, 1/6 cup uncooked cereal to 1 scant cup water (yield: approx. 3/4 cup)	133	28.0					177	37.3
Cream of Wheat, Instant, **Nabisco,** 14-oz. box	1400	254.0			100.0	21.00	(640)	(134.4)
1 serving prepared as directed for infants, 1 1/4 Tbsp. to 1/2 cup water (yield: approx. 1/2 cup)			50.0	10.50	(11.6)	(2.44)	(100)	(21.0)
28-oz. box	2800	588.0	100.0	21.00			(640)	(134.4)
1 serving prepared as directed for adults, 2 1/2 Tbsp. uncooked cereal to 1 cup water (yield: approx. 1 cup)	100	21.0			(11.6)	(2.44)	(100)	(21.0)
1 serving prepared as directed for adults, 2 1/2 Tbsp. uncooked cereal to 1 1/3 cup milk (yield: approx. 1 cup)	(312)	(37.0)			(36.3)	(4.30)	(312)	(37.0)
Cream of Wheat, Mix 'N Eat, **Nabisco,** Regular, 10-oz. box, 10 packets	1000	210.0	100.0	21.00			(640)	(134.4)
1 packet prepared as directed, 1 oz. uncooked cereal to 1 cup water (yield: approx. 1 cup)	100	21.0			(11.6)	(2.31)	(100)	(21.0)
Baked Apple with Cinnamon Flavor, 10-oz. box, 8 packets	1040	232.0	104.0	23.20			(666)	(148.5)
1 packet prepared as directed, 1 1/4 oz. uncooked cereal to 1 cup water (yield: approx. 1 cup)	130	29.0			(15.1)	(3.37)	(130)	(29.0)
Banana Artificial Flavor and Spice, 10-oz. box, 8 packets	867	193.3	86.7	19.33			(555)	(123.7)
1 packet prepared as directed, 1 1/4 oz. uncooked cereal to 1 cup water (yield: approx. 1 cup)	130	29.0			(15.1)	(3.37)	(130)	(29.0)
Maple Artificial Flavor and Brown Sugar, 10-oz. box, 8 packets	1040	232.0	104.0	23.20			(666)	(148.5)
1 packet prepared as directed, 1 1/4 oz. uncooked cereal to 1 cup water (yield: approx. 1 cup)	130	29.0			(15.1)	(3.37)	(130)	(29.0)
Cream of Wheat, Quick, **Nabisco,** 28-oz. box	2800	588.0	100.0	21.00			640	134.4
1 serving prepared as directed for adults, 2 1/2 Tbsp. uncooked cereal to 3/4 cup water (yield: approx. 3/4 cup)	100	21.0			15.3	3.18	130	26.7
Cream of Wheat, Regular, **Nabisco,** 28-oz. box	2800	616.0	100.0	21.00			640	140.8
1 serving prepared as directed for adults, 2 1/2 Tbsp. uncooked cereal to 3/4 cup water (yield: approx. 3/4 cup)	100	21.0			15.0	3.12	134	27.7
Farina, Chocolate Flavor with Toasted Malt Flakes, **Malt-O-Meal,** 22-oz. box	2200	462.0	100.0	21.00			607	128.3
1 serving prepared as directed, 1 oz. uncooked cereal to 1 scant cup water (yield: approx. 3/4 cup)	100	21.0			(15.5)	(3.26)	133	28.0
Farina, Cream Enriched, **H-O,** 14-oz. box	1440	312.0	103.1	22.39			640	139.0
1 serving prepared as directed, 3 Tbsp. uncooked cereal to 1 cup water (yield: approx. 1 cup)	120	26.0			14.0	3.02	120	26.0
Farina, enriched, **Pillsbury,** 13 1/2-oz. container	1440	306.0	106.7	22.67			(672)	(142.8)
27 1/2-oz. container	2800	612.0	106.7	22.67			(672)	(142.8)
1 serving prepared as directed for adults, 2 Tbsp. uncooked cereal to 3/4 cup water (yield: approx. 2/3 cup)	80	17.0			(14.0)	(2.97)	(120)	(25.5)
1 serving prepared as directed for adults, 2 Tbsp. uncooked cereal to 3/4 cup milk (yield: approx. 2/3 cup)	200	26.0			(34.9)	(3.02)	300	39.0
Farina, Hot N Creamy, **Quaker,** 14-oz. box	(1414)	(303.8)	101.0	21.70			(606)	(130.2)
1 serving prepared as directed, 1/6 cup uncooked cereal to 1 cup water (yield: approx. 1 cup)	101	21.7			(11.7)	(2.51)	(101)	(21.7)
Farina, Quick, **Malt-O-Meal,** 12-oz. box	1200	264.0	100.0	22.00			607	134.4
1 serving prepared as directed, 1 oz. uncooked cereal to 1 scant cup water (yield: approx. 1 cup)	100	22.0			(11.6)	(2.56)	100	22.0
Wheat Cereal & Soya, **Fearn,** 16-oz. (1-lb.) package	1605	278.2	100.3	17.39			600	104.0
1 serving prepared as directed, 1 1/4 cup uncooked cereal to 1 cup water (yield: approx. 3/4 cup)	230	32.0			(28.8)	(4.00)	(307)	(42.7)

	UNIT		1 OZ., BY WT. UN-PREPARED		1 OZ., BY WT. PREPARED		1 CUP	
	Cal.	Carb.	Cal.	Carb.	Cal.	Carb.	Cal.	Carb.
Wheatena, **Standard Milling,** 11-oz. package	1320	231.0	120.0	21.00				
22-oz. package	2640	462.0	120.0	21.00				
1 serving prepared as directed, ¼ cup uncooked cereal to 1 cup water (yield: approx. 1 cup)	120	21.0			(14.0)	(2.44)	(120)	(21.0)
Whole Wheat Cereal, Instant with added Wheat Germ, **Ralston,** 18-oz. box	1986	360.0	110.0	20.00			440	80.0
1 serving prepared as directed, ¼ cup uncooked cereal to ¾ cup water (yield: approx. ¾ cup)	110	20.0			(17.8)	(3.24)	(147)	(26.6)
Whole Wheat Cereal with added Wheat Germ, Regular, **Ralston,** 22-oz. box	2420	400.0	110.0	20.00			440	80.0
1 serving prepared as directed, ¼ cup uncooked cereal to ¾ cup water (yield: approx. ¾ cup)	110	20.0			(17.8)	(3.23)	(147)	(26.7)
Whole Wheat Hot Natural Cereal, **Quaker,** 14-oz. box	(1400)	(288.4)	100.0	20.60			(300)	(61.8)
1 serving prepared as directed, ⅓ cup uncooked cereal to ⅔ cup water (yield: approx. ⅔ cup)	100	20.6			(16.9)	(3.49)	(150)	(30.9)
MIXED AND UNSPECIFIED GRAINS								
Energy Cereal, Wheat Germ Added, with Date Nuggets, **Golden Harvest,** 16-oz. (1-lb.) box	1680	320.0	105.0	20.00			(210)	(40.0)
1 serving prepared as directed, based on 2 servings per cup uncooked cereal to 2½ cups water (yield: approx. 1 cup)	105	20.0			(12.7)	(2.41)	(105)	(20.0)
1 serving prepared as directed, based on 3 servings per 1 cup uncooked cereal to 2½ cups water (yield: approx. ⅔ cup)	70	13.3			(12.7)	(2.41)	(105)	(20.0)
5-Minute Cereal, **Roman Meal,** 28-oz. package	2800	560.0	100.0	20.00			300	60.0
1 serving prepared as package directs, ⅓ cup uncooked cereal to ⅔ cup water (yield: approx. ⅔ cup)	100	20.0			(19.1)	(3.81)	(150)	(30.0)
5-Minute Cereal with Oats, **Roman Meal,** 25-oz. package	2750	475.0	110.0	19.00			330	57.0
1 serving prepared as package directs, ⅓ cup uncooked cereal to ⅔ cup water (yield: approx. ⅔ cup)	110	19.0			(21.1)	(3.62)	(165)	(28.5)
Maltex Hot Cereal, Old Fashioned, **Standard Milling,** 20-oz. box	2340	420.0	117.0	21.00			468	84.0
1 serving prepared as directed, ¼ cup uncooked cereal to ¾ cup water (yield: approx. ¾ cup)	176	31.5			22.5	4.04	234	42.0
7 Grain Cereal, **Arrowhead Mills,** 24-oz. bag	2400	408.0	100.0	17.00			(320)	(54.4)
1 serving prepared as directed, ⅓ cup uncooked cereal to ⅔ cup water (yield: approx. ⅔ cup)	100	17.0			(16.7)	(2.83)	(150)	(25.5)
Swiss Shield, **Golden Harvest,** 12-oz. bag	1680	228.0	140.0	19.00			(420)	(57.0)
1 serving prepared as directed, ⅓ cup uncooked cereal to ¾ cup water (yield: approx. ¾ cup)	140	19.0			(20.0)	(2.71)	(187)	(25.3)
2-Minute Cereal, **Roman Meal,** 25-oz. package	2500	500.0	100.0	20.00			300	60.0
1 serving prepared as package directs, ⅓ cup uncooked cereal to ⅔ cup water (yield: approx. ⅔ cup)	100	20.0			(19.1)	(3.81)	(150)	(30.0)
Whole Grains, **Golden Harvest,** 16-oz. (1-lb.) bag	1760	166.0	110.0	10.00			440	40.0
1 serving prepared as directed, ¼ cup uncooked cereal to ⅝ cup water (yield: approx. ⅔ cup)	110	10.0			(20.0)	(1.82)	(165)	(15.0)

COLD BREAKFAST CEREALS

(With collections under the headings of Bran, Corn, Granola, Natural, Rice, and Wheat)

	UNIT		1 OZ., BY WT.		1 CUP	
	Cal.	Carb.	Cal.	Carb.	Cal.	Carb.
All-Bran, **Kellogg's,** 16-oz. (1-lb.) box	1120	336.0	70.0	21.00	(210)	(63.0)
Almond Crisp, **Back to Nature,** 22-oz. box	2200	462.0	100.0	21.00	(400)	(84.0)
Almond Granola, "Vita Crunch," **Back to Nature,** 32-oz. (2-lb.) box	3840	640.0	120.0	20.00	(480)	(80.0)
Alpen, Natural Cereal with Raisins, 12-oz. box	1320	240.0	110.0	20.00	(440)	(80.0)
Alpha-Bits, **Post,** single serving size, ¾-oz. box	90	18.0	110.0	24.00	(110)	(24.0)
13-oz. box	1430	312.0	110.0	24.00	(110)	(24.0)
Apple Bran Granola, **Golden Harvest,** 15-oz. box	1800	165.0	120.0	11.00	(480)	(44.0)
Apple Cinnamon 8-Grain Cereal N' Snack, **Good Shepherd,** 16-oz. (1-lb.) box	2000	304.0	125.0	19.00		
Applejacks, **Kellogg's,** single serving size, ⅝-oz. box	69	16.3	110.0	26.00	(110)	(26.0)
11-oz. box	1210	286.0	110.0	26.00	(110)	(26.0)
15-oz. box	1650	390.0	110.0	26.00	(110)	(26.0)
Banana Crisp, **Back to Nature,** 22-oz. box	2288	462.0	104.0	21.00	416	84.0
Barley Flaked Whole Grain Cereal, Nutri Grain, **(Kellogg's),** 12-oz. box	1320	276.0	110.0	23.00	147	30.7
Birchermuesli, see Familia, and Frutifort						
Booberry, **General Mills,** 12-oz. box	1320	288.0	110.0	24.00	(110)	(24.0)
***BRAN:* (see also the BASIC BAKING & COOKING INGREDIENTS chapter)**						
(This section is not meant to single out cereals with high bran content. Cereals listed under "BRAN" are cereals that incorporate the word "bran" in their names.)						
All-Bran, **Kellogg's,** 16-oz. (1-lb.) box	1120	352.0	70.0	22.00	(210)	(66.0)
Apple-Bran Granola, **Golden Harvest,** 15-oz. box	1800	165.0	120.0	11.00	(480)	(44.0)
Bran Buds, **Kellogg's,** 18-oz. box	1260	414.0	70.0	23.00	(210)	(69.0)
Bran Chex, **Ralston Purina,** 14-oz. box	1540	280.0	110.0	20.00	(165)	(30.0)
Branola Cinnamon Apple, **Hi-Protein,** 16-oz. (1-lb.) bag	1712	283.2	107.0	17.70	(428)	(70.8)
Branola Honey-Bran, **Hi-Protein,** 16-oz. (1-lb.) bag	1920	283.2	120.0	17.70	(480)	(70.8)
Branola Raisin, **Hi-Protein,** 16-oz. (1-lb.) bag	2352	316.8	147.0	19.80	(588)	(79.2)
Corn Bran, **Quaker,** 12-oz. box	1308	279.6	109.0	23.30	164	35.0
16-oz. (1-lb.) box	1744	372.8	109.0	23.30	164	35.0
Cracklin' Bran, **Kellogg's,** 11-oz. box	1210	209.0	110.0	19.00	(330)	(57.0)
16-oz. (1-lb.) box	1760	304.0	110.0	19.00	(330)	(57.0)
40% Bran Flakes, **Kellogg's,** 1-oz. box	90	22.0	90.0	22.00	135	33.0
16-oz. (1-lb.) box	1440	368.0	90.0	23.00	(135)	(34.5)
20-oz. box	1800	460.0	90.0	23.00	(135)	(34.5)
40% Bran Flakes, **Post,** single serving, 1-oz. box	90	22.0	90.0	22.00	(135)	(33.0)
16-oz. (1-lb.) box	1440	352.0	90.0	22.00	(135)	(33.0)
Natural Bran Cereal with Apples and Cinnamon, **Health Valley,** 12-oz. box	1200	276.0	100.0	23.00	(400)	(92.0)
Natural Bran Cereal with Raisins, **Health Valley,** 12-oz. box	1200	276.0	100.0	23.00	(400)	(92.0)
100% Bran Cereal, **Nabisco,** 16-oz. (1-lb.) box	1120	336.0	70.0	21.00	(140)	(42.0)
Pure Bran, **Golden Harvest,** 4-oz. bag	360	56.0	90.0	14.00	(190)	(29.6)
7-oz. bag	630	98.0	90.0	14.00	(190)	(29.6)
16-oz. (1-lb.) bag	1440	224.0	90.0	14.00	(190)	(29.6)
Raisin Bran, **A&P,** 20-oz. box	2000	440.0	100.0	22.00	(200)	(44.0)
Raisin Bran, **Kellogg's,** single serving, 1-oz. box	86	21.4	85.7	21.43	160	40.0
11-oz. box	943	235.7	85.7	21.43	160	40.0
15-oz. box	1286	321.5	85.7	21.43	160	40.0
20-oz. box	1714	428.6	85.7	21.43	160	40.0
Raisin Bran, **Post (General Foods),** 15-oz. box	1350	330.0	90.0	22.00	(180)	(44.0)
Raisin Bran, **Ralston Purina,** 20-oz. box	2000	440.0	100.0	22.00	(200)	(44.0)
Raisin Bran, **Safeway,** 20-oz. box	2000	440.0	100.0	22.00	(200)	(17.6)
Raisin Bran, **Skinner's,** 10-oz. box	1000	210.0	100.0	21.00	(200)	(42.0)
Raisin Bran Crunch (No Sugar Added), **Back to Nature,** 22-oz. box	1870	462.0	85.0	21.00	(340)	(84.0)
Raisin Bran Granola, **Golden Harvest,** 2-oz. bag	240	34.0	120.0	17.00	(480)	(68.0)
13-oz. bag	1560	221.0	120.0	17.00	(480)	(68.0)
(Pure) Rice Bran, Gluten Free, **Jolly Joan,** 8-oz. box	(421)	(116.6)	(52.6)	(14.57)	(130)	(36.0)
Toasted Bran, **Crawford's,** 8-oz. package	800	160.0	100.0	20.00	300	60.0
Wheat Bran, **Deaf Smith Farms,** 10-oz. package	1000	150.0	100.0	15.00	267	40.0
Unprocessed Bran, **Quaker,** 8-oz. box	640	128.0	80.0	16.00	(160)	(32.0)

	UNIT		1 OZ., BY WT.		1 CUP	
	Cal.	Carb.	Cal.	Carb.	Cal.	Carb.
Unprocessed Miller's Bran Flakes, **El Molino,** 12-oz. box	1080	180.0	90.0	15.00	(240)	(40.1)
Wheat Germ and Bran, **Golden Harvest,** 12-oz. box	1560	216.0	130.0	18.00	(273)	(37.8)
(END OF BRAN)						
Buc Wheats, **General Mills,** 10-oz. box	1100	230.2	110.0	23.00	(147)	(30.7)
15-oz. box	1650	345.0	110.0	23.00	(147)	(30.7)
Cap'n Crunch, **Quaker,** 8-oz. box	968	183.2	121.0	22.90	(161)	(30.5)
Cap'n Crunch's Crunchberries, **Quaker,** 11-oz. box	1320	251.9	120.0	22.90	(160)	(30.5)
Cap'n Crunch's Peanut Butter Cereal, **Quaker,** 12-oz. box	1524	250.8	127.0	20.90	(169)	(27.9)
Cheerios, **General Mills,** single serving, ¾-oz. box	83	15.0	110.0	20.00	(88)	(16.0)
7-oz. box	770	140.0	110.0	20.00	(88)	(16.0)
10-oz. box	1100	200.0	110.0	20.00	(88)	(16.0)
15-oz. box	1650	300.0	110.0	20.00	(88)	(16.0)
20-oz. box	2200	400.0	110.0	20.00	(88)	(16.0)
Cheerios, Honey Nut, **General Mills,** 14-oz. box	1540	322.0	110.0	23.00	(147)	(30.7)
Chex, Bran, **Ralston Purina,** 14-oz. box	1540	280.0	110.0	20.00	(165)	(30.0)
Chex, Corn, **Ralston Purina,** 12-oz. box	1320	300.0	110.0	25.00	(110)	(25.0)
Chex, Rice, **Ralston Purina,** 8-oz. box	880	200.0	110.0	25.00	(98)	(22.2)
Chex, Wheat, **Ralston Purina,** 15-oz. box	1650	345.0	110.0	23.00	(165)	(34.5)
Chex, Wheat and Raisin, **Ralston Purina,** 18-oz. box	1750	406.3	97.2	22.57	185	43.0
Cinnamon Life, **Quaker,** 15-oz. box	1575	295.5	105.0	19.70	156	29.6
20-oz. box	2100	394.0	105.0	19.70	156	29.6
Cocoa Krispies, **Kellogg's,** single serving, 1-oz. box	110	25.0	110.0	25.00	(147)	(33.3)
13-oz. box	1430	325.0	110.0	25.00	(147)	(33.3)
Cocoa Pebbles, **Post (General Foods),** 11-oz. box	1320	275.0	120.0	25.00	(137)	(28.6)
Cocoa Puffs, **General Mills,** 8-oz. box	880	200.0	110.0	25.00	(110)	(25.0)
12-oz. box	1320	300.0	110.0	25.00	(110)	(25.0)
17-oz. box	1870	425.0	110.0	25.00	(110)	(25.0)
Cookie Crisp, Chocolate Chip Flavor, **Ralston Purina,** 11-oz. box	1210	275.0	110.0	25.00	(110)	(25.0)
Cookie Crisp, Oatmeal Cookie Flavor, **Ralston Purina,** 11-oz. box	1320	264.0	120.0	24.00	120	24.0
Cookie Crisp, Vanilla Wafer Flavor, **Ralston Purina,** 11-oz. box	1210	275.0	110.0	25.00	(110)	(25.0)
CORN:						
(see also Puffed Corn)						
Corn Bran, **Quaker,** 12-oz. box	1308	279.6	109.0	23.30	164	35.0
Corn Chex, **Ralston Purina,** 12-oz. box	1320	300.0	110.0	25.00	(110)	(25.0)
(Country) Corn Flakes, **General Mills,** 10-oz. box	1100	240.0	110.0	24.00	(110)	(24.0)
15-oz. box	1650	360.0	110.0	24.00	(110)	(24.0)
Corn Flakes, **Kellogg's,** single serving, ¾-oz. box	80	18.0	110.0	24.00	(110)	(24.0)
8-oz. box	880	192.0	110.0	24.00	(110)	(24.0)
12-oz. box	1320	288.0	110.0	24.00	(110)	(24.0)
18-oz. box	1980	432.0	110.0	24.00	(110)	(24.0)
24-oz. box	2640	576.0	110.0	24.00	(110)	(24.0)
Corn Flakes, "Nutri-Grain" **Kellogg's,** 12-oz. box	1296	287.2	108.0	23.93	160	35.5
Corn Flakes, **Post Toasties,** 8-oz. box	880	192.0	110.0	24.00	(88)	(19.2)
12-oz. box	1320	288.0	110.0	24.00	(88)	(19.2)
18-oz. box	1980	432.0	110.0	24.00	(88)	(19.2)
Corn Flakes, **Ralston Purina,** 8-oz. box	880	192.0	110.0	24.00	(110)	(24.0)
Corn Flakes, **Safeway,** 18-oz. box	1980	432.0	110.0	24.00	(110)	(24.0)
Corn Flakes, Honey & Nut, **Kelloggs,** ⅞-oz. package	105	21.0	120.0	24.00	160	32.0
Corn Total, **General Mills,** 7-oz. box	770	168.0	110.0	24.00	(110)	(24.0)
Corney-Snaps, **Kellogg's,** 11-oz. box	1320	264.0	110.0	24.00	(110)	(24.0)
(END OF CORN)						
Count Chocula, **General Mills,** 12-oz. box	1320	288.0	110.0	24.00	(110)	(24.0)
Country Morning, **Kellogg's,** 15-oz. box	1950	270.0	130.0	18.00	(390)	(54.0)
Country Morning with Coconut, **Kellogg's,** 15-oz. box	1950	270.0	130.0	18.00	(390)	(54.0)
Country Morning with Raisins and Dates, **Kellogg's,** 15-oz. box	1950	285.0	130.0	19.00	(390)	(57.0)
Cracklin' Bran, see under BRAN						
Crazy Cow, Chocolate, **General Mills,** 12-oz. box	1320	288.0	110.0	24.00	(110)	(24.0)
Crazy Cow, Strawberry, **General Mills,** 12-oz. box	1320	300.0	110.0	24.00	(110)	(25.0)
Crispy Rice, see under RICE						
Crispy Wheats 'n Raisins, **General Mills,** 12-oz. package	1320	276.0	110.0	23.00	147	30.7
Crunch, **Arrowhead Mills,** 16-oz. (1-lb.) box	1920	288.0	120.0	18.00	(480)	(72.0)
48-oz. (3-lb.) box	5760	864.0	120.0	18.00	(480)	(72.0)

	UNIT		1 OZ., BY WT.		1 CUP	
	Cal.	Carb.	Cal.	Carb.	Cal.	Carb.
Crunchy Natural Cereal 'n' Snack, **Hearty Life,** 16-oz. (1-lb.) box	2080	272.0	130.0	17.00	(390)	(51.0)
C.W. Post, **General Mills,** 15-oz. box	1893	304.5	126.2	20.30	432	69.4
C.W. Post with Raisins, **General Mills,** 15-oz. box	1842	305.4	122.8	20.36	446	73.9
Dinky Donuts, **Ralston Purina,** 11-oz. package	1210	275.0	110.0	25.00	110	25.0
8-Grain Cereal 'n' Snack, Apple Cinnamon, **Good Shepherd,** 16-oz. (1-lb.) box	2000	304.0	125.0	19.00		
8-Grain Cereal 'n' Snack, Raisin Cinnamon, **Good Shepherd,** 16-oz. (1-lb.) box	1920	304.0	120.0	19.00		
Familia Mixed Cereal with Fruit and Nuts, **Richter Bros.,** 12-oz. box	1360	229.2	113.1	19.10	452	76.4
Familia with 25% Bran Mixed Cereal with Fruit and Nuts, **Richter Bros.,** 12-oz. box	1184	198.0	98.7	16.50	(395)	(66.0)
Familia Swiss Birchermuesli, Mixed Cereal with Fruit and Nuts, No Added Sugar, **Richter Bros.,** 11-oz. box	1144	212.9	104.0	19.35	(416)	(77.4)
Familia Swiss Granola, **Richter Bros.,** 24-oz. box	3077	421.9	128.2	17.58	(513)	(70.3)
Family Style Cereal, **Post (General Foods),** 15-oz. box	2100	285.0	140.0	19.00	(560)	(76.0)
Family Style Cereal with Raisins, **Post (General Foods),** 15-oz. box	1950	285.0	130.0	19.00	(520)	(76.0)
Frankenberry, **General Mills,** 12-oz. box	1320	288.0	110.0	24.00	(110)	(24.0)
Froot Loops, **Kellogg's,** single serving, ¾-oz. box	80	19.0	110.0	25.00	(110)	(25.0)
7-oz. box	770	175.0	110.0	25.00	(110)	(25.0)
15-oz. box	1650	375.0	110.0	25.00	(110)	(25.0)
Frosted Flakes (Sugar Frosted Flakes), **A&P,** 20-oz. box	2200	500.0	110.0	25.00	(147)	(33.3)
Frosted Flakes (Sugar Frosted Flakes), **Kellogg's,** single serving, 1-oz. box	110	26.0	110.0	26.00	(165)	(39.0)
10-oz. box	1100	260.0	110.0	26.00	(165)	(39.0)
15-oz. box	1650	390.0	110.0	26.00	(165)	(39.0)
20-oz. box	2200	520.0	110.0	26.00	(165)	(39.0)
Frosted Flakes (Sugar Frosted Flakes), **Ralston Purina,** 11-oz. box	1210	275.0	110.0	25.00	(147)	(33.3)
Frosted Mini-Wheats, **Kellogg's,** 16-oz. (1-lb.) box	1760	384.0	110.0	24.00		
1 biscuit (approx. 64 per 16-oz. box)	28	6.0	110.0	24.00		
Frosted Rice, **Kellogg's,** ⅞-oz. box	96	21.9	110.0	25.00	(110)	(25.0)
12-oz. box	1320	312.0	110.0	26.00	(110)	(26.0)
16-oz. (1-lb.) box	1760	416.0	110.0	26.00	(110)	(26.0)
Frosted Rice Krinkles, **Post (General Foods),** 11-oz. box	1210	286.0	110.0	26.00	(126)	(29.7)
Frosted Rice Krispies, **Kellogg's,** 14-oz. box	1520	359.2	108.6	25.66	95	22.5
Frosty O's, **General Mills,** 9-oz. box	990	216.0	110.0	24.00	(110)	(24.0)
Fruit & Nut, **Nature Valley (General Mills),** 16-oz. (1-lb.) box	2080	320.0	130.0	20.00	(390)	(60.0)
Fruit & Nut Natural 100 Cereal 'n' Snack, **Hearty Life,** 16-oz. (1-lb.) box	2080	272.0	130.0	17.00	(390)	(51.0)
Fruit Brute, **General Mills,** 12-oz. box	1320	288.0	110.0	24.00	(110)	(24.0)
Fruity Pebbles, **Post (General Foods),** single serving, ¾-oz. box	83	19.0	110.0	25.00	(126)	(28.6)
11-oz. box	1210	275.0	110.0	25.00	(126)	(28.6)
(Birchermuesli) Frutifort, **Zwicky,** 12-oz. box	(1340)	(151.2)	(111.6)	(12.60)	(446)	(50.4)
Golden Grahams, **General Mills,** 10-oz. box	1100	240.0	110.0	24.00	(110)	(24.0)
15-oz. box	1650	360.0	110.0	24.00	(110)	(24.0)
Good Farmer Cereal, **Golden Harvest,** 24-oz. box	3120	456.0	130.0	19.00		
Good Shepherd 8-Grain Cereal 'n' Snack Raisin Cinnamon **Sovex,** 16-oz. (1-lb.) bag	1920	304.0	120.0	19.00		
Good Shepherd Granola, Unsweetened Cereal, **Sovex,** 16-oz. (1-lb.) bag	2080	272.0	130.0	17.00	(520)	(68.0)
Good Shepherd Traditional Cereal, **Sovex,** 16-oz. (1-lb.) bag	2080	272.0	130.0	17.00	(520)	(68.0)
32-oz. (2-lb.) bag	4160	544.0	130.0	17.00	(520)	(68.0)
Graham Crackos, **Kellogg's,** ¾-oz. package	83	18.0	110.0	24.00	147	32.0
GRANOLA:						
Almond "Vita Crunch" Granola, **Back to Nature,** 32-oz. (2-lb.) box	3840	640.0	120.0	20.00	(480)	(80.0)
Apple Bran Granola, **Golden Harvest,** 15-oz. box	1800	165.0	120.0	11.00	(480)	(44.0)
Branola, see under BRAN						
Cinnamon & Raisin Granola, **Nature Valley (General Mills),** 16-oz. (1-lb.) box	2080	304.0	130.0	19.00	(390)	(57.0)
Coconut & Honey Granola, **Nature Valley (General Mills),** 16-oz. (1-lb.) box	2080	288.0	130.0	18.00	(390)	(54.0)
Crunchy Granola, **Golden Harvest,** 26-oz. box	3380	494.0	130.0	19.00	(520)	(76.0)
Granola with Almonds, **Sun Country (Kretschmer),** 16-oz. (1-lb.) box	2080	304.0	130.0	19.00	(520)	(96.0)
Granola Puffs, regular flavor, **Heartland (Pet),** 10-oz. box	1200	200.0	120.0	20.00	(240)	(40.0)
Granola Puffs, Cinnamon Spice Flavor, **Heartland (Pet),** 10-oz. box	1200	200.0	120.0	20.00	(240)	(40.0)

	UNIT Cal.	UNIT Carb.	1 OZ., BY WT. Cal.	1 OZ., BY WT. Carb.	1 CUP Cal.	1 CUP Carb.
Granola with Raisins, **Sun Country (Kretschmer),** 16-oz. (1-lb.) box	2080	320.0	130.0	20.00	(520)	(80.0)
High Fiber Granola, **Golden Harvest,** 14-oz. box	1820	294.0	130.0	21.00	(520)	(84.0)
High Protein Granola with Almonds and Seeds, Natural, **Better Way,** 16-oz. (1-lb.) box	1920	272.0	120.0	17.00	(480)	(68.0)
Honey Almond Granola, **Golden Harvest,** 26-oz. box	3380	468.0	130.0	18.00	(520)	(72.0)
Maple Nut Granola, **Old Mill (Arrowhead Mills),** 16-oz. (1-lb.) container	2080	272.0	130.0	17.00	(520)	(68.0)
Oats & Honey Granola, **Nature Valley (General Mills),** 16-oz. (1-lb.) box	2080	304.0	130.0	19.00	(390)	(57.0)
Old Fashioned Granola, **Golden Harvest,** 16-oz. (1-lb.) bag	1920	288.0	120.0	18.00	(480)	(72.0)
100% Natural Cereal Granola, **Premier,** 14-oz. box	1960	210.0	140.0	15.00	(560)	(60.0)
Proteinola, **Golden Harvest,** 16-oz. (1-lb.) box	2080	256.0	130.0	16.00	(520)	(64.0)
Raisin "Vitacrunch" Granola, **Back to Nature,** 32-oz. (2-lb.) box	3840	640.0	120.0	20.00	(480)	(80.0)
Traditional Cereal, **Good Shepherd (Sovex),** 1-lb. bag	2080	272.0	130.0	17.00	(520)	(68.0)
2-lb. bag	4160	544.0	130.0	17.00	(520)	(68.0)
Unsweetened Granola, **Good Shepherd (Sovex),** 16-oz. (1-lb.) bag	2080	272.0	130.0	17.00	(520)	(68.0)
(END OF GRANOLA)						
Grape-Nuts, **Post,** 16-oz. (1-lb.) box	1600	352.0	100.0	22.00	(400)	(88.0)
Grape-Nuts Flakes, **Post,** 12-oz. box	1200	276.0	100.0	23.00	(114)	(26.2)
Hi-Proteen Breakfast Food, **Hoffman,** 16-oz. (1-lb.) box	1440	160.0	90.0	10.00		
Hi-Proteen Breakfast Food with Fruit & Nut, **Hoffman,** 16-oz. (1-lb.) box	1600	192.0	100.0	12.00		
High Fiber Granola, **Golden Harvest,** 14-oz. box	1820	294.0	130.0	21.00	(520)	(84.0)
High Protein Granola with Almonds and Seeds, Natural, **Better Way,** 16-oz. (1-lb.) box	1920	272.0	120.0	17.00	(480)	(58.0)
Honey Almond Granola, **Golden Harvest,** 26-oz. box	3380	468.0	130.0	18.00	(520)	(72.0)
Honey and Almond Crunch, **Lassen,** 48-oz. (3-lb.) box	6240	864.0	130.0	18.00	(520)	(72.0)
Honey Bran Branola, **Hi-Protein,** 16-oz. (1-lb.) bag	1920	283.2	120.0	17.70	(480)	(70.8)
Honeycomb, **Post (General Foods),** 12-oz. box	1320	300.0	110.0	25.00	(83)	(18.8)
Honey Nut Cheerios, **General Mills,** 14-oz. box	1540	322.0	110.0	23.00	147	(30.7)
Honey & Nut Corn Flakes, **Kellogg's,** 7/8-oz. box	105	21.0	120.0	24.00	160	32.0
13-oz. box	1560	312.0	120.0	24.00	(160)	(32.0)
16-oz. (1-lb.) package	1920	384.0	120.0	24.00	160	32.0
Kaboom, **General Mills,** 6-oz. box	990	216.0	110.0	24.00	(110)	(24.0)
King Vitamin, **Quaker,** 9-oz. box	990	209.7	110.0	22.00	(147)	(31.1)
Kix, **General Mills,** 9-oz. box	990	216.0	110.0	24.00	(73)	(16.0)
Life, **Quaker,** 10-oz. box	1050	197.0	105.0	19.70	(158)	(29.6)
15-oz. box	1575	295.5	105.0	19.70	(158)	(29.6)
20-oz. box	2100	394.0	105.0	19.70	(158)	(29.6)
Life, Cinnamon, **Quaker,** 15-oz. box	1575	295.5	105.0	19.70	156	29.6
20-oz. box	2100	394.0	105.0	19.70	156	29.6
Lucky Charms, **General Mills,** single serving, 1-oz. box	110	24.0	110.0	24.00	(110)	(24.0)
9-oz. box	990	216.0	110.0	24.00	(110)	(24.0)
14-oz. box	1540	336.0	110.0	24.00	(110)	(24.0)
20-oz. box	2200	480.0	110.0	24.00	(110)	(24.0)
Maple Nut Granola, **Old Mill (Arrowhead Mills),** 16-oz. (1-lb.) container	2080	272.0	130.0	17.00	(520)	(68.0)
48-oz. (3-lb.) container	6240	816.0	130.0	17.00	(520)	(68.0)
Millet Flakes, **Zwicky,** 12-oz. box	776	249.9	64.6	20.82		
See also Puffed Millet						
Mini-Wheats, see under WHEAT						
Most, **Kellogg's,** 12-oz. box	1146	259.2	95.5	21.60	175	39.6
"NATURAL CEREAL":						
(This section is not meant to differentiate "natural" from "unnatural" cereals, whatever that means. Cereals listed in this section are cereals for which the word "natural" is an integral descriptive part of the label.)						
Coconut Natural Cereal, **Heartland,** 16-oz. (1-lb.) box	2080	288.0	130.0	18.00	(520)	(70.0)
Crunchy Natural Cereal 'n' Snack, **Hearty Life,** 16-oz. (1-lb.) box	2080	272.0	130.0	17.00	(390)	(51.0)
Fruit & Nut Natural 100 Cereal 'n' Snack, **Hearty Life,** 16-oz. (1-lb.) box	2080	272.0	130.0	17.00	(390)	(51.0)
Natural Cereal, Raisin, **Heartland,** 16-oz. (1-lb.) box	1920	288.0	120.0	18.00	(480)	(72.0)
Natural Cereal with Raisins, **Alpen,** 12-oz. box	1320	240.0	110.0	20.0	(440)	(80.0)
Natural Cereal, Rolled Oats, **Heartland,** 16-oz. (1-lb.) box	1920	288.0	120.0	18.00	(480)	(72.0)
100% Natural Cereal, **Golden Harvest,** 2-oz. bag	240	36.0	120.0	18.00		
32-oz. (2-lb.) bag	2160	576.0	120.0	18.00		
100% Natural Cereal, Granola, **Premier,** 14-oz. box	1960	210.0	140.0	15.00	(560)	(60.0)
100% Natural Cereal, **Quaker,** 16-oz. (1-lb.) box	2224	272.0	139.0	17.00	(556)	(68.0)
32-oz. (2-lb.) box	4448	544.0	139.0	17.00	(556)	(68.0)
100% Natural Cereal with Apple and Cinnamon, **Quaker,** 15-oz. box	2025	270.0	135.0	18.00	(640)	(72.0)
30-oz. box	4050	540.0	135.0	18.00	(640)	(72.0)
100% Natural Cereal with Raisins and Dates, **Quaker,** 16-oz. (1-lb.) box	2144	284.8	134.0	17.80	(536)	(71.2)
32-oz. (2-lb.) box	4288	569.6	134.0	17.80	(536)	(71.2)
100% Natural Cereal with Raisins & Dates, **Shopwell,** 16-oz. (1-lb.) package	2080	272.0	130.0	17.00	390	51.0
(END OF "NATURAL CEREAL")						
Oat Flakes, Fortified, **General Foods,** 12-oz. box	1320	240.0	110.0	20.00	(165)	(30.0)
Oats & Honey Granola, **Nature Valley (General Mills),** 16-oz. (1-lb.) box	2080	304.0	130.0	19.00	(390)	(57.0)
Pebbles, Cocoa, **Post (General Foods),** 11-oz. box	1320	275.0	120.0	25.00	(137)	(28.6)
Pebbles, Fruity, **Post (General Foods),** single serving, 3/4-oz. box	83	19.0	110.0	25.00	(126)	(28.6)
11-oz. box	1210	275.0	110.0	25.00	(126)	(28.6)
Pep, Wheat Flakes, **Kellogg's,** 10-oz. box	1000	240.0	100.0	24.00	(133)	(32.0)
Post Toasties, see Corn Flakes						
Product 19, **Kellogg's,** single serving, 1-oz. box	110	24.0	110.0	24.00	(147)	(32.0)
8-oz. box	880	192.0	110.0	24.00	(147)	(32.0)
12-oz. box	1320	288.0	110.0	24.00	(147)	(32.0)
17-oz. box	1870	408.0	110.0	24.00	(147)	(32.0)
Proteinola, **Golden Harvest,** 16-oz. (1-lb.) box	2080	256.0	130.0	16.00	(520)	(64.0)
Puffed Corn, **El Molino,** 6-oz. bag	600	132.0	100.0	22.00	(67)	14.7
Puffed Millet, **El Molino,** 6-oz. bag	600	132.0	100.0	22.00	(67)	14.7
Puffed Rice, **El Molino,** 6-oz. bag	600	144.0	100.0	24.00	(67)	(16.1)
Puffed Rice, **Kellogg's,** 3/8-oz. package	40	9.0	105.3	23.68		
Puffed Rice, **Malt-O-Meal,** 6-oz. bag	600	144.0	100.0	24.00	(67)	(16.1)
16-oz. (1 lb.) bag	1600	384.0	100.0	24.00	(67)	(16.1)
Puffed Rice, **Quaker,** 5-oz. box	550	127.0	110.0	25.40	(74)	(17.1)
7-oz. box	770	177.8	110.0	25.40	(74)	(17.1)
Puffed Wheat, "Wheat Puffs," **A&P,** 8-oz. box	800	176.0	100.0	22.00	(43)	(9.4)
Puffed Wheat, **El Molino,** 6-oz. bag	600	132.0	100.0	22.00	43	9.4
Puffed Wheat, **Kellogg's,** 5/16-oz. box	35	7.0	112.9	22.58		
Puffed Wheat, **Malt-O-Meal,** 6-oz. bag	600	120.0	100.0	20.00	43	8.6
16-oz. (1-lb.) bag	1600	320.0	100.0	20.00	43	8.6
Puffed Wheat, **Quaker,** 4-oz. box	400	88.0	100.0	22.00	(43)	(9.4)
6-oz. box	600	132.0	100.0	22.00	(43)	(9.4)
Quisp, **Quaker,** 9-oz. box	1089	207.9	121.0	23.10	(73)	(13.9)
Raisin Bran, see under BRAN						
Raisin Granola, "Vitacrunch," **Back to Nature,** 32-oz. (2-lb.) box	3840	640.0	120.0	20.00	(480)	(80.0)
Raisin Natural Cereal, **Heartland,** 16-oz. (1-lb.) box	1920	288.0	120.0	18.00	(480)	(72.0)
Raisins, Rice & Rye, **Kellogg's,** 13-oz. package	1239	314.7	95.3	24.21	155	39.3
RICE:						
(also see Puffed Rice)						
Crispy Rice, **Ralston Purina,** 13-oz. box	1430	325.5	110.0	25.00	(110)	(25.0)
Crispy Rice, **Safeway,** 10-oz. box	1100	250.0	110.0	25.00	(110)	(25.0)
Pure Rice Bran, Gluten Free, **Jolly Joan,** 8-oz. box	(421)	(116.6)	(52.6)	(14.57)	(130)	(36.0)
Rice Chex, **Ralston Purina,** 8-oz. box	880	200.0	110.0	25.00	(98)	(22.2)
Rice Krispies, **Kellogg's,** 5/8-oz. box	70	16.0	110.0	25.00	110	25.0
6-oz. box	660	150.0	110.0	25.00	(110)	(25.0)
10-oz. box	1100	250.0	110.0	25.00	(110)	(25.0)
13-oz. box	1430	325.0	110.0	25.00	(110)	(25.0)
Rice Puffs, **A&P,** 8-oz. bag	960	208.0	120.0	26.00	(60)	(13.0)
(END OF RICE)						
Rye Flaked Whole Grain Cereal, **Nutri Grain (Kellogg's),** 12-oz. box	1320	288.0	110.0	24.00	147	32.0
Shredded Wheat, **Nabisco,** 3/4-oz. package	68	14.3	90.0	19.00		
10-oz. package	900	190.0	90.0	19.00		
15-oz. box	1350	285.0	90.0	19.00	(130)	(29.8)

	UNIT Cal.	UNIT Carb.	1 OZ., BY WT. Cal.	1 OZ., BY WT. Carb.	1 CUP Cal.	1 CUP Carb.
Shredded Wheat (Spoon Size), **Nabisco,** 12-oz. box	1320	276.0	110.0	23.00	(165)	(34.5)
18-oz. box (approx. 450 biscuits per box)	1980	414.0	110.0	23.00	(165)	(34.5)
1 biscuit, approx. 0.03 oz.	3	0.7	110.0	23.00	(165)	(34.5)
Shredded Wheat, **Quaker,** 12-oz. box (approx. 18 biscuits per box)	936	198.0	78.0	16.50	(117)	(24.8)
1 biscuit, approx. ⅔ oz.	52	11.0	78.0	16.50	(117)	(24.8)
Shredded Wheat Biscuits, **Sunshine,** 10-oz. box, approx. 11–12 biscuits	1008	225.4	100.8	22.54		
1 biscuit, approx. 0.8 oz.	85	19.0	100.8	22.54		
Special K, **Kellogg's,** single serving, ⅝-oz. box	69	13.1	110.0	21.00	(88)	(16.8)
7-oz. box	770	147.0	110.0	21.00	(88)	(16.8)
11-oz. box	1210	231.0	110.0	21.00	(88)	(16.8)
15-oz. box	1650	315.0	110.0	21.00	(88)	(16.8)
Sprouted Seven Grain Natural Breakfast Cereal with Bananas & Honey (No Sugar Added), **Health Valley,** 12-oz. box	1320	276.0	110.0	23.00	(440)	(92.0)
Sprouted Seven Grain Natural Breakfast Cereal with Raisins, **Health Valley,** 12-oz. box	1320	264.0	110.0	22.00	(440)	(88.0)
Sugar Corn Pops (Sugar Pops), **Kellogg's,** single serving, ¾-oz. box	83	19.5	110.0	26.00	(110)	(26.0)
10-oz. box	1100	260.0	110.0	26.00	(110)	(26.0)
15-oz. box	1650	390.0	110.0	26.00	(110)	(26.0)
Sugar Frosted Flakes, see Frosted Flakes						
Sugar Puffs, **Malt-O-Meal,** 18-oz. bag	1980	468.0	110.0	26.00		
Sugar Smacks, **Kellogg's,** ⅞-oz. package	96	21.9	110.0	25.00	147	25.0
12-oz. box	1320	300.0	110.0	25.00	(147)	(33.3)
18-oz. box	1980	450.0	110.0	25.00	(147)	(33.3)
Super Sugar Crisp, **Post (General Foods),** single serving, 1-oz. box	110	25.0	110.0	25.00	(126)	(28.6)
12-oz. box	1320	300.0	110.0	25.00	(126)	(28.6)
Swiss Birchermuesli, see Familia and Frutifort						
Tasteeos, **Safeway,** 15-oz. box	1650	330.0	110.0	22.00	(88)	(17.6)
Team Flakes, **Nabisco,** 13-oz. box	1430	312.0	110.0	24.00	(110)	(24.0)
Toasty O's, **Malt-O-Meal,** 10-oz. bag	1100	200.0	110.0	20.00	(88)	(16.0)
15-oz. bag	1650	300.0	110.0	20.00	(88)	(16.0)
Total, **General Mills,** single serving, 1-oz. box	110	23.0	110.0	23.00	(110)	(23.0)
8-oz. box	880	184.0	110.0	23.00	(110)	(23.0)
12-oz. box	1320	276.0	110.0	23.00	(110)	(23.0)
18-oz. box	1980	414.0	110.0	23.00	(110)	(23.0)
Total (Corn), **General Mills,** 7-oz. box	770	168.0	110.0	24.00	(110)	(24.0)
Trix, **General Mills,** 8-oz. box	880	200.0	110.0	25.00	(110)	(25.0)
12-oz. box	1320	300.0	110.0	25.00	(110)	(25.0)
16-oz. (1 lb.) box	1760	400.0	110.0	25.00	(110)	(25.0)
Uncle Sam, "A Natural Laxative Cereal," 10-oz. box	1100	190.0	110.0	19.00	(220)	(38.0)
Vitagrain & Nuts, **Lassen,** 48-oz. (3-lb.) box	6240	912.0	130.0	19.00	(520)	(76.0)
Waffelos, **Ralston Purina,** 11-oz. package	1263	269.2	114.8	24.47	121	25.9
Waffelos, Blueberry, **Ralston Purina,** 11-oz. package	1210	275.0	110.0	25.00	110	25.0
WHEAT:						
(see also Puffed Wheat)						
Mini-Wheats, Toasted, **Kellogg's,** 16-oz. (1-lb.) box	1600	352.0	100.0	22.00		
Pep Wheat Flakes, **Kellogg's,** 10-oz. box	1000	240.0	100.0	24.00	(133)	(32.0)
Weetabix, 14-oz. box	1440	300.0	102.9	21.43		
1 biscuit, 0.58 oz.	60	12.5	102.9	21.43		
Wheat Chex, **Ralston Purina,** 15-oz. box	1650	345.0	110.0	23.00	(165)	(34.5)
Wheat Flakes, "Nutri-Grain," **Kellogg's,** 15-oz. box	1532	359.9	102.1	23.99	158	37.2
Wheat Flakes (Kollath), **Zwicky,** 12-oz. box	786	220.2	65.5	18.35		
Wheat Germ with Brown Sugar & Honey, **Kretschmer,** 10-oz. jar	1100	170.0	110.0	17.00	440	68.0
1 cup (approx. 4 oz.)	440	68.0	110.0	17.00	440	68.0
1 pound (approx. 4 cups)	1760	272.0	110.0	17.00	440	68.0
Wheat Germ, Natural, Not Toasted, **Fisher From Krustez,** 12-oz. package	1236	168.0	103.0	14.00	412	56.0
1 cup (approx. 4 oz.)	412	56.0	103.0	14.00	412	56.0
1 pound (approx. 4 cups)	1648	224.0	103.0	14.00	412	56.0
Wheat Germ, Raw, **Golden Harvest,** 16-oz. (1-lb.) jar	1600	240.0	100.0	15.00	300	45.0
Wheat Germ, Raw, **Naturfresh (Fearn),** 10-oz. pouch	1100	130.0	110.0	13.00	440	52.0
Wheat Germ, Regular, **Kretschmer,** 12-oz. jar	1320	156.0	110.0	13.00	440	52.0
Wheat and Raisin Chex, **Ralston Purina,** 18-oz. box	1750	406.3	97.2	22.57	185	43.0
Wheaties, **General Mills,** single serving, 1-oz. box	110	23.0	110.0	23.00	(110)	23.00
8-oz. box	880	184.0	110.0	23.00	(110)	(23.0)
12-oz. box	1320	276.0	110.0	23.00	(110)	(23.0)

	UNIT Cal.	UNIT Carb.	1 OZ., BY WT. Cal.	1 OZ., BY WT. Carb.	1 CUP Cal.	1 CUP Carb.
18-oz. box	1980	414.0	110.0	23.00	(110)	(23.0)
24-oz. box	2640	552.0	110.0	23.00	(110)	(23.0)
(END OF WHEAT)						
SINGLE SERVING MULTI-PACKS						
General Mills:						
8-Pack Cheerios (8 boxes, ¾ oz. each), 6-oz. package	640	120.0	106.7	20.00		
8-Pack Total (8 boxes, 1 oz. each), 8-oz. package	880	184.0	110.0	23.00		
8-Pack Variety: Wheaties (2 boxes, 1 oz. each), Cheerios (2 boxes, ¾ oz. each), Total (2 boxes, 1 oz. each), Lucky Charms (2 boxes, 1 oz. each)	826	172.0	110.0	22.90		
8-Pack Variety: Wheaties (2 boxes, 1 oz. each), Cheerios (2 boxes, ¾ oz. each), Total (2 boxes, 1 oz. each), Trix (2 boxes, 1 oz. each)	826	170.0	110.0	22.67		
Post-Tens (Assorted Cereals): Wheaties (2 boxes, 1 oz. each), Cheerios (2 boxes, ¾ oz. each), Total (2 boxes, 1 oz. each), Lucky Charms (2 boxes, 1 oz. each)	910	205.0	121.3	27.30		
Kellogg's:						
Corn Flakes Handi-Pak (8 boxes, ¾ oz. each), 6-oz. pak	640	152.0	106.7	25.33		
Frosted Flakes Handi-Pak (8 boxes, 1 oz. each), 8-oz. pak	880	208.0	110.0	26.00		
Product 19 Handi-Pak (8 boxes, 1 oz. each), 8-oz. pak	880	129.0	110.0	24.00		
Rice Krispies Handi-Pak (8 boxes, ⅝ oz. each), 5-oz. pak	560	128.0	112.0	25.60		
Special K Handi-Pak (8 boxes, ⅝ oz. each), 5-oz. pak	560	104.0	112.0	20.80		
Jumbo Assortment: Corn Flakes (3 boxes, ¾ oz. each), Raisin Bran (2 boxes, 1¼ oz. each), Froot Loops (1 box, ¾ oz.), Rice Krispies (2 boxes, ⅝ oz. each), Frosted Rice (1 box, ⅞ oz.), Product 19, (1 box, 1 oz.), Applejacks (1 box, ⅝ oz.), Sugar Smacks (2 boxes, ⅞ oz. each), Sugar Corn Pops (1 box, ¾ oz.), Sugar Frosted Flakes (2 boxes, 1 oz. each), Special K (2 boxes, ⅝ oz. each)	1570	352.0	104.7	23.47		
Request Pak: Corn Flakes (2 boxes, ¾ oz. each), Rice Krispies (1 box, ⅝ oz.) Special K (1 box, ⅝ oz.), Raisin Bran (1 box, 1¼ oz.), Product 19 (1 box, 1 oz.)	520	110.0	104.0	22.00		
Snack Pak: Applejacks, (1 box, ⅝ oz.), Cocoa Krispies, (1 box, 1 oz.), Froot Loops (1 box, ¾ oz.), Sugar Corn Pops (1 box, ¾ oz.), Frosted Flakes (1 box, 1 oz.), Sugar Smacks (1 box, ⅞ oz.)	540	128.0	108.0	25.60		
Variety: Rice Krispies, (1 box, ⅝ oz.), Corn Flakes (2 boxes, ¾ oz. each), Froot Loops (1 box, ¾ oz.), Raisin Bran (2 boxes, 1¼ oz. each), Special K (1 box, ⅝ oz.), Product 19 (1 box, 1 oz.), Frosted Flakes (1 box, 1 oz.), 40% Bran Flakes (1 box, 1 oz.)	910	213.0	101.1	23.70		

BREAKFAST BREADS MADE FROM SCRATCH, based on USDA home recipes

	UNIT Cal.	UNIT Carb.	ONE PANCAKE OR WAFFLE Cal.	ONE PANCAKE OR WAFFLE Carb.	1 OZ., BY WT. Cal.	1 OZ., BY WT. Carb.	1 CUP Cal.	1 CUP Carb.
PANCAKES made with enriched or unenriched flour								
Made with 1½ cups flour, 1 cup fluid skim milk, 2½ Tbsp. cooking fat, 1 large egg, 1 Tbsp. sugar, 1½ tsp. baking powder, ½ tsp. salt (yield: approx. 16 4" pancakes (approx. 15.1 oz., prepared)	(990)	(145.9)			65.5	9.67		
1 4" pancake as above, approx. 0.95 oz. prepared			62	9.2	65.5	9.67		
1 pound (approx. 17 4" pancakes) (2g/10g/2g/50%/120mg)	1048	154.7			65.5	9.67		
WAFFLES made with enriched or unenriched flour								
Made with 1½ cup flour, 1 cup milk, 2 Tbsp. cooking fat, 2 large eggs, 1 Tbsp. sugar, 1½ tsp. baking powder, ½ tsp. salt (yield: approx. 1.9 waffles, approx. 13.5 oz.)	(1068)	(143.5)			79.1	10.63		

	UNIT		ONE PANCAKE OR WAFFLE		1 OZ., BY WT.		1 CUP	
	Cal.	Carb.	Cal.	Carb.	Cal.	Carb.	Cal.	Carb.
1 waffle as above (approx. 9" square), approx. 7.1 oz.			558	75.0	79.1	10.63		
1 pound (approx. 2¼ waffles) (3g/11g/3g/41%/135mg)	1266	170.1			79.1	10.63		
BREAKFAST BREADS MADE FROM MIXES								
Breakfast Batters								
PANCAKES and WAFFLES								
PREMIXED, FROZEN:								
Aunt Jemima (Regular), 16-oz. (1-lb.) container (yield: approx. 12 4" pancakes)	840	168.8			52.5	10.55		
1 4" pancake, approx. 1.1 oz.			70	14.5	(62.5)	(12.95)		
Blueberry, 16-oz. (1-lb.) container (yield: 12 4" pancakes)	820	166.0			51.3	10.38		
1 4" pancake, approx. 1.1 oz.			68	13.8	60.7	12.32		
Buttermilk, 16-oz. (1-lb.) container (yield: approx. 12 4" pancakes)	848	170.4			53.0	10.65		
1 4" pancake, approx. 1.1 oz.			71	14.2	63.4	12.68		
DRY MIXES:								
Regular:								
Aunt Jemima Complete Pancake and Waffle Mix, 16-oz. (1-lb.) box	1667	321.7			104.2	20.11	594	114.6
Prepared as package directs (yield: approx. 24 4" pancakes or 5 waffles)	1667	321.7			(61.5)	(11.86)		
32-oz. (2-lb.) box	3335	643.4			104.2	20.11	594	114.6
Prepared as package directs (yield: approx. 48 4" pancakes or 10 waffles)	3335	643.4			(61.5)	(11.86)		
80-oz. (5-lb.) box	8335	1608.5			104.2	20.11	594	114.6
Prepared as package directs (yield: approx. 120 4" pancakes or 24 waffles)	8335	1608.5			(61.5)	(11.86)		
1 4" pancake, approx. 1.1 oz.			66	12.7	(61.5)	(11.86)		
1 waffle, approx. 4.8 oz.			(365)	(70.4)	(75.7)	(14.62)		
Original Pancake and Waffle Mix, 16-oz. (1-lb.) box	1571	327.2			98.2	20.45	432	90.0
Prepared as package directs (yield: approx. 42 4" pancakes or 10 waffles)	3142	369.9			(66.2)	(7.79)		
32-oz. (2-lb.) box	3142	654.4			98.2	20.45	432	90.0
Prepared as package directs (yield: approx. 84 4" pancakes or 19 waffles)	6284	1308.4			(66.2)	(7.79)		
52-oz. (3¼-lb.) box	5106	1063.4			98.2	20.45	432	90.0
Prepared as package directs (yield: approx. 137 4" pancakes or 32 waffles)	10212	2126.8			(66.2)	(7.75)		
96-oz. (4½-lb.) box	7070	1472.4			98.2	20.45	432	90.0
Prepared as package directs (yield: approx. 189 4" pancakes or 44 waffles)	14140	2944.8			(66.2)	(7.79)		
1 4" pancake, approx. 1.1 oz.			73	8.7	(66.2)	(7.79)		
1 waffle, approx. 3.9 oz.			(314)	(37.0)	(81.5)	(8.49)		
Hungry Jack Complete Pancake Mix, 24-oz. (1½-lb.) box	3080	588.0			128.3	24.51		
Prepared as package directs (yield: approx. 42 4" pancakes)	3080	588.0			(64.9)	(12.39)		
1 4" pancake, approx. 1.1 oz.			73	14.0	(64.9)	(12.39)		
1 waffle, approx. 4.3 oz.			(342)	(65.3)	(79.2)	(15.12)		
Extra Lights, Pancake and Waffle Mix, 16-oz. (1-lb.) box	1430	253.0			89.4	15.81		
Prepared as package directs (yield: approx. 39 4" pancakes)	2600	364.0			(59.0)	(8.26)		
1 4" pancake, approx. 1.1 oz.			67	9.3	(59.0)	(8.26)		
1 waffle, approx. 4.6 oz.			(333)	(46.7)	(72.9)	(10.08)		
Log Cabin Pancake and Waffle Mix, 32-oz. (2-lb.) box	2900	638.0			90.6	19.94		
Prepared as package directs (yield: approx. 87 4" pancakes)	(5510)	(728.6)			(60.7)	(8.02)		
1 4" pancake, approx. 1.1 oz.			(63)	(8.4)	(60.7)	(8.02)		
1 waffle, approx. 4.1 oz.			(329)	(33.1)	(81.0)	(9.78)		
Complete Pancake and Waffle Mix, 32-oz. (2-lb.) box	3230	627.0			100.9	19.59		
Prepared as package directs (yield: approx. 57 4" pancakes)	3230	627.0			(50.2)	(8.73)		
1 4" pancake, approx. 1.1 oz.			57	11.0	(50.2)	(8.73)		
1 waffle, approx. 3.7 oz.			(288)	(41.8)	(77.7)	(11.87)		
Tillie Lewis "Tasti-Diet" Low Calorie Pancake and Waffle Mix, 4-oz. box	390	78.0			97.5	19.50	390	78.0
Prepared as package directs (yield: approx. 9 4" pancakes)	390	78.0			(38.7)	(7.74)		
1 4" pancake, approx. 1.1 oz.			43	8.7	(38.7)	(7.74)		
1 waffle, approx. 2.7 oz.			130	26.0	(47.5)	(9.63)		
Blueberry:								
Hungry Jack Blueberry Pancake and Waffle Mix, 12-oz. box	900	195.0			75.0	16.25		
Prepared as package directs (yield: approx. 16 4" pancakes)	1700	215.0			(94.0)	(11.89)		
1 4" pancake, approx. 1.2 oz.			113	14.3	(94.0)	(11.89)		
1 waffle, approx. 3.7 oz.			425	53.8	(114.7)	(14.51)		
Buckwheat:								
Aunt Jemima "High Fiber" Buckwheat Pancake and Waffle Mix, 16-oz. (1-lb.) box	1556	309.8			97.3	19.36	428	85.2
Prepared as package directs (yield: approx. 42 4" pancakes)	2800	352.0			(59.0)	(7.42)		
32-oz. (2-lb.) box	3113	619.5			97.3	19.36	428	85.2
Prepared as package directs (yield: approx. 84 4" pancakes)	5600	704.0			(59.0)	(7.42)		
1 4" pancake, approx. 1.1 oz.			67	8.4	(59.0)	(7.42)		
1 waffle, approx. 4.6 oz.			(391)	(39.1)	(85.1)	(8.51)		
Fearn Buckwheat Pancake Mix, 16-oz. (1-lb.) package	1430	286.0						
Prepared as package directs (yield: approx. 33 4" pancakes)	2535	312.0			(69.0)	(8.50)		
1 4" pancake, approx. 1.1 oz.	78	9.6	89	17.8	(8.50)	(8.50)		
Golden Harvest, Buckwheat Pancake Mix, 16-oz. (1-lb.) package	1440	304.0						
Prepared as package directs (yield: approx. 28 4" pancakes)	2400	320.0			(73.9)	(9.85)		
1 4" pancake, approx. 1.1 oz.	(86)	(11.4)	90	19.0	(73.9)	(9.85)		
Vermont General Store & Grist Mill, Buckwheat Pancake Mix, Whole Grain, 19.9-oz. (1 lb. 3.9 oz.) bag	2300	420.0			115.0	21.00	690	126.0
Prepared as package directs (yield: 24 to 36 pancakes)	(3860)	(442.5)			(110.1)	(12.62)		
1 4" pancake, approx. 1.1 oz.			(124)	(14.2)	(110.0)	(12.62)		
Buttermilk:								
Aunt Jemima Buttermilk Pancake and Waffle Mix, 16-oz. (1-lb.) box	1556	324.5			97.2	20.28	525	109.8
Prepared as package directs (yield: approx. 38 4" pancakes)	2745	360.6			(65.2)	(8.56)		
32-oz. (2-lb.) box	3111	649.0			97.2	20.28	525	109.8
Prepared as package directs (yield: approx. 75 4" pancakes)	5490	721.2			(65.2)	(8.56)		
52-oz. (3¼-lb.) box	5057	1054.6			97.2	20.28	525	109.8
Prepared as package directs (yield: approx. 123 4" pancakes)	8921	1172.0			(65.2)	(8.56)		
80-oz. (5-lb.) box	7780	1622.5			97.2	20.28	525	109.8
Prepared as package directs (yield: approx. 189 4" pancakes)	13725	1803.0			(65.2)	(8.56)		

	UNIT Cal.	UNIT Carb.	ONE PANCAKE OR WAFFLE Cal.	ONE PANCAKE OR WAFFLE Carb.	1 OZ., BY WT. Cal.	1 OZ., BY WT. Carb.	1 CUP Cal.	1 CUP Carb.
1 4" pancake, approx. 1.1 oz.			(73)	(10.0)	(65.2)	(9.56)		
1 waffle, approx. 3.2 oz.			(287)	(32.5)	(91.2)	(10.44)		
Complete Buttermilk Pancake and Waffle Mix, 32-oz. (2-lb.) box	3284	644.2			102.6	20.13	708	138.6
Prepared as package directs (yield: approx. 38.5 4" pancakes)	3284	644.2			(69.9)	(13.63)		
1 4" pancake, approx. 1.1 oz.			79	15.4	(69.9)	(13.63)		
1 waffle, approx. 2.8 oz.			(354)	(46.0)	(128.7)	(16.73)		
Betty Crocker Buttermilk Pancake Mix, 28-oz. (1¾-lb.) box	2856	604.8			102.0	21.60	510	108.0
Prepared as package directs (yield: approx. 50 4" pancakes)	4536	655.2			(80.4)	(11.61)		
42-oz. box	4284	907.2			102.0	21.60	510	108.0
Prepared as package directs (yield: approx. 76 4" pancakes)	(6804)	(982.8)			(80.4)	(11.61)		
1 4" pancake, approx. 1.1 oz.			90	13.0	(80.4)	(11.61)		
Complete Buttermilk Pancake Mix, 26-oz. box	2730	533.0			105.0	20.50	420	82.0
Prepared as package directs (yield: approx. 39 4" pancakes)	2730	533.0			(62.0)	(12.10)		
1 4" pancake, approx. 1.1 oz.			70	13.7	(62.0)	(12.10)		
Hungry Jack Buttermilk Pancake Mix, 16-oz. (1-lb.) box	1560	324.0			97.5	20.25	(450)	(84.7)
Prepared as package directs (yield: approx. 36 4" pancakes)	2880	348.1			(66.9)	(8.08)		
1 4" pancake, approx. 1.1 oz.			(76)	(9.2)	(66.9)	(8.08)		
1 waffle, approx. 5.6 oz.	(554)	(60.4)	(554)	(60.5)	(78.9)	(10.80)		
Complete Buttermilk Pancake Mix, 16-oz. (1-lb.) box	1560	294.7			97.5	18.42		
Prepared as package directs (yield: approx. 26 4" pancakes)	1560	294.7						
1 4" pancake			60	11.3				
1 waffle, approx. ⅕ of mix			312	58.9				
Log Cabin Buttermilk Pancake & Waffle Mix, 32-oz. (2-lb.) box	3080	682.0			96.3	21.31	(420)	(92.9)
Prepared as package directs (yield: approx. 66 4" pancakes)	5060	748.0			(68.1)	(10.00)		
1 4" pancake, approx. 1.1 oz.)			77	11.3	(68.1)	(10.00)		
1 waffle, approx. 3.1 oz.			(271)	(34.2)	(87.4)	(11.00)		
Vermont General Store & Grist Mill Buttermilk, Whole Wheat & Corn Meal Pancake Mix, 20.6-oz. bag	2300	430.0			111.7	20.87	690	129.0
Prepared as package directs (yield: 24 to 36 4" pancakes)	3900	460.0			(106.3)	(12.53)		
1 4" pancake, approx. 1.4 oz.			(150)	(17.6)	(106.3)	(12.53)		
Low Sodium:								
Fearn Low Sodium Pancake Mix, 16-oz. (1-lb.) package	1430	286.0	89	17.9				
Prepared as package directs (yield: 33 4" pancakes)	2470	318.5			(67.3)	(8.61)		
1 4" pancake, approx. 1.1 oz.			76	9.8	(67.3)	(8.61)		
Mixed Grain:								
Arrowhead Mills Multigrain Pancake & Waffle Mix, 32-oz. (2-lb.) box	2800	560.0	88	17.5				
Prepared as package directs (yield: approx. 48 4" pancakes)	3280	560.0			(60.7)	(10.37)		
1 4" pancake, approx. 1.1 oz.			66	11.2	(60.7)	(10.37)		
Triticale:								
Fearn Triticale Pancake Mix, 16-oz. (1-lb.) package	1540	273.0	96	17.1				
Prepared as package directs (yield: approx. 35 4" pancakes)	2660	301.0			(67.3)	(7.61)		
1 4" pancake, approx. 1.1 oz.			76	8.6	(67.3)	(7.61)		
Unbleached Wheat Flour:								
Fearn Unbleached Wheat Flour & Soya Pancake Mix, 16-oz. (1-lb.) package	1430	286.0	89	17.9				
Prepared as package directs (yield: approx. 33 4" pancakes)	2470	318.5			(66.8)	(8.61)		
1 4" pancake, approx. 1.1 oz.			76	9.8	(66.8)	(8.61)		
Whole Wheat:								
Aunt Jemima Whole Wheat Pancake & Waffle Mix, 35-oz. box	3313	665.0			97.7	19.00	426	85.5
Prepared as package directs (yield: approx. 69 4" pancakes)	5931	733.8			(74.1)	(9.55)		
1 4" pancake, approx. 1.1 oz.			83	10.7	(74.1)	(9.55)		
1 waffle, approx. 3.3 oz.			(362)	(31.9)	(111.3)	(11.65)		
Fearn "Rich Earth" Stoneground Whole Wheat & Soya Pancake Mix, 16-oz. (1-lb.) package	1450	297.3			90.6	18.58	400	82.0
Prepared as package directs (yield: approx. 36 4" pancakes)	2755	340.8	76	9.4	(67.3)	(8.32)		
1 4" pancake, approx. 1.1 oz.			76	9.4	(67.3)	(8.32)		
Fearn Stone Ground Whole Wheat & Soya Pancake Mix, 16-oz. (1-lb.) package	1365	260.0			85.3	16.25		
Prepared as package directs (yield: approx. 33 4" pancakes)	2405	286.0			(65.0)	(7.73)		
1 4" pancake, approx. 1.1 oz.			74	8.8	(65.0)	(7.73)		
Golden Harvest Stone Ground Whole Wheat Pancake Mix, 20-oz. box	1880	384.0			94.0	19.20	470	96.0
Whole Wheat & Soy Pancake Mix With Lecithin, 20-oz. box	1840	376.0			92.0	18.00	460	94.0

	UNIT Cal.	UNIT Carb.	ONE CRÊPE Cal.	ONE CRÊPE Carb.	1 OZ., BY WT. Cal.	1 OZ., BY WT. Carb.	1 CUP Cal.	1 CUP Carb.
CRÊPE MIXES								
Aunt Jemima Crêpes, 14-oz. box	1519	253.8			108.6	18.14		
Prepared as package directs (yield: approx. 32 6" crêpes)	2089	271.9						
1 6" crêpe			55	7.5				
Sweet 'N Low Low Cholesterol & Sugar Restricted Crêpe Mix, 8-oz. carton	1120	192.0			140.0	24.00		
Prepared as package directs (yield: 16 7" crepes)	1120	192.0						
1 7" crêpe			70	12.0				

FROZEN FRENCH TOAST, PANCAKES, AND WAFFLES

	UNIT Cal.	UNIT Carb.	1 PANCAKE, WAFFLE, or SLICE Cal.	1 PANCAKE, WAFFLE, or SLICE Carb.	1 OZ., BY WT. Cal.	1 OZ., BY WT. Carb.
FROZEN FRENCH TOAST						
Aunt Jemima French Toast, 9-oz. box, 6 slices per box	510	79.2			56.7	8.80
1 slice, approx. 1.5 oz.			85	13.2	56.7	8.80
Cinnamon Swirl French Toast, 9-oz. box, 6 slices per box	579	81.9	97	13.7	64.3	9.10
Downyflake French Toast, 9-oz. box, 6 slices per box	810	90.0			90.0	10.00
1 slice, approx. 1.5 oz.			135	15.0	90.0	10.00
Eggo French Toast, 12-oz. box, 8 slices per box	640	96.0			53.3	8.00
1 slice, approx. 1.5 oz.			80	12.0	53.3	8.00
Swanson's "TV" Entrées, French Toast with Sausages, 4½-oz. tray	300	22.0			66.7	4.89
6-oz. tray	(400)	(29.3)			(66.7)	(4.89)

	UNIT		1 PANCAKE, WAFFLE, or SLICE		1 OZ., BY WT.	
	Cal.	Carb.	Cal.	Carb.	Cal.	Carb.
FROZEN PANCAKES						
Hungry Jack Apple Cinnamon Pancakes (microwave), 9-oz. container (yield: 8 4" pancakes)	700	106.0			77.8	11.78
1 pancake, approx. 1.1 oz.			88	13.3	77.8	11.78
Blueberry Pancakes (microwave), 9.1-oz. container (yield: 8 4" pancakes)	700	106.0			76.9	11.65
1 pancake, approx. 1.1 oz.			88	13.3	76.9	11.65
Maple Pancakes (microwave), 8.9-oz. container (yield: 8 4" pancakes)	740	110.0			81.3	12.36
1 pancake, approx. 1.1 oz.			93	13.8	81.3	12.36
Swanson's "TV" Entrées, Pancakes & Sausages, 6-oz. tray	500	50.0			83.3	8.33
FROZEN WAFFLES						
PLAIN:						
Ann Page (A&P) Pre-Baked Waffles, 10-oz. box, 12 waffles per box	720	120.0			72.0	12.00
5-oz. box, 6 waffles per box	360	80.0			72.0	12.00
1 waffle, approx. 0.8 oz.			60	10.0	72.0	12.00
Aunt Jemima Original "Jumbo" Waffles, 10-oz. box, 8 waffles per box	688	108.8			68.8	10.88
1 waffle, approx. 1½ oz.			86	13.6	68.8	10.88
Downyflake "Jumbo" Waffles, 14¼-oz. box, 12 waffles per box	1020	180.0			71.6	12.63
1 waffle, approx. 1.2 oz.			85	15.0	71.6	12.63
Eggo Waffles, 11-oz. box, 8 waffles per box	960	136.0			87.3	12.36
1 waffle, approx. 1.4 oz.			120	17.0	87.3	12.36
Fresh Pict Waffles, 5-oz. box, 6 waffles per box	360	60.0			72.0	12.00
1 waffle, approx. 0.8 oz.			60	10.0	72.0	12.00
Golden Delight 12-oz. box, 8 waffles per box	800	152.0			66.7	12.67
1 waffle, approx. 1½ oz.			100	19.0	66.7	12.67
Roman Meal Waffles, 14-oz. box, 8 waffles per box	1200	212.0			85.7	15.14
1 waffle, approx. 1¾ oz.			150	26.5	85.7	15.14
FLAVORED:						
Blueberry "Jumbo" Waffles, **Aunt Jemima,** 10-oz. box, 8 waffles per box	688	108.8			68.8	10.88
1 waffle, approx. 1¼ oz.			86	13.6	68.8	10.88
Imitation Blueberry Waffles, **Eggo,** 11-oz. box, 8 waffles per box	1040	144.0			94.5	13.09
1 waffle, approx. 1.4 oz.			130	16.0	94.5	13.09
Buttermilk "Jumbo" Waffles, **Aunt Jemima,** 10-oz. box, 8 waffles per box	688	108.8			68.8	10.88
1 waffle, approx. 1¼ oz.			86	13.6	68.8	10.88
Buttermilk Waffles, **Downyflake,** 12-oz. box, 10 waffles per box	850	150.0			70.8	12.50
1 waffle, approx. 1.2 oz.			85	15.0	70.8	12.50

FROZEN BLINTZES

	UNIT		1 BLINTZ		1 OZ., BY WT.	
	Cal.	Carb.	Cal.	Carb.	Cal.	Carb.
Golden cheese blintzes, 15-oz. box, 6 blintzes per box	(1278)	(23.2)			(85.2)	(1.55)
1 blintz, approx. 2.5 oz.			(213)	3.9	(85.2)	(1.55)

BREAKFAST BARS, SNACK BARS, AND FOOD STICKS

	UNIT		1 BAR or STICK		1 OZ., BY WT.	
	Cal.	Carb.	Cal.	Carb.	Cal.	Carb.
BREAKFAST BARS AND SNACK BARS						
Almond Crunch Breakfast Bar, **Carnation,** 9.1-oz. box, 6 bars	1260	120.0			138.2	13.16
1 bar, approx. 1.5 oz.			210	20.0	138.2	13.16
Almond Granola Bar, **Nature Valley,** 10-oz. box, 12 bars	1440	180.0			144.0	18.00
1 bar, approx. 0.8 oz.			120	15.0		
Blueberry Yogurt & Granola Bar, **Crunchola,** 7-oz box, 8 bars	952	119.0			136.0	17.60
1 bar, approx. ⅞ oz.			119	15.4	136.0	17.60
Butter Pecan Bar, **General Mills** "Breakfast Squares," 12-oz. box, 4 bars	1520	180.0			126.6	15.00
1 bar, approx. 3 oz.			380	45.0	126.6	15.00
Caramel Nut Bar, **Pillsbury** "Figurines," 7.05-oz. package, 8 bars	1100	84.0			156.0	11.91
1 bar, approx. 0.9 oz.			138	10.5	156.0	11.91
Cherry Yogurt & Granola Bar, **Crunchola,** 7-oz. box, 8 bars	952	119.0			136.0	17.60
1 bar, approx. ⅞ oz.			119	15.4	136.0	17.60
Chocolate Bar, **Carnation** "Slender," 1.98-oz. package, 2 bars	275	24.0			139.4	12.10
1 bar, approx. 1 oz.			138	12.0	139.4	12.10
Chocolate Bar, **Pillsbury** "Figurines," 7.05-oz. package, 8 bars	1100	84.0			156.0	11.91
1 bar, approx. 0.9 oz.			138	10.5	156.0	11.91
(Double Rich) Chocolate Bar, **Pillsbury** "Figurines," 7.05-oz. package, 8 bars	1100	84.0			156.0	11.91
1 bar, approx. 0.9 oz.			138	10.5	156.0	11.91
Chocolate Caramel Bar, **Pillsbury** "Figurines," 7.05-oz. package, 8 bars	1100	84.0			156.0	11.91
1 bar, approx. 0.9 oz.			138	10.5	156.0	11.91
Chocolate Chip Breakfast Bar, **Carnation,** 9.4-oz. box, 6 bars	1260	144.0			134.6	15.38
1 bar, approx. 1.6 oz.			210	24.0	134.6	15.38
Chocolate Chip Peanut Butter & Granola Bar, **Crunchola,** 8-oz. box, 8 bars	1200	120.0			150.0	15.00
1 bar, approx. 1 oz.			150	15.0	150.0	15.00
Chocolate Crunch Breakfast Bar, **Carnation,** 8.9-oz. box, 6 bars	1260	138.0			140.9	15.44
1 bar, approx. 1.5 oz.			210	23.0	140.9	15.44
Chocolate Malt Bar, **General Mills** "Breakfast Squares," 12-oz. box, 4 bars	1520	180.0			126.6	15.00
1 bar, approx. 3 oz.			380	45.0	126.6	15.00
Chocolate Mint Bar, **Pillsbury** "Figurines," 7.05-oz. package, 8 bars	1100	84.0			156.0	11.91
1 bar, approx. 0.9 oz.			138	10.5	156.0	11.91
Cinnamon Bar, **Carnation** "Slender," 1.98-oz. package, 2 bars	275	24.0			139.4	12.10
1 bar, approx. 1 oz.			138	12.0	139.4	12.10
Cinnamon Bar, **General Mills** "Breakfast Squares," 12-oz. box, 4 bars	1520	180.0			126.6	15.00
1 bar, approx. 3 oz.			380	45.0	126.6	15.00
Cinnamon Granola Bar, **Nature Valley,** 10-oz. box, 12 bars	1440	180.0			144.0	18.00
1 bar, approx. 0.8 oz.			120	15.0	144.0	18.00
Cinnamon Raisin Peanut Butter & Granola Bar, **Crunchola,** 8-oz. box, 8 bars	1120	136.0			140.0	17.00
1 bar, approx. 1 oz.			140	17.0	140.0	17.00
Coconut Granola Bar, **Nature Valley,** 10-oz. box, 12 bars	1440	180.0			144.0	18.00
1 bar, approx. 0.8 oz.			120	15.0	144.0	18.00
Granola Crunch Bar, **Hi-Energy,** 24-oz. package, 12 bars	2856	727.2			119.0	30.30
1 bar, approx. 2 oz.			238	60.6	119.0	30.30
Granola Grabber Bar, **Hi-Energy,** 24-oz. package, 12 bars	2760	718.8			115.0	29.95
1 bar, approx. 2 oz.			230	59.9	115.0	29.95
Granola with Peanut Crunch Breakfast Bar, **Carnation,** 8.9-oz. box, 6 bars	1200	126.0			137.0	14.38
1 bar, approx. 1.51 oz.			200	21.0	137.0	14.38
Granola with Raisins Breakfast Bar, **Carnation,** 8.3-oz. box, 6 bars	1140	114.0			136.7	13.67
1 bar, approx. 1.4 oz.			190	19.0	136.7	13.67
Honey Graham Honey Baked Granola Bar, **Crunchola,** 10-oz. box, 10 bars	1200	190.0			120.0	19.00
1 bar, approx. 1 oz.			120	19.0	120.0	19.00
Honey Nut Honey Baked Granola Bar, **Crunchola,** 10-oz. box, 10 bars	1200	190.0			120.0	19.00
1 bar, approx. 1 oz.			120	19.0	120.0	19.00
Lemon Crunch Bar, **Hi-Energy,** 24-oz. package, 12 bars	2976	700.8			124.0	29.20
1 bar, approx. 2 oz.			248	58.4	124.0	29.20
Maple Nut Bar, **Hi-Energy,** 24-oz. package, 12 bars	2760	757.2			115.0	31.55
1 bar, approx. 2 oz.			230	63.1	115.0	31.55
Oats 'N Honey Granola Bar, **Nature Valley,** 10-oz. box, 12 bars	1320	192.0			132.0	19.20
1 bar, approx. 0.8 oz.			110	16.0	132.0	19.20
Orange Yogurt & Granola Bar, **Crunchola,** 8-oz. box, 8 bars	1120	136.0			140.0	17.00
1 bar, approx. 1 oz.			140	17.0	140.0	17.00
Original Peanut Butter & Granola Bar, **Crunchola,** 8-oz. box, 8 bars	1120	112.0			140.0	14.00
1 bar, approx. 1 oz.			140	14.0	140.0	14.00
Peanut Butter Crunch Breakfast Bar, **Carnation,** 8.9-oz. box, 6 bars	1200	132.0			134.2	14.76
1 bar, approx. 1.5 oz.			200	22.0	134.2	14.76
Peanut Butter Crunch Bar, **Hi-Energy,** 24-oz. package, 12 bars	2820	584.4			117.5	24.35
1 bar, approx. 2 oz.			235	48.7	117.5	24.35

	UNIT Cal.	UNIT Carb.	1 BAR or STICK Cal.	1 BAR or STICK Carb.	1 OZ., BY WT. Cal.	1 OZ., BY WT. Carb.
Peanut Granola Bar, **Nature Valley,** 10-oz. box, 12 bars	1440	180.0			144.0	18.00
1 bar, approx. 0.8 oz.			120	15.0	144.0	18.00
Peanut & Raisin Bar, **Crunchola,** 7-oz. box, 8 bars	960	112.0			137.1	16.00
1 bar, approx. ⅞ oz.			120	14.0	137.1	16.00
Raisin Bran Bar, **Hi-Energy,** 24-oz. package, 12 bars	2808	390.0			117.0	16.25
1 bar, approx. 2 oz.			234	32.5	117.0	16.25
Raspberry Bar, **Pillsbury** "Figurines," 7.05-oz. package, 8 bars	1100	84.0			156.0	11.91
1 bar, approx. 0.9 oz.			138	10.5	156.0	11.91
Strawberry Yogurt & Granola Bar, **Crunchola,** 8-oz. box, 8 bars	1120	136.0			140.0	17.00
1 bar, approx. 1 oz.			140	17.0	140.0	17.00
Vanilla Bar (artificial flavor), **Carnation** "Slender," 1.96-oz. package, 2 bars	275	24.0			140.8	12.24
1 bar, approx. 1 oz.			138	12.0	140.8	12.24
Vanilla Bar, **Pillsbury** "Figurines," 7.05-oz. package, 8 bars	1100	84.0			156.0	11.91
1 bar, approx. 0.9 oz.			138	10.5	156.0	11.91

FOOD STICKS

	UNIT Cal.	UNIT Carb.	1 BAR or STICK Cal.	1 BAR or STICK Carb.	1 OZ., BY WT. Cal.	1 OZ., BY WT. Carb.
Caramel Food Sticks, **Pillsbury,** 4⅞-oz. box, 14 sticks	630	94.5			129.2	19.38
1 stick, approx. 0.4 oz.			45	6.8	129.2	19.38
Chocolate Food Sticks, **Pillsbury,** 4⅞-oz. box, 14 sticks	630	94.5			129.2	19.38
1 stick, approx. 0.4 oz.			45	6.8	129.2	19.38
Chocolate Malt Food Sticks, **Pillsbury,** 4⅞-oz. box, 14 sticks	630	94.5			129.2	19.38
1 stick, approx. 0.4 oz.			45	6.8	129.2	19.38
Chocolate Mint Food Sticks, **Pillsbury,** 4⅞-oz. box, 14 sticks	630	94.5			129.2	19.38
1 stick, approx. 0.4 oz.			45	6.8	129.2	19.38
Orange Food Sticks, **Pillsbury,** 4⅞-oz. box, 14 sticks	630	94.5			129.2	19.38
1 stick, approx. 0.4 oz.			45	6.8	129.2	19.38
Peanut Butter Food Sticks, **Pillsbury,** 4⅞-oz. box, 14 sticks	630	94.5			129.2	19.38
1 stick, approx. 0.4 oz.			45	6.8	129.2	19.38

21 CAKES, SNACK CAKES & PASTRIES •

CAKES, CUPCAKES, and PASTRIES MADE FROM SCRATCH, based on generic data

BASED ON USDA HOME RECIPES:

	UNIT		1 SLICE, CUPCAKE, OR PASTRY		1 OZ., BY WT.	
	Cal.	**Carb.**	**Cal.**	**Carb.**	**Cal.**	**Carb.**
ANGEL FOOD CAKE, baked in a tube pan, made from 1 cup cake flour, 1 cup sugar, 1 cup egg whites (7 to 8 large whites), ⅔ tsp. cream of tartar, ⅜ tsp. salt, 1 tsp. vanilla. Yield:						
1 cake, approx. 16.6 oz. (loss of 14% has been applied for evaporation in baking), 8½" diameter, 3½" high (vol. 164 cu. in.) (2g/17g/tr/32%/80mg)	1270	284.1			76.4	17.08
1 slice, 1/12 of cake, approx. 1.4 oz.			105	23.5	76.4	17.08
1 slice, 1/16 of cake, approx. 1.0 oz.			81	18.1	76.4	17.08
1 cubic inch (approx. 0.1 oz.)	8	1.7			76.4	17.08
For comparison: Angel Food Cake, **Duncan Hines,** 1 cake, approx. 22½ oz. net wt. (yield from 14.5-oz. box)	1680	360.0			(75.0)	(16.00)
BOSTON CREAM PIE, 2-layer cake with custard filling and powdered sugar topping, cake portion made from: 1⅔ cups cake flour, ½ cup milk, 1 cup sugar, ¼ cup cooking fat, 2 large eggs, 1½ tsp. baking powder, ¼ tsp. salt, 1 tsp. vanilla. Yield:						
1 cake, approx. 29.1 oz. (loss of 10% has been applied for evaporation in baking), 8" diameter, 3⅓" high (vol. 166 cu. in.) (1g/14g/3g/35%/53mg)	2492	411.7			84.4	13.96
1 slice, 1/12 of cake, approx. 2.4 oz.			208	34.4	84.4	13.96
1 slice, 1/16 of cake, approx. 1.8 oz.			156	25.7	84.4	13.96
1 cubic inch (approx. 0.2 oz.)	15	2.5			84.4	13.96
CARAMEL CAKE, 2 layers, made from: 1¾ cups cake flour, ½ cup milk, 1 cup brown sugar, ½ cup cooking fat, 2 large eggs, 1¾ tsp. baking powder, ½ tsp. salt, 1 tsp. vanilla. Yield:						
1 cake, approx. 24 oz. (loss of 7% has been applied for evaporation in baking), 8" diameter, 3" high (vol. 142 cu. in.) (1g/15g/5g/23%/86mg)	2618	365.2			109.1	15.22
1 slice, 1/12 of cake, approx. 2 oz.			218	30.4	109.1	15.22
1 slice, 1/16 of cake, approx. 1.5 oz.			164	22.8	109.1	15.22
Iced with ¾ cup caramel icing, approx. 35.3 oz. (vol. 156 cu. in.) (1g/17g/4g/21%/252mg)	3790	591.0			107.7	16.89
1 slice, 1/12 of cake, approx. 2.9 oz.			315	49.1	107.7	16.89
1 slice, 1/16 of cake, approx. 2.2 oz.			235	36.6	107.7	16.89
1 cake, approx. 30.5 oz. (loss of 7% has been applied for evaporation in baking), 9" diameter, 3" high (vol. 180 cu. in.)	3325	464.0			109.9	15.21
1 slice, 1/12 of cake, approx. 2.5 oz.			277	38.7	109.9	15.21
1 slice, 1/16 of cake, approx. 1.9 oz.			208	29.0	109.9	15.21
Iced with 1 cup caramel icing, approx. 44½ oz. (2.8 lbs.) (vol. 197 cu. in.)	4779	745.3			107.4	16.95
1 slice, 1/12 of cake, approx. 3.7 oz.			398	62.1	107.4	16.95
1 slice, 1/16 of cake, approx. 2.8 oz.			299	46.7	107.4	16.95
1 cubic inch (approx. 0.2 oz.)	18	2.6			109.9	15.21
Iced with 1/5 tsp. caramel icing; approx. 0.24 oz.	28	3.8			107.4	16.95
CHOCOLATE DEVIL'S FOOD CAKE, 2 layers, made from: 2 cups cake flour, 1 cup milk, 1½ cups sugar, ½ cup cooking fat, 2 large eggs, 3½ tsp. baking powder, ½ tsp. salt, 1 tsp. vanilla. Yield:						
1 cake, approx. 31.4 oz. (loss of 7% has been applied for evaporation in baking), 9" diameter, 3" high (vol. 180 cu. in.) (1g/15g/5g/25%/83mg)	3257	462.8			103.8	14.74
1 slice, 1/12 of cake, approx. 2.6 oz.			271	38.6	103.8	14.74
1 slice, 1/16 of cake, approx. 2.0 oz.			204	28.9	103.8	14.74
Iced with 1 cup chocolate icing, approx. 42 oz. (vol. 196 cu. in.) (1g/16g/5g/22%/67mg)	4402	665.7			107.4	16.24
1 slice, 1/12 of cake, approx. 3.5 oz.			365	55.2	107.4	16.24
1 slice, 1/16 of cake, approx. 2.6 oz.			275	41.6	107.4	16.24
1 cake, approx. 24.7 oz., 8" diameter, 3" high (vol. 142 cu. in.)	2562	364.0			103.8	14.74
1 slice, 1/12 of cake, approx. 2.1 oz.			214	30.3	103.8	14.74
1 slice, 1/16 of cake, approx. 1.5 oz.			160	22.8	103.8	14.74
Iced with 1¼ cups chocolate icing, approx. 33 oz. (vol. 155 cu. in.)	3461	523.4			104.9	15.86
1 slice, 1/12 of cake, approx. 2.8 oz.			288	43.5	104.9	15.86
1 slice, 1/16 of cake, approx. 2.1 oz.			218	32.9	104.9	15.86
1 cubic inch (approx. 0.2 oz.)	18	2.5			103.8	14.74
Iced with 1/3 tsp. chocolate icing: approx. 0.2 oz.	24	3.4			104.9	15.86
Cut from cake baked on a sheet:						
1 piece, approx. 2" × 2" × 2", approx. 1.4 oz.			143	20.3	103.8	14.74
Iced with 1/16 cup chocolate icing, approx. 1.9 oz.			196	29.6	103.1	15.58
1 piece, approx. 3" × 3" × 2", approx. 3.1 oz.			322	45.8	103.8	14.74
Iced with ⅛ cup chocolate icing, approx. 4.2 oz.			443	67.0	105.5	15.95
1 cupcake, 2½" diameter, 0.9 oz.	92	13.0			103.8	14.74
Iced with 0.2 oz. chocolate icing, approx. 1.2 oz.	122	19.5			104.2	15.83
1 cupcake, 2¾" diameter, 1.2 oz.	121	17.2			103.8	14.74
Iced with 1/32 cup chocolate icing; iced cupcake, approx. 1.6 oz.	162	24.6			105.2	15.97

	UNIT Cal.	UNIT Carb.	1 SLICE, CUPCAKE, OR PASTRY Cal.	1 SLICE, CUPCAKE, OR PASTRY Carb.	1 OZ., BY WT. Cal.	1 OZ., BY WT. Carb.
For comparison: Chocolate Fudge Cake/Vanilla Frosting, **Betty Crocker** "Stir n' Frost," 1 cake, approx. 17 oz. net wt. (yield from 13.5-oz. box)	1680	276.0			(98.8)	(16.24)
COTTAGE PUDDING CAKE, one sheet, made from: 1½ cups all-purpose flour, ½ cup milk, ½ cup sugar, 3 tsp. cooking fat, 1 large egg, 1½ Tbsp. baking powder, ¼ tsp. salt, 1 tsp. vanilla. Yield:						
1 cake, approx. 15.3 oz. (0.96 lb.) (loss of 10% has been applied for evaporation in baking) (8" × 8" × 1½") (vol. 96 cu. in.) (2g/15g/3g/27%/85mg)	1500	236.7			97.4	15.37
1 piece (2" × 4" × 1½"), approx. 1.9 oz.			186	29.3	97.4	15.37
With 1 Tbsp. chocolate sauce (weight of cake and sauce approx. 2.6 oz.) (2g/16g/3g/28%/66mg)			235	42.0	90.0	16.03
With 1 Tbsp. (strawberry) fruit sauce (weight of cake and sauce approx. 2½ oz.) (1g/14g/3g/37%/66mg)			204	33.9	82.8	13.75
1 piece (2¾" × 4" × 1½"), approx. 2.6 oz.			251	39.6	97.4	15.37
With 1⅓ Tbsp. chocolate sauce (weight of cake and sauce approx. 3½ oz.)			315	56.1	90.4	16.15
With 1⅓ Tbsp. (strawberry) fruit sauce (weight of cake and sauce, approx. 3.3 oz.)			274	45.5	81.6	13.56
CHARLOTTE RUSSE, made from: 24 ladyfingers, ½ cup water, 4 Tbsp. confectioner's sugar, 1½ Tbsp. gelatin, 1 tsp. vanilla, 2 cups whipping cream. Yield:						
6 servings (approx. 24.2 oz.) (2g/10g/4g/46%/12mg)	1959	229.5			81.0	9.50
1 serving, 4 ladyfingers (approx. 4.0 oz.)			326	38.2	81.0	9.50
CREAM PUFFS, with custard filling, ingredients as follows: Shell: 1¼ cups flour, 1 cup milk, 5 large eggs, 9⅔ Tbsp. butter, ⅛ tsp. salt. Filling: ¼ cup cornstarch, 2 cups milk, ½ cup sugar, 2 large eggs, ½ tsp. vanilla. Yield:						
9 cream puffs (approx. 42 oz.) (loss of 10% has been applied for evaporation in cooking) (2g/6g/4g/58%/24mg)	2756	242.7			66.1	5.82
1 cream puff (approx. 4.6 oz.)			303	26.7	66.1	5.82
ECLAIRS, with custard filling and chocolate icing, made from: Shell: 1¼ cups flour, 1 cup milk, 5 large eggs, 9⅔ Tbsp. butter, ⅛ tsp. salt. Filling: ¼ cup cornstarch, 2 cups milk, ½ cup sugar, 2 large eggs, 1 tsp. vanilla. Icing: 1⅓ cups milk, 1 cup sugar, 1 oz. chocolate, 1 Tbsp. corn syrup, 1 Tbsp. fat, ½ tsp. vanilla. Icing: 1⅓ cups milk, 1 cup sugar, 1 oz. bitter chocolate, 1 Tbsp. corn syrup, 1 Tbsp. butter, ½ tsp. vanilla. Yield:						
12 eclairs (approx. 42.5 oz.) (loss of 10% has been applied for evaporation in cooking of shell and custard; 18% for icing) (2g/7g/4g/56%/23mg);	2882	280.0			67.8	6.58
1 eclair (approx. 3.5 oz.)			239	23.2	67.8	6.58
FRUITCAKE, Dark, made from: 4 cups all-purpose flour, ½ cup cider, ½ cup light sour cream, 1 cup sugar, 1 cup cooking fat, 5 large eggs, 1 cup light molasses, 4 oz. citron, 1 lb. raisins, 1 lb. currants, 1 cup chopped almonds, ⅓ cup jelly, 2 tsp. baking powder, ½ tsp. soda, ⅞ tsp. salt, 1⅔ tsp. spices, 2 oz. candied cherries, 1 cup chopped pecans. Yield:						
1 cake, approx. 102 oz. (loss of 7% has been applied for evaporation in baking) (vol. 143 cu. in.) (1g/17g/4g/18%/45mg)	10955	1726.9			107.4	16.93
1 slice, 1/100 of cake, approx. 1.0 oz.			110	17.3	107.4	16.93
1 tube cake (7" diameter, 2¼" high, vol. 77 cu. in.), 3 pounds	5158	812.5			107.4	16.93
1 wedge, 1/32 of cake (⅔" arc, vol. 2.4 cu. in.), 1½ oz.			163	25.7	107.4	16.93
1-lb. loaf, 7½" × 2" × 2"	1719	270.8			107.4	16.93
1 slice (¼" × 2" × 1½", vol. 0.8 cu. in.), approx. 0.6 oz.			57	9.0	107.4	16.93
FRUITCAKE, Light, made from: 2 cups all-purpose flour, ½ cup light sour cream, ½ cup sugar, ½ cup cooking fat, whites of 5 medium eggs, ¼ tsp. salt, ¼ tsp. soda, 2 tsp. baking powder, 1 cup chopped almonds, 1 cup seedless or 1¼ cup seeded raisins, 4 oz. citron, 4 oz. candied pineapple, 1 tsp. vanilla. Yield:						
1 cake, approx. 44 oz. (loss of 7% has been applied for evaporation in baking), (vol. 62 cu. in.) (2g/16g/5g/19%/55mg)	4853	716.3			110.3	16.28
1 slice, 1/100 of cake, approx. 0.4 oz.			49	7.2	110.3	16.28

	UNIT Cal.	UNIT Carb.	1 SLICE, CUPCAKE, OR PASTRY Cal.	1 SLICE, CUPCAKE, OR PASTRY Carb.	1 OZ., BY WT. Cal.	1 OZ., BY WT. Carb.
1 tube cake (approx. 7" diameter, 2¼" high, vol. 77 cu. in.), 3 pounds	5294	781.2			110.3	16.28
1 slice, 1/32 of cake (⅔" arc, vol. 2.4 cu. in.), approx. 1½ oz.			163	25.7	110.3	16.28
1-lb. loaf, 7½" × 2" × 2"	1765	260.4			110.3	16.28
1 slice (approx. ¼" × 2" × 1½", vol. 0.8 cu. in.), approx. 0.6 oz.			58	8.6	110.3	16.28
GINGERBREAD, baked in a pan 9" × 9" × 2", made from: 2½ cups all-purpose flour, 1 cup water, ½ cup sugar, ½ cup cooking fat, 2 medium eggs, 1 tsp. baking powder, ⅜ tsp. salt, vanilla, ⅞ tsp. baking soda, 2½ tsp. spices. Yield:						
1 cake, approx. 37.1 oz. (2.3 lbs.) (loss of 7% has been applied for evaporation in baking) (vol. 162 cu. in.) (1g/15g/3g/31%/67mg)	3344	548.6			92.9	14.79
1 piece (approx. 3" × 3" × 2"), approx. 4.1 oz.			371	60.8	92.9	14.79
"PLAIN" CAKE, baked in a pan 9" × 9" × 2", made from: 2⅛ cups flour, ⅞ cup milk, 1¼ cups sugar, 7 tsp. cooking fat, 2 medium eggs, 2¼ tsp. baking powder, ½ tsp. salt, 1½ tsp. vanilla. Yield:						
1 cake, approx. 27.3 oz. (1.75 lbs.) (loss of 10% has been applied for evaporation in baking) (vol. 162 cu. in.) (1g/16g/4g/25%/85mg)	2828	434.3			101.0	15.51
Iced with 1⅛ cups chocolate icing, approx. 38.9 oz. (2.4 lbs.) (vol. 179 cu. in.) (1g/17g/4g/21%/65mg)	4081	658.7			104.6	16.89
Iced with 2⅓ cups coconut icing, approx. 38 oz. (1g/17g/3g/21%/71mg)	3994	648.3			105.1	17.06
Iced with 1⅛ cups boiled white icing, approx. 36 oz. (2.4 lbs.) (vol. 200 cu. in.) (1g/18g/3g/23%/74mg)	3619	635.3			100.6	17.66
Iced with 1⅛ cups uncooked white icing, approx. 36 oz. (1g/18g/3g/21%/64mg)	4022	693.8			104.8	18.09
1 piece, ⅑ of cake (approx. 3" × 3" × 2"), approx. 3.0 oz.			313	48.1	101.0	15.50
Iced with ⅛ cup chocolate icing, approx. 4.4 oz.			453	73.1	104.6	16.89
Iced with ¼ cup coconut icing, approx. 4.2 oz.			443	72.0	105.1	17.06
Iced with ⅛ cup boiled white icing, approx. 4 oz.			401	70.5	100.6	17.66
Iced with ⅛ cup uncooked white icing, approx. 4.2 oz.			444	76.6	104.8	18.09
1 cubic inch (approx. 0.17 oz.)	19	2.7			101.0	15.34
Iced with ⅓ tsp. chocolate icing, approx. 0.23 oz.	23	3.7			104.6	16.89
Iced with ½ tsp. coconut icing, approx. 0.19 oz.	20	3.2			105.1	17.06
Iced with ¼ tsp. boiled white icing, approx. 0.18 oz.	18	3.2			100.6	17.66
Iced with ⅓ tsp. uncooked white icing, approx. 0.22 oz.	23	3.9			104.8	18.09
1 cupcake; approx. 2½" diam., approx. 0.9 oz.			91	14.0	101.0	15.51
Iced with 2⅓ tsp. chocolate icing, approx. 1.3 oz.			132	21.4	104.6	16.46
Iced with 3½ tsp. coconut icing, approx. 1.2 oz.			123	19.9	105.1	17.06
Iced with 2 tsp. boiled white icing, approx. 1.2 oz.			116	20.4	100.6	17.66
Iced with 2⅓ tsp. uncooked white icing, approx. 1.2 oz.			128	22.2	104.9	18.09
1 cupcake; approx. 2¾" diam., 1.2 oz.			120	18.4	101.0	16.89
Iced with 1 Tbsp. chocolate icing, approx. 1.7 oz.			173	27.9	104.6	16.91
Iced with 4⅛ tsp. coconut icing, approx. 1.6 oz.			168	27.3	105.1	17.06
Iced with 2 tsp. boiled white icing, approx. 1.6 oz.			155	27.2	100.6	17.66
Iced with 1 Tbsp. uncooked white icing, approx. 1.7 oz.			172	29.8	104.8	18.09
POUND CAKE, "Modified" loaf, made from: 1½ cups flour, 2⅔ tsp. milk, ¾ cup sugar, ⅜ cup cooking fat, 3 large eggs, ⅝ tsp. baking powder, ⅙ tsp. salt, ⅛ tsp. flavoring: Yield:						
1 cake, approx. 17.6 oz. (loss of 12% has been applied for evaporation in baking) (8½" × 3½" × 3", vol. 89 cu. in.) (2g/16g/5g/19%/50mg)	2055	273.5			116.8	15.54
1 slice, 1/17 of loaf (3½" × 3" × ½"), approx. 1 oz.			119	15.9	116.8	15.54
1 cubic inch (approx. 0.2 oz.)	23	3.1			116.8	15.54

	UNIT		1 SLICE, CUPCAKE, OR PASTRY		1 OZ., BY WT.	
	Cal.	Carb.	Cal.	Carb.	Cal.	Carb.
POUND CAKE, "Old-Fashioned," made from: 4 cups flour, 2 cups sugar, 2 cups cooking fat, 9 large eggs, ½ tsp. salt, ½ tsp. flavoring: Yield:						
1 cake, approx. 54 oz. (3.4 lbs.) (loss of 7% has been applied for evaporation in baking) (vol. 89 cu. in.) (2g/13g/8g/17%/31mg)	7289	724.3			134.9	13.41
1 loaf made from ⅓ of recipe above (8½" × 3½" × 3", vol. 89 cu. in.), 18 oz.	2431	241.6			134.9	13.41
1 slice, 1/17 of loaf (3½" × 3" × ½"), approx. 1.1 oz.			142	14.1	134.9	13.41
1 cubic inch (approx. 0.2 oz.)	27	2.7			134.9	13.41
SPONGE CAKE, baked in a tube pan, made from: 1 cup flour, 1 cup sugar, 5 large eggs, ¼ tsp. salt, 2½ tsp. lemon juice. Yield:						
1 cake, approx. 18½ oz. (1.2 lbs.) (loss of 11% has been applied for evaporation in baking) 8½" diameter, 3½" high (vol. 164 cu. in) (2g/15g/2g/32%/47mg)	1556	283.5			83.8	15.26
1 slice, 1/12 of cake, approx. 1.6 oz.			131	23.8	83.8	15.26
1 slice, 1/16 of cake, approx. 1.2 oz.			98	17.9	83.8	15.26
1 cake, approx. 27⅔ oz. (1 lb. 11⅔ oz.), 9¾" diameter, 4" high (vol. 247 cu. in.)	2346	427.4			83.8	15.26
1 slice, 1/12 of cake, approx. 2.3 oz.			196	35.7	83.8	15.26
1 slice, 1/16 of cake, approx. 1.8 oz.			147	26.7	83.8	15.26
1 cubic inch (approx. 0.1 oz.)	9	1.7			83.8	15.26
WHITE CAKE, 2 layers, made from: 1¾ cups flour, ½ cup milk, 1 cup sugar, ½ cup cooking fat, 4 medium eggs, 3 tsp. baking powder, ¼ tsp. salt, 1½ tsp. flavoring. Yield:						
1 cake, approx. 23.4 oz. (1½ lbs.) (loss of 10% has been applied for evaporation in baking) 8" diameter, 3" high (vol. 142 cu. in.) (1g/15g/5g/24%/92mg)	2490	358.6			106.5	15.33
Iced with ¾ cups chocolate icing; approx. 31.2 oz.	(3320)	(510.4)			(106.4)	(16.36)
Iced with 2¼ cups coconut icing, approx. 34.5 oz. (2.1 lbs.) (vol. 169 cu. in.) (1g/17g/4g/21%/73mg)	3625	593.0			104.9	17.16
Iced with 1¾ cups boiled white icing, approx. 31.4 oz.	(2970)	(645.6)			(94.6)	(20.56)
1 slice, 1/12 of cake, approx. 2.0 oz.			208	29.9	106.5	15.33
Iced with 1 Tbsp. chocolate icing, approx. 2.6 oz.			(277)	(42.5)	(106.4)	(16.36)
Iced with 3 Tbsp. coconut icing, approx. 2.9 oz.			301	49.2	104.9	17.16
Iced with 2 Tbsp. boiled white icing, approx. 2.6 oz.			(248)	(53.8)	(94.6)	(20.56)
1 slice, 1/16 of cake, approx. 1.5 oz.			156	22.4	106.5	15.33
Iced with ¾ Tbsp. chocolate icing, approx. 2.0 oz.			(208)	(31.9)	(106.4)	(16.36)
Iced with 2¼ Tbsp. coconut icing, approx. 2.2 oz.			226	37.0	104.9	17.16
Iced with 1⅓ Tbsp. boiled white icing, approx. 2.0 oz.			(186)	(40.4)	(94.6)	(20.56)
1 cake, approx. 29.8 oz. (1.9 lbs.), 9" diameter, 3" high (vol. 180 cu. in.)	3173	456.8			106.5	15.33
Iced with 1 cup chocolate icing, approx. 41.6 oz.	(4426)	(686.5)			(106.4)	(16.36)
Iced with 3 cups coconut icing, approx. 43.9 oz. (2¾ lbs.) (vol. 214 cu. in.)	4615	755.1			104.9	17.16
Iced with 2½ cups boiled white icing, approx. 41.9 oz.	(3964)	(645.6)			(94.6)	(15.41)
Iced with ⅓ cup uncooked white icing; iced cake, approx. 33 oz.	3686	618.3			111.7	18.74
1 slice, 1/12 of cake, approx. 2.5 oz.			264	38.2	106.5	16.33
Iced with 1⅓ Tbsp. chocolate icing, approx. 3.5 oz.			(369)	(56.7)	(106.4)	(16.36)
Iced with 4 Tbsp. coconut icing, approx. 3.7 oz.			386	63.1	104.9	17.16
Iced with 3⅓ Tbsp. boiled white icing, approx. 3.5 oz.			(330)	(53.8)	(94.6)	(15.41)
Iced with ⅓ Tbsp. uncooked white icing, approx. 2.8 oz.			308	51.6	111.7	18.74
1 slice, 1/16 of cake, approx. 1.9 oz.			198	28.6	106.5	16.33
Iced with 1 Tbsp. chocolate icing, approx. 2.6 oz.			(277)	(42.5)	(106.4)	(16.36)
Iced with 3 Tbsp. coconut icing, approx. 2.8 oz.			289	47.3	104.9	17.16
Iced with 2⅓ Tbsp. boiled white icing, approx. 2.6 oz.			(248)	(40.4)	(94.6)	(15.41)
Iced with ⅓ Tbsp. uncooked white icing, approx. 2.1 oz.			229	38.4	111.7	18.74
1 cubic inch (approx. 0.17 oz.)	18	2.5			102.3	14.20
Iced with ⅓ tsp. chocolate icing; iced cake, approx. 0.23 oz.	23	3.7			109.5	17.62
Iced with ½ tsp. coconut icing; iced cake, approx. 0.19 oz.	22	3.5			103.6	16.94
Iced with ½ tsp. boiled white icing; iced cake, approx. 0.18 oz.	17	2.1			94.6	11.67
Iced with 1/10 tsp. uncooked white icing; iced cake, approx. 0.22 oz.	24	4.0			111.7	18.74
YELLOW CAKE, 2 layers, made from: 3 cups flour, 1 cup milk, ½ cup sugar, ½ cup cooking fat, 2 large eggs, 4 tsp. baking powder, ¼ tsp. salt, 1 tsp. flavoring. Yield:						
1 cake, approx. 24 oz. (1½ lbs.) (loss of 9% has been applied for evaporation in baking), 8" diameter, 3" high (vol. 142 cu. in.) (1g/17g/4g/24%/73mg)	2476	396.9			103.2	16.54
Iced with ¾ cups caramel icing, approx. 35.2 oz. (2.2 lbs.) (vol. 156 cu. in.) (1g/18g/3g/22%/64mg)	3678	622.8			102.2	17.79
Iced with ¾ cups chocolate icing; iced cake, approx. 33.2 oz. (1g/17g/4g/21%/59mg)	3442	569.6			104.0	17.30
Iced with 1 cup coconut icing, approx. 37.7 oz.	3611	631.3			95.8	16.74
Iced with ¾ cup boiled white icing, approx. 35.2 oz.	(3003)	(530.9)			(85.3)	(15.08)
Iced with ¾ cup uncooked white icing, approx. 35.2 oz.	(3272)	(570.2)			(93.0)	(16.20)
1 slice, 1/12 of cake, approx. 2.0 oz.			206	33.1	103.2	16.54
Iced with 1 Tbsp. caramel icing, approx. 3.0 oz.			308	52.1	102.2	17.79
Iced with 1 Tbsp. chocolate icing, approx. 2.8 oz.			288	47.7	104.0	17.30
Iced with 1⅓ Tbsp. coconut icing, approx. 3.1 oz.			301	52.6	95.8	16.74
Iced with 1 Tbsp. boiled white icing, approx. 2.9 oz.			(250)	(44.2)	(85.3)	(15.08)
Iced with 1 Tbsp. uncooked white icing, approx. 2.9 oz.			(273)	(47.5)	(93.0)	16.20)
1 slice, 1/16 of cake, approx. 1.5 oz.			155	24.8	103.2	16.54
Iced with ¾ Tbsp. caramel icing, approx. 2.3 oz.			232	39.2	102.2	17.79
Iced with ¾ Tbsp. chocolate icing, approx. 2.1 oz.			215	35.6	104.0	17.30
Iced with 1 Tbsp. coconut icing, approx. 2.4 oz.			226	39.4	95.8	16.74
Iced with ¾ Tbsp. boiled white icing, approx. 2.2 oz.			(188)	(33.2)	(85.3)	(15.08)
Iced with ¾ Tbsp. uncooked white icing, approx. 2.2 oz.			(205)	(35.0)	(93.0)	(16.20)
1 cake, approx. 31 oz. (1.15 lbs.), 9" diam., 3" high (vol. 180 cu. in.)	3158	506.3			101.9	16.33
Iced with ¾ cup caramel icing, approx. 45 oz. (2.6 lbs.) (vol. 197 cu. in.)	4692	794.4			104.3	17.65
Iced with 1⅛ cup chocolate icing, approx. 42.3 oz.	4391	726.6			104.5	17.30
Iced with 3 cups coconut icing, approx. 44.7 oz.	4280	740.7			95.8	16.57
Iced with 2⅓ cups boiled white icing, approx. 42.2 oz.	3600	636.4			(85.3)	(15.08)
Iced with 2⅓ cups uncooked white icing, approx. 42.2 oz.	3925	683.6			(93.0)	(16.20)
1 slice, 1/12 of cake, approx. 2.6 oz.			263	42.2	101.9	16.33
Iced with 1 Tbsp. caramel icing, approx. 3.7 oz.			391	66.2	102.2	17.79
Iced with 1½ Tbsp. chocolate icing, approx. 3.5 oz.			365	60.4	104.0	17.30
Iced with 4 Tbsp. coconut icing, approx. 3.7 oz.			357	61.7	95.8	16.57
Iced with 3 Tbsp. boiled white icing, approx. 3.5 oz.			300	53.0	(85.3)	(15.08)
Iced with 3 Tbsp. uncooked white icing, approx. 3.5 oz.			327	57.0	(93.0)	(16.20)
1 slice, 1/16 of cake, approx. 1.9 oz.			197	31.6	103.2	16.54
Iced with ¾ Tbsp. caramel icing, approx. 2.8 oz.			293	49.7	102.2	17.79
Iced with 1⅛ Tbsp. chocolate icing, approx. 2.6 oz.			274	45.3	104.0	17.30
Iced with 3 Tbsp. coconut icing, approx. 2.8 oz.			268	46.3	95.8	16.57
Iced with 2¼ Tbsp. boiled white icing, approx. 2.6 oz.			225	39.8	(85.3)	(15.08)
Iced with 2¼ Tbsp. uncooked white icing, approx. 2.6 oz.			245	42.7	(93.0)	(16.20)
1 cubic inch (approx. 0.17 oz.)	17	2.8			103.2	16.54
Iced with ¼ tsp. caramel icing, approx. 0.22 oz.	24	4.0			104.0	17.30
Iced with ¼ tsp. chocolate icing, approx. 0.21 oz.	22	3.7			104.5	17.30
Iced with ¼ tsp. coconut icing, approx. 0.19 oz.	21	3.5			110.4	17.98

	UNIT		1 SLICE, CUPCAKE, OR PASTRY		1 OZ., BY WT.	
	Cal.	Carb.	Cal.	Carb.	Cal.	Carb.
Iced with ¼ tsp. boiled white icing, approx. 0.18 oz.	16	2.1			85.3	12.42
Iced with ¼ tsp. uncooked white icing, approx. 0.22 oz.	23	4.0			(93.0)	(16.20)
BASED ON DATA FROM THE MIDDLE EAST:						
BAKLAVAH, 1 pound	2450	228.5			153.1	14.28

CAKE MIXES, by brand

	UNIT		1 SLICE, CUPCAKE, OR PASTRY		1 OZ., BY WT.	
	Cal.	Carb.	Cal.	Carb.	Cal.	Carb.
ANGEL FOOD						
Angel Food Cake, **Betty Crocker** "One-Step," 14-oz. box	1680	384.0			120.0	27.43
Prepared as package directs (yield: approx. 22.4 oz.)	1680	384.0			(75.0)	(17.14)
"Suggested" slice, 1/12 of cake (approx. 1.9 oz.)			140	32.0	(75.0)	(17.14)
Angel Food Cake, **Duncan Hines,** 14.5-oz. box	1680	360.0			115.9	24.83
Prepared as package directs (yield: approx. 22½ oz.)	1680	360.0			(75.0)	(16.00)
"Suggested" slice, 1/12 of cake (approx. 1.9 oz.)			140	30.0	(75.0)	(16.00)
Chocolate Angel Food Cake, **Betty Crocker,** 16-oz. (1-lb.) box	1680	384.0			120.0	24.00
Prepared as package directs (yield: approx. 22½ oz.)	1680	384.0			(74.7)	(17.07)
"Suggested" slice, 1/12 of cake (approx. 1.9 oz.)			140	32.0	(74.7)	(17.07)
Confetti Angel Food Cake, **Betty Crocker,** 17-oz. box	1800	408.0			105.9	24.00
Prepared as package directs (yield: approx. 22½ oz.)	1800	408.0			(80.0)	(18.13)
"Suggested" slice, 1/12 of cake (approx. 1.9 oz.)			150	34.0	(80.0)	(18.13)
Lemon Custard Angel Food Cake, **Betty Crocker,** 16-oz. (1-lb.) box	1680	384.0			105.0	24.00
Prepared as package directs (yield: approx. 22½ oz.)	1680	384.0			(74.7)	(17.07)
"Suggested" slice, 1/12 of cake (approx. 1.9 oz.)			140	32.0	(74.7)	(17.07)
Raspberry Angel Food Cake, **Pillsbury,** 16-oz. (1-lb.) box	1680	384.0			105.0	24.75
Prepared as package directs (yield: approx. 22½ oz.)	1680	384.0			(74.7)	(17.60)
"Suggested" slice, 1/12 of cake (approx. 1.9 oz.)			140	32.0	(74.7)	(17.60)
Strawberry Angel Food Cake, **Betty Crocker,** 17-oz. box	1800	408.0			105.9	24.00
Prepared as package directs (yield: approx. 23½ oz.)	1800	408.0			(76.6)	(17.36)
"Suggested" slice, 1/12 of cake (approx. 2.0 oz.)			150	34.0	(76.6)	(17.36)
Traditional White Angel Food Cake, **Betty Crocker,** 15-oz. box	1560	360.0			104.0	24.00
Prepared as package directs (yield: approx. 22½ oz.)	1560	360.0			(69.3)	(16.00)
"Suggested" slice, 1/12 of cake (approx. 1.9 oz.)			130	30.0	(69.3)	(16.00)
White Angel Food Cake, **Pillsbury,** 16-oz. (1-lb.) box	1680	396.0			105.0	24.75
Prepared as package directs (yield: approx. 23 oz.)	1680	396.0			73.0	17.20
"Suggested" slice, 1/12 of cake (approx. 1.9 oz.)			140	33.0	(74.7)	(17.60)
APPLE						
Apple Cake, **Duncan Hines** "Deluxe," 18.25-oz. box	2280	408.0			120.0	22.00
Prepared as package directs (yield: approx. 15 oz.)	2280	408.0			(108.0)	(19.80)
"Suggested" slice, 1/9 of cake (approx. 1⅔ oz.)			190	34.0	(108.0)	(19.80)
Applesauce Raisin Cake, **Betty Crocker** "Snackin' Cake," 13.5-oz. box	1620	297.0			120.0	22.00
Prepared as package directs (yield: approx. 19.5 oz.)	1620	297.0			(83.1)	(15.23)
"Suggested" slice, 1/9 of cake (approx. 2.2 oz.)			180	33.0	(83.1)	(15.23)
Applesauce Raisin Layer Cake, **Duncan Hines,** 18½-oz. box	2160	396.0			116.8	21.41
Prepared as package directs (yield: approx. 28 oz.)	2280	396.0			(81.4)	(14.10)
"Suggested" slice, 1/12 of cake (approx. 2⅓ oz.)			190	33.0	(81.4)	(14.10)
1 cupcake (approx. 1.2 oz., 24 to the box)			106	18.3	(81.4)	(14.10)

	UNIT		1 SLICE, CUPCAKE, OR PASTRY		1 OZ., BY WT.	
	Cal.	Carb.	Cal.	Carb.	Cal.	Carb.
BANANA						
Banana Cake, **Betty Crocker** "Supermoist," 18.5 oz. box	2160	432.0			116.8	23.35
Prepared as package directs (yield: approx. 30 oz.)	3120	432.0			(104.3)	(14.44)
"Suggested" slice, 1/12 of cake (approx. 2.5 oz.)			260	36.0	(104.3)	(14.44)
Banana Cake, **Fearn,** 8.6-oz. box	780	150.0			90.7	17.44
Prepared as package directs (yield: approx. 21.4 oz.)	(1858)	(289.8)			(86.8)	(13.54)
"Suggested" slice, 1/6 of cake (approx. 3.6 oz.)			(310)	(48.3)	(86.8)	(13.54)
Banana Cake, **Pillsbury** "Plus," 18½-oz. box	2160	408.0			116.8	22.05
Prepared as package directs (yield: approx. 32 oz., or 2 lb.)	3000	432.0			(97.5)	(12.75)
"Suggested" slice, 1/12 of cake (approx. 2.6 oz.)			250	36.0	(97.5)	(12.75)
1 cupcake (approx. 1.3 oz., 24 to the box)			125	18.0	(97.5)	(12.75)
Banana Cake, sugar restricted, **Sweet 'N Low,** 8-oz. box	900	160.0			112.5	20.00
Prepared as package directs (weight of yield not available)	900	160.0				
"Suggested" slice, 1/10 of cake			90	16.0		
Banana Supreme Cake, **Duncan Hines** "Deluxe," 18.25-oz. box	2280	432.0			123.2	22.05
Prepared as package directs (yield: approx. 28 oz.)	3120	432.0			(85.7)	(14.57)
"Suggested" slice, 1/12 of cake (approx. 2⅓ oz.)			260	36.0	(85.7)	(14.57)
1 cupcake (approx. 1.2 oz., 24 to the box)			100	17.0	(85.7)	(14.57)
Banana Walnut Cake, **Betty Crocker** "Snackin' Cake," 13.5-oz. box	1710	290.0			126.7	20.67
Prepared as package directs (yield: approx. 19 oz.)	1710	279.0			(90.0)	(14.68)
"Suggested" slice, 1/9 of cake (approx. 2.1 oz.)			190	31.0	(90.0)	(14.68)
BROWNIE MIXES, see the COOKIES & CRACKERS chapter						
BUNDT						
Chocolate Macaroon Bundt Cake and Glaze Mix, **Pillsbury** "Bundt," 27¼-oz. box	3520	592.0			123.3	20.70
Prepared as package directs (yield: approx. 39 oz.)	4000	592.0			(101.5)	(14.46)
"Suggested" slice, 1/16 of cake (approx. 3.3 oz.)			250	37.0	(101.5)	(14.46)
Fudge Nut Crown Bundt Cake and Glaze Mix, **Pillsbury** "Bundt," 22½-oz. box	2880	496.0			128.0	21.87
Prepared as package directs (yield: approx. 35 oz.)	3520	496.0			(99.4)	(14.06)
"Suggested" slice, 1/16 of cake (approx. 2.9 oz.)			220	31.0	(99.4)	(14.06)
Lemon Blueberry Bundt Cake and Glaze Mix, **Pillsbury** "Bundt," 23½-oz. box	2400	448.0			117.4	21.54
Prepared as package directs (yield: approx. 35 oz.)	3200	448.0			(96.0)	(14.40)
"Suggested" slice, 1/16 of cake (approx. 3 oz.)			200	28.0	(96.0)	(14.40)
Marble Supreme Bundt Cake and Glaze Mix, **Pillsbury** "Bundt," 27½-oz. box	3360	608.0			122.2	22.25
Prepared as package directs (yield: approx. 41 oz.)	4000	608.0			(96.6)	(14.93)
"Suggested" slice, 1/16 of cake (approx. 3.4 oz.)			250	38.0	(96.6)	(14.93)
Pound Cake Supreme Bundt Cake and Glaze Mix, **Pillsbury** "Bundt," 24¾-oz. box	3040	528.0			121.2	21.82
Prepared as package directs (yield: approx. 41 oz.)	3680	528.0			(90.7)	(13.17)
"Suggested" slice, 1/16 of cake (approx. 3.4 oz.)			230	33.0	(90.7)	(13.17)
BUTTER						
Butter Brickle Cake, **Betty Crocker,** "Supermoist," 18½-oz. box	2160	444.0			116.8	24.00
Prepared as package directs (yield: approx. 29.9 oz.)	3120	444.0			(104.3)	(14.84)
"Suggested" slice, 1/12 of cake, (approx. 2.5 oz.)			260	37.0	(104.3)	(14.84)
1 cupcake (approx. 1.2 oz., 24 to the box)			130	18.5	(104.3)	(14.84)
Butter Pecan Cake, **Betty Crocker** "Supermoist," 18-oz. box	2160	420.0			120.0	23.33
Prepared as package directs (yield: approx. 29 oz.)	3000	420.0			(102.0)	(14.28)
"Suggested" slice, 1/12 of cake (approx. 2.5 oz.)			250	35.0	(102.0)	(14.28)
1 cupcake (approx. 1.2 oz., 24 to the box)			125	17.5	(102.0)	(14.28)

	UNIT		1 SLICE, CUPCAKE, OR PASTRY		1 OZ., BY WT.	
	Cal.	Carb.	Cal.	Carb.	Cal.	Carb.
Butter Recipe Cake, **Pillsbury** "Plus," 18½-oz. box	2280	432.0			123.2	21.41
Prepared as package directs (yield: approx. 32 oz., or 2 lb.)	2880	432.0			(90.0)	(12.38)
"Suggested" slice, 1/12 of cake (approx. 2.7 oz.)			240	36.0	(90.0)	(12.38)
1 cupcake (approx. 1.3 oz., 24 to the box)			(120)	(16.5)	(90.0)	(12.38)
CAROB						
Carob Cake, **Fearn,** 8.2-oz. box	750	150.0			91.5	18.29
Prepared as package directs (yield: approx. 21.4 oz.)	(1828)	(289.8)			(85.4)	(13.54)
"Suggested" slice, 1/6 of cake, (approx. 3.6 oz.)			(305)	(48.3)	(85.4)	(13.54)
Whole Grain Carob, **Deaf Smith Farms,** 32-oz. (2-lb.) box	3200	608.0			100.0	19.00
1 cake prepared as package directs (yield: approx. 12.2 oz.)	2880	384.0			(73.9)	(13.14)
"Suggested" slice, 1/12 of cake (approx. 1.0 oz.)			240	32.0	(73.9)	(13.14)
CARROT						
Carrot Cake, **Betty Crocker** "Supermoist," 18.5-oz. box	2160	408.0			116.8	22.05
Prepared as package directs (yield: approx. 30 oz.)	3120	408.0			(104.3)	(13.64)
"Suggested" slice, 1/12 of cake (approx. 2.5 oz.)			260	34.0	(104.3)	(13.64)
Carrot Cake, **Duncan Hines** "Deluxe," 18.25-oz. box	2160	408.0			162.2	22.70
Prepared as package directs (yield: approx. 28 oz.)	3000	408.0			(107.1)	(15.00)
"Suggested" slice, 1/12 of cake (approx. 2.3 oz.)			250	34.0	(107.1)	(15.00)
Carrot Cake, **Fearn,** 8.6-oz. box	810	138.0			94.2	16.05
Prepared as package directs (yield: approx. 21.4 oz.)	(1888)	(278.0)			(88.2)	(12.99)
"Suggested" slice, 1/6 of cake (approx. 3.6 oz.)			(315)	(46.3)	(88.2)	(12.99)
Carrot Nut Cake, **Betty Crocker** "Snackin' Cake," 13.5-oz. package	1620	270.0			120.0	20.00
Prepared as package directs (yield: approx. 19 oz.)	1620	270.0			(85.3)	(14.21)
"Suggested" slice, 1/9 of cake (approx. 2.1 oz.)			180	30.0	(85.3)	(14.21)
CHERRY						
Cherry Chip Cake, **Betty Crocker** "Supermoist," 18½-oz. box	2160	432.0			116.8	23.35
Prepared as package directs (yield: approx. 27 oz.)	2160	432.0			(80.8)	(16.16)
"Suggested" slice, 1/12 of cake (approx. 2.3 oz.)			180	36.0	(80.8)	(16.16)
1 cupcake (approx. 1.1 oz., 24 to the box)			90	18.0	(80.8)	(16.16)
Cherry Supreme Layer Cake, **Duncan Hines,** 18½-oz. box	2280	408.0			123.2	22.05
Prepared as package directs (yield: approx. 28 oz.)	2280	408.0			(81.4)	(14.57)
CHOCOLATE						
Chocolate Cake, dietetic, **Batter-Lite,** 8-oz. box	960	140.0			120.0	17.50
Prepared as package directs (yield: approx. 11 oz.)	983	137.0			87.7	12.23
"Suggested" slice, 1/10 of cake (approx. 1.1 oz.)			98	13.7	87.7	12.23
1 cupcake (approx. 1.1 oz., 10 to the box)			98	13.7	87.7	12.23
Chocolate Cake, sugar restricted, **Sweet 'N Low,** 8-oz. box	900	160.0			112.5	20.00
Prepared as package directs (yield: approx. 12.2 oz.)	900	160.0			(73.9)	(13.14)
"Suggested" slice, 1/10 of cake (approx. 1.2 oz.)			90	16.0	(73.9)	(13.14)
Chocolate Almond Cake, **Betty Crocker** "Snackin' Cake," 13.5-oz. box	1710	279.0			126.7	20.67
Prepared as package directs (yield: approx. 20 oz.)	1710	279.0			(85.5)	(13.95)
"Suggested" slice, 1/9 of cake (approx. 2.3 oz.)			190	31.0	(85.5)	(13.95)
Chocolate Fudge Cake, **Betty Crocker** "Supermoist," 18½-oz. box	2160	420.0			116.8	22.70
Prepared as package directs (yield: approx. 30 oz.)	3000	420.0			(100.3)	(14.04)
"Suggested" slice, 1/12 of cake (approx. 2.5 oz.)			250	35.0	(100.3)	(14.04)
1 cupcake (approx. 1.2 oz., 24 to the box)			125	17.5	(100.3)	(14.04)
Chocolate Fudge Cake/Vanilla Frosting, **Betty Crocker** "Stir 'N Frost," 13.5-oz. package	1680	276.0			124.4	20.40

	UNIT		1 SLICE, CUPCAKE, OR PASTRY		1 OZ., BY WT.	
	Cal.	Carb.	Cal.	Carb.	Cal.	Carb.
Prepared as package directs (yield: approx. 17 oz.)	1680	276.0			(98.8)	(16.24)
"Suggested" slice, 1/6 of cake (approx. 2.8 oz.)			280	46.0	(98.8)	(16.24)
Chocolate Fudge Chip Cake, **Betty Crocker** "Snackin' Cake," 13.5-oz. box	1710	279.0			126.7	20.67
Prepared as package directs (yield: approx. 18.5 oz.)	1710	279.0			(92.4)	(15.08)
"Suggested" slice, 1/9 of cake (approx. 2.1 oz.)			190	31.0	(92.4)	(15.08)
Chocolate Macaroon Bundt Cake and Glaze Mix, **Pillsbury** "Bundt," 27¼-oz. box	3520	592.0			123.3	20.70
Prepared as package directs (yield: approx. 39 oz.)	4000	592.0			(101.5)	(14.46)
"Suggested" slice, 1/12 of cake (approx. 3.3 oz.)			250	37.0	(101.5)	(14.46)
Chocolate Pudding Cake, **Betty Crocker,** 11-oz. box	1320	270.0			120.0	24.55
Prepared as package directs (yield: approx. 17 oz.)	1380	270.0			(81.2)	(15.88)
"Suggested" slice, 1/6 of cake (approx. 2.8 oz.)			230	45.0	(81.2)	(15.88)
Dark Chocolate Cake, **Pillsbury** "Plus," 18½-oz. box	2160	420.0			123.2	22.70
Prepared as package directs (yield: approx. 33 oz.)	3120	420.0			(94.5)	(12.73)
"Suggested" slice, 1/12 of cake (approx. 2.8 oz.)			260	35.0	(94.5)	(12.73)
1 cupcake (approx. 1.4 oz., 24 to the box)			130	17.5	(94.5)	(12.73)
Deep Chocolate Cake, **Duncan Hines** "Deluxe," 18.25-oz. box	2280	396.0			123.2	21.41
Prepared as package directs (yield: approx. 28 oz.)	3360	396.0			(85.7)	(14.14)
"Suggested" slice, 1/12 of cake (approx. 2⅓ oz.)			280	33.0	(85.7)	(14.14)
1 cupcake (approx. 1.2 oz., 24 to the box)			100	16.5	(85.7)	(14.14)
German Chocolate Cake, **Betty Crocker** "Supermoist," 18½-oz. box	2160	432.0			116.8	23.25
Prepared as package directs (yield: approx. 30 oz.)	3120	432.0			(104.3)	(14.44)
"Suggested" slice, 1/12 of cake (approx. 2.5 oz.)			260	36.0	(104.3)	(14.44)
1 cupcake (approx. 1.2 oz., 24 to the box)			130	18.0	(104.3)	(14.44)
German Chocolate Cake, **Duncan Hines** "Pudding Recipe," 18½-oz. box	2160	408.0			116.8	22.05
Prepared as package directs (yield: approx. 30 oz.)	3000	408.0			(101.3)	(13.78)
"Suggested" serving, 1/12 of cake (approx. 2.5 oz.)			250	34.0	(101.3)	(13.78)
German Chocolate Cake, **Pillsbury** "Plus," 18½-oz. box	3000	432.0			123.2	22.70
Prepared as package directs (yield: approx. 33 oz.)	3000	432.0			(94.5)	(12.73)
"Suggested" slice, 1/12 of cake (approx. 2.8 oz.)			250	36.0	(94.5)	(12.73)
1 cupcake (approx. 1.4 oz., 24 to the box)			130	17.5	(94.5)	(12.73)
German Chocolate Cake, **Pillsbury** "Streusel Swirl," 27¼-oz. box	3360	576.0			114.5	21.14
Prepared as package directs (yield: approx. 39 oz.)	4160	576.0			(101.5)	(14.77)
"Suggested" slice, 1/16 of cake (approx. 2.5 oz.)			260	36.0	(101.5)	(14.77)
German Chocolate Coconut Pecan Cake, **Betty Crocker** "Snackin' Cake," 13.5-oz. box	1620	270.0			120.0	20.00
Prepared as package directs (yield: approx. 19 oz.)	1620	270.0			(85.3)	(14.21)
"Suggested" slice, 1/9 of cake (approx. 2.1 oz.)			180	30.0	(85.3)	(14.21)
Milk Chocolate Cake, **Betty Crocker** "Supermoist," 18½-oz. box	2160	420.0			116.8	22.70
Prepared as package directs (yield: approx. 30 oz.)	3120	420.0			(104.3)	(14.04)
"Suggested" slice, 1/12 of cake (approx. 2.5 oz.)			250	35.0	(104.3)	(14.04)
1 cupcake (each approx. 1.2 oz., 24 to the box)			125	17.5	(104.3)	(14.04)
Sour Cream Chocolate Cake, **Betty Crocker** "Supermoist," 18½-oz. box	2160	432.0			116.8	23.35
Prepared as package directs (yield: approx. 30 oz.)	3120	432.0			(104.3)	(14.44)
"Suggested" slice, 1/12 of cake (approx. 2.5 oz.)			260	36.0	(104.3)	(14.44)
1 cupcake (approx. 1.2 oz., 24 to the box)			130	18.0	(104.3)	(14.44)

	UNIT		1 SLICE, CUPCAKE, OR PASTRY		1 OZ., BY WT.	
	Cal.	Carb.	Cal.	Carb.	Cal.	Carb.
Sour Cream Chocolate Layer Cake, **Duncan Hines**, 18½-oz. box	2283	408.0			123.2	22.05
Prepared as package directs (yield: approx. 28 oz.)	2400	408.0			(85.7)	(14.57)
"Suggested" slice, 1/12 of cake (approx. 2⅓ oz.)			200	34.0	(85.7)	(14.57)
1 cupcake (approx. 1.2 oz., 24 to the box)			100	17.0	(85.7)	(14.57)
Swiss Chocolate Cake, **Duncan Hines** "Deluxe," 18.25-oz. box	2280	396.0			123.2	21.41
Prepared as package directs (yield: approx. 28 oz.)	3360	396.0			(85.7)	(14.14)
"Suggested" slice, 1/12 of cake (approx. 2⅓ oz.)			280	33.0	(85.7)	(14.14)
1 cupcake (approx. 1.2 oz., 24 to the box)			100	16.5	(85.7)	(14.14)
CHOCOLATE CHIP						
Double Chocolate Chip Cake, **Duncan Hines**, 13½-oz. box	1620	288.0			120.0	21.33
Prepared as package directs (yield: approx. 15 oz.)	1620	288.0			(108.0)	(19.20)
"Suggested" slice, 1/9 of cake (approx. 1⅔ oz.)			180	32.2	(108.0)	(19.20)
Golden Chocolate Chip Cake, **Betty Crocker** "Snackin' Cake," 14-oz. package	1710	306.0			122.0	21.86
Prepared as package directs (yield: approx. 19.5 oz.)	1710	306.0			(87.7)	(15.69)
"Suggested" slice, 1/9 of cake (approx. 2.2 oz.)			190	34.0	(87.7)	(15.69)
Golden Chocolate Chip Cake, **Duncan Hines**, 13½-oz. box	1710	288.0			126.7	21.33
Prepared as package directs (yield: approx. 15 oz.)	1710	288.0			(114.0)	(19.20)
"Suggested" slice, 1/9 of cake (approx. 1⅔ oz.)			190	32.0	(114.0)	(19.20)
CINNAMON						
Cinnamon Cake, **Pillsbury** "Streusel Swirl," 27¼-oz. box	3360	608.0			118.9	22.02
Prepared as package directs (yield: approx. 40 oz.)	4160	608.0			(98.9)	(14.54)
"Suggested" slice, 1/16 of cake (approx. 2.5 oz.)			260	38.0	(98.9)	(15.54)
COCONUT						
Coconut Pecan Cake, **Betty Crocker** "Snackin' Cake," 14½-oz. box	1890	279.0			130.3	19.24
Prepared as package directs (yield: approx. 20 oz.)	1890	279.0			(94.5)	(13.95)
"Suggested" slice, 1/9 of cake (approx. 2.3 oz.)			210	31.0	(94.5)	(13.95)
COFFEE						
Coffee Cake, **Aunt Jemima** "Easy Mix," 10½-oz. box	1309	231.8			124.6	22.08
Prepared as package directs (yield: approx. 14½ oz.)	1482	240.1			(102.2)	(16.56)
"Suggested" slice, 1/8 of cake (approx. 1.8 oz.)			185	30.0	(102.2)	(16.56)
Apple Cinnamon Coffee Cake, **Pillsbury,** 19-oz. box	1760	312.0			88.4	16.42
Prepared as package directs (yield: approx. 22 oz.)	1920	320.0			(85.5)	(14.55)
"Suggested" slice, 1/8 of cake (approx. 2.7 oz.)			240	40.0	(85.5)	(14.55)
Butter Pecan Coffee Cake, **Pillsbury,** 14-oz. box	1760	304.0			125.7	21.71
Prepared as package directs (yield: approx. 21 oz.)	2480	312.0			(118.1)	(14.86)
"Suggested" slice, 1/8 of cake (approx. 2.6 oz.)			310	39.0	(118.1)	(14.86)
Cinnamon Streusel Coffee Cake, **Pillsbury,** 14½-oz. box	1840	320.0			126.9	22.07
Prepared as package directs (yield: approx. 18 oz.)	2000	328.0			111.1	18.22
"Suggested" slice, 1/8 of cake (approx. 2.2 oz.)			250	41.0	111.1	18.22
Sour Cream Coffee Cake, **Pillsbury,** 14-oz. box	1920	272.0			137.1	19.40
Prepared as package directs (yield: approx. 19 oz.)	2160	280.0			113.7	14.74
"Suggested" slice, 1/8 of cake (approx. 2.4 oz.)			270	35.0	113.7	14.74
DATE NUT						
Date Nut Cake, **Betty Crocker** "Snackin' Cake," 13.5-oz. box	1710	288.0			127.7	21.33
Prepared as package directs (yield: approx. 19.5 oz.)	1710	288.0			(87.7)	(14.77)
"Suggested" slice, 1/9 of cake (approx. 2.2 oz.)			190	32.0	(87.7)	(14.77)
DEVIL'S FOOD						
Chocolate Devil's Food Cake/Chocolate Frosting, **Betty Crocker** "Stir N' Frost," 13.5-oz. package	1680	264.0			124.4	19.56
Prepared as package directs (yield: approx. 17.0 oz.)	1680	264.0			(98.8)	(15.53)
"Suggested" slice, 1/6 of cake (approx. 2.8 oz.)			280	44.0	(98.8)	(15.53)
Devil's Food Cake, **Ann Page (A&P)** "Deluxe," 18½-oz. box	2160	384.0			108.2	20.70
Prepared as package directs (yield: approx. 28 oz.)	2320	385.0			(82.9)	(13.75)
"Suggested" slice, 1/12 of cake (approx. 2⅓ oz.)			193	32.1	(82.9)	(13.75)
1 cupcake (approx. 1.2 oz., 24 to the box)			97	16.0	(82.9)	(13.75)
Devil's Food Cake, **Betty Crocker** "Supermoist," 18½-oz. box	2160	420.0			116.8	22.70
Prepared as package directs (yield: approx. 30 oz.)	3000	420.0			(100.3)	(14.04)
"Suggested" slice, 1/12 of cake (approx. 2.5 oz.)			250	35.0	(100.3)	(14.04)
Devil's Food Cake, **Duncan Hines** "Deluxe," 18.25-oz. box	2280	396.0			123.2	21.40
Prepared as package directs (yield: approx. 28 oz.)	3360	396.0			(85.7)	(14.14)
"Suggested" slice, 1/12 of cake (approx. 2⅓ oz.)			280	33.0	(85.7)	(14.14)
1 cupcake (approx. 1.2 oz., 24 to the box)			100	16.5	(85.7)	(14.14)
Devil's Food Cake, **Jiffy,** 9-oz. box	1050	200.0			116.7	22.22
Prepared as package directs (yield: approx. 13 oz.)	1050	203.0			(88.4)	(15.62)
"Suggested" serving, 1/10 of cake (approx. 1.3 oz.)			(96)	(16.9)	(88.4)	(15.62)
Devil's Food Cake, **Pillsbury** "Plus," 18½-oz. box	2280	420.0			123.2	22.70
Prepared as package directs (yield: approx. 33 oz.)	3240	420.0			(98.2)	(12.73)
"Suggested" slice, 1/12 of cake (approx. 2.8 oz.)			270	35.0	(98.2)	(12.73)
1 cupcake (approx. 1.4 oz., 24 to the box)			132	17.5	(98.2)	(12.73)
Devil's Food Cake, **Pillsbury** "Streusel Swirl," 27¼-oz. box	3360	600.0			123.3	22.02
Prepared as package directs (yield: approx. 40 oz.)	3960	600.0			99.0	15.00
"Suggested" slice, 1/12 of cake (approx. 3.3 oz.)			330	50.0	99.0	15.00
FUDGE						
Dark Fudge Cake, **Jiffy,** 9-oz. box	1040	200.0			119.5	22.22
Prepared as package directs (yield: approx. 12.3 oz.)	1070	(210.0)			87.0	(17.07)
"Suggested" slice, 1/10 of cake (approx. 1.23 oz.)			107	(21.0)	87.0	(17.07)
Fudge Cake, **Duncan Hines** "Butter Recipe," 18½-oz. box	2280	408.0			123.2	22.05
Prepared as package directs (yield: approx. 28 oz.)	3120	408.0			115.7	14.57
"Suggested" slice, 1/12 of cake (approx. 2⅓ oz.)			270	34.0	115.7	14.57
1 cupcake (approx. 1.2 oz., 24 to the box)			135	17.0	115.7	14.57
Fudge Marble Cake, **Ann Page** "Deluxe," 18½-oz. box	2160	408.0			116.8	22.05
Prepared as package directs (yield: approx. 28 oz.)	2160	408.0			(77.1)	(14.57)
"Suggested" slice, 1/12 of cake (approx. 2⅓ oz.)			180	34.0	(77.1)	(14.57)
1 cupcake (approx. 1.2 oz., 24 to the box)			90	17.0	(77.1)	(14.57)
Fudge Marble Cake, **Duncan Hines,** "Deluxe," 18.25-oz. box	2280	432.0			123.2	22.05
Prepared as package directs (yield: approx. 28 oz.)	3120	432.0			(85.7)	(14.57)
"Suggested" slice, 1/12 of cake (approx. 2.3 oz.)			260	36.0	(85.7)	(14.57)
1 cupcake (approx. 1.2 oz., 24 to the box)			100	17.0	(85.7)	(14.57)
Fudge Marble Cake, **Pillsbury** "Plus," 18½-oz. box	2280	420.0			123.2	22.70
Prepared as package directs (yield: approx. 28 oz.)	2400	420.0			(85.7)	(15.00)
"Suggested" slice, 1/12 of cake (approx. 2.3 oz.)			200	35.0	(85.7)	(15.00)
1 cupcake (approx. 1.4 oz., 24 to the box)			100	17.5	(85.7)	(15.00)
Fudge Marble Cake, **Pillsbury** "Streusel Swirl," 19¾-oz. box	2400	432.0			121.5	21.87
Prepared as package directs (yield: approx. 33 oz.)	3240	432.0			(98.2)	(13.09)
"Suggested" slice, 1/12 of cake (approx. 3.3 oz.)			270	36.0	(98.2)	(13.09)
Fudge Nut Crown Cake, **Pillsbury** "Bundt," 22½-oz. box	2880	492.0			128.0	21.87

	UNIT		1 SLICE, CUPCAKE, OR PASTRY		1 OZ., BY WT.	
	Cal.	Carb.	Cal.	Carb.	Cal.	Carb.
Prepared as package directs (yield: approx. 35 oz.)	3480	492.0			(99.4)	(14.06)
"Suggested" slice, 1/12 of cake (approx. 2.9 oz.)			290	41.0	(99.4)	(14.06)
GERMAN CHOCOLATE, see CHOCOLATE						
GINGERBREAD						
Gingerbread Mix, **Ann Page (A&P),** "Deluxe," 13½-oz. box	1560	432.0			115.6	32.00
Prepared as package directs (yield: 1 pan, approx. 20 oz.)	1560	432.0			(78.0)	(21.60)
Gingerbread Mix, **Betty Crocker,** 14.5-oz. box	1800	324.0			124.1	22.34
Prepared as package directs (yield: 1 pan, approx. 20 oz.)	1890	324.0			(94.5)	(16.20)
Gingerbread Mix, **Dromedary,** 14-oz. box	1600	320.0			114.3	22.86
Prepared as package directs (yield: 1 pan, approx. 20 oz.)	1600	320.0			(80.0)	(16.00)
Gingerbread Mix, **Pillsbury,** 14.5-oz. box	1710	324.0			117.9	22.34
Prepared as package directs (yield: 1 pan, approx. 20 oz.)	1710	324.0			(85.5)	(16.20)
Gingerbread Mix, Whole Wheat Old Fashioned, **Vermont General Store & Grist Mill,** 13.7-oz. bag	1270	286.7			92.7	20.93
Prepared as package directs (yield: 1 pan, approx. 25.2 oz.)	1764	288.0			(70.0)	(11.43)
GOLDEN						
Golden Cake, **Duncan Hines** "Butter Recipe," 18½-oz. box	2280	432.0			123.2	23.35
Prepared as package directs (yield: approx. 28 oz.)	3240	432.0			(115.7)	(15.43)
"Suggested" slice, 1/12 of cake (approx. 2⅓ oz.)			270	36.0	(115.7)	(15.43)
1 cupcake (approx. 1.2 oz., 24 to the box)			135	18.0	(115.7)	(15.43)
Golden Vanilla Cake, **Duncan Hines** "Deluxe," 18.25-oz. box	2280	432.0			116.8	23.35
Prepared as package directs (yield: approx. 30 oz.)	3120	432.0			101.3	14.58
"Suggested" slice, 1/12 of cake (approx. 2½ oz.)			260	36.0	101.3	14.58
LEMON						
Lemon Cake, artificial flavor, **Ann Page (A&P),** 18½-oz. box	2160	396.0			116.8	21.41
Prepared as package directs (yield: approx. 28 oz.)	2320	397.0			82.9	14.18
"Suggested" slice, 1/12 of cake (approx. 2⅓ oz.)			180	33.0	82.9	14.18
1 cupcake (approx. 1.2 oz., 24 to the box)			90	16.5	82.9	14.18
Lemon Cake, dietetic, **Batter-Lite,** 8-oz. box	979	149.0			122.4	18.63
Prepared as package directs (yield: approx. 12 oz.)	992	149.0			82.7	12.42
"Suggested" slice, 1/10 of cake (approx. 1.2 oz.)			99	14.9	82.7	12.42
1 cupcake (approx. 1.2 oz., 10 to the box)			99	14.9	82.7	12.42
Lemon Cake, **Betty Crocker** "Supermoist," 18½-oz. box	2160	432.0			116.8	23.35
Prepared as package directs (yield: approx. 32 oz., or 2 lb.)	3120	432.0			(98.5)	(13.64)
"Suggested" slice, 1/12 of cake (approx. 2.6 oz.)			260	36.0	(98.5)	(13.64)
1 cupcake (approx. 1.3 oz., 24 to the box)			130	18.0	(98.5)	(13.64)
Lemon Cake/Lemon Frosting, **Betty Crocker** "Stir N' Frost," 11-oz. box	1380	234.0			125.5	21.27
Prepared as package directs (yield: approx. 16.5 oz.)	1380	234.0			(83.6)	(14.18)
"Suggested" slice, 1/8 of cake (approx. 2.1 oz.)			173	29.3	(83.6)	(14.18)
Lemon Cake, **Duncan Hines,** "Deluxe," 18.25-oz. box	2280	432.0			116.8	23.35
Prepared as package directs (yield: approx. 30 oz.)	3120	432.0			101.3	14.58
"Suggested" slice, 1/12 of cake (approx. 2½ oz.)			260	36.0	101.3	14.58
Lemon Cake, **Pillsbury** "Plus," 18½-oz. box	2280	444.0			123.2	24.00
Prepared as package directs (yield: approx. 32 oz., or 2 lb.)	3240	444.0			(101.3)	(13.88)
"Suggested" slice, 1/12 of cake (approx. 2.6 oz.)			270	37.0	(101.3)	(13.88)
1 cupcake (approx. 1.3 oz., 24 to the box)			135	18.5	(101.3)	(13.88)
Lemon Cake, **Pillsbury** "Streusel Swirl," 27¼-oz. box	3240	600.0			118.9	22.02
Prepared as package directs (yield: approx. 40 oz.)	4200	600.0			(105.0)	(15.00)
"Suggested" slice, 1/12 of cake (approx. 3.3 oz.)			350	50.0	(105.0)	(15.00)
Lemon Cake, **Sweet 'N Low,** sugar restricted, 8-oz. box	900	160.0			112.5	20.00
Prepared as package directs (yield: approx. 12.2 oz.)	900	160.0			(73.9)	(13.14)
"Suggested" slice, 1/10 of cake (approx. 2.0 oz.)			90	16.0	(73.9)	(13.14)
Lemon Blueberry Cake, **Pillsbury** "Bundt," 23½-oz. box	2760	504.0			117.4	21.45
Prepared as package directs (yield: approx. 35 oz.)	3360	504.0			(96.0)	(14.40)
"Suggested" slice, 1/12 of cake (approx. 3.0 oz.)			280	42.0	(96.0)	(14.40)
Lemon Flavored Cake, dietetic, **Dia-Mel,** 8-oz. box	900	180.0			112.5	22.50
Prepared as package directs (yield: approx. 13 oz.)	1000	180.0			(76.9)	(13.85)
"Suggested" slice, 1/10 of cake (approx. 1.3 oz.)			100	18.0	(76.9)	(13.85)
1 cupcake (approx. 1.3 oz., 10 to a box)			100	18.0	(76.9)	(13.85)
Lemon Pudding Cake, **Betty Crocker,** 11-oz. box	1320	270.0			120.0	24.55
Prepared as package directs (yield: approx. 17 oz.)	1380	270.0			(81.2)	(15.88)
"Suggested" slice, 1/6 of cake (approx. 2.8 oz.)			230	45.0	(81.2)	(15.88)
1 cupcake (approx. 1.4 oz., 12 to the box)			115	22.5	(81.2)	(15.88)
Lemon Supreme Layer Cake, **Duncan Hines,** 18½-oz. box	2280	408.0			123.2	22.05
Prepared as package directs (yield: approx. 28 oz.)	2400	408.0			(85.7)	(14.57)
"Suggested" slice, 1/12 of cake (approx. 2⅓ oz.)			200	34.0	(85.7)	(14.57)
1 cupcake (approx. 1.2 oz., 24 to the box)			100	17.0	(85.7)	(14.57)
Sunkist Lemon Chiffon Layer Cake, **Betty Crocker,** 18½-oz. box	2160	420.0			116.8	22.70
Prepared as package directs (yield: approx. 28 oz.)	2280	420.0			(81.4)	(15.00)
"Suggested" slice, 1/12 of cake (approx. 2⅓ oz.)			190	35.0	(81.4)	(15.00)
1 cupcake (approx. 1.2 oz., 24 to the box)			95	17.5	(81.4)	(15.00)
MARBLE						
Marble Cake, **Betty Crocker** "Supermoist," 20-oz. box	2400	480.0			120.0	24.00
Prepared as package directs (yield: approx. 31 oz.)	3240	480.0			(103.1)	(15.28)
"Suggested" slice, 1/12 of cake (approx. 2.6 oz.)			270	40.0	(103.1)	(15.28)
1 cupcake (approx. 1.3 oz., 24 to the box)			135	20.0	(103.1)	(15.28)
ORANGE						
Orange Cake, **Betty Crocker** "Supermoist," 18½-oz. box	2160	432.0			116.8	23.35
Prepared as package directs (yield: approx. 30 oz.)	3120	432.0			(104.3)	(14.44)
"Suggested" slice, 1/12 of cake (approx. 1.5 oz.)			260	36.0	(104.3)	(14.44)
1 cupcake (approx. 1.2 oz., 24 to the box)			130	18.0	(104.3)	(14.44)
Orange Supreme Cake, **Duncan Hines,** "Deluxe," 18.25-oz. box	2280	432.0			123.2	22.05
Prepared as package directs (yield: approx. 28 oz.)	3120	432.0			(85.7)	(14.57)
"Suggested" slice, 1/12 of cake (approx. 2⅓ oz.)			260	36.0	(85.7)	(14.57)
1 cupcake (approx. 1.2 oz., 24 to the box)			100	17.0	(85.7)	(14.57)
PINEAPPLE						
Pineapple Supreme Cake, **Duncan Hines** "Deluxe," 18.25-oz. box	2280	432.0			123.2	22.05
Prepared as package directs (yield: approx. 28 oz.)	3120	432.0			(85.7)	(14.57)
"Suggested" slice, 1/12 of cake (approx. 2⅓ oz.)			260	36.0	(85.7)	(14.57)
1 cupcake (approx. 1.2 oz., 24 to the box)			100	17.0	(85.7)	(14.57)
Pineapple Upside Down Cake, **Betty Crocker,** 21½-oz. box	2070	387.0			96.3	18.00
Prepared as package directs (weight of yield not available)	2430	387.0				
"Suggested" slice, 1/9 of cake			270	43.0		

	UNIT Cal.	UNIT Carb.	1 SLICE, CUPCAKE, OR PASTRY Cal.	1 SLICE, CUPCAKE, OR PASTRY Carb.	1 OZ., BY WT. Cal.	1 OZ., BY WT. Carb.
POUND						
Golden Pound Cake, **Betty Crocker,** 16-oz. (1-lb.) box	2160	324.0			135.0	20.25
Prepared as package directs (weight of yield not available)	2400	324.0				
"Suggested" slice, 1/12 of cake			200	27.0		
Pound Cake, **Dromedary,** 17-oz. box	2240	348.0			131.8	20.47
Prepared as package directs (yield: approx. 27 oz.)	2560	372.0			(94.8)	(13.78)
"Suggested" slice, 1/8 of cake (approx. 3.4 oz.)			320	46.5	(94.8)	(13.78)
Pound Cake, **Pillsbury** "Bundt," 24¾-oz. box	3000	540.0			121.2	21.82
Prepared as package directs (yield: approx. 41 oz.)	3720	540.0			(90.7)	(13.17)
"Suggested" slice, 1/12 of cake (approx. 3.4 oz.)			310	45.0	(90.7)	(13.17)
Whole Wheat Pound Cake Flavored with Almond Oil, **Vermont General Store & Grist Mill,** 13.8-oz. bag	1400	300.0			101.4	21.70
Prepared as package directs (yield: approx. 24 oz.)	(2160)	(301.1)			(90.0)	(12.54)
"Suggested" slice, 1/20 of cake (approx. 1.2 oz.)			(108)	(15.1)	(90.0)	(12.54)
SOUR CREAM						
Sour Cream Chocolate Cake, **Betty Crocker** "Supermoist," 18½-oz. box	2160	432.0			116.8	22.35
Prepared as package directs (yield: approx. 30 oz.)	3120	432.0			(104.3)	(14.44)
"Suggested" slice, 1/12 of cake (approx. 2.5 oz.)			260	36.0	(104.3)	(14.44)
1 cupcake (approx. 1.2 oz., 24 to the box)			130	18.0	(104.3)	(14.44)
Sour Cream Chocolate Layer Cake, **Duncan Hines,** 18½-oz. box	2283	408.0			123.2	22.05
Prepared as package directs (yield: approx. 28 oz.)	2400	408.0			(85.7)	(14.57)
"Suggested" slice, 1/12 of cake (approx. 2⅓ oz.)			200	34.0	(85.7)	(14.57)
1 cupcake (approx. 1.2 oz., 24 to the box)			100	17.0	(85.7)	(14.57)
Sour Cream Coffee Cake, **Pillsbury,** 14-oz. box	1920	272.0			137.1	19.40
Prepared as package directs (yield: approx. 19 oz.)	2160	280.0			(113.7)	(14.74)
"Suggested" slice, 1/8 of cake (approx. 2.4 oz.)			270	35.0	(113.7)	(14.74)
Sour Cream White Cake, **Betty Crocker** "Supermoist," 18½-oz. box	2160	432.0			116.8	22.35
Prepared as package directs (yield: approx. 27 oz.)	2160	432.0			(80.8)	(16.16)
"Suggested" slice, 1/12 of cake (approx. 2.2 oz.)			180	36.0	(80.8)	(16.16)
1 cupcake (approx. 1.1 oz., 24 to the box)			90	18.0	(80.8)	(16.16)
SPICE						
Spice Cake/Vanilla Frosting, **Betty Crocker** "Stir N' Frost," 13½-oz. box	1620	282.0			120.0	20.89
Prepared as package directs (yield: approx. 17 oz.)	1620	282.0			(95.3)	(16.60)
"Suggested" slice, 1/6 of cake (approx. 2.8 oz.)			270	47.0	(95.3)	(16.60)
1 cupcake (approx. 1.4 oz., 12 to the box)			135	23.5	(95.3)	(16.60)
Spice Cake, **Betty Crocker** "Supermoist," 18½-oz. box	2160	432.0			116.8	23.35
Prepared as package directs (yield: approx. 30 oz.)	3120	432.0			(104.3)	(14.44)
"Suggested" slice, 1/12 of cake (approx. 2.5 oz.)			260	36.0	(104.3)	(14.44)
1 cupcake (approx. 1.2 oz., 24 to the box)			130	18.0	(104.3)	(14.44)
Spice Cake, **Fearn,** 8.6-oz. box	864	132.0			100.5	15.35
Prepared as package directs (yield: approx. 21.4 oz.)	(1942)	(272.0)			(90.7)	(12.71)
"Suggested" slice, 1/6 of cake (approx. 3.6 oz.)			(324)	(45.3)	(90.7)	(12.71)
Spice Cake, **Jiffy,** 9-oz. box	1060	207.0			117.8	23.00
Prepared as package directs (weight of yield not available)	1210	215.0				
"Suggested" slice, 1/10 of cake			121	21.5		
Spice Carob Cake, **Elf Liberty Natural Foods,** 12-oz. box	1320	204.0			110.0	17.00
Prepared as package directs (yield: approx. 29 oz.)	3000	336.0			(103.4)	(11.59)
"Suggested" slice, 1/12 of cake (approx. 2.4 oz.)			250	28.0	(103.4)	(11.59)
Spice Layer Cake, **Duncan Hines,** 18½-oz. box	2280	420.0			123.2	22.70
Prepared as package directs (yield: approx. 28 oz.)	2400	420.0			(85.7)	(15.00)
"Suggested" slice, 1/12 of cake (approx. 2⅓ oz.)			200	35.0	(85.7)	(15.00)
1 cupcake (approx. 1.2 oz., 24 to the box)			100	17.5	(85.7)	(15.00)
Spice Raisin Cake, **Betty Crocker** "Snackin' Cake," 13½-oz. box	1620	297.0			120.0	22.00
Prepared as package directs (yield: approx. 19 oz.)	1620	297.0			(85.3)	(15.63)
"Suggested" slice, 1/9 of cake (approx. 2.1 oz.)			180	33.0	(85.3)	(15.63)
STRAWBERRY						
Strawberry Cake, **Betty Crocker** "Supermoist," 18½-oz. box	2160	432.0			116.8	22.35
Prepared as package directs (yield: approx. 30 oz.)	3120	432.0			(104.3)	(14.44)
"Suggested" slice, 1/12 of cake (approx. 2.5 oz.)			260	36.0	(104.3)	(14.44)
1 cupcake (approx. 1.2 oz., 24 to the box)			130	18.0	(104.3)	(14.44)
Strawberry Cake, **Pillsbury** "Plus," 18¾-oz. box	2280	408.0			121.6	21.76
Prepared as package directs (yield: approx. 32 oz., or 2 lb.)	3120	408.0			(97.5)	(12.75)
"Suggested" slice, 1/12 of cake (approx. 2.6 oz.)			260	34.0	(97.5)	(12.75)
1 cupcake (approx. 1.3 oz., 24 to the box)			130	17.0	(97.5)	(12.75)
Strawberry Supreme Cake, **Duncan Hines** "Deluxe," 18.25-oz. box	2280	432.0			123.2	22.70
Prepared as package directs (yield: approx. 28 oz.)	3120	432.0			(85.7)	(15.00)
"Suggested" slice, 1/12 of cake (approx. 2⅓ oz.)			260	36.0	(85.7)	(15.00)
1 cupcake (approx. 1.2 oz., 24 to the box)			100	17.5	(85.7)	(15.00)
VANILLA						
Golden Vanilla Cake, **Duncan Hines** "Deluxe," 18.25-oz. box	2280	432.0			116.8	23.35
Prepared as package directs (yield: approx. 30 oz.)	3120	432.0			101.3	14.58
"Suggested" slice, 1/12 of cake (approx. 2½ oz.)			260	36.0	101.3	14.58
WHITE						
Sour Cream White Cake, **Betty Crocker** "Supermoist," 18½-oz. box	2160	432.0			116.8	23.35
Prepared as package directs (yield: approx. 27 oz.)	2160	432.0			(80.8)	(16.16)
"Suggested" slice, 1/12 of cake (approx. 2.2 oz.)			180	36.0	(80.8)	(16.16)
1 cupcake (approx. 1.1 oz., 24 to the box)			90	18.0	(80.8)	(16.16)
White Cake, **Ann Page (A&P)** "Deluxe," 18½-oz. box	2160	408.0			116.8	22.05
Prepared as package directs (yield: approx. 28 oz.)	2160	408.0			(77.1)	(14.57)
"Suggested" slice, 1/12 of cake (approx. 2⅓ oz.)			180	34.0	(77.1)	(14.57)
1 cupcake (approx. 1.2 oz., 24 to the box)			95	17.0	(77.1)	(14.57)
White Cake, dietetic, **Batter-Lite,** 8-oz. box	979	149.0			122.0	18.63
Prepared as package directs (yield: approx. 12 oz.)	992	149.0			82.7	12.42
"Suggested" slice, 1/10 of cake (approx. 1.2 oz.)			99	14.9	82.7	12.42
1 cupcake (approx. 1.2 oz., 10 to the box)			99	14.9	82.7	12.42
White Cake, **Betty Crocker** "Supermoist," 18½-oz. box	2160	432.0			116.8	23.35
Prepared as package directs (yield: approx. 27 oz.)	2160	432.0			(80.8)	(16.16)
"Suggested" slice, 1/12 of cake (approx. 2.2 oz.)			180	36.0	(80.8)	(16.16)
1 cupcake (approx. 1.1 oz., 24 to the box)			90	18.0	(80.8)	(16.16)
White Cake, **Duncan Hines** "Deluxe" 18.25-oz. box	2280	432.0			123.2	22.05
Prepared as package directs (yield: approx. 28 oz.)	3000	432.0			(81.4)	(14.57)
"Suggested" slice, 1/12 of cake (approx. 2⅓ oz.)			190	36.0	(81.4)	(14.57)
1 cupcake (approx. 1.2 oz., 24 to the box)			85	17.0	(81.4)	(14.57)
White Cake, **Jiffy,** 9-oz. box	978	200.0			108.7	22.22
Prepared as package directs (yield: approx. 11.5 oz.)	1060	203.0			92.2	17.65
"Suggested" slice, 1/10 of cake (approx. 1.15 oz.)			106	20.3	92.2	17.65

	UNIT		1 SLICE, CUPCAKE, OR PASTRY		1 OZ., BY WT.	
	Cal.	Carb.	Cal.	Carb.	Cal.	Carb.
White Cake, **Pillsbury** "Plus," 18½-oz. box	2400	432.0			129.7	23.35
Prepared as package directs (yield: approx. 33 oz.)	3000	432.0			(90.9)	(13.09)
"Suggested" slice, 1/12 of cake (approx. 2.3 oz.)			250	36.0	(90.9)	(13.09)
1 cupcake (approx. 1.4 oz., 24 to the box)			125	18.0	(90.9)	(13.09)
White Cake, sugar restricted, **Sweet 'N Low,** 8-oz. box	900	160.0			112.5	20.00
Prepared as package directs (yield: approx. 12.2 oz.)	900	160.0			(73.9)	(13.14)
"Suggested" slice, 1/10 of cake (approx. 2.0 oz.)			90	16.0	(73.9)	(13.14)
YELLOW						
Golden Yellow Cake, **Jiffy,** 9-oz. box	1050	204.0			116.7	22.67
Prepared as package directs (yield: approx. 12.5 oz.)	1080	(210.0)			86.4	(16.80)
"Suggested" slice, 1/10 of cake (approx. 1.25 oz.)			108	(21.0)	86.4	(16.80)
Yellow Cake, **Ann Page (A&P)** "Deluxe," 18½-oz. box	2160	396.0			116.8	21.41
Prepared as package directs (yield: approx. 28 oz.)	2320	397.0			(80.3)	(14.18)
"Suggested" slice, 1/12 of cake (approx. 2⅓ oz.)			193	33.1	(80.3)	(14.18)
1 cupcake (approx. 1.2 oz., 24 to the box)			97	16.6	(80.3)	(14.18)
Yellow Cake, **Betty Crocker** "Supermoist," 18½-oz. box	2160	444.0			116.8	24.00
Prepared as package directs (yield: approx. 30 oz.)	3000	444.0			(100.3)	(14.84)
"Suggested" slice, 1/12 of cake (approx. 2.5 oz.)			250	37.0	(100.3)	(14.84)
1 cupcake (approx. 1.2 oz., 24 to the box)			125	18.5	(100.3)	(14.84)
Yellow Cake/Chocolate Frosting, **Betty Crocker** "Stir N' Frost," 11-oz. box	1320	228.0			120.0	20.73
Prepared as package directs (yield: approx. 17 oz.)	1320	228.0			(77.6)	(13.41)
"Suggested" slice, 1/6 of cake (approx. 2.8 oz.)			220	38.0	(77.6)	(13.41)
Yellow Cake, **Duncan Hines** "Deluxe," 18½-oz. box	2280	432.0			123.2	22.05
Prepared as package directs (yield: approx. 28 oz.)	3120	432.0			(85.7)	(14.57)
"Suggested" slice, 1/12 of cake (approx. 2⅓ oz.)			260	36.0	(85.7)	(14.57)
1 cupcake (approx. 1.2 oz., 24 to the box)			100	17.0	(85.7)	(14.57)
Yellow Cake, **Pillsbury** "Plus," 18½-oz. box	2280	420.0			123.2	22.70
Prepared as package directs (yield: approx. 32 oz., or 2 lb.)	3120	420.0			(97.5)	(13.13)
"Suggested" slice, 1/12 of cake (approx. 2.6 oz.)			260	35.0	(97.5)	(13.13)
1 cupcake (approx. 1.3 oz., 24 to the box)			130	17.5	(97.5)	(13.13)
Yellow Cake, sugar restricted, **Sweet 'N Low,** 8-oz. box	900	160.0			112.5	20.00
Prepared as package directs (yield: approx. 12.2 oz.)	900	160.0			(73.9)	(13.14)
"Suggested" slice, 1/10 of cake (approx. 2.0 oz.)			90	16.0	(73.9)	(13.14)
Yellow Layer Cake, **Duncan Hines** "Butter Recipe," 18½-oz. box	2160	432.0			116.8	23.35
Prepared as package directs (yield: approx. 30 oz.)	2760	432.0			(92.3)	(14.44)
"Suggested" slice, 1/12 of cake (approx. 1.2 oz.)			230	36.0	(92.3)	(14.44)
1 cupcake (approx. 1.2 oz., 24 to the box)			115	18.0	(92.3)	(14.44)
NO-BAKE CAKE MIXES						
Boston Cream Pie, **Betty Crocker** "Dessert Mix," 15½-oz. box	1760	360.0			113.5	23.23
Prepared as package directs (yield: approx. 28 oz.)	2160	384.0			(77.0)	(13.71)
"Suggested" slice, 1/8 of cake (approx. 3½ oz.)			270	48.0	(77.0)	(13.71)
Creamy Cheesecake with Sour Cream Topping, **Pillsbury** "No Bakes," 14.8-oz. box	2080	272.0			141.0	18.38
Prepared as package directs (yield: 9″ cake, approx. 24 oz.)	1840	248.0			76.7	10.33
"Suggested" slice, 1/8 of cake (approx. 3 oz.)			230	31.0	76.7	10.33

PREPACKAGED CAKES

	UNIT		1 SLICE, CUPCAKE, OR PASTRY		1 OZ., BY WT.	
	Cal.	Carb.	Cal.	Carb.	Cal.	Carb.
BOSTON CREAM						
Boston Cream Cake, **Pepperidge Farm** "Cakes Supreme," 13-oz. cake	1215	193.5			93.5	14.88
"Suggested" serving, 1/9 of cake (1.44 oz.)			135	21.5	93.5	14.88
CARROT						
Carrot Cake, **Sara Lee,** 12¼-oz. cake	1223	151.4			99.8	12.36
"Suggested" serving, 1/8 of cake (approx. 1.53 oz.)			153	18.9	99.8	12.36
Old Fashioned Carrot Pound Cake, **Pepperidge Farm,** 14¼-oz. cake	1600	200.1			112.3	14.04
"Suggested" serving, 1/10 of cake (approx. 1.4 oz.			160	20.0	112.3	14.04
CHEESECAKE						
Cheesecake, **World's Best,** 16-oz. (1-lb.) cake	1578	126.1			98.6	7.88
2-lb. cake	3156	252.2			98.6	7.88
"Suggested" serving, 1/12 of 1-lb. cake (approx. 1.3 oz.)			131	10.5	98.6	7.88
Cherry Cheesecake, **Morton** "Great Little Desserts," 6-oz. cake	434	48.9			72.3	8.15
Cherry Cream Cheese Cake, **Sara Lee,** 19-oz. cake	1284	181.8			67.5	9.58
"Suggested" serving, 1/6 of cake (approx. 3.17 oz.)			214	30.3	67.5	9.58
Cream Cheesecake, **Morton** "Great Little Desserts," 6-oz. cake	443	38.8			73.8	6.46
Cream Cheese Cake, **Sara Lee,** Small, 10-oz. cake	861	84.9			86.1	8.49
"Suggested" serving, 1/3 of cake (approx. 3⅓ oz.)			287	28.3	86.1	8.49
Large, 17-oz. cake	1449	142.8			84.8	8.41
"Suggested" serving, 1/6 of cake (approx. 2.83 oz.)			240	23.8	84.8	8.41
French Cream Cheese Cake, **Sara Lee,** 23.5-oz. cake	2193	199.2			93.3	8.48
"Suggested" serving, 1/8 of cake (approx. 2.94 oz.)			274	24.9	93.2	8.48
Pineapple Cheesecake, **Morton** "Great Little Desserts," 6-oz. cake	434	50.8			72.3	8.46
Strawberry Cheesecake, **Morton** "Great Little Desserts," 6-oz. cake	443	53.5			73.8	8.92
Strawberry Cream Cheese Cake, **Sara Lee,** 19-oz. cake	1283	180.0			67.5	9.47
"Suggested" serving, 1/6 of cake (approx. 3.2 oz.)			214	30.0	67.5	9.47
CHOCOLATE						
Chocolate Bavarian Cake, **Sara Lee,** 22.5-oz. cake	2277	181.1			101.2	8.07
"Suggested" serving, 1/8 of cake (approx. 2.8 oz.)			285	22.6	101.2	8.07
Chocolate Brownies, **Sara Lee,** 13-oz. cake	1600	206.8			123.1	15.91
1 brownie, 1/8 of cake (approx. 1.6 oz.)			200	25.8	123.1	15.91
Chocolate Cake, **Pepperidge Farm** "Cakes Supreme," 11½-oz. cake	1189	164.9			103.4	14.34
"Suggested" serving, 1/9 of cake (approx. 1.27 oz.)			132	18.3	103.4	14.34
Chocolate Cake, **Sara Lee,** 13.25-oz. cake	1476	194.2			111.4	14.66
"Suggested" serving, 1/8 of cake (approx. 1.66 oz.)			185	24.3	111.4	14.66
Chocolate Fudge Cake, **Pepperidge Farm,** 17-oz. cake	1800	250.0			105.9	14.71
"Suggested" serving, 1/10 of cake (approx. 1.7 oz.)			180	25.0	105.9	14.71
"Half Cake," 8½-oz. cake	900	125.0			105.9	14.71
Chocolate 'N Cream Layer Cake, **Sara Lee,** 18-oz. cake	1674	190.4			93.0	10.58
"Suggested" serving, 1/8 of cake (approx. 2¼ oz.)			209	23.8	93.0	10.58
Double Chocolate Layer Cake, **Sara Lee,** 18-oz. cake	1710	192.4			95.0	10.69
"Suggested" serving, 1/8 of cake (approx. 2¼ oz.)			214	24.0	95.0	10.69
German Chocolate Cake, **Pepperidge Farm,** 17-oz. cake	1600	240.0			94.1	14.18
"Suggested" serving, 1/10 of cake (approx. 1.7 oz.)			160	24.0	94.1	14.18
Old Fashioned Chocolate Pound Cake, **Pepperidge Farm,** 10¾-oz. cake	1300	150.0			120.9	13.95
"Suggested" serving, 1/10 of cake (approx. 1.05 oz.)			130	15.0	120.9	13.95
COCONUT						
Coconut Cake, **Pepperidge Farm,** 17-oz. cake	1800	260.0			105.9	15.29

	UNIT		1 SLICE, CUPCAKE, OR PASTRY		1 OZ., BY WT.	
	Cal.	Carb.	Cal.	Carb.	Cal.	Carb.
"Suggested" serving, 1/10 of cake (approx. 1.7 oz.)			180	26.0	105.9	15.29
"Half Cake," 8½ oz.	900	130.0			105.9	15.29
Coconut Cake, **Sara Lee,** 10-oz. cake	1152	139.2			115.2	13.92
"Suggested" serving, 1/8 of cake (approx. 1¼ oz.)			144	17.4	115.2	13.92
Lemon Coconut Cake, **Pepperidge Farm** "Cakes Supreme," 12¼-oz. cake	1144	171.6			93.4	14.01
"Suggested" serving, 1/9 of cake (approx. 1.36 oz.)			127	19.1	93.4	14.01
COFFEE CAKES AND COFFEE RINGS						
Almond Coffee Cake, **Sara Lee,** 12-oz. cake	1352	154.4			112.7	12.87
"Suggested" serving, 1/8 of cake (approx. 1½ oz.)			169	19.3	112.7	12.87
Almond Coffee Ring, **Sara Lee,** 9½-oz. cake	1128	128.0			118.7	13.47
"Suggested" serving, 1/8 of cake (approx. 1.2 oz.)			141	16.0	118.7	13.47
Blueberry Coffee Ring, **Sara Lee,** 9¾-oz. cake	1064	140.8			109.1	14.44
"Suggested" serving, 1/8 of cake (approx. 1.2 oz.)			133	17.6	109.1	14.44
Maple Crunch Coffee Ring, **Sara Lee,** 9¾-oz. cake	1104	137.6			113.2	14.19
"Suggested" serving, 1/8 of cake (approx. 1.2 oz.)			138	17.2	113.2	14.19
Pecan Coffee Cake, **Sara Lee,** "small," 6½-oz. cake	764	83.2			117.5	12.80
"Suggested" serving, 1/4 of cake (approx. 1.6 oz.)			191	20.8	117.5	12.80
"Large," 11-oz. cake	1320	144.0			120.0	13.09
"Suggested" serving, 1/8 of cake (approx. 1.4 oz.)			165	18.0	120.0	13.09
Raspberry Coffee Ring, **Sara Lee,** 9½-oz. cake	1120	145.6			117.9	15.33
"Suggested" serving, 1/8 of cake (approx. 1.2 oz.)			140	18.2	117.9	15.33
DATE-NUT						
Date Nut, **Thomas',** 16-oz. (1-lb.) loaf	1360	268.8			85.1	16.80
"Suggested" serving, 1/15 of loaf (approx. 1.07 oz.)			91	17.9	85.1	16.80
DEVIL'S FOOD						
Devil's Food Cake, **Pepperidge Farm,** 17-oz. cake	1800	260.0			105.9	15.29
"Suggested" serving, 1/10 of cake (approx. 1.7 oz.)			180	26.0	105.9	15.29
GERMAN CHOCOLATE, see CHOCOLATE						
GOLDEN						
Golden Cake, **Sara Lee,** 14-oz. cake	1501	219.1			107.2	15.65
"Suggested" serving, 1/8 of cake (approx. 1¾ oz.)			188	27.4	107.2	15.65
Golden Layer Cake, **Pepperidge Farm,** 18-oz. cake	1800	250.0			100.0	13.89
"Suggested" serving, 1/10 of cake (approx. 1.8 oz.)			180	25.0	100.0	13.89
HONEY						
Honey Cake, unsalted, cholesterol free, **Holland Honey Cake,** approx. 7 slices	980	252.0				
1 slice			140	36.0		
LEMON						
Lemon Bavarian Cake, **Sara Lee,** 23½-oz. cake	2178	178.4			92.7	7.59
"Suggested" serving, 1/8 of cake (approx. 2.94 oz.)			272	22.3	92.7	7.59
Lemon Coconut Cake, **Pepperidge Farm** "Cakes Supreme," 12¼-oz. cake	1144	171.6			93.4	14.01
"Suggested" serving, 1/9 of cake (approx. 1.36 oz.)			127	19.1	93.4	14.01
MARBLE						
Marble Cake, **Chock Full O'Nuts,** 16-oz. (1-lb.) cake	1747	220.8			109.2	13.80
ORANGE						
Orange Cake, **Sara Lee,** 13¾-oz. cake	1400	202.3			101.8	14.72
"Suggested" serving, 1/8 of cake (approx. 1.72 oz.)			175	25.3	101.8	14.72
POUND CAKE						
Banana Nut Pound Cake, **Sara Lee,** 11-oz. cake	1166	150.6			106.0	13.69
"Suggested" serving, 1/10 of cake (approx. 1.1 oz.)			117	15.1	106.0	13.69
Chocolate Pound Cake, **Sara Lee,** 10¾-oz. cake	1222	130.2			113.7	12.11
"Suggested" serving, 1/10 of cake (approx. 1.08 oz.)			122	13.0	113.7	12.11
Chocolate Swirl Pound Cake, **Sara Lee,** 11¾-oz. cake	1300	179.2			110.6	15.25
"Suggested" serving, 1/10 of cake (approx. 1.18 oz.)			130	17.9	110.6	15.25
Home Style Pound Cake, **Sara Lee,** 9.5-oz. cake	1094	127.4			115.1	13.41
"Suggested" serving, 1/10 of cake (approx. 0.95 oz.)			109	12.7	115.1	13.41
Old Fashioned Apple Walnut Pound Cake With Raisins, **Pepperidge Farm,** 14¼-oz. cake	1300	200.0			92.2	14.18
"Suggested" serving, 1/10 of cake (approx. 1.4 oz.)			130	20.0	92.2	14.18
Old Fashioned Carrot Pound Cake, **Pepperidge Farm,** 17-oz. cake	1909	238.7			112.3	14.04
"Suggested" serving, 1/10 of cake (approx. 1.7 oz.)			191	23.9	112.3	14.04
Old Fashioned Chocolate Pound Cake, **Pepperidge Farm,** 10¾-oz. cake	1300	150.0			120.9	13.95
"Suggested" serving, 1/10 of cake (approx. 1.05 oz.)			130	15.0	120.9	13.95
Old Fashioned Pound Cake, **Pepperidge Farm,** 10¾-oz. cake	1300	150.0			120.9	13.95
"Suggested" serving, 1/10 of cake (approx. 1.05 oz.)			130	15.0	120.9	13.95
Pound Cake, **Chock Full O'Nuts,** 16-oz. (1-lb.) cake	1678	239.0			104.9	14.94
Pound Cake, **Sara Lee,** 10¾-oz. cake	1237	144.4			115.1	13.47
"Suggested" serving, 1/10 of cake (approx. 1.1 oz.)			124	14.4	115.1	13.47
Family Size, 16-oz. (1-lb.) cake	1842	215.5			115.1	13.47
"Suggested" serving, 1/15 of cake (approx. 1.1 oz.)			127	14.8	115.1	13.47
Pound Cake, **Stouffer's,** 12-oz. cake	1500	168.0			125.0	14.00
"Suggested" serving, 1/12 of cake (approx. 1 oz.)			125	14.0	125.0	14.00
Raisin Pound Cake, **Sara Lee,** 12⅞-oz. cake	1267	193.5			98.4	15.03
"Suggested" serving, 1/10 of cake (approx. 1.29 oz.)			127	19.3	98.4	15.03
STRAWBERRY						
Strawberries 'N Cream Layer Cake, **Sara Lee,** 20½-oz. cake	1703	219.1			83.1	10.69
"Suggested" serving, 1/8 of cake (approx. 2.7 oz.)			213	27.4	83.1	10.69
Strawberry Shortcake, **Sara Lee,** 21-oz. cake	1541	207.2			73.4	9.87
"Suggested" serving, 1/8 of cake (approx. 2.6 oz.)			193	25.9	73.4	9.87
VANILLA						
Vanilla Cake, **Pepperidge Farm,** 17-oz. cake	1900	270.0			111.8	15.88
"Suggested" serving, 1/10 of cake (approx. 1.7 oz.)			190	27.0	111.8	15.88
WALNUT						
Walnut Layer Cake, **Sara Lee,** 18-oz. cake	1689	178.6			93.8	9.92
"Suggested" serving, 1/8 of cake (approx. 2.2 oz.)			211	22.3	93.8	9.92

PREPACKAGED SNACK CAKES, CUPCAKES, DONUTS, TURNOVERS, SWEET ROLLS, AND OTHER PASTRIES

Snack cakes are differentiated from cakes in the preceding section by weight and by function. That is to say, if a cake weighs less than five ounces and is commonly sold to be eaten by one person at one time, I put it here. This section also includes pastries weighing less than five ounces that are commonly sold in multiple units, such as cupcakes sold 12 to the box.

	UNIT		1 SLICE, CUPCAKE, OR PASTRY		1 OZ., BY WT.	
	Cal.	Carb.	Cal.	Carb.	Cal.	Carb.
Drakes						
Cherry Pies, 16-oz. (1-lb.) box (8 pies)	1600	224.0			100.0	14.00
1 pie, approx. 2 oz.			200	28.0	100.0	14.00
Coffee Cake Jr., 17-oz. box (16 cakes)	1967	582.4			115.7	34.26
1 cake, approx. 1.06 oz.			125	37.0	115.7	34.26
Cupcakes, Fudgy Moist & Cremey, 12-oz. box (8 cupcakes)	1360	216.0			113.3	18.00
1 cupcake, approx. 1½ oz.			170	27.0	113.3	18.00
Sunny Doodles, 18-oz. box (18 Doodles)	1890	315.0			105.0	17.50
1 Doodle, approx. 1 oz.			105	17.5	105.0	17.50
Yankee Doodles, 18-oz. box (18 Doodles)	1890	279.0			105.0	15.50
1 Doodle, approx. 1 oz.			105	15.5	105.0	15.50

	UNIT		1 SLICE, CUPCAKE, OR PASTRY		1 OZ., BY WT.	
	Cal.	Carb.	Cal.	Carb.	Cal.	Carb.
El Molino						
Apricot Cake, 2-oz. package	250	36.0	250	36.0	125.0	18.00
Brownie, Carob Filled, 2-oz. package	220	40.0	220	40.0	110.0	20.00
Crumb Cake, Cinnamon, 2-oz. package	250	37.0	250	37.0	125.0	18.50
Crumb Cake, Raspberry, 2-oz. package	260	37.0	260	37.0	130.0	18.50
Date Cake, 2-oz. package	240	36.0	240	36.0	120.0	18.00
Fruit & Spice Cake, 2-oz. package	230	42.0	230	42.0	115.0	21.00
Granola Cake, 2-oz. package	220	40.0	220	40.0	110.0	20.00
Honey 'N Bran Cake, 1½-oz. package	160	28.0	160	28.0	106.7	18.67
Strawberry Filled Cake, 2-oz. package	240	37.0	240	37.0	120.0	18.50
Frito-Lay						
Pecan Pie, 3-oz. package	353	53.5	353	53.5	117.7	17.83
Hostess						
Big Wheels, 2⅔-oz. package (2 wheels)	340	42.0			127.5	15.75
1 wheel, approx. 1⅓-oz.			170	21.0	127.5	15.75
Brownie, Large, 2-oz. package	240	39.0	240	39.0	120.0	19.50
Brownie, Small, 2½-oz. package (2 brownies)	300	48.0			120.0	19.20
1 brownie, approx. 1¼ oz.			150	24.0	120.0	19.20
Choco-Diles, 2.2-oz. package	250	37.0	250	37.0	113.6	16.82
Crumb Cakes, 2½-oz. package (2 cakes)	260	44.0			104.0	17.60
1 cake, approx. 1¼ oz.			130	22.0	104.0	17.60
Cupcakes, Chocolate, 3½-oz. package (2 cupcakes)	320	60.0			91.4	17.14
1 cupcake, approx. 1¾ oz.			160	30.0	91.4	17.14
Cupcakes, Orange, 3-oz. package (2 cupcakes)	300	54.0			100.0	18.00
1 cupcake, approx. 1½ oz.			150	27.0	100.0	18.00
Ding-Dongs, 2⅔-oz. package (2 Ding-Dongs)	340	42.0			127.5	15.75
1 Ding-Dong, approx. 1⅓ oz.			170	21.0	127.5	15.75
Donuts:						
Cinnamon Donuts, 9-oz. multipack (8 donuts)	880	120.0			97.8	13.33
1 donut, approx. 1.1 oz.			110	15.0	97.8	13.33
Crunch Donuts, 12-oz. family pack (12 donuts)	1200	192.0			100.0	16.00
1 donut, approx. 1 oz.			100	16.0	100.0	16.00
Enrobed Donuts, 11-oz. multipack	1430	154.0			130.0	14.00
1 donut, approx. 1 oz.			130	14.0	130.0	14.00
Plain Donuts, 9-oz. package (8 donuts)	880	96.0			97.7	10.67
1 donut, approx. 1.1 oz.			110	12.0	97.7	10.67
Powdered Donuts, 9-oz. multipack (8 donuts)	880	120.0			97.7	13.33
1 donut, approx. 1.1 oz.			110	15.0	97.7	13.33
Fruit Pies						
Apple Fruit Pie, 4½-oz. package	400	54.0	400	54.0	88.9	12.00
Berry Fruit Pie, 4½-oz. package	400	51.0	400	51.0	88.9	11.33
Blueberry Fruit Pie, 4½-oz. package	390	49.0	390	49.0	86.7	10.89
Cherry Fruit Pie, 4½-oz. package	420	59.0	420	59.0	93.3	13.11
Lemon Fruit Pie, 4½-oz. package	420	53.0	420	53.0	93.3	11.78
Peach Fruit Pie, 4½-oz. package	400	53.0	400	53.0	88.9	11.78
Ho Hos, 2-oz. package (2 Ho Hos)	240	33.0			120.0	16.50
1 Ho Ho, approx. 1 oz.			120	16.5	120.0	16.50
Honey Bun, 4¾-oz. package	580	63.0	580	63.0	122.1	13.26
Sno Balls, 3-oz. package (2 Sno Balls)	280	50.0			93.3	16.67
1 Sno Ball, approx. 1½ oz.			140	25.0	93.3	16.67
Suzy Q's Banana, 4½-oz. package (2 Suzy Q's)	480	76.0			106.7	16.89
1 Suzy Q, approx. 2¼ oz.			240	38.0	106.7	16.89
Suzy Q's Chocolate, 4½-oz. package (2 Suzy Q's)	450	72.0			100.0	16.00
1 Suzy Q, approx. 2¼ oz.			225	36.0	100.0	16.00
Tiger Tails, 4.4-oz. package	430	76.0	430	76.0	97.7	17.27
Twinkies, 3-oz. package (2 Twinkies)	280	52.0			93.3	17.30
1 Twinkie, approx. 1½ oz.			140	26.0	93.3	17.30
Twinkies, Devil's Food, 3-oz. package (2 Twinkies)	280	50.0			93.3	16.67
1 Twinkie, approx. 1½ oz.			140	25.0	93.3	16.67
Little Debbie						
Apple Delight, 1.16-oz. package	135	22.7	135	22.7	115.4	19.46
Banana Twin Cakes, 13-oz. box (12 cakes)	1496	232.4			115.1	17.88
1 cake, approx. 1.09 oz.			125	19.4	115.1	17.88
Brownies, Fudge, with Cashews, 11-oz. package (12 brownies)	1363	212.0			123.9	19.27
1 brownie, approx. 0.92 oz.			114	17.7	123.9	19.27
Co-Co-Jel Cakes, 13-oz. box (12 cakes)	1691	235.3			130.1	18.10
1 cake, approx. 1.09 oz.			141	19.6	130.1	18.10
Coconut Rounds Cakes, 13-oz. box (12 cakes)	1780	236.0			136.9	18.15
1 cake, approx. 1.09 oz.			148	19.7	136.9	18.15
Devil Square Cakes, 13-oz. box (12 cakes)	1619	240.7			124.5	18.51
1 cake, approx. 1.09 oz.			135	20.1	124.5	18.51
Devil Twin Cakes, 13-oz. box (12 cakes)	1444	236.4			111.1	18.18
1 cake, approx. 1.09 oz.			120	19.7	111.1	18.18
Fudge Round Cakes, 10-oz. box (8 cakes)	1310	189.7			131.0	18.97
1 cake, approx. 1¼ oz.			164	23.7	131.0	18.97
Granola Bars, 11-oz. box (12 bars)	1525	193.4			138.6	17.67
1 bar, approx. 0.92 oz.			127	16.2	138.6	17.67
Jel-Creme Roll, 15-oz. box (12 rolls)	1688	282.3			112.3	18.82
1 roll, approx. 1.09 oz.			141	23.5	112.3	18.82
Nutty Bar Wafers with Peanut Butter, 12-oz. box (12 wafers)	1889	190.0			157.4	15.91
1 wafer, approx. 1 oz.			157	15.9	157.4	15.91
Oatmeal Creme Pies, 16-oz. (1-lb.) box (12 pies)	2059	286.4			128.7	17.90
1 pie, approx. 1.34 oz.			172	23.9	128.7	17.90
Raisin Creme Pies, 14-oz. package (12 pies)	1767	255.8			126.2	18.27
1 pie, approx. 1.16 oz.			147	21.3	126.2	18.27
Snak Cakes, 15-oz. box (12 cakes)	1935	266.9			129.0	17.79
1 cake, approx. 1¼ oz.			161	22.2	129.0	17.79
Star Crunch Cakes, 13-oz. box (12 cakes)	1773	262.6			136.4	20.20
1 cake, approx. 1.09 oz.			148	21.9	136.4	20.20
Swiss Cake Rolls, 13-oz. box (12 cakes)	1593	224.1			122.5	17.24
1 cake, approx. 1.09 oz.			133	18.7	122.5	17.24
Morton						
Donuts:						
Bavarian Creme Donuts, 12-oz. package (6 donuts)	1080	132.0			90.0	11.00
1 donut, approx. 2 oz.			180	22.0	90.0	11.00
Boston Creme Donuts, 14-oz. package (6 donuts)	1260	168.0			90.0	12.00
1 donut, approx. 2.33 oz.			210	28.0	90.0	12.00
Chocolate Iced Donuts, 9-oz. package (6 donuts)	900	120.0			100.0	13.33
1 donut, approx. 1½ oz.			150	20.0	100.0	13.33
Glazed Donuts, 9⅛-oz. package (6 donuts)	900	114.0			100.0	12.67
1 donut, approx. 1½ oz.			150	19.0	100.0	12.67
Jelly Donuts, 11-oz. package (6 donuts)	1080	138.0			98.2	12.55
1 donut, approx. 1.83 oz.			180	23.0	98.2	12.55
Sugar 'N Spice, Mini-Donuts, 10-oz. package (18 donuts)	1080	144.0			108.0	14.40
1 donut, approx. 0.55 oz.			60	8.0	108.0	14.40
Honey Buns, 9-oz. package (4 buns)	920	124.0			102.2	13.78
1 bun, approx. 2.25 oz.			230	31.0	100.0	13.48
Mini Honey Buns, 6-oz. package (6 buns)	613	81.7			102.1	13.61
1 bun, approx. 1 oz.			102	13.6	102.1	13.61
Nabisco						
Chocolate Pinwheels Cakes, 13-oz. box (12 cakes)	1680	252.0			127.3	19.09
1 cake, approx. 1.1 oz.			140	21.0	127.3	19.09
Devil's Food Cakes, 8½-oz. box (18 cakes)	900	189.0			111.1	23.33
1 cake, approx. 0.45 oz.			50	10.5	111.1	23.33
Mallomars Chocolate Cakes, 8-oz. box (18 cakes)	990	162.0			122.2	20.00
1 cake, approx. 0.45 oz.			55	9.0	122.2	20.00
Pepperidge Farm						
Apple Dumplings, 12¼-oz. box (4 dumplings)	1120	124.0			91.4	10.12
1 dumpling, approx. 3.06 oz.			280	31.0	91.4	10.12
Apple Strudel, 15-oz. box (5 strudels)	1250	155.0			83.3	10.33
1 strudel, approx. 3 oz.			250	31.0	83.3	10.33
Tarts:						
Apple Pie Tarts, 11½-oz. box (4 tarts)	1120	132.0			97.4	11.48
1 tart, approx. 2.88 oz.			280	33.0	97.4	11.48
Blueberry Pie Tarts, 11½-oz. box (4 tarts)	1120	140.0			97.4	12.17
1 tart, approx. 2.88 oz.			280	35.0	97.4	12.17
Cherry Pie Tarts, 11½-oz. box (4 tarts)	1120	140.0			97.4	12.17
1 tart, approx. 2.88 oz.			280	35.0	97.4	12.17
Lemon Pie Tarts, 11½-oz. box (4 tarts)	1280	148.0			111.3	12.87
1 tart, approx. 2.88 oz.			320	37.0	111.3	12.87
Raspberry Pie Tarts, 11½-oz. box (4 tarts)	1280	136.0			111.3	11.83
1 tart, approx. 2.88 oz.			320	34.0	111.3	11.83
Turnovers:						
Apple Turnover, 12¼-oz. package (4 turnovers)	1240	120.0			101.2	9.80
1 turnover, approx. 3.06 oz.			310	30.0	101.2	9.80
Blueberry Turnover, 12¼-oz. package (4 turnovers)	1280	128.0			104.5	10.45
1 turnover, approx. 3.06 oz.			320	32.0	104.5	10.45

	UNIT		1 SLICE, CUPCAKE, OR PASTRY		1 OZ., BY WT.	
	Cal.	Carb.	Cal.	Carb.	Cal.	Carb.
Cherry Turnover, 12¼-oz. package (4 turnovers)	1360	120.0			111.0	9.80
1 turnover, approx. 3.06 oz.			340	30.0	111.0	9.80
Peach Turnover, 12¼-oz. package (4 turnovers)	1280	132.0			104.5	10.78
1 turnover, approx. 3.06 oz.			320	33.0	104.5	10.78
Raspberry Turnover, 12¼-oz. package (4 turnovers)	1360	148.0			111.0	12.08
1 turnover, approx. 3.06 oz.			340	37.0	111.0	12.08
Rich's						
Bavarian Cream Puffs, 8-oz. package (6 puffs)	900	102.0			112.5	12.75
1 puff, 1⅓ oz.			150	17.0	112.5	12.75
Chocolate Cream Puffs, 8-oz. package (6 puffs)	900	102.0			112.5	12.75
1 puff, 1⅓ oz.			150	17.0	112.5	12.75
Chocolate Eclairs, 8½-oz. package (4 eclairs)	1160	148.0			136.5	17.41
Institutional pack, 6.4 pounds (48 eclairs)	13920	1776.0			136.5	17.41
1 eclair, approx. 2.13 oz.			290	37.0	136.5	17.41
Vanilla Puffs (package weight not available)					77.0	10.78
1 puff, approx. 2.17 oz.			167	23.4	77.0	10.78
Sara Lee						
Apple Crunch Rolls, 9-oz. package (9 rolls)	918	121.5			102.0	13.50
1 roll, approx. 1 oz.			102	13.5	102.0	13.50
Caramel Pecan Rolls, 10½-oz. package (8 or 9 rolls)	1244	117.9			118.5	11.23
1 roll, approx. 1.3 oz.			154	14.6	118.5	11.23
Caramel Sticky Buns, 9¼-oz. package (9 or 10 buns)	1092	138.8			118.0	15.00
1 bun, approx. 1 oz.			118	15.0	118.0	15.00
Cinnamon Rolls, 8¼-oz. package (9 or 10 rolls)	963	115.5			116.7	14.00
1 roll, approx. 0.9 oz.			105	12.6	116.7	14.00
Crumb Cakes, Blueberry, 10½-oz. package (6 cakes)	929	143.2			88.5	13.64
1 cake, approx. 1¾-oz.			155	23.9	88.5	13.64
Crumb Cakes, French, 10¼-oz. package (6 cakes)	1032	162.0			100.7	15.79
1 cake, approx. 1.7 oz.			172	27.0	100.7	15.79
Cupcakes, Yellow, 10½-oz. package (6 cupcakes)	1044	167.4			104.4	16.74
1 cupcake, approx. 1¾ oz.			174	27.9	104.4	16.74
Danish:						
Apple Danish, 7¾-oz. package (6 danish)	726	104.4			93.7	13.47
1 danish, approx. 1.29 oz.			121	17.4	93.7	13.47
Cinnamon Raisin Danish, 7¾-oz. package (6 danish)	906	108.0			117.1	14.03
1 danish, approx. 1.29 oz.			151	18.0	117.1	14.03
Cheese Danish, 7¾-oz. package (6 danish)	786	83.4			101.5	10.80
1 danish, approx. 1.29 oz.			131	13.9	101.5	10.80
Honey Rolls, 9-oz. package (9 rolls)	1008	131.4			112.0	14.60
1 roll, approx. 1 oz.			112	14.6	112.0	14.60
Stouffer's						
Crumb Cakes:						
Blueberry Crumb Cakes, 12-oz. package (6 cakes)	1260	192.0			105.0	16.00
1 cake, approx. 2 oz.			210	32.0	105.0	16.00
Chocolate Chip Crumb Cakes, 10½-oz. package (6 cakes)	1362	162.0			129.7	15.43
1 cake, approx. 1¾ oz.			227	27.0	129.7	15.43
French Crumb Cakes, 10.13-oz. package (6 cakes)	1200	180.0			118.5	17.78
1 cake, approx. 1 11/16 oz.			200	30.0	118.5	17.78
Cupcakes:						
Cream Filled Cupcakes, 12-oz. package (6 cupcakes)	1440	216.0			120.0	18.00
1 cupcake, approx. 2 oz.			240	36.0	120.0	18.00
Yellow Cupcakes, 10.125-oz. box (6 cupcakes)	1140	180.0			112.6	17.78
1 cupcake, approx. 1 11/16 oz.			190	30.0	112.6	17.78
Tastykake						
Butterscotch Krimpets, 1.75-oz. package (3 Krimpets)	192				110.0	
1 Krimpet, approx. 0.58 oz.			64		110.0	
Chocolate Creamies, 2.33-oz. package (1 Creamy)	257		257		110.2	
Chocolate Cupcakes, 2-oz. package (3 cupcakes)	200				100.2	
1 cupcake, approx. 0.66 oz.			66		100.2	
Chocolate Juniors, 2.75-oz. package (1 Junior)	307		307		111.7	

	UNIT		1 SLICE, CUPCAKE, OR PASTRY		1 OZ., BY WT.	
	Cal.	Carb.	Cal.	Carb.	Cal.	Carb.
Chocolate Kandy Kakes, 1.33-oz. package (3 Kakes)	181				136.0	
1 Kake, approx. 0.44 oz.			60		136.0	
Chocolate Tasty Klairs, 4-oz. package (1 Klair)	435		435		108.8	
Chocolate Teens, 2.17-oz. package (2 Teens)	225				104.1	
1 Teen, 1.08 oz.			112		104.1	
Coconut Juniors, 2.75-oz. package (1 Junior)	330		330		120.1	
Cream Filled Chocolate Butter Cream Cups, 2.25-oz. package, 2 cups	240				106.6	
1 cup, approx. 1.12 oz.			120		106.6	
Cream Filled Chocolate Cupcakes, 2.25-oz. package (2 cupcakes)	245				108.9	
1 cupcake, approx. 1.12 oz.			123		108.9	
Cream Filled Chocolate Krimpies, 2.33-oz. package (2 Krimpies)	252				108.1	
1 Krimpy, 1.17 oz.			126		108.1	
Cream Filled Koffee Kake, 2-oz. package (2 Kakes)	248				124.0	
1 Kake, approx. 1 oz.			124		124.0	
Jelly Krimpets, 1.75-oz. package (3 Krimpets)	168				96.2	
1 Krimpet, 0.58 oz.			56		96.2	
Koffee Kake Juniors, 2.5-oz. package (1 Junior)	313		313		125.5	
Lemon Juniors, 2.75-oz. package (1 Junior)	297		297		108.1	
Oatmeal Raisin Bars, 1.75-oz. package (1 bar)	267		267		152.9	
Peanut Butter Kandy Kakes, 1.33-oz. package (3 Kakes)	190				142.5	
1 Kake, approx. 0.44 oz.			63		142.5	
Pies:						
Apple Pie, 4-oz. package (1 pie)	348		348		87.0	
Blueberry Pie, 4-oz. package (1 pie)	366		366		91.5	
Cherry Pie, 4-oz. package (1 pie)	381		381		95.3	
French Apple Pie, 4.25-oz. package (1 pie)	405		405		95.4	
Lemon Pie, 4-oz. package (1 pie)	370		370		92.5	
Peach Pie, 4-oz. package (1 pie)	349		349		87.3	
Spice Creamies, 2.6-oz. package (1 Creamy)	272		272		104.2	
Vanilla Krimpies, 2.17-oz. package (2 Krimpies)	240				110.6	
1 Krimpy, 1.09 oz.			120		110.6	

TOASTER PASTRIES

	UNIT		1 SLICE, CUPCAKE, OR PASTRY		1 OZ., BY WT.	
Poptarts (Kellogg's)						
Blueberry, 11-oz. box (6 pastries)	1263	216.4			114.8	19.70
1 pastry, approx. 1.83 oz.			210	36.0	114.8	19.70
Blueberry, frosted, 11-oz. box (6 pastries)	1263	222.4			114.8	20.22
1 pastry, approx. 1.83 oz.			210	37.0	114.8	20.27
Brown Sugar-Cinnamon, 10½-oz. box (6 pastries)	1260	204.0			120.0	19.43
1 pastry, approx. 1¾ oz.			210	34.0	120.0	19.43
Brown Sugar-Cinnamon, frosted, 10½-oz. box (6 pastries)	1260	188.0			120.0	18.86
1 pastry, approx. 1¾ oz.			210	33.0	120.0	18.86
Cherry, 11-oz. box (6 pastries)	1263	210.4			114.8	19.13
1 pastry, approx. 1.33 oz.			210	35.0	114.8	19.13
Cherry, frosted, 10½-oz. box (6 pastries)	1263	216.4			114.8	19.70
1 pastry, approx. 1¾ oz.			210	36.0	114.8	19.70
Chocolate Fudge, frosted, 10½-oz. box (6 pastries)	1263	210.4			114.8	19.13
1 pastry, approx. 1¾ oz.			210	35.0	114.8	19.13
Chocolate-Peppermint, frosted, 10½-oz. box (6 pastries)	1263	210.4			114.8	19.13
1 pastry, approx. 1¾ oz.			210	35.0	114.8	19.13
Chocolate-Vanilla Cream, frosted, 10½-oz. box (6 pastries)	1263	204.4			114.8	18.58
1 pastry, approx. 1¾ oz.			210	34.0	114.8	18.58
Concord Grape, frosted, 10½-oz. box (6 pastries)	1263	222.4			114.8	20.22
1 pastry, approx. 1¾ oz.			210	37.0	114.8	20.22
Dutch Apple, frosted, 11-oz. box (6 pastries)	1263	216.4			114.8	19.70
1 pastry, approx. 1.83 oz.			210	36.0	114.8	19.70
Raspberry, frosted, 10½-oz. box (6 pastries)	1260	222.0			114.8	20.22
1 pastry, approx. 1¾ oz.			210	37.0	114.8	20.22
Strawberry, 10½-oz. box (6 pastries)	1263	216.4			114.8	19.67
1 pastry, approx. 1¾ oz.			210	36.0	114.8	19.67

	UNIT Cal.	UNIT Carb.	1 SLICE, CUPCAKE, OR PASTRY Cal.	1 SLICE, CUPCAKE, OR PASTRY Carb.	1 OZ., BY WT. Cal.	1 OZ., BY WT. Carb.
Strawberry, frosted, 10½-oz. box (6 pastries)	1263	216.4			114.8	19.67
1 pastry, approx. 1¾ oz.			210	36.0	114.8	19.67
Toast-R-Cakes (Thomas')						
Blueberry, 7.6-oz. package (6 cakes)	660	102.0			86.6	13.39
1 cake, approx. 1.3 oz.			110	17.0	86.6	13.39
Bran, 7.6-oz. package (6 cakes)	720	120.0			94.5	15.75
1 cake, approx. 1.3 oz.			120	20.0	94.5	15.75
Corn, 7-oz. package (6 cakes)	720	108.0			94.5	14.18
1 cake, approx. 1 oz.			120	18.0	94.5	14.18
Toastettes (Nabisco)						
Apple, 6½-oz. package (4 pastries)	760	140.0			118.8	20.59
1 pastry, approx. 1.6 oz.			190	35.0	118.8	20.59
Blueberry, 6½-oz. package (4 pastries)	760	140.0			118.8	20.59
1 pastry, approx. 1.6 oz.			190	35.0	118.8	20.59
Brown Sugar Cinnamon, 6½-oz. package (4 pastries)	760	140.0			118.8	20.59
1 pastry, approx. 1.6 oz.			190	35.0	118.8	20.59
Cherry, 6½-oz. package (4 pastries)	760	140.0			118.8	20.59
1 pastry, approx. 1.6 oz.			190	35.0	118.8	20.59
Strawberry, 6½-oz. package (4 pastries)	760	140.0			118.8	20.59
1 pastry, approx. 1.6 oz.			190	35.0	118.8	20.59

FROSTINGS

FROSTINGS (ICINGS), Made from Scratch, based on USDA home recipes

	UNIT Cal.	UNIT Carb.	FROSTING FOR 1 SLICE, 1/12 OF CAKE Cal.	FROSTING FOR 1 SLICE, 1/12 OF CAKE Carb.	1 OZ., BY WT. Cal.	1 OZ., BY WT. Carb.	1 CUP Cal.	1 CUP Carb.
CARAMEL ICING								
For 2-layer, 9″ cake. Icing made from: 1½ cups brown sugar, ⅔ cup milk, 2 Tbsp. table fat, ½ tsp. vanilla (yield: approx. 15 oz., 1¼ cups). (Loss of 17% has been applied for evaporation in cooking.) (tr/22g/2g/14%/24mg)	1534	325.8	128	27.2	102.3	21.72	1224	260.1
For 2-layer, 8″ cake, ¾ of recipe above (yield: approx. 11¼ oz., approx. 0.9 cups)	1151	244.4	96	20.4	102.3	21.72	1224	260.1
1 cup (approx. 12 oz.)	1224	260.1			102.3	21.72	1224	260.1
CHOCOLATE ICING								
For 2-layer, 8″ cake. Icing made from: 1 cup granulated cane sugar, ½ cup milk, 1 Tbsp. table fat, 2 oz. bitter chocolate, ½ tsp. vanilla (yield: approx. 11¾ oz., 1¼ cups). (Loss of 16% has been applied for evaporation in cooking.) (1g/20g/4g/14%/61mg)	1252	224.4	104	18.7	106.6	19.10	1034	185.4
1 cup (approx. 9.7 oz.)	1034	185.4			106.6	19.10	1034	185.4
COCONUT ICING								
For 2-layer, 8″ cake. Icing made from: 1 cup granulated cane sugar, ¼ cup water, 1 large egg white, ⅛ tsp. salt, 2 oz. sweetened dried coconut, ½ tsp. vanilla (yield: approx. 11 oz., 1⅞ cups). (Loss of 15% has been applied for evaporation in cooking.) (1g/21g/2g/15%/33mg)	1136	233.7	95	19.5	103.3	21.25	604	124.3
1 cup (approx. 5.9 oz.)	604	124.3			103.3	21.25	604	124.3
WHITE ICING								
Uncooked, for 2-layer, 8″ cake. Icing made from: 2 cups powdered cane sugar, 3 Tbsp. light cream, 1 Tbsp. table fat, 1 tsp. vanilla (yield: approx. 11¼ oz., 1 cup) (tr/23g/2g/11%/14mg)	1199	260.3	100	21.7	106.6	23.14	1199	260.3
Boiled, for 2-layer, 8″ cake. Icing made from 1 cup granulated cane sugar, ¼ cup water, 1 large egg white, ⅛ tsp. salt, ½ tsp. vanilla (yield: approx. 8⅞ oz., ⅔ cup). (Loss of 15% has been applied for evaporation in cooking.) (tr/23g/0g/18%/41mg)	796	202.4	66	16.9	89.7	22.81	1193	303.4
1 cup (approx. 13.3 oz.)	1193	303.4			89.7	22.81	1193	303.4

DRY FROSTING (ICING) MIXES, based on USDA data

	UNIT Cal.	UNIT Carb.	FROSTING FOR 1 SLICE, 1/12 OF CAKE Cal.	FROSTING FOR 1 SLICE, 1/12 OF CAKE Carb.	1 OZ., BY WT. Cal.	1 OZ., BY WT. Carb.	1 CUP Cal.	1 CUP Carb.
Chocolate Fudge, for 2-layer, 8″ cake, 14 oz. mix, 5 Tbsp. water, 3 Tbsp. table fat (yield: approx. 17.9 oz., 1.6 cups) (1g/19g/4g/15%/44mg)	(1924)	(341.2)	(160)	(28.4)	107.5	19.06	1172	207.7
1 cup (approx. 10.9 oz.)	1172	207.7			107.5	19.06	1172	207.7
Creamy Fudge (package contains nonfat dry milk), 13 oz. of mix with 4 Tbsp. water (yield: approx. 15 oz., 1.7 cup) (1g/17g/2g/15%/66mg)	(1454)	(318.3)	121	26.5	96.9	21.22	831	182.2
1 cup (approx. 8.6 oz.)	831	182.2			96.9	21.22	831	182.2
6½ oz. of mix with 2 Tbsp. water and 2 Tbsp. table fat (1g/15g/4g/15%/91mg)	(938)	(161.5)	(78)	(13.5)	109.1	18.78	938	161.5
1 cup (approx. 8.6 oz.)	938	161.5			109.1	18.78	938	161.5

FROSTINGS (ICINGS), Dry Mixes and Ready To Spread, by brand

	UNIT Cal.	UNIT Carb.	FROSTING FOR 1 SLICE, 1/12 OF CAKE Cal.	FROSTING FOR 1 SLICE, 1/12 OF CAKE Carb.	1 OZ., BY WT. Cal.	1 OZ., BY WT. Carb.	1 CUP Cal.	1 CUP Carb.
BANANA								
Chiquita Banana, **Betty Crocker** "Creamy Frosting," Dry Mix, 15.4-oz. box	1800	360.0			116.9	23.38		
Prepared as package directs, with butter	2040	360.0	170	30.0			(1020)	(180.0)
BUTTER								
Butter Brickle, **Betty Crocker** "Creamy Frosting," Dry Mix, 15.4-oz. box	1800	360.0			116.9	23.38		
Prepared as package directs, with butter	2040	360.0	170	30.0			(1020)	(180.0)
Butter Pecan, **Betty Crocker** "Creamy Deluxe," Ready To Spread, 16½-oz. can	2040	324.0	170	27.0	123.6	19.64	(1020)	(162.0)
Butter Pecan, **Betty Crocker** "Creamy Frosting," Dry Mix, 15.4-oz. box	1800	360.0			116.9	23.38		
Prepared as package directs, with butter	2040	360.0	170	30.0			(1020)	(180.0)
CARAMEL								
Caramel, **Jiffy,** Dry Mix, 7½-oz. box	950	173.0			126.7	23.07		
Prepared as package directs (for 1-layer cake)	950	173.0	79	14.4	(111.8)	(20.35)	(1014)	(184.5)
Caramel, **Pillsbury** "Rich and Easy," Dry Mix, 15.1-oz. box	2040	348.0			135.1	23.05		
Prepared as package directs	2040	348.0	170	29.0			(1020)	(174.0)
CHERRY								
Cherry, **Betty Crocker** "Creamy Deluxe," Ready To Spread, 16½-oz. can	2040	336.0	170	28.0	123.6	20.36	(1020)	(168.0)
Creamy Cherry, **Betty Crocker** "Creamy Frosting," Dry Mix, 15.4-oz. box	1800	360.0			116.9	23.38		
Prepared as package directs, with butter	2040	360.0	170	30.0			(1020)	(180.0)
CHOCOLATE								
Chocolate, **Batter Lite** "Frost Lite," low-calorie, low-sodium, Dry Mix, 5-oz. box, prepared as package directs	(460)	(125.0)	(38)	(10.4)	62.8	17.14	(460)	(125.0)
Chocolate, **Betty Crocker** "Creamy Deluxe," Ready To Spread, 16½-oz. can	2040	300.0	170	25.0	123.6	18.18	(1020)	(150.0)
Chocolate, **Hershey's,** Ready To Spread, 16½-oz. can	1920	276.0	160	23.0	116.4	16.73	(950)	(136.5)

	UNIT		FROSTING FOR 1 SLICE, 1/12 OF CAKE		1 OZ., BY WT.		1 CUP	
	Cal.	Carb.	Cal.	Carb.	Cal.	Carb.	Cal.	Carb.
Chocolate Flavored (Sugar Restricted), **Sweet 'N Low,** Frosting & Fudge Topping Dry Mix, 5¼-oz. box	900	90.0			171.4	17.14		
Prepared for frosting as package directs, with water	900	90.0						
Prepared for fudge topping as package directs, with water	900	90.0						
Chocolate Fudge, **Betty Crocker** "Creamy Frosting," Dry Mix, 15.4-oz. box	1800	360.0			116.9	23.38		
Prepared as package directs, with butter	2040	360.0	170	30.0	(123.6)	(21.82)	(1020)	(180.0)
Chocolate Fudge, **Pillsbury** "Frosting Supreme," Ready To Spread, 16.5-oz. can	1920	288.0	160	24.0	116.4	17.45	(960)	(144.0)
Chocolate Fudge, **Pillsbury** "Rich and Easy," Dry Mix, 15.1-oz. box	2040	360.0			135.1	23.84		
Prepared as package directs	2040	360.0	170	30.0			(1020)	(180.0)
Chocolate Fudge, **Pillsbury** "Smooth and Creamy," 15.5-oz. box	1920	372.0			123.9	24.00		
Prepared as package directs, with butter	2160	372.0	180	31.0	(130.9)	(22.55)	(1080)	(186.0)
Chocolate Nut, **Betty Crocker** "Creamy Deluxe," Ready To Spread, 16½-oz. can	2040	288.0	170	24.0	123.6	17.45	(1162)	(164.0)
Dark Chocolate Fudge, **Betty Crocker** "Creamy Frosting," Dry Mix, 15.4-oz. box	1800	360.0			116.9	23.38		
Prepared as package directs, with butter	2040	360.0	170	30.0			(1166)	(180.0)
Milk Chocolate, **Betty Crocker** "Creamy Deluxe," Ready To Spread, 16½-oz. can	2040	312.0	170	26.0	123.6	18.91	(1020)	(156.0)
Milk Chocolate, **Betty Crocker** "Creamy Frosting," Dry Mix, 15.4-oz. box	1800	360.0			116.9	23.38		
Prepared as package directs, with butter	2040	360.0	170	30.0			(1020)	(180.0)
Milk Chocolate, **Hershey's,** Ready To Spread, 16½-oz. can	1920	288.0	160	24.0	116.4	17.45	(950)	(142.4)
Milk Chocolate, **Pillsbury** "Frosting Supreme," Ready To Spread, 16.5-oz. box	1920	300.0	160	25.0	116.4	18.18	(960)	(150.0)
Milk Chocolate, **Pillsbury** "Rich and Easy," Dry Mix, 15.1-oz. box	2040	348.0			136.1	23.05		
Prepared as package directs	2040	348.0	170	29.0			(1020)	(174.0)
Milk Chocolate, **Pillsbury** "Smooth and Creamy," 15.5-oz. box	1920	360.0			123.9	23.23		
Prepared as package directs, with butter	2280	360.0	190	30.0	(138.2)	(21.82)	(1140)	(180.0)
Sour Cream Chocolate, **Betty Crocker** "Creamy Deluxe," Ready To Spread, 16½-oz. can	2040	300.0	170	25.0	123.6	18.18	(1020)	(150.0)
Sour Cream Chocolate Fudge, **Betty Crocker** "Creamy Frosting," Dry Mix, 15.4-oz. box	1800	360.0			116.9	23.38		
Prepared as package directs, with butter	2040	360.0	170	30.0	123.6	21.82	(907)	(160.0)
CHOCOLATE CHIP								
Chocolate Chip, **Betty Crocker** "Creamy Deluxe," Ready To Spread, 16½-oz. can	2040	324.0	170	27.0	123.6	19.64	(1020)	(162.0)
COCONUT								
Coconut Almond, **Pillsbury** "Frosting Supreme," Ready To Spread, 15-oz. can	1800	204.0	150	17.0	120.0	13.60	(900)	(102.0)
Coconut Almond, **Pillsbury** "Smooth and Creamy," Dry Mix, 9.9-oz. box	1440	192.0			145.5	19.39		
Prepared as package directs, with butter	2040	204.0	170	17.0			(1020)	(102.0)
Coconut Pecan, **Betty Crocker** "Creamy Frosting," Dry Mix. 9.9-oz. box	1320	216.0			133.3	21.82		
Prepared as package directs, with butter and milk	1680	216.0	140.0	18.0			(960)	(123.4)
Coconut Pecan, **Pillsbury** "Frosting Supreme," Ready To Spread, 15-oz. can	1920	204.0	160	17.0	128.0	13.60	(920)	(102.0)
Coconut Pecan, **Pillsbury** "Smooth and Creamy," Dry Mix, 9.9-oz. box	1320	228.0			133.3	23.03		
Prepared as package directs, with butter	1800	240.0	150	20.0			(900)	(120.0)
CREAM CHEESE								
Cream Cheese, **Betty Crocker** "Creamy Deluxe," Ready To Spread, 16.5-oz. can	1920	324.0	160	27.0	116.4	19.64	(920)	(162.0)
Cream Cheese, **Pillsbury** "Frosting Supreme," Ready To Spread, 16.5-oz. can	1920	324.0	160	27.0	116.4	19.64	(920)	(162.0)
DECORATOR ICING								
Decorator Icing, **Pillsbury**								
Blue, 4½-oz. container	560	96.0			124.4	21.33	1120	192.0
1 tablespoon (approx. 0.6 oz.)	70	12.0			124.4	21.33	1120	192.0
Green, 4½-oz. container	560	96.0			124.4	21.33	1120	192.0
1 tablespoon (approx. 0.6 oz.)	70	12.0			124.4	21.33	1120	192.0
Pink, 4½-oz. container	560	96.0			124.4	21.33	1120	192.0
1 tablespoon (approx. 0.6 oz.)	70	12.0			124.4	21.33	1120	192.0
Yellow, 4½-oz. container	560	96.0			124.4	21.33	1120	192.0
1 tablespoon (approx. 0.6 oz.)	70	12.0			124.4	21.33	1120	192.0
DUTCH								
Dark Dutch, **Betty Crocker** "Creamy Deluxe," Ready To Spread, 16½-oz. box	1920	288.0	160	24.0	116.4	17.45	(1097)	(164.6)
Double Dutch, **Pillsbury** "Frosting Supreme," Ready To Spread, 16.5-oz. can	1920	288.0	160	24.0	116.4	17.45	(1097)	(164.6)
Double Dutch, **Pillsbury** "Rich and Easy," Dry Mix, 15.1-oz. box	2040	360.0			135.1	23.84		
Prepared as package directs	2040	360.0	170	30.0			(1020)	(180.0)
FUDGE								
Fudge Frosting, **Jiffy,** Dry Mix, 7½-oz. box	942	172.0			125.6	22.93		
Prepared as package directs	942	172.0	79	14.3	(110.8)	(20.24)	(1005)	(183.5)
LEMON								
Lemon, **Pillsbury** "Frosting Supreme," Ready To Spread, 16.5-oz. can	1920	324.0	160	27.0	116.4	19.64	(960)	(162.0)
Lemon, **Pillsbury** "Rich and Easy," Dry Mix, 15.1-oz. box	2040	360.0			135.1	23.84		
Prepared as package directs	2040	360.0	170	30.0			(1020)	(180.0)
Sunkist Lemon, **Betty Crocker** "Creamy Deluxe," Ready To Spread, 16½-oz. can	2040	336.0	170	28.0	123.6	20.36	(1020)	(168.0)
Sunkist Lemon, **Betty Crocker** "Creamy Frosting," Dry Mix, 15.4-oz. box	1800	360.0			116.9	23.38		
Prepared as package directs, with butter	2040	360.0	170	30.0	123.6	21.82	(1020)	(180.0)
ORANGE								
Orange, **Betty Crocker** "Creamy Deluxe," Ready To Spread, 16½-oz. can	2040	336.0	170	28.0	123.6	20.36	(1020)	(168.0)
PEANUT BUTTER								
Peanut Butter Creme, **Hershey's** Ready To Spread, 16½-oz. can	1920	264.0	160	22.0	116.4	16.00	(950)	(132.0)
SOUR CREAM								
Sour Cream Chocolate, **Betty Crocker** "Creamy Deluxe," Ready To Spread, 16½-oz. can	2040	300.0	170	25.0	123.6	18.18	(1020)	(150.0)
Sour Cream Chocolate Fudge **Betty Crocker** "Creamy Frosting," Dry Mix, 15.4-oz. box	1800	360.0			116.9	23.38		
Prepared as package directs, with butter	2040	360.0	170	30.0	(123.6)	(21.82)	(1020)	(180.0)
Sour Cream Vanilla, **Pillsbury** "Frosting Supreme," Ready To Spread, 16.5-oz. can	1920	324.0	160	27.0	116.4	19.64	(960)	(144.0)

	UNIT		FROSTING FOR 1 SLICE, 1/12 OF CAKE		1 OZ., BY WT.		1 CUP	
	Cal.	Carb.	Cal.	Carb.	Cal.	Carb.	Cal.	Carb.
Sour Cream White, **Betty Crocker** "Creamy Deluxe," Ready To Spread, 16½-oz. can	1920	324.0	160	27.0	116.4	19.64	(960)	(162.0)
Sour Cream White, **Betty Crocker** "Creamy Frosting," Dry Mix, 15.4-oz. box	1800	372.0			116.9	24.16		
Prepared as package directs, with butter	2160	372.0	180	31.0	(130.9)	(22.55)	(1080)	(186.0)
STRAWBERRY								
Strawberry, **Pillsbury** "Frosting Supreme," Ready To Spread, 16.5-oz. can	1920	324.0	160	27.0	116.4	19.64	(960)	(102.0)
Strawberry, **Pillsbury** "Rich and Easy," Dry Mix, 15.1-oz. box	2040	348.0			135.1	23.05		
Prepared as package directs	2040	348.0	170	29.0			(1020)	(174.0)
Strawberry, **Pillsbury** "Smooth and Creamy," 15.5-oz. box	1920	396.0	160	33.0	123.9	25.55		
Prepared as package directs, with butter	2160	396.0	180	33.0	(130.9)	(24.00)	(1080)	(198.0)
VANILLA								
Sour Cream Vanilla, **Pillsbury** "Frosting Supreme," Ready To Spread, 16.5-oz. can	1920	324.0	160	27.0	116.4	19.64	(960)	(144.0)
Vanilla, **Betty Crocker** "Creamy Deluxe," Ready To Spread, 16½-oz. can	2040	336.0	170	28.0	123.6	20.36	(1020)	(168.0)
Vanilla, **Hershey's** Ready To Spread, 16½-oz. can	2040	300.0	170	25.0	123.8	18.18	(1020)	(150.0)
Vanilla, **Pillsbury** "Frosting Supreme," Ready To Spread, 16.5-oz. can	2040	336.0	170	28.0	123.6	20.36	(1020)	(168.0)
Vanilla, **Pillsbury** "Rich and Easy," Dry Mix, 15.1-oz. box	2040	348.0			135.1	23.05		
Prepared as package directs	2040	348.0	170	29.0			(1020)	(174.0)
Vanilla, **Pillsbury** "Smooth and Creamy," 15.5-oz. box	1920	396.0	160	33.0	123.9	25.55		
Prepared as package directs, with butter	2160	396.0	180	33.0	(130.9)	(24.00)	(1080)	(198.0)
WHITE								
Creamy White, **Ann Page (A&P),** Ready To Spread, 16½-oz. can	1920	300.0	160	25.0	116.4	18.18	(960)	(150.0)
Creamy White, **Betty Crocker** "Creamy Frosting," Dry Mix, 15.4-oz. box	1800	372.0			116.9	24.16		
Prepared as package directs, with butter	2160	372.0	180	31.0	(130.9)	(22.55)	(1080)	(186.0)
Fluffy White, **Betty Crocker** "Fluffy Frosting," Dry Mix, 7.2-oz. box	720	192.0			100.0	26.67		
Prepared as package directs	720	192.0	60	16.0			(360)	(96.0)
Fluffy White, **Pillsbury,** Dry Mix, 7.2-oz. box	840	204.0			116.7	28.33		
Prepared as package directs	840	204.0	70	17.0			(1120)	(260.0)
Sour Cream White, **Betty Crocker** "Creamy Deluxe," Ready To Spread, 16½-oz. can	1920	324.0	160	27.0	116.4	19.64	(960)	(162.0)
Sour Cream White, **Betty Crocker** "Creamy Frosting," Dry Mix, 15.4-oz. box	1800	372.0			116.9	24.16		
Prepared as package directs, with butter	2160	372.0	180	31.0	(130.9)	(22.55)	(1080)	(1860)
White, **Jiffy,** Dry Mix, 7½-oz. box	950	177.0			126.7	23.66		
Prepared as package directs (for a 1-layer cake)	950	177.0	79	14.8	111.8	20.82	(1014)	(188.8)
White, Sugar Restricted, **Sweet 'N Low,** Frosting Mix, 7-oz. box	1200	120.0			171.4	17.14		
Prepared as package directs, with water	1200	120.0	100	10.0	(130.4)	(13.04)	900	90.0

22 PIES •

PIES MADE FROM SCRATCH, based on USDA home recipes

	UNIT Cal.	UNIT Carb.	1 SLICE Cal.	1 SLICE Carb.	1 OZ., BY WT. Cal.	1 OZ., BY WT. Carb.
APPLE BROWN BETTY, prepared with 5⅓ cups apples, 3½ Tbsp. water, ½ cup sugar, ⅔ tsp. cinnamon, 3¾ cups soft breadcrumbs, 2 Tbsp. butter, ⅙ tsp. salt (yield: approx. 4¾ cups, or 36 oz.) (Loss of 10% applied for evaporation in cooking.) (tr/8g/1g/65%/43mg)	(1544)	(303.3)			42.9	8.43
1 cup (approx. 7.6 oz.)	325	63.9			42.9	8.43
1 slice, ⅙ of dish (approx. 6.0 oz.)			257	50.6	42.9	8.43
1 slice, ⅛ of dish (approx. 4.5 oz.)			193	37.9	42.9	8.43
APPLE PIE, 2-crust, with filling as follows: 3¼ cups sliced apples, ¾ cup sugar, ½ cup water, 1⅓ Tbsp. cornstarch, ⅛ tsp. salt, 1 tsp. table fat (yield: approx. 33⅓ oz., or 2 lbs. 1⅓ oz.) (Loss of 13% has been applied for evaporation in cooking.) (1g/11g/3g/48%/85mg)	2419	360.0			72.6	10.80
1 slice, ⅙ of pie (approx. 5.6 oz.)			404	60.2	72.6	10.80
1 slice, ⅛ of pie (approx. 4.2 oz.)			302	45.0	72.6	10.80
BANANA CUSTARD PIE, 1-crust, with filling as follows: 2 medium bananas, 2 medium eggs, ½ cup sugar, 1¾ cups milk, 2⅓ Tbsp. cornstarch (yield: approx. 32 oz., or 2 lbs.) (1g/9g/3g/54%/55mg)	2011	279.4			62.8	8.73
1 slice, ⅙ of pie (approx. 5.3 oz.)			336	46.7	62.8	8.73
1 slice, ⅛ of pie (approx. 4.0 oz.)			252	35.0	62.8	8.73
BLACKBERRY PIE, 2-crust, with filling as follows: 2½ cups canned blackberries (canned in water), 2 tsp. lemon juice, 9 Tbsp. sugar (½ cup plus 1 Tbsp.), 2⅓ Tbsp. cornstarch (yield: approx. 33⅓ oz., or 2 lbs. 1⅓ oz.) (Loss of 13% has been applied for evaporation in cooking.) (1g/10g/3g/51%/76mg)	2296	325.1			68.9	9.75
1 slice, ⅙ of pie (approx. 5.6 oz.)			384	54.4	68.9	9.75
1 slice, ⅛ of pie (approx. 4.2 oz.)			287	40.6	68.9	9.75
BLUEBERRY PIE, 2-crust, with filling as follows: 2½ cups canned blueberries (canned in water), 2 tsp. lemon juice, 9 Tbsp. sugar (½ cup plus 1 Tbsp.), 2⅓ Tbsps. cornstarch (yield: approx. 33⅓ oz., or 2 lbs. 1⅓ oz.) (Loss of 13% has been applied for evaporation in cooking.) (1g/10g/3g/51%/76mg)	2287	329.8			68.6	9.89
1 slice, ⅙ of pie (approx. 5.6 oz.)			382	55.1	68.6	9.89
1 slice, ⅛ of pie (approx. 4.2 oz.)			286	42.1	68.6	9.89
BOSTON CREAM PIE, see the CAKES chapter (Boston Cream Pie is a cake!)						
BUTTERSCOTCH PIE, 1-crust, with filling as follows: 2 large egg yolks, 1 cup brown sugar, 2 cups milk, ¾ cup water, ½ cup flour, 2 Tbsp. table fat (yield: approx. 32 oz., or 2 lbs.) (1g/11g/4g/45%/61mg)	2430	348.5			75.9	10.89
1 slice, ⅙ of pie (approx. 5.3 oz.)			406	58.2	75.9	10.89
1 slice, ⅛ of pie (approx. 4.0 oz.)			304	43.7	75.9	10.89
CHERRY PIE, 2-crust, with filling as follows: 2⅓ cups canned cherries (packed in water), 11⅓ Tbsp. sugar (¾ cup less ⅔ Tbsp.), 2⅔ tsp. cornstarch, ⅛ tsp. salt, ½ Tbsp. table fat (yield: approx. 33⅓ oz., or 2 lbs. 1⅓ oz.) (Loss of 13% has been applied for evaporation in cooking.) (1g/11g/3g/47%/86mg)	2466	362.9			74.0	10.88
1 slice, ⅙ of pie (approx. 5.6 oz.)			412	60.7	74.0	10.88
1 slice, ⅛ of pie (approx. 4.2 oz.)			308	45.3	74.0	10.88
CHOCOLATE CHIFFON PIE, 1-crust, with filling as follows: 4 medium eggs, 15 Tbsp. sugar (1 cup less 1 Tbsp.), ¾ cup water, 1 Tbsp. gelatin, 1½ oz. bitter chocolate, ¼ tsp. vanilla (yield: approx. 22.9 oz.) (Loss of 20% has been applied for evaporation in cooking.) (2g/12g/4g/33%/71mg)	2125	283.2			92.8	12.37
1 slice, ⅙ of pie (approx. 3.8 oz.)			354	47.2	92.8	12.37
1 slice, ⅛ of pie (approx. 2.9 oz.)			266	35.4	92.8	12.37
CHOCOLATE MERINGUE PIE, 1-crust, with filling as follows: 2 medium egg yolks, ¾ cup sugar, 2 cups milk, 1 Tbsp. water, 2 oz. bitter chocolate, 3 Tbsp. flour, ¼ tsp. salt, 1 tsp. vanilla; and with meringue as follows: 2 medium egg whites, ¼ cup sugar (yield: approx. 32 oz., or 2 lbs.) (Loss of 5% has been applied for evaporation in cooking.) (1g/10g/3g/48%/73mg)	2293	304.9			71.7	9.53
1 slice, ⅙ of pie (approx. 5.3 oz.)			383	50.9	71.7	9.53
1 slice, ⅛ of pie (approx. 4.0 oz.)			287	38.2	71.7	9.53
COCONUT CUSTARD PIE, 1-crust, with filling as follows: 1¼ oz. sweetened dried coconut, 3 large eggs, 7 Tbsp. sugar (½ cup less 1 Tbsp.), 2½ cups milk, 1⅔ Tbsp. cornstarch, ⅛ tsp. salt, 1¾ tsp. vanilla (yield: approx. 32 oz., or 2 lbs.) (Loss of 20% has been applied for evaporation in cooking.) (2g/7g/4g/55%/70mg)	2139	226.6			66.8	7.08
1 slice, ⅙ of pie (approx. 5.3 oz.)			357	37.8	66.8	7.08
1 slice, ⅛ of pie (approx. 4.0 oz.)			268	28.4	66.8	7.08
CUSTARD PIE, 1-crust, with filling as follows: 3 large eggs, 7 Tbsp. sugar (½ cup less 1 Tbsp.), 2⅝ cups milk, 1⅔ Tbsp. cornstarch, ⅓ tsp. salt, 1¾ tsp. vanilla (yield: approx. 32 oz., or 2 lbs.) (Loss of 20% has been applied for evaporation in cooking.) (2g/7g/3g/58%/81mg)	1984	212.9			62.0	6.65
1 slice, ⅙ of pie (approx. 5.3 oz.)			331	35.6	62.0	6.65
1 slice, ⅛ of pie (approx. 4.0 oz.)			249	26.7	62.0	6.65
LEMON CHIFFON PIE, 1-crust, with filling as follows: 5⅓ Tbsp. lemon juice, ½ tsp. grated lemon rind, 5 medium eggs, 1 cup sugar, 6 Tbsp. water, 1 Tbsp. gelatin, 1 tsp. cornstarch (yield: approx. 22.9 oz.) (Loss of 20% has been applied for evaporation in cooking.) (2g/12g/4g/36%/74mg)	2028	283.8			88.6	12.39
1 slice, ⅙ of pie (approx. 3.8 oz.)			338	47.3	88.6	12.39
1 slice, ⅛ of pie (approx. 2.9 oz.)			254	35.5	88.6	12.39

	UNIT Cal.	UNIT Carb.	1 SLICE Cal.	1 SLICE Carb.	1 OZ., BY WT. Cal.	1 OZ., BY WT. Carb.
LEMON MERINGUE PIE, 1-crust, with filling as follows: ¼ cup lemon juice, 3 large egg yolks, ¾ cup sugar, 1½ cups water, 4 Tbsp. cornstarch, ¼ tsp. salt, 1 Tbsp. butter; and with meringue as follows: 3 large egg whites, ¼ cup sugar (yield: approx. 29.6 oz.) (Loss of 20% has been applied for evaporation in cooking.) (1g/11g/3g/47%/80mg)	2142	316.7			72.4	10.70
1 slice, ⅙ of pie (approx. 4.9 oz.)			357	52.8	72.4	10.70
1 slice, ⅛ of pie (approx. 3.7 oz.)			268	39.6	72.4	10.70
MINCE PIE, 2-crust, with filling as follows: ½ cup sulfured dehydrated apples, ⅔ cup seeded or ⅝ cup seedless raisins, ½ Tbsp. grated lemon peel, ½ Tbsp. grated orange peel, ½ cup brown sugar, 1¾ cup water, 1⅓ tsp. vinegar, 2 tsp. flour, 2¼ teaspoon molasses, 1¾ tsp. spices, ¼ oz. suet, ⅔ tsp. salt (yield: approx. 33⅓ oz., or 2 lbs. 1⅓ oz.) (Loss of 11% has been applied for evaporation in cooking. This includes the loss of evaporation for preliminary cooking of filling.) (1g/12g/3g/43%/127mg)	2561	389.3			76.8	11.68
1 slice, ⅙ of pie (approx. 5.6 oz.)			428	65.1	76.8	11.68
1 slice, ⅛ of pie (approx. 4.2 oz.)			320	48.6	76.8	11.68
PEACH PIE, 2-crust, with filling as follows: 3½ cups sliced peaches (approx. 5¾ medium peaches), 11½ Tbsp. sugar (¾ cup less ½ Tbsp.), 2⅔ Tbsp. cornstarch (yield: approx. 33⅓ oz., or 2 lbs. 1⅓ oz.) (Loss of 13% has been applied for evaporation in cooking.) (1g/11g/3g/48%/76mg)	2410	361.0			72.3	10.83
1 slice, ⅙ of pie (approx. 5.6 oz.)			403	60.4	72.3	10.83
1 slice, ⅛ of pie (approx. 4.2 oz.)			301	45.1	72.3	10.83
PECAN PIE, 1-crust, with filling as follows: 1½ cups pecans, 2 large eggs, 4 tsp. sugar, 2⅓ Tbsp. water, 1⅓ Tbsp. flour, 19 Tbsp. corn syrup (1 cup plus 3 Tbsp. (yield: approx. 29.1 oz.) (Loss of 11% has been applied for evaporation in cooking.) (1g/15g/6g/20%/63mg)	3449	423.2			118.5	14.54
1 slice, ⅙ of pie (approx. 4.9 oz.)			577	70.8	118.5	14.54
1 slice, ⅛ of pie (approx. 3.6 oz.)			431	52.8	118.5	14.54
PINEAPPLE PIE, 2-crust, with filling as follows: 1¾ cups canned crushed pineapple (light-syrup pack), ½ cup sugar, 9 Tbsp. water, 2⅓ Tbsp. corn syrup, 2 Tbsp. cornstarch (yield: approx. 32 oz., or 2 lbs.) (Loss of 13% has been applied for evaporation in cooking. This includes the loss of evaporation for preliminary cooking of filling.) (1g/11g/3g/48%/77mg)	2391	360.0			72.3	10.88
1 slice, ⅙ of pie (approx. 5.3 oz.)			400	60.2	72.3	10.88
1 slice, ⅛ of pie (approx. 4.0 oz.)			299	45.0	72.3	10.88
PINEAPPLE CHIFFON PIE, 1-crust, with filling as follows: 11 Tbsp. unsweetened canned pineapple juice (¾ cup less 1 Tbsp.), 4 medium eggs, ¾ cup sugar, 4½ Tbsp. water, 1 Tbsp. gelatin (yield: approx. 22.9 oz.) (Loss of 20% has been applied for evaporation in cooking.) (2g/11g/3g/41%/73mg)	1866	253.4			82.3	11.09
1 slice, ⅙ of pie (approx. 3.8 oz.)			311	42.2	82.3	11.09
1 slice, ⅛ of pie (approx. 2.9 oz.)			233	31.7	82.3	11.09
PUMPKIN PIE, 1-crust, with filling as follows: 1½ cups canned pumpkin, 2 large eggs, ½ cup sugar, 1 cup milk, 2 Tbsp. table fat, 2¼ tsp. spices (yield: approx. 32 oz., or 2 lbs.) (Loss of 11% has been applied for evaporation in cooking.) (1g/7g/3g/59%/61mg)	1920	223.0			60.0	6.97
1 slice, ⅙ of pie (approx. 5.3 oz.)			321	37.2	60.0	6.97
1 slice, ⅛ of pie (approx. 4.0 oz.)			241	27.9	60.0	6.97
RAISIN PIE, 2-crust, with filling as follows: 1½ cups seeded or 1¼ cups seedless raisins, 1 Tbsp. lemon juice, ½ cup sugar, 1⅞ cups water, 1 Tbsp. cornstarch, dash salt (yield: approx. 33⅓ oz., or 2 lbs. 1⅓ oz.) (Loss of 16% has been applied for evaporation in cooking. This includes the loss of evaporation for preliminary cooking of filling.) (1g/13g/3g/43%/81mg)	2552	406.4			76.6	12.79
1 slice, ⅙ of pie (approx. 5.6 oz.)			427	67.9	76.6	12.79
1 slice, ⅛ of pie (approx. 4.2 oz.)			319	50.7	76.6	12.79
RHUBARB PIE, 2-crust, with filling as follows: 2½ cups (or 21 oz.) frozen rhubarb, 7 Tbsp. sugar, 2⅓ Tbsp. water, 2½ Tbsp. cornstarch (yield: approx. 33⅓ oz., or 2 lbs. 1⅓ oz.) (Loss of 13% has been applied for evaporation in cooking.) (1g/11g/3g/47%/77mg)	2391	361.0			71.7	10.83
1 slice, ⅙ of pie (approx. 5.6 oz.)			400	60.4	71.7	10.83
1 slice, ⅛ of pie (approx. 4.2 oz.)			299	45.1	71.7	10.83
STRAWBERRY PIE, 1-crust, with filling as follows: 3 cups strawberries, 1 Tbsp. lemon juice, ½ cup sugar, 1½ Tbsp. cornstarch (yield: approx. 26.2 oz.) (Loss of 2% has been applied for evaporation in cooking.) (1g/9g/2g/58%/55mg)	1469	229.3			56.1	8.75
1 slice, ⅙ of pie (approx. 4.4 oz.)			246	38.3	56.1	8.75
1 slice, ⅛ of pie (approx. 3.3 oz.)			184	28.7	56.1	8.75
SWEET POTATO PIE, 1-crust, with filling as follows: 1½ cups riced boiled sweet potatoes, 2 tsp. lemon juice, 2 large eggs, ¼ cup sugar, 2 cups milk, 2 Tbsp. table fat, ½ tsp. spices (yield: approx. 32 oz., or 2 lbs.) (Loss of 11% has been applied for evaporation in cooking.) (1g/7g/3g/59%/62mg)	1938	215.7			60.6	6.74
1 slice, ⅙ of pie (approx. 5.3 oz.)			324	36.0	60.6	6.74
1 slice, ⅛ of pie (approx. 4.0 oz.)			243	27.0	60.6	6.74

PIE MIXES, by brand

	UNIT Cal.	UNIT Carb.	1 SLICE Cal.	1 SLICE Carb.	1 OZ., BY WT. Cal.	1 OZ., BY WT. Carb.
Bavarian Chocolate Cream Pie Mix (includes pie crust, filling, and whipped cream topping), **Betty Crocker** "International Desserts," 12.75-oz. box	1680	232.0			131.8	18.20
1 pie, prepared as package directs using whole milk (yield: approx. 21.2 oz.)	2000	248.0			94.3	11.70
1 "suggested" slice, ⅛ of pie (approx. 2.6 oz.)			250	31.0	94.3	11.70
1 pie, prepared as package directs using skim milk (yield: approx. 21.2 oz.)	1790	247.6			84.4	11.68
1 "suggested" slice, ⅛ of pie (approx. 2.6 oz.)			219.4	30.4	84.4	11.68
Bavarian Cream Pie Mix (includes pie crust, filling, and apple topping), **Betty Crocker** "International Desserts," 16.8-oz. box	1920	296.0			114.3	17.62
1 pie, prepared as package directs using whole milk (yield: approx. 25.2 oz.)	2080	312.0			82.5	12.38
1 "suggested" slice, ⅛ of pie (approx. 3.2 oz.)			260	39.0	82.5	12.38
1 pie, prepared as package directs using skim milk (yield: approx. 25.2 oz.)	2034	312.2			80.7	12.39
1 "suggested" slice, ⅛ of pie (approx. 3.2 oz.)			258	39.6	80.7	12.39

PREPACKAGED PIES

	UNIT Cal.	UNIT Carb.	1 SLICE Cal.	1 SLICE Carb.	1 OZ., BY WT. Cal.	1 OZ., BY WT. Carb.
APPLE						
Apple Pie, **Banquet,** 20-oz. pie	1440	213.2			72.0	10.66
Apple Pie, **Morton** "Great Little Desserts," 8-oz. pie	590	88.0			73.8	11.00
Apple Pie, **Morton** "Pastry Shop" Family-Pie, 24-oz. pie	1740	246.0			72.5	10.25
"Suggested" serving, ⅙ of pie (approx. 4 oz.)			290	41.0	72.5	10.25
Apple Pie, **Sara Lee,** 31-oz. pie	2418	301.2			78.0	9.72
"Suggested" serving, ⅙ of pie (approx. 5.2 oz.)			403	50.2	78.0	9.72
Dutch Apple Pie, **Morton** "Great Little Desserts," 7¾-oz. pie	600	94.0			77.4	13.13
Dutch Apple Pie, **Sara Lee,** 30-oz. pie	1956	304.8			65.2	10.16
"Suggested" serving, ⅙ of pie (approx. 5 oz.)			326	50.8	65.2	10.16
BANANA						
Banana Pie, **Banquet,** 14-oz. pie	1032	118.6			73.7	8.47
Banana Cream Pie, **Morton** "Great Little Desserts," 3½-oz. pie	250	27.0			71.4	7.71
Banana Cream Pie, **Morton** "Pastry Shop," 14-oz. pie	961	114.0			68.7	8.14
Banana Cream Pie, **Rich's** "Freeze Flo," 22-oz. pie	2080	264.0			94.5	12.00
"Suggested" serving, ⅛ of pie (approx. 2¾ oz.)			260	33.0	94.5	12.00
Banana Light Pie, **Mrs. Smith's,** 14-oz. pie	1340	164.4			95.7	11.74
BLUEBERRY						
Blueberry Pie, **Banquet,** 20-oz. pie	1520	225.1			76.0	11.26
Blueberry Pie, **Morton** "Great Little Desserts," 8-oz. pie	580	86.0			72.5	10.75
Blueberry Pie, **Morton** "Pastry Shop," Family-Pie, 24-oz. pie	1680	234.0			70.0	9.75
"Suggested" serving, ⅙ of pie (approx. 4 oz.)			280	39.0	70.0	9.75
Blueberry Pie, **Sara Lee,** 31-oz. pie	2292	304.8			73.9	9.83
"Suggested" serving, ⅙ of pie (approx. 5.16 oz.)			382	50.8	73.9	9.83
CHERRY						
Cherry Pie, **Banquet,** 20-oz. pie	1366	203.0			68.3	10.15
Cherry Pie, **Morton** "Great Little Desserts," 8-oz. pie	590	87.0			73.8	10.88

	UNIT Cal.	UNIT Carb.	1 SLICE Cal.	1 SLICE Carb.	1 OZ., BY WT. Cal.	1 OZ., BY WT. Carb.
Cherry Pie, **Morton** "Pastry Shop" Family-Pie, 24-oz. pie	1800	252.0			75.0	10.50
"Suggested" serving, ⅙ of pie (approx. 4 oz.)			300	42.0	75.0	10.50
Cherry Pie, **Sara Lee,** 31-oz. pie	2112	278.4			68.1	8.98
"Suggested" serving, ⅙ of pie (approx. 5.16 oz.)			352	46.4	68.1	8.98
CHOCOLATE						
Chocolate Cream Pie, **Banquet,** 14-oz. pie	1064	131.0			76.0	9.36
Chocolate Cream Pie, **Morton** "Great Little Desserts," 3½-oz. pie	270	29.0			77.1	8.29
Chocolate Cream Pie, **Morton** "Pastry Shop," 14-oz. pie	1080	120.0			77.1	8.57
"Suggested" serving, ⅙ of pie, approx. 2.3 oz.			180	20.0	77.1	8.57
Chocolate Light Pie, **Mrs. Smith's,** 14-oz. pie	1522	188.7			108.7	13.48
"Suggested" serving, ⅙ of pie (approx. 2.3 oz.)			250	31.0	108.7	13.48
COCONUT						
Coconut Cream Pie, **Banquet,** 14-oz. pie	1044	114.7			74.6	8.19
Coconut Cream Pie, **Morton** "Great Little Desserts," 3½-oz. pie	270	25.0			77.1	7.14
Coconut Cream Pie, **Morton** "Pastry Shop," 14-oz. pie	1020	102.0			72.9	7.29
"Suggested" serving, ⅙ of pie (approx. 2.3 oz.)			170	38.7	72.9	10.50
Coconut Cream Pie, **Rich's** "Freeze Flo," 22-oz. pie	2080	232.0			94.5	10.50
"Suggested" serving, ⅛ of pie (approx. 2¾ oz.)			260	29.0	94.5	10.50
Coconut Custard Pie, **Banquet,** 20-oz. pie	1219	196.5			61.0	9.83
Coconut Custard Pie, **Morton** "Great Little Desserts," 6½-oz. pie	370	53.0			56.9	8.15
Coconut Light Pie, **Mrs. Smith's,** 14-oz. pie	1400	170.4			100.0	12.17
"Suggested" serving, ⅙ of pie (approx. 2.3 oz.)			230	28.0	100.0	12.17
CUSTARD						
Custard Pie, frozen, **Banquet,** 20-oz. pie	1236	190.5			61.8	9.53
Honey Carrot Raisin Custard Pie (no cane sugar), **Salaam,** 20-oz. pie	1800	205.0			90.0	10.25
"Suggested" serving, ⅕ of pie (approx. 4 oz.)			360	41.0	90.0	10.25
LEMON						
Lemon Cream Pie, **Banquet,** 14-oz. pie	1008	131.0			72.0	9.36
Lemon Cream Pie, **Rich's,** "Freeze Flo," 22-oz. pie	2000	240.0			90.9	10.90
"Suggested" serving, ⅛ of pie (approx. 2¾ oz.)			250	30.0	90.9	10.90
Lemon Cream Pie, **Morton** "Great Little Desserts," 3½-oz. pie	250	27.0			71.4	7.71
Lemon Cream Pie, **Morton** "Pastry Shop," 14-oz. pie	960	108.0			68.6	7.71
"Suggested" serving, ⅙ of pie (approx. 2.3 oz.)			160	18.0	68.6	7.71
Lemon Yogurt Pie, **Mrs. Smith's,** 16-oz. (1-lb.) pie	1230	166.1			76.9	10.38
1 serving, ⅙ of pie, approx. 2.6 oz.			200	27.0	76.9	10.38
MINCE						
Mince Pie, **Morton** "Pastry Shop" Family-Pie, 24 oz.	1860	276.0			77.5	11.50
"Suggested" serving, ⅙ of pie (approx. 4 oz.)			310	46.0	77.5	11.50
Mincemeat Pie, **Banquet,** 20-oz. pie	1514	230.8			75.7	11.54
PEACH						
Peach Pie, **Banquet,** 20-oz. pie	1315	179.2			65.8	8.96
Peach Pie, **Morton** "Great Little Desserts," 8-oz. pie	590	91.0			73.8	11.38
Peach Pie, **Morton** "Pastry Shop" Family-Pie, 24-oz. pie	1680	234.0			70.0	9.75
"Suggested" serving, ⅙ of pie (approx. 4 oz.)			280	39.0	70.0	9.75
Peach Pie, **Sara Lee,** 31-oz. pie	2364	325.2			76.3	10.49
"Suggested" serving, ⅙ of pie (approx. 5.16 oz.)			394	54.2	76.3	10.49
PECAN						
Pecan Pie, **Frito-Lay,** 3-oz. pie	353	53.5			117.7	17.83
Pecan Pie, **Morton** "Pastry Shop" Family-Pie, 16-oz. (1-lb.) pie	(1896)	(237.8)			(118.5)	(14.86)
PUMPKIN						
Pumpkin Pie, **Banquet,** 20-oz. pie	1236	193.9			61.8	9.70
Pumpkin Pie, **Morton** "Pastry Shop," Family-Pie, 24-oz. pie	1380	216.0			57.5	9.00
"Suggested" serving, ⅙ of pie (approx. 4 oz.)			230	36.0	57.5	9.00

	UNIT Cal.	UNIT Carb.	1 SLICE Cal.	1 SLICE Carb.	1 OZ., BY WT. Cal.	1 OZ., BY WT. Carb.
STRAWBERRY						
Strawberry Cream Pie, **Banquet,** 14-oz. pie	1016	135.2			72.6	9.66
Strawberry Yogurt Pie, **Mrs. Smith's,** 16-oz. (1-lb.) pie	1230	153.9			76.9	9.62
"Suggested" serving, ⅙ of pie (approx. 2.6 oz.)			200	25.0	76.9	9.62

PREPACKAGED SNACK PIES

	UNIT Cal.	UNIT Carb.	ONE PASTRY Cal.	ONE PASTRY Carb.	1 OZ., BY WT. Cal.	1 OZ., BY WT. Carb.
APPLE						
Apple Fruit Pie, **Hostess,** 4½-oz. package (1 pie)	400	54.0	400	54.0	88.9	12.00
Apple Pie, **Tastykake,** 4-oz. package (1 pie)	348		348		87.0	
Apple Pie Tarts, **Pepperidge Farm,** 11½-oz. box (4 tarts)	1120	132.0			97.4	11.48
1 tart, approx. 2.88 oz.			280	33.0	97.4	11.48
French Apple Pie, **Tastykake,** 4.25-oz. package (1 pie)	405		405		95.4	
BERRY						
Berry Fruit Pie, **Hostess,** 4½-oz. package (1 pie)	400	51.0	400	51.0	88.9	11.33
BLUEBERRY						
Blueberry Fruit Pie, **Hostess,** 4½-oz. package (1 pie)	390	49.0	390	49.0	86.7	10.89
Blueberry Pie, **Tastykake,** 4-oz. package (1 pie)	366		366		91.5	
Blueberry Pie Tarts, **Pepperidge Farm,** 11½-oz. box (4 tarts)	1120	140.0			97.4	12.17
1 tart, approx. 2.88 oz.			280	35.0	97.4	12.17
CHERRY						
Cherry Fruit Pie, **Hostess,** 4½-oz. package (1 pie)	420	59.0	420	59.0	93.3	13.11
Cherry Pies, **Drakes,** 16-oz. (1-lb.) box (8 pies)	1600	224.0			100.0	14.00
1 pie, approx. 2 oz.			200	28.0	100.0	14.00
Cherry Pie, **Tastykake,** 4-oz. package (1 pie)	381		381		95.3	
Cherry Pie Tarts, **Pepperidge Farm,** 11½-oz. box (4 tarts)	1120	140.0			97.4	12.17
1 tart, approx. 2.88 oz.			280	35.0	97.4	12.17
LEMON						
Lemon Fruit Pie, **Hostess,** 4½-oz. package (1 pie)	420	53.0	420	53.0	93.3	11.78
Lemon Pie, **Tastykake,** 4-oz. package (1 pie)	370		370		92.5	
Lemon Pie Tarts, **Pepperidge Farm,** 11½-oz. box (4 tarts)	1280	148.0			111.3	12.87
1 tart, approx. 2.88 oz.			320	37.0	111.3	12.87
OATMEAL						
Oatmeal Creme Pies, **Little Debbie,** 16-oz. (1-lb.) box (12 pies)	2059	286.4			128.7	17.90
1 pie, approx. 1.34 oz.			172	23.9	128.7	17.90
PEACH						
Peach Fruit Pie, **Hostess,** 4½-oz. package (1 pie)	400	53.0	400	53.0	88.9	11.78
Peach Pie, **Tastykake,** 4-oz. package (1 pie)	349		349		87.3	
PECAN						
Pecan Pie, **Frito-Lay,** 3-oz. package (1 pie)	353	53.5	353	53.3	117.7	17.83
RAISIN						
Raisin Creme Pies, **Little Debbie,** 14-oz. package (12 pies)	1767	255.8			126.2	18.27
1 pie, approx. 1.16 oz.			147	21.3	126.2	18.27
RASPBERRY						
Raspberry Pie Tarts, **Pepperidge Farm,** 11½-oz. box (4 tarts)	1280	136.0			111.3	11.83
1 tart, approx. 2.88 oz.			320	34.0	111.3	11.83

PIE CRUSTS AND OTHER PASTRY SHELLS

PIE CRUSTS MADE FROM SCRATCH, based on USDA home recipes

(Made with enriched or unenriched flour. Enriching flour does not affect the calorie or carbohydrate values.)

	UNIT Cal.	UNIT Carb.	CRUST FOR 1 SLICE Cal.	CRUST FOR 1 SLICE Carb.	1 OZ., BY WT. Cal.	1 OZ., BY WT. Carb.
Pie Crust for 2-crust pie: Made with 1 cup flour, 2 Tbsp. cooking fat, 2 Tbsp. water, ½ tsp. salt: Unbaked, approx. 6.8 oz. (2g/12g/9g/21%/161mg)	900	78.8			131.6	11.55

	UNIT Cal.	UNIT Carb.	CRUST FOR 1 SLICE Cal.	CRUST FOR 1 SLICE Carb.	1 OZ., BY WT. Cal.	1 OZ., BY WT. Carb.
Baked (yield: crust for 1-crust pie, approx. 6.4 oz.) (loss of approximately 7% has been applied for evaporation in baking) (2g/12g/9g/15%/173mg)	900	78.8			142.8	12.50
Crust for 1/6 of pie (approx. 1.1 oz.)			150	13.1	142.8	12.50
Crust for 1/8 of pie (approx. 0.8 oz.)			113	9.9	142.8	12.50
Pie crust for 2-crust pie: Made from mix (including stick form).						
1 package, 10 oz. net wt. (2g/14g/9g/9%/196mg)	1482	140.6			148.2	14.06
1 cup dry mix, not packed (approx. 4.2 oz.)	626	59.4			148.2	14.06
Packed (approx. 6.9 oz.)	1018	96.5			148.2	14.06
Entire package prepared as package directs (yield: crust for 2-crust pie, approx. 11.3 oz. baked)	1485	140.8			131.4	12.46
Crust for 1/6 of pie (approx. 1.9 oz.)			248	23.5	131.4	12.46
Crust for 1/8 of pie (approx. 1.4 oz.)			186	17.6	131.4	12.46
PIE CRUST MIXES						
Pie Crust Mix, **Bisquick,** 11-oz. box	1920	160.0			174.6	14.54
Prepared as package directs (yield: crust for one 9" 2-crust pie, approx. 13 oz. of crust)	1920	160.0			(147.7)	(12.31)
22-oz. box	3820	320.0			174.6	14.54
Prepared as package directs (yield: crust for two 9" 2-crust pies, approx. 26 oz. of crust)	3820	320.0			(147.7)	(12.31)
Crust for 1/6 pie (approx. 2.2 oz.)			320	26.7	(147.7)	(12.31)
Crust for 1/8 pie (approx. 1.6 oz.)			240	20.0	(147.7)	(12.31)
Pie Crust Mix, **Flako,** 10-oz. box	1435	147.1			143.5	14.71
Prepared as package directs (yield: crust for one 9" 2-crust pie, approx. 12 oz. of crust)	1435	147.1			119.6	12.26
Crust for 1/6 of pie (approx. 2.0 oz.)			239	24.5	119.6	12.26
Crust for 1/8 of pie (approx. 1.5 oz.)			179	18.4	119.6	12.26
Pie Crust Mix, **Jiffy,** 9-oz. box	1288	132.8			143.1	14.76
Prepared as package directs (yield: crust for one 9" 2-crust pie, approx. 11 oz. of crust)	1288	132.8			117.1	12.07
Crust for 1/6 of pie (approx. 1.8 oz.)			215	22.1	117.1	12.07
Crust for 1/8 of pie (approx. 1.4 oz.)			161	16.6	117.1	12.07
Pie Crust Mix, **Pillsbury,** 11-oz. box	1740	162.0			158.2	14.73
Prepared as package directs (yield: crust for one 9" 2-crust pie, approx. 13 oz. of crust)	1740	162.0			133.8	12.46
Crust for 1/6 of pie (approx. 2.2 oz.)			290	27.0	133.8	12.46
Crust for 1/8 of pie (approx. 1.6 oz.)			218	20.3	133.8	12.46
Pie Crust Sticks, **Bisquick,** 11-oz. box	1920	160.0			174.6	14.54
Prepared as package directs (yield: crust for one 9" 2-crust pie, approx. 13 oz.)	1920	160.0			(147.7)	(12.31)
22-oz. box	3820	320.0			174.6	14.54
Prepared as package directs (yield: crust for two 9" 2-crust pies, approx. 26 oz. of crust)	3820	320.0			(147.7)	(12.31)
Crust for 1/6 of pie (approx. 2.2 oz.)			320	26.7	(147.7)	(12.31)
Crust for 1/8 of pie (approx. 1.6 oz.)			240	20.0	(147.7)	(12.31)
Pie Crust Sticks, **Pillsbury,** 11-oz. box, 2 sticks	1740	162.0			158.2	14.73
Prepared as package directs (yield: crust for one 9" 2-crust pie, approx. 11 oz. of crust)	1740	162.0			133.8	12.46
Crust for 1/6 of pie (approx. 1.8 oz.)			290	27.0	133.8	12.46
Crust for 1/8 of pie (approx. 1.4 oz.)			218	20.3	133.8	12.46
PREPACKAGED PIE CRUSTS AND OTHER PASTRY SHELLS						
Pastry Sheets, **Pepperidge Farm,** 17¼-oz. package (4 sheets)	2280	144.0			132.0	8.35
1 sheet, approx. 4.3 oz.	570	36.0			132.0	8.35
Patty Shells, **Pepperidge Farm,** 10-oz. package (6 shells)	1440	90.0			144.0	9.00
1 shell, approx. 1.7 oz.	240	15.0			144.0	9.00
Pie Shell Bottoms, **Pepperidge Farm,** deep bottom, 17¾-oz. package (2 shells)	1040	80.0			58.6	4.51
1 shell for 1-crust pie, approx. 8.63 oz.	520	40.0			58.6	4.51
"Suggested serving," ¼ pie shell (approx. 2.2 oz)			130	10.0	58.6	4.51
Shallow bottom, 14½-oz. package (2 shells)	880	72.0			60.7	4.97
1 shell, approx. 7.25 oz.	440	36.0			60.7	4.97
"Suggested serving," ¼ pie shell (approx. 1.8 oz.)			110	9.0	60.7	4.97
Tart Shells, **Pepperidge Farm,** 4-oz. package (6 shells)	540	60.0			135.0	15.00
1 shell, approx. ⅔ oz.	90	10.0			135.0	15.00

PIE FILLINGS, canned and dry

	UNIT Cal.	UNIT Carb.	FILLING FOR 1 SLICE Cal.	FILLING FOR 1 SLICE Carb.	1 OZ., BY WT. Cal.	1 OZ., BY WT. Carb.	1 CUP Cal.	1 CUP Carb.
APPLE								
Apple Pie Filling, **Wilderness,** 21-oz. can	660	180.0			31.4	8.57	(257)	(70.2)
Filling for 1 slice, 1/6 of pie (approx. 3.5 oz.)			110	30.0	31.4	8.57	(257)	(70.2)
French Apple Pie Filling, **Wilderness,** 21-oz. can	660	180.0			31.4	8.57	(257)	(70.2)
Filling for 1 slice, 1/6 of pie (approx. 3.5 oz.)			110	30.0	31.4	8.57	(257)	(70.2)
APRICOT								
Apricot Pie Filling, **Wilderness,** 21-oz. can	720	180.0			34.3	8.57	(281)	(70.2)
Filling for 1 slice, 1/6 of pie (approx. 3.5 oz.)			120	30.0	34.3	8.57	(281)	(70.2)
BANANA								
Banana Pudding & Pie Filling, **Jell-Well,** 3.25-oz. box	240	56.0			73.9	17.23		
As prepared for pie filling (yield: approx. 2 cups, 20.8 oz, or enough to fill an 8" pie shell)	560	80			(26.9)	(3.85)	280	40.0
Filling for 1 slice, 1/6 of pie (approx. 3.4 oz.)			93	13.3	(26.9)	(3.85)	280	40.0
Banana Pudding & Pie Filling, **Jell-Well Instant,** 3.75-oz. box	400	100.0			106.7	26.67		
As prepared for pie filling (yield: approx. 2 cups, 21.3 oz., or enough to fill an 8" pie shell)	720	124.0			(33.8)	(5.82)	360	62.0
Filling for 1 slice, 1/6 of pie (approx. 3.6 oz.)			120	20.7	(33.8)	(5.82)	360	62.0
Banana Pudding & Pie Filling, **Royal,** 3.0-oz. box	320	80.0			106.7	26.67		
As prepared for pie filling (yield: approx. 2 cups, 20.5 oz., or enough to fill an 8" pie shell)	640	104.0			(31.2)	(5.07)	320	52.0
Filling for 1 slice, 1/6 of pie (approx. 3.4 oz.)			107	17.3	31.2	5.07	320	54.0
Banana Pudding & Pie Filling, **Royal Instant,** 3½-oz. box	400	96.0			114.3	27.43		
As prepared for pie filling (yield: approx. 2 cups, 21.0 oz., or enough to fill an 8" pie shell)	720	120.0			(34.3)	(5.71)	360	60.0
Filling for 1 slice, 1/6 of pie (approx. 3.5 oz.)			120	20.0	(34.3)	(5.71)	360	60.0
Banana Cream Pudding & Pie Filling, **Ann Page (A&P),** 3¼-oz. box	360	88.0			110.8	27.08		
As prepared for pie filling (yield: approx. 2 cups, 20.8 oz., or enough to fill an 8" pie shell)	680	112.0			(32.7)	(5.38)	340	56.0
Filling for 1 slice, 1/6 of pie (approx. 3.5 oz.)			113	18.7	(32.7)	(5.38)	340	56.0
Banana Cream Pudding & Pie Filling, **Jell-O,** 3⅛-oz. box	360	84.0			115.0	26.84		
As prepared for pie filling (yield: approx. 2 cups, 20.6 oz., or enough to fill an 8" pie shell)	680	108.0			(33.0)	(5.24)	340	54.0
Filling for 1 slice, 1/6 of pie (approx. 3.4 oz.)			113	18.0	(33.0)	(5.24)	340	54.0
Banana Cream Pudding & Pie Filling, **Jell-O Instant,** 3¾-oz. box	400	100.0			106.7	26.67		
As prepared for pie filling (yield: approx. 2 cups, 21.3-oz., or enough to fill an 8" pie shell)	720	124.0			(33.8)	(5.82)	360	62.0
Filling for 1 slice, 1/6 of pie (approx. 3.6 oz.)			120	20.6	(33.8)	(5.82)	360	62.0
Banana Pudding & Pie Filling, **Jell-O Instant,** sugar free, 1.1 oz. box	120	28.0			109.1	25.45		
As prepared for pie filling (using low-fat milk) (yield: approx. 2 cups, 18.3 oz., or enough to fill an 8" pie shell)	362	51.4			(19.8)	(2.81	181	25.7
Filling for 1 slice, 1/6 of pie (approx. 3.1 oz.)			60	8.6	(19.8)	(2.81)	181	25.7

	UNIT		FILLING FOR 1 SLICE		1 OZ., BY WT.		1 CUP	
	Cal.	Carb.	Cal.	Carb.	Cal.	Carb.	Cal.	Carb.
Banana Cream Pudding & Pie Filling, **Royal,** 3½-oz. box	400	96.0			114.3	27.43		
As prepared for pie filling (yield: approx. 2 cups, 21.0 oz., or enough to fill an 8" pie shell)	720	120.0			(34.3)	(5.71)	360	60.0
Filling for 1 slice, ⅙ of pie (approx. 3.5 oz.)			120	20.0	(34.3)	(5.71)	360	60.0
BLUEBERRY								
Blueberry Pie Filling, **Comstock Lite,** 20-oz. can	480	114.0			24.0	5.70		
Filling for 1 slice, ⅙ of pie (approx. 3.3 oz.)			80	19.0	24.0	5.70		
Blueberry Pie Filling, **Wilderness,** 21-oz. can	660	168.0			31.4	8.00	(257)	(65.6)
Filling for 1 slice, ⅙ of pie (approx. 3.5 oz.)			110	28.0	31.4	8.00	(257)	(65.6)
BUTTERSCOTCH								
Butterscotch Pudding & Pie Filling, **Ann Page (A&P),** 4.0-oz. box	400	104.0			100.0	26.00		
As prepared for pie filling (yield: approx. 2 cups, 21.5 oz., or enough to fill an 8" pie shell)	720	128.0			(33.5)	(5.95)	360	64.0
Filling for 1 slice, ⅙ of pie (approx. 3.6 oz.)			120	21.3	(33.5)	(5.95)	360	64.0
Butterscotch Pudding & Pie Filling, low calorie, **D-Zerta,** 2.125-oz. box (2 envelopes)	200	48.0			94.1	22.59		
As prepared for pie filling (using nonfat milk) (yield: approx. 2 cups, 19.4 oz., or enough to fill an 8" pie shell)	380	72.6			(19.6)	(3.74)	190	36.3
Filling for 1 slice, ⅙ of pie (approx. 3.2 oz.)			63	12.1	(19.6)	(3.74)	190	36.3
Butterscotch Pudding & Pie Filling, low calorie, **Featherweight,** 1.0-oz. box (2 envelopes)	96	24.0			96.0	24.00		
As prepared for pie filling (using skim milk) (yield: approx. 3 cups, 26.9 oz., or enough to fill a 9" pie shell)	(366)	(60.9)			(13.6)	(2.26)	122	20.3
Filling for 1 slice, ⅙ of pie (approx. 4.5 oz.)			61	10.2	(13.6)	(2.26)	122	20.3
Butterscotch Pudding & Pie Filling, **Jell-O,** 3⅝-oz. box	400	96.0			110.3	26.48		
As prepared for pie filling (yield: approx. 2 cups, 21.1 oz., or enough to fill an 8" pie shell)	720	120.0			(34.1)	(5.69)	360	60.0
Filling for 1 slice, ⅙ of pie (approx. 3.4 oz.)			120	20.0	(34.1)	(5.69)	360	60.0
Butterscotch Pudding & Pie Filling, **Jell-O Instant,** 3¾-oz. box	400	96.0			106.7	25.60		
As prepared for pie filling (yield: approx. 2 cups, 21.3 oz., or enough to fill an 8" pie shell)	720	120.0			(33.8)	(5.63)	360	60.0
Filling for 1 slice, ⅙ of pie (approx. 3.4 oz.)			120	20.0	(33.8)	(5.63)	360	60.0
Butterscotch Pudding & Pie Filling, **Jell-O Instant,** sugar free, 1.1 oz. box	120	28.0			109.1	25.45		
As prepared for pie filling (using low-fat milk) (yield: approx. 2 cups, 18.3 oz., or enough to fill an 8" pie shell)	362	51.4			(19.8)	(2.81)	181	25.7
Filling for 1 slice, ⅙ of pie (approx. 3.1 oz.)			60	8.6	(19.8)	(2.81)	181	25.7
Butterscotch Pudding & Pie Filling, **Jell-Well,** 3.75 oz. box	440	100.0			117.3	26.67		
As prepared for pie filling (yield: approx. 2 cups, 21.3 oz., or enough to fill an 8" pie shell)	760	124.0			(35.7)	(5.82)	380	62.0
Filling for 1 slice, ⅙ of pie (approx. 3.6 oz.)			127	20.7	(35.7)	(5.82)	380	62.0
Butterscotch Pudding & Pie Filling, **Jell-Well Instant,** 3.75-oz. box	400	100.0			106.7	26.67		
As prepared for pie filling (yield: approx. 2 cups, 21.3 oz., or enough to fill an 8" pie shell)	720	124.0			(35.7)	(5.82)	360	62.0
Filling for 1 slice, ⅙ of pie (approx. 3.6 oz.)			120	20.7	(35.7)	(5.82)	360	62.0
Butterscotch Pudding & Pie Filling, **My-T-Fine,** 3¼-oz. box	(360)	88.0			(110.8)	(27.08)		
As prepared for pie filling (yield: approx. 20.8 oz., or enough to fill an 8" pie shell)	680	112.0			(32.7)	(5.38)	340	56.0
Filling for 1 slice, ⅙ of pie (approx. 3.5 oz.)			113.3	18.7	32.7	(5.38)	340	56.0
Butterscotch Pudding & Pie Filling, **Royal,** 3⅝-oz. box	320	80.0			88.3	22.07		
As prepared for pie filling (yield: approx. 2 cups, 21.1 oz., or enough to fill an 8" pie shell)	640	104.0			(30.3)	(4.93)	320	52.0
Filling for 1 slice, ⅙ of pie (approx. 3.5 oz.)			107	17.3	(30.3)	(4.93)	320	52.0
Butterscotch Pudding & Pie Filling, **Royal Instant,** 3½-oz. box	400	96.0			114.3	27.43		
As prepared for pie filling (yield: approx. 2 cups, 21.0 oz., or enough to fill an 8" pie shell)	720	120.0			(34.3)	(5.71)	360	60.0
Filling for 1 slice, ⅙ of pie (approx. 3.5 oz.)			120	20.0	(34.3)	(5.71)	360	60.0
CHERRY								
Cherry Pie Filling, **Comstock Lite,** 20-oz. can	480	114.0			24.0	5.70		
Filling for 1 slice, ⅙ of pie (approx. 3.3 oz.)			80	19.0	24.0	5.70		
Cherry Pie Filling, **Wilderness,** 21-oz. can	660	174.0			31.4	8.29	(257)	(67.9)
Filling for 1 slice, ⅙ of pie (approx. 3.5 oz.)			110	29.0	31.4	8.29	(257)	(67.9)
Cherry-Plum Pudding & Pie Filling, **Junket Danish Dessert,** Danish-style pudding and pie filling mix, 4.75-oz. box	520	128.0			109.5	26.95		
As prepared for pie filling (yield: approx. 2 cups, 21.5 oz., or enough to fill an 8" pie shell)	520	128.0			(24.2)	(5.95)	260	64.0
Filling for 1 slice, ⅙ of pie (approx. 3.6 oz.)			87	21.3	(24.2)	(5.95)	260	64.0
CHOCOLATE								
Chocolate Pudding & Pie Filling, **Ann Page (A&P),** 6-oz. box	660	156.0			110.0	26.00		
As prepared for pie filling (yield: approx. 3 cups, 32.3 oz., or enough to fill a 9" pie shell)	1140	192.0			(35.3)	(5.94)	380	64.0
Filling for 1 slice, ⅙ of pie (approx. 5.4 oz.)			190	32.0	(35.3)	(5.94)	380	64.0
Chocolate Pudding & Pie Filling, **Ann Page (A&P) Instant,** 4-oz. box	440	104.0			110.0	26.00		
As prepared for pie filling (yield: approx. 2 cups, 21.0 oz., or enough to fill an 8" pie shell)	760	128.0			35.3	5.95	380	64.0
Filling for 1 slice, ⅙ of pie (approx. 3.5 oz.)			127	21.3	35.3	5.95	380	64.0
Chocolate Pudding & Pie Filling, low calorie, **Dia-Mel (Louis Sherry),** 0.85-oz. box (2 envelopes)	48	16.0			56.5	18.82		
As prepared for pie filling (using skim milk) (yield: approx. 1¾ cups, 16.0 oz., or enough to fill an 8" pie shell)	(206)	(37.5)			(12.8)	(2.35)	103	18.8
Filling for 1 slice, ⅙ of pie (approx. 2.7 oz.)			(34)	(6.3)	(12.8)	(2.35)	103	18.8
Chocolate Pudding & Pie Filling, **Dieter's Gourmet,** 1⅞-oz. box	200	48.0			106.7	25.60		
As prepared for pie filling (using skim milk) (yield: approx. 2 cups, 19.2 oz., or enough to fill an 8" pie shell)	380	72.6			(19.8)	(3.78)	190	36.3
Filling for 1 slice, ⅙ of pie (approx. 3.2 oz.)			63	12.1	(19.8)	(3.78)	190	36.3
Chocolate Pudding & Pie Filling, low calorie, **D-Zerta,** 2-oz. box (2 envelopes)	160	40.0			80.0	20.00		

	UNIT		FILLING FOR 1 SLICE		1 OZ., BY WT.		1 CUP	
	Cal.	Carb.	Cal.	Carb.	Cal.	Carb.	Cal.	Carb.
As prepared for pie filling (using nonfat milk) (yield: approx. 2 cups, 19.3 oz., or enough to fill an 8″ pie shell)	(340)	(64.6)			(17.6)	(3.35)	170	32.3
Filling for 1 slice, ⅙ of pie (approx. 3.2 oz.)			57	10.8	(17.6)	(3.35)	170	32.3
Chocolate Pudding & Pie Filling, low calorie, **Featherweight,** 1.0-oz. box (2 envelopes)	96	24.0			96.0	24.00		
As prepared for pie filling (using skim milk) (yield: approx. 3 cups, 26.9 oz., or enough to fill a 9″ pie shell)	(366)	(60.9)			(13.6)	(2.26)	122	20.3
Filling for 1 slice, ⅙ of pie (approx. 4.5 oz.)			61	10.2	(13.6)	(2.26)	122	20.3
Chocolate Pudding & Pie Filling, **Jell-O,** 3½-oz. box	360	88.0			102.9	25.14		
As prepared for pie filling (yield: approx. 2¼ cups, 23.2 oz., or enough to fill an 8″ pie shell)	720	115.0			(31.0)	(4.96)	320	51.1
Filling for 1 slice, ⅙ of pie (approx. 3.9 oz.)			120	19.2	(31.0)	(4.96)	320	51.1
Chocolate Pudding & Pie Filling, **Jell-O Instant,** 4½-oz. box	440	112.0			97.8	24.89		
As prepared for pie filling (yield: approx. 1¾ cups, 19.8 oz., or enough to fill an 8″ pie shell)	720	133.0			(36.4)	(6.72)	411	76.0
Filling for 1 slice, ⅙ of pie (approx. 3.3 oz.)			120	22.2	(36.4)	(6.72)	411	76.0
Chocolate Pudding & Pie Filling, **Jell-O Instant,** sugar free, 1.5 oz. box	140	32.0			93.3	21.33		
As prepared for pie filling (using low-fat milk) (yield: approx. 2 cups, 18.7 oz., or enough to fill an 8″ pie shell)	382	55.4			(20.4)	(2.96)	191	27.7
Filling for 1 slice, ⅙ of pie (approx. 3.1 oz.)			64	9.2	(20.4)	(2.96)	191	27.7
Chocolate Pudding & Pie Filling, **Jell-Well,** 3.75-oz. box	440	92.0			117.3	24.53		
As prepared for pie filling (yield: approx. 2 cups, 21.3 oz., or enough to fill an 8″ pie shell)	760	116.0			(35.7)	(5.45)	380	58.0
Filling for 1 slice, ⅙ of pie (approx. 3.6 oz.)			127	19.3	(35.7)	(5.45)	380	58.0
Chocolate Pudding & Pie Filling, **Jell-Well Instant,** 4.5-oz. box	440	104.0			97.8	23.11		
As prepared for pie filling (yield: approx. 2 cups, 22.0 oz., or enough to fill an 8″ pie shell)	760	128.0			(34.5)	(5.82)	380	64.0
Filling for 1 slice, ⅙ of pie (approx. 3.7 oz.)			127	21.3	(34.5)	(5.82)	380	64.0
Chocolate Pudding & Pie Filling, low calorie, **Louis Sherry,** 1¼-oz. box (2 envelopes)	100	15.6			80.0	12.48		
As prepared for pie filling (using skim milk) (yield: approx. 2 cups, 18.5 oz., or enough to fill an 8″ pie shell)	(280)	(40.2)			(15.1)	(2.17)	140	20.1
Filling for 1 slice, ⅙ of pie (approx. 3.1 oz.)			(47)	(6.7)	(15.1)	(2.17)	140	20.1
Chocolate Pudding & Pie Filling, **My-T-Fine,** 3⅝-oz. box	(400)	(92.0)			(110.3)	(25.38)		
As prepared for pie filling (yield: approx. 2 cups, 21.1 oz., or enough to fill an 8″ pie shell)	720	116.0			(34.1)	(5.50)	360	58.0
Filling for 1 slice, ⅙ of pie (approx. 3.4 oz.)			120	19.3	(34.1)	(5.50)	360	58.0
Chocolate Pudding & Pie Filling, **Royal,** 3⅝-oz. box	480	100.0			132.4	27.59		
As prepared for pie filling (yield: approx. 2 cups, 21.1 oz., or enough to fill an 8″ pie shell)	800	124.0			(37.9)	(5.88)	400	62.0
Filling for 1 slice, ⅙ of pie (approx. 3.5 oz.)			133	20.7	(37.9)	(5.88)	400	62.0
5½-oz. box	720	150.0			132.4	27.59		

	UNIT		FILLING FOR 1 SLICE		1 OZ., BY WT.		1 CUP	
	Cal.	Carb.	Cal.	Carb.	Cal.	Carb.	Cal.	Carb.
As prepared for pie filling (yield: approx. 3 cups, 31.8 oz., or enough to fill a 9″ pie shell)	1200	186.0			(37.7)	(5.85)	400	62.0
Filling for 1 slice, ⅙ of pie (approx. 5.3 oz.)			200	31.0	(37.7)	(5.85)	400	62.0
Chocolate Pudding & Pie Filling, **Royal Instant,** 4¼-oz. box	480	108.0			112.9	25.41		
As prepared for pie filling (yield: approx. 2 cups, 21.8 oz., or enough to fill an 8″ pie shell)	800	132.0			(36.7)	(6.06)	400	66.0
Filling for 1 slice, ⅙ of pie (approx. 3.6 oz.)			133	22.0	(36.7)	(6.06)	400	66.0
Chocolate Almond Pudding & Pie Filling, **My-T-Fine,** 3¾-oz. box	(400)	(92.0)			(106.7)	(24.53)		
As prepared for pie filling (yield: approx. 2 cups, 21.3 oz., or enough to fill an 8″ pie shell)	720	116.0			(33.8)	(5.45)	360	58.0
Filling for 1 slice, ⅙ of pie (approx. 3.5 oz.)			120	19.3	(33.8)	(5.45)	360	58.0
Chocolate Fudge Pudding & Pie Filling, **Jell-O,** 3⅝-oz. box	360	88.0			99.3	24.28		
As prepared for pie filling (yield: approx. 2 cups, 21.1 oz., or enough to fill an 8″ pie shell)	680	112.0			(32.2)	(5.31)	340	56.0
Filling for 1 slice, ⅙ of pie (approx. 3.5 oz.)			113	18.7	(32.2)	(5.31)	340	56.0
Chocolate Fudge Pudding & Pie Filling, **Jell-O Instant,** 3⅝-oz. box	440	108.0			121.4	29.79		
As prepared for pie filling (yield: approx. 2 cups, 21.1 oz., or enough to fill an 8″ pie shell)	760	132.0			(36.0)	(6.26)	380	66.0
Filling for 1 slice, ⅙ of pie (approx. 3.5 oz.)			127	22.0	(36.0)	(6.26)	380	66.0
Chocolate Fudge Pudding & Pie Filling, **Jell-O Instant,** sugar free, 1.7 oz. box	160	36.0			94.1	21.18		
As prepared for pie filling (using low-fat milk) (yield: approx. 2 cups, 18.9 oz., or enough to fill an 8″ pie shell)	402	59.4			(21.3)	(3.14)	201	29.7
Filling for 1 slice, ⅙ of pie (approx. 3.2 oz.)			67	9.9	(21.3)	(3.14)	201	29.7
Milk Chocolate Pudding & Pie Filling, **Jell-O,** 3⅝-oz. box	360	92.0			99.3	25.38		
As prepared for pie filling (yield: approx. 2 cups, 21.1 oz., or enough to fill an 8″ pie shell)	680	116.0			(32.3)	(5.50)	340	58.0
Filling for 1 slice, ⅙ of pie (approx. 3.5 oz.)			113	19.3	(32.3)	(5.50)	340	58.0
COCONUT								
Coconut Pudding & Pie Filling, **Jell-Well,** 3.25-oz. box	240	56.0			73.9	17.23		
As prepared for pie filling (yield: approx. 2 cups, 20.8 oz., or enough to fill an 8″ pie shell)	560	80.0			(26.9)	(3.85)	280	40.0
Filling for 1 slice, ⅙ of pie (approx. 3.5 oz.)			93	13.3	(26.9)	(3.85)	280	40.0
Coconut Pudding & Pie Filling, **Royal Instant,** 3½-oz. box	400	92.0			114.3	26.29		
As prepared for pie filling (yield: approx. 2 cups, 21.0 oz., or enough to fill an 8″ pie shell)	720	116.0			(34.3)	(5.52)	360	58.0
Filling for 1 slice, ⅙ of pie (approx. 3.5 oz.)			120	19.3	(34.3)	(5.52)	360	58.0
Coconut Cream Pudding & Pie Filling, **Ann Page (A&P),** 3¼-oz. box	400	76.0			123.1	23.38		
As prepared for pie filling (yield: approx. 2 cups, 20.8 oz., or enough to fill an 8″ pie shell)	720	100.0			(34.6)	(4.81)	360	50.0
Filling for 1 slice, ⅙ of pie (approx. 3.5 oz.)			120	16.7	(34.6)	(4.81)	360	50.0
4⅞-oz. box	600	114.0			123.1	23.38		
As prepared for pie filling (yield: approx. 3 cups, 31.1 oz., or enough to fill a 9″ pie shell)	1080	150.0			(34.7)	(4.82)	360	50.0

	UNIT		FILLING FOR 1 SLICE		1 OZ., BY WT.		1 CUP	
	Cal.	Carb.	Cal.	Carb.	Cal.	Carb.	Cal.	Carb.
Filling for 1 slice, 1/6 of pie (approx. 5.2 oz.)			180	25.0	34.7	(4.82)	360	50.0
Coconut Cream Pudding & Pie Filling, **Jell-O Instant,** 4⅛-oz. box	440	104.0			106.7	25.21		
As prepared for pie filling (yield: approx. 1¾ cups, 19.4 oz., or enough to fill an 8" pie shell)	720	125.0			(37.1)	(6.44)	411	71.4
Filling for 1 slice, 1/6 of pie (approx. 3.2 oz.)			120	20.8	(37.1)	(6.44)	411	71.4
Toasted Coconut Pudding & Pie Filling, **Ann Page (A&P) Instant,** 3¼-oz. box	400	65.0			123.0	20.00		
As prepared for pie filling (yield: approx. 2 cups, 20.8 oz., or enough to fill an 8" pie shell)	720	89			(34.6)	(4.28)	360	44.5
Filling for 1 slice, 1/6 of pie (approx. 3.5 oz.)			120	14.8	(34.6)	(4.28)	360	44.5
COFFEE								
Coffee Pudding & Pie Filling, **Royal Instant,** 3½-oz. box	400	96.0			114.3	27.43		
As prepared for pie filling (yield: approx. 2 cups, 21.0 oz., or enough to fill an 8" pie shell)	720	120.0			(34.3)	(5.71)	360	60.0
Filling for 1 slice, 1/6 of pie (approx. 3.5 oz.)			120	20.0	(34.3)	(5.71)	360	60.0
CUSTARD								
Custard Pudding & Pie Filling, **Royal,** 2¼-oz. box	240	60.0			106.7	26.67		
As prepared for pie filling (yield: approx. 2¼ cups, 21.9 oz., or enough to fill an 8" pie shell)	600	87.0			(27.4)	(3.97)	267	38.7
Filling for 1 slice, 1/6 of pie (approx. 3.7 oz.)			100	14.5	(27.4)	(3.97)	267	38.7
Golden Egg Custard, **Jell-O** "Americana," 3.0-oz. box	360	68.0			120.0	22.67		
As prepared for pie filling (yield: approx. 2 cups, 20.5 oz., or enough to fill an 8" pie shell)	680	92.0			(33.2)	(4.49)	340	46.0
Filling for 1 slice, 1/6 of pie (approx. 3.4 oz.)			113	15.3	(33.2)	(4.49)	340	46.0
4½ oz. box	540	102.0			120.0	22.67		
As prepared for pie filling (yield: approx. 3 cups, 30.8 oz., or enough to fill a 9" pie shell)	1020	138.0			(33.1)	(4.48)	340	46.0
Filling for 1 slice, 1/6 of pie (approx. 5.1 oz.)			170	23.0	(33.1)	(4.48)	340	46.0
DARK N' SWEET								
Dark N' Sweet Pudding & Pie Filling, **Royal,** 3⅝-oz. box	480	100.0			132.4	27.59		
As prepared for pie filling (yield: approx. 2 cups, 21.2 oz., or enough to fill an 8" pie shell)	800	124.0			37.7	5.85	400	62.0
Filling for 1 slice, 1/6 of pie (approx. 3.5 oz.)			133	20.7	37.7	5.85	400	62.0
Dark N' Sweet Pudding & Pie Filling, **Royal Instant,** 3⅝-oz. box	480	108.0			132.4	29.79		
As prepared for pie filling (yield: approx. 2 cups, 21.5 oz., or enough to fill an 8" pie shell)	800	132.0			(37.2)	(6.14)	400	66.0
Filling for 1 slice, 1/6 of pie (approx. 3.6 oz.)			133	22.0	(37.2)	(6.14)	400	66.0
FLAN								
Flan Pudding & Pie Filling, **Royal,** 2-oz. box	240	60.0			120.0	(30.00)		
As prepared for pie filling (yield: approx. 2 cups, 19.5 oz., or enough to fill an 8" pie shell)	560	84.0			(28.7)	(4.31)	280	42.0
Filling for 1 slice, 1/6 of pie (approx. 3.2 oz.)			93	14.0	(28.7)	(4.31)	280	42.0
FRENCH VANILLA, see VANILLA								
KEY LIME, see LIME								
LEMON								
Lemon Pudding & Pie Filling, **Ann Page (A&P),** 3.37-oz. box	240	60.0			71.2	17.80		
As prepared for pie filling (yield: approx. 2 cups, 20.9 oz., or enough for an 8" pie shell)	560	84.0			(26.8)	(4.02)	280	42.0

	UNIT		FILLING FOR 1 SLICE		1 OZ., BY WT.		1 CUP	
	Cal.	Carb.	Cal.	Carb.	Cal.	Carb.	Cal.	Carb.
Filling for 1 slice, 1/6 of pie (approx. 3.5 oz.)			93	14.0	(26.8)	(4.02)	280	42.0
Lemon Pudding & Pie Filling, low calorie, **Dia-Mel (Louis Sherry),** 1¼-oz. box	56	16.0			56.0	16.00		
As prepared for pie filling (yield: approx. 2 cups, 18.0 oz., or enough to fill an 8" pie shell)	56	16.0			(3.1)	(0.89)	28	8.0
Filling for 1 slice, 1/6 of pie (approx. 3.0 oz.)			9	2.7	(3.1)	(0.89)	28	8.0
Lemon Pudding & Pie Filling, **Jell-O,** 3-oz. box	300	78.0			100.0	26.00		
As prepared for pie filling (yield: approx. 2 cups, 20.5 oz., or enough to fill an 8" pie shell)	620	102.0			(30.2)	(4.98)	310	(51.0)
Filling for 1 slice, 1/6 of pie (approx. 3.4 oz.)			103	17.0	(30.2)	(4.98)	(310)	(51.0)
Lemon Pudding & Pie Filling, **Jell-O Instant,** 3¾-oz. box	400	100.0			106.7	26.67		
As prepared for pie filling (yield: approx. 2 cups, 21.3 oz., or enough to fill an 8" pie shell)	720	124.0			(33.8)	(5.82)	360	62.0
Filling for 1 slice, 1/6 of pie (approx. 3.6 oz.)			120	20.7	(33.8)	(5.82)	360	62.0
Lemon Pudding & Pie Filling, **Jell-Well,** 3.25-oz. box	240	56.0			73.9	17.23		
As prepared for pie filling (yield: approx. 21.8 oz., or enough to fill an 8" pie shell)	670	80.0			(30.7)	(3.67)	335	40.0
Filling for 1 slice, 1/6 of pie (approx. 3.6 oz.)			112	13.3	(30.7)	(3.67)	335	40.0
Lemon Pudding & Pie Filling, **Jell-Well Instant,** 3.75-oz. box	400	100.0			106.7	26.67		
As prepared for pie filling (yield: approx. 2 cups, 21.3 oz., or enough to fill an 8" pie shell)	720	124.0			(33.8)	(5.82)	360	62.0
Filling for 1 slice, 1/6 of pie (approx. 3.6 oz.)			120	20.7	(33.8)	(5.82)	360	62.0
Lemon Pudding & Pie Filling, **My-T-Fine,** 3⅜-oz. box	240	60.0	71.1	17.78				
As prepared for pie filling (yield: approx. 2 cups, 26.3 oz., or enough to fill an 8" pie shell)	735	159.5			(27.5)	(5.97)	368	79.8
Filling for 1 slice, 1/6 of pie (approx. 4.5 oz.)			123	26.6	(27.5)	(5.97)	368	79.8
Lemon Pudding & Pie Filling, **Royal,** 3.0-oz. box	300	78.0			100.0	26.00		
As prepared for pie filling (yield: approx. 3 cups, 29.3 oz., or enough to fill a 9" pie shell)	780	114.0			(26.6)	(3.89)	260	38.0
Filling for 1 slice, 1/6 of pie (approx. 4.9 oz.)			130	19.0	(26.6)	(3.89)	260	38.0
Lemon Pudding & Pie Filling, **Royal Instant,** 3½-oz. box	400	96.0			114.3	27.43		
As prepared for pie filling (yield: approx. 2 cups, 21.0 oz., or enough to fill an 8" pie shell)	720	120.0			(34.3)	(5.71)	360	60.0
Filling for 1 slice, 1/6 of pie (approx. 3.5 oz.)			120	20.0	(34.3)	(5.71)	360	60.0
LIME								
Key Lime Pudding & Pie Filling, **Royal,** 3-oz. box	300	78.0			100.0	26.00		
As prepared for pie filling (yield: approx. 3 cups, 29.3 oz., or enough to fill a 9" pie shell)	780	114.0			(26.6)	(3.89)	260	38.0
Filling for 1 slice, 1/6 of pie (approx. 4.4 oz.)			130	19.0	(26.6)	(3.89)	260	38.0
PINEAPPLE CREAM								
Pineapple Cream Pudding & Pie Filling, **Jell-O Instant,** 3¾-oz. box	400	100.0			106.7	26.67		
As prepared for pie filling (yield: approx. 2 cups, 21.3 oz., or enough to fill an 8" pie shell)	720	124.0			(33.8)	(5.82)	360	62.0
Filling for 1 slice, 1/6 of pie (approx. 3.6 oz.)			120	20.7	(33.8)	(5.82)	360	62.0
PISTACHIO								
Pistachio Pudding & Pie Filling, **Jell-O Instant,** 3¾-oz. box	440	96.0			106.7	25.60		

	UNIT		FILLING FOR 1 SLICE		1 OZ., BY WT.		1 CUP	
	Cal.	Carb.	Cal.	Carb.	Cal.	Carb.	Cal.	Carb.
As prepared for pie filling (yield: approx. 2 cups, 21.3 oz., or enough to fill an 8″ pie shell)	720	120.0			(33.8)	(5.63)	360	60.0
Filling for 1 slice, ⅙ of pie (approx. 3.6 oz.)			120	20.0	(33.8)	(5.63)	360	60.0
Pistachio Pudding & Pie Filling, **Jell-Well Instant,** 3.75-oz. box	400	96.0			106.7	25.60		
As prepared for pie filling (yield: approx. 2 cups, 21.3 oz., or enough to fill an 8″ pie shell)	720	120.0			(33.8)	(5.63)	360	60.0
Filling for 1 slice, ⅙ of pie (approx. 3.6 oz.)			120	20.0	(33.8)	(5.63)	360	60.0
Pistachio Nut Pudding & Pie Filling, **Royal Instant,** 3½-oz. box	400	92.0			114.3	26.29		
As prepared for pie filling (yield: approx. 2 cups, 21.0 oz., or enough to fill an 8″ pie shell)	720	116.0			(34.3)	(5.63)	360	58.0
Filling for 1 slice, ⅙ of pie (approx. 3.5 oz.)			120	19.3	(34.3)	(5.63)	360	58.0
PUMPKIN								
Pumpkin for Pie, **Libby's,** 30-oz. (1-lb. 14-oz.) can	(729)	(195.0)			(24.3)	(6.50)		
Filling for 1 slice, ⅙ of pie (approx. 5.0 oz.)			122	32.5	(24.3)	(6.50)		
Pumpkin Pie Filling, **Stokely,** 18-oz. can	700	168.3			38.9	9.35	370	89.0
Filling for 1 slice, ⅙ of pie (approx. 3.0 oz.)			117	28.1	38.9	9.35	370	89.0
RAISIN								
Raisin Pie Filling, **Wilderness,** 22-oz. can	720	186.0			32.7	8.46	(281)	(72.7)
Filling for 1 slice, ⅙ of pie (approx. 3.7 oz.)			120	31.0	32.7	8.46	(281)	(72.7)
RASPBERRY CURRANT								
Raspberry Currant Danish-Style Pudding & Pie Filling, **Junket Danish Dessert,** 4.75-oz. box	520	128.0			109.5	26.95		
As prepared for pie filling (yield: approx. 2 cups, 21.5 oz., or enough to fill an 8″ pie shell)	520	128.0			(24.2)	(5.95)	260	64.0
Filling for 1 slice, ⅙ of pie (approx 3.6 oz.)			87	21.3	(24.2)	(5.95)	260	64.0
STRAWBERRY								
Strawberry Pie Filling, **Wilderness,** 21-oz. can	720	186.0			34.3	8.86	(281)	(72.7)
Filling for 1 slice, ⅙ of pie (approx. 3.5 oz.)			120	31.0	34.3	8.86	(281)	(72.7)
Strawberry Danish-Style Pudding & Pie Filling, **Junket Danish Dessert,** 4.75-oz. box	520	128.0			109.5	26.95		
As prepared for pie filling (yield: approx. 2 cups, 21.5 oz., or enough to fill an 8″ pie shell)	520	128.0			(24.2)	(5.95)	260	64.0
Filling for 1 slice, ⅙ of pie (approx. 3.6 oz.)			87	21.3	(24.2)	(5.95)	260	64.0
VANILLA								
French Vanilla Pudding & Pie Filling, **Jell-O,** 3½-oz. box	400	96.0			114.3	27.4		
As prepared for pie filling (yield: approx. 2 cups, 21.0 oz., or enough to fill an 8″ pie shell)	720	120.0			(34.3)	(5.71)	360	60.0
Filling for 1 slice, ⅙ of pie (approx. 3.5 oz.)			120	20.0	(34.3)	(5.71)	360	60.0
French Vanilla Pudding & Pie Filling, **Jell-O Instant,** 3¾-oz. box	400	96.0			110.3	26.48		
As prepared for pie filling (yield: approx. 2 cups, 21.3 oz., or enough to fill an 8″ pie shell)	720	120.0			(33.8)	(5.63)	360	60.0
Filling for 1 slice, ⅙ of pie (approx. 3.6 oz.)			120	20.0	(33.8)	(5.63)	360	60.0
Vanilla Pudding & Pie Filling, **Ann Page (A&P),** 3¼-oz. box	360	88.0			110.8	27.08		
As prepared for pie filling (yield: approx. 2 cups, 20.8 oz., or enough to fill an 8″ pie shell)	680	112.0			(32.7)	(5.38)	340	56.0
Filling for 1 slice, ⅙ of pie (approx. 3.5 oz.)			113	18.7	(32.7)	(5.38)	340	56.0
4⅞-oz. box	540	132.0			110.8	27.08		
As prepared for pie filling (yield: approx. 3 cups, 31.1 oz., or enough to fill a 9″ pie shell)	1020	168.0			(32.8)	(5.40)	340	56.0
Filling or 1 slice, ⅙ of pie (approx. 5.2 oz.)			170	28.0	(32.8)	(5.38)	340	56.0
Vanilla Pudding & Pie Filling, **Ann Page (A&P) Instant,** 3¼-oz. box	360	88.0			110.8	27.08		
As prepared for pie filling (yield: approx. 2 cups, 20.8 oz., or enough to fill an 8″ pie shell)	680	112.0			(32.7)	(5.38)	340	56.0
Filling for 1 slice, ⅙ of pie (approx. 3.5 oz.)			113	18.7	(32.7)	(5.38)	340	56.0
Vanilla Pudding & Pie Filling, low calorie, **Dia-Mel (Louis Sherry),** 1-oz. box (2 envelopes)	40	12.0			40.0	12.00		
As prepared for pie filling (using skim milk) (yield: approx. 1¾ cups, 16.1 oz., or enough to fill an 8″ pie shell)	(198)	(33.5)			(12.3)	(2.08)	113	19.2
Filling for 1 slice, ⅙ of pie (approx. 2.7 oz.)			33	5.6	(12.3)	(2.08)	113	19.2
Vanilla Pudding & Pie Filling, low calorie, **D-Zerta,** 2⅛-oz. box (2 envelopes)	240	56.0			112.9	26.35		
As prepared for pie filling (using nonfat milk) (yield: approx. 2 cups, 19.4 oz., or enough to fill an 8″ pie shell)	420	80.6			(21.6)	(4.15)	210	40.3
Filling for 1 slice, ⅙ of pie (approx. 3.2 oz.)			70	13.4	(21.6)	(4.15)	210	40.3
Vanilla Pudding & Pie Filling, **Jell-O,** 3⅛-oz. box	320	84.0			102.4	26.88		
As prepared for pie filling (yield: approx. 2 cups, 20.6 oz., or enough to fill an 8″ pie shell)	640	108.0			(31.1)	(5.24)	320	54.0
Filling for 1 slice, ⅙ of pie (approx. 3.4 oz.)			107	18.0	(31.1)	(5.24)	320	54.0
Vanilla Pudding & Pie Filling, **Jell-O Instant,** 3¾-oz. box	400	100.0			106.7	26.67		
As prepared for pie filling (yield: approx. 2 cups, 21.3 oz., or enough to fill an 8″ pie shell)	720	124.0			(33.8)	(5.82)	360	62.0
Filling for 1 slice, ⅙ of pie (approx. 3.6 oz.)			120	20.7	(33.8)	(5.82)	360	62.0
Vanilla Pudding & Pie Filling, **Jell-O Instant,** sugar free, 1.1 oz. box	120	28.0			109.1	25.45		
As prepared for pie filling (using low-fat milk) (yield: approx. 2 cups, 18.3 oz., or enough to fill an 8″ pie shell)	362	52.0			(19.8)	(2.84)	181	26.0
Filling for 1 slice, ⅙ of pie (approx. 3.1 oz.)			60	8.7	(19.8)	(2.84)	181	26.0
Vanilla Pudding & Pie Filling, **Jell-Well,** 3.25-oz. box	360	88.0			110.8	27.05		
As prepared for pie filling (yield: approx. 2 cups, 20.8 oz., or enough to fill an 8″ pie shell)	680	112.0			(32.7)	(5.38)	340	56.0
Filling for 1 slice, ⅙ of pie (approx. 3.5 oz.)			113	18.7	(32.7)	(5.38)	340	56.0
Vanilla Pudding & Pie Filling, **Jell-Well Instant,** 3.75-oz. box	400	100.0			106.7	26.67		
As prepared for pie filling (yield: approx. 2 cups, 21.3 oz., or enough to fill an 8″ pie shell)	720	124.0			(33.8)	(5.82)	360	62.0
Filling for 1 slice, ⅙ of pie (approx. 3.6 oz.)			120	20.7	(33.8)	(5.82)	360	62.0
Vanilla Pudding & Pie Filling, **My-T-Fine,** 3¼-oz. box	(360)	88.0			(110.8)	(27.08)		
As prepared for pie filling (yield: approx. 2 cups, 20.8 oz., or enough to fill an 8″ pie shell)	680	112.0			(32.7)	(5.38)	340	56.0
Filling for 1 slice, ⅙ of pie (approx. 3.5 oz.)			113	18.7	(32.7)	(5.38)	340	56.0
Vanilla Pudding & Pie Filling, **Royal,** 3-oz. box	320	80.0			106.7	26.67		
As prepared for pie filling (yield: approx. 2 cups, 20.5 oz., or enough to fill an 8″ pie shell)	640	108.0			(31.2)	(5.27)	320	54.0

	UNIT		FILLING FOR 1 SLICE		1 OZ., BY WT.		1 CUP	
	Cal.	Carb.	Cal.	Carb.	Cal.	Carb.	Cal.	Carb.
Filling for 1 slice, ⅙ of pie (approx. 3.4 oz.)			107	18.0	(31.2)	(5.27)	320	54.0
4½-oz. box	480	120.0			106.7	26.67		
As prepared for pie filling (yield: approx. 3 cups. 30.8 oz., or enough to fill a 9″ pie shell)	960	156.0			(31.2)	(5.06)	320	52.0
Filling for 1 slice, ⅙ of pie (approx. 5.1 oz.)			160	26.0	(31.2)	(5.06)	320	52.0
Vanilla Pudding & Pie Filling, **Royal Instant,** 3½-oz. box	400	96.0			114.3	27.43		
As prepared for pie filling (yield: approx. 2 cups, 20.7 oz., or enough to fill an 8″ pie shell)	720	120.0			(34.3)	(5.71)	360	60.0
Filling for 1 slice, ⅙ of pie (approx. 3.5 oz.)			120	20.0	(34.3)	(5.71)	360	60.0
QUICHE FILLINGS								
Pour-A-Quiche, **Land O' Lakes**								
Bacon & Onion Quiche, 26-oz. container (fills 9″ pie crust)	1380	36.0			53.1	1.38		
Filling for 1 "suggested" serving, ⅙ of pie (4.3 oz before baking)			230	6.0	53.1	1.38		
Ham and Cheese Quiche, 26-oz. container (fills 9″ pie crust)	1260	24.0			41.5	0.92		
Filling for 1 "suggested" serving, ⅙ of pie (4.3 oz. before baking)			210	4.0	41.5	0.92		
Spinach & Onion Quiche ("Quiche Florentine"), 26-oz. container	1320	36.0			50.1	1.38		
Filling for 1 "suggested" serving, ⅙ of pie (4.3 oz. before baking)			220	6.0	50.1	1.38		
3-Cheese Quiche (Swiss, Cheddar, Monterey Jack), 26-oz. container	1380	24.0			53.1			
Filling for 1 "suggested" serving, ⅙ of pie (4.3 oz. before baking)			230	4.0	53.1			

23 COOKIES & CRACKERS •

COOKIES and BROWNIES MADE FROM SCRATCH, based on USDA home recipes

Item	UNIT Cal.	UNIT Carb.	1 COOKIE Cal.	1 COOKIE Carb.	1 OZ., BY WT. Cal.	1 OZ., BY WT. Carb.
BROWNIES, made with enriched flour, water, and nuts						
Made from 10½ oz. complete brownie mix, ⅓ cup water, ½ cup chopped pecans (yield: approx. 22 brownies, 15.2 oz.)	(2113)	(223.4)			139.0	14.70
1 brownie, approx. 0.7 oz.			97	10.2	139.0	14.70
1 pound (approx. 23 brownies) (1g/15g/5g/15%/62mg)	2224	235.2			139.0	14.70
BROWNIES, made with 16 oz. (1 lb.) incomplete brownie mix, ¼ cup water, 1 large egg, ½ cup chopped pecans (yield: approx. 31 brownies, 21.9 oz.)	(2652)	(394.5)			121.0	18.00
1 brownie, approx. 0.7 oz.			86	12.6	121.0	18.00
1 pound (approx. 23 brownies) (1g/18g/6g/11%/47mg)	1936	288.0			121.0	18.00
PLAIN COOKIES, made with unenriched flour, egg and water						
Made from 11 oz. plain cookie mix, 2 Tbsp. milk, 1⅛ tsp. flavoring (yield: approx. 60 cookies, 12.4 oz.)	(1730)	(222.5)			140.0	18.00
1 cookie, approx. 0.2 oz.			28	3.6	140.0	18.00
1 pound (approx. 80 cookies) (1g(18g(7g/5%/98mg)	2240	288.0			140.0	18.00

COOKIES BAKED FROM PREMIXED COOKIE DOUGH, based on USDA data

Item	UNIT Cal.	UNIT Carb.	1 COOKIE Cal.	1 COOKIE Carb.	1 OZ., BY WT. Cal.	1 OZ., BY WT. Carb.
Plain, chilled in 18-oz. roll, 10½" long, 1¾" diameter:						
Entire roll, unbaked	2290	300.0			127.2	16.67
Entire roll, baked (yield: 16.9 oz., approx. 40 cookies)					140.8	18.46
1 cookie, approx. 0.5 oz.			60	7.8	140.8	18.46
1 pound (approx. 38 cookies) (1g/18g/7g/5%/155mg)	2253	295.4			140.8	18.46

COOKIES and BROWNIES MADE FROM MIXES, by brand

BROWNIE MIX

Item	UNIT Cal.	UNIT Carb.	1 COOKIE Cal.	1 COOKIE Carb.	1 OZ., BY WT. Cal.	1 OZ., BY WT. Carb.
Brownie Mix, **Duncan Hines,** 15½-oz. box	2080	304.0			134.2	19.61
Prepared as package directs (suggested yield: 16 brownies)	2240	336.0				
1 brownie, 16 per box			140	21.0		
Carob-Cake Brownie Mix With Sunflower Seeds, **Arrowhead Mills,** 32-oz. (2-lb.) package	(4640)	(608.0)			(145.0)	(19.00)
Prepared as package directs (suggested yield: 39 brownies)	(3184)	(335.2)			(119.7)	(12.60)
1 brownie, 39 per box			(82)	(8.6)	(119.7)	(12.60)
Chocolate Chip Butterscotch Brownie Mix, **Betty Crocker,** 16-oz. (1-lb.) box						
Prepared as package directs (suggested yield: 16 brownies)	2080	320.0			(91.5)	(14.08)
1 brownie, 16 per box			130	20.0	(91.5)	(14.08)
Double-Fudge Brownie Mix, **Duncan Hines,** 15½-oz. box	2080	304.0			134.2	19.60
Prepared as package directs for "Chewy Fudge" brownies (suggested yield: 16 brownies)	2240	336.0			(101.8)	(15.21)
1 brownie, 16 per box			140	21.0	(101.8)	(15.21)
23-oz. box	3087	450.8			134.2	19.60
Prepared as package directs for "Chewy Fudge" brownies (suggested yield: 24 brownies)	3360	504.0			(102.9)	(15.42)
1 brownie, 24 per box			140	21.0	(102.9)	(15.43)
Fudge Brownie Mix, **Ann Page (A&P)** Deluxe 22-oz. box	(2480)	(478.0)			(112.7)	(21.73)
Prepared as package directs (suggested yield: 24 brownies)	2640	480.0			(84.5)	(15.36)
1 brownie, 24 per box			110	20.0	(84.5)	(15.36)
Fudge Brownie Mix, **Betty Crocker,** 15½-oz. box						
Prepared as package directs (suggested yield: 16 brownies)	1920	336.0			(87.2)	(15.27)
1 brownie, 16 per box			120	21.0	(87.2)	(15.27)
Fudge Brownie Mix, **Jiffy,** 8-oz. box	960	164.4			120.0	20.55
Prepared as package directs (suggested yield: 12 brownies)	108	168.0			112.5	17.50
1 brownie, 12 per box			90	14.0	112.5	17.50
Fudge Brownie Mix, **Pillsbury,** 15½-oz. box	1760	272.0			113.5	17.55
Prepared as package directs (suggested yield: 36 brownies)	2340	360.0			(106.3)	(16.36)
1 brownie, 36 per box			65	10.0	(106.3)	(16.36)
Fudge Brownie Mix (Family Size), **Pillsbury,** 22½-oz. box	2640	504.0			117.3	22.50
Prepared as package directs (suggested yield: 48 brownies)	3360	504.0			(105.2)	(15.77)
1 brownie, 48 per box			70	10.5	(105.2)	(15.77)
Fudge Brownie Supreme Mix, **Betty Crocker,** 23½-oz. box						
Prepared as package directs (suggested yield: 24 brownies)	2880	480.0			(88.8)	(14.38)
1 brownie, 24 per box			120	20.0	(88.8)	(14.38)
German Chocolate Brownie Mix, **Betty Crocker,** 19-oz. box						
Prepared as package directs (suggested yield: 16 brownies)	2400	416.0			(89.0)	(15.42)
1 brownie, 16 per box			150	26.0	(89.0)	(15.42)

	UNIT Cal.	UNIT Carb.	1 COOKIE Cal.	1 COOKIE Carb.	1 OZ., BY WT. Cal.	1 OZ., BY WT. Carb.
Walnut Brownie Mix, **Betty Crocker,** 16½-oz. box						
Prepared as package directs (suggested yield: 16 brownies)					(95.6)	(15.02)
1 brownie, 16 per box			140	22.0	(95.6)	(15.02)
Walnut Brownie Mix, **Pillsbury,** 17¼-oz. box	2160	360.0			125.2	20.87
Prepared as package directs (suggested yield: 36 brownies)	2700	360.0			(110.2)	(14.70)
1 brownie, 36 per box			75	10.0	(110.2)	(14.70)
(Family Size) 23¾-oz. box	2880	504.0			121.3	21.22
Prepared as package directs (suggested yield: 48 brownies)	3600	504.0			(106.8)	(14.96)
1 brownie, 48 per box			75	10.5	(106.8)	(14.96)
Wholegrain, Stone Ground, Brownie Mix, **Vermont General Store & Grist Mill,** 13.7-oz. bag	1620	324.0			118.2	(25.65)
Prepared as package directs (suggested yield: 18 brownies)	2500	324.5			(128.5)	(16.68)
1 brownie, 18 per box			139	18.0	(128.5)	(16.68)
COOKIE MIXES						
Butter Cookie Mix, Dietetic, **Batter-Lite,** 6¼-oz. box	754	117.0			120.6	18.72
Prepared as package directs (suggested yield: 18 cookies)	799	122.2			121.1	18.55
1 cookie, 18 per box			44	6.8	121.1	18.55
Carob Chip Stoneground Whole Wheat Cookie Mix, **Elam's,** 32-oz. (2-lb.) box	3874	627.8			121.1	19.62
Prepared as package directs (suggested yield: 55 cookies)	3874	627.8			(95.9)	(15.54)
1 cookie, 55 per box			(70)	(11.4)	(95.9)	(15.54)
Carob-Nut Cookie Mix (Carob-Cake Mix), **Arrowhead Mills,** 32-oz. package	(4640)	(608.0)			(145.0)	(19.00)
Prepared as package directs (suggested yield: 22 cookies)	(4058)	(375.4)			(143.4)	(13.27)
1 cookie, 22 per batch			(184)	(17.0)	123.8	20.25
Chocolate Cookie Mix, Dietetic, **Batter-Lite,** 6¼-oz. box	758	118.8			121.2	19.01
Prepared as package directs (suggested yield: 18 cookies)	864	124.2			116.8	16.78
1 cookie, 18 per box			48	6.9	116.8	16.78
Chocolate Chip Cookie Mix, **Betty Crocker** "Big Batch," 32-oz. (2-lb.) box, 2 pouches (each 1 lb.)	4320	648.0			135.0	20.25
Prepared as package directs, 1 pouch (suggested yield: 36 cookies)	2700	324.0			(136.8)	(16.41)
1 cookie, 36 per pouch			75	9.0	(136.8)	(16.41)
Chocolate Chip Cookie Mix, **Nestlé,** 14-oz. box	1980	276.0			141.4	19.29
Prepared as package directs (suggested yield: 36 cookies)	2160	270.0			(152.2)	(19.03)
1 cookie, 36 per box			60	7.5	(152.2)	(19.03)
Chocolate Chip Cookie Mix, **Quaker,** 15-oz. box	1800	288.0			120.0	19.20
Prepared as package directs (suggested yield: 36 cookies)	2700	288.0				
1 cookie, 36 per box			75	8.0		
Coconut Macaroon Cookie Mix, **Betty Crocker,** 13-oz. box						
Prepared as package directs (suggested yield: 24 macaroons)	1920	240.0			(120.0)	(15.00)
1 macaroon, 24 per box			80	10.0	(120.0)	(15.00)
Double Chocolate Cookie Mix, **Betty Crocker** "Big Batch," 32-oz. (2-lb.) box, 2 pouches, each 1 lb.	4320	648.0			135.0	20.25
Prepared as package directs, 1 pouch (suggested yield: 36 cookies)	(2700)	(324.0)			(136.8)	(16.41)
1 cookie, 36 per pouch			(75)	(9.0)	(136.8)	(16.41)
Fudge Chip Cookie Mix, **Quaker,** 15-oz. box	1725	341.3			115.0	22.75
Prepared as package directs (suggested yield: 36 cookies)	2588	341.3			(140.0)	(18.45)
1 cookie, 36 per box			72	9.5	(140.0)	(18.45)
Gingerbread Mix, **Betty Crocker,** 14.5-oz. box	1800	324.0			124.1	22.34
Prepared as package directs (suggested yield: 9 squares	1890	324.0				
1 piece, 9 per box			210	36.0		
Lemon Cookie Mix, Dietetic, **Batter-Lite,** 6¼-oz. box	754	117.0			120.6	18.72
Prepared as package directs (suggested yield: 18 cookies)	799	122.4			121.1	18.55
1 cookie, 18 per box			44	6.8	121.1	18.55
Oatmeal Cookie Mix, **Betty Crocker** "Big Batch," 32-oz. (2-lb.) box, 2 pouches	3960	648.0			123.8	20.25
Prepared as package directs (suggested yield: 72 cookies, 36 per pouch)	5040	648.0				
1 cookie, 72 per box			70	9.0		

	UNIT Cal.	UNIT Carb.	1 COOKIE Cal.	1 COOKIE Carb.	1 OZ., BY WT. Cal.	1 OZ., BY WT. Carb.
Oatmeal Cookie Mix, **Quaker,** 18-oz. box	2358	333.8			131.0	18.50
Prepared as package directs (suggested yield: 36 cookies)	2358	333.8			(119.7)	(16.94)
1 cookie, 36 per box			66	9.3	(119.7)	(16.94)
Oatmeal Molasses Cookie Mix, **Vermont General Store & Grist Mill,** 12½-oz. box	1620	324.0			118.2	23.60
Prepared as package directs (suggested yield: 36 cookies)					(120.8)	(15.70)
1 cookie, 36 per box			(69)	(9.0)	(120.8)	(15.70)
Oatmeal Raisin Cookie Mix, **Nestlé,** 15-oz. box	1800	306.0			120.0	20.40
Prepared as package directs (suggested yield: 36 cookies)	2160	324.0			(135.8)	(20.40)
1 cookie, 36 per box			60	9.0	(135.8)	(20.40)
Orange Bran Cookie Mix, **Vermont General Store & Grist Mill,** 12.7-oz. bag	1368	300.0			107.7	23.62
Prepared as package directs (suggested yield: 36 cookies)	(2248)	(300.5)			(132.7)	(17.74)
1 cookie, 36 per box			(62)	(8.3)	(132.7)	(17.74)
Peanut Butter Cookie Mix, **Quaker,** 15-oz. box	1875	279.5			125.0	18.63
Prepared as package directs (suggested yield: 36 cookies)	2813	279.5			(152.5)	(15.15)
1 cookie, 36 per box			78	7.8	(152.5)	(15.15)
Slice & Bake Sugar Cookies, **A&P,** 16-oz. (1-lb.) tube	2160	270.0			135.0	16.88
Prepared as package directs (suggested yield: 36 cookies)	2160	270.0			150.0	18.75
1 cookie, 36 per tube			60	7.5	150.0	18.75
Sugar Cookie Mix, **Quaker,** 17-oz. box	2267	338.1			133.3	19.89
Prepared as package directs (suggested yield: 36 cookies)	2790	338.1			(133.5)	(16.18)
1 cookie, 36 per box			77	9.4	(133.5)	(16.18)
Whole Grain Lemon Crisp Cookie Mix, **Vermont General Store & Grist Mill,** 11.6-oz. bag	1260	270.0			108.6	23.28
Prepared as package directs (suggested yield: 36 cookies)	(2140)	(270.5)			(133.8)	(16.93)
1 cookie, 36 per box			59	7.5	(133.8)	(16.93)

PREPACKAGED COOKIES, based on USDA data

	UNIT Cal.	UNIT Carb.	1 COOKIE OR CRACKER Cal.	1 COOKIE OR CRACKER Carb.	1 OZ., BY WT. Cal.	1 OZ., BY WT. Carb.	Fiber per oz. (GMS.)
ANIMAL CRACKERS, 1 package, 2 oz. net wt. (approx. 22 "Animals")	245	45.5			121.6	22.65	0.03
1 Animal, approx. 0.1 oz. (approx. 11 to the oz.)			11	2.1	121.6	22.65	0.03
1 pound (approx. 175 "Animals") (2g/23g/3g/3%/86mg)	1946	362.4			121.6	22.65	0.03
ASSORTED COOKIES, consisting of sandwich type, shortbread, sugar wafers, butter flavored, chocolate chip, coconut bars, etc. 1 package, 11 oz. net wt. (approx. 36 cookies)	1498	221.5			136.1	20.13	0.31
"Average" cookie, approx. 0.3 oz.			41	6.2	136.1	20.13	0.31
1 pound (approx. 52 cookies) (1g/20g/6g/3%/104mg)	2177	322.1			136.1	20.13	0.31
BROWNIES WITH NUTS, frozen with chocolate icing, 1 container, 13 oz. net wt.	1542	223.4			118.8	17.21	0.17
1 brownie, approx. ¹⁄₁₅ of 13-oz. container, 1½" × 1¾" × ⅞", approx. 0.9 oz.			103	14.9	118.8	17.21	0.17
1 pound (approx. 18 brownies) (1g/17g/6g/13%/200mg)	1901	275.4			118.8	17.21	0.17
BUTTER COOKIES, (thin rich butter-flavored cookies) 1 package, 8 oz. net wt. (approx. 45 cookies)	1037	160.9			129.6	20.11	0.03
1 cookie, approx. 2"-2⅛" diameter, ¼" thick, approx. 0.2 oz.			23	3.6	129.6	20.11	0.03
1 pound (approx. 90 cookies) (2g/20g/5g/5%/418mg)	2073	321.6			129.6	20.11	0.03
CHOCOLATE CHIP COOKIES, 1 package, 7¾ oz. net wt. (approx. 30 cookies)	1036	153.3			133.5	19.76	0.11
1 cookie, 1¾" diameter, ½" thick, approx. ¼ oz.			34	5.1	133.5	19.76	0.11
1 package, 14½ oz. net wt. (approx. 39 cookies)	1936	286.5			133.5	19.76	0.11
1 cookie, 2¼" diameter, ⅜" thick, approx. 0.4 oz.			50	7.3	133.5	19.76	0.11

	UNIT Cal.	UNIT Carb.	1 COOKIE OR CRACKER Cal.	1 COOKIE OR CRACKER Carb.	1 OZ., BY WT. Cal.	1 OZ., BY WT. Carb.	Fiber per oz. (GMS.)
1 package, 15 oz. net wt. (approx. 80 cookies)	2002	296.2			133.5	19.76	0.11
1 cookie, 1¾" diameter, ⅜" thick, approx. 0.2 oz.			25	3.7	133.5	19.76	0.11
1 pound (approx. 62 cookies from 7¾-oz. package as above, 43 cookies from 14½-oz. package as above, or 86 cookies from 15-oz. package as above) (2g/20g/6g/3%/114mg)	2136	316.2			133.5	19.76	0.11
COCONUT BARS, coconut bar, approx. 2⅜" × 1⅝" × ⅜", approx. 0.3 oz.	45	5.8			140.1	18.12	0.17
1 coconut bar, 3" × 1¼" × ¼", approx. 0.3 oz.			45	5.8	140.1	18.12	0.17
1 pound (2g/18g/7g/4%/42mg)	2241	289.9			140.1	18.12	0.17
FIG BARS, 1 package, 16 oz. (1 lb.) net wt. (approx. 32 bars)	1624	342.0			101.5	21.38	0.48
1 square bar, 1⅝" × 1⅝" × ⅜", approx. 0.5 oz.			50	10.6	101.5	21.38	0.48
1 rectangular bar, 1½" × 1¾" × ½", approx. 0.5 oz.			50	10.6	101.5	21.38	0.48
1 pound (approx. 32 bars) (1g/21g/2g/14%/71mg)	1624	342.1			101.5	21.38	0.48
GINGER SNAPS, 1 package 16 oz. (1 lb.) net wt. (approx. 65 snaps)	1905	362.0			119.1	22.63	0.03
1 snap, approx. 2" diameter, ¼" thick, approx. ¼ oz.			29	5.6	119.1	22.63	0.03
1 pound (approx. 65 snaps) (2g/23g/3g/3%/162mg)	1905	362.0	29	5.6	119.1	22.63	0.03
GRAHAM CRACKERS							
Plain:							
1 package, 16 oz. (1 lb.) [approx. 32 rectangular pieces, each 5" long, 2½" wide, 3/16" thick marked for division into 2 equal pieces (2½" square, 3/16" thick), or into 4 equal rectangular pieces (each 2½" long, 1¼" wide, 3/16" thick)]	1742	332.5			108.9	20.78	0.31
1 cracker, uncut rectangle (as described for package above), approx. 0.5 oz.	55	10.4			108.9	20.78	0.31
1 square, when uncut rectangle is broken along line into 2 equal pieces (as described for package above), approx. ¼ oz.	28	5.2			108.9	20.78	0.31
1 rectangle, when uncut rectangle is broken along line into 4 equal pieces (as described for package above), approx. 0.1 oz.			14	2.6	108.9	20.78	0.31
1 pound (approx. 32 uncut rectangles, or 64 squares, or 4 smaller rectangles, as described above for package) (2g/21g/3g/6%/190mg)	1742	332.5			108.9	20.78	0.31
Crumbled, finely crushed:							
1 cup							
not packed (approx. 3 oz.; 6 uncut rectangles)	326	62.3			108.9	20.78	0.31
packed (approx. 7¼ oz.; 3¾ uncut rectangles)	403	77.0			108.9	20.78	0.31
1 tablespoon (approx. 0.2 oz.; 4 uncut rectangles as described for package above)	251	4.8			108.9	20.78	0.31
Sugar Honey Graham Crackers:							
1 package, 16 oz. (1 lb.) net wt. [approx. 32 rectangular pieces, each 5" long, 2½" wide, 3/16" thick marked for division into 2 equal pieces (2½" square, 3/16" thick), or into 4 equal rectangular pieces (each 2½" long, 1¼" wide, 3/16" thick)]	1864	346.6			115.4	21.66	0.31
1 cracker, uncut rectangle (as described for package above), approx. 0.5 oz.			58	10.8	115.4	21.66	0.31
1 square, when uncut rectangle is broken along line into 2 equal pieces (as described for package above), approx. ¼ oz.			29	6.4	115.4	21.66	0.31
1 rectangle, when uncut rectangle is broken along line into 4 equal pieces (as described for package above), approx. 0.1 oz.			15	2.7	115.4	21.66	0.31
1 pound (approx. 32 uncut rectangles, or 64 squares, or 4 smaller rectangles, all as described above for package) (2g/22g/3g/3%/143mg)	1864	346.6			115.4	21.66	0.31
Crumbled, finely crushed:							
1 cup							
not packed (approx. 3 oz.; 6 uncut rectangles)	349	64.9			115.4	21.66	0.31
packed (approx. 7¼ oz.; 7½ uncut rectangles)	432	80.2			115.4	21.66	0.31
1 tablespoon (approx. 0.2 oz.; 0.4 uncut rectangles as described for package above)	27	5.0			115.4	21.66	0.31
Chocolate Coated Graham Crackers: (The dimensions and counts for chocolate graham crackers vary considerably.)							
1 pound (approx. 34 or 35 chocolate grahams) (1g/19g/7g/2%/115mg)	2155	308.0			134.7	19.25	0.45
1 cracker, 2½" long, 2" wide, ¼" thick, approx. 0.5 oz.			62	8.8	134.7	19.25	0.45
LADYFINGERS, 1 package, 3 oz. net wt. (approx. 8 ladyfingers split lengthwise)	306	54.8			102.1	18.29	0.03
1 ladyfinger, 3¼" x 1⅜" x 1⅛", dimensions before split lengthwise (approx. ⅓ oz.)			40	7.1	102.1	18.29	0.03
1 pound (approx. 41 ladyfingers) (2g/18g/2g/19%/20mg)	1633	292.6			102.1	18.29	0.03
MACAROONS, 1 package, 11 oz. net wt. (approx. 16 macaroons)	1482	206.2			134.7	18.74	0.60
1 macaroon, 2¾" diameter, ¼" thick, approx. ⅔ oz.			91	12.6	134.7	18.74	0.60
1 pound (approx. 24 macaroons) (2g/19g/7g/4%/10mg)	2155	299.8			134.7	18.74	0.60
MARSHMALLOW COOKIES							
Chocolate-Coated:							
1 package, 8 oz. net wt. (approx. 18 cookies)	928	164.1			115.9	20.50	0.17
1 cookie, 1¾" diameter, ¾" thick, approx. 0.5 oz.			53	9.4	115.9	20.50	0.17
1 pound (approx. 35 cookies) (1g/21g/4g/10%/59mg)	1855	328.0			115.9	20.50	0.17
Coconut-Coated:							
1 package, .74 oz. net wt. (approx. 12 cookies)	871	154.0			115.9	20.50	0.17
1 cookie, 2⅓" diameter, 1⅛" thick, approx. 0.6 oz.			74	13.0	115.9	20.50	0.17
1 pound (approx. 25 cookies) (1g/21g/4g/10%/59mg)	1855	328.0			115.9	20.50	0.17
MOLASSES COOKIES, 1 cookie, 3⅝" diameter, ⅜" thick, approx. 1.2 oz.			137	24.7	119.6	21.54	0.03
1 pound (approx. 14 cookies) (2g/22g/3g/4%/109mg)	1914	344.7			119.6	21.54	0.03
OATMEAL COOKIES, with Raisins, 1 package, 14 oz. net wt. (approx. 30 cookies)	1790	291.8			127.9	20.84	0.11
1 cookie, 2⅝" diameter, ¼" thick, approx. 0.5 oz.			59	9.6	127.9	20.84	0.11
1 pound (approx. 35 cookies) (2g/21g/4g/3%/46mg)	2046	333.4			127.9	20.84	0.11
PEANUT COOKIES (COOKIES WITH PEANUT FILLING)							
Sandwich Type:							
1 package, 10 oz. net wt. (approx. 23 cookies)	1343	190.3			134.1	18.99	0.23
1 cookie, 1¾" diameter, 1½" thick, approx. 0.4 oz.			58	8.2	134.1	18.99	0.23
1 pound (approx. 37 cookies) (3g/19g/5g/2%/49mg)	2146	303.9			134.1	18.99	0.23
Sugar Wafer Type:							
1 package, 6¾ oz. net wt., 3 rectangular blocks 8¾" × 2¾" × ⅜", each marked for splitting into 10 cookies	903	128.0			134.1	18.99	0.23
1 cookie, 1¾" × 1⅜" × ⅜", approx. ¼ oz.			33	4.7	134.1	18.99	0.23
1 package, 9 oz. net wt., 4 rectangular blocks 8¾" × 2¾" × ⅜", each marked for splitting into 10 cookies	1206	170.9			134.1	18.99	0.23
1 cookie, 1¾" × 1⅜" × ⅜", approx. ¼ oz.			33	4.7	134.1	18.99	0.23
1 pound (approx. 65 cookies) (1g/19g/6g/1%/54mg)	2146	303.9			134.1	18.99	0.23
RAISIN COOKIES, Biscuit Type, 1 package, 7½ oz. net wt., 3 rectangular blocks 10⅛" × 2¼" × ¼", each marked for cutting into 4 cookies	807	172.1			107.4	22.91	0.26
1 cookie, 2¼" × 2½" × ¼", approx. 0.6 oz.			67	14.4	107.4	22.91	0.26

	UNIT Cal.	UNIT Carb.	1 COOKIE OR CRACKER Cal.	1 COOKIE OR CRACKER Carb.	1 OZ., BY WT. Cal.	1 OZ., BY WT. Carb.	Fiber per oz. (GMS.)
1 package, 7½ oz. net wt., 3 rectangular blocks, 10⅛" × 2¼" × ¼", each marked for cutting into 5 cookies	807	172.1			107.4	22.91	0.26
1 cookie, 2¼" × 2" × ¼", approx. 0.5 oz.			54	11.5	107.4	22.91	0.26
1 pound (approx. 25½ cookies from 4-split cookies above, approx. 32 cookies from 5-split cookies above) (1g/23g/2g/8%/15mg)	1719	366.5			107.4	22.91	0.26
SANDWICH COOKIES, chocolate or vanilla, 1 package, 16 oz. (1 lb.) net wt. (approx. 31 oval cookies)	2245	314.3			140.3	19.64	0.03
1 oval cookie, cross sectioned, 3⅛" × 1¼" × ⅜", approx. ½ oz.			74	10.4	140.3	19.64	0.03
1 package, 16 oz. (1 lb.) net wt. (approx. 45 round cookies)	2245	314.3			140.3	19.64	0.03
1 round cookie, 1¾" diameter, ⅜" thick, approx. ⅓ oz.			50	6.9	140.3	19.64	0.03
1 pound (approx. 31 oval cookies or 45 round cookies) (1g/20g/6g/2%/137mg)	2245	314.3			140.3	19.64	0.03
SUGAR WAFERS, 1 package, 8½ oz. net wt. (approx. 69 cookies)	1169	176.9			137.5	20.80	0.26
1 cookie, 2½" × ¾" × ¼", approx. 0.1 oz.			17	2.6	137.5	20.80	0.26
1 package, 13¼ oz. net wt (approx. 40 cookies	1824	276.0			137.5	20.80	0.26
1 cookie, 3½" × 1" × ½", approx. ⅓ oz.			45	6.9	137.5	20.80	0.26
Sugar Wafer from Assorted Cookies package, 1 sugar wafer, 3½" × 1½" × ¼", approx. ¼ oz.			34	5.1	137.5	20.80	0.26
1 sugar wafer, 1¾" × 1½" × ¾", approx. 0.3 oz.			44	6.6	137.5	20.80	0.26
1 pound (approx. 128 cookies from 8½-oz. package above, 48 cookies from 13¼-oz. package above, 65 cookies from assorted cookies .25 oz. each, or 50 cookies from assorted cookies 0.3 oz. each) (1g/21g/6g/1%/54mg)	2200	332.9			137.5	20.80	0.26
VANILLA WAFERS							
Regular Type:							
1 package, 12 oz. net wt. (approx. 113 cookies)	1571	253.0			131.0	21.09	0.37
1 cookie, 1⅜" diameter, ¼" thick, approx. 0.11 oz.			14	22.3	131.0	21.09	0.37
1 package, 12 oz. net wt. (approx. 85 cookies)	1571	253.0			131.0	21.09	0.37
1 cookie, 1¾" diameter, ¼" thick, approx. 0.14 oz.			19	3.0	131.0	21.09	0.37
1 pound (approx. 151 cookies of the 0.11 oz. cookies as above, or 113 cookies of the 0.14 oz. cookies as above) (2g/21g/5g/3%/71mg)	2096	337.5			131.0	21.09	0.37
Brown Edge:							
1 package, 10 oz. net wt. (approx. 49 cookies)	1312	211.3			131.0	21.09	0.37
1 cookie, 2¾" diameter, ¼" thick, approx. 0.2 oz.			27	4.3	131.0	21.09	0.37
1 pound (approx. 78 cookies)	2096	337.5			131.0	21.09	0.37
Biscuit Type:							
1 package, 11 oz. net wt. (approx. 66 wafers)	1441	232.0			131.0	21.09	0.37
1 wafer, 2¼" × 1½" × ¼", approx. 0.2 oz.			22	3.5	131.0	21.09	0.37
1 pound (approx. 96 wafers)	2096	337.5			131.0	21.09	0.37
Crumbled:							
1 cup (approx. 2.8 oz.)	370	59.5			131.0	21.09	0.37

PREPACKAGED CRACKERS, based on USDA data

	UNIT Cal.	UNIT Carb.	1 COOKIE OR CRACKER Cal.	1 COOKIE OR CRACKER Carb.	1 OZ., BY WT. Cal.	1 OZ., BY WT. Carb.	Fiber per oz. (GMS.)
ANIMAL CRACKERS, see under PREPACKAGED COOKIES							
BUTTER CRACKERS							
Rectangular, 2½" long, 1⅜" wide, ⅛" thick:							
1 package, 11½ oz. net wt. (approx. 85 to 86 crackers)	1493	219.4			129.8	19.08	0.09
1 cracker, approx. 0.1 oz. (approx. 7 per ounce)			17	2.6	129.8	19.08	0.09
1 pound (approx. 138 crackers)	2401	353.3			129.8	19.08	0.09
Round, 1⅞" diameter, 3/16" thick:							
1 package, 10–12 oz. net wt., containing 3 inner packs (approx. 31–32 crackers per inner pack; approx. 95 crackers total)	1429	210.0	15	2.2	129.8	19.08	0.09

	UNIT Cal.	UNIT Carb.	1 COOKIE OR CRACKER Cal.	1 COOKIE OR CRACKER Carb.	1 OZ., BY WT. Cal.	1 OZ., BY WT. Carb.	Fiber per oz. (GMS.)
1 package, 16 oz. (1 lb.) net wt. loose pack (approx. 138 crackers)	2077	305.3	15	2.2	129.8	19.08	0.09
1 cracker (from 10–12 oz. or 16-oz. package), approx. 0.1 oz. (approx. 9 per ounce)			15	2.2	129.8	19.08	0.09
1 pound (approx. 138 crackers) (2g/19g/5g/5%/310mg)	2077	305.3			129.8	19.08	0.09
Crumbled, finely crushed, not packed:							
1 cup (approx. 2.8 oz.; 24 round crackers, or 21 rectangular crackers)	366	53.8			129.8	19.08	0.09
1 tablespoon (approx. 0.2 oz.; 1½ round crackers, or 1⅓ rectangular crackers)	23	3.4			129.8	19.08	0.09
CHEESE CRACKERS							
Assorted Shapes (such as hexagon, clover, etc.) approx. 1⅞" diameter at widest cross-section, 3/16" thick:							
1 package, 8½ oz. net wt. (approx. 77 crackers)	1154	145.6			135.8	17.01	0.06
1 cracker, approx. 0.1 oz. (approx. 9 per ounce)			15	1.9	135.8	17.01	0.06
1 pound (approx. 145 crackers) (3g/17g/6g/4%/295mg)	2173	274.0			135.8	17.01	0.06
Rectangular sticks, 1⅝" long, ¼" thick:							
1 package, 2¼ oz. net wt. (approx. 70 or 71 sticks)	307	38.7			135.8	17.01	0.06
1 package, 11 oz. net wt. (approx. 344 sticks)	1494	188.4			135.8	17.01	0.06
1 stick (from 2¼ oz. or 11 oz. package), approx. 0.03 oz.			4	0.6	135.8	17.01	0.06
1 pound (approx. 500 sticks)	2200	275.0			135.8	17.01	0.06
Round, 1⅞" diameter, 3/16" thick:							
1 package, 8 oz. net wt. (approx. 66 crackers)	1087	137.1			135.8	17.01	0.06
1 cracker, approx. 0.1 oz.			16	2.1	135.8	17.01	0.06
1 pound (approx. 132 crackers)	2173	274.0			135.8	17.01	0.06
Square, 1" × 1" × ⅛" thick:							
1 package, 2 oz. net wt. (approx. 52 or 53 crackers)	273	34.4			135.8	17.01	0.06
1 package, 6¼ oz. net wt. (approx. 163 or 164 crackers)	850	106.9			135.8	17.01	0.06
1 package, 10 oz. (approx. 263 crackers)	1360	171.5			135.8	17.01	0.06
1 cracker (from 2 oz., 6¼ oz., or 10 oz. package), approx. 0.04 oz.			5	0.6	135.8	17.01	0.06
1 pound (approx. 420 crackers)	2173	274.0			135.8	17.01	0.06
Crumbled, finely crushed, not packed:							
1 cup (approx. 3 oz.; approx. 25 round crackers, or 93 rectangular sticks, or 79 squares)	407	51.3			136.5	17.06	0.06
1 tablespoon (approx. 0.2 oz.; 5.8 rectangular sticks, or 1.6 round crackers; or 4.9 squares)	25	3.2			136.5	17.06	0.06
PEANUT BUTTER SANDWICHES (made with cheese-flavored Saltines)							
1 package, 6 oz. net wt. containing 4 packets (approx. 36 crackers, 6 sandwiches per packet) or 6 packets (approx. 36 crackers, 4 sandwiches per packet)	835	95.4			139.2	15.90	0.14
1 packet, approx. 1½ oz. net wt. (6 sandwiches)	209	23.8			139.2	15.90	0.14
1 sandwich, approx. ¼ oz.			35	4.0	139.2	15.90	0.14
1 packet, 1 oz. net wt. (4 sandwiches)	139	15.9			139.2	15.90	0.14
1 sandwich, approx. ¼ oz.			35	4.0	139.2	15.90	0.14
1 pound (approx. 64 sandwiches) (4g/16g/7g/2%/281mg)	2227	254.4			139.2	15.90	0.14
SALTINES							
Plain, Salted or Unsalted:							
1 package, 7⅛ oz. net wt. (approx. 72 crackers)	875	144.4			122.8	20.27	0.11
1 package, 16 oz. (1 lb.) net wt. (approx. 160 crackers)	1964	324.3			122.8	20.27	0.11
Common restaurant packet, 4 crackers (approx. 0.4 oz.)	48	8.0			122.8	20.27	0.11
1 cracker, 1⅞" square, ⅛" thick, approx. 1/10 oz.			12	2.0	122.8	20.27	0.11
1 pound (approx. 160 saltines) (3g/20g/3g/4%/312mg)	1964	324.3			122.8	20.27	0.11
Crumbled, finely crushed:							
1 cup:							
Not packed (approx. 2.5 oz.; 24½ crackers)	303	50.1			122.8	20.27	0.11
Packed (approx. 3 oz.; 30 crackers)	369	60.9			122.8	20.27	0.11

	UNIT		1 COOKIE OR CRACKER		1 OZ., BY WT.		Fiber per oz.
	Cal.	Carb.	Cal.	Carb.	Cal.	Carb.	(GMS.)
1 tablespoon (approx. 0.2 oz.; 1.7 crackers)	23	3.8			122.8	20.27	0.11
SODA CRACKERS							
Regular, 1⅞" square, ⅛" thick:							
1 package, 16 oz. (1 lb.) net wt. (approx. 160 crackers)	1991	320.2			124.4	20.01	0.06
1 cracker, approx. 0.1 oz.			13	2.0	124.4	20.01	0.06
1 pound (approx. 160 crackers) (3g/20g/4g/4%/312mg)	1991	320.2			124.4	20.01	0.06
Crumbled:							
1 cup, not packed (approx. 2½ oz.; 25 crackers)	307	49.4			124.4	20.01	0.06
Biscuit Type, 2⅜" × 2⅛" × ¼" thick:							
1 package, 3½ oz. net wt. (approx. 19 or 20 biscuits)	435	69.9			124.4	20.01	0.06
1 biscuit, approx. 0.2 oz.			22	3.6	124.4	20.01	0.06
1 pound (approx. 90 biscuits)	1991	320.2			124.4	20.01	0.06
Crumbled:							
1 cup, not packed (approx. 2½ oz.; 14 biscuits)	307	49.4			124.4	20.01	0.06
SOUP or OYSTER SODA CRACKERS:							
1 package, 16 oz. (1 lb.) net wt. (approx. 530 to 600 hexagon-shaped crackers, each with ½" sides, 3/16" to 7/16" thick, or approx. 650 round crackers, each ⅞" diameter, 7/16" thick)	1991	320.2			124.4	20.01	0.06
1 package, 5 oz. net wt. (approx. 165 to 188 hexagon-shaped crackers)	623	100.3			124.4	20.01	0.06
1 hexagon-shaped cracker, approx. 0.03 oz.			3	0.5	124.4	20.01	0.06
1 round cracker, approx. 0.02 oz.			3	0.5	124.4	20.01	0.06
1 pound (approx. 530 to 600 hexagon-shaped crackers as described for package above, or 650 round crackers as described for package above ((3g/20g/4g/4%/312mg)	1991	320.2			124.4	20.01	0.06
1 cup:							
Whole crackers (approx. 1.4 oz.; 52 to 60 hexagon-shaped crackers, or 63 to 66 round crackers)	185	27.6			124.4	20.01	0.06
Crumbled (approx. 2.5 oz.; 80 to 92 hexagon-shaped crackers, or 94 to 100 round crackers)	307	49.4			124.4	20.01	0.06
WHOLE WHEAT CRACKERS							
1 package, 16 oz. (1 lb.) net wt. (2g/19g/4g/7%/155mg)	1828	309.4			114.3	19.34	0.68

PREPACKAGED COOKIES and CRACKERS, by brand

	ENTIRE PACKAGE		1 COOKIE OR CRACKER		1 OZ., BY WT.		1 CUP CRUMBLED	
	Cal.	Carb.	Cal.	Carb.	Cal.	Carb.	Cal.	Carb.
ADELAIDE								
Adelaide Cookies, **Pepperidge Farm,** 5½-oz. package (approx. 15 cookies)	800	100.0			145.5	18.18	(436)	(54.5)
1 cookie, approx. 0.4 oz.			53	6.7	145.5	18.18	(436)	(54.5)
ALLGRANE								
Allgrane Wafers, **Devonsheer Melba,** 5-oz. package (approx. 71 or 72 wafers)	496	110.4			99.2	22.07		
1 wafer, approx. 0.07 oz.			7	1.5	99.2	22.07		
Allgrane Wafers, unsalted, **Devonsheer Melba,** 5-oz. package (approx. 71 or 72 wafers)	496	110.4			99.2	22.07		
1 wafer, approx. 0.07 oz.			7	1.5	99.2	22.07		
ALMOND								
Almond Mandel Toast, **Stella D'Oro,** 8-oz. package (approx. 16 toasts)	864	158.4			108.6	19.92	(380)	(69.7)
1 toast, approx. 0.5 oz.			54	9.9	108.6	19.92	(380)	(69.7)
Almond Windmill Cookies, **Nabisco,** 11-oz. package (approx. 33 cookies)	1540	231.0			140.0	21.00		
1 cookie, approx. 0.3 oz.			47	7.0	140.0	21.00		
AMERICAN								
American Harvest Snack Crackers, **Nabisco,** 9-oz. package (approx. 81 crackers)	1260	162.0			140.0	18.00	(420)	(54.0)
1 cracker, approx. 0.1 oz.			16	2.0	140.0	18.00	(420)	(54.0)
ANGEL								
Angel Puffs, sugar free, salt free, **Stella D'Oro,** 3-oz. package (approx. 27 puffs)	477	40.9			159.1	13.64		
1 puff, approx. 0.1 oz.			18	1.5	159.1	13.64		
ANGELICA								
Angelica Goodies, **Stella D'Oro,** 11.1-oz. package (approx. 14 Goodies)	1400	198.8			(127.5)	(18.11)	(446)	(63.4)
1 Goodie, approx. 0.8 oz.			100	14.2	(127.5)	(18.11)	(446)	(63.4)
ANGINETTI								
Anginetti Cookies, **Stella D'Oro,** 5-oz. package (approx. 25 cookies)	685	95.3			136.9	19.06	(411)	(57.2)
1 Anginetti, approx. 0.2 oz.			28	3.9	136.9	19.06	(411)	(57.2)
ANIMAL								
Animal Crackers, **A&P,** 13-oz. package (approx. 195 Animals)	1560	286.0			120.0	22.00	(487)	(89.2)
1 Animal, approx. 0.07 oz.			8	1.5	120.0	22.00	(487)	(89.2)
Animal Crackers, **Marx Bros.,** 16 millimeter, 8,897 feet, 97 minutes	0	0.0			0.0	0.00		
1-quart container (approx. 1.3 oz.) of large kernel popcorn, popped in oil	164	21.0			129.3	16.76		
Animal Crackers, **Sunshine,** 2-oz. package (approx. 22 Animals)	240	43.6			119.9	21.81	(486)	(88.5)
1 Animal, approx. 0.1 oz.			11	2.0	119.9	21.81	(486)	(88.5)
Animal-Shaped Cookies, **Gerber,** 5-oz. box (22 Animals)	618	93.7			123.6	18.74		
1 Animal, approx. 0.2 oz.			30	4.5	123.6	18.74		
Barnum's Animal Crackers, **Nabisco,** 2-oz. package (approx. 22 Animals)	260	42.0			130.0	21.00	(455)	(73.5)
1 Animal, approx. 0.1 oz.			12	1.9	130.0	21.00	(455)	(73.5)
8-oz. tin, approx. 87 Animals	1040	168.0			130.0	21.00	(455)	(73.5)
1 Animal, approx. 0.1 oz.			12	1.9	130.0	21.00	(455)	(73.5)
Carob Animal Cookies, **El Molino,** 6-oz. package (approx. 56 Animals)	780	126.0			130.0	21.00		
1 Animal, approx. 0.1 oz.			14	2.3	130.0	21.00		
Ginger Animal Cookies, **El Molino,** 6-oz, package (approx. 56 Animals)	780	126.0			130.0	21.00		
1 Animal, approx. 0.1 oz.			14	2.3	130.0	21.00		
Honey Animal Cookies, **El Molino,** 6-oz. package (approx. 54 Animals)	900	96.0			150.0	16.00	(608)	(64.9)
1 Animal, approx. 0.1 oz.			17	1.8	150.0	16.00	(608)	(64.9)
Iced Animal Cookies, **Keebler,** vended size, 1½-oz. package (14 Animals)	160	26.0			106.7	17.33		
1 Animal, approx. 0.1 oz.			11	1.9	106.7	17.33		
ANISETTE								
Anisette Sponge, **Stella D'Oro,** approx. 7.8-oz. package (approx. 16 sponges)	800	153.6			103.5	19.87	(362)	(69.6)
1 sponge, approx. 0.5 oz.			50	9.6	103.5	19.87	(362)	(69.6)
Anisette Toast, **Stella D'Oro,** 6.9-oz. package (approx. 16 toasts)	736	148.8			106.9	21.60	(394)	(75.6)
1 toast, approx. 0.4 oz.			46	9.3	106.9	21.60	(394)	(75.6)
APPLE								
Apple Crisp Cookies, **Nabisco,** 12½-oz. package (approx. 33 cookies)	1650	231.0			132.0	18.48		
1 cookie, approx. 0.4 oz.			50	7.0	132.0	18.48		
ARROWROOT								
Arrowroot Biscuit, National, **Nabisco,** 10½-oz. package (approx. 60 biscuits)	1200	180.0			114.3	17.14		
1 biscuit, approx. 0.2 oz.			20	3.0	114.3	17.14		
Arrowroot Cookies, **Gerber,** 5-oz. box (approx. 25 cookies)	639	98.1			127.9	19.62		
1 cookie, approx. 0.2 oz.			25	4.0	127.9	19.62		

	ENTIRE PACKAGE		1 COOKIE OR CRACKER		1 OZ., BY WT.		1 CUP CRUMBLED	
	Cal.	Carb.	Cal.	Carb.	Cal.	Carb.	Cal.	Carb.
ASSORTMENTS: Cookie assortments are listed at the end of this chapter.								
BACON								
Bacon Crackers, **Keebler,** Vended Size, 1.4-oz. bag (31 crackers)	200	25.0			142.9	17.90		
1 cracker, approx. 0.05 oz.			6	0.8	142.9	17.90		
Bacon Discos, **Devonsheer Melba,** 5-oz. box (approx. 35 discos)	455	(76.9)			91.0	(15.37)		
1 Disco, approx. 1/7 oz.			13	(2.2)	91.0	(15.37)		
Bacon Flavored Thins Crackers, **Nabisco,** 8-oz package (approx. 112 crackers)	1200	144.0			150.0	18.00	(450)	(54.0)
1 cracker, approx. 0.07 oz.			11	1.3	150.0	18.00	(450)	(54.0)
Bacon 'n Dip Snack Crackers, **Nabisco,** 9-oz. package (approx. 153 crackers)	1350	144.0			150.0	16.00		
1 cracker, approx. 0.06 oz.			9	0.9	150.0	16.00		
Bacon Rounds, see under ROUNDS								
BANQUET								
Banquet Wafers, **Sunshine,** 11-oz. package (approx. 110 wafers)	1364	233.9			124.0	21.26	(350)	(60.0)
1 wafer, approx. 0.1 oz.			14	2.4	124.0	21.26	(350)	(60.0)
BARONET								
Baronet Creme Sandwich, packaged as part of the Famous Cookie Assortment, **Nabisco**								
1 sandwich, approx. 0.4 oz.			53	8.0	133.3	20.00		
BISCOS								
Biscos Sugar Wafers, **Nabisco,** 8½-oz. package (approx. 68 to 72 wafers)	1350	180.0			150.0	20.00		
1 wafer, approx. ⅛ oz.			19	2.5	150.0	20.00		
Biscos Waffle Creams, **Nabisco,** 10-oz. package (approx. 36 cookies)	1560	216.0			156.0	21.60	(468)	(64.8)
1 cookie, approx. 0.3 oz.			43	6.0	156.0	21.60	(468)	(64.8)
BORDEAUX								
Bordeaux Cookies, **Pepperidge Farm,** 6¾-oz. package (approx. 27 cookies)	990	135.0			146.8	20.00	(440)	(60.0)
1 cookie, approx. ¼ oz.			37	5.0	146.8	20.00	(440)	(60.0)
BRAN								
Bran Breakfast Biscuits, **El Molino,** 7-oz. box (approx. 46 biscuits)	882	132.3			126.0	18.90		
1 biscuit, ⅙ oz.			20	3.0	126.0	18.90		
Bran Crispbread, **Scandinavian,** 1.6-oz. package (approx. 12 pieces)	168	24.0			103.4	14.77		
1 piece, approx. 0.1 oz.			14	2.0	103.4	14.77		
Bran & Honey Cookies with Raisins, **Tiger's Milk,** 8-oz. package (approx. 32 cookies)	960	136.0			120.0	17.00	(360)	(51.0)
1 cookie, approx. ¼ oz.			60	4.3	120.0	17.00	(360)	(51.0)
BREAKFAST								
Breakfast Treats, **Stella D'Oro,** 9.8-oz. package (approx. 12 treats)	1200	189.6			122.4	19.35		
1 treat, approx. 0.8 oz.	100	15.8	100	15.8	122.4	19.35		
BROWN EDGE								
Brown Edge Sandwich, **Nabisco,** 6¼-oz. package (approx. 12 cookies)	960	120.0			153.6	19.20		
1 cookie, approx. 0.5 oz.			80	10.0	153.6	19.20		
Brown Edge Wafers, **Nabisco,** 9½-oz. package (approx. 48 wafers)	1330	199.5			140.0	21.00		
1 wafer, approx. 0.2 oz.			28	4.2	140.0	21.00		
BROWN SUGAR								
Brown Sugar Cookies, **Pepperidge Farm,** 5¼-oz. package (approx. 15 cookies)	750	105.0			142.9	20.00	(428)	(60.0)
1 cookie, approx. ⅓ oz.			50	7.0	142.9	20.00	(428)	(60.0)
BROWNIES								
Brownies, **Pepperidge Farm,** 2¼-oz. package (2 brownies)	340	41.0			151.1	18.22		
1 brownie, approx. 1⅛ oz.			170	20.5	151.1	18.22		

	ENTIRE PACKAGE		1 COOKIE OR CRACKER		1 OZ., BY WT.		1 CUP CRUMBLED	
	Cal.	Carb.	Cal.	Carb.	Cal.	Carb.	Cal.	Carb.
BUSTER'S								
Buster's Cookies, **Sunshine,** 9-oz. package (approx. 12 cookies)	993	183.1			110.3	20.34	(331)	(61.2)
1 cookie, approx. ¾ oz.			84	15.5	110.3	20.34	(331)	(61.2)
BUTTER								
Butter Flavored Cookies, **Nabisco,** 8-oz. package (approx. 48 cookies)	1120	160.0			140.0	20.00	(490)	(70.0)
1 cookie, approx. ⅛ oz.			23	3.3	140.0	20.00	(490)	(70.0)
Butter Flavored Cookies, **Sunshine,** 8-oz. package (approx. 40 cookies)	1058	158.8			132.3	19.25	(397)	(57.8)
1 cookie, approx. 0.2 oz.			28	4.2	132.3	19.25	(397)	(57.8)
BUTTERCUP								
Buttercup Cookies, **Keebler,** 8-oz. package (approx. 44 cookies)	1134	181.4			141.8	22.68	(400)	(64.0)
1 cookie, approx. 0.2 oz.			25	4.0	141.8	22.68	(400)	(64.0)
BUTTERSCOTCH								
Butterscotch Chip Cookies, **Nabisco** "Bakers Bonus," 11-oz. package, (approx. 20 cookies)	1600	220.0			145.5	20.00		
1 cookie, approx. 0.6 oz.			80	11.0	145.5	20.00		
CAMEO								
Cameo Creme Sandwich Cookies, **Nabisco,** 13½-oz. package (approx. 28 cookies)	1960	294.0			140.0	21.00	(490)	(73.4)
1 cookie, approx. 0.5 oz.			70	10.5	140.0	21.00	(490)	(73.4)
CAPRI								
Capri Cookies, **Pepperidge Farm,** 6½-oz. package (approx. 12 cookies)	1020	120.0			156.9	18.50	(471)	(55.5)
1 cookie, approx. 0.5 oz.			85	10.0	156.9	18.50	(471)	(55.5)
CARAMEL								
Caramel Peanut Logs, **Nabisco** "Heyday," 10-oz. package (approx. 14 logs)	1680	182.0			168.0	18.20		
1 log, approx. 0.7 oz.			120	13.0	168.0	18.20		
CAROB								
Carob Animal Cookies, **El Molino,** 6-oz. package (approx. 56 Animals)	780	126.0			130.0	21.00		
1 Animal, approx. 0.1 oz.			14	2.3	130.0	21.00		
Carob Chip Cookies, **El Molino,** 7-oz. package (approx. 11 or 12 cookies)	933	128.3			133.3	18.33	(400)	(55.0)
1 cookie, approx. 0.6 oz.			80	11.0	133.3	18.33	(400)	(55.0)
Carob Chip Cookies, **Tiger's Milk,** 8-oz. package (approx. 32 cookies)	960	136.0			120.0	17.00	(360)	(55.0)
1 cookie, approx. ¼ oz.			30	4.3	120.0	17.00	(360)	(55.0)
Carob Wheat-Free Cookies, **El Molino,** 7-oz. package (approx. 12 cookies)	933	128.3			133.3	18.33	(400)	(55.0)
1 cookie, approx. 0.6 oz.			80	11.0	133.3	18.33	(400)	(55.0)
CARROT								
Carrot Cake Cookies, **Tiger's Milk,** 8-oz. package (approx. 32 cookies)	960	136.0			120.0	17.00	(360)	(51.0)
1 cookie, approx. ¼ oz.			30	4.3	120.0	17.00	(360)	(51.0)
CHEDDAR								
Cheddar Triangles Snack Crackers, **Nabisco,** 8-oz. package (approx. 136 crackers)	1200	128.0			150.0	16.00		
1 cracker, approx. 0.06 oz.			9	1.0	150.0	16.00		
Country Cheddar 'n Sesame Snack Crackers, **Nabisco,** 8½-oz. package (approx. 136 crackers)	1275	136.0			150.0	16.00		
1 cracker, approx. 0.06 oz.			9	1.0	150.0	16.00		
CHEESE (or CHEEZE)								
Cheese Artificially Flavored Sandwich, **Nabisco,** ⅞-oz. package (approx. 4 crackers)	110	13.0			110.0	13.00		
1 cracker, approx. 0.3 oz.			28	3.3	110.0	13.00		
1-oz. package (approx. 4 crackers)	140	17.0			140.0	17.00		
1 cracker, approx. 0.3 oz.			35	4.3	140.0	17.00		
Cheese Crackers, **A&P,** 10-oz. package (approx. 250 crackers)	1400	160.0			140.0	16.00	(395)	(45.1)
1 cracker, approx. 0.04 oz.			6	0.6	140.0	16.00	(395)	(45.1)

	ENTIRE PACKAGE		1 COOKIE OR CRACKER		1 OZ., BY WT.		1 CUP CRUMBLED	
	Cal.	Carb.	Cal.	Carb.	Cal.	Carb.	Cal.	Carb.
Cheese Crackers, **Keebler,** 1.4-oz. package (31 crackers)	200	24.0			142.9	17.10		
1 cracker, approx. 0.05 oz.			6	0.8	142.9	17.10		
Cheese Crackers, **Rokeach,** 10-oz. box (approx. 250 crackers)	1400	160.0			140.0	16.00		
1 cracker, approx. 0.04 oz.			6	0.6	140.0	16.00		
Cheese Crackers With Extra Peanut Butter, **Austin** "Big Shot," 1¾-oz. package	250	24.0			142.9	13.70		
Cheese 'N Crunch Cheese Flavored Snack, **Nabisco,** 7-oz. package	1120	98.0			160.0	14.00		
Cheese 'N' Peanut Butter Crackers, **Keebler,** 1½-oz. package (6 crackers)	210	24.0			140.0	16.00		
1 cracker, approx. 0.25 oz.			35	4.0	140.0	16.00		
Cheese Nips Crackers, **Nabisco,** 10-oz. package (approx. 260 crackers)	1500	180.0			150.0	18.00	(423)	(50.8)
1 cracker, approx. 0.04 oz.			6	0.7	150.0	18.00	(423)	(50.8)
15-oz. package (approx. 420 crackers)	2100	270.0			140.0	18.00		
1 cracker, approx. 0.04 oz.			5	0.7	140.0	18.00		
Cheese on Cheese Crackers, **Austin,** 1.2-oz. package	160	20.0			133.3	16.67		
Cheese Peanut Butter Artificially Flavored Sandwich, **Nabisco,** 1-oz. package (approx. 4 sandwiches)	140	17.0			140.0	17.00		
1 sandwich, approx. ¼ oz.			35	4.3	140.0	17.00		
Cheese Peanut Butter Sandwiches, **Austin,** 1½-oz. package	210	22.0			140.0	14.67		
Cheese Rounds, see under ROUNDS								
Cheese Smacker Crackers, **Austin,** 1⅛-oz. package	150	19.0			133.3	16.89		
Cheese Swirls Parmesan Snack Crackers, **Nabisco,** 7½-oz. package (approx. 97 or 98 crackers)	1050	120.0			140.0	16.00	(420)	(48.0)
1 cracker, approx. 0.08 oz.			11	1.2	140.0	16.00	(420)	(48.0)
Cheese Tid-Bit Crackers, **Nabisco,** 11-oz. package (approx. 320 crackers)	1500	160.0			136.4	14.55	(450)	(48.0)
1 cracker, approx. 0.03 oz.			5	0.5	136.4	14.55	(450)	(48.0)
Cheez-It Crackers, **Sunshine,** 2-oz. package (approx. 50 crackers)	309	30.9			154.6	15.46	(436)	(43.6)
6¼-oz. package, approx. 156 to 157 crackers	966	96.6			154.6	15.46	(436)	(43.6)
10-oz. package (approx. 250 crackers)	1546	154.6			154.6	15.46	(436)	(43.6)
1 cracker, approx. 0.04 oz.			6	0.6	154.6	15.46	(436)	(43.6)
Combo Cheese Crackers, **Austin,** 1.2-oz. package	160	20.0			133.3	16.67		
Jumbo Cheese 'N' Peanut Butter Crackers, **Keebler,** 1¾-oz. package (6 crackers)	240	28.0			137.1	16.00		
1 cracker, approx. 0.29 oz.			40	4.7	137.1	16.00		
CHESSMEN								
Chessmen, **Pepperidge Farm,** 7¼-oz. package (approx. 24 cookies)	1040	144.0			143.4	19.86	(430)	(59.5)
1 Chessman, approx. 0.3 oz.			43	6.0	143.4	19.86	(430)	(59.5)
CHICKEN								
Chicken in a Biskit, **Nabisco,** 8-oz. package (approx. 109 crackers)	1200	128.0			150.0	16.00		
1 cracker, approx. 0.07 oz.			11	1.1	150.0	16.00		
CHINESE								
Chinese Dessert Cookies, **Stella D'Oro,** 10½-oz. package (approx. 9 cookies)	1530	186.3			144.2	17.92	(515)	(62.7)
1 cookie, approx. 1.2 oz.			170	20.0	144.2	17.92	(515)	(62.7)
CHIPPERS								
Chippers Potato 'n' Cheese Snack Crackers, **Nabisco,** 8-oz. package (approx. 80 crackers)	1200	136.0			150.0	17.00		
1 cracker, approx. 0.1 oz.			15	1.7	140.0	17.00		
Chips Ahoy!, see Chocolate Chip under CHOCOLATE								
CHOCOLATE								
Chocolate Cakes, see MALLOMARS								
Chocolate Chip Cookies, **Ann Page (A&P),** 10-oz. package (approx. 36 cookies)	1296	201.6			129.6	20.16	(389)	(60.5)
1 cookie, approx. 0.3 oz.			36	5.6	129.6	20.16	(389)	(60.5)
Chocolate Chip Cookies, **Nabisco** "Chips Ahoy!" 21-oz. package (approx. 57 cookies)	3040	418.0			145.5	20.00	(459)	(70.0)
1 cookie, approx. 0.4 oz.			53	7.3	145.5	20.00	(459)	(70.0)
Chocolate Chip Cookies, **Nabisco** "Cookie Little," 7-oz. package (approx. 140 cookies)	980	140.0			140.0	20.00		
1 cookie, approx. 0.05 oz.			7	1.0	140.0	20.00		
Chocolate Chip Cookies, **Pepperidge Farm,** 5-oz. package (approx. 15 cookies)	650	85.0			130.0	17.00	(390)	(51.0)
1 cookie, approx. ⅓ oz.			43	5.7	130.0	17.00	(390)	(51.0)
Vended size, 2¼-oz. package (2 cookies)	330	44.0			146.7	19.56		
1 cookie, approx. 1⅛ oz.			165	22.0	146.7	19.56		
Chocolate Chip Cookies, **Sweet N Good,** 11-oz. package (approx. 24 cookies)	1596	225.6			145.1	20.51	(435)	(64.3)
1 cookie, approx. 0.5 oz.			67	9.4	145.1	20.51	(435)	(64.3)
Chocolate Chip Cookies, **Sunshine** "Chip-a-Roos," 12-oz. package (approx. 28 cookies)	1525	258.1			127.1	21.51	(381)	(64.5)
7½-oz. package (approx. 42 cookies)	2224	376.4			127.1	21.51	(381)	(64.5)
1 cookie, approx. 0.4 oz.			52	8.0	127.1	21.51	(381)	(64.5)
Chocolate Chip Flavored Cookies, Snack Wrapped, **Drake's,** 1½-oz. package (approx. 3 cookies)	210	29.1			140.0	19.40	(420)	(58.2)
3-oz. package (approx. 6 cookies)	420	58.0			140.0	19.40	(420)	(58.2)
12-oz. package (approx. 24 cookies)	1680	232.8			140.0	19.40	(420)	(58.2)
1 cookie, approx. 0.5 oz.			70	9.7	140.0	19.40	(420)	(58.2)
Chocolate Chip Snaps, **Nabisco,** 2¾-oz. package (approx. 18 cookies)	360	60.0			130.9	21.82		
1 cookie, approx. 0.2 oz.			20	3.3	130.9	21.82		
Chocolate Chip Wafers, dietetic, **Estee,** 7½-oz. package (approx. 32 wafers)	960	128.0			128.0	17.07	(470)	(62.6)
1 wafer, approx. 0.2 oz.			30	4.0	128.0	17.07	(470)	(62.6)
Chocolate Chocolate Chip Cookies, **Nabisco,** 13-oz. package (approx. 36 cookies)	1920	264.0			147.7	20.30		
1 cookie, approx. 0.4 oz.			53	7.3	147.7	20.30		
Chocolate Fudge Cookies, **Sunshine,** 15-oz. package (approx. 30 cookies)	2127	276.5			141.8	18.43	(425)	(55.3)
1 cookie, approx. 0.5 oz.			70	9.1	141.8	18.43	(425)	(55.3)
Chocolate Fudge Sandwiches, **Keebler,** 16-oz. (1-lb.) package (approx. 26 or 27 sandwiches)	2269	320.2			141.8	20.01		
1 sandwich, approx. 0.6 oz.			85	12.0	141.8	20.01		
Chocolate Grahams, **Nabisco,** 5½-oz. package (approx. 15 Grahams)	850	105.0			154.5	19.09	(464)	(57.3)
1 Graham, approx. ⅓ oz.			57	7.1	154.5	19.09	(464)	(57.3)
Chocolate Nuggets Cookies, **Sunshine,** 14-oz. package (approx. 88 cookies)	1764	299.9			126.0	21.42	(378)	(64.3)
1 cookie, approx. 0.2 oz.			20	3.4	126.0	21.42	(378)	(64.3)
Chocolate Nutter Butter Peanut Butter Sandwich Cookies, **Nabisco,** 15½-oz. package (approx. 39 cookies)	2210	286.0			142.6	18.45		
1 cookie, approx. 0.4 oz.			57	7.3	142.6	18.45		
Chocolate Peanut Bars, **Nabisco** "Ideal," 10½-oz. package (approx. 18 bars)	1710	180.0			162.9	17.14		
1 bar, approx. 0.6 oz.			95	10.0	162.9	17.14		
Chocolate Pinwheels Cakes, **Nabisco,** 12-oz. package (approx. 12 cakes)	1680	252.0			140.0	21.00		
1 cake, approx. 1 oz.			140	21.0	140.0	21.00		
Chocolate Snaps, **Nabisco,** 2½-oz. package (approx. 16 cookies)	260	44.0			104.0	17.60		
1 cookie, approx. 0.2 oz.			16	2.8	104.0	17.60		

	ENTIRE PACKAGE		1 COOKIE OR CRACKER		1 OZ., BY WT.		1 CUP CRUMBLED	
	Cal.	Carb.	Cal.	Carb.	Cal.	Carb.	Cal.	Carb.
Chocolate Swirl Cookies, **Keebler,** Vended size, 1½ oz. package, 14 cookies	170	23.0			113.3	15.33		
1 cookie, approx. 0.1 oz.			12	1.6	113.3	15.33		
Chocolate Wafers, **Nabisco** "Famous," 8½-oz. package (approx. 35–39 wafers)	980	168.0			127.3	21.82	(446)	(76.4)
1 wafer, approx. 0.2 oz.			28	4.8	127.3	21.82	(446)	(76.4)
Coconut Chocolate Chip Cookies, **Nabisco,** 13-oz. package (approx. 26 cookies)	1950	234.0			150.0	18.00		
1 cookie, approx. 0.5 oz.			75	9.0	150.0	18.00		
CHOWDER								
Chowder & Oyster Crackers, **Original Trenton Crackers,** 8-oz. bag (approx. 37 crackers)	956	169.2			119.4	21.15		
1 cracker, approx. 0.2 oz.			26	4.6	119.4	21.15		
CINNAMON								
Cinnamon Grahams, **Sunshine,** 16-oz. (1-lb.) package, (approx. 115 Grahams)	2029	346.2			126.8	21.64	(380)	(64.9)
1 Graham, approx. 0.1 oz.			17	2.9	126.8	21.64	(380)	(64.9)
Cinnamon Sugar Cookies, **Pepperidge Farm,** 5¼-oz. package (approx. 15 cookies)	800	105.0			152.4	20.00	(457)	(60.0)
1 cookie, approx. 0.4 oz.			53	7.0	152.4	20.00	(457)	(60.0)
Cinnamon Treats, **Nabisco,** 16-oz. (1-lb.) package (approx. 70 treats)	1980	360.0			123.8	22.50		
1 treat, approx. 0.2 oz.			28	5.0	123.8	22.50		
CLUB								
Club Crackers, **Keebler,** 16-oz. (1-lb.) package (approx. 133 or 134 crackers)	2405	344.7			150.3	21.48	(424)	(60.6)
1 cracker, approx. 0.1 oz.			18	2.5	150.3	21.48	(424)	(60.6)
COCONUT								
Coconut Bars, **Nabisco** "Bakers Bonus," 10-oz. package (approx. 33 cookies)	1430	176.0			143.0	17.60		
1 cookie, approx. 0.3 oz.			43	5.3	143.0	17.60		
Coconut Bars Cookies, **Nabisco,** 11-oz. package (approx. 33 cookies)	1540	209.0			140.0	19.00	(490)	(66.5)
1 cookie, approx. ⅓ oz.			47	6.3	140.0	19.00	(490)	(66.5)
Coconut Chocolate Chip Cookies, **Nabisco,** 13-oz. package (approx. 26 cookies)	1950	234.0			150.0	18.00		
1 cookie, approx. 0.5 oz.			75	9.0	150.0	18.00		
Coconut Cremers Cookies, **Sunshine,** 15-oz. package (approx. 41 or 42 cookies)	2106	289.1			140.4	19.27	(421)	(57.8)
1 cookie, approx. 0.4 oz.			51	7.0	140.4	19.27	(421)	(57.8)
Coconut Macaroon Soft Cakes, see under MACAROON								
Coconut Snack Wrapped Cookies, **Drake's,** 1½-oz. package (approx. 3 cookies)	201	29.1			134.0	19.40	(402)	(58.2)
3-oz. package (approx. 6 cookies)	402	58.2			134.0	19.40	(402)	(58.2)
12-oz. package (approx. 24 cookies)	1608	232.8			134.0	19.40	(402)	(58.2)
1 cookie, approx. 0.5 oz.			67	9.7	134.0	19.40	(402)	(58.2)
COMO								
Como Delight Cookies, **Stella D'Oro,** 10¼-oz. package (approx. 9 cookies)	1350	165.6			132.7	16.28	(464)	(57.0)
1 cookie, approx. 1.1 oz.			150	18.4	132.7	16.28	(464)	(57.0)
CRAQUELINS								
Craquelins snackbread crackers, **Croustipain,** 7.1-oz. box (approx. 40 crackers)	800	160.0			112.7	22.54		
1 cracker, approx. 0.2 oz.			20	4.0	112.7	22.54		
CREAM (or CREME)								
Many other cream (or creme) sandwiches are listed throughout this chapter under their brand names, such as Oreo, or under their flavors, such as French Vanilla Creme.								
Creme Sandwich, Vanilla **Nabisco** "Cookie Break," 19-oz. (approx. 51 sandwiches)	2550	374.0			134.2	19.68		
1 sandwich, approx. 0.4 oz.			50	7.3	134.2	19.68		
Creme Sticks, **Holland American** "Dutch Treat," 9-oz. package (approx. 38 sticks)	1350	171.0			150.0	19.00		
1 stick, approx. 0.2 oz.			36	4.5	150.0	19.00		
Creme Sticks, **Holland American** "Dutch Twin," 9-oz. package (approx. 38 sticks)	1314	171.0			146.0	19.00		
1 stick, approx. 0.2 oz.			35	4.6	146.0	19.00		
Creme Wafer Sticks, **Nabisco,** 9-oz. package (approx. 27 sticks)	1260	171.0			140.0	19.00		
1 stick, approx. ⅓ oz.			47	6.3	140.0	19.00		
Crunchy Creme Wafers, Twiddle Sticks, **Nabisco,** 9½-oz. package (approx. 27 wafers)	1440	189.0			151.6	19.89		
1 wafer, approx. 0.4 oz.			53	7.0	151.6	19.89		
Filigree Creme Sandwich, **Nabisco,** packaged as part of the Mayfair Assortment English Style								
1 sandwich, approx. 0.4 oz.			60	8.5	150.0	21.25		
Fudge Creme Sandwich, Gaiety, **Nabisco,** 15-oz. package (approx. 42 cookies)	2240	294.0			149.3	19.60		
1 cookie, approx. 0.4 oz.			53	7.0	149.3	19.60		
Mayfair Creme Sandwich, packaged as part of the Mayfair Assortment English Style, **Nabisco**								
1 sandwich, approx. 0.5 oz.			65	9.0	144.4	20.00		
Mixed Creme Sandwich, **Cookie Break,** 19-oz. package (approx. 51 sandwiches)	2720	374.0			143.2	19.68		
1 sandwich, approx. 0.4 oz.			53	7.3	143.2	19.68		
Tea Rose Creme Sandwich, packaged as part of the Mayfair Assortment English Style, **Nabisco**								
1 sandwich, approx. 0.4 oz.			53	7.7	145.5	20.91		
CRISP BREAD (also see under individual flavors)								
Bran Crisp Bread, **Scandinavian,** 1.6-oz. package (approx. 12 pieces)	168	24.0			103.4	14.77		
1 piece, approx. 0.1 oz.			14	2.0	103.4	14.77		
Sesame Crisp Bread, **Wasa,** 7-oz. package (approx. 16 or 17 pieces)	844	126.7			120.5	18.10		
1 piece, approx. 0.4 oz.			51	7.7	120.5	18.10		
Sourdough Toast Crisp Bread, **Wasa,** 7-oz. package (approx. 16 or 17 pieces)	758	156.8			108.3	22.40	(408)	(84.4)
1 piece, approx. 0.4 oz.			46	9.5	108.3	22.40	(408)	(84.4)
Whole Wheat Crisp Bread, **Dar-Vida (Hug),** 8¾-oz. package	1084	177.1			123.9	20.24		
CROWN								
Crown Creme Sandwich, packaged as part of the Mayfair Assortment English Style, **Nabisco**								
1 sandwich, approx. 0.4 oz.			53	8.0	133.4	20.00		
Crown Pilot Crackers, **Crown Pilot,** 14-oz. package (approx. 24 crackers)	1800	312.0			128.6	22.29		
1 cracker, approx. 0.6 oz., (2 per ounce)			75	13.0	128.6	22.29		
CUSTARD								
Cup Custard Cookies, Vanilla, **Sunshine,** 14-oz. package (approx. 31 cookies)	1970	260.5			140.7	18.61		
1 cookie, approx. 0.5 oz.			65	8.6	140.7	18.61		
DATE NUT								
Date Nut Granola Cookies, **Pepperidge Farm,** 5½-oz. package (approx. 15 cookies)	800	100.0			145.5	18.18	(436)	(54.5)
1 cookie, approx. 0.4 oz.			53	6.7	145.5	18.18	(436)	(54.5)
DEVIL'S FOOD								
Devil's Food Cakes, **Nabisco,** 8-oz. package (approx. 12 cakes)	840	186.0			105.0	23.25		
1 cake, approx. 0.7 oz.			70	15.5	105.0	23.25		

	ENTIRE PACKAGE		1 COOKIE OR CRACKER		1 OZ., BY WT.		1 CUP CRUMBLED	
	Cal.	Carb.	Cal.	Carb.	Cal.	Carb.	Cal.	Carb.
DIP IN A CHIP								
Dip In A Chip Cheese 'n Chive Snack Crackers, **Nabisco,** 10-oz. package (approx. 150 crackers)	1500	160.0			150.0	16.00		
1 cracker, approx. 0.07 oz.			10	1.1	150.0	16.00		
DIXIE(S)								
Dixie Vanilla Cookies, **Sunshine,** 12-oz. package (approx. 26 or 27 cookies)	1530	258.5			127.5	21.54	(383)	(64.6)
1 cookie, approx. 0.5 oz.			58	9.8	127.5	21.54	(383)	(64.6)
Dixies Drumstick Snack Crackers, **Nabisco,** 8-oz. package (approx. 144 crackers)	1120	136.0			140.0	17.00		
1 cracker, approx. 0.06 oz.			8	0.9	140.0	17.00		
DOUBLE CHIPS								
Double Chips Fudge & Butterscotch Chip Cookies, **Nabisco** "Bakers Bonus," 11-oz. package (approx. 20 cookies)	1600	220.0			145.5	20.00		
1 cookie, approx. 0.6 oz.			80	11.0	145.5	20.00		
DUTCH								
Dutch Apple Fingers, Iced, **Ann Page (A&P)** 10-oz. package (approx. 36 Fingers)	1420	200.0			142.0	20.00		
1 Finger, approx. 0.3 oz.			39	5.6	142.0	20.00		
Dutch Treat Creme Sticks, **Holland American,** 9-oz. package (approx. 38 sticks)	1350	171.0			150.0	19.00		
1 stick, approx. 0.2 oz.			36	4.5	150.0	19.00		
Dutch Treat Sugar Wafers, **Holland American,** 3¾-oz. package (approx. 15 wafers)	548	71.3			146.0	19.00		
1 wafer, approx. ¼ oz.			37	4.8	146.0	19.00		
1¾-oz. package (approx. 8 wafers)	256	33.3			146.0	19.00		
1 wafer, approx. 0.2 oz.			32	4.2	146.0	19.00		
12-oz. package (approx. 42 wafers)	1752	228.0			146.0	19.00		
1 wafer, approx. 0.3 oz.			42	5.4	146.0	19.00		
Dutch Treat Waffle Cremes, **Holland American,** 10-oz. package (approx. 24 cremes)	1460	190.0			146.0	19.00		
1 creme, approx. 0.4 oz.			61	7.9	146.0	19.00		
Dutch Twin Creme Sticks, **Holland American,** 9-oz. package (approx. 38 sticks)	1314	171.0			146.0	19.00		
1 stick, approx. 0.2 oz.			35	4.6	146.0	19.00		
Dutch Twin Sugar Wafers, **Holland American,** 4½-oz. package (approx. 18 wafers)	657	85.5			146.0	19.00		
1 wafer, approx. ¼ oz.			44	5.7	146.0	19.00		
6-oz. package (approx. 20 wafers)	876	114.0			146.0	19.00		
1 wafer, approx. 0.3 oz.			44	5.7	146.0	19.00		
8-oz. package (approx. 42 wafers)	1168	152.0			146.0	19.00		
1 wafer, approx. 0.2 oz.			28	3.6	146.0	19.00		
11-oz. package (approx. 54 wafers)	1606	209.0			146.0	19.00		
1 wafer, approx. 0.2 oz.			29	3.8	146.0	19.00		
EGG								
Egg Biscuits, salt free, **Stella D'Oro,** 6.4-oz. package (approx. 18 biscuits)	756	117.0			118.8	18.39	(415)	(64.4)
1 biscuit, approx. 0.4 oz.			42	6.5	118.8	18.39	(415)	(64.4)
Egg Biscuits, sugared, **Stella D'Oro,** 5-oz. package (approx. 9 biscuits)	523	104.5			104.5	20.90	(366)	(73.2)
1 biscuit, approx. 0.6 oz.			60	12.0	104.5	20.90	(366)	(73.2)
Egg Jumbo Cookies, **Stella D'Oro,** 7½-oz. package (approx. 18 cookies)	774	168.8			104.1	22.03	(364)	(77.1)
1 cookie, approx. 0.4 oz.			43	9.1	104.1	22.03	(364)	(77.1)
ELFWICH								
Elfwich, **Keebler,** 14-oz. package (approx. 35 or 36 Elfwiches)	1974	287.1			141.0	20.51	(423)	(61.5)
1 Elfwich, approx. 0.4 oz.			55	8.0	141.0	20.51	(423)	(61.5)
ESCORT								
Escort Crackers, **Nabisco,** 8-oz. package (approx. 57 crackers)	1200	144.0			150.0	18.00		
1 cracker, approx. 0.1 oz.			21	2.6	150.0	18.00		

	ENTIRE PACKAGE		1 COOKIE OR CRACKER		1 OZ., BY WT.		1 CUP CRUMBLED	
	Cal.	Carb.	Cal.	Carb.	Cal.	Carb.	Cal.	Carb.
FAMOUS								
Famous Chocolate Wafers, **Nabisco,** 8½-oz. package (approx. 35-39 wafers)	980	168.0			127.3	21.82	(446)	(76.4)
1 wafer, approx. 0.2 oz.			28	4.8	127.3	21.82	(446)	(76.4)
Famous Cookie Assortment, **Nabisco,** is with Cookie Assortments at the end of this chapter.								
FIG								
Fig Bars, **Tom's,** 1.8-oz. package	180	39.0	180	39.0	100.0	21.67		
Fig Bars Cookies, **Sunshine,** 16-oz. (1-lb.) package (approx. 40 cookies)	1659	339.2			103.7	21.20		
1 cookie, approx. 0.4 oz.			41	8.5	103.7	21.20		
Fig Newtons Cakes, **Nabisco,** 16-oz. (1-lb.) package (approx. 30 cakes)	1800	330.0			112.5	20.62		
1 cake, approx. 0.5 oz.			60	11.0	112.5	20.62		
Fig Wheats Whole Wheat Fig Bars, **Nabisco,** 16-oz. package (approx. 30 cookies)	1800	345.0			112.5	21.56		
1 cookie, approx. 0.5 oz.			60	11.5	112.5	21.56		
FLATBREAD								
Flatbread, Norwegian, **Mors Norwegian,** 9-oz. package (approx. 10 pieces)	(650)	(135.0)			(72.2)	(15.00)		
1 piece, approx. 0.9 oz.			65	13.5	(72.2)	(15.00)		
Flatbrod, Caraway Seasoned, **Ideal,** 8-oz. package (approx. 53 pieces)	873	181.9			109.1	22.74		
1 piece, approx. 1/7 oz.			16	3.4	109.1	22.74		
Flatbrod, Ultra-Thin, **Ideal,** 8-oz. package (approx. 79 crackers)	873	189.0			109.1	23.62		
1 cracker, approx. 0.1 oz.			11	2.4	109.1	23.62		
Flatbrod, Whole Grain, **Ideal,** 8-oz. package (approx. 53 crackers)	873	181.9			109.1	22.74		
1 cracker, approx. 1/7 oz.			16	3.4	109.1	22.74		
FRENCH								
French Onion Crackers, **Nabisco,** 8-oz. package (approx. 92 crackers)	1200	144.0			150.0	18.00		
1 cracker, approx. 0.1 oz.			13	1.5	150.0	18.00		
French Vanilla Creme Cookies, **Keebler,** 16-oz. (1-lb.) package (approx. 26 or 27 cookies)	2269	320.2			141.8	20.01	(425)	(60.0)
1 cookie, approx. 0.6 oz.			85	12.0	141.8	20.01	(425)	(60.0)
Vended size, 1¾ oz. (6 cookies)	230	33.0			131.4	18.86		
1 cookie, approx. 0.3 oz.			38	5.5	131.4	18.86		
FROSTED								
Frosted Cakes Cookies, **Sunshine,** 10½-oz. package (approx. 19 or 20 cookies)	1163	244.4			110.8	23.28		
1 cookie, approx. 0.5 oz.			59	12.4	110.8	23.28		
FRUIT								
Fruit Biscuits, **Familia,** 4¼-oz. package (approx. 17 biscuits)	561	76.2			132.4	17.92	(397)	(53.8)
1 biscuit, approx. ¼ oz.			33	4.5	132.4	17.92	(397)	(53.8)
FUDGE (or FUDGY)								
Fudge Chip Cookies, **Pepperidge Farm,** 5½-oz. package (approx. 15 or 16 cookies)	850	110.0			161.9	20.95	(486)	(62.8)
1 cookie, approx. ⅓ oz.			57	7.3	161.9	20.95	(486)	(62.8)
Fudge Cookies, **Sweet N Good,** 11-oz. package (approx. 24 cookies)	1598	225.6			145.3	20.51	(436)	(61.5)
1 cookie, approx. 0.5 oz.			67	9.4	145.3	20.51	(436)	(61.5)
Fudge Creme Sandwich, Gaiety, **Nabisco,** 15-oz. package (approx. 42 cookies)	2240	294.0			149.3	19.60		
1 cookie, approx. 0.4 oz.			53	7.0	149.3	19.60		
Fudgy Cookies, Iced, **Ann Page (A&P),** 10-oz. package (approx. 36 cookies)	1296	201.6			129.6	20.16		
1 cookie, approx. 0.3 oz.			36	5.6	129.6	20.16		
GARLIC								
Garlic Discos, **Devonsheer Melba,** 5-oz. box (approx. 35 slices)	455	(76.9)			91.0	(15.37)		
1 slice, approx. 0.14 oz.			13	(2.2)	91.0	(15.37)		

	ENTIRE PACKAGE		1 COOKIE OR CRACKER		1 OZ., BY WT.		1 CUP CRUMBLED	
	Cal.	Carb.	Cal.	Carb.	Cal.	Carb.	Cal.	Carb.
Garlic Rounds, see ROUNDS								
GINGER								
Ginger Animal Cookies, **El Molino,** 6-oz. package (approx. 56 Animals)	780	126.0			130.0	21.00		
1 Animal, approx. 0.1 oz.			14	2.3	130.0	21.00		
Gingerman, **Pepperidge Farm,** 5-oz. package (approx. 21 cookies)	700	112.0			140.0	22.40	(420)	(67.2)
1 Gingerman, approx. ¼ oz.			33	5.3	140.0	22.40	(420)	(67.2)
Ginger Snaps, Old Fashioned, **Nabisco,** 16-oz. (1-lb.) package (approx. 64 Snaps)	1920	352.0			120.0	22.00	(420)	(77.0)
1 Snap, approx. ¼ oz.			30	5.5	120.0	22.00	(420)	(77.0)
GITANA								
Gitana Soda Crackers, **Nabisco,** 24-oz. package (approx. 192 crackers)	2280	480.0			95.0	20.00		
1 cracker, approx. 0.1 oz.			15	2.5	95.0	20.00		
GOLDEN								
Golden Bars, **Stella D'Oro,** 11.3-oz. package (approx. 12 bars)	1320	190.8			117.7	17.01	(412)	(59.6)
1 bar, approx. 0.9 oz.			110	15.9	117.7	17.01	(412)	(59.6)
Golden Fruit Cookies, **Sunshine,** 7½-oz. package (approx. 11 or 12 cookies)	701	164.7			93.5	21.96		
1 cookie, approx. 0.7 oz.			60	14.1	93.5	21.96		
GOLDFISH								
Goldfish Crackers, Cheddar Cheese Flavored, **Pepperidge Farm,** 6-oz. package (approx. 300 Goldfish)	842	100.4			140.3	16.73		
Vended size, ¾-oz. package (approx. 42 Goldfish)	105	12.5			140.3	16.73		
1 Goldfish, approx. 0.02 oz.			(3)	(0.3)	140.3	16.73		
Goldfish Crackers, Lightly Salted, **Pepperidge Farm,** 6-oz. package (approx. 300 Goldfish)	825	108.9			137.5	18.15		
Vended size, ¾-oz. package (approx. 41 Goldfish)	103	13.6			137.5	18.15		
1 Goldfish, approx. 0.02 oz.			(3)	(0.3)	137.5	18.15		
Goldfish Crackers, Pizza Flavored, **Pepperidge Farm,** 6-oz. package (approx. 300 Goldfish)	841	100.4			140.1	16.73		
Vended size, ¾-oz. package (approx. 42 Goldfish)	105	12.5			140.1	16.73		
1 Goldfish, approx. 0.02 oz.			(3)	(0.3)	140.1	16.73		
Goldfish Pretzels, **Pepperidge Farm,** 6-oz. package (approx. 275 Goldfish)	697	122.5			116.2	20.41		
Vended size, ¾-oz. package (approx. 35 Goldfish)	87	15.3			116.2	20.41		
1 Goldfish, approx. 0.02 oz.			(3)	(0.3)	116.2	20.41		
GRAHAM								
Chocolate Grahams, **Nabisco,** 5½-oz. package (approx. 15 Grahams)	850	105.0			154.5	19.09	(464)	(57.3)
1 Graham, approx. ⅓ oz.			57	7.1	154.5	19.09	(464)	(57.3)
Cinnamon Grahams, **Sunshine,** 16-oz. (1-lb.) package, (approx. 115 Grahams)	2029	346.2			126.8	21.64	(380)	(64.9)
1 Graham, approx. 0.1 oz.			17	2.9	126.8	21.64	(380)	(64.9)
Fancy Dip Grahams, **Nabisco,** 11-oz. package (approx. 24 Grahams)	1560	192.0			141.8	17.45		
1 Graham, approx. 0.5 oz.			65	8.0	141.8	17.45		
Graham Crackers, **Nabisco,** 16-oz. (1-lb.) package (approx. 64 crackers)	1920	336.0			120.0	21.00	(360)	(63.0)
1 cracker, approx. ¼ oz.			30	5.3	120.0	21.00	(360)	(63.0)
Graham Crackers, **Nabisco** "Honey Maid," 16-oz. (1-lb.) package, (approx. 64 crackers)	1920	352.0			120.0	22.00	(360)	(66.0)
1 cracker, approx. ¼ oz.			30	5.5	120.0	22.00	(360)	(66.0)
Graham Crackers, **Rokeach,** 16-oz. (1-lb.) package (approx. 128 crackers)	1920	336.0			120.0	21.00		
1 cracker, approx. 0.1 oz.			15	2.6	120.0	21.00		
Honey Grahams, **Keebler,** 32-oz. (2-lb.) package (approx. 57 to 58 Grahams)	3968	680.4			124.0	21.26	(372)	(63.8)
1 Graham, approx. 0.6 oz.			70	12.0	124.0	21.26	(372)	(63.8)
Party Grahams, **Nabisco,** 12½-oz. package (approx. 42 Grahams)	1960	252.0			156.8	20.16		
1 Graham, approx. 0.3 oz.			47	6.0	156.8	20.16		
Peanut Butter Graham Crackers, **Austin,** 1.4-oz. package	180	27.0			128.6	19.29		
Sugar Honey Grahams, **Sunshine,** 16-oz. (1-lb.) package (approx. 124 Grahams)	1944	359.9			121.5	21.87	(365)	(65.6)
1 Graham, approx. 0.1 oz.			15	2.7	121.5	21.87	(365)	(65.6)
GRANOLA (also see individual flavors such as Date Nut Granola Cookies)								
Granola Cookies, **Pepperidge Farm,** 2¼-oz. package (2 cookies)	320	41.0			142.2	18.22		
1 cookie, approx. 1⅛ oz.			160	20.5	142.2	18.22		
HERBAL								
Herbal Crackers, Lightly Salted, **Golden Harvest,** 6-oz. package	840	120.0			140.0	20.00		
HI HO								
Hi Ho Crackers, **Sunshine,** 4-oz. package (approx. 31 or 32 crackers)	598	66.2			149.6	16.54	(419)	(46.3)
12-oz. package (approx. 94 or 95 crackers)	1795	198.5			149.6	16.54	(419)	(46.3)
16-oz. (1-lb.) package (approx. 126 or 127 crackers)	2394	264.6			149.6	16.54	(419)	(46.3)
1 cracker, approx. 0.1 oz.			19	2.1	149.6	16.54	(419)	(46.3)
HOLLAND								
Holland Rusk Cookies, **Nabisco,** 4-oz. package (approx. 12 cookies)	480	90.0			120.0	22.50		
1 cookie, approx. 0.3 oz.			40	7.5	120.0	22.50		
HONEY								
Honey Animal Cookies, **El Molino,** 6-oz. package (approx. 54 cookies)	900	96.0			150.0	16.00	(608)	(64.9)
1 cookie, approx. 0.1 oz.			17	1.8	150.0	16.00	(608)	(64.9)
Honey Bran Crackers, **El Molino,** 7-oz. package (approx. 44 crackers)	880	132.0			125.7	18.86		
1 cracker, approx. 0.2 oz.			20	3.0	125.7	18.86		
Honey Grahams, **Keebler,** 32-oz. (2-lb.) package (approx. 57 to 58 Grahams)	3968	680.4			124.0	21.26	(372)	(63.8)
1 Graham, approx. 0.6 oz.			70	12.0	124.0	21.26	(372)	(63.8)
Honey 'n Apricot Cookies, **El Molino,** 1 cookie per package, approx. 2 oz.	250	36.0	250	36.0	125.0	18.00		
Honey 'n Bran Cookies, **El Molino,** 1 cookie per package, approx. 2 oz.	210	37.0	210	36.0	105.0	18.50		
Honey 'n Carob Chip Cookies, **El Molino,** 16 oz. (1 lb.) package, (approx. 58 cookies)	2197	307.5			137.3	19.22		
1 cookie, approx. 0.3 oz.			38	5.3	137.3	19.22		
Honey 'n Carob Cookies, **El Molino,** 1 cookie per package, approx. 2 oz.	220	40.0	220	40.0	110.0	20.00		
Honey 'n Cinnamon Cookies, **El Molino,** 1 cookie per package, approx. 2 oz.	250	37.0	250	37.0	125.0	18.50		
Honey 'n Date Cookies, **El Molino,** 1 cookie per package, approx. 2 oz.	240	36.0	240	36.0	120.0	18.00		
Honey 'n Fruit & Spice Cookies, **El Molino,** 1 cookie per package, approx. 2 oz.	230	42.0	230	42.0	115.0	21.00		
Honey 'n Granola Cookies, **El Molino,** 1 cookie per package, approx. 2 oz.	220	40.0	220	40.0	110.0	20.00		
Honey 'n Oatmeal Cookies, **El Molino,** 16-oz. (1-lb.) package (approx. 58 cookies)	2197	322.2			137.3	20.14		
1 cookie, approx. 0.3 oz.			38	5.5	137.3	20.14		
Honey 'n Peanut Butter Cookies, **El Molino,** 7-oz. package (approx. 12 cookies)	960	132.0			137.1	18.86	(411)	(56.6)
1 cookie, approx. 0.3 oz.			80	11.0	137.1	18.86	(411)	(56.6)

	ENTIRE PACKAGE		1 COOKIE OR CRACKER		1 OZ., BY WT.		1 CUP CRUMBLED	
	Cal.	Carb.	Cal.	Carb.	Cal.	Carb.	Cal.	Carb.
Honey 'n Raspberry Cookies, **El Molino,** 1 cookie per package, approx. 2 oz.	260	37.0	260	37.0	130.0	18.50		
Honey 'n Strawberry Cookies, **El Molino,** 1 cookie per package, approx. 2 oz.	240	37.0	240	37.0	120.0	18.50		
HOSTESS								
Hostess With The Mostest Assorted Cookies, **Stella D'Oro,** 28-oz. package (approx. 93 or 94 cookies)	3805	527.0			135.9	18.82	(476)	(65.9)
1 cookie, approx. 0.3 oz.			39	5.4	135.9	18.82	(476)	(65.9)
HYDROX								
Hydrox Cookies, Chocolate, **Sunshine,** 15-oz. package (approx. 41 or 42 cookies)	2024	297.3			134.9	19.82	(405)	(59.5)
19-oz. package (approx. 52 or 53 cookies)	2563	376.6			134.9	19.82	(405)	(59.5)
1 cookie, approx. 0.4 oz.			49	7.2	134.9	19.82	(405)	(59.5)
Hydrox Cookies, Vanilla, **Sunshine,** 15-oz. package (approx. 41 or 42 cookies)	2106	297.3			140.4	19.82	(421)	(59.5)
19-oz. package (approx. 52 or 53 cookies)	2668	376.6			140.4	19.82	(421)	(59.5)
1 cookie, approx. 0.4 oz.			51	7.2	140.4	19.82	(421)	(59.5)
KEEBIE								
Keebie Cookies, **Keebler,** Vended size, 1¾-oz. package (6 cookies)	220	32.0			125.7	18.29	(355)	(51.6)
1 cookie, approx. 0.3 oz.			37	5.3	125.7	18.29	(355)	(51.6)
KETTLE								
Kettle Cookies, packaged as part of the Famous Cookie Assortment, **Nabisco**								
1 cookie, approx. ¼ oz.			35	5.3	140.0	21.00		
KICHEL								
Kichel, reduced sugar, salt free, **Stella D'Oro,** 3.6-oz. package (approx. 60 pieces)	480	39.0			145.2	11.79	(436)	(35.4)
1 piece, approx. 0.06 oz.			8	0.7	145.2	11.79	(436)	(35.4)
KRISP								
Krisp Kreem Crackers, **Keebler,** 11½-oz. package (approx. 60 or 61 crackers)	1778	266.8			154.6	23.20	(436)	(65.4)
1 cracker, approx. 0.2 oz.			30	4.5	154.6	23.20	(436)	(65.4)
KRISPY								
Krispy Crackers, **Sunshine,** 8-oz. package (approx. 80 crackers)	938	172.1			117.3	21.51	(328)	(60.2)
16-oz. (1-lb.) package (approx. 160 crackers)	1877	344.2			117.3	21.51	(328)	(60.2)
32-oz. (2-lb.) package (approx. 320 crackers)	3754	688.3			117.3	21.51	(328)	(60.2)
1 cracker, approx. 0.1 oz.			12	2.2	117.3	21.51	(328)	(60.2)
Krispy Crackers, unsalted, **Sunshine,** 16-oz. (1-lb.) package (approx. 160 crackers)	2034	344.2			127.1	21.51	(356)	(60.2)
1 cracker, approx. 0.1 oz.			13	2.2	127.1	21.51	(356)	(60.2)
LADY STELLA								
Lady Stella Assortment Cookies, **Stella D'Oro,** 15-oz. package (approx. 52 or 53 cookies)	1934	287.4			128.9	19.16	(451)	(67.1)
1 cookie, approx. 0.3 oz.			37	5.5	128.9	19.16	(451)	(67.1)
LEMON								
Lemon Coolers Cookies, **Sunshine,** 10-oz. package (approx. 46 or 47 cookies)	1348	209.1			134.8	20.91	(404)	(62.7)
1 cookie, approx. 0.2 oz.			29	4.5	134.8	20.91	(404)	(62.7)
Lemon Creme Cookies, **Keebler,** Vended size, 1¾-oz. package (6 cookies)	220	32.0			125.7	18.29	(355)	(51.6)
1 cookie, approx. 0.3 oz.			37	5.3	125.7	18.29	(355)	(51.6)
Lemon Nut Cookies, **Pepperidge Farm,** Vended size, 2¼-oz. package (2 cookies)	340	41.0			151.0	18.22		
1 cookie, approx. 1⅛ oz.			170	20.5	151.0	18.22		
Lemon Nut Crunch Cookies, **Pepperidge Farm,** 5½-oz. package (approx. 15 cookies)	900	100.0			163.6	18.18	(491)	(54.5)
1 cookie, approx. 0.4 oz.			60	6.7	163.6	18.18	(491)	(54.5)
Lemon Sandwich Cookies, dietetic, **Estee,** 5-oz. package (approx. 11 or 12 cookies)	720	96.0			144.0	19.20	(432)	(57.6)
1 cookie, approx. 0.4 oz.			60	8.1	144.0	19.20	(432)	(57.6)
LIDO								
Lido Cookies, **Pepperidge Farm,** 7-oz. package (approx. 12 cookies)	1140	120.0			162.9	17.14	(488)	(57.4)
1 cookie, approx. 0.6 oz.			95	10.0	162.9	17.14	(488)	(57.4)
LORNA DOONE								
Lorna Doone Shortbread, **Nabisco,** 10-oz. package (approx. 36 cookies)	1440	180.0			144.0	18.00		
1 cookie, approx. 0.3 oz.			40	5.0	144.0	18.00		
LOVE								
Love Cookies, reduced sugar, no salt, **Stella D'Oro,** (package weight and number of cookies not available)								
1 Love cookie, approx. 0.7 oz.			110	14.0	156.0	19.85	(468)	(59.6)
MACAROON								
Coconut Macaroon Soft Cakes, **Nabisco,** 8-oz. package (approx. 12 cakes)	1140	138.0			142.5	17.25		
1 cake, approx. 0.4 oz.			95	11.5	142.5	17.25		
MALLOMARS								
Mallomars Chocolate Cakes, **Mallomars,** 8-oz. package (18 cakes)	1080	153.0			135.0	19.12		
1 cake, approx. 0.4 oz.			60	8.5	135.0	19.12		
MALLOPUFFS								
Mallopuffs, **Sunshine,** 9-oz. package (approx. 15 or 16 pieces)	977	187.5			108.5	20.83		
1 piece, approx. 0.6 oz.			62	11.9	108.5	20.83		
MALTED								
Malted Milk Peanut Butter Sandwiches, **Nabisco,** 1-oz. package (4 sandwiches)	150	18.0			150.0	18.00		
1 sandwich, approx. ¼ oz.			38	4.5	150.0	18.00		
MANDEL								
Mandel Toast, Almond, **Stella D'Oro,** 8-oz. package (approx. 16 toasts)	864	158.4			108.6	19.92	(380)	(69.7)
1 toast, approx. 0.5 oz.			54	9.9	108.6	19.92	(380)	(69.7)
MARGHERITE								
Margherite Cookies, Combination, **Stella D'Oro,** 15.2-oz. package (approx. 27 cookies)	1971	283.5			130.4	18.75	(456)	(65.6)
1 cookie, approx. 0.6 oz.			73	10.5	130.4	18.75	(456)	(65.6)
Margherite Cookies, Vanilla, **Stella D'Oro,** 15.2-oz. package (approx. 27 cookies)	1971	288.9			130.4	19.11	(456)	(66.9)
1 cookie, approx. 0.6 oz.			73	10.7	130.4	19.11	(456)	(66.9)
MARSHMALLOW								
Marshmallow Bars, **Sunshine,** 10-oz. package (approx. 11 or 12 bars)	1078	208.4			107.8	20.84		
1 bar, approx. 0.9 oz.			92	17.8	107.8	20.84		
Marshmallow Puffs, **Nabisco,** 13½-oz. package (approx. 20 puffs)	1700	280.0			125.9	20.74		
1 puff, approx. 0.7 oz.			85	14.0	125.9	20.74		
Marshmallow Sandwich, **Nabisco,** 4-oz. package (16 sandwiches)	480	92.0			120.0	23.00		
1 sandwich, approx. ¼ oz.			30	5.8	120.0	23.00		
Marshmallow Twirls Cakes, **Nabisco,** 12-oz. package (approx. 12 cookies)	1560	240.0			130.0	20.00		
1 cookie, approx. 1 oz.			130	20.0	130.0	20.00		
MATZO								
For more extensive listings of Matzo, see the BREADS chapter.								
Matzo Crackers, Bite Size, **Goodman's,** 8½-oz. box (approx. 88 matzo crackers)	880	198.0			103.1	23.20	(389)	(87.5)
1 matzo cracker, approx. 0.1 oz.			10	2.3	103.1	23.20	(389)	(87.5)
Passover Matzo Cracker Miniatures, **Manischewitz,** 8-oz. box (approx. 99 matzo crackers)	891	198.0			111.4	24.75	(420)	(93.1)
1 matzo cracker, approx. 0.08 oz.			9	2.0	111.4	24.75	(420)	(93.1)
MAYFAIR ASSORTMENT								
Mayfair Assortment, English Style, **Nabisco,** is with Cookie Assortments at the end of this chapter.								

	ENTIRE PACKAGE		1 COOKIE OR CRACKER		1 OZ., BY WT.		1 CUP CRUMBLED	
	Cal.	Carb.	Cal.	Carb.	Cal.	Carb.	Cal.	Carb.
MEAL MATES								
Meal Mates Sesame Bread Wafers, **Nabisco,** 10-oz. package, approx. 60 wafers	1300	190.0			130.0	19.00		
1 wafer, approx. 0.2 oz.			22	3.2	130.0	19.00		
MELBA (also see under TOAST(Y))								
Plain Toast, **Devonsheer Melba,** 4½-oz. package (approx. 30 pieces)	480	94.8			106.7	21.06		
1 piece, approx . 0.2 oz.			16	3.2	106.7	21.06		
Pumpernickel Melba Toast, **Old London,** 5-oz. package (approx. 30 pieces)	500	100.0			100.0	20.00		
1 piece, approx. 0.17 oz.			17	3.3	100.0	20.00		
Sesame Melba Toast, **Devonsheer Melba,** 4½-oz. package (approx. 30 pieces)	480	88.6			106.7	19.69		
1 piece, approx. 0.2 oz.			16	3.0	106.7	19.69		
Wheat Melba Toast, **Old London,** 5-oz. package (approx. 30 pieces)	500	100.0			100.0	20.00		
1 piece, approx. 1.7 oz.			17	3.3	100.0	20.00		
White Melba Toast, **Old London,** 5-oz. package (approx. 30 pieces)	500	100.0			100.0	20.00		
1 piece, approx. 1.7 oz.			17	3.3	100.0	20.00		
White Melba Toast, unsalted, **Old London,** 5-oz. package (approx. 30 pieces)	500	100.0			100.0	20.00		
1 piece, approx. 1.7 oz.			17	3.3	100.0	20.00		
MILANO								
Milano Cookies, **Pepperidge Farm,** 6-oz. package (approx. 15 cookies)	950	110.0			155.3	18.83	(475)	(55.0)
1 cookie, approx. 0.4 oz.			63	7.2	155.3	18.33	(475)	(55.0)
MILK								
Milk Crackers, Royal Lunch, **Nabisco,** 15-oz. package (approx. 38 crackers)	2090	304.0			139.3	20.27		
1 cracker, approx. 0.4 oz.			55	8.0	139.3	20.27		
MINT								
Mint Sandwich Cookies, Mystic, **Nabisco,** 11½-oz. package (approx. 20 cookies)	1800	220.0			156.5	19.13		
1 cookie, approx. 0.6 oz.			90	11.0	156.5	19.13		
MOLASSES								
Molasses Cookies, **Nabisco** "Pantry," 12-oz. package (approx. 26 cookies)	1560	247.0			130.0	20.58		
1 cookie, approx. 0.5 oz.			60	9.5	130.0	20.58		
Molasses Crisps Cookies, **Pepperidge Farm,** 5¾-oz. package (approx. 27 cookies)	810	117.0			140.9	20.35	(422)	(61.0)
1 cookie, approx. 0.2 oz.			30	4.3	140.9	20.35	(422)	(61.0)
NASSAU								
Nassau Cookies, **Pepperidge Farm,** 6½-oz. package (approx. 12 cookies)	900	96.0			138.5	14.76	(415)	(44.3)
1 cookie, approx. 0.5 oz.			75	8.0	138.5	14.76	(415)	(44.3)
NILLA								
Nilla Wafers, **Nabisco,** 12-oz. package (approx. 84 wafers)	1560	252.0			130.0	21.00	(455)	(73.5)
1 wafer, approx. 0.1 oz.			19	3.0	130.0	21.00	(455)	(73.5)
NUT								
Nut Sundae Cookies, **Sunshine,** 10-oz. package (approx. 20 cookies)	1107	203.9			110.7	20.39	(332)	(61.2)
1 cookie, approx. 0.5 oz.			57	10.5	110.7	20.39	(332)	(61.2)
Nutter Butter Peanut Butter Sandwich Cookies, **Nabisco,** 13½-oz. package (approx. 27 cookies)	1890	243.0			140.0	18.00	(490)	(66.5)
1 cookie, approx. 0.5 oz.			70	9.0	140.0	18.00	(490)	(66.5)
Nutter Butter Peanut Butter Sandwich Cookies, Chocolate, **Nabisco,** 15½-oz. package (approx. 39 cookies)	2210	286.0			142.6	18.45		
1 cookie, approx. 0.4 oz.			57	7.3	142.6	18.45		
OATMEAL								
Oatmeal Cookies, **Nabisco** "Bakers Bonus," 14-oz. package (approx. 24 cookies)	1920	288.0			137.1	20.57		
1 cookie, approx. 0.6 oz.			80	12.0	137.1	20.57		
Oatmeal Cookies, **Nabisco** "Cookie Little," 7-oz. package (approx. 140 cookies)	910	140.0			130.0	20.00		
1 cookie, approx. 0.05 oz.			7	1.0	130.0	20.00		
Oatmeal Cookies, **Pepperidge Farm,** vended size, 2¼-oz. package (2 cookies)	310	45.0			137.8	20.00		
1 cookie, approx. 1⅛-oz.			155	22.5	137.8	20.00		
Oatmeal Cookies, **Sunshine,** 14-oz. package (approx. 29 or 30 cookies)	1807	278.5			129.1	19.89	(387)	(59.7)
20-oz. package (approx. 41 or 42 cookies)	2582	397.8			129.1	19.89	(387)	(59.7)
1 cookie, approx. 0.5 oz.			61	9.4	129.1	19.89	(387)	(59.7)
Oatmeal Cookies, **Sweet N Good,** 11-oz. package (approx. 24 cookies)	1598	225.6			145.3	20.51	(436)	(61.5)
1 cookie, approx. 0.5 oz.			67	9.4	145.3	20.51	(436)	(61.5)
Oatmeal Cookies, Irish, **Pepperidge Farm,** 5-oz. package (approx. 15 cookies)	750	105.0			150.0	21.00	(450)	(63.0)
1 cookie, approx. ⅓ oz.			50	7.0	150.0	21.00	(450)	(63.0)
Oatmeal Cookies, Old Fashioned, **Keebler,** 13-oz. package (approx. 20 or 21 cookies)	1741	255.9			133.9	19.69	(402)	(59.1)
1 cookie, approx. 0.6 oz.			85	12.5	133.9	19.69	(402)	(59.1)
Oatmeal Almond Cookies, **Pepperidge Farm,** 5½-oz. package (approx. 15 cookies)	800	95.0			145.5	17.27	(436)	(51.8)
1 cookie, approx. 0.4 oz.			53	6.3	145.5	17.27	(436)	(51.8)
Oatmeal Peanut Sandwich Cookies, **Sunshine,** 16-oz. (1-lb.) package (approx. 27 or 28 cookies)	2254	294.1			140.9	18.38	(423)	(55.1)
1 cookie, approx. 0.6 oz.			82	10.7	140.9	18.38	(423)	(55.1)
Oatmeal Raisin Cookies, dietetic, **Estee,** 7½-oz. package (approx. 32 or 33 cookies)	960	128.0			128.0	17.07	(384)	(51.2)
1 cookie, approx. 0.3 oz.			30	4.0	128.0	17.07	(384)	(51.2)
Oatmeal Raisin Cookies, **Pepperidge Farm,** 6-oz. package (approx. 15 cookies)	850	115.0			141.7	19.17	(425)	(57.5)
1 cookie, approx. 0.4 oz.			57	7.7	141.7	19.17	(425)	(57.5)
Oatmeal Snack Wrapped Cookies, **Drake's,** 1.5-oz. package (approx. 3 cookies)	201	30.0			134.0	20.00	(402)	(60.0)
3-oz. package (approx. 6 cookies)	402	60.0			134.0	20.00	(402)	(60.0)
12-oz. package (approx. 24 cookies)	1608	240.0			134.0	20.00	(402)	(60.0)
1 cookie, approx. 0.5 oz.			67	10.0	134.0	20.00	(402)	(60.0)
ONION								
Onion Crackers, **Keebler,** 1.4-oz. package (31 crackers)	200	25.0			142.9	17.90		
1 cracker, approx. 0.05 oz.			6	0.8	142.9	17.90		
Onion Discos, **Devonsheer Melba,** 5-oz. box (approx. 35 slices)	455	(76.9)			91.0	(15.37)		
1 Disco, approx. 0.1 oz.			13	(2.2)	91.0	(15.37)		
Onion Rounds, see under ROUNDS								
Onion Tams, see under TAMS								
Onion Toast, **Keebler,** 9-oz. package (approx. 81 or 82 toasts)	1215	202.5			135.0	22.50	(381)	(63.5)
1 toast, approx. 0.1 oz.			15	2.5	135.0	22.50	(381)	(63.5)
OREO								
Oreo Chocolate Sandwich Cookies, **Nabisco,** 15-oz. package (approx. 40 cookies)	2046	300.0			136.4	20.00	(477)	(70.0)
19-oz. package (approx. 54 cookies)	2700	396.0			136.4	20.00	(477)	(70.0)
1 cookie, approx. 0.4 oz.			50	7.3	136.4	20.00	(477)	(70.0)
Oreo Double Stuf Chocolate Sandwich Cookie, **Nabisco,** 15-oz. package (approx. 32 cookies)	2240	288.0			155.6	20.00	(545)	(70.0)
1 cookie, approx. 0.4 oz.			70	9.0	155.6	20.00	(545)	(70.0)
Oreo & Swiss Cream Sandwich Assortment, see under COOKIE ASSORTMENTS at the end of this chapter.								
OYSTER(ETTES)								
Chowder & Oyster Crackers, **Original Trenton Crackers,** 8-oz. package (approx. 37 crackers)	956	169.2			119.4	21.15		
1 cracker, approx. 0.2 oz.			26	4.6	119.4	21.15		

	ENTIRE PACKAGE		1 COOKIE OR CRACKER		1 OZ., BY WT.		1 CUP CRUMBLED	
	Cal.	Carb.	Cal.	Carb.	Cal.	Carb.	Cal.	Carb.
Dandy Soup and Oyster Crackers, **Nabisco,** 16-oz. (1-lb.) package (approx. 640 crackers)	1920	320.0			120.0	20.00		
1 cracker, approx. 0.03 oz.			3	0.5	120.0	20.00		
Oyster Crackers, **Keebler,** 12-oz. package (approx. 375 to 380 crackers)	1512	245.7			126.0	20.48	(353)	(57.3)
1 cracker, approx. 0.03 oz.			4	0.7	126.0	20.48	(353)	(57.3)
Oyster Crackers, **Sunshine,** 12-oz. package (approx. 375 to 380 crackers)	1512	264.6			126.0	22.05	(353)	(57.3)
1 cracker, approx. 0.03 oz.			4	0.7	126.0	22.05	(353)	(57.3)
Oysterettes Soup & Oyster Crackers, **Nabisco,** 5-oz. package (approx. 200 crackers)	600	100.0			120.0	20.00	(360)	(63.0)
16-oz. (1-lb.) package (approx. 576 crackers)	1920	336.0			120.0	20.00	(360)	(63.0)
1 cracker, approx. 0.3 oz.			3	0.6	120.0	20.00	(360)	(63.0)
O·T·C								
O·T·C Trenton Crackers, **Original Trenton Crackers,** 8-oz. package (approx. 24 or 25 crackers)	(558)	(98.4)			(69.8)	(12.30)	(195)	(34.4)
1 cracker, approx. ⅓ oz.			23	4.1	(69.8)	(12.30)	(195)	(34.4)
O·T·C Wine Crackers, **Original Trenton Crackers,** 8-oz. package (approx. 32 crackers)	(589)	(102.4)			(73.6)	(12.80)	(206)	(35.8)
1 cracker, approx. ¼ oz.			18	3.2	(73.6)	(12.80)	(206)	(35.8)
PEACH								
Peach Apricot Pastry, sugar free, salt free, **Stella D'Oro,** 12-oz. package (approx. 18 pastries)	1746	261.0			145.5	21.75		
1 pastry, approx. 0.8 oz.			97	14.5	145.5	21.75		
PEANUT (and PEANUT BUTTER)								
Cheese Crackers With Extra Peanut Butter, **Austin** "Big Shot," 1¾-oz. package	250	24.0			142.9	13.70		
Cheese Peanut Butter Sandwiches, **Austin,** 1½-oz. package	210	22.00			140.0	14.67		
Cheese Peanut Butter Artificially Flavored Sandwich, **Nabisco,** 1-oz. package (4 sandwiches)	140	17.0			140.0	17.00		
1 sandwich, approx. ¼ oz.			35	4.3	140.0	17.00		
Chocolate Nutter Butter Peanut Butter Sandwich Cookies, **Nabisco,** 15½-oz. package (approx. 39 cookies)	2210	286.0			142.6	18.45		
1 cookie, approx. 0.4 oz.			57	7.3	142.6	18.45		
Chocolate Peanut Bars, **Nabisco** "Ideal," 10½-oz. package (approx. 18 bars)	1710	180.0			162.9	17.14		
1 bar, approx. 0.6 oz.			95	10.0	162.9	17.14		
Honey 'n Peanut Butter Cookies, **El Molino,** 7-oz. package (approx. 12 cookies)	960	132.0			137.1	18.86	(411)	(56.6)
1 cookie, approx. 0.6 oz.			80	11.0	137.1	18.86	(411)	(56.6)
Malted Milk Peanut Butter Artificially Flavored Sandwiches, **Nabisco,** 1-oz. package (approx. 4 sandwiches)	150	18.0			150.0	18.00		
1 sandwich, approx. ¼ oz.			38	4.5	150.0	18.00		
Peanut Butter Cookies, **Tiger's Milk,** 8-oz. package	960	136.0			120.0	17.00	(360)	(51.0)
1 cookie, approx. ¼ oz.			30	4.3	120.0	17.00	(360)	(51.0)
Peanut Butter Fudge Cookies, **Nabisco,** 13-oz. package (approx. 36 cookies)	1800	240.0			138.5	18.46		
1 cookie, approx. 0.4 oz.			50	6.7	138.5	18.46		
Peanut Butter Graham Crackers, **Austin,** 1.4-oz. package	180	27.0			128.6	19.29		
Peanut Cookies, **Pepperidge Farm,** 5-oz. package (approx. 15 cookies)	700	80.0			140.0	16.00	(420)	(48.0)
1 cookie, approx. ⅓ oz.			47	5.3	140.0	16.00	(420)	(48.0)
Nutter Butter Peanut Butter Sandwich Cookies, **Nabisco,** 13½-oz. package (approx. 27 sandwiches)	1890	243.0			140.0	18.00	(490)	(66.5)
1 cookie, approx. 0.5 oz.			70	9.0	140.0	18.00	(490)	(66.5)
Nutter Butter Peanut Butter Sandwich Cookies, Chocolate, **Nabisco,** 15½-oz. package (approx. 39 cookies)	2210	286.0			142.6	18.45		
1 cookie, approx. 0.4 oz.			57	7.3	142.6	18.45		
Peanut Creme Patties, **Nabisco,** 10½-oz. package (approx. 48 patties)	1680	180.0			160.0	17.14		
1 pattie, approx. 0.2 oz.			35	3.8	160.0	17.14		
Peanut Logs, Caramel, **Nabisco** "Heyday," 10-oz. package (approx. 14 logs)	1680	182.0			168.0	18.20		
1 log, approx. 0.7 oz.			120	13.0	168.0	18.20		
Toast N' Peanut Butter Crackers, **Keebler,** 1½-oz. package (6 crackers)	230	25.0			153.3	16.67		
1 cracker, approx. 0.25 oz.			38	4.2	153.3	16.67		
Toast Peanut Butter Crackers, **Frito Lay's,** 1½-oz. package	214	24.1			142.7	16.07	(400)	(45.0)
Triple Decker Peanut Butter Sugar Wafers, **Nabisco,** "Biscos," 12-oz. package (approx. 36 cookies)	1680	204.0			140.0	17.00		
1 cookie, approx. 0.3 oz.			47	5.7	140.0	17.00		
PECAN								
Pecan Shortbread Cookies, **Nabisco,** 20-oz. package (approx. 40 cookies)	3200	340.0			160.0	17.00	(560)	(59.5)
1 cookie, approx. 0.5 oz.			80	8.5	160.0	17.00	(560)	(59.5)
PFEFFERNEUSE								
Pfeffernuese (Spice Drops), **Stella D'Oro,** 13-oz. package (approx. 43 or 44 pieces)	1945	300.7			149.7	23.13	(524)	(81.0)
1 piece, approx. 0.3 oz.			44	6.8	149.7	23.13	(524)	(81.0)
PICCOLO								
Piccolo Crepe Cookies, **Nabisco,** 4½-oz. package (approx. 30 cookies)	650	100.0			144.4	22.22		
1 cookie, approx. 0.2 oz.			22	3.3	144.4	22.22		
PIROUETTE								
Chocolate Laced Pirouette Cookies, **Pepperidge Farm,** 5½-oz. package (approx. 24 cookies)	960	112.0			174.5	20.36	(523)	(61.1)
1 cookie, approx. 0.2 oz.			40	4.7	174.5	20.36	(523)	(61.1)
Pirouette Cookies, **Pepperidge Farm,** 5½-oz. package (approx. 24 cookies)	960	112.0			174.5	20.36	(523)	(61.1)
1 cookie, approx. 0.2 oz.			40	4.7	174.5	20.36	(523)	(61.1)
PITTER PATTER								
Pitter Patter Cookies, **Keebler,** 16-oz. (1-lb.) package (approx. 25 or 26 cookies)	2333	297.6			145.8	18.60	(411)	(52.5)
1 cookie, approx. 0.6 oz.			90	11.5	145.8	18.60	(411)	(52.5)
PROTEIN								
Protein Cookies, **Tiger's Milk,** 8-oz. package (approx. 32 cookies)	960	136.0			120.0	17.00	(360)	(51.0)
1 cookie, approx. ¼ oz.			30	4.3	120.0	17.00	(360)	(51.0)
PRUNE								
Prune Pastry, sugar free, salt free, **Stella D'Oro,** 12.8-oz. package (approx. 18 pastries)	1710	245.0			134.7	19.14		
1 pastry, approx. 0.7 oz.			95	13.5	134.7	19.14		
RAISIN								
Raisin Bran Cookies, **Pepperidge Farm,** 5½-oz. package (approx. 15 cookies)	800	110.0			145.5	20.00	(436)	(60.0)
1 cookie, approx. 0.4 oz.			53	7.3	145.5	20.00	(436)	(60.0)
Raisin Fruit Biscuit, **Nabisco,** 7½-oz. package (approx. 14 biscuits)	840	168.0			112.0	22.40		
1 biscuit, approx. 0.5 oz.			60	12.0	112.0	22.40		
REGINA								
Regina Sesame Cookies, **Stella D'Oro,** 11-oz. package (approx. 28 cookies)	1372	165.2			125.0	15.05	(438)	(52.7)
1 cookie, approx. 0.4 oz.			49	5.9	125.0	15.05	(438)	(52.7)
RICE								
Rice Cakes, salted, **Chico-San,** 4-oz. box (approx. 11 rice cakes)	432	91.2			108.0	22.80		
1 rice cake, approx. 0.3 oz.			39	8.0	108.0	22.80		
Rice Cakes, unsalted, **Chico-San,** 4-oz. package (12 rice cakes)	432	91.2			108.0	22.80		
1 rice cake, approx. 0.3 oz.			36	7.6	108.0	22.80		

	ENTIRE PACKAGE		1 COOKIE OR CRACKER		1 OZ., BY WT.		1 CUP CRUMBLED	
	Cal.	Carb.	Cal.	Carb.	Cal.	Carb.	Cal.	Carb.
Rice Cakes, salted, **Feather River,** 4-oz. package (12 rice cakes)	420	90.0			105.0	22.50		
1 rice cake, approx. 0.3 oz.			35	7.5	105.0	22.50		
Rice Cakes, unsalted, **Feather River,** 4-oz. package (12 rice cakes)	432	91.2			108.0	22.80		
1 rice cake, approx. 0.3 oz.			36	7.6	108.0	22.80		
Rice Cakes, salted, **Spiral Brand,** 4¼-oz. package (13 rice cakes)	468	97.5			110.1	22.94		
1 rice cake, approx. 0.3 oz.			36	7.5	110.1	22.94		
Rice Cakes, unsalted, **Spiral Brand,** 4¼-oz. bag (13 rice cakes)	468	98.8			110.1	23.25		
1 rice cake, approx. 0.3 oz.			36	7.6	110.1	23.25		
Rice Cakes, salted, buckwheat added, **Chico-San,** 4-oz. package (12 rice cakes)	432	91.2			108.0	22.80		
1 rice cake, approx. 0.3 oz.			36	7.6	108.0	22.80		
Rice Cakes, unsalted, buckwheat added, **Chico-San,** 4-oz. package (12 rice cakes)	432	92.4			108.0	23.10		
1 rice cake, approx. 0.3 oz.			36	7.7	108.0	23.10		
Rice Cakes, salted, buckwheat added, **Feather River,** 4-oz. package (12 rice cakes)	480	108.0			120.0	27.00		
1 rice cake, approx. 0.3 oz.			40	9.0	120.0	27.00		
Rice Cakes, salted, buckwheat added, **Spiral Brand,** 4¼-oz. bag (13 rice cakes)	468	98.8			110.1	23.25		
1 rice cake, approx. 0.3 oz.			36	7.6	110.1	23.25		
Rice Cakes, salted, millet added, **Chico-San,** 4-oz. package (12 rice cakes)	480	108.0			120.0	27.00		
1 rice cake, approx. 0.3 oz.			40	9.0	120.0	27.00		
Rice Cakes, unsalted, millet added, **Chico-San,** 4-oz. package (12 rice cakes)	432	91.2			108.0	22.80		
1 rice cake, approx. 0.3 oz.			36	7.6	108.0	22.80		
Rice Cakes, salted, millet added, **Feather River,** 4-oz. package (12 rice cakes)	420	90.0			105.0	22.50		
1 rice cake, approx. 0.3 oz.			35	7.5	105.0	22.50		
Rice Cakes, salted, millet added, **Spiral Brand,** 4¼-oz. bag (13 rice cakes)	455	97.5			107.1	22.94		
1 rice cake, approx. 0.3 oz.			35	7.5	107.1	22.94		
Rice Cakes, unsalted, millet added, **Spiral Brand,** 4¼-oz. bag (13 rice cakes)	468	98.8			110.1	23.25		
1 rice cake, approx. 0.3 oz.			36	7.6	110.1	23.25		
Rice Wafers, **Devonsheer Melba,** 5-oz. package (approx. 58 to 60 rice wafers)	532	119.2			106.3	23.84		
1 wafer, approx. 0.1 oz.			9	2.0	106.3	23.84		
Rice Wafers, unsalted, **Devonsheer Melba,** 5-oz. package (approx. 58 to 60 rice wafers)	532	119.2			106.3	23.84		
1 wafer, approx. 0.1 oz.			9	2.0	106.3	23.84		
Rice Wafer-ets, Natural, salted, **Hol-Grain,** 5-oz. package (approx. 46 pieces)	553	118.4			110.6	23.67		
1 Wafer-et, approx. 0.1 oz.			12	2.6	110.6	23.67		
RITZ								
Ritz Crackers, **Nabisco,** 8-oz. box (approx. 71 crackers)	1200	144.0			150.0	18.00	(450)	(54.0)
12-oz. box (approx. 106 crackers)	1800	216.0			150.0	18.00	(450)	(54.0)
16-oz. (1-lb.) package (approx. 135 crackers)	2250	270.0			150.0	18.00	(450)	(54.0)
1 cracker, approx. 0.1 oz.			17	2.0	150.0	18.00	(450)	(54.0)
ROMAN								
Roman Egg Biscuits, Anise, **Stella D'Oro,** 12-oz. package (approx. 10 to 11 biscuits)	1421	200.8			118.4	16.73	(415)	(58.5)
1 biscuit, approx. 1.1 oz.			131	18.5	118.4	16.73	(415)	(58.5)
Roman Egg Biscuits, Rum & Brandy, **Stella D'Oro,** 13.4-oz. package (approx. 12 biscuits)	1572	222.0			118.4	16.73	(415)	(58.5)
1 biscuit, approx. 1.1 oz.			131	18.5	118.4	16.73	(415)	(58.5)
Roman Egg Biscuits, Vanilla, **Stella D'Oro,** 12-oz. package (approx. 10 or 11 biscuits)	1421	200.8			118.4	16.73	(415)	(58.5)
1 biscuit, approx. 1.1 oz.			131	18.5	118.4	16.73	(415)	(58.5)

	ENTIRE PACKAGE		1 COOKIE OR CRACKER		1 OZ., BY WT.		1 CUP CRUMBLED	
	Cal.	Carb.	Cal.	Carb.	Cal.	Carb.	Cal.	Carb.
ROUNDS								
Bacon Rounds, **Old London,** 6-oz. package (approx. 60 rounds)	720	108.0			120.0	18.00		
1 round, approx. 0.1 oz.			12	1.8	120.0	18.00		
Cheese Rounds, **Old London,** 6-oz. package (approx. 60 rounds)	720	108.0			120.0	18.00		
1 round, approx. 0.1 oz.			12	1.8	120.0	18.00		
Garlic Rounds, **Devonsheer Melba,** 6-oz. package (approx. 65 or 66 rounds)	718	114.2			119.6	19.03		
1 round, approx. 0.09 oz.			11	1.8	119.6	19.03		
Garlic Rounds, **Old London,** 6-oz. package (approx. 60 rounds)	600	108.0			100.0	18.00		
1 round, approx. 0.1 oz.			10	1.8	100.0	18.00		
Harvest Grains Melba Rounds, **Devonsheer Melba,** 5¼-oz. box (approx. 58 rounds)	522	116.0			99.4	22.10		
1 round, approx. 0.09 oz.			9	2.0	99.4	22.10		
Onion Rounds, **Devonsheer Melba,** 6-oz. package (approx. 75 rounds)	682	113.8			113.6	18.97		
1 round, approx. 0.08 oz.			10	1.5	113.6	18.97		
Onion Rounds, **Old London,** 6-oz. package (approx. 60 rounds)	600	108.0			100.0	18.00		
1 round, approx. 0.1 oz.			10	1.8	100.0	18.00		
Plain Rounds, **Devonsheer Melba,** 6-oz. package (approx. 65 or 66 rounds)	652	126.4			108.7	21.06		
1 round, approx. 0.9 oz.			10	1.9	108.7	21.06		
Rye Rounds, **Devonsheer Melba,** 6-oz. package (approx. 75 rounds)	682	127.9			113.6	21.31		
1 round, approx. 0.08 oz.			10	1.9	113.6	21.31		
Salty Rye Rounds, **Old London,** 6-oz. package (approx. 60 rounds)	600	108.0			100.0	18.00		
1 round, approx. 0.1 oz.			10	1.8	100.0	18.00		
Sea Rounds, Crackers, **Nabisco,** 14-oz. package (approx. 36 rounds)	1620	270.0			115.7	19.29		
1 round, approx. 0.4 oz.			45	7.5	115.7	19.29		
Sesame Rounds, **Old London,** 6-oz. package (approx. 60 rounds)	720	96.0			120.0	16.00		
1 round, approx. 0.1 oz.			12	1.6	120.0	16.00		
White Melba Rounds, **Old London,** 6-oz. package (approx. 60 rounds)	600	108.0			100.0	18.00		
1 round, approx. 0.1 oz.			10	1.8	100.0	18.00		
ROYAL								
Royal Lunch Milk Crackers, **Nabisco,** 15-oz. package (approx. 38 crackers)	2090	304.0			139.3	20.27		
1 cracker, approx. 0.4 oz.			55	8.0	139.3	20.27		
Royal Nuggets, **Stella D'Oro,** 3-oz. package (approx. 300 nuggets)	465	31.1			155.0	10.37	(465)	(31.1)
1 nugget, approx. 0.01 oz.			2	0.1	155.0	10.37	(465)	(31.1)
RY(E)								
Brown Rye Crisp Bread, **Wasa,** 8¼-oz. package (approx. 19 to 21 pieces)	840	177.8			101.8	21.55		
1 piece, approx. 0.4 oz.			43	9.0	101.8	21.55		
Golden Rye Crisp Bread, **Wasa,** 8½-oz. package (approx. 19 to 21 pieces)	884	187.9			104.0	22.11		
1 piece, approx. 0.4 oz.			44	9.4	104.0	22.11		
Hearty Rye Crisp Bread, **Wasa,** 8¼-oz. package (approx. 19 to 21 pieces)	840	177.8			101.8	21.55		
1 piece, approx. 0.4 oz.			43	9.1	101.8	21.55		
Lite Rye Crisp Bread, **Wasa,** 8¾-oz. package (approx. 20 or 21 pieces)	920	196.0			105.2	22.40		
1 piece, approx. 0.4 oz.			45	9.5	105.2	22.40		
Ry Krisp Snack Cracker, **Purina,** 8-oz. package (36 crackers)	810	176.4			101.3	22.05		
1 "triple" cracker, approx. 0.2 oz.			23	4.9	101.3	22.05		
Ry Krisp Snack Cracker, Seasoned, **Purina,** 8-oz. package (approx. 36 crackers)	925	169.0			110.0	19.88		
1 cracker, approx. 0.2 oz.			26	4.7	110.0	19.88		

	ENTIRE PACKAGE		1 COOKIE OR CRACKER		1 OZ., BY WT.		1 CUP CRUMBLED	
	Cal.	Carb.	Cal.	Carb.	Cal.	Carb.	Cal.	Carb.
Rye Crackers, **Austin,** vended size, 1.2-oz. package	150	21.0			125.0	17.50		
Rye Rounds, see under ROUNDS								
Rye Toast, **Devonsheer Melba,** 5-oz. package (approx. 31 or 32 pieces)	535	105.0			106.9	20.99		
1 piece, approx. 0.2 oz.			17	3.3	106.9	20.99		
Rye Toast, unsalted, **Devonsheer Melba,** 4½-oz. package (approx. 30 pieces)	480	95.6			106.7	21.24		
1 piece, approx. 0.2 oz.			16	3.2	106.7	21.24		
Rye Toast, **Keebler,** 9-oz. package (approx. 81 or 82 pieces)	1418	202.5			157.5	22.50	(444)	(63.5)
1 piece, approx. 0.1 oz.			18	2.5	157.5	22.50	(444)	(63.5)
Rye Wafers, **Nabisco,** 0.4-oz. package (2 wafers)	40	8.0			100.0	20.00	(300)	(60.0)
1 wafer, approx. 0.2 oz.			20	4.0	100.0	20.00	(300)	(60.0)
Rye Wafers, Seasoned, **Nabisco,** 0.4-oz. package (2 wafers)	45	9.0			112.5	22.50	(337)	(66.5)
1 wafer, approx. 0.2 oz.			23	4.5	112.5	22.50	(337)	(66.5)
Seasoned Rye Crisp Bread, **Wasa,** 8¾-oz. package (approx. 19 to 21 pieces)	938	195.9			107.2	22.39		
1 piece, approx. 0.4 oz.			45	9.5	107.2	22.39		
SALTINE(S) (also see under KRISPY)								
Saltine Crackers, **Austin,** vended size, ⅝-oz. package	70	12.0			110.0	20.00		
vended size, 1-oz. package	110	20.0			110.0	20.00		
Saltine Crackers, **Nabisco** "Premium," 16-oz. (1-lb.) package (approx. 160 crackers)	1920	320.0			120.0	20.00	(340)	(56.0)
1 cracker, approx. 0.1 oz.			12	2.0	120.0	20.00	(340)	(56.0)
Saltine Crackers, unsalted tops, **Nabisco** "Premium," 16-oz. (1-lb.) package (approx. 160 crackers)	1920	320.0			120.0	20.00	(340)	(56.0)
1 cracker, approx. 0.1 oz.			12	2.0	120.0	20.00	(340)	(56.0)
Saltines, Kosher, **Rokeach,** 8-oz. package (approx. 80 crackers)	960	160.0			120.0	20.00	(340)	(56.4)
1 cracker, approx. 0.1 oz.			12	2.0	120.0	20.00	(340)	(56.4)
SANDWICH COOKIES								
Many sandwich cookies are listed throughout this chapter under their brand names, such as Hydrox, or under their flavors, such as marshmallow. There are many sandwich cookies under the heading "CREAM (or CREME)."								
Sandwich Cookies, dietetic, **Estee,** 6-oz. package (approx. 15 cookies)	750	120.0			125.0	20.00	(375)	(60.0)
1 cookie, approx. 0.4 oz.			50	8.0	125.0	20.00	(375)	(60.0)
SESAME								
Regina Sesame Cookies, **Stella D'Oro,** 11-oz. package (approx. 28 cookies)	1372	165.2			125.0	15.05	(438)	(52.7)
1 cookie, approx. 0.4 oz.			49	5.9	125.0	15.05	(438)	(52.7)
Sesa Wheat Crackers With Extra Peanut Butter, **Austin's** "Big Shot," 1⅝-oz. package	230	22.0			141.5	13.54		
Sesame Bread Wafers, **Nabisco** "Meal Mates," 10-oz. package (approx. 60 wafers)	1300	190.0			130.0	19.00		
1 wafer, approx. 0.2 oz.			22	3.2	130.0	19.00		
Sesame/Cheese Snack Sticks, **Nabisco** "Twigs," 10-oz. package (approx. 100 sticks)	1400	160.0			140.0	16.00		
1 stick, approx. 0.1 oz.			14	1.6	140.0	16.00		
Sesame Crackers, lightly salted, **Golden Harvest,** 6-oz. package	840	114.0			140.0	19.00		
Sesame Crackers, low sodium, **Golden Harvest,** 6-oz. package	840	114.0			140.0	19.00		
Sesame Crisp Bread, see under CRISP BREAD								
Sesame Crisp Crackers, Teeko Glazed, **Nabisco,** 9-oz. package (approx. 54 crackers)	1170	162.0			130.0	18.00	(390)	(54.0)
1 cracker, approx. 0.2 oz.			22	3.0	130.0	18.00	(390)	(54.0)

	ENTIRE PACKAGE		1 COOKIE OR CRACKER		1 OZ., BY WT.		1 CUP CRUMBLED	
	Cal.	Carb.	Cal.	Carb.	Cal.	Carb.	Cal.	Carb.
Sesame Melba Toast, see under MELBA								
Sesame Rounds, see under ROUNDS								
Sesame Snack Crackers, buttery flavored, **Nabisco,** 8-oz. package (approx. 72 crackers)	1200	136.0			150.0	17.00	(450)	(57.0)
1 cracker, approx. 0.1 oz.			17	1.9	150.0	17.00	(450)	(57.0)
Sesame Toast, **Keebler,** 9-oz. package (approx. 81 or 82 pieces)	1215	202.5			135.0	22.50	(381)	(63.5)
1 piece, approx. 0.1 oz.			15	2.5	135.0	22.50	(381)	(63.5)
Sesame 'n Whole Wheat Snack Crackers, Sesame Wheats! **Nabisco,** 8½-oz. package (approx. 77 crackers)	1275	136.0			150.0	16.00		
1 cracker, approx. 0.1 oz.			17	1.8	150.0	16.00		
SHORTBREAD								
Fancy Shortbread Biscuits, packaged as part of the Mayfair Assortment, English Style, **Nabisco**								
1 biscuit, approx. 0.2 oz.			22	3.3	130.0	20.00		
Lorna Doone Shortbread, **Nabisco,** 10-oz. package (approx. 36 cookies)	1440	180.0			144.0	18.00		
1 cookie, approx. 0.3 oz.			40	5.0	144.0	18.00		
Shortbread Cookies, **Pepperidge Farm,** 5½-oz. package (approx. 12 cookies)	780	90.0			141.8	16.36	(425)	(49.1)
1 cookie, approx. 0.5 oz.			65	7.5	141.8	16.36	(425)	(49.1)
Shortbread Cookies, Pecan, **Nabisco,** 13-oz. package (approx. 26 cookies)	2080	221.0			160.0	17.00		
1 cookie, approx. 0.5 oz.			80	8.5	160.0	17.00		
Shortbread Cookies, Striped, **Nabisco,** 20-oz. package (approx. 40 cookies)	3200	340.0			150.0	19.00	(560)	(59.5)
1 cookie, approx. 0.3 oz.			50	6.3	150.0	19.00	(560)	(59.5)
SHORTCAKE								
Melt-A-Way Shortcake Cookies, **Nabisco,** 5¼-oz. package (approx. 12 cookies)	840	96.0			160.0	18.29		
1 cookie, approx. 0.4 oz.			70	8.0	160.0	18.29		
Shortcake Cookies, **Nabisco** "Cookie Little," 7-oz. package (approx. 140 cookies)	910	147.0			130.0	21.00		
1 cookie, approx. 0.05 oz.			7	1.1	130.0	21.00		
SKITTLE								
Skittle Chips Snack Crackers, **Nabisco,** 8½-oz. package (approx. 85 crackers)	1190	153.0			140.0	18.00	(420)	(54.0)
1 cracker, approx. 0.1 oz.			14	1.8	140.0	18.00	(420)	(54.0)
SNACK CRACKERS and SNACK STICKS								
Savory Snack Crackers, **Nabisco** "Snacks Ahoy," 7-oz. package (approx. 105 crackers)	980	119.0			140.0	17.00		
1 cracker, approx. 0.07 oz.			9	1.1	140.0	17.00		
Snack Crackers, **Rokeach,** 11-oz. package (approx. 99 crackers)	1430	209.0			130.0	19.00		
1 cracker, approx. 0.1 oz.			14	2.1	130.0	19.00		
Snack Crackers, Swiss Cheese, **Nabisco,** 8½-oz. package (approx. 128 crackers)	1275	144.5			150.0	17.00	(450)	(51.0)
1 cracker, approx. 0.07 oz.			10	1.1	150.0	17.00	(450)	(51.0)
Snack Sticks, lightly salted, **Pepperidge Farm,** 7½-oz. package (approx. 7 or 8 sticks)	900	135.0			120.0	18.00		
1 stick, approx. 1 oz.			120	18.0	120.0	18.00		
Snack Sticks, Pumpernickel, **Pepperidge Farm,** 7½-oz. package (approx. 7 or 8 sticks)	825	127.5			110.0	17.00		
1 stick, approx. 1 oz.			110	17.0	110.0	17.00		
Snack Sticks, Sesame, **Pepperidge Farm,** 7½-oz. package (approx. 7 or 8 sticks)	900	120.0			120.0	16.00		
1 stick, approx. 1 oz.			120	16.0	120.0	16.00		
Snack Sticks, Sesame/Cheese, **Nabisco,** "Twigs," 10-oz. package (approx. 100 sticks)	1400	160.0			140.0	16.00		
1 stick, approx. 0.1 oz.			14	1.6	140.0	16.00		
Snack Sticks, Whole Wheat, **Pepperidge Farm,** 7½-oz. package (approx. 7 or 8 sticks)	825	127.5			110.0	17.00		
1 stick, approx. 1 oz.			110	17.0	110.0	17.00		

	ENTIRE PACKAGE Cal.	ENTIRE PACKAGE Carb.	1 COOKIE OR CRACKER Cal.	1 COOKIE OR CRACKER Carb.	1 OZ., BY WT. Cal.	1 OZ., BY WT. Carb.	1 CUP CRUMBLED Cal.	1 CUP CRUMBLED Carb.
Vegetable Thins Snack Crackers, **Nabisco,** 8-oz. package (approx. 104 crackers)	1200	136.0			150.0	17.00		
1 cracker, approx. 0.08 oz.			12	1.3	150.0	17.00		
SOCIABLES								
Sociables Crackers, **Nabisco,** 8-oz. package (approx. 109 sociables)	1200	144.0			150.0	18.00		
1 sociable, approx. 0.07 oz.			11	1.2	150.0	18.00		
SOCIAL								
Social Tea Biscuit, **Nabisco,** 11-oz. package (approx. 65 biscuits)	1430	231.0			130.0	21.00		
1 biscuit, approx. 0.2 oz.			22	3.5	130.0	21.00		
SORRENTO								
Sorrento Cookies, **Stella D'Oro,** 10-oz. package (25 cookies)	1369	187.3			136.9	18.73	(480)	(65.5)
1 cookie, approx. 0.4 oz.			55	7.5	136.9	18.73	(480)	(65.5)
SOUP and OYSTER CRACKERS, see under OYSTER								
SPICE								
Spice Cookies, Iced, **Sweet N Good,** 11-oz. package (approx. 24 cookies)	1598	225.6			145.3	20.51	(436)	(61.5)
1 cookie, approx. 0.5 oz.			67	9.4	145.3	20.51	(436)	(61.5)
Spiced Wafers, **Nabisco,** 16-oz. (1-lb.) package (approx. 60 wafers)	1950	360.0			121.9	22.50		
1 wafer, approx. 0.3 oz.			33	6.0	121.9	22.50		
SPRINKLES								
Sprinkles Cookies, **Sunshine,** 9-oz. package (approx. 15 or 16 cookies)	930	181.2			103.3	20.13	(310)	(60.4)
1 cookie, approx. 0.6 oz.			59	11.5	103.3	20.13	(310)	(60.4)
SUGAR								
Sugar Cookies, **Pepperidge Farm,** 5¼-oz. (approx. 15 cookies)	800	105.0			152.4	20.00	(457)	(60.0)
1 cookie, approx. 0.4 oz.			53	7.0	152.4	20.00	(457)	(60.0)
Vended size, 2¼-oz. package (2 cookies)	320	45.0			142.0	20.00		
1 cookie, approx. 1⅛ oz.			160	22.5	142.0	20.00		
Sugar Cookies, Old Fashioned, **Keebler,** 13-oz. package (approx. 20 or 21 cookies)	1741	268.3			133.9	20.63	(402)	(61.9)
1 cookie, approx. 0.6 oz.			85	13.0	133.9	20.63	(402)	(61.9)
Sugar Honey Grahams, **Sunshine,** 16-oz. (1-lb.) package (approx. 124 Grahams)	1944	359.9			121.5	21.87	(365)	(65.6)
1 Graham, approx. 0.1 oz.			15	2.7	121.5	21.87	(365)	(65.6)
Sugar Rings, **Nabisco** "Bakers Bonus," 12-oz. package (approx. 24 cookies)	1680	252.0			140.0	21.00		
1 cookie, approx. 0.5 oz.			70	10.5	140.0	21.00		
Sugar Wafers, **Nabisco** "Bakers Bonus," 8½-oz. package (approx. 67 wafers)	1275	178.5			150.0	21.00	(525)	(70.0)
1 wafer, approx. 0.1 oz.			19	2.7	150.0	21.00	(525)	(70.0)
Sugar Wafers, **Nabisco,** "Biscos," 8½-oz. package (approx. 68 to 72 wafers)	1350	180.0			150.0	20.00		
1 wafer, approx. ⅛ oz.			19	2.5	150.0	20.00		
Sugar Wafers, **Holland American** "Dutch Treat," 1¾-oz. package (approx. 8 wafers)	256	33.3			146.0	19.00		
1 wafer, approx. 0.2 oz.			32	4.2	146.0	19.00		
3¾-oz. package (approx. 15 wafers)	548	71.3			146.0	19.00		
1 wafer, approx. ¼ oz.			37	4.8	146.0	19.00		
12-oz. package (approx. 42 wafers)	1752	228.0			146.0	19.00		
1 wafer, approx. 0.3 oz.			42	5.4	146.0	19.00		
Sugar Wafers, **Holland American** "Dutch Twin," 4½-oz. package (approx. 18 wafers)	657	85.5			146.0	19.00		
1 wafer, approx. ¼ oz.			44	5.7	146.0	19.00		
6-oz. package (approx. 20 wafers)	876	114.0			146.0	19.00		
1 wafer, approx. 0.3 oz.			44	5.7	146.0	19.00		
8-oz. package (approx. 42 wafers)	1168	152.0			146.0	19.00		
1 wafer, approx. 0.2 oz.			28	3.6	146.0	19.00		
11-oz. package (approx. 54 wafers)	1606	209.0			146.0	19.00		
1 wafer, approx. 0.2 oz.			29	3.8	146.0	19.00		
Sugar Wafers Cookies, **Sunshine,** 12-oz. package (approx. 40 cookies)	1643	250.3			136.9	20.86		
1 cookie, approx. 0.3 oz.			41	6.3	136.9	20.86		
SUNFLOWER								
Sunflower Raisin Cookies, **Pepperidge Farm,** 5½-oz. package (approx. 15 cookies)	800	90.0			145.5	16.36	(536)	(59.1)
1 cookie, approx. 0.4 oz.			53	6.0	145.5	16.36	(536)	(59.1)
SWISS								
Swiss Cheese Snack Crackers, **Nabisco,** 8½-oz. package (approx. 128 crackers)	1275	144.5			150.0	17.00	(450)	(51.0)
1 cracker, approx. 0.07 oz.			10	1.1	150.0	17.00	(450)	(51.0)
Swiss Creme Sandwich Cookies, **Nabisco,** 1.1-oz. package (approx. 3 cookies)	150	23.0			136.4	20.90	(477)	(73.2)
1 cookie, approx. 0.4 oz.			50	7.7	136.4	20.90	(477)	(73.2)
Swiss Fudge Cookies, **Stella D'Oro,** 9.2-oz. package (approx. 20 cookies)	1280	154.0			140.7	16.92	(492)	(59.2)
1 cookie, approx. 0.5 oz.			64	7.7	140.7	16.92	(492)	(59.2)
TAHITI								
Tahiti Cookies, **Pepperidge Farm,** 6¼-oz. package (approx. 12 cookies)	1020	108.0			163.2	17.28	(489)	(51.8)
1 cookie, approx. 0.5 oz.			85	9.0	163.2	17.28	(489)	(51.8)
TAMS								
Onion Tams, **Manischewitz,** 8-oz. package (approx. 80 Tams)	1078	154.7			134.7	19.34	(404)	(58.0)
1 tam, approx. 0.1 oz.			13	1.9	134.7	19.34	(404)	(58.0)
Tam Tams, **Manischewitz,** 8-oz. package (approx. 80 Tams)	1130	146.3			141.2	18.29	(424)	(54.9)
1 tam, approx. 0.1 oz.			14	1.8	141.2	18.29	(424)	(54.9)
TASTE OF VIENNA								
Taste of Vienna Cookies, **Stella D'Oro,** 11.9-oz. package (approx. 20 cookies)	1700	204.0			143.7	17.24	(503)	(60.4)
1 cookie, approx. 0.6 oz.			85	10.2	143.7	17.24	(503)	(60.4)
TATER								
Tater Puffs, Snack Crackers, **Nabisco,** 5-oz. package (approx. 105 crackers)	700	85.0			140.0	17.00	(420)	(51.0)
1 cracker, approx. 0.05 oz.			7	0.8	140.0	17.00	(420)	(51.0)
TEA TIME								
Tea Time Biscuit, **Nabisco,** approx. 0.7 oz., packaged as part of the Mayfair Assortment, English Style								
1 biscuit, approx. 0.2 oz.			25	4.3	142.9	24.29		
TEETHING								
Teething Biscuits, **Gerber,** 4-oz. box (approx. 20 Biscuits)	435	88.8			108.9	22.20		
1 Biscuit, approx. 0.2 oz.			25	4.5	108.9	22.20		
THINS (also see under individual flavors, such as VANILLA and VEGETABLE)								
Thins Crackers, Bacon Flavored, **Nabisco,** 8-oz. package (approx. 112 crackers)	1200	144.0			150.0	18.00	(450)	(54.0)
1 cracker, approx. 0.07 oz.			11	1.3	150.0	18.00	(450)	(54.0)
Thins Crackers, Butter Flavored, **Nabisco,** 8-oz. package (approx. 72 crackers)	1040	160.0			130.0	20.00	(390)	(60.0)
1 cracker, approx. 0.1 oz.			14	2.2	130.0	20.00	(390)	(60.0)
TOAST(Y) (also see under individual flavors and under MELBA)								
Plain Toast, ("Melba Toast"), **Devonsheer Melba,** 4½-oz. package (approx. 30 pieces)	480	94.8			106.7	21.06		
1 piece, approx. 0.2 oz.			16	3.2	106.7	21.06		
Plain Toast, unsalted, **Devonsheer Melba,** 4½-oz. package (approx. 30 pieces)	480	96.5			106.7	21.44		
1 piece, approx. 0.2 oz.			16	3.2	106.7	21.44		
Rye Toast, **Devonsheer Melba,** 4½-oz. package (approx. 30 pieces)	480	94.5			106.7	20.99		

	ENTIRE PACKAGE		1 COOKIE OR CRACKER		1 OZ., BY WT.		1 CUP CRUMBLED	
	Cal.	Carb.	Cal.	Carb.	Cal.	Carb.	Cal.	Carb.
1 piece, approx. 0.2 oz.			16	3.2	106.7	20.99		
Rye Toast, unsalted, **Devonsheer Melba,** 4½-oz. package (approx. 30 pieces)	480	95.6			106.7	21.24		
1 piece, approx. 0.2 oz.			16	3.2	106.7	21.24		
Sourdough Toast Crisp Bread, **Wasa,** 7-oz. package (approx. 16 or 17 pieces)	758	156.8			108.3	22.40	(408)	(84.4)
1 piece, approx. 0.4 oz.			46	9.5	108.3	22.40	(408)	(84.4)
Toast Peanut Butter Crackers, **Frito Lay's,** 1½-oz. package	214	24.1			142.7	16.07	(400)	(45.0)
Toasty Crackers with Peanut Butter, **Austin's,** 1½-oz. package	210	22.0			140.0	14.67		
Toasty Crackers with extra Peanut Butter, **Austin's** "Big Shot," 1¾-oz. package	250	24.0			142.9	13.71		
Wheat Melba Toast, **Old London,** 5-oz. package (approx. 30 pieces)	500	100.0			100.0	20.00		
1 piece, approx. 1.7 oz.			17	3.3	100.0	20.00		
Wheat Toast, **Keebler,** 9-oz. package (approx. 81 or 82 pieces)	1418	202.5			157.5	22.50	(444)	(63.5)
1 piece, approx. 0.1 oz.			18	2.5	157.5	22.50	(444)	(63.5)
White Melba Toast, **Old London,** 5-oz. package (approx. 30 pieces)	500	100.0			100.0	20.00		
1 piece, approx. 1.7 oz.			17	3.3	100.0	20.00		
White Melba Toast, unsalted, **Old London,** 5-oz. package (approx. 30 pieces)	500	100.0			100.0	20.00		
1 piece, approx. 1.7 oz.			17	3.3	100.0	20.00		
Whole Wheat Toast, unsalted, **Devonsheer Melba,** 4½-oz. package (approx. 30 pieces)	480	95.5			106.7	21.21		
1 piece, approx. 0.2 oz.			16	3.2	106.7	21.21		
TOWN HOUSE								
Town House Crackers, **Keebler,** 12-oz. package (approx. 109 crackers)	1890	216.0			157.5	18.00	(444)	(50.8)
1 cracker, approx. 0.1 oz.			17	2.0	157.5	18.00	(444)	(50.8)
TOY								
Toy Cookies, **Sunshine,** 2-oz. package (approx. 20 cookies)	263	42.5			131.6	21.26	(534)	(86.2)
9½-oz. package (approx. 95 cookies)	1250	202.0			131.6	21.26	(534)	(86.2)
1 cookie, approx. 0.1 oz.			13	2.1	131.6	21.26	(534)	(86.2)
TRISCUIT								
Triscuit Wafers, **Nabisco,** 9½-oz. package (approx. 61 to 63 wafers)	1260	189.0			127.3	19.09	(362)	(59.3)
1 wafer, approx. 0.2 oz.			20	3.0	127.3	19.09	(362)	(59.3)
UNEEDA								
Uneeda Biscuits, **Nabisco,** 3½-oz. package (approx. 18 biscuits)	390	66.0			118.2	20.00	(335)	(60.0)
1 biscuit, approx. 0.2 oz.			22	3.7	118.2	20.00	(335)	(60.0)
Uneeda Biscuits, unsalted tops, **Nabisco,** 3½-oz. package (approx. 18 biscuits)	390	66.0			118.2	20.00	(335)	(60.0)
1 biscuit, approx. 0.2 oz.			22	3.7	118.2	20.00	(335)	(60.0)
VANILLA								
Dixie Vanilla Cookies, **Sunshine,** 12-oz. package (approx. 26 or 27 cookies)	1530	258.5			127.5	21.54	(383)	(64.6)
1 cookie, approx. 0.5 oz.			58	9.8	127.5	21.54	(383)	(64.6)
Vanilla Thins, dietetic, **Estee,** 7½-oz. package (approx. 35 Thins)	875	140.0			116.7	18.67	(428)	(68.5)
1 thin, approx. 0.2 oz.			25	4.0	116.7	18.67	(428)	(68.5)
Vanilla Wafers, **A&P,** 8-oz. package (approx. 56 wafers)	1040	168.0			130.0	21.00	(477)	(63.0)
1 wafer, approx. 0.1 oz.			19	3.0	130.0	21.00	(477)	(63.0)
Vanilla Wafers, **Keebler** 12-oz. package (approx. 92 or 93 wafers)	1791	232.8			149.2	19.40	(547)	(71.1)
1 wafer, approx. 0.1 oz.			19	2.5	149.2	19.40	(547)	(71.1)
Vanilla Wafers, dietetic, **Estee,** 1⅞-oz. 3-pak (3 wafers)	270	31.5			144.0	16.80	(530)	(61.6)
1 wafer, approx. 0.6 oz.			90	10.5	144.0	16.80	(530)	(61.6)
4-oz. package (approx. 24 wafers)	600	72.0			150.0	18.00	(550)	(66.0)
1 wafer, approx. 0.2 oz.			25	3.0	150.0	18.00	(550)	(66.0)
Vanilla Wafers, **Sunshine,** 11-oz. package (approx. 100 wafers)	1455	218.4			132.3	19.85	(485)	(72.8)
1 wafer, approx. 0.1 oz.			15	2.2	132.3	19.85	(485)	(72.8)
VEGETABLE								
Vegetable Thins Snack Crackers, **Nabisco,** 8-oz. package (approx. 104 crackers)	1200	136.0			150.0	17.00		
1 cracker, approx. 0.08 oz.			12	1.3	150.0	17.00		
VIENNA								
Vienna Fingers cookies, **Sunshine,** 12-oz. package (approx. 24 cookies)	1630	243.4			135.8	20.28	(407)	(60.8)
15-oz. package (approx. 30 cookies)	2037	304.2			135.8	20.28	(407)	(60.8)
19-oz. package (approx. 38 cookies)	2580	385.3			135.8	20.28	(407)	(60.8)
1 cookie, approx. 0.5 oz.			68	10.3	135.8	20.28	(407)	(60.8)
WAFERS have been listed alphabetically under their flavor or brand name.								
WAFFLE								
Waffle Cremes, **Holland American** "Dutch Treat," 10-oz. package (approx. 24 Cremes)	1460	190.0			146.0	19.00		
1 creme, approx. 0.4 oz.			61	7.9	146.0	19.00		
Waffle Cremes, **Nabisco** "Biscos," 10-oz. package (approx. 36 cookies)	1560	216.0			156.0	21.60	(468)	(64.8)
1 cookie, approx. 0.3 oz.			43	6.0	156.0	21.60	(468)	(64.8)
WALDORF								
Waldorf Crackers, **Keebler,** 13-oz. package (approx. 118 crackers)	1728	288.0			132.9	22.15	(375)	(62.5)
1 cracker, approx. 0.1 oz.			15	2.5	132.9	22.15	(375)	(62.5)
Waldorf Crackers, Low Sodium, **Keebler,** 13-oz. package (approx. 118 crackers)	1728	288.0			132.9	22.15	(375)	(62.5)
1 cracker, approx. 0.1 oz.			15	2.5	132.9	22.50	(375)	(62.5)
WAVERLY								
Waverly Wafers, **Nabisco,** 11½-oz. package (approx. 88 wafers)	1540	231.0			133.9	20.09	469	70.3
1 wafer, approx. 0.1 oz.			18	2.6	133.9	20.09	469	70.3
WHEAT								
Wheat Chips Whole Grain Goodness, **Nabisco,** 4¾-oz. package (approx. 166 crackers)	713	80.8			150.0	17.00		
1 cracker, approx. 0.03 oz.			4	0.5	150.0	17.00		
Wheat Free Cookies, Carob, **El Molino,** 7-oz. package (approx. 12 cookies)	993	128.3			133.3	18.33	(400)	(55.0)
1 cookie, approx. 0.6 oz.			80	11.0	133.3	18.33	(400)	(55.0)
Wheat Germ & Cheese Flavored Crackers, **Golden Harvest,** 6-oz. package	840	126.0			140.0	21.00		
Wheat Germ Crackers, lightly salted, **Golden Harvest,** 6-oz. package	900	102.0			150.0	17.00		
Wheat Smackers Cracker Snacks, **Austin,** 1½-oz. package	230	25.0			153.3	16.67		
Wheat Thins crackers, **Nabisco,** 10-oz. package (approx. 160 crackers)	1400	190.0			140.0	19.00	(420)	(57.0)
1 cracker, approx. 0.06 oz.			9	1.2	140.0	19.00	(420)	(57.0)
Wheat Toast, **Keebler,** 9-oz. package (approx. 81 or 82 pieces)	1418	202.5			157.5	22.50	(444)	(63.5)
1 piece, approx. 0.1 oz.			18	2.5	157.5	22.50	(444)	(63.5)
Wheat Wafers, **Sunshine,** 11-oz. package (approx. 155 wafers)	1404	233.9			127.6	21.26	(383)	(63.8)
1 wafer,approx. 0.07 oz.			9	1.5	127.6	21.26	(383)	(63.8)
Wheat Wafers, Bite Size, **Venus,** 6-oz. package (approx. 56 wafers)	700	126.0			116.7	21.00	(350)	(63.0)
1 wafer, approx. 0.1 oz.			13	2.3	116.7	21.00	(350)	(63.0)
Wheat Wafers, low sodium, **Venus,** 7-oz. package (approx. 54 wafers)	972	162.0			138.9	23.14	(417)	(69.4)
1 wafer, approx. 0.1 oz.			18	3.0	138.9	23.14	(417)	(69.4)

	ENTIRE PACKAGE Cal.	ENTIRE PACKAGE Carb.	1 COOKIE OR CRACKER Cal.	1 COOKIE OR CRACKER Carb.	1 OZ., BY WT. Cal.	1 OZ., BY WT. Carb.	1 CUP CRUMBLED Cal.	1 CUP CRUMBLED Carb.
Wheatsworth Stone Ground Wheat Crackers, **Nabisco,** 11-oz. package (approx. 99 crackers)	1430	176.0			130.0	16.00		
1 cracker, approx. 0.1 oz.			14	1.8	130.0	16.00		
WHOLE WHEAT								
Whole Wheat Crackers, lightly salted, **Golden Harvest,** 6-oz. package	840	114.0			140.0	19.00		
Whole Wheat Crackers, low sodium. **Golden Harvest,** 6-oz. package	840	114.0			140.0	19.00		
Whole Wheat Crisp Bread, see under CRISP BREAD								
Whole Wheat Snack Sticks, **Pepperidge Farm,** 7½-oz. package (approx. 7 or 8 sticks)	825	127.5			110.0	17.00		
1 stick, approx. 1.0 oz.			110	17.0	110.0	17.00		
Whole Wheat Toast, **Devonsheer Melba,** 4½-oz. package (approx. 30 toasts)	480	94.8			106.7	21.06		
1 toast, approx. 0.7 oz.			16	3.2	106.7	21.06		
Whole Wheat Toast, unsalted, **Devonsheer Melba,** 4½-oz. package (approx. 30 toasts)	480	95.5			106.7	21.21		
1 toast, approx. 0.2 oz.			16	3.2	106.7	21.21		
Whole Wheat Wafer-ets, salted, **Hol-Grain,** 5-oz. package (approx. 85 wafer-ets)	563	113.0			112.6	22.60		
1 wafer-et, approx. 0.06 oz.			7	1.3	112.6	22.60		
WINE								
Wine Crackers, **O.T.C.,** 8-oz. bag (approx. 32 crackers)	(589)	(102.4)			(73.6)	(12.80)	(206)	(35.8)
1 cracker, approx. ¼ oz.			18	3.2	(73.6)	(12.80)	(206)	(35.8)
YOGURT								
Yogurt Crackers, lightly salted, **Golden Harvest,** 6-oz. package	840	120.0			140.0	20.00		
YUM YUMMS								
Yum Yumms cookies, **Sunshine,** 10-oz. package (approx. 20 cookies)	1558	195.3			155.8	19.53		
1 cookie, approx. 0.5 oz.			83	10.4	155.8	19.53		
ZESTA								
Zesta crackers, **Keebler,** 16-oz. (1-lb.) package (approx. 228 or 229 crackers)	1890	378.1			118.1	23.63	(333)	(66.7)
1 cracker, approx. 0.07 oz.			8	1.7	118.1	23.63	(333)	(66.7)
ZWEIBACK								
Zweiback Toast, **Gerber,** 4-oz. box (approx. 16 toasts)	483	82.4			120.8	20.61	(423)	(72.1)
1 toast, approx. ¼ oz.			30	5.0	120.8	20.61	(423)	(72.1)
Zweiback Toast, **Nabisco,** 6-oz. package (approx 24 toasts)	720	120.0			120.0	20.00	(420)	(70.0)
1 toast, approx. ¼ oz.			30	5.0	120.0	20.00	(420)	(70.0)
COOKIE ASSORTMENTS								
Famous Cookie Assortment, **Nabisco,** 11-oz. package (contains 5 Butter-flavored Cookies, 3 Biscos Sugar Wafers, 3 Baronet Creme Sandwiches, 6 Oreo Chocolate Sandwiches, 5 Lorna Doone Shortbread Cookies, 5 Kettle Cookies, and 7 Cameo Creme Sandwiches)	1546	220.0			140.5	20.0		
Baronet Creme Sandwich, 3 Sandwiches (approx. 1.2 oz.)	160	24.0			133.3	20.00		
1 sandwich, approx. 0.4 oz.			53	8.0	133.3	20.00		
Biscos Sugar Wafers, 3 wafers (approx. 1 oz.)	150	20.0			150.0	20.00		
1 wafer, approx. ⅓ oz.			50	6.7	150.0	20.00		

	ENTIRE PACKAGE Cal.	ENTIRE PACKAGE Carb.	1 COOKIE OR CRACKER Cal.	1 COOKIE OR CRACKER Carb.	1 OZ., BY WT. Cal.	1 OZ., BY WT. Carb.	1 CUP CRUMBLED Cal.	1 CUP CRUMBLED Carb.
Butter Flavored Cookies, 5 cookies (approx. 1.1 oz.)	154	22.0			140.0	20.00	(490)	(70.0)
1 cookie, approx. 0.2 oz.			31	4.4	140.0	20.00	(490)	(70.0)
Cameo Creme Sandwich, 7 Sandwiches (approx. 3¾ oz.)	525	77.0			140.0	21.00	(490)	(73.4)
1 sandwich, approx. 0.5 oz.			70	10.5	140.0	21.00	(490)	(73.4)
Kettle Cookies, 5 cookies (approx. 1¼ oz.)	175	26.3			140.0	21.00		
1 cookie, approx. ¼ oz.			35	5.3	140.0	21.00		
Lorna Doone Shortbread cookies, 5 cookies (approx. 1.4 oz.)	200	25.0			144.0	18.00		
1 cookie, approx. 0.3 oz.			40	5.0	144.0	18.00		
Oreo Chocolate Sandwich Cookies, 6 cookies (approx. 2.2 oz.)	300	44.0			136.4	20.00	(477)	(70.0)
1 cookie, approx. 0.4 oz.			50	7.3	136.4	20.00	(477)	(70.0)
Hostess With The Mostest Assorted Cookies, **Stella D'Oro,** 28-oz. package (approx. 93 or 94 cookies)	3805	527.0			135.9	18.82	(476)	(65.9)
1 cookie, approx. 0.3 oz.			39	5.4	135.9	18.82	(476)	(65.9)
Lady Stella Assortment Cookies, **Stella D'Oro,** 15-oz. package (approx. 52 or 53 cookies)	1934	287.4			128.9	19.16	(451)	(67.1)
1 cookie, approx. 0.3 oz.			37	5.5	128.9	19.16	(451)	(67.1)
Mayfair Assortment, English Style, **Nabisco,** 11½-oz. package (contains 8 Crown Creme Sandwiches, 7 Fancy Shortbread Biscuits, 4 Filigree Creme Sandwiches, 4 Mayfair Creme Sandwiches, 8 Tea Rose Creme Sandwiches, and 4 Tea Time Biscuits)	1605	233.6			139.6	20.32		
Crown Creme Sandwiches, 8 Sandwiches (approx. 3.2 oz.)	427	64.0			133.4	20.00		
1 sandwich, approx. 0.4 oz.			53	8.0	133.4	20.00		
Fancy Shortbread Biscuit, 7 Biscuits (approx. 1.2 oz.)	152	23.3			130.0	20.00		
1 biscuit, approx. 0.2 oz.			22	3.3	130.0	20.00		
Filigree Creme Sandwich, 4 Sandwiches (approx. 1.6 oz.)	240	34.0			150.0	21.25		
1 sandwich, approx. 0.4 oz.			60	8.5	150.0	21.25		
Mayfair Creme Sandwich, 4 Sandwiches (approx. 1.8 oz.)	260	36.0			144.4	20.00		
1 sandwich, approx. 0.5 oz.			65	9.0	144.4	20.00		
Tea Rose Creme Sandwiches, 8 Sandwiches (approx. 2.9 oz.)	427	61.3			145.5	20.91		
1 sandwich, approx. 0.4 oz.			53	7.7	145.5	20.91		
Tea Time Biscuits, 4 Biscuits (approx. 0.7 oz.)	100	17.0			142.9	24.29		
1 biscuit, approx. 0.2 oz.			25	4.3	142.9	24.29		
Oreo & Swiss Creme Sandwich Assortment, **Nabisco,** 15-oz. package (contains 27 Swiss Creme Sandwiches, and 15 Oreo Chocolate Sandwiches)	2100	308.0			136.4	20.53	(477)	(71.9)
Oreo Chocolate Sandwich Cookies, 15 cookies	750	110.0			136.4	20.00	(477)	(70.0)
1 cookie, approx. 0.4 oz.			50	7.3	136.4	20.00	(477)	(70.0)
Swiss Creme Sandwich Cookie, 27 cookies	1350	198.0			136.4	20.90	(477)	(73.2)
1 cookie, approx. 0.4 oz.			50	7.7	136.4	20.90	(477)	(73.2)

24 SWEET LITTLE NOTHINGS—CANDY •

	UNIT Cal.	UNIT Carb.	1 OZ., BY WT. Cal.	1 OZ., BY WT. Carb.	1 POUND Cal.	1 POUND Carb.
CANDY, based on generic data						
BUTTERSCOTCH						
1 pound (tr/27g/1g/2%/19mg)	1801	430.4	112.6	26.90	1801	430.4
CANDY CORN						
1 pound, approx. 320 candy corns (tr/25g/1g/8%/61mg)	1651	406.4	103.2	25.40	1651	406.4
1 cup, approx. 7.0 oz. (approx. 143 candy corns)	728	179.2	103.2	25.40	1651	406.4
1 candy corn, ⅞" long, ½" wide, ¼" thick, approx. 0.05 oz. (approx. 20 per ounce)	5	1.3	103.2	25.40	1651	406.4
CARAMELS						
Plain, 1 pound (1g/22g/3g/8%/65mg)	1810	347.5	113.1	21.70	1810	347.5
Chocolate, 1 pound (1g/22g/3g/8%/65mg)	1810	347.5	113.1	21.70	1810	347.5
Plain, with nuts (1g/20g/5g/7%/58mg)	1941	319.8	121.3	20.00	1941	319.8
Chocolate, with nuts (1g/20g/5g/7%/58mg)	1941	319.8	121.3	20.00	1941	319.8
CHOCOLATE						
Bittersweet, 1 pound (2g/13g/11g/2%/1mg)	2164	212.8	135.3	13.27	2164	212.8
Semisweet, 1 pound (1g/16g/10g/1%/1mg)	2304	258.6	144.0	16.17	2304	258.6
1 piece, approx. 0.01 oz. (approx. 60 per ounce)	(2)	(0.3)	144.0	16.16	2304	258.6
Small pieces, 1 cup (approx. 1 6-oz. package or about 360 pieces)	862	96.9	144.0	16.16	2304	258.6
Sweet, 1 pound (1g/16g/10g/1%/tr)	2395	258.1	149.7	16.13	2395	258.1
Milk Chocolate:						
Plain, 1 pound (2g/16g/10g/1%/27mg)	2359	258.1	147.4	16.13	2359	258.1
With almonds, 1 pound (3g/15g/9g/2%/23mg)	2413	232.7	150.8	14.54	2413	232.7
With peanuts, 1 pound (4g/13g/11g/1%/19mg)	2463	202.3	154.0	12.64	2463	202.3
CHOCOLATE-COATED NUTS AND CANDIES						
Chocolate-Coated Almonds:						
1 pound (approx. 96 to 128 almonds) (3g/11g/12g/2%/17mg)	2581	179.6	161.3	11.23	2581	179.6
1 cup comprised of single nuts that are not clustered (approx. 5.8 oz.)	939	65.3	161.3	11.23	2581	179.6
1 chocolate-coated almond (approx. 0.14 oz., approx. 7 per ounce)	23	1.6	161.3	11.23	2581	179.6
Chocolate-Coated Coconut Centered Candies:						
1 pound (1g/20g/5g/7%/56mg)	1987	326.6	124.2	20.41	1987	326.6
Chocolate-Coated Mints:						
1 pound (tr/23g/3g/6%/52mg)	1860	367.4	116.3	23.00	1860	367.4
1 large mint (approx. 1⅐ oz.)	132	26.3	116.3	23.00	1860	367.4
1 small mint (approx. 0.4 oz., approx. 2½ per ounce)	46	9.2	116.3	23.00	1860	367.4
1 miniature mint (approx. 0.08 oz., approx. 12 per ounce)	9	1.8	116.3	23.00	1860	367.4

	UNIT Cal.	UNIT Carb.	1 OZ., BY WT. Cal.	1 OZ., BY WT. Carb.	1 POUND Cal.	1 POUND Carb.
Chocolate-Coated Peanuts:						
1 pound (approx. 128 to 256 single coated peanuts) (5g/11g/12g/1%/17mg)	2545	177.4	159.1	11.06	2545	177.4
1 cup (approx. 6 oz., or 48 to 96 nuts)	954	66.6	159.1	11.06	2545	177.4
1 cluster (approx. ½ oz., or 4 to 8 nuts)	80	5.6	159.1	11.06	2545	177.4
Chocolate-Coated Raisins:						
1 pound (approx. 800 small coated raisins) (2g/20g/12g/5%/17mg)	1928	319.8	120.5	20.00	1928	319.8
1 cup (approx. 6.7 oz., or approx. 335 small coated raisins, or 228 to 448 large coated raisins)	808	134.0	120.5	20.00	1928	319.8
1 small coated raisin (approx. 0.02 oz., approx. 50 per ounce)	2	0.4	120.5	20.00	1928	319.8
1 large coated raisin (approx. 0.03–0.05 oz., approx. 18 to 28 per ounce)	5	0.8	120.5	20.00	1928	319.8
FUDGE						
Chocolate Fudge, plain, 1 pound (1g/21g/3g/8%/54mg)	1814	340.2	113.4	21.26	1814	340.2
1 cubic inch (approx. ¾ oz.)	84	15.8	113.4	21.26	1814	340.2
With nuts, 1 pound (1g/20g/5g/8%/49mg)	1932	313.0	120.8	19.56	1932	313.0
1 cubic inch (approx. ¾ oz.)	89	14.5	120.8	19.56	1932	313.0
Vanilla Fudge, plain, 1 pound (1g/21g/3g/10%/59mg)	1805	339.3	112.8	21.21	1805	339.3
1 cubic inch (approx. ¾ oz.)	84	15.7	112.8	21.21	1805	339.3
With nuts, 1 pound (1g/20g/5g/10%/53mg)	1923	312.1	120.2	19.51	1923	312.1
1 cubic inch (approx. ¾ oz.)	89	14.4	120.2	19.51	1923	312.1
GUM DROPS						
All flavors, 1 pound (tr/25g/tr/12%/10mg)	1576	396.4	98.5	24.78	1576	396.4
HALVA (based on data from the Middle East)						
1 pound	2341	257.6	146.3	16.10	2341	257.6
HARD CANDIES						
1 pound (tr/28g/tr/1%/9mg)	1751	440.9	109.4	27.56	1751	440.9
JELLY BEANS						
1 pound (approx. 160 jelly beans) (tr/26g/tr/6%/3mg)	1665	422.3	104.1	26.40	1665	422.3
1 cup, approx. 7.8 oz. (approx. 75 jelly beans as described above)	807	204.8	104.1	26.40	1665	422.3
1 Jelly Bean, approx. 0.1 oz., (approx. 10 jelly beans per ounce, approx. ¾" long and ½" wide)	10	2.6	104.1	26.40	1665	422.3
MARSHMALLOWS						
All sizes, "regular" and "soft" types, 1 pound (1g/23g/tr/17%/11mg)	1447	364.7	90.4	22.80	1447	364.7
1 marshmallow, large, regular type (1⅛" diameter, ¾" high, approx. ¼ oz., approx. 63 per pound)	23	5.8	90.4	22.80	1447	364.7
1 marshmallow, soft type, (1⅛" diameter, 1⅛ high, approx. 0.2 oz., approx. 76 per pound)	19	4.8	90.4	22.80	1447	364.7
1 miniature marshmallow, approx. 0.02 oz. (approx. 50 per ounce)	2	0.5	90.4	22.80	1447	364.7

	UNIT		1 OZ., BY WT.		1 POUND	
	Cal.	Carb.	Cal.	Carb.	Cal.	Carb.
MINTS						
Uncoated, 1 pound (tr/25g/1g/8%/60mg)	1651	406.4	103.2	25.40	1651	406.4
1 round mint, 1½" diameter, ½" thick, (approx. 0.3 oz., approx. 3 per ounce)	32	7.9	103.2	25.40	1651	406.4
1 square mint, ⅝" long, ⅝" wide and ⅜" high (approx. 0.06 oz., approx. 16½ per ounce)	6	1.6	103.2	25.40	1651	406.4
1 rectangular mint, ½" long, ⅜" wide and ⅜" high, (approx. 0.03 oz. each, approx. 39 per ounce)	3	0.7	103.2	25.40	1651	406.4
Chocolate-coated mints are listed with Chocolate-Coated Nuts and Candies						
PEANUT BRITTLE						
1 pound (2g/23g/3g/2%/9mg)	1910	367.4	119.4	23.00	1910	367.4
SUGAR-COATED NUTS AND CANDIES						
Sugar-Coated Almonds:						
1 pound (approx. 128 sugar-coated almonds) (2g/20g/5g/2%/6mg)	2068	318.4	129.3	19.90	2068	318.4
1 cup, approx. 6.9 oz. (approx. 55 sugar-coated almonds as described above)	889	136.7	129.3	19.90	2068	318.4
1 sugar-coated almond, 1" long and ⅝" wide (approx. 0.13 oz., approx. 8 per ounce)	17	2.6	129.3	19.90	2068	318.4
Sugar-Coated Chocolate Disks:						
1 pound (approx. 496 disks) (1g/21g/6g/1%/20mg)	2114	329.8	132.1	20.61	2114	329.8
1 cup, approx. 6.9 oz., (approx. 215 sugar-coated disks as described above)	918	143.2	132.1	20.61	2114	329.8
1 disk, ½" diameter (approx. 0.03 oz., approx. 31 disks per ounce)	4	0.7	132.1	20.61	2114	329.8

CANDY, by brand

	UNIT		1 OZ., BY WT.		1 POUND	
	Cal.	Carb.	Cal.	Carb.	Cal.	Carb.
After-dinner Mints, **Richardson:**						
1 jelly mint, approx. 0.11 oz. (approx. 9 per ounce)	12	2.9	106.0	26.51	1696	424.2
If you eat only the jelly center approx. 0.03 oz.	3	0.6	96.6	24.72	1546	395.5
If you eat only the outside, approx. 0.08 oz.	9	2.3	110.9	27.73	1760	443.7
Pastel mint, Midget cut, approx. 0.03 oz. (approx. 36 per ounce)	3	0.8	109.8	27.46	1757	439.4
1 striped mint, approx. 0.05 oz. (approx. 19½ per ounce)	6	1.4	109.5	27.37	1752	437.9
White mint, Planet Cut, approx. 0.07 oz. (approx. 13½ per ounce)	8	2.1	109.8	27.46	1757	439.4
For more information on after-dinner mints, see the listings under individual flavors, such as Anise.						
Alligator Eggs, **Clark,** 0.7-oz. box	80	17.7	114.1	25.25	1825	404.0
0.75-oz. box	86	18.9	114.1	25.25	1825	404.0
1.25-oz. box	143	31.6	114.1	25.25	1825	404.0
Almond Bar, **Nestlé:**						
Candy counter size, 1.06-oz. bar	159	18.1	150.0	17.00	2400	272.0
Supermarket and vending machine size, 5-oz. bar	750	85.0	150.0	17.00	2400	272.0
Almond Caramel Cluster, **Spangler,** 1 cluster, ½ oz. (approx. 2 per ounce)	68	8.9	133.3	17.39	2133	278.2
Almond Chocolate Fudge, **Spangler,** 4.1-oz. box	528	76.7	128.8	18.71	2061	299.4
Almond Cluster, **Schrafft's,** 5.5-oz. box	902	61.6	164.0	11.20	2624	179.2
Almond Joy, **Peter Paul:**						
Vending machine size, 1.1-oz. bar	166	20.4	151.0	18.50	2416	296.0
Candy counter and movie concession size, 1.5-oz. bar	227	17.8	151.0	18.50	2416	296.0
Miniatures, 7-oz. bag (approx. 15 miniatures)	1057	129.5	151.0	18.50	2416	296.0
12-oz. bag (approx. 26 miniatures)	1812	222.0	151.0	18.50	2416	296.0
1 miniature, 0.46 oz. (approx. 2 per ounce)	70	8.6	151.0	18.50	2416	296.0
Almonds, Rainbow Jordan, **Schrafft's,** 4½-oz. box	683	61.4	151.9	13.64	2430	218.2
1 Jordan Almond, approx. 0.06 oz. (17 per ounce)	9	0.8	151.9	13.64	2430	218.2
Anise After Dinner Mints, **Richardson:**						
Midget cut, 5-oz. bag (approx. 180 mints)	549	137.3	109.8	27.46	1757	439.4
8-oz. bag (approx. 295 mints)	878	219.7	109.8	27.46	1757	439.4
4-lb. carton (approx. 2130 mints)	7027	1757.4	109.8	27.46	1757	439.4
Restaurant size carton, 25 lb. (approx. 14,400 mints)	43920	10984.0	109.8	27.46	1757	439.4
1 mint, approx. 0.03 oz. (approx. 33½ per ounce)	3	0.1	109.8	27.46	1757	439.4
Planet cut, 8-oz. bag (approx. 108 mints)	878	219.7	109.8	27.46	1757	439.4
Restaurant size carton, 25 lb. (approx. 5,400 mints)	43920	10984.0	109.8	27.46	1757	439.4
1 mint, approx. 0.07 oz. (approx. 13½ per ounce)	8	2.1	109.8	27.46	1757	439.4
Apple Caramels, **Clark,** 0.7-oz. box	81	17.4	116.3	24.88	1862	398.1

	UNIT		1 OZ., BY WT.		1 POUND	
	Cal.	Carb.	Cal.	Carb.	Cal.	Carb.
Apple Kisses, **Jolly Rancher,** 7-oz. bag (approx. 33 or 34 kisses)	827		118.1		1890	
9-oz. bag (approx. 42 or 43 kisses)	1063		118.1		1890	
1 kiss, approx. 0.2 oz. (approx. 5 per ounce)	25		118.1		1890	
Apple Stix, **Jolly Rancher,** 1 stix, 1 oz.	148		148.0		2368	
For comparison: Apple Snack (Dehydrated Apples), **Weight Watchers,** ½-oz. package	50	13.0	100.0	26.00	1600	416.0
For comparison: Dried Apples, Honey Dipped, **Fruit Pac,** 4-oz. package	342	89.5	85.4	22.37	1366	357.9
Baby Ruth Bar, **Standard Brands:**						
Candy counter size, 1.8-oz. bar	260	31.0	144.4	17.22	2310	275.5
Vending machine size, 2-oz. bar	289	34.4	144.4	17.22	2310	275.5
Movie concession size, 3.2-oz. bar	462	55.1	144.4	17.22	2310	275.5
Barley Sugar, **Callard & Bowser,** 1.76-oz. package (8 pieces)	185	48.1	105.0	27.30	1680	436.8
1 piece, approx. 0.2 oz. (approx. 4½ per ounce)	23	6.0	105.0	27.30	1680	436.8
Bit-O-Honey, **Ward:**						
Vending machine size, small, 1.5-oz. bar (6 pieces)	176	39.0	117.0	26.00	1872	416.0
1 piece, approx. ¼ oz.	29	6.5	117.0	26.00	1872	416.0
Candy counter size, 1.7-oz. bar (6 pieces)	199	44.2	117.0	26.00	1872	416.0
1 piece, approx. 0.3 oz.	33	7.4	117.0	26.00	1872	416.0
Vending machine size, large, 2.1-oz. bar (6 pieces)	246	54.6	117.0	26.00	1872	416.0
1 piece, approx. 0.35 oz.	41	9.1	117.0	26.00	1872	416.0
Miniatures, 7-oz. bag (70 to 76 miniatures)	819	182.0	117.0	26.00	1872	416.0
1 miniature, approx. 0.11 oz. (approx. 9 per ounce)	13	2.9	117.0	26.00	1872	416.0
Institutional shipping size, 30-pound bag, 2,400 pieces	56160	12480.0	117.0	26.00	1872	416.0
1 piece, approx. 0.2 oz. (approx. 5 per ounce)	23	5.2	117.0	26.00	1872	416.0
"Penny candy" size, approx. 0.11 oz.	13	2.9	117.0	26.00	1872	416.0
Bits O' Peppermint, **Heath,** 7.8-oz. bag	970	175.0	124.8	22.40	1996	358.4
Black Cow Sucker, **Clark,** 0.25-oz. size	32	6.0	127.4	23.81	2039	381.0
0.7-oz. size	89	16.7	127.4	23.81	2039	381.0
0.75-oz. size	98	17.9	127.4	23.81	2039	381.0
1.25-oz. size	159	29.8	127.4	23.81	2039	381.0
Black Jack Kiss, **Clark,** 12-oz. bag	1394	306.7	116.2	25.56	1860	409.0
Blow Pops, see the LOLLIPOPS section, which follows the main Candy listings.						
Bonomo, assorted plain hard candy (cherry, lemon, and root beer):						
Movie concession and vending machine size, 1.5-oz. box (approx. 8 or 9 candies)	165	41.3	110.0	27.50	1760	440.0
1 candy, approx. 0.17 oz. (approx. 6 per ounce)	18	4.6	110.0	27.50	1760	440.0
Brazil, see Milk Brazil Bar						
Breath Savers, Peppermint, Sugar Free (12 tablets to the roll)	84	21.6				
1 Peppermint tablet	7	1.8				
Spearmint, Sugar Free (12 tablets to the roll)	84	21.6				
1 Spearmint tablet	7	1.8				
Wintergreen, Sugar Free (12 tablets to the roll)	84	21.6				
1 Wintergreen tablet	7	1.8				
Bryan Drops, Dark, **Spangler,** 1 drop, approx. 0.42 oz. (approx. 2½ per ounce)	45	9.8	107.1	23.24	1714	371.8
Bryan Drops, Milk, **Spangler,** 1 drop, approx. 0.42 oz. (approx. 2½ per ounce)	46	10.0	109.5	23.69	1752	379.0
Butter Almond Brickle, **Heath,** 8-oz. carton (approx. 26 pieces)	1202	129.3	150.3	16.16	2404	258.6
1 piece, approx. 0.31 oz. (approx. 3 per ounce)	46	5.0	150.3	16.16	2404	258.6
Butter Mints, **Kraft,** 8-oz. box (approx. 108 mints)	864	216.0	108.0	27.00	1728	432.0
1 mint, approx. 0.07 oz. (approx. 14 per ounce)	8	2.0	108.0	27.00	1728	432.0
Butter Mints, **Richardson,** 5-oz. package (approx. 68 pieces)	556	135.8	111.2	27.15	1779	434.4
8-oz. box (approx. 103 mints)	890	217.2	111.2	27.15	1779	434.4
Restaurant size, 25-lb. carton (approx. 5300 pieces)	44480	10860.0	111.2	27.15	1779	434.4
1 mint, approx. 0.08 oz. (approx. 12½ per ounce)	9	2.2	111.2	27.15	1779	434.4
Butterfinger Bar, **Standard Brands:**						
Candy counter size, 1.6-oz. bar	220	28.0	137.5	17.50	2200	280.0
Vending machine size, 1.8-oz. bar	248	31.5	137.5	17.50	2200	280.0
Butterscotch, **Callard & Bowser,** 3.52-oz. package (16 candies)	406	87.5	115.3	24.86	1845	397.7
1 candy, approx. 0.22 oz. (approx. 4½ per ounce)	25	5.5	115.3	24.86	1845	397.7
Butterscotch Candy, **Rothchild's,** approx. 1½-oz. roll (9 candies)	171	36.0	114.0	24.00	1824	384.0

	UNIT		1 OZ., BY WT.		1 POUND	
	Cal.	Carb.	Cal.	Carb.	Cal.	Carb.
1 candy, approx. 0.17 oz. (approx. 6 per ounce)	19	4.0	114.0	24.00	1824	384.0
Butterscotch Kisses, **Jolly Rancher,** 7-oz. bag (approx. 33 or 34 kisses)	827		118.1		1890	
9-oz. bag (approx. 42 or 43 kisses)	1063		118.1		1890	
1 kiss, approx. 0.21 oz. (approx. 5 per ounce)	25		118.1		1890	
Butterscotch Stix, **Jolly Rancher,** 1 Stix, approx. 1 oz.	148		148.0		2368	
Candy Corn, see the generic data at the beginning of this chapter.						
CaraCoa 'n Rice Snack, **CaraCoa (El Molino),** 1-oz. package	150	16.0	150.0	16.00		
Caramel Bar, **Cadbury Schweppes,** 1.76-oz. bar	244	31.9	138.4	18.06	2214	289.0
Caramel Creams, **Goetze's,** 8-oz. bag (approx. 21 or 22 creams)	861	180.0	107.7	22.55	1723	360.8
1 cream, approx. 0.38 oz. (approx. 2½ per ounce)	41	8.5	107.7	22.55	1723	360.8
Caramel, Diamond Back, **Spangler;** 1 caramel, approx. 0.51 oz. (approx. 2 per ounce)	68	8.9	133.3	17.35	2133	277.6
Caramel Kisses, **Yinnies,** 3.5-oz. bag (12 kisses)	360	72.0	102.9	20.57	1646	329.1
1 kiss, approx. 0.29 oz. (approx. 3½ per ounce)	30	6.0	102.9	20.57	1646	329.1
Caramel Nut Clusters, **Delson's,** 6-oz. box (20 clusters)	746	48.7	124.2	8.12	1989	129.8
1 cluster, approx. 0.3 oz. (approx. 3½ per ounce)	37	2.4	124.2	8.12	1989	129.8
Caramels, **Kraft,** 14-oz. bag	1715	294.0	122.5	21.00	1960	336.0
28-oz. bag	3430	588.0	122.5	21.00	1960	336.0
1 caramel, approx. 0.3 oz. (approx. 3½ per ounce)	35	6.0	122.5	21.00	1960	336.0
Caramels, Wildfire, **Clark,** 0.7-oz. box	80	17.6	114.6	25.18	1834	402.9
¾-oz. box	86	18.9	114.6	25.18	1834	402.9
1¼-oz. box	143	31.5	114.6	25.18	1834	402.9
Caravel Bar, **Peter Paul**:						
Vending machine size, 1.15-oz. bar	156	21.0	136.0	18.30	2176	292.8
Candy store and movie concession size, 1.25-oz. bar	170	22.9	136.0	18.30	2176	292.8
Miniatures, 7-oz. bag (approx. 13 bars)	952	128.1	136.0	18.30	2176	292.8
12-oz. bag (approx. 23 bars)	1632	219.6	136.0	18.30	2176	292.8
1 miniature, approx. 0.54 oz. (approx. 2 per ounce)	73	9.9	136.0	18.30	2176	292.8
Carob Cluster Bar, **Hoffman's,** 1-oz. bar	160	10.0	160.0	10.00	2560	160.0
Carob Coated Caramels, **CaraCoa (El Molino),** vending machine size, 1-oz. package	110	21.0	110.0	21.00	1760	336.0
1 caramel, approx. 0.22 oz. (approx. 4½ per ounce)	24	4.6	110.0	21.00	1760	336.0
Carob Coated Dates, **CaraCoa (El Molino),** 1-oz. package	125	18.0	125.0	18.00	2000	288.0
4-oz. box	500	72.0	125.0	18.00	2000	288.0
Carob Coated Fruit Nut Bar, **Frank Milina,** 1.25-oz. bar	140	19.5	112.0	15.61	1792	249.7
Carob Coated Nuggets, **CaraCoa (El Molino),** 6-oz. package	840	120.0	140.0	20.00	2240	320.0
1 nugget, approx. 0.01 oz. (approx. 100 per ounce)	1	0.2	140.0	20.00	2240	320.0
Carob Coated Peanuts, **CaraCoa (El Molino),** 1-oz. package	160	12.0	160.0	12.00	2560	192.0
4-oz. box	640	48.0	160.0	12.00	2560	192.0
For comparison: Chocolate-covered peanuts, Goobers, **Ward,** 1-oz. box	153	12.0	153.0	12.00	2448	192.0
Carob Coated Peppermint Bar, **Frank Milina,** 1.25-oz. bar	151	28.6	120.8	22.88	1933	366.1
Carob Coated Raisins, **CaraCoa (El Molino),** 1-oz. package	130	18.0	130.0	18.00	2080	288.0
4-oz. box	520	72.0	130.0	18.00	2080	288.0
For comparison: Raisinets, **Ward,** 1-oz. box	90	14.0	90.0	14.00	1440	224.0
Carob Coated Soybeans, **CaraCoa (El Molino),** 1-oz. package	145	12.0	145.0	12.00	2320	192.0
4½-oz. box	653	54.0	145.0	12.00	2320	192.0
Certs (Clear), Crystal, approx. 0.7-oz. package (10 mints)	82	20.5	117.1	29.29	1874	468.6
Fruit, approx. 0.7-oz. package (10 mints)	82	20.5	117.1	29.29	1874	468.6
Spice, approx. 0.7-oz. package (10 mints)	82	20.5	117.1	29.29	1874	468.6
Spring, approx. 0.7-oz. package (10 mints)	82	20.5	117.1	29.29	1874	468.6
1 mint, approx. 0.07 oz. (approx. 14 per ounce)	8	2.1	117.1	29.29	1874	468.6
Certs (Pressed), Fruit, approx. 0.63-oz. package (11 mints)	67	16.5	106.5	26.19	1704	419.0
Peppermint, approx. 0.63-oz. package (11 mints)	67	16.5	106.5	26.19	1704	419.0
Spearmint, approx. 0.63-oz. package (11 mints)	67	16.5	106.5	26.19	1704	419.0
Wintergreen, approx. 0.63-oz. package (11 mints)	67	16.5	106.5	26.19	1704	419.0

	UNIT		1 OZ., BY WT.		1 POUND	
	Cal.	Carb.	Cal.	Carb.	Cal.	Carb.
1 mint, approx. 0.06 oz. (approx. 17 per ounce)	6	1.5	106.5	26.19	1704	419.0
Charleston Chew, **Fox-Cross Candy Co.,** 2¹⁄₁₆-oz. bar	248	44.8	120.0	21.74	1920	347.8
Charms, Assorted, 8-piece package	107	24.9	109.1	25.45	1745	407.2
Cherry, 8-piece package	107	24.9	109.1	25.45	1745	407.2
1 Charm, approx. 0.12 oz.	13	3.03	109.1	25.45	1745	407.2
Cherry Bites, **Switzer,** 6-oz. package	576	136.0	96.0	22.68	1536	362.9
7-oz. package	672	158.8	96.0	22.68	1536	362.9
10-oz. package	960	226.8	96.0	22.68	1536	362.9
22-oz. package	2112	499.0	96.0	22.68	1536	362.9
33-oz. package	3168	748.4	96.0	22.68	1536	362.9
Cherry Kisses, **Jolly Rancher,** 7-oz. bag (approx. 33 or 34 kisses)	827		118.1		1890	
9-oz. bag (approx. 42 or 43 kisses)	1063		118.1		1890	
1 kiss, approx. 0.21 oz. (approx. 5 per ounce)	25		118.1		1890	
Cherry Stix, **Jolly Rancher,** 1 Stix, approx. 1 oz.	148		148.0		2368	
Cherry Stix, **Switzer,** 4-oz. package	384	90.7	96.0	22.68	1536	362.9
5-oz. package	480	113.4	96.0	22.68	1536	362.9
16-oz. (1-lb.) package	1536	362.9	96.0	22.68	1536	362.9
Cherry Twists, Chocolate Covered, **Joyva,** 1 twist, approx. ¾ oz.	85	15.8	113.4	21.08	1814	337.3
Cherry Whips, **Switzer,** 6-oz. package	576	136.1	96.0	22.68	1536	362.9
Chew-ets, **Goldenberg's,** see Goldenberg's						
Chocolate Babies, **Heide:**						
Candy counter and vending machine size, 1.8-oz. box (approx. 15 chocolate babies)	135		75.0		1200	
Supermarket size, 7-oz. box (approx. 58 chocolate babies)	525		75.0		1200	
1 chocolate baby, approx. 0.12 oz. (approx. 8⅓ per ounce)	9		75.0		1200	
Chocolate Bites, **Switzer,** 6-oz. package	630	137.3	105.0	22.89	1680	366.2
10-oz. package	1050	228.9	105.0	22.89	1680	366.2
Chocolate Drops, Dark, **Spangler,** 1 drop, approx. 0.64 oz.	73	13.8	114.1	21.50	1826	344.0
Chocolate Drops, Milk, **Spangler,** 1 drop, approx. 0.64 oz.	76	14.4	118.8	22.44	1901	359.0
Chocolate Fudgies, **Kraft,** 14-oz. bag (48 or 49 fudgies)	1715	294.0	122.5	21.00	1960	336.0
28-oz. bag (96 or 97 fudgies)	3430	588.0	122.5	21.00	1960	336.0
1 fudgie, approx. 0.29 oz. (approx. 3½ per ounce)	35	6.0	122.5	21.00	1960	336.0
Chocolate Stix, **Switzer,** 5-oz. package	525	114.5	105.0	22.89	1680	366.2
16-oz. (1-lb.) package	1680	366.2	105.0	22.89	1680	366.2
Chocolate Twists, **Y&S,** 4½-oz. package (approx. 15 twists)	650	110.0	144.4	24.40	2310	390.4
1 twist, approx. 0.3 oz. (approx. 3½ per ounce)	43	7.3	144.4	24.40	2310	390.4
Chocolate Winter Greens, **Delson,** 6-oz. box (20 candies)	659	138.1	109.8	23.01	1757	368.2
1 winter green, approx. 0.3 oz. (approx. 3½ per ounce)	33	6.6	109.8	23.01	1757	368.2
Choco' Lite Bar, **Nestlé,** candy counter size, 1-oz. bar	150	18.0	150.0	18.00	2400	288.0
Supermarket size, 5-oz. bar	750	90.0	150.0	18.00	2400	288.0
Miniatures, 10.15-oz. bag (29 miniatures)	1523	182.7	150.0	18.00	2400	288.0
1 miniature, approx. 0.35 oz.	53	6.3	150.0	18.00	2400	288.0
Chuckles, **Nabisco:**						
Vending machine size, 1¾-oz. package (5 Chuckles)	166		95.0		1520	
1 Chuckle, approx. 0.35 oz. (approx. 3 per ounce)	33		95.0		1520	
Candy counter and vending machine size, 2-oz. package (5 Chuckles)	190		95.0		1520	
1 Chuckle, approx. 0.4 oz. (approx. 2½ per ounce)	38		95.0		1520	
2¼-oz. package (5 Chuckles, each approx. 0.45 oz.)	214		95.0		1520	
1 Chuckle, approx. 0.45 oz. (approx. 2 per ounce)	43		95.0		1520	
Supermarket size, 8-oz. bag	760		95.0		1520	
9-oz. bag	855		95.0		1520	
Chunky Bar, Original, **Ward:**						
Candy counter and supermarket size, 1-oz. bar	145	15.7	145.0	15.70	2320	251.2
4-oz. bar	580	62.8	145.0	15.70	2320	251.2
6-oz. bar	870	94.2	145.0	15.70	2320	251.2
Vending machine size, Chunky "twin," 0.9-oz. bar	131	14.1	145.0	15.70	2320	251.2
Chunky "triple," 1.25-oz. bar	181	19.6	145.0	15.70	2320	251.2
Movie concession size, 2.5-oz. bar	363	39.3	145.0	15.70	2320	251.2
Miniatures, 8-oz. bag (18 pieces)	1160	125.6	145.0	15.70	2320	251.2
1 piece, approx. 0.45 oz. (approx. 2 per ounce)	65	7.1	145.0	15.70	2320	251.2

	UNIT		1 OZ., BY WT.		1 POUND	
	Cal.	Carb.	Cal.	Carb.	Cal.	Carb.
Clark Bar, **Clark:**						
0.7-oz. bar	94	14.2	134.0	20.23	2145	323.7
1.4-oz. bar	188	28.3	134.0	20.23	2145	323.7
1.65-oz. bar	221	33.4	134.0	20.23	2145	323.7
Vending machine size, 1.3-oz. bar	177	25.7	134.0	20.23	2145	323.7
1.6-oz. bar	217	31.7	134.0	20.23	2145	323.7
Candy counter size, 1¾-oz. bar	238	34.6	134.0	20.23	2145	323.7
Movie concession size, 2¼-oz. bar	306	44.5	134.0	20.23	2145	323.7
"Tiny Treats," 2¾-oz. bag (approx. 16 or 17 treats)	374	54.4	134.0	20.23	2145	323.7
1 treat, approx. 0.17 oz. (approx. 6 per ounce)	23	3.4	134.0	20.23	2145	323.7
Miniatures, "Juniors," 8-oz. bag (approx. 15 to 19 Juniors)	1086	158.3	134.0	20.23	2145	323.7
12-oz. bag (approx. 17 to 20 Juniors)	1630	237.5	134.0	20.23	2145	323.7
1 Junior, approx. 0.46 oz.	63	9.1	134.0	20.23	2145	323.7
Clorets, Mints, approx. 0.7-oz. package (10 mints)	60	1.6	85.7	2.29	1371	36.6
1 mint, approx. 0.07 oz. (approx. 14½ per ounce)	6	1.6	85.7	2.29	1371	36.6
Club Mints, Planet Cut, **Richardson,** 8-oz. bag (approx. 108 mints)	878	219.7	109.8	27.46	1757	439.4
1 mint, approx. 0.07 oz. (approx. 13½ per ounce)	8	2.1	109.8	27.46	1757	439.4
Coffee Chocs, **Callard & Bowser,** 7-oz. box (29 or 30 Chocs)	840	158.6	119.2	22.50	1907	360.0
1 Choc, approx. ¼ oz.	29	5.4	119.2	22.50	1907	360.0
Cough Drops are in their own section, following the main Candy listings.						
Cracker Jack candied popcorn and peanuts, ¾-oz. box	90	16.5	120.0	22.00	1920	352.0
1-oz. box	120	22.0	120.0	22.00	1920	352.0
2-oz. box	240	44.0	120.0	22.00	1920	352.0
4½-oz. box	540	99.0	120.0	22.00	1920	352.0
5⅝-oz. box	675	123.8	120.0	22.00	1920	352.0
6-oz. box	720	132.0	120.0	22.00	1920	352.0
1 piece, approx. 0.01 oz. (approx. 71 per ounce)	(2)	(0.3)	120.0	22.00	1920	352.0
Creme de Menthe, **Andes,** 1.1-oz. bar	167	17.1	151.7	15.57	2427	249.1
1 miniature, approx. 0.16 oz. (6½ per ounce)	25	2.6	151.7	15.57	2427	249.1
Crispy Bar, **Clark:**						
1.06-oz. bar	159	20.6	149.2	19.34	2388	309.4
1.3-oz. bar	194	25.1	149.2	19.34	2388	309.4
3.25-oz. bar	485	62.9	149.2	19.34	2388	309.4
Vending machine size, 1¼-oz. bar	186	23.0	149.2	19.34	2388	294.4
Candy counter size, 1.4-oz. bar	208	25.8	149.2	19.34	2388	294.4
Movie concession size, 2-oz. bar	298	36.8	149.2	19.34	2388	294.4
Supermarket size, 6¼-oz. 5-pack (each bar approx. 1¼ oz.)	931	115.0	149.2	19.34	2388	294.4
1 bar, approx. 1¼ oz.	186	23.0	149.2	19.34	2388	294.4
Crows, **Mason:**						
Movie concession and vending size, 1⅞-oz. box (approx. 16 or 17 Crows)	178	44.3	94.7	23.64	1515	378.2
Supermarket size, 8-oz. box (approx. 70 or 71 Crows)	758	189.1	94.7	23.64	1515	378.2
1 Crow, approx. 0.11 oz. (approx. 9 per ounce)	11	2.7	94.7	23.64	1515	378.2
Crunch Bar, **Nestlé:**						
Candy store size, 1¹⁄₁₆-oz. bar	159	19.1	150.0	18.00	2400	288.0
Vending machine size, 1.16-oz. bar	174	20.9	150.0	18.00	2400	288.0
Movie concession size, 2.5-oz. bar	375	45.0	150.0	18.00	2400	288.0
Supermarket size, 5-oz. bar	750	90.0	150.0	18.00	2400	288.0
Miniatures, approx. 16-oz. (1-lb.) bag	2400	288.0	150.0	18.00	2400	288.0
1 miniature, approx. 0.35 oz. (approx. 3 per ounce)	53	6.3	150.0	18.00	2400	288.0
Crunchy Candy Bar, **CaraCoa (El Molino),** vending machine size, ⅞-oz. bar	140	14.0	160.0	16.00	2560	256.0
3½-oz. bar	560	56.0	160.0	16.00	2560	256.0
Crystal Blue Mints, **Richardson,** 5-oz. bag (approx. 20 mints)	561	140.3	112.2	28.06	1795	449.0
7-oz. bag (approx. 28 mints)	785	196.4	112.2	28.06	1795	449.0
3.5-lb. container (approx. 233 mints)	6283	1571.4	112.2	28.06	1795	449.0
Restaurant size carton, 25 lb. (approx. 1664 mints)	44880	11224	112.2	28.06	1795	449.0
1 Mint, approx. 0.25 oz. (approx. 4 per ounce)	27	6.8	112.2	28.06	1795	449.0
Date-Bar, **Frank Milina,** 1¼-oz. bar	127	71.2	101.6	56.96	1626	911.4
Dates, Carob Coated, **CaraCoa (El Molino),** 1-oz. package	125	18.0	125.0	18.00	2000	288.0
4-oz. box	500	72.0	125.0	18.00	2000	288.0
For Comparison: Dried Dates, Honey Dipped, **Fruit Pac,** 16-oz. (1-lb.) package	1344	357.9	84.0	22.37	1344	357.9
Delite, Swiss Bittersweet Chocolate Flavored Bar, **Bartons,** ¾-oz. bar	120	10.0	160.0	13.33	2560	213.3

	UNIT		1 OZ., BY WT.		1 POUND	
	Cal.	Carb.	Cal.	Carb.	Cal.	Carb.
Swiss Milk Chocolate Flavored Bar, ¾-oz. bar	140	10.0	(197.1)	(12.40)	3154	198.4
1¾-oz. bar	360	21.0	(197.1)	(12.40)	3154	198.4
Vanilla Coconut Bar, 2-oz. bar	388	34.0	(194.0)	17.00	3104	272.0
Dots, Assorted (cherry, orange, lemon, and lime), **Mason:**						
Movie concession and vending machine size, 1⅞-oz. box (approx. 16 or 17 Dots)	178	44.0	95.0	23.50	1520	376.0
Supermarket size, 8-oz. box (approx. 70 or 71 Dots)	760	188.0	95.0	23.50	1520	376.0
8¾-oz. bag, 18 mini boxes each approx. ½ oz., containing 4 Dots	831	205.6	95.0	23.50	1520	376.0
1 Dot, approx. 0.113 oz. (approx. 9 per ounce)	11	2.7	95.0	23.50	1520	376.0
Dots, Cherry, **Mason,** movie concession size, 4-oz. box (approx. 35 or 36 Dots)	380	94.0	95.0	23.50	1520	376.0
1 Dot, approx. 0.113 oz. (approx. 9 per ounce)	11	2.7	95.0	23.50	1520	376.0
Dum Dum Fruit Rolls, **Spangler,** 0.2-oz. roll (5 per ounce)	21	5.5	105.0	27.58	1680	441.3
0.48-oz. roll (2 per ounce)	51	13.2	105.0	27.58	1680	441.3
Dynamints, **Dentyne,** Cinnamon flavor, approx. 0.55-oz. box	60	14.0	109.1	25.45	1745	407.2
Fruit flavor, approx. 0.55-oz. box	60	14.0	109.1	25.45	1745	407.2
Lemon/Lime flavor, approx. 0.55-oz. box	60	14.0	109.1	25.45	1745	407.2
Peppermint flavor, approx. 0.55-oz. box	60	14.0	109.1	25.45	1745	407.2
Spearmint Flavor, approx. 0.55-oz. box	60	14.0	109.1	25.45	1745	407.2
1 mint, approx. 0.01 oz. (approx. 100 per ounce)	1	0.4	109.1	25.45	1745	407.2
E Power, **Frank Milina,** 1½-oz. bar	184	59.6	122.7	39.73	1963	635.7
Estee-Ets Peanut Candy, Dietetic, **Estee,** 1.75-oz. box	259	223.8	148.0	13.60	2368	217.6
Fig Bar, **Toms,** 1.8-oz. package	180	39.0	100.0	21.67		
For comparison: Figs, Calimyrna, Honey Dipped, **Fruit Pac,** 12-oz. package	(1013)	(256.4)	(84.4)	(21.37)	(1350)	(341.9)
Fire Kisses, **Jolly Rancher,** 7-oz. bag (approx. 33 or 34 Kisses)	827		118.1		1890	
9-oz. bag (approx. 42 or 43 kisses)	1063		118.1		1890	
1 kiss, approx. 0.21 oz. (approx. 5 per ounce)	25		118.1		1890	
Fire Stix, **Jolly Rancher,** 1 Stix, approx. 1 oz.	148		148.0		2368	
Flat Pops see the LOLLIPOPS section, which follows the main Candy listings.						
Fruit Fondants, **Callard & Bowser,** 6½-oz. box (14 or 15 Fondants)	644	168.0	99.3	26.91	1589	414.5
1 Fondant, 0.42 oz. (2½ per ounce)	43	11.3	99.3	26.91	1589	414.5
Fruit and Nut Bar, Bournville, **Cadbury,** 3.52-oz. bar	513	61.7	145.4	17.49	2326	278.8
Fruit & Nut Bar, Milk, **Cadbury,** 1¾-oz. bar	234	28.7	132.4	16.27	2118	260.3
3½-oz. bar	467	56.9	132.4	16.27	2118	260.3
7-oz. bar	934	113.9	132.4	16.27	2118	260.3
Fruit 'n Nut Candy Bar, **CaraCoa (El Molino),** vending machine size, 1-oz. bar	160	16.0	160.0	16.00	2560	256.0
4-oz. bar	640	64.0	160.0	16.00	2560	256.0
Fruit Nut Bar, Uncoated, **Frank Milina,** 1¼-oz. bar	140	21.0	112.0	16.80	1792	268.8
Fruit Roll, Apple, **Grocer's Choice,** 1-oz. package	90	20.0	90.0	20.00	1440	320.0
Apricot, 1-oz. package	90	21.0	90.0	21.00	1440	336.0
Cherry, 1-oz. package	90	20.0	90.0	20.00	1440	320.0
Grape, 1-oz. package	90	21.0	90.0	21.00	1440	336.0
Plum, 1-oz. package	90	20.0	90.0	20.00	1440	320.0
Raspberry, 1-oz. package	90	21.0	90.0	21.00	1440	336.0
Strawberry, 1-oz. package	100	22.0	100.0	22.00	1600	352.0
For comparison: Fruit Snack, Artificially Cinnamon flavored (Dehydrated Apples), **Weight Watchers,** ½-oz. package	50	13.0	100.0	26.00	1600	416.0
Artificially Peach Flavored (Dehydrated Apples), ½-oz. package	50	13.0	100.0	26.00	1600	416.0
Artificially Strawberry Flavored, (Dehydrated Apples), ½-oz. package	50	13.0	100.0	26.00	1600	416.0
Fudge, Creamy, **Callard & Bowser,** 2.29-oz. package	273	48.4	119.2	21.11	1907	337.8
Fudge Bar, Milk Chocolate Covered, **Nabisco,** 1⅜-oz. package (2 pieces)	186	26.4	135.2	19.19	2163	307.0
1 piece, approx. 0.7 oz. (approx. 1½ per ounce)	93	13.2	135.2	19.19	2163	307.0
Golden Almond, **Hershey's,** 3.2-oz. bar	512	38.4	160.0	12.00	2560	192.0
1-lb. box	2560	192.0	160.0	12.00	2560	192.0
2-lb. box	5120	384.0	160.0	12.00	2560	192.0
Goldenberg's Chew-ets, **Goldenberg's,** 1.5-oz. bar	206	28.0	137.3	18.67	2197	298.7
1.6-oz. bar	218	30.0	137.3	18.67	2197	298.7
1.75-oz. bar	240	33.0	137.3	18.67	2197	298.7
2.0-oz. bar	270	37.0	137.3	18.67	2197	298.7
3.0-oz. bar	410	56.0	137.3	18.67	2197	298.7

	UNIT Cal.	UNIT Carb.	1 OZ., BY WT. Cal.	1 OZ., BY WT. Carb.	1 POUND Cal.	1 POUND Carb.
Goldenberg's Peanut Chews, **Goldenberg's:**	222	28.3	138.7	17.69	2219	283.0
Vending machine size, 1½-oz. bar (5 pieces)	208	27.0	138.7	17.69	2219	283.0
1 piece, approx. 0.32 oz. (approx. 3 per ounce)	42	5.4	138.7	17.69	2219	283.0
Candy counter and vending machine size, 1¾-oz. bar (5 pieces)	243	31.0	138.7	17.69	2219	283.0
1 piece, approx. 0.37 oz. (approx. 2½ per ounce)	49	6.2	138.7	17.69	2219	283.0
Candy counter size, 2-oz. bar (6 pieces)	278	35.0	138.7	17.69	2219	283.0
1 piece, approx. 0.36 oz. (approx. 3 per ounce)	46	5.8	138.7	17.69	2219	283.0
Movie concession and vending machine size, 3-oz. bar or box (8 pieces)	417	53.0	138.7	17.69	2219	283.0
1 piece, approx. 0.39 oz. (approx. 2½ per ounce)	52	6.6	138.7	17.69	2219	283.0
Supermarket size, 9.6-oz. 6-pack, 6 bars, each with 5 pieces	1332	168.0	138.7	17.69	2219	283.0
1 bar, approx. 1.6 oz.	222	28.0	138.7	17.69	2219	283.0
Goobers, **Ward:**						
Candy store and vending machine size, 1-oz. box	153	12.0	153.0	12.00	2448	192.0
Movie concession size, 2.3-oz. box	352	27.6	153.0	12.00	2448	192.0
Supermarket size, 8-oz. box	1224	96.0	153.0	12.00	2448	192.0
Miniatures, 7½-oz. bag (contains 12 Miniature boxes)	1148	90.0	153.0	12.00	2448	192.0
1 miniature, approx. 0.63 oz.	96	7.5	153.0	12.00	2448	192.0
Good 'N Fruity, **American Chicle,** 1.8-oz. box	163	40.8	90.7	22.67	1451	362.7
3.5-oz. box	317	79.3	90.7	22.67	1451	362.7
Good & Plenty, **American Chicle,** 1.8-oz. box (approx. 48 pieces)	163	41.9	90.7	23.27	1451	362.7
3.5-oz. box	318	31.4	90.7	23.27	1451	362.7
1 piece, approx. 0.04 oz. (approx. 27 per ounce)	3	0.9	90.7	23.27	1451	362.7
Granola Bars and Granola Snacks have their own section, which follows Cough Drops after the main Candy listings.						
Grape Kisses, **Jolly Rancher,** 7-oz. bag (approx. 33 or 34 kisses)	827		118.1		1890	
9-oz. bag (approx. 42 or 43 kisses)	1063		118.1		1890	
1 kiss, approx. 0.21 oz. (approx. 5 per ounce)	25		118.1		1890	
Grape Stix, **Jolly Rancher,** 1 Stix, approx. 1 oz.	148		148.0		2368	
Gum has its own section at the end of this chapter.						
Halvah, Chocolate, **Joyva,** 0.8-oz. bar	128	9.6	160.0	12.00	2560	192.0
1¼-oz. bar	200	15.0	160.0	12.00	2560	192.0
19-oz. can	3040	228.0	160.0	12.00	2560	192.0
Halvah, Chocolate, with Assorted Nuts, **Joyva,** 12½-lb. bulk "bucket"	32000	2400.0	160.0	12.00	2560	192.0
1-lb. block	2560	192.0	160.0	12.00	2560	192.0
Halvah, Marble, **Joyva,** 0.8-oz. bar	128	9.6	160.0	12.00	2560	192.0
1¼-oz. bar	200	15.0	160.0	12.00	2560	192.0
3½-oz. bar	560	42.0	160.0	12.00	2560	192.0
19-oz. can	3040	228.0	160.0	12.00	2560	192.0
Halvah, Marble, with Assorted Nuts, **Joyva,** 12½-lb. bulk "bucket"	32000	2400.0	160.0	12.00	2560	192.0
1-lb. block	2560	192.0	160.0	12.00	2560	192.0
Halvah, Vanilla, **Joyva,** 0.8-oz. bar	128	9.6	160.0	12.00	2560	192.0
1¼-oz. bar	200	15.0	160.0	12.00	2560	192.0
19-oz. can	3040	228.0	160.0	12.00	2560	192.0
Halvah, Vanilla, with Assorted Nuts, **Joyva,** 12½-lb. bulk "bucket"	32000	2400.0	160.0	12.00	2560	192.0
1-lb. block	2560	192.0	160.0	12.00	2560	192.0
Hard Candies, see individual brands, such as Charms and Life Savers, and individual flavors, such as Grape Kisses.						
Heath Bar, **Heath,** 1⅛-oz. bar	170	11.0	151.1	9.78	2418	156.4
"Little" Heath Bars, 10.1-oz. bag (28 miniature bars)	1604	169.0	158.8	16.73	2541	267.7
1 "Little" Heath, approx. 0.36 oz. (approx. 3 per ounce)	57	6.0	158.8	16.73	2541	267.7
Hershey's Milk Chocolate Bar:						
Vending machine size, 1.05-oz. bar	160	17.0	152.4	16.19	2438	259.0
Candy counter size, 1.2-oz. bar	183	19.4	152.4	16.19	2438	259.0
2-oz. bar	305	32.4	152.4	16.19	2438	259.0
Movie concession size, 4-oz. bar	610	64.8	152.4	16.19	2438	259.0
Supermarket size, 8-oz. bar	1219	129.5	152.4	16.19	2438	259.0
Miniatures, 10.5-oz. bag (30 in bag)	1523	162.4	152.4	16.19	2438	259.0
1 miniature, approx. 0.34 oz. (3 per ounce)	52	5.5	152.4	16.19	2438	259.0
Hershey's Milk Chocolate with Almonds Bar:						
Vending machine size, 1.05-oz. bar	160	17.0	152.4	16.19	2438	259.0
Candy counter size, 1.5-oz. bar	229	24.3	152.4	16.19	2438	259.0
2-oz. bar	309	32.4	152.4	16.19	2438	259.0
Movie concession size, 4-oz. bar	610	64.8	152.4	16.19	2438	259.0
Supermarket size, 8-oz. bar	1219	129.5	152.4	16.19	2438	259.0
Hi Proteen Energy Bar, Vanilla, **Hoffman's,** 1¾-oz. bar	210	24.0	120.0	13.71	1920	219.3
Hi Protein Bar, **Jack La Lanne,** 1.7-oz. bar	200	25.0	117.6	14.71	1882	235.3
Hi Protein Peanut Butter Confection Bar, Carob Coated, **Alfa,** 2-oz. bar	270	33.0	135.0	16.50	2160	264.0
Honey-Coconut Bar, **Jack La Lanne,** 1.7-oz. bar	210	31.0	123.5	18.24	1976	291.8
Honey-Peanut Butter Bar, **Jack La Lanne,** 1.7-oz. bar	200	26.0	117.6	15.29	1882	244.6
$100,000 Bar, **Nestlé,** 0.56-oz. bar	78	10.6	140.0	19.00		
1-oz. bar	140	19.0	140.0	19.00		
1⅛-oz. bar	158	21.4	140.0	19.00		
Ice Cream Pops, see the LOLLIPOPS section, which follows the main Candy listings.						
It's-A-Lift Fruit Protein Bar, **Frank Milina,** 1½-oz. bar	160	28.1	106.7	18.71	1707	299.4
Jell Bars, Candy Store Bulk, **Joyva,** 1 bar, approx. ½ oz.	55	11.8	110.6	23.57	1770	377.1
Jells, Mini, Candy Store Bulk, **Joyva,** 1 jell, approx. ½ oz.	55	11.8	110.6	23.57	1770	377.1
Jells, Orange, Candy Store Bulk, **Joyva,** 1 jell, approx. ½ oz.	55	11.8	110.6	23.57	1770	377.1
Jells, Raspberry, Candy Store Bulk, **Joyva,** 1 jell, approx. ½ oz.	55	11.8	110.6	23.57	1770	377.1
Jells, Ring, Candy Store Bulk, **Joyva,** 1 ring, approx. ½ oz.	55	11.8	110.6	23.57	1170	377.1
Jelly Egg, **Heide,** candy counter and supermarket size, 10-oz. bag (approx. 88 or 89 pieces)	799		79.9		1278	
12-oz. bag (approx. 106 or 107 pieces)	959		79.9		1278	
1 piece, approx. 0.11 oz. (approx. 9 per ounce)	9		79.9		1278	
Jordan Almonds, Rainbow, **Schrafft's,** 4½-oz. box	683	61.4	151.9	13.64	2430	218.2
1 Jordan Almond, approx. 0.06 oz. (17 per ounce)	9	0.8	151.9	13.64	2430	218.2
Juicy Jellies, **Callard & Bowser,** 14-oz. box (40 Jellies)	1240	322.4	88.0	22.87	1407	365.9
1 Jelly, approx. 0.35 oz. (approx. 3 per ounce)	31	8.1	88.0	22.87	1407	365.9
Ju Ju Bes, **Nabisco:**						
Candy counter and movie concession size, 1½-oz. box	(143)		(95.0)		(1520)	
Movie concession size, 3¾-oz. box	(356)		(95.0)		(1520)	
Supermarket size, 8-oz. bag	(760)		(95.0)		(1520)	
Jujyfruits, **Heide,** candy counter and vending machine size, 2.1-oz. box (approx. 23 or 24 Jujyfruits)	198		94.1		1505	
Movie concession size, 4-oz. box (approx. 44 or 45 Jujyfruits)	376		94.1		1505	
Supermarket size, 7-oz. box (approx. 77 or 78 Jujyfruits)	659		94.1		1505	
10-oz. box (approx. 111 or 112 Jujyfruits)	941		94.1		1505	
1 Jujyfruit, approx. 0.09 oz. (approx. 11 per ounce)	9		94.1		1505	
Junior Mints, **Nabisco:**						
Vending machine size, 1.43-oz. box	169	32.9	117.9	22.99	1886	367.8
Candy counter size, 1.52-oz. box	179	34.9	117.9	22.99	1886	367.8
Movie concession size, 3⅛-oz. box	368	71.8	117.9	22.99	1886	367.8
Supermarket size, 5½-oz. box	649	126.4	117.9	22.99	1886	367.8
9-oz. polybag, 16 boxes (each approx. 0.6 oz.)	1061	206.9	117.9	22.99	1886	367.8
Kisses, **Hershey's,** 6-oz. bag (36 kisses)	900	90.0	150.0	15.00	2400	240.0
9-oz. bag (54 kisses)	1350	135.0	150.0	15.00	2400	240.0
14-oz. bag (84 kisses)	2100	210.0	150.0	15.00	2400	240.0
1 Kiss, 0.17 oz. (approx. 6 per ounce)	25	2.5	150.0	15.00	2400	240.0
Kisses, **Jolly Rancher,** see individual flavors						
Kit Kat Candy Bar, **Hershey's,** 1.125-oz. bar	160	19.0	142.2	16.89	2275	270.2
Miniatures, 10.08-oz. bag (18 miniatures)	1440	162.0	142.9	16.07	2286	257.1
1 miniature, 0.56 oz. (approx. 2 per ounce)	80	9.0	142.9	16.07	2286	257.1
Krackel Candy Bar, **Hershey's,** 1.05-oz. box	160	18.0	152.4	17.14	2438	274.2
1.2-oz. bar	183	20.6	152.4	17.14	2438	274.2
1.8-oz. bar	274	30.9	152.4	17.14	2438	274.2
3⅜-oz. bar	513	57.8	152.4	17.14	2438	274.2
Lemon Kisses, **Jolly Rancher,** 7-oz. bag (approx. 33 or 34 kisses)	827		118.1		1890	
9-oz. bag (approx. 42 or 43 kisses)	1063		118.1		1890	
1 kiss, approx. 0.21 oz. (approx. 5 per ounce)	25		118.1		1890	
Lemon Stix, **Jolly Rancher,** 1 Stix, approx. 1 oz.	148		148.0		2368	

	UNIT		1 OZ., BY WT.		1 POUND	
	Cal.	Carb.	Cal.	Carb.	Cal.	Carb.
Licorice Bites, **Switzer:**						
6-oz. bag	564	131.0	94.0	21.83	1504	349.3
7-oz. bag	658	152.8	94.0	21.83	1504	349.3
10-oz. bag	940	218.3	94.0	21.83	1504	349.3
22-oz. bag	2068	480.3	94.0	21.83	1504	349.3
33-oz. bag	3102	720.4	94.0	21.83	1504	349.3
Licorice, Diamond, **Heide,** 5½-oz. box (approx. 44 pieces)	616		112.0		1792	
1 piece, approx. 0.13 oz. (approx. 8 per ounce)	14		112.0		1792	
Licorice Drops, Diamond, **Heide:**						
Supermarket size, 5½-oz. box (approx. 44 drops)	616		112.0		1792	
1 drop, approx. 0.13 oz. (approx. 8 per ounce)	14		112.0		1792	
Licorice Stix, **Switzer:**						
4-oz. bag	376	87.3	94.0	21.83	1504	349.3
5-oz. bag	470	109.2	94.0	21.83	1504	349.3
16-oz. (1-lb.) bag	1504	349.3	94.0	21.83	1504	349.3
Licorice Twists, **Y&S,** 5-oz. bag (approx. 15 twists)	500	110.0	100.0	22.00	1600	352.0
1 twist, approx. ⅓ oz. (approx. 3 per ounce)	33	7.3	100.0	22.00	1600	352.0
Licorice Whips, **Switzer,** 6-oz. bag	564	131.0	94.0	21.83	1504	349.3
Life Savers, Drops, Butterrum, 0.9-oz. roll (11 Life Savers)	99	24.2	110.0	26.89	1760	430.2
1 Life Saver	9	2.2	110.0	26.89	1760	430.2
Butterscotch, 0.9-oz. roll (11 Life Savers)	99	24.2	110.0	26.89	1760	430.2
1 Life Saver	9	2.2	110.0	26.89	1760	430.2
Cin-O-Mon, 0.7-oz. roll (12 Life Savers)	84	21.6	116.7	30.00	1856	480.0
1 Life Saver	7	1.8	116.7	30.00	1856	480.0
Cryst-O-Mint, 0.9-oz. roll (11 Life Savers)	99	24.2	110.0	26.89	1760	430.2
1 Life Saver	9	2.2	110.0	26.89	1760	430.2
Fancy Fruit, 0.9-oz. roll (11 Life Savers)	99	24.2	110.0	26.89	1760	430.2
1 Life Saver	9	2.2	110.0	26.89	1760	430.2
Five Flavor, 0.9-oz. roll (11 Life Savers)	99	24.2	110.0	26.89	1760	430.2
1 Life Saver	9	2.2	110.0	26.89	1760	430.2
Pep-O-Mint, 0.7-oz. roll (12 Life Savers)	84	21.6	116.7	30.00	1856	480.0
1 Life Saver	7	1.8	116.7	30.00	1856	480.0
Spear-O-Mint, 0.7-oz. roll (12 Life Savers)	84	21.6	116.7	30.00	1856	480.0
1 Life Saver	7	1.8	116.7	30.00	1856	480.0
Stik-O-Pep, 0.9-oz. roll (11 Life Savers)	99	24.2	110.0	26.89	1760	430.2
1 Life Saver	9	2.2	110.0	26.89	1760	430.2
Strawberry, 0.9 oz. roll (11 Life Savers)	99	24.2	110.0	26.89	1760	430.2
1 Life Saver	9	2.2	110.0	26.89	1760	430.2
Swirled, 0.9-oz. roll (11 Life Savers)	99	24.2	110.0	26.89	1760	430.2
1 Life Saver	9	2.2	110.0	26.89	1760	430.2
Tangerine, 0.9-oz. roll (11 Life Savers)	99	24.2	110.0	26.89	1760	430.2
1 Life Saver	9	2.2	110.0	26.89	1760	430.2
Tropical Fruits, 0.9-oz. roll (11 Life Savers)	99	24.2	110.0	26.89	1760	430.2
1 Life Saver	9	2.2	110.0	26.89	1760	430.2
Wild Cherry, 0.9-oz. roll (11 Life Savers)	99	24.2	110.0	26.89	1760	430.2
1 Life Saver	9	2.2	110.0	26.89	1760	430.2
Wint-O-Green, 0.9-oz. roll (12 Life Savers)	84	21.6	116.7	30.00	1856	480.0
1 Life Saver	7	1.8	116.7	30.00	1856	480.0
Life Savers Lollipops, see the LOLLIPOPS section, which follows the main Candy listings.						
Lite-Mints, **Spangler,** 1-oz. roll (12 mints)	115		115.0		1840	
1 mint, approx. 0.08 oz. (approx. 12½ per ounce)	9		115.0		1840	
M&M's Peanut Chocolate Candies, **M&M/Mars,** candy counter and vending machine size, 1.56-oz. bag	212	24.1	143.3	16.30	2293	260.8
Companion pack, 1.87-oz. bag	268	30.4	143.3	16.30	2293	260.8
Grocery pack, 16-oz. (1-lb.) bag	2293	260.8	143.3	16.30	2293	260.8
Miniatures, 12-oz. bag, 15 "fun size" bags, each approx. 0.8 oz.	1719	195.6	143.3	16.30	2293	260.8
1 "fun size" bag, approx. 0.8 oz.	115	13.0	143.3	16.30	2293	260.8
1 M&M, approx. 0.07 oz. (approx. 14 per ounce)	11	1.2	143.3	16.30	2293	260.8
M&M's Plain Chocolate Candies, **M&M/Mars** grocery pack, 1-oz. bag	138	19.3	138.0	19.30	2208	308.8
Candy store size, 1½-oz. bag	215	29.9	138.0	19.30	2208	308.8
Vending machine size, 1.56-oz. bag	215	29.9	138.0	19.30	2208	308.8
Companion pack, 1.87-oz. bag	261	36.0	138.0	19.30	2208	308.8
Miniatures, 12.6-oz. bag, 20 "fun size" bags, each approx. 0.6 oz.	1759	243.2	138.0	19.30	2208	308.8
1 "fun size" bag, approx. 0.63 oz.	88	12.1	138.0	19.30	2208	308.8
1 M&M, approx. 0.03 oz. (approx. 35 per ounce)	4	0.6	138.0	19.30	2208	308.8
Malty Crunch Bar, **Frank Milina,** 1-oz. bar	150	17.9	150.0	17.95	2400	287.2
Maple Brazils, **Callard & Bowser,** 8-oz. bag (approx. 15 pieces)	908	175.2	113.5	21.90	1816	350.5
1 piece, approx. 0.5 oz. (2 per ounce)	60	11.6	113.5	21.90	1816	350.5
Marathon Bar, **M&M/Mars:**						
Candy store and supermarket size, 1.37-oz. bar	179	26.5	130.7	19.34	2091	309.4
Miniatures, 16-oz. (1-lb.) bag (approx. 36 miniatures)	2091	309.4	130.7	19.34	2091	309.4
1 miniature, approx. 0.4 oz. (approx. 2 per ounce)	58	8.5	130.7	19.34	2091	309.4
Mars Bar, **M&M/Mars,** 1.52-oz. bar	208	26.4	136.8	17.36	2189	277.8
Marshmallow Twists, **Joyva,** 6-oz. box (approx. 11 Twists)	680	122.1	113.4	20.35	1815	325.6
1 marshmallow Twist, approx. 0.5 oz. (approx. 2 per ounce)	61	11.0	113.4	20.35	1815	325.6
Marshmallows, **Jets (Kraft),** 10-oz. bag (approx. 38 or 39 marshmallows)	945	236.3	94.5	23.63	1512	378.1
16-oz. (1-lb.) bag (approx. 63 marshmallows)	1512	378.1	94.5	23.63	1512	378.1
1 marshmallow, approx. ¼ oz. (approx. 4 per ounce)	24	6.0	94.5	23.63	1512	378.1
Marshmallows, Miniature, **Kraft,** 6¼-oz. bag (approx. 295 or 296 marshmallows)	591	147.7	94.5	23.63	1512	378.1
10½-oz. bag (approx. 496 or 497 marshmallows)	992	248.1	94.5	23.63	1512	378.1
1 miniature marshmallow, approx. 0.02 oz. (approx. 50 per ounce)	2	0.5	94.5	23.63	1512	378.1
Mary Jane Candy Bar, **Miller:**						
Candy store and supermarket size, 1½-oz. bar	108	19.5	72.0	13.00	1152	208.0
Vending machine size, 1⅝-oz. bar	117	21.1	72.0	13.00	1152	208.0
Movie concession size, 1⅔-oz. bar	120	21.7	72.0	13.00	1152	208.0
Miniatures, 16-oz. (1-lb.) bag	1152	208.0	72.0	13.00	1152	208.0
1 miniature, approx. ¼ oz. (approx. 4 per ounce)	18	3.3	72.0	13.00	1152	208.0
Merri-Mints, **Delson,** 6-oz. box (20 mints)	598	154.2	99.6	25.71	1594	411.3
1 mint, approx. 0.3 oz. (approx. 3½ per ounce)	30	7.7	99.6	25.71	1594	411.3
Mexican Hats, **Heide,** Supermarket size, 7-oz. box (approx. 77 Hats)	1116		159.4		2550	
10-oz. box (approx. 110 Hats)	1594		159.4		2550	
1 Hat, approx. 0.09 oz. (approx. 11 per ounce)	15		159.4		2550	
Milk Brazil Bar, **Cadbury,** 3½-oz. bar	546	50.3	154.8	14.26	2477	228.2
7-oz. bar	1092	100.6	154.8	14.26	2477	228.2
Milk Chocolate Almond Bar, **Heath,** 2-oz. bar	300	32.0	150.0	16.00	2400	256.0
Milk Chocolate Bar, **Heath,** 2-oz. bar	290	36.0	147.4	18.15	2359	290.3
Milk Chocolate and Peanuts, **Enjoy (Heath),** 1.7-oz. bar	255	27.2	150.0	16.00	2400	256.0
Milk Chocolate Petite Bar, **Andes,** 1.1-oz. bar	169	17.5	153.4	15.93	2454	254.9
1 miniature, approx. 0.15 oz. (approx. 6½ per ounce)	23	2.4	153.4	15.93	2454	254.9
Milk Duds, **Clark,** 0.7-oz. box	83	16.6	118.2	23.66	1892	378.6
1.2-oz. box	142	28.4	118.2	23.66	1892	378.6
1.5-oz. box	177	35.5	118.2	23.66	1892	378.6
1.65-oz. box	195	39.0	118.2	23.66	1892	378.6
2-oz. box	236	47.3	118.2	23.66	1892	378.6
2.3-oz. box	272	54.4	118.2	23.66	1892	378.6
2.75-oz. box	325	65.1	118.2	23.66	1892	378.6
Milk-Free Candy Bar, **CaraCoa (El Molino),** vending machine size, 1-oz. bar	145	18.0	145.0	18.00	2320	288.0
4-oz. bar	590	70.0	145.0	18.00	2320	288.0
Milk Mounds, **Peter Paul:**						
Vending machine size, 1.1-oz. bar	162	21.8	147.0	19.80	2352	316.8
Candy store and movie concession size, 1½-oz. bar	221	29.7	147.0	19.80	2352	316.8
Milky Way Bar, **M&M/Mars:**						
Candy store, vending machine, and supermarket size, 1.91-oz. bar	242	39.6	126.7	20.73	2027	331.7
Miniatures, 16-oz. (1-lb.) bag (approx. 19 miniatures)	2027	331.7	126.7	20.73	2027	331.7
1 miniature, approx. 0.84 oz., 19 per bag	106	17.4	126.7	20.73	2027	331.7
Mint Candy Bar, vending machine size, **CaraCoa (El Molino),** 1-oz. bar	160	16.0	160.0	16.00	2560	256.0
4-oz. bar	640	64.0	160.0	16.00	2560	256.0

	UNIT		1 OZ., BY WT.		1 POUND	
	Cal.	Carb.	Cal.	Carb.	Cal.	Carb.
Mint Chocolates, **Callard & Bowser,** 7-oz. box (29 or 30 chocolates)	840	158.6	119.2	22.50	1907	360.0
1 chocolate, approx. 0.24 oz. (approx. 4 per ounce)	29	5.4	119.2	22.50	1907	360.0
Mint Smiles, **Spangler,** 0.8-oz. roll (10 Smiles)	87		108.8		1741	
1 Smile, 0.08 oz. (approx. 12½ per ounce)	9		108.8		1741	
Mint Truffles, **Heath,** 1 Truffle, approx. 0.3 oz. (3½ per ounce)	43	4.2	155.9	15.31	2495	245.0
Mintoes, **Callard & Bowser,** 1⅓-oz. package (9 Mintoes)	144	34.0	107.8	25.24	1725	406.7
1 Minto, approx. 0.15 oz. (approx. 6½ per ounce)	16	3.8	107.8	25.24	1725	406.7
Mints, Dietetic, Assorted, **Estee,** 2¼-oz. 5-pak (60 mints)	240	60.0	106.7	26.67	1707	426.7
1 mint, approx. 0.04 oz. (approx. 25 per ounce)	4	1.0	106.7	26.67	1707	426.7
Mints, also see many that are listed under their flavor or other descriptive word, such as White Mints.						
Mounds Bar, **Peter Paul:**						
Vending machine size, 1.1-oz. bar	162	21.8	147.0	19.80	2352	316.8
Candy Store and movie concession size, 1½-oz. bar	221	29.7	147.0	19.80	2352	316.8
Miniatures, 7-oz. bag (approx. 15 pieces)	1029	138.6	147.0	19.80	2352	316.8
12-oz. bag (approx. 26 pieces)	1764	237.6	147.0	19.80	2352	316.8
1 miniature, approx. 0.46 oz.	68	9.1	147.0	19.80	2352	316.8
Mr. Goodbar, **Hershey's:**						
Candy counter size, 1½-oz. bar	242	20.8	161.5	13.85	2584	221.6
2-oz. bar	323	27.7	161.5	13.85	2584	221.6
Vending machine size, 1.3-oz. bar	210	18.0	161.5	13.85	2584	221.6
Movie concession size, 4-oz. bar	646	55.4	161.5	13.85	2584	221.6
Supermarket size, 8-oz. bar	1292	110.8	161.5	13.85	2584	221.6
Miniatures, 10.15-oz. bag (approx. 29 miniatures)	1639	14.1	161.5	13.85	2584	221.6
1 miniature, approx. 0.35 oz.	57	4.8	161.5	13.85	2584	221.6
Munch Peanut Bar, **M&M/Mars,** 1½-oz. bar	229	18.9	152.7	12.60	2443	201.6
Natural Candy Bar, vending machine size, **CaraCoa (El Molino),** 1-oz. bar	160	16.0	160.0	16.00	2560	256.0
4-oz. bar	640	64.0	160.0	16.00	2560	256.0
Nestlé Milk Chocolate Bar:						
Vending machine sizes, 1⅙-oz. bar	159	18.1	150.0	17.00	2400	272.0
3.2-oz. bar	474	19.7	150.0	17.00	2400	272.0
Candy counter and supermarket size, 2.5-oz. bar	375	42.9	150.0	17.00	2400	272.0
5-oz. bar	750	85.0	150.0	17.00	2400	272.0
Miniatures, 10.15-oz. bag	1523	172.6	150.0	17.00	2400	272.0
1 miniature, 0.35 oz. (approx. 3 per ounce)	53	6.0	150.0	17.00	2400	272.0
Nib Nax, **Y&S,** 1⅞-oz. box	188	45.0	100.0	24.00	1600	384.0
1 Nib, approx. 0.1 oz. (approx. 10 per ounce)	10	2.4	100.0	24.00	1600	384.0
Nibs, Cherry, **Y&S,** 1⅞-oz. box	200	45.0	106.7	24.00	1707	384.0
1 Nib, approx. 0.06 oz. (approx. 18 per ounce)	6	1.3	106.7	24.00	1707	384.0
Nibs, Fruit, **Y&S,** 1⅞-oz. box	200	45.0	106.7	24.00	1707	384.0
1 Nib, approx. 0.06 oz. (approx. 18 per ounce)	6	1.3	106.7	24.00	1707	384.0
Nibs, Licorice Flavored, **Y&S,** 1⅞-oz. box	200	45.0	106.7	24.00	1707	384.0
1 Nib, approx. 0.6 oz. (approx. 18 per ounce)	6	1.3	106.7	24.00	1707	384.0
Nougat, Dessert, **Callard & Bowser,** 5.29-oz. box (10 or 11 pieces)	600	110.3	113.5	20.86	1816	333.7
1 piece, approx. ½ oz. (approx. 2 per ounce)	56	10.3	113.5	20.86	1816	333.7
Nougat, French, **Schrafft's,** 8-oz. package	907	208.6	113.4	26.08	1814	417.3
Nutcracker Bar, **Clark,** 1.06-oz. bar	163	18.9	153.1	17.75	2450	284.0
1.3-oz. bar	199	23.1	153.1	17.75	2450	284.0
Orange Candy Bar, **CaraCoa (El Molino),** vending machine size, 1-oz. bar	160	16.0	160.0	16.00	2560	256.0
4-oz. bar	640	64.0	160.0	16.00	2560	256.0
Orange Chocolates, **Callard & Bowser,** 7-oz. package	820	156.8	116.3	22.25	1861	355.9
1 Chocolate, approx. 24 oz. (approx. 4 per ounce)	30	5.3	116.3	22.25	1861	355.9
Orange Flavored Bar, Meal Time, **Frank Milina,** 1½-oz. bar	150	24.8	100.0	16.52	1600	264.5
Orange Kisses, **Jolly Rancher,** 7-oz. bag (approx. 33 or 34 kisses)	827		118.1		1890	
9-oz. bag (approx. 42 or 43 kisses)	1063		118.1		1890	
1 kiss, approx. 0.2 oz. (approx. 5 per ounce)	25		118.1		1890	
Orange Slices, **Nabisco:**						
Candy counter and vending machine size, 2¼-oz. package	214		95.0		1520	
Supermarket size, 8-oz. bag	760		95.0		1520	

	UNIT		1 OZ., BY WT.		1 POUND	
	Cal.	Carb.	Cal.	Carb.	Cal.	Carb.
Orange Stix, **Jolly Rancher,** 1 Stix, approx. 1 oz.	148		148.0		2368	
Parfait Crème de Menthe, **Andes,** 1.1-oz. bar	175	17.7	159.1	16.13	2546	258.1
Pastel Mints, Midget Cut, **Richardson,** 5-oz. bag (approx. 166–167 mints)	549	137.0	109.8	27.46	1757	439.4
8-oz. bag (approx. 266–267 mints)	878	219.7	109.8	27.46	1757	439.4
1 mint, approx. 0.03 oz. (approx. 33 per ounce)	3	0.8	109.8	27.46	1757	439.4
Patties, **Richardson,** 8-oz. package (approx. 88 or 89 patties)	870	217.3	108.7	27.16	1739	434.6
Restaurant size, 25-pound carton (approx. 4444 or 4445 patties)	43480	10864.0	108.7	27.16	1739	434.6
1 pattie, approx. 0.09 oz.	10	2.5	108.7	27.16	1739	434.6
Peach Kisses, **Jolly Rancher,** 7-oz. bag (approx. 33 or 34 kisses)	827		118.1		1890	
9-oz. bag (approx. 42 or 43 kisses)	1063		118.1		1890	
1 kiss, approx. 0.2 oz. (approx. 5 per ounce)	25		118.1		1890	
Peach Stix, **Jolly Rancher,** 1 Stix, approx. 1 oz.	148		148.0		2368	
For comparison: Dried Peaches, Honey Dipped, **Fruit Pac,** 8-oz. package	660	172.4	82.5	21.55	1320	344.8
Peanut Blossom Kisses, **Clark,** 12-oz. bag	1320	288.0	110.0	24.00	1760	384.0
Peanut Butter Bar, **Frito-Lay,** 1¾-oz. bar	274	27.4	156.6	15.66	2506	250.6
Peanut Butter Bar, Hi Protein Carob Coated, **Hi-Protein,** 1-oz. bar	135	16.5	135.0	16.50	2160	264.0
2-oz. bar	270	33.0	135.0	16.50	2160	264.0
Peanut Butter Cups, Dietetic, **Estee,** 3¼-oz. box	540	34.8	166.2	10.71	2659	171.4
1 peanut butter cup, approx. 0.27 oz. (approx. 3.7 per ounce)	45	2.9	166.2	10.71	2659	171.4
Peanut Butter Cups, Plain, **Reese's (Hershey's),** 1.2-oz. package	190	18.0	158.3	15.00	2533	240.0
1 peanut butter cup, approx. 0.6 oz. (approx. 1½ per ounce)	95	9.0	158.3	15.00	2533	240.0
Peanut Butter Cups, Crunchy, **Reese's (Hershey's),** 1.2-oz. package (2 peanut butter cups)	190	18.0	158.3	15.00	2533	240.0
1 peanut butter cup, approx. 0.6 oz.	95	9.0	158.3	15.00	2533	240.0
Peanut Butter Fudge Bar, **Frank Milina,** 1¼-oz. bar	161	22.7	128.8	18.15	2061	290.3
Peanut Butter Hi Protein Bar, **Golden Harvest,** 2-oz. bar	270	33.0	135.0	16.50	2160	264.0
Peanut Butter Sesame Hi Protein Bar, **Frank Milina,** 1¼-oz. bar	188	13.8	150.4	11.06	2406	176.9
Peanut Candy Bar, **CaraCoa (El Molino),** 1-oz. bar	160	16.0	160.0	16.00	2560	256.0
4-oz. bar	640	64.0	160.0	16.00	2560	256.0
Peanut Candy Bar, Old Fashioned, **Planters:**						
1.3-oz. bar	182	19.5	140.0	15.00	2240	240.0
1.6-oz. bar	224	24.0	140.0	15.00	2240	240.0
4-oz. bar	560	60.0	140.0	15.00	2240	240.0
8-oz. bar	1120	120.0	140.0	15.00	2240	240.0
Peanut Chews, **Goldenberg's,** see Goldenberg's						
Peanut Chocolate Fudge, **Spangler,** 1 piece, approx. 3.2 oz.	410	59.7	127.3	18.53	2037	296.5
Peanut Clusters, **Schrafft's,** 5½-oz. box (12 clusters)	864	68.3	157.1	12.42	2514	198.7
1 cluster, approx. 0.46 oz. (approx 2 per ounce)	72	5.7	157.1	12.42	2514	198.7
Peanut Clusters, Caramel, **Spangler,** 1 cluster, approx. 0.67 oz. (approx. 1½ per ounce)	91	11.1	135.8	16.54	2173	264.6
Peanut Clusters, Creme, **Spangler,** 1 cluster, approx. 0.72 oz. (approx. 1½ per ounce)	96	12.4	133.3	17.17	2133	274.7
Peanut Clusters, Fudge, **Spangler,** 1 cluster, approx. 0.95 oz.	123	17.1	129.5	18.03	2072	288.5
Peanut Crunch, **Sahadi,** vending machine size, ¾-oz. bar	106	6.3	141.7	8.33	2267	133.3
6-oz. bar	850	50.0	141.7	8.33	2267	133.3
1 piece, approx. 0.06 oz. (approx. 17 per ounce)	9	0.5	141.7	8.33	2267	133.3
Pecan Chocolate Fudge, **Spangler,** 1 piece, approx. 4.1 oz.	531	76.6	129.5	18.68	2072	298.9
Peppermint Bar, Carob Coated, **Frank Milina,** approx. 1.25 oz.	151	28.6	120.8	22.88	1933	336.1
Peppermint Pattie, **Spangler,** 1 pattie, approx. 0.34 oz. (approx. 3 per ounce)	38	7.8	111.8	22.82	1789	365.1
Peppermint Patty, **York:**						
Vending machine size, 1.05-oz. bar	130	26.3	124.0	25.00	1984	400.0
Candy counter, supermarket, and candy concession size, 1.35-oz. bar	167	33.8	124.0	25.00	1984	400.0
Miniatures, 7-oz. bag (approx. 15 patties)	868	175.0	124.0	25.00	1984	400.0
12-oz. bag (approx. 28 patties)	1488	300.0	124.0	25.00	1984	400.0
1 miniature patty, approx. 0.47 oz. (approx. 2 per ounce)	58	11.8	124.0	25.00	1984	400.0

	UNIT		1 OZ., BY WT.		1 POUND	
	Cal.	Carb.	Cal.	Carb.	Cal.	Carb.
"Penny candy" size, approx. 0.32 oz. (approx. 3 per ounce)	40	8.1	124.0	25.00	1984	400.0
Pineapple Stix, **Jolly Rancher,** 1 Stix, approx. 1 oz.	148		148.0		2368	
For comparison: Dried Pineapple, Honey Dipped, **Fruit Pac,** 8-oz. package	675	178.1	84.4	22.26	1350	356.2
Raisins, Carob Coated, **CaraCoa (El Molino),** 1-oz. package	130	18.0	130.0	18.00	2080	288.0
4-oz. package	520	72.0	130.0	18.00	2080	288.0
Raisins, Chocolate Covered, 4.5-oz. box, **Estee**	576	65.6	128.0	14.58	2048	233.3
0.05-oz. box	6	2.7	128.0	14.58	2048	233.3
For comparison: Dried Thompson Raisins, Honey Dipped, **Fruit Pac,** 16-oz. (1-lb.) package	1379	369.8	86.2	23.11	1379	369.8
Raisinets, **Ward:**						
Candy store, vending machine, and supermarket size, 1-oz. box	90	14.0	90.0	14.00	1440	224.0
Movie concession size, 2.3-oz. box	207	32.2	90.0	14.00	1440	224.0
8-oz. box	720	112.0	90.0	14.00	1440	224.0
Miniatures, 7½-oz. bag (contains 12 miniature boxes)	675	105.0	90.0	14.00	1440	224.0
1 miniature box, approx. 0.63 oz. (1½ per ounce)	56	8.8	90.0	14.00	1440	224.0
Rally, **Hershey's,** 1½-oz. bar	210	22.0	140.0	14.67	2240	234.7
Red Hot Dollars, **Heide,** 7-oz. box (approx. 74 Dollars)	1116		159.4		2550	
1 Dollar, approx. 0.09 oz. (approx. 11 per ounce)	15		159.4		2550	
Reggie Bar, **Standard Brands:**						
1.6-oz. bar	232	23.2	145.0	14.50	2320	232.0
Vending machine size, 2-oz. bar	290	29.0	145.0	14.50	2320	232.0
Rolo, **Hershey's,** 1-oz. roll (5 Rolos)	140	19.0	140.0	19.00	2240	304.0
1.35-oz. roll (6 or 7 Rolos)	189	25.7	140.0	19.00	2240	304.0
1.55-oz. roll (7 or 8 Rolos)	217	29.5	140.0	19.00	2240	304.0
1 Rolo, approx. 0.2 oz. (approx. 5 per ounce)	28	3.8	140.0	19.00	2240	304.0
Rum Truffles, **Callard & Bowser,** 14-oz. box (40 Truffles)	1880	262.4	133.4	18.61	2134	297.8
1 Truffle, approx. 0.35 oz. (approx. 3 per ounce)	47	6.6	133.4	18.61	2134	297.8
Scotties, **Callard & Bowser,** 1.23-oz. bag (approx. 19 or 20 Scotties)	126	33.3	102.2	26.96	1634	431.3
1 Scottie, approx. 0.06 oz. (approx. 17 per ounce)	7	1.7	102.2	26.96	1634	431.3
Sesame Bar, **Joyva,** 1⅛-oz. bar	200	28.1	178.0	25.00	2848	400.0
Sesame Crunch, **Joyva,** 8-oz. bag (approx. 40 pieces)	1424	200.0	178.0	25.00	2848	400.0
16-oz. (1-lb.) bag (approx. 80 pieces)	2848	400.0	178.0	25.00	2848	400.0
1 piece, approx. 0.02 oz. (approx. 5 per ounce)	36	5.0	178.0	25.00	2848	400.0
Sesame Crunch, dry roasted, **Sahadi,** 6-oz. jar (approx. 100 pieces)	900	65.0	150.0	10.83	2400	173.3
1 piece, approx. 0.06 oz. (approx. 17 per ounce)	9	0.7	150.0	10.83	2400	173.3
Sesame Crunch Bar, dry roasted, **Sahadi,** ¾-oz. bar	113	8.1	150.0	10.83	2400	173.3
Sesame & Honey Crunch Bar, dry roasted, **Sahadi,** ¾-oz. bar	120	9.0	160.0	12.00	2560	192.0
Sesamettes, **Joyva,** 11-oz. can	1958	275.0	178.0	25.00	2848	400.0
Slo-Poke Sucker, **D. L. Clark,** 0.25-oz. size	31	6.1	123.7	24.54	1979	392.6
0.7-oz. size	87	17.2	123.7	24.54	1979	392.6
0.75-oz. size	93	18.4	123.7	24.54	1979	392.6
1.25-oz. size	155	30.7	123.7	24.54	1979	392.6
Soft Mints, **Callard & Bowser,** 3.9-oz. bag (approx. 27 or 28 mints)	407	107.4	102.2	26.96	1634	431.3
1 mint, approx. 0.15 oz. (approx. 6½ per ounce)	15	3.9	102.2	26.96	1634	431.3
Sour Bites, Cherry (36-tablet package)	144	36.0				
Lemon (36-tablet package)	144	36.0				
1 tablet	4	1.0				
Snickers, **M&M/Mars,** candy store and supermarket size, 1.91-oz. bar	248	49.1	129.8	25.70	2077	411.0
Snowcaps, **Ward:**						
Candy store and supermarket size, 1-oz. box	124	19.0	124.0	19.00	1984	304.0
Movie concession size, 2.3-oz. box	285	43.7	124.0	19.00	1984	304.0
Supermarket size, 8-oz. box	992	153.0	124.0	19.00	1984	304.0
Miniatures, 7½-oz. bag (contains 12 miniature boxes)	930	143.0	124.0	19.00	1984	304.0
1 miniature box, approx. 0.63 oz. (approx. 1½ per ounce)	78	11.9	124.0	19.00	1984	304.0
Soybeans, Carob Coated, **CaraCoa (El Molino),** 1-oz. box	145	12.0	145.0	12.00	2320	192.0
4.5-oz. box	653	54.0	145.0	12.00	2320	192.0
Spearmint Leaves, **Nabisco:**						
Vending machine size, 1½-oz. bag	(143)		95.0		1520	
Supermarket size, 8-oz. bag	(760)		95.0		1520	
16-oz. (1-lb.) bag	(1520)		95.0		1520	
Special Dark Chocolate Bar, **Hershey's,** vending machine size, 1.05-oz. bar	166	19.2	158.3	18.33	2533	293.3
2-oz. bar	317	36.7	158.3	18.33	2533	293.3
Starburst Fruit Chews, **M&M/Mars,** 1-oz. package	113	26.6	113.0	26.60	1808	425.6
1.68-oz. package	186	44.1	113.0	26.60	1808	425.6
Starlight Mints, **Richardson,** 5-oz. bag (approx. 28 mints)	563	140.7	112.6	28.14	1802	450.2
7-oz. bag (approx. 39 mints)	788	197.0	112.6	28.14	1802	450.2
1 mint, approx. 0.18 oz. (approx. 5½ per ounce)	20	5.0	112.6	28.14	1802	450.2
Stix, **Jolly Rancher,** see individual flavors						
Strawberry Bites, **Switzer,** 10-oz. bag	960	226.8	96.0	22.68	1536	362.9
Strawberry Stix, **Jolly Rancher,** 1 Stix, approx. 1 oz.	148		148.0		2368	
Strawberry Stix, **Switzer,** 4-oz. bag	384	90.7	96.0	22.68	1536	362.9
5-oz. bag	480	113.3	96.0	22.68	1536	362.9
16-oz. (1-lb.) bag	1536	362.9	96.0	22.68	1536	362.9
Strawberry Twists, **Y&S,** 5-oz. package (15 twists)	475	115.0	95.0	23.00	1520	368.0
1 twist, approx. 0.33 oz. (approx. 3 per ounce)	32	7.7	95.0	23.00	1520	368.0
Striped Mints, **Richardson,** 8-oz. bag	876	219.0	109.5	27.37	1752	437.9
1 mint, approx. 0.05 oz. (approx. 20 per ounce)	6	1.4	109.5	27.37	1752	437.9
Sugar Babies, **Nabisco:**						
Vending machine size, 1⅜-oz. pouch (approx. 25 Sugar Babies)	160	34.0	116.5	24.72	1864	395.5
Candy counter size, 1⅝-oz. pouch (approx. 29 or 30 Sugar Babies)	189	40.2	116.5	24.72	1864	395.5
Supermarket size, 7-oz. box (approx. 125 to 130 Sugar Babies)	816	173.0	116.5	24.72	1864	395.5
1 baby, approx. 0.055 oz. (approx. 18 per ounce)	6	1.4	116.5	24.72	1864	395.5
Sugar Daddy, **Nabisco,** 1.125-oz. pop	128	27.8	113.4	24.70	1814	395.2
Sugar Daddy Juniors, approx. 0.4 oz. (approx. 2½ per ounce)	45	9.9	113.4	24.70	1814	395.2
Summit Cookie Bar, **M&M/Mars,** 1.37-oz. bar	197	21.9	143.8	15.99	2301	255.8
"Cookie breaks" size, 0.44 oz. bar	63	7.0	143.8	15.99	2301	255.8
Sunpower Bar, **D. L. Clark,** 1.06-oz. bar	162	18.7	152.4	17.63	2438	282.1
1.3-oz. bar	198	22.9	152.4	17.63	2438	282.1
Super Hi-Protein Diet Bar, **Hoffman's,** 1¾-oz. bar	230	25.0	131.4	14.29	2102	228.6
Swiss Mints, **Delson,** 6-oz. box (20 mints)	674	136.4	112.4	22.73	1798	363.7
1 mint, approx. 0.3 oz. (approx. 3½ per ounce)	34	6.8	112.4	22.73	1798	363.7
T.V. Mix, Dietetic, **Estee,** 4-oz. box (approx. 72 candies)	648	46.8	162.0	11.70	2592	187.2
1 candy, approx. 0.06 oz. (approx. 18 per ounce)	9	0.7	162.0	11.70	2592	187.2
Taffy, **Jolly Rancher,** 14-oz. package (approx. 62 pieces)	1861		132.9		2126	
1 piece, approx. 0.23 oz. (approx. 4 per ounce)	30		132.9		2126	
Taffy Candy Kisses, **Yinnies,** 3½-oz. bag (12 kisses)	360	84.0	102.9	24.00	1646	384.0
1 kiss, approx. 0.29 oz. (approx. 3½ per ounce)	30	7.0	102.9	24.00	1646	384.0
Teeny Mints, **Callard & Bowser,** 1.23-oz. bag (approx. 19 or 20 mints)	126	33.3	102.2	26.96	1634	431.1
1 mint, approx. 0.06 oz. (approx. 16½ per ounce)	7	1.7	102.2	26.96	1634	431.1
Thin Mints, **Delson,** 6-oz. box (20 mints)	659	138.1	109.8	23.01	1757	368.2
1 mint, approx. 0.3 oz. (approx. 3½ per ounce)	33	6.6	109.8	23.01	1757	368.2
Thin Mints, **Schrafft's,** 6-oz. box (19 mints)	699	133.6	116.6	22.26	1866	356.2
1 mint, approx. 0.32 oz. (approx. 3 per ounce)	37	7.1	116.6	22.26	1866	356.2
3 Musketeers Bar, **M&M/Mars,** candy store and supermarket size, 2.06-oz. bar	254	44.3	123.3	21.50	1973	344.0
Tigers Milk, **Plus,** 170 Calorie Snack Carob Coated Bar, 1.5-oz. bar	170	23.0	113.3	15.33	1813	245.3
Carob Coated Bar, 2-oz. bar	250	35.0	125.0	17.50	2000	280.0
Carob Coated Bar with Peanut Butter, 1.7-oz. bar	210	28.0	123.5	16.47	1976	263.5
Carob Coated Bar with Peanut Butter and Honey, 1.7-oz. bar	210	28.0	123.5	16.47	1976	263.5
Carob Coated Bar with Peanut Butter and Jelly, 1.7-oz. bar	210	28.0	123.5	16.47	1976	263.5
Ting-A-Ling Crunch Chocolates, **Andes,** 1.1-oz. bar	164	18.8	149.1	17.13	2386	274.1
"Penny candy" size, approx. 0.15 oz. (approx. 7 per ounce)	22	2.6	149.1	17.13	2386	274.1
Toffee Candy, Chocolate, **Rothchild's,** approx. 1.3-oz. roll (8 pieces)	176	26.4	135.4	20.31	2166	325.0

	UNIT		1 OZ., BY WT.		1 POUND	
	Cal.	Carb.	Cal.	Carb.	Cal.	Carb.
1 toffee, approx. 0.16 oz. (approx. 6 per ounce)	22	3.3	135.4	20.31	2166	325.0
Toffee Candy, Creamy, **Rothchild's,** approx. 1.3-oz. roll (8 pieces)	176	26.4	135.4	20.31	2166	325.0
1 toffee, approx. 0.16 oz. (approx. 6 per ounce)	22	3.3	135.4	20.31	2166	325.0
Toffee Rolls, Chocolate, **Callard & Bowser,** 3-oz. bag (approx. 11 or 12 rolls)	391	60.3	130.5	20.12	2088	321.9
1 roll, approx. 0.26 oz. (approx. 4 per ounce)	34	5.2	130.5	20.12	2088	321.9
Toffee Rolls, Milk Chocolate, **Callard & Bowser,** 3-oz. bag (approx. 11 or 12 rolls)	383	59.2	127.7	19.75	2043	316.0
1 roll, approx. 0.26 oz. (approx. 4 per ounce)	33	5.2	127.7	19.75	2043	316.0
Toffees, Brazil Nut, **Callard & Bowser,** 3.23-oz. bag (approx. 10 or 11 toffees)	442	57.9	136.2	17.85	2179	285.6
1 toffee, approx. 0.3 oz. (approx. 3 per ounce)	40	5.3	136.2	17.85	2179	285.6
Toffees, Chocolate, **Callard & Bowser,** 3.1-oz. bag (approx. 10 or 11 toffees)	405	57.1	130.5	18.40	2088	294.6
1 toffee, approx. ⅓ oz. (approx. 3 per ounce)	39	5.5	130.5	18.40	2088	294.6
Toffees, Chocolate Hazelnut, **Callard & Bowser,** 3.1-oz. bag (approx. 11 or 12 toffees)	422	59.4	136.2	19.15	2179	306.5
1 toffee, approx. 0.29 oz. (approx. 3½ per ounce)	40	5.7	136.2	19.15	2179	306.5
Toffees, Coffee, **Callard & Bowser,** 3½-oz. bag (approx. 12 toffees)	470	66.5	133.3	18.87	2134	301.9
1 toffee, approx. 0.29 oz. (approx. 3½ per ounce)	39	5.5	133.3	18.87	2134	301.9
Toffees, Cream Line, **Callard & Bowser,** 1.4-oz. roll pack (8 toffees)	188	26.6	133.4	18.90	2134	302.4
1 toffee, approx. 0.18 oz. (approx. 5½ per ounce)	24	3.3	133.4	18.90	2134	302.4
3.9-oz. bag (approx. 13 toffees)	517	73.3	133.4	18.90	2134	302.4
1 toffee, approx. 0.3 oz. (approx. 3½ per ounce)	40	5.6	133.4	18.90	2134	302.4
Toffees, Fruit & Nut, **Callard & Bowser,** 3.1-oz. bag (approx. 10 or 11 toffees)	405	56.9	130.5	18.36	2088	293.7
1 toffee, approx. 0.3 oz. (approx. 3 per ounce)	39	5.4	130.5	18.36	2088	293.7
Toffees, Licorice, **Callard & Bowser,** 1.4-oz. roll pack (8 toffees)	188	26.1	133.4	18.53	2134	296.5
1 toffee, approx. 0.18 oz. (approx. 5½ per ounce)	24	3.3	133.4	18.53	2134	296.5
3½-oz. bag (approx. 12 toffees)	470	65.3	133.4	18.53	2134	296.5
1 toffee, approx. 0.3 oz. (approx. 3 per ounce)	39	5.4	133.4	18.53	2134	296.5
Toffees, Mint, **Callard & Bowser,** 1.4-oz. roll pack (8 toffees)	188	26.6	133.4	18.90	2134	302.4
1 toffee, approx. 0.18 oz. (approx. 5½ per ounce)	24	3.3	133.4	18.90	2134	302.4
3½-oz. bag (approx. 12 toffees)	470	66.6	133.4	18.90	2134	302.4
1 toffee, approx. 0.3 oz. (approx. 3 per ounce)	40	5.6	133.4	18.90	2134	302.4
Toffees, Plain Jane, **Callard & Bowser,** 3.4-oz. bag (approx. 11 or 12 toffees)	466	60.5	136.2	17.71	2179	283.3
1 toffee, approx. 0.3 oz. (approx. 3 per ounce)	40	5.2	136.2	17.71	2179	283.3
Toffees, Strawberry, **Callard & Bowser,** 3.1-oz. bag (approx. 10 or 11 toffees)	414	59.4	133.4	19.15	2134	306.5
1 toffee, approx. 0.3 oz. (approx. 3 per ounce)	40	5.7	133.4	19.15	2134	306.5
Toffees, Treacle, **Callard & Bowser,** 3½-oz. bag (approx. 12 toffees)	450	69.7	127.7	19.78	2043	316.4
1 toffee, approx. 0.3 oz. (approx. 3 per ounce)	37	5.7	127.7	19.78	2043	316.4
Tootsie Roll Bar, Chocolate, **Tootsie Roll,** one midget bar, approx. 0.23 oz.	26	5.2	113.7	22.60	1819	361.6
1 bar, approx. ⅝ oz.	71	14.1	113.7	22.60	1819	361.6
1 bar, approx. ¾ oz.	85	17.0	113.7	22.60	1819	361.6
1 bar, approx. 1.0 oz.	114	22.6	113.7	22.60	1819	361.6
1 bar, approx. 1¼ oz.	142	28.3	113.7	22.60	1819	361.6
1 bar, approx. 1¾ oz.	199	39.6	113.7	22.60	1819	361.6
Tootsie Roll Bar, flavored, **Tootsie Roll,** one midget bar, approx. 0.2 oz.	27	5.4	116.5	23.54	1864	376.6
1 "square," approx. 0.16 oz.	19	3.8	116.5	23.54	1864	376.6
Tootsie Roll Pop Drops, Caramel, **Tootsie Roll,** vending machine size, approx. 1.7 oz. roll (10 Pop Drops)	189	42.8	113.0	25.60	1808	409.6
1 Pop Drop, approx. 0.17 oz. (approx. 6 per ounce)	19	4.3	113.0	25.60	1808	409.6
Tootsie Roll Pop Drops, Chocolate, **Tootsie Roll,** vending machine size, 1.7-oz. roll (approx. 10 Pop Drops)	184	43.8	110.0	26.20	1760	419.2
1 Pop Drop, approx. 0.17 oz. (approx. 6 per ounce)	18	4.4	110.0	26.20	1760	419.2

	UNIT		1 OZ., BY WT.		1 POUND	
	Cal.	Carb.	Cal.	Carb.	Cal.	Carb.
Flavored Tootsie Roll Pop Drops (cherry, grape, orange, raspberry)						
Vending machine size, 1.7-oz. roll (approx. 10 Pop Drops)	185	44.4	111.0	26.60	1776	425.6
Tootsie Roll Pops, see the LOLLIPOPS section, which follows the main Candy listings.						
Trident Mints, Fruit, approx. 0.77-oz. roll (11 mints)	86	21.6	111.4	28.00	1782	448.0
Peppermint, approx. 0.77 oz. roll (11 mints)	86	21.6	111.4	28.00	1782	448.0
Spearmint, approx. 0.77 oz. roll (11 mints)	86	21.6	111.4	28.00	1782	448.0
Wintergreen, approx. 0.77 oz. roll (11 mints)	86	21.6	111.4	28.00	1782	448.0
1 mint, approx. 0.07 oz. (approx. 14 per ounce)	8	2.0	111.4	28.00	1782	448.0
Tropical Fruit Mix, **Golden Harvest,** 4-oz. package	440	80.0	110.0	20.00		
Turkish Taffy, Assorted Flavors, (banana, chocolate, strawberry, vanilla), **Bonomo,** 1-oz. bar	107	24.7	107.0	24.66	1712	390.1
Mini-piece, approx. 0.14 oz.	15	3.4	107.0	24.38	1712	390.1
Twists, Chocolate Covered Vanilla, **Joyva,** ¾-oz. bar	85	15.8	113.4	21.08	1814	337.3
Twix Cookie Bar, **M&M/Mars,** 1¾-oz. bar	245	30.9	140.0	17.66	2240	282.6
"Cookie breaks" size, approx. 0.6 oz.	80	10.1	140.0	17.66	2240	282.6
Twizzlers, Chocolate Flavored, **Y&S,** Supermarket size, 5-oz. bag	550	120.0	110.0	24.00	1760	384.0
1 Twizzler, approx. 0.3 oz.	(34)	(8.0)	110.0	24.00	1760	384.0
Twizzlers, Licorice Flavored, **Y&S,** Supermarket size, 1¼-oz. bag	125	30.0	100.0	24.00	1600	384.0
1¾-oz. bag	175	42.0	100.0	24.00	1600	384.0
2⅛-oz. bag	213	51.0	100.0	24.00	1600	384.0
5-oz. bag	500	120.0	100.0	24.00	1600	384.0
1 Twizzler, approx. 0.3 oz.	(34)	(8.0)	100.0	24.00	1600	384.0
Twizzlers, Strawberry Flavored, **Y&S,** Supermarket size, 1¼-oz. bag	125	30.0	100.0	24.00	1600	384.0
1¾-oz. bag	175	42.0	100.0	24.00	1600	384.0
2⅛-oz. bag	213	51.0	100.0	24.00	1600	384.0
5-oz. bag	500	120.0	100.0	24.00	1600	384.0
1 Twizzler, approx. 0.3 oz.	(34)	(8.0)	100.0	24.00	1600	384.0
Watermelon Stix, **Jolly Rancher,** 1 Stix. approx. 1 oz.	148		148.0		2368	
Whatchamacallit Bar, **Hershey's,** 1.15-oz. bar	170	18.0	147.8	15.65	2365	250.4
Whistler Bar, **Cadbury,** 1.76-oz. bar	220	29.7	124.5	16.84	1992	269.4
White Mints, **Richardson:**						
Midget cut, 5-oz. bag (approx. 180 mints)	549	137.3	109.8	27.46	1757	439.4
8-oz. bag (approx. 295 mints)	878	219.7	109.8	27.46	1757	439.4
4-pound carton (approx. 2,360 mints)	7027	1757.4	109.8	27.46	1757	439.4
Restaurant size carton, 25-lb. (approx. 14,400 mints)	43920	10984.0	109.8	27.46	1757	439.4
1 mint, approx. 0.03 oz. (approx. 33½ per ounce)	3	0.8	109.8	27.46	1757	439.4
Planet cut, 8-oz. bag (approx. 108 mints)	878	219.7	109.8	27.46	1757	439.4
Restaurant size carton, 25-lb. (approx. 5,400 mints)	43920	10984.0	109.8	27.46	1757	439.4
1 mint, approx. 0.07 oz. (approx. 13½ per ounce)	8	2.1	109.8	27.46	1757	439.4
Yogurt Candy Bar, **Frank Milina,** 1¼-oz. bar	150	18.2	120.0	14.58	1920	233.2
Yogurt Candy Bar, Strawberry Flavor, **Frank Milina,** 1½-oz. bar	171	21.9	114.0	14.58	1824	233.2
Zagnut Bar, **Clark:**						
0.7-oz. bar	92	14.6	131.1	20.83	2097	333.3
1⅜-oz. bar	180	28.6	131.1	20.83	2097	333.3
1⅝-oz. bar	213	33.8	131.1	20.83	2097	333.3
Candy counter size, 1.3-oz. bar	170	27.1	131.1	20.83	2097	333.3
Vending machine size, 1.6-oz. bar	210	33.3	131.1	20,83	2097	333.3
Movie concession size, 2¾-oz. box (approx. 17 or 18 "Tiny Treats")	360	57.3	131.1	20.83	2097	333.3
1 "Tiny Treat," approx. 0.16 oz. (approx. 6 per ounce)	21	3.3	131.1	20.83	2097	333.3
Supermarket size, 8-oz. bag (approx. 16 to 20 "Juniors")	1049	166.6	131.1	20.83	2097	333.3
12-oz. bag (approx. 24 to 30 "Juniors")	1573	250.0	131.1	20.83	2097	333.3
1 "Junior," approx. 0.4 oz. (approx. 2 per ounce)	58	9.3	131.1	20.83	2097	333.3

COUGH DROPS

	UNIT		1 OZ., BY WT.		1 POUND	
	Cal.	Carb.	Cal.	Carb.	Cal.	Carb.
Beech-Nut Black, 11-tablet roll	110	27.5				
1 tablet	10	2.5				
Menthol, 11-tablet roll	110	27.5				
1 tablet	10	2.5				

	UNIT Cal.	UNIT Carb.	1 OZ., BY WT. Cal.	1 OZ., BY WT. Carb.	1 POUND Cal.	1 POUND Carb.
Wild Cherry, 11-tablet roll	110	27.5				
1 tablet	10	2.5				
Halls Cherry, 9-tablet package	135	33.3				
30-tablet bag	450	111.0				
1 tablet	15	3.7				
Lemon, 9-tablet package	135	33.3				
30-tablet bag	450	111.0				
1 tablet	15	3.7				
Mentho-Lyptus, 9-tablet package	135	33.3				
1 tablet	15	3.7				
Pine Bros. Honey, 14-drop box	112	28.0				
1 cough drop	8	2.0				
Wild Cherry, 14-drop box	112	28.0				
1 cough drop	8	2.0				

GRANOLA BARS and GRANOLA SNACKS

	UNIT Cal.	UNIT Carb.	1 OZ., BY WT. Cal.	1 OZ., BY WT. Carb.	1 POUND Cal.	1 POUND Carb.
Granola Bar, Cherry Yogurt, **Crunchola,** 1¼-oz. bar	170	22.0	136.0	17.60	2176	281.6
Granola Bar, Chocolate Chip, **Crunchola,** 1½-oz. bar	210	24.0	140.0	16.00	2240	256.0
Granola Bar, Chocolate Chip, **Nature Valley,** 8-oz. box (8 bars)	1040	160.0	130.0	20.00	2080	320.0
1 bar, approx. 1 oz.	130	20.0	130.0	20.00	2080	320.0
Granola Bar, Peanut Butter, **Nature Valley,** 8-oz. box (8 bars)	1152	144.0	144.0	18.00	2304	288.0
1 bar, approx. 1 oz.	144	18.0	144.0	18.00	2304	288.0
Granola Bar, Raisin & Cinnamon, **Quaker,** 8-oz. box (8 bars)	1040	152.0	130.0	19.00	2080	304.0
1 bar, approx. 1 oz.	130	19.0	130.0	19.00	2080	304.0
Granola Bar, Strawberry Yogurt, **Crunchola,** 1¼-oz. bar	175	21.3	140.0	17.00	2240	272.0
Granola Snack, Peanut Butter, Light & Crunchy, **Nature Valley,** 6-oz. box (6 pouches)	840	102.0	140.0	17.00	2240	272.0
1 pouch, approx. 1 oz.	140	17.0	140.0	17.00	2240	272.0
Granola Clusters, Raisin, **Nature Valley,** approx. 7.25-oz. package (6 rolls)	840	168.0	115.9	23.17	1854	370.7
1 roll, approx. 1.2 oz.	140	28.0	115.9	23.17	1854	370.7
Granola Snack, Cinnamon, Light & Crunchy, **Nature Valley,** 6-oz. box (6 pouches)	840	114.0	140.0	19.00	2240	304.0
1 pouch, approx. 1 oz.	140	19.0	140.0	19.00	2240	304.0
Granola Snack, Oats & Honey, Light & Crunchy, **Nature Valley,** 6-oz. box (6 pouches)	840	108.0	140.0	18.00	2240	288.0
1 pouch, approx. 1 oz.	140	18.0	140.0	18.00	2240	288.0

LOLLIPOPS

	UNIT Cal.	UNIT Carb.	1 OZ., BY WT. Cal.	1 OZ., BY WT. Carb.	1 POUND Cal.	1 POUND Carb.
Blow Pops, "5¢," Cherry, approx. 0.65 oz.	71	(18.2)	109.2	(28.00)	1748	(448.2)
Cinnamon, approx. 0.65 oz.	71	(18.2)	109.2	(28.00)	1748	(448.2)
Grape, approx. 0.65 oz.	71	(18.2)	109.2	(28.00)	1748	(448.2)
Sour Apple, approx. 0.65 oz.	71	(18.2)	109.2	(28.00)	1748	(448.2)
Watermelon, approx. 0.65 oz.	71	(18.2)	109.2	(28.00)	1748	(448.2)
Blow Pops, "10¢," Cherry, approx. 1.05 oz.	114	(29.2)	108.6	(27.80)	1737	(445.4)
Cinnamon, approx. 1.05 oz.	114	(29.2)	108.6	(27.80)	1737	(445.4)
Grape, approx. 1.05 oz.	114	(29.2)	108.6	(27.80)	1737	(445.4)
Sour Apple, approx. 1.05 oz.	114	(29.2)	108.6	(27.80)	1737	(445.4)
Watermelon, approx. 1.05 oz.	114	(29.2)	108.6	(27.80)	1737	(445.4)
Flat Pops, "5¢," Cherry, Sour, approx. 0.65 oz.	74	(19.0)	113.9	(28.30)	1822	(453.0)
Cherry, Sweet, approx. 0.64 oz.	74	(19.0)	113.9	(28.30)	1822	(453.0)
Cherry, Sweet & Sour, approx. 0.65 oz.	74	(19.0)	113.9	(28.30)	1822	(453.0)
Grape, Sour, approx. 0.65 oz.	74	(19.0)	113.9	(28.30)	1822	(453.0)
Grape, Sweet, approx. 0.65 oz.	74	(19.0)	113.9	(28.30)	1822	(453.0)
Grape, Sweet & Sour, approx. 0.65 oz.	74	(19.0)	113.9	(28.30)	1822	(453.0)
Lime, Sour, approx. 0.65 oz.	74	(19.0)	113.9	(28.30)	1822	(453.0)
Lime, Sweet, approx. 0.65 oz.	74	(19.0)	113.9	(28.30)	1822	(453.0)
Lime, Sweet & Sour, approx. 0.65 oz.	74	(19.0)	113.9	(28.30)	1822	(453.0)
Orange, Sour, approx. 0.65 oz.	74	(19.0)	113.9	(28.30)	1822	(453.0)
Orange, Sweet, approx. 0.65 oz.	74	(19.0)	113.9	(28.30)	1822	(453.0)
Orange, Sweet & Sour, approx. 0.65 oz.	74	(19.0)	113.9	(28.30)	1822	(453.0)
Flat Pops, "10¢," Cherry, Sour, approx. 1.05 oz.	119	(29.7)	113.9	(28.30)	1822	(453.0)
Cherry, Sweet, approx. 1.05 oz.	119	(29.7)	113.9	(28.30)	1822	(453.0)
Cherry, Sweet & Sour, approx. 1.05 oz.	119	(29.7)	113.9	(28.30)	1822	(453.0)
Grape, Sour, approx. 1.05 oz.	119	(29.7)	113.9	(28.30)	1822	(453.0)
Grape, Sweet, approx. 1.05 oz.	119	(29.7)	113.9	(28.30)	1822	(453.0)
Grape, Sweet & Sour, approx. 1.05 oz.	119	(29.7)	113.9	(28.30)	1822	(453.0)
Lime, Sour, approx. 1.05 oz.	119	(29.7)	113.9	(28.30)	1822	(453.0)
Lime, Sweet, approx. 1.05 oz.	119	(29.7)	113.9	(28.30)	1822	(453.0)
Lime, Sweet & Sour, approx. 1.05 oz.	119	(29.7)	113.9	(28.30)	1822	(453.0)
Orange, Sour, approx. 1.05 oz.	119	(29.7)	113.9	(28.30)	1822	(453.0)
Orange, Sweet, approx. 1.05 oz.	119	(29.7)	113.9	(28.30)	1822	(453.0)
Orange, Sweet & Sour, approx. 1.05 oz.	119	(29.7)	113.9	(28.30)	1822	(453.0)
Flat Pops, Junior, Cherry, Sour, approx. 0.54 oz.	61	(15.6)	113.9	(28.30)	1822	(453.0)
Cherry, Sweet, approx. 0.54 oz.	61	(15.6)	113.9	(28.30)	1822	(453.0)
Cherry, Sweet & Sour, approx. 0.54 oz.	61	(15.6)	113.9	(28.30)	1822	(453.0)
Grape, Sour, approx. 0.54 oz.	61	(15.6)	113.9	(28.30)	1822	(453.0)
Grape, Sweet, approx. 0.54 oz.	61	(15.6)	113.9	(28.30)	1822	(453.0)
Grape, Sweet & Sour, approx. 0.54 oz.	61	(15.6)	113.9	(28.30)	1822	(453.0)
Lime, Sour, approx. 0.54 oz.	61	(15.5)	113.9	(28.30)	1822	(453.0)
Lime, Sweet, approx. 0.54 oz.	61	(15.6)	113.9	(28.30)	1822	(453.0)
Lime, Sweet & Sour, approx. 0.54 oz.	61	(15.6)	113.9	(28.30)	1822	(453.0)
Orange, Sour, approx. 0.54 oz.	61	(15.6)	113.9	(28.30)	1822	(453.0)
Orange, Sweet, approx. 0.54 oz.	61	(15.6)	113.9	(28.30)	1822	(453.0)
Orange, Sweet & Sour, approx. 0.54 oz.	61	(15.6)	113.9	(28.30)	1822	(453.0)
Ice Cream Pops, "5¢," Buttermint, approx. 0.65 oz.	74	(19.0)	113.9	(28.30)	1822	(453.0)
Cherry/Vanilla, approx. 0.65 oz.	74	(19.0)	113.9	(28.30)	1822	(453.0)
Chocolate/Vanilla, approx. 0.65 oz.	74	(19.0)	113.9	(28.30)	1822	(453.0)
Coconut, approx. 0.65 oz.	74	(19.0)	113.9	(28.30)	1822	(453.0)
Pineapple/Coconut, approx. 0.65 oz.	74	(19.0)	113.9	(28.30)	1822	(453.0)
Strawberry, approx. 0.65 oz.	74	(19.0)	113.9	(28.30)	1822	(453.0)
Strawberry/Vanilla, approx. 0.65 oz.	74	(19.0)	113.9	(28.30)	1822	(453.0)
Tutti Frutti, approx. 0.65 oz.	74	(19.0)	113.9	(28.30)	1822	(453.0)
Vanilla, approx. 0.65 oz.	74	(19.0)	113.9	(28.30)	1822	(453.0)
Ice Cream Pops, "10¢," Buttermint, approx. 1.05 oz.	119	(29.7)	113.9	(28.30)	1822	(453.0)
Cherry/Vanilla, approx. 1.05 oz.	119	(29.7)	113.9	(28.30)	1822	(453.0)
Chocolate/Vanilla, approx. 1.05 oz.	119	(29.7)	113.9	(28.30)	1822	(453.0)
Coconut, approx. 1.05 oz.	119	(29.7)	113.9	(28.30)	1822	(453.0)
Pineapple/Coconut, approx. 1.05 oz.	119	(29.7)	113.9	(28.30)	1822	(453.0)
Strawberry, approx. 1.05 oz.	119	(29.7)	113.9	(28.30)	1822	(453.0)
Strawberry/Vanilla, approx. 1.05 oz.	119	(29.7)	113.9	(28.30)	1822	(453.0)
Tutti Frutti, approx. 1.05 oz.	119	(29.7)	113.9	(28.30)	1822	(453.0)
Vanilla, approx. 1.05 oz.	119	(29.7)	113.9	(28.30)	1822	(453.0)
Life Savers, Chocolate Swirled Pops, 18-oz. package (36 pieces)	2808		156.0		2496	
Chocolate Cherry Swirl, approx. 0.5 oz.	78		156.0		2496	
Chocolate Mint Swirl, approx. 0.5 oz.	78		156.0		2496	
Chocolate Vanilla Swirl, approx. 0.5 oz.	78		156.0		2496	
Life Savers, Assorted Flavor Pops, 5.25-oz. package (15 assorted pieces)	660		127.6		2042	
7.0-oz. package (20 assorted pieces)	880		127.6		2042	
Grape, approx. 0.35 oz.	44		127.6		2042	
Lime, approx. 0.35 oz.	44		127.6		2042	
Orange, approx. 0.35 oz.	44		127.6		2042	
Wild Cherry, approx. 0.35 oz.	44		127.6		2042	
Life Savers, Swirled Flavor Pops, 7.5-oz. package (15 pieces)	945		126.0		2016	
10-oz. package (20 pieces)	1260		126.0		2016	
Blueberry Banana Swirl, approx. 0.5 oz.	63		126.0		2016	
Cherry Vanilla Swirl, approx. 0.5 oz.	63		126.0		2016	
Orange Vanilla Swirl, approx. 0.5 oz	63		126.0		2016	
Strawberry Vanilla Swirl, approx. 0.5 oz.	63		126.0		2016	
Life Savers, Swirled Flavor Pops, 18-oz. package (36 pieces)	2268		126.0		2016	
Cherry Banana Swirl, approx. 0.5 oz.	63		126.0		2016	
Orange Vanilla Swirl, approx. 0.5 oz.	63		126.0		2016	
Strawberry Vanilla Swirl, approx. 0.5 oz.	63		126.0		2016	
Tootsie Roll, Caramel Tootsie Roll Pops:						
Candy counter size, 0.49-oz. pop	55	12.5	113.0	25.60	1808	409.6
Supermarket size, 5¼-oz. bag (approx. 10 or 11 pops)	593	134.4	113.0	25.60	1808	409.6
1 pop, approx. 0.49 oz. (approx. 2 per ounce)	55	12.5	113.0	25.60	1808	409.6
Tootsie Roll, Chocolate Tootsie Roll Pops, candy counter size, 0.49-oz. pop (approx. 2 per ounce)	54	12.8	111.0	26.60	1776	425.6
Tootsie Roll, Flavored Tootsie Roll Pops (cherry, grape, orange, raspberry), 0.49-oz. pop	54	13.0	111.0	26.60	1776	425.6
Supermarket size, 5¾-oz. bag (approx. 11 or 12 pops)	638	153.0	111.0	26.60	1776	425.6
8-oz. bag (approx. 16 or 17 pops)	888	212.8	111.0	26.60	1776	425.6
10¹⁄₁₆-oz. bag (approx. 20 or 21 pops)	1117	267.7	111.0	26.60	1776	425.6
1 pop, approx. 0.49 oz. (approx. 2 per ounce)	54	13.0	111.0	26.60	1776	425.6

GUM

	UNIT Cal.	UNIT Carb.
Adams Sour Apple Gum, 7-stick package	64	16.1
1 stick	9	2.3
Sour Cherry Gum, 7-stick package	64	16.1
1 stick	9	2.3
Sour Grape Gum, 7-stick package	64	16.1
1 stick	9	2.3
Sour Lemon Gum, 7-stick package	64	16.1
1 stick	9	2.3
Sour Orange Gum, 7-stick package	64	16.1
1 stick	9	2.3
Sour Raspberry Gum, 7-stick package	64	16.1
1 stick	9	2.3
Sour Strawberry Gum, 7-stick package	64	16.1
1 stick	9	2.3
Wild Berry Gum, 7-stick package	64	16.1
1 stick	9	2.3
Beech-Nut Cinnamon Gum, 5-stick package	45	11.0
7-stick package	63	15.4
17-stick package	153	37.4
1 stick	9	2.2
Fruit Stripe Gum, 5-stick package	45	11.0
7-stick package	63	15.4
17-stick package	153	37.4
1 stick	9	2.2
Peppermint Gum, 5-stick package	45	11.0
7-stick package	63	15.4
17-stick package	153	37.4
1 stick	9	2.2
Spearmint Gum, 5-stick package	45	11.0
7-stick package	63	15.4
17-stick package	153	37.4
1 stick	9	2.2
Beechies (Beach-Nut), Gum Fetti, 12-piece package	72	18.0
1 piece	6	1.5
Mixed Fruit Gum, 12-piece package	72	18.0
1 piece	6	1.5
Peppermint Gum, 12-piece package	72	18.0
1 piece	6	1.5
Pepsin Gum, 12-piece package	72	18.0
1 piece	6	1.5
Spearmint Gum, 12-piece package	72	18.0
1 piece	6	1.5
Big Red 5-stick vending size package	49	11.5
6-stick vending size package	59	13.8
7-stick package	69	16.1
17-stick Plen-t-pack	167	39.1
1 stick	10	2.3
Bubble Yum, Regular Fruit Flavor, Bubble Gum, 4-piece package	108	28.0
5-piece package	135	35.0
1 piece	27	7.0
Grape Bubble Gum, 4-piece package	108	28.0
5-piece package	135	35.0
1 piece	27	7.0
Spearmint Bubble Gum, 4-piece package	108	28.0
5-piece package	135	35.0
1 piece	27	7.0
Tropical Punch Bubble Gum, 5-piece package	108	28.0
1 piece	27	7.0
Bubblicious Soft Bubble Gum, Orange, 5-piece package	125	31.0
1 piece	25	6.2
Strawberry Bubble Gum, 5-piece package	125	31.0
1 piece	25	6.2
Carefree Sugarless Gum, Cinnamon, 5-stick package	39	8.5
17-stick package	133	28.9
1 stick	7	1.7
Fruit Gum, 5-stick package	39	8.5
17-stick package	133	28.9
1 stick	7	1.7
Peppermint Gum, 5-stick package	39	8.5
17-stick package	133	28.9
1 stick	7	1.7
Spearmint Gum, 5-stick package	39	8.5
17-stick package	133	28.9
1 stick	7	1.7
Carefree Sugarless Bubble Gum, Regular Flavor, 5-piece package	39	10.0
17-piece package	133	34.0
1 piece	8	2.0
Strawberry Bubble Gum, 5-piece package	39	10.0
1 piece	8	2.0
Wintergreen Bubble Gum, 5-piece package	39	10.0
1 piece	8	2.0
Chiclets Bubble Gum, 12-piece package	72	18.0
1 piece	6	1.5
Cherry Bubble Gum, 12-piece package	72	18.0
1 piece	6	1.5
Cinnamon Bubble Gum, 12-piece package	72	18.0
1 piece	6	1.5
Fruit Bubble Gum, 12-piece package	72	18.0
1 piece	6	1.5
Peppermint Bubble Gum, 12-piece package	72	18.0
1 piece	6	1.5
Spearmint Bubble Gum, 12-piece package	72	18.0
1 piece	6	1.5
Clorets Gum, 12-piece package	72	18.0
1 piece	6	1.5
Dentyne Regular Flavor Gum, 8-stick package	40	10.4
1 stick	5	1.3
Spearmint Gum, 8-stick package	40	10.4
1 stick	5	1.3
Doublemint Gum, 5-stick vending size	49	11.5
6-stick vending size	59	13.8
7-stick package	69	16.1
17-stick Plen-t-pack	167	39.1
1 stick	10	2.3
Estee Regular Flavor Bubble Gum, 5-stick package	15	4.8
6-Pak, 30 sticks	90	28.5
10-Pak, 50 sticks	150	47.5
1 stick	3	1.0
Cherry Bubble Gum, 5-stick package	15	4.8
6-Pak, 30 sticks	90	28.5
10-Pak, 50 sticks	150	47.5
1 stick	3	1.0
Fruit Bubble Gum, 5-stick package	15	4.8
6-Pak, 30 sticks	90	28.5
10-Pak, 50 sticks	150	47.5
1 stick	3	1.0
Grape Bubble Gum, 5-stick package	15	4.8
6-Pak, 30 sticks	90	28.5
10-Pak, 50 sticks	150	47.5
1 stick	3	1.0
Peppermint Bubble Gum, 5-stick package	15	4.8
6-Pak, 30 sticks	90	28.5
10-Pak, 50 sticks	150	47.5
1 stick	3	1.0
Spearmint Bubble Gum, 5-stick package	15	4.8
6-Pak, 30 sticks	90	28.5
10-Pak, 50 sticks	150	47.5
1 stick	3	1.0
Freedent Gum, 5-stick package	49	11.5
1 stick	10	2.3
Freshen Up Bubble Gum, 7-piece package	70	16.8
1 piece	10	2.4
Cinnamon Bubble Gum, 7-piece package	70	16.8
1 piece	10	2.4
Peppermint Bubble Gum, 7-piece package	70	16.8
1 piece	10	2.4
Spearmint Bubble Gum, 7-piece package	70	16.8
1 piece	10	2.4
Juicy Fruit Gum, 5-stick vending size	49	11.5
6-stick vending size	59	13.8
7-stick package	69	16.1
1 stick	10	2.3
Orbit Bubble Gum, 5-stick package	40	trace
1 stick	8	trace
Cinnamon Bubble Gum, 5-stick package	40	trace
1 stick	8	trace
Peppermint Bubble Gum, 5-stick package	40	trace
1 stick	8	trace
Spearmint Bubble Gum, 5-stick package	40	trace
1 stick	8	trace
Spearmint Gum, 5-stick vending size	49	11.5
6-stick vending size	59	13.8
7-stick package	69	16.1
17-stick Plen-t-pack	167	39.1
1 stick	10	2.3

	UNIT Cal.	UNIT Carb.
Trident Original Flavor Gum, 5-piece package	23	6.0
1 piece	5	1.2
Bubble Gum, 5-piece package	23	6.0
1 piece	5	1.2
Cinnamon Gum, 5-piece package	23	6.0
1 piece	5	1.2
Fruit Gum, 5-piece package	23	6.0
1 piece	5	1.2
Spearmint Gum, 5-piece package	23	6.0
1 piece	5	1.2
Xylitol Peppermint Gum, 5-piece package	24	(6.0)
1 piece	5	(1.2)
Spearmint Gum, 5-piece package	24	(6.0)
1 piece	5	(1.2)

25 FROZEN CONFECTIONS •

	UNIT		1 OZ., BY WT.		1 FLUID OZ.		1 CUP, PACKED	
	Cal.	Carb.	Cal.	Carb.	Cal.	Carb.	Cal.	Carb.
ICE CREAM, ICE MILK, SHERBET, and ICE, based on generic data								
ICE CREAM								
Vanilla, regular (10.8% fat), ½ gallon (2 lb. 5½ oz.)	2153	253.8	57.3	6.76	33.6	3.96	269	31.7
1 cup (approx. 4.7 oz.)	269	31.7	57.3	6.76	33.6	3.96	269	31.7
Vanilla, rich (16.0% fat), ½ gallon (approx. 2 lb. 10 oz.)	2805	256.5	66.9	6.12	43.6	4.00	349	32.0
1 cup (approx. 5.2 oz.)	349	32.0	66.9	6.12	43.6	4.00	349	32.0
French Vanilla, Soft Serve (13% fat), ½ gallon (approx. 3 lb. 1 oz.)	3014	306.3	61.8	6.27	47.1	4.78	377	38.2
1 cup (approx. 3.5 oz.)	377	38.2	61.8	6.27	47.1	4.78	377	38.2
ICE MILK								
Vanilla (4.3% fat), ½ gallon (2 lb. 5 oz.)	1469	231.7	39.7	6.27	23.0	3.62	184	29.0
1 cup (approx. 4.6 oz.)	184	29.0	39.7	6.27	23.0	3.62	184	29.0
Vanilla, Soft Serve (2.6% fat), ½ gallon (approx. 3 lb. 1 oz.)	1787	307.0	36.2	6.22	27.9	4.80	223	38.4
1 cup (approx. 6.2 oz.)	223	38.4	36.2	6.22	27.9	4.80	223	38.4
SHERBET								
Orange (2.0% fat), ½ gallon (approx. 3 lb. 6½ oz.)	2158	469.2	39.7	8.63	33.8	7.34	270	58.7
1 cup (approx. 6.8 oz.)	270	58.7	39.7	8.63	33.8	7.34	270	58.7
ICE								
Lime-flavored, 1 cup (approx. 6.8 oz.)	247	62.9	36.3	9.24	30.9	7.86	247	62.9

ICE CREAM, ICE MILK, FROZEN YOGURT, SHERBET, and SIMILAR FROZEN DESSERTS, by brand

The list that follows is alphabetized by the main descriptive fruit or flavor. A list alphabetized by brand follows this one.

Containers with more than one flavor, such as chocolate/vanilla/strawberry, are listed at the end of this section.

	UNIT		1 OZ., BY WT.		1 FLUID OZ.		1 CUP, PACKED	
	Cal.	Carb.	Cal.	Carb.	Cal.	Carb.	Cal.	Carb.
ALMOND (see Butter Almond, Maple Almond, Toasted Almond and Vanilla Almond Bark)								
APPLE								
Apple Sunshine Bars, **Hood,** Apple Water Ice on Stick, 2-fl.-oz. bar	50	13.0			25.0	6.50	200	52.0
BANANA								
Danny-in-a-Cup Hard Frozen Yogurt, 8-fl.-oz. container	210	42.0	35.0	7.00	26.3	5.25	210	42.0
Frozfruit Ice Milk Confection, 16-fl.-oz. (1 pint) container	480	79.6			30.0	4.98	240	39.8
Fudgesicle, 30-fl.-oz. box (12 pops)	1224	282.0			40.8	9.40	326	75.2
1 pop, approx. 2½ fl. oz.	102	23.5			40.8	9.40	326	75.2
Jell-O Banana Pudding Pop, 19.8-fl.-oz. box (12 bars)	1080	180.0			54.5	9.09	436	72.7
1 bar, approx. 1.65 fl. oz.	90	15.0			54.5	9.09	436	72.7
Natural Nectar Ice Cream, 3-gallon tub	(16128)	(1931.5)	64.4	7.71	(42.0)	(5.03)	(336)	(40.2)
Popsicle, 36-fl.-oz. box (12 pops)	840	198.0			23.3	5.50	187	44.0
1 pop, approx. 3 fl. oz.	70	16.5			23.3	5.50	187	44.0
Weight Watchers Frosted Treat, 7-fl.-oz. serving	120	22.0	28.6	5.24	17.1	3.14	137	25.1
Banana-Red Raspberry Twirl, **Breyers** Ice Cream, pint container	600	84.0	57.5	8.05	37.5	5.25	300	42.0
½-gallon container	2400	336.0	57.5	8,05	37.5	5.25	300	42.0
Banana-Red Raspberry Twirl, **Light n' Lively (Sealtest)** Ice Milk, ½-gallon container	1760	336.0	47.3	9.02	27.5	5.25	220	42.0
Banana Split, **Dairy Queen,** 13½ oz.	540	91.0	40.0	7.63				
Banana Strawberry Twirl, **Breyers** Ice Cream, quart container	1200	168.0	57.5	8,05	37.5	5.25	300	42.0
½-gallon container	2400	336.0	57.5	8.05	37.5	5.25	300	42.0
Banana Strawberry Twirl, **Light n' Lively (Sealtest)** Ice Milk, ½-gallon container	1760	336.0	47.2	9.01	27.5	5.25	220	42.0
BLACK CHERRY								
Good Humor Ice Cream, ½-gallon container	2080	224.0			32.5	3.50	260	28.0
Tuscan Soft Frozen Yogurt, pint container	460	96.0	28.8	6.00	28.8	6.00	230	48.0
Bordeaux Black Cherry, **Weight Watchers** Frosted Treat, 7-fl.-oz. serving	120	22.0	28.6	5.24	17.1	3.14	137	25.1

	UNIT		1 OZ., BY WT.		1 FLUID OZ.		1 CUP, PACKED	
	Cal.	Carb.	Cal.	Carb.	Cal.	Carb.	Cal.	Carb.
BLACK WALNUT								
Meadow Gold Ice Cream, quart container	1280	128.0	68.3	6.83	40.0	4.00	320	32.0
BLACKBERRY								
Weight Watchers Frosted Treat, 7-fl.-oz. serving	120	22.0	28.6	5.24	17.1	3.14	137	25.1
BLUEBERRY								
Beautiful Day Frozen Yogurt bars, uncoated Frozen Yogurt, 15-fl.-oz. box (6 bars)	240	30.0			16.0	2.00	128	16.0
1 bar, approx. 2½ fl. oz.	40	5.0			16.0	2.00	128	16.0
Carvel Sherbet, 3-fl.-oz. container	105	23.4	39.7	8.84	35.0	7.80	280	62.4
Weight Watchers Frosted Treat, 7-fl.-oz. serving	120	22.0	28.6	5.24	17.1	3.14	137	25.1
BLUE GRAPE								
Popsicle, 36-fl.-oz. box (12 pops)	840	198.0			23.3	5.50	187	44.0
1 pop, approx. 3 fl. oz.	70	16.5			23.3	5.50	187	44.0
BLUE RASPBERRY								
Popsicle, 36-fl. oz. box (12 pops)	840	198.0			23.3	5.50	187	44.0
1 pop, approx. 3 fl. oz.	70	16.5			23.3	5.50	187	44.0
BOYSENBERRY								
Danny-in-a-Cup Hard Frozen Yogurt, 8-fl.-oz. (1 cup) container	210	42.0	35.0	7.00	26.3	5.25	210	42.0
Danny-on-a-Stick, uncoated, 15-fl.-oz. box (6 bars)	420	78.0			28.0	5.20	224	41.6
1 bar, approx. 2½ fl. oz.	70	13.0			28.0	5.20	224	41.6
Danny-on-a-Stick, carob-coated, 15-fl.-oz. box (6 bars)	840	90.0			56.0	6.00	448	48.0
1 bar, approx. 2½ fl. oz.	140	15.0			56.0	6.00	448	48.0
BRANDY ALEXANDER								
Meadow Gold, Parfait, 1 serving	307	21.5						
BUTTER ALMOND								
Breyers Ice Cream, pint container	680	60.0	68.8	6.07	42.5	3.75	340	30.0
½-gallon container	2720	240.0	68.8	6.07	42.5	3.75	340	30.0
BUTTER BRICKLE								
Johnston Hard Frozen Yogurt, 8-fl.-oz. container	220	42.0	(36.7)	(7.00)	27.5	5.25	220	42.0
Sealtest Ice Cream, quart container	1200	152.0			37.5	4.75	300	38.0
½-gallon container	2400	304.0			37.5	4.75	300	38.0
BUTTER PECAN								
Breyers Ice Cream, pint container	720	60.0	72.9	6.07	45.0	3.75	360	30.0
½-gallon container	2880	240.0	72.9	6.07	45.0	3.75	360	30.0
Good Humor Ice Cream, ½-gallon container	2080	224.0			32.5	3.50	260	28.0
Harbison's Ice Cream, ½-gallon container	2240	256.0			35.0	4.00	280	32.0
Meadow Gold Ice Cream, quart container	1200	128.0	64.1	6.83	37.5	4.00	300	32.0
Weight Watchers Frosted Treat, 7-fl.-oz. serving	120	22.0	28.6	5.24	17.1	3.14	137	25.1
CANTALOUPE								
le sorbet, Sherbet, 4-fl.-oz. container	72	16.8			18.0	4.20	144	33.6
CARAMEL								
Caramel Nut, **Light n' Lively (Sealtest)** Ice Milk, 4-fl.-oz. container	120	18.0	51.5	7.73	30.0	4.50	240	36.0
pint container	480	72.0	51.5	7.73	30.0	4.50	240	36.0
½-gallon container	1920	288.0	51.5	7.73	30.0	4.50	240	36.0
Caramel Pecan, **Johnston** Hard Frozen Yogurt, 8-fl.-oz. container	200	37.0	(33.3)	(6.17)	25.0	4.63	200	37.0
Caramel Sundae, **Meadow Gold,** 5.1 oz.	282	50.8	55.3	9.96				
CAROB								
Häagen-Dazs Ice Cream, pint container	1013	80.2	64.3	5.09	63.3	5.01	507	40.1
CHERRY								
Carvel Sherbet, 3-fl.-oz. container	105	23.4	39.7	8.84	35.0	7.80	280	62.4
Chicquita Fruit & Juice Pops, 16-fl.-oz. (1-pint) box (8 pops)	400	104.0			25.0	6.50	200	52.0
1 pop, approx. 2 fl. oz.	50	13.0			25.0	6.50	200	52.0
Popsicle, 36-fl.-oz. box (12 pops)	840	198.0			23.3	5.50	187	44.0
1 pop, approx. 3 fl. oz.	70	16.5			23.3	5.50	187	44.0

	UNIT		1 OZ., BY WT.		1 FLUID OZ.		1 CUP, PACKED	
	Cal.	Carb.	Cal.	Carb.	Cal.	Carb.	Cal.	Carb.
Cherry Nugget, **Sealtest** Ice Cream, quart container	1120	128.0			35.0	4.00	280	32.0
½-gallon container	2240	256.0			35.0	4.00	280	32.0
CHERRY VANILLA								
Breyers Ice Cream, pint container	560	68.0	56.7	6.89	35.0	4.25	280	34.0
½-gallon container	2240	272.0	56.7	6.89	35.0	4.25	280	34.0
Meadow Gold Ice Cream, quart container	1120	144.0	59.7	7.69	35.0	4.50	280	36.0
Sealtest Ice Cream, pint container	520	68.0	52.6	6.89	32.5	4.25	260	34.0
½-gallon container	2080	272.0	52.6	6.89	32.5	4.25	260	34.0
CHIP CRUNCH								
Good Humor Whammy bars, 12.8-oz. box (8 bars)	880	80.0	68.8	6.25				
1 bar, approx. 1.6 oz.	110	10.0	68.8	6.25				
CHOCOLATE								
Armel Frozen Dietary Dairy Dessert, pint container	480	52.0			30.0	3.25	240	26.0
Baskin Robbins Ice Cream, 1 scoop, approx. 2.5 oz.	165	20.4	66.0	8.16	(55.0)	(6.80)	(440)	(54.4)
Bi-Sicle, 30-fl.-oz. box (12 pops)	1344	256.8			44.8	8.56	358	68.5
1 pop, approx. 2½ fl. oz.	112	21.4			44.8	8.56	358	68.5
Breyers Ice Cream, pint container	640	76.0	64.8	7.70	40.0	4.75	320	38.0
½-gallon container	2560	304.0	64.8	7.70	40.0	4.75	320	38.0
Carnation, Ice Cream Bon Bons, 1.7-oz. package	120	10.9	70.7	6.37	48.0	4.36		
3.42-oz. package	240	21.8	70.7	6.37	48.0	4.36		
13.69-oz. package	960	87.2	70.7	6.37	48.0	4.36		
1 bon bon, 0.34 oz.	24	2.2	70.7	6.37	48.0	4.36		
Carvel, Sherbet, 3-fl.-oz. container	105	23.4	39.7	8.84	35.0	7.80	280	62.4
Carvel "Thinny-Thin," 3-fl.-oz. container	56	10.4	30.9	5.82	18.7	3.47	149	27.7
Colombo bar, chocolate-coated, 15-fl.-oz. box (6 bars)	870	102.0			58.0	6.80	464	54.4
1 bar, approx. 2½ fl. oz.	145	17.0			58.0	6.80	464	54.4
Dairy Queen Sundae								
Small, 3¾ oz.	190	33.0	51.4	8.92				
Regular, 6¼ oz.	310	56.0	50.0	9.03				
Large, 8¾ oz.	440	78.0	50.6	8.97				
Danny-in-a-Cup Hard Frozen Yogurt, 8-fl.-oz. (1-cup) container	190	32.0	31.7	5.33	23.8	4.00	190	32.0
Danny-on-a-Stick, uncoated, 15-fl.-oz. box (6 bars)	360	60.0			24.0	4.00	192	32.0
1 bar, approx. 2½ fl. oz.	60	10.0			24.0	4.00	192	32.0
Danny-on-a-Stick, chocolate-coated, 15-fl.-oz. box (6 bars)	780	72.0			52.0	4.80	416	38.4
1 bar, approx. 2½ fl. oz.	130	12.0			52.0	4.80	416	38.4
Danny-Yo Soft Frozen Yogurt, 3½-fl.-oz. container	140	26.0			40.0	7.43	320	59.4
Friendly's Cake Cones filled with chocolate ice cream:								
regular, approx. 4.2 oz. (4 oz. ice cream, 0.2 oz. cone)	260	32.0	61.9	7.62				
double dip, approx. 7.2 oz. (7 oz. ice cream, 0.2 oz. cone)	440	54.0	61.1	7.50				
Friendly's Sugar Cones filled with chocolate ice cream:								
regular, approx. 4½ oz. (4 oz. ice cream, ½ oz. cone)	310	41.0	68.9	9.11				
double dip, approx. 7½ oz. (7 oz. ice cream, ½ oz. cone)	490	63.0	65.3	8.40				
Fudgsicle, 30-fl.-oz. box (12 pops)	1224	284.4			40.8	9.48	236	75.8
1 pop, approx. 2½ fl. oz.	102	23.7			40.8	9.48	236	75.8
Good Humor Ice Cream, ½-gallon container	2080	240.0			32.5	3.75	260	30.0
Good Humor Chocolate Eclair Bars, 18-oz. box (6 bars)	1320	150.0	73.3	8.33				
1 bar, approx. 3 oz.	220	25.0	73.3	8.33				
Good Humor Whammy Bars, 12.8-oz. box (8 bars)	800	72.0	62.5	5.63				
1 bar, approx. 1.6 oz.	100	9.0	62.5	5.63				
Häagen-Dazs Ice Cream, pint container	1073	96.2	70.9	6.36	67.0	6.01	536	48.1
Harbison's Ice Cream, ½-gallon container	2080	256.0			32.5	4.00	260	32.0

	UNIT		1 OZ., BY WT.		1 FLUID OZ.		1 CUP, PACKED	
	Cal.	Carb.	Cal.	Carb.	Cal.	Carb.	Cal.	Carb.
Hood Chocolate Pudding Stix, 1.9-fl.-oz. bar	100	17.0			52.6	8.95	421	71.6
Howard Johnson's Ice Cream, pint container	884	(71.4)	(89.5)	(7.23)	55.3	(4.46)	442	(35.7)
quart container	1768	(142.5)	(89.5)	(7.23)	55.3	(4.46)	442	(35.7)
Jell-O Chocolate Pudding Pop, 24-fl.-oz. box (12 bars)	1200	192.0			50.0	8.00	400	64.0
1 bar, approx. 2 fl. oz.	100	16.0			50.0	8.00	400	64.0
Johnston Hard Frozen Yogurt, 8-fl.-oz. container	240	47.0	(40.0)	(7.83)	30.0	5.88	240	47.0
Johnston Soft Frozen Yogurt, 8-fl.-oz. container	203	36.0			25.4	4.50	203	36.0
Light n' Lively (Sealtest) Ice Milk, 4-fl.-oz. container	100	19.0	43.0	8.16	25.0	4.75	200	38.0
pint container	400	76.0	43.0	8.16	25.0	4.75	200	38.0
½-gallon container	1600	304.0	43.0	8.16	25.0	4.75	200	38.0
Lucerne Dietetic Ice Cream, pint container	479		51.0		29.9		239	
Luxury Ice Cream, ½-gallon container	2080	256.0	55.4	6.82	32.5	4.00	260	32.0
Meadow Gold Ice Cream, quart container	1120	144.0	59.8	7.69	35.0	4.50	280	36.0
Popsicle, 36-fl.-oz. box (12 pops)	840	198.0			23.3	5.50	187	44.0
1 pop, approx. 3 fl. oz.	70	16.5			23.3	5.50	187	44.0
Schrafft's Think Thin Ice Milk, pint container	540	104.0			33.8	6.50	270	52.0
quart container	1080	208.0			33.8	6.50	270	52.0
Schrafft's Light Chocolate All Natural Ice Milk, pint container	540	104.0			33.8	6.50	270	52.0
Sealtest Ice Cream, pint container	560	72.0	56.7	7.29	35.0	4.50	280	36.0
½-gallon container	2240	288.0	56.7	7.29	35.0	4.50	280	36.0
Swift's Ice Cream, ½-gallon container	2080	256.0	57.8	7.11	32.5	4.00	260	32.0
Tuscan bars, uncoated, 15-fl.-oz. box (6 bars)	510	96.0			34.0	6.40	272	51.2
1 bar, approx. 2½ fl. oz.	85	16.0			34.0	6.40	272	51.2
Tuscan bars, chocolate-coated, 15-fl.-oz. box (6 bars)	900	102.0			60.0	6.80	480	54.4
1 bar, approx. 2½ fl. oz.	150	17.0			60.0	6.80	480	54.4
Tuscan Soft Frozen Yogurt, pint container	504	96.0	31.5	6.00	31.5	6.00	252	48.0
Weight Watchers Chocolate Treat Frozen Confection, 16.5-fl.-oz. box (6 bars)	600	114.0			36.4	6.91	291	55.3
1 bar, approx. 2.75 fl. oz.	100	19.0			36.4	6.91	291	55.3
Weight Watchers Chocolate Mint Treat Frozen Confection, 16.5-fl.-oz. box (6 bars)	600	114.0			36.4	6.91	291	55.3
1 bar, approx. 2.75 fl. oz.	100	19.0			36.4	6.91	291	55.3
Weight Watchers Frosted Treat, 7-fl.-oz. serving	120	22.0	28.6	5.24	17.1	3.14	137	25.1
Weight Watchers Frozen Dietary Dessert, 5-fl.-oz. container	100	19.0	32.3	6.18	20.0	3.80	160	30.4
Chocolate Chip, **Good Humor** Ice Cream, ½-gallon container	2400	240.0			37.5	3.75	300	30.0
Chocolate Chip, **Meadow Gold** Ice Cream, quart container	1200	136.0	64.0	7.26	37.5	4.25	300	34.0
Chocolate Chip, **Sealtest** Ice Cream, quart container	1200	136.0			37.5	4.25	300	34.0
½-gallon container	2400	272.0			37.5	4.25	300	34.0
Chocolate Fudge, **Baskin Robbins** Ice Cream, 1 scoop, approx. 2.5 oz.	178	21.5	71.7	8.52	(59.3)	(7.17)	(475)	(57.3)
Chocolate Marshmallow Twirl, **Light n' Lively (Sealtest)** Ice Milk, 4-fl.-oz. container	120	23.0	51.5	9.88	30.0	5.75	240	46.0
pint container	480	92.0	51.5	9.88	30.0	5.75	240	46.0
½-gallon container	1920	368.0	51.5	9.88	30.0	5.75	240	46.0
Chocolate Mint, **Carvel** "Thinny-Thin," 3-fl.-oz. container	56	10.4	30.9	5.82	18.7	3.47	149	27.7
Chocolate Revel, **Meadow Gold** Ice Cream, quart container	1120	152.0	59.8	8.11	35.0	4.75	280	38.0
Chocolate Sundae, **Luxury** ½-gallon container	2400	304.0	63.9	8.10	37.5	4.75	300	38.0
Dutch Chocolate Almond, **Breyers** Ice Cream, quart container	1440	144.0			45.0	4.50	360	36.0
½-gallon container	2880	288.0			45.0	4.50	360	36.0
Mint Chocolate Chip, **Breyers** Ice Cream, pint container	680	72.0	68.9	7.29	42.5	4.50	340	36.0
½-gallon container	2720	288.0	68.9	7.29	42.5	4.50	340	36.0

	UNIT		1 OZ., BY WT.		1 FLUID OZ.		1 CUP, PACKED	
	Cal.	Carb.	Cal.	Carb.	Cal.	Carb.	Cal.	Carb.
Mint Chocolate Chip, **Luxury** Ice Cream, ½-gallon container	2720	256.0	72.5	6.82	42.5	4.00	340	32.0
COCOA								
Royal Dutch Cocoa, **Natural Nectar** Ice Cream, pint container	(672)	(80.5)	64.4	7.71	(42.0)	(5.03)	(336)	(40.2)
quart container	(1345)	(161.0)	64.4	7.71	(42.0)	(5.03)	(366)	(40.2)
COCONUT								
Coconut Pineapple, **Weight Watchers** Frosted Treat, 7-fl.-oz. serving	120	22.0	28.6	5.24	17.1	3.14	137	25.1
COFFEE								
Breyers Ice Cream, pint container	560	60.0	56.7	6.07	35.0	3.75	280	30.0
½-gallon container	2240	240.0	56.7	6.07	35.0	3.75	280	30.0
Häagen-Dazs Ice Cream, pint container	1033	91.6	68.3	6.03	64.6	5.73	517	45.8
Light n' Lively (Sealtest) Ice Milk, 4-fl.-oz. container	100	17.0	43.0	7.30	25.0	4.25	200	34.0
pint container	400	68.0	43.0	7.30	25.0	4.25	200	34.0
½-gallon container	1600	272.0	43.0	7.30	25.0	4.25	200	34.0
Schrafft's Sugar-Less Frozen Dietary Dairy Dessert, pint container	600	56.0	(47.6)	(4.44)	37.5	3.50	300	28.0
Sealtest Ice Cream, ½-gallon container	2240	256.0	56.7	6.40	35.0	4.00	280	32.0
Tuscan bars (uncoated), 15-fl.-oz. box (6 bars)	420	84.0			28.0	5.60	224	44.8
1 bar, approx. 2½ fl. oz.	70	14.0			28.0	5.60	224	44.8
Tuscan bars, Chocolate-coated, 15-fl.-oz. box (6 bars)	780	102.0			52.0	6.80	416	54.4
1 bar, approx. 2½ fl. oz.	130	17.0			52.0	6.80	416	54.4
Tuscan Soft Frozen Yogurt, pint container	440	88.0	36.7	7.33	27.5	5.50	220	44.0
Weight Watchers Frosted Treat, 7-fl.-oz. serving	120	22.0	28.6	5.24	17.1	3.14	137	25.1
Weight Watchers Frozen Dietary Dessert, quart container	700	133.0	33.0	6.30	21.9	4.16	175	33.3
CRAN•GRAPE								
Ocean Spray Juice & Fruit Bars, 15-fl.-oz. box (6 bars)	480	120.0			32.0	8.00	256	64.0
1 bar, approx. 2½ fl. oz.	80	200			32.0	8.00	256	64.0
CRAN•RASPBERRY								
Ocean Spray Juice & Fruit Bars, 15-fl.-oz. box (6 bars)	420	114.0			28.0	7.60	224	60.8
1 bar, approx. 2½ fl. oz.	70	19.0			28.0	7.60	224	60.8
CREAMSICLE								
Creamsicle, Ice Cream Center Deluxe, 30-fl.-oz. box (12 pops)	936	153.6			31.2	5.12	250	41.0
1 pop, approx. 2½ fl. oz.	78	12.8			31.2	5.12	250	41.0
DAIQUIRI ICE								
Baskin Robbins, 1 scoop, approx. 2.5 oz.	84	20.9	33.6	8.36	(28.0)	(6.97)	(224)	(55.7)
DREAMSICLE								
Dreamsicle, Ice Milk Center Deluxe, 30-fl.-oz. box (12 pops)	840	157.2			28.0	5.24	224	41.9
1 pop, approx. 2½ fl. oz.	70	13.1			28.0	5.24	224	41.9
EGG NOG								
Breyers Ice Cream, quart container	1200	128.0			37.5	4.00	300	32.0
½-gallon container	2400	256.0			37.5	4.00	300	32.0
ENGLISH WALNUT								
Roasted English Walnut, **Breyers** Ice Cream, quart container	1360	120.0			42.5	3.75	340	30.0
½-gallon container	2720	240.0			42.5	3.75	340	30.0
FIESTA								
Fiesta Sundae, **Dairy Queen,** 9.5 oz.	570	84.0	60.0	8.84				
FREEZE								
Dairy Queen, 14.0 oz.	500	89.0	35.7	6.36				
FUDGE								
Fudge Royale, **Sealtest** Ice Cream, pint container	600	80.0	60.8	8.10	37.5	5.00	300	40.0
½-gallon container	2400	320.0	60.8	8,10	37.5	5.00	300	40.0
Fudge-Vanilla Ice Cream Sundae, **Friendly's,** approx. 6.3 oz.	420	50.0	66.7	7.94				
Hot Fudge Sundae, **Friendly's,** approx. 5⅓ oz.	290	44.6	54.4	8.36				
Hot Fudge Sundae, **Meadow Gold,** 5⅓-oz.	290	44.6	54.4	8.36				
Royal Fudge Ice Cream, **Good Humor,** ½-gallon container	1920	224.0			30.0	3.50	240	28.0

	UNIT		1 OZ., BY WT.		1 FLUID OZ.		1 CUP, PACKED	
	Cal.	Carb.	Cal.	Carb.	Cal.	Carb.	Cal.	Carb.
GRAPE								
Good Humor Ice Whammy, 18-oz. box (12 pops)	600	156.0	33.3	8.67				
1 pop, approx. 1½ oz.	50	13.0	33.3	8.67				
Popsicle, 36-fl.-oz. box (12 pops)	840	198.0			23.3	5.50	187	44.0
1 pop, approx. 3 fl. oz.	70	16.5			23.3	5.50	187	44.0
Super Juice Frozen Juice Bars, 24-fl.-oz. box (8 bars)	480	112.0			20.0	4.67	160	37.4
1 bar, approx. 3 fl. oz.	60	14.0			20.0	4.67	160	37.4
GUANABANA								
Carvel Sherbet, 3-fl.-oz. container	105	23.4	39.7	8.84	35.0	7.80	280	62.4
HEAVENLY HASH								
Light n' Lively Sealtest Ice Milk, ½-gallon container	1920	320.0			30.0	8.59	240	40.0
Sealtest Ice Cream, ½-gallon container	2400	304.0			37.5	4.75	300	38.0
HONEY								
Häagen-Dazs Ice Cream, pint container	1004	69.9	64.4	4.48	62.8	4.37	502	35.0
Natural Nectar Ice Cream Sandwich with Honey, 18-fl.-oz. box (6 sandwiches)	1236	174.6			68.7	9.70	550	77.6
1 sandwich, approx. 3 fl. oz.	206	29.1			68.7	9.70	550	77.6
LEMON								
Beautiful Day Frozen Yogurt bars, uncoated, 15-fl.-oz. box (6 bars)	240	30.0			16.0	2.00	128	16.0
1 bar, approx. 2½ fl. oz.	40	5.0			16.0	2.00	128	16.0
Carvel Sherbet, 3-fl.-oz. container	105	23.4	39.7	8.84	35.0	7.80	280	62.4
le sorbet Sherbet, 4-fl.-oz. container	96	22.1			24.0	5.53	192	44.2
Schrafft's Sugar-Less Frozen Dietary Dairy Dessert, pint container	600	56.0	(47.6)	(4.44)	37.5	3.50	300	28.0
Sealtest Sherbet, quart container	1040	240.0	(38.5)	(8.88)	32.5	7.50	260	60.0
½-gallon container	2080	480.0	(38.5)	(8.88)	32.5	7.50	260	60.0
Hood, Lemonade Sunshine Bars, Lemonade Water Ice on Stick, 2-fl.-oz. bar	50	13.0			25.0	6.50	200	520
Lemon Chiffon, **Light n' Lively (Sealtest)** Ice Milk, 4-fl.-oz. container	120	23.0	51.5	9.88	30.0	5.75	240	46.0
pint container	480	92.0	51.5	9.88	30.0	5.75	240	46.0
½-gallon container	1920	368.0	51.5	9.88	30.0	5.75	240	46.0
Lemon Chiffon, **Weight Watchers** Frozen Dietary Dessert, 5-fl.-oz. container	100	19.0	32.3	6.18	20.0	3.80	160	30.4
Lemon Custard, **Weight Watchers** Frosted Treat, 7-fl.-oz. serving	120	22.0	28.6	5.24	17.1	3.14	137	25.1
White Lemon, **Popsicle,** 36-fl.-oz. box (12 pops)	840	198.0			23.3	5.50	187	44.0
1 pop, approx. 3 fl. oz.	70	16.5			23.3	5.50	187	44.0
LIME								
Carvel Sherbet, 3-fl.-oz. container	105	23.4	39.7	8.84	35.0	7.80	280	62.4
Meadow Gold, quart container	960	216.0	35.3	7.95	30.0	6.75	240	54.0
Popsicle, 36-fl.-oz. box (12 pops)	840	198.0			23.3	5.50	187	44.0
1 pop, approx. 3 fl. oz.	70	16.5			23.3	5.50	187	44.0
Sealtest Sherbet, quart container	1040	240.0	(38.5)	(8.88)	32.5	7.50	260	60.0
½-gallon container	2080	480.0	(38.5)	(8.8)	32.5	7.50	260	60.0
LOVE DROPS								
Tofutti Chocolate Supreme with Chocolate-Covered Graham Cookies, Non-dairy Frozen Dessert, pint container	920	104.0			57.5	6.50	460	52.0
MAMEY								
Carvel Sherbet, 3-fl.-oz. container	105	23.4	39.7	8.84	35.0	7.80	280	62.4
MANDARIN ORANGE								
Tuscan Soft Frozen Yogurt, pint container	460	96.0	38.3	8.00	28.8	6.00	230	48.0
MANGO								
Carvel Sherbet, 3-fl.-oz. container	105	23.4	39.7	8.84	35.0	7.80	280	62.4
Weight Watchers Frosted Treat, 7-fl.-oz. serving	120	22.0	28.6	5.24	17.1	3.14	137	25.1
MAPLE								
Maple Almond, **Natural Nectar** Ice Cream, pint container	(672)	(80.5)	64.7	7.71	(42.0)	(5.03)	(336)	(40.2)
quart container	(1345)	(161.0)	64.7	7.71	(42.0)	(5.03)	(336)	(40.2)

	UNIT		1 OZ., BY WT.		1 FLUID OZ.		1 CUP, PACKED	
	Cal.	Carb.	Cal.	Carb.	Cal.	Carb.	Cal.	Carb.
Old Fashioned Maple, **Weight Watchers** Frozen Dietary Dessert, 5-fl.-oz. container	100	19.0	32.3	6.18	20.0	3.80	160	30.4
MINT								
Alpine Mint, **Weight Watchers** Frozen Dietary Dessert, 5-fl.-oz. container	100	19.0	32.3	6.18	20.0	3.80	160	30.4
Mint Chocolate Chip, **Breyers** Ice Cream, pint container	680	72.0	68.9	7.29	42.5	4.50	340	36.0
½-gallon container	2720	288.0	68.9	7.29	42.5	4.50	340	36.0
Mint Chocolate Chip, **Luxury** Ice Cream, ½-gallon container	2720	256.0	72.5	6.82	42.5	4.00	340	32.0
True Mint, **Weight Watchers** Frosted Treat, 7-fl.-oz. serving	120	22.0	28.6	5.24	17.1	3.14	137	25.1
MOCHA								
Brazilian Mocha, **Natural Nectar** Ice Cream, pint container	(672)	(80.5)	64.4	7.71	(42.0)	(5.03)	(336)	(40.2)
quart container	(1345)	(161.0)	64.4	7.71	(42.0)	(5.03)	(336)	(40.2)
Mocha Pie, **Natural Nectar,** 12-fl.-oz. box (3 pies)	1023	110.1			85.3	9.18	682	73.4
1 pie, approx. 4 fl. oz.	341	36.7			85.3	9.18	682	73.4
MR. MISTY								
Dairy Queen "Mr. Misty" Float, 14½-oz.	390	74.0	26.9	5.10				
"Mr. Misty" Freeze, 14½ oz.	500	91.0	34.5	6.28				
"Mr. Misty" Kiss, 3⅛ oz.	70	17.0	22.4	5.43				
NECTAR								
Natural Nectar Nectar Pie, 12-fl.-oz. box (3 pies)	1023	110.1			85.3	9.18	682	73.4
1 pie, approx. 4 fl. oz.	341	36.7			85.3	9.18	682	73.4
ORANGE								
Baskin-Robbins Sherbet, 1 scoop, approx. 2.5 oz.	99	20.9	39.6	8.36	(33.0)	(6.97)	(264)	(55.7)
Carvel Sherbet, 3-fl.-oz. container	105	23.4	39.7	8.84	35.0	7.80	280	62.4
Dolly Madison Frozen Yogurt, ½-gallon container	1704	336.0			26.6	5.25	213	42.0
Good Humor, Orange Ice Whammy, 18-oz. box (12 pops)	600	156.0	33.3	8.67				
1 pop, approx. 1½ oz.	50	13.0	33.3	8.67				
Häagen-Dazs Sorbet & Cream, Orange Fruit Ice and Vanilla Ice Cream, pint container	880	124.0			55.0	7.75	440	62.0
Hood, Orange Foam Cup, Orange Water Ice, 4-fl.-oz. cup	110	25.0			27.5	6.25	220	50.0
Hood, Orange Sunshine Cup, Orange Water Ice, 3-fl.-oz. cup	80	19.0			26.7	6.33	213	50.7
Howard Johnson's Sherbet, pint container	528	(112.1)	(38.7)	(8.22)	33.0	(7.01)	264	(56.1)
quart container	1056	(224.2)	(38.7)	(8.22)	33.0	(7.01)	264	(56.1)
le sorbet Sherbet, 4-fl.-oz. container	71	18.1			17.8	4.53	142	36.2
Meadow Gold Sherbet, quart container	960	216.0	35.3	7.95	30.0	6.75	240	54.0
Popsicle, 36-fl.-oz. box (12 pops)	840	198.0			23.3	5.50	187	44.0
1 pop, approx. 3 fl. oz.	70	16.5			23.3	5.50	187	44.0
Sealtest Sherbet, quart container	1040	240.0	(38.5)	(8.88)	32.5	7.50	260	60.0
½-gallon container	2080	480.0	(38.5)	(8.88)	32.5	7.50	260	60.0
Weight Watchers Frosted Treat, 7-fl.-oz. serving	120	22.0	28.6	5.24	17.1	3.14	137	25.1
ORANGE-PINEAPPLE								
Breyers Ice Cream, ½-gallon container	2240	272.0	56.7	6.80	35.0	4.25	280	34.0
Carvel Sherbet, 3-fl.-oz. container	105	23.4	39.7	8.84	35.0	7.80	280	62.4
Danny-in-a-Cup Hard Frozen Yogurt, 8-fl.-oz. container	210	42.0	35.0	7.00	26.3	5.25	210	42.0
Light n' Lively (Sealtest) Ice Milk, 4-fl.-oz. container	100	18.0	43.0	7.73	25.0	4.50	200	36.0
pint container	400	72.0	43.0	7.73	25.0	4.50	200	36.0
½-gallon container	1600	288.0	43.0	7.73	25.0	4.50	200	36.0
PAPAYA								
Weight Watchers Frosted Treat, 7-fl.-oz. serving	120	22.0	28.6	5.24	17.1	3.14	137	25.1
PARFAIT								
Dairy Queen Parfait, 10 oz.	430	76.0	43.0	7.60				
PEACH								
Beautiful Day Frozen Yogurt bars, uncoated, 15-fl.-oz. box (6 bars)	240	30.0			16.0	2.00	128	16.0
1 bar, approx. 2½ fl. oz.	40	5.0			16.0	2.00	128	16.0

	UNIT		1 OZ., BY WT.		1 FLUID OZ.		1 CUP, PACKED	
	Cal.	Carb.	Cal.	Carb.	Cal.	Carb.	Cal.	Carb.
Breyers Ice Cream, pint container	520	72.0	52.6	7.29	32.5	4.50	260	36.0
½-gallon container	2080	288.0	52.6	7.29	32.5	4.50	260	36.0
Carvel Sherbet, 3-fl.-oz. container	105	23.4	39.7	8.84	35.0	7.80	280	62.4
Danny-in-a-Cup Hard Frozen Yogurt, 8-fl.-oz. container	210	42.0	35.0	7.00	26.3	5.25	210	42.0
Johnston Hard Frozen Yogurt, 8-fl.-oz. container	180	34.0	(30.0)	(5.67)	22.5	4.25	180	34.0
Light n' Lively (Sealtest) Ice Milk, 4-fl.-oz. container	100	18.0	43.0	7.73	25.0	4.50	200	36.0
pint container	400	72.0	43.0	7.73	25.0	4.50	200	36.0
½-gallon container	1600	288.0	43.0	7.73	25.0	4.50	200	36.0
Meadow Gold Ice Cream, quart container	1040	128.0	55.5	6.83	32.5	4.00	260	32.0
Sealtest Old Fashioned Ice Cream, pint container	520	76.0	52.6	7.69	32.5	4.75	260	38.0
½-gallon container	2080	304.0	52.6	7.69	32.5	4.75	260	38.0
Weight Watchers Frosted Treat, 7-fl.-oz. serving	120	22.0	28.6	5.24	17.1	3.14	137	25.1
PASSION FRUIT								
le sorbet French Fruit Ice, pint container	320	72.0			20.0	4.50	160	36.0
PEANUT BUTTER								
Dairy Queen Parfait, 10.8 oz.	740	94.0	68.5	8.70				
PECAN CRUNCH								
Luxury Ice Cream, ½-gallon container	2240	288.0	59.7	7.67	35.0	4.50	280	36.0
PINA COLADA								
Colombo Frozen Yogurt, pint container	440	80.0			27.5	5.00	220	40.0
Danny-in-a-Cup Hard Frozen Yogurt, 8-fl.-oz. container	210	42.0	35.0	7.00	26.3	5.25	210	42.0
Danny-on-a-Stick uncoated, 15-fl.-oz. box (6 bars)	420	84.0			28.0	5.60	224	44.8
1 bar, approx. 2½ fl. oz.	70	14.0			28.0	5.60	224	44.8
PINEAPPLE								
Carvel Sherbet, 3-fl.-oz. container	105	23.4	39.7	8.84	35.0	7.80	280	62.4
Dole Frozen Fruit in Juice, 10-fl.-oz. box (4 bars)	280	72.0			28.0	7.20	224	57.6
1 bar, approx. 2½ fl. oz.	70	18.0			28.0	7.20	224	57.6
Frozfruit Frozen Fruit Bars, 16-fl.-oz. (1-pint) box (4 bars)	272	67.2			17.0	4.20	136	33.6
1 bar, approx. 4 fl. oz.	68	16.8			17.0	4.20	136	33.6
Meadow Gold Sherbet, quart container	1040	232.0	38.3	8.54	32.5	7.25	260	58.0
Weight Watchers Frosted Treat, 7-fl.-oz. serving	120	22.0	28.6	5.24	17.1	3.14	137	25.1
Pineapple Sundae, **Meadow Gold,** 5 oz.	230	42.9	46.0	8.58				
PISTACHIO								
Weight Watchers Frosted Treat, 7-fl.-oz. serving	120	22.0	28.6	5.24	17.1	3.14	137	25.1
PLAIN								
"Plain," **Carvel,** Lo-Yo, 3-fl.-oz. container	110	20.1	40.6	7.39	36.7	6.70	293	53.6
PRALINES 'N CREAM								
Baskin Robbins, 1 scoop, approx. 2.5 oz.	177	23.7	70.8	9.48	(59.0)	(7.90)	(472)	(62.4)
RASPBERRY								
Beautiful Day Frozen Yogurt bars, uncoated, 15-fl.-oz. box (6 bars)	240	30.0			16.0	2.00	128	16.0
1 bar, approx. 2½ fl. oz.	40	5.0			16.0	2.00	128	16.0
Danny-Yo Soft Frozen Yogurt, 3½-fl.-oz. container	110	21.0	44.0	8.40	31.4	6.00	251	48.0
Häagen-Dazs Sorbet & Cream, Raspberry Fruit Ice and Vanilla Ice Cream, pint container	760	100.0			47.5	6.25	380	50.0
le sorbet Sherbet, 4-fl.-oz. container	78	22.2			19.5	5.55	156	44.4
Popsicle, 36-fl.-oz. box (12 pops)	840	198.0			23.3	5.50	187	44.0
1 pop, approx. 3 fl. oz.	70	16.5			23.3	5.50	187	44.0
Black Raspberry, **Carvel** Sherbet, 3-fl.-oz. container	105	23.4	39.7	8.84	35.0	7.80	280	62.4
Blue Raspberry, **Popsicle,** 36-fl.-oz. box (12 pops)	840	198.0			23.3	5.50	187	44.0
1 pop, approx. 3 fl. oz.	70	16.5			23.3	5.50	187	44.0
RED RASPBERRY								
Danny-in-a-Cup Hard Frozen Yogurt, 8-fl.-oz. container	210	42.0	35.0	7.00	26.3	5.25	210	42.0

	UNIT		1 OZ., BY WT.		1 FLUID OZ.		1 CUP, PACKED	
	Cal.	Carb.	Cal.	Carb.	Cal.	Carb.	Cal.	Carb.
Danny-on-a-Stick, uncoated, 15-fl.-oz. box (6 bars)	420	78.0			28.0	5.20	224	41.6
1 bar, approx. 2½ fl. oz.	70	13.0			28.0	5.20	224	41.6
Danny-on-a-Stick, Chocolate-coated, 15-fl.-oz. box (6 bars)	780	90.0			52.0	6.00	416	48.0
1 bar, approx. 2½ fl. oz.	130	15.0			52.0	6.00	416	48.0
Sealtest Ice Cream, pint container	520		52.6		32.5		260	
½-gallon container	2080		52.6		32.5		260	
Sealtest Sherbet, quart container	1040	240.0	(38.5)	(8.88)	32.5	7.50	260	60.0
½-gallon container	2080	480.0	(38.5)	(8.88)	32.5	7.50	260	60.0
ROOT BEER								
Popsicle, 36-fl.-oz. box (12 pops)	840	198.0			23.3	5.50	187	44.0
1 pop, approx. 3 fl. oz.	70	16.5			23.3	5.50	187	44.0
RUM								
Weight Watchers Frosted Treat, 7-fl.-oz. serving	120	22.0	28.6	5.24	17.1	3.14	137	25.1
Rum Raisin, **Häagen-Dazs** Ice Cream, pint container	1023	98.0	66.0	6.33	64.0	6.13	517	49.0
STRAWBERRY								
Baskin-Robbins Ice Cream, 1 scoop, approx. 2.5 oz.	141	15.6	56.4	6.24	(47.0)	(5.20)	(376)	(41.6)
Beautiful Day Frozen Yogurt bars, uncoated, 15-fl.-oz. box (6 bars)	240	30.0			16.0	2.00	128	16.0
1 bar, approx. 2½ fl. oz.	40	5.0			16.0	2.00	128	16.0
Breyers Ice Cream, pint container	520	68.0	52.6	6.88	32.5	4.25	260	34.0
½-gallon container	2080	272.0	52.6	6.88	32.5	4.25	260	34.0
Carnation Frozen Yogurt Bon Bons, 1.7-oz. package	120	10.9	70.7	6.37	48.0	4.36		
3.42-oz. package	240	21.8	70.7	6.37	48.0	4.36		
13.69-oz. package	960	87.2	70.7	6.37	48.0	4.36		
1 bon bon, 0.34 oz.	24	2.2	70.7	6.37	48.0	4.36		
Carvel Sherbet, 3-fl.-oz. container	105	23.4	39.7	8.84	35.0	7.80	280	62.4
Chicquita, Fruit & Juice Pops, 16-fl.-oz. (1-pint) box (8 pops)	400	96.0			25.0	7.50	200	48.00
1 pop, approx. 2 fl. oz.	50	12.0			25.0	7.50	200	48.00
Colombo Frozen Yogurt, pint container	440	80.0			27.5	5.00	220	40.0
Colombo bar, uncoated, 15-fl.-oz. box (6 bars)	480	84.0			32.0	5.60	256	44.8
1 bar, approx. 2½ fl. oz.	80	14.0			32.0	5.60	256	44.8
Danny-in-a-Cup Hard Frozen Yogurt, 8-fl.-oz. container	210	42.0	35.0	7.00	26.3	5.25	210	42.0
Danny-on-a-Stick, uncoated, 15-fl.-oz. box (6 bars)	420	78.0			28.0	5.20	224	41.6
1 bar, approx. 2½ fl. oz.	70	13.0			28.0	5.20	224	41.6
Danny-on-a-Stick, chocolate-coated, 15-fl.-oz. box (6 bars)	780	90.0			52.0	6.00	416	48.0
1 bar, approx. 2½ fl. oz.	130	15.0			52.0	6.00	416	48.0
Danny-Yo Soft Frozen Yogurt, 3½-fl.-oz. container	110	21.0	44.0	8.40	31.4	6.00	251	48.0
Dole Frozen Fruit in Juice, 10-fl.-oz. box (4 bars)	280	64.0			28.0	6.40	224	51.2
1 bar, approx. 2½ fl. oz.	70	16.0			28.0	6.40	224	51.2
Dole Fruit Sorbet, pint container	440	112.0			27.5	7.00	220	56.0
Frozfruit Frozen Fruit Bars, 16-fl.-oz. (1-pint) box (4 bars)	280	64.0			17.5	4.00	140	32.0
1 bar, approx. 4 fl. oz.	70	16.0			17.5	4.00	140	32.0
Good Humor Ice Cream, ½-gallon container	1920	240.0			30.0	3.75	240	30.0
Good Humor Whammy Bars, 12.8-oz. box (8 bars)	800	72.0	62.5	5.63				
1 bar, approx. 1.6 oz.	100	9.0	62.5	5.63				
Häagen-Dazs Ice Cream, pint container	1032	95.7	66.6	6.18	64.5	5.98	516	47.9
Howard Johnson's Ice Cream, pint container	748	(65.3)	(75.7)	(6.61)	46.8	(4.09)	374	(32.7)
quart container	1496	(130.6)	(75.7)	(6.61)	46.8	(4.09)	374	(32.7)
Johnston Hard Frozen Yogurt, 8-fl.-oz. container	180	34.0	(30.0)	(5.67)	22.5	4.25	180	34.0
Soft Frozen Yogurt, 8-fl.-oz. container	208	37.0			26.0	4.63	208	37.0
le sorbet Sherbet, 4-fl.-oz. container	86	21.7			21.5	5.43	172	43.4

	UNIT		1 OZ., BY WT.		1 FLUID OZ.		1 CUP, PACKED	
	Cal.	Carb.	Cal.	Carb.	Cal.	Carb.	Cal.	Carb.
Light n' Lively (Sealtest) Ice Milk, 4-fl.-oz. container	100	18.0	43.0	7.73	25.0	4.50	200	36.0
pint container	400	72.0	43.0	7.73	25.0	4.50	200	36.0
Popsicle, 36-fl.-oz. box (12 pops)	840	198.0			23.3	5.50	187	44.0
1 pop, approx. 3 fl. oz.	70	16.5			23.3	5.50	187	44.0
Schrafft's Light, Strawberry All Natural Ice Milk, pint container	540	104.0			33.8	6.50	270	52.0
Schrafft's Think Thin Ice Milk, pint container	540	104.0	(42.9)	(8.25)	33.8	6.50	270	52.0
quart container	1080	208.0	(42.9)	(8.25)	33.8	6.50	270	52.0
Sealtest Ice Cream, pint container	520	76.0	52.6	7.69	32.5	4.75	260	38.0
Sealtest Sherbet, quart container	1040	240.0	(38.5)	(8.88)	32.5	7.50	260	60.0
½-gallon container	2080	480.0	(38.5)	(8.88)	32.5	7.50	260	60.0
Tuscan bars, uncoated, 15-fl.-oz. box (6 bars)	420	84.0			28.0	5.60	224	44.8
1 bar, approx. 2½ fl. oz.	70	14.0			28.0	5.60	224	44.8
Tuscan bars, chocolate-coated, 15-fl.-oz. box (6 bars)	780	96.0			52.0	6.40	416	51.2
1 bar, approx. 2½ fl. oz.	130	16.0			52.0	6.40	416	51.2
Weight Watchers Frosted Treat, 7-fl.-oz. serving	120	22.0	28.6	5.24	17.1	3.14	137	25.1
Strawberry Shortcake Bars, **Good Humor,** 18-oz. box (6 bars)	1200	126.0	66.7	7.00				
1 bar, approx. 3 oz.	200	21.0	66.7	7.00				
Strawberry Sundae, Meadow Gold, 5-oz. container	229	44.1	45.6	8.82				
TOASTED ALMOND								
Good Humor, Ice Cream, 18-oz. box (6 bars)	1320	126.0	73.3	7.00				
1 bar, approx. 3 oz.	220	21.0	73.3	7.00				
TOFFEE								
Toffee Crunch, **Light n' Lively (Sealtest)** Ice Milk, 4-fl.-oz. container	120	19.0	51.5	8.16	30.0	4.75	240	38.0
pint container	480	76.0	51.5	8.16	30.0	4.75	240	38.0
½-gallon container	1920	304.0	51.5	8.16	30.0	4.75	240	38.0
Toffee Fudge Swirl Ice Cream, **Good Humor,** ½-gallon container	2080	288.0			32.5	4.50	260	36.0
Toffee Ice Cream Bar, **Heath,** 18-fl.-oz. box (6 bars)	1020	96.0			56.7	5.33	454	42.6
1 bar, approx. 3 fl. oz	170	16.0			56.7	5.33	454	42.6
Toffee, Old Fashioned, **Weight Watchers** Frosted Treat, 7-fl.-oz. serving	120	22.0	28.6	5.24	17.1	3.14	137	25.1
VANILLA								
Ann Page (A&P) Ice Cream, ½-gallon	2080	224.0			32.5	3.50	260	28.0
Baskin Robbins Ice Cream, 1 scoop, approx. 2.5 oz.	147	15.8	58.8	6.24	(49.0)	(5.27)	(392)	(42.1)
Breyers Ice Cream, pint container	600	64.0	60.7	6.48	37.5	4.00	300	32.0
½-gallon container	2400	256.0	60.7	6.48	37.5	4.00	300	32.0
Carnation Ice Cream Bon Bons, 1.7-oz. package	120	10.9	70.7	6.37	48.0	4.36		
3.42-oz. package	240	21.8	70.7	6.37	48.0	4.36		
13.69-oz. package	960	87.2	70.7	6.37	48.0	4.36		
1 bon bon, approx. 0.34 oz.	24	2.2	70.7	6.37	48.0	4.36		
Carvel Ice Cream, 3-fl.-oz. container	148	15.9	55.9	6.02	49.3	5.30	395	42.4
Carvel "Thinny Thin," 3-fl.-oz. container	56	10.2	30.9	5.68	18.7	3.40	149	27.2
Colombo bar, chocolate-coated, 15-fl.-oz. box (6 bars)	870	102.0			58.0	6.80	464	54.4
1 bar, approx. 2½ fl. oz.	145	17.0			58.0	6.80	464	54.4
Colombo Frozen Yogurt, pint container	440	80.0			27.5	5.00	220	40.0
Coronet Ice Cream, ½-gallon container	2400	240.0			37.5	3.75	300	30.0
Danny-in-a-Cup Hard Frozen Yogurt, 8-fl.-oz. container	180	20.0	30.0	3.33	22.5	2.50	180	20.0
Danny-on-a-Stick uncoated, 15-fl.-oz. box (6 bars)	360	66.0			24.0	4.40	192	35.2
1 bar, approx. 2½ fl. oz.	60	11.0			24.0	4.40	192	35.2
Danny-on-a-Stick, carob-coated, 15-fl.-oz. box (6 bars)	720	60.0			48.0	4.00	384	32.0
1 bar, approx. 2½ fl. oz.	120	10.0			48.0	4.00	384	32.0
Danny-Yo Soft Frozen Yogurt, 3½-fl.-oz. container	110	21.0	44.0	8.40	31.4	6.00	251	48.0
Dolly Madison Dietary Dairy Dessert, ¼-pint container	140	15.0			35.0	3.75	280	30.0
Friendly's Cake Cones filled with vanilla ice cream:								
regular, approx. 4.2 oz. (4 oz. ice cream, 0.2 oz. cone)	250	29.0	59.5	6.95				
double dip, approx. 7.2 oz. (7 oz. ice cream, 0.2 oz. cone)	420	49.0	58.3	6.81				
Friendly's Sugar Cones filled with vanilla ice cream:								
regular, approx. 4½ oz. (4 oz. ice cream, ½ oz. cone)	290	38.0	64.4	8.44				
double dip, approx. 7½ oz. (7 oz. ice cream, ½ oz. cone)	460	57.0	61.3	7.60				
Good Humor Ice Cream, ½-gallon container	2240	224.0			35.0	3.50	280	28.0
Good Humor Ice Cream Sandwich, 15-oz. box (6 sandwiches)	1200	204.0	80.0	13.60				
1 sandwich, approx. 2½ oz.	200	34.0	80.0	13.60				
Good Humor Chocolate-Coated Ice Cream Bars, 18-oz. box (6 bars)	1020	72.0	56.7	4.00				
1 bar, approx. 3 oz.	170	12.0	56.7	4.00				
Good Humor Whammy Bars, 12.8-oz. box (8 bars)	800	72.0	62.5	5.63				
1 bar, approx. 1.6 oz.	100	9.0	62.5	5.63				
Häagen-Dazs Ice Cream, pint container	1027	92.0	66.0	5.97	64.2	5.75	513	46.0
Harbison's Ice Cream, ½-gallon container	2240	240.0			35.0	3.75	280	30.0
Hood Ice Cream, ½-gallon container	2080	256.0			32.5	4.00	260	32.0
Howard Johnson's Ice Cream, pint container	840	(59.7)	(85.0)	(6.04)	52.5	(3.73)	420	(29.8)
quart container	1680	(119.4)	(85.0)	(6.04)	52.5	(3.73)	420	(29.8)
Jell-O, Vanilla Pudding Pop, 24-fl.-oz. box (12 bars)	1080	192.0			45.0	8.00	384	64.0
1 bar, approx. 2 fl. oz.	90	16.0			45.0	8.00	384	64.0
Johnston Soft Frozen Yogurt, 8-fl.-oz. container	181	31.0			22.6	3.88	181	31.0
Light n' Lively (Sealtest) Ice Milk, 4-fl.-oz. container	100	17.0	43.0	7.30	25.0	4.25	200	34.0
pint container	400	68.0	43.0	7.30	25.0	4.25	200	34.0
½-gallon container	1600	272.0	43.0	7.30	25.0	4.25	200	34.0
Lucerne Dietetic Ice Cream, pint container	519		55.3		32.4		259	
Luxury Ice Cream, ½-gallon container	1920	224.0	(51.2)	(5.96)	30.0	3.50	240	28.0
Nuform Ice Milk, ½-gallon container	1760	272.0			27.5	4.25	220	34.0
Popsicle, 36-fl.-oz. box (12 pops)	840	198.0			23.3	5.50	187	44.0
1 pop, approx. 3 fl. oz.	70	16.5			23.3	5.50	187	44.0
Schrafft's Light, Vanilla All Natural Ice Milk, pint container	540	104.0			33.8	6.50	270	52.0
Schrafft's Sugar-Less Frozen Dietary Dairy Dessert, pint container	600	56.0	(56.7)	(5.28)	37.5	3.50	300	28.0
Schrafft's Think Thin Ice Milk, pint container	540	104.0			33.8	6.50	270	52.0
quart container	1080	208.0			33.8	6.50	270	52.0
Sealtest Ice Cream, pint container	560	64.0	56.6	6.47	35.0	4.00	280	32.0
½-gallon container	2240	256.0	56.6	6.47	35.0	4.00	280	32.0
Sweet 'n Low Frozen Dietary Dairy Dessert bar (chocolate flavor coated), 15-fl.-oz. box (6 bars)	780	72.0			52.0	4.80	416	38.4
1 bar, approx. 2½ fl. oz.	130	12.0			52.0	4.80	416	38.4
Swift's Ice Cream, ½-gallon container	2080	256.0	57.8	7.11	32.5	4.00	260	32.0
Tofutti Non-dairy Frozen Dessert, pint container	800	84.0			50.0	5.25	400	42.0
Tuscan bars, chocolate-coated, 15-fl.-oz. box (6 bars)	780	102.0			52.0	6.80	416	54.4
1 bar, approx. 2½ fl. oz.	130	17.0			52.0	6.80	416	54.4
Tuscan Soft Frozen Yogurt, pint container	440	92.0	27.5	5.75	27.5	5.75	220	46.0
Weight Watchers Frosted Treat, 7-fl.-oz. serving	120	22.0	28.6	5.24	17.1	3.14	137	25.1
Yulovit (Natural Nectar), 12-fl.-oz. box (3 pies)	807	92.4			67.3	7.70	538	61.6
1 pie, approx. 4 fl. oz.	269	30.8			67.3	7.70	538	61.6
French Vanilla, **Baskin Robbins** Ice Cream, 1 scoop, approx. 2.5 oz.	181	15.9	72.4	6.36	(60.3)	(5.30)	(483)	(42.4)

	UNIT		1 OZ., BY WT.		1 FLUID OZ.		1 CUP, PACKED	
	Cal.	Carb.	Cal.	Carb.	Cal.	Carb.	Cal.	Carb.
Golden Vanilla, **Meadow Gold** Ice Cream, quart container	1120	128.0	59.7	6.83	35.0	4.00	280	32.0
VANILLA ALMOND BARK								
Tofutti Non-dairy Frozen Dessert, pint container	920	92.0			57.5	5.75	460	46.0
VANILLA BUTTERSCOTCH								
Breyers Ice Cream, quart container	1360	184.0			42.5	5.75	340	46.0
½-gallon container	2720	368.0			42.5	5.75	340	46.0
VANILLA FUDGE								
Armel Frozen Dietary Dairy Dessert, pint container	520	60.0			32.5	3.75	260	30.0
Natural Nectar Ice Cream, pint container	(672)	(80.5)	64.4	7.71	(42.0)	(5.03)	(336)	(40.2)
quart container	(1345)	(161.0)	64.4	7.71	(42.0)	(5.03)	(336)	(40.2)
Schrafft's Sugar-Less Frozen Dietary Dairy Dessert, pint container	600	56.0	56.7	5.28	37.5	3.50	300	28.0
Vanilla Fudge Swirl Ice Cream, **Good Humor,** ½-gallon container	2240	240.0			35.0	3.75	280	30.0
Vanilla Fudge Twirl, **Breyers** Ice Cream, pint container	640	76.0	64.8	7.70	40.0	4.75	320	38.0
gallon container	5120	608.0	64.8	7.70	40.0	4.75	320	38.0
Vanilla Fudge Twirl **Light n' Lively (Sealtest)** Ice Milk, 4-fl.-oz. container	110	20.0	47.3	8.59	27.5	5.00	220	40.0
pint container	440	80.0	47.3	8.59	27.5	5.00	220	40.0
½-gallon container	1760	320.0	47.3	8.59	27.5	5.00	220	40.0
WALNUT (see English Walnut and Black Walnut)								
WHITE CHOCOLATE CHIP								
Glacé Lite (Sweet Victory) Lowfat Frozen Dairy Dessert, pint container	400	76.0			25.0	4.75	200	38.0
WILDBERRY SUPREME								
Tofutti Non-dairy Frozen Dessert, pint container	840	88.0			52.5	5.50	420	44.0

Containers With More Than 1 Flavor

	UNIT Cal.	UNIT Carb.	1 OZ., BY WT. Cal.	1 OZ., BY WT. Carb.	1 FLUID OZ. Cal.	1 FLUID OZ. Carb.	1 CUP, PACKED Cal.	1 CUP, PACKED Carb.
Butter Almond/Chocolate, **Breyers** Ice Cream, quart container	1280	136.0			40.0	4.25	320	34.0
½-gallon container	2560	272.0			40.0	4.25	320	34.0
Chocolate/Vanilla, **Weight Watchers** Frozen Dietary Dessert, 5-fl.-oz. container	100	19.0	32.3	6.18	20.0	3.80	160	30.4
Chocolate/Vanilla/Strawberry, **Harbison's** Ice Cream, ½-gallon container	2080	256.0			32.5	4.00	260	32.0
Chocolate/Vanilla/Strawberry, **Luxury** Ice Cream, ½-gallon container	1920	240.0	(51.2)	(6.39)	30.0	3.75	240	30.0
Coffee, Strawberry & Mint, **Carvel,** "Thinny-Thin," 3-fl.-oz. container	56	10.2	30.9	5.68	18.7	3.40	149	27.2
Strawberry/Vanilla, **Friendly's,** Ice Cream Sundae, 6.3 oz.	340	39.0	54.0	6.19				
Strawberry/Vanilla, **Weight Watchers** Frozen Dietary Dessert, 5-fl.-oz. container	100	19.0	32.3	6.18	20.0	3.80	160	30.4
"Stripes" (grape, orange, cherry, lemon), **Good Humor** Whammy Bars, 18-oz. box (12 pops)	600	156.0	33.3	8.67				
1 pop, approx. 1½ oz.	50	13.0	33.3	8.67				
Vanilla/Chocolate, **Breyers** Ice Cream, ½-gallon container	2560	272.0	64.8	6.88	40.0	4.25	320	34.0
Vanilla/Chocolate, **Luxury** Ice Cream, ½-gallon container	1920	224.0	(51.2)	(5.97)	30.0	3.50	240	28.0
Vanilla/Chocolate/Strawberry, **Breyers** Ice Cream, ½-gallon container	2400	272.0	60.0	6.88	37.5	4.25	300	34.0
Vanilla/Chocolate/Strawberry, **Good Humor** Ice Cream, ½-gallon container	2080	224.0			32.5	3.50	260	28.0
Vanilla/Chocolate/Strawberry, **Light n' Lively (Sealtest)** Ice Milk, 4-fl.-oz. container	100	18.0	43.0	7.73	25.0	4.50	200	36.0
pint container	400	72.0	43.0	7.73	25.0	4.50	200	36.0
½-gallon container	1600	288.0	43.0	7.73	25.0	4.50	200	36.0
Vanilla/Chocolate/Strawberry, **Sealtest** Ice Cream, pint container	520	72.0	52.6	7.28	32.5	4.50	260	36.0
½-gallon container	2080	288.0	52.6	7.28	32.5	4.50	260	36.0
Vanilla/Strawberry, **Weight Watchers** Frozen Dietary Dessert, 5-fl.-oz. container	100	19.0	32.3	6.18	20.0	3.80	160	30.4

ICE CREAM, ICE MILK, FROZEN YOGURT, SHERBET, and SIMILAR FROZEN DESSERTS, by brand

The list that follows is alphabetized by brand. A list alphabetized by the main descriptive fruit or flavor precedes this one.

	UNIT Cal.	UNIT Carb.	1 OZ., BY WT. Cal.	1 OZ., BY WT. Carb.	1 FLUID OZ. Cal.	1 FLUID OZ. Carb.	1 CUP, PACKED Cal.	1 CUP, PACKED Carb.
Ann Page (A&P) Ice Cream								
Vanilla, ½ gallon	2080	224.0			32.5	3.50	260	28.0
Armel Frozen Dietary Dairy Dessert								
Chocolate, pint container	480	52.0			30.0	3.25	240	26.0
Vanilla Fudge, pint container	520	60.0			32.5	3.75	260	30.0
Baskin-Robbins Ice Cream								
Chocolate, 1 scoop, approx. 2.5 oz.	165	20.4	66.0	8.16	(55.0)	(6.80)	(440)	(54.4)
Chocolate Fudge, 1 scoop, approx. 2.5 oz.	178	21.5	71.7	8.52	(59.3)	(7.17)	(475)	(57.3)
Daiquiri Ice, 1 scoop, approx. 2.5 oz.	84	20.9	33.6	8.36	(28.0)	(6.97)	(224)	(55.7)
French Vanilla, 1 scoop, approx. 2.5 oz.	181	15.9	72.4	6.36	(60.3)	(5.30)	(483)	(42.4)
Orange Sherbet, 1 scoop, approx. 2.5 oz.	99	20.9	39.6	8.36	(33.0)	(6.97)	(264)	(55.7)
Pralines 'n Cream, 1 scoop, approx. 2.5 oz.	177	23.7	70.8	9.48	(59.0)	(7.90)	(472)	(62.4)
Strawberry, 1 scoop, approx. 2.5 oz.	141	15.6	56.4	6.24	(47.0)	(5.20)	(376)	(41.6)
Vanilla, 1 scoop, approx. 2.5 oz.	147	15.8	58.8	6.24	(49.0)	(5.27)	(392)	(42.1)
Beautiful Day Frozen Yogurt Bars								
Blueberry, uncoated, 15-fl.-oz. box (6 bars)	240	30.0			16.0	2.00	128	16.0
1 bar, approx. 2½ fl. oz.	40	5.0			16.0	2.00	128	16.0
Lemon, uncoated, 15-fl.-oz. box (6 bars)	240	30.0			16.0	2.00	128	16.0
1 bar, approx. 2½ fl. oz.	40	5.0			16.0	2.00	128	16.0
Peach, uncoated, 15-fl.-oz. box (6 bars)	240	30.0			16.0	2.00	128	16.0
1 bar, approx. 2½ fl. oz.	40	5.0			16.0	2.00	128	16.0
Raspberry, uncoated, 15-fl.-oz. box (6 bars)	240	30.0			16.0	2.00	128	16.0
1 bar, approx. 2½ fl. oz.	40	5.0			16.0	2.00	128	16.0
Strawberry, uncoated, 15-fl.-oz. box (6 bars)	240	30.0			16.0	2.00	128	16.0
1 bar, approx. 2½ fl. oz.	40	5.0			16.0	2.00	128	16.0
Bi-Sicle Pops								
Chocolate, 30-fl.-oz. box (12 pops)	1344	256.8			44.8	8.56	358	68.5
1 pop, approx. 2½ fl. oz.	112	21.4			44.8	8.56	358	68.5
Breyers Ice Cream								
Banana-Red Raspberry Twirl, pint container	600	84.0	57.5	8.05	37.5	5.25	300	42.0
½-gallon container	2400	336.0	57.5	8.05	37.5	5.25	300	42.0
Banana Strawberry Twirl, quart container	1200	168.0	57.5	8,05	37.5	5.25	300	42.0
½-gallon container	2400	336.0	57.5	8,05	37.5	5.25	300	42.0
Butter Almond, pint container	680	60.0	68.8	6.07	42.5	3.75	340	30.0
½-gallon container	2720	240.0	68.8	6.07	42.5	3.75	340	30.0
Butter Almond/Chocolate, quart container	1280	136.0			40.0	4.25	320	34.0
½-gallon container	2560	272.0			40.0	4.25	320	34.0
Butter Pecan, pint container	720	60.0	72.9	6.07	45.0	3.75	360	30.0
½-gallon container	2880	240.0	72.9	6.07	45.0	3.75	360	30.0
Cherry Vanilla, pint container	560	68.0	56.7	6.89	35.0	4.25	280	34.0
½-gallon container	2240	272.0	56.7	6.89	35.0	4.25	280	34.0
Chocolate, pint container	640	76.0	64.8	7.70	40.0	4.75	320	38.0
½-gallon container	2560	304.0	64.8	7.70	40.0	4.75	320	38.0
Coffee, pint container	560	60.0	56.7	6.07	35.0	3.75	280	30.0
½-gallon container	2240	240.0	56.7	6.07	35.0	3.75	280	30.0
Dutch Chocolate Almond, quart container	1440	144.0			45.0	4.50	360	36.0
½-gallon container	2880	288.0			45.0	4.50	360	36.0

	UNIT		1 OZ., BY WT.		1 FLUID OZ.		1 CUP, PACKED	
	Cal.	Carb.	Cal.	Carb.	Cal.	Carb.	Cal.	Carb.
Egg Nog, quart container	1200	128.0			37.5	4.00	300	32.0
½-gallon container	2400	256.0			37.5	4.00	300	32.0
(Roasted) English Walnut, quart container	1360	120.0			42.5	3.75	340	30.0
½-gallon container	2720	240.0			42.5	3.75	340	30.0
Mint Chocolate Chip, pint container	680	72.0	68.9	7.29	42.5	4.50	340	36.0
½-gallon container	2720	288.0	68.9	7.29	42.5	4.50	340	36.0
Orange-Pineapple, ½-gallon container	2240	272.0	56.7	6.80	35.0	4.25	280	34.0
Peach, pint container	520	72.0	52.6	7.29	32.5	4.50	260	36.0
½-gallon container	2080	288.0	52.6	7.29	32.5	4.50	260	36.0
Strawberry, pint container	520	68.0	52.6	6.88	32.5	4.25	260	34.0
½-gallon container	2080	272.0	52.6	6.88	32.5	4.25	260	34.0
Vanilla, pint container	600	64.0	60.7	6.48	37.5	4.00	300	32.0
½-gallon container	2400	256.0	60.7	6.48	37.5	4.00	300	32.0
Vanilla Butterscotch, quart container	1360	184.0			42.5	5.75	340	46.0
½-gallon container	2720	368.0			42.5	5.75	340	46.0
Vanilla/Chocolate, ½-gallon container	2560	272.0	64.8	6.88	40.0	4.25	320	34.0
Vanilla/Chocolate/ Strawberry, ½-gallon container	2400	272.0	60.0	6.88	37.5	4.25	300	34.0
Vanilla Fudge ("Twirl"), pint container	640	76.0	64.8	7.70	40.0	4.75	320	38.0
gallon container	5120	608.0	64.8	7.70	40.0	4.75	320	38.0
Carnation Bon Bons								
Chocolate Ice Cream Bon Bons, 1.7-oz. package	120	10.9	70.7	6.37	48.0	4.36		
3.42-oz. package	240	21.8	70.7	6.37	48.0	4.36		
13.69-oz. package	960	87.2	70.7	6.37	48.0	4.36		
1 bon bon, approx. 0.34 oz.	24	2.2	70.7	6.37	48.0	4.36		
Strawberry Frozen Yogurt Bon Bons, 1.7-oz. package	120	10.9	70.7	6.37	48.0	4.36		
3.42-oz. package	240	21.8	70.7	6.37	48.0	4.36		
13.69-oz. package	960	87.2	70.7	6.37	48.0	4.36		
1 bon bon, approx. 0.34 oz.	24	2.2	70.7	6.37	48.0	4.36		
Vanilla Ice Cream Bon Bons, 1.7-oz. package	120	10.9	70.7	6.37	48.0	4.36		
3.42-oz. package	240	21.8	70.7	6.37	48.0	4.36		
13.69-oz. package	960	87.2	70.7	6.37	48.0	4.36		
1 bon bon, approx. 0.34 oz.	24	2.2	70.7	6.37	48.0	4.36		
Carvel								
Ice Cream:								
Chocolate, 3-fl.-oz. container	147	16.8	55.9	6.34	49.0	5.60	392	44.8
Vanilla, 3-fl.-oz. container	148	15.9	55.9	6.02	49.3	5.30	395	42.4
Thinny-Thin Frozen Dessert:								
Chocolate, 3-fl.-oz. container	56	10.4	30.9	5.82	18.7	3.47	149	27.7
Chocolate Mint, 3-fl.-oz. container	56	10.4	30.9	5.82	18.7	3.47	149	27.7
Coffee, Strawberry & Mint, 3-fl.-oz. container	56	10.2	30.9	5.68	18.7	3.40	149	27.2
Vanilla, 3-fl.-oz. container	56	10.2	30.9	5.68	18.7	3.40	149	27.2
Frozen Yogurt:								
"Plain" Lo-Yo, 3-fl.-oz. container	110	20.1	40.6	7.39	36.7	6.70	293	53.6
Sherbet:								
Black Raspberry, 3-fl.-oz. container	105	23.4	39.7	8.84	35.0	7.80	280	62.4
Blueberry, 3-fl.-oz. container	105	23.4	39.7	8.84	35.0	7.80	280	62.4
Cherry, 3-fl.-oz. container	105	23.4	39.7	8.84	35.0	7.80	280	62.4
Chocolate, 3-fl.-oz. container	105	23.4	39.7	8.84	35.0	7.80	280	62.4
Guanabana, 3-fl.-oz. container	105	23.4	39.7	8.84	35.0	7.80	280	62.4
Lemon, 3-fl.-oz. container	105	23.4	39.7	8.84	35.0	7.80	280	62.4
Lime, 3-fl.-oz. container	105	23.4	39.7	8.84	35.0	7.80	280	62.4
Mamey, 3-fl.-oz. container	105	23.4	39.7	8.84	35.0	7.80	280	62.4
Mango, 3-fl.-oz. container	105	23.4	39.7	8.84	35.0	7.80	280	62.4
Orange, 3-fl.-oz. container	105	23.4	39.7	8.84	35.0	7.80	280	62.4
Orange-Pineapple, 3-fl.-oz. container	105	23.4	39.7	8.84	35.0	7.80	280	62.4
Peach, 3-fl.-oz. container	105	23.4	39.7	8.84	35.0	7.80	280	62.4
Pineapple, 3-fl.-oz. container	105	23.4	39.7	8.84	35.0	7.80	280	62.4
Strawberry, 3-fl.-oz. container	105	23.4	39.7	8.84	35.0	7.80	280	62.4
Chicquita								
Fruit & Juice Pops:								
Cherry, 16-fl.-oz. (1-pint) box (8 pops)	400	104.0			25.0	6.50	200	52.0
1 pop, approx. 2 fl. oz.	50	13.0			25.0	6.50	200	52.0
Strawberry, 16-fl.-oz. (1-pint) box (8 pops)	400	96.0			25.0	7.50	200	48.0
1 pop, approx. 2 fl. oz.	50	12.0			25.0	7.50	200	48.0
Colombo Frozen Yogurt								
Containers:								
Piña Colada, pint container	440	80.0			27.5	5.00	220	40.0
Strawberry, pint container	440	80.0			27.5	5.00	220	40.0
Vanilla, pint container	440	80.0			27.5	5.00	220	40.0
Bars:								
Chocolate, chocolate-coated bar, 15-fl.-oz. box (6 bars)	870	102.0			58.0	6.80	464	54.4
1 bar, approx. 2½ fl. oz.	145	17.0			58.0	6.80	464	54.4
Strawberry, uncoated bar, 15-fl.-oz. box (6 bars)	480	84.0			32.0	5.60	256	44.8
1 bar, approx. 2½ fl. oz.	80	14.0			32.0	5.60	256	44.8
Vanilla, chocolate-coated bar, 15-fl.-oz. box (6 bars)	870	102.0			58.0	6.80	464	54.4
1 bar, approx. 2½ fl. oz.	145	17.0			58.0	6.80	464	54.4
Coronet Ice Cream								
Vanilla, ½-gallon container	2400	240.0			37.5	3.75	300	30.0
Creamsicle								
Ice Cream Center Deluxe, 30-fl.-oz. box (12 pops)	936	153.6			31.2	5.12	250	41.0
1 pop, approx. 2½ fl. oz.	78	12.8			31.2	5.12	250	41.0
Dairy Queen								
Banana Split, 13½ oz.	540	103.0	40.0	7.63				
Cones:								
Small, 2½ oz.	117	18.3	46.7	7.33				
Regular, 5.0 oz.	240	38.0	48.0	7.60				
Large, 7½ oz.	340	57.0	45.3	7.60				
Cones, dipped in Chocolate:								
Small, 2¾ oz.	163	21.5	59.4	7.81				
Regular, 5½ oz.	340	42.0	61.8	7.64				
Large, 8¼ oz.	510	64.0	61.4	7.71				
"Dilly" bar, 3 oz.	210	21.0	70.0	7.00				
"DQ" Sandwich, 2⅛ oz.	140	24.0	66.0	11.32				
"Fiesta" Sundae, 9.5 oz.	570	84.0	60.0	8.84				
Freeze, 14.0 oz.	500	89.0	35.7	6.36				
Mr. Misty Float, 14½ oz.	390	74.0	26.9	5.10				
Freeze, 14½ oz.	500	91.0	34.5	6.28				
Kiss, 3⅛ oz.	70	17.0	22.4	5.43				
Parfait, 10 oz.	430	76.0	43.0	7.60				
Peanut Butter Parfait, 10.8 oz.	740	94.0	68.5	8.70				
Sundaes, Chocolate:								
Small, 3¾ oz.	190	33.0	51.4	8.92				
Regular, 6¼ oz.	310	56.0	50.0	9.03				
Large, 8¾ oz.	440	78.0	50.6	8.97				
Dannon Frozen Yogurt								
Danny-in-a-Cup (hard frozen yogurt)								
Banana, 8-fl.-oz. container	210	42.0	35.0	7.00	26.3	5.25	210	42.0
Boysenberry, 8-fl.-oz. container	210	42.0	35.0	7.00	26.3	5.25	210	42.0
Chocolate, 8-fl.-oz. container	190	32.0	31.7	5.33	23.8	4.00	190	32.0
Orange-Pineapple, 8-fl.-oz. container	210	42.0	35.0	7.00	26.3	5.25	210	42.0
Peach, 8-fl.-oz. container	210	42.0	35.0	7.00	26.3	5.25	210	42.0
Piña Colada, 8-fl.-oz. container	210	42.0	35.0	7.00	26.3	5.25	210	42.0
Red Raspberry, 8-fl.-oz. container	210	42.0	35.0	7.00	26.3	5.25	210	42.0
Strawberry, 8-fl.-oz. container	210	42.0	35.0	7.00	26.3	5.25	210	42.0
Vanilla, 8-fl.-oz. container	180	20.0	30.0	3.33	22.5	2.50	180	20.0
Danny-on-a-Stick:								
Boysenberry, (uncoated), 15-fl.-oz. box (6 bars)	420	78.0			28.0	5.20	224	41.6
1 bar, approx. 2½ fl. oz.	70	13.0			28.0	5.20	224	41.6
Boysenberry, carob-coated, 15-fl.-oz. box (6 bars)	840	90.0			56.0	6.00	448	48.0
1 bar, approx. 2½ fl. oz.	140	15.0			56.0	6.00	448	48.0
Chocolate, (uncoated), 15-fl.-oz. box (6 bars)	360	60.0			24.0	4.00	192	32.0
1 bar, approx. 2½ fl. oz.	60	10.0			24.0	4.00	192	32.0
Chocolate, chocolate-coated, 15-fl.-oz. box (6 bars)	780	72.0			52.0	4.80	416	38.4
1 bar, approx. 2½ fl. oz.	130	12.0			52.0	4.80	416	38.4
Piña Colada, (uncoated), 15-fl.-oz. box (6 bars)	420	84.0			28.0	5.60	224	44.8
1 bar, approx. 2½ fl. oz.	70	14.0			28.0	5.60	224	44.8
Red Raspberry, (uncoated), 15-fl.-oz. box (6 bars)	420	78.0			28.0	5.20	224	41.6
1 bar, approx. 2½ fl. oz.	70	13.0			28.0	5.20	224	41.6

	UNIT		1 OZ., BY WT.		1 FLUID OZ.		1 CUP, PACKED	
	Cal.	Carb.	Cal.	Carb.	Cal.	Carb.	Cal.	Carb.
Red Raspberry, chocolate-coated, 15-fl.-oz. box (6 bars)	780	90.0			52.0	6.00	416	48.0
1 bar, approx. 2½ fl. oz.	130	15.0			52.0	6.00	416	48.0
Strawberry, (uncoated), 15-fl.-oz. box (6 bars)	420	78.0			28.0	5.20	224	41.6
1 bar, approx. 2½ fl. oz.	70	13.0			28.0	5.20	224	41.6
Strawberry, chocolate-coated, 15-fl.-oz. box (6 bars)	780	90.0			52.0	6.00	416	48.0
1 bar, approx. 2½ fl. oz.	130	15.0			52.0	6.00	416	48.0
Vanilla, (uncoated), 15-fl.-oz. box (6 bars)	360	66.0			24.0	4.40	192	35.2
1 bar, approx. 2½ fl. oz.	60	11.0			24.0	4.40	192	35.2
Vanilla, carob-coated, 15-fl.-oz. box (6 bars)	720	60.0			48.0	4.00	384	32.0
1 bar, approx. 2½ fl. oz.	120	10.0			48.0	4.00	384	32.0
Danny-Yo (soft frozen yogurt)								
Chocolate, 3½-fl.-oz. container	140	26.0			40.0	7.43	320	59.4
Raspberry, 3½-fl.-oz. container	110	21.0	44.0	8.40	31.4	6.00	251	48.0
Strawberry, 3½-fl.-oz. container	110	21.0	44.0	8.40	31.4	6.00	251	48.0
Vanilla, 3½-fl.-oz. container	110	21.0	44.0	8.40	31.4	6.00	251	48.0
Dole								
Frozen Fruit in Juice:								
Pineapple, 10-fl.-oz. box (4 bars)	280	72.0			28.0	7.20	224	57.6
1 bar, approx. 2½ fl. oz.	70	18.0			28.0	7.20	224	57.6
Strawberry, 10-fl.-oz. box (4 bars)	280	64.0			28.0	6.40	224	51.2
1 bar, approx. 2½ fl. oz.	70	16.0			28.0	6.40	224	51.2
Fruit Sorbet:								
Strawberry, pint container	440	112.0			27.5	7.00	220	56.0
Dolly Madison								
Orange, Frozen Yogurt, ½-gallon container	1704	336.0			26.6	5.25	213	42.0
Vanilla Dietary Dairy Dessert, ¼ pint container	140	15.0			35.0	3.75	280	30.0
Dreamsicle								
Ice Milk Center Deluxe, 30-fl.-oz. box (12 pops)	840	157.2			28.0	5.24	224	41.9
1 pop, approx. 2½ fl. oz.	70	13.1			28.0	5.24	224	41.9
Friendly's								
Cake Cones:								
Chocolate, Regular, approx. 4.2 oz. (4 oz. ice cream, 0.2 oz. cone)	260	32.0	61.9	7.62				
Double Dip, approx. 7.2 oz. (7 oz. ice cream, 0.2 oz. cone)	440	54.0	61.1	7.50				
Vanilla, Regular, approx. 4.2 oz. (4 oz. ice cream, 0.2 oz. cone)	250	29.0	59.5	6.95				
Double Dip, approx. 7.2 oz. (7 oz. ice cream, 0.2 oz. cone)	420	49.0	58.3	6.81				
Sugar Cones:								
Chocolate, Regular, approx. 4½ oz. (4 oz. ice cream, ½ oz. cone)	310	41.0	68.9	9.11				
Double Dip, approx. 7½ oz. (7 oz. ice cream, ½ oz. cone)	490	63.0	65.3	8.40				
Vanilla, Regular, approx. 4½ oz. (4 oz. ice cream, ½ oz. cone)	290	38.0	64.4	8.44				
Double Dip, approx. 7½ oz. (7 oz. ice cream, ½ oz. cone)	460	57.0	61.3	7.60				
Sundaes:								
Fudge-Vanilla Ice Cream, 6.3 oz.	420	50.0	66.7	7.94				
Hot Fudge Sundae, approx. 5⅓ oz.	290	44.6	54.4	8.36				
Strawberry/Vanilla Ice Cream, approx. 6.3 oz.	340	39.0	54.0	6.19				
Frozfruit								
Frozen Fruit Bars:								
Pineapple, 16-fl.-oz. (1-pint) box (4 bars)	272	67.2			17.0	4.20	136	33.6
1 bar, approx. 4 fl. oz.	68	16.8			17.0	4.20	136	33.6
Strawberry, 16-fl.-oz. (1-pint) box (4 bars)	280	64.0			17.5	4.00	140	32.0
1 bar, approx. 4 fl. oz.	70	16.0			17.5	4.00	140	32.0
Ice Milk Confection:								
Banana, 16-fl.-oz. (1-pint) container	480	79.6			30.0	4.98	240	39.8

	UNIT		1 OZ., BY WT.		1 FLUID OZ.		1 CUP, PACKED	
	Cal.	Carb.	Cal.	Carb.	Cal.	Carb.	Cal.	Carb.
Fudgsicle								
Banana, 30-fl.-oz. box (12 pops)	1224	282.0			40.8	9.40	326	75.2
1 pop, approx. 2½ fl. oz.	102	23.5			40.8	9.40	326	75.2
Chocolate, 30-fl.-oz. box (12 pops)	1224	284.4			40.8	9.48	236	75.8
1 pop, approx. 2½ fl. oz.	102	23.7			40.8	9.48	236	75.8
Glacé Lite (Sweet Victory)								
White Chocolate Chip Lowfat Frozen Dairy Dessert, pint container	400	76.0			25.0	4.75	200	38.0
Good Humor								
Bars:								
Chip Crunch Whammy Bars, 12.8-oz. box (8 bars)	880	80.0	68.8	6.25				
1 bar, approx. 1.6 oz.	110	10.0	68.8	6.25				
Chocolate Eclair Bars, 18-oz. box (6 bars)	1320	150.0	73.3	8.33				
1 bar, approx. 3 oz.	220	25.0	73.3	8.33				
Chocolate Whammy Bars, 12.8-oz. box (8 bars)	800	72.0	62.5	5.63				
1 bar, approx. 1.6 oz.	100	9.0	62.5	5.63				
Grape Ice Whammy, 18-oz. box (12 pops)	600	156.0	33.3	8.67				
1 pop, approx. 1½ oz.	50	13.0	33.3	8.67				
Orange Ice Whammy, 18-oz. box (12 pops)	600	156.0	33.3	8.67				
1 pop, approx. 1½ oz.	50	13.0	33.3	8.67				
Strawberry Shortcake Bars, 18-oz. box (6 bars)	1200	126.0	66.7	7.00				
1 bar, approx. 3 oz.	200	21.0	66.7	7.00				
Strawberry Whammy Bars, 12.8-oz. box (8 bars)	800	72.0	62.5	5.63				
1 bar, approx. 1.6 oz.	100	9.0	62.5	5.63				
"Stripes" (grape, orange, cherry, lemon), 18-oz. box (12 pops)	600	156.0	33.3	8.67				
1 pop, approx. 1½ oz.	50	13.0	33.3	8.67				
Toasted Almond, 18-oz. box (6 bars)	1320	126.0	73.3	7.00				
1 bar, approx. 3 oz.	220	21.0	73.3	7.00				
Vanilla, Chocolate-Coated, 18-oz. box (6 bars)	1020	72.0	56.7	4.00				
1 bar, approx. 3 oz.	170	12.0	56.7	4.00				
Vanilla Whammy Bars, 12.8-oz. box (8 bars)	800	72.0	62.5	5.63				
1 bar, approx. 1.6 oz.	100	9.0	62.5	5.63				
Containers, Ice Cream:								
Black Cherry, ½-gallon container	2080	224.0			32.5	3.50	260	28.0
Butter Pecan, ½-gallon container	2080	224.0			32.5	3.50	260	28.0
Chocolate, ½-gallon container	2080	240.0			32.5	3.75	260	30.0
Chocolate Chip, ½-gallon container	2400	240.0			37.5	3.75	300	30.0
Royal Fudge, ½-gallon container	1920	224.0			30.0	3.50	240	28.0
Strawberry, ½-gallon container	1920	240.0			30.0	3.75	240	30.0
Toffee Fudge Swirl, ½-gallon container	2080	288.0			32.5	4.50	260	36.0
Vanilla, ½-gallon container	2240	224.0			35.0	3.50	280	28.0
Vanilla/Chocolate/Strawberry, ½-gallon container	2080	224.0			32.5	3.50	260	28.0
Vanilla Fudge Swirl, ½-gallon container	2240	240.0			35.0	3.75	280	30.0
Sandwiches:								
Vanilla Ice Cream Sandwich, 15-oz. box (6 sandwiches)	1200	204.0	80.0	13.60				
1 sandwich, approx. 2½ oz.	200	34.0	80.0	13.60				
Häagen-Dazs								
Ice Cream								
Carob, pint container	1013	80.2	64.3	5.09	63.3	5.01	507	40.1
Chocolate, pint container	1073	96.2	70.9	6.36	67.0	6.01	536	48.1
Coffee, pint container	1033	91.6	68.3	6.06	64.6	5.73	517	45.8
Honey, pint container	1004	69.9	64.4	4.48	62.8	4.37	502	35.0
Rum Raisin, pint container	1023	98.0	66.0	6.33	64.0	6.13	517	49.0
Strawberry, pint container	1032	95.7	66.6	6.18	64.5	5.98	516	47.9
Vanilla, pint container	1027	92.0	66.0	5.97	64.2	5.75	513	46.0
Sorbet & Cream:								
Raspberry Fruit Ice and Vanilla Ice Cream, pint container	760	100.0			47.5	6.25	380	50.0

	UNIT		1 OZ., BY WT.		1 FLUID OZ.		1 CUP, PACKED	
	Cal.	Carb.	Cal.	Carb.	Cal.	Carb.	Cal.	Carb.
Orange Fruit Ice and Vanilla Ice Cream, pint container	880	124.0			55.0	7.75	440	62.0
Harbison's Ice Cream								
Butter Pecan, ½-gallon container	2240	256.0			35.0	4.00	280	32.0
Chocolate, ½-gallon container	2080	256.0			32.5	4.00	260	32.0
Chocolate/Vanilla/ Strawberry, ½-gallon container	2080	256.0			32.5	4.00	260	32.0
Vanilla, ½-gallon container	2240	240.0			35.0	3.75	280	30.0
Heath								
Toffee Ice Cream Bar, 18-fl.-oz. box (6 bars)	1020	96.0			56.7	5.33	454	42.6
1 bar, approx. 3 fl. oz.	170	16.0			56.7	5.33	454	42.6
Hood								
Apple Sunshine Bars, Apple Water Ice on Stick, 2-fl.-oz. bar	50	13.0			25.0	6.50	200	52.0
Chocolate Pudding Stix, 1.9-fl.-oz. bar	100	17.0			52.6	8.95	421	71.6
Lemonade Sunshine Bars, Lemonade Water Ice on Stick, 2-fl.-oz. bar	50	13.0			25.0	6.50	200	52.0
Orange Foam Cup, Orange Water Ice, 4-fl.-oz. cup	110	25.0			27.5	6.25	220	50.0
Orange Sunshine Bars, Orange Water Ice on Stick, 2-fl.-oz. bar	50	13.0			25.0	6.50	200	52.0
Orange Sunshine Cup, Orange Water Ice, 3-fl.-oz. cup	80	19.0			26.7	6.33	213	50.7
Vanilla Ice Cream, ½-gallon container	2080	256.0			32.5	4.00	260	32.0
Howard Johnson's								
Ice Cream:								
Chocolate, pint container	884	(71.4)	(89.5)	(7.23)	55.3	(4.46)	442	(35.7)
quart container	1768	(142.5)	(89.5)	(7.23)	55.3	(4.46)	442	(35.7)
Strawberry, pint container	748	(65.3)	(75.7)	(6.61)	46.8	(4.09)	374	(32.7)
quart container	1496	(130.6)	(75.7)	(6.61)	46.8	(4.09)	374	(32.7)
Vanilla, pint container	840	(59.7)	(85.0)	(6.04)	52.5	(3.73)	420	(29.8)
quart container	1680	(119.4)	(85.0)	(6.04)	52.5	(3.73)	420	(29.8)
Sherbet:								
Orange, pint container	528	(112.1)	(38.7)	(8.22)	33.0	(7.01)	264	(56.1)
quart container	1056	(224.2)	(38.7)	(8.22)	33.0	(7.01)	264	(56.1)
Jell-O Pudding Pops								
Banana, 19.8-fl.-oz. box (12 bars)	1080	180.0			54.5	9.09	436	72.7
1 bar, approx. 1.65 fl. oz.	90	15.0			54.5	9.09	436	72.7
Chocolate, 24-fl.-oz. box (12 bars)	1200	192.0			50.0	8.00	400	64.0
1 bar, approx. 2 fl. oz.	100	16.0			50.0	8.00	400	64.0
Vanilla, 24-fl.-oz. box (12 bars)	1080	192.0			45.0	8.00	384	64.0
1 bar, approx. 2 fl. oz.	90	16.0			45.0	8.00	384	64.0
Pudding Pop Variety Pack, 2 Banana, 2 Chocolate, 2 Vanilla, 12-oz. net wt. box (6 bars)	560	96.0						
Johnston Frozen Yogurt								
Butter Brickle, Hard Frozen Yogurt, 8-fl.-oz. container	220	42.0	(36.7)	(7.00)	27.5	5.25	220	42.0
Caramel Pecan, Hard Frozen Yogurt, 8-fl.-oz. container	200	37.0	(33.3)	(6.17)	25.0	4.63	200	37.0
Chocolate, Hard Frozen Yogurt, 8-fl.-oz. container	240	47.0	(40.0)	(7.83)	30.0	5.88	240	47.0
Chocolate, Soft Frozen Yogurt, 8-fl.-oz. container	203	36.0			25.4	4.50	203	36.0
Peach, Hard Frozen Yogurt, 8-fl.-oz. container	180	34.0	(30.0)	(5.67)	22.5	4.25	180	34.0
Strawberry, Hard Frozen Yogurt, 8-fl.-oz. container	180	34.0	(30.0)	(5.67)	22.5	4.25	180	34.0
Strawberry, Soft Frozen Yogurt, 8-fl.-oz. container	208	37.0			26.0	4.63	208	37.0
Vanilla, Soft Frozen Yogurt, 8-fl.-oz. container	181	31.0			22.6	3.88	181	31.0
le sorbet								
Sherbet:								
Cantaloupe, 4-fl.-oz. container	72	16.8			18.0	4.20	144	33.6
Lemon, 4-fl.-oz. container	96	22.1			24.0	5.53	192	44.2
Orange, 4-fl.-oz. container	71	18.1			17.8	4.53	142	36.2
Raspberry, 4-fl.-oz. container	78	22.2			19.5	5.55	156	44.4
Strawberry, 4-fl.-oz. container	86	21.7			21.5	5.43	172	43.4
French Fruit Ice:								
Passion Fruit, 1-pint container	320	720			20.0	4.50	160	36.0

	UNIT		1 OZ., BY WT.		1 FLUID OZ.		1 CUP, PACKED	
	Cal.	Carb.	Cal.	Carb.	Cal.	Carb.	Cal.	Carb.
Light n' Lively (Sealtest) Ice Milk								
Banana-Red Raspberry Twirl, ½-gallon container	1760	336.0	47.3	9.02	27.5	5.25	220	42.0
Banana Strawberry Twirl, ½-gallon container	1760	336.0	47.2	9.01	27.5	5.25	220	42.0
Caramel Nut, 4-fl.-oz. container	120	18.0	51.5	7.73	30.0	4.50	240	36.0
pint container	480	72.0	51.5	7.73	30.0	4.50	240	36.0
½-gallon container	1920	288.0	51.5	7.73	30.0	4.50	240	36.0
Chocolate, 4-fl.-oz. container	100	19.0	43.0	8.16	25.0	4.75	200	38.0
pint container	400	76.0	43.0	8.16	25.0	4.75	200	38.0
½-gallon container	1600	304.0	43.0	8.16	25.0	4.75	200	38.0
Chocolate Marshmallow Twirl, 4-fl.-oz. container	120	23.0	51.5	9.88	30.0	5.75	240	46.0
pint container	480	92.0	51.5	9.88	30.0	5.75	240	46.0
½-gallon container	1920	368.0	51.5	9.88	30.0	5.75	240	46.0
Coffee, 4-fl.-oz. container	100	17.0	43.0	7.30	25.0	4.25	200	34.0
pint container	400	68.0	43.0	7.30	25.0	4.25	200	34.0
½-gallon container	1600	272.0	43.0	7.30	25.0	4.25	200	34.0
Heavenly Hash, ½-gallon container	1920	320.0	30.0	8.59	240	40.0		
Lemon Chiffon, 4-fl.-oz. container	120	23.0	51.5	9.88	30.0	5.75	240	46.0
pint container	480	92.0	51.5	9.88	30.0	5.75	240	46.0
½-gallon container	1920	368.0	51.5	9.88	30.0	5.75	240	46.0
Orange-Pineapple, 4-fl.-oz. container	100	18.0	43.0	7.73	25.0	4.50	200	36.0
pint container	400	72.0	43.0	7.73	25.0	4.50	200	36.0
½-gallon container	1600	288.0	43.0	7.73	25.0	4.50	200	36.0
Peach, 4-fl.-oz. container	100	18.0	43.0	7.73	25.0	4.50	200	36.0
pint container	400	72.0	43.0	7.73	25.0	4.50	200	36.0
½-gallon container	1600	288.0	43.0	7.73	25.0	4.50	200	36.0
Strawberry, 4-fl.-oz. container	100	18.0	43.0	7.73	25.0	4.50	200	36.0
pint container	400	72.0	43.0	7.73	25.0	4.50	200	36.0
½-gallon container	1600	288.0	43.0	7.73	25.0	4.50	200	36.0
Toffee Crunch, 4-fl.-oz. container	120	19.0	51.5	8.16	30.0	4.75	240	38.0
pint container	480	76.0	51.5	8.16	30.0	4.75	240	38.0
½-gallon container	1920	304.0	51.5	8.16	30.0	4.75	240	38.0
Vanilla, 4-fl.-oz. container	100	17.0	43.0	7.30	25.0	4.25	200	34.0
pint container	400	68.0	43.0	7.30	25.0	4.25	200	34.0
½-gallon container	1600	272.0	43.0	7.30	25.0	4.25	200	34.0
Vanilla/Chocolate/ Strawberry, 4-fl.-oz. container	100	18.0	43.0	7.73	25.0	4.50	200	36.0
pint container	400	72.0	43.0	7.73	25.0	4.50	200	36.0
½-gallon container	1600	288.0	43.0	7.73	25.0	4.50	200	36.0
Vanilla Fudge Twirl, 4-fl.-oz. container	110	20.0	47.3	8.59	27.5	5.00	220	40.0
pint container	440	80.0	47.3	8.59	27.5	5.00	220	40.0
½-gallon container	1760	320.0	47.3	8.59	27.5	5.00	220	40.0
Lucerne Dietetic Ice Cream								
Chocolate, pint container	479		51.0		29.9		239	
Vanilla, pint container	519		55.3		32.4		259	
Luxury Ice Cream								
Chocolate, ½-gallon container	2080	256.0	55.4	6.82	32.5	4.00	260	32.0
Chocolate Sundae, ½-gallon container	2400	304.0	63.9	8.10	37.5	4.75	300	38.0
Chocolate/Vanilla/ Strawberry, ½-gallon container	1920	240.0	(51.2)	(6.39)	30.0	3.75	240	30.0
Mint Chocolate Chip, ½-gallon container	2720	256.0	72.5	6.82	42.5	4.00	340	32.0
Pecan Crunch, ½-gallon container	2240	288.0	59.7	7.67	35.0	4.50	280	36.0
Vanilla, ½-gallon container	1920	224.0	(51.2)	(5.96)	30.0	3.50	240	28.0
Vanilla/Chocolate, ½-gallon container	1920	224.0	(51.2)	(5.97)	30.0	3.50	240	28.0
Meadow Gold								
Ice Cream:								
Black Walnut, quart container	1280	128.0	68.3	6.83	40.0	4.00	320	32.0
Butter Pecan, quart container	1200	128.0	64.1	6.83	37.5	4.00	300	32.0
Cherry Vanilla, quart container	1120	144.0	59.7	7.69	35.0	4.50	280	36.0
Chocolate, quart container	1120	144.0	59.8	7.69	35.0	4.50	280	36.0
Chocolate Chip, quart container	1200	136.0	64.0	7.26	37.5	4.25	300	34.0
Chocolate Revel, quart container	1120	152.0	59.8	8.11	35.0	4.75	280	38.0

	UNIT		1 OZ., BY WT.		1 FLUID OZ.		1 CUP, PACKED	
	Cal.	Carb.	Cal.	Carb.	Cal.	Carb.	Cal.	Carb.
Golden Vanilla, quart container	1120	128.0	59.7	6.83	35.0	4.00	280	32.0
Peach, quart container	1040	128.0	55.5	6.83	32.5	4.00	260	32.0
Strawberry, quart container	1120	152.0	59.8	8.11	35.0	4.75	280	38.0
Sherbet:								
Lime, quart container	960	216.0	35.3	7.95	30.0	6.75	240	54.0
Orange, quart container	960	216.0	35.3	7.95	30.0	6.75	240	54.0
Pineapple, quart container	1040	232.0	38.3	8.54	32.5	7.25	260	58.0
Parfait:								
Brandy Alexander Parfait, 1 serving	307	21.5						
Sundaes:								
Caramel Sundae, 5.1 oz. container	282	50.8	55.3	9.96				
Hot Fudge Sundae, 5⅓ oz. container	290	44.6	54.4	8.36				
Pineapple Sundae, 5 oz. container	230	42.9	46.0	8.58				
Strawberry Sundae, 5 oz. container	229	44.1	45.6	8.82				
Natural Nectar Ice Cream								
Banana, 3-gallon tub	(16128)	(1931.5)	64.4	7.71	(42.0)	(5.03)	(336)	(40.2)
Brazilian Mocha, pint container	(672)	(80.5)	64.4	7.71	(42.0)	(5.03)	(336)	(40.2)
quart container	(1345)	(161.0)	64.4	7.71	(42.0)	(5.03)	(336)	(40.2)
Ice Cream Sandwich with Honey, 18-fl.-oz. box (6 sandwiches)	1236	174.6			68.7	9.70	550	77.6
1 sandwich, approx. 3 fl. oz.	206	29.1			68.7	9.70	550	77.6
Maple Almond, pint container	(672)	(80.5)	64.7	7.71	(42.0)	(5.03)	(336)	(40.2)
quart container	(1345)	(161.0)	64.7	7.71	(42.0)	(5.03)	(336)	(40.2)
Mocha Pie, 12-fl.-oz. box (3 pies)	1023	110.1			85.3	9.18	682	73.4
1 pie, approx. 4 fl. oz.	341	36.7			85.3	9.18	682	73.4
Nectar Pie, 12-fl.-oz. box (3 pies)	1023	110.1			85.3	9.18	682	73.4
1 pie, approx. 4 fl. oz.	341	36.7			85.3	9.18	682	73.4
Royal Dutch Cocoa, pint container	(672)	(80.5)	64.4	7.71	(42.0)	(5.03)	(336)	(40.2)
quart container	(1345)	(161.0)	64.4	7.71	(42.0)	(5.03)	(336)	(40.2)
Vanilla Fudge, pint container	(672)	(80.5)	64.4	7.71	(42.0)	(5.03)	(336)	(40.2)
quart container	(1345)	(161.0)	64.4	7.71	(42.0)	(5.03)	(336)	(40.2)
Yulovit, 12-fl.-oz. box (3 pies)	807	92.4			67.3	7.70	538	61.6
1 pie, approx. 4 fl. oz.	269	30.8			67.3	7.70	538	61.6
Nuform Ice Milk								
Vanilla, ½-gallon container	1760	272.0			27.5	4.25	220	34.0
Ocean Spray								
Juice & Fruit Bars:								
Cran•Grape, 15-fl.-oz. box (6 bars)	480	120.0			32.0	8.00	256	64.0
1 bar, approx. 2½ fl. oz.	80	20.0			32.0	8.00	256	64.0
Cran•Raspberry, 15-fl.-oz. box (6 bars)	420	114.0			28.0	7.60	224	60.8
1 bar, approx. 2½ fl. oz.	70	19.0			28.0	7.60	224	60.8
Popsicle								
Banana, 36-fl.-oz. box (12 pops)	840	198.0			23.3	5.50	187	44.0
1 pop, approx. 3 fl. oz.	70	16.5			23.3	5.50	187	44.0
Blue Grape, 36-fl.-oz. box (12 pops)	840	198.0			23.3	5.50	187	44.0
1 pop, approx. 3 fl. oz.	70	16.5			23.3	5.50	187	44.0
Blue Raspberry, 36-fl.-oz. box (12 pops)	840	198.0			23.3	5.50	187	44.0
1 pop, approx. 3 fl. oz.	70	16.5			23.3	5.50	187	44.0
Cherry, 36-fl.-oz. box (12 pops)	840	198.0			23.3	5.50	187	44.0
1 pop, approx. 3 fl. oz.	70	16.5			23.3	5.50	187	44.0
Chocolate, 36-fl.-oz. box (12 pops)	840	198.0			23.3	5.50	187	44.0
1 pop, approx. 3 fl. oz.	70	16.5			23.3	5.50	187	44.0
Grape, 36-fl.-oz. box (12 pops)	840	198.0			23.3	5.50	187	44.0
1 pop, approx. 3 fl. oz.	70	16.5			23.3	5.50	187	44.0
Lime, 36-fl.-oz. box (12 pops)	840	198.0			23.3	5.50	187	44.0
1 pop, approx. 3 fl. oz.	70	16.5			23.3	5.50	187	44.0
Orange, 36-fl.-oz. box (12 pops)	840	198.0			23.3	5.50	187	44.0
1 pop, approx. 3 fl. oz.	70	16.5			23.3	5.50	187	44.0
Raspberry, 36-fl.-oz. box (12 pops)	840	198.0			23.3	5.50	187	44.0
1 pop, approx. 3 fl. oz.	70	16.5			23.3	5.50	187	44.0

	UNIT		1 OZ., BY WT.		1 FLUID OZ.		1 CUP, PACKED	
	Cal.	Carb.	Cal.	Carb.	Cal.	Carb.	Cal.	Carb.
Root Beer, 36-fl.-oz. box (12 pops)	840	198.0			23.3	5.50	187	44.0
1 pop, approx. 3 fl. oz.	70	16.5			23.3	5.50	187	44.0
Strawberry, 36-fl.-oz. box (12 pops)	840	198.0			23.3	5.50	187	44.0
1 pop, approx. 3 fl. oz.	70	16.5			23.3	5.50	187	44.0
Vanilla, 36-fl.-oz. box (12 pops)	840	198.0			23.3	5.50	187	44.0
1 pop, approx. 3 fl. oz.	70	16.5			23.3	5.50	187	44.0
White Lemon, 36-fl.-oz. box (12 pops)	840	198.0			23.3	5.50	187	44.0
1 pop, approx. 3 fl. oz.	70	16.5			23.3	5.50	187	44.0
Schrafft's								
Chocolate Think Thin Ice Milk, pint container	540	104.0			33.8	6.50	270	52.0
quart container	1080	208.0			33.8	6.50	270	52.0
Coffee Sugar-Less Frozen Dietary Dairy Dessert, pint container	600	56.0	(47.6)	(4.44)	37.5	3.50	300	28.0
Lemon Sugar-Less Frozen Dietary Dairy Dessert, pint container	600	56.0	(47.6)	(4.44)	37.5	3.50	300	28.0
Strawberry Think Thin Ice Milk, pint container	540	104.0	(42.9)	(8.25)	33.8	6.50	270	52.0
quart container	1080	208.0	(42.9)	(8.25)	33.8	6.50	270	52.0
Vanilla Sugar-Less Frozen Dietary Dairy Dessert, pint container	600	56.0	(56.7)	(5.28)	37.5	3.50	300	28.0
Vanilla Think Thin Ice Milk, pint container	540	104.0			33.8	6.50	270	52.0
quart container	1080	208.0			33.8	6.50	270	52.0
Vanilla Fudge Sugar-Less Frozen Dietary Dairy Dessert, pint container	600	56.0	(56.7)	(5.28)	37.5	3.50	300	28.0
Schrafft's Light								
Chocolate All Natural Ice Milk, pint container	540	104.0			33.8	6.50	270	52.0
Strawberry All Natural Ice Milk, pint container	540	104.0			33.8	6.50	270	52.0
Vanilla All Natural Ice Milk, pint container	540	104.0			33.8	6.50	270	52.0
Sealtest								
Ice Cream:								
Butter Brickle, quart container	1200	152.0			37.5	4.75	300	38.0
½-gallon container	2400	304.0			37.5	4.75	300	38.0
Cherry Nugget, quart container	1120	128.0			35.0	4.00	280	32.0
½-gallon container	2240	256.0			35.0	4.00	280	32.0
Cherry Vanilla, pint container	520	68.0	52.6	6.89	32.5	4.25	260	34.0
½-gallon container	2080	272.0	52.6	6.89	32.5	4.25	260	34.0
Chocolate, pint container	560	72.0	56.7	7.29	35.0	4.50	280	36.0
½-gallon container	2240	288.0	56.7	7.29	35.0	4.50	280	36.0
Chocolate Chip, quart container	1200	136.0			37.5	4.25	300	34.0
½-gallon container	2400	272.0			37.5	4.25	300	34.0
Coffee, ½-gallon container	2240	256.0	56.7	6.40	35.0	4.00	280	32.0
Fudge Royale, pint container	600	80.0	60.8	8.10	37.5	5.00	300	40.0
½-gallon container	2400	320.0	60.8	8.10	37.5	5.00	300	40.0
Heavenly Hash, ½-gallon container	2400	304.0		37.5	4.75	300	38.0	
Peach, Old Fashioned, pint container	520	76.0	52.6	7.69	32.5	4.75	260	38.0
½-gallon container	2080	304.0	52.6	7.69	32.5	4.75	260	38.0
Red Raspberry, pint container	520		52.6		32.5		260	
½-gallon container	2080		52.6		32.5		260	
Strawberry, pint container	520	76.0	52.6	7.69	32.5	4.75	260	38.0
½-gallon container	2080	304.0	52.6	7.69	32.5	4.75	260	38.0
Vanilla, pint container	560	64.0	56.6	6.47	35.0	4.00	280	32.0
½-gallon container	2240	256.0	56.6	6.47	35.0	4.00	280	32.0
Vanilla/Chocolate/Strawberry, pint container	520	72.0	52.6	7.28	32.5	4.50	260	36.0
½-gallon container	2080	288.0	52.6	7.28	32.5	4.50	260	36.0
Sherbet:								
Lemon Sherbet, quart container	1040	240.0	(38.5)	(8.88)	32.5	7.50	260	60.0
½-gallon container	2080	480.0	(38.5)	(8.88)	32.5	7.50	260	60.0
Lime Sherbet, quart container	1040	240.0	(38.5)	(8.88)	32.5	7.50	260	60.0
½-gallon container	2080	480.0	(38.5)	(8.88)	32.5	7.50	260	60.0
Orange Sherbet, quart container	1040	240.0	(38.5)	(8.88)	32.5	7.50	260	60.0
½-gallon container	2080	480.0	(38.5)	(8.88)	32.5	7.50	260	60.0

	UNIT		1 OZ., BY WT.		1 FLUID OZ.		1 CUP, PACKED	
	Cal.	Carb.	Cal.	Carb.	Cal.	Carb.	Cal.	Carb.
Red Raspberry Sherbet, quart container	1040	240.0	(38.5)	(8.88)	32.5	7.50	260	60.0
½-gallon container	2080	480.0	(38.5)	(8.88)	32.5	7.50	260	60.0
Strawberry Sherbet, quart container	1040	240.0	(38.5)	(8.88)	32.5	7.50	260	60.0
½-gallon container	2080	480.0	(38.5)	(8.88)	32.5	7.50	260	60.0
Super Juice								
Grape Frozen Juice Bars, 24-fl.-oz. box (8 bars)	480	112.0			20.0	4.67	160	37.4
1 bar, approx. 3 fl. oz.	60	14.0			20.0	4.67	160	37.4
Sweet 'n Low								
Vanilla, Frozen Dietary Dairy Dessert bar (chocolate flavor coated), 15-fl.-oz. box (6 bars)	780	72.0			52.0	4.80	416	38.4
1 bar, approx. 2½ fl. oz.	130	12.0			52.0	4.80	416	38.4
Swift's Ice Cream								
Chocolate, ½-gallon container	2080	256.0	57.8	7.11	32.5	4.00	260	32.0
Vanilla, ½-gallon container	2080	256.0	57.8	7.11	32.5	4.00	260	32.0
Tofutti								
Non-Dairy Frozen Dessert:								
Love Drops Chocolate Supreme with Chocolate-Covered Graham Cookies, pint container	920	104.0			57.5	6.50	460	52.0
Vanilla, pint container	800	84.0			50.0	5.25	400	42.0
Vanilla Almond Bark, pint container	920	92.0			57.5	5.75	460	46.0
Wildberry Supreme, pint container	840	88.0			52.5	5.50	420	44.0
Tuscan Frozen Yogurt								
Bars:								
Chocolate, (uncoated), 15-fl.-oz. box (6 bars)	510	96.0			34.0	6.40	272	51.2
1 bar, approx. 2½ fl. oz.	85	16.0			34.0	6.40	272	51.2
Chocolate, chocolate-coated bars, 15-fl.-oz. box (6 bars)	900	102.0			60.0	6.80	480	54.4
1 bar, approx. 2½ fl. oz.	150	17.0			60.0	6.80	480	54.4
Coffee (uncoated), 15-fl.-oz. box (6 bars)	420	84.0			28.0	5.60	224	44.8
1 bar, approx. 2½ fl. oz.	70	14.0			28.0	5.60	224	44.8
Coffee, chocolate-coated bars, 15-fl.-oz. box (6 bars)	780	102.0			52.0	6.80	416	54.4
1 bar, approx. 2½ fl. oz.	130	17.0			52.0	6.80	416	54.4
Strawberry (uncoated), 15-fl.-oz. box (6 bars)	420	84.0			28.0	5.60	224	44.8
1 bar, approx. 2½ fl. oz.	70	14.0			28.0	5.60	224	44.8
Strawberry, chocolate-coated, 15-fl.-oz. box (6 bars)	780	96.0			52.0	6.40	416	51.2
1 bar, approx. 2½ fl. oz.	130	16.0			52.0	6.40	416	51.2
Vanilla, chocolate-coated, 15-fl.-oz. box (6 bars)	780	102.0			52.0	6.80	416	54.4
1 bar, approx. 2½ fl. oz.	130	17.0			52.0	6.80	416	54.4
Containers (Soft Frozen Yogurt):								
Black Cherry, pint container	460	96.0	28.8	6..00	28.8	6.00	230	48.0
Chocolate, pint container	504	96.0	31.5	6.00	31.5	6.00	252	48.0
Coffee, pint container	440	88.0	36.7	7.33	27.5	5.50	220	44.0
Mandarin Orange, pint container	460	96.0	38.3	8.00	28.8	6.00	230	48.0
Vanilla, pint container	440	92.0	27.5	5.75	27.5	5.75	220	46.0
Weight Watchers								
Alpine Mint, Frozen Dietary Dessert, 5-fl.-oz. container	100	19.0	32.3	6.18	20.0	3.80	160	30.4
Banana, Frosted Treat, 7-fl.-oz. serving	120	22.0	28.6	5.24	17.1	3.14	137	25.1
Blackberry, Frosted Treat, 7-fl.-oz. serving	120	22.0	28.6	5.24	17.1	3.14	137	25.1
Blueberry, Frosted Treat, 7-fl.-oz. serving	120	22.0	28.6	5.24	17.1	3.14	137	25.1
Bordeaux Black Cherry, Frosted Treat, 7-fl.-oz. serving	120	22.0	28.6	5.24	17.1	3.14	137	25.1
Butter Pecan, Frosted Treat, 7-fl.-oz. serving	120	22.0	28.6	5.24	17.1	3.14	137	25.1
Chocolate, Frosted Treat, 7-fl.-oz. serving	120	22.0	28.6	5.24	17.1	3.14	137	25.1
Chocolate, Frozen Dietary Dessert, 5-fl.-oz. container	100	19.0	32.3	6.18	20.0	3.80	160	30.4
Chocolate Treat Frozen Confection, 16.5-fl.-oz. box (6 bars)	600	114.0			36.4	6.91	291	55.3
1 bar, approx. 2.75 fl. oz.	100	19.0			36.4	6.91	291	55.3
Chocolate Mint Treat Frozen Confection, 16.5-fl.-oz. box (6 bars)	600	114.0			36.4	6.91	291	55.3
1 bar, approx. 2.75 fl. oz.	100	19.0			36.4	6.91	291	55.3
Chocolate/Vanilla, Frozen Dietary Dessert, 5-fl.-oz. container	100	19.0	32.3	6.18	20.0	3.80	160	30.4
Coconut Pineapple, Frosted Treat, 7-fl.-oz. serving	120	22.0	28.6	5.24	17.1	3.14	137	25.1
Coffee, Frosted Treat, 7-fl.-oz. serving	120	22.0	28.6	5.24	17.1	3.14	137	25.1
Coffee, Frozen Dietary Dessert, quart container	700	133.0	33.0	6.30	21.9	4.16	175	33.3
Lemon Chiffon, Frozen Dietary Dessert, 5-fl.-oz. container	100	19.0	32.3	6.18	20.0	3.80	160	30.4
Lemon Custard, Frosted Treat, 7-fl.-oz. serving	120	22.0	28.6	5.24	17.1	3.14	137	25.1
Mango, Frosted Treat, 7-fl.-oz. serving	120	22.0	28.6	5.24	17.1	3.14	137	25.1
Maple Old Fashioned, Frozen Dietary Dessert, 5-fl.-oz. container	100	19.0	32.3	6.18	20.0	3.80	160	30.4
Orange, Frosted Treat, 7-fl.-oz. serving	120	22.0	28.6	5.24	17.1	3.14	137	25.1
Papaya, Frosted Treat, 7-fl.-oz. serving	120	22.0	28.6	5.24	17.1	3.14	137	25.1
Peach, Frosted Treat, 7-fl.-oz. serving	120	22.0	28.6	5.24	17.1	3.14	137	25.1
Pineapple, Frosted Treat, 7-fl.-oz. serving	120	22.0	28.6	5.24	17.1	3.14	137	25.1
Pistachio, Frosted Treat, 7-fl.-oz. serving	120	22.0	28.6	5.24	17.1	3.14	137	25.1
Rum, Frosted Treat, 7-fl.-oz. serving	120	22.0	28.6	5.24	17.1	3.14	137	25.1
Strawberry, Frosted Treat, 7-fl.-oz. serving	120	22.0	28.6	5.24	17.1	3.14	137	25.1
Strawberry/Vanilla, Frozen Dietary Dessert, 5-fl.-oz. container	100	19.0	32.3	6.18	20.0	3.80	160	30.4
Toffee, Old Fashioned, Frosted Treat, 7-fl.-oz. serving	120	22.0	28.6	5.24	17.1	3.14	137	25.1
True Mint, Frosted Treat, 7-fl.-oz. serving	120	22.0	28.6	5.24	17.1	3.14	137	25.1
Vanilla, Frosted Treat, 7-fl.-oz. serving	120	22.0	28.6	5.24	17.1	3.14	137	25.1
Vanilla/Strawberry, Frozen Dietary Dessert, 5-fl.-oz. container	100	19.0	32.3	6.18	20.0	3.80	160	30.4

HARD and SOFT FROZEN YOGURT

	UNIT		1 OZ., BY WT.		1 FLUID OZ.		1 CUP, PACKED	
	Cal.	Carb.	Cal.	Carb.	Cal.	Carb.	Cal.	Carb.
BANANA								
Banana, Hard Frozen **Danny-in-a-Cup,** 8-fl.-oz. container	210	42.0			26.3	5.25	210	42.0
BLACK CHERRY								
Black Cherry, Soft Frozen **Tuscan,** 16-fl.-oz. (1-pint) container	460	96.0			28.8	6.00	230	48.0
BOYSENBERRY								
Boysenberry, Hard Frozen **Danny-in-a-Cup,** 8-fl.-oz. container	210	42.0			26.3	5.25	210	42.0
BUTTER BRICKLE								
Butter Brickle, Hard Frozen **Johnston,** 8-oz. container	220	42.0			27.5	5.25	220	42.0
CARAMEL-PECAN								
Caramel-Pecan, Hard Frozen **Johnston,** 8-oz. container	200	37.0			25.0	4.63	200	37.0
CHOCOLATE								
Chocolate, Hard Frozen **Danny-in-a-Cup,** 8-fl.-oz. container	190	32.0			23.8	4.00	190	32.0
Chocolate, Soft Frozen **Danny-Yo,** 3½-fl.-oz. container	140	26.0			40.0	7.43	320	59.4
Chocolate, Hard Frozen **Johnston,** 8-oz. container	240	47.0			30.0	5.88	240	47.0
Chocolate, Soft Frozen **Johnston,** 8-oz. container	203	36.0			25.4	4.50	203	36.0
Chocolate, Soft Frozen **Tuscan,** 16-fl.-oz. (1-pint) container	504	96.0			31.5	6.00	252	48.0
MANDARIN ORANGE								
Mandarin Orange, Soft Frozen **Tuscan,** 16-fl.-oz. (1-pint) container	460	96.0	38.3	8.00	28.8	6.00	230	48.0

	UNIT Cal.	UNIT Carb.	1 OZ., BY WT. Cal.	1 OZ., BY WT. Carb.	1 FLUID OZ. Cal.	1 FLUID OZ. Carb.	1 CUP, PACKED Cal.	1 CUP, PACKED Carb.
ORANGE								
Orange, **Dolly Madison,** ½-gallon container	1704	336.0			26.6	5.25	213	42.0
ORANGE-PINEAPPLE								
Orange-Pineapple, Hard Frozen **Danny-in-a-Cup,** 8-fl.-oz. container	210	42.0			26.3	5.25	210	42.0
PEACH								
Peach, Hard Frozen **Danny-in-a-Cup,** 8-fl.-oz. container	210	42.0			26.3	5.25	210	42.0
Peach, Hard Frozen **Johnston,** 8-oz. container	180	34.0			22.5	4.25	180	34.0
PINA COLADA								
Piña Colada, **Colombo,** pint container	440	80.0			27.5	5.00	220	40.0
Piña Colada, Hard Frozen **Danny-in-a-Cup,** 8-fl.-oz. container	210	42.0			26.3	5.25	210	42.0
PLAIN								
"Plain," **Carvel,** Lo-Yo, 3-fl.-oz. container	110	20.1	40.6	7.39	36.7	6.70	293	53.6
RASPBERRY								
Raspberry, Hard Frozen **Danny-in-a-Cup,** 8-fl.-oz. container	210	42.0			26.3	5.25	210	42.0
Raspberry, Soft Frozen **Danny-Yo,** 3½-fl.-oz. container	110	21.0	44.0	8.40	31.4	6.00	251	48.0
STRAWBERRY								
Strawberry, **Colombo,** pint container	440	80.0			27.5	5.00	220	40.0
Strawberry, Hard Frozen **Danny-in-a-Cup,** 8-fl.-oz. container	210	42.0			26.3	5.25	210	42.0
Strawberry, Soft Frozen **Danny-Yo,** 3½-fl.-oz. container	110	21.0			31.4	6.00	251	48.0
Strawberry, Hard Frozen **Johnston,** 8-oz. container	180	34.0			22.5	4.25	180	34.0
Strawberry, Soft Frozen **Johnston,** 8-oz. container	208	37.0			26.0	4.63	208	37.0
Strawberry, Soft Frozen **Tuscan,** 16-fl.-oz. (1-pint) container	460	96.0			28.8	6.00	230	48.0
VANILLA								
Vanilla, **Colombo,** pint container	440	80.0			27.5	5.00	220	40.0
Vanilla, Hard Frozen **Danny-in-a-Cup,** 8-fl.-oz. container	180	20.0			22.5	2.50	180	20.0
Vanilla, Soft Frozen **Danny-Yo,** 3½-fl.-oz. container	110	21.0			31.4	6.00	251	48.0
Vanilla, Soft Frozen **Johnston,** 8-oz. container	181	31.0			22.6	3.88	181	31.0
Vanilla, Soft Frozen **Tuscan,** 16-fl.-oz. (1-pint) container	440	92.0			27.5	5.75	220	46.0

ICE CREAM BARS

	ENTIRE CONTAINER Cal.	ENTIRE CONTAINER Carb.	1 BAR Cal.	1 BAR Carb.	1 FLUID OZ. Cal.	1 FLUID OZ. Carb.	1 CUP, PACKED Cal.	1 CUP, PACKED Carb.
Dairy Queen								
"Dilly" bar, 3 oz.			210	21.0				
Good Humor								
(Good Humor bars are sold by weight, not by fluid ounces. No fluid-ounce information was available.)								
Chip Crunch Whammy Bars, 12.8-oz. box (8 bars)	880	80.0						
1 bar, approx. 1.6 oz.			110	10.0				
Chocolate Eclair Bars, 18-oz. box (6 bars)	1320	150.0						
1 bar, approx. 3 oz.			220	25.0				
Chocolate Whammy Bars, 12.8-oz. box (8 bars)	800	72.0						
1 bar, approx. 1.6 oz.			100	9.0				
Strawberry Shortcake Bars, 18-oz. box (6 bars)	1200	126.0						
1 bar, approx. 3 oz.			200	21.0				
Strawberry Whammy Bars, 12.8-oz. box (8 bars)	800	72.0						
1 bar, approx. 1.6 oz.			100	9.0				
Toasted Almond, 18-oz. box (6 bars)	1320	126.0						
1 bar, approx. 3 oz.			220	21.0				
Vanilla, Chocolate-coated, 18-oz. box (6 bars)	1020	72.0						
1 bar, approx. 3 oz.			170	12.0				
Vanilla Whammy Bars, 12.8-oz. box (8 bars)	800	72.0						
1 bar, approx. 1.6 oz.			100	9.0				
Heath								
Toffee Ice Cream Bar, 18-fl.-oz. box (6 bars)	1020	96.0						
1 bar, approx. 3 fl. oz.			170	16.0				
Sweet 'N Low								
Vanilla, Frozen Dietary Dairy Dessert bar (chocolate flavor coated), 15-fl.-oz. box (6 bars)	780	72.0			52.0	4.80	416	38.4
1 bar, approx. 2½ fl. oz.			130	12.0	52.0	4.80	416	38.4

FROZEN YOGURT BARS

	ENTIRE CONTAINER Cal.	ENTIRE CONTAINER Carb.	1 BAR Cal.	1 BAR Carb.	1 FLUID OZ. Cal.	1 FLUID OZ. Carb.	1 CUP, PACKED Cal.	1 CUP, PACKED Carb.
Blueberry (uncoated) **Beautiful Day** bars, 15-fl.-oz. box (6 bars)	240	30.0			16.0	2.00	128	16.0
1 bar, approx. 2½ fl. oz.			40	5.0	16.0	2.00	128	16.0
Boysenberry (uncoated) **Danny-on-a-Stick,** 15-fl.-oz. box (6 bars)	420	78.0			28.0	5.20	224	41.6
1 bar, approx. 2½ fl. oz.			70	13.0	28.0	5.20	224	41.6
Boysenberry, carob-coated **Danny-on-a-Stick,** 15-fl.-oz. box (6 bars)	840	90.0			56.0	6.00	448	48.0
1 bar, approx. 2½ fl. oz.			140	15.0	56.0	6.00	448	48.0
Chocolate, chocolate-coated **Colombo** bar, 15-fl.-oz. box (6 bars)	870	102.0			58.0	6.80	464	54.4
1 bar, approx. 2½ fl. oz.			145	17.0	58.0	6.80	464	54.4
Chocolate (uncoated) **Danny-on-a-Stick,** 15-fl.-oz. box (6 bars)	360	60.0			24.0	4.00	192	32.0
1 bar, approx. 2½ fl. oz.			60	10.0	24.0	4.00	192	32.0
Chocolate, chocolate-coated **Danny-on-a-Stick,** 15-fl.-oz. box (6 bars)	780	72.0			52.0	4.80	416	38.4
1 bar, approx. 2½ fl. oz.			130	12.0	52.0	4.80	416	38.4
Chocolate (uncoated) **Tuscan** bars, 15-fl.-oz. box (6 bars)	510	96.0			34.0	6.40	272	51.2
1 bar, approx. 2½ fl. oz.			85	16.0	34.0	6.40	272	51.2
Chocolate, chocolate-coated **Tuscan** bars, 15-fl.-oz. box (6 bars)	900	102.0			60.0	6.80	480	54.4
1 bar, approx. 2½ fl. oz.			150	17.0	60.0	6.80	480	54.4
Coffee (uncoated) **Tuscan** bars, 15-fl.-oz. box (6 bars)	420	84.0			28.0	5.60	224	44.8
1 bar, approx. 2½ fl. oz.			70	14.0	28.0	5.60	224	44.8
Coffee, chocolate-coated **Tuscan** bars, 15-fl.-oz. box (6 bars)	780	102.0			52.0	6.80	416	54.4
1 bar, approx. 2½ fl. oz.			130	17.0	52.0	6.80	416	54.4
Lemon (uncoated) **Beautiful Day** bars, 15-fl.-oz. box (6 bars)	240	30.0			16.0	2.00	128	16.0
1 bar, approx. 2½ fl. oz.			40	5.0	16.0	2.00	128	16.0
Peach (uncoated) **Beautiful Day** bars, 15-fl.-oz. box (6 bars)	240	30.0			16.0	2.00	128	16.0
1 bar, approx. 2½ fl. oz.			40	5.0	16.0	2.00	128	16.0
Piña Colada (uncoated) **Danny-on-a-Stick,** 15-fl.-oz. box (6 bars)	420	84.0			28.0	5.60	224	44.8
1 bar, approx. 2½ fl. oz.			70	14.0	28.0	5.60	224	44.8
Raspberry (uncoated) **Beautiful Day** bars, 15-fl.-oz. box (6 bars)	240	30.0			16.0	2.00	128	16.0
1 bar, approx. 2½ fl. oz.			40	5.0	16.0	2.00	128	16.0
Red Raspberry (uncoated) **Danny-on-a-Stick,** 15-fl.-oz. box (6 bars)	420	78.0			28.0	5.20	224	41.6
1 bar, approx. 2½ fl. oz.			70	13.0	28.0	5.20	224	41.6
Red Raspberry, chocolate-coated **Danny-on-a-Stick,** 15-fl.-oz. box (6 bars)	780	90.0			52.0	6.00	416	48.0
1 bar, approx. 2½ fl. oz.			130	15.0	52.0	6.00	416	48.0
Strawberry (uncoated) **Beautiful Day** bars, 15-fl.-oz. box (6 bars)	240	30.0			16.0	2.00	128	16.0
1 bar, approx. 2½ fl. oz.			40	5.0	16.0	2.00	128	16.0

	ENTIRE CONTAINER		1 BAR		1 FLUID OZ.		1 CUP, PACKED	
	Cal.	Carb.	Cal.	Carb.	Cal.	Carb.	Cal.	Carb.
Strawberry (uncoated) **Colombo** bar, 15-fl.-oz. box (6 bars)	480	84.0			32.0	5.60	256	44.8
1 bar, approx. 2½ fl. oz.			80	14.0	32.0	5.60	256	44.8
Strawberry (uncoated) **Danny-on-a-Stick,** 15-fl.-oz. box (6 bars)	420	78.0			28.0	5.20	224	41.6
1 bar, approx. 2½ fl. oz.			70	13.0	28.0	5.20	224	41.6
Strawberry, chocolate-coated **Danny-on-a-Stick,** 15-fl.-oz. box (6 bars)	780	90.0			52.0	6.00	416	48.0
1 bar, approx. 2½ fl. oz.			130	15.0	52.0	6.00	416	48.0
Strawberry (uncoated) **Tuscan** bars, 15-fl.-oz. box (6 bars)	420	84.0			28.0	5.60	224	44.8
1 bar, approx. 2½ fl. oz.			70	14.0	28.0	5.60	224	44.8
Strawberry, chocolate-coated **Tuscan** bars, 15-fl.-oz. box (6 bars)	780	96.0			52.0	6.40	416	51.2
1 bar, approx. 2½ fl. oz.			130	16.0	52.0	6.40	416	51.2
Vanilla (uncoated) **Danny-on-a-Stick,** 15-fl.-oz. box (6 bars)	360	66.0			24.0	4.40	192	35.2
1 bar, approx. 2½ fl. oz.			60	11.0	24.0	4.40	192	35.2
Vanilla, carob-coated **Danny-on-a-Stick,** 15-fl.-oz. box (6 bars)	720	60.0			48.0	4.00	384	32.0
1 bar, approx. 2½ fl. oz.			120	10.0	48.0	4.00	384	32.0
Vanilla, chocolate-coated **Colombo** bar, 15-fl.-oz. box (6 bars)	870	102.0			58.0	6.80	464	54.4
1 bar, approx. 2½ fl. oz.			145	17.0	24.0	4.40	192	35.2
Vanilla, chocolate-coated **Tuscan** bars, 15-fl.-oz. box (6 bars)	780	102.0			52.0	6.80	416	54.4
1 bar, approx. 2½ fl. oz.			130	17.0	52.0	6.80	416	54.4
PUDDING BARS								
Hood, Chocolate Pudding Stix, 1.9-fl.-oz. bar	100	17.0			52.6	8.95	421	71.6
Jell-O Pudding Pops Banana, 19.8-fl.-oz. box (12 bars)	1080	180.0			54.5	9.09	436	72.7
1 bar, approx. 1.65 fl. oz.			90	15.0	54.5	9.09	436	72.7
Chocolate, 24-fl.-oz. box (12 bars)	1200	192.0			50.0	8.00	400	64.0
1 bar, approx. 2 fl. oz.			100	16.0	50.0	8.00	400	64.0
Vanilla, 24-fl.-oz. box (12 bars)	1080	192.0			45.5	8.00	384	64.0
1 bar, approx. 2 fl. oz.			90	16.0	45.5	8.00	384	64.0
Pudding Pop Variety Pack, 2 Banana, 2 Chocolate, 2 Vanilla, 12-oz. net wt. box (6 bars)	560	96.0						
SHERBET BARS and ICE POPS								
Bi-Sicle Chocolate, 30-fl.-oz. box (12 pops)	1344	256.8			44.8	8.56	358	68.5
1 pop, approx. 2½ fl. oz.			112	21.4	44.8	8.56	358	68.5
Chicquita Fruit & Juice Bars, Cherry, 16-fl.-oz. (1-pint) box (8 pops)	400	104.0			25.0	6.50	200	52.0
1 pop, approx. 2 fl. oz.			50	13.0	25.0	6.50	200	52.0
Strawberry, 16-fl.-oz. (1-pint) box (8 pops)	400	96.0			25.0	7.50	200	48.0
1 pop, approx. 2 fl. oz.			50	12.0	25.0	7.50	200	48.0
Creamsicle Ice Cream Center Deluxe, 30-fl.-oz. box (12 pops)	936	153.6			31.2	5.12	250	41.0
1 pop, approx. 2½ fl. oz.			78	12.8	31.2	5.12	250	41.0
Dole Frozen Fruit in Juice, Pineapple, 10-fl.-oz. box (4 bars)	280	72.0			28.0	7.20	224	57.6
1 bar, approx. 2½ fl. oz.			70	18.0	28.0	7.20	224	57.6
Strawberry, 10-fl.-oz. box (4 bars)	280	64.0			28.0	6.40	224	51.2
1 bar, approx. 2½ fl. oz.			70	16.0	28.0	6.40	224	51.2
Dreamsicle Ice Milk Center Deluxe, 30-fl.-oz. box (12 pops)	840	157.2			28.0	5.24	224	41.9
1 pop, approx. 2½ fl. oz.			70	13.1	28.0	5.24	224	41.9
Frozfruit Frozen Fruit Bars, Pineapple, 16-fl.-oz. (1-pint) box (4 bars)	272	67.2			17.0	4.20	136	33.6
1 bar, approx. 4 fl. oz.			68	16.8	17.0	4.20	136	33.6
Strawberry, 16-fl.-oz. (1-pint) box (4 bars)	280	64.0			17.5	4.00	140	32.0
1 bar, approx. 4 fl. oz.			70	16.0	17.5	4.00	140	32.0
1 bar, approx. 4 fl. oz.			70	16.0	17.5	4.00	140	32.0
Fudgesicle Banana, 30-fl.-oz. box (12 pops)	1224	282.0			40.8	9.40	326	75.2
1 pop, approx. 2½ fl. oz.			102	23.5	40.8	9.40	326	75.2
Chocolate, 30-fl.-oz. box (12 pops)	1224	284.4			40.8	9.48	326	75.8
1 pop, approx. 2½ fl. oz.			102	23.7	40.8	9.48	326	75.8
Good Humor Ice Whammy, Grape, 18-oz. box (12 pops)	600	156.0						
1 pop, approx. 1½ oz.			50	13.0				
Orange, 18-oz. box (12 pops)	600	156.0						
1 pop, approx. 1½ oz.			50	13.0				
"Stripes" (grape, orange, cherry, lemon), 18-oz. box (12 pops)	600	156.0						
1 pop, approx. 1½ oz.			50	13.0				
Hood Apple Sunshine Bars, Apple Water Ice on Stick, 2-fl.-oz. bar			50	13.0	25.0	6.50	200	52.0
Lemonade Sunshine Bars, Lemonade Water Ice on Stick, 2-fl.-oz. bar			50	13.0	25.0	6.50	200	52.0
Orange Sunshine Bars, Orange Water Ice on Stick, 2-fl.-oz. bar			50	13.0	25.0	6.50	200	52.0
Ocean Spray Juice & Fruit Bars, Cran•Grape, 15-fl.-oz. box (6 bars)	480	120.0			32.0	8.00	256	64.0
1 bar, approx. 2½ fl. oz.			80.0	20.0	32.0	8.00	256	64.0
Cran•Raspberry, 15-fl.-oz. box (6 bars)	420	114.0			28.0	7.60	224	60.8
1 bar, approx. 2½ fl. oz.			70.0	19.0	28.0	7.60	224	60.8
Popsicle, Banana, 36-fl.-oz. box (12 pops)	840	198.0			23.3	5.50	187	44.0
1 pop, approx. 3 fl. oz.			70	16.5	23.3	5.50	187	44.0
Blue Grape, 36-fl.-oz. box (12 pops)	840	198.0			23.3	5.50	187	44.0
1 pop, approx. 3 fl. oz.			70	16.5	23.3	5.50	187	44.0
Blue Raspberry, 36-fl.-oz. box (12 pops)	840	198.0			23.3	5.50	187	44.0
1 pop, approx. 3 fl. oz.			70	16.5	23.3	5.50	187	44.0
Cherry, 36-fl.-oz. box (12 pops)	840	198.0			23.3	5.50	187	44.0
1 pop, approx. 3 fl. oz.			70	16.5	23.3	5.50	187	44.0
Chocolate, 36-fl.-oz. box (12 pops)	840	198.0			23.3	5.50	187	44.0
1 pop, approx. 3 fl. oz.			70	16.5	23.3	5.50	187	44.0
Grape, 36-fl.-oz. box (12 pops)	840	198.0			23.3	5.50	187	44.0
1 pop, approx. 3 fl. oz.			70	16.5	23.3	5.50	187	44.0
Lime, 36-fl.-oz. box (12 pops)	840	198.0			23.3	5.50	187	44.0
1 pop, approx. 3 fl. oz.			70	16.5	23.3	5.50	187	44.0
Orange, 36-fl.-oz. box (12 pops)	840	198.0			23.3	5.50	187	44.0
1 pop, approx. 3 fl. oz.			70	16.5	23.3	5.50	187	44.0
Raspberry, 36-fl.-oz. box (12 pops)	840	198.0			23.3	5.50	187	44.0
1 pop, approx. 3 fl. oz.			70	16.5	23.3	5.50	187	44.0
Root Beer, 36-fl.-oz. box (12 pops)	840	198.0			23.3	5.50	187	44.0
1 pop, approx. 3 fl. oz.			70	16.5	23.3	5.50	187	44.0
Strawberry, 36-fl.-oz. box (12 pops)	840	198.0			23.3	5.50	187	44.0
1 pop, approx. 3 fl. oz.			70	16.5	23.3	5.50	187	44.0
Vanilla, 36-fl.-oz. box (12 pops)	840	198.0			23.3	5.50	187	44.0
1 pop, approx. 3 fl. oz.			70	16.5	23.3	5.50	187	44.0
White Lemon, 36-fl.-oz. box (12 pops)	840	198.0			23.3	5.50	187	44.0
1 pop, approx. 3 fl. oz.			70	16.5	23.3	5.50	187	44.0
Super Juice Frozen Fruit Bars, Grape, 24-fl.-oz. box (8 bars)	480	112.0			20.0	4.67	160	37.4
1 bar, approx. 3 fl. oz.			60	14.0	20.0	4.67	160	37.4

OTHER BARS

	ENTIRE CONTAINER Cal.	ENTIRE CONTAINER Carb.	1 BAR Cal.	1 BAR Carb.	1 FLUID OZ. Cal.	1 FLUID OZ. Carb.	1 CUP, PACKED Cal.	1 CUP, PACKED Carb.
Sweet 'n Low Frozen Dietary Dairy Dessert bar, Vanilla (chocolate flavor coated), 15-fl.-oz. box (6 bars)	780	72.0			52.0	4.80	416	38.4
1 bar, approx. 2½ fl. oz.			130	12.0	52.0	4.80	416	38.4
Weight Watchers Treat Frozen Confection, Chocolate, 16.5-fl.-oz. box (6 bars)	600	114.0			36.4	6.91	291	55.3
1 bar, approx. 2.75 fl. oz.			100	19.0	36.4	6.91	291	55.3
Chocolate Mint, 16.5-fl.-oz. box (6 bars)	600	114.0			36.4	6.91	291	55.3
1 bar, approx. 2.75 fl. oz.			100	19.0	36.4	6.91	291	55.3

ICE CREAM SANDWICHES

	ENTIRE CONTAINER Cal.	ENTIRE CONTAINER Carb.	1 BAR Cal.	1 BAR Carb.	1 FLUID OZ. Cal.	1 FLUID OZ. Carb.	1 CUP, PACKED Cal.	1 CUP, PACKED Carb.
Good Humor Vanilla Ice Cream Sandwich, 15-oz. box, 6 sandwiches	1200	204.0						
1 sandwich, approx. 2½ oz.			200	34.0				
Natural Nectar Ice Cream Sandwich with Honey, 18-fl.-oz. box (6 sandwiches)	1236	174.6			68.7	9.70	550	77.6
1 sandwich, approx. 3 fl. oz.			206	29.1	68.7	9.70	550	77.6
Mocha Pie, 12-fl.-oz. box (3 pies)	1023	110.1			85.3	9.18	682	73.4
1 pie, approx. 4 fl. oz.			341	36.7	85.3	9.18	682	73.4
Nectar Pie, 12-fl.-oz. box (3 pies)	1023	110.1			85.3	9.18	682	73.4
1 pie, approx. 4 fl. oz.			341	36.7	85.3	9.18	682	73.4
Yulovit, 12-fl.-oz. box (3 pies)	807	92.4			67.3	7.70	538	61.6
1 pie, approx. 4 fl. oz.			269	30.8	67.3	7.70	538	61.6

ICE CREAM and YOGURT BON BONS

	UNIT Cal.	UNIT Carb.	1 OZ., BY WT. Cal.	1 OZ., BY WT. Carb.	1 FLUID OZ. Cal.	1 FLUID OZ. Carb.	1 CUP, PACKED Cal.	1 CUP, PACKED Carb.
Carnation Chocolate Ice Cream Bon Bons, 1.7-oz. package	120	10.9	70.7	6.37	48.0	4.36		
3.42-oz. package	240	21.8	70.7	6.37	48.0	4.36		
13.69-oz. package	960	87.2	70.7	6.37	48.0	4.36		
1 bon bon, approx. 0.34 oz.	24	2.2	70.7	6.37	48.0	4.36		
Strawberry Frozen Yogurt Bon Bons. 1.7-oz. package	120	10.9	70.7	6.37	48.0	4.36		
3.42-oz. package	240	21.8	70.7	6.37	48.0	4.36		
13.69-oz. package	960	87.2	70.7	6.37	48.0	4.36		
1 bon bon, approx. 0.34 oz.	24	2.2	70.7	6.37	48.0	4.36		
Vanilla Ice Cream Bon Bons, 1.7-oz. package	120	10.9	70.7	6.37	48.0	4.36		
3.42-oz. package	240	21.8	70.7	6.37	48.0	4.36		
13.69-oz. package	960	87.2	70.7	6.37	48.0	4.36		
1 bon bon, approx. 0.34 oz.	24	2.2	70.7	6.37	48.0	4.36		
Dairy Queen "DQ" Sandwich, 2⅛ oz.	140	24.0	66.0	11.32				

EMPTY CONES

	UNIT Cal.	UNIT Carb.	1 OZ., BY WT. Cal.	1 OZ., BY WT. Carb.	1 FLUID OZ. Cal.	1 FLUID OZ. Carb.	1 CUP, PACKED Cal.	1 CUP, PACKED Carb.
Comet Cones, 1¾-oz. package (12 cones)	240	48.0	137.1	27.43				
1 cone, approx. 0.15 oz.	20	4.0	137.1	27.43				
Cups, 1¾-oz. package (12 cups)	240	48.0	137.1	27.43				
1 cup, approx. 0.15 oz.	20	4.0	137.1	27.43				
Sugar Cones, 4-oz. package (12 cones)	480	108.0	120.0	27.00				
1 sugar cone, approx. 0.33 oz.	40	9.0	120.0	27.00				

ICE CREAM FLAVORINGS

Concentrated pellets used to give ice cream its flavor.

The following flavorings are sold by Heath (makers of the Heath candy bar). Heath ships these chips to ice cream manufacturers in containers holding about 45 pounds. Names for these flavors apply to the pellets as they are shipped by Heath. Manufacturers use their own descriptive names for these flavors for sale to the consumer.

	UNIT Cal.	UNIT Carb.	1 OZ., BY WT. Cal.	1 OZ., BY WT. Carb.	1 FLUID OZ. Cal.	1 FLUID OZ. Carb.	1 CUP, PACKED Cal.	1 CUP, PACKED Carb.
Butter Brickle, Modified, 45-lb. container	85725	14697	119.1	20.41				
Cherry Canada, 45-lb. container	87795	16128	121.9	22.40				
Chocolate Almond Crunch, 45-lb. container	95940	12658	133.3	17.58				
Cinnamon Chip, 45-lb. container	87795	16128	121.9	22.40				
Coffee Brickle, 45-lb. container	77580	16740	107.7	23.25				
English Toffee, 45-lb. container	93915	15309	130.4	21.26				
Hazelnut Toffee, 45-lb. container	128610	3470.4	178.6	4.82				
Honey Toffee, 45-lb. container	61245	16740	85.1	23.25				
Lemon Candy, 45-lb. container	87795	16128	121.9	22.40				
Pecan Crisp, 45-lb. container	95940	13882	133.3	19.28				
Peppermint Candy, 45-lb. container	8982	16128	124.8	22.40				
Red Raspberry Candy, 45-lb. container	89415	16128	124.2	22.40				
Sesame Seed Toffee, 45-lb. container	114300	4491	158.8	6.24				

AND TO "TOP IT OFF" . . .

	UNIT Cal.	UNIT Carb.	1 OZ., BY WT. Cal.	1 OZ., BY WT. Carb.	1 FLUID OZ. Cal.	1 FLUID OZ. Carb.	1 CUP, PACKED Cal.	1 CUP, PACKED Carb.
Ice Cream Bar Chocolate Coating, **Heath**			190.0	10.77				

26 GELATINS, PUDDINGS & CUSTARDS •

	UNIT		1 OZ., BY WT.		1 CUP		1 TABLE-SPOON	
	Cal.	Carb.	Cal.	Carb.	Cal.	Carb.	Cal.	Carb.
CUSTARD and CUSTARD-FILLED PASTRIES, based on USDA home recipes								
BAKED CUSTARD, made with 2 cups milk, 3 Tbsp. sugar, 2 large eggs, a dash of salt, ¼ tsp. vanilla (yield: approx. 2 cups, approx. 17.8 oz.) (loss of 10% has been applied for evaporation in cooking) (2g/3g/2g/77%/22mg)	581	56.1	32.6	3.15	305	29.4	19	1.8
CREAM PUFFS with custard filling Shell: made with 1¼ cups flour, 1 cup milk, 5 large eggs, 9⅔ Tbsp. butter, ⅛ tsp. salt. Filling: made with ¼ cup cornstarch, 2 cups milk, ½ cup sugar, 2 large eggs, ½ tsp. vanilla (yield: approx. 9 cream puffs, approx. 42 oz.) (loss of 10% has been applied for evaporation in cooking) (2g/6g/4g/58%/24mg)	2756	242.7	66.1	5.82				
1 cream puff, approx. 4.6 oz.	303	26.7	66.1	5.82				
ECLAIRS with custard filling and chocolate icing Shell: made with 1¼ cups flour, 1 cup milk, 5 large eggs, 9⅔ Tbsp. butter, ⅛ tsp. salt. Filling: made with ¼ cup cornstarch, 2 cups milk, ½ cup sugar, 2 large eggs, 1 tsp. vanilla Icing: made with 1⅓ cups milk, 1 cup sugar, 1 oz. bitter chocolate, 1 Tbsp. corn syrup, 1 Tbsp. butter, ½ tsp. vanilla (yield: approx. 12 eclairs, approx. 42.5 oz.) (loss of 10% has been applied for evaporation in cooking of shell and custard; 18% for icing) (2g/7g/4g/56%/23mg)	2882	280.0	67.8	6.58				
1 eclair, approx. 3.5 oz.	239	23.2	67.8	6.58				
GELATINS, based on generic data								
UNFLAVORED GELATINS:								
1 package, approx. 8 oz. (32 .25 oz. envelopes)	760	0.0	95.0	0.00				
1 envelope, approx. ¼ oz. (24g/0g/tr/13%/na)	24	0.0	95.0	0.00				
1 capsule, approx. .02 oz.	2	0.0	95.0	0.00				
FLAVORED GELATINS, ALL FLAVORS:								
Dessert powder, 3-oz. box (3g/25g/0g/2%/90mg)	315	74.8	105.0	24.93				
Prepared as package directs, add 2 cups water (yield: approx. 2¼ cups, approx. 19.1 oz.) (tr/4g/0g/84%/14mg)	315	74.8	16.5	3.93	142	33.8	9	2.1
Prepared with fruit as package directs, add 1 cup of sliced bananas, 1 cup grapes, 2 cups water (yield: approx. 3½ cups, approx. 29.6 oz.)	563	137.8	19.0	4.66	161	39.4	10	2.5
PUDDINGS MADE FROM SCRATCH, based on USDA home recipes								
BREAD PUDDING with raisins, made from 2 cups dry, grated breadcrumbs, 4 cups milk, ½ cup sugar. 3 large eggs, 1 cup raisins, 2 Tbsp. butter or margarine, ¼ tsp. salt, and 1 tsp. vanilla (yield: approx. 5 cups, approx. 48 oz.) (loss of 10% has been applied for evaporation in cooking) (2g/8g/2g/59%/57mg)	2549	386.9	53.1	8.06	496	75.3	31	4.7
CHARLOTTE RUSSE, made with 24 ladyfingers and whipped cream filling with ingredients as follows: ½ cup water, 4 Tbsp. confectioner's sugar, 1½ tsp. gelatin, 1 tsp. vanilla, 2 cups whipping cream, whipped (yield: approx. 6 servings, approx. 24.2 oz.) (2g/10g/4g/46%/12mg)	1959	229.5	81.1	9.50				
1 serving, 4 ladyfingers, approx. 4 oz.	326	38.2	81.1	9.50				
CHOCOLATE PUDDING, regular starch base mix, 4-oz. box	408	103.4	102.0	25.85				
Prepared as package directs, add 2 cups of whole milk (yield: approx. 2¼ cups, approx. 20.6 oz.) (1g/6g/1g/70%/37mg)	723	132.9	35.1	6.45	322	59.3	20	3.7
CHOCOLATE PUDDING, instant, 4½-oz. box	457	116.2	101.6	25.82				

	UNIT Cal.	UNIT Carb.	1 OZ., BY WT. Cal.	1 OZ., BY WT. Carb.	1 CUP Cal.	1 CUP Carb.	1 TABLESPOON Cal.	1 TABLESPOON Carb.
Prepared as package directs, add 2 cups of whole milk (yield: approx. 2⅓ cups, approx. 21.7 oz.) (1g/7g/1g/69%/35mg)	770	150.3	35.4	6.92	325	63.4	20	4.0
TAPIOCA DESSERTS								
Apple Tapioca, made with ½ cup granulated tapioca, 2 cups water, ½ cup sugar, 1 cup diced apples, ⅛ tsp. salt (yield: approx. 2½ cups, approx. 22 oz.) (loss of 20% has been applied for evaporation in cooking) (tr/8g/tr/70%/14mg)	733	183.9	33.2	8.33	293	73.5	18	4.6
Tapioca Cream, made with 1½ Tbsp. granulated tapioca, 2 cups milk, ⅓ cup sugar, 2 large eggs, ¼ tsp. salt, 1 tsp. vanilla (yield: approx. 3 cups, approx. 19.4 oz.) (loss of 10% has been applied for evaporation in cooking) (1g/5g/1g/72%/44mg)	737	94.1	38.0	4.85	221	28.2	14	1.8

RENNIN and RENNIN DESSERTS, based on generic data

	UNIT Cal.	UNIT Carb.	1 OZ., BY WT. Cal.	1 OZ., BY WT. Carb.	1 CUP Cal.	1 CUP Carb.	1 TABLESPOON Cal.	1 TABLESPOON Carb.
RENNIN Tablet (salts, starch, rennin enzyme), ⅝" diameter, ⅛" thick, .035 oz., package of 12 tablets (tr/8g/tr/9%/6323mg)	12	2.7	34.3	7.71				
1 tablet (approx. 0.003 oz.)	1	0.2	34.3	7.71				
RENNIN DESSERT, home prepared, mixing 1 tablet with 2 cups milk, 1 Tbsp. water, 3 Tbsp. sugar, and 1 tsp. vanilla (yield: approx. 2⅛ cup (1g/3g/1g/81%/23mg)	485	63.2	25.2	3.29	227	29.6	14	1.9
1 cup (approx. 9 oz.)	227	29.6	25.2	3.29	227	29.6	14	1.9
RENNIN DESSERT MIXES:								
Chocolate								
Mix, dry form, 2-oz. package	221	52.2	110.5	26.00				
1 tablespoon (approx. 0.32 oz.)	35	8.2	110.5	26.00	560	131.2	35	8.2
Prepared with 2 cups milk added to 2 oz. dry mix (yield: approx. 2⅛ cup) (1g/4g/1g/78%/15mg)	556	76.8	28.9	4.00	260	36.0	16	2.3
1 cup (approx. 9 oz.)	260	36.0	28.9	4.00	260	36.0	16	2.3
Other Flavors (vanilla, caramel, and fruit flavorings)								
Mix, dry form, 1½-oz. package	165	42.6	110.0	28.40				
1 tablespoon (approx. 0.35 oz.)	38	9.9	110.0	28.40	608	158.4	38	9.9
Prepared with 2 cups of milk added to 1½ oz. dry mix (yield: approx. 2⅛ cup) (1g/4g/1g/80%/13mg)	504	67.8	27.0	3.63	238	32.0	15	2.0
1 cup (approx. 8.8 oz.)	238	32.0	27.0	3.63	238	32.0	15	2.0

GELATINS, and gelatin-like products, by brand

Unflavored

	UNIT Cal.	UNIT Carb.	1 OZ., BY WT. Cal.	1 OZ., BY WT. Carb.	1 CUP Cal.	1 CUP Carb.	1 TABLESPOON Cal.	1 TABLESPOON Carb.
Ann Page (A&P), 1-oz. box (4 envelopes)	96	0.0	96.0	0.00	(480)	0.0	(30)	0.0
8-oz. box, 32 envelopes	768	0.0	96.0	0.00	(480)	0.0	(30)	0.0
1 envelope, approx. ¼ oz.	24	0.0	96.0	0.00	(480)	0.0	(30)	0.0
Carmel Kosher, ¾-oz. box (3 envelopes)	90	0.0	120.0	0.00	(480)	0.0	(30)	0.0
1 envelope, approx. ¼ oz.	30	0.0	120.0	0.00	(480)	0.0	(30)	0.0
Knox, 1-oz. box (4 envelopes)	120	0.0	120.0	0.00	(480)	0.0	(30)	0.0
8-oz. box (32 envelopes)	960	0.0	120.0	0.00	(480)	0.0	(30)	0.0
1 envelope, approx. ¼ oz.	30	0.0	120.0	0.00	(480)	0.0	(30)	0.0

Flavored

	UNIT Cal.	UNIT Carb.	1 OZ., BY WT. Cal.	1 OZ., BY WT. Carb.	1 CUP Cal.	1 CUP Carb.	1 TABLESPOON Cal.	1 TABLESPOON Carb.
APPLE								
Candy Apple, **Royal,** 3-oz. box	320	76.0	106.7	25.33				
Prepared as package directs, adding 2 cups of water (yield: approx. 2 cups, 19 oz.)	320	76.0	(16.8)	(4.00)	160	38.0	10	2.4
Golden Apple, **Royal,** 3-oz. box	320	76.0	106.7	25.33				
Prepared as package directs, adding 2 cups of water (yield: approx. 2 cups, 19 oz.)	320	76.0	(16.8)	(4.00)	160	38.0	10	2.4
APRICOT								
Ann Page (A&P), 3-oz. box	320	76.0	106.7	25.33				
Prepared as package directs, adding 2 cups of water (yield: approx. 2 cups, 19 oz.)	320	76.0	(16.8)	(4.00)	160	38.0	10	2.4
6-oz. box	640	152.0	106.7	25.33				
Prepared as package directs, adding 4 cups of water (yield: approx. 4 cups, 38 oz.)	640	152.0	(16.8)	(4.00)	160	38.0	10	2.4
BLACKBERRY								
Royal, 3-oz. box	320	76.0	106.7	25.33				
Prepared as package directs, adding 2 cups of water (yield: approx. 2 cups, 19 oz.)	320	76.0	(16.8)	(4.00)	160	38.0	10	2.4
6-oz. box	640	152.0	106.7	25.33				
Prepared as package directs, adding 4 cups of water (yield: approx. 4 cups, 38 oz.)	640	152.0	(16.8)	(4.00)	160	38.0	10	2.4
BLACK CHERRY								
Ann Page (A&P), 3-oz. box	320	76.0	106.7	25.33				
Prepared as package directs, adding 2 cups of water (yield: approx. 2 cups, 19 oz.)	320	76.0	(16.8)	(4.00)	160	38.0	10	2.4
6-oz. box	640	152.0	106.7	25.33				
Prepared as package directs, adding 4 cups of water (yield: approx. 4 cups, 38 oz.)	640	152.0	(16.8)	(4.00)	160	38.0	10	2.4
Carmel Kosher, 3-oz. box	320	80.0	106.7	26.67				
Prepared as package directs, adding 2 cups of water (yield: approx. 2 cups, 19 oz.)	320	80.0	(16.8)	(4.21)	160	40.0	10	2.5
Jell-O, 3-oz. box	320	76.0	106.7	25.33				
Prepared as package directs, adding 2 cups of water (yield: approx. 2 cups, 19 oz.)	320	76.0	(16.8)	(4.00)	160	38.0	10	2.4
BLACK RASPBERRY								
Ann Page (A&P), 6-oz. box	640	152.0	106.7	25.33				
Prepared as package directs, adding 4 cups of water (yield: approx. 4 cups, 38 oz.)	640	152.0	(16.8)	(4.00)	160	38.0	10	2.4
Carmel Kosher, 3-oz. box	320	80.0	106.7	26.67				
Prepared as package directs, adding 2 cups of water (yield: approx. 2 cups, 19 oz.)	320	80.0	(16.8)	(4.21)	160	40.0	10	2.5
Jell-O, 3-oz. box	320	76.0	106.7	25.33				
Prepared as package directs, adding 2 cups of water (yield: approx. 2 cups, 19 oz.)	320	76.0	(16.8)	(4.00)	160	38.0	10	2.4
Louis Sherry "Shimmer," low calorie, ¼-oz. box	40	4.0	160.0	16.00				
Prepared as package directs, adding 2 cups of water (yield: approx. 2 cups, 16.3 oz.)	40	4.0	(2.5)	(0.25)	20	2.0	1	0.1
BLACK RASPBERRY & CONCORD GRAPE								
Jell-O, 3-oz. box	320	76.0	106.7	25.33				
Prepared as package directs, adding 2 cups of water (yield: approx. 2 cups, 19 oz.)	320	76.0	(16.8)	(4.00)	160	38.0	10	2.4
CANDY APPLE, see under APPLE								
CHERRY (also see BLACK CHERRY and WILD CHERRY)								
Ann Page (A&P), 3-oz. box	320	76.0	106.7	25.33				
Prepared as package directs, adding 2 cups of water (yield: approx. 2 cups, 19 oz.)	320	76.0	(16.8)	(4.00)	160	38.0	10	2.4

	UNIT		1 OZ., BY WT.		1 CUP		1 TABLESPOON	
	Cal.	Carb.	Cal.	Carb.	Cal.	Carb.	Cal.	Carb.
Carmel Kosher, 3-oz. box	320	80.0	106.7	26.67				
Prepared as package directs, adding 2 cups of water (yield: approx. 2 cups, 19 oz.)	320	80.0	(16.8)	(4.21)	160	40.0	10	2.5
Carmel Kosher, low calorie, 0.53-oz. box (3 envelopes)	48		90.7					
1 envelope, approx. 0.18 oz., prepared as package directs adding 1 cup of water (yield: approx. 1 cup, 8.20 oz.)	16		(2.0)		16			
Dia-Mel (Louis Sherry) "Gel-a-Thin," low calorie, ½-oz. box (2 envelopes)	80	8.0	160.0	16.00				
1 envelope, approx. ¼ oz., prepared as package directs adding 2 cups of water (yield: approx. 2 cups, 16.3 oz.)	40	4.0	(2.5)	(0.25)	20	2.0	1	0.1
Ready-to-eat dessert, 4-oz. package (2 containers)	1	0.2	0.3	0.05	2	(0.4)	trace	trace
1 container, approx. 4 oz.	1	0.2	0.3	0.05	(2)	(0.4)	trace	trace
D-Zerta, low calorie, ⅝-oz. box, 2 envelopes	64	0.0	102.4	0.00				
1 envelope, approx. 0.31 oz., prepared as package directs adding 2 cups of water (yield: approx. 2 cups, 16.3 oz.)	32	0.0	(2.0)	0.00	32	0.0	2	0.0
Estee, low calorie, 1⅔-oz. box	160	36.0	95.8	21.55				
Prepared as package directs, adding 2 cups of water (yield: approx. 2 cups, 17.5 oz.)	160	36.0	(9.1)	(2.06)	80	18.0	5	1.1
Featherweight, low calorie, 0.8-oz. box	80	8.0	100.0	10.00				
Prepared as package directs, adding 4 cups of water (yield: approx. 4 cups, 34 oz.)	80	8.0	2.4	0.24	20	2.0	1	0.1
Jell-O, 3-oz. box	320	72.0	106.7	24.00				
Prepared as package directs, adding 2 cups of water (yield: approx. 2 cups, 19 oz.)	320	72.0	(16.8)	(3.79)	160	36.0	10	2.3
Jello-O, sugar-free, 3-oz. box	32	0.0	10.7	0.00				
Prepared as package directs, adding 2 cups of water (yield: approx. 2 cups, 19 oz.	32	0.0	(1.7)	0.00	16	0.0	1	0.0
Louis Sherry "Shimmer," low calorie, ¼-oz. box	40	4.0	160.0	16.00				
Prepared as package directs, adding 2 cups of water (yield: approx. 2 cups, 16.3 oz.)	40	4.0	(2.5)	(0.25)	20	2.0	1	0.1
FRUIT PUNCH								
Carmel Kosher, 3-oz. box	320	80.0	106.7	26.67				
Prepared as package directs, adding 2 cups of water (yield: approx. 2 cups, 19 oz.)	320	80.0	(16.8)	(4.21)	160	40.0	10	2.5
GOLDEN APPLE, see under APPLE								
GRAPE								
Carmel Kosher, 3-oz. box	320	80.0	106.7	26.67				
Prepared as package directs, adding 2 cups of water (yield: approx. 2 cups, 19 oz.)	320	80.0	(16.8)	(4.21)	160	40.0	10	2.5
HAWAIIAN PINEAPPLE								
Jell-O, sugar-free, 3-oz. box	32	0.0	10.7	0.0				
Prepared as package directs, adding 2 cups of water (yield: approx. 2 cups, 19 oz.)	32	0.0	(1.7)	0.00	16	0.0	1	0.0
LEMON								
Ann Page (A&P), 6-oz. box	640	152.0	106.7	25.33				
Prepared as package directs, adding 4 cups of water (yield: approx. 4 cups, 38 oz.)	600	152.0	(16.8)	(4.00)	160	40.0	10	2.5
Carmel Kosher, 3-oz. box	320	80.0	106.7	26.67				
Prepared as package directs, adding 2 cups of water (yield: approx. 2 cups, 19 oz.)	320	80.0	(16.8)	(4.21)	160	40.0	10	2.5
D-Zerta, low calorie, ⅝-oz. box, 2 envelopes	64	0.0	102.4	0.00				
1 envelope, approx. 0.31 oz., prepared as package directs, adding 2 cups of water (yield: approx. 2 cups, 16.3 oz.)	32	0.0	(2.0)	0.00	32	0.0	2	0.0
Featherweight, low calorie, 0.8-oz. box	80	8.0	100.0	10.00				
Prepared as package directs, adding 4 cups of water (yield: approx. 4 cups, 34 oz.)	80	8.0	2.4	0.24	20	2.0	1	0.1
Jell-O, 3-oz. box	320	72.0	106.7	24.00				
Prepared as package directs, adding 2 cups of water (yield: approx. 2 cups, 19 oz.)	320	72.0	(16.8)	(3.79)	160	36.0	10	2.3
Royal, 3-oz. box	320	76.0	106.7	25.33				
Prepared as package directs, adding 2 cups of water (yield: approx. 2 cups, 19 oz.)	320	76.0	(16.8)	(4.00)	160	38.0	10	2.4
6-oz. box	640	152.0	106.7	25.33				
Prepared as package directs, adding 4 cups of water (yield: approx. 4 cups, 38 oz.)	640	152.0	(16.8)	(4.00)	160	38.0	10	2.4
LEMON/LIME								
Dia-Mel (Louis Sherry) "Gel-a-Thin," low calorie, 0.42 oz. box (2 envelopes)	32	0.0	76.2	0.00				
1 envelope, approx. ¼-oz., prepared as package directs, adding 2 cups of water (yield: approx. 2 cups, 16.3 oz.)	32	0.0	(2.0)	0.00	16	0.0	1	0.0
Louis Sherry "Shimmer," low calorie, ¼-oz. box	40	4.0	(2.5)	(0.25)				
Prepared as package directs, adding 2 cups of water (yield: approx. 2 cups, 16.3 oz.)	40	4.0	(2.5)	(0.25)	20	2.0	1	0.1
LIME								
Ann Page (A&P), 6-oz. box	640	152.0	106.7	25.33				
Prepared as package directs, adding 4 cups of water (yield: approx. 4 cups, 38 oz.)	640	152.0	(16.8)	(4.00)	160	38.0	10	2.4
Carmel Kosher, 3-oz. box	320	80.0	106.7	26.67				
Prepared as package directs, adding 2 cups of water (yield: approx. 2 cups, 19 oz.)	320	80.0	(16.8)	(4.21)	160	40.0	10	2.5
Carmel Kosher, low calorie, 0.53-oz. box (3 envelopes)	48		90.7					
1 envelope, approx. 0.18 oz., prepared as package directs, adding 1 cup water (yield: approx. 1 cup, 8.2 oz.)	16		(2.0)		16		1	
D-Zerta, low calorie, ⅝-oz. box (2 envelopes)	64	0.0	102.4	0.00				
1 envelope, approx. 0.31 oz., prepared as package directs, adding 2 cups of water (yield: approx. 2 cups, 16.3 oz.)	32	0.0	(2.0)	0.00	16	0.0	1	0.0
Featherweight, low calorie, 0.8-oz. box	80	0.0	100.0	10.00				
Prepared as package directs, adding 4 cups of water (yield: approx. 4 cups, 34 oz.)	80	8.0	2.4	0.24	20	2.0	1	0.1
Jell-O, 3-oz. box	320	76.0	106.7	25.33				
Prepared as package directs, adding 2 cups of water (yield: approx. 2 cups, 19 oz.)	320	76.0	(16.8)	(4.00)	160	38.0	10	2.4
Royal, 3-oz. box	320	76.0	106.7	25.33				
Prepared as package directs, adding 2 cups of water (yield: approx. 2 cups, 19 oz.)	320	76.0	(16.8)	(4.00)	160	38.0	10	2.4
6-oz. box	640	152.0	106.7	25.30				
Prepared as package directs, adding 4 cups of water (yield: approx. 4 cups, 38 oz.)	640	152.0	(16.8)	(4.00)	160	38.0	10	2.4
MIXED FRUIT								
Jello, 3-oz. box	320	76.0	106.7	25.33				
Prepared as package directs, adding 2 cups of water (yield: approx. 2 cups. 19 oz.)	320	76.0	(16.8)	(4.00)	160	38.0	10	2.4

	UNIT		1 OZ., BY WT.		1 CUP		1 TABLE-SPOON	
	Cal.	Carb.	Cal.	Carb.	Cal.	Carb.	Cal.	Carb.
Jell-O, sugar-free, 3-oz. box	32	0.0	10.7	0.00				
Prepared as package directs, adding 2 cups of water (yield: approx. 2 cups, 19 oz.)	32	0.0	(1.7)	0.00	16	0.0	1	0.0
ORANGE								
Ann Page (A&P), 6-oz. box	640	152.0	106.7	25.33				
Prepared as package directs, adding 4 cups of water (yield: approx. 4 cups, 38 oz.)	640	152.0	(16.8)	(4.00)	160	38.0	10	2.4
Carmel Kosher, 3-oz. box	320	80.0	106.7	26.67				
Prepared as package directs, adding 2 cups of water (yield: approx. 2 cups, 17 oz.)	320	80.0	(16.8)	(4.21)	160	40.0	10	2.5
Carmel Kosher, low calorie, 0.53-oz. box (3 envelopes)	48	0.0	90.0	0.00				
1 envelope, approx. 0.18 oz., prepared as package directs, adding 1 cup of water (yield: approx. 1 cup, 8.2 oz.)	16	0.0	(2.0)	0.00	16	0.0	2	0.0
Dia-Mel (Louis Sherry) "Gel-a-Thin," low calorie, ½-oz. box (2 envelopes)	80	8.0	160.0	16.00				
1 envelope, prepared as package directs, adding 2 cups of water (yield: approx. 2 cups, 16.3 oz.)	40	4.0	(2.5)	(0.25)	20	2.0	1	0.1
D-Zerta, low calorie, ⅝-oz. box (2 envelopes)	64	0.0	102.4	0.00				
1 envelope, approx. 0.31 oz., prepared as package directs, adding 2 cups of water (yield: approx. 2 cups, 16.3 oz.)	32	0.0	(2.0)	0.00	16	0.0	1.0	0.0
Featherweight, low calorie, 0.8-oz. box	80	8.0	100.0	10.00				
Prepared as package directs, adding 4 cups of water (yield: approx. 4 cups, 38 oz.)	80	8.0	2.4	0.24	20	2.0	1	0.1
Jell-O, 3-oz. box	320	76.0	106.7	25.30				
Prepared as package directs, adding 2 cups of water (yield: approx. 2 cups, 19 oz.)	320	76.0	(16.8)	(4.00)	160	38.0	10	2.4
Jell-O, sugar-free, 3-oz. box	32	0.0	10.7	0.00				
Prepared as package directs, adding 2 cups of water (yield: approx. 2 cups, 19 oz.)	32	0.0	(1.7)	0.00	16	0.0	1	0.0
Knox drinking gelatin, 0.61-oz. envelope	70	10.0	114.0	16.39				
Prepared as package directs, adding ½ cup of water (yield: approx. ½ cup, 4.8 oz.)	70	10.0	(14.7)	(2.10)	141	20.0	1	0.1
Louis Sherry "Shimmer," low calorie, ¼-oz. box	40	4.0	160.0	16.00				
Prepared as package directs, adding 2 cups of water (yield: approx. 2 cups, 16.3 oz.)	40	4.0	(2.5)	(0.25)	20	2.0	1	0.1
Royal, 3-oz. box	320	76.0	106.7	25.33				
Prepared as package directs, adding 2 cups of water (yield: approx. 2 cups, 19 oz.)	320	76.0	(16.8)	(4.00)	160	38.0	10	2.4
ORANGE-PINEAPPLE & LIME								
Jell-O, 3-oz. box	320	76.0	106.7	25.33				
Prepared as package directs, adding 2 cups of water (yield: approx. 2 cups, 19 oz.)	320	76.0	(16.8)	(4.00)	160	38.0	10	2.4
ORANGE & RASPBERRY								
Jell-O, 3-oz. box	320	76.0	106.7	25.33				
Prepared as package directs, adding 2 cups of water (yield: approx. 2 cups, 19 oz.)	320	76.0	(16.8)	(4.00)	160	38.0	10	2.4
PEACH								
Jell-O, 3-oz. box	320	76.0	106.7	25.33				
Prepared as package directs, adding 2 cups of water (yield: approx. 2 cups, 19 oz.)	320	76.0	(16.8)	(4.00)	160	38.0	10	2.4

	UNIT		1 OZ., BY WT.		1 CUP		1 TABLE-SPOON	
	Cal.	Carb.	Cal.	Carb.	Cal.	Carb.	Cal.	Carb.
Royal, 3-oz. box	320	76.0	106.7	25.33				
Prepared as package directs, adding 2 cups of water (yield: approx. 2 cups, 19 oz.)	320	76.0	(16.8)	(4.00)	160	38.0	10	2.4
6-oz. box	640	152.0	106.7	25.33				
Prepared as package directs, adding 4 cups of water (yield: approx. 4 cups, 38 oz.)	640	152.0	(16.8)	(4.00)	160	38.0	10	2.4
PINEAPPLE								
Royal, 3-oz. box	320	76.0	106.7	25.33				
Prepared as package directs, adding 2 cups of water (yield: approx. 2 cups, 19 oz.)	320	76.0	(16.8)	(4.00)	160	38.0	10	2.4
RASPBERRY (also see BLACK RASPBERRY, RED RASPBERRY, and WILD RASPBERRY)								
Carmel Kosher, 3-oz. box	320	80.0	106.7	26.67				
Prepared as package directs, adding 2 cups of water (yield: approx. 2 cups, 19 oz.)	320	80.0	(16.8)	(4.21)	160	40.0	10	2.5
Carmel Kosher, low calorie, 0.53-oz. box (3 envelopes)	48	0.0	90.7	0.00				
1 envelope, approx. 0.18 oz., prepared as package directs, adding 1 cup of water (yield: approx. 1 cup, 8.2 oz.)	16	0.0	(2.0)	0.00	16	0.0	1	0.0
Dia-Mel (Louis Sherry) "Gel-A-Thin," low calorie, ½-oz. box (2 envelopes)	80	8.0	160.0	16.00				
1 envelope, approx. ¼ oz., prepared as package directs, adding 2 cups of water (yield: approx. 2 cups, 16.3 oz.)	40	4.0	(2.5)	(0.25)	20	2.0	1	0.1
D-Zerta, low calorie, ⅝-oz. box (2 envelopes)	64	0.0	102.4	0.00				
1 envelope, 0.31 oz., prepared as package directs, adding 2 cups of water (yield: approx. 2 cups, 16.3 oz.)	32	0.0	(2.0)	0.00	16	0.0	1	0.0
Featherweight, low calorie, 0.8-oz. box	80	8.0	100.0	10.00				
Prepared as package directs, adding 4 cups of water (yield: approx. 4 cups, 34 oz.)	80	8.0	2.4	0.24	20	2.0	1	0.1
Jell-O, 3-oz. box	320	76.0	106.7	25.30				
Prepared as package directs, adding 2 cups of water (yield: approx. 2 cup, 19 oz.)	320	76.0	(16.8)	(4.00)	160	38.0	10	0.3
Royal, 3-oz. box	320	76.0	106.7	25.30				
Prepared as package directs, adding 2 cups of water (yield: approx. 2 cups, 19 oz.)	320	76.0	(16.8)	(4.00)	160	38.0	10	0.3
6-oz. box	640	152.0	106.7	25.30				
Prepared as package directs, adding 4 cups of water (yield: approx. 4 cups, 38 oz.)	640	152.0	(16.8)	(4.00)	160	38.0	10	0.3
RED RASPBERRY								
Louis Sherry "Shimmer," low calorie, ¼-oz. box	40	4.0	160.0	16.00				
Prepared as package directs, adding 2 cups of water (yield: approx. 2 cups, 16.3 oz.)	40	4.0	(2.5)	(0.25)	20	2.0	1	0.1
STRAWBERRY								
Ann Page (A&P), 3-oz. box	320	76.0	106.7	25.33				
Prepared as package directs, adding 2 cups of water (yield: approx. 2 cups, 19 oz.)	320	76.0	(16.8)	(4.00)	160	38.0	10	0.3
Carmel Kosher, 3-oz. box	320	80.0	106.7	26.67				
Prepared as package directs, adding 2 cups of water (yield: approx. 2 cups, 19 oz.)	320	80.0	(16.8)	(4.21)	160	40.0	10	2.5
Dia-Mel (Louis Sherry) "Gel-A-Thin," low calorie, ½-oz. box (2 envelopes)	80	8,0	160.0	16.00				

	UNIT		1 OZ., BY WT.		1 CUP		1 TABLE-SPOON	
	Cal.	Carb.	Cal.	Carb.	Cal.	Carb.	Cal.	Carb.
1 envelope, approx. ¼ oz., prepared as package directs, adding 2 cups of water (yield: approx. 2 cups, 16.3 oz.)	40	4.0	(2.5)	(0.25)	20	2.0	1	0.1
Ready-to-eat, 8-oz. package (2 containers)	2	0.4	0.3	0.05	(2)	(0.4)	trace	trace
1 container, approx. 4 oz.	1	0.2	0.3	0.05	(2)	(0.4)	trace	trace
D-Zerta, low calorie, ⅝-oz. box (2 envelopes)	64	0.0	102.4	0.00				
1 envelope, approx. 0.31 oz., prepared as package directs, adding 2 cups of water (yield: approx. 2 cups, 16.3 oz.)	32	0.0	(2.0)	0.00	32	0.0	2	0.0
Estee, low calorie, 1⅔-oz. box	160	36.0	95.8	21.56				
Prepared as package directs, adding 2 cups of water (yield: approx. 2 cups, 19 oz.)	160	36.0	(9.1)	(2.06)	80	18.0	5	1.1
Featherweight, low calorie, 0.8-oz. box	80	8.0	100.0	10.00				
Prepared as package directs, adding 4 cups of water (yield: approx. 4 cups, 38 oz.)	80	8.0	(2.4)	(0.24)	20	0.2	1	0.1
Jell-O, 3-oz. box	320	76.0	106.7	25.30				
Prepared as package directs, adding 2 cups of water (yield: approx. 2 cups, 19 oz.)	320	76.0	(16.8)	(4.00)	160	38.0	10	2.4
Jell-O, sugar-free, 3-oz. box	32	0.0	10.7	0.00				
Prepared as package directs, adding 2 cups of water (yield: approx. 2 cups, 19 oz.)	32	0.0	(1.7)	0.00	16	0.0	1	0.0
Louis Sherry "Shimmer," low calorie, ¼-oz. box	40	4.0	160.0	16.00				
Prepared as package directs, adding 2 cups of water (yield: approx. 2 cups, 16.3 oz.)	40	4.0	(2.5)	(0.25)	20	2.0	1	0.1
Royal, 3-oz. box	320	76.0	106.7	25.30				
Prepared as package directs, adding 2 cups of water (yield: approx. 2 cups, 19 oz.)	320	76.0	(16.8)	(4.00)	160	38.0	10	2.4
6-oz. box	640	152.0	106.7	25.30				
Prepared as package directs, adding 4 cups of water (yield: approx. 4 cups, 38 oz.)	640	152.0	(16.8)	(4.00)	160	38.0	10	2.4
STRAWBERRY-BANANA								
Jell-O, sugar-free, 3-oz. box	32	0.0	10.7	0.00				
Prepared as package directs, adding 2 cups of water (yield: approx. 2 cups, 19 oz.)	32	0.0	(1.7)	0.00	16	0.0	1	0.0
Dia-Mel (Louis Sherry) "Gel-A-Thin," low calorie, 0.4-oz. box (2 envelopes)	32	0.0	80.0	0.00				
1 envelope, approx. ¼ oz., prepared as package directs, adding 2 cups of water (yield: approx. 2 cups, 16.3 oz.)	32	0.0	(2.0)	0.00	16	0.0	1	0.0
Louis Sherry "Shimmer," low calorie, ¼-oz. box	40	4.0	160.0	16.00				
Prepared as package directs, adding 2 cups of water (yield: approx. 2 cups, 16.3 oz.)	40	4.0	(2.5)	(0.25)	20	2.0	1	0.1
Royal, 3-oz. box	320	76.0	106.7	25.33				
Prepared as package directs, adding 2 cups of water (yield: approx. 2 cups, 19 oz.)	320	76.0	(16.8)	(4.00)	160	38.0	10	2.4
6-oz. box	640	152.0	106.7	25.33				
Prepared as package directs, adding 4 cups of water (yield: approx. 4 cups, 38 oz.)	640	152.0	(16.8)	(4.00)	160	38.0	10	2.4
TROPICAL FRUIT								
Royal, 3-oz. box	320	76.0	106.7	25.33				
Prepared as package directs, adding 2 cups of water (yield: approx. 2 cups, 19 oz.)	320	76.0	(16.8)	(4.00)	160	38.0	10	2.4
WILD CHERRY								
Jell-O, 3-oz. box	320	76.0	106.7	25.33				

	UNIT		1 OZ., BY WT.		1 CUP		1 TABLE-SPOON	
	Cal.	Carb.	Cal.	Carb.	Cal.	Carb.	Cal.	Carb.
Prepared as package directs, adding 2 cups of water (yield: approx. 2 cups, 19 oz.)	320	76.0	(16.8)	(4.00)	160	36.0	10	2.3
WILD RASPBERRY								
Jell-O, 3-oz. box	320	72.0	106.7	24.00				
Prepared as package directs, adding 2 cups of water (yield: approx. 2 cups, 19 oz.)	320	72.0	(16.8)	(3.79)	160	36.0	10	0.3
WILD STRAWBERRY								
Jell-O, 3-oz. box	320	72.0	106.7	24.00				
Prepared as package directs, adding 2 cups of water (yield: approx. 2 cups, 19 oz.)	320	72.0	(16.8)	(4.00)	160	36.0	10	2.3

PUDDINGS and CUSTARDS, by brand

	UNIT		1 OZ., BY WT.		1 CUP		1 TABLE-SPOON	
	Cal.	Carb.	Cal.	Carb.	Cal.	Carb.	Cal.	Carb.
BANANA								
Jell-O Instant, sugar-free, 1.1 oz. box	120	28.0	109.1	25.45				
Prepared as package directs: For pudding or pie filling, add 2 cups of lowfat (2% fat) milk (yield: approx. 2 cups, 18.3 oz., or enough to fill an 8″ pie shell)	362	51.4	(19.8)	(2.81)	181	25.7	11	1.6
Jell-Well, 3.25-oz. box	240	56.0	73.9	17.23				
Prepared as package directs: For pudding or pie filling, add 2 cups of whole milk (yield: approx. 2 cups, 20.8 oz., or enough to fill an 8″ pie shell)	560	80.0	(26.9)	(3.85)	280	40.0	18	2.5
Jell-Well Instant, 3.75-oz. box	400	100.0	106.7	26.67				
Prepared as package directs: For pudding or pie filling, add 2 cups of whole milk (yield: approx. 2 cups, 21.3 oz., or enough to fill an 8″ pie shell)	720	124.0	(33.8)	(5.82)	360	62.0	23	3.9
Royal, 3.0-oz. box	320	80.0	106.7	26.67				
Prepared as package directs: For pudding or pie filling, add 2 cups of whole milk (yield: approx. 2 cups, 20.5 oz., or enough to fill an 8″ pie shell)	640	104.0	(31.2)	(5.07)	320	52.0	20	3.3
Royal Instant, 3½-oz. box	400	96.0	114.3	27.43				
Prepared as package directs: For pudding or pie filling, add 2 cups of whole milk (yield: approx. 2 cups, 21.0 oz., or enough to fill an 8″ pie shell)	720	120.0	(34.3)	(5.71)	360	60.0	23	3.8
BANANA CREAM								
Ann Page (A&P), 3¼-oz. box	360	88.0	110.8	27.08				
Prepared as package directs: For pudding or pie filling, add 2 cups of whole milk (yield: approx. 2 cups, 20.8 oz., or enough to fill an 8″ pie shell)	680	112.0	(32.7)	(5.38)	340	56.0	21	3.5
Jell-O, 3⅛-oz. box	360	84.0	115.0	26.84				
Prepared as package directs: For pudding or pie filling, add 2 cups of whole milk (yield: approx. 2 cups, 20.6 oz., or enough to fill an 8″ pie shell)	680	108.0	(33.0)	(5.24)	340	54.0	21	3.4
Jell-O Instant, 3¾-oz. box	400	100.0	106.7	26.67				
Prepared as package directs: For pudding or pie filling, add 2 cups of whole milk (yield: approx. 2 cups, 21.3 oz., or enough to fill an 8″ pie shell)	720	124.0	(33.8)	(5.82)	360	62.0	23	3.9
Royal, 3½-oz. box	400	96.0	114.3	27.43				
Prepared as package directs: For pudding or pie filling, add 2 cups of whole milk (yield: approx. 2 cups, 21.0 oz., or enough to fill an 8″ pie shell)	720	120.0	(34.3)	(5.71)	360	60.0	23	3.8
BUTTERSCOTCH								
Ann Page (A&P), 4.0-oz. box	400	104.0	100.0	26.00				

	UNIT		1 OZ., BY WT.		1 CUP		1 TABLESPOON	
	Cal.	Carb.	Cal.	Carb.	Cal.	Carb.	Cal.	Carb.
Prepared as package directs: For pudding or pie filling, add 2 cups of whole milk (yield: approx. 2 cups, 21.5 oz., or enough to fill an 8″ pie shell)	720	128.0	(33.5)	(5.95)	360	64.0	23	4.0
D-Zerta, low calorie, 2.125-oz. box (2 envelopes)	200	48.0	94.1	22.59				
Prepared as package directs: For pudding, add 2 cups of nonfat milk to 1 envelope (yield: approx. 2 cups, 18.3 oz.)	280	48.6	(15.3)	(2.66)	140	24.3	9	1.5
For pie filling, add 2 cups of nonfat milk to 2 envelopes (yield: approx. 2 cups, 19.4 oz., or enough to fill an 8″ pie shell)	380	72.6	(19.6)	(3.74)	190	36.3	12	2.3
Featherweight, low calorie, 1.0-oz. box (2 envelopes)	96	24.0	96.0	24.00				
Prepared as package directs: For pudding, add 2 cups of skim milk to 1 envelope (yield: approx. 2 cups, 17.8 oz.)	228	36.6	(12.8)	(2.06)	114	18.3	7	1.1
For pie filling, add 3 cups of skim milk to 2 envelopes (yield: approx. 3 cups, 26.9 oz., or enough to fill a 9″ pie shell)	366	60.9	(13.6)	(2.26)	122	20.3	8	1.3
Jell-O, 3⅝-oz. box	400	96.0	110.3	26.48				
Prepared as package directs: For pudding or pie filling, add 2 cups of whole milk (yield: approx. 2 cups, 21.1 oz., or enough to fill an 8″ pie shell)	720	120.0	(34.1)	(5.69)	360	60.0	23	3.8
Jell-O Instant, 3¾-oz. box	400	96.0	106.7	25.60				
Prepared as package directs: For pudding or pie filling, add 2 cups of whole milk (yield: approx. 2 cups, 21.3 oz., or enough to fill an 8″ pie shell)	720	120.0	33.8	5.63	360	60.0		
Jell-O Instant, sugar-free, 1.1 oz. box	120	28.0	109.1	25.45				
Prepared as package directs: For pudding or pie filling, add 2 cups of lowfat (2% fat) milk (yield: approx. 2 cups, 18.3 oz., or enough to fill an 8″ pie shell)	362	51.4	(19.8)	(2.81)	181	25.7	11	1.6
Jell-Well, 3.75-oz. box	440	100.0	117.3	26.67				
Prepared as package directs: For pudding or pie filling, add 2 cups of whole milk (yield: approx. 2 cups, 21.3 oz., or enough to fill an 8″ pie shell)	760	124.0	(35.7)	(5.82)	380	62.0	24	3.9
Jell-Well Instant, 3.75-oz. box	400	100.0	106.7	26.67				
Prepared as package directs: For pudding or pie filling, add 2 cups of whole milk (yield: approx. 2 cups, 21.3 oz., or enough to fill an 8″ pie shell)	720	124.0	(35.7)	(5.82)	360	62.0	23	3.9
My-T-Fine, 3¼-oz. box	360	88.0	110.8	27.08				
Prepared as package directs: For pudding or pie filling, add 2 cups of whole milk (yield: approx. 2 cups, 20.8 oz., or enough to fill an 8″ pie shell)	680	112.0	32.7	(5.38)	340	56.0	21	3.5
Rich's ready-to-serve, 3-oz. container	133	18.2	44.2	6.07	(392)	(54.3)	(25)	(3.4)
Royal, 3⅝-oz. box	320	80.0	88.3	22.07				
Prepared as package directs: For pudding or pie filling, add 2 cups of whole milk (yield: approx. 2 cups, 21.1 oz., or enough to fill an 8″ pie shell)	640	104.0	(30.3)	(4.93)	320	52.0	20	3.3
Royal Instant, 3½-oz. box	400	96.0	114.3	27.43				
Prepared as package directs: For pudding or pie filling, add 2 cups of whole milk (yield: approx. 2 cups, 21.0 oz., or enough to fill an 8″ pie shell)	720	120.0	(34.3)	(5.71)	360	60.0	23	3.8
Town House ready-to-serve, 20-oz. package (4 containers)	720	120.0	36.0	6.00	(330)	(55.0)	(21)	(3.4)
1 container, approx. 5 oz.	180	30.0	36.0	6.00	(330)	(55.0)	(21)	(3.4)

	UNIT		1 OZ., BY WT.		1 CUP		1 TABLESPOON	
	Cal.	Carb.	Cal.	Carb.	Cal.	Carb.	Cal.	Carb.
CHERRY-PLUM								
Junket Danish Dessert, Danish-style pudding and pie filling mix, 4.75-oz. box	520	128.0	109.5	26.95				
Prepared as package directs: For pudding or pie filling, add 2 cups of water (yield: approx. 2 cups, 24.2 oz., or enough to fill an 8″ pie shell)	520	128.0	(24.2)	(5.95)	260	64.0	16	4.0
CHOCOLATE (see also CHOCOLATE ALMOND, CHOCOLATE FUDGE, DARK CHOCOLATE, and MILK CHOCOLATE)								
Ann Page (A&P), 6.0-oz. box	660	156.0	110.0	26.00				
Prepared as package directs: For pudding or pie filling add 3 cups of whole milk (yield: approx. 3 cups, 32.3 oz., or enough to fill a 9″ pie shell)	1140	192.0	(35.3)	(5.94)	380	64.0	24	4.0
Ann Page (A&P) Instant, 4.0-oz. box	440	104.0	110.0	26.00				
Prepared as package directs: For pudding or pie filling, add 2 cups of whole milk (yield: approx. 2 cups, 21.5 oz., or enough to fill an 8″ pie shell)	760	128.0	(35.3)	(5.95)	380	64.0	24	4.0
Dia-Mel (Louis Sherry), low calorie, .85-oz. box (2 envelopes)	48	16.0	56.5	18.82				
Prepared as package directs: For pudding, add 2 cups of skim milk to 1 envelope (yield: approx. 2 cups, 17.7 oz.)	204	32.6	(11.5)	(1.84)	102	16.3	6	1.0
For pie filling, add 1¾ cups of skim milk to 2 envelopes (yield: approx. 1¾ cups, 16.0 oz., or enough to fill an 8″ pie shell)	206	37.5	(12.8)	(2.35)	103	18.8	6	1.2
Dieter's Gourmet, 1⅞-oz. box	200	48.0	106.7	25.60				
Prepared as package directs: For pudding, add 2 cups of skim milk (yield: approx. 2 cups, 19.2 oz., or enough to fill an 8″ pie shell)	380	72.6	(19.8)	(3.78)	190	36.3	12	2.3
D-Zerta, low calorie, 2.0-oz. box (2 envelopes)	160	40.0	80.0	20.00				
Prepared as package directs: For pudding, add 2 cups of nonfat milk to 1 envelope (yield: approx. 2 cups, 18.3 oz.)	260	44.6	(14.2)	(2.44)	130	22.3	8	1.4
For pie filling, add 2 cups of nonfat milk to 2 envelopes (yield: approx. 2 cups, 19.3 oz., or enough to fill an 8″ pie shell)	340	64.6	(17.6)	(3.35)	170	32.3	11	2.0
Estee, low calorie, 1⅞-oz. box	160	40.0	85.3	21.33				
Prepared as package directs, adding 2 cups of skim milk (yield: approx. 2 cups, 19.2 oz.)	340	64.6	(17.7)	(3.36)	170	32.3	11	2.0
Featherweight, low calorie, 1.0-oz. box (2 envelopes)	96	24.0	96.0	24.00				
Prepared as package directs: For pudding, add 2 cups of skim milk to 1 envelope (yield: approx. 2 cups, 17.8 oz.)	228	36.6	(12.8)	(2.06)	114	18.3	7	1.1
For pie filling, add 3 cups of skim milk to 2 envelopes (yield: approx. 3 cups, 26.9 oz., or enough to fill a 9″ pie shell)	366	60.9	(13.6)	(2.26)	122	20.3	8	1.3
Jell-O, 3½-oz. box	360	88.0	102.9	25.14				
Prepared as package directs: For pudding, add 2 cups of whole milk (yield: approx. 2 cups, 21.0 oz.)	680	112.0	(32.4)	(5.33)	340	56.0	21	3.5
For pie filling, add 2¼ cups of whole milk (yield: approx. 2¼ cups, 23.2 oz., or enough to fill an 8″ pie shell)	720	115.0	(31.0)	(4.96)	320	51.1	20	3.2

	UNIT		1 OZ., BY WT.		1 CUP		1 TABLESPOON	
	Cal.	Carb.	Cal.	Carb.	Cal.	Carb.	Cal.	Carb.
Jell-O Instant, 4½-oz. box	440	112.0	97.8	24.89				
Prepared as package directs: For pudding, add 2 cups of whole milk (yield: approx. 2 cups, 22.0 oz.)	760	136.0	(34.5)	(6.18)	380	68.0	24	4.3
For pie filling, add 1¾ cups of whole milk (yield: approx. 1¾ cups, 19.8 oz., or enough to fill an 8" pie shell)	720	133.0	(36.4)	(6.72)	411	76.0	26	4.8
Jell-O Instant, sugar-free, 1.5 oz. box	140	32.0	93.3	21.33				
Prepared as package directs: For pudding or pie filling, add 2 cups of lowfat (2% fat) milk (yield: approx. 2 cups, 18.5 oz., or enough to fill an 8" pie shell)	382	55.4	(20.4)	(2.96)	191	27.7	12	1.7
Jell-Well, 3.75-oz. box	440	92.0	117.3	24.53				
Prepared as package directs: For pudding or pie filling, add 2 cups of whole milk (yield: approx. 2 cups, 21.3 oz., or enough to fill an 8" pie shell)	760	116.0	(35.7)	(5.45)	380	58.0	24	3.6
Jell-Well Instant, 4.5-oz. box	440	104.0	97.8	23.11				
Prepared as package directs: For pudding or pie filling, add 2 cups of whole milk (yield: approx. 2 cups, 22.0 oz., or enough to fill an 8" pie shell)	760	128.0	(34.5)	(5.82)	380	64.0	24	4.0
Louis Sherry, low calorie, 1¼-oz. box (2 envelopes)	100	15.6	80.0	12.48				
Prepared as package directs: For pudding, add 2 cups of skim milk to 1 envelope (yield: approx. 2 cups, 17.9 oz.)	230	32.4	(12.8)	(1.81)	115	16.2	7	1.0
For pie filling, add 2 cups of skim milk to 2 envelopes (yield: approx. 2 cups, 18.5 oz., or enough to fill an 8" pie shell)	280	40.2	(15.1)	(2.17)	140	20.1	8	1.3
My-T-Fine, 3⅝-oz. box	400	92.0	110.3	25.38				
Prepared as package directs: For pudding or pie filling, add 2 cups of whole milk (yield: approx. 2 cups, 21.1 oz., or enough to fill an 8" pie shell)	720	116.0	(34.1)	(5.50)	360	58.0	23	3.6
Rich's ready-to-serve, 3-oz. container	140	18.0	46.7	6.00	(392)	(54.3)	(25)	(3.4)
Royal, 3⅝-oz. box	480	100.0	132.4	27.59				
Prepared as package directs: For pudding or pie filling, add 2 cups of whole milk (yield: approx. 2 cups, 21.1 oz., or enough to fill an 8" pie shell)	800	124.0	(37.9)	(5.88)	400	62.0	25	3.9
5½-oz. box	720	150.0	132.4	27.59				
Prepared as package directs: For pudding or pie filling, add 3 cups of whole milk (yield: approx. 3 cups, 31.8 oz., or enough to fill a 9" pie shell)	1200	186.0	(37.7)	(5.85)	400	62.0	25	3.9
Royal Instant, 4¼-oz. box	480	108.0	112.9	25.41				
Prepared as package directs: For pudding or pie filling, add 2 cups of whole milk (yield: approx. 2 cups, 21.8 oz., or enough to fill an 8" pie shell)	800	132.0	(36.7)	(6.06)	400	66.0	25	4.1
CHOCOLATE ALMOND								
My-T-Fine, 3¾-oz. box	400	92.0	106.7	24.53				
Prepared as package directs, adding 2 cups of whole milk (yield: approx. 2 cups, 21.3 oz.)	720	116.0	(33.8)	(5.45)	360	58.0	23	3.6
CHOCOLATE FUDGE								
Jell-O, 3⅝-oz. box	360	88.0	99.3	24.28				
Prepared as package directs: For pudding or pie filling, add 2 cups of whole milk (yield: approx. 2 cups, 21.1 oz., or enough to fill an 8" pie shell)	680	112.0	(32.2)	(5.31)	340	56.0	21	3.5
Jell-O Instant, 3⅝-oz. box	440	108.0	121.4	29.79				

	UNIT		1 OZ., BY WT.		1 CUP		1 TABLESPOON	
	Cal.	Carb.	Cal.	Carb.	Cal.	Carb.	Cal.	Carb.
Prepared as package directs: For pudding or pie filling, add 2 cups of whole milk (yield: approx. 2 cups, 21.1 oz., or enough to fill an 8" pie shell)	760	132.0	(36.0)	(6.26)	380	66.0	24	4.1
Jell-O Instant, sugar-free, 1.7 oz. box	160	36.0	94.1	21.18				
Prepared as package directs: For pudding or pie filling, add 2 cups of lowfat (2% fat) milk (yield: approx. 2 cups, 18.9 oz., or enough to fill an 8" pie shell)	402	59.4	(21.3)	(3.14)	201	29.7	13	1.9
Town House ready-to-serve, 20-oz. package (4 containers)	760	128.0	38.0	6.40	(348)	(58.7)	(22)	(3.7)
1 container, 5 oz.	190	32.0	38.0	6.40	(348)	(58.7)	(22)	(3.7)
COCONUT								
Jell-Well, 3.25-oz. box	240	56.0	73.9	17.23				
Prepared as package directs: For pudding or pie filling, add 2 cups of whole milk (yield: approx. 2 cups, 20.8 oz., or enough to fill an 8" pie shell)	560	80.0	(26.9)	(3.85)	280	40.0	18	2.5
Royal Instant, 3½-oz. box	400	92.0	114.3	26.29				
Prepared as package directs: For pudding or pie filling, add 2 cups of whole milk (yield: approx. 2 cups, 21.0 oz., or enough to fill an 8" pie shell)	720	116.0	(34.3)	(5.52)	360	58.0	23	3.6
Coconut Cream, **Ann Page (A&P),** 3¼-oz. box	400	76.0	123.1	23.38				
Prepared as package directs: For pudding or pie filling, add 2 cups of whole milk (yield: approx. 2 cups, 20.8 oz., or enough to fill an 8" pie shell)	720	100.0	(34.6)	(4.81)	360	50.0	23	3.1
4⅞-oz. box	600	114.0	123.1	23.38				
Prepared as package directs: For pudding or pie filling, add 3 cups of whole milk (yield: approx. 3 cups, 31.1 oz., or enough to fill a 9" pie shell)	1080	150.0	(34.7)	(4.82)	360	50	23	3.1
Coconut Cream, **Jell-O Instant,** 4⅛-oz. box	440	104.0	106.7	25.21				
Prepared as package directs: For pudding, add 2 cups of whole milk (yield: approx. 2 cups, 21.6 oz.)	760	128.0	(35.2)	(5.93)	380	64.0	24	4.0
For pie filling, add 1¾ cups of whole milk (yield: approx. 1¾ cups, 19.4 oz., or enough to fill an 8" pie shell)	720	125.0	(37.1)	(6.44)	411	71.4	26	4.5
Toasted Coconut, **Ann Page (A&P) Instant,** 3¼-oz. box	400	65.0	123.0	20.00				
Prepared as package directs: For pudding or pie filling, add 2 cups of whole milk (yield: approx. 2 cups, 20.8 oz., or enough to fill an 8" pie shell)	720	89.0	(34.6)	(4.28)	360	44.5	23	2.8
COCONUT CREAM, see under COCONUT								
COFFEE								
Royal Instant, 3½-oz. box	400	96.0	114.3	27.43				
Prepared as package directs: For pudding or pie filling, add 2 cups of whole milk (yield: approx. 2 cups, 21.0 oz., or enough to fill an 8" pie shell)	720	120.0	(34.3)	(5.71)	360	60.0	23	3.8
CUSTARD								
Royal, 2¼-oz. box	240	60.0	106.7	26.67				
Prepared as package directs: For pudding or pie filling, add 2¼ cups of whole milk (yield: approx. 2¼ cups, 21.9 oz., or enough to fill an 8" pie shell)	600	87.0	(27.4)	(3.97)	267	38.7	17	2.4
Chocolate-flavored Custard Mix, **Sweet 'n Low,** 1½-oz. box	200	32.0	133.3	21.33				
Prepared as package directs, adding 4 cups of skim milk (yield: approx. 4 cups, 36.1 oz.)	560	81.2	(15.5)	(2.25)	140	20.3	9	1.3

	UNIT		1 OZ., BY WT.		1 CUP		1 TABLESPOON	
	Cal.	Carb.	Cal.	Carb.	Cal.	Carb.	Cal.	Carb.
Golden Egg Custard, **Jell-O** "Americana," 3.0-oz. box	360	68.0	120.0	22.67				
Prepared as package directs, add 2 cups of whole milk (yield: approx. 2 cups, 20.5 oz., or enough to fill an 8" pie shell)	680	92.0	(33.2)	(4.49)	340	46.0	21	2.9
4½-oz. box	540	102.0	120.0	22.67				
Prepared as package directs, add 3 cups of whole milk (yield: approx. 3 cups, 33.1 oz., or enough to fill a 9" pie shell)	1020	138.0	(33.1)	(4.48)	340	46.0	21	2.9
Vanilla Custard, **Sweet 'n Low,** 2.0-oz. box	240	40.0	120.0	20.00				
Prepared as package directs, adding 4 cups of skim milk (yield: approx. 4 cups, 36.6 oz.)	600	89.2	(16.4)	(2.48)	150	22.3	9	1.4
DARK CHOCOLATE								
Rich's ready-to-serve, 3-oz. container	140	18.0	46.7	6.00	(422)	(54.3)	(26)	(3.4)
DARK N' SWEET								
Royal, 3⅝-oz. box	480	100.0	132.4	27.59				
Prepared as package directs: For pudding or pie filling, add 2 cups of whole milk (yield: approx. 2 cups, 21.1 oz., or enough to fill an 8" pie shell)	800	124.0	37.9	5.88	400	62.0	25	3.9
Royal Instant, 3⅝-oz. box	480	108.0	132.4	29.79				
Prepared as package directs: For pudding or pie filling, add 2 cups of whole milk (yield: approx. 2 cups, 21.1 oz., or enough to fill an 8" pie shell)	800	132.0	(37.9)	(6.26)	400	66.0	25	4.1
FLAN								
Royal, 2.0-oz. box	240	60.0	120.0	30.00				
Prepared as package directs: For pudding or pie filling, add 2 cups of whole milk (yield: approx. 2 cups, 19.5 oz., or enough to fill an 8" pie shell)	560	84.0	(28.7)	(4.31)	280	42.0	18	2.6
FRENCH VANILLA, see under VANILLA								
KEY LIME, see LIME								
LEMON								
Ann Page (A&P), 3.37-oz. box	240	60.0	71.2	17.80				
Prepared as package directs: For pudding or pie filling, add 2 cups of whole milk (yield: approx. 2 cups, 20.9 oz., or enough to fill an 8" pie shell)	560	84.0	(26.8)	(4.02)	280	42.0	18	2.6
Dia-Mel (Louis Sherry), low calorie, 1¼-oz. box	56	16.0	56.0	16.00				
Prepared as package directs: For pudding or pie filling, add 2 cups of water (yield: approx. 2 cups, 18.0 oz., or enough to fill an 8" pie shell)	56	16.0	(3.1)	(0.89)	28	8.0	2	0.5
Jell-O, 3-oz. box	300	78.0	100.0	26.00				
Prepared as package directs for pudding or pie filling, add 2 cups of whole milk (yield: approx. 2 cups, 20.5 oz., or enough to fill an 8" pie shell)	620	102.0	(30.2)	(4.98)	310	51.0	19	3.2
Jell-O Instant, 3¾-oz. box	400	100.0	106.7	26.67				
Prepared as package directs: For pudding or pie filling, add 2 cups of whole milk (yield: approx. 2 cups, 21.3 oz., or enough to fill an 8" pie shell)	720	124.0	(33.8)	(5.82)	360	62.0	23	3.9
Jell-Well, 3.25-oz. box	240	56.0	73.9	17.23				
Prepared as package directs: For pudding or pie filling, add 2 cups of whole milk and 2 egg yolks (yield: approx. 2 cups, 21.8 oz., or enough to fill an 8" pie shell)	670	80.0	(30.7)	(3.67)	335	40.0	21	2.5
Jell-Well Instant, 3.75-oz. box	400	100.0	106.7	26.67				
Prepared as package directs: For pudding or pie filling, add 2 cups of whole milk (yield: approx. 2 cups, 21.3 oz., or enough to fill an 8" pie shell)	720	124.0	(33.8)	(5.82)	360	62.0	23	3.9
My-T-Fine, 3⅜-oz. box	240	60.0	71.1	17.78				
Prepared as package directs: For pudding or pie filling, add 2¼ cups of water, ½ cup sugar, and 2 egg yolks (yield: approx. 2 cups, 26.7 oz., or enough to fill an 8" pie shell)	735	159.5	(27.5)	(5.97)	368	79.8	23	5.0
Royal, 3.0-oz. box	300	78.0	100.0	26.00				
Prepared as package directs: For pudding or pie filling, add 3 cups of whole milk (yield: approx. 3 cups, 29.3 oz., or enough to fill a 9" pie shell)	780	114.0	(26.6)	(3.89)	260	38.0	16	2.4
Royal Instant, 3½-oz. box	400	96.0	114.3	27.43				
Prepared as package directs: For pudding or pie filling, add 2 cups of whole milk, (yield: approx. 2 cups, 21.0 oz., or enough to fill an 8" pie shell)	720	120.0	(34.3)	(5.71)	360	60.0	23	3.8
LIME								
Key Lime, **Royal,** 3.0-oz. box	300	78.0	100.0	26.00				
Prepared as package directs: For pudding or pie filling, add 3 cups of whole milk (yield: approx. 3 cups, 29.3 oz., or enough to fill a 9" pie shell)	780	114.0	(26.6)	(3.89)	260	38.0	16	2.4
MILK CHOCOLATE								
Jell-O, 3⅝-oz. box	360	92.0	99.3	25.38				
Prepared as package directs: For pudding or pie filling, add 2 cups of whole milk (yield: approx. 2 cups, 21.1 oz., or enough to fill an 8" pie shell)	680	116.0	(32.3)	(5.50)	340	58.0	21	3.6
MOUSSE								
Chocolate French Mousse Mix, **Betty Crocker** "International Desserts," 11.25-oz. box	1400	240.0	124.4	21.33				
Prepared as package directs: For "Light and Creamy" Mousse, add 2 cups of whole milk (yield: approx. 2 cups, 28.5 oz.) (The manufacturer's information considers whole milk as having 200 calories per cup, which is higher than the figure of 160 used by other manufacturers whose products appear in this chapter.	1800	270.0	(63.3)	(9.49)	(900)	(135.0)	(56)	(8.4)
Prepared as package directs: For "Light and Creamy" Mousse, using 2 cups of skim milk instead of whole milk (yield: approx. 1¼ cups, 28.5 oz.)	1572	263.8	(55.2)	(9.27)	(786)	(131.9)	(49)	(8.2)
Prepared as package directs: For "Thick and Rich" Mousse, add 1¼ cups of whole milk (yield: approx. 1¼ cups, 19.9 oz.)	1650	258.8	(83.1)	(13.04)	(1320)	(207.0)	(83)	(12.9)
Prepared as package directs: For "Thick and Rich" Mousse, using 1¼ cups of skim milk instead of whole milk (yield: approx. 1¼ cups, 19.9 oz.)	1580	254.9	(75.9)	(12.84)	(754)	(127.4)	(47)	(8.0)
PINEAPPLE CREAM								
Jell-O Instant, 3¾-oz. box	400	100.0	106.7	26.67				
Prepared as package directs: For pudding or pie filling, add 2 cups of whole milk (yield: approx. 2 cups, 21.3 oz., or enough to fill an 8" pie shell)	720	124.0	(33.8)	(5.82)	360	62.0	23	3.9
PISTACHIO								
Jell-O Instant, 3¾-oz. box	400	96.0	106.7	25.60				
Prepared as package directs: For pudding or pie filling, add 2 cups of whole milk (yield: approx. 2 cups, 21.3 oz., or enough to fill an 8" pie shell)	720	120.0	(33.8)	(5.63)	360	60.0	23	3.8

	UNIT		1 OZ., BY WT.		1 CUP		1 TABLESPOON	
	Cal.	Carb.	Cal.	Carb.	Cal.	Carb.	Cal.	Carb.
Jell-Well Instant, 3.75-oz. box	400	96.0	106.7	25.60				
Prepared as package directs: For pudding or pie filling, add 2 cups of whole milk (yield: approx. 2 cups, 21.3 oz., or enough to fill an 8" pie shell)	720	120.0	(33.8)	(5.63)	360	60.0	23	3.8
Pistachio Nut, **Royal Instant,** 3½-oz. box	400	92.0	114.3	26.29				
Prepared as package directs: For pudding or pie filling, add 2 cups of whole milk (yield: approx. 2 cups, 21.0 oz., or enough to fill an 8" pie shell)	720	116.0	(34.3)	(5.63)	360	58.0	23	3.6
RASPBERRY CURRANT								
Junket Danish Dessert, Danish-style pudding and pie filling mix, 4.75-oz. box	520	128.0	109.5	26.95				
Prepared as package directs: For pudding or pie filling, add 2 cups of water (yield: approx. 2 cups, 21.5 oz., or enough to fill an 8" pie shell)	520	128.0	(24.2)	(5.95)	260	64.0	16	4.0
RICE PUDDING								
Jell-O, 3¾-oz. box	400	96.0	106.7	25.60				
Prepared as package directs: For pudding, add 2 cups of whole milk (yield: approx. 2 cups, 21.3 oz.)	720	120.0	(33.8)	(5.63)	360	60.0	23	3.8
STRAWBERRY								
Junket Danish Dessert, Danish-style pudding & pie filling, 4.75-oz. box	520	128.0	109.5	26.95				
Prepared as package directs, adding 2 cups of water (yield: approx. 2 cups, 21.5 oz., or enough to fill an 8" pie shell)	520	128.0	(24.2)	(5.95)	260	64.0	16	4.0
TAPIOCA								
Chocolate Tapioca, **Ann Page (A&P),** 5¼-oz. box	540	138.0	102.6	26.29				
Prepared as package directs, adding 3 cups of whole milk (yield: approx. 3 cups, 31.5 oz.)	1020	174.0	(32.4)	(5.52)	340	58.0	21	3.6
Chocolate Tapioca, **Jell-O,** Americana, 3½-oz. box	360	88.0	102.9	25.10				
Prepared as package directs, adding 2 cups of whole milk (yield: approx. 2 cups, 21.0 oz.)	680	112.0	(32.4)	(5.33)	340	56.0	21	3.5
Chocolate Tapioca, **Royal,** 3⅝-oz. box	480	100.0	132.4	27.59				
Prepared as package directs, adding 2 cups of whole milk (yield: approx. 2 cups, 21.1 oz.)	800	124.0	(37.9)	(5.88)	400	62.0	25	3.9
Vanilla Tapioca, **Jell-O,** Americana, 3¼-oz. box	360	88.0	110.8	27.08				
Prepared as package directs, adding 2 cups of whole milk (yield: approx. 2 cups, 20.8 oz.)	680	112.0	(32.7)	(5.38)	340	56.0	21	3.5
Vanilla Tapioca, **My-T-Fine,** 3¼-oz. box	360	84.0	110.8	27.08				
Prepared as package directs, adding 2 cups of whole milk (yield: approx. 2 cups, 20.8 oz.)	680	108.0	(32.7)	(5.19)	340	54.0	21	3.4
Vanilla Tapioca, **Royal,** 3¼-oz. box	320	80.0	98.5	24.62				
Prepared as package directs, adding 2 cups of whole milk (yield: approx. 2 cups, 20.8 oz.)	640	104.0	(30.8)	(5.00)	320	52.0	20	3.3
TOASTED COCONUT, see under COCONUT								
VANILLA								
Ann Page (A&P), 3¼-oz. box	360	88.0	110.8	27.08				
Prepared as package directs: For pudding or pie filling, add 2 cups of whole milk (yield: approx. 2 cups, 20.8 oz., or enough to fill an 8" pie shell)	680	112.0	(32.7)	(5.38)	340	56.0	21	3.5
4⅞-oz. box	540	132.0	110.8	27.08				

	UNIT		1 OZ., BY WT.		1 CUP		1 TABLESPOON	
	Cal.	Carb.	Cal.	Carb.	Cal.	Carb.	Cal.	Carb.
Prepared as package directs: For pudding or pie filling, add 3 cups of whole milk (yield: approx. 3 cups, 31.1 oz., or enough to fill a 9" pie shell)	1020	168.0	(32.8)	(5.40)	340	56.0	21	3.5
Ann Page (A&P) Instant, 3¼-oz. box	360	88.0	110.8	27.08				
Prepared as package directs: For pudding or pie filling, add 2 cups of whole milk (yield: approx. 2 cups, 20.8 oz., or enough to fill an 8" pie shell)	680	112.0	(32.7)	(5.38)	340	56.0	21	3.5
Dia-Mel (Louis Sherry), low calorie, 1.0-oz. box (2 envelopes)	40	12.0	40.0	12.00				
Prepared as package directs: For pudding, add 2 cups of skim milk to 1 envelope (yield: approx. 2 cups, 17.8 oz.)	200	30.6	(11.4)	(1.72)	100	15.3	6	1.0
For pie filling, add 1¾ cups of skim milk to 2 envelopes (yield: approx. 1¾ cups, 16.1 oz., or enough to fill an 8" pie shell)	198	33.5	(12.3)	(2.08)	113	19.2	7	1.2
D-Zerta, low calorie, 2⅛-oz. box (2 envelopes)	240	56.0	112.9	26.35				
Prepared as package directs: For pudding, add 2 cups of nonfat milk to 1 envelope (yield: approx. 2 cups, 18.3 oz.)	300	52.6	(16.4)	(2.87)	150	26.3	9	1.6
For pie filling, add 2 cups of nonfat milk to 2 envelopes (yield: approx. 2 cups, 19.4 oz., or enough to fill an 8" pie shell)	420	80.6	(21.6)	(4.15)	210	40.3	13	2.5
Estee, low calorie, 1⅞-oz. box	85	16.0	45.2	8.51				
Prepared as package directs, adding 2 cups of skim milk (yield: approx. 2 cups, 19.2 oz.)	265	40.6	(13.8)	(2.11)	133	20.3	8	1.3
Jell-O, 3⅛-oz. box	320	84.0	102.4	26.88				
Prepared as package directs: For pudding or pie filling, add 2 cups of whole milk (yield: approx. 2 cups, 20.6 oz., or enough to fill an 8" pie shell)	640	108.0	(31.1)	(5.24)	320	54.0	20	3.4
Jell-O Instant, 3¾-oz. box	400	100.0	106.7	26.67				
Prepared as package directs: For pudding or pie filling, add 2 cups of whole milk (yield: approx. 2 cups, 21.3 oz., or enough to fill an 8" pie shell)	720	124.0	(33.8)	(5.82)	360	62.0	23	3.9
Jell-O Instant, sugar-free, 1.1 oz. box	120	28.0	109.1	25.45				
Prepared as package directs: For pudding or pie filling, add 2 cups of lowfat (2% fat) milk (yield: approx. 2 cups, 18.3 oz., or enough to fill an 8" pie shell)	362	52.0	(19.8)	(2.84)	181	26.0	11	1.6
Jell-Well, 3.25-oz. box	360	88.0	110.8	27.05				
Prepared as package directs: For pudding or pie filling, add 2 cups of whole milk (yield: approx. 2 cups, 20.8 oz., or enough to fill an 8" pie shell)	680	112.0	(32.7)	(5.38)	340	56.0	21	3.5
Jell-Well Instant, 3.75-oz. box	400	100.0	106.7	26.67				
Prepared as package directs: For pudding or pie filling, add 2 cups of whole milk (yield: approx. 2 cups, 21.3 oz., or enough to fill an 8" pie shell)	720	124.0	(33.8)	(5.82)	360	62.0	23	3.9
My-T-Fine, 3¼-oz. box	360	88.0	110.8	27.08				
Prepared as package directs: For pudding or pie filling, add 2 cups of whole milk (yield: approx. 2 cups, 20.8 oz., or enough to fill an 8" pie shell)	680	112.0	(32.7)	(5.38)	340	56.0	21	3.5
Rich's ready-to-eat, 3-oz. container	130	18.0	43.3	6.00	(392)	(54.3)	(25)	(3.4)
Royal, 3.0-oz. box	320	80.0	106.7	26.67				

	UNIT		1 OZ., BY WT.		1 CUP		1 TABLESPOON	
	Cal.	Carb.	Cal.	Carb.	Cal.	Carb.	Cal.	Carb.
Prepared as package directs: For pudding or pie filling, add 2 cups of whole milk (yield: approx. 2 cups, 20.5 oz., or enough to fill an 8″ pie shell)	640	108.0	(31.2)	(5.27)	320	54.0	20	3.4
4½-oz. box	480	120.0	106.7	26.67				
Prepared as package directs: For pudding or pie filling, add 3 cups of whole milk (yield: approx. 3 cups, 30.8 oz., or enough to fill a 9″ pie shell)	960	156	(31.2)	(5.06)	320	52.0	20	3.3
Royal Instant, 3½-oz. box	400	96.0	114.3	27.43				
Prepared as package directs: For pudding or pie filling, add 2 cups of whole milk (yield: approx. 2 cups, 21.0 oz., or enough to fill an 8″ pie shell)	720	120.0	(34.3)	(5.71)	360	60.0	23	3.8
French Vanilla, **Jell-O,** 3½-oz. box	400	96.0	114.3	27.4				
Prepared as package directs: For pudding or pie filling, add 2 cups of whole milk (yield: approx. 2 cups, 21.0 oz., or enough to fill an 8″ pie shell)	720	120.0	(34.3)	(5.71)	360	60.0	23	3.8
French Vanilla, **Jell-O Instant,** 3¾-oz. box	400	96.0	110.3	26.48				
Prepared as package directs: For pudding or pie filling, add 2 cups of whole milk (yield: approx. 2 cups, 21.3 oz., or enough to fill an 8″ pie shell)	720	120.0	(33.8)	(5.63)	360	60.0	23	3.8
RENNIN DESSERTS								
Chocolate-flavored Rennet Custard, **Junket,** 1.5-oz. box	160	40.0	106.7	26.67				
Prepared as package directs: For custard, add 2 cups of whole milk (yield: approx. 2 cups, 19.0 oz., or enough to fill an 8″ pie shell)	480	64.0	(25.3)	(3.37)	240	32.0	15	2.0
Prepared with skim milk (yield: approx. 2 cups, 18.8 oz., or enough to fill an 8″ pie shell)	340	64.6	(18.1)	(3.44)	170	32.3	11	2.0
Raspberry-flavored Rennet Custard, **Junket,** 1.5-oz. box	160	40.0	106.7	26.67				
Prepared as package directs: For custard, add 2 cups of whole milk (yield: approx. 2 cups, 19.0 oz., or enough to fill an 8″ pie shell)	480	64.0	(25.3)	(3.37)	240	32.0	15	2.0
Prepared with skim milk (yield: approx. 2 cups, 18.8 oz., or enough to fill an 8″ pie shell)	360	64.6	(18.1)	(3.44)	170	32.3	11	2.0
Strawberry-flavored Rennet Custard, **Junket,** 1.5-oz. box	160	40.0	106.7	26.67				
Prepared as package directs: For custard, add 2 cups of whole milk (yield: approx. 2 cups, 19.0 oz., or enough to fill an 8″ pie shell)	480	64.0	(25.3)	(3.37)	240	32.0	15	2.0
Prepared with skim milk (yield: approx. 2 cups, 18.8 oz., or enough to fill an 8″ pie shell)	360	64.6	(18.1)	(3.44)	170	32.3	11	2.0
Vanilla-flavored Rennet Custard, **Junket,** 1.5-oz. box	160	40.0	106.7	26.67				
Prepared as package directs: For custard, add 2 cups of whole milk (yield: approx. 2 cups, 19.0 oz., or enough to fill an 8″ pie shell)	480	64.0	(25.3)	(3.37)	240	32.0	15	2.0
Prepared with skim milk (yield: approx. 2 cups, 18.8 oz., or enough to fill an 8″ pie shell)	360	64.6	(18.1)	(3.44)	170	32.3	11	2.0

27 YOGURT •

(For Frozen Yogurt, see the FROZEN CONFECTIONS chapter.)

	CONTAINER		1 OZ., BY WT.		1 CUP		1 TABLE-SPOON	
	Cal.	Carb.	Cal.	Carb.	Cal.	Carb.	Cal.	Carb.
PLAIN YOGURT, based on generic data								
Arranged in ascending order of fat content:								
Skim milk yogurt (0.18% fat), 8-oz. container	127	17.4	15.9	2.18	(139)	(19.1)	(8.7)	(1.19)
1 cup (approx. 8.8 oz.)	(139)	(19.1)	15.9	2.18	(139)	(19.1)	(8.7)	(1.19)
Low-fat yogurt (1.55% fat), 8-oz. container	144	16.0	17.9	2.00	(158)	(17.5)	(9.9)	(1.09)
1 cup (approx. 8.8 oz.)	(158)	(17.5)	17.9	2.00	(158)	(17.5)	(9.9)	(1.09)
Whole milk yogurt (3.25% fat), 8-oz. container	139	10.6	17.3	1.32	(150)	(11.4)	(9.4)	(0.69)
1 cup (approx. 8.6 oz.)	(150)	(11.4)	17.3	1.32	(150)	(11.4)	(9.4)	(0.69)
For comparison: Sour Cream, **Friendship,** 8-oz. container	440	5.9	55.0	0.74	(445)	(6.0)	(27.9)	(0.37)
For comparison: Low-Fat and Whole-Milk Yogurts from other parts of the world								
Africa: 5.5% fat yogurt, 8 oz.	193	10.9	24.1	1.36	(210)	(11.8)	(13.1)	(0.74)
East Asia: 0.8% fat yogurt, 8 oz.	204	39.9	25.5	4.99	(224)	(43.9)	(14.0)	(2.74)
France: 0% fat yogurt, 8 oz.	84	11.4	10.5	1.42	(91)	(12.4)	(5.7)	(0.77)
1.0% fat yogurt, 8 oz.	105	11.4	13.0	1.42	(114)	(12.5)	(7.2)	(0.78)
3.1% fat yogurt, 8 oz.	136	10.9	17.0	1.36	(148)	(11.8)	(9.2)	(0.74)
1.6% fat yogurt with fruit, 8 oz.	209	36.3	26.1	4.54	(227)	(39.5)	(14.2)	(2.46)
Great Britain: **St. Ivel,** 5-oz. container	85	9.5	17.0	1.90	(148)	(16.5)	(9.2)	(1.03)
16-oz. (1-lb.) container	272	30.4	17.0	1.90	(148)	(16.5)	(9.2)	(1.03)
YOGURT, by brand								
The list that follows is alphabetized by the descriptive fruit or flavor. A list alphabetized by brand follows this one.								
Plain Yogurt								
LOW-FAT:								
A&P, 32-oz. (2-lb.) container	600	68.0	18.8	2.13	(165)	(18.7)	(10.3)	(1.17)
Axelrod's "Easy-Dieter," 8-oz. container	150	18.0	18.8	2.25	(165)	(19.8)	(10.3)	(1.24)
16-oz. (1-lb.) container	300	36.0	18.8	2.25	(165)	(19.8)	(10.3)	(1.24)
32-oz. (2-lb.) container	600	72.0	18.8	2.25	(165)	(19.8)	(10.3)	(1.24)
Bison, 8-oz. container	160	17.0	20.0	2.13	(176)	(18.7)	(11.0)	(1.17)
Continental, 32-oz. (2-lb.) container	720	80.0	22.5	2.50	(198)	(22.0)	(12.4)	(1.38)
Dannon, 8-oz. container	150	17.0	18.8	2.12	(165)	(18.7)	(10.3)	(1.17)
16-oz. (1-lb.) container	300	34.0	18.8	2.12	(165)	(18.7)	(10.3)	(1.17)
Johnston's, 8-oz. container	140	15.0	17.5	1.88	(154)	(16.5)	(9.6)	(1.03)
Knudsen, 8-oz. container	150	16.0	18.8	2.00	166	17.7	10.3	1.10
Lacto, 32-oz. (2-lb.) container	600	56.0	18.8	1.75	(165)	(16.3)	(10.3)	(1.02)
Light n' Lively (Sealtest), 8-oz. container	134	16.8	16.8	2.10	(148)	(19.5)	(9.2)	(1.22)
Look-Fit (A&P), 8-oz. container	140	19.0	17.5	2.38	(154)	(20.9)	(9.6)	(1.31)
Lucerne (Safeway), 8-oz. container	160	17.0	20.0	2.13	(176)	(18.7)	(11.0)	(1.17)
32-oz. (2-lb.) container	640	68.0	20.0	2.13	(176)	(18.7)	(11.0)	(1.17)
Ralph's, 8-oz. container	160	28.3	20.0	3.54	(176)	(31.2)	(11.0)	(1.95)
16-oz. (1-lb.) container	320	56.6	20.0	3.54	(176)	(31.2)	(11.0)	(1.95)
32-oz. (2-lb.) container	640	113.2	20.0	3.54	(176)	(31.2)	(11.0)	(1.95)
White Rose, 32-oz. (2-lb.) container	440	68.0	13.8	2.13	(121)	(18.7)	(7.6)	(1.17)
Zausner, Plain Yogurt with Cottage Cheese, 12-oz. container	249	9.0	20.8	0.75	(184)	(7.0)	(11.5)	(0.44)
WHOLE-MILK:								
Breyers, 8-oz. container	160	14.0	20.0	1.75	(174)	(15.2)	(10.9)	(0.95)
Brown Cow Farm, 8-oz. container	190	13.0	23.8	1.63	(207)	(15.2)	(12.9)	(0.95)
16-oz. (1-lb.) container	380	26.1	23.8	1.63	(207)	(15.2)	(12.9)	(0.95)
Colombo, 8-oz. container	150	13.0	18.8	1.63	(164)	(14.2)	(10.2)	(0.89)
16-oz. (1-lb.) container	300	26.0	18.8	1.63	(164)	(14.2)	(10.2)	(0.89)
32-oz. (2-lb.) container	600	52.0	18.8	1.63	(164)	(14.2)	(10.2)	(0.89)
Continental, 8-oz. container	240	17.0	30.0	2.13	(261)	(18.5)	(16.3)	(1.16)
Erewhon, 8-oz. container	159	11.8	19.9	1.48	(173)	(12.9)	(10.8)	(0.80)
32-oz. (2-lb.) container	636	47.2	19.9	1.48	(173)	(12.9)	(10.8)	(0.80)
Europa, 6-oz. container	130	11.0	21.7	1.83	(189)	(15.9)	(11.8)	(1.00)
Knudsen, 8-oz. container	180	15.0	22.5	1.88	195	16.3	12.2	1.02
16-oz. (1-lb.) container	360	30.0	22.5	1.88	195	16.3	12.2	1.02
32-oz. (2-lb.) container	720	60.0	22.5	1.88	195	16.3	12.2	1.02
La Yogurt, 6-oz. container	130	12.0	21.7	2.00	(189)	(16.4)	(11.8)	(1.02)
Maya, 8-oz. container	210	18.0	26.3	2.25	(228)	(19.5)	(14.2)	(1.22)
Natural & Kosher, 8-oz. container	200	16.0	25.0	2.00	(218)	(17.4)	(13.6)	(1.09)
16-oz. (1-lb.) container	400	32.0	25.0	2.00	(218)	(17.4)	(13.6)	(1.09)
Vermont, 8-oz. container	190	16.0	23.8	2.00	(207)	(17.4)	(12.9)	(1.09)
Yoplait, 6-oz. container	130	14.0	20.1	2.16	(175)	(19.0)	(10.9)	(1.19)
Fruit- and Extract-Flavored Yogurt								
APPLE								
Dannon Mélangé, low-fat, 6-oz. container	180	31.0	30.0	5.17	(279)	(48.1)	(17.4)	(3.01)

	CONTAINER		1 OZ., BY WT.		1 CUP		1 TABLESPOON	
	Cal.	Carb.	Cal.	Carb.	Cal.	Carb.	Cal.	Carb.
Yoplait, whole milk, 6-oz. container	190	32.0	29.3	4.94	(272)	(45.9)	(17.0)	(2.87)
Apple Crisp, **New Country,** low-fat, 8-oz. container	240	42.0	30.0	5.25	(279)	(48.8)	(17.4)	(3.05)
Apple with Granola, **Knudsen,** Yogurt Plus, low-fat, 8-oz. container	260	52.0	32.5	6.50	302	60.5	18.9	3.78
Dutch Apple, **Bison,** low-fat, 8-oz. container	250	46.0	31.3	5.75	(291)	(53.5)	(18.2)	(3.34)
Dutch Apple, **Dannon,** low-fat, 8-oz. container	260	49.0	32.5	6.13	(302)	(57.0)	(18.9)	(3.56)
French Apple, **Johnston's,** low-fat, 8-oz. container	260	53.0	32.5	6.63	(302)	(61.6)	(18.9)	(3.85)
French Apple, **Light n' Lively (Sealtest),** low-fat, 8-oz. container	245	47.2	30.6	5.90	(285)	(54.9)	(17.8)	(3.43)
French Apple, **Lucerne (Safeway),** low-fat, 8-oz. container	250	46.0	31.3	5.75	(291)	(53.5)	(18.2)	(3.34)
Spiced Apple, **Axelrod's,** Sundae Style, low-fat, 8-oz. container	250	50.0	31.3	6.25	(291)	(58.1)	(18.2)	(3.63)
Spiced Apple, **Colombo,** whole milk, 8-oz. container	240	39.0	30.0	4.88	(279)	(45.4)	(17.4)	(2.84)
Spiced Apple, **Knudsen,** Fruit-On-The-Bottom, low-fat, 8-oz. container	250	45.0	31.3	5.63	291	52.3	18.2	3.27
Spiced Apple, **Knudsen,** Pre-stirred, low-fat, 8-oz. container	260	45.0	32.5	5.63	302	52.3	18.9	3.27
Spiced Apple, **Ralph's,** low-fat, 8-oz. container	200	34.0	25.0	4.25	(233)	(39.5)	(14.5)	(2.47)
APRICOT								
Axelrod's, Sundae Style, low-fat, 8-oz. container	250	50.0	31.3	6.25	(291)	(58.1)	(18.2)	(3.63)
Bison, low-fat, 8-oz. container	250	46.0	31.3	5.75	(291)	(53.5)	(18.2)	(3.34)
Breakstone's, Parfait, low-fat, 8-oz. container	250	18.9	31.3	2.36	(291)	(21.9)	(18.2)	(1.37)
Dannon, low-fat, 8-oz. container	260	49.0	32.5	6.13	(302)	(57.0)	(18.9)	(3.56)
Light n' Lively (Sealtest), low-fat, 8-oz. container	240	46.0	30.0	5.75	(279)	(53.5)	(17.4)	(3.34)
Look-Fit (A&P), Swiss Style, low-fat, 8-oz. container	220	42.0	27.5	5.25	(256)	(48.8)	(16.0)	(3.05)
Viva, Swiss Style, skim milk, 8-oz. container	250	47.0	31.3	5.88	(291)	(54.6)	(18.2)	(3.41)
For comparison: Apricot Fruit Yogurt, **Prize (St. Ivel),** (sold in Great Britain), 5-oz. container	110	19.8	22.0	3.97	(205)	(36.9)	(12.8)	(2.31)
Apricot Pineapple, **Knudsen,** Pre-stirred, low-fat, 8-oz. container	260	48.0	32.5	6.00	302	55.8	18.9	3.49
32-oz. (2-lb.) container	1040	192.0	32.5	6.00	302	55.8	18.9	3.49
Apricot-Pineapple, **Lucerne (Safeway),** low-fat, 8-oz. container	260	46.0	32.5	5.75	(302)	(53.5)	(18.9)	(3.34)
Apricot-Pineapple, **Ralph's,** low-fat, 8-oz. container	180	29.0	22.5	3.63	(209)	(33.7)	(13.1)	(2.11)
BANANA								
Colombo, Sundae Style, whole milk, 5-oz. container	140	23.0	28.0	4.60	(260)	(42.8)	(16.3)	(2.67)
Dannon, low-fat, 8-oz. container	260	49.0	32.5	6.13	(302)	(57.0)	(18.9)	(3.56)
Knudsen, Fruit-On-The-Bottom, low-fat, 8-oz. container	270	49.0	33.8	6.13	314	56.9	19.7	3.56
Le Shake, low-fat, 8-oz. container	200	35.0	25.0	4.38	(233)	(40.7)	(14.5)	(2.55)
Lucerne (Safeway), low-fat, 8-oz. container	260	46.0	32.5	5.75	(302)	(53.5)	(18.9)	(3.34)
Banana Colada, **Knudsen,** Pre-stirred, low-fat, 8-oz. container	260	48.0	32.5	6.00	302	55.8	18.9	3.49
Banana-Strawberry, **Colombo,** whole milk, 8-oz. container	235	38.0	29.4	4.75	(273)	(44.2)	(17.1)	(2.76)
Banana-Strawberry, **Colombo Lite,** nonfat, 8-oz. container	190	40.0	23.8	5.00	(221)	(46.5)	(13.8)	(2.91)
BLACKBERRY								
Knudsen Fruit-On-The-Bottom, low-fat, 8-oz. container	270	49.0	33.8	6.13	314	56.9	19.7	3.56
Knudsen, Pre-stirred, low-fat, 8-oz. container	260	48.0	32.5	6.00	302	55.8	18.9	3.49
Lucerne (Safeway), low-fat, 8-oz. container	260	46.0	32.5	5.75	(302)	(53.5)	(18.9)	(3.34)
Viva, Swiss Style, skim milk, 8-oz. container	250	47.0	31.3	5.88	(291)	(54.6)	(18.2)	(3.41)

	CONTAINER		1 OZ., BY WT.		1 CUP		1 TABLESPOON	
	Cal.	Carb.	Cal.	Carb.	Cal.	Carb.	Cal.	Carb.
BLACK CHERRY								
Axelrod's, Sundae Style, low-fat, 8-oz. container	250	50.0	31.3	6.25	(291)	(58.1)	(18.2)	(3.63)
Bison, low-fat, 8-oz. container	250	46.0	31.3	5.75	(291)	(53.5)	(18.2)	(3.34)
Breakstone's, Parfait, low-fat, 8-oz. container	256	19.8	32.0	2.48	(298)	(23.1)	(18.6)	(1.44)
Breyers, whole milk, 8-oz. container	270	47.0	33.8	5.89	(314)	(54.6)	(19.6)	(3.41)
Colombo, whole milk, 8-oz. container	230	34.0	28.8	4.25	(268)	(39.5)	(16.7)	(2.47)
Light n' Lively (Sealtest), low-fat, 8-oz. container	240	44.0	30.0	5.50	(279)	(51.2)	(17.4)	(3.20)
Viva, Swiss Style, skim milk, 8-oz. container	250	47.0	31.3	5.88	(291)	(54.6)	(18.2)	(3.41)
BLUEBERRY								
A & P, low-fat, 8-oz. container	270	52.0	33.8	6.50	(314)	(60.5)	(19.6)	(3.78)
Axelrod's, Sundae Style, low-fat, 8-oz. container	250	50.0	31.3	6.25	(291)	(58.1)	(18.2)	(3.63)
Bison, low-fat, 8-oz. container	250	46.0	31.3	5.75	(291)	(53.5)	(18.2)	(3.34)
Breakstone's, Parfait, low-fat, 8-oz. container	286	23.4	35.8	2.93	(333)	(27.2)	(20.8)	(1.70)
Breyers, whole milk, 8-oz. container	270	47.0	33.8	5.89	(314)	(54.6)	(19.6)	(3.41)
Brown Cow Farm, whole milk, 8-oz. container	230	30.0	28.8	3.75	(268)	(34.9)	(16.7)	(2.18)
Chambourcy, whole milk, French style (Yoghourt à la Française), 6-oz. container	190	31.0	23.8	3.88	(221)	(36.0)	(13.8)	(2.25)
Colombo, whole milk, 8-oz. container	250	38.0	31.3	4.75	(291)	(44.2)	(18.2)	(2.76)
Colombo, Sundae Style, whole milk, 5-oz. container	140	23.0	28.0	4.60	(260)	(42.8)	(16.3)	(2.67)
Colombo Lite, nonfat, 8-oz. container	190	40.0	23.8	5.00	(221)	(46.5)	(13.8)	(2.91)
Dannon, low-fat, 8-oz. container	260	49.0	32.5	6.13	(302)	(57.0)	(18.9)	(3.56)
Dannon Mélangé, low-fat, 6-oz. container	180	31.0	30.0	5.17	(279)	(48.1)	(17.4)	(3.01)
Europa, whole milk, 6-oz. container	210	37.0	35.0	6.17	(326)	(57.4)	(20.3)	(3.59)
Johnston's, low-fat, 8-oz. container	250	50.0	31.3	6.25	(291)	(58.1)	(18.2)	(3.63)
Knudsen, Fruit-On-The-Bottom, low-fat, 8-oz. container	270	49.0	33.8	6.13	314	56.9	19.7	3.56
Knudsen, Pre-stirred, low-fat, 8-oz. container	260	49.0	32.5	6.13	302	56.9	18.9	3.56
La Yogurt, whole milk, 6-oz. container	200	32.0	33.3	5.33	(310)	(49.6)	(19.4)	(3.10)
Le Shake, low-fat, 8-oz. container	180	31.0	22.5	3.88	(209)	(36.1)	(13.1)	(2.26)
Light n' Lively (Sealtest), low-fat, 8-oz. container	240	46.0	30.0	5.75	(279)	(53.5)	(17.4)	(3.34)
Look-Fit (A&P), Swiss Style, low-fat, 8-oz. container	240	47.0	30.0	5.88	(279)	(54.7)	(17.4)	(3.41)
Lucerne (Safeway), low-fat, 8-oz. container	260	46.0	32.5	5.75	(302)	(53.5)	(18.9)	(3.34)
Maya, whole milk, 8-oz. container	280	39.0	35.0	4.88	(326)	(45.4)	(20.3)	(2.84)
Meadow Gold, Western Sundae Style, skim milk, 8-oz. container	270	49.0	33.8	6.13	(314)	(57.0)	(19.6)	(3.56)
Ralph's, low-fat, 8-oz. container	190	31.0	23.8	3.88	(221)	(36.1)	(13.8)	(2.26)
Sippity, nonfat, 8-oz. container	150	29.0	18.8	3.60	(175)	(33.5)	(10.9)	(2.09)
Sweet 'N Low, nonfat, 8-oz. container	150	33.0	18.8	4.13	(174)	(38.3)	(10.9)	(2.39)
Viva, Swiss Style, skim milk, 8-oz. container	250	47.0	31.3	5.88	(291)	(54.6)	(18.2)	(3.41)
White Rose, low-fat, 8-oz. container	250	48.0	31.3	6.00	(291)	(55.8)	(18.2)	(3.49)
Yoplait, whole milk, 6-oz. container	190	32.0	29.3	4.94	(272)	(45.9)	(17.0)	(2.87)
For comparison: Blueberry Frosted Treat, **Weight Watchers,** 7-fl.-oz. serving	120	22.0	28.6	5.24	137	25.1	8.6	1.57
Blueberry Yogurt with Cottage Cheese, **Zausner,** low-fat, 12-oz. container	276	21.0	23.0	1.75	(214)	(16.3)	(13.8)	(1.02)
Blueberry with Granola, **Knudsen,** Yogurt Plus, low-fat, 8-oz. container	260	52.0	32.5	6.50	302	60.5	18.9	3.78
Blueberry Ripple, **New Country,** low-fat, 8-oz. container	240	43.0	30.0	5.38	(279)	(50.0)	(17.4)	(3.13)

	CONTAINER		1 OZ., BY WT.		1 CUP		1 TABLESPOON	
	Cal.	Carb.	Cal.	Carb.	Cal.	Carb.	Cal.	Carb.
BOYSENBERRY								
Dannon, low-fat, 8-oz. container	260	49.0	32.5	6.13	(302)	(57.0)	(18.9)	(3.56)
Fresh 'N Fruity, Original Style, low-fat, 6-oz. container	190	30.0	31.7	5.00	(295)	(46.5)	(18.4)	(2.91)
Johnston's, low-fat, 8-oz. container	250	49.0	30.3	6.13	(282)	(57.0)	(17.6)	(3.56)
Knudsen, Fruit-On-The-Bottom, low-fat, 8-oz. container	260	47.0	32.5	5.88	302	54.6	18.9	3.41
Knudsen, Pre-stirred, low-fat, 8-oz. container	270	50.0	33.8	6.25	314	58.1	19.6	3.63
32-oz. (2-lb.) container	1080	200.0	33.8	6.25	314	58.1	19.6	3.63
Lucerne (Safeway), low-fat, 8-oz. container	260	46.0	32.5	5.75	(302)	(53.5)	(18.9)	(3.34)
Meadow Gold, Western Sundae Style, skim milk, 8-oz. container	270	49.0	33.8	6.13	(314)	(57.0)	(19.6)	(3.56)
Viva, Swiss Style, skim milk, 8-oz. container	250	47.0	31.3	5.88	(291)	(54.6)	(18.2)	(3.41)
Yoplait, whole milk, 6-oz. container	190	32.0	29.3	4.94	(272)	(45.9)	(17.0)	(2.87)
CARAMEL								
Caramel Nut, **Ralph's,** low-fat, 8-oz. container	220	38.0	27.5	4.75	(256)	(44.2)	(16.0)	(2.76)
Caramel-Pecan, **Johnston's,** low-fat, 8-oz. container	290	60.0	36.3	7.50	(340)	(69.8)	(21.3)	(4.36)
CHERRY								
Brown Cow Farm, whole milk, 8-oz. container	245	32.0	30.6	4.00	(285)	(37.2)	(17.8)	(2.33)
Colombo Lite, nonfat, 8-oz. container	180	36.0	22.5	4.50	(209)	(41.9)	(13.1)	(2.62)
Continental, whole milk, 8-oz. container	310	39.0	38.8	4.88	(361)	(45.4)	(22.6)	(2.84)
Dannon, low-fat, 8-oz. container	260	49.0	32.5	6.13	(302)	(57.0)	(18.9)	(3.56)
Dannon Mélangé, low-fat, 6-oz. container	180	31.0	30.0	5.17	(279)	(48.1)	(17.4)	(3.01)
Europa, whole milk, 6-oz. container	210	37.0	35.0	6.17	(326)	(57.4)	(20.3)	(3.59)
Johnston's, low-fat, 8-oz. container	250	49.0	31.3	6.13	(291)	(57.0)	(18.2)	(3.56)
Knudsen, Fruit-On-The-Bottom, low-fat, 8-oz. container	260	47.0	32.5	5.88	302	54.6	18.9	3.41
Knudsen, Pre-stirred, low-fat, 8-oz. container	260	45.0	32.5	5.63	302	52.3	18.9	3.27
La Yogurt, whole milk, 6-oz. container	190	29.0	31.7	4.83	(295)	(44.9)	(18.4)	(2.81)
Le Shake, low-fat, 8-oz. container	180	31.0	22.5	3.88	(209)	(36.1)	(13.1)	(2.26)
Lucerne (Safeway), low-fat, 8-oz. container	260	46.0	32.5	5.75	(302)	(53.5)	(18.9)	(3.34)
Sweet 'N Low, nonfat, 8-oz. container	150	33.0	18.8	4.13	(174)	(38.3)	(10.9)	(2.39)
Yoplait, whole milk, 6-oz. container	190	32.0	29.3	4.94	(272)	(45.9)	(17.0)	(2.87)
Cherries Jubilee, **Johnston's,** low-fat, 8-oz. container	260	54.0	32.5	6.75	(302)	(62.8)	(18.9)	(3.92)
Cherry-Coconut, **Lucerne (Safeway),** low-fat, 8-oz. container	260	46.0	32.5	5.75	(302)	(53.5)	(18.9)	(3.34)
Cherry Supreme, **New Country,** low-fat, 8-oz. container	240	44.0	30.0	5.50	(279)	(51.2)	(17.4)	(3.20)
Cherry Vanilla, **Colombo,** whole milk, 8-oz. container	250	40.0	31.3	5.00	(291)	(46.5)	(18.2)	(2.91)
Dark Cherry, **Sugar Lo,** nonfat, 8-oz. container	130	26.0	16.3	3.25	(152)	(30.2)	(9.5)	(1.89)
Red Cherry, **Look-Fit (A&P),** Swiss Style, low-fat, 8-oz. container	220	42.0	27.5	5.25	(256)	(48.8)	(16.0)	(3.05)
Red Cherry, **Viva,** Swiss Style, skim milk, 8-oz. container	250	47.0	31.3	5.88	(291)	(54.6)	(18.2)	(3.41)
COFFEE								
Colombo, whole milk, 8-oz. container	200	29.0	25.0	3.63	(233)	(33.8)	(14.5)	(2.11)
Dannon, low-fat, 8-oz. container	200	32.0	25.0	4.00	(233)	(37.2)	(14.5)	(2.33)
Knudsen, Pre-stirred, low-fat, 8-oz. container	240	40.0	30.0	5.00	279	46.5	17.4	2.90
Yoplait, Custard Style, whole milk, 6-oz. container	180	30.0	30.0	5.00	(279)	(46.5)	(17.4)	(2.91)
Creamy Coffee, **Brown Cow Farm,** whole milk, 8-oz. container	230	30.0	28.8	3.75	(268)	(34.9)	(16.7)	(2.18)
COTTAGE CHEESE and YOGURT								
Cottage Cheese and Plain Yogurt, **Zausner,** low-fat, 12-oz. container	249	9.0	20.8	0.75	(184)	(7.0)	(11.5)	(0.44)
Cottage Cheese with Blueberry Yogurt, **Zausner,** low-fat, 12-oz. container	276	21.0	23.0	1.75	(221)	(16.3)	(13.8)	(1.02)
Cottage Cheese with Pineapple Yogurt, **Zausner,** low-fat, 12-oz. container	276	21.0	23.0	1.75	(214)	(16.3)	(13.4)	(1.02)
Cottage Cheese with Raspberry Yogurt, **Zausner,** low-fat, 12-oz. container	276	21.0	23.0	1.75	(214)	(16.3)	(13.4)	(1.02)
Cottage Cheese with Strawberry Yogurt, **Zausner,** low-fat, 12-oz. container	276	21.0	23.0	1.75	(214)	(16.3)	(13.4)	(1.02)
CRANBERRY-APPLE								
Knudsen, Pre-stirred, low-fat, 8-oz. container	260	50.0	32.5	6.25	302	58.1	18.9	3.63
FRUIT CRUNCH								
New Country, low-fat, 8-oz. container	240	42.0	30.0	5.25	(279)	(48.8)	(17.4)	(3.05)
FRUIT SALAD								
Viva, Swiss Style, skim milk, 8-oz. container	250	47.0	31.3	5.88	(291)	(54.6)	(18.2)	(3.41)
GRAPE								
Light n' Lively (Sealtest), low-fat, 8-oz. container	245	42.4	30.6	5.30	(285)	(49.3)	(17.8)	(3.08)
GUAVA								
Dannon, low-fat, 8-oz. container	260	49.0	32.5	6.13	(302)	(57.0)	(18.9)	(3.56)
HAWAIIAN SALAD								
New Country, low-fat, 8-oz. container	250	42.0	31.3	5.25	(291)	(48.8)	(18.2)	(3.05)
HONEY								
Dannon, low-fat, 8-oz. container	260	49.0	32.5	6.13	(302)	(57.0)	(18.9)	(3.56)
Honey Banana, **Colombo,** whole milk, 8-oz. container	220	30.4	27.5	3.80	(256)	(35.3)	(16.0)	(2.21)
Honey 'N Pear, **Dannon,** low-fat, 8-oz. container	260	49.0	32.5	6.13	(302)	(57.0)	(18.9)	(3.56)
Honey Vanilla, **Colombo,** Sundae Style, whole milk, 5-oz. container	138	19.0	27.6	3.80	(257)	(35.3)	(16.0)	(2.21)
Honey Vanilla, **Colombo Lite,** low-fat, 8-oz. container	160	32.0	20.0	4.00	(186)	(37.2)	(11.6)	(2.33)
Plain with Honey, **Yoplait,** Custard Style whole milk, 6-oz. container	160	23.0	26.7	3.83	(232)	(33.3)	(14.5)	(2.08)
Tupelo Honey, **Brown Cow Farm,** whole milk, 8-oz. container	240	27.0	30.0	3.38	(279)	(31.4)	(17.4)	(2.00)
LEMON								
Bison, low-fat, 8-oz. container	250	46.0	31.3	5.75	(291)	(53.5)	(18.2)	(3.34)
Breakstone's, Parfait, low-fat, 8-oz. container	254	19.8	31.8	2.48	(296)	(23.1)	(18.5)	(1.44)
Breyers, whole milk, 8-oz. container	230	32.0	28.8	4.00	(268)	(37.2)	(16.7)	(2.33)
Brown Cow Farm, whole milk, 8-oz. container	250	30.0	31.3	3.75	(291)	(34.9)	(18.2)	(2.18)
32-oz. (2-lb.) container	1000	120.0	31.3	3.75	(291)	(34.9)	(18.2)	(2.18)
Colombo, whole milk, 8-oz. container	220	30.0	27.5	3.75	(256)	(34.9)	(16.0)	(2.18)
Dannon, low-fat, 8-oz. container	200	32.0	25.0	4.00	(233)	(37.2)	(14.5)	(2.33)
Knudsen, Pre-stirred, low-fat, 8-oz. container	250	46.0	31.3	5.75	290	53.4	18.1	3.34
32-oz. (2-lb.) container	1000	184.0	31.3	5.75	290	53.4	18.1	3.34
Le Shake, low-fat, 8-oz. container	200	35.0	25.0	4.38	(233)	(40.7)	(14.5)	(2.55)
Light n' Lively (Sealtest), low-fat, 8-oz. container	240	46.0	30.0	5.75	(279)	(53.5)	(17.4)	(3.34)
Ralph's, low-fat, 8-oz. container	230	40.0	28.8	5.00	(268)	(46.5)	(16.7)	(2.91)
Viva, Swiss Style, skim milk, 8-oz. container	250	49.0	31.3	6.13	(291)	(57.0)	(18.2)	(3.56)
Yoplait, whole milk, 6-oz. container	190	32.0	29.3	4.94	(272)	(45.9)	(17.0)	(2.87)
Lemon Chiffon, **Knudsen,** Fruit-On-The-Bottom, low-fat, 8-oz. container	260	47.0	32.5	5.88	302	54.6	18.9	3.41
Lemon-Coconut, **Ralph's,** low-fat, 8-oz. container	210	36.0	26.3	4.50	(255)	(41.9)	(15.3)	(2.62)
Lemon-Lime, **Viva,** Swiss Style, skim milk, 8-oz. container	250	49.0	31.3	6.13	(291)	(57.0)	(18.2)	(3.56)

	CONTAINER		1 OZ., BY WT.		1 CUP		1 TABLE-SPOON	
	Cal.	Carb.	Cal.	Carb.	Cal.	Carb.	Cal.	Carb.
Lemon Ripple, **New Country,** low-fat, 8-oz. container	240	43.0	30.0	5.38	(279)	(50.0)	(17.4)	(3.13)
Plain Yogurt with Lemon Puree & Other Natural Flavors, **Yoplait,** Custard Style, 6-oz. container	180	30.0	30.0	5.00	(279)	(46.5)	(17.4)	(2.91)
LEMON-LIME								
Breakstone's, Parfait, low-fat, 8-oz. container	242	17.7	30.3	2.21	(282)	(20.6)	(17.6)	(1.28)
Viva, Swiss Style, skim milk, 8-oz. container	250	49.0	31.3	6.13	(291)	(57.0)	(18.2)	(3.56)
LIME								
Knudsen, Pre-stirred, low-fat, 8-oz. container	260	47.0	32.5	5.88	302	54.6	18.9	3.41
Lucerne (Safeway), low-fat, 8-oz. container	260	46.0	32.5	5.75	(302)	(53.5)	(18.9)	(3.34)
Ralph's, low-fat, 8-oz. container	220	38.0	27.5	4.75	(256)	(44.2)	(16.0)	(2.76)
Lime Margarita, **Knudsen,** Pre-stirred, low-fat, 8-oz. container	270	49.0	33.8	6.13	314	56.9	19.6	3.56
LOGANBERRY								
Ralph's, low-fat, 8-oz. container	220	38.0	27.5	4.75	(256)	(44.2)	(16.0)	(2.76)
MANDARIN ORANGE								
Breakstone's, Parfait, low-fat, 8-oz. container	264	21.3	33.0	2.66	(307)	(24.7)	(19.2)	(1.55)
Breyers, whole milk, 8-oz. container	240	45.0	30.0	5.63	(279)	(52.4)	(17.4)	(3.27)
Light n' Lively (Sealtest), low-fat, 8-oz. container	234	44.9	29.3	5.61	(272)	(52.2)	(17.0)	(3.26)
Meadow Gold, Western Sundae Style, skim milk, 8-oz. container	260	47.0	32.5	5.88	(302)	(54.6)	(18.9)	(3.41)
Viva, Swiss Style, skim milk, 8-oz. container	240	44.0	30.0	5.50	(279)	(51.2)	(17.4)	(3.20)
MAPLE								
Brown Cow Farm, whole milk, 8-oz. container	250	30.0	31.3	3.75	(291)	(34.9)	(18.2)	(2.18)
MIXED BERRIES								
Dannon, low-fat, 8-oz. container	260	49.0	32.5	6.13	(302)	(57.0)	(18.9)	(3.56)
Yoplait, whole milk, 6-oz. container	190	32.0	29.3	4.94	(272)	(45.9)	(17.0)	(2.87)
ORANGE								
Le Shake, low-fat, 8-oz. container	200	35.0	25.0	4.38	(233)	(40.7)	(14.5)	(2.55)
Lucerne (Safeway), low-fat, 8-oz. container	260	46.0	32.5	5.75	(302)	(53.5)	(18.9)	(3.34)
Yoplait, whole milk, 6-oz. container	190	32.0	29.3	4.94	(272)	(45.9)	(17.0)	(2.87)
Orange Supreme, **New Country,** low-fat, 8-oz. container	240	43.0	30.0	5.38	(279)	(50.0)	(17.4)	(3.13)
ORANGE-PINEAPPLE								
Orange-Pineapple, **Axelrod's,** Sundae Style, low-fat, 8-oz. container	250	50.0	31.3	6.25	(291)	(58.1)	(18.2)	(3.63)
Orange-Pineapple, **Johnston's,** low-fat, 8-oz. container	270	55.0	33.8	6.88	(314)	(64.0)	(19.6)	(4.00)
PEACH								
Bison, low-fat, 8-oz. container	250	46.0	31.3	5.75	(291)	(53.5)	(18.2)	(3.34)
Breakstone's, Parfait, low-fat, 8-oz. container	254	20.9	31.8	2.61	(296)	(24.3)	(18.5)	(1.52)
Breyers, whole milk, 8-oz. container	270	47.0	33.8	5.89	(314)	(54.8)	(19.6)	(3.42)
Brown Cow Farm, whole milk, 8-oz. container	225	30.0	28.1	3.75	(261)	(34.9)	(16.3)	(2.18)
Colombo Lite, nonfat, 8-oz. container	190	40.0	23.8	5.00	(221)	(46.5)	(13.8)	(2.91)
Dannon, low-fat, 8-oz. container	260	49.0	32.5	6.13	(302)	(57.0)	(18.9)	(3.56)
Europa, whole milk, 6-oz. container	210	37.0	35.0	6.17	(326)	(57.4)	(20.3)	(3.59)
Friendship, low-fat, 8-oz. container	230	57.0	28.8	7.13	(268)	(66.3)	(16.7)	(4.14)
Johnston's, low-fat, 8-oz. container	260	53.0	32.5	6.63	(302)	(61.6)	(18.9)	(3.85)
Knudsen, Fruit-On-The-Bottom, low-fat, 8-oz. container	260	48.0	32.5	6.00	302	55.8	18.9	3.49
Knudsen, Pre-stirred, low-fat, 8-oz. container	260	50.0	32.5	6.25	302	58.1	18.9	3.63
32-oz. (2-lb.) container	1040	200.0	32.5	6.25	302	58.1	18.9	3.63
Light n' Lively (Sealtest), low-fat, 8-oz. container	240	46.0	30.0	5.75	(279)	(53.3)	(17.4)	(3.33)

	CONTAINER		1 OZ., BY WT.		1 CUP		1 TABLE-SPOON	
	Cal.	Carb.	Cal.	Carb.	Cal.	Carb.	Cal.	Carb.
Look-Fit (A&P), Swiss Style, low-fat, 8-oz. container	240	47.0	30.0	5.88	(279)	(54.7)	(17.4)	(3.41)
Maya, whole milk, 8-oz. container	280	39.0	35.0	4.88	(326)	(45.4)	(20.3)	(2.84)
Meadow Gold, Western Sundae Style, skim milk, 8-oz. container	260	47.0	32.5	5.88	(302)	(54.6)	(18.9)	(3.41)
Ralph's, low-fat, 8-oz. container	210	36.0	26.3	4.50	(255)	(41.9)	(15.3)	(2.62)
Viva, Swiss style, skim milk, 8-oz. container	240	44.0	30.0	5.50	(279)	(51.2)	(17.4)	(3.20)
White Rose, low-fat, 8-oz. container	250	48.0	31.3	6.00	(291)	(55.8)	(18.2)	(3.49)
Yoplait whole milk, 6-oz. container	190	32.0	29.3	4.94	(272)	(45.9)	(17.0)	(2.87)
For comparison: Peach frozen yogurt, **Danny-in-a-Cup,** 8-fl.-oz. container	210	42.0	35.0	7.00	210	42.0	13.1	2.63
Peaches 'n' Cream, low-fat, **New Country,** 8-oz. container	240	43.0	30.0	5.38	(279)	(50.0)	(17.4)	(3.13)
Peach with Granola, **Knudsen,** Yogurt Plus, low-fat, 8-oz. container	260	52.0	32.5	6.50	302	60.5	18.9	3.78
Peach with Peaches and Nectarines, **Sugar Lo,** nonfat, 8-oz. container	130	26.0	16.3	3.25	(152)	(30.2)	(9.5)	(1.89)
Peach-Pineapple, **Natural & Kosher,** whole milk, 8-oz. container	240	35.0	30.0	4.38	(279)	(40.7)	(17.4)	(2.55)
PEACH MELBA								
Peach Melba, **Breakstone's,** Parfait, low-fat, 8-oz. container	268	21.8	33.5	2.73	(312)	(25.4)	(19.5)	(1.59)
Peach Melba, **Colombo,** Sundae Style, whole milk, 5-oz. container	140	23.0	28.0	4.60	(260)	(42.8)	(16.3)	(2.67)
Peach Melba, **Light n' Lively (Sealtest),** low-fat, 8-oz. container	250	47.0	31.3	5.89	(291)	(54.6)	(18.2)	(3.41)
PIÑA COLADA								
Colombo, whole milk, 8-oz. container	240	40.0	30.0	5.00	(279)	(46.5)	(17.4)	(2.91)
Dannon, low-fat, 8-oz. container	260	49.0	32.5	6.13	(302)	(57.0)	(18.9)	(3.56)
Friendship, low-fat, 8-oz. container	240	59.0	30.0	7.38	(279)	(68.6)	(17.4)	(4.29)
Johnston's, low-fat, 8-oz. container	270	53.0	33.8	6.63	(314)	(61.6)	(19.6)	(3.85)
Knudsen, Fruit-On-The-Bottom, low-fat, 8-oz. container	260	48.0	32.5	6.00	302	55.8	18.9	3.49
Knudsen, Pre-stirred, low-fat, 8-oz. container	260	48.0	32.5	6.00	302	55.8	18.9	3.49
Yoplait, whole milk, 6-oz. container	190	32.0	29.3	4.94	(272)	(45.9)	(17.0)	(2.87)
PINEAPPLE								
Breyers, whole milk, 8-oz. container	270	47.0	33.8	5.89	(314)	(54.8)	(19.6)	(3.42)
Colombo Lite, nonfat, 8-oz. container	190	38.0	23.8	4.75	(221)	(44.2)	(13.8)	(2.76)
Dannon Mélangé, low-fat, 6-oz. container	180	31.0	30.0	5.17	(279)	(48.1)	(17.4)	(3.01)
Knudsen, Pre-stirred, low-fat, 8-oz. container	270	50.0	33.8	6.25	314	58.1	19.6	3.63
Light n' Lively (Sealtest), low-fat, 8-oz. container	240	47.0	30.0	5.88	(279)	(54.7)	(17.4)	(3.42)
Lucerne (Safeway), low-fat, 8-oz. container	260	46.0	32.5	5.75	(302)	(53.5)	(18.9)	(3.34)
Meadow Gold, Western Sundae Style, skim milk, 8-oz. container	270	49.0	33.8	6.13	(314)	(57.0)	(19.6)	(3.56)
Ralph's, low-fat, 8-oz. container	230	41.0	28.8	5.13	(268)	(47.7)	(16.7)	(2.98)
Sugar Lo, nonfat, 8-oz. container	130	26.0	16.3	3.25	(152)	(30.2)	(9.5)	(1.89)
Yoplait, whole milk, 6-oz. container	190	32.0	29.3	4.94	(272)	(45.9)	(17.0)	(2.87)
Pineapple Coconut, **Viva,** Swiss Style, skim milk, 8-oz. container	250	47.0	31.3	5.88	(291)	(54.6)	(18.2)	(3.41)
Pineapple Yogurt with Cottage Cheese, **Zausner,** low-fat, 12-oz. container	276	21.0	23.0	1.75	(214)	(16.3)	(13.4)	(1.02)
PINEAPPLE-ORANGE								
Pineapple-Orange, **Dannon,** low-fat, 8-oz. container	260	49.0	32.5	6.13	(302)	(57.0)	(18.9)	(3.56)
Pineapple-Orange, **Viva,** Swiss Style, skim milk, 8-oz. container	250	47.0	31.3	5.88	(291)	(54.6)	(18.2)	(3.41)

	CONTAINER Cal.	CONTAINER Carb.	1 OZ., BY WT. Cal.	1 OZ., BY WT. Carb.	1 CUP Cal.	1 CUP Carb.	1 TABLE-SPOON Cal.	1 TABLE-SPOON Carb.
PRUNE								
Lucerne (Safeway), low-fat, 8-oz. container	260	46.0	32.5	5.75	(302)	(53.5)	(18.9)	(3.34)
RASPBERRY								
Axelrod's, Sundae Style, low-fat, 8-oz. container	250	50.0	31.3	6.25	(291)	(58.1)	(18.2)	(3.63)
Bison, low-fat, 8-oz. container	250	46.0	31.3	5.75	(291)	(53.5)	(18.2)	(3.34)
Colombo, whole milk, 8-oz. container	250	39.0	31.3	4.88	(291)	(45.4)	(18.2)	(2.84)
Colombo Lite, nonfat, 8-oz. container	190	40.0	23.8	5.00	(221)	(46.5)	(13.8)	(2.91)
Dannon, low-fat, 8-oz. container	260	49.0	32.5	6.13	(302)	(57.0)	(18.9)	(3.56)
Dannon Mélangé, low-fat, 6-oz. container	180	31.0	30.0	5.17	(279)	(48.1)	(17.4)	(3.01)
Europa, whole milk, 6-oz. container	210	37.0	35.0	6.17	(326)	(57.4)	(20.3)	(3.59)
Fresh 'N Fruity, Original Style, low-fat, 6-oz. container	190	30.0	31.7	5.00	(295)	(46.5)	(18.4)	(2.91)
La Yogurt, whole milk, 6-oz. container	210	34.0	35.0	5.67	(326)	(52.7)	(20.3)	(3.30)
Le Shake, low-fat, 8-oz. container	190	32.0	23.8	4.00	(221)	(37.2)	(13.8)	(2.33)
Sugar Lo, nonfat, 8-oz. container	130	26.0	16.3	3.25	(152)	(30.2)	(9.5)	(1.89)
Sweet 'n Low, nonfat, 8-oz. container	150	33.0	18.8	4.13	(174)	(38.3)	(10.9)	(2.39)
Viva, Swiss Style, skim milk, 8-oz. container	250	47.0	31.3	5.88	(291)	(54.6)	(18.2)	(3.41)
White Rose, low-fat, 8-oz. container	250	48.0	31.3	6.00	(291)	(55.8)	(18.2)	(3.49)
Yoplait, whole milk, 6-oz. container	190	32.0	29.3	4.94	(272)	(45.9)	(17.0)	(2.87)
Raspberry Ripple, **New Country,** low-fat, 8-oz. container	240	43.0	30.0	5.38	(279)	(50.0)	(17.4)	(3.13)
Raspberry Yogurt with Cottage Cheese, **Zausner,** low-fat, 12-oz. container	276	21.0	23.0	1.75	(214)	(16.3)	(13.4)	(1.02)
For comparison: Raspberry Fruit Yogurt, **Prize (St. Ivel)** (sold in Great Britain), 5-oz. container	110	19.8	22.0	3.97	(205)	(36.9)	(12.8)	(2.31)
RED RASPBERRY								
Breakstone's, Parfait, low-fat, 8-oz. container	264	20.5	33.0	2.56	(307)	(23.8)	(19.2)	(1.49)
Breyers, whole milk, 8-oz. container	270	47.0	33.8	5.89	(314)	(54.8)	(19.6)	(3.42)
Colombo, Sundae Style, whole milk, 5-oz. container	140	23.0	28.0	4.60	(260)	(42.8)	(16.3)	(2.67)
Knudsen, Fruit-On-The-Bottom, low-fat, 8-oz. container	270	49.0	33.8	6.13	314	56.9	19.7	3.56
Knudsen, Pre-stirred, low-fat, 8-oz. container	250	46.0	31.3	5.75	290	53.4	18.1	3.34
Light n' Lively (Sealtest), low-fat, 8-oz. container	230	43.0	28.8	5.38	(268)	(50.0)	(16.7)	(3.12)
Look-Fit (A&P), Swiss Style, low-fat, 8-oz. container	210	42.0	26.3	5.25	(245)	(48.8)	(15.3)	(3.05)
Lucerne (Safeway), low-fat, 8-oz. container	260	46.0	32.5	5.75	(302)	(53.5)	(18.9)	(3.34)
16-oz. (1-lb.) container	520	92.0	32.5	5.75	(302)	(53.5)	(18.9)	(3.34)
32-oz. (2-lb.) container	1040	184.0	32.5	5.75	(302)	(53.5)	(18.9)	(3.34)
Meadow Gold, Western Sundae Style, skim milk, 8-oz. container	270	49.0	33.8	6.13	(314)	(57.0)	(19.6)	(3.56)
Red Raspberry with Granola, Knudsen, Yogurt Plus, low-fat, 8-oz. container	260	52.0	32.5	6.50	302	60.5	18.9	3.78
STRAWBERRY								
Axelrod's, Sundae Style, low-fat, 8-oz. container	250	50.0	31.3	6.25	(291)	(58.1)	(18.2)	(3.63)
Bison, low-fat, 8-oz. container	250	46.0	31.3	5.75	(291)	(53.5)	(18.2)	(3.34)
Breakstone's, Parfait, low-fat, 8-oz. container	260	22.3	32.5	2.79	(302)	(26.0)	(18.9)	(1.62)
Breyers, whole milk, 8-oz. container	270	47.0	33.8	5.89	(314)	(54.8)	(19.6)	(3.42)
Brown Cow Farm, whole milk, 8-oz. container	223	30.0	27.9	3.75	(259)	(34.9)	(16.2)	(2.18)
Chambourcy, whole milk, French style (Yoghourt à la Française), 6-oz. container	190	31.0	(23.8)	(3.88)	(221)	(36.0)	(13.8)	(2.25)
Colombo, whole milk, 8-oz. container	230	36.0	28.8	4.50	(268)	(41.9)	(16.7)	(2.62)
Colombo, Sundae Style, whole milk, 5-oz. container	140	23.0	28.0	4.60	(260)	(42.8)	(16.3)	(2.67)
Colombo Lite, nonfat, 8-oz. container	190	40.0	23.8	5.00	(221)	(46.5)	(13.8)	(2.91)

	CONTAINER Cal.	CONTAINER Carb.	1 OZ., BY WT. Cal.	1 OZ., BY WT. Carb.	1 CUP Cal.	1 CUP Carb.	1 TABLE-SPOON Cal.	1 TABLE-SPOON Carb.
Dannon, low-fat, 8-oz. container	260	49.0	32.5	6.13	(302)	(57.0)	(18.9)	(3.56)
Dannon Mélangé, low-fat, 6-oz. container	180	31.0	30.0	5.17	(279)	(48.1)	(17.4)	(3.01)
Europa, whole milk, 6-oz. container	210	37.0	35.0	6.17	(326)	(57.4)	(20.3)	(3.59)
Fresh 'N Fruity, Original Style, low-fat, 6-oz. container	190	30.0	31.7	5.00	(295)	(46.5)	(18.4)	(2.91)
Friendship, low-fat, 8-oz. container	230	57.0	28.8	7.13	(268)	(66.3)	(16.7)	(4.14)
Johnston's, low-fat, 8-oz. container	250	51.0	31.3	6.38	(291)	(59.3)	(18.2)	(3.71)
Knudsen, Fruit-On-The-Bottom, low-fat, 8-oz. container	260	47.0	32.5	5.88	302	54.6	18.9	3.41
Knudsen, Pre-stirred, low-fat, 8-oz. container	250	46.0	31.3	5.75	290	53.4	18.1	3.34
32-oz. (2-lb.) container	1000	184.0	31.3	5.75	290	53.4	18.1	3.34
Le Shake, low-fat, 8-oz. container	180	30.0	22.5	3.75	(209)	(34.8)	(13.1)	(2.20)
Light n' Lively (Sealtest), low-fat, 8-oz. container	240	46.0	30.0	5.75	(279)	(53.5)	(17.4)	(3.34)
Look-Fit (A&P), Swiss Style, low-fat, 8-oz. container	220	42.0	27.5	5.25	(256)	(48.8)	(16.0)	(3.05)
Lucerne (Safeway), low-fat, 8-oz. container	260	46.0	32.5	5.75	(302)	(53.5)	(18.9)	(3.34)
Maya, whole milk, 8-oz. container	280	39.0	35.0	4.88	(326)	(45.4)	(20.3)	(2.84)
Meadow Gold, Western Sundae Style, skim milk, 8-oz. container	270	49.0	33.8	6.13	(314)	(57.0)	(19.6)	(3.56)
Ralph's, low-fat, 8-oz. container	190	31.0	23.8	3.88	(221)	(36.1)	(13.8)	(2.26)
Sippity, nonfat, 8-oz. container	150	29.0	18.8	3.60	(175)	(33.5)	(10.9)	(2.09)
Sugar Lo, nonfat, 8-oz. container	130	26.0	16.3	3.25	(152)	(30.2)	(9.5)	(1.89)
Sweet 'n Low, nonfat, 8-oz. container	150	33.0	18.8	4.13	(174)	(38.3)	(10.9)	(2.39)
Viva, Swiss Style, skim milk, 8-oz. container	250	47.0	31.3	5.88	(291)	(54.6)	(18.2)	(3.41)
White Rose, low-fat, 8-oz. container	250	48.0	31.3	6.00	(291)	(55.8)	(18.2)	(3.49)
Yoplait, whole milk, 6-oz. container	190	32.0	29.3	4.94	(272)	(45.9)	(17.0)	(2.87)
For comparison: Strawberry ice cream, **Häagen-Dazs,** 1-pint container	1032	95.7	66.6	6.18	516	47.9	32.3	2.99
Strawberry Banana, **Light n' Lively (Sealtest),** low-fat, 8-oz. container	260	52.0	32.5	6.50	(302)	(60.5)	(18.9)	(3.78)
Strawberry-Banana, **Sweet 'n Low,** nonfat, 8-oz. container	150	33.0	18.8	4.13	(174)	(38.3)	(10.9)	(2.39)
Strawberry-Banana, **Yoplait,** whole milk, 6-oz. container	190	32.0	29.3	4.94	(272)	(45.9)	(17.0)	(2.87)
Strawberry Daiquiri, **Knudsen,** Pre-stirred, low-fat, 8-oz. container	270	49.0	33.8	6.13	314	56.9	19.6	3.56
Strawberry Fruit Cup, **Light n' Lively (Sealtest),** low-fat, 8-oz. container	250	47.0	31.3	5.89	(291)	(54.6)	(18.2)	(3.41)
Strawberry with Granola, **Knudsen,** Yogurt Plus, low-fat, 8-oz. container	260	52.0	32.5	6.50	302	60.5	18.9	3.78
Strawberry Supreme, **New Country,** low-fat, 8-oz. container	240	43.0	30.0	5.38	(279)	(30.0)	(17.4)	(3.13)
Strawberry Walnut, **Breyers,** whole milk, 8-oz. container	240	39.0	30.0	4.88	(279)	(45.3)	(17.4)	(2.84)
Strawberry Yogurt with Cottage Cheese, **Zausner,** low-fat, 12-oz. container	276	21.0	23.0	1.75	(214)	(16.3)	(13.4)	(1.02)
VANILLA								
A&P, low-fat, 8-oz. container	200	32.0	25.0	4.00	(233)	(37.2)	(14.5)	(2.33)
Bison, low-fat, 8-oz. container	200	39.0	25.0	4.88	(233)	(45.3)	(14.5)	(2.83)
Brown Cow Farm, whole milk, 8-oz. container	250	30.0	31.2	3.75	(290)	(34.9)	(18.1)	(2.18)
Dannon, low-fat, 8-oz. container	200	32.0	25.0	4.00	(233)	(37.2)	(14.5)	(2.33)
16-oz. (1-lb.) container	400	64.0	25.0	4.00	(233)	(37.2)	(14.5)	(2.33)
Knudsen, Pre-stirred, low-fat, 8-oz. container	240	44.0	30.0	5.50	279	51.1	17.4	3.19
32-oz. (2-lb.) container	960	176.0	30.0	5.50	279	51.1	17.4	3.19
Le Shake, low-fat, 8-oz. container	190	33.0	23.8	4.13	(221)	(38.4)	(13.8)	(2.40)
Light n' Lively (Sealtest), low-fat, 8-oz. container	195	32.7	24.4	4.09	(227)	(38.0)	(14.2)	(2.38)

	CONTAINER		1 OZ., BY WT.		1 CUP		1 TABLE-SPOON	
	Cal.	Carb.	Cal.	Carb.	Cal.	Carb.	Cal.	Carb.
French Vanilla, **New Country,** low-fat, 8-oz. container	210	40.0	26.3	5.00	(245)	(46.5)	(15.3)	(2.91)
French Vanilla Ripple, **New Country,** low-fat, 8-oz. container	240	42.0	30.0	5.25	(279)	(48.8)	(17.4)	(3.05)
Vanilla Bean, **Breyers,** whole milk, 8-oz. container	230	32.0	28.8	4.00	(268)	(37.2)	(16.7)	(2.33)
Vanilla Honey, **Colombo,** whole milk, 8-oz. container	250	40.0	31.3	5.00	(291)	(46.5)	(18.2)	(2.91)
For comparison: Vanilla frozen yogurt, **Danny-in-a-Cup,** 8-fl.-oz. container	180	20.0	30.0	3.33	180	20.0	11.3	1.25
WALNUT RAISIN								
Bison, low-fat, 8-oz. container	250	46.0	31.3	5.75	(291)	(53.5)	(18.2)	(3.34)

YOGURT, by brand

The list that follows is alphabetized by brand name. A list alphabetized by the main descriptive fruit or flavor precedes this one.

	CONTAINER		1 OZ., BY WT.		1 CUP		1 TABLE-SPOON	
	Cal.	Carb.	Cal.	Carb.	Cal.	Carb.	Cal.	Carb.
A&P low-fat yogurt								
Plain, 32-oz. (2-lb.) container	600	68.0	18.8	2.13	(165)	(18.7)	(10.3)	(1.17)
Blueberry, 8-oz. container	270	52.0	33.8	6.50	(314)	(60.5)	(19.6)	(3.78)
Vanilla, 8-oz. container	200	32.0	25.0	4.00	(233)	(37.2)	(14.5)	(2.33)
Axelrod's "Easy Dieter" low-fat yogurt								
Plain, 8-oz. container	150	18.0	18.8	2.25	(165)	(19.8)	(10.3)	(1.24)
16-oz. (1-lb.) container	300	36.0	18.8	2.25	(165)	(19.8)	(10.3)	(1.24)
32-oz. (2-lb.) container	600	72.0	18.8	2.25	(165)	(19.8)	(10.3)	(1.24)
Axelrod's Sundae Style low-fat yogurt								
Apricot, 8-oz. container	250	50.0	31.3	6.25	(291)	(58.1)	(18.2)	(3.63)
Black Cherry, 8-oz. container	250	50.0	31.3	6.25	(291)	(58.1)	(18.2)	(3.63)
Blueberry, 8-oz. container	250	50.0	31.3	6.25	(291)	(58.1)	(18.2)	(3.63)
Orange-Pineapple, 8-oz. container	250	50.0	31.3	6.25	(291)	(58.1)	(18.2)	(3.63)
Raspberry, 8-oz. container	250	50.0	31.3	6.25	(291)	(58.1)	(18.2)	(3.63)
Spiced Apple, 8-oz. container	250	50.0	31.3	6.25	(291)	(58.1)	(18.2)	(3.63)
Strawberry, 8-oz. container	250	50.0	31.3	6.25	(291)	(58.1)	(18.2)	(3.63)
Bison low-fat yogurt								
Plain, 8-oz. container	160	17.0	20.0	2.13	(176)	(18.7)	(11.0)	(1.17)
Apricot, 8-oz. container	250	46.0	31.3	5.75	(291)	(53.5)	(18.2)	(3.34)
Black Cherry, 8-oz. container	250	46.0	31.3	5.75	(291)	(53.5)	(18.2)	(3.34)
Blueberry, 8-oz. container	250	46.0	31.3	5.75	(291)	(53.5)	(18.2)	(3.34)
Dutch Apple, 8-oz. container	250	46.0	31.3	5.75	(291)	(53.5)	(18.2)	(3.34)
Lemon, 8-oz. container	250	46.0	31.3	5.75	(291)	(53.5)	(18.2)	(3.34)
Peach, 8-oz. container	250	46.0	31.3	5.75	(291)	(53.5)	(18.2)	(3.34)
Raspberry, 8-oz. container	250	46.0	31.3	5.75	(291)	(53.5)	(18.2)	(3.34)
Strawberry, 8-oz. container	250	46.0	31.3	5.75	(291)	(53.5)	(18.2)	(3.34)
Vanilla, 8-oz. container	200	39.0	25.0	4.88	(233)	(45.3)	(14.5)	(2.83)
Walnut Raisin, 8-oz. container	250	46.0	31.3	5.75	(291)	(53.5)	(18.2)	(3.34)
Breakstone's, Parfait low-fat yogurt								
Apricot, 8-oz. container	250	18.9	31.3	2.36	(291)	(21.9)	(18.2)	(1.37)
Black Cherry, 8-oz. container	256	19.8	32.0	2.48	(298)	(23.1)	(18.6)	(1.44)
Blueberry, 8-oz. container	286	23.4	35.8	2.93	(333)	(27.2)	(20.8)	(1.70)
Lemon, 8-oz. container	254	19.8	31.8	2.48	(296)	(23.1)	(18.5)	(1.44)
Lemon-Lime, 8-oz. container	242	17.7	30.3	2.21	(282)	(20.6)	(17.6)	(1.28)
Mandarin Orange, 8-oz. container	264	21.3	33.0	2.66	(307)	(24.7)	(19.2)	(1.55)
Peach, 8-oz. container	254	20.9	31.8	2.61	(296)	(24.3)	(18.5)	(1.52)
Peach Melba, 8-oz. container	268	21.8	33.5	2.73	(312)	(25.4)	(19.5)	(1.59)
Red Raspberry, 8-oz. container	264	20.5	33.0	2.56	(307)	(23.8)	(19.2)	(1.49)
Strawberry, 8-oz. container	260	22.3	32.5	2.79	(302)	(26.0)	(18.9)	(1.62)
Breyers whole milk yogurt								
Plain, 8-oz. container	160	14.0	20.0	1.75	(174)	(15.2)	(10.9)	(0.95)
Black Cherry, 8-oz. container	270	47.0	33.8	5.89	(314)	(54.6)	(19.6)	(3.41)
Blueberry, 8-oz. container	270	47.0	33.8	5.89	(314)	(54.6)	(19.6)	(3.41)
Lemon, 8-oz. container	230	32.0	28.8	4.00	(268)	(37.2)	(16.7)	(2.33)
Mandarin Orange, 8-oz. container	240	45.0	30.0	5.63	(279)	(52.4)	(17.4)	(3.27)
Peach, 8-oz. container	270	47.0	33.8	5.89	(314)	(54.8)	(19.6)	(3.42)
Pineapple, 8-oz. container	270	47.0	33.8	5.89	(314)	(54.8)	(19.6)	(3.42)

	CONTAINER		1 OZ., BY WT.		1 CUP		1 TABLE-SPOON	
	Cal.	Carb.	Cal.	Carb.	Cal.	Carb.	Cal.	Carb.
Red Raspberry, 8-oz. container	270	47.0	33.8	5.89	(314)	(54.8)	(19.6)	(3.42)
Strawberry, 8-oz. container	270	47.0	33.8	5.89	(314)	(54.8)	(19.6)	(3.42)
Strawberry Walnut, 8-oz. container	240	39.0	30.0	4.88	(279)	(45.3)	(17.4)	(2.84)
Vanilla Bean, 8-oz. container	230	32.0	28.8	4.00	(268)	(37.2)	(16.7)	(2.33)
Brown Cow Farm whole milk yogurt								
Plain, 8-oz. container	190	13.0	23.8	1.63	(207)	(15.2)	(12.9)	(0.95)
16-oz. (1-lb.) container	380	26.1	23.8	1.63	(207)	(15.2)	(12.9)	(0.95)
Blueberry, 8-oz. container	230	30.0	28.8	3.75	(268)	(34.9)	(16.7)	(2.18)
Cherry, 8-oz. container	245	32.0	30.6	4.00	(285)	(37.2)	(17.8)	(2.33)
Creamy Coffee, 8-oz. container	230	30.0	28.8	3.75	(268)	(34.9)	(16.7)	(2.18)
Lemon, 8-oz. container	250	30.0	31.3	3.75	(291)	(34.9)	(18.2)	(2.18)
Maple, 8-oz. container	250	30.0	31.3	3.75	(291)	(34.9)	(18.2)	(2.18)
Peach, 8-oz. container	225	30.0	28.1	3.75	(261)	(34.9)	(16.3)	(2.18)
Strawberry, 8-oz. container	223	30.0	27.9	3.75	(259)	(34.9)	(16.2)	(2.18)
Tupelo Honey, 8-oz. container	240	27.0	30.0	3.38	(279)	(31.4)	(17.4)	(2.00)
Vanilla, 8-oz. container	250	30.0	31.2	3.75	(290)	(34.9)	(18.1)	(2.18)
Chambourcy whole milk yogurt (Yoghourt à la Française)								
Blueberry and other natural flavors, 6-oz. container	190	31.0	23.8	3.88	(221)	(36.0)	(13.8)	(2.25)
Strawberry and other natural flavors, 6-oz. container	190	31.0	23.8	3.88	(221)	(36.0)	(13.8)	(2.25)
Colombo whole milk yogurt								
Plain, 8-oz. container	150	13.0	18.8	1.63	(164)	(14.2)	(10.2)	(0.89)
16-oz. (1-lb.) container	300	26.0	18.8	1.63	(164)	(14.2)	(10.2)	(0.89)
32-oz. (2-lb.) container	600	52.0	18.8	1.63	(164)	(14.2)	(10.2)	(0.89)
Banana-Strawberry, 8-oz. container	235	38.0	29.4	4.75	(273)	(44.2)	(17.1)	(2.76)
Black Cherry, 8-oz. container	230	34.0	28.8	4.25	(268)	(39.5)	(16.7)	(2.47)
Blueberry, 8-oz. container	250	38.0	31.3	4.75	(291)	(44.2)	(18.2)	(2.76)
Cherry Vanilla, 8-oz. container	250	40.0	31.3	5.00	(291)	(46.5)	(18.2)	(2.91)
Coffee, 8-oz. container	200	29.0	25.0	3.63	(233)	(33.8)	(14.5)	(2.11)
Honey Banana, 8-oz. container	220	30.4	27.5	3.80	(256)	(35.3)	(16.0)	(2.21)
Lemon, 8-oz. container	220	30.0	27.5	3.75	(256)	(34.9)	(16.0)	(2.18)
Piña Colada, 8-oz. container	240	40.0	30.0	5.00	(279)	(46.5)	(17.4)	(2.91)
Raspberry, 8-oz. container	250	39.0	31.3	4.88	(291)	(45.4)	(18.2)	(2.84)
Spiced Apple, 8-oz. container	240	39.0	30.0	4.88	(279)	(45.4)	(17.4)	(2.84)
Strawberry, 8-oz. container	230	36.0	28.8	4.50	(268)	(41.9)	(16.7)	(2.62)
Vanilla Honey, 8-oz. container	250	40.0	31.3	5.00	(291)	(46.5)	(18.2)	(2.91)
Colombo Sundae Style whole milk yogurt								
Banana, 5-oz. container	140	23.0	28.0	4.60	(260)	(42.8)	(16.3)	(2.67)
Blueberry, 5-oz. container	140	23.0	28.0	4.60	(260)	(42.8)	(16.3)	(2.67)
Honey Vanilla, 5-oz. container	138	19.0	27.6	3.80	(257)	(35.3)	(16.0)	(2.21)
Peach Melba, 5-oz. container	140	23.0	28.0	4.60	(260)	(42.8)	(16.3)	(2.67)
Red Raspberry, 5-oz. container	140	23.0	28.0	4.60	(260)	(42.8)	(16.3)	(2.67)
Strawberry, 5-oz. container	140	23.0	28.0	4.60	(260)	(42.8)	(16.3)	(2.67)
Colombo-Lite nonfat yogurt								
Banana-Strawberry, 8-oz. container	190	40.0	23.8	5.00	(221)	(46.5)	(13.8)	(2.91)
Blueberry, 8-oz. container	190	40.0	23.8	5.00	(221)	(46.5)	(13.8)	(2.91)
Cherry, 8-oz. container	180	36.0	22.5	4.50	(209)	(41.9)	(13.1)	(2.62)
Honey Vanilla, 8-oz. container	160	32.0	20.0	4.00	(186)	(37.2)	(11.6)	(2.33)
Peach, 8-oz. container	190	40.0	23.8	5.00	(221)	(46.5)	(13.8)	(2.91)
Pineapple, 8-oz. container	190	38.0	23.8	4.75	(221)	(44.2)	(13.8)	(2.76)
Raspberry, 8-oz. container	190	40.0	23.8	5.00	(221)	(46.5)	(13.8)	(2.91)
Strawberry, 8-oz. container	190	40.0	23.8	5.00	(221)	(46.5)	(13.8)	(2.91)
Continental low-fat yogurt								
Plain, 32-oz. (2-lb.) container	720	80.0	22.5	2.50	(198)	(22.0)	(12.4)	(1.38)
Continental whole milk yogurt								
Plain, 8-oz. container	240	17.0	30.0	2.13	(261)	(18.5)	(16.3)	(1.16)
Cherry, 8-oz. container	310	39.0	38.8	4.88	(361)	(45.4)	(22.6)	(2.84)
Dannon low-fat yogurt								
Plain, 8-oz. container	150	17.0	18.8	2.12	(165)	(18.7)	(10.3)	(1.17)
16-oz. (1-lb.) container	300	34.0	18.8	2.12	(165)	(18.7)	(10.3)	(1.17)
Apricot, 8-oz. container	260	49.0	32.5	6.13	(302)	(57.0)	(18.9)	(3.56)
Banana, 8-oz. container	260	49.0	32.5	6.13	(302)	(57.0)	(18.9)	(3.56)

	CONTAINER		1 OZ., BY WT.		1 CUP		1 TABLESPOON	
	Cal.	Carb.	Cal.	Carb.	Cal.	Carb.	Cal.	Carb.
Blueberry, 8-oz. container	260	49.0	32.5	6.13	(302)	(57.0)	(18.9)	(3.56)
Boysenberry, 8-oz. container	260	49.0	32.5	6.13	(302)	(57.0)	(18.9)	(3.56)
Cherry, 8-oz. container	260	49.0	32.5	6.13	(302)	(57.0)	(18.9)	(3.56)
Coffee, 8-oz. container	200	32.0	25.0	4.00	(233)	(37.2)	(14.5)	(2.33)
Dutch Apple, 8-oz. container	260	49.0	32.5	6.13	(302)	(57.0)	(18.9)	(3.56)
Guava, 8-oz. container	260	49.0	32.5	6.13	(302)	(57.0)	(18.9)	(3.56)
Honey, 8-oz. container	260	49.0	32.5	6.13	(302)	(57.0)	(18.9)	(3.56)
Honey 'n Pear, 8-oz. container	260	49.0	32.5	6.13	(302)	(57.0)	(18.9)	(3.56)
Lemon, 8-oz. container	200	32.0	25.0	4.00	(233)	(37.2)	(14.5)	(2.33)
Mixed Berries, 8-oz. container	260	49.0	32.5	6.13	(302)	(57.0)	(18.9)	(3.56)
Peach, 8-oz. container	260	49.0	32.5	6.13	(302)	(57.0)	(18.9)	(3.56)
Piña Colada, 8-oz. container	260	49.0	32.5	6.13	(302)	(57.0)	(18.9)	(3.56)
Pineapple-Orange, 8-oz. container	260	49.0	32.5	6.13	(302)	(57.0)	(18.9)	(3.56)
Raspberry, 8-oz. container	260	49.0	32.5	6.13	(302)	(57.0)	(18.9)	(3.56)
Strawberry, 8-oz. container	260	49.0	32.5	6.13	(302)	(57.0)	(18.9)	(3.56)
Vanilla, 8-oz. container	200	32.0	25.0	4.00	(233)	(37.2)	(14.5)	(2.33)
16-oz. (1-lb.) container	400	64.0	25.0	4.00	(233)	(37.2)	(14.5)	(2.33)
Dannon Mélangé blended low-fat yogurt								
Apple, 6-oz. container	180	31.0	30.0	5.17	(279)	(48.1)	(17.4)	(3.01)
Blueberry, 6-oz. container	180	31.0	30.0	5.17	(279)	(48.1)	(17.4)	(3.01)
Cherry, 6-oz. container	180	31.0	30.0	5.17	(279)	(48.1)	(17.4)	(3.01)
Pineapple, 6-oz. container	180	31.0	30.0	5.17	(279)	(48.1)	(17.4)	(3.01)
Raspberry, 6-oz. container	180	31.0	30.0	5.17	(279)	(48.1)	(17.4)	(3.01)
Strawberry, 6-oz. container	180	31.0	30.0	5.17	(279)	(48.1)	(17.4)	(3.01)
Erewhon whole milk yogurt								
Plain, 8-oz. container	159	11.8	19.9	1.48	(173)	(12.9)	(10.8)	(0.80)
32-oz. (2-lb.) container	636	47.2	19.9	1.48	(173)	(12.9)	(10.8)	(0.80)
Europa whole milk yogurt								
Plain, 6-oz. container	130	11.0	21.7	1.83	(189)	(15.9)	(11.8)	(1.00)
Blueberry, 6-oz. container	210	37.0	35.0	6.17	(326)	(57.4)	(20.3)	(3.59)
Cherry, 6-oz. container	210	37.0	35.0	6.17	(326)	(57.4)	(20.3)	(3.59)
Peach, 6-oz. container	210	37.0	35.0	6.17	(326)	(57.4)	(20.3)	(3.59)
Raspberry, 6-oz. container	210	37.0	35.0	6.17	(326)	(57.4)	(20.3)	(3.59)
Strawberry, 6-oz. container	210	37.0	35.0	6.17	(326)	(57.4)	(20.3)	(3.59)
Fresh 'N Fruity Original Style low-fat yogurt								
Boysenberry, 6-oz. container	190	30.0	31.7	5.00	(295)	(46.5)	(18.4)	(2.91)
Raspberry, 6-oz. container	190	30.0	31.7	5.00	(295)	(46.5)	(18.4)	(2.91)
Strawberry, 6-oz. container	190	30.0	31.7	5.00	(295)	(46.5)	(18.4)	(2.91)
Friendship low-fat yogurt								
Peach, 8-oz. container	230	57.0	28.8	7.13	(268)	(66.3)	(16.7)	(4.14)
Piña Colada, 8-oz. container	240	59.0	30.0	7.38	(279)	(68.6)	(17.4)	(4.29)
Strawberry, 8-oz. container	230	57.0	28.8	7.13	(268)	(66.3)	(16.7)	(4.14)
Johnston's low-fat yogurt								
Plain, 8-oz. container	140	15.0	17.5	1.88	(154)	(16.5)	(9.6)	(1.03)
Blueberry, 8-oz. container	250	50.0	31.3	6.25	(291)	(58.1)	(18.2)	(3.63)
Boysenberry, 8-oz. container	250	49.0	30.3	6.13	(282)	(57.0)	(17.6)	(3.56)
Caramel Pecan, 8-oz. container	290	60.0	36.6	7.50	(340)	(69.8)	(21.3)	(4.36)
Cherries Jubilee, 8-oz. container	260	54.0	32.5	6.75	(302)	(62.8)	(18.9)	(3.92)
Cherry, 8-oz. container	250	49.0	31.3	6.13	(291)	(57.0)	(18.2)	(3.56)
French Apple, 8-oz. container	260	53.0	32.5	6.63	(302)	(61.6)	(18.9)	(3.85)
Orange-Pineapple, 8-oz. container	270	55.0	33.8	6.88	(314)	(64.0)	(19.6)	(4.00)
Peach, 8-oz. container	260	53.0	32.5	6.63	(302)	(61.6)	(18.9)	(3.85)
Piña Colada, 8-oz. container	270	53.0	33.8	6.63	(314)	(61.6)	(19.6)	(3.85)
Strawberry, 8-oz. container	250	51.0	31.3	6.38	(291)	(59.3)	(18.2)	(3.71)
Knudsen low-fat yogurt								
Plain, 8-oz. container	150	16.0	18.8	2.00	166	17.7	10.3	1.10
Knudsen Fruit-On-The-Bottom low-fat yogurt								
Banana, 8-oz. container	270	49.0	33.8	6.13	314	56.9	19.7	3.56
Blackberry, 8-oz. container	270	49.0	33.8	6.13	314	56.9	19.7	3.56
Blueberry, 8-oz. container	270	49.0	33.8	6.13	314	56.9	19.7	3.56
Boysenberry, 8-oz. container	260	47.0	32.5	5.88	302	54.6	18.9	3.41
Cherry, 8-oz. container	260	47.0	32.5	5.88	302	54.6	18.9	3.41
Lemon Chiffon, 8-oz. container	260	47.0	32.5	5.88	302	54.6	18.9	3.41
Peach, 8-oz. container	260	48.0	32.5	6.00	302	55.8	18.9	3.49
Piña Colada, 8-oz. container	260	48.0	32.5	6.00	302	55.8	18.9	3.49
Red Raspberry, 8-oz. container	270	49.0	33.8	6.13	314	56.9	19.7	3.56
Spiced Apple, 8-oz. container	250	45.0	31.3	5.63	291	52.3	18.2	3.27
Strawberry, 8-oz. container	260	47.0	32.5	5.88	302	54.6	18.9	3.41

	CONTAINER		1 OZ., BY WT.		1 CUP		1 TABLESPOON	
	Cal.	Carb.	Cal.	Carb.	Cal.	Carb.	Cal.	Carb.
Knudsen Pre-stirred low-fat yogurt								
Apricot Pineapple, 8-oz. container	260	48.0	32.5	6.00	302	55.8	18.9	3.49
32-oz. (2-lb.) container	1040	192.0	32.5	6.00	302	55.8	18.9	3.49
Banana Colada, 8-oz. container	260	48.0	32.5	6.00	302	55.8	18.9	3.49
Blackberry, 8-oz. container	260	48.0	32.5	6.00	302	55.8	18.9	3.49
Blueberry, 8-oz. container	260	49.0	32.5	6.13	302	56.9	18.9	3.56
Boysenberry, 8-oz. container	270	50.0	33.8	6.25	314	58.1	19.6	3.63
32-oz. (2-lb.) container	1088	200.0	33.8	6.25	314	58.1	19.6	3.63
Cherry, 8-oz. container	260	45.0	32.5	5.63	302	52.3	18.9	3.63
Coffee, 8-oz. container	240	40.0	30.0	5.00	299	46.5	17.4	2.90
Cranberry-Apple, 8-oz. container	260	50.0	32.5	6.25	302	58.1	18.9	3.63
Lemon, 8-oz. container	250	46.0	31.3	5.75	290	53.4	18.1	3.34
32-oz. (2-lb.) container	1000	184.0	31.3	5.75	290	53.4	18.1	3.34
Lime, 8-oz. container	260	47.0	32.5	5.88	302	54.6	18.9	3.41
Lime Margarita, 8-oz. container	270	49.0	33.8	6.13	314	56.9	19.6	3.56
Peach, 8-oz. container	260	50.0	32.5	6.25	302	58.1	18.9	3.63
32-oz. (2-lb.) container	1040	200.0	32.5	6.25	302	58.1	18.9	3.63
Piña Colada, 8-oz. container	260	48.0	32.5	6.00	302	55.8	18.9	3.49
Pineapple, 8-oz. container	270	50.0	33.8	6.25	314	58.1	19.6	3.63
Red Raspberry, 8-oz. container	250	46.0	31.3	5.75	290	53.4	18.1	3.34
Spiced Apple, 8-oz. container	260	45.0	32.5	5.63	302	52.3	18.9	3.27
Strawberry, 8-oz. container	250	46.0	31.3	5.75	290	53.4	18.1	3.34
32-oz. (2-lb.) container	1000	184.0	31.3	5.75	290	53.4	18.1	3.34
Strawberry Daiquiri, 8-oz. container	270	49.0	33.8	6.13	314	56.9	19.6	3.56
Vanilla, 8-oz. container	240	44.0	30.0	5.50	27	51.1	17.4	3.19
32-oz. (2-lb.) container	960	176.0	30.0	5.50	27	51.1	17.4	3.19
Knudsen "Yogurt Plus" low-fat yogurt								
Apple with Granola, 8-oz. container	260	52.0	32.5	6.50	302	60.5	18.9	3.78
Blueberry with Granola, 8-oz. container	260	52.0	32.5	6.50	302	60.5	18.9	3.78
Peach with Granola, 8-oz. container	260	52.0	32.5	6.50	302	60.5	18.9	3.78
Red Raspberry with Granola, 8-oz. container	260	52.0	32.5	6.50	302	60.5	18.9	3.78
Strawberry with Granola, 8-oz. container	260	52.0	32.5	6.50	302	60.5	18.9	3.78
Knudsen whole milk yogurt								
Plain, 8-oz. container	180	15.0	22.5	1.88	195	16.3	12.2	1.02
16-oz. (1-lb.) container	360	30.0	22.5	1.88	195	16.3	12.2	1.02
32-oz. (2-lb.) container	720	60.0	22.5	1.88	195	16.3	12.2	1.02
Lacto low-fat yogurt								
Plain, 32-oz. (2-lb.) container	600	56.0	18.8	1.75	(165)	(16.3)	(10.3)	(1.02)
La Yogurt whole milk yogurt								
Plain, 6-oz. container	130	12.0	21.7	2.00	(189)	(16.4)	(11.8)	(1.02)
Blueberry, 6-oz. container	200	32.0	33.3	5.33	(310)	(49.6)	(19.4)	(3.10)
Cherry, 6-oz. container	190	29.0	31.7	4.83	(295)	(44.9)	(18.4)	(2.81)
Raspberry, 6-oz. container	210	34.0	35.0	5.67	(326)	(52.7)	(20.3)	(3.30)
Le Shake low-fat yogurt								
Banana, 8-oz. container	200	35.0	25.0	4.38	(233)	(40.7)	(14.5)	(2.55)
Blueberry, 8-oz. container	180	31.0	22.5	3.88	(209)	(36.1)	(13.1)	(2.26)
Cherry, 8-oz. container	180	31.0	22.5	3.88	(209)	(36.1)	(13.1)	(2.26)
Lemon, 8-oz. container	200	35.0	25.0	4.38	(233)	(40.7)	(14.5)	(2.55)
Orange, 8-oz. container	200	35.0	25.0	4.38	(233)	(40.7)	(14.5)	(2.55)
Raspberry, 8-oz. container	190	32.0	23.8	4.00	(221)	(37.2)	(13.8)	(2.33)
Strawberry, 8-oz. container	180	30.0	22.5	3.75	(209)	(34.8)	(13.1)	(2.20)
Vanilla, 8-oz. container	190	33.0	23.8	4.13	(221)	(38.4)	(13.8)	(2.40)
Light n' Lively (Sealtest), low-fat yogurt								
Plain, 8-oz. container	134	16.8	16.8	2.10	(148)	(19.5)	(9.2)	(1.22)
Apricot, 8-oz. container	240	46.0	30.0	5.75	(279)	(53.5)	(17.4)	(3.34)
Black Cherry, 8-oz. container	240	44.0	30.0	5.50	(279)	(51.2)	(17.4)	(3.20)
Blueberry, 8-oz. container	240	46.0	30.0	5.75	(279)	(53.5)	(17.4)	(3.34)
French Apple, 8-oz. container	245	47.2	30.6	5.90	(285)	(54.9)	(17.8)	(3.43)
Grape, 8-oz. container	245	42.4	30.6	5.30	(285)	(49.3)	(17.8)	(3.08)
Lemon, 8-oz. container	240	46.0	30.0	5.75	(279)	(53.5)	(17.4)	(3.34)
Mandarin Orange, 8-oz. container	234	44.9	29.3	5.61	(272)	(52.2)	(17.0)	(3.26)
Peach, 8-oz. container	240	46.0	30.0	5.75	(279)	(53.3)	(17.4)	(3.33)
Peach Melba, 8-oz. container	250	47.0	31.3	5.89	(291)	(54.6)	(18.2)	(3.41)
Pineapple, 8-oz. container	240	47.0	30.0	5.88	(279)	(54.7)	(17.4)	(3.42)

	CONTAINER		1 OZ., BY WT.		1 CUP		1 TABLESPOON	
	Cal.	Carb.	Cal.	Carb.	Cal.	Carb.	Cal.	Carb.
Red Raspberry, 8-oz. container	230	43.0	28.8	5.38	(268)	(50.0)	(16.7)	(3.12)
Strawberry, 8-oz. container	240	46.0	30.0	5.75	(279)	(53.5)	(17.4)	(3.34)
Strawberry Banana, 8-oz. container	260	52.0	32.5	6.50	(302)	(60.5)	(18.9)	(3.78)
Strawberry Fruit Cup, 8-oz. container	250	47.0	31.3	5.89	(291)	(54.6)	(18.2)	(3.41)
Vanilla, 8-oz. container	195	32.7	24.4	4.09	(277)	(38.0)	(14.2)	(2.38)
Look-Fit (A&P) low-fat yogurt								
Plain, 8-oz. container	140	19.0	17.5	2.38	(154)	(20.9)	(9.6)	(1.31)
Look-Fit (A&P) Swiss Style low-fat yogurt								
Apricot, 8-oz. container	220	42.0	27.5	5.25	(256)	(48.8)	(16.0)	(3.05)
Blueberry, 8-oz. container	240	47.0	30.0	5.88	(279)	(54.7)	(17.4)	(3.41)
Peach, 8-oz. container	240	47.0	30.0	5.88	(279)	(54.7)	(17.4)	(3.41)
Red Cherry, 8-oz. container	220	42.0	27.5	5.25	(256)	(48.8)	(16.0)	(3.05)
Red Raspberry, 8-oz. container	210	42.0	26.3	5.25	(245)	(48.8)	(15.3)	(3.05)
Strawberry, 8-oz. container	220	42.0	27.5	5.25	(256)	(48.8)	(16.0)	(3.05)
Lucerne (Safeway) low-fat yogurt								
Plain, 8-oz. container	160	17.0	20.0	2.13	(176)	(18.7)	(11.0)	(1.17)
32-oz. (2-lb.) container	640	68.0	20.0	2.13	(176)	(18.7)	(11.0)	(1.17)
Apricot-Pineapple, 8-oz. container	260	46.0	32.5	5.75	(302)	(53.5)	(18.9)	(3.34)
Banana, 8-oz. container	260	46.0	32.5	5.75	(302)	(53.5)	(18.9)	(3.34)
Blackberry, 8-oz. container	260	46.0	32.5	5.75	(302)	(53.5)	(18.9)	(3.34)
Blueberry, 8-oz. container	260	46.0	32.5	5.75	(302)	(53.5)	(18.9)	(3.34)
Boysenberry, 8-oz. container	260	46.0	32.5	5.75	(302)	(53.5)	(18.9)	(3.34)
Cherry, 8-oz. container	260	46.0	32.5	5.75	(302)	(53.5)	(18.9)	(3.34)
Cherry-Coconut, 8-oz. container	260	46.0	32.5	5.75	(302)	(53.5)	(18.9)	(3.34)
French Apple, 8-oz. container	250	46.0	31.3	5.75	(291)	(53.5)	(18.2)	(3.34)
Lime, 8-oz. container	260	46.0	32.5	5.75	(302)	(53.5)	(18.9)	(3.34)
Orange, 8-oz. container	260	46.0	32.5	5.75	(302)	(53.5)	(18.9)	(3.34)
Pineapple, 8-oz. container	260	46.0	32.5	5.75	(302)	(53.5)	(18.9)	(3.34)
Prune, 8-oz. container	260	46.0	32.5	5.75	(302)	(53.5)	(18.9)	(3.34)
Red Raspberry, 8-oz. container	260	46.0	32.5	5.75	(302)	(53.5)	(18.9)	(3.34)
16-oz (1-lb.) container	520	92.0	32.5	5.75	(302)	(53.5)	(18.9)	(3.34)
32-oz. (2-lb.) container	1040	184.0	32.5	5.75	(302)	(53.5)	(18.9)	(3.34)
Strawberry, 8-oz. container	260	46.0	32.5	5.75	(302)	(53.5)	(18.9)	(3.34)
Maya whole milk yogurt								
Plain, 8-oz. container	210	18.0	26.3	2.25	(228)	(19.5)	(14.2)	(1.22)
Blueberry, 8-oz. container	280	39.0	35.0	4.88	(326)	(45.4)	(20.3)	(2.84)
Peach, 8-oz. container	280	39.0	35.0	4.88	(326)	(45.4)	(20.3)	(2.84)
Strawberry, 8-oz. container	280	39.0	35.0	4.88	(326)	(45.4)	(20.3)	(2.84)
Meadow Gold Western Sundae Style skim milk yogurt								
Blueberry, 8-oz. container	270	49.0	33.8	6.13	(314)	(57.0)	(19.6)	(3.56)
Boysenberry, 8-oz. container	270	49.0	33.8	6.13	(314)	(57.0)	(19.6)	(3.56)
Mandarin Orange, 8-oz. container	260	47.0	32.5	5.88	(302)	(54.6)	(18.9)	(3.41)
Peach, 8-oz. container	260	47.0	32.5	5.88	(302)	(54.6)	(18.9)	(3.41)
Pineapple, 8-oz. container	270	49.0	33.8	6.13	(314)	(57.0)	(19.6)	(3.56)
Red Raspberry, 8-oz. container	270	49.0	33.8	6.13	(314)	(57.0)	(19.6)	(3.56)
Strawberry, 8-oz. container	270	49.0	33.8	6.13	(314)	(57.0)	(19.6)	(3.56)
Natural & Kosher whole milk yogurt								
Plain, 8-oz. container	200	16.0	25.0	2.00	(218)	(17.4)	(13.6)	(1.09)
16-oz. (1-lb.) container	400	32.0	25.0	2.00	(218)	(17.4)	(13.6)	(1.09)
Peach-Pineapple, 8-oz. container	240	35.0	30.0	4.38	(279)	(40.7)	(17.4)	(2.55)
New Country low-fat yogurt								
Apple Crisp, 8-oz. container	240	42.0	30.0	5.25	(279)	(48.8)	(17.4)	(3.05)
Blueberry Ripple, 8-oz. container	240	43.0	30.0	5.38	(279)	(50.0)	(17.4)	(3.13)
Cherry Supreme, 8-oz. container	240	44.0	30.0	5.50	(279)	(51.2)	(17.4)	(3.20)
French Vanilla, 8-oz. container	210	40.0	26.3	5.00	(245)	(46.5)	(15.3)	(2.91)
French Vanilla Ripple, 8-oz. container	240	42.0	30.0	5.25	(279)	(48.8)	(17.4)	(3.05)
Fruit Crunch, 8-oz. container	240	42.0	30.0	5.25	(279)	(48.8)	(17.4)	(3.05)
Hawaiian Salad, 8-oz. container	250	42.0	31.3	5.25	(291)	(48.8)	(18.2)	(3.05)
Lemon Ripple, 8-oz. container	240	43.0	30.0	5.38	(279)	(50.0)	(17.4)	(3.13)
Orange Supreme, 8-oz. container	240	43.0	30.0	5.38	(279)	(50.0)	(17.4)	(3.13)

	CONTAINER		1 OZ., BY WT.		1 CUP		1 TABLESPOON	
	Cal.	Carb.	Cal.	Carb.	Cal.	Carb.	Cal.	Carb.
Peaches 'n Cream, 8-oz. container	240	43.0	30.0	5.38	(279)	(50.0)	(17.4)	(3.13)
Raspberry Ripple, 8-oz. container	240	43.0	30.0	5.38	(279)	(50.0)	(17.4)	(3.13)
Strawberry Supreme, 8-oz. container	240	43.0	30.0	5.38	(279)	(30.0)	(17.4)	(3.13)
Ralph's low-fat yogurt								
Plain, 8-oz. container	160	28.3	20.0	3.54	(176)	(31.2)	(11.0)	(1.95)
16-oz. (1-lb.) container	320	56.6	20.0	3.54	(176)	(31.2)	(11.0)	(1.95)
32-oz. (2-lb.) container	640	113.2	20.0	3.54	(176)	(31.2)	(11.0)	(1.95)
Apricot-Pineapple, 8-oz. container	180	29.0	22.5	3.63	(209)	(33.7)	(13.1)	(2.11)
Blueberry, 8-oz. container	190	31.0	23.8	3.88	(221)	(36.1)	(13.8)	(2.26)
Caramel Nut, 8-oz. container	220	38.0	27.5	4.75	(256)	(44.2)	(16.0)	(2.76)
Lemon, 8-oz. container	230	40.0	28.8	5.00	(268)	(46.5)	(16.7)	(2.91)
Lemon-Coconut, 8-oz. container	210	36.0	26.3	4.50	(255)	(41.9)	(15.3)	(2.62)
Lime, 8-oz. container	220	38.0	27.5	4.75	(256)	(44.2)	(16.0)	(2.76)
Loganberry, 8-oz. container	220	38.0	27.5	4.75	(256)	(44.2)	(16.0)	(2.76)
Peach, 8-oz. container	210	36.0	26.3	4.50	(255)	(41.9)	(15.3)	(2.62)
Pineapple, 8-oz. container	230	41.0	28.8	5.13	(268)	(47.7)	(16.7)	(2.98)
Spiced Apple, 8-oz. container	200	34.0	25.0	4.25	(233)	(39.5)	(14.5)	(2.47)
Strawberry, 8-oz. container	190	31.0	23.8	3.88	(221)	(36.1)	(13.8)	(2.26)
Sippity nonfat yogurt								
Blueberry, 8-oz. container	150	29.0	18.8	3.60	(175)	(33.5)	(10.9)	(2.09)
Strawberry, 8-oz. container	150	29.0	18.8	3.60	(175)	(33.5)	(10.9)	(2.09)
Sugar Lo nonfat yogurt								
Dark Cherry, 8-oz. container	130	26.0	16.3	3.25	(152)	(30.2)	(9.5)	(1.89)
Peach with Peaches and Nectarines, 8-oz. container	130	26.0	16.3	3.25	(152)	(30.2)	(9.5)	(1.89)
Pineapple, 8-oz. container	130	26.0	16.3	3.25	(152)	(30.2)	(9.5)	(1.89)
Raspberry, 8-oz. container	130	26.0	16.3	3.25	(152)	(30.2)	(9.5)	(1.89)
Strawberry, 8-oz. container	130	26.0	16.3	3.25	(152)	(30.2)	(9.5)	(1.89)
Sweet 'n Low nonfat yogurt								
Blueberry, 8-oz. container	150	33.0	18.8	4.13	(174)	(38.3)	(10.9)	(2.39)
Cherry, 8-oz. container	150	33.0	18.8	4.13	(174)	(38.3)	(10.9)	(2.39)
Raspberry, 8-oz. container	150	33.0	18.8	4.13	(174)	(38.3)	(10.9)	(2.39)
Strawberry, 8-oz. container	150	33.0	18.8	4.13	(174)	(38.3)	(10.9)	(2.39)
Strawberry-Banana, 8-oz. container	150	33.0	18.8	4.13	(174)	(38.3)	(10.9)	(2.39)
Vermont whole milk yogurt								
Plain, 8-oz. container	190	16.0	23.8	2.00	(207)	(17.4)	(12.9)	(1.09)
Viva Swiss Style skim milk yogurt								
Apricot, 8-oz. container	250	47.0	31.3	5.88	(291)	(54.6)	(18.2)	(3.41)
Blackberry, 8-oz. container	250	47.0	31.3	5.88	(291)	(54.6)	(18.2)	(3.41)
Black Cherry, 8-oz. container	250	47.0	31.3	5.88	(291)	(54.6)	(18.2)	(3.41)
Blueberry, 8-oz. container	250	47.0	31.3	5.88	(291)	(54.6)	(18.2)	(3.41)
Boysenberry, 8-oz. container	250	47.0	31.3	5.88	(291)	(54.6)	(18.2)	(3.41)
Fruit Salad, 8-oz. container	250	47.0	31.3	5.88	(291)	(54.6)	(18.2)	(3.41)
Lemon, 8-oz. container	250	49.0	31.3	6.13	(291)	(57.0)	(18.2)	(3.56)
Lemon-Lime, 8-oz. container	250	49.0	31.3	6.13	(291)	(57.0)	(18.2)	(3.56)
Mandarin Orange, 8-oz. container	240	44.0	30.0	5.50	(279)	(51.2)	(17.4)	(3.20)
Peach, 8-oz. container	240	44.0	30.0	5.50	(279)	(51.2)	(17.4)	(3.20)
Pineapple Coconut, 8-oz. container	250	47.0	31.3	5.88	(291)	(54.6)	(18.2)	(3.41)
Pineapple-Orange, 8-oz. container	250	47.0	31.3	5.88	(291)	(54.6)	(18.2)	(3.41)
Raspberry, 8-oz. container	250	47.0	31.3	5.88	(291)	(54.6)	(18.2)	(3.41)
Red Cherry, 8-oz. container	250	47.0	31.3	5.88	(291)	(54.6)	(18.2)	(3.41)
Strawberry, 8-oz. container	250	47.0	31.3	5.88	(291)	(54.6)	(18.2)	(3.41)
White Rose low-fat yogurt								
Plain, 32-oz. (2-lb.) container	440	68.0	13.8	2.13	(121)	(18.7)	(7.6)	(1.17)
Blueberry, 8-oz. container	250	48.0	31.3	6.00	(291)	(55.8)	(18.2)	(3.49)
Peach, 8-oz. container	250	48.0	31.3	6.00	(291)	(55.8)	(18.2)	(3.49)
Raspberry, 8-oz. container	250	48.0	31.3	6.00	(291)	(55.8)	(18.2)	(3.49)
Strawberry, 8-oz. container	250	48.0	31.3	6.00	(291)	(55.8)	(18.2)	(3.49)
Yoplait "Original" whole milk yogurt								
Plain, 6-oz. container	130	14.0	20.1	2.16	(175)	(19.0)	(10.9)	(1.19)
Apple, 6-oz. container	190	32.0	29.3	4.94	(272)	(45.9)	(17.0)	(2.87)
Blueberry, 6-oz. container	190	32.0	29.3	4.94	(272)	(45.9)	(17.0)	(2.87)
Boysenberry, 6-oz. container	190	32.0	29.3	4.94	(272)	(45.9)	(17.0)	(2.87)
Cherry, 6-oz. container	190	32.0	29.3	4.94	(272)	(45.9)	(17.0)	(2.87)
Lemon, 6-oz. container	190	32.0	29.3	4.94	(272)	(45.9)	(17.0)	(2.87)

	CONTAINER		1 OZ., BY WT.		1 CUP		1 TABLE-SPOON	
	Cal.	Carb.	Cal.	Carb.	Cal.	Carb.	Cal.	Carb.
Mixed Berries, 6-oz. container	190	32.0	29.3	4.94	(272)	(45.9)	(17.0)	(2.87)
Orange, 6-oz. container	190	32.0	29.3	4.94	(272)	(45.9)	(17.0)	(2.87)
Peach, 6-oz. container	190	32.0	29.3	4.94	(272)	(45.9)	(17.0)	(2.87)
Piña Colada	190	32.0	29.3	4.94	(272)	(45.9)	(17.0)	(2.87)
Pineapple, 6-oz. container	190	32.0	29.3	4.94	(272)	(45.9)	(17.0)	(2.87)
Raspberry, 6-oz. container	190	32.0	29.3	4.94	(272)	(45.9)	(17.0)	(2.87)
Strawberry, 6-oz. container	190	32.0	29.3	4.94	(272)	(45.9)	(17.0)	(2.87)
Strawberry-Banana, 6-oz. container	190	32.0	29.3	4.94	(272)	(45.9)	(17.0)	(2.87)
Yoplait custard style whole milk yogurt								
Plain with Honey, 6-oz. container	160	23.0	26.7	3.83	(232)	(33.3)	(14.5)	(2.08)
Plain with Lemon Purée and other natural flavors, 6-oz. container	180	30.0	30.0	5.00	(279)	(46.5)	(17.4)	(2.91)
Coffee, 6-oz. container	180	30.0	30.0	5.00	(279)	(46.5)	(17.4)	(2.91)
Zausner low-fat yogurt with Cottage Cheese								
Plain, 12-oz. container	249	9.0	20.8	0.75	(184)	(7.0)	(11.5)	(0.44)
Blueberry, 12-oz. container	276	21.0	23.0	1.75	(214)	(16.3)	(13.8)	(1.02)
Pineapple, 12-oz. container	276	21.0	23.0	1.75	(214)	(16.3)	(13.4)	(1.02)
Raspberry, 12-oz. container	276	21.0	23.0	1.75	(214)	(16.3)	(13.4)	(1.02)
Strawberry, 12-oz. container	276	21.0	23.0	1.75	(214)	(16.3)	(13.4)	(1.02)

28 CONDIMENTS •

	UNIT		1 OZ., BY WT.		1 CUP		1 TABLE-SPOON	
	Cal.	Carb.	Cal.	Carb.	Cal.	Carb.	Cal.	Carb.
MARINATED VEGETABLES, PICKLED VEGETABLES, and VEGETABLE SALADS								
Artichoke Hearts								
Marinated in Oil, **Cara Mia,** 6-oz. jar	(174)	(6.6)	(29.0)	(1.10)				
Cole Slaw, based on generic data								
Prepared with homemade French dressing, based on USDA home recipe with ingredients as follows: 4 cups shredded cabbage, 4 Tbsp. oil, 1 Tbsp. vinegar, ½ tsp. sugar, and spices (yield: approx. 4 cups, approx. 17 oz.)	620	24.4	36.6	1.46	155	6.1	10	0.4
1 cup (approx. 4.2 oz.)	155	6.1	36.6	1.46	155	6.1	10	0.4
1 pound (approx. 3.8 cups) (tr/1g/3g/81%/37mg)	586	23.4	36.6	1.46	155	6.1	10	0.4
Prepared with commercial French dressing:								
1 cup (approx. 4.2 oz.)	(114)	(9.1)	(26.9)	(2.15)	(114)	(9.1)	(7)	(0.6)
1 pound (approx. 3.8 cups) (tr/2g/2g/83%/76mg)	(430)	(34.4)	(26.9)	(2.15)	(114)	(9.1)	(7)	(0.6)
Prepared with mayonnaise:								
1 cup (approx. 4.2 oz.)	(173)	(5.8)	(42.1)	(1.37)	(173)	(5.8)	(11)	(0.4)
1 pound (approx. 3.8 cups) (tr/1g/4g/79%/56mg)	(674)	(21.9)	(42.1)	(1.37)	(173)	(5.8)	(11)	(0.4)
Prepared with mayonnaise-type salad dressing:								
1 cup (approx. 4.2 oz.)	(119)	(8.5)	(28.1)	(2.01)	(119)	(8.5)	(7)	(0.5)
1 pound (approx. 3.8 cups) (tr/2g/2g/83%/54mg)	(450)	(32.2)	(28.1)	(2.01)	(119)	(8.5)	(7)	(0.5)
Cucumber and Yogurt Salad (based on data from the Middle East)								
Prepared with 1 quart yogurt, 1¾ lb. sliced cucumber, garlic paste, and mint (yield: approx. 4 lbs., 64 oz.)	672	49.2	10.5	0.77				
1 pound	168	12.3	10.5	0.77				

	UNIT		1 OZ., BY WT.		1 CUP		1 TABLE-SPOON	
	Cal.	Carb.	Cal.	Carb.	Cal.	Carb.	Cal.	Carb.
Olives, pickled, canned or bottled, based on generic data								
GREEN OLIVES								
Whole [refuse: pits, approx. 16%]:								
Small, Select, or Standard (approx. 10/16" diam., 13/16" long, 135 per pound), 1 pound	446	5.4	27.6	0.31				
1 small, select, or standard olive (approx. 0.12 oz., 8.3 to the ounce)	3	trace	27.6	0.31				
Large (approx. 12/16" diam., 15/16" long, 98 per pound), 1 pound	441	4.9	27.6	0.31				
1 large olive (approx. 0.16 oz., 6 to the ounce)	5	0.1	27.6	0.31				
Giant (approx. 14/16" diam., 1 2/16" long, 53 to 64 per pound), 1 pound	445	5.3	27.6	0.31				
1 giant olive (approx. 0.27 oz., 3.7 to the ounce)	8	0.1	27.6	0.31				
Pitted:								
1 pound (approx. 161 small, select, or standard, 117 large, or 63 to 76 giant) (tr/tr/4g/78%/680mg)	526	5.9	32.9	0.37				
1 cup, sliced (approx. 4.7 oz.)	(154)	(1.7)	32.9	0.37	(154)	(1.7)	(10)	(0.1)
RIPE OLIVES								
ASCOLANO:								
Whole [refuse: pits, approx. 14%]:								
Extra Large (approx. ¾" diam., 1" long, 82 per pound), 1 pound	500	9.8	31.5	0.63				
1 extra large olive (approx. 0.20 oz., 5 to the ounce)	6	0.1	31.5	0.63				
Mammoth (approx. 13/16" diameter, 1 1/16" long, 70 per pound, 1 pound	504	10.5	31.5	0.63				
1 mammoth olive (approx. 0.23 oz., 4.3 to the ounce)	7	0.2	31.5	0.63				
Giant (approx. 13/16" diam., 1 2/16" long, 53 to 60 per pound), 1 pound	504	10.2	31.5	0.63				
1 giant olive (approx. 0.28 oz., 3.6 to the ounce)	9	0.2	31.5	0.63				

	UNIT		1 OZ., BY WT.		1 CUP		1 TABLESPOON	
	Cal.	Carb.	Cal.	Carb.	Cal.	Carb.	Cal.	Carb.
Jumbo (approx. 15/16″ diameter, 1 3/16″ long, 46 to 50 per pound), 1 pound	504	10.1	31.5	0.63				
1 jumbo olive (approx. 0.33 oz., 3.0 to the ounce)	11	0.2	31.5	0.63				
Pitted:								
1 pound (approx. 95 extra large, 81 mammoth, 62 to 70 giant, 53 to 58 jumbo (tr/1g/4g/80%/231mg)	585	11.8	36.6	0.73				
1 cup, sliced, (approx. 4.8 oz.)	174	3.5	36.6	0.73	174	3.5	11	0.2
MANZANILLO:								
Whole [refuse: pits, approx. 14%]:								
Small (approx. 10/16″ diameter, 13/16″ long, 135 per pound), 1 pound	500	10.2	31.5	0.63				
1 small olive (approx. 0.12 oz., 8.3 to the ounce)	4	0.1	31.5	0.63				
Medium (approx. 11/16″ diameter, 14/16″ long, 113 per pound), 1 pound	500	10.2	31.5	0.63				
1 medium olive (approx. 0.14 oz., 7.1 to the ounce)	4	0.1	31.5	0.63				
Large (approx. 12/16″ diameter, 15/16″ long, 98 per pound), 1 pound	500	10.2	31.5	0.63				
1 large olive (approx. 0.16 oz., 6 to the ounce)	5	0.1	31.5	0.63				
Extra Large (approx. 12/16″ diameter, 1″ long; 82 per pound), 1 pound	500	10.2	31.5	0.63				
1 extra large olive (approx. 0.20 oz., 5 to the ounce)	6	0.1	31.5	0.63				
Pitted:								
1 pound (approx. 157 small, 131 medium, 114 large, or 95 extra large) (tr/1g/4g/80%/231mg)	585	11.8	36.6	0.74				
1 cup, sliced (approx. 4.8 oz.)	174	3.5	36.6	0.74	174	3.5	11	0.2
MISSION:								
Whole [refuse: pits, approx. 14%]:								
Small (approx. 10/16″ diameter, 13/16″ long; 135 per pound), 1 pound	712	12.4	44.5	0.78				
1 small olive (approx. 0.12 oz., 8.3 to the ounce)	5	0.1	44.5	0.78				
Medium (approx. 11/16″ diameter, 14/16″ long; 113 per pound), 1 pound	712	12.4	44.5	0.78				
1 medium olive (approx. 0.14 oz., 7.1 to the ounce)	6	0.1	44.5	0.78				
Large (approx. 12/16″ diameter, 15/16″ long; 98 per pound), 1 pound	712	12.4	44.5	0.78				
1 large olive (approx. 0.16 oz., 6.3 to the ounce)	7	0.1	44.5	0.78				
Extra large (approx. 12/16″ diameter, 15/16″ long; 82 per pound), 1 pound	712	12.4	44.5	0.78				
1 extra large olive (approx. 0.20 oz., 5 to the ounce)	9	0.2	44.5	0.78				
Pitted:								
1 pound (approx. 157 small, 131 medium, 114 large, or 95 extra large) (tr/1g/6g/73%/213mg)	835	14.5	52.2	0.91				
1 cup, sliced (approx. 4.8 oz.)	(251)	(4.4)	52.2	0.91				
SEVILLANO:								
Whole [refuse: pits, approx. 14%]:								
Giant (approx. 13/16″ diameter, 1 2/16″ long; 53 to 60 per pound), 1 pound	355	10.2	22.2	0.64				
1 giant olive (approx. 0.28 oz., 3.6 to the ounce)	6	0.2						
Jumbo (approx. 15/16″ diameter, 1 3/16″ long; 46 to 50 per pound), 1 pound	355	10.2	22.2	0.64				
1 jumbo olive (approx. 0.33 oz., 3 to the ounce)	8	0.2						
Colossal (approx. 1″ diameter, 1 4/16″ long; 36 to 40 per pound), 1 pound	355	10.2	22.2	0.64				
1 colossal olive (approx. 0.42 oz., 2.4 to the ounce)	10	0.3						

	UNIT		1 OZ., BY WT.		1 CUP		1 TABLESPOON	
	Cal.	Carb.	Cal.	Carb.	Cal.	Carb.	Cal.	Carb.
Supercolossal (approx. 1 1/16″ diameter, 1 6/16″ long; 32 per pound), 1 pound	355	10.2	22.2	0.64				
1 supercolossal olive (approx. 0.50 oz., 2 to the ounce)	11	0.3						
Pitted:								
1 pound (approx. 62 to 70 giant, 53 to 58 jumbo, 42 to 47 colossal or 37 supercolossal) (tr/1g/3g/84%/235mg)	422	12.2	26.4	0.76				
1 cup, sliced (approx. 4.8 oz.)	126	3.6	26.4	0.76	126	3.6	(8)	(0.1)
GREEK OLIVES, ripe, salt cured, oil coated								
Whole [refuse: pits, approx. 20%]:								
Medium (approx. 188 per pound), 1 pound	1226	31.6	76.6	1.98				
1 medium olive (approx. 0.09 oz., 11.7 to the ounce)	7	0.2	76.6	1.98				
Extra Large (approx. 137 per pound), 1 pound	1226	31.6	76.6	1.98				
1 extra large olive (approx. 0.17 oz., 5.9 to the ounce)	13	0.3	76.6	1.98				
Pitted:								
1 pound (approx. 235 medium, or 171 extra large) (1g/2g/10g/44%/932mg)	1533	39.5	95.8	2.47				
1 cup, sliced (approx. 4.8 oz.)	(460)	(11.9)	95.8	2.47	(460)	(11.9)	(29)	(0.8)

Olives, based on data from the Middle East

	UNIT		1 OZ., BY WT.		1 CUP		1 TABLESPOON	
	Cal.	Carb.	Cal.	Carb.	Cal.	Carb.	Cal.	Carb.
BLACK OLIVES								
1 pound	939	5.0	58.7	0.31				
GREEN OLIVES								
1 pound	653	12.7	40.8	0.79				

Olives, by brand

(The label weight for canned olives customarily does not include the weight of the packing liquid.)

	UNIT		1 OZ., BY WT.		1 CUP		1 TABLESPOON	
	Cal.	Carb.	Cal.	Carb.	Cal.	Carb.	Cal.	Carb.
GREEN OLIVES								
Lindsay California Green Ripe Olives, Whole, 6-oz. (drained weight) can	281	0.0	46.8	0.00				
9-oz. (drained weight) can	421	0.0	46.8	0.00				
Chopped, 4.25-oz. (drained weight) can	231	0.0	54.4	0.00				
Pitted, small, 6-oz. (drained weight) can (approx. 102 olives)	326	0.0	54.4	0.00				
1 small olive (approx. 0.06 oz.)	(3)	0.0	54.4	0.00				
Medium, 6-oz. (drained weight) can (approx. 84 olives)	326	0.0	54.4	0.00				
1 medium olive (approx. 0.07 oz.)	(4)	0.0	54.4	0.00				
Large, 6-oz. (drained weight) can (approx. 60 olives)	326	0.0	54.4	0.00				
1 large olive (approx. 0.10 oz.)	(6)	0.0	54.4	0.00				
Extra large, 5.7-oz. (drained weight) can (approx. 51 olives)	310	0.0	54.4	0.00				
1 extra large olive (approx. 0.11 oz.)	(6)	0.0	54.4	0.00				
Colossal, 5.6-oz. (drained weight) can (approx. 22 olives)	305	0.0	54.4	0.00				
1 colossal olive (approx. 0.25 oz.)	(14)	0.0	54.4	0.00				
Sliced, 2.25-oz. (drained weight) can	122	0.0	54.4	0.00				
RIPE OLIVES								
Lindsay California Ripe Olives, Whole, Small Size, 7.8-oz. (drained weight) can (approx. 109 olives)	365	0.0	46.8	0.00				
1 small olive (approx. 0.07 oz.)	(3)	0.0	46.8	0.00				

	UNIT Cal.	UNIT Carb.	1 OZ., BY WT. Cal.	1 OZ., BY WT. Carb.	1 CUP Cal.	1 CUP Carb.	1 TABLE-SPOON Cal.	1 TABLE-SPOON Carb.
Medium, 7.7-oz. (drained weight) can (approx. 92 olives)	360	0.0	46.8	0.00				
1 medium olive (approx. 0.09 oz.)	(4)	0.0	46.8	0.00				
Large, 7.4-oz. (drained weight) can (approx. 67 olives)	346	0.0	46.8	0.00				
1 large olive (approx. 0.12 oz.)	(6)	0.0	46.8	0.00				
Extra Large, 7.25-oz. (drained weight) can (approx. 58 olives)	339	0.0	46.8	0.00				
1 extra large olive (approx. 0.13 oz.)	(6)	0.0	46.8	0.00				
Colossal, 7.2-oz. (drained weight) can (approx. 25 olives)	337	0.0	46.8	0.00				
1 colossal olive (approx. 0.29 oz.)	(14)	0.0	46.8	0.00				

Pickled Beets

Additional listings for pickled beets can be found in the VEGETABLES chapter.

	UNIT Cal.	UNIT Carb.	1 OZ., BY WT. Cal.	1 OZ., BY WT. Carb.	1 CUP Cal.	1 CUP Carb.	1 TABLE-SPOON Cal.	1 TABLE-SPOON Carb.
Pickled Beets, **Blue Boy,** 16-oz. (1-lb.) jar	376	84.6	23.5	5.29	200	45.0	13	2.8
104-oz can	2444	550.2	23.5	5.29	200	45.0	13	2.8
Pickled Beets with Onions, **Blue Boy,** 16-oz. (1-lb.) jar	376	84.6	23.5	5.29	200	45.0	13	2.8
104-oz. can	2444	550.2	23.5	5.29	200	45.0	13	2.8

Pickled Onions

	UNIT Cal.	UNIT Carb.	1 OZ., BY WT. Cal.	1 OZ., BY WT. Carb.	1 CUP Cal.	1 CUP Carb.	1 TABLE-SPOON Cal.	1 TABLE-SPOON Carb.
Cocktail Onions, **Crosse & Blackwell,** 3-oz. jar	2	trace	0.6	trace				
8.5-oz. jar	5	trace	0.6	trace				
1 onion (approx. 0.1 oz.)	trace	trace	0.6	trace				

Pickled Red Cabbage

	UNIT Cal.	UNIT Carb.	1 OZ., BY WT. Cal.	1 OZ., BY WT. Carb.	1 CUP Cal.	1 CUP Carb.	1 TABLE-SPOON Cal.	1 TABLE-SPOON Carb.
Red Cabbage, Sweet-Sour, **Greenwood,** 8-oz. jar								
Drained (yield: approx. 5.9 oz.)	120	25.0	20.3	4.24	120	25.0	8	1.6
Red Cabbage, **Lohmanns,** 32-oz. (2-lb.) jar	450	90.0	14.1	2.80	113	23.0	7	1.4
Drained (yield: approx. 24 oz.)	(426)	(85.2)	(17.8)	(3.55)				

Pickles, based on generic data

	UNIT Cal.	UNIT Carb.	1 OZ., BY WT. Cal.	1 OZ., BY WT. Carb.	1 CUP Cal.	1 CUP Carb.	1 TABLE-SPOON Cal.	1 TABLE-SPOON Carb.
BREAD AND BUTTER or FRESH PICKLES (sugar added)								
Crosscut slices, each approx. 1½" diameter, ¼" thick:								
1 slice (approx. 0.3 oz.)	5	1.3	20.7	5.08	124	30.4		
1 cup (approx. 23 slices, 6 oz.)	124	30.4	20.7	5.08	124	30.4		
1 pound (approx. 2.7 cups) (tr/5g/tr/79%/192mg)	331	81.2	20.7	5.08	124	30.4		
CHOWCHOW or MUSTARD PICKLES (cucumber with added cauliflower, onion, and mustard)								
Sour chowchow or mustard pickles:								
1 cup (approx. 8.4 oz.)	70	9.8	8.3	1.16	70	9.8		
1 pound (approx. 1.9 cups) (tr/1g/tr/88%/382mg)	132	18.6	8.3	1.16	70	9.8		
Sweet chowchow or mustard pickles:								
1 cup (approx. 8.6 oz.)	284	66.2	32.9	7.66	284	66.2		
1 pound (approx. 1.9 cups) (tr/8g/tr/69%/151mg)	526	122.5	32.9	7.66	284	66.2		
DILL PICKLES								
Whole:								
1 medium dill pickle (approx. 3¾" long, 1¼" diameter, 2.2 oz.)	7	1.4	3.1	0.63				
1 large dill pickle (approx. 4" long, 1¾" diameter, 4.8 oz.)	15	3.0	3.1	0.63				
1 pound (approx. 3.3 large or 7.3 medium pickles) (tr/1g/tr/93%/408mg)	50	10.0	3.1	0.63				
Sliced:								
Sliced lengthwise with triangular-shaped cross section (spears or sticks), approx. 6" long, 1"–1½" across:								
1 slice, approx. 1.1 oz.	3	0.7	3.1	0.63				
1 pound (approx. 15 slices)	50	10.1	3.1	0.63				
Sliced crosswise, 1½" diameter, ¼" thick:								
1 slice (approx. 0.22 oz.)	1	0.1	3.1	0.63	17	3.4		
1 cup (approx. 23 slices, 5½ oz.)	17	3.4	3.1	0.63	17	3.4		
1 pound (approx. 72 slices)	50	10.1	3.1	0.63				
SOUR PICKLES								
1 medium Sour Pickle (approx. 3¾" long, 1¼" diameter, 2.3 oz.)	7	1.3	2.8	0.57				
1 large Sour Pickle (approx. 4" long, 1¾" diameter, 4.8 oz.)	14	2.7	2.8	0.57				
1 pound (approx. 3.3 large or 7 medium pickles) (tr/1g/tr/95%/386mg)	45	9.1	2.8	0.57				
SWEET PICKLES (sugar has been added)								
1 midget Gherkin (approx. 2⅛" long, ⅜" diameter, 0.21 oz.)	9	2.2	41.4	10.35				
1 small Gherkin (approx. 2½" long, ¾" diameter, 0.53 oz.)	22	5.5	41.4	10.35				
1 large Gherkin (approx. 3" long, 1" diameter, 1.23 oz.)	51	12.8	41.4	10.35				
1 pound (approx. 13 large, 30 small, or 76 midget Gherkins) (tr/10g/tr/61%/na)	662	165.6	41.4	10.35				
Sliced lengthwise with triangular-shaped cross section, 4½" long, 1½" across:								
1 slice, approx. 0.71 oz.	29	7.3	41.4	10.35				
1 pound (approx. 22½ slices)	662	165.6	41.4	10.35				
Chopped into ¼" cubes:								
1 cup (approx. 5.6 oz.)	234	58.4	41.4	10.35	234	58.4		
1 pound (approx. 2.9 cups)	662	165.6	41.4	10.35	234	58.4		

Pickles, by brand

	UNIT Cal.	UNIT Carb.	1 OZ., BY WT. Cal.	1 OZ., BY WT. Carb.	1 CUP Cal.	1 CUP Carb.	1 TABLE-SPOON Cal.	1 TABLE-SPOON Carb.
BREAD AND BUTTER PICKLES								
Bread and Butter Pickles, **Fanning's,** 14-fl.-oz. jar, entire contents of jar, including liquid	190	48.9	13.6	3.49				
DILL PICKLES								
Dill Pickles, Whole, **Featherweight,** low sodium, 16-oz. (1-lb.) jar, entire contents of jar, including liquid	80	14.4	5.0	0.90				
Drained pickles, approx. 19.6 oz.	(81)	(9.4)	(4.1)	(0.48)				
1 small pickle, 17 per jar (each approx. 1.2 oz.)	(5)	(0.6)	(4.1)	(0.48)				
1 large pickle, 7 per jar (each approx. 2.8 oz.)	(12)	(1.3)	(4.1)	(0.48)				
KOSHER PICKLES								
Kosher Pickles, Halves, **Claussen,** 32-fl.-oz. (1 quart) jar (7 to 13 pickles depending upon size), entire contents of jar, including liquid	(117)	(19.8)	3.7	0.62				
Drained pickles, approx. 18.9 oz.	(79)	(10.8)	(4.2)	(0.57)				
1 small half pickle, 13 per jar (each approx. 1.5 oz.)	(6)	(0.8)	(4.2)	(0.57)				
1 large half pickle, 7 per jar (each approx. 2.7 oz.)	(11)	(1.5)	(4.2)	(0.57)				
Kosher Pickles, Slices, **Claussen,** 24-fl.-oz. jar (approx. 60 slices) entire contents of jar, including liquid	(89)	(13.5)	3.7	0.57				
Drained pickles, approx. 7.8 oz.	(40)	(2.4)	(5.2)	(0.31)				
1 slice, approx. 0.1 oz.	(1)	trace	(5.2)	(0.31)				
Kosher Pickles, Whole, **Claussen,** 32-fl.-oz. (1-quart) jar (7 to 17 pickles depending on size), entire contents of jar, including liquid	(117)	(18.1)	(3.7)	(0.57)				

	UNIT Cal.	UNIT Carb.	1 OZ., BY WT. Cal.	1 OZ., BY WT. Carb.	1 CUP Cal.	1 CUP Carb.	1 TABLESPOON Cal.	1 TABLESPOON Carb.
SWEET AND SOUR PICKLES								
Sweet 'n Sour Pickles, Slices, **Claussen,** 24-fl.-oz. jar (approx. 60 slices) entire contents of jar, including liquid	(89)	(13.5)	3.7	0.57				
Drained pickles, approx. 7.8 oz.	(40)	(2.4)	(5.2)	(0.31)				
1 slice, approx. 0.1 oz.	(1)	trace	(5.2)	(0.31)				
Pimientos, based on generic data								
2-oz. jar	15	3.3	7.5	1.65				
4-oz. can	31	6.6	7.5	1.65				
Pimientos, by brand								
Pimientos, **Dromedary,** 4-oz. jar	40	8.0	10.0	2.00				
Potato Salad, based on USDA home recipes								
Prepared with 4 boiled medium potatoes, 1 Tbsp. chopped onion, ¾ cup cooked salad dressing, and salt (yield: approx. 2¾ cups, 24.1 oz.) (1g/5g/1g/76%/150mg)	676	111.3	28.1	4.62	248	40.8	16	2.6
1 cup (approx. 8.8 oz.)	248	40.8	28.1	4.62	248	40.8	16	2.6
1 pound (approx. 1.8 cups)	450	73.9	28.1	4.62	248	40.8	16	2.6
Prepared with 4 boiled medium potatoes, ½ cup celery, ¼ cup pickles, 1 Tbsp. chopped onion, ¼ cup French dressing, ¼ cup mayonnaise, and salt (yield: approx. 3⅔ cups, 32.3 oz.) (1g/4g/3g/72%/136mg)	1328	122.7	41.1	3.80	363	33.5	23	2.1
1 cup (approx. 8.8 oz.)	363	33.5	41.1	3.80	363	33.5	23	2.1
1 pound (approx. 1.8 cups)	658	60.8	41.1	3.80	363	33.5	23	2.1
Relishes, based on generic data								
CRANBERRY-ORANGE RELISH								
Made-from-scratch, based on USDA home recipe, with ingredients as follows: 1 lb. (approx. 4 cups) cranberries, 1 3" diameter (approx. 7 oz.) orange, including peel, 2 cups sugar (yield: approx. 3½ cups, approx. 35 oz.) (tr/13g/tr/54%/na)	(1758)	(448.1)	50.5	12.88	490	124.9	31	7.8
1 teaspoon (approx. 0.2 oz.)	10	2.6	50.5	12.88	490	124.9	31	7.8
1 cup (approx. 9.7 oz.)	490	124.9	50.5	12.88	490	124.9	31	7.8
Cranberry Sauce is with Sauces at the end of this chapter.								
SWEET PICKLE RELISH								
Commercially prepared; finely cut or chopped:								
1 teaspoon (approx. 0.2 oz.)	7	1.7	39.1	9.64	338	83.3	21	5.1
1 packet (approx. ¾ tablespoon, approx. 0.4 oz.)	14	3.4	39.1	9.64	338	83.3	21	5.1
1 tablespoon (approx. 0.6 oz.)	21	5.1	39.1	9.64	338	83.3	21	5.1
1 cup (approx. 8.6 oz.)	338	83.3	39.1	9.64	338	83.3	21	5.1
Relishes, by brand								
CranOrange Relish, **Ocean Spray,** 14-oz. jar	700	182.0	50.0	13.00	485	126.1	30	7.9
1 teaspoon (approx. 0.2 oz.)	10	2.6	50.0	13.00	485	126.1	30	7.9
Cucumber Relish, low calorie, **Featherweight,** 8-oz. jar	85	18.4	10.6	2.30	(92)	(19.9)	(6)	(1.2)
1 teaspoon (approx. 0.2 oz.)	(2)	(0.4)	10.6	2.30	(92)	(19.9)	(6)	(1.2)
Relish Sandwich Spread, **Hellmans,** 8-fl.-oz. jar	800	32.0	(100.0)	(4.00)	800	32.0	50	2.0
1 teaspoon (approx. 0.2 oz.)	17	0.7	(100.0)	(4.00)	800	32.0	50	2.0
Relish Sandwich Spread, **Numade,** 16-fl.-oz. (1-pint) jar	1800	120.0	112.5	7.50	960	64.0	60	4.0
1 teaspoon (approx. 0.2 oz.)	20	1.3	112.5	7.50	960	64.0	60	4.0

	UNIT Cal.	UNIT Carb.	1 OZ., BY WT. Cal.	1 OZ., BY WT. Carb.	1 CUP Cal.	1 CUP Carb.	1 TABLESPOON Cal.	1 TABLESPOON Carb.
Sauerkraut, based on generic data								
1 Can, #303; 16 oz. (1 lb.) net wt.:								
Solids and liquid, 16 oz. (approx. 1.9 cups) (1g/1g/tr/93%/212mg)	82	18.1	5.1	1.13	42	9.4	3	0.6
Drained sauerkraut (approx. 14.1 oz., 1.9 cup) (1g/1g/tr/na/na)	(77)	(16.8)	(5.4)	(1.19)	(40)	(8.8)	(3)	(0.6)
Sauerkraut juice (approx. 1.9 oz.) (tr/1g/tr/95%/223mg)	(5)	(1.3)	2.8	0.66	24	5.6	2	0.4
1 Can, #10; 99 oz. (6 lb. 3 oz.) net wt.:								
Solids and liquid, 99 oz. (approx. 11.9 cups)	505	112.3	5.1	1.13	42	9.4	3	0.6
Drained sauerkraut (approx. 87.1 oz., 11.9 cups)	(472)	(103.6)	(5.4)	(1.19)	(40)	(8.8)	(3)	(0.6)
Sauerkraut juice (approx. 11.9 oz.)	33	8.7	2.8	0.66	24	5.6	2	0.4
1 pound:								
Solids and liquid (approx. 1.9 cups)	82	18.1	5.1	1.13	42	9.4	3	0.6
Drained sauerkraut (approx. 2.2 cups)	(86)	(19.0)	(5.4)	(1.19)	(40)	(8.8)	(3)	(0.6)
Sauerkraut juice (approx. 1.9 cups)	45	10.6	2.8	0.66	24	5.6	2	0.4
1 cup:								
Solids and liquid (approx. 8.3 oz.)	42	9.4	5.1	1.13	42	9.4	3	0.6
Drained sauerkraut (approx. 7.4 oz.)	(40)	(8.8)	(5.4)	(1.19)	(40)	(8.8)	(3)	(0.6)
Sauerkraut juice (approx. 8.5 oz.)	24	5.6	2.8	0.66	24	5.6	2	0.4
Sauerkraut, by brand								
Blue Boy, 8-oz. can, solids and liquid	55	7.3	6.9	0.91	60	8.0	4	0.5
16-oz. (1-lb.) can, solids and liquid	110	14.5	6.9	0.91	60	8.0	4	0.5
99-oz. (6-lb. 3-oz.) can, solids and liquid	683	90.1	6.9	0.91	60	8.0	4	0.5
Claussen, 32-fl.-oz. (2-lb.) jar (yield: 24.9 oz. drained solids)	141	26.1	5.7	1.05	(47)	(8.7)	(3)	(0.5)
Stokely, Bavarian Style Sauerkraut, 16-oz. (1-lb.) can	113	26.5	7.1	1.65	60	14.0	(3)	(0.9)
Chopped Sauerkraut, 16-oz. (1-lb.) can	76	17.0	4.7	1.06	40	9.0	(3)	(0.6)
Shredded Sauerkraut, 8-oz. can	38	8.5	4.7	1.06	40	9.0	(3)	(0.6)
Three Bean Salad								
Green Giant, 17-oz. can	362	79.6	21.3	4.68	190	42.0	2	2.6
Hanover, 8-oz. can	250	48.0	31.3	6.00	(270)	(51.0)	(17)	(3.2)
52-oz. can	1628	312.0	31.3	6.00	(270)	(51.0)	(17)	(3.2)
SALAD DRESSING								
Salad Dressing, based on generic data								
BLUE CHEESE DRESSING								
Regular, 1 cup (approx. 8.6 oz.) (1g/2g/15g/32%/310mg)	1235	18.1	142.9	2.09	1235	18.1	77.1	1.13
Low-fat (approx. 5 cal. per teaspoon), 1 cup (approx. 9 oz.) (1g/1g/2g/84%/314mg)	194	10.5	21.6	1.17	194	10.5	12.1	0.66
Very low-fat (approx. 1 cal. per teaspoon), 1 cup (approx. 8.6 oz.) (tr/tr/tr/93%/322mg)	47	3.4	5.4	0.39	47	3.4	2.7	0.21
FRENCH DRESSING								
Made from scratch, based on USDA home recipe with ingredients as follows: ¼ cup vinegar, ¾ cup cooking oil, 1 tsp. sugar, 1 tsp. salt, ½ tsp. paprika, ½ tsp. dry mustard, 1 dash pepper (tr/1g/20g/24%/187mg) Yield: approx.:								
1 cup (approx. 7.8 oz.)	1390	7.9	178.2	1.01	1390	7.9	88.0	0.50

	UNIT		1 OZ., BY WT.		1 CUP		1 TABLE-SPOON	
	Cal.	Carb.	Cal.	Carb.	Cal.	Carb.	Cal.	Carb.
1 tablespoon (approx. 0.5 oz.; a loss of 10% has been applied for evaporation in cooking)	88	0.5	178.2	1.01	1390	7.9	88.0	0.50
Regular, 1 cup (approx. 8.8 oz.) (tr/5g/11g/39%/388mg)	1025	43.8	116.2	4.97	1025	43.8	64.1	2.74
Low-Calorie (approx. 5 cal. per teaspoon), 1 cup (approx. 9.2 oz.) (tr/4g/1g/77%/233mg)	250	40.6	27.3	4.43	250	40.6	15.6	2.54
ITALIAN DRESSING								
Regular, 1 cup (approx. 8.3 oz.) (tr/2g/17g/28%/593mg)	1297	16.2	156.5	1.95	1297	16.2	81.1	1.01
Low-Calorie (approx. 2 cal. per teaspoon), 1 cup (approx. 8.5 oz.) (tr/1g/1g/90%/223mg)	120	6.2	14.2	0.73	120	6.2	7.5	0.39
RUSSIAN DRESSING								
Regular, 1 cup (approx. 8.6 oz.) (tr/3g/14g/35%/246mg)	1210	25.5	140.0	2.95	1210	25.5	75.6	1.59
THOUSAND ISLAND DRESSING								
Regular, 1 cup (approx. 8.8 oz.) (tr/4g/14g/32%/198mg)	1255	38.5	142.3	4.37	1255	38.5	78.4	2.41
Low-Calorie (approx. 10 cal. per teaspoon), 1 cup (approx. 8.6 oz.) (tr/4g/4g/68%/198mg)	441	38.2	51.0	4.42	441	38.2	27.6	2.39
Salad Dressing, by brand								
AVOCADO								
Kraft, Avocado Dressing, 8-fl.-oz. bottle	1120	32.0	132.3	4.00	1120	32.0	70.0	2.00
BLEU OR BLUE CHEESE								
Dia-Mel, Lo-Cal Bleu Cheese Dressing, 8-oz. box, 16 envelopes	320	16.0	40.0	2.00	(336)	(16.8)	(21.0)	(1.05)
1 envelope, approx. 0.5 oz.	20	1.0	40.0	2.00	(336)	(16.8)	(21.0)	(1.05)
Dieter's Gourmet, Bleu Cheese Dressing for Salads, 9-oz. box, 18 envelopes	252	36.0	28.0	4.00	224	32.0	14.0	2.00
1 envelope (ready to serve), approx. 0.5 oz.	14	2.0	28.0	4.00	224	32.0	14.0	2.00
Featherweight, Low Calorie Imitation Neu Bleu Cheese Dressing, 8-fl.-oz. bottle	64	16.0	(7.6)	(1.91)	64	16.0	4.0	1.00
Frenchette, Low Calorie Blue Cheese Dressing, 8-fl.-oz. bottle	336	32.0	(40.0)	(3.80)	336	32.0	7.0	0.66
Good Seasons, Bleu Cheese Salad Dressing Mix, 0.78-oz. envelope	63	3.3	80.8	4.20	646	33.3	40.4	2.08
As prepared (yield: approx. 8.4 fl. oz.)	1440	16.0	(171.4)	(1.90)	1440	16.0	90.0	1.00
Thick 'N Creamy Bleu Cheese Salad Dressing Mix, 0.78-oz. envelope	97	3.1	138.6	4.40	1109	35.2	69.3	2.20
As prepared (yield: approx. 8.4 fl. oz.)	1280	8.0	(152.4)	(1.00)	1280	8.0	80.0	0.50
Henri's, Yogurt Bleu Cheese Dressing, 8-fl.-oz. bottle	480	64.0	(57.1)	(7.62)	480	64.0	30.0	4.00
Hidden Valley Ranch, Blue Cheese Flavor Salad Dressing Mix, 0.4-oz. package								
As prepared with milk (yield: approx. 1 pint)	1720	19.2	(103.6)	(1.16)	860	9.6	53.8	0.60
As prepared with buttermilk (yield: approx. 1 pint)	(1650)	(18.2)	(99.4)	(1.10)	(825)	(9.1)	(51.6)	(0.57)
Milk Recipe Blue Cheese Flavor Salad Dressing Mix, 1.1-oz. package								
As prepared with milk and mayonnaise (yield: approx. 1 pint)	1811	24.6	(104.7)	(1.42)	905	12.3	56.6	0.77
As prepared with buttermilk (yield: approx. 1 pint)	(1741)	(23.6)	(100.6)	(1.36)	(871)	(11.8)	(54.4)	(0.74)
Kraft, Chunky Blue Cheese Dressing, 8-fl.-oz. bottle	1120	32.0	(133.3)	(3.80)	1120	32.0	70.0	2.00
Low Calorie Blue Cheese Dressing, 8-fl.-oz. bottle	224	16.0	(26.7)	(1.90)	224	16.0	14.0	1.00
Roka Blue Cheese Dressing, 8-fl.-oz. bottle	960	16.0	114.3	1.90	960	16.0	60.0	1.00
16-fl.-oz. (1-pint) bottle	1920	32.0	114.3	1.90	960	16.0	60.0	1.00
Ralph's, Bleu Cheese Dressing, 16-fl.-oz. (1-pint) bottle	2400	32.0	(141.2)	(1.88)	1200	16.0	75.0	1.00

	UNIT		1 OZ., BY WT.		1 CUP		1 TABLE-SPOON	
	Cal.	Carb.	Cal.	Carb.	Cal.	Carb.	Cal.	Carb.
Seven Seas, Real Blue Cheese Dressing, 8-fl.-oz. bottle	1120	16.0	(133.3)	(1.90)	1120	16.0	70.0	1.00
Tillie Lewis "Tasti Diet," Artificially Flavored Blue Cheese Dressing, 8-fl.-oz. bottle	224	16.0	(26.7)	(1.90)	224	16.0	14.0	1.00
Walden Farms, Chunky Style Blue Cheese Dressing, 12-fl.-oz. jar	216	40.7	(17.1)	(3.23)	144	27.1	9.0	1.70
Weight Watchers, Blue Cheese-Flavored Salad Dressing and Dip Mix, 0.6-oz. envelope	80	8.0	133.3	13.33	1067	106.7	66.7	6.67
As prepared (for dressing) with water (yield: approx. ½ cup, 4 fl. oz.)	80	8.0	(17.4)	(1.74)	160	16.0	10.0	1.00
Wish-Bone, Chunky Blue Cheese Dressing, 8-fl.-oz. bottle	1120	16.0	(133.4)	(1.90)	1120	16.0	70.0	1.00
16-fl.-oz. (1-pint) bottle	2240	32.0	(133.4)	(1.90)	1120	16.0	70.0	1.00
Lite Chunky Blue Cheese Dressing, 8-fl.-oz. bottle	640	48.0	(80.0)	(6.00)	640	48.0	40.0	3.00
BUTTERMILK								
Good Seasons, Buttermilk Farm Style Salad Dressing Mix, dry mix, 1.4-oz. envelope	105	14.6	75.0	10.43				
As prepared (yield: approx. 2 cups, 16.8 oz.)	1920	32.0	(114.3)	(1.90)	1920	32.0	60.0	1.00
CAESAR								
Dia-Mel, Lo Cal Caesar Dressing, 8-oz. box, 16 envelopes	384	16.0	48.0	2.00	(408)	(17.0)	25.5	1.06
1 envelope, approx. 0.5 oz.	24	1.0	48.0	2.00	(408)	(17.0)	25.5	1.06
Dieter's Gourmet, Caesar Dressing for Salads, 9-oz. box, 18 envelopes	720	18.0	80.0	2.00	(680)	(17.0)	(42.3)	(1.06)
1 envelope (ready to serve), 0.5 oz.	40	1.0	80.0	2.00	(680)	(17.0)	(42.3)	(1.06)
Hain, Natural Caesar Dressing, 12-fl.-oz. bottle	1512	48.0	(118.0)	(3.76)	1008	32.0	63.0	2.00
Hollywood, Caesar Dressing, 12-fl.-oz. bottle	1512	48.0	(118.0)	(3.76)	1008	32.0	63.0	2.00
Hunza, Caesar Dressing, 12-fl.-oz. bottle	1512	48.0	(118.0)	(3.76)	1008	32.0	63.0	2.00
Kraft, Golden Caesar Dressing, 8-fl.-oz. bottle	1120	16.0	132.3	2.00	1120	16.0	70.0	1.00
16-fl.-oz. (1-pint) bottle	2240	32.0	132.3	2.00	1120	16.0	70.0	1.00
Louis Sherry, Lo Cal Caesar Dressing, 8-oz. bottle	(408)	(17.0)	48.0	2.00	(408)	(17.0)	(25.5)	(1.06)
Pfeiffer, Caesar Salad Dressing, 8-fl.-oz. bottle	1120	8.0	140.0	1.00	(1190)	(8.5)	(74.1)	(0.53)
Low calorie Caesar Salad Dressing, 8-fl.-oz. bottle	160	16.0	20.0	2.00	(170)	(17.0)	(10.6)	(1.06)
Seven Seas, Caesar Dressing, 8-fl.-oz. bottle	1120	16.0	(131.8)	(1.88)	1120	16.0	70.0	1.00
16-fl.-oz. (1-pint) bottle	2240	32.0	(131.8)	(1.88)	(1120)	(16.0)	70.0	1.00
Wish-Bone, Caesar Dressing, 8-fl.-oz. bottle	1280	16.0	(150.0)	(1.90)	1280	16.0	80.0	1.00
CASABLANCA								
Dieter's Gourmet, Casablanca Zestfully Continental Dressing for Salads, 9-oz. box, 18 individual envelopes	540	36.0	60.0	4.00	(510)	(34.0)	(31.7)	(2.11)
1 envelope (ready to serve), approx. 0.5 oz.	30	2.0	60.0	4.00	(510)	(34.0)	(31.7)	(2.11)
CHEF								
Kraft, Chef Style Dressing, low calorie, 8-fl.-oz. bottle	288	48.0	34.0	6.00	288	48.0	18.0	3.00
Tillie Lewis, Chef's Dressing, "Tasti Diet," 8-fl.-oz. bottle	32	0.0	(4.0)	0.00	32	0.0	2.0	0.00
COLESLAW								
Kraft, Coleslaw Dressing, 8-fl.-oz. bottle	1128	64.0	132.3	8.00	1120	64.0	70.0	4.00
Coleslaw Dressing, low calorie, 8-fl.-oz. bottle	480	64.0	56.7	8.00	480	64.0	30.0	4.00
COUNTRY STYLE								
Ralph's, Country Style Dressing, 16-fl.-oz. (1-pint) bottle	1629	128.0	(95.8)	(7.53)	814	64.0	50.9	4.00
CUCUMBER								
Kraft, Creamy Cucumber Dressing, 8-fl.-oz. bottle	1280	16.0	151.2	2.00	1280	16.0	80.0	1.00
16-fl.-oz. (1-pint) bottle	2560	32.0	151.2	2.00	2560	32.0	80.0	1.00
Creamy Cucumber Dressing, low calorie, 8-fl.-oz. bottle	480	16.0	56.7	2.00	480	16.0	30.0	1.00

	UNIT		1 OZ., BY WT.		1 CUP		1 TABLESPOON	
	Cal.	Carb.	Cal.	Carb.	Cal.	Carb.	Cal.	Carb.
Featherweight, Creamy Cucumber-Onion Dressing, low calorie, 8-fl.-oz. bottle	64	16.0	8.0	2.00	64	16.0	4.0	1.00
Henri's, Yogurt Cucumber 'N Onion Creamy Dressing, 8-fl.-oz.	320	64.0	(37.8)	(7.56)	320	64.0	20.0	4.00
DILL								
Herb Magic, Dill Salad Dressing, no oil, 12-fl.-oz. bottle	144	48.0	12.0	4.00	96	32.0	6.0	2.00
FRENCH								
Catalina, French Dressing, 8-fl.-oz. bottle	960	64.0	112.9	7.53	960	64.0	60.0	4.00
Dia-Mel, Lo-Cal French Salad Dressing, 8-oz. box, 16 envelopes	288	0.0	36.0	0.00	(320)	0.0	20.0	0.00
1 ½-oz. envelope	18	0.0	36.0	0.00	(320)	0.0	20.0	0.00
Dieter's Gourmet, Low Oil French Style Dressing, 9-oz. package, 18 packets	252	36.0	28.0	4.00	224	32.0	14.0	2.00
1 packet, 0.5 oz.	14	2.0	28.0	4.00	224	32.0	14.0	2.00
Featherweight, French Dressing, low-sodium, 8-fl.-oz. bottle	960	96.0	(109.3)	(10.93)	960	96.0	60.0	6.00
French Style Dressing, 8-fl.-oz. bottle	96	16.0	(11.4)	(1.91)	96	16.0	6.0	1.00
Good Seasons, French Salad Dressing Mix, Old Fashioned, 0.6-oz. envelope	32	9.0	53.3	1.50				
As prepared (yield: approx. 1 cup, 8.6 oz.)	1280	16.0	(148.8)	(1.86)	1280	16.0	80.0	1.00
French Salad Dressing Mix, Riviera, 1.8-oz. envelope	149	36.3	82.8	20.17				
As prepared (yield: approx. 1 cup, 8.6 oz.)	1440	48.0	(167.4)	(5.58)	1440	48.0	90.0	3.00
French Style Dressing Mix, 2.3-oz. envelope	232	45.2	100.9	19.68				
As prepared (yield: 1 cup, or 8 fl. oz.)	1280	48.0	(148.8)	(5.58)	1280	48.0	80.0	3.00
Hain, Natural Creamy French Dressing, 12-fl.-oz. bottle	1512	72.0	(117.2)	(5.58)	1008	48.0	63.0	3.00
Henri's, Yogurt French Style Dressing, 8-fl.-oz. bottle	640	96.0	(74.4)	(11.16)	640	96.0	40.0	6.00
Hollywood, French Dressing, 12-fl.-oz. bottle	1512	72.0	(117.2)	(5.58)	1008	48.0	63.0	3.00
Hunza, French Dressing, 12-fl.-oz. bottle	1512	72.6	(117.2)	(5.58)	1008	48.0	63.0	3.00
Kraft, French Dressing, 8-fl.-oz. bottle	960	32.0	(112.9)	(3.76)	960	32.0	60.0	2.00
French Style Dressing, low calorie, 8-fl.-oz. bottle	400	32.0	(47.1)	(3.76)	400	32.0	25.0	2.00
Garlic French Dressing, 8-fl.-oz. bottle	1120	48.0	(131.8)	(5.65)	1120	48.0	70.0	3.00
Herb & Garlic French Dressing, 8-fl.-oz. bottle	1440	0.0	(169.4)	0.00	1440	0.0	90.0	0.00
Miracle, French Dressing, 8-fl.-oz. bottle	1120	48.0	(131.8)	(5.65)	1120	48.0	70.0	3.00
16-fl.-oz. (1-pint) bottle	2240	96.0	(131.8)	(5.65)	1120	48.0	70.0	3.00
Numade, Low Cal French Dressing, 8-fl.-oz. bottle	320	48.0	(37.8)	(5.67)	320	48.0	20.0	3.00
Pfeiffer, French Dressing, 8-fl.-oz. bottle	880	56.0	(110.0)	7.00	(943)	(60.0)	(58.9)	(3.75)
16-fl.-oz. (1-pint) bottle	1760	112.0	(110.0)	7.00	(943)	(60.0)	(58.9)	(3.75)
French Style Dressing, Low Calorie, 8-fl.-oz. bottle	280	40.0	(35.0)	5.00	(312)	(44.5)	(19.5)	(2.79)
Saffola, French Salad Dressing, 12-fl.-oz. bottle	1200	48.0	(94.5)	(3.78)	800	32.0	50.0	2.00
French Dressing, Low Calorie, 8-fl.-oz. bottle	960	32.0	(111.6)	(3.72)	960	32.0	60.0	2.00
Seven Seas, Family Style French Dressing, 8-fl.-oz. bottle	960	48.0	(111.6)	(5.58)	960	48.0	60.0	3.00
Creamy French Dressing, 8-fl.-oz. bottle	960	48.0	(111.6)	(5.58)	960	48.0	60.0	3.00
Tillie Lewis "Tasti Diet," French Dressing Substitute, 8-fl.-oz. bottle	96	32.0	(10.9)	(3.64)	96	32.0	6.0	2.00
Walden Farms, Creamy French Dressing, 12-fl.-oz. jar	264	67.1	(19.7)	(5.01)	176	44.8	11.0	2.80
Weight Watchers, French Style Dressing Mix, Salad Surprise, 0.35-oz. envelope	32	8.0	91.4	22.85				
As prepared, add ½ cup water (yield: approx. ½ cup, 4.3 oz.)	32	8.0	(7.4)	(1.84)	64	16.0	4.0	1.00
Wish-Bone, French Dressing, DeLuxe, 8-fl.-oz. bottle	960	48.0	(112.0)	(5.60)	960	48.0	60.0	3.00
French Style Salad Dressing, Lite, 8-fl.-oz. bottle	480	32.0	(60.0)	(4.00)	480	32.0	30.0	2.00
Garlic French Dressing, 8-fl.-oz. bottle	960	32.0	(112.0)	(3.73)	960	32.0	60.0	2.00

	UNIT		1 OZ., BY WT.		1 CUP		1 TABLESPOON	
	Cal.	Carb.	Cal.	Carb.	Cal.	Carb.	Cal.	Carb.
Sweet 'N Spice French Dressing, 8-fl.-oz. bottle	960	48.0	(112.0)	(5.60)	960	48.0	60.0	3.00
GARLIC								
Dieter's Gourmet, Cream Garlic Dressing for Salads, 9-oz. box, 18 envelopes	252	36.0	28.0	4.00	224	32.0	14.0	2.00
1 envelope (ready to serve), approx. ½ oz.	14	2.0	28.0	4.00	224	32.0	14.0	2.00
Good Seasons, Cheese Garlic Salad Dressing Mix, 0.7-oz. envelope	57	7.0	81.4	10.00				
As prepared (yield: approx. 1 cup, 8 oz.)	1440	16.0	(171.4)	(1.90)	1440	16.0	90.0	1.00
Garlic Salad Dressing Mix, 0.7-oz. envelope	45	7.1	64.3	10.14				
As prepared (yield: approx. 1 cup, 8 oz.)	1280	16.0	(160.0)	(2.00)	1280	16.0	80.0	1.00
Kraft, Creamy Garlic Dressing, 8-fl.-oz. bottle	800	16.0	(94.1)	(1.88)	800	16.0	50.0	1.00
16-fl.-oz. (1-pint) bottle	1600	32.0	(94.1)	(1.88)	800	16.0	50.0	1.00
Wish-Bone, Creamy Garlic Dressing, 8-fl.-oz. bottle	1280	32.0	(149.4)	(3.74)	1280	32.0	80.0	2.00
GREEN GODDESS								
Hidden Valley Ranch, Green Goddess Flavor Salad Dressing Mix, 0.6-oz. package								
As prepared with milk (yield: approx. 1 pint)	1707	23.5	(101.6)	(1.40)	854	11.8	53.4	0.74
As prepared with buttermilk (yield: approx. 1 pint)	(1637)	(22.5)	(97.4)	(1.34)	(819)	(11.3)	(51.2)	(0.70)
Kraft, Green Goddess Dressing, 8-fl.-oz. bottle	1280	16.0	(150.6)	(1.88)	1280	16.0	80.0	1.00
Seven Seas, Green Goddess Dressing, 8-fl.-oz. bottle	1120	0.0	(130.0)	0.00	1120	0.0	70.0	0.00
16-fl.-oz. (1-pint) bottle	2240	0.0	(130.0)	0.00	1120	0.0	70.0	0.00
Wish-Bone, Green Goddess Dressing, 8-fl.-oz. bottle	1120	16.0	(140.0)	2.00	1120	16.0	70.0	1.00
HERB								
Dieter's Gourmet, Herb Dressing, 9-oz. box, 18 individual envelopes	252	36.0	28.0	4.00	224	32.0	14.0	2.00
1 envelope (ready to serve), approx. 0.5 oz.	14	2.0	28.0	4.00	224	32.0	14.0	2.00
Herb Magic, Herb Basket Salad Dressing, no oil, 12-fl.-oz. bottle	144	48.0	12.0	4.00	96	32.0	6.0	2.00
Hidden Valley Ranch, Vintage Herb Flavor Salad Dressing Mix, Milk Recipe, 0.9-oz. package								
As prepared with mayonnaise and milk (yield: approx. 1 pint)	1821	32.0	(106.5)	(1.87)	910	16.0	56.9	1.00
As prepared with buttermilk (yield: approx. 1 pint)	(1751)	(31.0)	(102.4)	(1.81)	(876)	(15.5)	(54.7)	(0.97)
ITALIAN								
Ann Page (A&P), Low Calorie Italian Dressing, 8-fl.-oz. bottle	224	16.0	(27.7)	(1.98)	224	16.0	14.0	1.00
Dia-Mel, Lo-Cal Italian Dressing, 8-oz. box, 16 envelopes	32	0.0	4.0	0.00	(32)	0.0	(2.0)	0.00
1 envelope (½ oz.)	2	0.0	4.0	0.00	(32)	0.0	(2.0)	0.00
Featherweight, Low Calorie Italian Dressing, 8-fl.-oz. bottle	64	16.0	(7.9)	(1.98)	64	16.0	4.0	1.00
Frenchette, Low Calorie Italian Dressing, 8-fl.-oz. bottle	96	32.0	(11.9)	(3.95)	96	32.0	6.0	2.00
Good Seasons, Italian Salad Dressing Mix, 0.6-oz. envelope	42	9.3	70.0	15.50				
As prepared (yield: approx. 1 cup, 8 oz.)	1280	16.0	(160.0)	(2.00)	1280	16.0	80.0	1.00
Cheese Italian Salad Dressing Mix, 1-oz. envelope	79	14.4	79.0	14.40				
As prepared (yield: approx. 1 cup, 8.4 oz.)	1440	16.0	(171.4)	(1.90)	1440	16.0	90.0	1.00
Low Calorie Italian Salad Dressing Mix, 1.4-oz. envelope	120	29.6	85.7	21.14				
As prepared (yield: approx. 1 cup, 8 oz.)	1280	32.0	(160.0)	(4.00)	1280	32.0	8.0	2.00
Mild Italian Salad Dressing Mix, 1-oz. envelope	84	20.4	84.0	20.40				
As prepared (yield: approx. 1 cup, 8 oz.)	1440	16.0	(180.0)	(2.00)	1440	16.0	90.0	1.00
Thick 'N Creamy Italian Salad Dressing Mix, 0.7-oz. envelope	68	10.9	97.1	15.57				
As prepared (yield: approx. 1 cup, 8.6 oz.)	1360	16.0	(158.1)	(1.86)	1360	16.0	85.0	1.00

	UNIT		1 OZ., BY WT.		1 CUP		1 TABLESPOON	
	Cal.	Carb.	Cal.	Carb.	Cal.	Carb.	Cal.	Carb.
Hain, Natural Italian Dressing, 12-fl.-oz. bottle	2304	trace	192.0	trace	1024	trace	64.0	trace
Henri's, Yogurt Italian Dressing, 8-fl.-oz. bottle	560	64.0	(65.9)	(7.53)	560	64.0	35.0	4.00
Herb Magic, no oil Italian Dressing, 12-fl.-oz. bottle	96	24.0	8.0	2.00	64	16.0	4.0	1.00
Hidden Valley Ranch, Creamy Italian Flavor Salad Dressing Mix, 0.5-oz. package								
As prepared with milk (yield: approx. 1 pint)	1696	21.8	(101.6)	(1.31)	848	10.9	53.0	0.68
As prepared with buttermilk (yield: approx. 1 pint)	(1626)	(20.8)	(97.4)	(1.25)	(813)	(10.4)	(50.8)	(0.65)
Milk Recipe Creamy Italian Flavor Salad Dressing Mix, 1.18-oz. package	1846	39.7	(106.1)	(2.28)	923	19.8	57.7	1.24
As prepared with milk (yield: approx. 1 pint)	1846	38.7	(106.1)	(2.28)	923	19.8	57.7	1.24
As prepared with buttermilk (yield: approx. 1 pint)	(1776)	(38.7)	(102.1)	(2.22)	(888)	(19.4)	(55.5)	(1.21)
Hollywood, Italian Dressing, 12-fl.-oz.	1536	trace	(128.0)	trace	1024	trace	64.0	trace
Hunza, Italian Dressing, 12-fl.-oz.	1536	trace	(128.0)	trace	1024	trace	64.0	trace
Kraft, Creamy Italian Dressing, 8-fl.-oz. bottle	800	16.0	(94.1)	(1.88)	800	16.0	50.0	1.00
Italian Dressing, 8-fl.-oz. bottle	1280	16.0	(150.0)	(1.88)	1280	16.0	80.0	1.00
Italian Dressing, Low Calorie, 8-fl.-oz. bottle	96	16.0	(11.3)	(1.88)	96	16.0	6.0	1.00
Zesty Italian Dressing, Low Calorie, 8-fl.-oz. bottle	96	16.0	(11.3)	(1.88)	96	16.0	6.0	1.00
Nu Made, Low Cal Italian Dressing, 8-fl.-oz. bottle	256	16.0	(30.2)	(1.89)	256	16.0	16.0	1.00
Pfeiffer, Chef Italian Dressing, 8-fl.-oz. bottle	960	8.0	120.0	1.00	(972)	(8.1)	(60.8)	(0.51)
16-fl.-oz. (1-pint) bottle	1920	16.0	120.0	1.00	(972)	(8.1)	(60.8)	(0.51)
Italian Dressing, Low Calorie, 8-fl.-oz. bottle	160	(24.0)	20.0	3.00	(162)	(24.3)	(10.2)	(1.53)
Saffola, Italian Salad Dressing, 12-fl.-oz. bottle	1200	24.0	(94.5)	(1.89)	800	16.0	50.0	1.00
Seven Seas, Creamy Italian Dressing, 8-fl.-oz. bottle	1120	16.0	(133.3)	(1.90)	1120	16.0	70.0	1.00
16-fl.-oz. (1-pint) bottle	2240	32.0	(133.3)	(1.90)	1120	16.0	70.0	1.00
Italian Dressing, 8-fl.-oz. bottle	1120	16.0	(140.0)	(2.00)	1120	16.0	70.0	1.00
Italian Dressing, Low Calorie, 8-fl.-oz. bottle	600	24.0	(75.0)	(3.00)	600	24.0	37.5	1.50
Viva Italian Dressing, 8-fl.-oz. bottle	1120	16.0	(140.0)	(2.00)	1120	16.0	70.0	1.00
16-fl.-oz. (1-pint) bottle	2240	32.0	(140.0)	(2.00)	1120	16.0	70.0	1.00
Viva Italian Dressing, Mild, 8-fl.-oz. bottle	1120	16.0	(140.0)	(2.00)	1120	16.0	70.0	1.00
Tillie Lewis "Tasti Diet," Italian Dressing, 8-fl.-oz. bottle	32	0.0	(4.0)	0.00	32	0.0	2.0	0.00
Walden Farms, Classic Italian Dressing, 12-fl.-oz. jar	216	34.1	(18.0)	(2.84)	144	22.7	9.0	1.40
Weight Watchers, Creamy Italian Dressing, 16-fl.-oz. (1-pint) bottle	1600	64.0	(94.5)	(3.78)	800	32.0	50.0	2.00
Creamy Italian Dressing Mix, 0.6-oz. envelope	48	12.0	80.0	20.00				
As prepared, add 3/4 cups water (yield: approx. 3/4 cups, 6 fl. oz.)	48	12.0	(7.5)	(1.88)	64	16.0	4.0	1.00
Wish-Bone, Creamy Italian Salad Dressing, 8-fl.-oz.	1280	32.0	(160.0)	(4.00)	1280	32.0	80.0	2.00
Creamy Italian Salad Dressing, Lite, 8-fl.-oz. bottle	480	16.0	(60.0)	(2.00)	480	16.0	30.0	1.00
Italian Salad Dressing, 8-fl.-oz. bottle	1280	16.0	(160.0)	(2.00)	1280	16.0	80.0	1.00
LOW CALORIE								
Many low-calorie salad dressings are listed under their flavors, such as Blue Cheese, Caesar, and French.								
Catalina, Dressing, low calorie, 8-fl.-oz. bottle	400	32.0	(47.2)	(3.78)	400	32.0	25.0	2.00
Kraft, Green Onion Dressing, 8-fl.-oz. bottle	1280	16.0	151.2	2.00	1280	16.0	80.0	1.00
MAYONNAISE								
Mayonnaise has its own section directly following this one. Also see the products in this listing called "Salad Dressing."								

	UNIT		1 OZ., BY WT.		1 CUP		1 TABLESPOON	
	Cal.	Carb.	Cal.	Carb.	Cal.	Carb.	Cal.	Carb.
OIL & VINEGAR (Vinaigrette)								
Featherweight, Red Wine & Vinegar Dressing, dietetic, 8-fl.-oz. bottle	96	16.0	12.0	2.00	96	16.0	6.0	1.00
Herb Magic, Vinaigrette Salad Dressing, no oil, 12-fl.-oz. bottle	144	24.0	12.0	2.00	96	16.0	6.0	1.00
Kraft, Oil & Vinegar Dressing, 8-fl.-oz. bottle	1120	16.0	(140.0)	(2.00)	1120	16.0	70.0	1.00
Red Wine Vinegar & Oil Dressing, 8-fl.-oz. bottle	960	64.0	(120.0)	(8.00)	960	64.0	60.0	4.00
Pfeiffer's, Lo-Cal Red Wine Dressing, 8-fl.-oz. bottle	160	16.0	20.0	2.00	170	17.0	10.6	1.06
Seven Seas, Viva Red Wine Vinegar & Oil Dressing, 8-fl.-oz. bottle	1120	16.0	(140.0)	(2.00)	1120	16.0	70.0	1.00
ONION								
16-fl.-oz. (1-pint) bottle	2560	32.0	151.0	(1.90)	1280	16.0	80.0	1.00
Good Seasons, Onion Salad Dressing Mix, dry mix, 0.6-oz. envelope	(31)	(6.4)	(52.0)	(10.70)				
As prepared (yield: approx. 1 cup, 8 oz.)	1280	16.0	(160.0)	(2.00)	1280	16.0	80.0	1.00
Herb Magic, Onion-Chive Salad Dressing, no oil, 12-fl.-oz. bottle	144	48.0	12.0	4.00	96	32.0	6.0	2.00
Wish-Bone, California Onion Salad Dressing, 8-fl.-oz. bottle	1280	16.0	(151.0)	(1.90)	1280	16.0	80.0	1.00
Wish-Bone, Onion and Chives Salad Dressing, 8-fl.-oz. bottle	1120		(132.1)		1120		70.0	
Onion and Chives Salad Dressing, Lite, 8-fl.-oz. bottle	640	48.0	(80.0)	(6.00)	640	48.0	40.0	3.00
RANCH								
Hidden Valley Ranch, Ranch Original Flavor Salad Dressing Mix, 0.4-oz. package								
As prepared with milk (yield: approx. 1 pint)	1704	17.8	(102.7)	(1.07)	852	8.9	53.3	0.56
As prepared with buttermilk (yield: approx. 1 pint)	(1634)	(16.8)	(98.4)	(1.01)	(817)	(8.4)	(51.1)	(0.52)
Ranch Original Flavor Salad Dressing Mix, Milk Recipe, 1.0-oz. package								
As prepared with milk (yield: approx. 1 pint)	1780	75.2	(103.5)	(4.37)	890	37.6	55.6	2.35
As prepared with buttermilk (yield: approx. 1 pint)	(1710)	(74.2)	(99.4)	(4.31)	(855)	(37.1)	(53.4)	(2.32)
ROQUEFORT								
Ralph's Roquefort Salad Dressing, 16-fl.-oz. (1-pint) bottle	2240	32.0	(131.8)	(1.88)	1120	16.0	70.0	1.00
RUSSIAN								
Dia-Mel, Lo-Cal Russian Salad Dressing, 8-oz. box, 16 envelopes	320	0.0	40.0	0.00	(348)	0.0	(21.8)	0.00
1/2-oz. envelope	20	0.0	40.0	0.00	(348)	0.0	(21.8)	0.00
Featherweight, low calorie Creamy Russian Dressing, 8-fl.-oz. bottle	96	16.0	(11.0)	(1.83)	96	16.0	6.0	1.00
Hain, Natural Russian Dressing, 12-fl.-oz. bottle	1584	72.0	(120.9)	(5.50)	1056	48.0	66.0	3.00
Hollywood, Russian Dressing, 12-fl.-oz. bottle	1584	72.0	(120.9)	(5.50)	1056	48.0	66.0	3.00
Hunza, Russian Dressing, 12-fl.-oz. bottle	1584	72.0	(120.9)	(5.50)	1056	48.0	66.0	3.00
Kraft, Creamy Russian Dressing, 8-fl.-oz. bottle	960	32.0	113.4	4.00	960	32.0	60.0	2.00
Russian Dressing, Low Calorie, 8-fl.-oz. bottle	480	64.0	56.7	8.00	480	64.0	30.0	4.00
Russian Dressing With Pure Honey, 8-fl.-oz. bottle	960	80.0	113.4	10.00	960	80.0	60.0	5.00
Nickabood's, "Fisherman's Wharf," Louis Russian Dressing, 8-fl.-oz. bottle	1296	16.8	(152.8)	(1.98)	1296	16.8	81.0	1.05
Pfeiffer, Russian Dressing, 8-fl.-oz. bottle	1040	32.0	130.0	4.00	(1131)	(34.8)	(70.8)	(2.18)
16-fl.-oz. (1-pint) bottle	2080	64.0	130.0	4.00	(1131)	(34.8)	(70.8)	(2.18)
Russian Dressing, Low-Cal, 8-fl.-oz. bottle	240	32.0	30.0	4.00	(261)	(34.8)	(16.3)	(2.18)
Seven Seas, Creamy Russian, 8-fl.-oz. bottle	1280	16.0	(147.1)	(1.84)	1280	160.0	80.0	1.00
16-fl.-oz. (1-pint) bottle	2560	32.0	(147.1)	(1.84)	1280	160.0	80.0	1.00
Weight Watchers, Russian Salad Dressing, 16-fl.-oz. (1-pint) jar	1600	64.0	(94.3)	(3.77)	800	32.0	50.0	2.00
Russian Salad Dressing Mix, 0.34-oz. envelope	24	0.0	70.6	0.00				

	UNIT		1 OZ., BY WT.		1 CUP		1 TABLE-SPOON	
	Cal.	Carb.	Cal.	Carb.	Cal.	Carb.	Cal.	Carb.
As prepared (yield: approx. ¾ cup, 6 fl. oz.)	48	12.0	(7.4)	(1.85)	64	16.0	4.0	1.00
Wish-Bone, Russian Dressing, 8-fl.-oz. bottle	800	112.0	(91.9)	(12.87)	800	112.0	50.0	7.00
16-fl.-oz. (1-pint) bottle	1600	224.0	(91.9)	(12.87)	800	112.0	50.0	7.00
Russian Dressing, Lite, 8-fl.-oz. bottle	400	80.0	(50.0)	(10.00)	400	8.0	25.0	5.00
"SALAD DRESSING"								
Ann Page (A&P), Salad Dressing, 8-fl.-oz. jar	1120	32.0	(132.2)	(3.78)	1120	32.0	70.0	2.00
16-fl.-oz. (1-pint) jar	2240	64.0	(132.2)	(3.78)	1120	32.0	70.0	2.00
Bright Day, Salad Dressing, 16-fl.-oz. (1-pint) jar	1920	64.0	113.3	(3.78)	960	32.0	60.0	2.00
Featherweight, Salad Dressing, Imitation, low calorie, 7.75-fl.-oz. bottle	231	0.0	(29.7)	0.00	256	0.0	16.0	0.00
Mrs. Filbert's, Salad Dressing, 16-fl.-oz. (1-pint) jar	2080	64.0	(123.1)	(3.79)	1040	32.0	65.0	2.00
Nu Made, Salad Dressing, 32-fl.-oz. (1-quart) jar	4800	120.0	150.0	3.75	1280	32.0	80.0	2.00
Piedmont, Salad Dressing, 16-fl.-oz. (1-pint) bottle	2100	60.0	131.3	3.75	1120	32.0	70.0	2.00
Saffola, Salad Dressing, 24-fl.-oz. bottle	2880	144.0	120.0	6.00	960	48.0	60.0	3.00
Scotch Buy, Salad Dressing, 32-fl.-oz. (1-quart) jar	4200	120.0	131.3	3.75	1120	32.0	70.0	2.00
Hellmann's, Spin Blend Salad Dressing, 32-oz. (1-quart) jar	3840	192.0	120.0	6.00	960	48.0	60.0	3.00
SESAME								
Sahadi, Creamy Sesame Salad Dressing, 8-fl.-oz. bottle	960	32.0	(113.3)	(3.78)	960	32.0	60.0	2.00
Spice Sesame Salad Dressing, 8-fl.-oz. bottle	1280	16.0	(160.0)	(2.00)	1280	16.0	80.0	1.00
TARRAGON								
Herb Magic, Tarragon Green Pepper Salad Dressing, no oil, 12-fl.-oz. bottle	192	48.0	16.0	4.00	128	32.0	8.0	2.00
THIN								
Mary's, Thin Dressing, 12-fl.-oz. bottle	96	24.0	(8.0)	(2.00)	64	16.0	4.0	1.00
THOUSAND ISLAND								
Dia-Mel, Lo-Cal 1000 Island Salad Dressing, 8-oz. box, 16 envelopes	320	0.0	40.0	0.00	(344)	0.0	(21.5)	0.00
1 envelope, approx. ½ oz.	20	0.0	40.0	0.00	(344)	0.0	(21.5)	0.00
Dieter's Gourmet, Thousand Island Dressing for Salads, 9-oz. box, 18 envelopes	252	36.0	28.0	4.00	224	32.0	14.0	2.00
1 envelope (ready to serve), approx. 0.5 oz.	14	2.0	28.0	4.00	224	32.0	14.0	2.00
Featherweight, Low Calorie Thousand Island Dressing, 7.75-fl.-oz. bottle	248	15.5	29.8	1.86	256	16.0	16.0	1.00
Frenchette, Low Calorie Thousand Island Dressing, 8-fl.-oz. bottle	336	48.0	(39.7)	(5.67)	336	48.0	21.0	3.00
Hain, Natural Creamy Thousand Island Dressing, 12-fl.-oz. bottle	1980	108.0	(152.7)	(8.33)	880	48.0	55.0	3.00
Henri's, Yogurt 1000 Island Dressing, 8-fl.-oz. bottle	320	64.0	(37.8)	(7.56)	320	64.0	20.0	4.00
Hidden Valley Ranch, Thousand Island Flavor Salad Dressing Mix, 0.5-oz. package								
As prepared with milk (yield: approx. 1 pint)	1760	25.3	(105.4)	(1.51)	880	12.6	55.0	0.79
As prepared with buttermilk (yield: approx. 1 pint)	(1690)	(24.3)	(10.2)	(1.46)	(845)	(12.2)	(52.8)	(0.76)
Kraft, Thousand Island Dressing, 8-fl.-oz. bottle	960	32.0	113.4	3.70	960	32.0	60.0	2.00
16-fl.-oz. (1-pint) bottle	1920	64.0	113.4	3.70	1920	64.0	60.0	2.00
Thousand Island Dressing, Low Calorie, 8-fl.-oz. bottle	480	32.0	56.7	3.70	480	32.0	30.0	2.00
16-fl.-oz. (1-pint) bottle	960	64.0	56.7	3.70	480	32.0	30.0	2.00
Nu Made, Reduced Calorie 1000 Island Dressing, 8-fl.-oz. bottle	480	32.0	(56.7)	(3.78)	480	32.0	30.0	2.00
Pfeiffer, 1000 Island Dressing, 8-fl.-oz. bottle	1040	32.0	(120.4)	(3.70)	1040	32.0	65.0	2.00
16-fl.-oz. (1-pint) bottle	2080	64.0	(120.4)	(3.70)	1040	32.0	65.0	2.00
Ralph's, 1000 Island Dressing, 16-fl.-oz. (1-pint) bottle	2400	48.0	(141.2)	(2.82)	1200	24.0	75.0	1.50
Seven Seas, Thousand Island, 8-fl.-oz. bottle	800	32.0	(92.6)	(3.70)	800	32.0	50.0	2.00
Tillie Lewis "Tasti Diet," Thousand Island Dressing, 8-fl.-oz. bottle	224	16.0	(25.9)	(1.85)	224	16.0	14.0	1.00

	UNIT		1 OZ., BY WT.		1 CUP		1 TABLE-SPOON	
	Cal.	Carb.	Cal.	Carb.	Cal.	Carb.	Cal.	Carb.
Walden Farms, Low Calorie Tangy Thousand Island Dressing, 12-fl.-oz. jar	576	(75.9)	(44.3)	(5.80)	386	50.6	24.0	3.20
Weight Watchers, Thousand Island Dressing, imitation 16-fl.-oz. (1-pint) jar	1600	64.0	(94.3)	(3.77)	800	32.0	50.0	2.00
Thousand Island Dressing Mix, 0.4-oz. envelope	24	0.0	60.0	0.00				
As prepared, add ¾ cup water (yield: approx. ¾ cup, 6 fl. oz.)	144	12.0	24.0	2.00	192	16.0	12.0	1.00
Wish-Bone, Thousand Island Dressing, 8-fl.-oz. bottle	960	48.0	(111.0)	(5.55)	960	48.0	60.0	3.00
16-fl.-oz. (1-pint) bottle	1920	96.0	(111.0)	(5.55)	960	48.0	60.0	3.00
Thousand Island Dressing, Lite, 8-fl.-oz. bottle	400	48.0	46.3	5.56	400	48.0	25.0	3.00
TWO-CALORIE								
Featherweight, Two-Calorie Dressing, low sodium, 8-fl.-oz. bottle	30	0.0	(3.8)	0.00	32	0.0	2.0	0.00
VINAIGRETTE								
Dieter's Gourmet, Creamy Vinaigrette Dressing, low oil, 9-oz. package	252	36.0	28.0	4.00	224	32.0	14.0	2.00
1 packet, approx. 0.5 oz.	14	2.0	28.0	4.00	224	32.0	14.0	2.00
WHIPPED								
Dia-Mel, Whipped Salad Dressing, Lo-Cal, Diet, 8-fl.-oz. bottle	352	33.9	44.0	4.24	352	33.9	22.0	2.12
Tillie Lewis, Whipped Dressing Salad Dressing Substitute, "Tasti Diet," 8-fl.-oz. bottle	640	32.0	(75.7)	(3.78)	640	32.0	40.0	2.00
YOGURT								
For Yogurt Bleu Cheese Dressing, look under "Bleu Cheese"; for Yogurt French Style Dressing, look under "French"; etc.								
MAYONNAISE								
MAYONNAISE, based on generic data								
1 teaspoon (approx. 0.2 oz.)	33	0.1	203.6	0.62	1580	4.8	101	0.3
1 tablespoon (approx. 0.5 oz.)	101	0.3	203.6	0.62	1580	4.8	101	0.3
1 cup (approx. 7.8 oz.)	1580	4.8	203.6	0.62	1580	4.8	101	0.3
1 pound (approx. 2.1 cups) (tr/1g/23g/15%/169mg)	3258	9.9	203.6	0.62	1580	4.8	101	0.3
MAYONNAISE, by brand								
Ann Page (A&P), Really Fine Mayonnaise, 16-fl.-oz. (1-pint) jar	3200	0.0	(202.5)	0.00	1600	0.0	100	0.0
1 teaspoon (approx. 0.2 oz.)	33	0.0	(202.5)	0.00	1600	0.0	100	0.0
Balanced, Balanaise Pure Mayonnaise (soy bean oil), 8-fl.-oz. jar	1600	0.0	(202.5)	0.00	1600	0.0	100	0.0
32-fl.-oz. (1-quart) jar	3200	0.0	(202.5)	0.00	1600	0.0	100	0.0
1 teaspoon (approx. 0.2 oz.)	33	0.0	(202.5)	0.00	1600	0.0	100	0.0
Hain, Mayonnaise, Sweetened with Honey, unsalted, no sugar, 24-fl.-oz. bottle	4800	0.0	(202.5)	0.00	1600	0.0	100	0.0
1 teaspoon (approx. 0.2 oz.)	33	0.0	(202.5)	0.00	1600	0.0	100	0.0
Safflower Mayonnaise, Sweetened with Honey, no sugar, 11-fl.-oz. jar	2200	0.0	(202.5)	0.00	1600	0.0	100	0.0
1 teaspoon (approx. 0.2 oz.)	33	0.0	(202.5)	0.00	1600	0.0	100	0.0
Hellman's, Mayonnaise, 8-fl.-oz. jar	1600	0.0	202.5	0.00	1600	0.0	100	0.0
16-fl.-oz. (1-pint) jar	3200	0.0	202.5	0.00	1600	0.0	100	0.0
32-fl.-oz. (1-quart) jar	6400	0.0	202.5	0.00	1600	0.0	100	0.0
1 teaspoon (approx. 0.2 oz.)	33	0.0	202.5	0.00	1600	0.0	100	0.0
Hollywood, unsalted Mayonnaise, 11-fl.-oz. jar	2200	0.0	200.0	0.00	1600	0.0	100	0.0
1 teaspoon (approx. 0.2 oz.)	33	0.0	200.0	0.00	1600	0.0	100	0.0
Safflower Mayonnaise, 11-fl.-oz. jar	2200	0.0	200.0	0.00	1600	0.0	100	0.0
24-fl.-oz. jar	4800	0.0	200.0	0.00	1600	0.0	100	0.0
1 teaspoon (approx. 0.2 oz.)	33	0.0	200.0	0.00	1600	0.0	100	0.0
Hunza, Safflower Mayonnaise, 11-fl.-oz. jar	2200	0.0	200.0	0.00	1600	0.0	100	0.0
1 teaspoon (approx. 0.2 oz.)	33	0.0	200.0	0.00	1600	0.0	100	0.0

	UNIT		1 OZ., BY WT.		1 CUP		1 TABLE-SPOON	
	Cal.	Carb.	Cal.	Carb.	Cal.	Carb.	Cal.	Carb.
Kraft, Real Mayonnaise, 16-fl.-oz. (1-pint) bottle	3200	0.0	202.5	0.00	1600	0.0	100	0.0
32-fl.-oz. (1-quart) bottle	6400	0.0	202.5	0.00	1600	0.0	100	0.0
1 teaspoon (approx. 0.2 oz.)	33	0.0	202.5	0.00	1600	0.0	100	0.0
Laura Scudder's, Mayonnaise, 32-fl.-oz. (1-quart) jar	6718	9.6	212.1	0.30	1672	2.4	105	0.2
1 teaspoon (approx. 0.2 oz.)	35	0.1	212.1	0.30	1672	2.4	105	0.2
Mrs. Filberts, Real Mayonnaise, 32-fl.-oz. (1-quart) jar	6400	0.0	200.0	0.00	1600	0.0	100	0.0
1 teaspoon (approx. 0.2 oz.)	33	0.0	200.0	0.00	1600	0.0	100	0.0
Nu Made, Real Mayonnaise, 32-fl.-oz. (1-quart) jar	6400	0.0	200.0	0.00	1600	0.0	100	0.0
Saffola, Mayonnaise, 24-fl.-oz. jar	4800	0.0	(205.1)	0.00	1600	0.0	100	0.0
1 teaspoon (approx. 0.2 oz.)	33	0.0	(205.1)	0.00	1600	0.0	100	0.0
Scotch Buy, Mayonnaise, 32-fl.-oz. (1-quart) jar	6400	0.0	200.0	0.00	1600	0.0	100	0.0

Mayonnaise Substitutes

	Cal.	Carb.	Cal.	Carb.	Cal.	Carb.	Cal.	Carb.
Bright Day, Imitation Mayonnaise Dressing, 16-fl.-oz. (1-pint) jar	1920	64.9	(120.0)	(4.00)	960	32.0	60	2.0
1 teaspoon (approx. 0.2 oz.)	20	0.7	(120.0)	(4.00)	960	32.0	60	2.0
Dia-Mel, Low Calorie Mayonnaise, 8-fl.-oz. jar	1696	0.0	(205.6)	0.00	1696	0.0	106	0.2
1 teaspoon (approx. 0.2 oz.)	35	0.0	(205.6)	0.00	1696	0.0	106	0.2
Featherweight, Low Sodium Soyamaise, 7.75-oz. jar	(1550)	0.0	(200.0)	0.00	1600	0.0	100	0.0
1 teaspoon (approx. 0.2 oz.)	33	0.0	(200.0)	0.00	1600	0.0	100	0.0
Hain, Eggless Imitation Mayonnaise, 11-fl.-oz. jar	1870	44.0	170.0	4.00	1360	32.0	85	2.0
1 teaspoon (approx. 0.2 oz.)	28	0.7	170.0	4.00	1360	32.0	85	2.0
Henri's, Yogonaise, 32-fl.-oz. (1-quart) jar	3840	128.0	(120.0)	(4.00)	960	32.0	60	2.0
Yogowip, 32-fl.-oz. (1-quart) jar	3840	192.0	(120.0)	(6.00)	960	48.0	60	3.0
Hollywood, Egg-Free Mayonnaise, 11-fl.-oz. jar	1870	44.0	170.0	4.00	1360	32.0	85	2.0
1 teaspoon (approx. 0.2 oz.)	28	0.7	170.0	4.00	1360	32.0	85	2.0
Kraft, Miracle Whip, 16-fl.-oz. (1-pint) bottle	2240	64.0	(132.3)	4.00	1120	32.0	70	2.0
32-fl.-oz. (1-quart) bottle	4480	128.0	(132.3)	4.00	1120	32.0	70	2.0
1 teaspoon (approx. 0.2 oz.)	23	0.7	(132.3)	4.00	1120	32.0	70	2.0
Light N' Lively, Reduced Calorie Mayonnaise, 32-fl.-oz. (1-quart) jar	2560	64.0	(80.0)	(2.00)	640	16.0	40	1.0
Mrs. Filberts, Imitation Mayonnaise, 16-fl.-oz. (1-pint) jar	1280	32.0	(80.0)	(2.00)	640	16.0	40	1.0
1 teaspoon (approx. 0.2 oz.)	13	0.3	(80.0)	(2.00)	640	16.0	40	1.0
Saffola. Imitation Mayonnaise, 16-fl.-oz. (1-pint) jar	1920	32.0	(123.1)	(2.05)	960	16.0	60	1.0
1 teaspoon (approx. 0.2 oz.)	20	0.3	(123.1)	(2.05)	960	16.0	60	1.0
Scotch Buy, Imitation Mayonnaise, 32-fl.-oz. (1-quart) jar	3200	0.0	100.0	0.00	800	0.0	50	0.0
Spredlite (Batter-Lite), Mayonnaise, 8-fl.-oz. jar	(704)	(16.0)	(88.0)	(2.00)	704	16.0	44	1.0
1 teaspoon (approx. 0.2 oz.)	15	0.3	(88.0)	(2.00)	704	16.0	44	1.0
Tillie Lewis "Tasti Diet," Low Calorie May-Lo-Naise, 8-fl.-oz. jar	400	16.0	(48.5)	(1.94)	400	16.0	25	1.0
1 teaspoon (approx. 0.2 oz.)	8	0.3	(48.5)	(1.94)	400	16.0	25	1.0
Weight Watchers, Imitation Mayonnaise, 16-fl.-oz. (1-pint) jar	1280	128.0	(80.0)	(8.00)	640	64.0	40	4.0
1 teaspoon (approx. 0.2 oz.)	13	1.3	(80.0)	(8.00)	640	64.0	40	4.0
Reduced Calorie Mayonnaise, 32-fl.-oz. (1-quart) jar	2560	64.0	(80.0)	(2.00)	640	16.0	40	1.0
1 teaspoon (approx. 0.2 oz.)	13	0.3	(80.0)	(2.00)	640	16.0	40	1.0

SOUR CREAM

	Cal.	Carb.	Cal.	Carb.	Cal.	Carb.	Cal.	Carb.
HALF AND HALF SOUR CREAM, based on generic data (12% fat)								
1 cup (approx. 8.5 oz.)	320	28.8	38.3	3.40	320	28.8	31	0.6
1 pound (approx. 1.9 cups)	613	54.4	38.3	3.40	320	28.8	31	0.6
1 teaspoon (approx. 0.2 oz.)	7	0.6	38.3	3.40	320	28.8	20	1.8
SOUR CREAM, based on generic data (20.96% fat)								
1 cup (approx. 8.1 oz.)	492	9.8	60.7	1.21	492	9.8	31	0.6
1 pound (approx. 2 cups)	971	19.4	60.7	1.21	492	9.8	31	0.6
1 teaspoon (approx. 0.2 oz.)	10	0.2	60.7	1.21	492	9.8	31	0.6
SOUR CREAM, by brand								
Axelrod, Cultured (17.6% fat), 8-oz. container	400	8.0	50.0	1.00	(400)	(8.0)	(25)	(0.5)
16-oz. (1-lb.) container	800	16.0	50.0	1.00	(400)	(8.0)	(25)	(0.5)
Country Fresh (20.5% fat), 8-oz. container	485	10.0	60.6	1.25	(485)	(10.0)	(30)	(0.6)
Dairy Barn (20.5% fat), 16-oz. (1-lb.) container	970	20.0	60.6	1.25	(485)	(10.0)	(30)	(0.6)
Fikes (20.5% fat), 8-oz. container	485	10.0	60.6	1.25	(485)	(10.0)	(30)	(0.6)
Foodland (20.5% fat), 8-oz. container	485	10.0	60.6	1.25	(485)	(10.0)	(30)	(0.6)
Friendship (18% fat), 8-oz. container	440	5.9	55.0	0.74	(440)	(5.9)	(28)	(0.4)
16-oz. (1-lb.) container	880	11.8	55.0	0.74	(440)	(5.9)	(28)	(0.4)
Knudsen, real Hampshire Sour Cream, 8-fl.-oz. container	480	8.0	60.0	1.00	480	8.0	30	0.5
Sealtest "All Natural" (18% fat), 16-oz. (1-lb.) container	960	24.0	60.0	1.50	(450)	(11.3)	(30)	(0.7)
Zausner (20.5% fat), 8-oz. container	485	10.0	60.6	1.25	(485)	(10.0)	(30)	(0.6)
16-oz. (1-lb.) container	970	20.0	60.6	1.25	(485)	(10.0)	(30)	(0.6)

Sour Cream, Imitation, and Non-Butterfat Sour Dressing

	Cal.	Carb.	Cal.	Carb.	Cal.	Carb.	Cal.	Carb.
FILLED CREAM-TYPE NON-BUTTERFAT SOUR DRESSING, based on generic data (16.6% fat)								
1 cup (approx. 8.3 oz.)	417	11.0	50.5	1.33	417	11.0	21	0.6
1 pound (approx. 1.9 cups)	806	21.2	50.5	1.33	417	11.0	21	0.6
1 teaspoon (approx. 0.2 oz.)	7	0.2	50.5	1.33	417	11.0	21	0.6
NONDAIRY IMITATION SOUR CREAM, based on generic data								
1 cup (approx. 8.1 oz.)	479	15.3	59.9	1.88	479	15.3	30	1.0
1 pound (approx. 2 cups)	946	30.1	59.9	1.88	479	15.3	30	1.0
1 teaspoon (approx. 0.2 oz.)	10	0.3	59.9	1.88	479	15.3	30	1.0
NONDAIRY IMITATION SOUR CREAM, by brand								
Friendship Sour Treat, 16-oz. (1-lb.) container	784	24.0	49.0	1.50	(392)	(12.0)	(25)	(0.8)
King Sour Non-Butterfat Sour Dressing, 16-fl.-oz. (1-lb.) container	560	16.0	(35.0)	(1.00)	280	8.0	18	0.5
Ralph's Imitation Sour Cream, 16-fl.-oz. (1-lb.) container	1040	24.0	65.0	1.50	520	12.0	33	0.8

YOGURT, PLAIN, based on generic data

(Yogurt has its own chapter, directly preceding this one.)

	Cal.	Carb.	Cal.	Carb.	Cal.	Carb.	Cal.	Carb.
Low-fat yogurt, 1 teaspoon (approx. 0.2 oz.)	(3)	(0.4)	17.9	2.00	(158)	(17.5)	(10)	(1.1)
Skim-milk yogurt, 1 teaspoon (approx. 0.2 oz.)	(3)	(0.4)	15.9	2.18	(139)	(19.1)	(9)	(1.2)
Whole-milk yogurt, 1 teaspoon (approx. 0.2 oz.)	(3)	trace	17.3	1.32	(150)	(11.4)	(9)	(0.7)

SAUCES, SPREADS, and SEASONINGS

Many other sauces can be found in the BASIC BAKING & COOKING INGREDIENTS chapter.

A-1, see STEAK SAUCE

APPLESAUCE

Additional applesauces are in the FRUITS chapter.

	Cal.	Carb.	Cal.	Carb.	Cal.	Carb.	Cal.	Carb.
Applesauce, **Blue Boy,** 8½-oz. jar	215	53.8	25.3	6.33	200	50.0	13	3.1
16-oz. (1-lb.) jar	405	101.3	25.3	6.33	200	50.0	13	3.1
50-oz. jar	1265	316.5	25.3	6.33	200	50.0	13	3.1
1 teaspoon (approx. 0.2 oz.)	4	1.0	25.3	6.33	200	50.0	13	3.1

	UNIT		1 OZ., BY WT.		1 CUP		1 TABLESPOON	
	Cal.	Carb.	Cal.	Carb.	Cal.	Carb.	Cal.	Carb.
Applesauce, **Del Monte,** 8½-oz. jar	181	49.9	21.3	5.88	170	47.0	11	2.9
16-oz. (1-lb.) jar	340	94.0	21.3	5.88	170	47.0	11	2.9
Applesauce, Prepared without sugar or salt, **Featherweight,** 8-oz. can	100	24.0	12.5	3.00	100	24.0	6	1.5
16-oz. (1-lb.) can	200	48.0	12.5	3.00	100	24.0	6	1.5
Applesauce, **Golden Harvest,** 16-oz. (1-lb.) jar	240	60.0	15.0	3.75	120	30.0	8	1.9
25-oz. jar	375	93.8	15.0	3.75	120	30.0	8	1.9
1 teaspoon (approx. 0.2 oz.)	3	0.6	15.0	3.75	120	30.0	8	1.9
Applesauce, Regular, **Musselman's,** 8-oz. jar	(170)	(41.5)	(21.3)	(5.18)	193	47.0	12	2.9
Natural Style, 16½-oz. jar	(200)	(48.0)	(12.1)	(2.91)	100	24.0	6	1.5
25-oz. jar	(303)	(72.8)	(12.1)	(2.91)	100	24.0	6	1.5
Apple Barrel Sauce, **Seneca,** 35-oz. jar	810	198.0	23.1	5.60	180	44.0	11	2.8
Applesauce, 100% Natural, **Seneca,** 24-oz. jar	275	66.0	11.5	2.75	100	24.0	6	1.5
1 teaspoon (approx. 0.2 oz.)	2	0.5	11.5	2.75	100	24.0	6	1.5
Cinnamon Applesauce, **Seneca,** 35-oz. jar	698	170.5	20.0	4.90	180	44.0	11	2.8
McIntosh Applesauce, **Seneca,** 15-oz. jar	300	73.3	20.0	4.90	180	44.0	11	2.8
Applesauce, Unsweetened, **Tillie Lewis** "Tasti Diet," 8¼-oz. can	120	30.0	14.5	3.64	120	30.0	8	1.9
AVOCADO SAUCE								
Avocado Sauce, **Nickabood's** "Fisherman's Wharf," 8-fl.-oz. bottle	1088	4.8	128.3	0.57	1088	4.8	68	0.3
1 teaspoon (approx. 0.2 oz.)	23	0.1	128.3	0.57	1088	4.8	68	0.3
BURGER SAUCE								
"Big H" Burger Sauce, **Hellman's,** 12-fl.-oz. jar	1610	46.0	132.0	3.77	1120	32.0	70	2.0
18-fl.-oz. jar	2415	69.0	132.0	3.77	1120	32.0	70	2.0
1 teaspoon (approx. 0.2 oz.)	23	0.7	132.0	3.77	1120	32.0	70	2.0
BUTTER, based on generic data								
1 teaspoon (approx. 0.2 oz.)	34	trace	203.0	0.11	1625	0.1	102	0.1
1 tablespoon (approx. 0.5 oz.)	102	0.1	203.0	0.11	1625	0.1	102	0.1
1 pat (approx. 0.18 oz.)	36	trace	203.0	0.11	1625	0.1	102	0.1
More on Butter is in the FATS & OILS chapter.								
CATSUP, based on generic data								
1 pound (approx. 1⅔ cups) (tr/7g/tr/69%/295mg)	481	115.2	30.1	7.20	289	69.3	18	4.3
1 cup (approx. 9.6 oz.)	289	69.3	30.1	7.20	289	69.3	18	4.3
1 teaspoon (approx. 0.2 oz.)	6	1.4	30.1	7.20	289	69.3	18	4.3
1 bottle, 12 oz. net wt.	361	86.4	30.1	7.20	289	69.3	18	4.3
14 oz. net wt.	421	100.8	30.1	7.20	289	69.3	18	4.3
20 oz. net wt.	602	144.0	30.1	7.20	289	69.3	18	4.3
Restaurant packet, ½ oz. (approx. 1 tablespoon)	(18)	(4.3)	30.1	7.20	289	69.3	18	4.3
CATSUP, by brand								
Catsup, **Blue Boy,** 14-oz. bottle	497	126.9	35.4	9.07	250	64.0	16	4.0
20-oz. bottle	708	181.4	35.4	9.07	250	64.0	16	4.0
24-oz. bottle	850	217.7	35.4	9.07	250	64.0	16	4.0
1 teaspoon (approx. 0.2 oz.)	5	1.3	35.4	9.07	250	64.0	16	4.0
Catsup, low calorie, no salt, **Featherweight,** 11-oz. bottle	132	22.0	12.0	2.00	(120)	(20.0)	(8)	(1.3)
1 teaspoon (approx. 0.2 oz.)	3	0.4	12.0	2.00	(120)	(20.0)	(8)	(1.3)
Catsup Substitute, dry mix, **Weight Watchers,** 0.64-oz. package prepared (yield: 1 cup, 8.6 oz.)	64	16.0	(7.4)	(1.86)	64	16.0	4	1.0
Prepared, 1 teaspoon (approx. 0.2 oz.)	1	0.3	(7.4)	(1.86)	64	16.0	4	1.0
Tomato Catsup, **Del Monte,** 14-fl.-oz. bottle	420	112.0	30.0	8.00	240	64.0	15	4.0
24-fl.-oz. bottle	720	192.0	30.0	8.00	240	64.0	15	4.0
1 teaspoon (approx. 0.2 oz.)	5	1.3	30.0	8.00	240	64.0	15	4.0
Tomato Catsup, imitation, **Dia-Mel,** 13-oz. bottle	(146)	(31.1)	(11.2)	(2.40)	112	24.0	7	1.5
1 teaspoon (approx. 0.2 oz.)	2	0.5	(11.2)	(2.40)	112	24.0	7	1.5
Tomato Catsup, imitation, no salt added, **Tillie Lewis** "Tasti Diet," 12½-oz. bottle	420	126.0	33.6	10.10	320	96.0	20	6.0
1 teaspoon (approx. 0.2 oz.)	7	2.0	33.6	10.10	320	96.0	20	6.0
CHILI SAUCE, based on generic data								
1 cup, 8.7 oz. (tr/1g/tr/94%/na)	50	12.4	5.7	1.42	50	12.4	3	0.8
1 teaspoon (approx. 0.2 oz.)	1	0.3	5.7	1.42	50	12.4	3	0.8

	UNIT		1 OZ., BY WT.		1 CUP		1 TABLESPOON	
	Cal.	Carb.	Cal.	Carb.	Cal.	Carb.	Cal.	Carb.
CHILE SAUCE, by brand								
Chili Hot Dog Sauce, **Gebhardt,** 10-oz. can	(115)	26.1	(11.5)	2.61				
Chili Sauce, low sodium, **Featherweight,** 11-oz. container	176	33.0	16.0	3.00	(139)	(26.1)	(9)	(1.6)
1 teaspoon (approx. 0.2 oz.)	(3)	(0.5)	16.0	3.00	(139)	(26.1)	(9)	(1.6)
Chutney Chile Sauce, **Smithers,** 12-oz. bottle	589	94.9	49.1	7.91	397	63.2	25	4.0
1 teaspoon (approx. 0.2 oz.)	8	1.3	49.1	7.91	397	63.2	25	4.0
CHUTNEY								
Chutney, (Major Grey's), **Crosse & Blackwell,** 9-oz. jar	273	64.0	30.3	7.11				
22-oz. jar	668	156.6	30.3	7.11				
COCKTAIL SAUCE								
Cocktail Sauce, **Nickabood's** "Fisherman's Wharf," 8-fl.-oz. bottle	264	54.4	31.1	6.46	264	54.4	17	3.4
1 teaspoon (approx. 0.2 oz.)	6	1.1	31.1	6.46	264	54.4	17	3.4
Seafood Cocktail Sauce, **Smither's,** 12-oz. bottle	420	102.0	(35.0)	(8.50)	280	68.0	18	4.3
1 teaspoon (approx. 0.2 oz.)	6	1.4	(35.0)	(8.50)	280	68.0	18	4.3
CRANBERRY SAUCE, based on generic data								
Made-from-scratch, based on USDA home recipe, with ingredients as follows: 1 lb. (approx. 4 cups) cranberries, 1 cup water, 2 cups sugar, unstrained (yield: approx. 3½ cups, approx. 34 oz.) (tr/13g/tr/54%/tr)	(1730)	(442.3)	53.0	12.89	493	126.0	31	7.9
1 cup (approx. 9.8 oz.)	493	126.0	53.0	12.89	493	126.0	31	7.9
CRANBERRY SAUCE, by brand								
Cranberry Sauce, Jellied, **Ocean Spray,** 16-oz. (1-lb.) can	720	176.0	45.0	11.00	(430)	(105.1)	(27)	(6.6)
Cranberry Sauce, Jellied, **Town House,** 16-oz. (1-lb.) can	800	200.0	50.0	12.50	478	119.4	30	7.5
Cranberry Sauce, Whole, **Ocean Spray,** 16-oz. (1-lb.) can	720	168.0	45.0	10.50	(430)	(105.1)	(27)	(6.6)
Cranberry Sauce, Whole Berry, **Ocean Spray,** 16-oz. (1-lb.) jar	720	176.0	45.0	11.00	(430)	(105.1)	(27)	(6.6)
Cran-Raspberry Jellied Sauce, **Ocean Spray,** 16-oz. (1-lb.) jar	720	168.0	45.0	10.50	(430)	(105.1)	(27)	(6.6)
DIABLE								
Sauce Diable, **Escoffier,** 6-oz. bottle	(200)	(42.0)	(33.3)	(7.00)	320	67.2	20	4.2
1 teaspoon (approx. 0.2 oz.)	7	1.4	(33.3)	(7.00)	320	67.2	20	4.2
DUCK SAUCE								
Plum Duck Sauce, **China Bowl,** 6-oz. bottle	330	46.3	55.0	7.71	(611)	(85.7)	(38)	(5.4)
1 teaspoon (approx. 0.2 oz.)	(13)	(1.8)	55.0	7.71	(611)	(85.7)	(38)	(5.4)
ENGLISH SAUCE								
English Sauce, **Smithers,** 5½-oz. bottle	124	27.8	22.6	5.05	184	40.0	12	2.5
1 teaspoon (approx. 0.2 oz.)	4	0.8	22.6	5.05	184	40.0	12	2.5
FISH SAUCE								
Fish Sauce, **China Bowl,** 6-oz. bottle	87	1.9	14.5	0.31	(120)	(2.6)	(8)	(0.2)
1 teaspoon (approx. 0.2 oz.)	(3)	(0.1)	14.5	0.31	(120)	(2.6)	(8)	(0.2)
Fish Sauce, **Dieter's Gourmet,** 18-oz. box, 18 packets	252	36.0	14.0	2.00	(113)	(16.2)	(7)	(1.0)
1 packet, approx. 1 oz.	14	2.0	14.0	2.00	(113)	(16.2)	(7)	(1.0)
1 teaspoon (approx. 0.2 oz.)	(2)	(0.3)	14.0	2.00	(113)	(16.2)	(7)	(1.0)
GREEN CHILE SALSA								
Green Chile Salsa, **Ortega,** 7-oz. can	42	7.0	6.0	1.00	(58)	(9.6)	(4)	(0.6)
12-oz. jar	72	12.0	6.0	1.00	(58)	(9.6)	(4)	(0.6)
24-oz. jar	144	24.0	6.0	1.00	(58)	(9.6)	(4)	(0.6)
28-oz. jar	168	28.0	6.0	1.00	(58)	(9.6)	(4)	(0.6)
102-oz. can	612	102.0	6.0	1.00	(58)	(9.6)	(4)	(0.6)
1 teaspoon (approx. 0.2 oz.)	1	0.2	6.0	1.00	(58)	(9.6)	(4)	(0.6)
HORSERADISH								
Horseradish, **Gold's,** 4-oz. jar	50	10.5	12.5	2.63	100	21.0	6	1.3
6-oz. jar	76	15.8	12.5	2.63	100	21.0	6	1.3
8-oz. jar	100	21.0	12.5	2.63	100	21.0	6	1.3
1 teaspoon (approx. 0.2 oz.)	2	0.4	12.5	2.63	100	21.0	6	1.3
Horseradish Sauce, **Kraft,** 9-oz. jar	900	90.0	100.0	10.00	800	80.0	50	5.0
1 teaspoon (approx. 0.2 oz.)	17	1.7	100.0	10.00	800	80.0	50	5.0

	UNIT		1 OZ., BY WT.		1 CUP		1 TABLESPOON	
	Cal.	Carb.	Cal.	Carb.	Cal.	Carb.	Cal.	Carb.
Horseradish Sauce, **Nickabood's,** "Fisherman's Wharf," 8-fl.-oz. bottle	944	15.2	(111.3)	(1.79)	944	15.2	59	1.0
1 teaspoon (approx. 0.2 oz.)	20	0.3	111.3	1.79	944	15.2	59	1.0
HOT OIL								
Hot Oil, **China Bowl,** 5-oz. bottle	1252	0.0	250.4	0.00	(1927)	0.0	(120)	0.0
1 teaspoon (approx. 0.2 oz.)	(40)	0.0	250.4	0.00	(1927)	0.0	(120)	0.0
HOT SAUCE								
Hot Sauce, **Frank's,** 12-oz. can	672	112.0	56.0	9.33	576	96.0	36	6.0
1 teaspoon (approx. 0.2 oz.)	12	2.0	56.0	9.33	576	96.0	36	6.0
LEMON JUICE, based on generic data								
Juice of 1 medium lemon (approx. 3 tablespoons, approx. 1.7 oz.)	(12)	(3.8)	7.1	2.27	61	19.5	4	1.2
Juice of 1 1⅝" arc wedge, ¼ of fruit (approx. 1 tablespoon, 0.4 oz.)	(3)	(1.0)	7.1	2.27	61	19.9	4	1.2
Juice of 1 1⅛" arc wedge, ⅙ of fruit (approx. 0.5 tablespoon, 0.3 oz.)	(2)	(0.6)	7.1	2.27	61	19.9	4	1.2
1 teaspoon	1	0.4	7.1	2.27	61	19.9	4	1.2
MARGARINE, based on generic data								
1 teaspoon (approx. 0.2 oz.)	34	trace	204.1	0.11	1634	0.9	102	0.1
1 tablespoon (approx. ½ oz.)	102	0.1	204.1	0.11	1634	0.9	102	0.1
1 pat (approx. 0.18 oz.)	36	trace	204.1	0.11	1634	0.9	102	0.1
More on Margarine is in the FATS & OILS chapter.								
MAYONNAISE has its own section earlier in this chapter.								
MUSTARD, based on generic data								
Brown Mustard, 6-oz. jar (2g/2g/2g/78%/371mg)	155	9.1	25.9	1.51	228	13.3	14	0.8
1 teaspoon (approx. 0.2 oz.)	5	0.3	25.9	1.51	288	13.3	14	0.8
Yellow Mustard, 6-oz. jar (1g/2g/1g/80%/355mg)	128	10.9	21.3	1.81	188	16.0	12	1.0
1 teaspoon (approx. 0.2 oz.)	4	0.3	21.3	1.81	188	16.0	12	1.0
MUSTARD, by brand								
Brown 'N Spicy Mustard, **French's,** 6-oz. jar	160	10.6	26.6	1.77	240	16.0	15	1.0
1 teaspoon (approx. 0.2 oz.)	5	0.3	26.6	1.77	240	16.0	15	1.0
Cream Salad Mustard, **French's,** 6-oz. jar	113	11.3	18.9	1.89	160	16.0	10	1.0
12-oz. jar	227	22.7	18.9	1.89	160	16.0	10	1.0
24-oz. jar	454	45.4	18.9	1.89	160	16.0	10	1.0
1 teaspoon (approx. 0.2 oz.)	3	0.3	18.9	1.89	160	16.0	10	1.0
Diablo Mustard, **Gulden's,** 5-oz. jar	160	0.0	32.0	0.00	(283)	0.0	(18)	0.0
1 teaspoon (approx. 0.2 oz.)	(6)	0.0	32.0	0.00	(283)	0.0	(18)	0.0
Dijon Mustard, **Grey Poupon,** 8-oz. jar	240	(9.9)	30.0	(1.24)	288	(11.0)	18	(0.7)
1 teaspoon (approx. 0.2 oz.)	6	(0.2)	30.0	(1.24)	288	(11.0)	18	(0.7)
Dijon Mustard, salt free, **Reine,** 7¼-oz. jar	259	0.0	35.7	0.00	(316)	0.0	(20)	0.0
1 teaspoon (approx. 0.2 oz.)	(7)	0.0	35.7	0.00	(316)	0.0	(20)	0.0
Low Sodium Mustard, **Featherweight,** 6-oz. jar	0	0.0	0.0	0.00	0	0.0	0	0.0
1 teaspoon (approx. 0.2 oz.)	0	0.0	0.0	0.00	0	0.0	0	0.0
Medford Mustard, **French's,** 16-oz. (1-lb.) jar	454	28.3	28.4	1.77	256	16.0	16	1.0
1 teaspoon (approx. 0.2 oz.)	5	0.3	28.4	1.77	256	16.0	16	1.0
Mr. Mustard, **Mr. Mustard,** 5-oz. jar	264	9.6	52.8	1.92	528	19.2	33	1.2
1 teaspoon (approx. 0.2 oz.)	11	0.4	52.8	1.92	528	19.2	33	1.2
Mustard with Horseradish, **French's,** 6-oz. jar	160	10.6	26.6	1.77	240	16.0	15	1.0
1 teaspoon (approx. 0.2 oz.)	5	0.3	26.6	1.77	240	16.0	15	1.0
Mustard with Onions, **French's,** 6-oz. jar	250	50.0	41.7	8.34	400	80.0	25	5.0
1 teaspoon (approx. 0.2 oz.)	8	1.7	41.7	8.34	400	80.0	25	5.0
For Mustard Powder, see the SALTS & SPICES chapter.								
OYSTER SAUCE								
Oyster Sauce, **China Bowl,** 8-oz. bottle	256	39.7	32.0	4.96	(256)	(39.7)	(16)	(2.5)
1 teaspoon (approx. 0.2 oz.)	(5)	(0.8)	32.0	4.96	(256)	(39.7)	(16)	(2.5)
PICANTE SAUCE								
Picante Sauce, **Picante, Inc.,** 16-oz. (1-lb.) jar	180	30.0	11.3	1.88	96	16.0	6	1.0
1 teaspoon (approx. 0.2 oz.)	2	0.3	11.3	1.88	96	16.0	6	1.0
Picante Sauce, Tostitos, **Frito-Lay,** 10½-oz. tin	150	26.7	14.3	2.54	(121)	(21.6)	(8)	(1.3)
1 teaspoon (approx. 0.2 oz.)	(3)	(0.4)	14.3	2.54	(121)	(21.6)	(8)	(1.3)
ROBERT								
Sauce Robert, **Escoffier,** 6-oz. bottle	(190)	(45.0)	(31.7)	(7.50)	304	72.0	19	4.5
1 teaspoon (approx. 0.2 oz.)	6	1.5	(31.7)	(7.50)	304	72.0	19	4.5
SALAD DRESSINGS have their own section earlier in this chapter.								
SEAFOOD COCKTAIL SAUCE, see COCKTAIL SAUCE								
SESAME								
Sesame Oil, **China Bowl,** 5-oz. bottle	1250	0.2	250.0	0.03	(1927)	(0.2)	(120)	trace
1 teaspoon (approx. 0.2 oz.)	(40)	trace	250.0	0.03	(1927)	(0.2)	(120)	trace
SOUR CREAM, based on generic data								
Sour Cream, 1 teaspoon (approx. 0.2 oz.)	10	0.2	60.7	1.21	493	9.8	31	0.6
Sour Cream, Imitation, 1 teaspoon (approx. 0.2 oz.)	10	0.3	59.0	1.88	479	15.3	30	1.0
More on Sour Cream can be found in the SOUR CREAM section, which immediately precedes this list.								
SOY SAUCE, based on generic data								
1 cup, 10.2 oz. (tr/3g/2g/63%/2077mg)	197	29.6	19.3	2.69	197	29.6	12	1.9
1 teaspoon (approx. 0.2 oz.)	4	0.6	19.3	2.69	197	29.6	12	1.9
SOY SAUCE, by brand								
Soy Sauce, **La Choy,** 5-oz. bottle	83	9.1	16.6	1.81	(170)	(18.5)	(11)	(1.2)
10-oz. bottle	166	18.1	16.6	1.81	(170)	(18.5)	(11)	(1.2)
16-oz. (1-lb.) bottle	266	29.0	16.6	1.81	(170)	(18.5)	(11)	(1.2)
1 teaspoon (approx. 0.2 oz.)	(4)	(0.4)	16.6	1.81	(170)	(18.5)	(11)	(1.2)
Dark Soy Sauce, **China Bowl,** 5-oz. bottle	122	21.4	24.4	4.28	(249)	(43.8)	(16)	(2.7)
12-oz. bottle	293	51.4	24.4	4.28	(249)	(43.8)	(16)	(2.7)
1 teaspoon (approx. 0.2 oz.)	(5)	(0.9)	24.4	4.28	(249)	(43.8)	(16)	(2.7)
Light Soy Sauce, **China Bowl,** 5-oz. bottle	78	11.5	15.6	2.30	(160)	(23.5)	(10)	(1.5)
12-oz. bottle	187	27.6	15.6	2.30	(160)	(23.5)	(10)	(1.5)
1 teaspoon (approx. 0.2 oz.)	(3)	(0.5)	15.6	2.30	(160)	(23.5)	(10)	(1.5)
Tamari, **Arrowhead Mills,** 16-fl.-oz. (1-pint) bottle	480	64.0	(30.0)	(4.00)	240	32.0	15	2.0
1 teaspoon (approx. 0.2 oz.)	5	0.7	(30.0)	(4.00)	240	32.0	15	2.0
STEAK SAUCE								
Steak Sauce, **A-1,** 5-oz. bottle	(100)	(23.4)	(20.0)	(4.7)	192	44.8	12	2.8
10-oz. bottle	(200)	(46.7)	(20.0)	(4.67)	192	44.8	12	2.8
1 teaspoon (approx. 0.2 oz.)	4	0.9	(20.0)	(4.67)	192	44.8	12	2.8
Steak Sauce, **Steak Supreme,** 5-oz. bottle	167	(39.9)	33.3	(7.97)	320	(76.5)	20	(4.8)
10-oz. bottle	333	(79.7)	33.3	(7.97)	320	(76.5)	20	(4.8)
1 teaspoon (approx. 0.2 oz.)	7	(1.6)	33.3	(7.97)	320	(76.5)	20	(4.8)
SWEET AND SOUR SAUCE								
Sweet and Sour Sauce, **La Choy,** 10-oz. can	514	125.7	51.4	12.57	(450)	(110.0)	(28)	(6.9)
1 teaspoon (approx. 0.2 oz.)	(9)	(2.3)	51.4	12.57	(450)	(110.0)	(28)	(6.9)
TABASCO								
Tabasco Pepper Sauce, **Tabasco,** 2-fl.-oz. bottle	7	0.7	3.1	0.31	26	2.7	2	0.2
12-fl.-oz. bottle	40	4.0	3.1	0.31	26	2.7	2	0.2
1 teaspoon (approx. 0.2 oz.)	1	0.1	3.1	0.31	26	2.7	2	0.2
TACO SAUCE								
Taco Sauce, Regular, **Ortega,** 1-oz. pouch	37	8.3	36.7	8.34	352	80.0	22	5.0
8-fl.-oz. bottle	352	80.0	36.7	8.34	352	80.0	22	5.0
102-oz. can	3742	850.5	36.7	8.34	352	80.0	22	5.0
1 teaspoon (approx. 0.2 oz.)	7	1.7	36.7	8.34	352	80.0	22	5.0
Taco Sauce, Hot, **Ortega,** 8-fl.-oz. bottle	352	80.0	36.7	8.34	352	80.0	22	5.0
102-oz. can	3742	850.5	36.7	8.34	352	80.0	22	5.0
1 teaspoon (approx. 0.2 oz.)	7	1.7	36.7	8.34	352	80.0	22	5.0
TAHINI (based on data from the Middle East)								
Tehineh (Tahini) (based on data from the Middle East), 1 pound (6g/3g/18g/3%/na)	3139	46.3	196.2	2.89				
TAHINI, by brand								
Tahini (Sesame Butter), **Protein Aide,** 1 tablespoon (approx. 0.5 oz.)	101	2.3	180.0	4.00	1620	36.0	101	2.3
1 teaspoon (approx. 0.2 oz.)	34	0.8	180.0	4.00	1620	36.0	101	2.3

	UNIT		1 OZ., BY WT.		1 CUP		1 TABLE-SPOON	
	Cal.	Carb.	Cal.	Carb.	Cal.	Carb.	Cal.	Carb.
TAMARI, see SOY SAUCE								
TARTAR SAUCE, based on generic data								
Tartar Sauce, Regular, 1 cup, 8.1-oz. (tr/1g/16g/34%/200mg)	1221	9.7	150.6	1.19	1221	9.7	74	0.6
1 teaspoon (approx. 0.2 oz.)	25	0.2	150.6	1.19	1221	9.7	74	0.6
Low-Calorie, 1 cup (approx. 8 oz. (tr/2g/6g/68%/200mg)	(496)	(14.4)	63.5	1.90	515	15.4	31	0.9
1 teaspoon (approx. 0.2 oz.)	11	0.3	63.5	1.90	515	15.4	31	0.9
TARTAR SAUCE, by brand								
Tartar Sauce, **Best Foods,** 16-oz. jar	2314	6.4	144.6	0.40	1125	3.1	70	0.2
6-fl.-oz. jar	868	2.4	144.6	0.40	1125	3.1	70	0.2
1 teaspoon (approx. 0.2 oz.)	23	0.1	144.6	0.40	1125	3.1	70	0.2
Tartar Sauce, **Seven Seas,** 8-fl.-oz. bottle	1280	16.0	(160.0)	(2.00)	1280	16.0	80	1.0
1 teaspoon (approx. 0.2 oz.)	27	0.3	(160.0)	(2.00)	1280	16.0	80	1.0
Tartar Sauce, **Shopwell,** 8-fl.-oz. jar	1280	16.0	(160.0)	(2.00)	1280	16.0	80	1.0
1 teaspoon (approx. 0.2 oz.)	27	0.3	(160.0)	(2.00)	1280	16.0	80	1.0
TIGER SAUCE								
Tiger Sauce, **Tulkoffs,** 8-oz. jar	1120	16.0	140.0	2.00	1120	16.0	70	1.0
1 teaspoon (approx. 0.2 oz.)	23	0.3	140.0	2.00	1120	16.0	70	1.0
VINEGAR, based on generic data								
Cider Vinegar, 1 quart (32 fl. oz.; 33.9 oz. by weight) (0g/2g/0g/94%/tr)	134	56.6	4.0	1.67	34	14.2	2	0.9
1 teaspoon (approx. 0.2 oz.)	1	0.3	4.0	1.67	34	14.2	2	0.9
Distilled Vinegar, 1 quart (32 fl. oz.; 33.9 oz. by weight) (0g/1g/0g/95%/tr)	115	48.0	3.4	1.42	29	12.0	2	0.8
1 teaspoon (approx. 0.2 oz.)	1	0.3	3.4	1.42	29	12.0	2	0.8
VINEGAR, by brand								
Champagne Vinegar, **Regina,** 12-fl.-oz. bottle	48	(1.4)	3.8	(0.11)	32	(1.0)	2	(0.1)
1 teaspoon (approx. 0.2 oz.)	1	trace	3.8	(0.11)	32	(1.0)	2	(0.1)
Chinese Red Vinegar, **China Bowl,** 12-oz. bottle	34	14.6	2.7	1.15	22	9.8	1	0.6
1 teaspoon (approx. 0.2 oz.)	trace	0.2	2.7	1.15	22	9.8	1	0.6
Chinese White Vinegar, **China Bowl,** 12-oz. bottle	34	14.6	2.7	1.15	22	9.8	1	0.6
1 teaspoon (approx. 0.2 oz.)	trace	0.2	2.7	1.15	22	9.8	1	0.6
Red Wine Vinegar, **Regina,** 12-fl.-oz. bottle	48	1.8	3.8	0.14	32	1.2	2	0.1
24-fl.-oz. bottle	96	3.6	3.8	0.14	32	1.2	2	0.1
1 teaspoon (approx. 0.2 oz.)	1	trace	3.8	0.14	32	1.2	2	0.1
Red Wine Vinegar with Garlic, **Regina,** 12-fl.-oz. bottle	48	1.8	3.8	0.14	32	1.2	2	0.1
24-fl.-oz. bottle	96	3.6	3.8	0.14	32	1.2	2	0.1
1 teaspoon (approx. 0.2 oz.)	1	trace	3.8	0.14	32	1.2	2	0.1
WORCESTERSHIRE SAUCE, based on generic data								
1 teaspoon (approx. 0.2 oz.)	4	1.0	20.0	5.00	192	48.0	12	3.0
WORCESTERSHIRE SAUCE, by brand								
Worcestershire Sauce, Regular, **French's,** 5-oz. bottle	89	17.7	17.7	3.54	160	32.0	10	2.0
Worcestershire Sauce, Smoky, **French's,** 5-oz. bottle	89	17.7	17.7	3.54	160	32.0	10	2.0
1 teaspoon (approx. 0.2 oz.)	3	0.7	17.7	3.54	160	32.0	10	2.0
YOGURT, PLAIN, based on generic data								
Low-fat yogurt, 1 teaspoon (approx. 0.2 oz.)	(3)	(04)	17.9	2.00	(158)	(17.5)	(10)	(1.1)
Skim-milk yogurt, 1 teaspoon (approx. 0.2 oz.)	(3)	(0.4)	15.9	2.18	(139)	(19.1)	(9)	(1.2)
Whole-milk yogurt, 1 teaspoon (approx. 0.2 oz.)	(3)	trace	17.3	1.32	(150)	(11.4)	(9)	(0.7)
(Yogurt has its own chapter, directly preceding this one.)								

SALAD SEASONINGS

	UNIT		1 OZ., BY WT.		1 CUP		1 TABLE-SPOON	
	Cal.	Carb.	Cal.	Carb.	Cal.	Carb.	Cal.	Carb.
Bac Os, **General Mills,** 3.25-oz. package	480	24.0	147.7	7.38	640	32.0	40	2.0
1 teaspoon, (approx. 0.1 oz.)	13	0.7	147.7	7.38	640	32.0	40	2.0
Bacon Bits, **Oscar Mayer,** 3-oz. can	274	4.1	91.4	1.36	(1200)	(17.8)	(75)	(1.1)
1 teaspoon (approx. 0.3 oz.)	(25)	(0.4)	91.4	1.36	(1200)	(17.8)	(75)	(1.1)
Bacon Bits, imitation, **Durkee,** 2¾-oz. container	384	24.0	139.6	8.73	384	24.0	24	1.5
1 teaspoon (approx. 0.1 oz.)	8	0.4	139.6	8.73	384	24.0	24	1.5
Bacon Crumbles, imitation, **French's,** 2-oz. jar	212	trace	106.3	trace	288	trace	18	trace
1 teaspoon (approx. 0.1 oz.)	6	trace	106.3	trace	288	trace	18	trace
Parmesan Cheese, grated (based on generic data)	453	3.7	129.3	1.06	453	3.7	28	0.2
1 teaspoon (approx. 0.07 oz.)	9	0.1	129.3	1.06	453	3.7	28	0.2
Parmesan Cheese, grated, **Borden,** 3-oz. canister (approx. ¾ cup)	420	9.0	140.0	3.00	(560)	(12.0)	(35)	(0.8)
8-oz. canister (approx. 2 cups)	1120	24.0	140.0	3.00	(560)	(12.0)	(35)	(0.8)
1 teaspoon (approx. 0.08 oz.)	(12)	(0.3)	140.0	3.00	(560)	(12.0)	(35)	(0.8)
Parmesan and Romano Cheese, grated, **Borden,** 3-oz. canister (approx. ¾ cup)	420	9.0	140.0	3.00	(560)	(12.0)	(35)	(0.8)
8-oz. canister (approx. 2 cups)	1120	24.0	140.0	3.00	(560)	(12.0)	(35)	(0.8)
16-oz. (1-lb.) canister (approx. 4 cups)	2240	48.0	140.0	3.00	(560)	(12.0)	(35)	(0.8)
1 teaspoon (approx. 0.08 oz.)	(12)	(0.3)	140.0	3.00	(560)	(12.0)	(35)	(0.8)
Romano Cheese, grated, **Kraft,** 3-oz. jar	390	3.0	130.0	1.00				
6-oz. jar	780	6.0	130.0	1.00				
Salad Crunchies, **NSB,** 2-oz. bag	240	24.0	120.0	12.00	(1080)	108.0	(68)	(6.8)
1 teaspoon (approx. 0.2 oz.)	23	2.3	120.0	12.00	(1080)	108.0	(68)	(6.8)
Salad Lift, **French's,** 2½-oz. jar	118	19.7	47.3	7.88	288	48.0	18	3.0
1 teaspoon (approx. 0.1 oz.)	6	1.0	47.3	7.88	288	48.0	18	3.0
Salad Onions, Instant, **French's,** 2⅛-oz. bottle	181	36.1	85.0	17.01	240	48.0	15	3.0
1 teaspoon (approx. 0.1 oz.)	5	1.0	85.0	17.01	240	48.0	15	3.0
Salad Seasoning, **Durkee,** 2½-oz. container	192	33.6	76.8	13.40	192	33.6	12	2.1
1 teaspoon (approx. 0.1 oz.)	4	0.7	76.8	13.40	192	33.6	12	2.1
Salad Seasoning with Cheese, **Durkee,** 2⅛-oz. container	480	19.2	225.9	9.04	480	19.2	30	1.2
1 teaspoon (approx. ¹⁄₂₀ oz.)	10	0.4	225.9	9.04	480	19.2	30	1.2

CROUTONS

	UNIT		1 OZ., BY WT.		1 CUP		1 TABLE-SPOON	
	Cal.	Carb.	Cal.	Carb.	Cal.	Carb.	Cal.	Carb.
Artificial Bacon Croutons, **Bel Air,** 2¾-oz. box	320	48.0	116.4	17.45	(160)	(24.0)		
Buttery Toasted Croutons, **Brownberry,** 6-oz. box	793	109.0	132.2	18.16	(331)	(45.5)		
Caesar Seasoned Croutons, **Brownberry,** 6-oz. box	800	95.5	133.4	15.92	(334)	(39.8)		
Cheddar Cheese Croutons, **Brownberry,** 6-oz. box	827	97.2	137.9	16.20	(345)	(40.5)		
Cheddar Cheese Croutons, **Pepperidge Farm,** 6½-oz. package	845	123.5	130.0	19.00	(193)	(28.1)		
Cheese & Garlic Croutons, **Bel Air,** 3-oz. box	400	48.0	133.3	16.00	(200)	(24.0)		
Cheese-Garlic Croutons, **Pepperidge Farm,** 6-oz. package	840	102.0	140.0	17.00	(207)	(25.2)		
Croutettes, Herb Seasoned Croutons, **Kellogg's** 7-oz. box	700	150.0	100.0	21.43	(141)	(30.2)		
French Style Garlic Croutons, **Arnold,** 6-oz. box	792	109.6	132.0	18.26	(165)	(22.8)		
Garlic Croutons, **Bel Air,** 2¾-oz. box	320	48.0	116.4	17.45	(160)	(24.0)		
Italian Cheese Croutons, **Bel Air,** 3-oz. box	400	48.0	133.3	16.00	(200)	(24.0)		
Italian Style Seasoned Croutons, **Arnold,** 6-oz. box	786	108.4	131.0	18.07	(164)	(22.6)		
Onion & Garlic Croutons, **Brownberry,** 6-oz. box	797	101.1	132.8	16.85	(332)	(42.1)		
Onion-Garlic Croutons, **Pepperidge Farm,** 6-oz. package	840	114.0	140.0	19.00	(207)	(28.1)		
"Plain" Croutons, **Bel Air,** 2½-oz. box	240	56.0	96.0	22.40	(120)	(28.0)		
"Plain" Croutons, **Pepperidge Farm,** 6½-oz. package	910	130.0	140.0	20.00	(207)	(29.6)		

	UNIT		1 OZ., BY WT.		1 CUP		1 TABLESPOON	
	Cal.	Carb.	Cal.	Carb.	Cal.	Carb.	Cal.	Carb.
Seasoned Croutons, **Bel Air,** 2¾-oz. box	360	48.0	130.9	17.45	(180)	(24.0)		
Seasoned Croutons, **Brownberry,** 6-oz. box	788	107.8	131.4	17.96	(329)	(44.9)		
Seasoned Croutons, **Pepperidge Farm,** 6-oz. package	840	114.0	140.0	19.00	(207)	(28.1)		
"Something Better Than Croutons," **NSB,** 3.6-oz. package	320	16.0	88.9	4.44	(111)	(5.8)		

	UNIT		1 OZ., BY WT.		1 CUP		1 TABLESPOON	
	Cal.	Carb.	Cal.	Carb.	Cal.	Carb.	Cal.	Carb.
Sour Cream & Chives Croutons, **Pepperidge Farm,** 6-oz. package	840	102.0	140.0	17.00	(207)	(25.2)		
Sourdough Croutons, no sugar, no oils, **Pioneer,** 8-oz. box	560	112.0	70.0	14.00	(103)	(20.8)		

29 SALTY SNACKS •

	ENTIRE PACKAGE		1 PIECE		1 QUART		1 OZ., BY WT.	
	Cal.	Carb.	Cal.	Carb.	Cal.	Carb.	Cal.	Carb.
CHEESE SNACKS								
Cheddar Bitz, **Frito-Lay,** 1⅜-oz. bag	177	26.0					129.0	18.90
Cheddar Cheese with Sesame Chips, **Flavor Tree,** 5-oz. box	750	70.0					150.0	14.00
Cheddar Fries, **Andy Capp's,** ⅝-oz. bag	93	10.2					149.4	16.33
Cheese Corn, **Ann Page,** 4-oz. bag	720	56.0					180.0	14.00
Cheese Corn Twists, Baked, **Jax (Bachman)** ¾-oz. package	113	12.8	(6)	(0.7)	(312)	(35.4)	150.0	17.00
⅜-oz. package	56	6.3	(6)	(0.7)	(312)	(35.4)	150.0	17.00
1½-oz. package	225	25.5	(6)	(0.7)	(312)	(35.4)	150.0	17.00
5-oz. bag	750	85.0	(6)	(0.7)	(312)	(35.4)	150.0	17.00
8-oz. bag	1200	136.0	(6)	(0.7)	(312)	(35.4)	150.0	17.00
1 Twist, approx. 0.04 oz. (approx. 24 per oz.)			(6)	(0.7)	(312)	(35.4)	150.0	17.00
1 quart, approx. 2.1 oz. (approx. 50 Twists)					(312)	(35.4)	150.0	17.00
Cheese Corn Twists, Fried, **Jax (Bachman)** 8-oz. bag	1264	112.0					158.0	14.00
1½-oz. package	237	21.0					158.0	14.00
Cheese Flavored Curls, Flings, **Nabisco,** 5¾-oz. package	880	71.5	(10)	(0.8)			160.0	13.00
1 Curl, approx. 0.06 oz. (approx. 16 per oz.)			(10)	(0.8)			160.0	13.00
Cheese 'n Crunch, **Nabisco,** 7-oz. bag	1120	98.0					160.0	14.00
Cheese Nibbles, **Granny Goose,** 1-oz. bag	167	14.2					167.6	14.15
1¼-oz. bag	209	17.7					167.6	14.15
1¾-oz. bag	293	24.8					167.6	14.15
7-oz. bag	1341	99.0					167.6	14.15
Cheese Puffs, **Laura Scudder's,** 1¼-oz. bag	180	21.4					144.0	17.10
1⅓-oz. bag	192	22.8					144.0	17.10
6-oz. bag	864	102.6					144.0	17.10
1-lb. bag	2304	273.6					144.0	17.10
Cheese Sticks, **Bachman,** 10-oz. bag	1100	210.0					110.0	32.00
Cheese Twists (Baked), **Sloan's,** 8-oz. bag	1200	136.0					150.0	17.00
Cheese Waffles, **Wise,** ¾-oz. bag	105	10.5					140.0	14.00
3¾-oz. bag	525	52.5					140.0	14.00
Chee•tos, cheese flavored snacks, Crunchy, **Frito-Lay,** 1¼-oz. bag	200	18.7	(4)	(0.8)	(448)	(42.0)	160.0	15.00
1½-oz. bag	240	23.1	(5)	(0.5)	(896)	(84.0)	160.0	15.00
5-oz. bag	800	77.0	(5)	(0.5)	(896)	(84.0)	160.0	15.00
8-oz. bag	1280	123.2	(5)	(0.5)	(896)	(84.0)	160.0	15.00
1 Chee•to, approx. 0.03 oz. (approx. 29 per oz.)			(5)	(0.5)	(896)	(84.0)	160.0	15.00
1 quart, approx. 5.6 oz. (approx. 162 Chee•tos)					(896)	(84.0)	160.0	15.00
Chee•tos, cheese-flavored snacks, Puffed, **Frito-Lay,** 1-oz. bag	160	15.0	(4)	(0.8)	(448)	(42.0)	160.0	15.00
1¼-oz. bag	200	18.3	(9)	(0.8)	(448)	(42.0)	160.0	15.00
1 Chee•to, approx. 0.06 oz. (approx. 18 per oz.)			(9)	(0.8)	(448)	(42.0)	160.0	15.00
1 quart, approx. 2.8 oz. (approx. 50 Chee•tos)					(448)	(42.0)	160.0	15.00
Chee•tos, Nacho Cheese flavored snacks, **Frito-Lay,** 1-oz. bag	160	15.0					160.0	15.00
Cheez Balls, **Planters,** 5-oz. package	800	75.0	(4)	(0.4)	(640)	(60.0)	160.0	15.00
1 Cheez Ball, approx. 0.03 oz. (approx. 39 per oz.)			(4)	(0.4)	(640)	(60.0)	160.0	15.00
1 quart, approx. 4.0 oz. (approx. 156 Cheez Balls)					(640)	(60.0)	160.0	15.00
Cheez Curls, **Planters,** 6½-oz. package	1040	97.5	(7)	(0.6)	(704)	(66.0)	160.0	15.00
1 Cheez Curl, approx. 0.04 oz. (approx. 24 per oz.)			(7)	(0.6)	(704)	(66.0)	160.0	15.00
1 quart, approx. 4.4 oz. (approx. 106 Cheez Curls)					(704)	(66.0)	160.0	15.00
Cheez Doodles, cheese flavored corn puffs, Baked, **Old London (Wise),** ¾-oz. bag	120	12.0					160.0	16.00
Cheez Doodles, cheese flavored corn puffs, Crunchy Fried, **Old London (Wise),** 1-oz. bag	160	16.0	(6)	(0.6)	(1244)	(124.4)	160.0	16.00
1¼-oz. bag	200	20.0	(6)	(0.6)	(1244)	(124.4)	160.0	16.00
2¼-oz. bag	360	36.0	(6)	(0.6)	(1244)	(124.4)	160.0	16.00
5-oz. bag	800	80.0	(6)	(0.6)	(1244)	(124.4)	160.0	16.00
6-oz. bag	960	96.0	(6)	(0.6)	(1244)	(124.4)	160.0	16.00
9-oz. bag	1440	144.0	(6)	(0.6)	(1244)	(124.4)	160.0	16.00
1 Puff, approx. 0.04 oz. (approx. 27 per ounce)			(6)	(0.6)	(1244)	(124.4)	160.0	16.00
1 quart, approx. 7.8 oz. (approx. 211 Puffs)					(1244)	(124.4)	160.0	16.00
Cheez Doodles, cheese flavored corn puffs, Oven Baked, **Old London (Wise),** ¾-oz. bag	120	12.0	(6)	(0.6)	(1048)	(104.0)	160.0	16.00
1½-oz. bag	240	24.0	(6)	(0.6)	(1048)	(104.0)	160.0	16.00
4-oz. bag	640	64.0	(6)	(0.6)	(1048)	(104.0)	160.0	16.00

	ENTIRE PACKAGE		1 PIECE		1 QUART		1 OZ., BY WT.	
	Cal.	Carb.	Cal.	Carb.	Cal.	Carb.	Cal.	Carb.
5-oz. bag	800	80.0	(6)	(0.6)	(1048)	(104.0)	160.0	16.00
8-oz. bag	1280	128.0	(6)	(0.6)	(1048)	(104.0)	160.0	16.00
1 Puff, approx. 0.04 oz. (approx. 27 per ounce)			(6)	(0.6)	(1048)	(104.0)	160.0	16.00
1 quart, approx. 6.4 oz. (approx. 173 Puffs)					(1048)	(104.0)	160.0	16.00
Cheez Waffles, waffle crackers with cheese filling, **Old London (Wise)**, ¾-oz. bag	105	10.5					140.0	14.00
3¼-oz. bag	455	45.5					140.0	14.00
5-oz. bag	700	70.0					140.0	14.00
Nacho Cheese Flavor, Wheatwists, **Spicer's**, 3-oz. bag	360	50.0	(3)	(0.4)	(384)	(54.0)	120.0	16.67
1 Wheatwist, approx. 0.03 oz. (approx. 40 per ounce)			(3)	(0.4)	(384)	(54.0)	120.0	16.67
1 quart, approx. 3.2 oz. (approx. 128 Wheatwists)	360	50.0	(3)	(0.4)	(384)	(54.0)	120.0	16.67

CORN CHIPS, TACO CHIPS, and TORTILLA CHIPS

	ENTIRE PACKAGE		1 PIECE		1 QUART		1 OZ., BY WT.	
	Cal.	Carb.	Cal.	Carb.	Cal.	Carb.	Cal.	Carb.
Ann Page (A&P)								
Corn Chips, 8-oz. bag	1280	136.0					160.0	17.00
Nacho Cheese Flavor Tortilla Chips, 8-oz. bag	1200	136.0					150.0	17.00
Bachman								
Corn Chips, 8-oz. bag	1200	120.0			(825)	(82.5)	150.0	15.00
BBQ Corn Chips, 9-oz. bag	1350	135.0	(8)	(0.8)	(825)	(82.5)	150.0	15.00
1 Chip, approx. 0.05 oz. (approx. 20 per ounce)			(8)	(0.8)	(825)	(82.5)	150.0	15.00
1 quart, approx. 5.5 oz. (approx. 110 Chips)					(825)	(82.5)	150.0	15.00
Indian Corn Chips, 9-oz. bag	1350	135.0					150.0	15.00
11-oz. bag	1650	165.0					150.0	15.00
Bachman, Tor'tico								
Nacho Tortilla Chips, 8-oz. bag	1200	136.0					150.0	17.00
Nacho Cheese Flavor Tortilla Chips, 7-oz. bag	952	119.0			(769)	(96.1)	136.0	17.00
1 Chip, approx. 0.07 oz. (approx. 14 per ounce)			(10)	(2.4)	(769)	(96.1)	136.0	17.00
1 quart, approx. 5.7 oz. (approx. 80 Chips)					(769)	(96.1)	136.0	17.00
Taco Tortilla Chips, 8-oz. bag	1200	136.0					150.0	17.00
Taco Flavor Tortilla Chips, 7-oz. bag	966	119.0			(780)	(96.1)	138.0	17.00
1 Chip, approx. 0.07 oz. (approx. 15 per ounce)			(10)	(1.2)	(780)	(96.1)	138.0	17.00
1 quart, approx. 5.7 oz. (approx. 86 Chips)					(780)	(96.1)	138.0	17.00
Toasted Tortilla Chips, 8-oz. bag	1144	128.0					143.0	16.00
Frito-Lay, Doritos								
Tortilla Chips, 1⅛-oz. bag	157	21.3	(8)	(1.1)	(472)	(64.1)	140.0	19.00
8-oz. bag	1120	152.0	(8)	(1.1)	(472)	(64.1)	140.0	19.00
12-oz. bag	1680	228.0	(8)	(1.1)	(472)	(64.1)	140.0	19.00
1 Chip, approx. 0.06 oz. (approx. 17 per ounce)			(8)	(1.1)	(472)	(64.1)	140.0	19.00
1 quart, approx. 3.4 oz. (approx. 58 Chips)					(472)	(64.1)	140.0	19.00
Cool Ranch Flavor Tortilla Chips, 11-oz. bag	1540	198.0					140.0	18.00
Nacho Cheese Flavor Tortilla Chips, 1½-oz. bag	210	27.0	(9)	(1.1)	(616)	(79.2)	140.0	18.00
4¼-oz. bag	630	81.0	(9)	(1.1)	(616)	(79.2)	140.0	18.00
7-oz. bag	980	126.0	(9)	(1.1)	(616)	(79.2)	140.0	18.00
11-oz. bag	1540	198.0	(9)	(1.1)	(616)	(79.2)	140.0	18.00
1 Chip, approx. 0.06 oz. (approx. 16 per ounce)			(9)	(1.1)	(616)	(79.2)	140.0	18.00
1 quart, approx. 4.4 oz. (approx. 70 Chips)					(616)	(79.2)	140.0	18.00
Sour Cream and Onion Tortilla Chips, 1⅛-oz. bag	158	20.3					140.0	18.00
Taco Flavor Tortilla Chips, 4½-oz. bag	630	81.0					140.0	18.00
7-oz. bag	980	126.0					140.0	18.00
Toasted Corn Flavor Tortilla Chips, 11-oz. bag	1540	209.0					140.0	19.00
Frito-Lay, Fritos								
Corn Chips, ½-oz. bag	80	8.0	(8)	(0.8)	(992)	(99.2)	160.0	16.00
¾-oz. bag	120	12.0	(8)	(0.8)	(992)	(99.2)	160.0	16.00
1½-oz. bag	240	24.0	(8)	(0.8)	(992)	(99.1)	160.0	16.00
2-oz. bag	320	32.0	(8)	(0.8)	(992)	(99.2)	160.0	16.00

	ENTIRE PACKAGE		1 PIECE		1 QUART		1 OZ., BY WT.	
	Cal.	Carb.	Cal.	Carb.	Cal.	Carb.	Cal.	Carb.
6½-oz. bag	1040	104.0	(8)	(0.8)	(992)	(99.2)	160.0	16.00
10½-oz. bag	1680	168.0	(8)	(0.8)	(992)	(99.2)	160.0	16.00
15-oz. bag	2400	240.0	(8)	(0.8)	(992)	(99.2)	160.0	16.00
1 Chip, approx. 0.05 oz. (approx. 21 per ounce)			(8)	(0.8)	(992)	(99.2)	160.0	16.00
1 quart, approx. 6.2 oz. (approx. 130 Chips)					(992)	(99.2)	160.0	16.00
Barbecue Flavored Corn Chips, 1⅞-oz. bag	300	30.0					160.0	16.00
9-oz. bag	1440	144.0					160.0	16.00
Chili Cheese Flavored Corn Chips, 8-oz. bag	1280	128.0					160.0	16.00
Dip Size Corn Chips, 8-oz. bag	1200	128.0					150.0	16.00
Light Corn Chips, 1¼-oz. bag	200	20.0			(812)	(81.2)	160.0	16.00
8-oz. bag	1280	128.0			(812)	(81.2)	160.0	16.00
1 Chip, approx. 0.05 oz. (approx. 22 per ounce)					(812)	(81.2)	160.0	16.00
1 quart, approx. 5.1 oz. (approx. 112 Chips)					(812)	(81.2)	160.0	16.00
Frito-Lay, Tostitos								
Crispy Round Tortilla Chips, 1⅛-oz. bag	158	20.3					140.0	18.00
Nacho Flavored Round Tortilla Chips, 1⅛-oz. bag	169	19.1					150.0	17.00
Granny Goose								
Corn Chips:								
Corn Chips, 1-oz. bag	159	15.4					158.8	15.37
2-oz. bag	318	30.7					158.8	15.37
9-oz. bag	1429	138.3					158.8	15.37
Native American style Corn Chips, 8-oz. bag	1243	128.8	(12)	(1.3)	(1380)	(143.0)	155.4	16.10
1 Chip, approx. 0.08 oz. (approx. 13 per ounce)			(12)	(1.3)	(1380)	(143.0)	155.4	16.10
1 quart, approx. 8.9 oz. (approx. 116 Chips)					(1380)	(143.0)	155.4	16.10
Tortilla Chips and Tortillos:								
Tortilla Chips, 1-oz. bag	140	17.9					139.8	17.86
1⅛-oz. bag	157	20.1					139.8	17.86
1¼-oz. bag	175	22.3					139.8	17.86
Barbecue Flavored Tortilla Chips, 1¼-oz. bag	175	21.8					140.3	17.46
6-oz. bag	842	104.8					140.3	17.46
Barbecue Flavor Stone Ground Tortillas, 6-oz. bag	856	108.2					142.6	18.03
Cheese Tortilla Chips, 1⅛-oz. bag	164	19.9					145.4	17.66
1⅜-oz. bag	200	24.3					145.4	17.66
6-oz. bag	872	106.0					145.4	18 77
Nacho Cheese Tortillos, 1-oz. bag	140	17.4					140.0	17.40
1¼-oz. bag	175	21.8					140.0	17.40
Stone Ground Tortilla Chips, 1¼-oz. bag	183	22.2					146.9	17.72
Stone Ground Nacho Cheese Tortillos, 5½-oz. canister	784	99.2	(19)	(2.3)	(800)	(101.1)	142.6	18.03
1 Chip, approx. 0.13 oz. (approx. 8 per ounce)			(19)	(2.3)	(800)	(101.1)	142.6	18.03
1 quart, approx. 5.6 oz. (approx. 45 Chips)					(800)	(101.1)	142.6	18.03
Laura Scudder's								
Corn Chips, 1½-oz. bag	237	22.7					158.0	15.20
1⅞-oz. bag	296	28.5					158.0	15.20
9½-oz. bag	1501	144.4					158.0	15.20
Sold bulk, 1-lb.	2528	243.2					158.0	15.20
Mini Tacos, 7-oz. bag	924	133.0					132.0	19.00
Tortilla Chips, 6-oz. bag	822	111.6					137.0	18.60
8-oz. bag	1096	148.8					137.0	18.60
9-oz. bag	1233	167.4					137.0	18.60
Nabisco								
Corn & Sesame Chips, 7-oz. bag	1120	105.0					160.0	15.00
Tortilla Chips, 7-oz. bag	1050	133.0	(11)	(1.4)			150.0	19.00
1 Chip, approx. 0.07 oz. (approx. 14 per ounce)			(11)	(1.4)			150.0	19.00
Nacho Cheese Tortilla Chips, 6-oz. bag	900	102.0	(12)	(7.9)			150.0	17.00
1 Chip, approx. 0.08 oz. (approx. 13 per ounce)			(12)	(7.9)			150.0	17.00
Old London (see under Wise)								
Planters								
Corn Chips, 8-oz. package	1360	120.0					170.0	15.00
7½-oz. canister	1275	112.5					170.0	15.00

	ENTIRE PACKAGE		1 PIECE		1 QUART		1 OZ., BY WT.	
	Cal.	Carb.	Cal.	Carb.	Cal.	Carb.	Cal.	Carb.
Nacho Tortilla Chips, 8-oz. bag	1040	112.0					130.0	14.00
Taco Tortilla Chips, 5½-oz. bag	715	77.0					130.0	14.00
Torteros								
Nacho Cheese Tortilla Chips, 7-oz. bag	1050	119.0	(8)	(0.9)	(676)	(76.6)	150.0	17.00
1 Chip, approx. 0.05 oz. (approx. 20 per ounce)			(8)	(0.9)	(676)	(76.6)	150.0	17.00
1 quart, approx. 4.5 oz. (approx. 90 Chips)					(676)	(76.6)	150.0	17.00
Toasted Corn Flavor Tortilla Chips, 7-oz. bag	1050	119.0					150.0	17.00
Wise								
Barbecue Flavored Corn Chips, 1⅜-oz. bag	206	23.4					150.0	17.00
2½-oz. bag	375	42.5					150.0	17.00
7-oz. bag	1050	119.0					150.0	17.00
Nacho Cheese Tortilla Chips, 2-oz. bag	300	34.0					150.0	17.00
5-oz. bag	750	85.0					150.0	17.00
7½-oz. bag	1125	127.5					150.0	17.00
Taco Flavored Tortilla Chips, 1-oz. bag	150	17.0					150.0	17.00
2-oz. bag	300	34.0					150.0	17.00
5-oz. bag	750	85.0					150.0	17.00
Wise, Bravos								
Crispy Round Nacho Cheese Tortilla Chips, 7-oz. bag	1050	119.0	(18)	(2.0)	(901)	(102.1)	150.0	17.00
1 Chip, approx. 0.12 oz. (approx. 9 per ounce)			(18)	(2.0)	(901)	(102.1)	150.0	17.00
1 quart, approx. 6.0 oz. (approx. 54 Chips)					(901)	(102.1)	150.0	17.00
Nacho Cheese Flavor Triangles Tortilla Chips, 1-oz. bag	150	18.0					150.0	18.00
Toasted Corn Flavor Tortilla Chips, 7-oz. bag	1050	126.0	(18)	(2.2)	(901)	(102.1)	150.0	18.00
1 Chip, approx. 0.12 oz. (approx. 9 per ounce)			(18)	(2.2)	(901)	(102.1)	150.0	18.00
1 quart, approx. 6.0 oz. (approx. 54 Chips)					(901)	(102.1)	150.0	18.00
Wise, Buenos								
Nacho Cheese Tortilla Chips, 6-oz. bag	900	102.0					150.0	17.00
Sour Cream and Onion Tortilla Chips, 6-oz. bag	900	108.0					150.0	17.00
Wise, Dipsy Doodles								
Rippled Corn Chips, 1.2-oz. bag	192	19.2	(8)	(0.8)	(800)	(80.0)	160.0	16.00
7.5-oz. bag	1200	120.0	(8)	(0.8)	(800)	(80.0)	160.0	16.00
1 Chip, approx. 0.05 oz. (approx. 20 per ounce)			(8)	(0.8)	(800)	(80.0)	160.0	16.00
1 quart, approx. 5.0 oz. (approx. 100 Chips)					(800)	(80.0)	160.0	16.00
Wise, Old London								
Barbecue Flavored Corn Chips, 1⅜-oz. bag	206	23.4					150.0	17.00
NUTS, see the NUTS & SEEDS chapter.								
POPCORN								
POPCORN, based on generic data								
Unpopped, 1 pound	1642	327.0					102.6	20.44
1 cup (approx. 7.2 oz.)	742	147.8					102.6	20.44
Popped, 1 pound (approx. 19 quarts)	1751	347.9			92	18.4	109.4	21.74
1 quart, large kernel (approx. 0.8 oz., smaller kernels may weigh twice as much per cup)					92	18.4	109.4	21.74
Popped with 1 tablespoon oil added per ¼ cup unpopped kernels, salt added, 1 pound (approx. 13 quarts)	2068	268.1			164	21.0	129.3	16.76
1 quart, large kernel (approx. 1.3 oz.)					164	21.0	129.3	16.76
Sugar-coated popcorn, 1 pound (approx. 3¼ quarts)	1737	387.4			536	119.6	108.6	24.21
1 quart (approx. 4.8 oz.)					536	119.6	108.6	24.21
POPCORN, by brand								
Ann Page (A&P), Cheese Corn, 4-oz. bag	720	56.0					180.0	14.00

	ENTIRE PACKAGE		1 PIECE		1 QUART		1 OZ., BY WT.	
	Cal.	Carb.	Cal.	Carb.	Cal.	Carb.	Cal.	Carb.
Bachman, Pop Corn, 1⅛-oz. package	180	14.6					160.0	13.00
4½-oz. bag	720	58.5	(1)	(0.1)	(238)	(19.6)	160.0	13.00
1 piece, approx. 0.01 oz. (approx. 148 per ounce)			(1)	(0.1)	(238)	(19.6)	160.0	13.00
1 quart, approx. 1.5 oz. (approx. 222 pieces)					(238)	(19.6)	160.0	13.00
Caramel Corn, 1¼-oz. package	140	31.2					112.0	25.00
7-oz. bag	784	175.0					112.0	25.00
9½-oz. bag	1064	237.5					112.0	25.00
Cheese Popcorn, 1-oz. package	180	14.0					180.0	14.00
4-oz. package	720	56.0					180.0	14.00
Corn Diggers, Nabisco, Popcorn Tastin' Snacks, 5-oz. package	750	85.0	(4)	(0.5)	(600)	(68.0)	150.0	17.00
1 piece, approx. 0.03 oz. (approx. 38 per ounce)			(4)	(0.5)	(600)	(68.0)	150.0	17.00
1 quart, approx. 4.0 oz. (approx. 152 Diggers)					(600)	(68.0)	150.0	17.00
Cracker Jack, candied popcorn and peanuts, ¾-oz. box	90	16.5	(2)	(0.3)	(688)	(123.2)	120.0	22.00
1-oz. box	120	22.0	(2)	(0.3)	(688)	(123.2)	120.0	22.00
2-oz. box	240	44.0	(2)	(0.3)	(688)	(123.2)	120.0	22.00
4½-oz. box	540	99.0	(2)	(0.3)	(688)	(123.2)	120.0	22.00
5⅝-oz. box	675	123.8	(2)	(0.3)	(688)	(123.2)	120.0	22.00
6-oz. box	720	132.0	(2)	(0.3)	(688)	(123.2)	120.0	22.00
1 Cracker Jack, approx. 0.01 oz. (approx. 71 per ounce)			(2)	(0.3)	(688)	(123.2)	120.0	22.00
1 quart, approx. 5.7 oz. (approx. 405 Cracker Jacks)					(688)	(123.2)	120.0	22.00
Golden Pop, Cheese Popcorn, 4½-oz. package	720	56.0					180.0	14.00
Regular Popcorn, 4-oz. package	720	58.5					160.0	13.00
Hungry Jack, Microwave Popcorn, 2.5-oz. package	380	34.0					152.0	13.60
Jolly Time								
Popcorn, white, hulless, 10-oz. can	1094	217.5				109.4	21.75	
(yield: approx. 5 quarts, popped)	1094	217.5			(219)	(43.5)	(109.4)	(21.75)
20-oz. bag	2188	217.5					109.4	21.75
(yield: approx. 10 quarts, popped)	2188	217.5			(219)	(43.5)	(109.4)	(21.75)
1 quart, popped, approx. 2.0 oz.					(219)	(43.5)	(109.4)	(21.75)
Popcorn, yellow, hulless, 10-oz. can	1094	21.8					109.4	21.75
(yield: approx. 5 quarts, popped)	1094	217.5			(219)	(43.5)	(109.4)	(21.75)
20-oz. can	2188	435.0					109.4	21.75
(yield: approx. 10 quarts, popped)	2188	435.0			(219)	(43.5)	(109.4)	(21.75)
1 quart, popped, approx. 2.0 oz.					(219)	(43.5)	(109.4)	(21.75)
Laura Scudder's, Caramel Corn, 1½-oz. bag	183	32.9					122.0	21.90
Korn Kernels, 1¼-oz. bag	159	26.4					127.0	21.10
3¼-oz. bag	413	68.6					127.0	21.10
Munch Mates, Caramel Corn, 7½-oz. bag	975	172.5					130.0	23.00
Sloan's, Popcorn, 1-oz. bag	160	13.0					160.0	13.00
Wise, Popcorn, Butter Flavored, ½-oz. bag	70	8.0	(1)	(0.1)	(172)	(20.0)	140.0	16.00
⅞-oz. bag	123	14.0	(1)	(0.1)	(172)	(20.0)	140.0	16.00
3-oz. bag	420	48.0	(1)	(0.1)	(172)	(20.0)	140.0	16.00
4-oz. bag	560	64.0	(1)	(0.1)	(172)	(20.0)	140.0	16.00
1 piece, approx. 0.01 oz. (approx. 189 per ounce)			(1)	(0.1)	(172)	(20.0)	140.0	16.00
1 quart, approx. 1.2 oz. (approx. 227 pieces)					(172)	(20.0)	140.0	16.00
Popcorn, Cheese Flavored, ¾-oz. bag	105	12.0						
4-oz. bag	560	64.0						
POTATO CHIPS								
Ann Page (A&P), Ripple Potato Chips, 7½-oz. bag	1125	105.0					150.0	14.00
Bachman, Potato Chips, regular, 4½-oz. bag	720	63.0					160.0	14.00
7-oz. bag	1120	98.0					160.0	14.00
11-oz. bag	1760	154.0					160.0	14.00

	ENTIRE PACKAGE Cal.	ENTIRE PACKAGE Carb.	1 PIECE Cal.	1 PIECE Carb.	1 QUART Cal.	1 QUART Carb.	1 OZ., BY WT. Cal.	1 OZ., BY WT. Carb.
16-oz. (1-lb.) bag	2560	224.0					160.0	14.00
BBQ Potato Chips, 4½-oz. bag	675	63.0					150.0	14.00
Sour Cream & Onion Potato Chips, 4½-oz. bag	675	63.0					150.0	14.00
Chicago Dietetic, Potato Chips, Unsalted, 6-oz. bag	960	84.0					160.0	14.00
Commissary, Potato Chips, 7½-oz. twin pack	1125	105.0					150.0	14.00
Golden Crisp (Bachman) Potato Chips, 4-oz. bag	600	56.0					150.0	14.00
Golden Ridges (Bachman) Potato Chips, 7½-oz. twin pack	1125	105.0					150.0	14.00
Granny Goose, Potato Chips, Natural, 1⅛-oz. bag	176	18.6					156.2	14.91
6-oz. bag	937	89.6					156.2	14.91
Potato Chips, regular, 1¼-oz. bag	198	17.8					158.8	14.20
4¼-oz. bag	675	60.4					158.8	14.20
Barbecue Flavored Potato Chips, 1⅛-oz. bag	171	16.3					152.3	14.50
4¾-oz. bag	723	68.7					152.3	14.50
7½-oz. bag	1142	108.8					152.3	14.50
Dip Potato Chips, 8-oz. twin pak	1211	122.3					151.4	15.28
Sold bulk, 1-lb.	2422	244.5					151.4	15.28
100% Natural Dip Chips, 6-oz. bag	900	94.1	(13)	(1.3)	(384)	(40.1)	150.0	15.68
1 Chip, approx. 0.1 oz. (approx. 12 per ounce)			(13)	(1.3)	(384)	(40.1)	150.0	15.68
1 quart, approx. 2.6 oz. (approx. 31 Chips)					(384)	(40.1)	150.0	15.68
Pan Fries Double Thick Potato Chips, 1¼-oz. bag	179	20.1	(9)	(0.9)	(380)	(42.5)	143.5	16.05
6-oz. bag	861	96.3	(9)	(0.9)	(380)	(42.5)	143.5	16.05
1 Chip, approx. 0.6 oz. (approx. 17 per ounce)			(9)	(0.9)	(380)	(42.5)	143.5	16.05
1 quart, approx. 2.6 oz. (approx. 44 Chips)					(380)	(42.5)	143.5	16.05
Sour Cream & Onion Potato Chips, ⅞-oz. bag	133	12.7	(15)	(1.5)			152.0	14.52
1⅛-oz. bag	171	16.3	(15)	(1.5)			152.0	14.52
4¾-oz. bag	723	69.0	(15)	(1.5)			152.0	14.52
1 Chip, approx. 0.1 oz. (approx. 10 per ounce)			(15)	(1.5)			152.0	14.52
Laura Scudder's, Potato Chips, 1-oz. bag	150	15.1					150.0	15.10
2½-oz. bag	375	37.8					150.0	15.10
3-oz. bag	450	45.3					150.0	15.10
1-lb. bag	2400	241.6					150.0	15.10
Barbecue Flavored Potato Chips, 1-oz. bag	146	15.7					146.0	15.70
3-oz. bag	438	47.1					146.0	15.70
5-oz. bag	730	78.5					146.0	15.70
8-oz. bag	1168	125.6					146.0	15.70
Lay's (Frito-Lay), Potato Chips, ½-oz. bag	75	7.0	(6)	(0.6)	(380)	(35.5)	150.0	14.00
1-oz. bag	150	14.0	(6)	(0.6)	(380)	(35.5)	150.0	14.00
1½-oz. bag	225	21.0	(6)	(0.6)	(380)	(35.5)	150.0	14.00
3-oz. bag	450	42.0	(6)	(0.6)	(380)	(35.5)	150.0	14.00
4-oz. bag	600	56.0	(6)	(0.6)	(380)	(35.5)	150.0	14.00
4½-oz. bag	675	63.0	(6)	(0.6)	(380)	(35.5)	150.0	14.00
7½-oz. bag	1125	205.0	(6)	(0.6)	(380)	(35.5)	150.0	14.00
8-oz. bag	1200	112.0	(6)	(0.6)	(380)	(35.5)	150.0	14.00
12½-oz. bag	1875	175.0	(6)	(0.6)	(380)	(35.5)	150.0	14.00
1 Chip, approx. 0.04 oz. (approx. 25 per ounce)			(6)	(0.6)	(380)	(35.5)	150.0	14.00
1 quart, approx. 2.5 oz. (approx. 63 Chips)					(380)	(35.5)	150.0	14.00
Bar-B-Q Flavored Potato Chips, 1-oz. bag	150	14.0	(6)	(0.6)	(380)	(35.5)	150.0	14.00
1½-oz. bag	225	21.3	(6)	(0.6)	(380)	(35.5)	150.0	14.00
6-oz. bag	900	85.2	(6)	(0.6)	(380)	(35.5)	150.0	14.00
1 Chip, approx. 0.04 oz. (approx. 25 per ounce)			(6)	(0.6)	(380)	(35.5)	150.0	14.00
1 quart, approx. 2.5 oz. (approx. 63 Chips)					(380)	(35.5)	150.0	14.00
Jalapeno & Cheddar Potato Chips, 6½ oz. bag	975	97.5					150.0	15.00
Sour Cream & Onion Flavor Potato Chips, 1¼-oz. bag	200	17.5	(6)	(0.6)	(404)	(35.5)	160.0	14.00
6-oz. bag	960	84.0	(6)	(0.6)	(404)	(35.5)	160.0	14.00
1 Chip, approx. 0.04 oz. (approx. 25 per ounce)			(6)	(0.6)	(404)	(35.5)	160.0	14.00
1 quart, approx. 2.5 oz. (approx. 63 Chips)					(404)	(35.5)	160.0	14.00
Zesty Cheese Flavored Potato Chips, 1¼-oz. bag	200	17.5	(6)	(0.6)	(404)	(35.5)	160.0	14.00
6-oz. bag	960	84.0	(6)	(0.6)	(404)	(35.5)	160.0	14.00
1 Chip, approx. 0.04 oz. (approx. 25 per ounce)			(6)	(0.6)	(404)	(35.5)	160.0	14.00
1 quart, approx. 2.5 oz. (approx. 63 Chips)					(404)	(35.5)	160.0	14.00
Munchos, Potato Crisps, 1-oz. bag	154	15.2	(7)	(0.8)	(784)	(89.2)	154.0	15.20
1⅛-oz. bag	173	17.1	(7)	(0.8)	(784)	(89.2)	154.0	15.20
1 Chip, approx. 0.05 oz. (approx. 21 per ounce)			(7)	(0.8)	(784)	(89.2)	154.0	15.20
1 quart, approx. 5.1 oz. (approx. 107 Chips)					(784)	(89.2)	154.0	15.20
Nabisco, Potato Chipsters, 4¾-oz. bag	618	90.3	(2)	(0.3)			130.0	19.00
1 Chip, approx. 0.02 oz. (approx. 57 per ounce)			(2)	(0.3)			130.0	19.00
O'Grady's, Au•Gratin Potato Chips, 6½-oz. bag	975	97.5					150.0	15.00
Extra Thick & Crunchy Potato Chips, 7 oz. bag	1050	112.0					150.0	16.00
Planters, Potato Chips, stackable, 4-oz. package	600	68.0					150.0	17.00
4½-oz. package	675	76.5					150.0	17.00
8-oz. package	1200	136.0					150.0	17.00
12-oz. package	1800	204.0					150.0	17.00
Pringles, Potato Chips, 4½-oz. container	675	67.5					150.0	15.00
9-oz. container	1350	135.0					150.0	15.00
13½-oz. container	2025	202.5					150.0	15.00
Country Style Potato Chips, 4½-oz. container	675	67.5					150.0	15.00
9-oz. container	1350	135.0					150.0	15.00
Extra Ripple Potato Chips, 4-oz. container	600	60.0			(600)	(60.0)	150.0	15.00
8-oz. container	1200	120.0	(11)	(1.1)	(600)	(60.0)	150.0	15.00
1 Chip, approx. 0.07 oz. (approx. 14 per ounce)			(11)	(1.1)	(600)	(60.0)	150.0	15.00
1 quart, approx. 4.0 oz. (approx. 5.6 Chips)					(600)	(60.0)	150.0	15.00
Ridgies (Wise), Natural Flavor Rippled Potato Chips, 1¾-oz. bag	298	22.8	(10)	(0.8)	(556)	(42.8)	170.0	13.00
4½-oz. bag	765	58.5	(10)	(0.8)	(556)	(42.8)	170.0	13.00
7½-oz. bag	1275	97.5	(10)	(0.8)	(556)	(42.8)	170.0	13.00
4-lb. box	10880	832.0	(10)	(0.8)	(556)	(42.8)	170.0	13.00
1 Chip, approx. 0.06 oz. (approx. 16 per ounce)			(10)	(0.8)	(566)	(42.8)	170.0	13.00
1 quart, approx. 3.3 oz. (approx. 53 Chips)					(556)	(42.8)	170.0	13.00
Rippled Sour Cream and Onion Potato Chips, 1¾-oz. bag	298	22.8	(10)	(0.8)	(556)	(42.8)	170.0	13.00
4½-oz. bag	765	58.5	(10)	(0.8)	(556)	(42.8)	170.0	13.00
6½-oz. bag	1105	84.5	(10)	(0.8)	(556)	(42.8)	170.0	13.00
7½-oz. bag	1275	97.5	(10)	(0.8)	(556)	(42.8)	170.0	13.00
1 Chip, approx. 0.06 oz. (approx. 17 per ounce)			(10)	(0.8)	(556)	(42.8)	170.0	13.00
1 quart, approx. 3.3 oz. (approx. 56 Chips)					(556)	(42.8)	170.0	13.00
Ruffles (Frito-Lay), Potato Chips, 1-oz. bag	150	15.0	(6)	(0.6)	(452)	(45.2)	150.0	15.00
1¼-oz. bag	188	18.8	(6)	(0.6)	(452)	(45.2)	150.0	15.00
4-oz. bag	600	60.0	(6)	(0.6)	(452)	(45.2)	150.0	15.00
7-oz. bag	1050	105.0	(6)	(0.6)	(452)	(45.2)	150.0	15.00
7½-oz. bag	1125	112.5	(6)	(0.6)	(452)	(45.2)	150.0	15.00
12-oz. bag	1800	180.0	(6)	(0.6)	(452)	(45.2)	150.0	15.00
1 Chip, approx. 0.04 oz. (approx. 25 per ounce)			(6)	(0.6)	(452)	(45.2)	150.0	15.00
1 quart, approx. 3.0 oz. (approx. 75 Chips)					(452)	(45.2)	150.0	15.00
Bar-B-Que Flavor Potato Chips, 1-oz. bag	150	15.0	(6)	(0.6)	(452)	(45.2)	150.0	15.00
7-oz. bag	1050	105.0	(6)	(0.6)	(452)	(45.2)	150.0	15.00
1 Chip, approx. 0.04 oz. (approx. 25 per ounce)			(6)	(0.6)	(452)	(45.2)	150.0	15.00
1 quart, approx. 3.0 oz. (approx. 75 Chips)					(452)	(45.2)	150.0	15.00
Sloan's, Ripple Potato Chips, 1-oz. bag	160	14.0					160.0	14.00
Wise, Potato Chips, 1-oz. bag	150	14.0	(7)	(0.6)	(492)	(46.0)	150.0	14.00
1½-oz. bag	225	21.0	(7)	(0.6)	(492)	(46.0)	150.0	14.00
1¾-oz. bag	263	24.5	(7)	(0.6)	(492)	(46.0)	150.0	14.00
4-oz. bag	600	56.0	(7)	(0.6)	(492)	(46.0)	150.0	14.00
5-oz. bag	750	70.0	(7)	(0.6)	(492)	(46.0)	150.0	14.00

	ENTIRE PACKAGE		1 PIECE		1 QUART		1 OZ., BY WT.	
	Cal.	Carb.	Cal.	Carb.	Cal.	Carb.	Cal.	Carb.
7½-oz. twinpak	1125	105.0	(7)	(0.6)	(492)	(46.0)	150.0	14.00
8-oz. bag	1200	112.0	(7)	(0.6)	(492)	(46.0)	150.0	14.00
13-oz. bag	1950	182.0	(7)	(0.6)	(492)	(46.0)	150.0	14.00
16-oz. (1-lb.) bag	2400	224.0	(7)	(0.6)	(492)	(46.0)	150.0	14.00
4-lb. box	9600	896.0	(7)	(0.6)	(492)	(46.0)	150.0	14.00
1 Chip, approx. 0.04 oz. (approx. 23 per ounce)			(7)	(0.6)	(492)	(46.0)	150.0	14.00
1 quart, approx. 3.0 oz. (approx. 69 Chips)					(492)	(46.0)	150.0	14.00
Barbecue Flavored Potato Chips, 1¼-oz. bag	188	18.8	(9)	(0.8)	(564)	(55.2)	150.0	15.00
5½-oz. bag	825	82.5	(9)		(564)	(55.2)	150.0	15.00
1 Chip, approx. 0.06 oz. (approx. 17 per ounce)			(9)	(0.8)	(564)	(55.2)	150.0	15.00
1 quart, approx. 3.8 oz. (approx. 65 Chips)					(564)	(55.2)	150.0	15.00
Lightly Salted Potato Chips, 6½ oz. bag	1040	91.0					160.0	14.00
Onion Garlic Flavored Potato Chips, 1½-oz. bag	225	21.0			(564)	(52.8)	150.0	14.00
1¾-oz. bag	263	24.5			(564)	(52.8)	150.0	14.00
4-oz. bag	600	56.0			(564)	(52.8)	150.0	14.00
4½-oz. bag	675	63.0			(564)	(52.8)	150.0	14.00
1 Chip, approx. 0.06 oz. (approx. 17 per ounce)					(564)	(52.8)	150.0	14.00
1 quart, approx. 3.8 oz. (approx. 65 Chips)					(564)	(52.8)	150.0	14.00
Salt & Vinegar Potato Chips, 6-oz. bag	960	84.0					160.0	14.00
Sour Cream & Onion Rippled Potato Chips, 1¾-oz. bag	280	24.5					160.0	14.00
Potato Sticks, see OTHER SALTY SNACKS at the end of this chapter.								

PRETZELS

	ENTIRE PACKAGE		1 PIECE		1 QUART		1 OZ., BY WT.	
	Cal.	Carb.	Cal.	Carb.	Cal.	Carb.	Cal.	Carb.
Anderson, Bavarian Dutch Style Pretzels, 7½-oz. box	825	150.0	(64)	(11.7)	(828)	(151.2)	110.0	20.00
1 Pretzel, approx. 0.6 oz. (approx. 2 per ounce)			(64)	(11.7)	(828)	(151.2)	110.0	20.00
1 quart, approx. 7.5 oz. (approx. 15 Pretzels)					(828)	(151.2)	110.0	20.00
Thin Style Pretzels, 14-oz. box	1540	280.0	(22)	(4.5)	(1072)	(223.2)	110.0	20.00
1 Pretzel, approx. 0.2 oz. (approx. 5 per ounce)			(22)	(4.5)	(1072)	(223.2)	110.0	20.00
1 quart, approx. 9.7 oz. (approx. 49 Pretzels)					(1072)	(223.2)	110.0	20.00
Ann Page (A&P), Pretzel Teenees, 13-oz. bag	1430	286.0					110.0	22.00
Twist Pretzels, 8½-oz. bag	935	18.7	(22)	(4.5)	(396)	(80.0)	110.0	22.00
1 Pretzel, approx. 0.2 oz. (approx. 5 per oz.)			(22)	(4.5)	(396)	(80.0)	110.0	22.00
1 quart, approx. 3.6 oz. (approx. 18 Pretzels)					(396)	(80.0)	110.0	22.00
Bachman, Butter Pretzels, enriched, 8-oz. bag	880	168.0					110.0	21.00
9-oz. bag	990	189.0					110.0	21.00
11-oz. bag	1210	231.0					110.0	21.00
Nutzels (bite-size Pretzels), 9-oz. bag	990	189.0	(6)	(1.1)	(836)	(159.6)	110.0	21.00
1 Pretzel, approx. 0.05 oz. (approx. 20 per ounce)			(6)	(1.1)	(836)	(159.6)	110.0	21.00
1 quart, approx. 7.6 oz. (approx. 152 Pretzels)					(836)	(159.6)	110.0	21.00
Petite Pretzels, 11-oz. bag	1023	209.0					110.0	21.00
Plain Pretzels, 8-oz. bag	880	(168.0)					110.0	21.00
9-oz. bag	990	189.0					110.0	21.00
11-oz. bag	1210	231.0					110.0	21.00
Plain Pretzels, enriched, 12-oz. bag	1320	252.0					110.0	21.00
Baldies (Anderson), Pretzels, 7¼-oz. bag	798	145.0	(64)	(11.7)	(768)	(140.0)	110.0	20.00
1 Pretzel, approx. 0.6 oz.			(64)	(11.7)	(768)	(35.0)	110.0	20.00
1 quart, approx. 7.0 oz.					(768)	(35.0)	110.0	20.00
Drakes, bite-size Mini Pretzels, 1¼-oz. bag	125	27.5					100.0	22.00
Granny Goose, Bavarian Pretzels, 1-oz. bag	112	23.4					112.0	23.40
2-oz. bag	224	46.9					112.0	23.40
3-oz. bag	336	70.3					112.0	23.40
3½-oz. bag	395	82.7					112.0	23.40
4-oz. bag	448	93.8					112.0	23.40
8½-oz. bag	952	198.9					112.0	23.40

	ENTIRE PACKAGE		1 PIECE		1 QUART		1 OZ., BY WT.	
	Cal.	Carb.	Cal.	Carb.	Cal.	Carb.	Cal.	Carb.
Mini Pretzels, 1-oz. bag	110	22.9					110.0	22.90
2-oz. bag	221	45.8					110.0	22.90
3-oz. bag	331	68.7					110.0	22.90
3½-oz. bag	385	80.2					110.0	22.90
4-oz. bag	441	91.6					110.0	22.90
8½-oz. bag	935	194.7					110.0	22.90
Ring Pretzels, 1-oz. bag	112	23.0					112.0	23.00
2-oz. bag	224	46.0					112.0	23.00
3-oz. bag	337	68.9					112.0	23.00
3⅓-oz. bag	373	76.7					112.0	23.00
4-oz. bag	449	92.0					112.0	23.00
8½-oz. bag	952	195.5					112.0	23.00
Stick Pretzels, 1-oz. bag	108	22.9					108.0	22.90
2-oz. bag	215	45.9					108.0	22.90
3-oz. bag	323	68.8					108.0	22.90
3⅓-oz. bag	360	76.3					108.0	22.90
4-oz. bag	431	91.7					108.0	22.90
8½-oz. bag	918	194.7					108.0	22.90
Twist Pretzels, 1-oz. bag	109	22.7					109.0	22.70
2-oz. bag	217	45.3					109.0	22.70
3-oz. bag	326	68.0					109.0	22.70
3½-oz. bag	383	79.9					109.0	22.70
4-oz. bag	434	90.6					109.0	22.70
8½-oz. bag	927	193.0					109.0	22.70
Mister Salty (Nabisco), Pretzels, 10-oz. box	1100	220.0	(20)	(4.0)			110.0	22.00
1 Pretzel, approx. 0.2 oz. (approx. 5 per ounce)			(20)	(4.0)			110.0	22.00
Dutch Pretzels, 8-oz. box	880	176.0	(55)	(11.0)			110.0	22.00
1 Pretzel, approx. 0.5 oz.			(55)	(11.0)			110.0	22.00
Little Shapes Pretzels, 8-oz. box	880	176.0	(6)	(1.2)			110.0	22.00
1 Pretzel, approx. 0.05 oz. (approx. 19 per ounce)			(6)	(1.2)			110.0	22.00
Pretzel Sticks, 10-oz. box	1100	220.0	(1)	(0.2)			110.0	22.00
1 Pretzel stick, approx. 0.01 oz. (approx. 94 per ounce)			(1)	(0.2)			110.0	22.00
Pretzelets, 5¾-oz. box	605	121.0	(7)	(1.3)			110.0	22.00
1 Pretzel, approx. 0.06 oz. (approx. 17 per ounce)			(7)	(1.3)			110.0	22.00
Veri-Thin Pretzels, 10-oz. box	1100	220.0	(20)	(4.0)	(512)	(102.4)	111.1	22.22
1 Pretzel, approx. 0.2 oz. (approx. 6 per ounce)			(20)	(4.0)	(512)	(102.4)	111.1	22.22
1 quart, approx. 4.6 oz. (approx. 28 Pretzels)					(512)	(102.4)	111.1	22.22
Old London (Wise), Pretz-l Nuggets, 1⅛-oz. bag	124	24.8					110.0	22.00
1⅞-oz. bag	206	41.3					110.0	22.00
3½-oz. bag	385	77.0					110.0	22.00
9-oz. bag	990	198.0					110.0	22.00
6-lb. box	10560	2112.0					110.0	22.00
Pepperidge Farm, see the VENDING MACHINES chapter.								
Planters, Pretzel Sticks, 6½-oz. package	715	143.0					110.0	22.00
Pretzel Twists, 6½-oz. package	715	143.0					110.0	22.00
7-oz. package	770	154.0					110.0	22.00
Rold Gold (Frito-Lay), Pretzel Twists, 1⅝-oz. bag	180	36.7	(11)	(2.3)	(292)	(59.6)	111.0	22.60
9-oz. bag	999	203.4	(11)	(2.3)	(292)	(59.6)	111.0	22.60
12-oz. bag	1332	271.2	(11)	(2.3)	(292)	(59.6)	111.0	22.60
1 pretzel, approx. 0.1 oz. (approx. 10 per ounce)			(11)	(2.3)	(292)	(59.6)	111.0	22.60
1 quart, approx. 2.6 oz. (approx. 26 Pretzels)					(292)	(59.6)	111.0	22.60
Sloan's, Petite Pretzels, unsalted, 11-oz. bag	1210	231.0					110.0	21.00
Thin Pretzels, 11-oz. bag	1210	231.0					110.0	21.00
Wise, Pretzel Nuggets, 1⅛-oz. bag	124	24.8	(8)	(1.6)	(1032)	(207.2)	110.0	22.00
1⅞-oz. bag	206	41.3	(8)	(1.6)	(1032)	(207.2)	110.0	22.00
3½-oz. bag	385	77.0	(8)	(1.6)	(1032)	(207.2)	110.0	22.00
9-oz. bag	990	198.0	(8)	(1.6)	(1032)	(207.2)	110.0	22.00
11-oz. bag	1210	242.0	(8)	(1.6)	(1032)	(207.2)	110.0	22.00
6-lb. box	10560	2112.0	(8)	(1.6)	(1032)	(207.2)	110.0	22.00
1 Pretzel, approx. 0.07 oz. (approx. 14 per ounce)			(8)	(1.6)	(1032)	(207.2)	110.0	22.00
1 quart, approx. 9.4 oz. (approx. 132 Pretzels)					(1032)	(207.2)	110.0	22.00

	ENTIRE PACKAGE		1 PIECE		1 QUART		1 OZ., BY WT.	
	Cal.	Carb.	Cal.	Carb.	Cal.	Carb.	Cal.	Carb.
SEEDS, see the NUTS & SEEDS chapter.								
SESAME SNACKS								
Flavor Tree, Sesame Chips, 5-oz. box	800	65.0					160.0	13.00
Sesame Sticks, 5-oz. box	800	65.0					160.0	13.00
Unsalted Sesame Sticks, 5-oz. box	750	65.0					150.0	13.00
Joyva, Sesame Crunch, 16-oz. (1-lb.) bag	2848	400.0	(35)	(5.0)			178.0	25.00
1 Chip, approx. 0.2 oz. (approx. 5 per ounce)			(35)	(5.0)			178.0	25.00
Sesamettes, 11-oz. can	1958	275.0					178.0	25.00
Pepperidge Farm, Sesame Snack Sticks, 7½-oz. box	900	135.0					120.0	16.00
Planters, Sesame Nut Mix, 11½-oz. tin	1840	92.0					160.0	8.00
Twigs (sesame/cheese flavored snacks), 10-oz. package	1400	160.0					140.0	16.00
SOYBEAN SNACKS, see the NUTS & SEEDS chapter and the VEGETABLES chapter.								
OTHER SALTY SNACKS								
Bacon Shindigs, **Keebler,** 1.59-oz. package	230	30.0					144.7	18.87
8-oz. package	1158	150.9					144.7	18.87
Baken-ets, see Pork Rinds								
Chicken In A Biskit, **Nabisco,** 8-oz. box	1120	128.0					140.0	16.00
1 cracker, approx. 0.07 oz. (approx. 14 per ounce)			(10)	(1.1)			140.0	16.00
Corn Crunchies, **Wise,** 10-oz. bag	1600	160.0	(6)	(0.6)	(832)	(83.2)	160.0	16.00
1 Corn Crunchie, approx. 0.04 oz. (approx. 29 per ounce)			(6)	(0.6)	(832)	(83.2)	160.0	16.00
1 quart, approx. 5.2 oz. (approx. 151 Corn Crunchies)					(832)	(83.2)	160.0	16.00
Corn Diggers, **Nabisco,** 4½-oz. box	675	76.5	(4)	(0.5)	(450)	(51.0)	150.0	17.00
1 Corn Digger, approx. 0.03 oz. (approx. 36 per ounce)			(4)	(0.5)	(450)	(51.0)	150.0	17.00
1 quart, approx. 3.0 oz. (approx. 108 Corn Diggers)					(450)	(51.0)	150.0	17.00
Corn Nuggets, **Frito-Lay,** 1⅜-oz. bag	176	29.2					128.0	21.24
Corn Snacks, **Laura Scudder's** "Scudderings," 2⅜-oz. bag	373	36.8					157.0	15.50
4-oz. bag	628	62.0					157.0	15.50
Corn Twists, **Korkers (Nabisco),** 6-oz. package	960	96.0	(8)	(0.8)			160.0	16.00
7-oz. package	1120	112.0	(8)	(0.8)			160.0	16.00
1 Twist, approx. 0.05 oz. (approx. 20 per ounce)			(8)	(0.8)			160.0	16.00
Cracker Jack, ¾-oz. box	90	16.5	(2)	(0.3)	(688)	(123.2)	120.0	22.00
1-oz. box	120	22.0	(2)	(0.3)	(688)	(123.2)	120.0	22.00
2-oz. box	240	44.0	(2)	(0.3)	(688)	(123.2)	120.0	22.00
4½-oz. box	540	99.0	(2)	(0.3)	(688)	(123.2)	120.0	22.00
5⅝-oz. box	675	123.8	(2)	(0.3)	(688)	(123.2)	120.0	22.00
6-oz. bag	720	132.0	(2)	(0.3)	(688)	(123.2)	120.0	22.00
1 Cracker Jack, approx. 0.01 oz. (approx. 71 per ounce)			(2)	(0.3)	(688)	(123.2)	120.0	22.00
1 quart, approx. 5.7 oz. (approx. 405 Cracker Jacks)					(688)	(123.2)	120.0	22.00
Doo Dads, **Nabisco,** 7-oz. bag	980	119.0	(3)	(0.3)			140.0	17.00
8-oz. bag	1120	136.0	(3)	(0.3)			140.0	17.00
1 Dad, approx. 0.02 oz. (approx. 57 per ounce)			(3)	(0.3)			140.0	17.00
Funyuns, Onion Flavored snacks, **Frito-Lay,** ⅞-oz. bag	120	16.4					138.0	18.80

	ENTIRE PACKAGE		1 PIECE		1 QUART		1 OZ., BY WT.	
	Cal.	Carb.	Cal.	Carb.	Cal.	Carb.	Cal.	Carb.
1¼-oz. bag	173	23.5					138.0	18.80
4¼-oz. bag	587	79.9					138.0	18.80
High Fiber Chips, **Golden Harvest,** 7-oz. bag	980	105.0					140.0	15.00
High Protein Chips, **Golden Harvest,** 7-oz. bag	1050	98.0					150.0	14.00
Hot Fries, **Andy Capp's,** ⅝-oz. bag	93	10.2					149.4	16.33
Lil' Loaf Snack Sticks, **Nabisco,** 8-oz. package	1120	144.0	(14)	(1.8)			140.0	18.00
1-oz. bag	154	15.2	(7)	(0.8)	(784)	(89.2)	154.0	15.20
1 Stick, approx. 0.1 oz. (approx. 10 per ounce)			(14)	(1.8)			140.0	18.00
Onion Crisps, French, **Flavor Tree,** 5-oz. box	750	65.0					150.0	13.00
Onion Flavored Rings, **Old London (Wise),** ¾-oz. bag	98	16.5					130.0	22.00
3-oz. bag	390	66.0					130.0	22.00
Onion Flavored Rings, **Wise,** ½-oz. bag	65	11.0	(5)	(0.8)	(188)	(31.8)	130.0	22.00
¾-oz. bag	98	16.5	(5)	(0.8)	(188)	(31.8)	130.0	22.00
3½-oz. bag	455	77.0	(5)	(0.8)	(188)	(31.8)	130.0	22.00
1 Ring, approx. 0.04 oz. (approx. 29 per ounce)			(5)	(0.8)	(188)	(31.8)	130.0	22.00
1 quart, approx. 1.4 oz.					(188)	(31.8)	130.0	22.00
Pizza Flavor Wheatwists, **Spicer's,** 3-oz. bag	360	50.0	(3)	(0.4)	(384)	(54.0)	120.0	16.67
1 Wheatwist, approx. 0.03 oz. (approx. 40 per ounce)			(3)	(0.4)	(384)	(54.0)	120.0	16.67
1 quart, approx. 3.2 oz. (approx. 128 Wheatwists)					(384)	(54.0)		
Platanitos Plantain Chips, **Chiffles,** 6-oz. bag	1056		(5)		(1180)		176.0	
1 Chip, approx. 0.03 oz. (approx. 35 per ounce)			(5)		(1180)		176.0	
1 quart, approx. 6.7 oz. (approx. 235 Chips)					(1180)		176.0	
Pork Rinds, Fried, **Baken-ets,** ⅝-oz. bag	94	0.6					150.0	1.00
2½-oz. bag	375	2.5					150.0	1.00
5-oz. bag	750	5.0					150.0	1.00
Pork Rinds, **Granny Goose,** 1-oz. bag	152	0.0					152.0	0.00
2-oz. bag	305	0.0					152.0	0.00
3-oz. bag	458	0.0					152.0	0.00
3.3-oz. bag	502	0.0					152.0	0.00
4-oz. bag	610	0.0					152.0	0.00
Pork Rinds, Fried, **Wise,** ⅜-oz. bag	56	0.0					150.0	0.00
Potato Sticks, **Dali-Fresh,** 4½-oz. bag	675	63.0	(1)	(0.1)	(900)	(8.4)	150.0	14.00
1 stick, approx. 0.01 oz. (approx. 163 per ounce)			(1)	(0.1)	(900)	(8.4)	150.0	14.00
1 quart, approx. 6.0 oz.					(900)	(8.4)	150.0	14.00
Potato Sticks, **O&C,** 1½-oz. canister	231	22.0					154.0	14.67
Pumpernickel Snack Sticks, **Pepperidge Farm,** 7½-oz. box	825	127.5					110.0	17.00
Seaweed Crunch, **Soken,** 2.1-oz. bag	277		(8)				131.8	
1 Chip, approx. 0.07 oz. (approx. 16 per ounce)			(8)				131.8	
Seven ("7") Grain Chips, **Hain,** 4-oz. bag	524	80.0					131.0	20.00
Sour Cream and Onion Flavor Wheatwists, **Spicer's,** 3-oz. bag	360	50.0	(3)	(0.4)	(384)	(54.0)	120.0	16.67
1 Wheatwist, approx. 0.03 oz. (approx. 40 per ounce)			(3)	(0.4)	(384)	(54.0)	120.0	16.67
1 quart, approx. 3.2 oz. (approx. 128 Wheatwists)					(384)	(54.0)	120.0	6.67
Vegetable Chips, **Soken,** 2.1-oz. bag	271		(8)				129.0	
1 Chip, approx. 0.07 oz. (approx. 16 per ounce)			(8)				129.0	
Whole Grain Goodness Wheat Chips, **Nabisco,** 4¾-oz. package	713	80.8	(4)	(0.5)			150.0	17.00
1 Chip, approx. 0.03 oz. (approx. 33 per ounce)			(4)	(0.5)			15.00	17.00
Whole Wheat Snack Sticks, **Pepperidge Farm,** 7½-oz. box	825	127.5					110.0	17.00
Yogurt Chips, **Hain,** 4-oz. bag	576	60.0					144.0	15.00

30 HORS D'OEUVRES, DIPS & SPREADS •

As the Chapter Preface for HORS D'OEUVRES warns you, "the arrangement of HORS D'OEUVRES looks like a tray of hors d'oeuvres—distinctly non-alphabetical."

M.F.

HORS D'OEUVRES

NUTS, POPCORN, POTATO CHIPS, PRETZELS

	UNIT Cal.	UNIT Carb.	1 OZ., BY WT. Cal.	1 OZ., BY WT. Carb.
Cashews, roasted, (based on generic data), 1 cup (approx. 4.9 oz.)	785	41.0	159.0	8.30
1 medium cashew (approx. 0.06 oz., 18 to the ounce)	9	0.5	159.0	8.30
Peanuts, Virginia, salted, (based on generic data), 1 cup (approx. 5.1 oz.)	842	27.1	165.9	5.33
1 Virginia peanut (approx. 0.04 oz., 30 to the ounce)	6	0.2	165.9	5.33
Popcorn, **Bachman,** 1 quart (approx. 1.5 oz.)	(238)	(19.6)	160.0	13.00
1 piece, approx. 0.01 oz.	(1)	(0.1)	160.0	13.00
Potato Chips, **Ruffles (Frito-Lay),** 1 quart (approx. 3.0 oz.)	(452)	(45.2)	150.0	15.00
1 chip, approx. 0.04 oz.	(6)	(0.6)	150.0	15.00
Pretzels, Twist, **Ann Page (A&P),** 1 quart (approx. 3.6 oz.	(396)	(80.0)	110.0	22.00
1 pretzel twist, approx. 0.2 oz.	(22)	(4.5)	110.0	22.00

More in the NUTS & SEEDS chapter and the SALTY SNACKS chapter.

CRACKERS

	UNIT Cal.	UNIT Carb.	1 OZ., BY WT. Cal.	1 OZ., BY WT. Carb.
Flatbrod, Ultra Thin, **Ideal,** 1 cracker, approx. 0.1 oz.	11	2.4	109.1	23.62
Garlic Discos, **Devonsheer Melba,** 1 cracker, approx. 0.14 oz.	13	(2.2)	91.0	(15.37)
Ritz Crackers, **Nabisco,** 1 cracker, approx. 0.1 oz.	17	2.0	150.0	18.00
Saltine Crackers, **Nabisco "Premium,"** 1 cracker, approx. 0.1 oz.	12	2.0	120.0	20.00
Town House Crackers, **Keebler,** 1 cracker, approx. 0.1 oz.	17	2.0	157.5	18.00

More in the COOKIES & CRACKERS chapter.

COCKTAIL BREADS (PARTY SLICED)

	UNIT Cal.	UNIT Carb.	1 OZ., BY WT. Cal.	1 OZ., BY WT. Carb.
Pumpernickel (Party Sliced), **Pepperidge Farm,** 1 slice, approx. 0.21 oz.	23	3.5	106.9	16.60
Pumpernickel (Cocktail), **Rubschlager,** 1 slice, approx. 0.38 oz.	29	5.0	75.6	13.06
Rye (Party Sliced), **Pepperidge Farm,** 1 slice, approx. 0.21 oz.	18	3.0	83.1	14.25
Rye (Cocktail), **Rubschlager,** 1 slice, approx. 0.38 oz.	25	4.5	68.8	12.38

More in the BREADS chapter.

HARD CHEESES

Cheese spreads are in their own section at the end of this chapter.

	UNIT Cal.	UNIT Carb.	1 OZ., BY WT. Cal.	1 OZ., BY WT. Carb.
Cheddar Cheese (based on generic data), Domestic, 1 chunk measuring 1 cu in., approx. 0.6 oz.	69	0.2	114.4	0.36
Laughing Cow Cheese, 1 wedge, approx. 1 oz.	72	0.7	72.3	0.71
1 Cheezbit, approx. 0.18 oz.	13	0.1	72.3	0.71
Swiss Cheese (based on generic data), Domestic, 1 chunk measuring 1 cu. in., approx. 0.5 oz.	56	0.5	106.7	0.95

More (and how!) in the CHEESE chapter.

EGGS

	UNIT Cal.	UNIT Carb.	1 OZ., BY WT. Cal.	1 OZ., BY WT. Carb.
Hard Boiled Egg, 1 medium egg (based on generic data), shelled (approx. 1.5 oz.)	69	0.5	44.8	0.34
Deviled Eggs (based on a U.S. Army recipe; more Army recipes are in the MESS chapter): ½ hard cooked egg hollowed, with stuffing as follows: ½ yolk, 1 tsp. salad dressing, ½ tsp. drained sweet pickle relish, ½ tsp. prepared mustard, pinches of ground paprika and salt	114	2.5	60.2	1.30

More in the EGGS chapter.

RAW VEGETABLES (Crudités)

	UNIT Cal.	UNIT Carb.	1 OZ., BY WT. Cal.	1 OZ., BY WT. Carb.
Broccoli, 1 segment, approx. 3″ long, 1½″ diameter at head, approx. 0.4 oz.	3	0.6	9.1	1.70
Carrot Strips (based on generic data), 1 strip, approx. ⅜″ wide, 3″ long, approx. 0.2 oz.	2	0.5	11.9	2.75
Cauliflower, 1 segment, approx. 2″ long, 1½″ diameter at head, approx. 0.7 oz.	5	1.0	7.6	1.48
Celery Stalks, trimmed (based on generic data), 1 stalk, approx. 5″ long × ¾″ wide at root end, approx. 0.6 oz.	3	0.7	4.9	1.14
Celery, Stuffed (based on U.S. Army recipes; more Army recipes are in the MESS chapter):				
Blue-veined Cheese Stuffed Celery Stalk, 2″–3″ stalk stuffed as follows: 0.1 oz. blue-veined natural cheese, 0.3 Tbsp. cottage cheese blended with 0.1 tsp. reconstituted nonfat dry milk; sprinkle with paprika	(16)	(0.8)	(22.0)	(1.08)
Cheddar Cheese Stuffed Celery Stalk, 2″–3″ stalk stuffed as follows: 0.3 oz. of shredded processed Cheddar cheese, 0.4 tsp. chopped pimientoes, ¼ tsp. salad dressing with a drop of Worcestershire sauce and a pinch of cayenne pepper	(35)	(0.9)	(42.5)	(1.15)
Cottage Cheese Stuffed Celery Stalk, 2″–3″ stalk stuffed as follows: 1 tsp. cottage cheese, dash tomato catsup, 1 tsp. prepared horseradish, pinch of grated dry onions	(8)	(0.8)	(11.7)	(1.21)
Peanut Butter Stuffed Celery Stalk, 2″–3″ stalk stuffed as follows: 0.5 tsp. peanut butter thoroughly blended with ½ tsp. honey	(24)	(2.8)	(37.0)	(4.37)
Cherry Tomatoes (based on generic data), 1 medium tomato, approx. 0.7 oz.	(4)	(0.9)	(6.2)	(1.33)
Cucumber Slices, pared (based on generic data), 1 slice, approx. ⅛″ thick, approx. 0.1 oz.	trace	0.1	3.9	0.91
Green Pepper Rings (based on generic data), 1 ring, approx. 3″ diameter × ¼″ thick, approx. 0.35 oz.	2	0.5	6.2	1.36
Red Radishes, trimmed (based on generic data), medium, ¾″–1″ diameter; 1 radish, approx. 0.2 oz.	1	0.2	4.8	1.02
Scallions trimmed (based on generic data), tops of 1 bulb, approx. 1.3 oz.	10	2.0	7.7	1.56

More in the VEGETABLES chapter.

PICKLED and MARINATED VEGETABLES

	UNIT Cal.	UNIT Carb.	1 OZ., BY WT. Cal.	1 OZ., BY WT. Carb.
Artichoke Hearts, marinated in oil, **Cara Mia,** 6-oz. jar	(174)	(6.6)	(29.0)	(1.10)
Dill Pickles, large (approx. 4″ long × 1¾″ diameter) (based on generic data); 1 pickle, approx. 4.8 oz.	15	3.0	3.1	0.63
Gherkin Pickles, small (approx. 2½″ long × ¾″ diameter) (based on generic data); 1 pickle, approx. 0.5 oz.	22	5.5	41.4	10.35
Green Olives, large, with pits (approx. 12/16″ diameter x 15/16″ long) (based on generic data); 1 olive (approx. 0.2 oz.)	5	trace	27.6	0.31
Ripe Greek Olives, medium-size, with pits (approx. 12 per ounce) (based on generic data); 1 olive	7	0.2	76.4	2.00

More in the CONDIMENTS chapter.

FRUITS, based on generic data

	UNIT Cal.	UNIT Carb.	1 OZ., BY WT. Cal.	1 OZ., BY WT. Carb.
Apricots, 1 apricot, approx. 1.3 oz. (weighed with pit)	18	4.5	13.6	3.41
Dates, 1 date, approx. ⅓ oz. (weighed with pit)	21	5.8	67.6	17.98
Figs, 1 medium fig, approx. 1.8 oz.	40	10.2	22.7	5.76
Pineapple, 1 slice, approx. 3 oz.	44	11.5	14.8	3.88
Prunes, dried, 1 large prune, approx. ⅓ oz. (weighed with pit)	22	5.7	62.9	16.63

(For prunes at parties, see The Monologue, page 16.)

More in the FRUITS chapter.

COLD MEATS and SAUSAGES, based on generic data

	UNIT Cal.	UNIT Carb.	1 OZ., BY WT. Cal.	1 OZ., BY WT. Carb.
Bologna, beef, approx. 4″ diameter × ⅛″ thick; 1 slice, approx. 0.8 oz.	72	0.5	89.0	0.55
Braunschweiger (smoked Liverwurst), approx. 3⅛″ diameter × ¼″ thick; 1 slice, approx. 1 oz.	90	0.7	90.4	0.65
Chicken Roll, light meat, 1 slice, approx. 1 oz.	45	0.7	45.1	0.69
Frankfurters, approx. 5″ long × ⅞″ diameter; 1 frank, approx. 2 oz.	170	0.9	86.2	0.45
Ham, Boiled, approx. 4¼″ × 4¼″ × 1⁄16″ thick; 1 slice, approx. ¾ oz.	49	0.0	66.3	0.00
Kielbasa, approx. 5⅜″ long × 1″ diameter; 1 sausage, approx. 2.7 oz.	231	0.9	86.2	0.34
Knockwurst, approx. 4″ long × 1⅛″ diameter; 1 link, approx. 2.4 oz.	189	1.5	78.8	0.63
Pepperoni, approx. 1⅜″ diameter × ⅛″ thick, 1 slice, approx. 0.2 oz.	27	0.2	140.9	0.81
Pork Sausage, cooked, approx. 4″ long × ⅞″ diameter, 1 link, approx. 0.5 oz.	48	0.1	104.6	0.29
Roast Beef, trimmed of separable fat before cooking, 1 slice, approx. 1 oz.	68	0.0	68.4	0.00
Salami, beef, approx. 4″ diameter, × ⅛″ thick, 1 slice, approx. 0.8 oz.	58	0.6	72.0	0.71
Tongue, beef, 1 slice, approx. ¾ oz.	61	0.1	81.7	0.11
Turkey Roll, light meat, 1 slice, approx. 1 oz.	42	0.2	41.7	0.15

More in the SAUSAGES & COLD CUTS chapter and in the MEATS & GAME chapter.

SEAFOOD

	UNIT Cal.	UNIT Carb.	1 OZ., BY WT. Cal.	1 OZ., BY WT. Carb.
Anchovies (based on generic data), flat, 4″ long × ½″ wide × ⅛″ thick, or roll, ½″–¾″ diameter × ½″ thick; 1 fillet (approx. 0.14 oz.)	7	0.1	49.9	0.60
Caviar (based on generic data):				
Granular, 1 tablespoon (approx. 0.6 oz.)	42	0.5	74.0	0.90
Pressed, 1 tablespoon (approx. 0.6 oz.)	54	0.8	90.0	1.34
Clams, frozen, stuffed, **Matlaw's** Casino Hors d'Oeuvres, 1 clam, approx. 0.9 oz. weighed without shell	40	4.3	43.6	4.73
Clams, frozen, stuffed, New England Style, **Matlaw's** Casino Hors d'Oeuvres, 1 clam, approx. 1.8 oz. weighed without shell	90	9.0	49.1	4.91
Herring, smoked, kippered, canned (based on generic data), 1 fillet, approx. 0.7 oz.	42	0.0	60.4	0.00
Mussels, smoked, **Pacific Pearl,** 1 oz.	72	1.9	72.3	1.93
Oysters, smoked, **Pacific Pearl,** 1 oz.	81	4.1	80.5	4.05
Salmon, smoked (based on generic data), 1 slice, approx. 3 oz.	150	0.0	49.9	0.00
Sardines, Norway, **King Oscar,** 1 sardine, approx. 0.15 oz.	(13)	(0.1)	(87.8)	(0.34)
Shrimp, medium, canned (based on generic data), approx. 2½″ long; 1 shrimp, approx. 0.1 oz.	4	trace	32.9	0.20

More in the FISH, SHELLFISH & WATERLIFE chapter.

EGG ROLLS and SEAFOOD ROLLS

	UNIT Cal.	UNIT Carb.	1 OZ., BY WT. Cal.	1 OZ., BY WT. Carb.
Chicken Egg Roll, **La Choy,** 6½-oz. container, 15 egg rolls	447	54.2	68.7	8.34
1 egg roll, approx. 0.4 oz.	(28)	(3.3)	68.7	8.34
Lobster Egg Roll, **La Choy,** 6½-oz. container, 15 egg rolls	400	57.2	61.6	8.80
1 lobster egg roll, approx. 0.4 oz.	25	3.5	61.6	8.80
Lobster Rolls, **Matlaw's,** 15-oz. package, 6 rolls	1080	120.0	72.0	8.00
1 lobster roll, approx. 2½ oz.	180	20.0	72.0	8.00
Meat and Shrimp Egg Roll, **La Choy,** 6½-oz. container, 15 egg rolls	402	52.4	61.9	8.06
1 meat & shrimp egg roll, approx. 0.4 oz.	25	3.2	61.9	8.06
7½-oz. container, 30 egg rolls	519	70.2	69.2	9.36
1 meat & shrimp egg roll, approx. 0.25 oz.	17	2.3	69.2	9.36
Shrimp Egg Roll, **La Choy,** 5-oz. container, 2 egg rolls	216	29.8	43.1	5.96
1 shrimp egg roll, approx. 2½ oz.	108	14.9	43.1	5.96
6½-oz. container, 15 egg rolls	387	55.5	59.6	8.54
1 shrimp egg roll, approx. 0.4 oz.	24	3.4	59.6	8.54

PIZZA NOVELTIES

	UNIT Cal.	UNIT Carb.	1 OZ., BY WT. Cal.	1 OZ., BY WT. Carb.
Cheese Pizza Bagels, **Lender's,** 12-oz. box, 6 bagels	840	102.0	70.0	8.50
1 bagel, approx. 2 oz.	140	17.0	70.0	8.50
Cheeseburger Pizza Rolls, **Jeno's,** 6-oz. package, 12 rolls	540	54.0	90.0	9.00
1 roll, approx. ½ oz.	45	4.5	90.0	9.00
Mushroom Pizza Bagels, **Lender's,** 13½-oz. box, 6 bagels	900	108.0	66.7	8.00
1 bagel, approx. 2¼ oz.	150	18.0	66.7	8.00
Onion Pizza Bagels, **Lender's,** 13½-oz. box, 6 bagels	840	114.0	62.2	8.44
1 bagel, approx. 2¼ oz.	140	19	62.2	8.44
Pepperoni & Cheese Pizza Rolls, **Jeno's,** 6-oz. package, 12 rolls	520	50.0	86.7	8.33
1 roll, approx. ½ oz.	43	4.2	86.7	8.33
Sausage & Cheese Pizza Rolls, **Jeno's,** 6-oz. package, 12 rolls	520	50.0	86.7	8.33
1 roll, approx. ½ oz.	43	4.2	86.7	8.33
Shrimp & Cheese Pizza Rolls, **Jeno's,** 6-oz. package, 12 rolls	440	46.0	73.3	7.67
1 roll, approx. ½ oz.	37	3.8	73.3	7.67
"The Works," Onions, Peppers & Mushrooms Pizza Bagels, **Lender's,** 16½-oz. box, 6 bagels	1020	137.9	61.8	8.36
1 bagel, approx. 2¾ oz.	170	23.0	61.8	8.36

For PIZZAS, see the COMBINATION MAIN DISHES chapter.

DIPS and SPREADS

COTTAGE CHEESE, based on generic data

	UNIT Cal.	UNIT Carb.	1 OZ., BY WT. Cal.	1 OZ., BY WT. Carb.	1 CUP Cal.	1 CUP Carb.	1 TEASPOON Cal.	1 TEASPOON Carb.
Creamed Cottage Cheese, small curd, (4.51% fat), 8-oz. container	234	6.1	29.2	0.76	216	5.6	5	0.1
1 tablespoon (approx. 0.5 oz.)	15	0.4	29.2	0.76	216	5.6	5	0.1
Low-Fat Cottage Cheese (1% fat), 8-oz. container	164	6.2	20.4	0.77	163	6.1	3	0.1
1 tablespoon (approx. 0.5 oz.)	10	0.4	20.4	0.77	163	6.1	3	0.1

More in the CHEESE chapter.

CREAM CHEESE, based on generic data

	UNIT Cal.	UNIT Carb.	1 OZ., BY WT. Cal.	1 OZ., BY WT. Carb.	1 CUP Cal.	1 CUP Carb.	1 TEASPOON Cal.	1 TEASPOON Carb.
Regular or Whipped, (34.87% fat) 1 pound	1584	12.1	99.0	0.75				
Regular, 1 tablespoon (approx. 0.51 oz.)	51	0.4	99.0	0.75	812	6.2	17	0.1
1 teaspoon (approx. 0.2 oz.)	17	0.1	99.0	0.75	812	6.2	17	0.1
Whipped, 1 tablespoon (approx. 0.34 oz.)	34	0.3	99.0	0.75	545	4.1	11	0.1
1 teaspoon (approx. 0.1 oz.)	11	0.1	99.0	0.75	545	4.1	11	0.1

More in the CHEESE chapter.

Cream Cheese, Imitation

	UNIT Cal.	UNIT Carb.	1 OZ., BY WT. Cal.	1 OZ., BY WT. Carb.	1 CUP Cal.	1 CUP Carb.	1 TEASPOON Cal.	1 TEASPOON Carb.
Imitation Cream Cheese, **Philadelphia,** 8-oz. package	400	16.0	50.0	2.00	410	16.4	9	0.3
1 tablespoon (approx. 0.5 oz.)	26	1.0	50.0	2.00	410	16.4	9	0.3
1 teaspoon (approx. 0.2 oz.)	9	0.3	50.0	2.00	410	16.4	9	0.3

	UNIT Cal.	UNIT Carb.	1 OZ., BY WT. Cal.	1 OZ., BY WT. Carb.	1 CUP Cal.	1 CUP Carb.	1 TEASPOON Cal.	1 TEASPOON Carb.
Cream Cheese Product								
Pasteurized Process Cream Cheese Product, **Philadelphia** "Light," 8-oz. container	480	16.0	60.0	2.00	423	14.1	9	0.3
1 tablespoon (approx. 0.4 oz.)	26	0.9	60.0	2.00	423	14.1	9	0.3
1 teaspoon (approx. 0.1 oz.)	9	0.3	60.0	2.00	423	14.1	9	0.3
MAYONNAISE, based on generic data								
1 cup (approx. 7.8 oz.)	1580	4.8	203.6	0.62	1580	4.8	33	0.1
1 tablespoon (approx. 0.5 oz.)	99	0.3	203.6	0.62	1580	4.8	33	0.1
1 teaspoon (approx. 0.2 oz.)	33	0.1	203.6	0.62	1580	4.8	33	0.1
More in the CONDIMENTS chapter.								
Mayonnaise, Imitation								
Imitation Mayonnaise, **Mrs. Filberts,** 16-fl.-oz. (1-pint) jar	1280	32.0	(80.0)	(2.00)	640	16.0	13	0.3
1 tablespoon (approx. 0.5 oz.)	40	1.0	(80.0)	(2.00)	640	16.0	13	0.3
1 teaspoon (approx. 0.2 oz.)	13	0.3	(80.0)	(2.00)	640	16.0	13	0.3
More in the CONDIMENTS chapter.								
SOUR CREAM								
HALF AND HALF SOUR CREAM, based on generic data								
12% fat, 1 pound (approx. 1.9 cups)	613	54.4	38.3	3.40	320	28.8	7	0.6
1 cup (approx. 8.5 oz.)	320	28.8	38.3	3.40	320	28.8	7	0.6
1 tablespoon (approx. 0.5 oz.)	20	1.8	38.3	3.40	320	28.8	7	0.6
SOUR CREAM, based on generic data								
20.96% fat, 1 pound (approx. 2 cups)	971	19.4	60.7	1.21	492	9.8	10	0.2
1 cup (approx. 8.1 oz.)	492	9.8	60.7	1.21	492	9.8	10	0.2
1 tablespoon (approx. 0.4 oz.)	31	0.6	60.7	1.21	492	9.8	10	0.2
More in the CONDIMENTS chapter.								
Sour Cream, Imitation, and Non-Butterfat Sour Dressing								
NONDAIRY IMITATION SOUR CREAM, based on generic data								
19.5% fat, 1 pound (approx. 2 cups)	946	30.1	59.9	1.88	479	15.3	10	0.3
1 cup (approx. 8.1 oz.)	479	15.3	59.9	1.88	479	15.3	10	0.3
1 tablespoon (approx. 0.4 oz.)	30	1.0	59.9	1.88	479	15.3	10	0.3
FILLED CREAM-TYPE NON-BUTTERFAT SOUR DRESSING, based on generic data								
16.6% fat, 1 pound (approx. 1.9 cups)	806	21.2	50.5	1.33	417	11.0	7	0.2
1 cup (approx. 8.3 oz.)	417	11.0	50.5	1.33	417	11.0	7	0.2
1 tablespoon (approx. 0.4 oz.)	21	0.6	50.5	1.33	417	11.0	7	0.2
More in the CONDIMENTS chapter.								
YOGURT, based on generic data								
Low-Fat Yogurt, 1 teaspoon (approx. 0.2 oz.)	(3)	(0.4)	17.9	2.00	(158)	(17.5)	(3)	(0.4)
Skim-Milk Yogurt, 1 teaspoon (approx. 0.2 oz.)	(3)	(0.4)	15.9	2.18	(139)	(19.1)	(3)	(0.4)
Whole-Milk Yogurt, 1 teaspoon (approx. 0.2 oz.)	(3)	(0.2)	17.3	1.32	(150)	(11.4)	(3)	(0.2)

	UNIT Cal.	UNIT Carb.	1 OZ., BY WT. Cal.	1 OZ., BY WT. Carb.	1 CUP Cal.	1 CUP Carb.	1 TEASPOON Cal.	1 TEASPOON Carb.
More in the YOGURT chapter.								
DIPS								
DIPS, based on data from the Middle East								
Eggplant Dip (Baba Gannuj), 1 pound	481	66.2	30.1	4.14				
Hummus (Hommous or Humus), 1 pound	1361	95.5	85.1	5.97				
Tahini, 1 pound	3139	46.3	196.2	2.89				
DIPS, by brand								
Bacon and Horseradish Sour Cream Dip, **Kraft,** 8-oz. container	263	22.5	32.8	2.81	280	24.0	6	0.5
1 cup (approx. 8.5 oz.)	280	24.0	32.8	2.81	280	24.0	6	0.5
1 tablespoon (approx. 0.5 oz.)	18	1.5	32.8	2.81	280	24.0	6	0.5
Bacon and Horseradish Yogurt Dip, **Light n' Lively,** 8-oz. container	263	22.5	32.8	2.81	280	24.0	6	0.5
1 cup (approx. 8.5 oz.)	280	24.0	32.8	2.81	280	24.0	6	0.5
1 tablespoon (approx. 0.5 oz.)	18	1.5	32.8	2.81	280	24.0	6	0.5
Blue Cheese Chip-Dip, **Granny Goose,** 1-oz. container	108	14.0	108.0	14.00	(922)	(119.5)	(19)	(2.5)
2-oz. container	217	28.0	108.0	14.00	(922)	(119.5)	(19)	(2.5)
3-oz. container	326	41.9	108.0	14.00	(922)	(119.5)	(19)	(2.5)
3.3-oz. container	383	49.3	108.0	14.00	(922)	(119.5)	(19)	(2.5)
4-oz. container	434	55.9	108.0	14.00	(922)	(119.5)	(19)	(2.5)
1 cup (approx. 8.5 oz.)	(922)	(119.5)	108.0	14.00	(922)	(119.5)	(19)	(2.5)
1 tablespoon (approx. 0.5 oz.)	(58)	(7.5)	108.0	14.00	(922)	(119.5)	(19)	(2.5)
Blue Cheese Dip, **Kraft,** 8-oz. container	454	121.0	56.7	15.12	480	121.0	10	0.3
1 cup (approx. 8.5 oz.)	480	16.0	56.7	15.12	480	121.0	10	0.3
1 tablespoon (approx. 0.5 oz.)	30	1.0	56.7	15.12	480	121.0	10	0.3
Blue Cheese Dressing & Chip Mix, **Weight Watchers,** 6-oz. envelope	80	8.0	133.3	13.33				
Prepared as directed, add 6 tablespoons water (yield: 3 fl. oz., or 3.6 oz. by weight)	80	8.0	(22.2)	(2.22)	214	21.4	4	0.4
1 cup (approx. 9.6 oz.)	214	21.4	(22.2)	(2.22)	214	21.4	4	0.4
1 tablespoon (approx. 0.6 oz.)	13	1.3	(22.2)	(2.22)	214	21.4	4	0.4
Blue Cheese Yogurt Dip, **Light n' Lively,** 8-oz. container	338	22.5	42.9	2.81	360	24.0	8	0.5
1 cup (approx. 8.4 oz.)	360	24.0	42.9	2.81	360	24.0	8	0.5
1 tablespoon (approx. 0.5 oz.)	23	1.5	42.9	2.81	360	24.0	8	0.5
California Dip, see Sour Cream & Onion Dip								
Cucumber & Onion Yogurt Dip, **Light n' Lively,** 8-oz. container	263	22.5	32.8	2.81	280	24.0	6	0.5
1 cup (approx. 8.5 oz.)	280	24.0	32.8	2.81	280	24.0	6	0.5
1 tablespoon (approx. 0.5 oz.)	18	1.5	32.8	2.81	280	24.0	6	0.5
Enchilada Dip, **Fritos,** 10½-oz. container	387	43.3	37.1	4.13	(317)	(35.1)	(7)	(0.7)
1 cup (approx. 8.5 oz.)	(317)	(35.1)	37.1	4.13	(317)	(35.1)	(7)	(0.7)
1 tablespoon (approx. 0.5 oz.)	(20)	(2.1)	37.1	4.13	(317)	(35.1)	(7)	(0.7)
French Onion Yogurt Dip, **Light n' Lively,** 8-oz. container	263	22.5	32.8	2.81	280	24.0	6	0.5
1 cup (approx. 8.5 oz.)	280	24.0	32.8	2.81	280	24.0	6	0.5
1 tablespoon (approx. 0.5 oz.)	18	1.5	32.8	2.81	280	24.0	6	0.5
Garlic Chip Dip, **Granny Goose,** 1-oz. container	101	15.7	101.0	15.70	(862)	(134.0)	(18)	(2.8)
2-oz. container	203	31.2	101.0	15.70	(862)	(134.0)	(18)	(2.8)
3-oz. container	304	47.2	101.0	15.70	(862)	(134.0)	(18)	(2.8)
3.3-oz. container	358	55.5	101.0	15.70	(862)	(134.0)	(18)	(2.8)
4-oz. container	405	62.9	101.0	15.70	(862)	(134.0)	(18)	(2.8)
1 cup (approx. 8.5 oz.)	(862)	(134.0)	101.0	15.70	(862)	(134.0)	(18)	(2.8)
1 tablespoon (approx. 0.5 oz.)	(54)	(8.4)	101.0	15.70	(862)	(134.0)	(18)	(2.8)
Green Onion Chip Dip, **Granny Goose,** 1-oz. container	105	16.3	105.0	16.30	(896)	(139.0)	(19)	(2.9)
2-oz. container	210	32.7	105.0	16.30	(896)	(139.0)	(19)	(2.9)
3-oz. container	314	49.0	105.0	16.30	(896)	(139.0)	(19)	(2.9)

	UNIT Cal.	UNIT Carb.	1 OZ., BY WT. Cal.	1 OZ., BY WT. Carb.	1 CUP Cal.	1 CUP Carb.	1 TEASPOON Cal.	1 TEASPOON Carb.
3.3-oz. container	370	57.7	105.0	16.30	(896)	(139.0)	(19)	(2.9)
4-oz. container	418	65.2	105.0	16.30	(896)	(139.0)	(19)	(2.9)
1 cup (approx. 8.5 oz.)	(896)	(139.0)	105.0	16.30	(896)	(139.0)	(19)	(2.9)
1 tablespoon (approx. 0.5 oz.)	(56)	(8.7)	105.0	16.30	(896)	(139.0)	(19)	(2.9)
Jalapeño Bean Dip, **Fritos,** 10½-oz. tin	333	43.3	31.7	4.12	(270)	(35.1)	(6)	(0.7)
1 cup (approx. 8.5 oz.)	(270)	(35.1)	31.7	4.12	(270)	(35.1)	(6)	(0.7)
1 tablespoon (approx. 0.5 oz.)	(17)	(2.2)	31.7	4.12	(270)	(35.1)	(6)	(0.7)
Jalapeño Bean Dip, **Granny Goose,** 1-oz. container	37	4.8	37.0	4.80	(316)	(40.9)	(7)	(0.9)
2-oz. container	74	9.6	37.0	4.80	(316)	(40.9)	(7)	(0.9)
3-oz. container	111	14.4	37.0	4.80	(316)	(40.9)	(7)	(0.9)
3.3-oz. container	131	17.0	37.0	4.80	(316)	(40.9)	(7)	(0.9)
4-oz. container	148	19.3	37.0	4.80	(316)	(40.9)	(7)	(0.9)
1 cup (approx. 8.5 oz.)	(316)	(40.9)	37.0	4.80	(316)	(40.9)	(7)	(0.9)
1 tablespoon (approx. 0.5 oz.)	(20)	(2.6)	37.0	4.80	(316)	(40.9)	(7)	(0.9)
Jalapeño Pepper Dip, **Kraft,** 8-oz. container	378	22.7	47.3	2.84	400	24.0	8	0.5
1 cup (approx. 8.5 oz.)	400	24.0	47.3	2.84	400	24.0	8	0.5
1 tablespoon (approx. 0.5 oz.)	25	1.5	47.3	2.84	400	24.0	8	0.5
Sour Cream & Onion Dip ("California Dip"), made from **Lipton's** Onion Soup Mix:								
1 envelope prepared as directed with 2 cups sour cream (yield: 2 cups dip, approx. 19 oz.)	1110	43.8	58.5	2.31	555	21.9	12	0.5
Entire package prepared (yield: 4 cups, approx. 38 oz.)	2220	87.6	58.5	2.31	555	21.9	12	0.5
1 cup (approx. 9.5 oz.)	555	21.9	58.5	2.31	555	21.9	12	0.5
1 tablespoon (approx. 0.6 oz.)	35	1.4	58.5	2.31	555	21.9	12	0.5
Tostitos Picante Sauce, **Frito-Lay,** 10½-oz. tin	150	26.7	14.3	2.54	(121)	(21.6)	(3)	(0.4)
1 cup (approx. 8.5 oz.)	(121)	(21.6)	14.3	2.54	(121)	(21.6)	(3)	(0.4)
1 tablespoon (approx. 0.5 oz.)	(8)	(1.3)	14.3	2.54	(121)	(21.6)	(3)	(0.4)

CHEESE SPREADS

	UNIT Cal.	UNIT Carb.	1 OZ., BY WT. Cal.	1 OZ., BY WT. Carb.	1 CUP Cal.	1 CUP Carb.	1 TEASPOON Cal.	1 TEASPOON Carb.
Neufchâtel Blue Cheese, **Kraft,** 1 tablespoon (approx. 0.5 oz.)	(37)	(1.1)	70.0	2.00	(592)	(17.6)	(12)	(0.4)
Neufchâtel Cheese Spread with Bacon & Horseradish, **Kraft,** 1 tablespoon (approx. 0.5 oz.)	(37)	(0.5)	70.0	1.00	(592)	(8.0)	(12)	(0.2)
Neufchâtel Cheese Spread with Clams, **Kraft,** 1 tablespoon (approx. 0.5 oz.)	(37)	(1.1)	70.0	2.00	(592)	(17.6)	(12)	(0.4)
Neufchâtel Cheese Spread with Dill Pickles, **Kraft,** 1 tablespoon (approx. 0.5 oz.)	(37)	(1.1)	70.0	2.00	(592)	(17.6)	(12)	(0.4)
Neufchâtel Cheese Spread with Garlic & Onions, **Kraft,** 1 tablespoon (approx. 0.5 oz.)	(37)	(1.1)	70.0	2.00	(592)	(17.6)	(12)	(0.4)
Neufchâtel Cheese Spread with Onions, **Kraft,** 1 tablespoon (approx. 0.5 oz.)	(37)	(1.6)	70.0	3.00	(592)	(25.6)	(12)	(0.5)

SANDWICH SPREADS

	UNIT Cal.	UNIT Carb.	1 OZ., BY WT. Cal.	1 OZ., BY WT. Carb.	1 CUP Cal.	1 CUP Carb.	1 TEASPOON Cal.	1 TEASPOON Carb.
SANDWICH SPREADS, based on generic data								
Chicken Spread, canned, 1 pound (4g/2g/3g/na/na)	880	24.5	55.0	1.53	400	11.2	8	0.2
1 tablespoon (approx. 0.5 oz.)	25	0.7	55.0	1.53	400	11.2	8	0.2
Ham & Cheese Spread, 1 pound (5g/1g/5g/59%/339mg)	1104	10.2	69.0	0.64	592	5.5	12	0.1
1 tablespoon (approx. 0.5 oz.)	37	0.3	69.0	0.64	592	5.5	12	0.1
Ham Salad Spread, 1 pound (2g/3g/4g/63%/259mg)	976	48.3	61.0	3.02	976	25.6	11	0.5
1 tablespoon (approx. 0.5 oz.)	32	1.6	61.0	3.02	976	25.6	11	0.5
Poultry Salad Sandwich Spread, 1 pound (3g/2g/4g/na/107mg)	912	33.6	57.0	2.10	416	16.0	9	0.3
1 tablespoon (approx. 0.5 oz.)	26	1.0	57.0	2.10	416	16.0	9	0.3
Sandwich Spread made with pork and beef, 1 pound (2g/3g/5g/60%/287mg)	1072	54.2	67.0	3.39	560	28.8	12	0.6

	UNIT Cal.	UNIT Carb.	1 OZ., BY WT. Cal.	1 OZ., BY WT. Carb.	1 CUP Cal.	1 CUP Carb.	1 TEASPOON Cal.	1 TEASPOON Carb.
1 tablespoon (approx. 0.5 oz.)	35	1.8	67.0	3.39	560	28.8	12	0.6
SANDWICH SPREADS, by brand								
Chicken Salad Sandwich Spread, **Carnation,** 7½-oz. can	470	13.0	62.7	1.73	544	15.0	11	0.3
1 tablespoon (approx. 0.5 oz.)	34	0.9	62.7	1.73	544	15.0	11	0.3
Chicken Spread, **Swanson,** 5-oz. can	350	5.0	70.0	1.00	(560)	(8.0)	(12)	(0.2)
1 tablespoon (approx. 0.5 oz.)	35	0.5	70.0	1.00	(560)	(8.0)	(12)	(0.2)
Chicken Spread, **Underwood,** 4¾-oz. can	299	5.2	63.0	1.05	(547)	(9.5)	(11)	(0.2)
1 tablespoon (approx. 0.5 oz.)	(34)	(0.6)	63.0	1.05	(547)	(9.5)	(11)	(0.2)
Corned Beef Spread, **Underwood,** 4½-oz. can	247		54.8		(475)		(10)	
1 tablespoon (approx. 0.5 oz.)	(30)		54.8		(475)		(10)	
Ham, Deviled, **Armour,** 3-oz. can	220	0.0	73.3	0.00	(633)	0.0	(13)	0.0
4½-oz. can	330	0.0	73.3	0.00	(633)	0.0	(13)	0.0
1 tablespoon (approx. 0.5 oz.)	(40)	0.0	73.3	0.00	(633)	0.0	(13)	10.0
Ham, Deviled, **Hormel,** 3-oz. can	222	0.0	74.0	0.00	(639)	0.0	(13)	0.0
1 tablespoon (approx. 0.5 oz.)	(40)	0.0	74.0	0.00	(639)	0.0	(13)	0.0
Ham, Deviled, **Libby's,** 3-oz. can	(222)	(0.9)	(74.1)	(0.29)	640	2.5	13	0.1
5¼-oz. can	(389)	(1.5)	(74.1)	(0.29)	640	2.5	13	0.1
1 tablespoon (approx. 0.5 oz.)	40	0.2	(74.1)	(0.29)	640	2.5	13	0.1
Ham, Deviled, **Underwood,** 4½-oz. can	437		97.0	trace	(839)		(17)	trace
1 tablespoon (approx. 0.5 oz.)	(52)	trace	97.0	trace	(839)		(17)	trace
Ham & Cheese Spread, **Oscar Mayer,** 6-oz. tube	437	3.2	72.9	0.54	(365)	(2.7)	(8)	(0.1)
1 tablespoon (approx. 0.5 oz.)	23	0.2	72.9	0.54	(365)	(2.7)	(8)	(0.1)
Ham Salad Sandwich Spread, **Carnation,** 7½-oz. can	390	17.0	52.0	2.27	451	19.7	9	0.4
1 tablespoon (approx. 0.5 oz.)	28	1.2	52.0	2.27	451	19.7	9	0.4
Ham Salad Spread, **Oscar Mayer,** 6-oz. tube	367	16.8	61.2	2.81	(306)	(14.1)	(6)	(0.3)
1 tablespoon (approx. 0.5 oz.)	19	0.9	61.2	2.81	(306)	(14.1)	(6)	(0.3)
Liverwurst Spread, **Underwood,** 4¾-oz. can	437	5.2	92.0	1.10	(795)	(9.5)	(17)	(0.2)
1 tablespoon (approx. 0.5 oz.)	(49)	(0.6)	92.0	1.10	(795)	(9.5)	(17)	(0.2)
Relish Sandwich Spread, **Numade,** 16-fl.-oz. (1-pint) jar	1800	120.0	112.5	7.50	960	64.0	20	1.3
24-fl.-oz. jar	2700	180.0	112.5	7.50	960	64.0	20	1.3
1 tablespoon (approx. 0.2 oz.)	20	1.3	112.5	7.50	960	64.0	20	1.3
Roast Beef Spread, **Underwood,** 4¾-oz. can	276	1.4	58.0	0.30	(501)	(2.6)	(10)	(0.1)
1 tablespoon (approx. 0.5 oz.)	(31)	(0.7)	58.0	0.30	(501)	(2.6)	(10)	(0.1)
Sandwich Spread, **Oscar Mayer,** 8-oz. tube	488	32.2	61.0	4.03	(527)	(34.8)	(11)	(0.7)
1 tablespoon (approx. 0.5 oz.)	(33)	(2.2)	61.0	4.03	(527)	(34.8)	(11)	(0.7)
Spam Luncheon Meat, Deviled, **Spam (Hormel),** 2-oz. can	160	0.0	80.0	0.00	560	0.0	12	0.0
4½-oz. can	360	0.0	80.0	0.00	560	0.0	12	0.0
1 tablespoon (approx. 0.4 oz.)	35	0.0	80.0	0.00	560	0.0	12	0.0
Treet, Deviled, **Armour,** 3-oz. can	240	0.0	80.0	0.00				
Tuna Salad Sandwich Spread, **Carnation,** 7½-oz. can	405	16.0	54.0	2.13	468	18.5	10	0.4
1 tablespoon (approx. 0.5 oz.)	29	1.1	54.0	2.13	468	18.5	10	0.4
Tuno Spread (vegetarian tuna fish substitute), frozen, **Worthington,** 12-oz. roll	540	18.0	45.0	1.50	(357)	(11.9)	(7)	(0.2)
1 tablespoon (approx. 0.5 oz.)	(22)	(0.7)	45.0	1.50	(357)	(11.9)	(7)	(0.2)
Turkey Salad Sandwich Spread, **Carnation,** 7½-oz. can	430	15.0	57.3	2.00	497	17.3	10	0.4
1 tablespoon (approx. 0.5 oz.)	31	1.1	57.3	2.00	497	17.3	10	0.4

	UNIT		1 OZ., BY WT.		1 CUP		1 TEASPOON	
	Cal.	Carb.	Cal.	Carb.	Cal.	Carb.	Cal.	Carb.
VEGETABLE SPREADS								
Vegetable Spread, Curry, **Tartex,** 4-oz. tin	272	13.6	68.0	3.40	(495)	(24.3)	(10)	(0.5)
Vegetable Spread, Deluxe, **Tartex,** 2⅛-oz. tin	174	6.8	80.2	3.12	(588)	(22.9)	(12)	(0.5)
4-oz. tin	321	12.5	80.2	3.12	(588)	(22.9)	(12)	(0.5)
Vegetable Spread with Herbs, **Tartex,** 2⅛-oz. tin	149	6.8	68.3	3.12	(501)	(22.9)	(10)	(0.5)
4-oz. tin	273	12.5	68.3	3.12	(501)	(22.9)	(10)	(0.5)
Vegetable Spread, Plain, **Tartex,** 2⅛-oz. tin	149	6.8	68.3	3.12	(501)	(22.9)	(10)	(0.5)
4-oz. tin	273	12.5	68.3	3.12	(501)	(22.9)	(10)	(0.5)
PÂTÉS, based on generic data								
Chicken Liver Pâté, canned, 1 pound (4g/2g/4g/na/na)	912	29.8	57.0	1.86	416	14.4	9	0.3
1 tablespoon (approx. 0.5 oz.)	26	0.9	57.0	1.86	416	14.4	9	0.3
Goose Liver Pâté, Smoked (Pâté de Foie Gras), canned; 1 pound (3g/1g/12g/37%/na)	2096	21.1	131.0	1.32	960	9.6	20	0.2
1 tablespoon (approx. 0.5 oz.)	60	0.6	131.0	1.32	960	9.6	20	0.2
Liver Pâté (type of liver not specified), canned; 1 pound (4g/tr/8g/54%/198mg)	1440	6.9	90.0	0.43	656	3.2	14	0.1
1 tablespoon (approx. 0.5 oz.)	41	0.2	90.0	0.43	656	3.2	14	0.1

31 ALCOHOLIC BEVERAGES •

	UNIT		1 FLUID OZ.		1 CUP		1 TABLE-SPOON	
	Cal.	Carb.	Cal.	Carb.	Cal.	Carb.	Cal.	Carb.
BEER AND ALE, based on generic data								
Based on data from the University of California:								
Ale, mild, 12-fl.-oz. bottle	148	12.0	12.3	1.00	99	8.0	6.2	0.50
Beer, 12-fl.-oz. can or bottle	156	13.2	13.0	1.10	104	8.8	6.5	0.55
Based on data from Africa:								
Maize Beer, 12 fl. oz.	(122)	(13.1)	(10.2)	(1.09)	(82)	(8.7)	(5.1)	(0.54)
BEER AND ALE, by brand								
Amstel Light Bier, 12-fl.-oz. container	95	5.0	7.9	0.42	63	3.3	3.9	0.21
For comparison: **Birell "Near Beer,"** 12-fl.-oz. bottle	75	15.6	6.3	1.30	50	10.4	3.1	0.65
Budweiser Beer, 7-fl.-oz. can	88	7.6	12.5	1.08	100	8.7	6.3	0.54
12-fl.-oz. can or bottle	150	13.0	12.5	1.08	100	8.7	6.3	0.54
16-fl.-oz. (1-pint) can	200	17.3	12.5	1.08	100	8.7	6.3	0.54
32-fl.-oz. (1-quart) bottle	400	34.6	12.5	1.08	100	8.7	6.3	0.54
Budweiser Light Beer, 12-fl.-oz. can	108	8.8	9.0	0.73	72	5.9	4.5	0.37
Busch Beer, 12-fl.-oz. can or bottle	145	12.0	12.1	1.00	97	8.0	6.1	0.50
32-fl.-oz. (1-quart) bottle	390	32.0	12.1	1.00	97	8.0	6.1	0.50
Carling Black Label Light Beer, 12-fl.-oz. bottle or can	96	3.2	8.0	0.27	64	2.1	4.0	0.13
Coors Light Beer, 12-fl.-oz. can	103	4.5	8.6	0.37	69	3.0	4.3	0.19
Coors Premium Beer, 12-fl.-oz. can or bottle	143	12.3	12.0	1.02	96	8.2	6.0	0.51
Delight Beer, reduced calorie, 12-fl.-oz. can or bottle	96	4.1	8.0	0.34	64	2.7	4.0	0.17
Erlanger Beer, 12-fl.-oz. container	161	15.6	13.4	1.30	107	10.4	6.7	0.65
Kirin Beer, 12-fl.-oz. bottle	150	12.0	12.5	1.00	100	8.0	6.3	0.50
Michelob Beer, 7-fl.-oz. bottle	95	8.7	13.8	1.24	110	9.9	6.8	0.62
12-fl.-oz. can or bottle	166	14.9	13.8	1.24	110	9.9	6.8	0.62
Michelob Light Beer, 12-fl.-oz. can or bottle	134	12.0	11.2	1.00	90	8.0	5.6	0.50
Miller High Life Beer, 12-fl.-oz. bottle or can	150	14.0	12.5	1.17	100	9.3	6.3	0.58
Miller Lite Beer, 12-fl.-oz. can or bottle	96	2.8	8.0	0.23	64	1.8	4.0	0.11
Natural Light Beer, 12-fl.-oz. can or bottle	97	5.5	8.1	0.46	65	3.7	4.1	0.23

	UNIT		1 FLUID OZ.		1 CUP		1 TABLE-SPOON	
	Cal.	Carb.	Cal.	Carb.	Cal.	Carb.	Cal.	Carb.
For comparison: **"Near Beer," (Kingsbury Brew),** 12-fl.-oz. can	63		5.3		42		2.6	
Old Milwaukee Beer, 12-fl.-oz. can	144	13.5	12.0	1.13	96	9.0	6.0	0.57
Old Milwaukee Light Beer, 12-fl.-oz. can	120		10.0		80		5.0	
Olympia Gold Light Beer, 12-fl.-oz. bottle	70		5.8		47		2.9	
Pabst Blue Ribbon Beer, 7-oz. bottle	88	7.6	12.5	1.08	100	8.6	6.3	0.54
Pabst Extra Light Beer, 12-oz. bottle	70	5.1	5.8	0.43	47	3.4	2.9	0.21
Pripps Kalback Lager, 12-fl.-oz. container	110	3.3	9.2	0.28	73	2.2	4.6	0.14
Rheingold Extra Light Beer, 12-fl.-oz. bottle or can	96	3.0	8.0	0.25	64	2.0	4.0	0.13
Schaefer Light Lager, 12-fl.-oz. can	115	8.0	9.6	0.67	77	5.3	4.8	0.33
Schlitz Beer, 12-fl.-oz. bottle or can	148	13.4	12.3	1.12	98	9.0	6.1	0.56
Schlitz Light Beer, 12-fl.-oz. bottle or can	96	5.0	8.0	0.42	64	3.3	4.0	0.21
Schlitz Malt Liquor, 12-fl.-oz. can	175	13.5	14.6	1.12	117	9.0	7.3	0.56
Schlitz Repeal, 12-fl.-oz. container	121	10.6	10.1	0.88	81	7.0	5.1	0.44
Schmidt's Beer, 12-fl.-oz. bottle or can	145	12.9	12.1	1.08	97	8.6	6.1	0.54
Schmidt's Bavarian Beer, 12-fl.-oz. bottle or can	140	12.6	11.7	1.05	93	8.4	5.8	0.53
Schmidt's Light Beer, 12-fl.-oz. bottle or can	96	2.6	8.0	0.22	64	1.7	4.0	0.11
Schmidt's Tiger Head Ale, 12-fl.-oz. bottle	150	12.7	12.5	1.06	100	8.5	6.3	0.53
Stroh's Bock Beer, 12-fl.-oz. bottle or can	157	14.1	13.1	1.18	105	9.4	6.6	0.59
Stroh's Bohemian Beer, 12-fl.-oz. bottle or can	148	13.6	12.3	1.13	99	9.1	6.2	0.57
Stroh's Bohemian "3.2" Beer, 12-fl.-oz. bottle or can	126	11.6	10.5	0.97	84	7.7	5.3	0.48
Stroh's Goebel Lager, 12-fl.-oz. bottle or can	145	13.4	12.1	1.12	97	8.9	6.1	0.56
Stroh's Light Beer, 12-fl.-oz. bottle or can	115	7.1	9.6	0.59	77	4.7	4.8	0.29
CHAMPALE								
Champale, 12-fl.-oz. bottle	180	12.0	15.0	1.00	120	8.0	7.5	0.50
Golden Champale, 12-fl.-oz. bottle	240	18.0	20.0	1.50	160	12.0	10.0	0.75
Pink Champale, 12-fl.-oz. bottle	217	15.0	18.1	1.25	145	10.0	9.1	0.63

WINES, based on generic data

	UNIT Cal.	UNIT Carb.	1 FLUID OZ. Cal.	1 FLUID OZ. Carb.	1 CUP Cal.	1 CUP Carb.	1 TABLE-SPOON Cal.	1 TABLE-SPOON Carb.
Dessert Wine (Dessert Wine includes those wines that are more than 15% alcohol by volume, such as apple, muscatel, sherry, port, and tokay; it also includes aperitif wine and vermouth), 18.8% alcohol by volume; 15.3% by weight, 750-ml (25.4-fl.-oz.) bottle	1041	58.4	41.0	2.30	328	18.4	20.5	1.15
Table Wine (Table Wine includes those wines that are less than 15% alcohol by volume, such as burgundy, cabernet, chablis, champagne, chianti, claret, Rhine wine, rosé, and sauterne. Cherry, peach, berry, and varietal wines usually fall into this category though some may have alcoholic content high enough to be classified as dessert wine), 12.2% alcohol by volume; 9.9% by weight, 750-ml (25.4-fl.-oz.) bottle	635	30.5	25.0	1.20	200	9.6	12.5	0.60
Based on data from Africa:								
Banana Wine (alcohol content 1.7%), 750-ml (25.4-fl.-oz.) bottle	(346)	(74.0)	(13.6)	(2.91)	(109)	(23.3)	(6.8)	(1.46)
Honey Wine (alcohol content 4.9%), 750-ml (25.4-fl.-oz.) bottle	(433)	(53.5)	(17.1)	(2.11)	(136)	(16.9)	(8.5)	(1.05)

WINES, by brand

Table or Dinner Wines

RED TABLE OR DINNER WINES

	UNIT Cal.	UNIT Carb.	1 FLUID OZ. Cal.	1 FLUID OZ. Carb.	1 CUP Cal.	1 CUP Carb.	1 TABLE-SPOON Cal.	1 TABLE-SPOON Carb.
Baco Noir, **Great Western** (alcohol content 13%), 750-ml (25.4-fl.-oz.) bottle	597	4.5	23.6	0.18	188	1.4	11.8	0.09
Barbera, **Gallo** (alcohol content 12.5%), 750-ml (25.4-fl.-oz.) bottle	535	7.2	21.0	0.30	168	2.4	10.5	0.15
1.5-liter (50.7-fl.-oz.) bottle	1069	14.4	21.0	0.30	168	2.4	10.5	0.15
Burgundy, **Gallo** (alcohol content 12.5%), 750-ml (25.4-fl.-oz.) bottle	580	10.1	23.0	0.40	184	3.2	11.5	0.20
1.5-liter (50.7-fl.-oz.) bottle	1159	20.2	23.0	0.40	184	3.2	11.5	0.20
3-liter (101.4-fl.-oz.) bottle	2318	40.4	23.0	0.40	184	3.2	11.5	0.20
Burgundy, **Great Western** (alcohol content 12.5%), 750-ml (25.4-fl.-oz.) bottle	596	7.5	23.5	0.30	188	2.4	11.8	0.15
Burgundy, **Taylor** (alcohol content 12.5%), 187-ml (6.3-fl.-oz.) bottle	159	6.9	25.0	1.09	200	8.7	12.5	0.55
750-ml (25.4-fl.-oz.) bottle	635	27.7	25.0	1.09	200	8.7	12.5	0.55
1.5-liter (50.7 fl.-oz.) bottle	1268	55.3	25.0	1.09	200	8.7	12.5	0.55
Burgundy, Hearty, **Gallo** (alcohol content 12.5%), 750-ml (25.4-fl.-oz.) bottle	580	10.1	23.0	0.40	184	3.2	11.5	0.20
1.5-liter (50.7-fl.-oz.) bottle	1159	20.2	23.0	0.40	184	3.2	11.5	0.20
3-liter (101.4-fl.-oz.) bottle	2318	40.4	23.0	0.40	184	3.2	11.5	0.20
Burgundy, Mellow, **Meier's** (alcohol content 12%), 750-ml (25.4-fl.-oz.) bottle	(635)	(30.5)	(25.0)	(1.20)	(200)	(9.6)	(12.5)	(0.60)
1.5-liter (50.7-fl.-oz.) bottle	(1268)	(60.8)	(25.0)	(1.20)	(200)	(9.6)	(12.5)	(0.60)
Cabernet, Ruby, **Gallo** (alcohol content 12.5%), 750-ml (25.4-fl.-oz.) bottle	529	2.5	21.0	0.10	168	0.8	10.5	0.05
1.5-liter (50.7-fl.-oz.) bottle	1058	5.0	21.0	0.10	168	0.8	10.5	0.05
Chianti, **Gallo** (alcohol content 12.5%), 750-ml (25.4-fl.-oz.) bottle	1084	12.6	43.0	0.50	344	4.0	21.5	0.25
1.5-liter (50.7-fl.-oz.) bottle	2167	25.2	43.0	0.50	344	4.0	21.5	0.25
4-liter (135.3-fl.-oz.) bottle	5777	67.2	43.0	0.50	344	4.0	21.5	0.25
Claret, **Taylor** (alcohol content 12.5%), 750-ml (25.4-fl.-oz.) bottle	610	20.3	24.0	0.80	192	6.4	12.0	0.40
De Chaunac, **Great Western** (alcohol content 12.5%), 750-ml (25.4-fl.-oz.) bottle	566	3.0	22.3	0.12	178	0.9	11.1	0.06
Paisano, **Gallo** (alcohol content 12.5%), 750-ml (25.4-fl.-oz.) bottle	580	12.6	23.0	0.50	184	4.0	11.5	0.25
1.5-liter (50.7-fl.-oz.) bottle	1159	25.2	23.0	0.50	184	4.0	11.5	0.25
Red, Island, **Meier's** (alcohol content 12%), 750-ml (25.4-fl.-oz.) bottle	(635)	(30.5)	(25.0)	(1.20)	(200)	(9.6)	(12.5)	(0.60)
1.5-liter (50.7-fl.-oz.) bottle	(1268)	(60.8)	(25.0)	(1.20)	(200)	(9.6)	(12.5)	(0.60)
Red, Lake Country, **Taylor** (alcohol content 12.5%), 375-ml (12.7-fl.-oz.) bottle	343	20.3	27.0	1.60	216	12.8	13.5	0.80
750-ml (25.4-fl.-oz.) bottle	686	40.6	27.0	1.60	216	12.8	13.5	0.80
1.5-liter (50.7-fl.-oz.) bottle	1369	81.1	27.0	1.60	216	12.8	13.5	0.80
3-liter (101.4-fl.-oz.) bottle	2738	162.2	27.0	1.60	216	12.8	13.5	0.80
Sangria, **Taylor** (alcohol content 11.6%), 750-ml (25.4-fl.-oz.) bottle	838	91.7	33.0	3.61	264	28.9	17.5	1.81
1.5-liter (50.7-fl.-oz.) bottle	1673	183.0	33.0	3.61	264	28.9	17.5	1.81
Zinfandel, **Gallo** (alcohol content 12.5%), 750-ml (25.4-fl.-oz.) bottle	529	5.5	21.0	0.20	168	1.6	10.5	0.10
1.5-liter (50.7-fl.-oz.) bottle	1058	10.1	21.0	0.20	168	1.6	10.5	0.10

ROSÉ TABLE OR DINNER WINES

	UNIT Cal.	UNIT Carb.	1 FLUID OZ. Cal.	1 FLUID OZ. Carb.	1 CUP Cal.	1 CUP Carb.	1 TABLE-SPOON Cal.	1 TABLE-SPOON Carb.
Catawba, Pink, **Great Western** (alcohol content 12.0%), 750-ml (25.4-fl.-oz.) bottle	820	57.8	32.3	2.28	259	18.2	16.2	1.14
Catawba, Pink, **Taylor** (alcohol content 12.0%), 750-ml (25.4-fl.-oz.) bottle	813	75.9	32.0	2.99	256	23.9	16.0	1.50
1.5-liter (50.7-fl.-oz.) bottle	1622	151.6	32.0	2.99	256	23.9	16.0	1.50
Chablis, Pink, **Gallo** (alcohol content 11.5%), 750-ml (25.4-fl.-oz.) bottle	580	22.7	23.0	0.90	184	7.2	11.5	0.45
1.5-liter (50.7-fl.-oz.) bottle	1159	45.4	23.0	0.90	184	7.2	11.5	0.45
3-liter (101.4-fl.-oz.) bottle	2318	90.8	23.0	0.90	184	7.2	11.5	0.45
Lake Country, Pink, **Taylor** (alcohol content 12.5%), 375-ml (12.7-fl.-oz.) bottle	343	20.3	27.0	1.60	216	12.8	13.5	0.80
750-ml (25.4-fl.-oz.) bottle	686	40.6	27.0	1.60	216	12.8	13.5	0.80
1.5-liter (50.7-fl.-oz.) bottle	1369	81.1	27.0	1.60	216	12.8	13.5	0.80
3-liter (101.4-fl.-oz.) bottle	2738	162.2	27.0	1.60	216	12.8	13.5	0.80
Rosé, **Gallo** (alcohol content 11.5%), 750-ml (25.4-fl.-oz.) bottle	580	22.7	23.0	0.90	184	7.2	11.5	0.45
1.5-liter (50.7-fl.-oz.) bottle	1159	45.4	23.0	0.90	184	7.2	11.5	0.45
Rosé, **Great Western** (alcohol content 12%), 750-ml (25.4-fl.-oz.) bottle	611	15.8	24.1	0.62	193	5.0	12.1	0.31
Rosé, **Taylor** (alcohol content 12.5%), 375-ml (12.7-fl.-oz.) bottle	320	16.5	24.0	1.30	192	10.4	12.0	0.65
750-ml (25.4-fl.-oz.) bottle	610	33.0	24.0	1.30	192	10.4	12.0	0.65
1.5-liter (50.7-fl.-oz.) bottle	1220	66.0	24.0	1.30	192	10.4	12.0	0.65
Rosé, American, **Meier's** (alcohol content 12%), 750-ml (25.4-fl.-oz.) bottle	(635)	(30.5)	(25.0)	(1.20)	(200)	(9.6)	(12.5)	(0.60)
1.5-liter (50.7-fl.-oz.) bottle	(1268)	(60.8)	(25.0)	(1.20)	(200)	(9.6)	(12.5)	(0.60)
Rosé DeChaunac, **Great Western** (alcohol content 12%), 750-ml (25.4-fl.-oz.) bottle	566	6.0	22.3	0.24	178	1.9	11.1	0.12
Rosé of Isabella, **Great Western** (alcohol content 12%), 750-ml (25.4-fl.-oz.) bottle	655	27.0	25.8	1.07	207	8.5	12.9	0.53
Rosé, Island, **Meier's** (alcohol content 11.5%), 750-ml (25.4-fl.-oz.) bottle	(635)	(30.5)	(25.0)	(1.20)	(200)	(1.2)	(12.5)	(0.60)
Rosé, Isle St. George, **Meier's** (alcohol content 12%), 750-ml (25.4-fl.-oz.) bottle	(635)	(30.5)	(25.0)	(1.20)	(200)	(9.6)	(12.5)	(0.60)
1.5-liter (50.7-fl.-oz.) bottle	(1268)	(60.8)	(25.0)	(1.20)	(200)	(9.6)	(12.5)	(0.60)
Rosé, Light, **Masson Light Premium** (alcohol content 7.1%), 1.5-liter (50.7-fl.-oz.) bottle	810	64.5	16.0	1.27	128	10.2	8.0	0.64
Rosé, Light, **Taylor** (alcohol content 8.6%), 750-ml (25.4-fl.-oz.) bottle	435	12.0	17.2	0.47	138	3.8	8.6	0.24
1.5-liter (50.7-fl.-oz.) bottle	870	24.0	17.2	0.47	138	3.8	8.6	0.24
Rosé, Red, **Gallo** (alcohol content 12.5%), 750-ml (25.4-fl.-oz.) bottle	630	42.8	25.0	1.70	200	13.6	12.5	0.85
1.5-liter (50.7-fl.-oz.) bottle	1260	85.6	25.0	1.70	200	13.6	12.5	0.85
3-liter (101.4-fl.-oz.) bottle	2520	171.2	25.0	1.70	200	13.6	12.5	0.85
Vin Rosé, **Gallo** (alcohol content 12%), 750-ml (25.4-fl.-oz.) bottle	555	15.1	22.0	0.60	176	4.8	11.0	0.30
1.5-liter (50.7-fl.-oz.) bottle	1109	30.2	22.0	0.60	176	4.8	11.0	0.30
4-liter (135.3-fl.-oz.) bottle	2976	80.6	22.0	0.60	176	4.8	11.0	0.30

	UNIT		1 FLUID OZ.		1 CUP		1 TABLESPOON	
	Cal.	Carb.	Cal.	Carb.	Cal.	Carb.	Cal.	Carb.
WHITE TABLE OR DINNER WINES								
Aurora, **Great Western** (alcohol content 11.5%), 750-ml (25.4-fl.-oz.) bottle	584	15.8	23.0	0.62	184	5.0	11.5	0.31
Aurora Blanc, **Great Western** (alcohol content 12%), 750-ml (25.4-fl.-oz.) bottle	566	6.0	22.3	0.24	178	1.9	11.1	0.12
Catawba Dry and Light, **Gold Seal** (alcohol content 9.5%), 1.5-liter (50.7-fl.-oz.) bottle	1140	52.5	22.5	1.04	180	8.3	11.3	0.52
Catawba, "Light and Delicate," **Meier's** (alcohol content 12%), 750-ml (25.4-fl.-oz.) bottle	(635)	(30.5)	(25.0)	(1.20)	(200)	(9.6)	(12.5)	(0.60)
Catawba, "Special Selection," **Meier's** (alcohol content 12%), 750-ml (25.4-fl.-oz.) bottle	(635)	(30.5)	(25.0)	(1.20)	(200)	(9.6)	(12.5)	(0.60)
Cayuga White, **Great Western** (alcohol content 11%), 750-ml (25.4-fl.-oz.) bottle	533	9.8	21.0	0.38	168	3.1	10.5	0.19
Chablis, **Great Western** (alcohol content 11.5%), 750-ml (25.4-fl.-oz.) bottle	536	6.0	21.2	0.24	169	1.9	10.6	0.12
Chablis, **Taylor** (alcohol content 12.0%), 187-ml (6.3-fl.-oz.) bottle	152	6.9	24.0	1.09	192	8.7	12.0	0.55
375-ml (12.7-fl.-oz.) bottle	304	13.8	24.0	1.09	192	8.7	12.0	0.55
750-ml (25.4-fl.-oz.) bottle	608	27.6	24.0	1.09	192	8.7	12.0	0.55
1.5-liter (50.7-fl.-oz.) bottle	1220	55.4	24.0	1.09	192	8.7	12.0	0.55
Chablis, Almaden Light, **Paul Masson** (alcohol content 7.0%), 1.5-liter (50.7-fl.-oz.) bottle	720	37.5	14.2	0.74	114	5.9	7.1	0.37
Chablis Blanc, **Gallo** (alcohol content 11.5%), 750-ml (25.4-fl.-oz.) bottle	529	10.2	21.0	0.40	168	3.2	10.5	0.20
1.5-liter (50.7-fl.-oz.) bottle	1058	20.2	21.0	0.40	168	3.2	10.5	0.20
Chablis, California Light, **Paul Masson Light Premium** (alcohol content 7.1%), 750-ml (25.4-fl.-oz.) bottle	368	22.5	14.5	0.89	116	7.1	7.3	0.45
Chablis, Isle St. George, **Meier's** (alcohol content 12%), 750-ml (25.4-fl.-oz.) bottle	(635)	(30.9)	(25.0)	(1.20)	(200)	(9.6)	(12.5)	(0.60)
1.5-liter (50.7-fl.-oz.) bottle	(1268)	(60.8)	(25.0)	(1.20)	(200)	(9.6)	(12.5)	(0.60)
Chablis, Light, **Taylor** (alcohol content 8.2%), 750-ml (25.4-fl.-oz.) bottle	398	9.8	15.7	0.38	126	3.0	7.9	0.19
Chablis, "Special Selection," **Meier's** (alcohol content 11.5%), 750-ml (25.4-fl.-oz.) bottle	(635)	(30.9)	(25.0)	(1.20)	(200)	(9.6)	(12.5)	(0.60)
Chenin Blanc, **Gallo** (alcohol content 11.5%), 750-ml (25.4-fl.-oz.) bottle	529	12.6	21.0	0.50	168	4.0	10.5	0.25
1.5-liter (25.4-fl.-oz.) bottle	1058	25.2	21.0	0.50	168	4.0	10.5	0.25
Colombard, French, **Gallo** (alcohol content 11.5%), 750-ml (25.4-fl.-oz.) bottle	529	12.6	21.0	0.50	168	4.0	10.5	0.25
1.5-liter (25.4-fl.-oz.) bottle	1058	25.2	21.0	0.50	168	4.0	10.5	0.25
Delaware, **Great Western** (alcohol content 11.5%), 750-ml (25.4-fl.-oz.) bottle	574	12.8	22.6	0.50	181	4.0	11.3	0.25
Diamond Ventura, **Great Western** (alcohol content 11.5%), 750-ml (25.4-fl.-oz.) bottle	560	10.5	22.1	0.41	177	3.3	11.1	0.21
Dutchess, **Great Western** (alcohol content 11.5%), 750-ml (25.4-fl.-oz.) bottle	534	4.5	21.1	0.18	169	1.4	10.6	0.09
Gold, Lake Country, **Taylor** (alcohol content 12%), 750-ml (25.4-fl.-oz.) bottle	660	45.7	26.0	1.80	208	14.4	13.0	0.90
1.5-liter (25.4-fl.-oz.) bottle	1318	91.3	26.0	1.80	208	14.4	13.0	0.90
3-liter (101.4-fl.-oz.) bottle	2636	182.9	26.0	1.80	208	14.4	13.0	0.90
La Brusca Rubio, **Meier's** (alcohol content 12%), 750-ml (25.4-fl.-oz.) bottle	(635)	(30.5)	(25.0)	(1.20)	(200)	(9.6)	(12.5)	(9.60)
Rhine, **Gallo** (alcohol content 11.5%), 750-ml (25.4-fl.-oz.) bottle	605	25.2	24.0	1.00	192	8.0	12.0	0.50
1.5-liter (50.7-fl.-oz.) bottle	1210	50.4	24.0	1.00	192	8.0	12.0	0.50
3-liter (101.4-fl.-oz.) bottle	2420	100.8	24.0	1.00	192	8.0	12.0	0.50
Rhine, **Great Western** (alcohol content 11.5%), 750-ml (25.4-fl.-oz.) bottle	551	8.3	21.7	0.33	174	2.6	10.9	0.16

	UNIT		1 FLUID OZ.		1 CUP		1 TABLESPOON	
	Cal.	Carb.	Cal.	Carb.	Cal.	Carb.	Cal.	Carb.
Rhine, American, **Meier's** (alcohol content 12%), 750-ml (25.4-fl.-oz.) bottle	(635)	(30.5)	(25.0)	(1.20)	(200)	(9.6)	(12.5)	(0.60)
1.5-liter (50.7-fl.-oz.) bottle	(1268)	(60.8)	(25.0)	(1.20)	(200)	(9.6)	(12.5)	(0.60)
Rhine Garten, **Gallo** (alcohol content 11.5%), 750-ml (25.4-fl.-oz.) bottle	605	25.2	24.0	1.00	192	8.0	12.0	0.50
1.5-liter (50.7-fl.-oz.) bottle	1210	50.4	24.0	1.00	192	8.0	12.0	0.50
Rhine, Light, **Taylor** (alcohol content 7.9%), 750-ml (25.4-fl.-oz.) bottle	413	15.8	16.3	0.62	130	5.0	8.2	0.31
1.5-liter (50.7-fl.-oz.) bottle	825	31.5	16.3	0.62	130	5.0	8.2	0.31
Riesling, **Gallo** (alcohol content 11.5%), 750-ml (25.4-fl.-oz.) bottle	504	7.6	20.0	0.30	160	2.4	10.0	0.15
1.5-liter (50.7-fl.-oz.) bottle	1008	15.1	20.0	0.30	160	2.4	10.0	0.15
Sauterne, **Taylor** (alcohol content 12.5%), 375-ml (12.7-fl.-oz.) bottle	343	20.3	27.0	1.60	216	12.8	13.5	0.80
750-ml (25.4-fl.-oz.) bottle	686	40.6	27.0	1.60	216	12.8	13.5	0.80
1.5-liter (50.7-fl.-oz.) bottle	1369	81.1	27.0	1.60	216	12.8	13.5	0.80
Sauternes, Haut, Isle St. George, **Meier's** (alcohol content 12%), 750-ml (25.4-fl.-oz.) bottle	(635)	(30.5)	(25.0)	(1.20)	(200)	(9.6)	(12.5)	(0.60)
1.5-liter (50.7-fl.-oz.) bottle	(1268)	(60.8)	(25.0)	(1.20)	(200)	(9.6)	(12.5)	(0.60)
Sauvignon Blanc, **Gallo** (alcohol content 11.5%), 750-ml (25.4-fl.-oz.) bottle	484	5.1	19.0	0.20	152	1.6	9.5	0.10
1.5-liter (50.7-fl.-oz.) bottle	968	10.2	19.0	0.20	152	1.6	9.5	0.10
Seyval Blanc, **Great Western** (alcohol content 11.5%), 750-ml (25.4-fl.-oz.) bottle	566	12.0	22.3	0.47	178	3.8	11.1	0.24
Verdelet, **Great Western** (alcohol content 12.5%), 750-ml (25.4-fl.-oz.) bottle	568	4.5	22.4	0.18	179	1.4	11.2	0.09
Vidal Blanc, **Great Western** (alcohol content 10%), 750-ml (25.4-fl.-oz.) bottle	521	17.3	20.5	0.68	164	5.4	10.3	0.34
White, Island, **Meier's** (alcohol content 12%), 750-ml (25.4-fl.-oz.) bottle	(635)	(30.5)	(25.0)	(1.20)	(200)	(9.6)	(12.5)	(0.60)
White, Lake Country, **Taylor** (alcohol content 12.5%), 750-ml (25.4-fl.-oz.) bottle	660	35.3	26.0	1.39	208	11.1	13.0	0.70
1.5-liter (50.7-fl.-oz.) bottle	1318	70.5	26.0	1.39	208	11.1	13.0	0.70
3-liter (101.4-fl.-oz.) bottle	2636	140.9	26.0	1.39	208	11.1	13.0	0.70

Champagne and Other Sparkling Wines

	UNIT		1 FLUID OZ.		1 CUP		1 TABLESPOON	
	Cal.	Carb.	Cal.	Carb.	Cal.	Carb.	Cal.	Carb.
CHAMPAGNE								
Champagne, Blanc de Blanc, **Meier's** (alcohol content 12%), 750-ml (25.4-fl.-oz.) bottle	(635)	(30.5)	(25.0)	(1.20)	(200)	(9.6)	(12.5)	(0.60)
Champagne, Brut, **Great Western** (alcohol content 12%), 750-ml (25.4-fl.-oz.) bottle	569	6.8	22.4	0.27	179	2.1	11.2	0.13
Champagne, Brut, **Taylor** (alcohol content 12.5%), 375-ml (12.7-fl.-oz.) bottle	318	13.9	25.0	1.09	200	8.7	12.5	0.55
750-ml (25.4-fl.-oz.) bottle	635	27.7	25.0	1.09	200	8.7	12.5	0.55
1.5-liter (50.7-fl.-oz.) bottle	1268	55.3	25.0	1.09	200	8.7	12.5	0.55
Champagne, Chateau Reiém, **Meier's** (alcohol content 12%), 750-ml (25.4-fl.-oz.) bottle	(635)	(30.5	(25.0)	(1.20)	(200)	(9.6)	(12.5)	(0.60)
Champagne, Chateau Reiém Pink, **Meier's** (alcohol content 12%), 750-ml (25.4-fl.-oz.) bottle	(635)	(30.5)	(25.0)	(1.20)	(200)	(9.6)	(12.5)	(0.60)
Champagne, Dry, **Taylor** (alcohol content 12.5%), 375-ml (12.7-fl.-oz.) bottle	330	16.5	26.0	1.30	208	10.4	13.0	0.65
750-ml (25.4-fl.-oz.) bottle	660	33.0	26.0	1.30	208	10.4	13.0	0.65
1.5-liter (50.7-fl.-oz.) bottle	1318	65.9	26.0	1.30	208	10.4	13.0	0.65
Champagne, Extra Dry, **Great Western** (alcohol content 12%), 750-ml (25.4-fl.-oz.) bottle	610	15.0	24.0	0.59	192	4.7	12.0	0.29
Champagne, Naturel, **Great Western** (alcohol content 12%), 750-ml (25.4-fl.-oz.) bottle	539	0.0	21.2	0.00	170	0.0	10.6	0.00
Champagne, Pink, **Great Western** (alcohol content 12%), 750-ml (25.4-fl.-oz.) bottle	611	15.8	24.1	0.62	193	5.0	12.1	0.31

	UNIT		1 FLUID OZ.		1 CUP		1 TABLE-SPOON	
	Cal.	Carb.	Cal.	Carb.	Cal.	Carb.	Cal.	Carb.
Champagne, Pink, **Meier's** (alcohol content 12%), 750-ml (25.4-fl.-oz.) bottle	(635)	(30.5)	(25.0)	(1.20)	(200)	(9.6)	(12.5)	(0.60)
Champagne, Pink, **Taylor** (alcohol content 12.5%), 375-ml (12.7-fl.-oz.) bottle	342	20.3	27.0	1.60	216	12.8	13.5	0.80
750-ml (25.4-fl.-oz.) bottle	686	40.6	27.0	1.60	216	12.8	13.5	0.80
1.5-liter (50.7-fl.-oz.) bottle	1369	81.1	27.0	1.60	216	12.8	13.5	0.80
COLD DUCK								
Cold Duck, **Meier's** (alcohol content 12%), 750-ml (25.4-fl.-oz.) bottle	(635)	(30.5)	(25.0)	(1.20)	(200)	(9.6)	(12.5)	(0.60)
Cold Duck, **Taylor** (alcohol content 12.5%), 375-ml (12.7-fl.-oz.) bottle	380	27.8	30.0	2.19	240	17.5	15.0	1.10
750-ml (25.4-fl.-oz.) bottle	762	55.6	30.0	2.19	240	17.5	15.0	1.10
Cold Duck, Pink, **Great Western** (alcohol content 12%), 750-ml (25.4-fl.-oz.) bottle	682	30.0	26.9	1.18	215	9.5	13.4	0.59
SPARKLING BURGUNDY								
Sparkling Burgundy, **Great Western** (alcohol content 12%), 750-ml (25.4-fl.-oz.) bottle	635	21.0	25.1	0.83	200	6.6	12.5	0.41
Sparkling Burgundy, Chateau Reiém, **Meier's** (alcohol content 12%), 750-ml (25.4-fl.-oz.) bottle	(635)	(30.5)	(25.0)	(1.20)	(200)	(9.6)	(12.5)	(0.60)
Sparkling Burgundy, **Taylor** (alcohol content 12.5%), 750-ml (25.4-fl.-oz.) bottle	660	35.3	26.0	1.39	208	11.1	13.0	0.70
SPUMANTE								
Spumante, Sparkling White Wine, **Meier's** (alcohol content 12%), 750-ml (25.4-fl.-oz.) bottle	(635)	(30.5)	(25.0)	(1.20)	(200)	(9.6)	(12.5)	(0.60)
Aromatized, Fortified, and Other Wines								
PORT								
Port, **Great Western** (alcohol content 18%), 750-ml (25.4-fl.-oz.) bottle	1112	83.3	43.9	3.28	351	26.3	21.9	1.64
Port, **Meier's** (alcohol content 19%), 750-ml (25.4-fl.-oz.) bottle	(1041)	(58.4)	(41.0)	(2.30)	(328)	(18.4)	(20.5)	(1.15)
1.5-liter (50.7-fl.-oz.) bottle	(2079)	(116.6)	(41.0)	(2.30)	(328)	(18.4)	(20.5)	(1.15)
Port, **Taylor** (alcohol content 18.5%), 750-ml (25.4-fl.-oz.) bottle	1219	112.0	48.0	4.41	384	35.3	24.0	2.21
1.5-liter (50.7-fl.-oz.) bottle	2434	223.5	48.0	4.41	384	35.8	24.0	2.21
Porto Branco, **Hiram Walker** (alcohol content 20%), 750-ml (25.4-fl.-oz.) bottle	1168	108.0	46.0	4.25	368	34.0	23.0	2.13
Ruby Port, **Hiram Walker** (alcohol content 20%), 750-ml (25.4-fl.-oz.) bottle	1168	108.0	46.0	4.25	368	34.0	23.0	2.13
Tawny Port, **Great Western** (alcohol content 18%), 750-ml (25.4-fl.-oz.) bottle	1094	78.8	43.2	3.11	345	24.9	21.6	1.56
Tawny Port, **Hiram Walker** (alcohol content 20%), 750-ml (25.4-fl.-oz.) bottle	1168	108.0	46.0	4.25	368	34.0	23.0	2.13
Tawny Port, **Meier's** (alcohol content 19%), 750-ml (25.4-fl.-oz.) bottle	(1041)	(58.4)	(41.0)	(2.30)	(328)	(18.4)	(20.5)	(1.15)
1.5-liter (50.7-fl.-oz.) bottle	(2079)	(116.6)	(41.0)	(2.30)	(328)	(18.4)	(20.5)	(1.15)
White Port, **Meier's** (alcohol content 19%), 750-ml (25.4-fl.-oz.) bottle	(1041)	(58.4)	(41.0)	(2.30)	(328)	(18.4)	(20.5)	(1.15)
1.5-liter (50.7-fl.-oz.) bottle	(2079)	(116.6)	(41.0)	(2.30)	(328)	(18.4)	(20.5)	(1.15)
SHERRY								
Amontillado Sherry, **Hiram Walker** (alcohol content 19%), 750-ml (25.4-fl.-oz.) bottle	940	38.1	37.0	1.50	296	12.0	18.5	0.75
Armada Cream Sherry, **Hiram Walker** (alcohol content 19%), 750-ml (25.4-fl.-oz.) bottle	1041	63.5	41.0	2.50	328	20.0	20.5	1.25
one "tenth" (12.8-fl.-oz.) bottle	525	32.0	41.0	2.50	328	20.0	20.5	1.25
Cocktail Sherry, **Hiram Walker** (alcohol content 18%), 750-ml (25.4-fl.-oz.) bottle	889	31.8	35.0	1.25	280	10.0	17.5	0.63
Cream Sherry, **Taylor** (alcohol content 17.5%), 750-ml (25.4-fl.-oz.) bottle	1168	112.0	46.0	4.41	368	35.3	23.0	2.21
1.5-liter (50.7-fl.-oz.) bottle	2332	223.5	46.0	4.41	368	35.3	23.0	2.21
Dry Sherry, **Taylor** (alcohol content 17.5%), 750-ml (25.4-fl.-oz.) bottle	889	38.4	35.0	1.51	280	12.1	17.5	0.76
1.5-liter (50.7-fl.-oz.) bottle	1775	76.6	35.0	1.51	280	12.1	17.5	0.76
No. 11 Pale Dry Cocktail Sherry, **Meier's** (alcohol content 19%), 750-ml (25.4-fl.-oz.) bottle	(1041)	(58.4)	(41.0)	(2.30)	(328)	(18.4)	(20.5)	(1.15)
1.5-liter (50.7-fl.-oz.) bottle	(2079)	(116.6)	(41.0)	(2.30)	(328)	(18.4)	(20.5)	(1.15)
Solera Cream Sherry, **Great Western** (alcohol content 18%), 750-ml (25.4-fl.-oz.) bottle	1126	87.0	44.4	3.43	355	27.5	22.2	1.72
Solera Dry Sherry, **Great Western** (alcohol content 18%), 750-ml (25.4-fl.-oz.) bottle	867	23.3	34.2	0.92	274	7.3	17.1	0.46
Solera Regular Sherry, **Great Western** (alcohol content 18%), 750-ml (25.4-fl.-oz.) bottle	1006	57.0	39.7	2.25	317	18.0	19.8	1.13
VERMOUTH								
Dry Vermouth, **Great Western** (alcohol content 16%), 750-ml (25.4-fl.-oz.) bottle	686	0.0	27.1	0.00	217	0.0	13.6	0.00
Dry Vermouth, **Taylor** (alcohol content 17%), 750-ml (25.4-fl.-oz.) bottle	838	25.7	33.0	1.01	264	8.1	16.5	0.51
Sweet Vermouth, **Great Western** (alcohol content 16%), 750-ml (25.4-fl.-oz.) bottle	1035	72.8	40.8	2.87	327	23.0	20.4	1.44
Sweet Vermouth, **Taylor** (alcohol content 17%), 750-ml (25.4-fl.-oz.) bottle	1118	104.4	44.0	4.11	352	32.9	22.0	2.06
1-liter (33.8-fl.-oz.) bottle	1487	138.9	44.0	4.11	352	32.9	22.0	2.06
OTHER WINES								
Blackberry Wine, **Meier's** (alcohol content 19%), 750-ml (25.4-fl.-oz.) bottle	(1041)	(58.4)	(41.0)	(2.30)	(328)	(18.4)	(20.5)	(1.15)
1.5-liter (50.7-fl.-oz.) bottle	(2079)	(116.6)	(41.0)	(2.30)	(328)	(18.4)	(20.5)	(1.15)
Concord Wine, **Meier's** (alcohol content 19%), 750-ml (25.4-fl.-oz.) bottle	(1041)	(58.4)	(41.0)	(2.30)	(328)	(18.4)	(20.5)	(1.15)
1.5-liter (50.7-fl.-oz.) bottle	(2079)	(116.6)	(41.0)	(2.30)	(328)	(18.4)	(20.5)	(1.15)
Madiera, **Hiram Walker** (alcohol content 19%), 750-ml (25.4-fl.-oz.) bottle	1067	69.9	42.0	2.75	336	22.0	21.0	1.38
Sweet Catawba Wine, **Meier's** (alcohol content 19%), 750-ml (25.4-fl.-oz.) bottle	(1041)	(58.4)	(41.0)	(2.30)	(328)	(18.4)	(20.5)	(1.15)
1.5-liter (50.7-fl.-oz.) bottle	(2079)	(116.6)	(41.0)	(2.30)	(328)	(18.4)	(20.5)	(1.15)

CORDIALS, LIQUEURS, and FLAVORED BRANDIES

	UNIT		1 FLUID OZ.		1 TABLE-SPOON		1 JIGGER	
	Cal.	Carb.	Cal.	Carb.	Cal.	Carb.	Cal.	Carb.
Amaretto Delight, **Mr. Boston**, 750-ml (25.4-fl.-oz.) bottle	1727	233.7	68.0	9.20	34.0	4.60	102	13.8
Amaretto di Saranno, **Glenmore**, 750-ml (25.4-fl.-oz.) bottle	2083	228.6	82.0	9.00	41.0	4.50	123	13.5
Anisette, Red or White (60-proof), **Hiram Walker**, 200-ml (6.8-fl.-oz.) bottle	623	72.7	92.0	10.75	46.0	5.38	138	16.1
500-ml (16.9-fl.-oz.) bottle	1555	181.7	92.0	10.75	46.0	5.38	138	16.1
750-ml (25.4-fl.-oz.) bottle	2332	272.5	92.0	10.75	46.0	5.38	138	16.1
1-liter (33.8-fl.-oz.) bottle	3110	363.4	92.0	10.75	46.0	5.38	138	16.1
Anisette, **Mr. Boston**, 750-ml (25.4-fl.-oz.) bottle	2235	274.3	88.0	10.80	44.0	5.40	132	16.2
Apricot Cordial (60-proof), **Hiram Walker**, 200-ml (6.8-fl.-oz.) bottle	534	50.7	79.0	7.50	39.5	3.75	119	11.3
500-ml (16.9-fl.-oz.) bottle	1335	126.8	79.0	7.50	39.5	3.75	119	11.3
750-ml (25.4-fl.-oz.) bottle	2003	190.1	79.0	7.50	39.5	3.75	119	11.3

	UNIT		1 FLUID OZ.		1 TABLESPOON		1 JIGGER	
	Cal.	Carb.	Cal.	Carb.	Cal.	Carb.	Cal.	Carb.
Apricot Flavored Brandy (70-proof), **Hiram Walker,** 200-ml (6.8-fl.-oz.) bottle	595	50.7	88.0	7.50	44.0	3.75	132	11.3
500-ml (16.9-fl.-oz.) bottle	1487	126.8	88.0	7.50	44.0	3.75	132	11.3
750-ml (25.4-fl.-oz.) bottle	2231	190.1	88.0	7.50	44.0	3.75	132	11.3
1-liter (33.8-fl.-oz.) bottle	2974	253.5	88.0	7.50	44.0	3.75	132	11.3
1.75-liter (59.2-fl.-oz.) bottle	5205	443.6	88.0	7.50	44.0	3.75	132	11.3
Apricot Flavored Brandy, **Mr. Boston,** 750-ml (25.4-fl.-oz.) bottle	2388	226.1	94.0	8.90	47.0	4.45	141	13.4
Blackberry Cordial (60-proof), **Hiram Walker,** 200-ml (6.8-fl.-oz.) bottle	629	74.4	93.0	11.00	46.5	5.50	140	16.5
500-ml (16.9-fl.-oz.) bottle	1572	185.9	93.0	11.00	46.5	5.50	140	16.5
750-ml (25.4-fl.-oz.) bottle	2358	278.9	93.0	11.00	46.5	5.50	140	16.5
Blackberry Flavored Brandy (70-proof), **Hiram Walker,** 200-ml (6.8-fl.-oz.) bottle	595	50.7	88.0	7.50	44.0	3.75	132	11.3
500-ml (16.9-fl.-oz.) bottle	1487	126.8	88.0	7.50	44.0	3.75	132	11.3
750-ml (25.4-fl.-oz.) bottle	2231	190.1	88.0	7.50	44.0	3.75	132	11.3
1-liter (33.8-fl.-oz.) bottle	2974	253.5	88.0	7.50	44.0	3.75	132	11.3
Blackberry Flavored Brandy, **Mr. Boston,** 750-ml (25.4-fl.-oz.) bottle	2337	226.1	92.0	8.60	46.0	4.30	138	12.9
Cherry Brandy, Kirchwasser (90-proof), **Hiram Walker,** 200-ml (6.8-fl.-oz.) bottle	503	0.0	74.0	0.00	37.0	0.00	111	0.0
750-ml (25.4-fl.-oz.) bottle	1876	0.0	74.0	0.00	37.0	0.00	111	0.0
Cherry Flavored Brandy (70-proof), **Hiram Walker,** 200-ml (6.8-fl.-oz.) bottle	595	50.7	88.0	7.50	44.0	3.75	132	11.3
500-ml (16.9-fl.-oz.) bottle	1487	126.8	88.0	7.50	44.0	3.75	132	11.3
750-ml (25.4-fl.-oz.) bottle	2231	190.1	88.0	7.50	44.0	3.75	132	11.3
1-liter (33.8-fl.-oz.) bottle	2974	253.5	88.0	7.50	44.0	3.75	132	11.3
Cherry Flavored Brandy, **Mr. Boston,** 750-ml (25.4-fl.-oz.) bottle	2210	188.0	87.0	7.40	43.5	3.70	131	11.1
Cherry Heering (49-proof), **Hiram Walker,** 500-ml (16.9-fl.-oz.) bottle	1352	169.0	80.0	10.00	40.0	5.00	120	15.0
750-ml (25.4-fl.-oz.) bottle	2028	253.5	80.0	10.00	40.0	5.00	120	15.0
1-liter (33.8-fl.-oz.) bottle	2704	338.0	80.0	10.00	40.0	5.00	120	15.0
1.75-liter (59.2-fl.-oz.) bottle	4732	592.0	80.0	10.00	40.0	5.00	120	15.0
Chocolate Cherry Cordial (54-proof), **Hiram Walker,** 200-ml (6.8-fl.-oz.) bottle	615	79.4	91.0	11.75	45.5	5.88	137	17.6
500-ml (16.9-fl.-oz.) bottle	1538	198.6	91.0	11.75	45.5	5.88	137	17.6
750-ml (25.4-fl.-oz.) bottle	2307	297.9	91.0	11.75	45.5	5.88	137	17.6
Chocolate Mint Cordial (54-proof), **Hiram Walker,** 200-ml (6.8-fl.-oz.) bottle	615	79.4	91.0	11.75	45.5	5.88	137	17.6
500-ml (16.9-fl.-oz.) bottle	1538	198.6	91.0	11.75	45.5	5.88	137	17.6
750-ml (25.4-fl.-oz.) bottle	2307	297.9	91.0	11.75	45.5	5.88	137	17.6
Coffee Flavored Brandy (70-proof), **Hiram Walker,** 200-ml (6.8-fl.-oz.) bottle	649	64.2	96.0	9.50	48.0	4.75	144	14.3
500-ml (16.9-fl.-oz.) bottle	1622	160.6	96.0	9.50	48.0	4.75	144	14.3
750-ml (25.4-fl.-oz.) bottle	2434	240.8	96.0	9.50	48.0	4.75	144	14.3
1-liter (33.8-fl.-oz.) bottle	3245	321.1	96.0	9.50	48.0	4.75	144	14.3
Coffee Flavored Brandy, **Mr. Boston,** 750-ml (25.4-fl.-oz.) bottle	2540	269.2	100.0	10.60	50.0	5.30	150	15.9
Coffee Liqueur (53-proof), **Kahlua,** 200-ml (6.8-fl.-oz.) bottle	717	104.8	106.0	15.50	53.0	7.75	159	23.3
500-ml (16.9-fl.-oz.) bottle	1792	262.0	106.0	15.50	53.0	7.75	159	23.3
750-ml (25.4-fl.-oz.) bottle	2687	392.9	106.0	15.50	53.0	7.75	159	23.3
1-liter (33.8-fl.-oz.) bottle	3583	523.9	106.0	15.50	53.0	7.75	159	23.3
Crème de Banana (56-proof), **Hiram Walker,** 200-ml (6.8-fl.-oz.) bottle	696	96.3	103.0	14.25	51.5	7.13	155	21.4
500-ml (16.9-fl.-oz.) bottle	1741	240.8	103.0	14.25	51.5	7.13	155	21.4
750-ml (25.4-fl.-oz.) bottle	2611	361.2	103.0	14.25	51.5	7.13	155	21.4
1-liter (33.8-fl.-oz.) bottle	3481	481.7	103.0	14.25	51.5	7.13	155	21.4
Crème de Banana, **Mr. Boston,** 750-ml (25.4-fl.-oz.) bottle	2362	304.8	93.0	12.00	46.5	6.00	140	21.4
Crème de Cacao, Brown, **Mr. Boston,** 750-ml (25.4-fl.-oz.) bottle	2591	36.2	102.0	14.30	51.0	7.15	153	21.5
Crème de Cacao, Regular (54-proof), **Hiram Walker,** 200-ml (6.8-fl.-oz.) bottle	690	98.0	102.0	14.50	51.0	7.25	153	21.8
500-ml (16.9-fl.-oz.) bottle	1724	245.1	102.0	14.50	51.0	7.25	153	21.8
750-ml (25.4-fl.-oz.) bottle	2586	367.6	102.0	14.50	51.0	7.25	153	21.8
1-liter (33.8-fl.-oz.) bottle	3448	490.1	102.0	14.50	51.0	7.25	153	21.8
Crème de Cacao, White (54-proof), **Hiram Walker,** 200-ml (6.8-fl.-oz.) bottle	649	87.9	96.0	13.00	48.0	6.50	144	19.5

	UNIT		1 FLUID OZ.		1 TABLESPOON		1 JIGGER	
	Cal.	Carb.	Cal.	Carb.	Cal.	Carb.	Cal.	Carb.
500-ml (16.9-fl.-oz.) bottle	1622	219.7	96.0	13.00	48.0	6.50	144	19.5
750-ml (25.4-fl.-oz.) bottle	2434	329.6	96.0	13.00	48.0	6.50	144	19.5
1-liter (33.8-fl.-oz.) bottle	3245	439.4	96.0	13.00	48.0	6.50	144	19.5
Crème de Cacao, White, **Mr. Boston,** 750-ml (25.4-fl.-oz.) bottle	2362	304.8	93.0	12.00	46.5	6.00	140	18.0
Crème de Cassis, Black Currant (40-proof), **Hiram Walker,** 200-ml (6.8-fl.-oz.) bottle	642	104.8	95.0	15.50	47.5	7.75	143	23.3
500-ml (16.9-fl.-oz.) bottle	1606	262.0	95.0	15.50	47.5	7.75	143	23.3
750-ml (25.4-fl.-oz.) bottle	2408	392.9	95.0	15.50	47.5	7.75	143	23.3
Crème de Cassis, **Mr. Boston,** 750-ml (25.4-fl.-oz.) bottle	2159	458.1	85.0	14.10	42.5	7.05	128	21.2
Crème de Curacao, Orange (60-proof), **Hiram Walker,** 500-ml (16.9-fl.-oz.) bottle	1606	194.4	95.0	11.50	47.5	5.75	143	17.3
750-ml (25.4-fl.-oz.) bottle	2408	291.5	95.0	11.50	47.5	5.75	143	17.3
1-liter (33.8-fl.-oz.) bottle	3211	388.7	95.0	11.50	47.5	5.75	143	17.3
Crème de Menthe, Green (60-proof), **Hiram Walker,** 200-ml (6.8-fl.-oz.) bottle	649	79.4	96.0	11.75	48.0	5.88	144	17.6
500-ml (16.9-fl.-oz.) bottle	1622	198.6	96.0	11.75	48.0	5.88	144	17.6
750-ml (25.4-fl.-oz.) bottle	2434	297.9	96.0	11.75	48.0	5.88	144	17.6
1-liter (33.8-fl.-oz.) bottle	3245	397.2	96.0	11.75	48.0	5.88	144	17.6
Crème de Menthe, Green, **Mr. Boston,** 750-ml (25.4-fl.-oz.) bottle	2669	406.4	109.0	16.00	54.5	8.00	163	24.0
Crème de Menthe, White (60-proof), **Hiram Walker,** 200-ml (6.8-fl.-oz.) bottle	649	79.4	96.0	11.75	48.0	5.88	144	17.6
500-ml (16.9-fl.-oz.) bottle	1622	198.6	96.0	11.75	48.0	5.88	144	17.6
750-ml (25.4-fl.-oz.) bottle	2434	297.9	96.0	11.75	48.0	5.88	144	17.6
1-liter (33.0-fl.-oz.)	3245	397.2	96.0	11.75	48.0	5.88	144	17.6
Crème de Menthe, White, **Mr. Boston,** 750-ml (25.4-fl.-oz.) bottle	2464	330.2	97.0	13.00	48.5	6.50	146	19.5
Crème de Noyaux, **Mr. Boston,** 750-ml (25.4-fl.-oz.) bottle	2515	342.9	99.0	13.50	49.5	6.75	149	20.3
Crème de Noyaux, Almond, (56-proof), **Hiram Walker,** 200-ml (6.8-fl.-oz.) bottle	669	89.6	99.0	13.25	49.5	6.63	149	19.9
500-ml (16.9-fl.-oz.) bottle	1673	223.9	99.0	13.25	49.5	6.63	149	19.9
750-ml (25.4-fl.-oz.) bottle	2510	335.9	99.0	13.25	49.5	6.63	149	19.9
Drambuie (80-proof), **Hiram Walker,** 200-ml (6.8-fl.-oz.) bottle	744	74.4	110.0	11.00	55.0	5.50	165	16.5
500-ml (16.9-fl.-oz.) bottle	1859	185.9	110.0	11.00	55.0	5.50	165	16.5
750-ml (25.4-fl.-oz.) bottle	2788	278.9	110.0	11.00	55.0	5.50	165	16.5
1-liter (33.8-fl.-oz.) bottle	3718	371.8	110.0	11.00	55.0	5.50	165	16.5
Espresso Coffee Liqueur, **Mr. Boston,** 750-ml (25.4-fl.-oz.) bottle	2642	381.0	104.0	15.00	52.0	7.50	156	22.5
Ginger Flavored Brandy (70-proof), **Hiram Walker,** 200-ml (6.8-fl.-oz.) bottle	480	22.0	71.0	3.25	35.5	1.63	107	4.9
500-ml (16.9-fl.-oz.) bottle	1200	54.9	71.0	3.25	35.5	1.63	107	4.9
750-ml (25.4-fl.-oz.) bottle	1800	82.4	71.0	3.25	35.5	1.63	107	4.9
1-liter (33.8-fl.-oz.) bottle	2400	110.0	71.0	3.25	35.5	1.63	107	4.9
Ginger Flavored Brandy, **Mr. Boston,** 750-ml (25.4-fl.-oz.) bottle	1829	88.9	72.0	3.50	36.0	1.75	108	5.3
Kahlua, see Coffee Liqueur.								
Kummel (70-proof), **Hiram Walker,** 200-ml (6.8-fl.-oz.) bottle	480	22.0	71.0	3.25	35.5	1.63	107	4.9
500-ml (16.9-fl.-oz.) bottle	1200	54.9	71.0	3.25	35.5	1.63	107	4.9
750-ml (25.4-fl.-oz.) bottle	1800	82.4	71.0	3.25	35.5	1.63	107	4.9
Peach Cordial, **Hiram Walker,** 200-ml (6.8-fl.-oz.) bottle	534	50.7	79.0	7.50	39.5	3.75	119	11.3
500-ml (16.9-fl.-oz.) bottle	1335	126.8	79.0	7.50	39.5	3.75	119	11.3
750-ml (25.4-fl.-oz.) bottle	2003	190.1	79.0	7.50	39.5	3.75	119	11.3
Peach Flavored Brandy (70-proof), **Hiram Walker,** 200-ml (6.8-fl.-oz.) bottle	595	50.7	88.0	7.50	44.0	3.75	132	11.3
500-ml (16.9-fl.-oz.) bottle	1487	126.8	88.0	7.50	44.0	3.75	132	11.3
750-ml (25.4-fl.-oz.) bottle	2231	190.1	88.0	7.50	44.0	3.75	132	11.3
1-liter (33.8-fl.-oz.) bottle	2974	253.5	88.0	7.50	44.0	3.75	132	11.3
Peach Flavored Brandy, **Mr. Boston,** 750-ml (25.4-fl.-oz.) bottle	2388	226.1	94.0	8.90	47.0	4.45	141	13.4
Peppermint Schnapps, **Hiram Walker,** 200-ml (6.8-fl.-oz.) bottle	541	52.4	80.0	7.75	40.0	3.88	120	11.6
500-ml (16.9-fl.-oz.) bottle	1352	131.0	80.0	7.75	40.0	3.88	120	11.6
750-ml (25.4-fl.-oz.) bottle	2028	200.3	80.0	7.75	40.0	3.88	120	11.6

	UNIT		1 FLUID OZ.		1 TABLE-SPOON		1 JIGGER	
	Cal.	Carb.	Cal.	Carb.	Cal.	Carb.	Cal.	Carb.
1-liter (33.8-fl.-oz.) bottle	2704	262.0	80.0	7.75	40.0	3.88	120	11.6
1.75-liter (59.2-fl.-oz.) bottle	4732	467.3	80.0	7.75	40.0	3.88	120	11.6
Peppermint Schnapps, **Mr. Boston,** 750-ml (25.4-fl.-oz.) bottle	1956	203.2	77.0	8.00	38.5	4.00	116	12.0
Raspberry Flavored Brandy, (70-proof), **Hiram Walker,** 200-ml (6.8-fl.-oz.) bottle	595	50.7	88.0	7.50	44.0	3.75	132	11.3
500-ml (16.9-fl.-oz.) bottle	1487	126.8	88.0	7.50	44.0	3.75	132	11.3
750-ml (25.4-fl.-oz.) bottle	2231	190.1	88.0	7.50	44.0	3.75	132	11.3
Rock and Rye, **Mr. Boston,** 750-ml (25.4-fl.-oz.) bottle	1880	182.9	74.0	7.20	37.0	3.60	111	10.8
Sloe Gin, **Mr. Boston,** 750-ml (25.4-fl.-oz.) bottle	1727	119.4	68.0	4.70	34.0	2.35	102	7.1
Swiss Chocolate Almond Cordial (54-proof), **Hiram Walker,** 200-ml (6.8-fl.-oz.) bottle	615	79.4	91.0	11.75	45.5	5.88	137	17.6
500-ml (16.9-fl.-oz.) bottle	1538	198.6	91.0	11.75	45.5	5.88	137	17.6
750-ml (25.4-fl.-oz.) bottle	2307	297.9	91.0	11.75	45.5	5.88	137	17.6
Triple Sec, **Mr. Boston,** 750-ml (25.4-fl.-oz.) bottle	2007	215.9	79.0	8.50	39.5	4.25	119	12.8
HARD LIQUOR (GIN, RUM, VODKA, and WHISKEY), based on generic data								
100-proof, 750-ml (25.4-fl.-oz.) bottle	2108	trace	83.0	trace	41.5	trace	124	trace
94-proof, 750-ml (25.4-fl.-oz.) bottle	1956	trace	77.0	trace	38.5	trace	116	trace
90-proof, 750-ml (25.4-fl.-oz.) bottle	1880	trace	74.0	trace	37.0	trace	110	trace
86-proof, 750-ml (25.4-fl.-oz.) bottle	1778	trace	70.0	trace	35.0	trace	105	trace
80-proof, 750-ml (25.4-fl.-oz.) bottle	1651	trace	65.0	trace	32.5	trace	97	trace
HARD LIQUOR, by brand								
BOURBON								
Ten High Bourbon (86-proof), 500-ml (16.9-fl.-oz.) bottle	1200	0.0	71.0	0.00	35.5	0.00	107	0.0
750-ml (25.4-fl.-oz.) bottle	1800	0.0	71.0	0.00	35.5	0.00	107	0.0
1-liter (33.8-fl.-oz.) bottle	2400	0.0	71.0	0.00	35.5	0.00	107	0.0
Walker's Deluxe Bourbon (86-proof), 500-ml (16.9-fl.-oz.) bottle	1200	0.0	71.0	0.00	35.5	0.00	107	0.0
750-ml (25.4-fl.-oz.) bottle	1800	0.0	71.0	0.00	35.5	0.00	107	0.0
1-liter (33.8-fl.-oz.) bottle	2400	0.0	71.0	0.00	35.5	0.00	107	0.0
BRANDY								
Walker's Brandy (80-proof), 500-ml (16.9-fl.-oz.) bottle	1115	0.0	66.0	0.00	33.0	0.00	99	0.0
750-ml (25.4-fl.-oz.) bottle	1673	0.0	66.0	0.00	33.0	0.00	99	0.0
1-liter (33.8-fl.-oz.) bottle	2231	0.0	66.0	0.00	33.0	0.00	99	0.0
GIN								
London Dry Gin (90-proof), 500-ml (16.9-fl.-oz.) bottle	1251	0.0	74.0	0.00	37.0	0.00	111	0.0
750-ml (25.4-fl.-oz.) bottle	1876	0.0	74.0	0.00	37.0	0.00	111	0.0
1-liter (33.8-fl.-oz.) bottle	2501	0.0	74.0	0.00	37.0	0.00	111	0.0
RUM								
White and Gold Label Rum (80-proof), 500-ml (16.9-fl.-oz.) bottle	1115	0.0	66.0	0.00	33.0	0.00	99	0.0
750-ml (25.4-fl.-oz.) bottle	1673	0.0	66.0	0.00	33.0	0.00	99	0.0
1-liter (33.8-fl.-oz.) bottle	2231	0.0	66.0	0.00	33.0	0.00	99	0.0
RYE								
Meadow Brook Rye (86-proof), 500-ml (16.9-fl.-oz.) bottle	1200	0.0	71.0	0.00	35.5	0.00	107	0.0
750-ml (25.4-fl.-oz.) bottle	1800	0.0	71.0	0.00	35.5	0.00	107	0.0
1-liter (33.8-fl.-oz.) bottle	2400	0.0	71.0	0.00	35.5	0.00	107	0.0
SCOTCH								
Grand Macnish Scotch (86-proof), 500-ml (16.9-fl.-oz.) bottle	1200	0.0	71.0	0.00	35.5	0.00	107	0.0
750-ml (25.4-fl.-oz.) bottle	1800	0.0	71.0	0.00	35.5	0.00	107	0.0
1-liter (33.8-fl.-oz.) bottle	2400	0.0	71.0	0.00	35.5	0.00	107	0.0
Old Smuggler Scotch (86-proof), 500-ml (16.9-fl.-oz.) bottle	1200	0.0	71.0	0.00	35.5	0.00	107	0.0
750-ml (25.4-fl.-oz.) bottle	1800	0.0	71.0	0.00	35.5	0.00	107	0.0
1-liter (33.8-fl.-oz.) bottle	2400	0.0	71.0	0.00	35.5	0.00	107	0.0
Thorne's Scotch (86.8-proof), 750-ml (25.4-fl.-oz.) bottle	1800	0.0	71.0	0.00	35.5	0.00	107	0.0
VODKA								
Hiram Walker Vodka (80-proof), 500-ml (16.9-fl.-oz.) bottle	1115	0.0	66.0	0.00	33.0	0.00	99	0.0
750-ml (25.4-fl.-oz.) bottle	1673	0.0	66.0	0.00	33.0	0.00	99	0.0
1-liter (33.8-fl.-oz.) bottle	2231	0.0	66.0	0.00	33.0	0.00	99	0.0
(100-proof), 500-ml (16.9-fl.-oz.) bottle	1386	0.0	82.0	0.00	41.0	0.00	123	0.0
750-ml (25.4-fl.-oz.) bottle	2080	0.0	82.0	0.00	41.0	0.00	123	0.0
1-liter (33.8-fl.-oz.) bottle	2772	0.0	82.0	0.00	41.0	0.00	123	0.0
WHISKEY (also see BOURBON, RYE, and SCOTCH)								
Canadian Club Whiskey (86.8-proof), 500-ml (16.9-fl.-oz.) bottle	1200	0.0	71.0	0.00	35.5	0.00	107	0.0
750-ml (25.4-fl.-oz.) bottle	1800	0.0	71.0	0.00	35.5	0.00	107	0.0
1-liter (33.8-fl.-oz.) bottle	2400	0.0	71.0	0.00	35.5	0.00	107	0.0
Corby's Reserve Blended Whiskey (80-proof), 750-ml (25.4-fl.-oz.) bottle	1676	0.0	66.0	0.00	33.0	0.00	99	0.0
1-liter (33.8-fl.-oz.) bottle	2237	0.0	66.0	0.00	33.0	0.00	99	0.0
1.75-liter (59.0-fl.-oz.) bottle	3914	0.0	66.0	0.00	33.0	0.00	99	0.0
Imperial Blended Whiskey (86-proof), 500-ml (16.9-fl.-oz.) bottle	1200	0.0	71.0	0.00	35.5	0.00	107	0.0
750-ml (25.4-fl.-oz.) bottle	1800	0.0	71.0	0.00	35.5	0.00	107	0.0
1-liter (33.8-fl.-oz.) bottle	2400	0.0	71.0	0.00	35.5	0.00	107	0.0
Jack Daniels Tennessee Sourmash Whiskey (90-proof), 750-ml (25.4-fl.-oz.) bottle	(1778)	0.0	(70.0)	0.00	(35.0)	0.00	(105)	0.0
Private Cellar Bonded Whiskey (100-proof), 500-ml (16.9-fl.-oz.) bottle	1386	0.0	82.0	0.00	41.0	0.00	123	0.0
750-ml (25.4-fl.-oz.) bottle	2080	0.0	82.0	0.00	41.0	0.00	123	0.0
1-liter (33.8-fl.-oz.) bottle	2777	0.0	82.0	0.00	41.0	0.00	123	0.0
Royal Canadian Whiskey (80-proof), 500-ml (16.9-fl.-oz.) bottle	1115	0.0	66.0	0.00	33.0	0.00	99	0.0
750-ml (25.4-fl.-oz.) bottle	1673	0.0	66.0	0.00	33.0	0.00	99	0.0
1-liter (33.8-fl.-oz.) bottle	2231	0.0	66.0	0.00	33.0	0.00	99	0.0
Ten High Bonded Whiskey (100-proof), 500-ml (16.9-fl.-oz.) bottle	1386	0.0	82.0	0.00	41.0	0.00	123	0.0
750-ml (25.4-fl.-oz.) bottle	2080	0.0	82.0	0.00	41.0	0.00	123	0.0
1-liter (33.8-fl.-oz.) bottle	2772	0.0	82.0	0.00	41.0	0.00	123	0.0

COCKTAILS AND MIXED DRINKS AS SERVED AT SARDI'S, NEW YORK

	1 DRINK	
	Cal.	Carb.
ALEXANDER, made with ½ fl. oz. gin, ½ fl. oz. crème de cacao, and 1½ fl. oz. heavy cream; topped with nutmeg	244	7.5
BACARDI, made with 1 fl. oz. Bacardi White Label rum, 1 tsp. superfine sugar, 1½ fl. oz. lime juice, and ½ fl. oz. grenadine	144	18.7
BETWEEN THE SHEETS, made with ½ fl. oz. brandy, ½ fl. oz. rum, ½ fl. oz. Triple Sec or Cointreau, and 1½ fl. oz. fresh lemon juice	141	9.8
BLACK RUSSIAN, made with ½ fl. oz. vodka and 1 fl. oz. Kahlua	137	15.0
BLOODY MARY, made with 1 fl. oz. vodka, 3 oz. tomato juice, 1 drop tabasco sauce, 2 drops Worcestershire sauce, and two dashes each of salt and pepper; sprinkle with celery salt	86	4.4
BOCCI BALL, made with 1½ fl. oz. Amaretto, 3 fl. oz. orange juice, 3 fl. oz. club soda	135	18.8
BRANDY ALEXANDER, made with ½ fl. oz. brandy, ½ fl. oz. dark crème de cacao, and 1½ fl. oz. heavy cream; topped with nutmeg	253	11.8
BRONX, made with 1½ fl. oz. gin, ½ fl. oz. sweet vermouth, ½ fl. oz. dry vermouth, ½ fl. oz. orange juice, and 1 strip lemon peel	191	7.1
BULL SHOT, made with 1 fl. oz. vodka, 5–6 oz. beef bouillon, and a dash each of salt, and pepper, Tabasco sauce and Worcestershire sauce	91	1.3
CUBA LIBRE (Rum & Cola), made with 1 fl. oz. light or dark rum and 5 fl. oz. cola, with a squeeze of lime	127	16.7
DAIQUIRI, made with 1½ fl. oz. light rum, 1 tsp. superfine sugar, and 1 fl. oz. lime juice	125	5.8
DUBONNET COCKTAIL, made with 1½ fl. oz. red Dubonnet and 1½ fl. oz. gin	173	5.1
FRENCH 75, made with 1 fl. oz. gin, 3 fl. oz. champagne, 1 tsp. superfine sugar, and 2 fl. oz. lemon juice	170	12.5
GIBSON, made with 3 fl. oz. gin and a dash (5 drops, or ⅕ fl. oz.) dry vermouth; garnished with a cocktail onion	207	0.7
GIMLET, unsweetened, made with 1½ fl. oz. gin or vodka and ½ fl. oz. Rose's Lime Juice	110	1.8
sweetened Gimlet: add 1 fl. oz. of Cointreau	210	15.7
GIN AND BITTER LEMON, made with 1½ fl. oz. gin, 3 fl. oz. tonic water, and 3 fl. oz. bitter lemon	181	16.4

	1 DRINK Cal.	Carb.
GIN FIZZ, made with 1½ fl. oz. gin, 1 tsp. superfine sugar, and 2 fl. oz. fresh lemon juice, club soda to fill glass	130	7.0
GIN RICKEY, made with 1½ fl. oz. gin, club soda, and 1 slice lime, squeezed	104	1.8
GIN AND TONIC, made with 1½ fl. oz. gin, 6 fl. oz. tonic, and a squeeze of lime	175	16.1
GOLDEN CADILLAC, made with 1 fl. oz. Galiano, 1 fl. oz. white Crème de Cacao, and 1 fl. oz. heavy cream	250	27.5
GOLDEN DREAM, made with 1 fl. oz. Galiano, 1 fl. oz. Cointreau, 1 fl. oz. orange juice, 1 fl. oz. heavy cream	269	32.7
GRASSHOPPER, made with ½ fl. oz. green crème de menthe, ½ fl. oz. white crème de cacao, and 1½ fl. oz. heavy cream	255	12.0
HARVEY WALLBANGER, made with 1½ fl. oz. vodka, 6 fl. oz. orange juice, and ½ fl. oz. Galiano liqueur	258	27.0
HOT BUTTERED RUM, made with 1½ fl. oz. dark or light rum, 4 fl. oz. boiling water, 1 pat butter, 2 cinnamon sticks, pinch of nutmeg, cloves, 1 tsp. superfine sugar, and a slice of lemon with cloves	158	3.9
IRISH COFFEE, made with 1½ fl. oz. Irish whiskey, very hot, strong black coffee to fill glass, 2 heaping tablespoons whipped cream, and 1 tsp. sugar	218	4.4
KIR, made with 6½ fl. oz. chilled dry white chablis wine and ½ fl. oz. crème de cassis; garnished with lemon peel	121	27.1
MADRAS, made with 1½ fl. oz. vodka, 2 fl. oz. cranberry juice, 2 fl. oz. orange juice	123	6.6
MAI TAI, made with 1½ fl. oz. light rum, 1 fl. oz. Triple Sec, 1½ fl. oz. fresh lemon juice, and 1 tsp. superfine sugar; garnished with a cherry and a slice of orange	209	17.6
Or: made with 1 fl. oz. light rum, 1 fl. oz. dark rum, ½ fl. oz. Curacao, ½ fl. oz. orgeat, 1 fl. oz. grenadine, ½ tsp. sugar, ½ fl. oz. lime juice; garnished with fresh pineapple and a cherry	310	36.1
MANHATTAN, made with 2 fl. oz. rye or blended whiskey, 1 fl. oz. sweet vermouth; garnished with a cherry	183	4.8
MARGARITA, made with 1½ fl. oz. Tequila, 1 fl. oz. Triple Sec, and 1 fl. oz. fresh lemon juice	185	11.2
MARTINI, (15 to 1) made with 3 fl. oz. gin and a dash (5 drops, or ⅕ fl. oz.) dry vermouth; garnished with a medium green olive	210	0.7
MIMOSA, made with 3½ fl. oz. champagne and 3½ fl. oz. orange juice	137	14.2
MINT JULEP, made with 5–8 mint leaves, muddled; one tsp. superfine sugar, 1½ fl. oz. bourbon, club soda; garnished with a mint sprig and sprinkled with sugar	115	4.4
OLD FASHIONED, made with 2 fl. oz. whiskey, ½ tsp. superfine sugar, 1 twist lemon peel, and 2 dashes of aromatic bitters; garnished with a cherry and a slice of orange	156	6.4
PIÑA COLADA, made with 1½ fl. oz. light rum, 1½ fl. oz. cream of coconut, 1 fl. oz. heavy cream, 3 tbsp. crushed pineapple	342	13.8
PLANTER'S PUNCH, made with 1½ fl. oz. Jamaican rum, 1 fl. oz. orange juice, 1 fl. oz. fresh lemon juice, 1 tsp. superfine sugar, ½ fl. oz. grenadine; topped with club soda	184	21.6
ROB ROY, sweet, made with 2 fl. oz. scotch whiskey, 1½ fl. oz. sweet vermouth	194	6.2
dry Rob Roy: made with 1½ fl. oz. scotch whiskey and dry vermouth	176	0.6
RUM & COLA, see CUBA LIBRE		
RUM SOUR, made with 1½ fl. oz. rum, 2 oz. lemon juice, and 1 tsp. sugar	128	8.0
RUM SWIZZLE, made with 1½ fl. oz. light or dark rum, club soda, soda water, and ½ tsp. superfine sugar	102	1.3
RUM TODDY, made with 1½ fl. oz. rum, boiling water, 1 tsp. superfine sugar, garnished with ground nutmeg, 4 or 5 cloves, and a slice of lemon	114	2.9
RUSTY NAIL, made with 1½ fl. oz. scotch whiskey and 1 fl. oz. Drambuie	223	11.0
SANGRIA, 4 fl. oz. red wine, ½ fl. oz. brandy, ½ fl. oz. Triple Sec, 1 fl. oz. orange juice, 1 tsp. superfine sugar, soda water; garnished with lemon slice, orange spiral, strawberries, and a few drops cherry brandy	225	19.2
SCREWDRIVER, made with 1½ fl. oz. vodka and 6 fl. oz. orange juice	181	19.4
SHERRY FLIP, made with 3 fl. oz. sweet sherry, yolk of 1 medium egg, and 1 tsp. superfine sugar	195	10.9
SIDE CAR, made with 1½ fl. oz. brandy, 1 fl. oz. Triple Sec (Cointreau), and 1½ fl. oz. fresh lemon juice	225	23.0
SILVER BULLET, made with 3 fl. oz. vodka and a few drops scotch, with a medium green olive	210	0.7
SINGAPORE SLING, made with 1½ fl. oz. gin, 1 fl. oz. cherry liqueur, 2 fl. oz. fresh lemon juice, club soda, 1 tsp. superfine sugar; garnished with a cherry and a slice of orange	241	11.2
SLOE GIN FIZZ, made with 2 fl. oz. sloe gin, 2 fl. oz. fresh lemon juice, soda water, and 1 tsp. superfine sugar	167	17.4
SOMBRERO, made with 1 fl. oz. Kahlua, 1 fl. oz. Triple Sec (Cointreau), and 1 fl. oz. heavy cream	232	17.5
STINGER, made with 2 fl. oz. brandy and ½ fl. oz. white crème de menthe	235	30.5
STRAWBERRY DAIQUIRI, made with 1½ fl. oz. light rum, 1 tsp. superfine sugar, 1 fl. oz. lime juice, and 6 fresh strawberries, blended	150	12.1
STRAWBERRY MARGARITA, made with 1½ fl. oz. Tequila, 1 fl. oz. Triple Sec, 1 fl. oz. fresh lemon juice, and 6 fresh strawberries	210	17.5
TEQUILA SUNRISE, made with 1½ fl. oz. Tequila, 5 fl. oz. orange juice, and ½ fl. oz. grenadine	219	24.2
TOASTED ALMOND, made with 1 fl. oz. Kahlua, 1 fl. oz. Amaretto, and 1 fl. oz. heavy cream	286	25.3
TOM COLLINS, made with 2 fl. oz. gin, 1½ fl. oz. fresh lemon juice, club soda, and 1 tsp. superfine sugar; garnished with a cherry and a slice of orange	169	10.2
TOM AND JERRY, made with 1½ fl. oz. brandy, 1 tsp. dark rum, 1 tsp. egg yolk, 1 tsp. egg white, 1 tsp. superfine sugar, and 5 fl. oz. hot milk; garnished with nutmeg	252	11.2

	1 DRINK Cal.	Carb.
VODKA AND BITTER LEMON, made with 1½ fl. oz. vodka, 3 fl. oz. 7-Up, and 3 fl. oz. tonic water; garnished with a slice of lime	178	17.4
VODKA AND COLA, made with 1½ fl. oz. vodka and 4 fl. oz. cola	145	12.4
VODKA AND TONIC, made with 1½ fl. oz. vodka, 6 fl. oz. tonic water, and a slice of lime	175	16.1
VODKA MARTINI, made with 3 fl. oz. vodka, a dash (5 drops, or ⅕ fl. oz.) dry vermouth, and a medium green olive	210	0.7
WHISKEY SOUR, made with 1½ fl. oz. rye whiskey, 1½ fl. oz. lemon juice, and 1 tsp. superfine sugar; garnished with a cherry and a slice of orange	126	7.8
WHITE RUSSIAN, made with ½ fl. oz. vodka, 1 fl. oz. Kahlua, and ½ fl. oz. heavy cream	190	15.5
ZOMBIE, made with 1 fl. oz. fresh lemon juice, 1 fl. oz. orange juice, 1 tsp. sugar, 1½ fl. oz. white rum, ½ fl. oz. Triple Sec, a few dashes of 151 proof lemon hart; garnished with a cherry and a slice of orange	254	12.3

PRE-MIXED COCKTAILS

	UNIT Cal.	UNIT Carb.	1 FLUID OZ. Cal.	1 FLUID OZ. Carb.	1 COCKTAIL Cal.	1 COCKTAIL Carb.
Amaretto Sour, **Mr. Boston,** 750-ml (25.4-fl.-oz.) bottle	1041	132.1	41.0	5.20		
1 cocktail, approx. 3 fl. oz.	123	15.6	41.0	5.20	123	15.6
Daiquiri, **Mr. Boston,** 750-ml (25.4-fl.-oz.) bottle	838	76.2	33.0	3.00		
1 cocktail, approx. 3 fl. oz.	99	9.0	33.0	3.00	99	9.0
Daiquiri, **The Club,** (3.5 fl. oz.)	129	15.7	36.6	4.46	129	15.7
Egg Nog, **Mr. Boston,** 750-ml (25.4-fl.-oz.) bottle	1524	160.0	60.0	6.30		
1 cocktail, approx. 4 fl. oz.	240	25.2	60.0	6.30	240	18.9
Mai Tai, **Mr. Boston,** 750-ml (25.4-fl.-oz.) bottle	940	104.1	37.0	4.10		
1 cocktail, approx. 5 fl. oz.	185	20.5	37.0	4.10	185	20.5
Manhattan, **Mr. Boston,** 750-ml (25.4-fl.-oz.) bottle	1041	53.3	41.0	2.10		
1 cocktail, approx. 2½ fl. oz.	103	5.3	41.0	2.10	103	5.3
Margarita, **Mr. Boston,** 750-ml (25.4-fl.-oz.) bottle	889	91.4	35.0	3.60		
1 cocktail, approx. 3 fl. oz.	105	10.8	35.0	3.60	105	10.8
Martini, Extra Dry, **Mr. Boston,** 750-ml (25.4-fl.-oz.) bottle	838	0.0	33.0	0.00		
1 cocktail, approx. 3 fl. oz.	99	0.0	33.0	0.00	99	0.0
Piña Colada, **Mr. Boston,** 750-ml (25.4-fl.-oz.) bottle	2032	289.6	80.0	11.40		
1 cocktail, approx. 4½ fl. oz.	360	51.3	80.0	11.40	360	51.3
Piña Colada, **The Club,** 3.5-fl.-oz. can	243	27.6	68.8	7.82	243	27.6
Screwdriver, **Mr. Boston,** 750-ml (25.4-fl.-oz.) bottle	940	101.6	37.0	4.00		
1 cocktail, approx. 6 fl. oz.	222	24.0	37.0	4.00	222	24.0
Strawberry Daiquiri, **Mr. Boston,** 750-ml (25.4-fl.-oz.) bottle	940	101.6	37.0	4.00		
1 cocktail, approx. 3 fl. oz.	111	12.0	37.0	4.00	111	12.0
Strawberry Margarita, **Mr. Boston,** 750-ml (25.4-fl.-oz.) bottle	1168	160.0	46.0	6.30		
1 cocktail, approx. 3 fl. oz.	138	18.9	46.0	6.30	138	18.9
Tequila Sunrise, **Mr. Boston,** 750-ml (25.4-fl.-oz.) bottle	1016	121.9	40.0	4.80		
1 cocktail, approx. 6 fl. oz.	240	28.8	40.0	4.80	240	28.8
Tequila Sunrise, **The Club,** 3.5 fl. oz.	112	11.7	31.8	3.32	112	11.7
Vodka Martini, **Mr. Boston,** 750-ml (25.4-fl.-oz.) bottle	864	7.6	34.0	0.30		
1 cocktail, approx. 3 fl. oz.	102	0.9	34.0	0.30	102	0.9
Wallbanger, **Mr. Boston,** 750-ml (25.4-fl.-oz.) bottle	864	81.3	34.0	3.20		
1 cocktail, approx. 3 fl. oz.	102	9.6	34.0	3.20	102	9.6
Whiskey Sour, **Mr. Boston,** 750-ml (25.4-fl.-oz.) bottle	1016	121.9	40.0	4.80		
1 cocktail, approx. 3 fl. oz.	120	14.4	40.0	4.80	120	14.4
Whiskey Sour, **The Club,** 3.5-fl.-oz. can	120	13.5	34.1	3.84	120	13.5

COCKTAIL MIXES

	UNIT Cal.	UNIT Carb.	1 FLUID OZ. Cal.	1 FLUID OZ. Carb.	1 COCKTAIL Cal.	1 COCKTAIL Carb.
Cocktail Host, cocktail mixes						
In order to facilitate comparisons, I have calculated all mixed drinks on the basis of 80-proof alcohol.						
Cocktail Mix, 16-fl.-oz. (1-pint) bottle	752	192.0	47.0	12.00		
Collins: One cocktail prepared as directed, combine 1 jigger mix with 8 oz. club soda and:						
1 jigger bourbon, rye, or scotch (yield: approx. 11 fl. oz.)	(168)	(18.0)	(15.3)	(1.64)	(168)	(18.0)
1 jigger gin or vodka (yield: approx. 11 fl. oz.)	(168)	(18.0)	(15.3)	(1.64)	(168)	(18.0)

	UNIT		1 FLUID OZ.		1 COCKTAIL	
	Cal.	Carb.	Cal.	Carb.	Cal.	Carb.
Daiquiri: One cocktail prepared as directed, combine 1 jigger mix with:						
1½ jiggers light rum (yield: approx. 3¾ fl. oz.)	(217)	(18.0)	(57.8)	(4.80)	(217)	(18.0)
2 jiggers light rum (yield: approx. 4.5 fl. oz.)	(267)	(18.0)	(59.0)	(4.00)	(267)	(18.0)
Fruit Brandy Sour: One cocktail prepared as directed, combine 1 jigger mix with:						
1 jigger apricot brandy liqueur (yield: approx. 3 fl. oz.)	(203)	(18.0)	(67.5)	(6.00)	(203)	(18.0)
1½ jiggers apricot brandy liqueur (yield: approx. 3¾ fl. oz.)	(269)	(18.0)	(71.6)	(4.80)	(269)	(18.0)
Gimlet: One cocktail prepared as directed, combine 1 jigger mix with:						
2 jiggers gin or vodka (yield: approx. 4.5 fl. oz.)	(266)	(18.0)	(59.0)	(4.00)	(266)	(18.0)
3 jiggers gin or vodka (yield: approx. 6 fl. oz.)	(363)	(18.0)	(60.5)	(3.00)	(363)	(18.0)
Sour: 1 cocktail prepared as directed, combine 1 jigger mix with:						
1 jigger bourbon, rye, or scotch (yield: approx. 3 fl. oz.)	(168)	(18.0)	(56.0)	(6.00)	(168)	(18.0)
1 jigger gin or vodka (yield: approx. 3 fl. oz.)	(168)	(18.0)	(56.0)	(6.00)	(168)	(18.0)
1½ jiggers bourbon, rye, or scotch (yield: approx. 3¾ fl. oz.)	(217)	(18.0)	(57.8)	(4.80)	(217)	(18.0)
1½ jiggers gin or vodka (yield: approx. 3¾ fl. oz.)	(217)	(18.0)	(57.8)	(4.80)	(217)	(18.0)
Coco Casa, cocktail mixes						
Banana Colada Mix, 16-fl.-oz. (1-pint) can	1776	352.0	111.0	22.00		
1 cocktail prepared as directed, combine ⅔ jigger mix with ⅔ jigger water and ⅔ jigger rum (yield: approx. 3 fl. oz.)	(176)	(22.0)	(58.7)	(7.33)	(176)	(22.0)
Chocolate Colada Mix, 16-fl.-oz. (1-pint) can	1728	352.0	108.0	22.00		
1 cocktail prepared as directed, combine 1 jigger mix with 1 jigger water and 1 jigger rum (yield: approx. 4½ fl. oz.)	(260)	(33.0)	(57.8)	(7.33)	(260)	(33.0)
Coconut Colada Mix, 16-fl.-oz. (1-pint) can	1824	352.0	114.0	22.00		
1 cocktail prepared as directed, combine ⅔ jigger mix with ⅔ jigger water and ⅔ jigger rum (yield: approx. 3 fl. oz.)	(179)	(22.0)	(59.8)	(7.33)	(179)	(22.0)
Cream of Coconut, 16-fl-oz. (1-pint) can	1814	352.0	117.0	22.00		
1 cocktail prepared as directed, combine ⅔ fl. oz. mix with 1⅓ fl. oz. unsweetened pineapple juice and ⅔ jigger rum (yield: approx. 3 fl. oz.)	(204)	(27.3)	(68.0)	(9.10)	(204)	(27.3)
Piña Colada Mix, 16-fl.-oz. (1-pint) can	1872	416.0	117.0	26.00		
1 cocktail prepared as directed, combine 1 jigger mix with 1 jigger water and 1 jigger rum (yield: approx. 4½ fl. oz.)	(273)	(39.0)	(60.7)	(8.67)	(273)	(39.0)
Strawberry Colada Mix, 16-fl.-oz. (1-pint) can	1772	352.0	107.0	22.00		
1 cocktail prepared as directed, combine 1 jigger mix with 1 jigger water and 1 jigger rum (yield: approx. 4½ fl. oz.)	(259)	(33.0)	(57.6)	(7.33)	(259)	(33.0)
Holland House, bottled cocktail mixes						
Alexander: 1 cocktail prepared as directed, combine 1 jigger mix and 1 jigger brandy and:						
1 jigger light cream (yield: approx. 4.5 fl. oz.)	(366)	(48.8)	(81.3)	(10.83)	(366)	(48.8)
1 jigger milk (yield: approx. 4.5 fl. oz.)	(303)	(49.2)	(67.3)	(10.93)	(303)	(49.2)
Amaretto Cocktail Mix, 16-fl.-oz. (1-pint) bottle	1264	264.0	79.0	16.50		
1 cocktail prepared as directed, combine 1 jigger mix with 1 jigger vodka (yield: approx. 3 fl. oz.)	(216)	(24.8)	(72.0)	(16.50)	(216)	(24.8)
Apricot Sour Cocktail Mix, 16-fl.-oz. (1-pint) bottle	768	192.0	48.0	12.00		
1 cocktail prepared as directed, combine 1 jigger mix with 1 jigger vodka (yield: approx. 3 fl. oz.)	(146)	(12.0)	(48.6)	(4.00)	(146)	(12.0)
Black Russian Cocktail Mix, 16-fl.-oz. (1-pint) bottle	1472	368.0	92.0	23.00		
1 cocktail prepared as directed, combine 1 jigger mix with 2 jiggers vodka (yield: approx. 4.5 fl. oz.)	(332)	(34.5)	(73.8)	(7.67)	(332)	(34.5)
Also from Black Russian mix:						
White Russian: 1 cocktail prepared as directed, combine 1 jigger mix with 1 jigger vodka and:						
1 jigger light cream (yield: approx. 4.5 fl. oz.)	(331)	(36.3)	(73.6)	(8.07)	(331)	(36.3)
1 jigger milk (yield: approx. 4.5 fl. oz.)	(265)	(36.8)	(58.9)	(8.17)	(265)	(36.8)
Blackberry Sour Cocktail Mix, 16-fl.-oz. (1-pint) bottle	800	192.0	50.0	12.00		
1 cocktail prepared as directed, combine 1 jigger mix with 2 jiggers vodka (yield: approx. 4.5 fl. oz.)	(269)	(18.0)	(59.8)	(4.00)	(269)	(18.0)

	UNIT		1 FLUID OZ.		1 COCKTAIL	
	Cal.	Carb.	Cal.	Carb.	Cal.	Carb.
Bloody Mary Cocktail Mix, Regular, 24-fl.-oz. bottle	240	60.0	10.0	2.50		
1 cocktail prepared as directed, combine 1 jigger vodka or gin with:						
3 jiggers mix (yield: approx. 6 fl. oz.)	(143)	(11.4)	(23.8)	(1.90)	(143)	(11.4)
4 jiggers mix (yield: approx. 7.5 fl. oz.)	(158)	(14.9)	(21.0)	(1.99)	(158)	(14.9)
Bloody Mary Cocktail Mix, Extra Tangy, 24-fl.-oz. bottle	240	60.0	10.0	2.50		
1 cocktail prepared as directed, combine 1 jigger vodka or gin with:						
3 jiggers mix (yield: approx. 6 fl. oz.)	(143)	(11.4)	(23.8)	(1.90)	(143)	(11.4)
4 jiggers mix (yield: approx. 7.5 fl. oz.)	(158)	(14.9)	(21.0)	(1.99)	(158)	(14.9)
Bloody Mary Cocktail Mix, Smooth 'N Spicy, 32-fl.-oz. (1-quart) bottle	192	48.0	6.0	1.50		
1 cocktail prepared as directed, combine 1 jigger vodka or gin with:						
3 jiggers mix (yield: approx. 6 fl. oz.)	(125)	(6.9)	(20.8)	(1.15)	(125)	(6.9)
4 jiggers mix (yield: approx. 7.5 fl. oz.)	(134)	(9.2)	(17.8)	(1.23)	(134)	(9.2)
Chi Chi is an alternate recipe under Piña Colada Mix.						
Daiquiri Cocktail mix, 16-fl.-oz. (1-pint) bottle	816	208.0	51.0	13.00		
1 cocktail prepared as directed, combine 1 jigger mix with 1 jigger light rum (yield: approx. 3 fl. oz.)	(174)	(19.5)	(58.0)	(6.50)	(174)	(19.5)
Dry Martini Cocktail Mix, 16-fl.-oz. (1-pint) bottle	160	40.0	10.0	2.50		
1 cocktail prepared as directed, combine ⅓ jigger mix with 1⅓ jigger dry gin or vodka (yield: approx. 2.5 fl. oz.)	(134)	1.3	(53.6)	(0.51)	(134)	(1.3)
Extra Dry Martini, or Gibson Cocktail: 1 cocktail prepared as directed, combine ⅓ jigger mix with:						
1⅓ jiggers gin or vodka (yield: approx. 2.5 fl. oz.)	(134)	(1.3)	(53.6)	(0.42)	(134)	(1.3)
2 jiggers gin or vodka (yield: approx. 3.5 fl. oz.)	(199)	(1.3)	(56.8)	(0.42)	(199)	(1.3)
Gimlet Cocktail Mix, 16-fl.-oz. (1-pint) bottle	640	160.0	40.0	10.00		
1 cocktail prepared as directed, combine ½ jigger mix with 1⅔ jiggers dry gin or vodka (yield: approx. 3.5 fl. oz.)	(192)	(7.5)	(59.0)	(2.31)	(192)	(7.5)
Mai-Tai Cocktail Mix, 16-fl.-oz. (1-pint) bottle	53	128.0	33.0	8.00		
1 cocktail prepared as directed, combine 1 jigger rum with:						
1 jigger mix (yield: approx. 3 fl. oz.)	(147)	(12.0)	(49.0)	(4.00)	(147)	(12.0)
2 jiggers mix (yield: approx. 4.5 fl. oz.)	(197)	(24.0)	(43.8)	(5.33)	(197)	(24.0)
Manhattan Cocktail Mix, 16-fl.-oz. (1-pint) bottle	46	112.0	29.0	7.00		
1 cocktail prepared as directed, combine ½ jigger mix with 1 jigger bourbon, rye, scotch (yield: approx. 2.25 fl. oz.)	(119)	(5.3)	(52.9)	(2.33)	(119)	(5.3)
Margarita Cocktail Mix, 16-fl.-oz. (1-pint) bottle	624	152.0	39.0	9.50		
1 cocktail prepared as directed, combine 1 jigger mix with 1 jigger Tequila (yield: approx. 3 fl. oz.)	(156)	(14.3)	(52.0)	(4.76)	(156)	(14.3)
Old Fashioned Cocktail Mix, 16-fl.-oz. (1-pint) bottle	576	144.0	36.0	9.00		
1 cocktail prepared as directed, combine ½ jigger mix with 1 jigger bourbon, rye, or scotch (yield: approx. 2.25 fl. oz.)	(115)	(4.5)	(53.5)	(2.00)	(115)	(4.5)
Piña Colada Cocktail Mix, 16-fl.-oz. (1-pint) bottle	960	240.0	60.0	15.00		
1 cocktail prepared as directed, combine 2 jiggers mix with 1 jigger rum and 1 jigger water (yield: approx. 6 fl. oz.)	(277)	(45.0)	(46.2)	(7.50)	(277)	(45.0)
Also from Piña Colada mix:						
Chi Chi: 1 cocktail prepared as directed, combine 2 jiggers mix with 1 jigger vodka and 1 jigger water (yield: approx. 6 fl. oz.)	(277)	(4.0)	(46.2)	(7.50)	(277)	(4.0)
Sip 'n Slim Cocktail Mix, reduced calorie, 16-fl.-oz. (1-pint) bottle	144	40.0	9.0	2.50		
1 cocktail prepared as directed, combine 1 jigger mix with:						
1 jigger gin, rum, vodka, or whiskey (yield: approx. 3 fl. oz.)	(111)	(3.8)	(37.0)	(1.25)	(111)	(3.8)
1 jigger brandy (yield: approx. 3 fl. oz.)	(148)	(3.8)	(48.7)	(1.25)	(148)	(3.8)
Strawberry Sting Cocktail Mix, 16-fl.-oz. (1-pint) bottle	560	128.0	35.0	8.00		
1 cocktail prepared as directed, combine 1⅓ jiggers mix with ⅔ jigger Canadian whiskey (yield: approx. 3 fl. oz.)	(135)	(16.0)	(45.1)	(5.33)	(135)	(16.0)
Tom Collins Cocktail Mix, 16-fl.-oz. (1-pint) bottle	1072	264.0	67.0	16.50		
1 cocktail prepared as directed, combine 1⅓ jiggers mix with 1 jigger dry gin or vodka (yield: approx. 3.5 fl. oz.)	(231)	(33.1)	(66.2)	(9.45)	(231)	(33.1)
Whiskey Sour Cocktail Mix, 16-fl.-oz. (1-pint) bottle	880	208.0	55.0	13.00		

	UNIT Cal.	UNIT Carb.	1 FLUID OZ. Cal.	1 FLUID OZ. Carb.	1 COCKTAIL Cal.	1 COCKTAIL Carb.
1 cocktail prepared as directed, combine 1 jigger mix with 1 jigger bourbon, rye, or scotch (yield: approx. 3 fl. oz.)	(180)	(19.5)	(60.0)	(6.50)	(180)	(19.5)
White Russian is an alternate recipe under Black Russian Cocktail Mix.						
Holland House, dry cocktail mixes						
(One packet of dry mix is meant to make one drink.)						
Alexander Cocktail Mix, 4½-oz. box, 8 packets	552	128.0				
1 packet, approx. 9/16 oz.	69	16.0				
1 cocktail prepared as directed, combine 1 jigger vodka, 1 envelope mix, and:						
1 jigger milk (yield: approx. 3 fl. oz.)	(196)	(18.3)	(65.3)	(6.10)	(196)	(18.3)
1 jigger cream (yield: approx. 3 fl. oz.)	(261)	(17.9)	(87.0)	(5.97)	(261)	(17.9)
1 cocktail prepared as directed, combine 1 jigger brandy, 1 envelope mix and:						
1 jigger milk (yield: approx. 3 fl. oz.)	(231)	(18.3)	(77.0)	(6.10)	(231)	(18.3)
1 jigger cream (yield: approx. 3 fl. oz.)	(296)	(17.9)	(98.5)	(5.97)	(296)	(17.9)
Also from Alexander mix:						
Brown Cow: 1 cocktail prepared as directed, combine 1 jigger vodka, 1 envelope mix, and:						
1½ jiggers milk (yield: approx. 3¾ fl. oz.)	(211)	(19.4)	(56.3)	(5.17)	(211)	(19.4)
1½ jiggers cream (yield: approx. 3¾ fl. oz.)	(308)	(18.9)	(82.1)	(5.04)	(308)	(18.9)
1 cocktail prepared as directed, combine 1 jigger brandy, 1 envelope mix, and:						
1½ jiggers milk (yield: approx. 3¾ fl. oz.)	(240)	(19.4)	(65.5)	(5.17)	(246)	(19.4)
1½ jiggers cream (yield: approx. 3¾ fl. oz.)	(343)	(18.9)	(91.5)	(5.04)	(343)	(18.9)
Banana Daiquiri Cocktail Mix, 4½-oz. box, 8 packets	528	138.0				
1 packet, approx. 9/16 oz.	66	16.0				
1 cocktail prepared as directed, combine 1 jigger rum with 1 envelope mix, 1 jigger water, and 1 rounded teaspoon sugar (yield: 3 fl. oz.)	(178)	(20.0)	(59.3)	(6.66)	(178)	(20.0)
Bloody Mary Cocktail Mix, 3-oz. box, 6 packets	336	84.0				
1 packet, approx. ½ oz.	56	14.0				
1 cocktail prepared as directed, combine 1 jigger vodka or gin with 1 envelope mix and:						
2 jiggers water (yield: approx. 4½ fl. oz.)	(154)	(14.0)	(34.2)	(3.10)	(154)	(14.0)
3 jiggers water (yield: approx. 6 fl. oz.)	(154)	(14.0)	(25.7)	(2.33)	(154)	(14.0)
Brown Cow is an alternate recipe under Alexander Mix.						
Chi Chi is an alternate recipe under Piña Colada Mix.						
Daiquiri Cocktail Mix, 4½-oz. box, 8 packets	552	(136.0)				
1 packet, approx. 9/16 oz.	69	(17.0)				
1 cocktail prepared as directed, combine 1 jigger light rum with 1 envelope mix and 1 jigger water (yield: approx. 3 fl. oz.)	(166)	(17.0)	(55.3)	(5.67)	(166)	(17.0)
Gimlet Cocktail Mix, 4½-oz. box, 8 packets	552	136.0				
1 packet, approx. 9/16 oz.	69	17.0				
1 cocktail prepared as directed, combine 1 jigger gin or vodka with 1 envelope mix and 1 jigger water (yield: approx. 3 fl. oz.)	(166)	(17.0)	(55.3)	(5.67)	166	17.0
Grasshopper Cocktail Mix, 4½-oz. box, 8 packets	552	136.0				
1 packet, approx. 9/16 oz.	69	17.0				
1 cocktail prepared as directed, combine 1 jigger vodka with 1 envelope mix and 1 jigger:						
milk (yield: approx. 3 fl. oz.)	(196)	(18.5)	(65.3)	(6.17)	(196)	(18.5)
half & half (yield: approx. 3 fl. oz.)	(226)	(19.1)	(75.3)	(6.37)	(226)	(19.1)
Also from Grasshopper mix:						
Mint Cow: 1 cocktail prepared as directed, combine 1 jigger vodka with one envelope mix, ½ jigger water, and 2 heaping tablespoons (2 oz.) vanilla ice cream (yield: approx. 4¼ fl. oz.)	(231)	(23.9)	(54.4)	(5.63)	(231)	(23.9)
Mai-Tai Cocktail Mix, 4½-oz. box, 8 packets	552	136.0				
1 packet, approx. 9/16 oz.	69	17.0				
1 cocktail prepared as directed, combine 1 jigger light or dark rum with 1 envelope mix and 2 jiggers water (yield: approx. 4½ fl. oz.)	(166)	(17.0)	(36.9)	(3.78)	(166)	(17.0)
Margarita Cocktail Mix, 4½-oz. box, 8 packets	552	136.0				
1 packet, approx. 9/16 oz.	69	17.0				
1 cocktail prepared as directed, combine 1 jigger Tequila with 1 envelope mix and 1 jigger water (yield: approx. 3½ fl. oz.)	(167)	(17.0)	(55.7)	(5.67)	(167)	(17.0)

	UNIT Cal.	UNIT Carb.	1 FLUID OZ. Cal.	1 FLUID OZ. Carb.	1 COCKTAIL Cal.	1 COCKTAIL Carb.
Mint Cow is an alternate recipe under Grasshopper Mix.						
Mint Julep Cocktail Mix, 4½-oz. box, 8 packets	536	136.0				
1 packet, approx. 9/16 oz.	67	17.0				
1 cocktail prepared as directed, combine 1 jigger bourbon with 1 envelope mix and 1⅓ jiggers water (yield: approx. 3½ fl. oz.)	(165)	(17.0)	(47.0)	(4.86)	(165)	(17.0)
Piña Colada Cocktail Mix, 4½-oz. box, 8 packets	528	128.0				
1 packet, approx. 9/16 oz.	66	16.0				
1 cocktail prepared as directed, combine 1 jigger rum with 1 envelope mix, 2 jiggers water, and 1 rounded teaspoon sugar (yield: approx. 4½ fl. oz.)	(178)	(20.0)	(39.6)	(4.44)	(178)	(20.0)
Also from Piña Colada mix:						
Chi Chi: 1 cocktail prepared as directed, combine 1 jigger vodka with 1 envelope mix, 2 jiggers water, and 1 rounded tsp. sugar (yield: approx. 4½ fl. oz.)	(178)	(20.0)	(39.5)	(4.44)	(178)	(20.0)
Pink Cow is an alternate recipe under Pink Squirrel Cocktail Mix.						
Pink Squirrel Cocktail Mix, 4½-oz. box, 8 packets	552	136.0				
1 packet, approx. 9/16 oz.	69	17.0				
1 cocktail prepared as directed, combine 1 jigger vodka and 1 envelope mix, 1 rounded teaspoon sugar and:						
1 jigger milk (yield: approx. 3 fl. oz.)	(211)	(23.3)	(70.3)	(7.77)	(211)	(23.3)
1 jigger half & half (yield: approx. 3 fl. oz.)	(241)	(23.1)	(80.3)	(7.70)	(241)	(23.1)
Also from Pink Squirrel mix:						
Pink Cow: 1 cocktail prepared as directed, combine 1 jigger vodka with 1 envelope mix, 1 rounded teaspoon sugar, and:						
1½ jiggers milk (yield: approx. 3¾ fl. oz.)	(226)	(21.0)	(60.3)	(5.60)	(226)	(21.0)
1½ jiggers ice cream (yield: approx. 3¾ fl. oz.)	(271)	(24.4)	(72.3)	(6.51)	(271)	(24.4)
Strawberry Margarita Cocktail Mix, 4½-oz. box, 8 packets	496	120.0				
1 packet, approx. 9/16 oz.	62	15.0				
1 cocktail prepared as directed, combine ⅔ jigger Tequila with 1 envelope mix and 1 jigger water (yield: approx. 2½ fl. oz.)	(127)	(15.0)	(50.8)	(6.00)	(127)	(15.0)
Strawberry Sting Cocktail Mix, 4½-oz. box, 8 packets	592	144.0				
1 packet, approx. 9/16 oz.	74	18.0				
1 cocktail prepared as directed, combine ⅔ jigger Canadian whiskey with 1 envelope mix and 1⅓ jiggers water (yield: approx. 3 fl. oz.)	(139)	(18.0)	(46.4)	(6.00)	(139)	(18.0)
Tequila Sunrise Cocktail Mix, 4½-oz. box, 8 packets	504	120.0				
1 packet, approx. 9/16 oz.	63	15.0				
1 cocktail prepared as directed, combine 1⅓ jiggers Tequila with 1 envelope mix, 2⅔ jiggers water, and 1 rounded teaspoon sugar (yield: approx. 6 fl. oz.)	(193)	(15.0)	(32.2)	(2.50)	(193)	(15.0)
Tom Collins Cocktail Mix, 4½-oz. box, 8 packets	552	136.0				
1 packet, approx. 9/16 oz.	69	17.0				
1 cocktail prepared as directed, combine 1 jigger gin or vodka with 1 envelope mix and 1 jigger water (yield: approx. 3 fl. oz.)	(166)	(17.0)	(55.3)	(5.67)	(166)	(17.0)
Vodka Sour Cocktail Mix, 4½-oz. box, 8 packets	520	128.0				
1 packet, approx. 9/16 oz.	65	16.0				
1 cocktail prepared as directed, combine 1 jigger vodka with 1 envelope mix and 1 jigger water (yield: approx. 3 fl. oz.)	(162)	(16.0)	(54.0)	(5.33)	(162)	(16.0)
Wallbanger Cocktail Mix, 4½-oz. box, 8 packets	520	128.0				
1 packet, approx. 9/16 oz.	65	16.0				
1 cocktail prepared as directed, combine 1 jigger vodka with 1 envelope mix, 1 rounded teaspoon sugar, and 2⅔ jiggers water (yield: approx. 5½ fl. oz.)	(177)	(20.0)	(32.2)	(3.64)	(177)	(20.0)
Sacramento						
Bloody Mary Cocktail Mix, 33-fl.-oz. 6-pack	271	60.0	8.2	1.82		
1 can, 5½ fl. oz.	45	10.0	8.2	1.82		
1 cocktail prepared as directed, combine 1 can mix with 1 jigger vodka or gin (yield: approx. 7 fl. oz.)	(142)	(10.0)	(20.3)	(1.43)	(142)	(10.0)
Snap-E-Tom						
Tomato (Bloody Mary) Cocktail Mix, 6-fl.-oz. can	38	6.8	6.3	1.13		
10-fl.-oz. can	63	11.3	6.3	1.13		
32-fl.-oz. (1-quart) bottle	203	36.3	6.3	1.13		

	UNIT Cal.	UNIT Carb.	1 FLUID OZ. Cal.	1 FLUID OZ. Carb.	1 COCKTAIL Cal.	1 COCKTAIL Carb.
1 cocktail prepared as directed, combine 1 can mix with 1 jigger vodka or gin (yield: approx. 7½ fl. oz.)	(135)	(6.8)	(18.0)	(0.91)	(135)	(6.8)

MIXERS

	UNIT Cal.	UNIT Carb.	1 FLUID OZ. Cal.	1 FLUID OZ. Carb.
CARBONATED BEVERAGES				
Bitter Lemon, **Schweppe's,** 6 fl. oz.	84	20.3	14.0	3.38
Club Soda (based on generic data), 6 fl. oz.	0	0.0	0.0	0.00
Cola (based on generic data), 6 fl. oz.	72	18.6	12.0	3.10
Ginger Ale (based on generic data), 6 fl. oz.	57	14.7	9.4	2.44
7-Up, 6 fl. oz.	72	18.1	12.0	3.02
Tonic Water, **Schweppe's,** 6 fl. oz.	66	16.5	11.0	2.75
JUICE AND BOUILLON				
Beef Bouillon (based on generic data), yield from 1 0.2-oz. packet: approx. 6 fl. oz.	14	1.4	2.3	0.23
Orange Juice, fresh (based on generic data), 6 fl. oz.	83	19.3	13.9	3.22
Tomato Juice, **Libby's,** 1 can, 5½ fl. oz.	32	7.3	5.8	1.33

GARNISHES

	UNIT Cal.	UNIT Carb.
Aromatic Bitters, **Angostura,** 1 teaspoon (approx. 0.2 oz.)	13	0.1
Lemon (based on generic data), ¼ slice, ¼" thick (approx. 0.2 oz.)	1	0.3
Lemon Peel (based on generic data), 1 "twist" (approx. 0.1 oz.)	(2)	0.3
Lime (based on generic data), 1 slice, ¼" thick (approx. 0.6 oz.)	4	1.4
1 wedge, approx. ⅛ lime (approx. 0.3 oz.)	2	0.8
Maraschino Cherry (based on generic data), 1 medium (approx. 0.2 oz.)	(6)	(1.4)
Mint (based on data from the Middle East), 1 sprig	trace	trace
Olive (based on generic data), 1 small green (approx. 0.12 oz.)	3	trace
Onion (cocktail onion), **Crosse & Blackwell,** (approx. 0.1 oz.)	trace	trace
Orange (based on generic data), 1 slice, 2¼" diameter, ¼" thick (approx. 0.6 oz.)	7	2.6

32 VEGETARIAN FOODS •

PREPACKAGED VEGETARIAN FOODS

	UNIT		1 SLICE, PATTY, OR PIECE		1 OZ., BY WT.		1 POUND	
	Cal.	Carb.	Cal.	Carb.	Cal.	Carb.	Cal.	Carb.
CAMPBELL'S								
Vegetarian Vegetable Soup, Condensed, 10½-oz. can	176	29.1			16.7	2.77	267	44.3
Prepared with an equal amount of water (yield: approx. 20 fl. oz.)	176	29.1			8.5	1.41	136	22.6
FAMILIA								
Swiss Mix for vegetable patties								
Plain, 7-oz. package	694	118.3			99.2	16.90	1587	270.4
Curry, 7-oz. package	694	118.3			99.2	16.90	1587	270.4
Herb, 7-oz. package	694	118.3			99.2	16.90	1587	270.4
Paprika, 7-oz. package	694	118.3			99.2	16.90	1587	270.4
FARM FOODS								
Texturized Vegetable Protein, 1-lb. 8-oz. foil pouch	2204	224.5			91.8	9.35	1469	149.7
FEARN								
Brazil Nut Burger Mix, 3.8-oz. foil pouch	416	28.0			109.5	7.37	1752	117.9
Breakfast Patty Mix, 3.7-oz. foil pouch	448	40.0			121.1	10.81	1938	173.0
Sesame Burger Mix, 10-oz. package	1276	63.8			127.6	6.38	2042	102.1
Sunflower Burger Mix, 4.2-oz. foil pouch	484	60.0			115.2	14.29	1845	228.6
LIBBY'S								
Deep Brown Vegetarian Beans in Tomato Sauce, 14-oz. can	(405)	(79.3)			(28.9)	(5.67)	(462)	(90.7)
LOMA LINDA								
FROZEN:								
(Meatless) Bologna, 8-oz. package, 8 slices	526	16.6			65.8	2.07	1053	33.1
1 slice, approx. 1 oz.	66	2.1	66	2.1	65.8	2.07	1053	33.1
(Meatless) Burgers, sizzle, 10-oz. package, 4 patties	720	40.0			72.0	4.00	1152	64.0
1 patty, approx. 2½ oz.	180	10.0	180	10.0	72.0	4.00	1152	64.0
(Meatless) Breakfast Links, 14-oz. package	909	29.0			64.9	2.07	1038	33.1
(Meatless) Breakfast Sausage, 16-oz. (1-lb.) package	1112	25.9			69.5	1.62	1112	25.9
1 patty, approx. 1 oz.	(70)	(1.6)	(70)	(1.6)	69.5	1.62	1112	25.9
(Meatless) Chicken, 8-oz. package, 8 slices	478	14.7			59.8	1.84	1136	29.4
1 slice, approx. 1 oz.	60	1.8	60	1.8	59.8	1.84	1136	29.4

	UNIT		1 SLICE, PATTY, OR PIECE		1 OZ., BY WT.		1 POUND	
	Cal.	Carb.	Cal.	Carb.	Cal.	Carb.	Cal.	Carb.
(Meatless) Meatballs, 1-pound tub	989	46.2			61.8	2.89	989	46.2
(Meatless) Roast Beef, 8-oz. package, 8 slices	517	10.2			64.6	1.28	1034	20.5
1 slice, approx. 1 oz.	65	1.3	65	1.3	64.6	1.28	1034	20.5
(Meatless) Salami, 8-oz. package, 8 slices	551	13.1			68.9	1.64	1102	26.2
1 slice, approx. 1 oz.	69	1.6	69	1.6	68.9	1.64	1102	26.2
(Meatless) Turkey, 8-oz. package, 8 slices	483	12.7			60.4	1.59	966	25.4
1 slice, approx. 1 oz.	60	1.6	60	1.6	60.4	1.59	966	25.4
CANNED:								
(Meatless) Big Franks, 19-oz. can (15.2 oz. drained weight), 8 franks	800	32.0			52.6	2.11	842	33.8
1 frank, approx. 1.9 oz.	100	4.0	100	4.0	52.6	2.11	842	33.8
(Meatless) Chili with Beans, 15-oz. can	468	68.1			31.2	4.54	499	72.6
Dinner Cuts, 13-oz. can	450	22.5			34.6	1.73	554	27.7
19-oz. can	657	32.9			34.6	1.73	554	27.7
36-oz. can	1246	62.3			34.6	1.73	554	27.7
Linketts, 19-oz. can (13 oz. drained weight), 10 linketts	900	50.0			69.2	3.85	1107	61.5
1 linkett, approx. 1.3 oz.	90	5.0	90	5.0	69.2	3.85	1107	61.5
Little Links, 14-oz. can	723	24.6			51.6	1.76	826	28.2
1 little link, approx. 0.8 oz.	44	1.4	44	1.4	51.6	1.76	889	29.1
Nuteena, 14-oz. can	1092	43.7			78.0	3.12	1248	49.9
19-oz. can	1482	59.3			78.0	3.12	1248	49.9
28-oz. can	2184	87.4			78.0	3.12	1248	49.9
Proteena, 20-oz. can	1214	43.0			60.7	2.15	971	34.4
Redi-Burger, 19-oz. can	1153	40.9			60.7	2.15	971	34.4
Sandwich Spread, 14-oz. can	679	50.4			48.5	3.60	776	57.6
Savorex, 9-oz. tub	455	40.1			50.5	4.45	808	71.2
Soy Beans, Boston, 15-oz. can	455	57.9			30.3	3.86	485	61.8
Soy Beans, Green, 15-oz. can	378	35.7			25.2	2.38	403	38.1
Stew Pac, 37-oz. can	1269	105.1			34.3	2.84	549	45.4
(Meatless) Swiss Steak with Gravy, 28-oz. can, 8 patties	1120	48.0			39.7	1.70	635	27.2
1 patty, approx. 2¾ oz.	140	6.0	140	6.0	39.7	1.70	635	27.2
Tender Bits, 13-oz. can	416	46.0			32.0	3.54	512	56.6
19-oz. can	608	67.3			32.0	3.54	512	56.6
36-oz. can	1152	127.4			32.0	3.54	512	56.6
Tender Rounds, 19-oz. can	895	49.6			47.1	2.61	754	41.8
Vege-Burger, 13½-oz. can	432	26.7			47.1	2.61	754	41.8
19-oz. can	608	37.6			32.0	1.98	512	31.7
Vege-Lona, 19-oz. can	899	71.6			47.3	3.77	757	60.3
Vita-Burger Mix, 16-oz. (1-lb.) can	(1492)	136.2			(93.3)	8.51	(1492)	136.2

	UNIT Cal.	UNIT Carb.	1 SLICE, PATTY, OR PIECE Cal.	1 SLICE, PATTY, OR PIECE Carb.	1 OZ., BY WT. Cal.	1 OZ., BY WT. Carb.	1 POUND Cal.	1 POUND Carb.
MORNINGSTAR FARMS								
Bacon-Like breakfast strips, 5½-oz. package, 19 strips, raw	660	12.0			125.7	2.29	2011	36.6
Cooked (yield: approx. 3¼ oz.)	684	3.6			198.2	1.11	3171	17.8
1 strip, approx. 0.29 oz., raw	37	0.7	37	0.7	125.7	2.29	2011	36.6
1 strip, cooked (yield: approx. 0.19 oz.)	38	0.2	38	0.2	198.2	1.11	3171	17.8
Hamburger-Like Grillers, 10-oz. package, 4 patties, raw	840	24.0			84.0	2.40	1344	38.4
Cooked (yield: approx. 9½-oz.)	844	12.5			89.3	1.32	1429	21.1
1 patty, raw approx. 2.5 oz.	210	6.0	210	6.0	84.0	2.40	1344	38.4
1 patty, cooked (yield: approx. 2.4 oz.)	211	5.0	211	5.0	89.3	1.32	1429	21.2
Ham-Like luncheon slices, 6-oz. package, 8 slices	197	10.9			32.9	1.81	526	29.0
1 slice, approx. 0.75 oz.	25	0.9	25	0.9	32.9	1.81	526	29.0
Sausage-Like Breakfast Links, 8-oz. package, 10 links, raw	730	13.3			91.3	1.66	1461	26.6
Cooked (yield: approx. 7.6-oz.)	634	8.0			83.4	1.07	1334	17.1
1 link, approx. 0.80 oz., raw	73	1.3	73	1.3	91.3	1.66	1461	26.6
1 link, cooked (yield: approx. 0.76 oz.)	63	0.8	63	0.8	83.4	1.07	1334	17.1
Sausage-Like Breakfast Patties, 8-oz. package, 6 patties, raw	600	21.0			75.0	2.63	1200	42.1
Cooked: (yield: approx. 7.5-oz.)	470	13.4			62.7	1.79	1003	28.6
1 patty, raw, approx. 1.33 oz.	100	3.5	100	3.5	75.0	2.63	1200	42.1
1 patty, cooked (yield: 1.25 oz.)	78	2.2	78	2.2	62.7	1.79	1402	28.6
WORTHINGTON								
FROZEN:								
Smoked Beef-Like luncheon slices, 8-oz. package, 12 slices	526	24.3			65.8	3.04	1053	48.6
1 slice, approx. 0.67 oz.	22	1.0	22	1.0	65.8	3.04	1053	48.6
Bologna-Like Bolono, 6-oz. package, 8 slices	280	12.0			46.7	2.00	747	32.0
1 slice, approx. 0.74 oz.	35	1.5	35	1.5	46.7	2.00	747	32.0
Chicken-Like slices, 8-oz. package, 8 slices	560	8.0			70.0	1.00	1120	16.0
1 slice, approx. 0.99 oz.	70	1.0	70	1.0	70.0	1.00	1120	16.0
Chic-ketts, 16-oz. (1-lb.) roll	973	32.4			60.8	2.03	973	32.5
Corned Beef-Like luncheon slices, 8-oz. package, 4-5 slices	640	20.0			80.0	2.50	1280	40.0
1 slice, approx. 1.76 oz.	140	1.3	140	1.3	80.0	2.50	1280	40.0
Fri-Pats, 10½-oz. package, 6 fillets	645	30.0			61.4	2.86	982	45.8
1 fillet, approx. 1.76 oz.	108	5.0	108	5.0	61.4	2.86	982	45.8
Luncheon Slices, see Corned Beef-like and Turkey-like								
Pot Pie, Beef-Like, 8-oz. pie	470	51.0			58.8	6.38	941	102.1
Pot Pie, Chicken-Like, 8-oz. pie	450	42.0			56.3	5.25	901	84.0
Prosage, 16-oz. (1-lb.) package, 13-14 slices	1134	46.7			70.9	2.92	(700)	(29.0)
1 slice, ⅜", approx. 1.19 oz.	85	3.5	85	3.5	70.9	2.92	(700)	(29.0)
Prosage Links, 8-oz. package, 8 links	600	16.7			75.0	2.08	(375)	10.4
1 link, approx. 0.99 oz.	75	2.1	75	2.1	75.0	2.08	(375)	10.4
Salami, Meatless 6-oz. package, 8 slices	400	12.0			66.7	0.50	1067	8.0
1 slice, approx. 0.74 oz.	50	1.5	50	1.5	66.7	0.50	1067	8.0

	UNIT Cal.	UNIT Carb.	1 SLICE, PATTY, OR PIECE Cal.	1 SLICE, PATTY, OR PIECE Carb.	1 OZ., BY WT. Cal.	1 OZ., BY WT. Carb.	1 POUND Cal.	1 POUND Carb.
Stakelets, 12-oz. package, 4 stakelets	720	32.0			60.0	2.67	960	42.7
1 stakelet, approx. 3.00 oz.	180	8.0	180	8.0	60.0	2.67	960	42.7
Stripples, 5-oz. package, 18 slices	425	12.8			85.0	2.55	1360	40.8
1 slice, approx. 0.28 oz.	25	0.8	25	0.8	85.0	2.55	1360	40.8
Tuno, 12-oz. roll, approx. 24 tablespoons	540	18.0			45.0	1.50	720	24.0
1 tablespoon (approx. ½ oz.)	(22)	(0.7)	(22)	(0.7)	45.0	1.50	720	24.0
Smoked Turkey-Like luncheon slices, 8-oz. package, 12 slices	600	9.0			75.0	1.12	1200	17.9
1 slice, approx. 0.67 oz.	50	0.8	50	0.8	75.0	1.12	1200	17.9
Wham Ham-Like Flavor slices, 8-oz. package, 10 slices	467	13.3			58.4	1.66	934	26.6
1 slice, approx. 0.81 oz.	47	1.3	47	1.3	58.4	1.66	934	26.6
CANNED:								
Chili, 20-oz. can	770	81.0			38.5	4.05	616	64.8
1 tablespoon	24	2.5	24	2.5	38.5	4.05	616	64.8
Choplets, 20-oz. can, 12 slices	616	33.0			30.8	1.84	493	29.4
1 slice, approx. 1.62 oz.	50	3.0	50	3.0	30.8	1.84	493	29.4
Cutlets, 50-oz. can, 23-24 slices	1450	61.6			29.0	1.23	464	19.7
1 slice, approx. 2.15 oz.	63	2.7	63	2.7	29.0	1.23	464	19.7
Fri-Chik, 13-oz. can, 8 pieces	779	8.2			59.9	0.63	958	10.1
1 piece, approx. 1.59 oz.	85	1.0	85	1.0	59.9	0.63	958	10.1
Non-Meat Balls, 19-oz. can, 30 "meatballs"	1197	69.8			63.0	3.68	1008	58.9
1 "meatball", approx. 0.64 oz.	40	2.3	40	2.3	63.0	3.68	1008	58.9
Numete, 19-oz. can, 8 slices	1267	71.3			66.7	3.75	1067	60.0
1 slice, ½", approx. 2.45 oz.	160	9.0	160	9.0	66.7	3.75	1067	60.0
Protose, 19-oz. can, 7 slices	1347	49.6			70.9	2.61	1134	41.8
1 slice, ½", approx. 2.68 oz.	190	7.0	190	7.0	70.9	2.61	1134	41.8
Saucettes, 12-oz. can, 10 links	650	15.0			54.2	1.25	867	20.0
1 link, approx. 1.20 oz.	65	1.5	65	1.5	54.2	1.25	867	20.0
Skallops, 20-oz. can	450	20.0			23.3	1.00	373	16.0
Soyameat Beef-Like slices, 13-oz. can, 13 slices	724	19.7			55.7	1.52	891	24.3
1 slice, approx. 1 oz.	55	1.5	55	1.5	55.7	1.52	891	24.3
Soyameat Chicken-Like, diced, 13-oz. can	763	12.7			58.7	0.98	939	15.7
Soyameat Chicken-Like slices with Sauce, 13-oz. can, 12 slices	798	12.4			61.4	0.95	982	15.2
1 slice, approx. 1.06 oz.	65	1.0	65	1.0	61.4	0.95	982	15.2
Soyameat Salisbury Steak-Like slices, 13½-oz. can, 6 slices	960	12.0			71.1	0.89	1138	14.2
1 slice, approx. 2.26 oz.	160	2.0	160	2.0	71.1	0.89	1138	14.2
Super Links, 15-oz. can, 8 links	960	32.0			64.0	2.13	1024	40.5
1 link, approx. 1.90 oz.	120	4.0	120	4.0	64.0	2.13	1024	50.5
Turkey-Like Flavor slices, 13-oz. can, 12 slices	877	17.6			67.5	1.35	1080	21.6
1 slice, approx. 1.13 oz.	75	1.5	75	1.5	67.5	1.35	1080	21.6
Vegetable Steaks, 20-oz. can, 2½ pieces	630	44.1			31.5	2.21	504	35.4
1 piece, approx. 1.27 oz.	40	2.8	40	2.8	31.5	2.21	504	35.4
Vegetarian Burger, 20-oz. can	784	36.2			39.2	1.81	627	29.0
Veja-Bits, 13-oz. can	201	12.0			15.5	0.92	248	14.7
Veja-Links, 19-oz. can, 17-18 links	1216	26.1			64.0	1.37	1024	21.9
1 link, approx. 1.09 oz.	70	1.5	70	1.5	64.0	1.37	1024	21.9
DRY:								
Granburger Beef-Like Granules, 10-oz. package	1053	97.2			105.3	9.72	1684	155.5

33 INFANT FORMULAS & BABY FOODS •

My publisher says that I should include a warning right here that you shouldn't put a baby on a diet without competent medical advice. But you knew that all along.

M.F.

INFANTS

Breast Milk

	UNIT		1 FLUID OZ.		1 CUP		1 TEASPOON	
	Cal.	Carb.	Cal.	Carb.	Cal.	Carb.	Cal.	Carb.
Based on data from the United States, 4.38% fat, 1 oz. by weight	20	2.0	21.4	2.11	171	17.0	4	0.4
Based on data from:								
Africa, 3.1% fat, 1 oz. by weight	19	2.6	(20.6)	(2.80)	(165)	(22.4)	(3)	(0.5)
Canada (percentage of fat unavailable), 1 oz. by weight	(20)	(1.8)	(22.1)	(2.00)	(177)	(16.0)	(4)	(0.3)
East Asia, 3.2% fat, 1 oz. by weight	18	2.0	(19.1)	(2.16)	(153)	(17.3)	(3)	(0.4)
France, 5.0% fat, 1 oz. by weight	22	1.8	(23.4)	(2.00)	(187)	(16.0)	(4)	(0.3)

Infant Feeding Formulas

	UNIT		1 FLUID OZ.		1 CUP		1 TEASPOON	
	Cal.	Carb.	Cal.	Carb.	Cal.	Carb.	Cal.	Carb.
Enfamil, Infant Formula, ready-to-use, 8-fl.-oz. can	160	56.0	20.0	7.00	160	56.0	3	1.2
32-fl.-oz. (1-quart) can	640	224.0	20.0	7.00	160	56.0	3	1.2
Infant Formula, concentrated liquid, 13-fl.-oz. can	520	182.0	40.0	14.0	320	112.0	7	2.3
Standard dilution: equal amounts formula and water (yield: approx. 26 fl. oz.)	520	182.0	20.0	7.00	160	56.0	3	1.2
Infant Formula with Iron, ready-to-use, 32-fl.-oz. (1-quart) can	640	224.0	20.0	7.00	160	56.0	3	1.2
Infant Formula with Iron, concentrated liquid, 13-fl.-oz. can	520	182.0	40.0	14.00	320	112.0	7	2.3
Standard dilution: equal amounts formula and water (yield: approx. 26 fl. oz.)	520	182.0	20.0	7.00	160	5.0	3	1.2
Infant Formula with Iron, powdered, 16-oz. (1-lb.) can	1280	448.0						
Standard dilution: 2 quarts water (yield: approx. 2 quarts)	1280	448.0	20.0	7.00	160	56.0	3	1.2
Enfamil Nursette, Infant Formula, ready-to-use, 4-fl.-oz. bottle	80	28.0	20.0	7.00	160	56.0	3	1.2
6-fl.-oz. bottle	120	42.0	20.0	7.00	160	56.0	3	1.2

	UNIT		1 FLUID OZ.		1 CUP		1 TEASPOON	
	Cal.	Carb.	Cal.	Carb.	Cal.	Carb.	Cal.	Carb.
Isomil, Milk-Free Soy Protein Formula, ready-to-use, 8-fl.-oz. can	160	16.1	20.0	2.01	160	16.1	3	0.3
32-fl.-oz. (1-quart) can	640	64.4	20.0	2.01	160	16.1	3	0.3
PM 60/40, powdered, 16-oz. (1-lb.) can	2320	260.8	(80.0)	(16.30)	1280	260.8	13	2.7
Standard dilution: 1 measuring cup formula to 3½ cups water (yield: approx. 1 quart)	640	71.7	20.0	2.24	160	17.9	3	0.4
Multi-Soy, Milk-Free Soy Food, concentrated liquid, 14-fl.-oz. can	560	154.0	40.0	11.00	320	88.0	7	1.8
Standard dilution: equal amounts formula and water (yield: approx. 28 fl. oz.)	560	154.0	20.0	5.50	160	44.0	3	0.9
Nursoy, Milk-Free Soy-Protein Formula, ready-to-use, 32-fl.-oz. (1-quart) can	640	62.6	20.0	1.96	160	15.7	3	0.3
Pro-Sobee, Milk-Free Formula with Soy Protein Isolate, ready-to-use, 32-fl.-oz. (1-quart) can	640	217.6	20.0	6.80	160	54.4	3	1.1
Lactose-Free, Milk-Free Formula with Soy Protein Isolate, concentrated liquid, 13-fl.-oz. can	520	175.5	40.0	13.50	320	108.0	20	6.8
Standard dilution: equal amounts formula and water (yield: approx. 26 fl. oz.)	520	175.5	20.0	6.80	160	54.0	10	3.4
Similac, Infant Formula, ready-to-use, 8-fl.-oz. bottle	160	17.4	20.0	2.17	160	17.4	3	0.4
32-fl.-oz. (1-quart) can	640	69.4	20.0	2.17	160	17.4	3	0.4
Infant Formula, concentrated liquid, 13-fl.-oz. can	520	55.6	40.0	4.28	320	34.2	7	0.7
Standard dilution: equal amounts formula and water (yield: approx. 26 fl. oz.)	520	55.6	20.0	2.14	160	17.1	3	0.4
Infant Formula with Iron, ready-to-use, 32-fl.-oz. (1-quart) can	640	69.4	20.0	2.17	160	17.4	3	0.4
Infant Formula with Iron, concentrated liquid, 13-fl.-oz. can	520	55.6	40.0	4.28	320	34.2	7	0.7
Standard dilution: equal amounts formula and water (yield: approx. 26 fl. oz.)	520	55.6	20.0	2.14	160	17.1	3	0.4
SMA, Iron Fortified Infant Formula, ready-to-use, 32-fl.-oz. (1-quart) can	640	65.3	20.0	7.20	160	16.3	3	0.3
Iron Fortified Infant Formula, concentrated liquid, 13-fl.-oz. can	520	53.1	40.0	4.08	320	32.7	7	0.7

	UNIT		1 FLUID OZ.		1 CUP		1 TEASPOON	
	Cal.	Carb.	Cal.	Carb.	Cal.	Carb.	Cal.	Carb.
Standard dilution: equal amounts formula and water (yield: approx. 26 fl. oz.)	520	53.1	20.0	2.04	160	16.3	3	0.4
Soyalac, Milk-Free Fortified Soy Formula, ready-to-use, 32-fl.-oz. (1-quart) can	640	60.5	20.0	1.89	160	15.1	3	0.3
Milk-Free Fortified Soy Formula, concentrated, 14-fl.-oz. can	560	52.8	40.0	3.77	320	30.2	7	0.6
Standard dilution: equal amounts formula and water (yield: approx. 28 fl. oz.)	560	52.8	20.0	1.89	160	15.1	10	0.9
Milk-Free Fortified Soy Formula, powdered, 16-oz. (1-lb.) can (yield: approx. 15 cups)	2341	223.6	80.0	7.45	1280	119.2	13	1.2
Standard dilution: 4 level tablespoons to 1 cup water (yield: approx. 1 cup)	160	14.9	20.0	1.85	160	14.9	3	0.3
Corn-Free, Milk-Free Fortified Soy Isolate Formula, concentrated liquid, 14-fl.-oz. can	560	52.8	40.0	3.77	320	30.2	7	0.6
Standard dilution: equal amounts formula and water (yield: approx. 28 fl. oz.)	560	52.8	20.0	1.89	160	15.1	3	0.3

BABY FOODS

	UNIT		1 OZ., BY WT.		1 TABLESPOON		Fiber per oz. (GMS.)
	Cal.	Carb.	Cal.	Carb.	Cal.	Carb.	
Baked Goods							
Animal-Shaped Cookies, **Gerber,** 5-oz. box, 22 cookies	618	93.7	123.6	18.74			0.30
1 Animal, approx. 0.2 oz.	30	4.5	123.6	18.74			0.30
Arrowroot Biscuit, National, **Nabisco,** 10½-oz. box, 60 biscuits	1200	180.0	114.3	17.14			
1 Arrowroot biscuit, approx. 0.2 oz.	20	3.0	114.3	17.14			
Arrowroot Cookies, **Gerber,** 5-oz. box, 25 cookies	639	98.1	127.9	19.62			0.20
1 Arrowroot cookie, approx. 0.2 oz.	25	4.0	127.9	19.62			0.20
Biscuits, **Gerber,** 4-oz. package	500	90.0	125.0	22.50			
Pretzels, **Gerber,** 6½-oz. box, 30 pretzels	706	145.4	108.6	22.37			0.10
1 pretzel, approx. 0.2 oz.	23	5.0	108.6	22.37			0.10
Teething Biscuits, **Gerber,** 4-oz. box, approx. 20 biscuits	435	88.8	108.9	22.20			0.20
1 biscuit, approx. 0.2 oz.	25	4.5	108.9	22.20			0.20
Zweiback Toast, **Gerber,** 4-oz. box, 16 toasts	483	82.4	120.8	20.61			
1 Zweiback toast, approx. ¼ oz.	30	5.0	120.8	20.61			
Zweiback Toast, **Nabisco,** 6-oz. box, 24 toasts	720	120.0	120.0	20.00			
1 Zweiback toast, approx. ¼ oz.	30	5.0	120.0	20.00			
Cereals, Dry Mixes							
Barley, **Beech-Nut,** 1-oz. box	100	20.0	100.0	20.00	13	2.5	0.17
8-oz. box	800	160.0	100.0	20.00	13	2.5	0.17
Barley, **Gerber,** 1-oz. box	120	22.0	120.0	22.00	15	2.8	0.37
8-oz. box	960	176.0	120.0	22.00	15	2.8	0.37
16-oz. (1-lb.) box	1920	352.0	120.0	22.00	15	2.8	0.37
Barley, **Heinz,** 8-oz. box	857	164.9	107.2	20.61	(13)	(2.5)	
Hi Protein Cereal, **Beech-Nut,** 1-oz. box	100	12.0	100.0	12.00	13	1.5	0.23
8-oz. box	800	96.0	100.0	12.00	13	1.5	0.23
High Protein Cereal, **Gerber,** 1-oz. box	100	12.0	100.0	12.00	13	1.5	0.65
8-oz. box	800	96.0	100.0	12.00	13	1.5	0.65
16-oz. (1-lb.) box	1600	192.0	100.0	12.00	13	1.5	0.65
High Protein Cereal, **Heinz,** 8-oz. box	823	101.2	102.9	12.65	(13)	(1.6)	
High Protein Cereal with Apple & Orange, **Gerber,** 1-oz. box	120	16.0	120.0	16.00	15	2.0	0.40
8-oz. box	960	128.0	120.0	16.00	15	2.0	0.40
16-oz. (1-lb.) box	1920	256.0	120.0	16.00	15	2.0	0.40
Mixed Cereal, **Beech-Nut,** 1-oz. box	100	20.0	100.0	20.00	13	2.5	
8-oz. box	800	160.0	100.0	20.00	13	2.5	
16-oz. (1-lb.) box	1600	320.0	100.0	20.00	13	2.5	
Mixed Cereal, **Gerber,** 1-oz. box	120	20.0	120.0	20.00	15	2.5	0.31
8-oz. box	960	160.0	120.0	20.00	15	2.5	0.31
16-oz. (1-lb.) box	1920	320.0	120.0	20.00	15	2.5	0.31
Mixed Cereal, **Heinz,** 8-oz. box	855	157.6	106.9	19.71	(13)	(2.5)	
Mixed Cereal with Banana, **Gerber,** 1-oz. box	120	22.0	120.0	22.00	15	2.8	0.28
8-oz. box	960	176.0	120.0	22.00	15	2.8	0.28
16-oz. (1-lb.) box	1920	352.0	120.0	22.00	15	2.8	0.28
Mixed Cereal with Fruit, Nuts and Honey, **Familia,** 12-oz. box	1360	256.0	113.0	21.00			
Oatmeal, **Beech-Nut,** 1-oz. box	100	18.0	100.0	18.00	13	2.3	0.17
8-oz. box	800	144.0	100.0	18.00	13	2.3	0.17
16-oz. (1-lb.) box	1600	288.0	100.0	18.00	13	2.3	0.17
Oatmeal, **Gerber,** 1-oz. box	100	18.0	100.0	18.00	13	2.3	0.40
8-oz. box	800	144.0	100.0	18.00	13	2.3	0.40
16-oz. (1-lb.) box	1600	288.0	100.0	18.00	13	2.3	0.40
Oatmeal, **Heinz,** 8-oz. box	860	151.1	107.5	18.89	(13)	(2.4)	
Oatmeal with Banana, **Gerber,** 1-oz. box	120	20.0	120.0	20.00	15	2.5	0.31
8-oz. box	960	160.0	120.0	20.00	15	2.5	0.31
16-oz. (1-lb.) box	1920	320.0	120.0	20.00	15	2.5	0.31
Rice Cereal, **Beech-Nut,** 1-oz. box	100	20.0	100.0	20.00	13	2.5	
8-oz. box	800	160.0	100.0	20.00	13	2.5	
16-oz. (1-lb.) box	1600	320.0	100.0	20.00	13	2.5	
Rice Cereal, **Gerber,** 1-oz. box	120	22.0	120.0	22.00	15	2.8	0.26
8-oz. box	960	176.0	120.0	22.00	15	2.8	0.26
16-oz. (1-lb.) box	1920	352.0	120.0	22.00	15	2.8	0.26
Rice Cereal, **Heinz,** 8-oz. box	855	106.9	106.9	13.36	(13)	(1.6)	
Rice Cereal with Banana, **Gerber,** 1-oz. box	120	22.0	120.0	22.00	15	2.8	0.26
8-oz. box	960	176.0	120.0	22.00	15	2.8	0.26
16-oz. (1-lb.) box	1920	352.0	120.0	22.00	15	2.8	0.26
Strained Baby Foods							
CEREALS							
Cereal & Eggs, **Heinz,** 4½-oz. jar	74	11.7	16.4	2.61	(8)	(1.3)	
Cereal & Egg Yolk, **Gerber,** 4½-oz. jar	70	9.6	15.6	2.13	8	1.1	0.03
Cereal, Egg Yolks & Bacon, **Beech-Nut,** 4½-oz. jar	110	9.0	24.4	2.00	12	1.0	
Mixed Cereal with Apples & Bananas, **Heinz,** 4¾-oz. jar	92	20.4	19.3	4.28	(10)	(2.2)	
Mixed Cereal with Apples & Bananas, **Beech-Nut,** 4¾-oz. jar	80	18.0	18.0	4.00	9	2.0	
Oatmeal with Apples & Bananas, **Beech-Nut,** 4¾-oz. jar	90	17.0	20.0	3.81	10	1.9	
Oatmeal with Apples & Bananas, **Gerber,** 4¾-oz. jar	100	20.0	21.1	4.21	11	2.0	
Oatmeal with Apples & Bananas, **Heinz,** 4¾-oz. jar	100	21.4	21.0	4.51	(11)	(2.3)	
Rice Cereal with Apples & Bananas, **Beech-Nut,** 4¾-oz. jar	90	20.0	20.0	4.50	10	2.3	
Rice Cereal with Apples & Bananas, **Heinz,** 4¾-oz. jar	108	24.5	22.7	5.16	(12)	(2.7)	
Rice Cereal With Applesauce & Bananas, **Gerber,** 4¾-oz. jar	96	21.3	20.1	4.48	10	2.3	0.09
JUICES							
Apple Juice, **Beech-Nut,** 4.2-fl.-oz. jar	60	14.0	(14.0)	(3.20)	7	1.7	
Apple Juice, **Gerber,** 4.2-fl.-oz. jar	60	16.0	13.9	3.32	7	1.9	0.03
Apple Juice, **Heinz,** 4.2-fl.-oz. jar	70	17.0	13.3	3.26	8	2.0	
Apple-Apricot Juice, **Heinz,** 4.2-fl.-oz. jar	70	18.0	13.6	3.32	8	2.2	
Apple-Banana Juice, **Gerber,** 4.2-fl.-oz. jar	60	15.0	13.9	3.26	7	1.8	0.03
Apple-Cherry Juice, **Beech-Nut,** 4.2-fl.-oz. jar	50	12.0	(12.0)	(2.70)	6	1.5	
Apple-Cherry Juice, **Gerber,** 4.2-fl.-oz. jar	60	16.0	13.6	3.26	7	1.9	0.03
Apple-Cherry Juice, **Heinz,** 4.2-fl.-oz. jar	60	16.0	13.3	3.18	7	1.9	
Apple-Cranberry Juice, **Beech-Nut,** 4.2-fl.-oz. jar	60	14.0	(14.0)	(3.20)	7	1.7	
Apple-Grape Juice, **Beech-Nut,** 4.2-fl.-oz. jar	60	14.0	(14.0)	(3.20)	7	1.7	
Apple-Grape Juice, **Gerber,** 4.2-fl.-oz. jar	60	16.0	13.9	3.32	7	1.9	0.03
Apple-Grape Juice, **Heinz,** 4.2-fl.-oz. jar	70	17.0	14.4	3.46	8	2.0	
Apple-Peach Juice, **Beech-Nut,** 4.2-fl.-oz. jar	60	15.0	(14.0)	(3.40)	7	1.8	
Apple-Peach Juice, **Gerber,** 4.2-fl.-oz. jar	60	15.0	13.3	3.18	7	1.8	0.03
Apple-Pineapple Juice, **Heinz,** 4.2-fl.-oz. jar	80	18.0	14.5	3.43	10	2.2	

	UNIT		1 OZ., BY WT.		1 TABLE-SPOON		Fiber per oz.
	Cal.	Carb.	Cal.	Carb.	Cal.	Carb.	(GMS.)
Apple-Plum Juice, **Gerber,** 4.2-fl.-oz. jar	60	16.0	14.2	3.43	7	1.9	
Apple-Prune Juice, **Beech-Nut,** 4.2-fl.-oz. jar	70	17.0	(16.0)	(3.90)	8	2.0	0.03
Apple-Prune Juice, **Gerber,** 4.2-fl.-oz. jar	60	16.0	14.5	3.49	7	1.9	
Apple-Prune Juice, **Heinz,** 4.2-fl.-oz. jar	100	24.0	14.5	3.43	12	2.9	
Mixed Fruit Juice, **Beech-Nut,** 4.2-fl.-oz. jar	60	15.0	(14.0)	(3.40)	7	1.8	
Mixed Fruit Juice, **Gerber,** 4.2-fl.-oz. jar	70	16.0	13.9	3.23	8	1.9	0.03
Mixed Fruit Juice, **Heinz,** 4.2-fl.-oz. jar	90	21.0	15.3	3.63	11	2.5	
Orange Juice, **Beech-Nut,** 4.2-fl.-oz. jar	60	14.0	(14.0)	(3.20)	7	1.7	
Orange Juice, **Gerber,** 4.2-fl.-oz. jar	70	14.0	13.6	2.98	8	1.7	0.03
Orange Juice, **Heinz,** 4.2-fl.-oz. jar	60	15.0	13.3	3.01	7	1.8	
Orange-Apple Juice, **Beech-Nut,** 4.2-fl.-oz. jar	60	14.0	(14.0)	(3.20)	7	1.7	
Orange-Apple Juice, **Gerber,** 4.2-fl.-oz. jar	70	15.0	14.2	3.20	8	1.8	0.03
Orange-Apple-Banana Juice, **Heinz,** 4.2-fl.-oz. jar	70	18.0	14.2	3.35	8	2.2	
Orange-Apricot Juice, **Gerber,** 4.2-fl.-oz. jar	70	15.0	14.2	3.15	8	1.8	0.03
Orange-Banana Juice, **Beech-Nut,** 4.2-fl.-oz. jar	60	14.0	(14.0)	(3.20)	7	1.7	
Orange-Pineapple Juice, **Beech-Nut,** 4.2-fl.-oz. jar	60	14.0	(14.0)	(3.20)	7	1.7	
Orange-Pineapple Juice, **Gerber,** 4.2-fl.-oz. jar	80	17.0	15.3	3.52	10	2.0	0.03
FRUITS							
Apple Blueberry, **Gerber,** 4½-oz. jar	75	17.5	16.7	3.88	8	2.0	0.17
Apples & Cranberries with Tapioca, **Heinz,** 4¾-oz. jar	81	19.0	17.0	4.02	(9)	(2.0)	
Apples, Mandarin Oranges & Banana, **Beech-Nut,** 4½-oz. jar	90	22.0	20.0	4.90	10	2.5	
Apple & Nonfat Yogurt, **Gerber,** 4½-oz.	97	21.2	21.5	4.71	11	2.4	0.06
Apples, Peaches & Strawberries, **Beech-Nut,** 4½-oz. jar	100	24.0	22.0	5.30	11	2.7	
Apples & Pears, **Heinz,** 4½-oz. jar	73	16.6	16.1	3.69	(8)	(1.8)	
Apples, Pears & Banana, **Beech-Nut,** 4½-oz. jar	100	24.0	22.0	5.30	11	2.7	
Apples, Pears & Pineapple, **Beech-Nut,** 4½-oz. jar	100	24.0	22.0	5.30	11	2.7	
Apples & Strawberries, **Beech-Nut,** 4½-oz. jar	100	24.0	22.0	5.30	11	2.7	
Applesauce, **Beech-Nut,** 4½-oz. jar	60	14.0	13.0	3.10	7	1.6	0.03
Applesauce, **Gerber,** 4½-oz. jar	59	13.8	13.0	3.06	7	1.5	0.20
Applesauce, **Heinz,** 4½-oz. jar	68	15.2	15.0	3.37	(8)	(1.7)	
Applesauce & Apricots, **Beech-Nut,** 4½-oz. jar	60	14.0	13.0	3.10	7	1.6	
Applesauce & Apricots, **Gerber,** 4½-oz. jar	66	15.4	14.7	3.43	7	1.7	0.20
Applesauce & Apricots, **Heinz,** 4¾-oz. jar	100	25.0	21.1	5.26	(11)	(2.6)	
Applesauce & Bananas, **Beech-Nut,** 4½-oz. jar	60	15.0	13.0	3.30	7	1.7	
Applesauce & Cherries, **Beech-Nut,** 4½-oz. jar	68	17.0	15.0	3.80	8	1.9	
Applesauce with Pineapple, **Gerber,** 4½-oz. jar	63	14.8	13.9	3.29	7	1.7	0.17
Applesauce & Raspberries, **Beech-Nut,** 4½-oz. jar	60	15.0	13.0	3.30	7	1.9	
Apricots with Tapioca, **Beech-Nut,** 4½-oz. jar	80	20.0	18.0	4.50	9	2.3	
Apricots with Tapioca, **Gerber,** 4¾-oz. jar	97	23.2	20.4	4.88	0	2.5	0.09
Apricots with Tapioca, **Heinz,** 4¾-oz. jar	78	18.9	16.5	3.97	(8)	(2.0)	
Bananas with Tapioca, **Beech-Nut,** 4½-oz. jar	80	19.0	18.9	4.20	9	2.1	0.03
Bananas with Tapioca, **Gerber,** 4½-oz. jar	85	20.5	18.0	4.56	10	2.3	0.06
Bananas with Tapioca, **Heinz,** 4¾-oz. jar	100	22.9	21.1	5.82	(11)	(2.4)	
Bananas & Pineapple, **Beech-Nut,** 4½-oz. jar	70	16.0	16.0	3.60	8	1.8	
Bananas & Pineapple with Tapioca, **Gerber,** 4½-oz. jar	64	14.7	14.2	3.26	7	1.6	0.03
Bananas & Pineapple with Tapioca, **Heinz,** 4¾-oz. jar	90	21.6	18.9	4.54	(9)	(2.2)	
Guava, **Gerber,** 4½-oz. jar	84	19.9	18.7	4.42	9	2.2	0.06
Guava & Papaya, **Gerber,** 4½-oz. jar	85	20.3	19.0	4.51	10	2.3	0.06
Mango, **Gerber,** 4¾-oz. jar	92	22.1	20.4	4.91	10	2.5	0.06
Mixed Fruit & Nonfat Yogurt, **Gerber,** 4½-oz. jar	101	21.6	22.4	4.79	11	2.4	0.06
Papaya & Applesauce, **Gerber,** 4½-oz.	83	19.9	18.4	4.42	9	2.2	
Peaches, **Beech-Nut,** 4½-oz. jar	90	23.0	20.0	5.10	10	2.6	0.09
Peaches, **Gerber,** 4¾-oz. jar	98	23.2	20.7	4.88	10	2.4	0.23
Peaches, **Heinz,** 4½-oz. jar	60	13.0	13.3	2.89	(9)	(1.4)	
Pears, **Beech-Nut,** 4½-oz. jar	90	22.0	20.0	4.90	10	2.5	
Pears, **Gerber,** 4½-oz. jar	70	15.0	15.6	3.33	8	1.9	0.43
Pears, **Heinz,** 4½-oz. jar	80	19.0	17.9	4.23	(9)	(2.1)	
Pears & Pineapple, **Beech-Nut,** 4½-oz. jar	100	25.0	22.0	5.60	11	2.8	0.20
Pears & Pineapple, **Gerber,** 4½-oz. jar	68	15.7	15.0	3.49	13	3.4	0.37
Pears & Pineapple, **Heinz,** 4½-oz. jar	77	18.4	17.0	4.09	(9)	(2.0)	
Plums with Tapioca, **Beech-Nut,** 4½-oz. jar	90	22.0	20.0	4.90	10	2.5	
Plums with Tapioca, **Gerber,** 4¾-oz. jar	90	22.2	19.0	4.68	10	2.4	0.11
Plums with Tapioca, **Heinz,** 4½-oz. jar	79	18.8	17.6	4.17	(9)	(2.1)	
Prunes with Tapioca, **Beech-Nut,** 4½-oz. jar	100	24.0	22.0	5.30	11	2.7	
Prunes with Tapioca, **Gerber,** 4¾-oz. jar	97	22.6	20.4	4.76	10	2.4	0.17
Prunes with Tapioca, **Heinz,** 4¾-oz. jar	120	28.8	25.3	6.07	(13)	(3.0)	
EGGS							
Egg Yolks with Water, **Heinz,** 3¼-oz. jar	180	2.0	55.4	1.00	(28)	(0.3)	
SOUPS							
Chicken Soup, **Heinz,** 4½-oz. jar	66	10.0	14.7	2.21	(7)	(1.1)	
Cream of Chicken Soup, **Gerber,** 4½-oz. jar	77	11.1	17.0	2.47	9	1.2	0.09
VEGETABLES							
Beets, **Beech-Nut,** 4½-oz. jar	50	10.0	11.0	2.20	6	1.1	
Beets, **Gerber,** 4½-oz. jar	47	10.0	10.5	2.21	5	1.1	0.17
Beets, **Heinz,** 4½-oz. jar	50	10.5	11.1	2.32	(6)	(1.2)	
Carrots, **Beech-Nut,** 4½-oz. jar	40	8.0	8.9	1.78	5	0.9	
Carrots, **Gerber,** 4½-oz. jar	31	6.3	6.8	1.39	3	0.7	0.20
Carrots, **Heinz,** 4½-oz. jar	29	6.3	6.5	1.39	(3)	(0.7)	
For comparison: Buttered Carrots, **Cow & Gate** (sold in Great Britain), 4½-oz. jar	44	5.4	9.8	1.20	5	6.0	
Creamed Corn, **Beech-Nut,** 4½-oz. jar	90	19.0	20.0	2.40	10	1.2	
Creamed Corn, **Gerber,** 4½-oz. jar	83	16.7	18.4	3.71	9	1.9	
Creamed Corn, **Heinz,** 4½-oz. jar	91	20.0	20.1	4.45	(10)	(2.2)	
Creamed Peas, **Heinz,** 4½-oz. jar	73	11.0	16.2	2.44	(8)	(1.2)	
Creamed Spinach, **Gerber,** 4½-oz. jar	56	6.9	12.5	1.53	6	0.8	0.11
Garden Vegetables, **Beech-Nut,** 4½-oz. jar	60	12.0	13.0	2.70	7	1.4	
Garden Vegetables, **Gerber,** 4½-oz. jar	43	6.9	9.6	1.53	5	0.8	0.23
Green Beans, **Beech-Nut,** 4½-oz. jar	40	8.0	8.9	1.78	5	0.9	
Green Beans, **Gerber,** 4½-oz. jar	31	5.9	6.8	1.30	3	0.7	0.26
Green Beans, **Heinz,** 4½-oz. jar	31	5.7	6.8	1.28	(3)	(0.6)	
Mixed Vegetables, **Beech-Nut,** 4½-oz. jar	50	12.0	11.0	2.70	6	1.4	
Peas, **Beech-Nut,** 4½-oz. jar	70	12.0	16.0	2.70	8	1.4	
Peas, **Gerber,** 4½-oz. jar	56	8.5	12.5	1.90	6	1.0	0.03
Peas and Carrots, **Beech-Nut,** 4½-oz. jar	60	11.0	13.0	2.40	7	1.2	
Squash, **Beech-Nut,** 4½-oz. jar	30	7.0	7.0	1.60	4	0.8	
Squash, **Gerber,** 4½-oz. jar	33	6.6	7.4	1.47	4	0.7	0.23
Squash, **Heinz,** 4½-oz. jar	37	7.8	8.2	1.73	(4)	(0.9)	
Sweet Potatoes, **Beech-Nut,** 4¾-oz. jar	70	16.0	16.0	3.60	8	1.8	
Sweet Potatoes, **Gerber,** 4¾-oz. jar	81	18.2	17.0	3.83	9	1.9	0.14
Sweet Potatoes, **Heinz,** 4¾-oz. jar	97	22.2	20.4	4.68	(10)	(2.3)	
PASTA DINNERS							
Beef & Egg Noodles, **Heinz,** 4½-oz. jar	55	7.9	12.2	1.76	(6)	(0.9)	
Beef & Egg Noodles with Vegetables, **Gerber,** 4½-oz. jar	84	11.9	18.7	2.64	9	1.3	0.09
Chicken & Noodles, **Gerber,** 4½-oz. jar	77	11.1	17.0	2.47	9	1.2	0.09
Chicken Noodle, **Beech-Nut,** 4½-oz. jar	70	10.0	16.0	2.22	8	1.1	
Chicken Noodle Dinner, **Heinz,** 4½-oz. jar	71	9.6	15.9	2.13	(8)	(1.1)	
Macaroni & Cheese, **Gerber,** 4½-oz. jar	80	10.8	17.9	2.41	9	1.2	

	UNIT		1 OZ., BY WT.		1 TABLE-SPOON		Fiber per oz.
	Cal.	Carb.	Cal.	Carb.	Cal.	Carb.	(GMS.)
Macaroni, Tomato & Beef, **Beech-Nut,** 4½-oz. jar	90	11.0	20.0	2.44	10	1.2	
Macaroni, Tomato with Beef, **Gerber,** 4½-oz. jar	70	11.5	15.6	2.55	8	1.3	
Macaroni, Tomatoes & Beef, **Heinz,** 4½-oz. jar	68	11.4	15.0	2.52	(8)	(1.2)	
Vegetables, Egg Noodles & Chicken, **Heinz,** 4½-oz. jar	82	11.9	18.1	2.64	(9)	(1.3)	
Vegetables, Egg Noodles & Turkey, **Heinz,** 4½-oz. jar	64	10.2	14.2	2.27	(7)	(1.1)	
VEGETABLES WITH MEAT OR POULTRY							
Chicken Rice, **Beech-Nut,** 4½-oz. jar	70	12.0	16.0	2.70	8	1.4	
Turkey Rice, **Beech-Nut,** 4½-oz. jar	70	12.0	16.0	2.70	8	1.4	
Turkey Rice Dinner with Vegetables, **Heinz,** 4½-oz. jar	57	10.5	12.8	2.32	(6)	(1.2)	
Vegetable Bacon, **Beech-Nut,** 4½-oz. jar	90	10.0	20.0	2.20	10	1.1	
Vegetables & Bacon, **Gerber,** 4½-oz. jar	96	10.6	21.3	2.35	11	1.2	0.11
Vegetables & Bacon, **Heinz,** 4½-oz. jar	68	8.0	15.0	1.79	(8)	(0.9)	0.11
Vegetable Beef, **Beech-Nut,** 4½-oz. jar	90	11.0	20.0	2.40	10	1.2	
Vegetables & Beef, **Gerber,** 4½-oz. jar	85	10.6	19.0	2.35	10	1.2	0.11
Vegetables & Beef, **Heinz,** 4½-oz. jar	73	10.1	16.2	2.24	(8)	(1.1)	
Vegetable Chicken, **Beech-Nut,** 4½-oz. jar	80	12.0	18.0	2.70	9	1.4	
Vegetables & Chicken, **Gerber,** 4½-oz. jar	61	8.5	13.6	1.90	7	1.0	0.06
Vegetables, Dumplings & Beef, **Heinz,** 4½-oz. jar	69	11.1	15.3	2.47	(8)	(1.2)	
Vegetable Ham, **Beech-Nut,** 4½-oz. jar	90	13.0	20.0	2.90	10	1.5	
Vegetables & Ham, **Gerber,** 4½-oz. jar	73	10.7	16.2	2.38	8	1.2	0.06
Vegetables & Ham, **Heinz,** 4½-oz. jar	53	8.7	11.9	1.93	(6)	(1.0)	
Vegetable Lamb, **Beech-Nut,** 4½-oz. jar	80	10.0	18.0	2.20	9	1.1	0.09
Vegetables & Lamb, **Gerber,** 4½-oz. jar	73	9.1	16.2	2.01	8	1.0	0.09
Vegetables & Lamb, **Heinz,** 4½-oz. jar	60	8.2	13.3	1.81	(7)	(0.9)	
Vegetable Liver, **Beech-Nut,** 4½-oz. jar	70	12.0	16.0	2.70	(8)	(1.4)	0.06
Vegetables & Liver, **Gerber,** 4½-oz. jar	70	9.7	13.3	2.15	7	1.1	0.09
Vegetable Turkey, **Beech-Nut,** 4½-oz. jar	70	12.0	16.0	2.70	8	1.4	
Vegetables & Turkey, **Gerber,** 4½-oz. jar	65	9.3	14.5	2.07	7	1.0	0.06
MEATS							
Beef, **Gerber,** 3½-oz. jar	93	0.3	26.7	0.09	13	trace	
Beef & Beef Broth, **Beech-Nut,** 3½-oz. jar	120	1.0	34.0	0.10	17	0.1	
Beef & Beef Broth, **Heinz,** 3½-oz. jar	133	0.7	38.0	0.20	(19)	(0.1)	
Beef with Beef Heart, **Gerber,** 3½-oz. jar	90	0.5	25.8	0.14	13	0.1	
Beef Liver, **Gerber,** 3½-oz. jar	98	2.9	28.1	0.82	14	0.4	
Chicken, **Gerber,** 3½-oz. jar	139	0.3	39.7	0.09	20	trace	
Chicken & Chicken Broth, **Beech-Nut,** 3½-oz. jar	110	1.0	31.0	0.10	16	0.1	
Chicken & Chicken Broth, **Heinz,** 3½-oz. jar	132	0.1	37.7	0.03	(19)	trace	
Ham, **Gerber,** 3½-oz. jar	105	0.5	30.1	0.14	15	0.1	
Ham & Ham Broth, **Beech-Nut,** 3½-oz. jar	120	1.0	34.0	0.10	17	0.1	
Lamb, **Gerber,** 3½-oz. jar	98	0.6	28.1	0.17	14	0.1	
Lamb & Lamb Broth, **Beech-Nut,** 3½-oz. jar	130	1.0	37.0	0.10	19	0.1	
Lamb & Lamb Broth, **Heinz,** 3½-oz. jar	135	0.3	38.6	0.09	(19)	trace	
Liver & Liver Broth, **Heinz,** 3½-oz. jar	91	3.6	26.1	1.02	(13)	(0.5)	
Pork, **Gerber,** 3½-oz. jar	106	0.3	30.3	0.09	15	trace	
Turkey, **Gerber,** 3½-oz. jar	126	0.3	36.0	0.09	18	trace	
Turkey & Turkey Broth, **Beech-Nut,** 3½-oz. jar	120	1.0	34.0	0.10	17	0.1	
Veal, **Gerber,** 3½-oz. jar	90	0.2	25.8	0.06	13	trace	
Veal & Veal Broth, **Beech-Nut,** 3½-oz. jar	120	1.0	34.0	0.10	17	0.1	
Veal & Veal Broth, **Heinz,** 3½-oz. jar	108	0.5	30.9	0.14	(16)	(0.1)	

	UNIT		1 OZ., BY WT.		1 TABLE-SPOON		Fiber per oz.
	Cal.	Carb.	Cal.	Carb.	Cal.	Carb.	(GMS.)
For comparison: Liver, Beef & Bacon Savoury, **Cow & Gate** "Teatime Treats" (sold in Great Britain), 2¼-oz. jar	61	5.7	27.0	2.55	14	1.3	
For comparison: Oxtail & Beef Casserole, **Cow & Gate** (sold in Great Britain), 2¼-oz. jar	48	5.4	21.5	2.39	11	1.1	
For comparison: Steak & Kidney Dinner, **Cow & Gate** (sold in Great Britain), 2¼-oz. jar	46	5.0	20.3	2.24	10	1.1	
HIGH-MEAT DINNERS and CHEESE FOODS							
Beef, **Beech-Nut,** 4½-oz. jar	130	8.0	28.9	1.78	16	1.0	
Beef with Vegetables, **Gerber,** 4½-oz. jar	111	7.4	24.7	1.64	12	0.8	0.09
Beef with Vegetables, **Heinz,** 4½-oz. jar	85	6.1	19.0	1.36	(10)	(0.7)	
Chicken, **Beech-Nut,** 4½-oz. jar	90	9.0	20.0	2.00	10	1.0	
Chicken with Vegetables, **Gerber,** 4½-oz. jar	125	7.8	27.8	1.73	14	0.9	0.06
Chicken with Vegetables, **Heinz,** 4½-oz. jar	106	5.6	23.5	1.25	(12)	(0.6)	
Cottage Cheese with Bananas, **Heinz,** 4½-oz. jar	91	17.2	20.4	3.83	(10)	(1.9)	
Cottage Cheese with Pineapple, **Gerber,** 4¾-oz. jar	121	18.2	25.5	3.83	13	1.9	0.03
Cottage Cheese with Pineapple Juice, **Beech-Nut,** 4¾-oz. jar	120	21.0	27.0	4.70	14	2.4	
Ham, **Beech-Nut,** 4½-oz. jar	130	8.0	28.9	1.78	16	1.0	
Ham with Vegetables, **Gerber,** 4½-oz. jar	100	8.3	22.1	1.84	11	0.9	0.06
Turkey, **Beech-Nut,** 4½-oz. jar	110	9.0	22.0	1.80	11	0.9	
Turkey with Vegetables, **Gerber,** 4½-oz. jar	128	7.4	28.4	1.64	14	0.8	0.03
Turkey with Vegetables, **Heinz,** 4½-oz. jar	116	8.4	25.8	1.87	(13)	(0.9)	
Veal, **Beech-Nut,** 4½-oz. jar	100	8.0	22.2	1.78	16	1.0	
Veal with Vegetables, **Gerber,** 4½-oz. jar	85	7.8	19.0	1.13	10	0.9	0.09
DESSERTS							
Apple Betty, **Beech-Nut,** 4¾-oz. jar	100	24.0	22.0	5.30	11	2.7	
Apple Custard Pudding, **Beech-Nut,** 4½-oz. jar	100	20.0	22.0	4.40	11	2.2	
Apricots with Tapioca, **Gerber,** 4¾-oz. jar	97	23.2	20.4	4.88	10	2.5	0.09
Banana-Apple Dessert, **Gerber,** 4¾-oz. jar	96	22.6	20.1	4.76	10	2.4	0.09
Banana-Apple Dessert, **Heinz,** 4¾-oz. jar	96	22.6	20.1	4.76	(10)	(2.4)	0.09
Banana Custard Pudding, **Beech-Nut,** 4½-oz. jar	90	18.0	20.0	4.00	10	2.0	
Banana Pudding, **Heinz,** 4¾-oz. jar	105	23.2	22.1	4.88	(11)	(2.5)	
Cherry Vanilla Pudding, **Gerber,** 4¾-oz. jar	92	19.9	19.3	4.20	10	2.1	0.09
Chocolate Custard, **Beech-Nut,** 4½-oz. jar	120	21.0	27.0	4.70	14	2.4	
Chocolate Custard Pudding, **Gerber,** 4½-oz. jar	106	19.3	23.5	4.28	12	2.2	0.26
Custard Pudding, **Heinz,** 4½-oz. jar	98	17.9	21.8	3.97	(9)	(1.6)	
Dutch Apple Dessert, **Gerber,** 4¾-oz. jar	97	21.1	20.4	4.45	10	2.2	0.11
Dutch Apple Dessert, **Heinz,** 4¾-oz. jar	93	22.5	19.6	4.74	(10)	(2.4)	
Fruit Dessert, **Beech-Nut,** 4¾-oz. jar	100	24.0	22.0	5.30	11	2.7	
Fruit Dessert, **Gerber,** 4¾-oz. jar	92	22.0	19.3	4.62	10	2.2	0.06
Fruit Dessert, **Heinz,** 4¾-oz. jar	90	21.4	19.0	4.51	(10)	(2.4)	
Hawaiian Delight, **Gerber,** 4½-oz. jar	111	24.2	24.7	5.39	12	2.7	
Mixed Fruit Yogurt, **Beech-Nut,** 4½-oz. jar	70	17.0	16.0	3.80	8	1.9	
Orange Pineapple Dessert, **Beech-Nut,** 4¾-oz. jar	100	25.0	22.0	5.60	11	2.8	
Orange Pudding, **Gerber,** 4¾-oz. jar	114	24.0	24.1	5.05	12	2.5	0.09
Peach-Apple Yogurt, **Beech-Nut,** 4½-oz. jar	70	15.0	16.0	3.30	8	1.7	
Peach Cobbler, **Gerber,** 4¾-oz. jar	94	24.0	19.8	5.05	12	2.3	0.14
Peach Cobbler, **Heinz,** 4¾-oz. jar	93	21.8	20.7	4.60	(10)	(2.2)	
Peach Melba, **Beech-Nut,** 4¾-oz. jar	90	23.0	20.0	5.10	10	2.6	
Pineapple Dessert, **Beech-Nut,** 4¾-oz. jar	100	25.0	22.0	5.60	11	2.8	
Pineapple and Non-Fat Yogurt, **Beech-Nut,** 4½-oz. jar	80	18.0	18.0	4.00	9	2.0	
Pineapple Orange, **Heinz,** 4½-oz.	92	22.1	20.4	4.91	(20)	(4.9)	
Plums with Tapioca, **Gerber,** 4¾-oz.	90	22.2	19.0	4.68	10	2.4	0.06
Raspberry Dessert with Yogurt, **Gerber,** 4½-oz. jar	87	20.2	19.3	4.48	10	2.3	0.03
Rice Pudding, **Beech-Nut,** 4½-oz. jar	100	18.0	22.0	4.00	11	2.0	
Tutti Frutti, **Heinz,** 4½-oz. jar	96	21.8	21.3	4.85	(11)	(2.4)	

	UNIT Cal.	UNIT Carb.	1 OZ., BY WT. Cal.	1 OZ., BY WT. Carb.	1 TABLE-SPOON Cal.	1 TABLE-SPOON Carb.	Fiber per oz. (GMS.)
Vanilla Custard Pudding, **Beech-Nut,** 4½-oz. jar	100	16.0	22.0	3.60	11	1.8	
Vanilla Custard Pudding, **Gerber,** 4½-oz. jar	105	19.5	23.2	4.34	12	2.2	0.26
Junior Baby Foods							
CEREALS							
Cereal & Eggs, **Heinz,** 7½-oz. jar	111	15.5	14.7	2.07	(7)	(1.0)	
Cereal & Egg Yolk, **Gerber,** 7½-oz. jar	70	10.0	9.3	1.33	5	0.7	0.03
Mixed Cereal with Applesauce & Bananas, **Gerber,** 7¾-oz. jar	130	25.3	17.3	3.52	9	1.8	0.06
Oatmeal with Applesauce & Bananas, **Gerber,** 7¾-oz. jar	119	23.0	15.9	3.06	8	1.5	0.09
Rice Cereal with Mixed Fruit, **Gerber,** 7¾-oz. jar	160	27.2	20.7	3.52	9	1.8	0.03
FRUITS							
Apples & Apricots, **Beech-Nut,** 7½-oz. jar	90	23.0	12.0	3.10	6	1.6	
Apple Blueberry, **Gerber,** 7½-oz. jar	111	26.2	14.7	3.49	7	1.5	0.11
Apples & Cranberries with Tapioca, **Heinz,** 7¾-oz. jar	132	31.2	17.0	4.03	(9)	(2.0)	
Apples, Oranges & Bananas, **Beech-Nut,** 7½-oz. jar	150	37.0	20.0	4.90	10	2.5	
Apples, Peaches, & Strawberries, **Beech-Nut,** 7½-oz. jar	160	40.0	21.0	5.30	11	2.7	
Apples & Pears, **Heinz,** 7¾-oz. jar	125	28.6	16.2	3.69	(8)	(1.9)	
Apples, Pears & Bananas, **Beech-Nut,** 7½-oz. jar	160	40.0	21.0	5.30	11	2.7	
Apples, Pears & Pineapple, **Beech-Nut,** 7½-oz. jar	160	40.0	21.0	5.30	11	2.7	
Apples & Strawberries, **Beech-Nut,** 7½-oz. jar	160	40.0	21.0	5.30	11	2.7	
Applesauce, **Beech-Nut,** 7½-oz. jar	100	24.0	13.0	2.20	7	1.1	
Applesauce, **Gerber,** 7½-oz. jar	94	22.3	12.5	2.98	6	1.5	0.20
Applesauce, **Heinz,** 7½-oz. jar	112	25.3	15.0	3.37	(8)	(1.7)	
Applesauce & Apricots, **Gerber,** 7½-oz. jar	98	22.8	13.0	3.03	7	1.5	0.20
Applesauce & Apricots, **Heinz,** 7¾-oz. jar	151	34.9	20.1	4.65	(10)	(2.3)	
Applesauce & Banana, **Beech-Nut,** 7½-oz. jar	110	26.0	15.0	3.50	8	1.8	
Applesauce & Cherries, **Beech-Nut,** 7¼-oz. jar	110	28.0	15.0	3.70	8	1.9	
Applesauce & Raspberries, **Beech-Nut,** 7¼-oz. jar	100	24.0	14.0	3.20	7	1.6	0.11
Apricots with Tapioca, **Beech-Nut,** 7½-oz. jar	140	33.0	19.0	4.40	10	2.2	
Apricots with Tapioca, **Gerber,** 7¾-oz. jar	160	38.0	20.7	4.90	10	2.5	0.09
Apricots with Tapioca, **Heinz,** 7¾-oz. jar	147	35.6	19.0	4.59	(10)	(2.3)	
Banana, **Beech-Nut,** 7½-oz. jar	130	32.0	17.0	4.30	9	2.2	
Banana & Pineapple, **Beech-Nut,** 7½-oz. jar	120	29.0	16.0	3.90	8	2.0	
Bananas & Pineapple with Tapioca, **Heinz,** 7¾-oz. jar	147	35.2	19.0	4.54	(10)	(2.3)	
Bananas with Pineapple and Tapioca, **Gerber,** 7½-oz. jar	113	25.9	15.0	3.46	8	1.7	0.09
Bananas with Tapioca, **Gerber,** 7½-oz. jar	142	34.2	19.0	4.56	10	2.3	0.06
Peaches, **Beech-Nut,** 7½-oz. jar	150	37.0	20.0	4.90	10	2.5	
Peaches, **Gerber,** 7¾-oz. jar	156	36.9	20.1	4.76	10	2.4	0.26
Peaches, **Heinz,** 7½-oz. jar	100	21.7	13.3	2.89	(7)	(1.5)	
Pears, **Beech-Nut,** 7½-oz. jar	140	35.0	19.0	4.70	10	2.4	
Pears, **Gerber,** 7½-oz. jar	111	25.3	14.7	3.37	7	1.7	0.37
Pears, **Heinz,** 7½-oz. jar	134	31.7	17.9	4.22	(9)	(2.1)	
Pears & Pineapple, **Beech-Nut,** 7½-oz. jar	160	40.0	21.0	5.30	11	2.7	
Pears & Pineapple, **Gerber,** 7½-oz. jar	113	25.3	15.0	3.37	8	1.7	0.34
Pears & Pineapple, **Heinz,** 7½-oz. jar	128	30.6	17.0	4.08	(9)	(2.1)	
For comparison: Pears in Chocolate Sauce, Toddler Babymeal, **Cow & Gate** (sold in Great Britain), 6-oz. jar	151	34.0	25.2	5.68	13	2.8	
Plums with Tapioca, **Beech-Nut,** 7½-oz. jar	150	36.0	20.0	4.80	10	2.4	
Plums with Tapioca, **Gerber,** 7¾-oz. jar	154	37.4	19.8	4.82	10	2.4	0.11
Prunes with Tapioca, **Gerber,** 7¾-oz. jar	169	40.0	21.8	5.16	11	2.6	0.20
VEGETABLES							
Carrots, **Beech-Nut,** 7½-oz. jar	60	14.0	8.0	1.90	4	1.0	
Carrots, **Gerber,** 7½-oz. jar	53	10.6	7.1	1.42	4	0.7	0.20
Carrots, **Heinz,** 7½-oz. jar	49	10.4	6.5	1.39	(3)	(0.7)	
Creamed Corn, **Beech-Nut,** 7½-oz. jar	150	32.0	20.0	4.30	10	2.2	
Creamed Corn, **Gerber,** 7½-oz. jar	128	26.2	17.0	3.49	9	1.8	0.06
Creamed Corn, **Heinz,** 7¾-oz. jar	152	33.6	19.6	4.34	(10)	(2.2)	
Creamed Green Beans, **Gerber,** 7½-oz. jar	89	17.6	11.9	2.35	6	1.2	0.09
Creamed Green Beans, **Heinz,** 7½-oz. jar	83	12.3	11.1	1.64	(6)	(0.8)	
Creamed Peas, **Heinz,** 7¾-oz. jar	132	20.6	17.6	2.75	(9)	(1.4)	
Green Beans, **Beech-Nut,** 7¼-oz. jar	60	13.0	8.0	1.70	4	0.9	
Mixed Vegetables, **Beech-Nut,** 4½-oz. jar	80	17.0	11.0	2.30	6	1.2	
Mixed Vegetables, **Gerber,** 7½-oz. jar	85	17.0	11.3	2.27	6	1.1	0.14
Mixed Vegetables, **Heinz,** 4½-oz. jar	56	11.7	12.5	2.61	(6)	(1.3)	
Peas, **Beech-Nut,** 7½-oz. jar	110	20.0	15.0	2.70	8	1.4	
Peas, **Gerber,** 7½-oz. jar	128	21.5	17.0	2.86	9	1.4	
Squash, **Beech-Nut,** 7½-oz. jar	50	12.0	7.0	1.60	4	0.8	
Squash, **Gerber,** 7½-oz. jar	57	11.1	7.7	1.47	4	0.7	0.23
Sweet Potatoes, **Beech-Nut,** 7¾-oz. jar	120	27.0	16.0	3.60	8	1.8	
Sweet Potatoes, **Gerber,** 7¾-oz. jar	132	29.4	17.0	3.80	9	1.9	0.23
Sweet Potatoes, **Heinz,** 7½-oz. jar	153	35.1	20.4	4.68	(10)	(2.4)	
PASTA DINNERS							
Beef & Egg Noodle, **Beech-Nut,** 7½-oz. jar	130	18.0	17.0	2.40	9	1.2	
Beef & Egg Noodles with Vegetables, **Gerber,** 7½-oz. jar	138	18.9	18.4	2.52	9	1.3	0.06
Beef Lasagna, **Gerber** Toddler Meals, 6¼-oz. jar	110	15.6	17.6	2.49	9	1.3	0.06
Chicken & Noodles, **Gerber,** 7½-oz. jar	115	16.8	15.3	2.24	8	1.1	0.09
Chicken Noodle, **Beech-Nut,** 7½-oz. jar	120	18.0	16.0	2.40	8	1.2	
Chicken Noodle Dinner, **Heinz,** 7½-oz. jar	134	19.8	17.9	2.64	(9)	(1.3)	
Egg Noodles & Beef, **Heinz,** 7½-oz. jar	106	17.0	14.2	2.27	(7)	(1.1)	
Macaroni & Cheese, **Gerber,** 7½-oz. jar	136	18.7	18.1	2.50	9	1.3	
Macaroni, Tomato & Beef, **Beech-Nut,** 7½-oz. jar	120	16.0	16.0	2.10	8	1.3	
Macaroni, Tomato with Beef, **Gerber,** 7½-oz. jar	119	21.3	15.9	2.84	8	1.4	0.09
Macaroni, Tomatoes & Beef, **Heinz,** 7½-oz. jar	104	16.8	13.9	2.24	(7)	(1.1)	
Spaghetti & Meat Balls, **Gerber** Toddler Meals, 6¼-oz. jar	126	18.6	20.1	2.98	10	1.5	0.11
Spaghetti, Tomato & Beef, **Beech-Nut,** 7½-oz. jar	140	20.0	19.0	2.70	10	1.4	
Spaghetti, Tomato Sauce & Beef, **Gerber,** 7½-oz. jar	136	22.1	18.1	2.95	9	1.5	0.11
Spaghetti, Tomato Sauce & Meat, **Heinz,** 7½-oz. jar	102	21.1	13.6	2.81	(7)	(1.4)	
Vegetables, Egg Noodles & Chicken, **Heinz,** 7½-oz. jar	136	18.7	18.1	2.50	(9)	(1.3)	
Vegetables, Egg Noodles & Turkey, **Heinz,** 7½-oz. jar	113	15.3	15.0	2.04	(8)	(1.0)	
VEGETABLES WITH MEAT OR POULTRY							
Beef & Rice with Tomato Sauce, **Gerber** Toddler Meals, 6¼-oz. jar	131	17.0	21.0	2.72	11	1.4	0.09
Beef Stew, **Gerber** Toddler Meals, 6-oz. jar	111	12.4	18.4	2.07	9	1.0	0.09
Chicken Stew, **Gerber** Toddler Meals, 6-oz. jar	145	12.2	24.1	2.04	12	1.0	0.09
Green Beans, Potatoes & Ham Casserole, **Gerber** Toddler Meals, 6¼-oz. jar	131	14.5	21.0	2.32	11	1.2	0.11
Split Peas & Ham, **Beech-Nut,** 7½-oz. jar	140	24.0	19.0	3.20	10	1.6	
Split Peas with Ham, **Gerber,** 7½-oz. jar	153	23.8	20.4	3.18	10	1.6	0.09
Turkey & Rice with Vegetables, **Gerber,** 7½-oz. jar	130	17.4	17.3	2.32	9	1.2	0.06
Turkey Rice, **Beech-Nut,** 7½-oz. jar	130	21.0	17.0	2.80	9	1.4	
Turkey Rice Dinner with Vegetables, **Heinz,** 74-oz. jar	106	18.3	14.2	2.44	(7)	(1.2)	
Vegetable Bacon, **Beech-Nut,** 7½-oz. jar	140	19.0	19.0	2.50	10	1.3	
Vegetables & Bacon, **Gerber,** 7½-oz. jar	166	19.1	22.1	2.55	11	1.3	0.06
Vegetables & Bacon, **Heinz,** 7½-oz. jar	130	17.2	17.3	2.30	(9)	(1.2)	
Vegetable Beef, **Beech-Nut,** 7½-oz. jar	140	21.0	19.0	2.40	10	1.2	
Vegetables & Beef, **Gerber,** 7½-oz. jar	140	20.5	18.7	2.75	9	1.4	0.06

	UNIT		1 OZ., BY WT.		1 TABLE-SPOON		Fiber per oz. (GMS.)
	Cal.	Carb.	Cal.	Carb.	Cal.	Carb.	
Vegetables & Beef, **Heinz,** 7½-oz. jar	111	15.5	14.7	2.07	(7)	(1.0)	
Vegetable Chicken, **Beech-Nut,** 7½-oz. jar	140	20.0	19.0	2.70	10	1.4	
Vegetables & Chicken, **Gerber,** 7½-oz. jar	108	16.8	14.5	2.24	7	1.1	0.06
Vegetables, Dumplings & Beef, **Heinz,** 7½-oz. jar	104	17.4	13.9	2.32	(7)	(1.2)	
Vegetables & Ham, **Gerber,** 7½-oz. jar	120	18.0	16.0	2.40	8	1.0	0.06
Vegetables & Ham, **Heinz,** 7½-oz. jar	117	18.5	15.6	2.47	(8)	(1.2)	
Vegetable Lamb, **Beech-Nut,** 7½-oz. jar	120	17.0	16.0	2.30	8	1.2	
Vegetables & Lamb, **Gerber,** 7½-oz. jar	128	16.4	17.0	2.18	9	1.1	0.06
Vegetable Liver, **Beech-Nut,** 7½-oz. jar	120	21.0	16.0	2.80	8	1.4	
Vegetables & Liver, **Gerber,** 7½-oz. jar	91	16.4	12.2	2.18	6	1.1	0.09
Vegetables & Turkey, **Gerber,** 7½-oz. jar	113	18.3	15.0	2.44	8	1.2	0.06
Vegetables & Turkey Casserole, **Gerber** Toddler Meals, 6¼-oz. jar	147	14.2	23.5	2.27	11	1.1	0.14
For comparison: Grilled Bacon Breakfast With Vegetables, Toddler Babymeal, **Cow & Gate** (sold in Great Britain), 6-oz. jar	181	15.3	30.1	2.55	15	1.3	
MEATS							
Beef, **Gerber,** 3½-oz. jar	97	0.4	27.8	0.11	14	0.1	
Beef & Beef Broth, **Beech-Nut,** 3½-oz. jar	120	1.0	34.0	0.10	17	0.1	
Beef & Beef Broth, **Heinz,** 3½-oz. jar	133	0.7	38.0	0.20	(19)	(0.1)	
Chicken, **Gerber,** 3½-oz. jar	136	0.7	38.8	0.06	20	trace	
Chicken & Chicken Broth, **Beech-Nut,** 3½-oz. jar	110	1.0	31.0	0.10	16	0.1	
Chicken & Chicken Broth, **Heinz,** 3½-oz. jar	132	0.1	37.7	0.03	(19)	trace	
Chicken Sticks, **Gerber,** 2½-oz. jar	120	1.0	47.9	0.40	24	0.2	0.06
Ham, **Gerber,** 3½-oz. jar	114	0.4	32.6	0.11	16	0.1	
Lamb, **Gerber,** 3½-oz. jar	98	0.5	28.1	0.14	14	0.1	
Lamb & Lamb Broth, **Beech-Nut,** 3½-oz. jar	130	1.0	37.0	0.10	19	0.1	
Lamb & Lamb Broth, **Heinz,** 3½-oz. jar	135	0.3	38.6	0.09	(19)	trace	
Meat Sticks, **Gerber,** 2½-oz. jar	103	0.9	41.4	0.34	21	0.2	
Turkey, **Gerber,** 3½-oz. jar	130	0.0	37.1	0.00	19	0.0	
Turkey Sticks, **Gerber,** 2½-oz. jar	122	1.1	48.8	0.43	25	0.2	0.03
Veal, **Gerber,** 3½-oz. jar	98	0.1	28.1	0.03	14	trace	
Veal & Veal Broth, **Heinz,** 3½-oz. jar	108	0.5	30.9	0.14	(16)	(0.1)	
HIGH-MEAT DINNERS and CHEESE FOODS							
Beef, **Beech-Nut,** 4½-oz. jar	130	8.0	29.0	1.80	15	0.9	
Beef with Vegetables, **Gerber,** 4½-oz. jar	125	8.4	27.8	1.87	14	0.9	0.09
Beef with Vegetables & Cereal, **Heinz,** 4½-oz. jar	101	7.5	22.4	1.67	(11)	(0.8)	
Chicken, **Beech-Nut,** 4½-oz. jar	90	9.0	20.0	2.00	10	1.0	0.03
Chicken with Vegetables, **Gerber,** 4½-oz. jar	131	7.5	29.2	1.67	15	0.8	0.06
Chicken with Vegetables, **Heinz,** 4½-oz. jar	120	8.0	26.7	1.79	(13)	(0.9)	
Cottage Cheese with Bananas, **Heinz,** 7¾-oz. jar	158	29.7	20.4	3.83	(10)	(1.9)	
Cottage Cheese with Pineapple, **Beech-Nut,** 7-oz. jar	180	31.0	24.0	4.10	12	2.0	0.03
Ham, **Beech-Nut,** 4½-oz. jar	130	8.0	29.0	1.80	15	0.9	0.06
Ham with Vegetables, **Gerber,** 4½-oz. jar	105	9.4	23.2	2.10	12	1.1	0.06
Turkey, **Beech-Nut,** 4½-oz. jar	110	9.0	24.0	2.00	12	1.0	0.03
Turkey with Vegetables, **Gerber,** 4½-oz. jar	131	8.4	29.2	1.87	15	0.9	0.06
Turkey with Vegetables, **Heinz,** 4½-oz. jar	120	8.5	26.7	1.90	(13)	(1.0)	
Veal with Vegetables, **Gerber,** 4½-oz. jar	92	9.2	9.2	2.04	10	1.0	0.09
DESSERTS							
Apple Betty, **Beech-Nut,** 7-oz. jar	160	40.0	21.0	5.30	(11)	(2.6)	0.06
Apple Custard Pudding, **Beech-Nut,** 7½-oz. jar	170	33.0	23.0	4.40	(12)	(2.2)	0.03
Bananas with Tapioca, **Heinz,** 7¾-oz. jar	163	37.4	21.0	4.82	(11)	(2.4)	
Banana Custard Pudding, **Beech-Nut,** 7½-oz. jar	150	30.0	20.0	4.00	(10)	(2.0)	
Banana Dessert, **Beech-Nut,** 7-oz. jar	160	40.0	21.0	5.30	(11)	(2.6)	0.03
Cherry Vanilla Pudding, **Gerber,** 7-oz. jar	147	31.9	19.6	4.25	10	2.1	0.09
Cottage Cheese with Bananas and with Pineapple, see HIGH-MEAT DINNERS AND CHEESE FOODS, above							
Custard Pudding, **Heinz,** 7¾-oz. jar	169	30.8	21.8	3.97	(11)	(2.0)	
Dutch Apple Dessert, **Gerber,** 7¾-oz. jar	160	34.9	20.7	4.51	10	2.3	0.11
Dutch Apple Dessert, **Heinz,** 7¾-oz. jar	152	36.7	19.6	4.73	(10)	(2.4)	
Fruit Dessert, **Beech-Nut,** 7-oz. jar	160	39.0	21.0	5.20	(11)	(2.6)	0.03
Fruit Dessert, **Gerber,** 7¾-oz. jar	160	38.2	20.7	4.93	10	2.5	0.06
Fruit Dessert, **Heinz,** 7¾-oz. jar	152	35.6	19.6	4.59	(10)	(2.3)	
Hawaiian Delight, **Gerber,** 7¾-oz. jar	185	40.7	23.8	5.25	12	2.6	0.20
Mixed Fruit Yogurt, **Beech-Nut,** 7½-oz. jar	120	28.0	16.0	3.70	(8)	(1.9)	
Peach-Apple Yogurt, **Beech-Nut,** 7½-oz. jar	110	28.0	24.0	3.30	(12)	(1.7)	
Peach Cobbler, **Gerber,** 7¾-oz. jar	156	36.7	20.1	4.73	10	2.4	0.06
Peach Cobbler, **Heinz,** 7¾-oz. jar	160	35.6	20.7	4.59	(10)	(2.3)	
Pineapple Orange, **Heinz,** 7¾-oz. jar	158	38.0	20.4	4.91	(10)	(2.5)	
Raspberry Dessert with Yogurt, **Gerber,** 7½-oz. jar	145	33.6	19.3	4.48	10	2.3	
Rice Pudding, **Beech-Nut,** 7½-oz. jar	200	38.0	27.0	5.10	(14)	(2.6)	
Tropical Fruit Dessert, **Beech-Nut,** 7¾-oz. jar	140	33.0	19.0	4.40	(9)	(2.2)	
Tutti Frutti, **Heinz,** 7¾-oz. jar	156	35.4	20.1	4.56	(10)	(2.3)	
Vanilla Custard Pudding, **Beech-Nut,** 7½-oz. jar	170	20.0	23.0	2.70	(12)	(1.4)	
Vanilla Custard Pudding, **Gerber,** 7¾-oz. jar	187	33.6	24.1	4.34	12	2.2	0.51

PUREED VEGETABLES

	UNIT		1 OZ., BY WT.		1 TABLE-SPOON		1 CUP (8 fl. oz.)	
	Cal.	Carb.	Cal.	Carb.	Cal.	Carb.	Cal.	Carb.
Cellu								
low sodium Asparagus Puree, 16½-oz. jar	(100)	(14.0)	(6.1)	(0.85)	3.1	0.44	50.0	7.00
low sodium Bean Puree, 16-oz. (1-lb.) jar	(140)	(30.0)	(8.8)	(1.88)	4.4	0.94	70.0	15.00
low sodium Beet Puree, 16-oz. (1-lb.) jar	(200)	(40.0)	(12.5)	(2.50)	6.3	1.25	100.0	20.00
low sodium Carrot Puree, 17-oz. can	(140)	(30.0)	(8.3)	(1.76)	4.4	0.94	70.0	15.00
low sodium Pea Puree, 16-oz. (1-lb.) jar	(280)	(58.0)	(17.5)	(3.63)	8.8	1.81	140.0	29.00
low sodium Spinach Puree, 16½-oz. jar	900	14.0	(5.5)	(0.85)	2.8	0.44	45.0	7.00
low sodium Squash Puree, 16-oz. (1-lb.) jar	(200)	(38.0)	(12.5)	(2.38)	6.3	1.20	100.0	19.00
low sodium Tomato Puree, 19-oz. jar	(160)	(40.0)	(8.4)	(2.11)	5.0	1.25	80.0	20.00

34 WEIGHT LOSS AND WEIGHT GAIN PREPARATIONS, SUPPLEMENTS & BOOSTERS •

WEIGHT LOSS PRODUCTS

	UNIT		1 OZ., BY WT.		1 FLUID OZ.		1 CUP	
	Cal.	Carb.	Cal.	Carb.	Cal.	Carb.	Cal.	Carb.
All Star, High Protein Reducing Formula, 28-oz. container	3080	224.0	110.0	8.00				
Suggested serving: 2 tablespoons (approx. 1 oz.)	110	8.0	110.0	8.00				
Prepared as package directs, mixing 1 suggested serving with 1 cup (8 fl. oz.) non-fat milk (0.1% fat) (yield: approx. 8 fl. oz.)	190	17.0			23.8	2.13	190	17.0
Hoffman's, Hi-Proteen Reducing Plan Formula, Chocolate Flavor, 10-oz. canister	1050	130.0	105.0	13.00				
16-oz. (1-lb.) canister	1680	208.0	105.0	13.00				
Suggested serving: 4 oz. powder mix	420	52.0	105.0	13.00				
Prepared as package directs, mixing 1 suggested serving with 1 cup (8 fl. oz.) liquid (yield: approx. 8 fl. oz.):								
Prepared with skim milk (0.1% fat)	510	64.5			63.8	8,06	510	64.5
Prepared with water	420	52.0			52.5	6.50	420	52.0
Hoffman's, Hi-Proteen Reducing Plan Formula, Vanilla Flavor, 10-oz. can	1000	135.0	100.0	13.50				
16-oz. (1-lb.) can	1600	216.0	100.0	13.50				
Suggested serving: 2 oz. powder mix	200	27.0	100.0	13.50				
Prepared as package directs, mixing 1 suggested serving with 1 cup (8 fl. oz.) liquid (yield: approx. 8 fl. oz.):								
Prepared with skim milk (0.1% fat)	288	39.5			36.0	4.94	288	39.5
Prepared with water	200	27.0			25.0	3.38	200	27.0
Naturade, Weight Reduction Program, N-R-G Natural Powder, 18-oz. can	1548	198.0	86.0	11.00	43.0	5.50	688	88.0
36-oz. can	3096	396.0	86.0	11.00	43.0	5.50	688	88.0
Suggested serving: 2 tablespoons (approx. 1 oz.)	86	11.0	86.0	11.00	43.0	5.50	688	88.0
Prepared as package directs, mixing 1 suggested serving with 1 cup (8 fl. oz.) non-fat milk (yield: approx. 8 fl. oz.)	273	23.5			34.1	2.94	273	23.5
Nature's Inn, Protein Natural Slimmer Drink, Banana, 10-fl.-oz. can	180	15.0			18.0	1.50	144	12.0
Chocolate, 10-fl.-oz. can	160	10.0			16.0	1.00	128	8.0
Vanilla, 10-fl.-oz. can	180	15.0			18.0	1.50	144	12.0
Rich Life, Super Trim Formula 1 Protein Powder, 18-oz. can	1840	46.0	102.2	2.56				
Suggested serving: 2 tablespoons (approx. 0.78 oz.)	80	2.0	102.2	2.56				
Prepared as package directs, mixing 1 suggested serving with 1 cup (8 fl. oz.) liquid (yield: approx. 8 fl. oz.):								
Prepared with whole milk (3.5% fat)	239	14.5			28.9	1.81	239	14.5
Prepared with non-fat milk (0.1% fat)	168	11.0			21.0	1.38	168	11.0
Prepared with apple juice	197	31.5			24.6	3.94	197	31.5
Thompson, Weight Loss Plan, 16-oz. (1-lb.) can	1800	60.0	112.5	3.75				
Suggested serving: 2 heaping tablespoons (approx. 0.53 oz.)	60	2.0	112.5	3.75				
Prepared as package directs, mixing 1 suggested serving with liquid:								
Prepared with 8 oz. non-fat milk (0.1% fat) (yield: approx. 8 fl. oz.)	148	11.0			18.5	1.38	148	11.0
Prepared with 6 oz. apple juice (yield: approx. 6 fl. oz.)	177	31.5			22.1	3.94	177	31.5
Weider, Weight Loss Drink Mix, Chocolate Flavored, 12-oz. box, 12 envelopes	1320	96.0	110.0	8.00				
Suggested serving: 1 envelope, approx. 1 oz.	110	8.0	110.0	8.00				
Prepared as package directs, mixing 1 suggested serving with 1 cup (8 fl. oz.) non-fat milk (0.1% fat) (yield: approx. 8 fl. oz.)	198	17.0			24.8	2.13	198	17.0

WEIGHT GAIN PRODUCTS

	UNIT		1 OZ., BY WT.		1 FLUID OZ.		1 CUP	
	Cal.	Carb.	Cal.	Carb.	Cal.	Carb.	Cal.	Carb.
All Star, Rapid Weight Gain, Instant Nutrition Shake, Chocolate, 16-oz. (1-lb.) container	1920	176.0	120.0	11.00				
Suggested serving: ½ cup (approx. 2 oz.)	240	22.0	120.0	11.00				

	UNIT Cal.	UNIT Carb.	1 OZ., BY WT. Cal.	1 OZ., BY WT. Carb.	1 FLUID OZ. Cal.	1 FLUID OZ. Carb.	1 CUP Cal.	1 CUP Carb.
Prepared as package directs, mixing 1 suggested serving with 1 cup (8 fl. oz.) liquid (yield: approx. 8 fl. oz.):								
Prepared with whole milk (3.5% fat)	398	33.8	(37.5)	(3.19)	49.7	4.22	398	33.8
Vanilla, 16-oz. (1-lb.) container	1920	196.0	120.0	12.25				
Suggested serving: ½ cup (approx. 2 oz.)	240	24.5	120.0	12.25				
Prepared as package directs, mixing 1 suggested serving with 1 cup (8 fl. oz.) liquid (yield: approx. 8 fl. oz.):								
Prepared with whole milk (3.5% fat)	398	36.3	(37.5)	(3.42)	49.8	4.53	398	36.3
Hoffman's, Quick Gain Weight, Chocolate Flavored Powder, 64-oz. (4-lb.) can	8320	736.0	130.0	11.50				
Suggested serving: 4 oz. powder	520	46.0	130.0	11.50				
Prepared as package directs, mixing 1 suggested serving with 2 cups (16 fl. oz.) liquid (yield: approx. 16 fl. oz.):								
Prepared with whole milk (3.5% fat)	838	70.0			52.4	4.38	419	35.0
Quick Gain Weight, Vanilla Flavored Powder, 64-oz. (4-lb.) can	8320	736.0	130.0	11.50				
Suggested serving: 4 oz. powder	520	46.0	130.0	11.50				
Prepared as package directs, mixing 1 suggested serving with 2 cups (16 fl. oz.) liquid (yield: approx. 16 fl. oz.):								
Prepared with whole milk (3.5% fat)	838	70.0			52.4	4.38	419	35.0
Weight Gain Hi-Proteen, 300-tablet can (8½ oz.)	1105	119.0	130.0	14.00				
400-tablet can (10 oz.)	1300	140.0	130.0	14.00				
Suggested serving: 40 tablets (approx. 1 oz.)	130	14.0	130.0	14.00				
Weight Gain Hi-Proteen Powder, 16-oz. (1-lb.) can	1760	64.0	110.0	4.00				
Suggested serving: 2 oz. powder	220	8.0	110.0	4.00				
Prepared as package directs, mixing 1 suggested serving with 1 cup (8 fl. oz.) liquid (yield: approx. 8 fl. oz.):								
Prepared with whole milk (3.5% fat)	379	20.0			47.5	2.50	379	20.0
Prepared with water	220	8.0			27.5	1.00	220	8.0
Prepared with apple juice	337	37.5			42.1	4.69	337	37.5
Prepared with tomato juice	266	18.4			33.3	2.30	266	18.4
M-L-O (Tillmore Foods), 24-oz. can, Banana	2720	424.0	113.3	17.67				
Strawberry	2720	424.0	113.3	17.67				
Vanilla	2720	424.0	113.3	17.67				
Suggested serving: 5 heaping tablespoons (approx. 3 oz.)	340	53.0	113.3	17.67				
Prepared as package directs, mixing 1 suggested serving with 2 cups (16 fl. oz.) whole milk (3.5% fat) (yield: approx. 16 fl. oz.)	660	76.0			41.3	4.75	330	38.0
Naturade, Weight Gain Program, N-R-G Natural Powder, 16-oz. (1-lb.) can	2808	69.4	175.5	4.34	93.0	2.30	1488	36.8
32-oz. (2-lb.) can	5616	138.9	175.5	4.34	93.0	2.30	1488	36.8
64-oz. (4-lb.) can	11232	277.7	175.5	4.34	93.0	2.30	1488	36.8
Suggested serving: 3 tablespoons (approx. 1.6 oz.)	279	6.9	175.5	4.34	93.0	2.30	1488	36.8
Prepared as package directs, mixing 1 suggested serving with 1 cup (8 fl. oz.) whole milk (3.5% fat) (yield: approx. 8 fl. oz.)	439	16.0			54.9	2.00	439	16.0
Nature's Inn, Natural Weight Plus Drink, 10-fl.-oz. can, Banana	601	22.0			60.1	2.20	481	17.6
Chocolate	601	22.0			60.1	2.20	481	17.6
Vanilla	600	34.1			60.0	3.40	480	27.2

	UNIT Cal.	UNIT Carb.	1 OZ., BY WT. Cal.	1 OZ., BY WT. Carb.	1 FLUID OZ. Cal.	1 FLUID OZ. Carb.	1 CUP Cal.	1 CUP Carb.
Weider, Crash Weight Gain Formula #7 Powder, 64-oz. (4-lb.) canister	7200	122.4	112.5	19.13				
Suggested serving: 4 rounded tablespoons (approx. 2⅔ oz.)	300	51.0	112.5	19.13				
Prepared as package directs, mixing 1 suggested serving with 2 cups (16 fl. oz.) whole milk (3.5% fat) (yield: approx. 16 fl. oz.)	610	74.0			38.1	4.63	305	37.0

SUPPLEMENTS and BOOSTERS

PROTEIN

	UNIT Cal.	UNIT Carb.	1 OZ., BY WT. Cal.	1 OZ., BY WT. Carb.	1 FLUID OZ. Cal.	1 FLUID OZ. Carb.	1 CUP Cal.	1 CUP Carb.
All-Star, Body Builder's Protein, 16-oz. (1-lb.) container	1600		100.0	trace				
Suggested serving: 2 heaping tablespoons (approx. 1 oz.)	100	trace	100.0	trace				
Prepared as package directs, mixing 1 suggested serving with 1 cup (8 fl. oz.) liquid (yield: approx. 8 fl. oz.):								
Prepared with whole milk (3.5% fat)	260	12.0	(27.1)	(1.25)	32.5	1.50	260	12.0
Milk & Egg Protein, 16-oz. (1-lb.) container	1760	16.0	110.0	1.00				
Suggested serving: 2 heaping tablespoons (approx. 1 oz.)	110	1.0	110.0	1.00				
Prepared as package directs, mixing 1 suggested serving with 1 cup (8 fl. oz.) liquid (yield: approx. 8 fl. oz.):								
Prepared with whole milk (3.5% fat)	270	13.0	(28.1)	(1.35)	33.8	1.63	270	13.0
Prepared with apple juice	220	29.0	(23.7)	(3.12)	27.5	3.63	220	29.0
90% Instant High Protein Powder with Lecithin and Papain, 64-oz. (4-lb.) tub	6400	25.6	100.0	0.40				
Suggested serving: 2 heaping tablespoons (approx. 1 oz.)	100	0.4	100.0	0.40				
Prepared as package directs, mixing 1 suggested serving with 1 cup (8 fl. oz.) liquid (yield: approx. 8 fl. oz.):								
Prepared with whole milk (3.5% fat)	259	12.4			32.4	1.55	259	12.4
Prepared with apple juice	217	29.9			27.1	3.74	217	29.9
95% Protein, No Sugar, No Starch, No Fat, 64-oz. (4-lb.) tub	6400	0.0	100.0	0.00				
Suggested serving: 2 tablespoons (approx. 1 oz.)	100	0.0	100.0	0.00				
Prepared as package directs, mixing 1 suggested serving with 1 cup (8 fl. oz.) liquid (yield: approx. 8 fl. oz.):								
Prepared with whole milk (3.5% fat)	259	12.0			32.4	1.50	259	12.0
Prepared with apple juice	217	29.5			27.1	3.69	217	29.5
95% Protein Supreme with Lecithin and Papain, 64-oz. (4-lb.) tub	6400	0.0	100.0	0.00				
Suggested serving: 2 tablespoons (approx. 1 oz.)	100	0.0	100.0	0.00				
Prepared as package directs, mixing 1 suggested serving with 1 cup (8 fl. oz.) liquid (yield: approx. 8 fl. oz.):								
Prepared with whole milk (3.5% fat)	259	12.0			32.4	1.50	259	12.0
Prepared with apple juice	217	29.5			27.1	3.69	217	29.5
American Dietaids, Tasty Protein Crunchy Delicious Wafers, 1 package (120 wafers)	576	72.0						
Suggested serving: 12 wafers daily	58	7.2						
1 wafer	5	0.6						
Cher Amino, Cher-Amino Predigested Liquid Protein, 16-fl.-oz. (1-pint) bottle	960	0.0			60.0	0.00	480	0.0
32-fl.-oz. (1-quart) bottle	1920	0.0			60.0	0.00	480	0.0

	UNIT		1 OZ., BY WT.		1 FLUID OZ.		1 CUP	
	Cal.	Carb.	Cal.	Carb.	Cal.	Carb.	Cal.	Carb.
Suggested serving: 2 tablespoons	60	0.0			60.0	0.00	480	0.0
Citramino, Citramino Predigested Liquid Protein, Orange Flavored, 16-fl.-oz. (1-pint) bottle	960	0.0			60.0	0.00	480	0,0
32-fl.-oz. (1-quart) bottle	1920	0.0			60.0	0.00	480	0.0
Suggested serving: 2 tablespoons (1 fl. oz.)	60	0.0			60.0	0.00	480	0.0
Dr. Donsbach, Athletic Formula Protein Powder, 16-oz. (1-lb.) can	1680	30.0	105.0	1.90	105.0	1.90	1680	30.4
Suggested serving: 1 tablespoon (approx. 0.53 oz.)	56	1.0	105.0	1.90	105.0	1.90	1680	30.4
Prepared as package directs, mixing 1 suggested serving with 1 cup (8 fl. oz.) liquid (yield: approx. 8 fl. oz.):								
Prepared with whole milk (3.5% fat)	215	12.0			26.9	1.50	215	12.0
Prepared with apple juice	173	30.5			21.6	3.80	173	30.5
EMF, Concentrated Predigested Liquid Protein Supplement, Cherry Flavor, 16 fl. oz. (1 pint)	1152	48.0			72.0	3.00	576	24.0
32 fl. oz. (1 quart)	2304	96.0			72.0	3.00	576	24.0
Grapefruit Flavor, 16 fl. oz. (1 pint)	1152	48.0			72.0	3.00	576	24.0
32 fl. oz. (1 quart)	2304	96.0			72.0	3.00	576	24.0
Orange Flavor, 16 fl. oz. (1 pint)	1152	48.0			72.0	3.00	576	24.0
32 fl. oz. (1 quart)	2304	96.0			72.0	3.00	576	24.0
Suggested serving: 2 tablespoons	72	3.0			72.0	3.00	576	24.0
Fearn, Low Cal Protein Drink								
Prepared as package directs, mixing 1 suggested serving with 12 oz. tomato juice (yield: approx. 12 fl. oz.)	120	49.0			15.0	6.13	120	49.0
Qualipro, 80% Protein Drink Mix, 12-oz. can, Vanilla	1276	21.3	186.3	1.77				
Suggested serving: ⅓ cup (approx. 1 oz.)	186	1.8	186.3	1.77				
Prepared as package directs, mixing 1 suggested serving with 1 cup (8 fl. oz.) liquid (yield: approx. 8 fl. oz.):								
Prepared with whole milk (3.5% fat)	219	13.0			27.4	1.63	219	13.0
Prepared with apple juice	177	30.5			22.1	3.81	177	30.5
Soya Protein Isolate 91% Protein, 10-oz. canister	975	na	97.5	trace	25.0	trace	200	na
16-oz. (1-lb.) canister	1560	na	97.5	trace	25.0	trace	200	na
40-oz. canister	3900	na	97.5	trace	25.0	trace	200	na
Suggested serving: 4 level tablespoons	50	na	97.5	trace	25.0	trace	200	na
Whole Milk High Cal Drink								
Prepared as package directs, mixing 1 suggested serving with 2 cups whole milk, 2 eggs, 3 tablespoons honey and 1 tablespoon vegetable oil (yield: approx. 8 fl. oz.)	880	49.0			110.0	6.13	880	49.0
Golden California Co., Golden Cal Instant Protein, 16-oz. (1-lb.) can	1600	0.0	100.0	0.00				
Suggested serving: 1 oz.	100	0.0	100.0	0.00				
Prepared as package directs, mixing 1 suggested serving with 1 cup (8 fl. oz.) liquid (yield: approx. 8 fl. oz.):								
Prepared with whole milk (3.5% fat)	259	0.0			32.4	0.00	259	0.0
Prepared with water	100	0.0			12.5	0.00	100	0.0
Natural Soya Powder, 11-oz. box	1248	74.9	113.5	6.81				
Suggested serving: ¼ cup (approx. 0.9 oz.)	100	6.0	113.5	6.81				
Prepared as package directs, mixing 1 suggested serving with 1 cup (8 fl. oz.) liquid (yield: approx. 8 fl. oz.)	100	6.0			12.5	0.75	100	6.0
Hoffman's, Hi-Proteen Instant Broth, 8-oz. can	720	48.0	90.0	6.00	90.0	6.00	720	48.0
Suggested serving: 1 oz. (approx. 2 tablespoons)	90	6.0	90.0	6.00	90.0	6.00	720	48.0
Prepared as package directs, mixing 1 suggested serving with 1 cup (8 fl. oz.) boiling water (yield: approx. 8 fl. oz.)	90	6.0			11.3	0.75	90	6.0
Hi-Proteen Instant Powder, Plain, 16-oz. (1-lb.) can	1600	192.0	100.0	12.00				
Suggested serving: 1 oz. (approx. 2 tablespoons)	100	12.0	100.0	12.00				
Prepared as package directs, mixing 1 suggested serving with 1 cup (8 fl. oz.) liquid (yield: approx. 8 fl. oz.):								
Prepared with whole milk (3.5% fat)	259	24.0			32.4	3.00	259	24.0
Prepared with water	100	12.0			12.5	1.50	100	12.0
Prepared with apple juice	217	41.5			27.1	5.19	217	41.5
Hi-Proteen Instant Powder, Carob Flavor, 16-oz. (1-lb.) can	1760	240.0	110.0	15.00				
Suggested serving: 1 oz. (approx. 2 tablespoons)	110	15.0	110.0	15.00				
Prepared as package directs, mixing 1 suggested serving with 1 cup (8 fl. oz.) liquid (yield: approx. 8 fl. oz.):								
Prepared with whole milk (3.5% fat)	269	27.0			33.6	3.38	269	27.0
Prepared with water	110	15.0			13.8	1.88	110	15.0
Hi-Proteen Instant Powder, Chocolate Flavor, 16-oz. (1-lb.) canister	1920	208.0	120.0	13.00				
Suggested serving: 1 oz. (approx. 2 tablespoons)	120	13.0	120.0	13.00				
Prepared as package directs, mixing 1 suggested serving with 1 cup (8 fl. oz.) liquid (yield: approx. 8 fl. oz.):								
Prepared with whole milk (3.5% fat)	279	25.0			34.9	3.13	279	25.0
Prepared with water	120	13.0			15.0	1.63	120	13.0
Hi-Proteen Instant Powder, Vanilla Flavor, 16-oz. (1-lb.) canister	1920	192.0	120.0	12.00				
Suggested serving: 1 oz. (approx. 2 tablespoons)	120	12.0	120.0	12.00				
Prepared as package directs, mixing 1 suggested serving with 1 cup (8 fl. oz.) liquid (yield: approx. 8 fl. oz.):								
Prepared with whole milk (3.5% fat)	279	24.0			34.9	3.00	279	24.0
Prepared with water	120	12.0			15.0	1.50	120	12.0
Hi-Proteen Instant Powder, Vegetable Flavor, 16-oz. (1-lb.) canister	1760	96.0	110.0	6.00				
Suggested serving: 1 oz. (approx. 2 tablespoons)	110	6.0	110.0	6.00				
Prepared as package directs, mixing 1 suggested serving with 1 cup (8 fl. oz.) liquid (yield: approx. 8 fl. oz.):								
Prepared with whole milk (3.5% fat)	269	18.0			33.6	2.25	269	15.0
Prepared with water	110	6.0			13.8	0.75	110	6.0
Hi-Proteen Tablets, 8½-oz. (280-tablet) canister, Chocolate	910	126.0	107.1	14.82				
Suggested serving: 40 tablets (approx. 1.2 oz.)	130	18.0	107.1	14.82				
Vanilla	910	112.0	107.1	13.18				
Suggested serving: 40 tablets (approx. 1.2 oz.)	130	16.0	107.1	13.18				
Special Hi-Proteen with Lecithin and Papain, 16-oz. (1-lb.) can	1600	0.0	100.0	0.00				
Suggested serving: 1 oz. (approx. 2 tablespoons)	100	0.0	100.0	0.00				
Prepared as package directs, mixing 1 suggested serving with 1 cup (8 fl. oz.) liquid (yield: approx. 8 fl. oz.):								
Prepared with whole milk (3.5% fat)	259	12.0			32.4	1.50	259	12.0
Prepared with water	100	0.0			12.5	0.00	100	0.0

	UNIT		1 OZ., BY WT.		1 FLUID OZ.		1 CUP	
	Cal.	Carb.	Cal.	Carb.	Cal.	Carb.	Cal.	Carb.
Super Hi-Proteen Instant, more than 90% protein, 16-oz. (1-lb.) can	1600	0.0	100.0	0.00				
Suggested serving: 1 oz. (approx. 2 tablespoons)	100	0.0	100.0	0.00				
Prepared as package directs, mixing 1 suggested serving with 1 cup (8 fl. oz.) liquid (yield: approx. 8 fl. oz.):								
Prepared with whole milk (3.5% fat)	259	9.0			32.4	1.13	259	9.0
Prepared with water	100	0.0			12.5	0.00	100	0.0
Tablets, Formula 90, 10-oz. (400-tablet) canister	1400	80.0	140.0	8.00				
Suggested serving: 20 tablets (approx. ½ oz.)	70	4.0	140.0	8.00				
LPP, Predigested Collagen Protein with Honey, 16-fl.-oz. (1-pint) bottle	1120	40.0			70.0	2.50	560	20.0
32-fl.-oz. (1-quart) bottle	2240	80.0			70.0	2.50	560	20.0
210-fl.-oz. bottle	14700	525.0			70.0	2.50	560	20.0
Suggested serving: 1 fl. oz. (2 tablespoons)	70	2.5			70.0	2.50	560	20.0
Protein, 16-fl.-oz. (1-pint) bottle	960	0.0			60.0	0.00	480	0.0
Suggested serving: 1 fl. oz. (2 tablespoons)	60	0.0			60.0	0.00	480	0.0
Tablets, 50-tablet bottle	2500							
Suggested serving: 1 tablet	50							
M-L-O (Tillmore Foods), All Vegetable Protein, 16-oz. (1-lb.) can	1540	0.0	96.3	0.00				
Suggested serving: 1 fl. oz. (2 tablespoons, approx. 0.73 oz.)	70	0.0	96.3	0.00				
Prepared as package directs, mixing 1 suggested serving with 1 cup (8 fl. oz.) liquid (yield: approx. 8 fl. oz.):								
Prepared with non-fat milk (0.1% fat)	158	12.5			19.8	1.56	158	12.5
Prepared with water	70	0.0			8.8	0.00	70	0.0
Naturade, N-R-G Protein Powder, 8-oz. (½-lb.) can	754	30.2	94.3	3.77	50.0	2.00	800	32.0
16-oz. (1-lb.) can	1509	60.4	94.3	3.77	50.0	2.00	800	32.0
32-oz. (2-lb.) can	3018	120.8	94.3	3.77	50.0	2.00	800	32.0
64-oz. (4-lb.) can	6035	241.6	94.3	3.77	50.0	2.00	800	32.0
Suggested serving: 1 tablespoon (approx. 0.53 oz.)	50	2.0	94.3	3.77	50.0	2.00	800	32.0
Prepared as package directs, mixing 1 suggested serving with 1 cup (8 fl. oz.) liquid (yield: approx. 8 fl. oz.):								
Prepared with whole milk (3.5% fat)	209	14.0			26.1	1.75	209	14.0
Prepared with non-fat milk (0.1% fat)	140	14.5			17.5	1.81	140	14.5
Vegetable Protein, 1-lb. (16-oz.) can	1661	15.1	103.8	0.94	110.0	1.00	880	8.0
2-lb. (32-oz.) can	3322	30.2	103.8	0.94	110.0	1.00	880	8.0
Suggested serving: 1 tablespoon (approx. 0.53 oz.)	55	0.5	103.8	0.94	110.0	1.00	880	8.6
Prepared as package directs, mixing 1 suggested serving with 1 cup (8 fl. oz.) liquid (yield: approx. 8 fl. oz.):								
Prepared with whole milk (3.5% fat)	269	13.0			33.6	1.63	269	13.0
Prepared with skim milk (0.1% fat)	200	13.5			25.0	1.69	200	13.5
Nature's Inn, Natural Protein Density Drink, 10-fl.-oz. can, Banana	125	trace			12.5	trace	100	trace
Strawberry	125	trace			12.5	trace	100	trace
Vanilla	125	trace			12.5	trace	100	trace
Protein Power Drink, 10-fl.-oz. can, Chocolate	258	30.0			25.8	3.00	206	24.0
Vanilla	258	30.0			25.8	3.00	206	24.0
Nature's Way, 95% Protein, 16-oz. (1-lb.) container	1600	0.0	100.0	0.00				
Suggested serving: 2 tablespoons (approx. 1 oz.)	100	0.0	100.0	0.00				
Prepared as package directs, mixing 1 suggested serving with 1 cup (8 fl. oz.) liquid (yield: approx. 8 fl. oz.):								
Prepared with whole milk (3.5% fat)	260	12.0	(27.1)	(1.25)	32.5	1.50	260	12.0
Prepared with non-fat milk (0.1% fat)	190	12.5	(20.2)	(1.33)	23.8	1.56	190	12.5
Prepared with apple juice	217	29.5	(23.3)	(3.17)	27.1	3.69	217	29.5
NF Factors, Protesoy Instant Protein Powder w/B Complex, 16-oz. (1-lb.) can	1600		100.0					
Carob, 56-oz. can	5600		100.0					
Suggested serving: 6 tablespoons (approx. 0.7 oz.)	70		100.0					
Prepared as package directs, mixing 1 suggested serving with 1 cup (8 fl. oz.) liquid (yield: approx. 8 fl. oz.):								
Prepared with whole milk (3.5% fat)	182				22.8		182	
Prepared with apple juice	187				23.4		187	
Nu-Life, Nutra Pro Finest Milk & Egg Protein, 16-oz. (1-lb.) can	1680	16.0	105.0	1.00				
Suggested serving: 1 heaping tablespoon (approx. 0.53 oz.)	56	1.0	105.0	1.00				
Prepared as package directs, mixing 1 suggested serving with 1 cup (8 fl. oz.) liquid (yield: approx. 8 fl. oz.):								
Prepared with whole milk (3.5% fat)	215	13.0			26.9	1.63	215	13.0
Prepared with apple juice	173	30.5			21.6	3.81	173	30.5
Qualipro, 80% Protein Drink Mix, 12-oz. can, Vanilla	1276	21.3	136.3	1.77	30.0	0.50	240	4.0
Suggested serving: ¼ cup (approx. 0.44 oz.)	60	1.0	136.3	1.77	30.0	0.50	240	4.0
Prepared as package directs, mixing 1 suggested serving with 1 cup (8 fl. oz.) liquid (yield: approx. 8 fl. oz.):								
Prepared with whole milk (3.5% fat)	220	13.0			27.5	1.63	220	13.0
Prepared with apple juice	177	13.5			22.1	1.69	177	13.5
Squibb, Golden Bounty Protein Powder, bottle, 16-fl.-oz. (1 pint)	1920	128.0			120.0	8.00	960	64.0
Suggested serving: 1 tablespoon (approx. ½ oz.)	60	4.0			120.0	8.00	960	64.0
Tablets, bottle of 500	1950	16.7						
Suggested daily serving: 30 tablets	117	1.0						
Staminex RDA, Especially Recommended for Vegetarians, 16-oz. (1-lb.) can	1650	15.0	103.1	0.94				
Suggested serving: 3 rounded tablespoons (approx. 1.1 oz.)	(118)	(1.1)	103.1	0.94				
Stamigen, 16-oz. (1-lb.) can	1820	98.0	113.8	6.13				
Suggested serving: 3 rounded tablespoons (approx. 1.1 oz.)	130	7.0	113.8	6.13				
Staminex, 16-oz. (1-lb.) can	(1680)	(42.0)	(105.0)	(2.63)				
Suggested serving: 3 rounded tablespoons (approx. 1.1 oz.)	120	3.0	(105.0)	(2.63)				
Staminex with Ginseng, 16-oz. (1-lb.) can	1800	60.0	112.5	3.75				
Suggested serving: 3 rounded tablespoons			112.5	3.75				
Superior Health, Super Pro Gest Predigested Protein Liquid, 16-fl.-oz. (1-pint) bottle	960	trace	(60.0)	trace	60.0	trace	480	trace
Suggested serving: 2 tablespoons (approx. 1 oz.)	60	trace	(60.0)	trace	60.0	trace	480	trace
Thompson, 90% Protein Powder, 16-oz. (1-lb.) can	1575	0.0	98.4	0.00				
Suggested serving: 2 heaping tablespoons (approx. 0.7 oz.)	70	0.0	98.4	0.00				

	UNIT		1 OZ., BY WT.		1 FLUID OZ.		1 CUP	
	Cal.	Carb.	Cal.	Carb.	Cal.	Carb.	Cal.	Carb.
Prepared as package directs, mixing 1 suggested serving with 1 cup (8 fl. oz.) liquid (yield: approx. 8 fl. oz.):								
Prepared with whole milk (3.5% fat)	229	12.0			28.6	1.50	229	12.0
Prepared with apple juice	187	29.5			23.4	3.69	187	29.5
Prepared with lemonade	177	28.3			22.1	3.54	177	28.3
Vanguard, Liquid Protein, Wild Cherry Flavor, 32 fl. oz. (1 quart)	1920	0.0			60.0	0.00	480	0.0
Suggested serving: 2 tablespoons	60	0.0			60.0	0.00	480	0.0
Weider, High Protein Powder, 16-oz. (1-lb.) canister	1600	128.0	100.0	8.00				
Suggested serving: 2 heaping tablespoons (approx. 1 oz.)	100	8.0	100.0	8.00				
Prepared as package directs, mixing 1 suggested serving with 1 cup (8 fl. oz.) liquid (yield: approx. 8 fl. oz.):								
Prepared with non-fat milk (0.1% fat)	188	20.5			23.5	2.56	188	20.5
Sugar Free 90% Plus Protein, 16-oz. (1-lb.) canister	1600	16.0	100.0	1.00				
Suggested serving: 3 heaping tablespoons (approx. 1 oz.)	100	1.0	100.0	1.00				
Prepared as package directs, mixing 1 suggested serving with 1 cup (8 fl. oz.) liquid (yield: approx. 8 fl. oz.):								
Prepared with non-fat milk (0.1% fat)	188	13.5			23.5	1.69	188	13.5
Super Pro "101" Drink Mix, 18-oz. box	1920	216.0	106.7	12.00				
Suggested serving: 1 envelope (approx. 1½ oz.)	160	12.0	106.7	12.00				
Prepared as package directs, mixing 1 suggested serving with 1 cup (8 fl. oz.) liquid (yield: approx. 8 fl. oz.):								
Prepared with non-fat milk (0.1% fat)	248	24.5			31.0	3.06	248	24.5
Super Protein Powder, 16-oz. (1-lb.) canister	1600	64.0	100.0	4.00				
Suggested serving: 3 heaping tablespoons (approx. 1 oz.)	100	4.0	100.0	4.00				
Prepared as package directs, mixing 1 suggested serving with 1 cup (8 fl. oz.) liquid (yield: approx. 8 fl. oz.):								
Prepared with non-fat milk (0.1% fat)	188	16.5			23.5	2.06	188	16.5
Super Protein Tablets, 18½-oz. canister	2160	108.0	116.8	5.84				
Suggested serving: 10 tablets (approx. ½ oz.)	60	3.0	116.8	5.84				
OTHER BOOSTERS								
Arica, Dragons Milk, 16-oz. (1-lb.) can	1512	141.1	94.5	8.82				
Suggested serving: approx. 2 tablespoons (approx. 0.6 oz.)	60	2.8	94.5	8.82				
Prepared as package directs, mixing 1 suggested serving with 1 cup (8 fl. oz.) whole milk (3.5% fat) plus 1 tablespoon honey and ½ tablespoon molasses (yield: approx. 9 fl. oz.)	273	42.3			(30.3)	(4.70)	(243)	(37.6)
Fearn, Liquid Lecithin, 16-fl.-oz. (1-pint) bottle	3616	32.0			226.0	2.00	1808	16.0
32-fl.-oz. (1-quart) bottle	7232	640.0			226.0	2.00	1808	16.0
Suggested serving: 1 tablespoon	113	1.0			226.0	2.00	1808	16.0
Golden Harvest, Soy Lecithin Granules, 20-oz. package	2820	188.0	141.0	9.40	120.0	8.00	960	64.0
Suggested serving: 1 level tablespoon (approx. 0.43 oz.)	60	4.0	141.0	9.40	120.0	8.00	960	64.0

	UNIT		1 OZ., BY WT.		1 FLUID OZ.		1 CUP	
	Cal.	Carb.	Cal.	Carb.	Cal.	Carb.	Cal.	Carb.
Hoffman's, Energol Capsules, 2.7-oz. bottle (100 capsules, each approx. 0.8 grams)	500	0.0	185.2	0.00				
Suggested serving: 6 capsules (approx. 4.8 grams, 1.7 oz.)	30	0.0	185.2	0.00				
Isocal, Liquid Diet, 8-fl.-oz. can	250	31.3			31.3	3.91	250	31.3
32-fl.-oz. can (1 quart)	1000	125.0			31.3	3.91	250	31.3
64-fl.-oz. can (½ gallon)	2000	250.0			31.3	3.91	250	31.3
Joe Weider Olympians, Dynamic Stamina Builder, 4-lb. canister	5950	1360.0	93.0	21.25				
Suggested serving: 2 level tablespoons (approx. ¾ oz.)	70	16.0	93.0	21.25				
Prepared as package directs, mixing 1 suggested serving with 1 cup (8 fl. oz.) liquid (yield: approx. 8 fl. oz.):								
Prepared with water	70	16.0			8.8	2.00	70	16.0
Lonalac, Low Sodium, High Protein Food, 32-fl.-oz. (1-quart) container	649	48.0			20.3	1.50	162	12.0
Suggested serving: 8 fl. oz.	162	12.0			20.3	1.50	162	12.0
Naturade, Instant Nutrition Drink, Vegetable, 6¼-oz. jar	150	29.0	24.0	4.64				
Suggested serving: 1 tablespoon	30	5.8	24.0	4.64				
Prepared as package directs, mixing 1 suggested serving with 1 cup (8 fl. oz.) water (yield: approx. 8 fl. oz.)	30	5.8			3.8	0.73	30	5.8
Sport Shake, 18 oz. container	1620	144.0	90.0	8.00	90.0	8.00	720	4.0
Suggested serving: 1 tablespoon (approx. ½ oz.)	45	4.0	90.0	8.00	90.0	8.00	720	64.0
Prepared as package directs, mixing 1 suggested serving with 1 cup (8 fl. oz.) liquid (yield: approx. 8 fl. oz.):								
Prepared with whole milk (3.5% fat)	195	16.0			24.4	2.00	195	16.0
Natural Brand, Soy Lecithin Granules, 16-oz. (1-lb.) package	3600	60.0	225.0	3.75	120.0	2.00	960	16.0
Suggested serving: 1 tablespoon (approx. 0.3 oz.)	60	1.0	225.0	3.75	120.0	2.00	960	16.0
Naura Hayden's, Dynamite Milk Shake, 24-oz. canister								
Suggested serving: 4 heaping tablespoons	230	16.0						
Prepared as package directs, mixing 1 suggested serving with 2 cups (16 fl. oz.) liquid (yield: approx. 16 fl. oz.):								
Prepared with skim milk (0.1% fat)	400	40.0			25.0	2.50	200	20.0
Prepared with apple juice	320	28.5			20.0	1.78	160	14.2
Nutrament, Body Building Energy Food, 12-fl.-oz. container	360	52.0			30.0	4.33	240	34.6
Suggested serving: 1 tablespoon	15	2.7			30.0	4.33	240	34.6
Portagen, Complete Dietary, 32-fl.-oz. (1-quart) container	960	112.4			30.0	3.51	240	28.1
Suggested serving: 8 fl. oz.	240	28.1			30.0	3.51	240	28.1
Qualipro, Carob Shake Mix, 12-oz. container	1260	126.0	104.0	10.50	37.5	3.75	300	30.0
Suggested serving: ⅓ cup (approx. 1 oz.)	100	10.0	104.0	10.50	37.5	3.75	300	30.0
Prepared as package directs, mixing 1 suggested serving with 1 cup (8 fl. oz.) liquid (yield: approx. 8 fl. oz.):								
Prepared with whole milk (3.5% fat)	259	22.0			32.4	2.75	259	22.0
Prepared with skim milk (0.1% fat)	188	22.5			23.5	2.81	188	22.5
Prepared with water	100	10.0			12.5	1.25	100	10.0
Chocolate Shake Mix, 12-oz. container	1260	113.4	104.0	9.45	18.8	1.68	300	27.0
Suggested serving: ⅓ cup (approx. 1 oz.)	100	9.0	105.0	9.45	18.8	1.68	300	27.0

	UNIT		1 OZ., BY WT.		1 FLUID OZ.		1 CUP	
	Cal.	Carb.	Cal.	Carb.	Cal.	Carb.	Cal.	Carb.
Prepared as package directs, mixing 1 suggested serving with 1 cup (8 fl. oz.) liquid (yield: approx. 8 fl. oz.):								
Prepared with whole milk (3.5% fat)	259	21.0			32.4	2.63	259	21.0
Prepared with skim milk (0.1% fat)	188	21.5			23.5	2.69	188	21.5
Prepared with water	100	9.0			12.5	1.13	100	9.0
Vanilla Shake Mix, 12-oz. container	1260	126.0	105.0	10.50	37.5	3.75	300	30.0
Suggested serving: ⅓ cup (approx. 1 oz.)	100	10.0	105.0	10.50	37.5	3.75	300	30.0
Prepared as package directs, mixing 1 suggested serving with 1 cup (8 fl. oz.) liquid (yield: approx. 8 fl. oz.):								
Prepared with whole milk (3.5% fat)	259	22.0			32.4	2.75	259	22.0
Prepared with skim milk (0.1% fat)	188	22.5			23.5	2.81	188	22.5
Prepared with water	100	10.0			12.5	1.25	100	10.0
Sustacal, Chocolate Liquid, 8-fl.-oz. can	240	33.0			30.0	4.13	240	33.0
12-fl.-oz. can	360	49.5			30.0	4.13	240	33.0
32-fl.-oz. (1-quart) can	960	132.0			30.0	4.13	240	33.0
Suggested serving: 6 fl. oz.	180	27.8			30.0	4.13	240	33.0
Chocolate Powder, Suggested serving: 1 1.9-oz. packet	199	35.4	104.7	18.63				
Prepare as package directs, mixing 1 packet with 8 fl. oz. whole milk (3.5% fat) (yield: approx. 8 fl. oz.)	360	47.4			45.0	5.93	360	47.4
Vanilla Liquid, 8-fl.-oz. can	240	33.0			30.0	4.13	240	33.0
12-fl.-oz. can	360	49.5			30.0	4.13	240	33.0
32-fl.-oz. (1-quart) can	960	132.0			30.0	4.13	240	33.0
Suggested serving: 6 fl. oz.	180	24.8			30.0	4.13	240	33.0
Vanilla Powder, Suggested serving: 1 1.9-oz. packet	199	36.4	104.7	19.16				
Prepare as package directs, mixing 1 suggested serving with 1 cup (8 fl. oz.) liquid (yield: approx. 8 fl. oz.):								
Prepared with whole milk (3.5% fat)	360	48.4			45.0	6.05	360	48.4
Sustagen, Chocolate Complete Nutriment Powder, 16-oz. (1-lb.) can	1750	300.0	109.4	18.75	72.9	12.50	583	100.0
Suggested serving: 3.5 oz. (approx. ⅔ cup)	390	66.5	109.4	18.75	72.9	12.50	583	100.0
Prepared as package directs, mixing 1 suggested serving with ⅔ cup water (yield: approx. 8 fl. oz.)	390	66.5			48.8	8.31	390	66.5
Vanilla Complete Nutriment Powder, 32-fl.-oz. (1-quart) can	1750	300.0	109.4	18.75	72.9	12.50	583	100.0
Suggested serving: 3.5 oz. (approx. ⅔ cup)	390	66.5	109.4	18.75	72.9	12.50	583	100.0
Prepared as package directs, mixing 1 suggested serving with ⅔ cup water (yield: approx. 8 fl. oz.)	390	66.5			48.8	8.31	390	66.5
Tigers Milk, Nutrition Booster, Plain, 10-oz. container	974	111.5	97.4	11.15	25.8	2.95	206	23.6
16-oz. (1-lb.) container	1558	178.4	97.4	11.15	25.8	2.95	206	23.6
32-oz. container	3505	401.4	97.4	11.15	25.8	2.95	206	23.6
Suggested serving: ½ cup (approx. 1.05 oz.)	103	11.8	97.4	11.15	25.8	2.95	206	23.6
Prepared as package directs, mixing 1 suggested serving with 1 cup whole milk (3.5% fat) (yield: approx. 8 fl. oz.)	262	23.8			32.8	2.98	262	23.8
Natural Carob Flavor, 10-oz. can	1004	145.0	100.4	14.50	31.0	4.48	248	35.8
16-oz. (1-lb.) can	1607	232.0	100.4	14.50	31.0	4.48	248	35.8
Suggested serving: ½ cup (approx. 1¼ oz.)	124	17.9	100.4	14.50	31.0	4.48	248	35.8
Prepared as package directs, mixing 1 suggested serving with 1 cup (8 fl. oz.) liquid (yield: approx. 8 fl. oz.):								
Prepared with whole milk (3.5% fat)	283	26.9			35.4	3.36	283	26.9
Natural Vanilla Flavor, 10-oz. can	964	141.8	96.4	14.18	29.8	4.38	238	35.0
16-oz. (1-lb.) can	1542	226.8	96.4	14.18	29.8	4.38	238	35.0
Suggested serving: ½ cup (approx. 1¼ oz.)	119	17.5	96.4	14.18	29.8	4.38	238	35.0
Prepared as package directs, mixing 1 suggested serving with 1 cup (8 fl. oz.) liquid (yield: approx. 8 fl. oz.):								
Prepared with whole milk (3.5% fat)	278	26.5			34.8	3.31	278	26.5

YEAST

POWDERS and FLAKES

	UNIT		1 OZ., BY WT.		1 FLUID OZ.		1 CUP	
	Cal.	Carb.	Cal.	Carb.	Cal.	Carb.	Cal.	Carb.
Golden Harvest, Debittered Brewer's Yeast, Dried Flakes, 16-oz. (1-lb.) package	1600	192.0	100.0	12.00				
Suggested serving: 4 heaping teaspoons (approx. ½ oz.)	50	6.0	100.0	12.00				
Debittered Brewer's Yeast, Powder, 20-oz. (1-lb. 4-oz.) package	2000	240.0	100.0	12.00	75.0	9.00	600	72.0
Suggested serving: 4 level teaspoons (approx. ½ oz.)	50	6.0	100.0	12.00	75.0	9.00	600	72.0
Potent Yeast, 18-oz. package	2240	256.0	124.4	14.22				
Suggested serving: 1 heaping tablespoon (approx. 0.56 oz.)	70	8.0	124.4	14.22				
Primary Grown Brewer's Yeast, Dried Flakes, 16-oz. (1-lb.) package	1800	180.0	112.5	11.25				
Suggested serving: 3 heaping teaspoons (approx. 0.27 oz.)	30	3.0	112.5	11.25				
Naturade, Yeast Flakes, 8-oz. package	744	0.0	93.0	0.00				
Suggested serving: 3 heaping tablespoons (approx. 1.05 oz.)	98	0.0	93.0	0.00				
Yeast Powder, 8-oz. package	744	0.0	93.0	0.00				
Suggested serving: 2 heaping tablespoons (approx. 1.05 oz.)	98	0.0	93.0	0.00				
Plus, Super Yeast Formula 300, 32-oz. (2-lb.) can	1400	112.0	43.8	3.50				
Suggested serving: approx. 1 heaping tablespoon (approx. 1.1 oz.)	50	4.0	43.8	3.50				
Yeast Plus Formula 250, 32-oz. (2-lb.) can	3080	308.0	96.3	9.63				
Suggested serving: 2 heaping tablespoons (approx. 1.14 oz.)	110	11.0	96.3	9.63				
Schiff, Delecta Yeast Flakes, 9-oz. jar	750	75.0	83.3	8.33	30.0	3.00	240	24.0
Suggested serving: 2 tablespoons (approx. 0.36 oz.)	30	3.0	83.3	8.33	30.0	3.00	240	24.0
Natural Brewer's Yeast, 16-oz. (1-lb.) bottle	1650	165.0	103.1	10.31	50.0	5.00	400	40.0
Suggested serving: 1 tablespoon (approx. 0.24 oz.)	25	2.5	103.1	10.31	50.0	5.00	400	40.0
Nucle-Yeast, Powder, 8-oz. bottle	810	48.6	101.3	6.08	50.0	3.00	400	24.0
Suggested serving: 1 tablespoon (approx. 0.24 oz.)	25	1.5	101.3	6.08	50.0	3.00	400	24.0
Squibb, Yeast, Flavored, 5-oz. bottle								
Suggested serving: 1 teaspoon	17	2.0			102.0	12.00	816	96.0
Twin Lab, Genuine Brewer's Debittered Yeast, 9-oz. jar	768	80.0	85.3	8.89	96.0	10.00	768	80.0
Suggested serving: 1 heaping tablespoon (approx. 0.56 oz.)	48	5.0	85.3	8.89	96.0	10.00	768	80.0
Herbal Yeast, 9-oz. container	768	80.0	85.3	8.89	96.0	10.00	768	80.0
Suggested serving: 1 heaping tablespoon (approx. 0.56 oz.)	48	5.0	85.3	8.89	96.0	10.00	768	80.0
Natural Nutritional Yeast, 9-oz. bottle	644	98.0	71.6	10.89				
Suggested serving: 1 heaping tablespoon (approx. 0.64 oz.)	46	7.0	71.6	10.89				
Super Rich Yeast, 8-oz. container	560	77.0	70.0	9.63				

	UNIT Cal.	UNIT Carb.	1 OZ., BY WT. Cal.	1 OZ., BY WT. Carb.	1 FLUID OZ. Cal.	1 FLUID OZ. Carb.	1 CUP Cal.	1 CUP Carb.
Suggested serving: 1 heaping tablespoon (approx. 0.57 oz.)	40	5.5	70.0	9.63				
Super Rich Yeast Plus, 9-oz. bottle	640	88.0	71.1	9.78				
Suggested serving: 1 heaping tablespoon (approx. 0.56 oz.)	40	5.5	71.1	9.78				
Vita-Food, Green Label Non-Debittered Brewer's Yeast, 16-oz. (1-lb.) can	1600	171.2	100.0	10.70				
Suggested serving: 1 rounded tablespoon	50	5.4	100.0	10.70				
Red Label Debittered Genuine Grain Grown Brewer's Yeast, 8-oz. can	750	75.0	93.8	9.38				
Suggested serving: 1 rounded tablespoon (approx. 0.53 oz.)	50	5.0	93.8	9.38				
TABLETS								
Naturade, Yeast Tablets, 100-tablet bottle	200	(30.0)						
250-tablet bottle	500	(7.5)						
500-tablet bottle	1000	(150.0)						
Suggested serving: 1 tablet	2	(0.3)						
Plus, Super Yeast Tablets Formula 299, 250-tablet bottle	875	70.0						
Suggested serving: 7 tablets	25	2.0						
Squibb, Yeast Tablets, 100-tablet bottle	200	30.0						
250-tablet bottle	500	75.0						
500-tablet bottle	1000	150.0						
Suggested serving: 10 tablets	20	3.0						
LIQUID								
Twin Lab, B Complex Liquid Enzymatic Digested Yeast, 16-fl.-oz. (1-pint) container	1120	96.0			70.0	6.00	560	48.0
Suggested serving: 2 tablespoons	70	6.0			70.0	6.00	560	48.0

35 PHARMACEUTICALS •

VITAMINS and DIETARY SUPPLEMENTS

	ENTIRE BOTTLE OR PACKAGE Cal.	ENTIRE BOTTLE OR PACKAGE Carb.	1 TABLET OR CAPSULE Cal.	1 TABLET OR CAPSULE Carb.
Calcium, Phosphate & Vitamin D Tablets, **Squibb,** 90-tablet bottle	28	6.6		
180-tablet bottle	56	13.1		
360-tablet bottle	112	26.3		
1 tablet			0.3	0.07
Cod Liver Oil Capsules Formula #220, **Plus,** 100-capsule bottle	400			
1 capsule			4.0	
Iron With Vitamin C Tablets, **Squibb,** 100-tablet bottle	170	40.0	1.7	0.40
Lecithin Capsules, 19 Grain Formula #93A, **Plus,** 100-capsule bottle	1100			
250-capsule bottle	2750			
500-capsule bottle	5900			
1 capsule			11.0	
Monsters, **Bristol-Myers,** 60-tablet bottle	162	37.0		
100-tablet bottle	270	61.6		
1 tablet			2.7	0.62
Monsters With Iron, **Bristol-Myers,** 60-tablet bottle	150	33.0		
100-tablet bottle	250	55.0		
1 tablet			2.5	0.55
Multi-Vitamin Supplement With Iron Tablets, **Golden Bounty,** 100-tablet bottle	97	23.2		
1 tablet			1.0	0.23
Niacin, 25-mg tablets, **Squibb,** 100-tablet bottle	19	4.0		
1 tablet			0.2	0.04
Niacin, 50-mg Tablets, **Squibb,** 100-tablet bottle	33	7.9		
1,000-tablet bottle	330	79.0		
1 tablet			0.3	0.08
Niacin, 100-mg Tablets, **Squibb,** 100-tablet bottle	5	1.2		
1,000-tablet bottle	50	12.0		
1 tablet			0.1	0.01
Niacin, 500-mg Tablets, **Squibb,** 100-tablet bottle	14	3.3		
1 tablet			0.1	0.03
Pals, **Bristol-Myers,** 60-tablet bottle	162	37.0		
100-tablet bottle	270	61.6		
1 tablet			2.7	0.62
Pals With Iron, **Bristol-Myers,** 60-tablet bottle	150	33.0		
100-tablet bottle	250	55.0		
1 tablet			2.5	0.55
Rose Hips With Vitamin C, 125-mg. tablets, **Golden Bounty,** 100-tablet bottle	340	79.8		
1 tablet			3.4	0.80
Rose Hips With Vitamin C, 250-mg. tablets, **Golden Bounty,** 100-tablet bottle	320	75.8		
1 tablet			32.0	0.76

	ENTIRE BOTTLE OR PACKAGE Cal.	ENTIRE BOTTLE OR PACKAGE Carb.	1 TABLET OR CAPSULE Cal.	1 TABLET OR CAPSULE Carb.
Rose Hips With Vitamin C, 500-mg tablets, **Golden Bounty,** 60-tablet bottle	165	39.2		
90-tablet bottle	248	58.9		
1 tablet			2.8	0.65
Theragran Tablets, **Squibb,** "handy pack" of 30 tablets	39	9.4		
"handy pack" of 60 tablets	78	18.8		
"handy pack" of 100 tablets	130	31.3		
"handy pack" of 180 tablets	234	56.3		
unimatic carton of 100 tablets	130	31.3		
1,000-tablet bottle	1300	313.0		
1 tablet			1.3	0.31
Theragran Hematinic Tablets, **Squibb,** 90-tablet bottle	76	18.0		
1 tablet			0.8	0.20
Theragran-M Tablets, **Squibb,** "handy pack" of 30 tablets	45	10.6		
"handy pack" of 60 tablets	90	21.2		
"handy pack" of 100 tablets	150	35.3		
"handy pack" of 180 tablets	270	63.5		
unimatic carton of 100 tablets	150	35.3		
1,000-tablet bottle	1500	353.0		
1 tablet			1.5	0.35
Vigran Chewable Tablets, **Squibb,** 60-tablet bottle	129	30.6		
1 tablet			2.2	0.51
Vigran Plus Iron Tablets, **Squibb,** 90-tablet bottle	120	29.0		
1 tablet			1.3	0.32
Vitamin B, 50-mg Tablets, **Squibb,** 100-tablet bottle	104	24.7		
1 tablet			1.0	0.25
Vitamin B_1, 100-mg tablets, **Squibb,** 100-tablet bottle	124	29.5		
1 tablet			1.2	0.30
Vitamin B_{12}, 25-mg tablets, **Squibb,** 100-tablet bottle	107	25.5		
1 tablet			1.1	0.26
Vitamin B Complex Tablets, **Squibb,** 30-tablet bottle	39	9.5		
100-tablet bottle	130	31.5		
1 tablet			1.3	0.32
Vitamin B Complex with C, **Squibb,** 100-tablet bottle	160	37.3		
1 tablet			1.6	0.37
Vitamin C, 100-mg Tablets, **Squibb,** 100-tablet bottle	52	12.3		
1 tablet			0.5	0.12
Vitamin C, 250-mg Tablets, **Squibb,** 100-tablet bottle	35	8.5		
1 tablet			0.4	0.08
Vitamin C, 250-mg Orange-Flavored Tablets, **Squibb,** 100-tablet bottle	250	60.5		
1 tablet			2.5	0.61
Vitamin C, 500-mg Tablets, **Squibb,** 100-tablet bottle	46	10.9		
1 tablet			0.5	0.11
Vitamin E Walnut-Flavored Tablets, 200-i.u. tablets, **Squibb,** 100-tablet bottle	150	36.0		
1 tablet			1.5	0.36
400-i.u. tablets, 50-tablet bottle	75	18.0		
1 tablet			1.5	0.36

	ENTIRE BOTTLE OR PACKAGE		1 TABLET OR CAPSULE	
	Cal.	Carb.	Cal.	Carb.
Wheat Germ Oil Capsules, Formula #150, **Plus**, 100-capsule bottle, 760-mg capsules	700			
250-capsule bottle	1750			
1 capsule			7.0	

TABLETS and CAPSULES

	ENTIRE BOTTLE OR PACKAGE		1 TABLET OR CAPSULE	
	Cal.	Carb.	Cal.	Carb.
Amnestrogen, **Squibb**, 0.625-mg tablets, 100-tablet bottle	28	6.7		
1 tablet			0.3	0.07
1.25-mg tablets, 100-tablet bottle	55	12.9		
1 tablet			0.6	0.13
2.5-mg tablets, 100-tablet bottle	73	17.3		
1 tablet			0.7	0.17
Aspirin, **Squibb**, 250-tablet bottle, 5-grain tablets	65	15.5		
1 tablet			0.3	0.06
1,000-tablet bottle	260	62.0		
1 tablet			0.3	0.06
BQ Cold Tablets, **Bristol-Myers**, 16-tablet tin, 445-mg tablets	3	0.5		
30-tablet bottle	6	0.9		
50-tablet bottle	10	1.5		
1 tablet			0.2	0.03
Bufferin, **Bristol-Myers**, 12-tablet bottle, 7.25-grain tablets	4	1.0		
100-tablet bottle	33	8.0		
375-tablet bottle	124	30.0		
1 tablet			0.3	0.08
Bufferin, Arthritis Strength, **Bristol-Myers**, 40-tablet bottle, 10.9-grain tablets	20	4.8		
100-tablet bottle	50	12.4		
1 tablet			0.5	0.12
Comtrex Tablets, **Bristol-Myers**, 24-tablet bottle, 550-mg tablets	5	1.2		
50-tablet bottle	11	2.5		
100-tablet bottle	22	5.0		
1 tablet			0.2	0.05
Congespirin Tablets for Children, **Bristol-Myers**, 36-tablet bottle, 90-mg tablets	33	8.3		
1 tablet			0.9	0.23
Datril Tablets, **Bristol-Myers**, 24-tablet bottle, 5-grain tablets	6	1.3		
100-tablet bottle	24	5.5		
250-tablet bottle	60	13.8		
1 tablet			0.2	0.06
Datril 500 Tablets, **Bristol-Myers**, 24-tablet bottle, 7.5-grain tablets	6	1.3		
50-tablet bottle	12	2.8		
72-tablet bottle	17	4.0		
1 tablet			0.2	0.06
Excedrin Tablets, **Bristol-Myers**, 12-tablet tin, 7.5-grain tablets	2	0.5		
36-tablet bottle	7	1.4		
100-tablet bottle	19	4.0		
1 tablet			0.2	0.04
Excedrin-PM Tablets, **Bristol-Myers**, 10-tablet bottle, 7.5-grain tablets	2	0.4		
30-tablet bottle	5	1.2		
50-tablet bottle	8	2.0		
80-tablet bottle	12	3.2		
1 tablet			0.2	0.04
Fedrazil Tablets, **Burroughs Wellcome**, 24-tablet vial, 55-mg tablets	10			
1 tablet			0.4	
Florinef Acetate Tablets, **Squibb**, 100-tablet bottle, 0.1-mg tablets	33	7.8		
1 tablet			0.3	0.08
4-Way Cold Tablets, **Bristol-Myers**, 15-tablet box, 138-mg tablets	12	3.0		
60-tablet bottle	48	12.0		
1 tablet			0.8	0.20
Gelusil Tablets, **Warner Lambert**, 100-tablet bottle	(320)	(73.5)		
1 tablet			(3.2)	(0.74)
Gelusil II Tablets, **Warner Lambert**, 100-tablet bottle	(350)	8.2		
1 tablet			(3.5)	(0.82)
Hydrea Capsules, **Squibb**, 100-tablet bottle, 500-mg tablets	100	24.3		
1 tablet			1.0	0.24
Kenacort, 1-mg Tablets, **Squibb**, 50-tablet bottle	37	8.7		
1 tablet			0.7	0.17
Kenacort, 2-mg Tablets, **Squibb**, 50-tablet bottle	37	8.0		
1 tablet			0.7	0.17
Kenacort, 4-mg Tablets, **Squibb**, 30-tablet bottle	36	8.6		
100-tablet bottle	120	28.8		

	ENTIRE BOTTLE OR PACKAGE		1 TABLET OR CAPSULE	
	Cal.	Carb.	Cal.	Carb.
1,000-tablet bottle	1200	288.0		
1 tablet			1.2	0.29
Kenacort, 8-mg Tablets, **Squibb**, 50-tablet bottle	41	9.8		
1 tablet			0.8	0.20
Leukeran Tablets, **Burroughs Wellcome**, 50-tablet bottle, 2-mg tablets	10			
1 tablet			0.2	
Lomotil Tablets, **Searle**, 100-tablet bottle, 2.5-mg tablets	22	5.4		
500-tablet bottle	110	2.7		
1 tablet			0.2	0.05
Migral Tablets, **Burroughs Wellcome**, 100-tablet bottle, 76-mg tablets	30			
1 tablet			0.3	
Milk of Magnesia Tablets, **Squibb**, 80-tablet bottle, 324-mg tablets	96	22.4		
1 tablet			1.2	0.28
Mycostatin Oral Tablets, **Squibb**, 100-tablet bottle, 500,000-unit tablets	35	8.4		
1 tablet			0.4	0.08
Naturetin, 2.5-mg Tablets, **Squibb**, 100-tablet bottle	50	5.8		
1 tablet			0.5	0.12
Naturetin, 5-mg Tablets, **Squibb**, 100-tablet bottle	70	16.3		
1,000-tablet bottle	700	163.0		
1 tablet			0.7	0.16
Naturetin 10-mg Tablets, **Squibb**, 100-tablet bottle	113	27.0		
1 tablet			1.1	0.27
Naturetin K 2.5/500 Tablets (2.5 mg Naturetin + 500 mg potassium chloride), **Squibb**, 100-tablet bottle	98	23.3		
1 tablet			1.0	0.22
Naturetin K 5/500 Tablets, **Squibb**, 100-tablet bottle	97	23.0		
1,000-tablet bottle	970	230.0		
1 tablet			1.0	0.23
Neomycin Sulfate Tablets, **Squibb**, 100-tablet bottle, 500-mg tablets	4	1.0		
1 tablet			trace	0.01
No Doz Tablets, **Bristol-Myers**, 15-tablet box, 361-mg tablets	8			
60-tablet bottle	30			
1 tablet			0.5	
Nydrazid Tablets, **Squibb**, 100-tablet bottle, 100-mg tablets	80	19.2		
1 tablet			0.8	0.20
Ora-Testryl Tablets, **Squibb**, 50-tablet bottle, 5-mg tablets	55	13.2		
1 tablet			1.1	0.26
Pentids Tablets, **Squibb**, 100-tablet bottle, 125-mg tablets	31	7.3		
1 tablet			0.3	0.07
Pentids '400' Tablets, **Squibb**, 16-tablet bottle, 250-mg tablets	9	2.0		
100-tablet bottle	53	12.7		
unimatic carton of 100	53	12.7		
1 tablet			0.5	0.13
Pentids '800' Tablets, **Squibb**, 30-tablet bottle, 500-mg tablets	5	1.1		
100-tablet bottle	16	3.8		
1 tablet			0.2	0.04
Principin '250' Capsules, **Squibb**, 100-tablet bottle, 250-mg tablets	4	1.1		
500-tablet bottle	22	5.3		
unimatic carton of 100	4	1.1		
unimatic carton of 500	22	5.3		
1 tablet			trace	0.01
Principin '500' Capsules, **Squibb**, 16-tablet bottle, 500-mg tablets	0.02	trace		
100-tablet bottle	0.10	trace		
unimatic carton of 100	0.10	trace		
1 tablet			trace	trace
Prolixin, 1-mg Tablets, **Squibb**, 50-tablet bottle	30	7.0		
500-tablet bottle	300	70.0		
1 tablet			0.6	0.14
Prolixin, 2.5-mg Tablets, **Squibb**, 50-tablet bottle	41	9.8		
1 tablet			0.8	0.20
Prolixin, 5-mg Tablets, **Squibb**, 50-tablet bottle	70	16.4		
500-tablet bottle	700	164.0		
unimatic carton of 100	140	32.8		
1 tablet			1.4	0.33
Prolixin, 10-mg Tablets, **Squibb**, 50-tablet bottle	75	17.8		
500-tablet bottle	750	178.0		
1 tablet			1.5	0.36
Raudixin, 50-mg Tablets, **Squibb**, 100-tablet bottle	66	15.6		
1,000-tablet bottle	660	156.0		
1 tablet			0.7	0.16
Raudixin, 100-mg Tablets, **Squibb**, 100-tablet bottle	66	15.6		

	ENTIRE BOTTLE OR PACKAGE		1 TABLET OR CAPSULE	
	Cal.	Carb.	Cal.	Carb.
1,000-tablet bottle	660	156.0		
1 tablet			0.7	0.16
Rau-Sed Tablets, **Squibb,** 100-tablet bottle, 0.25-mg tablets	36	8.6		
1 tablet			0.4	0.09
Rautrax Tablets, **Squibb,** 100-tablet bottle, 850-mg tablets	105	25.0		
1 tablet			1.1	0.25
Rautrax-N Tablets, **Squibb,** 100-tablet bottle, 454-mg tablets	142	33.9		
1,000-tablet bottle	1420	339.0		
1 tablet			1.4	0.34
Rautrax-N Modified Tablets, **Squibb,** 100-tablet bottle, 454-mg tablets	108	25.7		
1 tablet			1.1	0.26
Rauzide Tablets, **Squibb,** 100-tablet bottle, 54-mg tablets	106	25.2		
1,000-tablet bottle	1060	252.0		
1 tablet			1.1	0.25
Rolaids, **American Chicle,** 1 tablet (approx. 1.2 grams)			4.4	1.10
Serenium Tablets, **Squibb,** 50-tablet bottle	43	10.3		
1 tablet			0.9	0.21
Sine-Aid Tablets, **McNeil,** 24-tablet bottle, 350-mg tablets	(11)	2.4		
50-tablet bottle	(23)	5.0		
100-tablet bottle	(45)	10.0		
1 tablet			(0.4)	0.10
Sudafed, 30-mg Tablets, **Burroughs Wellcome,** 24-tablet box	7			
100-tablet bottle	30			
1 tablet			0.3	
Sumycin, 250-mg Capsules, **Squibb,** 100-capsule bottle	61	14.5		
1,000 capsule bottle	610	145.0		
unimatic carton of 100	61	14.5		
1 capsule			0.6	0.15
Sumycin, 500-mg Capsules, **Squibb,** 100-capsule bottle	16	3.7		
500-capsule bottle	80	18.5		
unimatic carton of 100	16	3.7		
1 capsule			0.2	0.04
Sumycin, 500-mg Tablets, **Squibb,** 100-tablet bottle	25	6.0		
500-tablet bottle	125	30.0		
1 tablet			0.3	0.06
Terfonyl Tablets, **Squibb,** 100-tablet bottle, 500-mg tablets	50	11.9		
1 tablet			0.5	0.12
Teslac, 50-mg Tablets, **Squibb,** 100-tablet bottle	90	21.4		
1 tablet			0.9	0.21
Titralac Antacid Tablets, **Riker,** 100-tablet bottle	(100)			
1 tablet			(1)	
Trigesic Tablets, **Squibb,** 100-tablet bottle, 6-grain tablets	10.0	2.2		
1 tablet			0.1	0.02
Trimox "250" Capsules, **Squibb,** 100-capsule bottle, 250-mg capsules	880	210.0		
500-capsule bottle	4400	1050.0		
1 capsule			8.8	2.10
Tylenol Acetaminophen Tablets, **McNeil,** 12-tablet tin, 325-mg tablets	(5)	1.2		
24-tablet bottle	(10)	2.4		
50-tablet bottle	(20)	5.0		
100-tablet bottle	(40)	10.0		
250-tablet bottle	(100)	25.0		
1 tablet			(0.4)	0.10
Tylenol Acetaminophen Capsules, Extra Strength, **McNeil,** 30-capsule bottle, 500-mg capsules	(12)	3.0		
60-capsule bottle	(24)	6.0		
100-capsule bottle	(40)	10.0		
1 capsule			(0.4)	0.10
Tylenol Acetaminophen Chewable Tablets, Children's, **McNeil,** 30-tablet bottle, 80-mg tablets	(66)	15.0		
1 tablet			(2.2)	0.50
Tylenol Acetaminophen Tablets, Extra Strength, **McNeil,** 24-tablet bottle, 500-mg tablets	(17)	3.8		
50-tablet bottle	(34)	8.0		
100-tablet bottle	(69)	16.0		
1 tablet			(0.7)	0.16
Valadal Tablets, **Squibb,** 100-tablet bottle, 325-mg tablets	48	11.3		
1 tablet			0.5	0.11
Veetids '250' Capsules or Tablets, **Squibb,** 100-capsule/tablet bottle, 250-mg capsule/tablets	23	5.6		
1 capsule or tablet			0.2	0.06
Veetids '500' Capsules or Tablets, **Squibb,** 100-capsule/tablet bottle, 500-mg capsule/tablets	46	11.1		
1 capsule or tablet			0.5	0.11
Velosef '250' Capsules, **Squibb,** 24-capsule bottle, 250-mg capsules	31	7.3		
100-capsule bottle	128	30.5		
1 capsule			1.3	0.31
Velosef '500' Capsules, **Squibb,** 24-capsule bottle, 500-mg capsules	61	14.6		
100-capsule bottle	256	61.0		
1 capsule			2.6	0.61
Vesprin, 10-mg Tablets, **Squibb,** 50-tablet bottle	44	10.1		
500-tablet bottle	440	100.5		
1 tablet			0.9	0.20
Vesprin, 25-mg Tablets, **Squibb,** 50-tablet bottle	41	9.6		
500-tablet bottle	405	96.0		
1 tablet			0.8	0.19
Vesprin, 50-mg Tablets, **Squibb,** 50-tablet bottle	70	16.4		
500-tablet bottle	700	164.0		
1 tablet			1.4	0.33

LIQUIDS—SYRUPS, ELIXIRS, DROPS

	ENTIRE BOTTLE		1 TEASPOON		1 TABLESPOON	
	Cal.	Carb.	Cal.	Carb.	Cal.	Carb.
Actidil Syrup, **Burroughs Wellcome,** 16-fl.-oz. (1-pint) bottle	787	(167.4)	8.2	(1.74)	24.6	(5.23)
Actifed Syrup, **Burroughs Wellcome,** 4-fl.-oz. bottle	324	(68.9)	13.5	(2.87)	40.5	(8.61)
16-fl.-oz. (1-pint) bottle	1296	(275.7)	13.5	(2.87)	40.5	(8.61)
Antepar Syrup, **Burroughs Wellcome,** 16-fl.-oz. (1-pint) bottle	931	(198.1)	9.7	(2.06)	29.1	(6.19)
Asbron Elixir, **Dorsey,** 4-fl.-oz. bottle	451	(96.0)	18.8	(4.00)	56.4	(12.00)
8-fl.-oz. bottle	902	(191.9)	18.8	(4.00)	56.4	(12.00)
Chicken Soup, **Margo Schab's** home recipe, 1 quart	(156)	(3.7)	(0.8)	(0.02)	(2.4)	(0.06)
Coca-Cola Syrup, concentrated, 1 cup (see Monologue, page 18.)	(640)	(160.0)	(13.3)	(3.33)	(40.0)	(10.00)
Cod Liver Oil, Norwegian, high potency, **Hain,** 8-fl.-oz. bottle	1920	0.0	40.0	0.00	120.0	0.00
Cod Liver Oil, Cherry, Norwegian, high potency, **Hain,** 8-fl.-oz. bottle	1920	0.0	40.0	0.00	120.0	0.00
Comtrex Liquid, **Bristol-Myers,** 6-fl.-oz. bottle	248	61.8	13.8	3.43	41.3	10.30
10-fl.-oz. bottle	413	103.0	13.8	3.43	41.3	10.30
Congespirin Cough Syrup for Children, **Bristol-Myers,** 3-fl.-oz. bottle	284	71.1	15.8	3.95	47.4	11.90
Congespirin Liquid Cold Medicine, **Bristol-Myers,** 3-fl.-oz. bottle	231	57.6	12.8	3.20	38.4	9.60
CoTylenol Liquid Cold Formula, **McNeil,** 4-fl.-oz. bottle	408	86.4	17.0	3.60	51.0	10.80
Dorcol Pediatric Cough Syrup, **Dorsey,** 4-fl.-oz. bottle	326	(69.4)	13.6	(2.89)	40.8	(8.68)
8-fl.-oz. bottle	653	(138.9)	13.6	(2.89)	40.8	(8.68)
Gelusil Liquid, **Warner Lambert,** 6-fl.-oz. bottle	(86)	(18.0)	(2.4)	(0.50)	(7.2)	(1.50)
12-fl.-oz. bottle	(173)	(36.0)	(2.4)	(0.50)	(7.2)	(1.50)
Gelusil-II Liquid, **Warner Lambert,** 6-fl.-oz. bottle	(43)	(9.0)	(1.2)	(0.25)	(3.6)	(0.75)
12-fl.-oz. bottle	(86)	(18.0)	(1.2)	(0.25)	(3.6)	(0.75)
Klorvess Liquid, **Dorsey,** 4-fl.-oz. bottle	222	(47.2)	9.2	(1.96)	27.6	(5.87)
8-fl.-oz. bottle	444	(94.5)	9.2	(1.96)	27.6	(5.87)
Lanoxin Elixir, **Burroughs Wellcome,** 2-fl.-oz. bottle	70	(14.9)	5.9	(1.25)	17.7	(3.76)
Metaprel Syrup, **Dorsey,** 16-fl.-oz. (1-pint) bottle	537	(114.3)	5.6	(1.19)	16.8	(3.57)
Mycostatin Oral Suspension, **Squibb,** 10-fl.-oz. bottle	630	150.0	10.5	2.50	31.5	7.50
Neo-Calglucon Syrup, **Dorsey,** 16-fl.-oz. (1-pint) bottle	397	(84.5)	4.1	(0.88)	12.4	(2.64)
Noctec Syrup, **Squibb,** 16-fl.-oz. (1-pint) bottle	1440	336.0	15.0	3.50	45.0	10.50
128-fl.-oz. (1-gallon) bottle	11520	2688.0	15.0	3.50	45.0	10.50
Principin '125' for Oral Suspension, **Squibb,** 80-ml bottle	195	46.4	12.2	2.90	36.6	8.70
100-ml bottle	244	58.0	12.2	2.90	36.6	8.70
150-ml bottle	366	87.0	12.2	2.90	36.6	8.70
200-ml bottle	488	116.0	12.2	2.90	36.6	8.70
Principin '250' for Oral Suspension, **Squibb,** 80-ml bottle	195	0.1	12.2	0.01	36.6	0.01
100-ml bottle	244	0.1	12.2	0.01	36.6	0.01
150-ml bottle	366	0.1	12.2	0.01	36.6	0.01
200-ml bottle	488	0.1	12.2	0.01	36.6	0.01
Prolixin Elixir, **Squibb,** 60-ml dropper bottle	151	trace	12.6	trace	37.8	0.01
473-ml dropper bottle	1192	0.3	12.6	trace	37.8	0.01
Septra Suspension, **Burroughs Wellcome,** 15.21-fl.-oz. bottle	885	(188.3)	9.7	(2.06)	29.1	(6.19)

	ENTIRE BOTTLE		1 TEASPOON		1 TABLE-SPOON	
	Cal.	Carb.	Cal.	Carb.	Cal.	Carb.
Sudafed Syrup, **Burroughs Wellcome,** 4-fl.-oz. bottle	324	(68.9)	13.5	(2.87)	40.5	(8.61)
16-fl.-oz. (1-pint) bottle	5184	(1102.6)	13.5	(2.87)	40.5	(8.61)
Sumycin Syrup, **Squibb,** 60-ml bottle	112	26.4	9.3	2.20	27.9	6.60
473-ml (1-pint) bottle	880	208.1	9.3	2.20	27.9	6.60
Terfonyl Suspension, **Squibb,** 473-ml (1-pint) bottle	501	120.6	5.3	1.27	15.9	3.81
Triaminic Expectorant, **Dorsey,** 4-fl.-oz. bottle	384		16.0		48.0	
8-fl.-oz. bottle	768		16.0		48.0	
Triaminic Expectorant DH, **Dorsey,** 8-fl.-oz. bottle	538		11.2		33.6	
Triaminic Expectorant with Codeine, **Dorsey,** 4-fl.-oz. bottle	415		17.3		51.9	
8-fl.-oz. bottle	828		17.3		51.9	
Triaminic Syrup, **Dorsey,** 8-fl.-oz. bottle	739	(157.2)	15.4	(3.28)	46.2	(9.83)
Triaminicol, **Dorsey,** 8-fl.-oz. bottle	682		14.2		42.6	
Trimox '125' for Oral Suspension, **Squibb,** 80-ml bottle	155	36.8	9.7	2.30	29.1	6.90
100-ml bottle	194	46.0	9.7	2.30	29.1	6.90
150-ml bottle	291	69.0	9.7	2.30	29.1	6.90
Trimox '250' for Oral Suspension, **Squibb,** 80-ml bottle	141	33.6	8.8	2.10	26.4	6.30
100-ml bottle	176	42.0	8.8	2.10	26.4	6.30
150-ml bottle	264	63.0	8.8	2.10	26.4	6.30
Tussagesic Suspension, **Dorsey,** 8-fl.-oz. bottle	787		16.4		49.2	
Children's Tylenol Acetaminophen Elixir, **McNeil,** 2-fl.-oz. bottle	102	21.6	17.0	3.60	51.0	10.80
4-fl.-oz. bottle	204	43.2	17.0	3.60	51.0	10.80
Extra-Strength Tylenol Acetaminophen Liquid, **McNeil,** 16-fl.-oz. (1-pint) bottle	518	147.8	10.8	3.08	32.4	9.24
Infants Tylenol Acetaminophen Drops, **McNeil,** ½-fl.-oz. bottle	(59)	12.6	(19.5)	4.20	(58.7)	12.60
Valadol Liquid, **Squibb,** 4-fl.-oz. bottle	25	6.0	1.1	0.25	3.2	0.75
Veetids '125' for Oral Solution, **Squibb,** 100-ml bottle	240	57.0	12.0	2.85	36.0	8.55
200-ml bottle	480	114.0	12.0	2.85	36.0	8.55
Veetids '250' for Oral Solution, **Squibb,** 100-ml bottle	228	54.0	11.4	2.70	34.2	8.10
200-ml bottle	456	108.0	11.4	2.70	34.2	8.10
Velosef '125' for Oral Suspension, **Squibb,** 100-ml bottle	260	0.1	13.0	0.01	39.0	0.02
200-ml bottle	520	0.1	13.0	0.01	39.0	0.02
Velosef '250' for Oral Suspension, **Squibb,** 100-ml bottle	244	0.1	12.2	0.01	36.6	0.02
200-ml bottle	488	0.1	12.2	0.01	36.6	0.02

POWDERS and GRANULES

	ENTIRE BOTTLE		1 TEASPOON		1 TABLE-SPOON		1 OZ., BY WT.	
	Cal.	Carb.	Cal.	Carb.	Cal.	Carb.	Cal.	Carb.
Metamucil, Instant Mix, **Searle,** 16-packet carton	48						13.3	
30-packet carton	90						13.3	
1 packet, approx. 6.4 grams	3						13.3	
Metamucil Powder, **Searle,** 7-oz. container	397		(14.0)		(42.0)		56.7	
14-oz. container	794		(14.0)		(42.0)		56.7	
Oragrafin Calcium Granules, **Squibb,** 1 packet, approx. 8 grams	20	4.9					70.9	17.36

	ENTIRE BOTTLE		1 TEASPOON		1 TABLE-SPOON		1 OZ., BY WT.	
	Cal.	Carb.	Cal.	Carb.	Cal.	Carb.	Cal.	Carb.
Pentids for Syrup, **Squibb,** in bottles for reconstitution, 100-ml bottle	240	56.0	12.0	2.80	36.0	8.40		
200-ml bottle	480	112.0	12.0	2.80	36.0	8.40		
Pentids '400' for Syrup, **Squibb,** in bottles for reconstitution, 100-ml bottle	240	56.0	12.0	2.80	36.0	8.40		
Pentids '200'-ml bottle	480	112.0	12.0	2.80	36.0	8.40		
Psyllium Seed, Blond, **Golden Harvest,** 16-oz. (1-lb.) package	1350	225.0	9.0	1.50	27.0	4.50	84.4	14.06
1 tablespoon (approx. 0.32 oz.)	27	4.5			27.0	4.50	84.4	14.06

LOZENGES and COUGH DROPS

	ENTIRE PACKAGE		1 LOZENGE OR COUGH DROP		1 OZ., BY WT.	
	Cal.	Carb.	Cal.	Carb.	Cal.	Carb.
Beech-Nut, Black, 11-tablet roll	110	27.5				
1 cough tablet			10.0	2.50		
Menthol, 11-tablet roll	110	27.5				
1 cough tablet			10.0	2.50		
Wild Cherry, 11-tablet roll	110	27.5				
1 cough tablet			10.0	2.50		
Hall's Cough Tablets, Cherry, bag of 30	450	111.0				
stick pack of 9	135	33.3				
1 cough tablet			15.0	3.70		
Lemon, bag of 30	450	111.0				
stick pack of 9	135	33.3				
1 cough tablet			15.0	3.70		
Mentho-Lyptus, bag of 30	450	111.0				
stick pack of 9	135	33.3				
1 cough tablet			15.0	3.70		
Listerine Throat Lozenges, **American Chicle,** 24-lozenge box	204	48.0			111.6	26.25
1 lozenge, approx. 2.2 grams			8.5	2.00	111.6	26.25
Pine Bros., Honey, 14-drop box	112	28.0				
1 cough drop			8.0	2.00		
Wild Cherry, 14-drop box	112	28.0				
1 cough drop			8.0	2.00		
Squibb, Cough Suppressant Lozenges, 1 stick or flat pack of 10	158	37.5				
1 lozenge			15.8	0.04		
Squibb, Decongestant Lozenges, 1 stick pack of 10	158	37.5				
1 lozenge			15.8	0.04		
Squibb, Spec T Sore Throat Anesthetic Lozenges, 1 stick or flat pack of 10	158	37.5				
1 lozenge			15.8	0.04		
Sucrets Children's Cherry Flavored Lozenges, **Beecham,** 24-tablet tin	240	0.1			118.1	0.24
1 lozenge, approx. 2.4 grams			10.0	0.02	118.1	0.24
Cold Decongestant Formula Lozenges, 12-tablet tin	108	0.0			110.9	0.00
1 lozenge, approx. 2.3 grams			9.0	0.00	110.9	0.00
Cough Control Formula Lozenges, 24-tablet tin	240	0.6			123.3	0.00
1 lozenge, approx. 2.3 grams			10.0	0.00	123.3	0.00
Mentholated Sore Throat Lozenges, 24-tablet tin	240	0.1			118.1	0.24
1 lozenge, approx. 2.4 grams			10.0	0.02	118.1	0.24
Sore Throat Lozenges, 24-tablet tin	240	0.1			118.1	0.24
1 lozenge, approx. 2.4 grams			10.0	0.02	118.1	0.24

36 PET FOODS •

	UNIT		1 OZ., BY WT.	
	Cal.	Carb.	Cal.	Carb.
CATS				
Cadillac				
Chicken Dinner, 14½-oz. can	469	1.5	32.3	0.10
Chicken & Fish, 14½-oz. can	489	0.5	33.8	0.03
Chicken & Liver, 14½-oz. can	448	2.3	30.9	0.16
"6 in 1," 14½-oz. can	448	2.5	30.9	0.17
Figaro				
Tuna, 6-oz. can	200	2.0	33.3	0.33
Kal Kan				
Beef & Heart Dinner, 6½-oz. can	221	6.8	34.0	1.04
Bits O'Beef Dinner, 6½-oz. can	221	6.8	34.0	1.04
Bits O'Kidney, 6½-oz. can	221	6.8	34.0	1.04
Kidney 'n Tuna Platter, 6½-oz. can	221	6.8	34.0	1.04
Kitty Stew, 6½-oz. can	221	6.8	34.0	1.04
Liver 'n Beef, 6½-oz. can	221	6.8	34.0	1.04
Mealtime, 6½-oz. can	221	6.8	34.0	1.04
Moist & Tender Bits, 6½-oz. can	221	6.8	34.0	1.04
Pick of the Ocean, 6½-oz. can	221	6.8	34.0	1.04
Poultry Dinner, 6½-oz. can	221	6.8	34.0	1.04
Seaside Supper, 6½-oz. can	221	6.8	34.0	1.04
Simmered Supper, 6½-oz. can	221	6.8	34.0	1.04
Tuna, 6½-oz. can	221	6.8	34.0	1.04
Tuna 'n Chicken with Sauce, 6½-oz. can	221	6.8	34.0	1.04
Purina				
Chef's Delight, 6½-oz. can	200	1.8	30.8	0.28
Chicken, 6½-oz. can	240	1.8	26.9	0.28
Chicken & Kidney, 6½-oz. can	230	1.8	35.4	0.28
Chicken & Liver, 6½-oz. can	220	1.8	33.8	0.28
Country Dinner, 6½-oz. can	200	1.8	30.8	0.28
Fish & Liver, 6½-oz. can	200	1.8	30.8	0.28
Fish & Shrimp, 6½-oz. can	200	1.8	30.8	0.28
Hearty Feast, 6½-oz. can	200	1.8	30.8	0.28
Kidney, 6½-oz. can	180	1.8	27.7	0.28
Liver, 6½-oz. can	180	1.8	27.7	0.28
Mackerel, 6½-oz. can	200	1.8	30.8	0.28
Sardines, 6½-oz. can	240	1.8	36.9	0.28
Southern Style, 6½-oz. can	240	1.8	36.9	0.28
Super Stew, 6½-oz. can	180	1.8	27.7	0.28
Tasty Treat, 6½-oz. can	200	1.8	30.8	0.28
Tender Meat By-Products, 6½-oz. can	220	1.8	33.8	0.28
Tuna, 6-oz. can	185	1.8	28.5	0.28
Tuna & Chicken, 6½-oz. can	200	1.8	30.8	0.28
Tuna & Egg, 6½-oz. can	200	1.8	30.8	0.28
Turkey & Giblets, 6½-oz. can	220	1.8	33.8	0.28
Lovin' Spoonfuls:				
Beef Dish, 12½-oz. can	390	3.6	31.2	0.28
Beef, Bacon & Cheese Dish, 6½-oz. can	220	1.8	33.8	0.28

	UNIT		1 OZ., BY WT.	
	Cal.	Carb.	Cal.	Carb.
Chicken Dish, 12½-oz. can	350	3.5	28.0	0.28
Chicken & Liver Dish, 12½-oz. can	350	3.5	28.0	0.28
Kidney Dish, 12½-oz. can	310	3.5	24.8	0.28
Liver Dish, 12½-oz. can	390	3.5	31.2	0.28
Savory Combo, 6½-oz. can	200	1.8	30.8	0.28
Seafare Supper, 6½-oz. can	180	1.8	27.7	0.28
Tuna, 6½-oz. can	200	1.8	30.8	0.28
Tuna Dish, 12½-oz. can	310	3.5	24.8	0.28
Tender Vittles:				
Beef, Chicken, Liver & Seafood Flavor, box of eight 1½-oz. packets	1000	(81.6)	83.3	(6.80)
1 1½-oz. packet	125	(10.2)	83.3	(6.80)
Gourmet Flavor, box of eight 1½-oz. packets	1000	(81.6)	83.3	(6.80)
1 1½-oz. packet	125	(10.2)	83.3	(6.80)
Cat Chow, Country Blend, 22-oz. box	(1971)	(221.3)	(89.6)	(10.06)
1 cup (approx. 3.3 oz.)	(300)	(33.2)	(89.6)	(10.06)
Cat Chow, Original Blend, 22-oz. box	(1971)	(221.3)	(89.6)	(10.06)
1 cup (approx. 3.3 oz.)	(300)	(33.2)	(89.6)	(10.06)
Kitten Chow, 18-oz. box	(1613)	(153.2)	(89.6)	(8.51)
1 cup (approx. 3.3 oz.)	(300)	(28.5)	(89.6)	(8.51)
Meow Mix, Seafood Blend, 22-oz. box	(1971)	(221.3)	(89.6)	(1.06)
1 cup (approx. 3.3 oz.)	(300)	(33.2)	(89.6)	(10.06)
Meow Mix, Tuna, Chicken & Liver Flavor, 18-oz. box	(1424)	(178.4)	(79.1)	(9.91)
1 cup (approx. 3.3 oz.)	(300)	(33.2)	(89.6)	(1.06)
Special Dinners, 18-oz. box	(1531)	(181.1)	(85.1)	(10.01)
1 cup (approx. 3.3 oz.)	(285)	(33.2)	(85.1)	(10.01)
Thrive, 22-oz. box	(1971)	(221.3)	(89.6)	(10.06)
1 cup (approx. 3.3 oz.)	(300)	(33.2)	(89.6)	(10.06)
Whisker Lickin's, box of four 1½-oz. packets	500	42.5	83.3	7.09
1 1½-oz. packet	125	10.6	83.3	7.09
Skippy				
Canned Dog Food for Dogs & Cats, 15-oz. can	378	51.0	25.1	3.50
Dog & Cat Food, 15-oz. can	378	51.0	25.1	3.50
Pet Stew for Dogs & Cats, 14-oz. can	392	39.7	28.0	2.80
DOGS				
Alpo				
Beef Chunks Dinner, 14½-oz. can	440	11.4	30.3	0.79
23¾-oz. can	712	18.6	30.3	0.79
Beef Dinner, 23½-oz. can	712	18.6	30.3	0.79
Beef & Liver Dinner, 14½-oz. can	425	10.9	29.3	0.75
Beef Stew, 14½-oz. can	380	20.5	26.2	1.41
23¾-oz. can	616	33.1	26.2	1.41
Chicken Dinner, 14½-oz. can	560	6.3	38.6	0.43
23¾-oz. can	916	10.2	38.6	0.43
Chicken & Liver Dinner, 14½-oz. can	495	9.4	34.1	0.65
Chopped Beef Dinner, 14½-oz. can	450	9.9	31.0	0.68
Chopped Horsemeat Dinner, 14½-oz. can	400	9.4	27.6	0.65
Chopped Rib of Veal Dinner, 14½-oz. can	450	12.6	31.0	0.87

	UNIT		1 OZ., BY WT.	
	Cal.	Carb.	Cal.	Carb.
Eggs 'N Beef Dinner, 14½-oz. can	435	21.8	30.6	1.50
Horsemeat Chunks Dinner, 14½-oz. can	445	12.9	30.7	0.86
Lamb Chunks Dinner, 14½-oz. can	445	11.3	30.7	0.78
Liver Chunks Dinner, 14½-oz. can	440	13.8	30.3	0.95
Liver Dinner, 23½-oz. can	712	22.3	30.3	0.95
23¾-oz. can	719	23.0	30.3	0.95
Trio Dinner, 14½-oz. can	560	11.8	38.6	0.81
23½-oz. can	907	19.0	38.6	0.81
Cadillac				
Beef Dinner, 14½-oz. can	428	3.5	29.5	0.24
Chicken Dinner, 14½-oz. can	487	1.5	33.6	0.10
Chicken & Liver, 14½-oz. can	469	1.5	32.3	0.10
"5 in 1," 14½-oz. can	448	2.5	30.9	0.17
Home Style Stew, 14½-oz. can	448	2.5	30.9	0.17
Horsemeat & Meat, 14½-oz. can	428	3.5	29.5	0.24
Lamb & Meat By-Products, 14½-oz. can	428	3.5	29.5	0.24
Liver, Bacon & Egg, 14½-oz. can	428	3.5	29.5	0.24
Liver & Meat, 14½-oz. can	428	3.5	29.5	0.24
Puppy Meat, 14½-oz. can	448	2.5	30.9	0.17
Turkey Dinner, 14½-oz. can	448	2.5	30.9	0.17
French's Dog "Treats"				
Doggie Donuts, 4½-oz. box (approx. 42 donuts)	(585)		(130.0)	
1 donut, approx. 0.11 oz.	(14)		(130.0)	
People Crackers, 4¼-oz. box (approx. 46 crackers)	(382)		(90.0)	
1 person, approx. 0.09 oz.	(8)		(90.0)	
Say Cheese, 6½-oz. box (approx. 47 crackers)	(520)		(80.0)	
1 cracker, approx. 0.14 oz.	(11)		(80.0)	
Gaines				
CANNED:				
Cycle 1, Moist, 14-oz. can	638		45.5	
Cycle 2, Moist, 14-oz. can	602		43.0	
Cycle 3, Moist, 14-oz. can	516		36.0	
Cycle 4, Moist, 14-oz. can	555		39.0	
DRY:				
Cycle 1, 5-lb. bag	10135		126.0	
1 cup (approx. 3 oz.)	380		126.0	
1 pound (approx. 5⅓ cups)	2027		126.0	
Cycle 2, 5-lb. bag	9575		119.0	
1 cup (approx. 3 oz.)	359		119.0	
1 pound (approx. 5⅓ cups)	1915		119.0	
Cycle 3, 5-lb. bag	9545		119.0	
1 cup (approx. 3 oz.)	358		119.0	
1 pound (approx. 5⅓ cups)	1909		119.0	
Cycle 4, 5-lb. bag	9440		118.0	
1 cup (approx. 3 oz.)	356		118.0	
1 pound (approx. 5⅓ cups)	1888		118.0	
Gaines Burgers				
Regular Flavor, 12-burger package (36 oz.)	3672		102.0	
1 burger, approx. 3 oz.	306		102.0	
Bacon & Egg Flavor, 12-burger package (36 oz.)	3672		102.0	
1 burger, approx. 3 oz.	306		102.0	
Cheese Flavor, 12-burger package (36 oz.)	3672		102.0	
1 burger, approx. 3 oz.	306		102.0	
Gaines Meal, 5-lb. box	9865		123.0	
1 cup (approx. 3 oz.)	370		123.0	
1 pound (approx. 5⅓ cups)	1973		123.0	
Gravy Train, 5-lb. box	10050		125.0	
1 cup (approx. 3 oz.)	377		125.0	
1 pound (approx. 5⅓ cups)	2010		125.0	
Prime, 36-oz. package (containing 6 6-oz. packets)	3672		102.0	
1 6-oz. packet	612		102.0	
Prime Variety, 36-oz. package (containing 6 6-oz. packets)	3672		102.0	
1 6-oz. packet	612		102.0	
Puppy Choice, 36-oz. package (containing 6 6-oz. packets)	3732		103.0	
1 6-oz. packet	622		103.0	
Top Choice				
Regular Flavor, 36-oz. package (containing 6 6-oz. packets)	3504		97.0	
1 6-oz. packet	584		97.0	
Egg & Cheese Flavors, 36-oz. package (containing 6 6-oz. packets)	3504		97.0	
1 6-oz. packet	584		97.0	
Liver & Bacon Flavors, 36-oz. package (containing 6 6-oz. packets)	3504		97.0	
1 6-oz. packet	584		97.0	
Hills				
Prescription Diet:				
d/d (Allergy), 15¾-oz. can	595	51.3	37.8	3.26
p/d (Growth/Recovery), 15¾-oz. can	660	43.2	42.0	2.74
h/d (Heart), 15¾-oz. can	635	51.6	40.3	3.28
i/d (Intestinal), 15¾-oz. can	560	60.0	35.5	3.81
k/d (Kidney), 15¾-oz. can	660	53.5	42.0	3.40
r/d (Reducing), 15¾-oz. can	330	36.9	21.0	2.34
Science Diet:				
Growth, 25-pound bag	(72000)	(6600.0)	(180.0)	(16.50)
1 cup (approx. 2 oz.)	(360)	(33.0)	(180.0)	(16.50)
Lactation, 25-pound bag	(74000)	(6700.0)	(185.0)	(16.75)
1 cup (approx. 2 oz.)	(370)	(33.5)	(185.0)	(16.75)
Maintenance, 25-pound bag	(66000)	(7200.0)	(165.0)	(18.00)
1 cup (approx. 2 oz.)	(330)	(36.0)	(165.0)	(18.00)
Maximum Stress, 25-pound bag	(116000)	(6180.0)	(290.0)	(15.45)
1 cup (approx. 2 oz.)	(580)	(30.9)	(290.0)	(15.45)
Performance, 25-pound bag	(122000)	(5940.0)	(305.0)	(14.85)
1 cup (approx. 2 oz.)	(610)	(29.7)	(305.0)	(14.85)
Kal-Kan				
CANNED:				
Chunky Beef Dinner, 14-oz. can	405	17.9	25.3	1.12
Chunky Meat Stew, 14-oz. can	405	17.9	25.3	1.12
Horsemeat & Beef, 14-oz. can	405	17.9	25.3	1.12
M.P.S., 14-oz. can	405	17.9	25.3	1.12
Thoro-Fed, 14-oz. can	405	17.9	25.3	1.12
DRY:				
Crave, 7-lb. bag	23352	2968.0	208.5	26.50
1 cup (approx. 3½-oz.)	730	93.0	208.5	26.50
1 pound (approx. 4.6 cups)	3340	424.0	208.5	26.50
Mealtime Small Crunchy Bites, 5-lb. bag	19680	2928.0	246.0	36.30
1 cup (approx. 3 oz.)	738	109.0	246.0	36.30
1 pound (approx. 5⅓ cups)	3936	585.6	246.0	36.30
Mealtime Large Crunchy Bites, 5-lb. bag	19680	2928.0	246.0	36.30
1 cup (approx. 3 oz.)	738	109.0	246.0	36.30
1 pound (approx. 5⅓ cups)	3936	585.6	246.0	36.30
Purina				
Chuck Wagon, 5-lb. bag	7500	36.4	93.8	0.46
1 cup (approx. 2.9 oz.)	275	1.4	93.8	0.46
1 pound (approx. 5½ cups)	1500	7.3	93.8	0.46
Recommended daily feeding portion for a 35-pound dog: 4 cups (approx. 11.7 oz.)	1100	5.4	93.8	0.46
Dog Chow, 5-lb. bag	8000	36.4	100.0	0.46
1 cup (approx. 3 oz.)	300	1.4	100.0	0.46
1 pound (approx. 5⅓ cups)	1600	7.3	100.0	0.46
Recommended daily feeding portion for a 35-pound dog: 4 cups (approx. 12 oz.)	1200	5.5	100.0	0.46
Field 'n Farm, 5-lb. bag	8000	36.4	100.0	0.46
1 cup (approx. 3.4 oz.)	340	1.6	100.0	0.46
1 pound (approx. 4.7 cups)	1600	7.3	100.0	0.46
Recommended daily feeding portion for a 35-pound dog: 4 cups (approx. 13.6 oz.)	1360	6.3	100.0	0.46
Fit & Trim, 5-lb. bag	7000	38.4	87.5	0.48
1 cup (approx. 3 oz.)	263	1.4	87.5	0.48
1 pound (approx. 5⅓ cups)	1400	7.7	87.5	0.48
Recommended daily feeding portion for a 35-pound dog: 4 cups (approx. 12 oz.)	1052	5.8	87.5	0.48
High Protein Dog Meal, 5-lb. bag	8250	32.0	103.0	0.40
1 cup (approx. 4.1 oz.)	425	1.7	103.0	0.40
1 pound (approx. 3.9 cups)	1650	6.4	103.0	0.40
Recommended daily feeding portion for a 35-pound dog: 4 cups (approx. 16.5 oz.)	1700	6.6	103.0	0.40
Lab Canine Diet, 1 pound	1995	193.3	124.7	12.08
Puppy Chow, 5-lb. bag	8000	30.4	100.0	0.36
1 pound	1600	6.1	100.0	0.38
Skippy				
Beef & Cheese Flavored Dog Food, 15-oz. can	378	51.0	25.1	3.50
Beef Flavored Dog Food, 15-oz. can	378	51.0	25.1	3.50
Canned Dog Food for Dogs & Cats, 15-oz. can	378	51.0	25.1	3.50
Chicken Flavored Dog Food, 15-oz. can	378	51.0	25.1	3.50
Dog & Cat Food, 15-oz. can	378	51.0	25.1	3.50
Liver Flavored Dog Food, 15-oz. can	378	51.0	25.1	3.50
Pet Stew for Dogs & Cats, 14-oz. can	392	39.7	28.0	2.80
"7 in 1" Variety Dinner Dog Food, 15-oz. can	378	51.0	25.1	3.50
Vegetables & Beef Flavored Dog Food, 15-oz. can	378	51.0	25.1	3.50
Premium:				
Beef & Chicken Dinner for Dogs, 14½-oz. can	420	41.1	28.9	2.30
Burgers with Cheese Flavored Chunks for Dogs, 14½-oz. can	420	41.1	28.9	2.80
Chunky Beef Dinner for Dogs, 14½-oz. can	420	41.1	28.9	2.80
Chunky Liver & Meat By-Products Dinner for Dogs, 14½-oz. can	420	41.1	28.9	2.80
Chunky Stew for Dogs, 14½-oz. can	380	51.0	26.2	3.40
Picnic Dinner (Burgers and Frank Style Chunks) for Dogs, 14½-oz. can	420	41.1	28.9	2.80
"3 in 1" Dinner made with Chicken, Beef & Liver for Dogs, 14½-oz. can	420	41.1	28.9	2.80

	UNIT Cal.	UNIT Carb.	1 OZ., BY WT. Cal.	1 OZ., BY WT. Carb.
BEARS				
Hill's				
Zu-Preem Omnivore Diet, Dry (for all bears except polar bears), 25-lb. bag	42600	3412.5	106.5	8.53
1 pound	1704	136.5	106.5	8.53
BIG CATS: Bobcats, Jaguars, Leopards, Lions, Ocelots, Panthers, Pumas, Tigers, etc.				
Hill's				
Zu-Preem Feline Diet (for non-domestic carnivores in the family Felidae, e.g., bobcats, jaguars, leopards, lions, ocelots, panthers, pumas, tigers), 14-oz. can	961	10.3	68.7	0.74
1 pound	1100	11.8	68.7	0.74
CHICKENS				
Purina				
Cage Layer Chow, 1 pound	1300	243.2	81.2	15.20
Recommended daily feeding portion ranges from 3.9 oz. to 8.8 oz., depending on body weight and temperature:				
3.9 oz.	316	59.2	81.2	15.20
8.8 oz.	714	133.8	81.2	15.20
Chick Chow, 1 pound	1300	234.1	81.2	14.63
Recommended daily feeding portion ranges from 3.9 oz. to 8.8 oz., depending on body weight and temperature:				
3.9 oz.	316	57.0	81.2	14.63
8.8 oz.	714	128.7	81.2	14.63
HYENAS, WOLVES, COYOTES, DINGOS, etc.				
Hill's				
Zu-Preem Feline Diet (for non-domestic carnivores in the family Hyaenidae), 14-oz. can	961	10.3	68.7	0.74
1 pound	1100	11.8	68.7	0.74
RATITE BIRDS: Ostriches, Emus, Cassowaries, and Rheas				
Hill's				
Zu-Preem Ratite Diet (for growing and adult ratite birds), 50-lb. bag	71500	10000.0	89.4	12.50
1 pound	1430	200.0	89.4	12.50
PRIMATES: Chimpanzees, Marmosets, Tamarins, Monkeys, etc.				
Hill's				
Zu-Preem Marmoset Diet (for marmosets and tamarins), 15½-oz. can	764	111.7	49.3	7.21
1 pound	790	115.3	49.3	7.21
Zu-Preem Primate Diet (for growing and mature primates), 20-lb. bag	35720	3340.0	111.6	10.44
1 pound	1786	167.0	111.6	10.44
Zu-Preem Primate Diet, Canned (for all primates except marmosets and tamarins), 15½-oz. can	750	110.2	48.4	7.11
1 pound	775	113.7	48.4	7.11

	UNIT Cal.	UNIT Carb.	1 OZ., BY WT. Cal.	1 OZ., BY WT. Carb.
Purina				
Monkey Chow, 1 pound	1896	282.1	118.5	17.63
Recommended daily feeding portion ranges from 5 oz. for a 10-lb. monkey to 15 oz. for a 30-lb. monkey depending on species, activity level, body weight and temperature:				
5 oz.	592	88.1	118.5	17.63
15 oz.	1777	264.4	118.5	17.63
Monkey Chow, High Protein, 1 pound	1906	233.1	119.1	14.57
Recommended daily feeding portion ranges from 5 oz. for a 10-lb. monkey to 15 oz. for a 30-lb. monkey depending on species, activity level, body weight and temperature:				
5 oz.	595	72.8	119.1	14.57
15 oz.	1786	218.5	119.1	14.57
RABBITS				
Purina				
Rabbit Chow, 1 pound	1808	235.8	113.0	14.74
Recommended daily feeding portion ranges from 3.9 oz. to 8.8 oz. depending on species and size:				
3.9 oz.	441	57.4	113.0	14.74
8.8 oz.	994	129.7	113.0	14.74
Rabbit Chow, High Fiber, 1 pound	1770	192.2	110.6	12.01
Recommended daily feeding portion ranges from 3.9 oz. to 8.8 oz. depending on species and size:				
3.9 oz.	431	46.8	110.6	12.01
8.8 oz.	973	105.6	110.6	12.01
RODENTS: Guinea Pigs, Hamsters, Mice, and Rats				
Purina				
Formulab Chow (for rats, hamsters and many mouse strains), 1 pound	1906	224.0	119.1	14.00
Recommended daily feeding portion ranges from 0.14 oz. to 0.53 oz. depending on species, body weight and temperature:				
0.14 oz.	16	1.9	119.1	14.00
0.53 oz.	63	7.4	119.1	14.00
Guinea Pig Chow, 1 pound	1906	215.5	119.1	13.47
Recommended daily feeding portion: 1.2 oz.	142	16.1	119.1	13.47
Mouse Chow, 1 pound	1958	244.5	122.4	15.28
Recommended daily feeding portion ranges from 0.14 oz. to 0.18 oz. depending on body weight and temperature:				
0.14 oz.	17	2.1	122.4	15.28
0.18 oz.	22	2.7	122.4	15.28
Rat Chow, 1 pound	1886	240.0	117.9	15.00
Recommended daily feeding portion ranges from 0.4 oz. to 0.5 oz. depending on species and size:				
0.4 oz.	49	6.3	117.9	15.00
0.5 oz.	62	7.9	117.9	15.00
Rodent Chow, 1 pound	1928	225.9	120.5	14.12
Recommended daily feeding portion ranges from 0.14 oz. to 0.53 oz. depending on species and size:				
0.14 oz.	16	1.9	120.5	14.12
0.53 oz.	64	7.4	120.5	14.12

37 FAST FOOD •

ARBY'S

	UNIT Cal.	UNIT Carb.	1 OZ., BY WT. Cal.	1 OZ., BY WT. Carb.
SANDWICHES				
Ham & Cheese, approx. 5½ oz.	380	33.6	69.1	6.00
Roast Beef, Regular, approx. 5 oz.	350	32.0	70.0	6.40
Roast Beef, Junior, approx. 3 oz.	220	21.0	73.3	7.00
Roast Beef, Super, approx. 9¾ oz.	620	61.0	63.6	6.26
Turkey De Luxe, approx. 6 oz.	510	46.0	85.0	7.61

ARTHUR TREACHER'S FISH & CHIPS

	UNIT Cal.	UNIT Carb.	1 OZ., BY WT. Cal.	1 OZ., BY WT. Carb.
FISH AND SEAFOOD PLATTERS				
Cabin Boy, approx. 13.5 oz. Components and their approximate weights: same as for "Fish Sandwich," plus chips (3 oz.), 2 hush puppies (2 oz.), cole slaw (3 oz.), parsley	(1040)	(97.4)	(77.2)	(7.21)
Captain, approx. 13.2 oz. Components and their approximate weights: same as for "Original Fish Fillet," plus cole slaw (3 oz.)	(957)	(83.4)	(72.5)	(6.32)
Family Boat, approx. 25.6 oz. Components and their approximate weights: 6 fish fillets (15.6 oz.), chips (10 oz.)	1755	163.5	68.6	6.39
Fish Sandwich, approx. 5.5 oz. Components and their approximate weights: 1 fish fillet (2.6 oz.), toasted bun (1.4 oz.), cheese (1 oz.), tartar sauce (½ oz.)	440	39.4	80.0	7.16
Fish & Shrimp Platter, approx. 12.4 oz. Components and their approximate weights: 1 fish fillet (2.6 oz.), 3 shrimps (1¾ oz.), chips (3 oz.), 2 hush puppies (2 oz.), cole slaw (3 oz.), parsley	(667)	(47.3)	(53.8)	(3.81)
Mate, approx. 15.8 oz. Components and their approximate weights: same as for "Original Fish Fillet," plus 1 additional fish fillet (2.6 oz., total 7.8 oz. fish) and cole slaw (3 oz.)	(1135)	(96.1)	(71.8)	(6.08)
Original Fish Fillet, approx. 10.2 oz. Components and their approximate weights: 2 fish fillets (2.6 oz. each), chips (3 oz.), 2 hush puppies (2 oz.), parsley	(834)	(72.3)	(81.8)	(7.05)
Party Boat, approx. 33.4 oz. Components and their approximate weights: 9 fish fillets (23.4 oz.), chips (10 oz.)	2288	201.6	68.5	6.04
Shrimp Boat, approx. 18.7 oz. Components and their approximate weights: 15 shrimps (8.7 oz.), chips (10 oz.)	1506	145.5	80.5	7.78
Shrimp & Chips, approx. 9.1 oz. Components and their approximate weights: 7 shrimp (4.06 oz.), chips (3 oz.), 2 hush puppies (2 oz.), parsley	(860)	(74.1)	(94.5)	(8.14)
Shrimp Platter, approx. 7.4 oz. Components and their approximate weights: same as for "Shrimp & Chips," except 4 shrimp (2⅓ oz.) instead of 7	697	62.4	94.2	8.43
Trawler, approx. 26 oz. Components and their approximate weights: 10 fish fillets (26 oz.)	1775	127.0	68.3	4.88
CHICKEN PLATTERS				
Chicken Basket, approx. 21.6 oz. Components and their approximate weights: 9 chicken fillets (21.6 oz.)	1661	74.3	76.9	3.44
Chicken Boat, approx. 24.4 oz. Components and their approximate weights: 6 chicken fillets (14.4 oz.), chips (10 oz.)	1797	136.8	73.6	5.61
Chicken & Chips, approx. 7.8 oz. Components and their approximate weights: 2 chicken fillets (4.8 oz.), chips (3 oz.), parsley	620	70.2	8.0	9.00
Chicken Sandwich, approx. 5.5 oz. Components and their approximate weights: 1 chicken fillet (2.4 oz.), toasted bun (1.4 oz.), cole slaw (1 oz.), Russian dressing (0.7 oz.)	413	44.0	75.1	8.00
HOT DOG PLATTERS				
Krunch Pup, approx. 2 oz. Components and their approximate weights: 1 batter-dipped hot dog (2 oz.), parsley	203	12.0	101.5	6.00
Krunch Pup & Chips, approx. 5 oz. Components and their approximate weights: same as for "Krunch Pup," plus chips (3 oz.)	410	38.2	82.0	7.64
COMBINATION PLATTERS				
Family Sampler, approx. 26 oz. Components and their approximate weights: 2 fish fillets (5.2 oz.), 2 chicken fillets (4.8 oz.), 2 shrimps (4.06 oz.), 1 krunch pup (2 oz.), chips (10 oz.)	(1998)	(156.4)	(76.8)	(6.02)
SIDE ORDERS				
Chips, approx. 3 oz.	207	26.7	69.0	8.75
DESSERTS				
Lemon Luv (lemon-filled pie), approx. 3 oz.	276	35.1	92.0	11.70

BASKIN-ROBBINS

	UNIT Cal.	UNIT Carb.	1 OZ., BY WT. Cal.	1 OZ., BY WT. Carb.
ICE CREAM				
Chocolate, 1 scoop (approx. 2.5 oz.)	165	20.4	66.0	8.16
Chocolate Fudge, 1 scoop (approx. 2.5 oz.)	178	21.5	71.7	8.52
French Vanilla, 1 scoop (approx. 2.5 oz.)	181	15.9	72.4	6.36
Pralines 'n Cream, 1 scoop (approx. 2.5 oz.)	177	23.7	70.8	9.48
Strawberry, 1 scoop (approx. 2.5 oz.)	141	15.6	56.4	6.24
Vanilla, 1 scoop (approx. 2.5 oz.)	147	15.8	58.8	6.24
OTHER FROZEN DESSERTS				
Daiquiri Ice, 1 scoop (approx. 2.5 oz.)	84	20.9	33.6	8.36
Orange Sherbet, 1 scoop (approx. 2.5 oz.)	99	20.9	39.6	8.36

BURGER CHEF

The weights of most servings were not available.

	UNIT Cal.	UNIT Carb.	1 OZ., BY WT. Cal.	1 OZ., BY WT. Carb.
HAMBURGERS				
Big Shef	569	38.1		

	UNIT Cal.	UNIT Carb.	1 OZ., BY WT. Cal.	1 OZ., BY WT. Carb.
Cheeseburger	290	29.3		
Double Cheeseburger	420	29.5		
Hamburger	244	29.1		
Super Shef	563	44.3		
Top Shef	661	36.4		
OTHER SANDWICHES				
Bacon Sunrise, approx. 4⅔ oz.	437		93.6	
Biscuit & Sausage, approx. 4⅔ oz.	530		113.5	
Chicken Club Sandwich	539			
Fish Filet	547	45.6		
Sausage Sunrise	652			
PLATTERS				
Bacon Platter	582			
2 small grade A eggs, 3 strips bacon, approx. 2 oz. hash browns, 2 slices white bread lightly brushed with margarine				
Mariner Platter	734	78.3		
Rancher Platter	640	33.1		
Sausage Platter	764			
2 small grade A eggs, approx. 2⅔ oz. sausage, approx. 2 oz. hash browns, 2 slices of white bread lightly brushed with margarine				
SIDE ORDERS				
Fries, Regular, approx. 2½ oz.	250	19.9	100.1	7.95
Fries, Large, approx. 3½ oz.	351	27.8	100.1	7.95
Hash Rounds, approx. 2 oz.	189		94.5	
Salad (Lettuce and Carrots)	18	4.1		
DESSERT				
Donut	185			
COLD DRINKS				
Chocolate Shake, approx. 12-oz. (by weight) cup	401	72.0	33.4	6.00
Orange Juice, approx. 7-oz. (by weight) cup	96		13.7	
approx. 12-oz. (by weight) cup	165		13.7	
Vanilla Shake, approx. 12-oz. (by weight) cup	380	60.4	31.7	5.03

BURGER KING

	UNIT Cal.	UNIT Carb.	1 OZ., BY WT. Cal.	1 OZ., BY WT. Carb.
HAMBURGERS				
Hamburger, approx. 4.1 oz.	310	30.0	75.8	7.33
Hamburger with Cheese, approx. 4.6 oz.	360	31.0	78.4	6.75
Hamburger, Double Meat, approx. 5.6 oz.	440	32.0	78.7	5.72
Hamburger with Cheese, Double Meat, approx. 6.6 oz.	540	33.0	81.9	5.01
Whopper, approx. 9.4 oz.	680	51.0	72.0	5.40
Whopper with Cheese, approx. 10.4 oz.	760	54.0	72.8	5.17
Whopper, Double Beef, approx. 12 oz.	850	54.0	70.8	4.50
Whopper with Cheese, Double Beef, approx. 13 oz.	970	55.0	74.6	4.23
Whopper Jr., approx. 5.0 oz.	360	31.0	71.6	6.76
Whopper Jr. with Cheese, approx. 5.5 oz.	420	32.0	75.9	5.79
Whopper Jr., Double Meat, approx. 6.5 oz.	490	32.0	75.0	4.90
Whopper Jr. with Cheese, Double Meat, approx. 7.0 oz.	550	33.0	78.2	4.69
OTHER SANDWICHES				
Steak Sandwich, approx. 8.6 oz.	600	64.0	69.8	7.44
Whaler, approx. 8.7 oz.	660	54.0	76.3	6.24
Whaler with Cheese, approx. 9.7 oz.	770	55.0	79.8	5.70
SIDE ORDERS				
French Fries, Regular, approx. 2¾ oz.	240	28.0	87.3	10.18
French Fries, Large, approx. 4⅛ oz.	360	42.0	87.3	10.18
Onion Rings, Regular, approx. 2¼ oz.	230	24.0	102.2	10.67
Onion Rings, Large, approx. 3⅜ oz.	330	36.0	97.8	10.67
COLD DRINKS				
Chocolate Milk Shake, approx. 10½-oz. (by weight) cup	380	62.0	36.2	5.80
Vanilla Milk Shake, approx. 10½-oz. (by weight) cup	360	55.0	34.3	5.24
DESSERT				
Apple Pie, approx. 3 oz.	240	32.0	80.0	10.87

CARL'S JR.

	UNIT Cal.	UNIT Carb.	1 OZ., BY WT. Cal.	1 OZ., BY WT. Carb.
HAMBURGERS				
Famous Star, approx. 10.1 oz.				
Components and their approximate weights: patty (3.6 oz. raw, 3 oz. cooked), bun (2½ oz.), lettuce (¼ oz.), 2 tomato slices (1.1 oz.), fresh onion (½ oz.), 3 dill pickle chips (½ oz.), mayonnaise (⅝ oz.), special sauce (⅝ oz.)	480	35.0	47.5	3.47
Famous Star with Cheese, approx. 10.6 oz.				
Components and their approximate weights: same as for "Famous Star," plus 1 slice American process cheese (0.44 oz.)	520	36.0	49.3	3.41
Happy Star, approx. 4½ oz.				
Components and their approximate weights: patty (2 oz. raw, 1⅔ oz. cooked), bun (2 oz.), 2 dill pickle chips (⅓ oz.), catsup (½ oz.)	290	31.0	64.4	6.89
Old Time Star, approx. 7¾ oz.				
Components and their approximate weights: patty (3.6 oz. raw, 3 oz. cooked), bun (2½ oz.), fresh onion (½ oz.), 3 dill pickle chips (½ oz.), catsup (1 oz.)	440	42.0	56.8	5.42
Super Star, approx. 13.1 oz.				
Components and their approximate weights: same as for "Famous Star," plus 1 additional meat patty (3.6 oz. raw, 3 oz. cooked)	660	44.0	50.4	3.36
HOT DOGS				
Original Hot Dog, approx. 5.4 oz.				
Components and their approximate weights: frank (2 oz. raw, 1¾ oz. cooked), bun (2.33 oz.), 3 dill pickle chips (½ oz.), 2 tomato wedges (½ oz.), mustard (¼ oz.)	340	28.0	63.0	5.19
Chili Dog, approx. 5.9 oz.				
Components and their approximate weights: same as for "Original Hot Dog," plus chili (1¼ oz.), 1 chili pepper (⅛ to ¼ oz.)	360	34.0	61.0	5.76
Chili Cheese Dog, approx. 6.4 oz.				
Components and their approximate weights: same as for "Chili Dog," plus grated cheddar process cheese (6½ oz.)	400	36.0	62.5	5.63
OTHER SANDWICHES				
California Roast Beef Sandwich, approx. 7¼ oz.				
Components and their approximate weights: roast beef (2½ oz.), 1 slice Swiss process cheese (1½ oz.), bun (2½ oz.), 1 tomato slice (0.55 oz.), 1 whole Ortega green chili (¾ oz.)	380	43.0	52.4	5.93
Fish Fillet, approx. 8.3 oz.				
Components and their approximate weights: breaded fish (3 oz. uncooked), 1 slice American process cheese (0.44 oz.), bun (2½ oz.), lettuce (¼ oz.), 2 tomato slices (1.1 oz.), tartar sauce (1 oz.)	550	59.0	66.3	7.11
Steak Sandwich, approx. 12.1 oz.				
Components and their approximate weights: steak (4 oz. raw), bun (4 oz.), lettuce (½ oz.), 2 tomato slices (1.1 oz.), 2 fried onion rings (1¼ oz.), beef spread (½ oz.)	630	65.0	52.1	5.37
SALADS				
Salad, Regular, with Condiments, approx. 11 oz.	170	26.0	15.5	2.36
Blue Cheese Dressing, approx. 2 oz.	200	trace	100.0	trace
1000 Island Dressing, approx. 2 oz.	190	5.0	95.0	2.50
Lo-Cal Italian Dressing, approx. 2 oz.	48	1.0	24.0	0.50
SIDE ORDERS				
French Fries, Regular, approx. 3 oz.	220	33.0	73.3	11.00
French Fries, Large, approx. 4 oz.	(293)	(44.0)	(73.3)	(11.00)
Onion Rings, approx. 4 oz.	320	35.0	80.0	8.75
DESSERTS				
Apple Turnover, approx. 4 oz.	330	44.0	82.5	11.00
Carrot Cake, approx. 3 oz.	380	46.0	126.7	15.33
COLD DRINKS				
SHAKES:				
Chocolate, approx. 20 fl. oz. (approx. 10 oz. by weight)	(310)	(59.0)	(31.0)	(5.90)
Strawberry, approx. 20 fl. oz. (approx. 10 oz. by weight)	(310)	(59.0)	(31.0)	(5.90)
Vanilla, approx. 20 fl. oz. (approx. 10 oz. by weight)	(310)	(59.0)	(31.0)	(5.90)
SODA:				
Diet Pepsi, approx. 20-oz. (by weight) cup	0	0.0	0.0	0.00
Dr. Pepper, approx. 20-oz. (by weight) cup	(229)	(60.5)	(11.4)	(3.03)
Pepsi, approx. 20-oz. (by weight) cup	(241)	(60.7)	(12.1)	(3.04)
7-Up, approx. 20-oz. (by weight) cup	(219)	(55.2)	(11.0)	(2.76)

CARVEL

	UNIT Cal.	UNIT Carb.	1 OZ., BY WT. Cal.	1 OZ., BY WT. Carb.
ICE CREAM				
Chocolate, approx. 3 fl. oz.	147	16.8	55.9	6.34
Vanilla, approx. 3 fl. oz.	148	15.9	55.9	6.02
THINNY-THIN FROZEN DESSERT				
Chocolate, approx. 3 fl. oz.	56	10.4	30.9	5.82
Chocolate Mint, approx. 3 fl. oz.	56	10.4	30.9	5.82
Coffee, Strawberry & Mint, approx. 3 fl. oz.	56	10.2	30.9	5.68
Vanilla, approx. 3 fl. oz.	56	10.2	30.9	5.68
FROZEN YOGURT				
"Plain" Lo-Yo, approx. 3 fl. oz.	110	20.1	40.6	7.39
SHERBET				
Black Raspberry, approx. 3 fl. oz.	105	23.4	39.7	8.84
Blueberry, approx. 3 fl. oz.	105	23.4	39.7	8.84
Cherry, approx. 3 fl. oz.	105	23.4	39.7	8.84
Chocolate, approx. 3 fl. oz.	105	23.4	39.7	8.84
Guanabana, approx. 3 fl. oz.	105	23.4	39.7	8.84
Lemon, approx. 3 fl. oz.	105	23.4	39.7	8.84
Lime, approx. 3 fl. oz.	105	23.4	39.7	8.84
Mamey, approx. 3 fl. oz.	105	23.4	39.7	8.84
Mango, approx. 3 fl. oz.	105	23.4	39.7	8.84
Orange, approx. 3 fl. oz.	105	23.4	39.7	8.84
Orange-Pineapple, approx. 3 fl. oz.	105	23.4	39.7	8.84

	UNIT Cal.	UNIT Carb.	1 OZ., BY WT. Cal.	1 OZ., BY WT. Carb.
Peach, approx. 3 fl. oz.	105	23.4	39.7	8.84
Pineapple, approx. 3 fl. oz.	105	23.4	39.7	8.84
Strawberry, approx. 3 fl. oz.	105	23.4	39.7	8.84

DAIRY QUEEN

	UNIT Cal.	UNIT Carb.	1 OZ., BY WT. Cal.	1 OZ., BY WT. Carb.
HAMBURGERS				
Cooked weights were not available, but a loss of 15–35% can be expected after cooking.				
Cheeseburger, approx. 5.7 oz.	410	33.0	71.9	5.79
Double Cheeseburger, approx. 8.4 oz.	650	34.0	77.4	4.05
Triple Cheeseburger, approx. 10.6 oz.	820	34.0	77.4	3.21
Hamburger, Single, approx. 5.2 oz.	360	33.0	69.2	6.35
Double Hamburger, approx. 7.4 oz.	530	33.0	71.6	4.46
Triple Hamburger, approx. 9.6 oz.	710	33.0	74.0	3.44
HOT DOGS				
Hot Dog, approx. 3½ oz.	280	21.0	80.0	6.00
Hot Dog with Cheese, approx. 4.0 oz.	330	21.0	82.5	5.25
Hot Dog with Chili, approx. 4½ oz.	320	23.0	71.1	5.11
Super Hot Dog, approx. 6.2 oz.	520	44.0	83.9	7.10
Super Hot Dog with Chili, approx. 7.8 oz.	570	47.0	73.1	6.03
Super Hot Dog with Cheese, approx. 6.9 oz.	580	45.0	84.1	6.52
FISH SANDWICHES				
Fish Sandwich, approx. 6.0 oz.	400	41.0	66.7	6.83
Fish Sandwich with Cheese, approx. 6¼ oz.	440	39.0	71.0	6.24
SIDE ORDERS				
French Fries, approx. 2½ oz.	200	25.0	80.0	10.00
French Fries, Large, approx. 4.0 oz.	320	40.0	80.0	10.00
Onion Rings, approx. 3.0 oz.	280	31.0	93.3	10.33
ICE CREAM and OTHER DESSERTS				
Banana Split, approx. 13½ oz.	540	103.0	40.0	7.63
Buster Bar, approx. 5.3 oz.	460	41.0	86.8	7.74
Dilly Bar, approx. 3 oz.	210	21.0	70.0	7.00
Double Delight, approx. 9.0 oz.	490	69.0	54.4	7.67
DQ Sandwich, approx. 2⅛ oz.	140	24.0	66.0	11.32
Fiesta Sundae, approx. 9.5 oz.	570	84.0	60.0	8.84
Freeze, approx. 14.0 oz.	500	89.0	35.7	6.36
Hot Fudge "Brownie Delight," approx. 9.4 oz.	600	85.0	63.8	9.04
CONES:				
Small, approx. 2½ oz.	117	18.3	46.7	7.33
Regular, approx. 5.0 oz.	240	38.0	48.0	7.60
Large, approx. 7½ oz.	340	57.0	45.3	7.60
CONES, DIPPED IN CHOCOLATE:				
Small, approx. 2¾ oz.	163	21.5	59.4	7.81
Regular, approx. 5½ oz.	340	42.0	61.8	7.64
Large, approx. 8¼ oz.	510	64.0	61.4	7.71
MALTS, CHOCOLATE:				
Small, approx. 10¼ oz.	520	91.0	50.5	8.83
Regular, approx. 14¾ oz.	760	134.0	51.7	9.12
Large, approx. 20¾ oz.	1060	187.0	51.2	9.03
MR. MISTY				
Mr. Misty Float, approx. 14½ oz.	390	74.0	26.9	5.10
Mr. Misty Freeze, approx. 14½ oz.	500	91.0	34.5	6.28
Mr. Misty Kiss, approx. 3⅛ oz.	70	17.0	22.4	5.43
PARFAIT				
Parfait, approx. 10 oz.	430	76.0	43.0	7.60
Peanut Butter Parfait, approx. 10.8 oz.	740	94.0	68.5	8.70
SHAKES:				
Small, approx. 10.3 oz.	490	82.0	47.6	7.96
Regular, approx. 14.7 oz.	710	120.0	48.3	8.16
Large, approx. 20.7 oz.	990	168.0	47.8	8.12
Strawberry Shortcake Shake, approx. 11.0 oz.	540	100.0	49.1	9.09
SUNDAES, CHOCOLATE:				
Small, approx. 3¾ oz.	190	33.0	51.4	8.92
Regular, approx. 6¼ oz.	310	56.0	50.0	9.03
Large, approx. 8¾ oz.	440	78.0	50.6	8.97

DUNKIN' DONUTS

	UNIT Cal.	UNIT Carb.	1 OZ., BY WT. Cal.	1 OZ., BY WT. Carb.
DONUTS				
Honey Dip Glazed Donut, approx. 1.8 oz.	226	na	125.6	na

FRIENDLY'S

	UNIT Cal.	UNIT Carb.	1 OZ., BY WT. Cal.	1 OZ., BY WT. Carb.
HAMBURGERS				
Big Beef Cheeseburger, approx. 7.8 oz.	480	34.0	61.5	4.36
Big Beef Hamburger, approx. 7.3 oz.	420	33.0	57.5	4.52
Bounty Burger, approx. 12.2 oz.	570	40.0	46.7	3.28
Hamburger, approx. 4.4 oz.	260	29.0	59.1	6.59
OTHER SANDWICHES				
Fish, approx. 6 oz.	340	31.0	56.7	5.17
Ham & Cheese, approx. 5.9 oz.	400	26.0	67.8	4.41
Tuna Salad, approx. 5.8 oz.	320	32.0	55.2	5.52
SIDE ORDERS				
Cole Slaw, approx. 3 oz.	80	6.0	26.7	2.00
French Fries, approx. 2.5 oz.	125	16.0	50.0	6.40
BREAKFAST MENU				
Eggwich, approx. 2.7 oz.	260	27.0	96.3	10.00
Pancakes (information for unprepared mix only), approx. 0.9 oz.	110	16.0	122.2	17.18
DESSERTS				
FRIBBLES:				
Chocolate, approx. 11.7 oz.	420	73.0	39.9	6.24
Strawberry, approx. 11 oz.	470	86.0	42.7	7.82
Vanilla, approx. 11 oz.	470	86.0	42.7	7.87
SUNDAES:				
Fudge-Vanilla Ice Cream, approx. 6.3 oz.	420	50.0	66.7	7.94
Strawberry-Vanilla Ice Cream, approx. 6.3 oz.	340	39.0	54.0	6.19
ICE CREAM CONES				
SUGAR CONES:				
Chocolate, regular, approx. 4½ oz. (4 oz. ice cream, ½ oz. cone)	310	41.0	68.9	9.11
Chocolate, double dip, approx. 7½ oz. (7 oz. ice cream, ½ oz. cone)	490	63.0	65.3	8.40
Vanilla, regular, approx. 4½ oz. (4 oz. ice cream, ½ oz. cone)	290	38.0	64.4	8.44
Vanilla, double dip, approx. 7½ oz. (7 oz. ice cream, ½ oz. cone)	460	57.0	61.3	7.60
CAKE CONES:				
Chocolate, regular, approx. 4.2 oz. (4 oz. ice cream, 0.2 oz. cone)	260	32.0	61.9	7.62
Chocolate, double dip, approx. 7.2 oz. (7 oz. ice cream, 0.2 oz. cone)	440	54.0	61.1	7.50
Vanilla, regular, approx. 4.2 oz. (4 oz. ice cream, 0.2 oz. cone)	250	29.0	59.5	6.95
Vanilla, double dip, approx. 7.2 oz. (7 oz. ice cream, 0.2 oz. cone)	420	49.0	58.3	6.81
COLD DRINKS				
Cola, approx. 12-oz. (by weight) cup	120	30.0	10.0	2.50
approx. 16-oz. (1-lb.) (by weight) cup	160	40.0	10.0	2.50
Cola, Sugar-Free, approx. 12-oz. (by weight) cup	1	trace	0.1	trace
approx. 16-oz. (1-lb.) (by weight) cup	1	trace	0.1	trace
Milk, approx. 8-oz. (by weight) cup	160	12.0	20.0	1.50

HARDEE'S

	UNIT Cal.	UNIT Carb.	1 OZ., BY WT. Cal.	1 OZ., BY WT. Carb.
HAMBURGERS				
Big Cheese, approx. 6 oz.	495	27.5	82.5	4.58
Big Deluxe, approx. 8.9 oz.	675	45.8	75.8	5.15
Big Twin, approx. 5.8 oz.	447	29.4	77.1	5.07
Cheeseburger, approx. 4.1 oz.	335	28.7	81.7	6.99
Hamburger, approx. 3.9 oz.	305	29.4	78.2	7.53
HOT DOGS				
Hot Dog, approx. 4.2 oz.	346	25.8	82.4	6.14
OTHER SANDWICHES				
Fish Sandwich, approx. 5.1 oz.	468	41.9	91.8	8.22
Roast Beef, approx. 5.1 oz.	390	44.2	76.5	8.67
SIDE DISHES				
French Fries, Small, approx. 2.5 oz.	239	27.6	95.6	11.02
French Fries, Large, approx. 4.0 oz.	381	43.8	95.3	10.96
COLD DRINKS				
Milk Shake, approx. 11.5 oz.	391	62.9	34.0	5.47
DESSERTS				
Apple Turnover, approx. 3.1 oz.	282	36.9	91.0	11.90

KENTUCKY FRIED CHICKEN

	UNIT Cal.	UNIT Carb.	1 OZ., BY WT. Cal.	1 OZ., BY WT. Carb.
CHICKEN BY THE PIECE:				
Edible Portion:				
1 Drumstick, Original Recipe, approx. 1.66 oz.	117	2.6	70.5	1.56
Extra Crispy, approx. 2.04 oz.	155	5.1	76.0	2.50
1 Keel, Original Recipe, approx. 3.35 oz.	236	7.4	70.5	2.21
Extra Crispy, approx. 3.67 oz.	297	13.6	80.9	3.71
1 Side Breast, Original Recipe, approx. 2.43 oz.	199	7.1	81.9	2.92
Extra Crispy, approx. 2.98 oz.	286	14.1	96.0	4.73
1 Thigh, Original Recipe, approx. 3.10 oz.	257	6.5	82.9	2.10
Extra Crispy, approx. 3.77 oz.	343	12.6	91.0	3.34
1 Wing, Original Recipe, approx. 1.48 oz.	136	4.2	91.9	2.84
Extra Crispy, approx. 1.86 oz.	201	8.7	108.1	4.68
CHICKEN COMBINATIONS:				
2-PIECE SNACK				
All Dark				
Components and their approximate weights: 1 drumstick (2.64 oz.), 1 thigh (4.26 oz.), and 1 roll (0.6 oz.), 1 box, 7.5 oz., as purchased	463	23.2	61.7	3.09
Edible portion, approx. 5.9 oz.	463	23.2	78.5	3.93

	UNIT		1 OZ., BY WT.	
	Cal.	Carb.	Cal.	Carb.
All White				
Components and their approximate weights: 1 rib (3.71 oz.), 1 keel (3.70 oz.), and 1 roll (0.6 oz.), 1 box, 8 oz., as purchased	525	22.3	65.6	2.79
Edible portion, approx. 6.9 oz.	525	22.3	76.1	3.23
Or: 2 ribs (7.42 oz.), and 1 roll (0.6 oz.), 1 box, 8 oz., as purchased	534	24.2	66.7	3.02
Edible portion, approx. 6.9 oz.	534	24.2	83.4	3.78
Combo				
Components and their approximate weights: 1 rib (3.71 oz.), 1 wing (2.21 oz.), and 1 roll (0.6 oz.), 1 box, 6.5 oz., as purchased	444	20.5	68.2	3.15
Edible portion, approx. 5.5 oz.	444	20.5	80.7	3.72
Or: 1 wing (2.21 oz.), 1 thigh (4.26 oz.), and 1 roll (0.6 oz.), 1 box, 7.1 oz., as purchased	478	24.9	67.3	3.51
Edible portion, approx. 4.6 oz.	478	24.9	85.4	4.45
3-PIECE SNACK				
All Dark				
Components and their approximate weights: 2 drumsticks (5.28 oz.), 1 thigh (4.26 oz.), and 1 roll (0.6 oz.), 1 box, 10.1 oz., as purchased	599	25.6	59.3	2.56
Edible portion, approx. 7.8 oz.	599	25.6	76.8	3.28
Or: 1 drumstick (2.64 oz.), 2 thighs (8.56 oz.), and 1 roll (0.6 oz.), 1 box, 11.8 oz., as purchased	739	35.4	62.6	3.00
Edible portion, approx. 8.7 oz.	739	35.4	84.9	4.07
All White				
Components and their approximate weights: 2 ribs (7.42 oz.), 1 keel (3.70 oz.), and 1 roll (0.6 oz.), 1 box, 11.7 oz., as purchased	817	30.1	69.8	2.57
Edible portion, approx. 9.2 oz.	817	30.1	88.8	3.27
Combo				
Components and their approximate weights: 1 wing (2.21 oz.), 1 rib (3.71 oz.), 1 thigh (4.26 oz.), and 1 roll (0.6 oz.), 1 box, 10.8 oz., as purchased	719	32.7	66.6	3.03
Edible portion, approx. 8.5 oz.	719	32.7	84.6	3.85
Or: 1 wing (2.21 oz.), 1 drumstick (2.64 oz.), 1 thigh (4.26 oz.), and 1 roll (0.6 oz.), 1 box, 9.7 oz., as purchased	614	27.3	63.3	2.81
Edible portion, approx. 7.5 oz.	614	27.3	81.9	3.64
Combo				
Components and their approximate weights: 1 rib (3.71 oz.), 1 drumstick (2.64 oz.), 1 thigh (4.26 oz.), and 1 roll (0.6 oz.), 1 box, 11.2 oz. as purchased	704	31.0	62.9	2.77
Edible portion, approx. 8.2 oz.	704	31.0	85.9	3.78
9-PIECE THRIFT BOX				
Components and their approximate weights: 2 wings (4.42 oz.), 2 ribs (7.42 oz.), 1 keel (3.70 oz.), 2 drumsticks (2.64 oz.), 2 thighs (8.56 oz.), 1 box, 26.7 oz., as purchased	1892	59.0	70.9	2.21
Edible portion, approx. 20.9 oz.	1892	59.0	90.5	2.82
15-PIECE CARRY PACK				
Components and their approximate weights: 4 wings (8.84 oz.), 3 ribs (11.13 oz.), 1 keel (3.70 oz.), 4 drumsticks (10.56 oz.), 3 thighs (12.78 oz.), 1 box, 47.0 oz., as purchased	2984	92.0	63.5	1.96
Edible portion, approx. 36.3 oz.	2984	92.0	82.2	2.53
Components and their approximate weights: 3 wings (6.63 oz.), 2 ribs (7.42 oz.), 3 keels (11.10 oz.), 3 drumsticks (7.92 oz.), 4 thighs (17.04 oz.), 1 box, 50.1 oz., as purchased	3297	101.8	65.8	2.03
Edible portion, approx. 40.1 oz.	3297	101.8	82.2	2.54
Or: 4 wings (8.84 oz.), 3 ribs (11.13 oz.), 1 keel (3.70 oz.), 3 drumsticks (7.92 oz.), 3 thighs (12.78 oz.), 1 box, 44.4 oz., as purchased	2848	89.6	64.1	2.02
Edible portion, approx. 34.4 oz.	2848	89.6	82.8	2.60
21-PIECE BARREL				
Components and their approximate weights: 5 wings (11.05 oz.), 4 drumsticks (10.56 oz.), 2 keels (7.40 oz.), 5 ribs (18.55 oz.), 5 thighs (21.30 oz.), 1 box, 68.9 oz., as purchased	4453	142.1	64.6	2.06
Edible portion, approx. 53.9 oz.	4453	142.1	82.6	2.64
Or: 5 wings (11.05 oz.), 5 drumsticks (13.20 oz.), 2 keels (7.40 oz.), 5 ribs (18.55 oz.), 4 thighs (17.04 oz.), 1 box, 67.2 oz., as purchased	4313	132.3	64.2	1.97
Edible portion, approx. 52.4 oz.	4313	132.3	82.3	2.52
Or: 5 wings (11.05 oz.), 5 drumsticks (13.20 oz.), 2 keels (7.40 oz.), 4 ribs (14.84 oz.), 5 thighs (21.30 oz.), 1 box, 67.8 oz., as purchased	4348	136.7	64.1	2.02
Edible portion, approx. 51.3 oz.	4348	136.7	84.8	2.66
MEALS:				
2-PIECE COLONEL'S SPECIAL				
All Dark				
Components and their approximate weights: 1 drumstick (2.64 oz.), 1 thigh (4.26 oz.), 1 individual potatoes and gravy (4.0 oz.), 1 individual cole slaw (3.2 oz.), and 1 roll, (0.6 oz.), 1 box, 14.7 oz., as purchased	650	42.2	44.2	2.87
Edible portion, approx. 13.1 oz.	650	42.2	49.6	3.22
All White				
Components and their approximate weights: 1 rib (3.71 oz.), 1 keel (3.70 oz.), 1 individual potatoes and gravy (4.0 oz.), 1 individual cole slaw (3.2 oz.), and 1 roll, (0.6 oz.), 1 box, 15.2 oz., as purchased	763	41.3	50.2	2.71
Edible portion, approx. 14.1 oz.	763	41.3	54.1	2.93
Or: 2 ribs (7.42 oz.), 1 individual potatoes and gravy (4.0 oz.), 1 individual cole slaw (3.2 oz.), and 1 roll (0.6 oz.), 1 box, 15.2 oz., as purchased	721	43.1	47.4	2.84
Edible portion, approx. 13.6 oz.	721	43.1	53.0	3.17
Combo				
Components and their approximate weights: 1 wing (2.21 oz.), 1 thigh (4.26 oz.), 1 individual potatoes and gravy (4.0 oz.), 1 individual cole slaw (3.2 oz.), and 1 roll (0.6 oz.), 1 box, 14.3 oz., as purchased	665	43.9	46.5	3.07
Edible portion, approx. 12.8 oz.	665	43.9	52.0	3.43
Combo				
Components and their approximate weights: 1 rib (3.71 oz.), 1 wing (2.21 oz.), 1 individual potatoes and gravy (4.0 oz.), 1 individual cole slaw (3.2 oz.), and 1 roll (0.6 oz.), 1 box, 13.7 oz., as purchased	631	39.5	46.0	2.88
Edible portion, approx. 12.3 oz.	631	39.5	51.3	3.21
3-PIECE COLONEL'S CHOICE				
All Dark				
Components and their approximate weights: 2 drumsticks (5.28 oz.), 1 thigh (4.26 oz.), 1 individual potatoes and gravy (4.0 oz.), 1 individual cole slaw (3.2 oz.), and 1 roll (0.6 oz.), 1 box, 17.3 oz., as purchased	786	44.5	45.4	2.57
Edible portion, approx. 15.0 oz.	786	44.5	52.4	2.97
Or: 1 drumstick (2.64 oz.), 2 thighs (8.56 oz.), 1 individual potatoes and gravy (4.0 oz.), 1 individual cole slaw (3.2 oz.), and 1 roll (0.6 oz.), 1 box, 19.0 oz., as purchased	926	54.4	48.7	2.86
Edible portion, approx. 16.5 oz.	926	54.4	56.1	3.30
All White				
Components and their approximate weights: 2 ribs (7.42 oz.), 1 keel (3.70 oz.), 1 individual potatoes and gravy (4.0 oz.), 1 individual cole slaw (3.2 oz.), and 1 roll (0.6 oz.), 1 box, 18.9 oz., as purchased	1004	49.1	53.1	2.60
Edible portion, approx. 17.0 oz.	1004	49.1	59.1	2.89
Combo				
Components and their approximate weights: 1 wing (2.21 oz.), 1 rib (3.71 oz.), 1 thigh (4.26 oz.), 1 individual potatoes and gravy (4.0 oz.), 1 individual cole slaw (3.2 oz.), and 1 roll (0.6 oz.), 1 box, 18.2 oz., as purchased	906	51.7	50.4	2.87
Edible portion, approx. 15.7 oz.	906	51.7	57.7	3.29
Combo				
Components and their approximate weights: 1 wing (2.21 oz.), 1 drumstick (2.64 oz.), 1 thigh (4.26 oz.), 1 individual potatoes and gravy (4.0 oz.), 1 individual cole slaw (3.2 oz.), and 1 roll (0.6 oz.), 1 box, 16.9 oz., as purchased	801	46.3	47.4	2.74
Edible portion, approx. 14.7 oz.	801	46.3	54.5	31.50
Or: 1 rib (3.71 oz.), 1 drumstick (2.64 oz.), 1 thigh (4.26 oz.), 1 individual potatoes and gravy (4.0 oz.), 1 individual cole slaw, (3.2 oz.), and 1 roll (0.6 oz.), 1 box, 18.4 oz., as purchased	891	50.0	48.4	2.72
Edible portion, approx. 16.0 oz.	891	50.0	55.7	3.13
4-PIECE WING DINNER				
Components and their approximate weights: 4 wings (8.84 oz.), 1 individual potatoes and gravy (4.0 oz.), 1 individual cole slaw (3.2 oz.), and 1 roll (0.6 oz.), 1 box, 16.6 oz., as purchased	843	44.0	50.8	2.65
Edible portion, approx. 14.2 oz.	843	44.0	59.4	3.10
6-PIECE JUMBO FOR TWO				
All Dark				
Components and their approximate weights: 3 drumsticks (7.96 oz.), 3 thighs (12.78 oz.), 2 individual potatoes and gravy (8.0 oz.), 2 individual cole slaw (6.4 oz.), and 2 rolls (1.2 oz.), 1 box, 36.3 oz., as purchased	1712	98.9	47.2	2.73
Edible portion, approx. 31.5 oz.	1712	98.9	54.3	3.14
All White				
Components and their approximate weights: 4 ribs (14.84 oz.), 2 keels (7.40 oz.), 2 individual potatoes and gravy (8.0 oz.), 2 individual cole slaw (6.4 oz.), and 2 rolls (1.2 oz.), 1 box, 37.8 oz., as purchased	2008	98.1	53.1	2.60
Edible portion, approx. 34.0 oz.	2008	98.1	59.1	2.89
Combo				
Components and their approximate weights: 2 wings (4.42 oz.), 1 rib (3.17 oz.), 1 drumstick (2.64 oz.), 2 thighs (8.52 oz.), 2 individual potatoes and gravy (8.0 oz.), 2 individual cole slaw (6.4 oz.), and 2 rolls (1.2 oz.), 1 box, 34.9 oz., as purchased	1807	97.0	51.8	2.81
Edible portion, approx. 30.4 oz.	1807	97.0	59.4	3.22

	UNIT Cal.	UNIT Carb.	1 OZ., BY WT. Cal.	1 OZ., BY WT. Carb.
Or: 2 wings (4.42 oz.), 1 keel (3.70 oz.), 1 drumstick (2.64 oz.), 2 thighs (8.52 oz.), 2 individual potatoes and gravy (8.0 oz.), 2 individual cole slaw (6.4 oz.), and 2 rolls (1.2 oz.), 1 box, 34.9 oz., as purchased	1749	92.0	50.1	2.64
Edible portion, approx. 30.9 oz.	1749	92.0	56.6	2.98
SIDE ORDERS:				
Cole Slaw, 1 serving, approx. 3.2 oz.	121	12.7	37.8	3.97
Corn, one 5½-inch ear, edible portion, approx. 4.8 oz.	169	31.2	35.5	6.55
Gravy, 1 serving, approx. 0.5 oz.	23	1.3	45.4	2.60
Mashed Potatoes, 1 serving, approx. 3 oz.	64	12.2	21.3	4.07
Roll, approx. ¾ oz.	61	10.9	81.3	14.53

LONG JOHN SILVER'S

	UNIT Cal.	UNIT Carb.	1 OZ., BY WT. Cal.	1 OZ., BY WT. Carb.
FISH and SEAFOOD PLATTERS				
Breaded Clams, approx. 5.01 oz.	617	61.3	123.4	12.26
Breaded Oysters, 6 pieces, approx. 5.50 oz.	441	53.2	80.2	9.67
Fish with Batter, 2 pieces, approx. 4.80 oz.	366	21.4	76.3	4.46
Fish with Batter, 3 pieces, approx. 7.30 oz.	549	32.1	75.2	4.40
Ocean Scallops, 6 pieces, approx. 4.23 oz.	283	29.5	66.9	6.97
Peg Legs with Batter, 5 pieces, approx. 4.41 oz.	350	25.5	79.5	5.80
Shrimp with Batter, 6 pieces, approx. 3.10 oz.	268	30.4	86.5	9.81
Treasure Chest, 2 pieces fish, 2 peg legs, approx. 5.04 oz.	506	31.6	101.2	6.27
CHICKEN PLATTERS				
Chicken Planks, 4 pieces, approx. 5.86 oz.	457	34.7	78.0	5.92
SIDE ORDERS				
Clam Chowder, approx. 8 oz.	107	14.9	13.4	1.86
Cole Slaw, approx. 4 oz.	138	15.6	34.5	3.90
Corn on the Cob, 1 ear, approx. 5.30 oz.	176	28.7	33.2	5.42
French Fries, approx. 3 oz.	288	33.2	96.0	11.07
Hush Puppies, 3 pieces, approx. 1.59 oz.	153	20.3	95.6	12.69

McDONALD'S

	UNIT Cal.	UNIT Carb.	1 OZ., BY WT. Cal.	1 OZ., BY WT. Carb.
HAMBURGERS				
Big Mac, approx. 6½ oz.	541	39.0	83.3	6.00
Cheeseburger, approx. 4 oz.	306	30.8	76.5	7.70
Hamburger, approx. 3½ oz.	257	30.2	73.4	8.63
Quarter Pounder, approx. 5.7 oz.	418	32.9	73.3	5.77
Quarter Pounder with Cheese, approx. 6¾ oz.	518	34.2	76.7	5.07
OTHER SANDWICHES				
Fillet-O-Fish, approx. 4.6 oz.	402	34.3	87.4	7.46
McChicken, approx. 6 oz.	475	39.8	79.2	6.63
McRib, approx. 6.7 oz.	461	43.7	68.8	6.52
SIDE ORDERS				
French Fries, Regular, approx. 2.4 oz.	211	25.8	87.9	10.75
French Fries, Large, approx. 4.2 oz.	369	45.2	87.9	10.75
Hashbrown Potatoes, approx. 2 oz.	130	13.8	65.0	6.90
BREAKFAST MENU				
Egg McMuffin, approx. 4⅔ oz.	352	26.0	75.4	5.57
Buttered English Muffin, approx. 2.2 oz.	186	28.3	84.5	12.86
Hotcakes with Butter & Syrup, approx. 7¼ oz.	472	88.9	65.1	12.30
Pork Sausage, approx. 1.7 oz.	184	0.1	108.2	0.06
Scrambled Eggs, approx. 2¾ oz.	162	1.9	58.9	0.69
OTHER				
Chicken McNuggets, approx. 4.3 oz.	332	17.6	77.2	4.09
Sauces for Chicken McNuggets:				
Barbeque, approx. 1 oz.	41	9.6	41.0	9.60
Honey, approx. 0.5 oz.	100	24.8	200.0	49.60
Hot Mustard, approx. 1 oz.	57	8.1	57.0	8.10
Steak Sauce, approx. 0.6 oz.	29	6.8	48.3	11.30
Sweet & Sour, approx. 1 oz.	56	13.5	56.0	13.50
Ham Biscuit, approx. 4.2 oz.	422	43.0	100.5	10.24
Sausage Biscuit, approx. 4.8 oz.	582	42.5	121.3	8.85
COLD DRINKS				
SHAKES:				
Chocolate, approx. 10.2 oz.	360	60.0	35.3	5.88
Strawberry, approx. 10.3 oz.	340	57.0	33.0	5.53
Vanilla, approx. 10.2 oz.	320	52.0	31.4	5.10
OTHER DRINKS:				
Milk, approx. 8 fl. oz. (8.6 oz. net wt.)	159	12.0	18.5	1.40
Orange Juice, approx. 6 fl. oz. (approx. 6.45 oz. net wt.)	82	19.6	12.7	3.04
DESSERTS				
Apple Pie, approx. 3.2 oz.	300	31.0	93.8	9.69
Cherry Pie, approx. 3.3 oz.	310	33.0	93.8	10.30
McDonaldland Cookies, approx. 2¼ oz.	290	45.0	128.9	20.00
SUNDAES				
Caramel, approx. 5.1 oz.	282	50.8	55.3	9.96
Hot Fudge, approx. 5⅓ oz.	290	44.6	54.4	8.36
Pineapple, approx. 5 oz.	230	42.9	46.0	8.58
Strawberry, approx. 5-oz.	229	44.1	45.6	8.82

PONDEROSA

	UNIT Cal.	UNIT Carb.	1 OZ., BY WT. Cal.	1 OZ., BY WT. Carb.
COMBINATION PLATTERS				
Chopped Beef Dinner, approx. 21.6 oz.	691	73.5	32.0	3.40
Chopped Beef (approx. 5.3 oz.)	324	0.0	61.1	0.00
Baked Potato (approx. 7.2 oz.)	145	32.8	20.1	4.56
Lettuce (approx. 3 oz.)	12	2.1	3.9	0.70
Tomato, 1 small (approx. 3.5 oz.)	22	4.7	6.3	1.34
Onion, chopped, 1 tablespoon (approx. 0.4 oz.)	4	0.9	10.0	2.25
Kaiser Roll (approx. 2.2 oz.)	184	33.0	83.6	15.00
Filet of Sole Dinner, approx. 22.3 oz.	618	82.3	27.7	3.69
Filet of Sole, 2 pieces (approx. 6 oz.)	251	8.8	41.7	1.47
Baked Potato (approx. 7.2 oz.)	145	32.8	20.1	4.56
Lettuce (approx. 3 oz.)	12	2.1	3.9	0.70
Tomato, 1 small (approx. 3.5 oz.)	22	4.7	6.3	1.34
Onion, chopped, 1 tablespoon (approx. 0.4 oz.)	4	0.9	10.0	2.25
Kaiser Roll (approx. 2.2 oz.)	184	33.0	83.6	15.00
Prime Rib Dinner, approx. 20.5 oz.	653	73.5	31.8	3.58
Prime Rib (approx. 4.2 oz.)	286	0.0	68.1	0.00
Baked Potato (approx. 7.2 oz.)	145	32.8	20.1	4.56
Lettuce (approx. 3 oz.)	12	2.1	3.9	0.70
Tomato, 1 small (approx. 3.5 oz.)	22	4.7	6.3	1.34
Onion, chopped, 1 tablespoon (approx. 0.4 oz.)	4	0.9	10.0	2.25
Kaiser Roll (approx. 2.2 oz.)	184	33.0	83.6	15.00
Rib Eye Dinner, approx. 20.1 oz.	626	73.5	31.1	3.65
Rib Eye (approx. 3.8 oz.)	259	0.0	68.2	0.00
Baked Potato (approx. 7.2 oz.)	145	32.8	20.1	4.56
Lettuce (approx. 3 oz.)	12	2.1	3.9	0.70
Tomato, 1 small (approx. 3.5 oz.)	22	4.7	6.3	1.34
Onion, chopped, 1 tablespoon (approx. 0.4 oz.)	4	0.9	10.0	2.25
Kaiser Roll (approx. 2.2 oz.)	184	33.0	83.6	15.00
Rib Eye & Shrimp Dinner, approx. 22.3 oz.	765	79.7	34.3	3.57
Rib Eye (approx. 3.8 oz.)	259	0.0	68.2	0.00
Shrimp, 4 pieces (approx. 2.2 oz.)	139	6.2	63.2	2.82
Baked Potato (approx. 7.2 oz.)	145	32.8	20.1	4.56
Lettuce (approx. 3 oz.)	12	2.1	3.9	0.70
Tomato, 1 small (approx. 3.5 oz.)	22	4.7	6.3	1.34
Onion, chopped, 1 tablespoon (approx. 0.4 oz.)	4	0.9	10.0	2.25
Kaiser Roll (approx. 2.2 oz.)	184	33.0	83.6	15.00
Shrimp Dinner, approx. 19.8 oz.	587	83.3	29.6	4.21
Shrimp, 7 pieces (approx. 3.5 oz.)	220	9.8	62.9	2.80
Baked Potato (approx. 7.2 oz.)	145	32.8	20.1	4.56
Lettuce (approx. 3 oz.)	12	2.1	3.9	0.70
Tomato, 1 small (approx. 3.5 oz.)	22	4.7	6.3	1.34
Onion, chopped, 1 tablespoon (approx. 0.4 oz.)	4	0.9	10.0	2.25
Kaiser Roll (approx. 2.2 oz.)	184	33.0	83.6	15.00
Strip Sirloin Dinner, approx. 21 oz.	644	73.5	30.6	3.50
Strip Sirloin (approx. 4.7 oz.)	227	0.0	48.3	0.00
Baked Potato (approx. 7.2 oz.)	145	32.8	20.1	4.56
Lettuce (approx. 3 oz.)	12	2.1	3.9	0.70
Tomato, 1 small (approx. 3.5 oz.)	22	4.7	6.3	1.34
Onion, chopped, 1 tablespoon (approx. 0.4 oz.)	4	0.9	10.0	2.25
Kaiser Roll (approx. 2.2 oz.)	184	33.0	83.6	15.00
Super Sirloin Dinner, approx. 22.8 oz.	750	73.5	32.9	3.22
Sirloin (approx. 6.5 oz.)	383	0.0	58.9	0.00
Baked Potato (approx. 7.2 oz.)	145	32.8	20.1	4.56
Lettuce (approx. 3 oz.)	12	2.1	3.9	0.70
Tomato, 1 small (approx. 3.5 oz.)	22	4.7	6.3	1.34
Onion, chopped, 1 tablespoon (approx. 0.4 oz.)	4	0.9	10.0	2.25
Kaiser Roll (approx. 2.2 oz.)	184	33.0	83.7	15.00
T-Bone Dinner, approx. 23 oz.	741	73.5	32.2	3.19
T-Bone (approx. 6.7 oz.)	374	0.0	55.8	0.00
Baked Potato (approx. 7.2 oz.)	145	32.8	20.1	4.56
Lettuce (approx. 3 oz.)	12	2.1	3.9	0.70
Tomato, 1 small (approx. 3.5 oz.)	22	4.7	6.3	1.34
Onion, chopped 1 tablespoon (approx. 0.4 oz.)	4	0.9	10.0	2.25
Kaiser Roll (approx. 2.2 oz.)	184	33.0	83.6	15.00
X-Tra-Cut Rib Eye Dinner, approx. 22.5 oz.	725	73.5	32.2	3.26
X-Tra-Cut Rib Eye (approx. 6.2 oz.)	358	0.0	57.7	0.00
Baked Potato (approx. 7.2 oz.)	145	32.8	20.1	4.56
Lettuce (approx. 3 oz.)	12	2.1	3.9	0.70
Tomato, 1 small (approx. 3.5 oz.)	22	4.7	6.3	1.34
Onion, chopped, 1 tablespoon (approx. 0.4 oz.)	4	0.9	10.0	2.25
Kaiser Roll (approx. 2.2 oz.)	184	33.0	83.6	15.00
SANDWICHES				
Double Deluxe Sandwich, approx. 13.3 oz.	792	67.3	59.5	5.06
Double Deluxe Steak (approx. 5.9 oz.)	362	0.0	61.4	0.00
Steakhouse Deluxe Bun (approx. 2.4 oz.)	190	35.0	79.2	14.60
French Fries (approx. 3 oz.)	230	30.2	76.7	10.07
Dill Pickles, 3 slices (approx. 0.7 oz.)	2	0.5	2.1	0.64

	UNIT Cal.	UNIT Carb.	1 OZ., BY WT. Cal.	1 OZ., BY WT. Carb.
Lettuce (approx. 0.5 oz.)	2	0.4	3.8	0.70
Tomato Slices, 2 (approx. 0.8 oz.)	6	1.2	6.2	1.36
Filet of Sole Sandwich, approx. 9.2 oz.	550	72.3	59.7	7.85
Filet of Sole, 1 piece (approx. 3 oz.)	125	4.4	41.7	1.47
Steakhouse Deluxe Bun (approx. 2.4 oz.)	190	35.0	79.2	14.58
French Fries (approx. 3 oz.)	230	30.2	76.7	10.07
Lemon Wedge (approx. 0.8 oz.)	5	2.7	5.7	3.06
Junior Patty, approx. 6 oz.	446	51.2	74.3	8.53
(Child's Portion–Dinner)				
Patty (approx. 1.6 oz.)	98	0.0	61.3	0.00
Junior Bun (approx. 1.4 oz.)	118	21.0	83.6	15.00
French Fries (approx. 3 oz.)	230	30.2	76.7	10.07
Steakhouse Deluxe Sandwich, approx. 10.36 oz.	611	67.3	59.0	6.48
Steakhouse Deluxe Steak (approx. 2.96 oz.)	181	0.0	61.1	0.00
Steakhouse Deluxe Bun (approx. 2.4 oz.)	190	35.0	79.2	14.58
French Fries (approx. 3 oz.)	230	30.2	76.7	10.07
Dill Pickles, 3 slices (approx. 0.7 oz.)	2	0.5	2.1	0.64
Lettuce (approx. 0.5 oz.)	2	0.4	3.8	0.70
Tomato Slices, 2 (approx. 0.8 oz.)	6	1.2	6.2	1.36
SALAD DRESSINGS and SAUCES				
Blue Cheese Salad Dressing (approx. 7/16 oz.)	56	0.9	128.0	2.06
Catsup, 1 tablespoon (approx. 0.6 oz.)	18	4.3	30.1	6.78
Cocktail Sauce (approx. 1½ oz.)	57	14.5	38.0	9.67
Creamy Italian Salad Dressing (approx. 7/16 oz.)	60	1.2	137.0	2.70
French Salad Dressing (approx. 7/16 oz.)	56	4.0	128.0	9.14
Mayonnaise, 1 tablespoon (approx. 0.5 oz.)	101	0.3	204.7	0.61
Mustard, 1 teaspoon (approx. 0.2 oz.)	4	0.3	22.7	1.70
Oil-Vinegar Dressing (approx. 7/16 oz.)	54	0.4	123.0	0.91
Steak Sauce (approx. 7/16 oz.)	10	2.0	22.8	4.57
Tartar Sauce, 1 tablespoon (approx. 0.7 oz.)	95	1.5	134.8	2.13
Thousand Island Dressing (approx. 7/16 oz.)	51	0.9	126.6	6.63
Worcestershire Sauce, 1 teaspoon (approx. 0.2 oz.)	4	0.9	22.7	5.11

ROY ROGERS

	UNIT Cal.	UNIT Carb.	1 OZ., BY WT. Cal.	1 OZ., BY WT. Carb.
HAMBURGERS				
Cheeseburger, approx. 3¾ oz.	475		126.7	
Double-R Bar Burger, approx. 3¾ oz.	565		150.7	
Hamburger, approx. 3¾ oz.	425		113.3	
OTHER SANDWICHES				
Roast Beef Sandwich, approx. 3½ oz.	450		128.6	
SIDE ORDERS				
French Fries, approx. 3-oz. serving	240		80.0	
Cole Slaw, approx. 3-oz. serving	90		30.0	
COLD DRINKS				
Cola, approx. 12 fl. oz.	130		10.8	
approx. 16 fl. oz. (1 pt.)	175		10.8	
Milk, approx. 8 fl. oz. (approx. 8.6 oz. by weight)	160	12.0	18.5	1.40

TACO BELL

	UNIT Cal.	UNIT Carb.	1 OZ., BY WT. Cal.	1 OZ., BY WT. Carb.
Bean Burrito, approx. 5.9 oz.	343	48.0	58.6	8.20
Beef Burrito, approx. 6.5 oz.	466	37.0	71.8	5.70
Beefy Tostado, approx. 6.5 oz.	291	21.0	44.8	3.24
Bellbeefer, approx. 4.3 oz.	221	23.0	50.9	5.30
Bellbeefer With Cheese, approx. 4.8 oz.	278	23.0	57.5	4.76
Burrito Supreme, approx. 7.9 oz.	457	43.0	57.6	5.42
Combination Burrito, approx. 6.2 oz.	404	43.0	65.4	6.97
Enchirito, approx. 7.3 oz.	454	42.0	62.2	5.75
Taco, approx. 2.9 oz.	186	14.0	63.5	4.78
Tostada, approx. 4.9 oz.	179	25.0	36.8	5.14

WENDY'S

	UNIT Cal.	UNIT Carb.	1 OZ., BY WT. Cal.	1 OZ., BY WT. Carb.
HAMBURGERS				
Cheeseburger, approx. 8.4 oz.	577	34.1	68.7	4.06
Double Cheeseburger, approx. 11.5 oz.	797	40.9	69.6	3.56
Triple Cheeseburger, approx. 14 oz.	1035	35.0	73.4	2.50
Hamburger, approx. 7 oz.	472	33.6	67.4	4.80
Double Hamburger, approx. 10 oz.	669	34.0	67.0	3.40
Triple Hamburger, approx. 12.7 oz.	853	33.1	67.2	2.61
SIDE ORDERS				
Chili, approx. 3.8 oz.	229	20.6	26.0	2.34
French Fries, approx. 4.2 oz.	327	41.0	77.9	9.80
COLD DRINKS				
Frosty, approx. 8.8 oz.	391	53.6	44.4	6.10

WHITE CASTLE

	UNIT Cal.	UNIT Carb.	1 OZ., BY WT. Cal.	1 OZ., BY WT. Carb.
HAMBURGERS				
Cheeseburger, approx. 2.2 oz.	198		90.0	
Hamburger, with Onion & Pickle, approx. 1.9 oz.	165	13.3	86.8	7.00
OTHER SANDWICHES				
Fish Sandwich, approx. 2.4 oz.	200		88.3	
SIDE ORDERS				
French Fries, Regular, approx. 2.7 oz.	219		81.1	
Onion Rings, approx. 3.3 oz.	341		103.3	
COLD DRINKS				
Shake (flavor not specified), approx. 4.9 oz.	213		43.5	

38 VENDING MACHINES •

SOUPS

This list is only a sampling. See the SOUPS chapter for more.

	UNIT Cal.	UNIT Carb.	1 OZ., BY WT. Cal.	1 OZ., BY WT. Carb.
Campbell's Individual Service Size Soups, Ready-To-Serve:				
Bean Soup, 7½-oz. can	150	21.0	20.0	2.80
Beef Noodle Soup, 7¼-oz. can	70	8.0	9.7	1.10
Chicken Noodle Soup, 7¼-oz. can	70	8.0	9.7	1.10
Chicken with Rice Soup, 7¼-oz. can	60	7.0	8.3	0.97
Chili Beef Soup, 7½-oz. can	140	17.0	18.7	2.27
Clam Chowder Soup (Manhattan Style), 7¼-oz. can	80	12.0	11.0	1.66
Cream of Chicken Soup, 7¼-oz. can	90	7.0	12.4	0.97
Cream of Mushroom Soup, 7¼-oz. can	100	8.0	13.3	1.10
Green Pea Soup, 7½-oz. can	140	22.0	18.7	2.93
Minestrone Soup, 7¼-oz. can	80	11.0	11.0	1.52
Tomato Soup, 7¼-oz. can	110	20.0	15.2	2.76
Vegetable Soup, 7¼-oz. can	80	12.0	11.0	1.66
Vegetable Beef Soup, 7¼-oz. can	70	7.0	9.7	0.97
Campbell's "Chunky Soups," Individual Service Size, Ready-To-Serve:				
Chunky Chicken Soup, 7½-oz. can	160	16.0	21.3	2.13
Chunky Old Fashioned Bean with Ham Soup, 7½-oz. can	210	24.0	28.0	3.20
Chunky Sirloin Burger Soup, 7½-oz. can	160	16.0	21.3	2.13
Chunky Vegetable Soup, 7½-oz. can	100	17.0	13.3	2.27

ONE-DISH MEALS

This list is only a sampling. See the COMBINATION MAIN DISHES chapter for more.

	UNIT Cal.	UNIT Carb.	1 OZ., BY WT. Cal.	1 OZ., BY WT. Carb.
Bounty Individual Service Size:				
Beef Stew, 7½-oz. can	150	17.0	20.0	2.27
Chicken Stew, 7½-oz. can	170	16.0	22.7	2.13
Chili Con Carne With Beans, 7¾-oz. can	300	28.0	38.7	3.61
Chili Mac, 7¾-oz. can	240	25.0	31.0	3.23
Dumplings & Chicken, 7½-oz. can	200	19.0	26.7	2.53
Hot Chili Con Carne, 7¾-oz. can	300	28.0	38.7	3.61
Noodles with Chicken, 7½-oz. can	210	17.0	28.0	2.27
Potatoes & Beef in Gravy, 7½-oz. can	140	24.0	18.7	3.20
Campbell's Individual Service Size Bean Products:				
Beans & Franks in Tomato & Molasses Sauce, 8-oz. can	360	42.0	45.0	5.25
Beans 'n Beef in Tomato & Molasses Sauce, 8-oz. can	270	37.0	33.8	4.63
Beans 'n Rice, Mexican Style, 7½-oz. can	180	30.0	24.0	4.00
Pork & Beans with Tomato Sauce, 8-oz. can	260	44.0	32.5	5.50
Dinty Moore "Short Orders":				
Beef Stew, 7½-oz. can	180	14.0	24.0	1.87
Brunswick Stew, 7½-oz. can	230	14.0	30.7	1.87
Hashed Potatoes 'n Beef, 7½-oz. can	250	25.0	33.3	3.33
Noodles 'n Chicken, 7½-oz. can	210	15.0	28.0	2.00
Franco-American Individual Serving Size:				
Beef Raviolios in Meat Sauce, 7¾-oz. can	220	35.0	28.4	4.52
Beefy Mac—Macaroni 'n Beef in Tomato Sauce, 7½-oz. can	210	29.0	28.0	3.87
Elbow Macaroni & Cheese, 7½-oz. can	170	23.0	22.7	3.07
Spaghetti 'n Beef in Tomato Sauce, 7½-oz. can	220	26.0	29.3	3.47
Spaghetti with Meatballs in Tomato Sauce, 7¼-oz. can	210	26.0	29.0	3.59
Hormel "Short Orders":				
Au Gratin Potatoes 'n Bacon, 7½-oz. can	230	20.0	30.7	2.67
Beans 'n Bacon, 7½-oz. can	340	40.0	45.3	5.33
Beans 'n Wieners, 7½-oz. can	290	29.0	38.7	3.87
Beef Goulash, 7½-oz. can	230	16.0	30.7	2.13
Beef Tamales, 7½-oz. can	270	17.0	36.0	2.27
Beef 'n Vegetable Chowder, 7½-oz. can	120	15.0	16.0	2.00
Chicken 'n Corn Chowder, 7½-oz. can	130	15.0	17.3	2.00
Chili Mac, 7½-oz. can	200	16.0	26.7	2.13
Chili No Beans, 7½-oz. can	370	11.0	49.3	1.47
Chili With Beans, 7½-oz. can	300	24.0	40.0	3.20
German Potato Salad, 7½-oz. can	220	35.0	29.3	4.67
Ham 'n Potato Chowder, 7½-oz. can	130	14.0	17.3	1.87
Hot Chili With Beans, 7½-oz. can	300	23.0	40.0	3.07
Lasagne, 7½-oz. can	260	24.0	34.7	3.20
Macaroni 'n Cheese, 7½-oz. can	170	22.0	22.7	2.93
Noodles 'n Beef, 7½-oz. can	230	15.0	30.7	2.00
Pork Chow Mein, 7½-oz. can	140	13.0	18.7	1.73
Scalloped Potatoes 'n Ham, 7½-oz. can	250	18.0	33.3	2.40
Spaghetti 'n Beef, 7½-oz. can	240	23.0	32.0	3.07
Spaghetti and Meatballs, 7½-oz. can	210	24.0	28.0	3.20
Mary Kitchen "Short Orders":				
Corned Beef Hash, 7½-oz. can	370	16.0	49.3	2.13
Roast Beef Hash, 7½-oz. can	370	19.0	49.3	2.53

BREAKFAST CEREALS

This list is only a sampling. See the BREAKFAST CEREALS chapter for more.

	UNIT Cal.	UNIT Carb.	1 OZ., BY WT. Cal.	1 OZ., BY WT. Carb.
Kellogg's Individual Self-Serve Bowl:				
Apple Jacks, ⅝-oz. box	69	16.3	110.0	26.00
Cocoa Krispies, 1-oz. box	110	25.0	110.0	25.00
Corn Flakes, ¾-oz. box	80	18.0	110	24.00
40% Bran Flakes, 1-oz. box	90	22.0	90.0	22.00
Froot Loops, ¾-oz. box	80	19.0	110.0	25.00
Frosted Flakes, see Sugar Frosted Flakes				
Frosted Rice, ⅞-oz. box	96	21.9	110.0	25.00
Graham Crackos, ¾-oz. box	83	18.0	110.0	24.00

	UNIT		1 OZ., BY WT.	
	Cal.	Carb.	Cal.	Carb.
Honey & Nut Corn Flakes, 7/8-oz. box	105	21.0	120.0	24.00
Product 19, 1-oz. box	110	24.0	110.0	24.00
Puffed Rice, 3/8-oz. box	40	9.0	105.3	23.68
Puffed Wheat, 5/16-oz. box	35	7.0	112.9	22.58
Raisin Bran, 1 1/4-oz. box	120	30.0	85.7	21.42
Rice Krispies, 5/8-oz. box	70	16.0	110.0	25.00
Special K, 5/8-oz. box	69	13.1	110.0	21.00
Sugar Corn Pops (Sugar Pops), 3/4-oz. box	83	19.5	110.0	26.00
Sugar Frosted Flakes, 1-oz. box	110	26.0	110.0	26.00
Sugar Smacks, 7/8-oz. box	96	21.9	110.0	25.00

BREAKFAST BARS

This list is only a sampling. See the BREAKFAST CEREALS chapter for more.

	UNIT		1 OZ., BY WT.	
	Cal.	Carb.	Cal.	Carb.
Chocolate Chip Breakfast Bar, **Carnation,** 1.56-oz. bar	210	24.0	134.6	15.38
Peanut Butter Crunch Breakfast Bar, **Carnation,** 1.5-oz. bar	200	22.0	134.2	14.76

BEEF JERKY

This list is only a sampling. See the SAUSAGES & COLD CUTS chapter for more.

	UNIT		1 OZ., BY WT.	
	Cal.	Carb.	Cal.	Carb.
Pemmican Tender Beef Jerky Tomahawk Stick, 0.25-oz. stick	22	0.5	85.9	2.18

BEVERAGES

This list is only a sampling. See the BEVERAGES chapter for more.

	UNIT		1 FLUID OZ.	
	Cal.	Carb.	Cal.	Carb.
JUICE				
Tomato Juice, **Campbells,** 6-fl.-oz. can	35	8.0	5.8	1.33
V-8 Cocktail Vegetable Juice, **Campbells,** 6-fl.-oz. can	35	8.0	5.8	1.33
SODA				
(Red) Apple Soda, **Shasta,** 12-fl.-oz. can	168	42.5	14.0	3.54
(Red) Apple Soda, diet, **Shasta,** 12-fl.-oz. bottle	2	0.5	0.2	0.05
Birch Beer, **Canada Dry,** 12-fl.-oz. can	165	42.0	13.8	3.50
Black Cherry Soda, **Kirsch,** 12-fl.-oz. can	175	43.8	14.6	3.65
Black Cherry Soda, **Shasta,** 12-fl.-oz. can	168	42.5	14.0	3.54
Black Cherry Soda, **White Rock,** 12-fl.-oz. can	178	45.0	14.8	3.75
Black Cherry Soda, diet, **Canada Dry,** 12-fl.-oz. can	3	0.5	0.3	0.04
Black Cherry Soda, diet, **Shasta,** 12-fl.-oz. bottle	1	trace	trace	trace
Black Cherry Soda, diet, **Tab,** 12-fl.-oz. can	3	0.0	0.3	0.00
Cactus Cooler Soda, **Canada Dry,** 12-fl.-oz. can	180	43.5	15.0	3.63
(Wild) Cherry Soda, **Canada Dry,** 12-fl.-oz. can	195	48.0	16.3	4.00
Coca-Cola, 12-fl.-oz. can	144	36.0	12.0	3.00
Dr Pepper, 12-fl.-oz. can	150	39.7	12.5	3.31
Mountain Dew, 12-fl.-oz. can	176	43.9	14.7	3.66
Pepsi Cola, 12-fl.-oz. can	157	39.6	13.1	3.30
7-Up, 12-fl.-oz. can	144	36.3	12.0	3.02
Sprite, 12-fl.-oz. can	143	36.0	11.9	3.00
NON-CARBONATED SOFT DRINKS				
Yoo Hoo, 9 1/2-fl.-oz. bottle	180	40.0	18.9	4.21

YOGURT

This list is only a sampling. See the YOGURT chapter for more.

Dannon:

All flavors of Dannon Yogurt are vendable. The range of flavors available will depend upon the individual vendor. Here are some examples.

	UNIT		1 OZ., BY WT.	
	Cal.	Carb.	Cal.	Carb.
Plain Yogurt, 8-oz. container	150	17.0	18.8	2.12
Cherry Yogurt, 8-oz. container	260	49.0	32.5	6.13
Coffee Yogurt, 8-oz. container	200	32.0	25.0	4.00
Dutch Apple Yogurt, 8-oz. container	260	49.0	32.5	6.13
Lemon Yogurt, 8-oz. container	200	32.0	25.0	4.00
Strawberry Yogurt, 8-oz. container	260	49.0	32.5	6.13
Vanilla Yogurt, 8-oz. container	200	32.0	25.0	4.00

COOKIES And CRACKERS

This list is only a sampling. See the COOKIES and CRACKERS chapter for more.

	UNIT		1 OZ., BY WT.	
	Cal.	Carb.	Cal.	Carb.
Austin Foods Co.:				
Cheese on Cheese Crackers, 1.2-oz. package	160	20.0	133.3	16.67
Cheese Peanut Butter Sandwiches, 1 1/2-oz. package	210	22.0	140.0	14.67
Cheese Smacker Crackers, 1 1/8-oz. package	150	19.0	133.3	16.89
Combo Cheese Crackers, 1.2-oz. package	160	20.0	133.3	16.67
Peanut Butter Graham Crackers, 1.4-oz. package	180	27.0	128.6	19.29
Rye Crackers, 1.2-oz. package	150	21.0	125.0	17.50
Saltine Crackers, 1-oz. package	110	20.0	110.0	20.00
5/8-oz. package	70	12.0	110.0	20.00
Keebler:				
BAG COOKIES				
Chocolate Swirl Cookies, 1 1/2-oz. package (14 cookies)	170	23.0	113.3	15.33
Iced Animal Cookies, 1 1/2-oz. package (14 cookies)	160	26.0	106.7	17.33
BAG SNACK CRACKERS				
Bacon Crackers, 1.4-oz. package (31 crackers)	200	25.0	142.9	17.90
Cheese Crackers, 1.4-oz. package (31 crackers)	200	24.0	142.9	17.10
Onion Crackers, 1.4-oz. package (31 crackers)	200	25.0	142.9	17.90
SANDWICH COOKIES				
French Vanilla Creme Cookies, 1 3/4-oz. package (6 cookies)	230	33.0	131.4	18.86
Keebie Cookies, 1 3/4-oz. package (6 cookies)	220	32.0	125.7	18.29
Lemon Creme Cookies, 1 3/4-oz. package (6 cookies)	220	32.0	125.7	18.29
SANDWICH CRACKERS				
Cheese 'N' Peanut Butter Crackers, 1 1/2-oz. package (6 crackers)	210	24.0	140.0	16.00
Jumbo Cheese 'N' Peanut Butter Crackers, 1 3/4-oz. package (6 crackers)	240	28.0	137.1	16.00
Toast N' Peanut Butter Crackers, 1 1/2-oz. package (6 crackers)	230	25.0	153.3	16.67
Pepperidge Farm:				
COOKIES				
Brownies, 2 1/4-oz. package (2 brownies)	340	41.0	151.1	18.22
Chocolate Chip Cookies, 2 1/4-oz. package (2 cookies)	330	44.0	146.7	19.56
Granola Cookies, 2 1/4-oz. package (2 cookies)	320	41.0	142.2	18.22
Lemon Nut Cookies, 2 1/4-oz. package (2 cookies)	340	41.0	151.1	18.22
Oatmeal Cookies, 2 1/4-oz. package (2 cookies)	310	45.0	137.8	20.00
Sugar Cookies, 2 1/4-oz. package (2 cookies)	320	45.0	142.0	20.00
GOLDFISH CRACKERS				
Cheddar Cheese Flavored Goldfish Crackers, 3/4-oz. package (approx. 42 crackers)	105	12.5	140.3	16.73
Lightly Salted Goldfish Crackers, 3/4-oz. package (approx. 41 crackers)	103	13.6	137.5	18.15
Pizza Flavored Goldfish Crackers, 3/4-oz. package (approx. 42 crackers)	105	12.5	140.1	16.73
Pretzel Goldfish Crackers, 3/4-oz. package (approx. 35 crackers)	87	15.3	116.2	20.41

CANDY BARS and SNACK BARS

This list is only a sampling. See the SWEET LITTLE NOTHINGS chapter for more.

	UNIT		1 OZ., BY WT.	
	Cal.	Carb.	Cal.	Carb.
Almond Bar, **Nestlé,** 5-oz. bar	750	85.0	150.0	17.00
Almond Joy, **Peter Paul,** 1.1-oz. bar	166	20.4	151.0	18.50
Baby Ruth Bar, **Standard Brands,** 2-oz. bar	289	34.4	144.4	17.22
Bit-O-Honey, **Ward Foods,** 1.5-oz. bar (6 pieces)	176	39.0	117.0	26.00
1 piece, approx. 1/4 oz.	29	6.5	117.0	26.00
2.1-oz. bar (6 pieces)	246	54.6	117.0	26.00
1 piece, approx. 0.35 oz.	41	9.1	117.0	26.00
Butterfinger Bar, **Standard Brands,** 1.8-oz. bar	248	31.5	137.5	17.50
CaraCoa Crunchy Candy Bar, 7/8-oz. bar	140	14.0	160.0	16.00
3 1/2-oz. bar	560	56.0	160.0	16.00
Fruit 'n Nut Candy Bar, 1-oz. bar	160	16.0	160.0	16.00
4-oz. bar	640	64.0	160.0	16.00
Milk-Free Candy Bar, 1-oz. bar	145	18.0	145.0	18.00
4-oz. bar	590	70.0	145.0	18.00
Mint Candy Bar, 1-oz. bar	160	16.0	160.0	16.00
4-oz. bar	640	64.0	160.0	16.00
Natural Candy Bar, 1-oz. bar	160	16.0	160.0	16.00
4-oz. bar	640	64.0	160.0	16.00
Orange Candy Bar, 1-oz. bar	160	16.0	160.0	16.00
4-oz. bar	640	64.0	160.0	16.00
Peanut Candy Bar, 1-oz. bar	160	16.0	160.0	16.00
4-oz. bar	640	64.0	160.0	16.00
Carob Coated Caramels, 1-oz. package	110	21.0	110.0	21.00

	UNIT Cal.	UNIT Carb.	1 OZ., BY WT. Cal.	1 OZ., BY WT. Carb.
Dates, 1-oz. package	125	18.0	125.0	18.00
4-oz. box	500	72.0	125.0	18.00
Peanuts, 1-oz. package	160	12.0	160.0	12.00
4-oz. box	640	48.0	160.0	12.00
Raisins, 1-oz. package	130	18.0	130.0	18.00
4-oz. box	520	72.0	130.0	18.00
Soybeans, 1-oz. package	145	12.0	145.0	12.00
4½-oz. box	653	54.0	145.0	12.00
Caravel, **Peter Paul,** 1.15-oz. bar	156	21.0	136.0	18.30
Charleston Chew, **Fox-Cross Candy Co.,** 2¹⁄₁₆-oz. bar	248	44.8	120.0	21.74
Choco'Lite Bar, **Nestlé,** 1-oz. bar	150	18.0	150.0	18.00
5-oz. bar	750	90.0	150.0	18.00
Chunky, original, **Ward,** 1.25-oz. "Triple" bar	181	19.6	145.0	15.70
0.9-oz. "Twin" bar	131	14.1	145.0	15.70
Crunch Bar, **Nestlé,** 1¹⁄₁₆-oz. bar	174	20.9	150.0	18.00
Goobers, **Ward,** 1-oz. box	153	12.0	153.0	12.00
Granola Bar, Cherry Yogurt, **Crunchola,** 1¼-oz. bar	170	22.0	136.0	17.60
Granola Bar, Chocolate Chip, **Crunchola,** 1½-oz. bar	210	24.0	140.0	16.00
Granola Bar, Strawberry Yogurt, **Crunchola,** 1¼-oz. bar	175	21.3	140.0	17.00
Granola Crunch, Honey Almond, **Sun Country,** 1½-oz. package	150	19.0	100.0	12.67
Cinnamon Apple, **Sun Country,** 1½-oz. package	140	20.0	93.3	13.33
Cinnamon Raisin, **Sun Country,** 1½-oz. package	150	18.0	100.0	12.00
Kit Kat, **Hershey's,** 1.125-oz. bar	160	19.0	142.2	16.89
Krackel Candy Bar, **Hershey's,** 1.05-oz. bar	160	18.0	152.4	17.14
M&M's Peanut Chocolate Candies, 1.56-oz. bag	212	24.1	143.3	16.30
M&M's Plain Chocolate Candies, 1.56-oz. bag	215	29.9	138.0	19.30
Mary Jane Candy Bar, **Miller,** 1⅝-oz. bar	117	21.1	72.0	13.00
Milk Chocolate, **Hershey's,** 1.05-oz. bar	160	17.0	152.4	16.19
Milk Chocolate with Almonds, **Hershey's,** 1.05-oz. bar	160	17.0	152.4	16.19
Milk Chocolate Bar, **Nestlé,** 3.2-oz. bar	474	19.7	150.0	17.00
Milk Mounds, **Peter Paul,** 1.1-oz. bar	162	21.8	147.0	19.80
Milky Way, **M&M/Mars,** 1.91-oz. bar	242	39.6	126.7	20.73
Mounds, **Peter Paul,** 1.1-oz. bar	162	21.8	147.0	19.80
Mr. Goodbar, **Hershey's,** 1.3-oz. bar	210	18.0	161.5	13.85
Nibs, Cherry Artificial Flavor, **Y & S,** 1⅞-oz. bag	200	45.0	106.7	24.00
Fruit Artificial Flavor, 1⅞-oz. bag	200	45.0	106.7	24.00
Licorice Flavored, 1⅞-oz. bag	200	45.0	106.7	24.00
$100,000 Bar, **Nestlé,** 0.56-oz. bar	78	10.6	140.0	19.00
1-oz. bar	140	19.0	140.0	19.00
1⅛-oz. bar	158	21.4	140.0	19.00
Peanut Butter Cups, **Reese's (Hershey's),** 1.2-oz. package	190	18.0	158.3	15.00
Peanut Crunch, **Sahadi,** ¾-oz. bar	106	6.3	141.7	8.33
Peppermint Patty, **York,** 1.05-oz. patty	130	26.3	124.0	25.00
Raisinets, **Ward Foods,** 1-oz. box	90	14.0	90.0	14.00
Rally, **Hershey's,** 1.5-oz. bar	210	22.0	140.0	14.67
Reggie Bar, **Standard Brands,** 1.6-oz. bar	232	23.2	145.0	14.50
2-oz. bar	290	29.0	145.0	14.50
Rolo, **Hershey's,** 1-oz. roll	140	19.0	140.0	19.00
Sesame Crunch, dry-roasted, **Sahadi,** ¾-oz. bar	113	8.1	150.0	10.83
Sesame & Honey Crunch Bar, dry roasted, **Sahadi,** ¾-oz. bar	120	9.0	160.0	12.00
Special Dark chocolate bar, **Hershey's,** 1.05-oz. bar	166	19.2	158.3	18.33
Stix, Apple, **Jolly Rancher,** 1-oz. Stix	148		148.0	
Butterscotch, 1-oz. Stix	148		148.0	
Cherry, 1-oz. Stix	148		148.0	
Fire, 1-oz. Stix	148		148.0	
Grape, 1-oz. Stix	148		148.0	
Lemon, 1-oz. Stix	148		148.0	
Orange, 1-oz. Stix	148		148.0	
Peach, 1-oz. Stix	148		148.0	
Pineapple, 1-oz. Stix	148		148.0	
Strawberry, 1-oz. Stix	148		148.0	
Watermelon, 1-oz. Stix	148		148.0	
Twists, Chocolate, **Y & S,** 4.5-oz. package	650	110.0	144.4	24.40
1 piece, approx. 0.3 oz.	43	7.3	144.4	24.40
Licorice, 5-oz. package	500	110.0	100.0	22.00
1 piece, approx. 0.3 oz.	33	7.3	100.0	22.00
Strawberry, 5-oz. package	475	115.0	95.0	23.00
1 piece, approx. 0.33 oz.	32	7.7	95.0	23.00
Twizzlers, Chocolate Flavored, **Y & S,** 5-oz. package	550	120.0	110.0	24.00
1 piece, approx. 0.3 oz.	34	8.0	110.0	24.00
Licorice Flavored, 1¼-oz. package	125	30.0	100.0	24.00
1¾-oz. package	175	42.0	100.0	24.00
2⅛-oz. package	213	51.0	100.0	24.00
5-oz. package	500	120.0	100.0	24.00
Strawberry, Artificial Flavored, 1¼-oz. package	125	30.0	100.0	24.00
1¾-oz. package	175	42.0	100.0	24.00
2⅛-oz. package	213	51.0	100.0	24.00
5-oz. package	500	120.0	100.0	24.00

SALTY SNACKS

This list is only a sampling. See the SALTY SNACKS chapter for more.

	UNIT Cal.	UNIT Carb.	1 OZ., BY WT. Cal.	1 OZ., BY WT. Carb.
Andy Capp's:				
Cheddar Fries, ⅝-oz. bag	93	10.2	149.4	16.33
Hot Fries, ⅝-oz. bag	93	10.2	149.4	16.33
Bachman:				
CHEESE TWISTS				
Jax Cheese Corn Twists, Baked, ¾-oz. package	113	12.8	150.0	17.00
⅜-oz. package	56	6.3	150.0	17.00
1½-oz. package	225	25.5	150.0	17.00
Jax Cheese Corn Twists, Fried, 1½-oz. package	237	21.0	158.0	14.00
CORN CHIPS				
Corn Chips, 1¼-oz. bag	188	18.8	150.0	15.00
2-oz. bag	300	30.0	150.0	15.00
BBQ Corn Chips, 1-oz. bag	150	15.0	150.0	15.00
1⅞-oz. bag	281	28.1	150.0	15.00
POPCORN				
Popcorn, 1⅛-oz. package	180	14.6	160.0	13.00
Caramel Corn, 1¼-oz. package	140	31.2	112.0	25.00
Cheese Popcorn, 1-oz. package	180	14.0	180.0	14.00
POTATO CHIPS				
BBQ Potato Chips, ¾-oz. bag	112	10.5	150.0	14.00
1¼-oz. bag	188	17.5	150.0	14.00
Golden Crisp Fries, ¾-oz. bag	112	10.5	150.0	14.00
1¼-oz. bag	188	17.5	150.0	14.00
Golden Crisp Potato Chips, ½-oz. bag	75	7.0	150.0	14.00
¾-oz. bag	113	10.5	150.0	14.00
1¼-oz. bag	188	17.5	150.0	14.00
Golden Ridges Potato Chips, 1¼-oz. bag	188	17.5	150.0	14.00
Sour Cream and Onion Potato Chips, ¾-oz. bag	113	10.5	150.0	14.00
1¼-oz. bag	188	17.5	150.0	14.00
PRETZELS:				
Petite Pretzels, 1-oz. bag	110	21.0	110.0	21.00
Stix Pretzels, 1-oz. bag	110	21.0	110.0	21.00
Twist Pretzels, 1½-oz. bag	165	31.5	110.0	21.00
TORTILLA CHIPS:				
Tortilla Chips, Nacho Cheese Flavor, 1-oz. bag	136	17.0	136.0	17.00
1½-oz. bag	204	25.5	136.0	17.00
Tortilla Chips, Taco Flavor, 1-oz. bag	138	17.0	138.0	17.00
1½-oz. bag	207	25.5	138.0	17.00
Frito-Lay:				
Baken-Ets Fried Pork Rinds, ⅝-oz. bag	93	0.6	150.0	1.00
Chee•Tos Cheese Flavored Snacks, Crunchy, 1¼-oz. bag	200	18.7	160.0	15.00
Chee•Tos Cheese Flavored Snacks, Puffed, 1-oz. bag	160	15.0	160.0	15.00
Doritos Tortilla Chips, 1⅛-oz. bag	157	21.3	140.0	19.00
Doritos Tortilla Chips, Nacho Cheese Flavor, 1⅛-oz. bag	157	20.2	140.0	18.00
Fritos Corn Chips, 1½-oz. bag	240	24.0	160.0	16.00
Funyuns Onion Flavored Snacks, ⅞-oz. bag	120	16.4	138.0	18.80
Lay's Potato Chips, 1-oz. bag	150	14.0	150.0	14.00
Lay's Potato Chips, Bar-B-Q Flavor, 1-oz. bag	150	14.0	150.0	14.00
Lay's Potato Chips, Sour Cream & Onion Flavor, 1-oz. bag	160	14.0	160.0	14.00
Munchos Potato Crisps, 1-oz. bag	154	15.2	154.0	15.20
Ruffles Potato Chips, 1-oz. bag	150	15.0	150,0	15.00
Ruffles Potato Chips, Bar-B-Q Flavor, 1-oz. bag	150	15.0	150.0	15.00
Granny Goose:				
Cheese Nibbles, 1-oz. foil package	167	14.2	167.6	14.15
Cheese Tortilla Chips, 1⅜-oz. foil package	200	24.3	145.4	17.66
Corn Chips, 1-oz. foil package	159	15.4	158.8	15.37
Mini Pretzels, 1-oz. package	110	22.9	110.0	22.90
Potato Chips, Regular, ⅞-oz. foil package	140	12.4	158.8	14.20
Potato Chips, Barbecue Flavored, 1⅛-oz. foil package	171	16.3	152.3	14.50
Potato Chips, Sour Cream & Onion, ⅞-oz. foil package	133	12.7	152.0	14.52
Tortilla Chips, 1-oz. foil package	140	17.9	139.8	17.86
Pepperidge Farm Vending Pretzels:				
Nuggets, 1⅛-oz. package	150	27.0	120.0	21.60
Thin Sticks, 1¼-oz. package	150	30.0	120.0	24.00
Tiny Twists, 1-oz. package	120	22.0	120.0	22.00
Wise:				
Cheez Doodles, Baked, Puffed, ¾-oz. bag	120	12.0	160.0	16.00
Cheez Doodles, Fried, Crunchy, 1¼-oz. bag	200	20.0	160.0	16.00
Corn Crunchies, 1⅛-oz. bag	180	18.0	160.0	16.00
Onion Flavored Rings, ½-oz. bag	65	11.0	130.0	22.00
Popcorn, Butter Flavored, ½-oz. bag	70	8.0	140.0	16.00
Pork Rinds, Fried, ⅜-oz. bag	56	0.0	150.0	0.00
Potato Chips, 1-oz. bag	150	14.0	150.0	14.00

	UNIT Cal.	UNIT Carb.	1 OZ., BY WT. Cal.	1 OZ., BY WT. Carb.
Potato Chips, Barbeque Flavored, 7/8-oz. bag	131	13.1	150.0	15.00
Potato Chips, Sour Cream & Onion Rippled, 1¾-oz. bag	280	24.5	160.0	14.00
Pretzel Mini, 1-oz. bag	100	22.0	100.0	22.00
Pretzel Nuggets, 1⅛-oz. bag	124	24.8	110.0	22.00
Tortilla Chips, Nacho Cheese, 1-oz. bag	150	17.0	150.0	17.00
NUTS & SEEDS				
This list is only a sampling. See the NUTS & SEED chapter for more.				
David's:				
Pumpkin Seeds, 1-oz. package	120	1.0	120.0	1.00
Snack 'n Wheat, Cheese Flavored, 1-oz. package	150	15.0	150.0	15.00
Sunflower Kernels, 1-oz. package	180	4.0	180.0	4.00
Sunflower Seeds, roasted and salted in the shell, 1-oz. package	90	2.0	90.0	2.00
Granny Goose:				
Cashews, 1-oz. package	169	7.0	169.0	7.00
Goobers, 1-oz. package	166	4.9	166.0	4.90
Spanish Peanuts, 1-oz. package	168	4.0	168.0	4.00
Virginia Peanuts, 1-oz. package	166	4.6	166.0	4.60
Planters:				
Peanuts, ½-oz. foil pack	85	2.5	170.0	5.00
Peanuts, dry-roasted, ½-oz. cello-pak	85	2.5	170.0	5.00

39 AIRLINE FARE •

BRANIFF INTERNATIONAL

Regular Meals

	UNIT Cal.	UNIT Carb.
BEEF DINNER (#SP10)		
3 oz. boiled beef, 2 oz. vegetable, 2 oz. potatoes, choice of chocolate brownie, apple, or banana:		
1 dinner with apple or banana	(307)	(36.7)
1 dinner with brownie	(342)	(29.4)
1 dinner without dessert	(208)	(12.2)
CHICKEN DINNER (#SP42)		
½ broiled chicken (1 lb.), 2 oz. vegetable, 2 oz. boiled or baked potato, choice of chocolate brownie, apple, or banana:		
1 dinner with apple or banana	(545)	(36.7)
1 dinner with brownie	(565)	(29.5)
1 dinner without dessert	(445)	(12.2)
FISH DINNER (#SP41)		
5 oz. broiled or boiled fish, 2 oz. vegetable, 2 oz. boiled or baked potato, choice of chocolate brownie, apple, or banana:		
1 dinner with apple or banana	(388)	(44.9)
1 dinner with brownie	(408)	(37.6)
1 dinner without dessert	(288)	(10.4)
FRESH FRUIT PLATE (#SP44)		
12 to 15 oz. fresh sliced fruits such as melons, oranges, apples, or pears:		
1 plate	(164-205)	(41.6-52.0)
SEAFOOD PLATTER (#SP34)		
Flaked crab meat, shrimp, egg slices, tomatoes, lettuce, celery, remoulade sauce, cocktail sauce, lemon wedge, garnish (rolls, butter and dessert not included in calculations):		
1 platter	(250)	(34.0)

Children's Meals

	UNIT Cal.	UNIT Carb.
HAMBURGER MEAL (#SP36)		
4 oz. chopped beef on a 4" bun with 2 slices tomato and lettuce leaf, 1 packet mustard, 1 packet catsup, 1 packet pickle relish, 1 oz. potato chips, 1 Ding Dong, 8 fl. oz. chocolate-flavored milk:		
1 meal	(890)	(95.8)
HOT DOG MEAL (#SP37)		
1 frankfurter on 5" bun, 1 packet mustard, 1 packet catsup, 1 packet pickle relish, 1 oz. potato chips, 1 Ding Dong, 8 fl. oz. chocolate-flavored milk:		
1 meal	(830)	(95.0)

Special Meals

	UNIT Cal.	UNIT Carb.
BLAND OR ULCER		
LUNCH or DINNER (#SP77)		
2 oz. cottage cheese, 2 peach halves, 5 oz. boneless roast chicken, 3 oz. mashed potatoes, 2 oz. baby carrots, 1 roll with 1 pat butter, choice of plain Jell-O, rice pudding, or custard:		
1 lunch or dinner with Jell-O	(672)	(72.2)
1 lunch or dinner with rice pudding or custard	(743)	(68.7)
BREAKFAST (#SP75)		
4 oz. orange juice, 2 poached eggs on English muffin, 1 peach half, 1 sweet roll or muffin, 1 pat butter, 1 tablespoon marmalade:		
1 breakfast	(660)	(82.3)
GLUTEN FREE		
BREAKFAST (#SP20)		
4 oz. orange juice, 2 eggs with cheese omelet, 2 oz. broiled ham steak, 4 oz. fruit salad:		
1 breakfast	(505)	(31.5)
SNACK (#SP23)		
3 oz. cold roast beef on lettuce, 2 oz. cottage cheese, 3 oz. orange sections, 5 oz. gelatin dessert:		
1 snack	(355)	(28.9)
HYPOGLYCEMIC OR LOW CARBOHYDRATE		
LUNCH or DINNER (#SP53)		
4 oz. broiled fillet, 3 oz. green beans, 2 oz. cottage cheese, lettuce, 3 tomato wedges, lemon wedge, 1 fresh fruit:		
1 lunch or dinner	(309)	(23.3)
BREAKFAST (#SP51)		
4 oz. orange juice, 4 oz. filet mignon, omelet made with 4 oz. "Eggbeaters," 1 fresh fruit, 8 fl. oz. skim milk:		
1 breakfast if fresh fruit is peach	(549)	(35.9)
1 breakfast if fresh fruit is banana	(612)	(52.7)
LACTOSE RESTRICTED		
LUNCH or DINNER (#SP26)		
4 oz. broiled fillet, 2 oz. green vegetable, 2 oz. boiled potatoes, #3 mixed green salad, lemon wedges, fresh fruit, soda crackers and 1 tablespoon margarine:		
1 lunch or dinner	(493)	(52.2)
1 lunch or dinner without the crackers and margarine	(345)	(44.3)
BREAKFAST (#SP24)		
4 oz. orange juice, 2 poached eggs, 3 strips bacon, fruit, soda crackers and margarine:		
1 breakfast	(586)	(46.9)
1 breakfast without the crackers and margarine	(438)	(39.0)

	UNIT Cal.	Carb.
SNACK (#SP27)		
1 oz. roast beef, 1 oz. ham, 1 oz. turkey, fresh fruit, soda crackers and 1 tablespoon margarine:		
1 snack	(297)	(32.4)
1 snack without the crackers and margarine	(149)	(24.5)
"LOW CALORIE"		
LUNCH or DINNER (#SP32)		
5 oz. fillet mignon, 3 oz. baked potato, 2 oz. green peas, #2 mixed salad with oil and vinegar dressing, 1 baked apple, 8 fl. oz. skim milk:		
1 lunch or dinner	(557)	(65.0)
BREAKFAST (#SP30)		
4 oz. unsweetened grapefruit juice, omelet made with 4 oz. "Eggbeaters," 2 beef patties, 2 pieces melba toast or zwieback with 1 tablespoon margarine, 8 fl. oz. skim milk:		
1 breakfast	(669)	(30.7)
BREAKFAST SNACK (#SP31)		
1½-oz. low-fat cheese, 3 pieces melba toast or zwieback, 8 fl. oz. skim milk:		
1 snack	(238)	(21.4)
SNACK (#SP33)		
2 oz. roast beef, 2 oz. turkey breast, 2 oz. cottage cheese, 2 pieces melba toast, 1 fresh fruit:		
1 snack	(351)	(31.1)
LOW CHOLESTEROL		
LUNCH or DINNER (#SP57)		
5 oz. chicken breast, 2 oz. green peas with almonds, small baked potato, mixed green salad with 1 oz. oil and vinegar dressing, 1 roll with 1 tablespoon margarine, 4 oz. fruit salad:		
1 lunch or dinner	(644)	(60.4)
BREAKFAST (#SP55)		
4 oz. orange juice, omelet made with 4 oz. "Eggbeaters," 3 oz. "very lean" ham steak, 1 biscuit with 1 tablespoon margarine and 1 tablespoon jelly, 8 fl. oz. skim milk:		
1 breakfast	(794)	(53.2)
SNACK (#SP58)		
Cold roast beef sandwich on white bread, 2 oz. cottage cheese with peach half, bowl of raw carrots, celery, cherry tomatoes, and olives:		
1 snack	(396)	(36.0)
LOW SODIUM		
LUNCH or DINNER (#SP61)		
4 oz. fruit salad, 5 oz. filet mignon, 1½ oz. carrots, 1½ oz. corn, 1 small baked potato, 1 dinner roll and 1 pat butter, 4 oz. Jell-O:		
1 lunch or dinner	(740)	(82.0)
BREAKFAST (#SP59)		
4 oz. orange juice, 2 poached eggs on English muffin, 2 oz. hash brown potatoes, 1 peach half, 3" sweet roll with 1 pat butter, 1 tablespoon marmalade:		
1 breakfast	(787)	(98.8)
SNACK (#SP62)		
3 oz. cold roast beef, 2 oz. cottage cheese, 5 oz. orange slices, 2 celery sticks, 2 carrot sticks, 2 cherry tomatoes, 2 pieces raw cauliflower, 1 dinner roll with 1 pat butter, 4 oz. Jell-O:		
1 snack	(513)	(48.7)
SUGAR FREE OR DIABETIC		
LUNCH or DINNER (#SP73)		
5 oz. fillet mignon, 2 oz. green peas, 3 oz. boiled potatoes, lettuce & tomato salad with 1 oz. oil and vinegar dressing, 1 roll with 1 pat margarine, 1 fresh apple:		
1 lunch or dinner	(664)	(58.4)
BREAKFAST (#SP71)		
Orange sections, 2-egg omelet, 1 slice of toast with 1 tablespoon margarine, 1 dinner roll, 8 fl. oz. skim milk:		
1 breakfast	(618)	(59.8)
BREAKFAST SNACK (#SP72)		
1 fresh orange, 2 slices of toast with margarine, 8 fl. oz. skim milk:		
1 breakfast snack	(409)	(58.8)
SNACK (#SP74)		
Roast beef sandwich, ¾-oz. cheese wedge, 1 fresh apple, 1 cherry tomato, 1 pickle, 1 olive:		
1 snack	(496)	(54.6)
VEGETARIAN		
Lacto/Ovo Vegetarian		
LUNCH or DINNER (#SP65)		
4 oz. imitation meat, vegetables "du jour" (including a starchy vegetable), #2 mixed greens, ¾ oz. chef's dressing, 1 roll with 1 tablespoon margarine, dessert "du jour":		
1 lunch or dinner	(521)	(47.8)
BREAKFAST (#SP63)		
4 oz. orange juice, 2-egg omelet, 2 soy patties, 1 buttermilk biscuit, 1 tablespoon margarine, 1 roll, 8 oz. nonfat milk:		
1 breakfast	(820)	(60.5)
Pure Vegetarian		
LUNCH or DINNER (#SP69)		
4 oz. imitation meat, vegetables "du jour" (including a starchy vegetable), #2 mixed greens, ¾ oz. oil and vinegar dressing, 1 roll with 1 tablespoon margarine, 4 oz. fresh fruit salad:		
1 lunch or dinner	(521)	(47.8)

	UNIT Cal.	Carb.
BREAKFAST (#SP67)		
4 oz. orange juice, a 1-oz. box cereal (Special "K," Bran Flakes, Product 19, or Funky Granola), 16 fl. oz. soy milk, 1 banana or 3 oz. fresh berries, 2 soy patties, 1 biscuit or muffin with 1 tablespoon margarine, 1 roll:		
1 breakfast with banana	(900)	(106.0)
1 breakfast with berries	(832)	(87.2)

LUFTHANSA

Hors d'Oeuvres

	Cal.	Carb.
Smoked Loin of Pork, 1 serving	(155)	(2.7)
Smoked Trout, 1 serving	(480)	(8.1)
Stuffed Green Pepper, Beef Salad, 1 serving	(81)	(3.9)
Stuffed Tomatoes with Rice Salad, 1 serving (½ tomato)	(104)	(10.2)

Soup

	Cal.	Carb.
Consomme "Princess," served with 1 oz. cheese sticks, ⅓ oz. diced chicken, and ⅓ oz. white asparagus spear, 1 serving	(155)	(3.4)
Consommé alone	(32)	(3.4)
Garnish alone	(123)	(0.0)

Main Course

	Cal.	Carb.
Bay Scallops in White Wine Sauce, 1 serving	(473)	(11.2)
Braised Veal in Cream Sauce and Carrots Spaetzle, 1 serving	(708)	(31.1)
Fillet Stroganoff, Buttered Carrots, Spaetzle, 1 serving	(565)	(28.9)
Hanseatic "Fischtopf" (a fish stew), 1 serving	(588)	(30.8)
Koenigbergers Klopse (meatballs, caper sauce), 1 serving	(831)	(29.1)
Shrimp Newburg, 1 serving	(416)	(12.0)
Stuffed Beef Roll, Peas & Carrots, Duchess Potatoes, 1 serving	(665)	(26.9)

Salad

	Cal.	Carb.
Puszta Salad, with Oil and Vinegar Dressing, 1 serving	(37)	(4.1)

Desserts

	Cal.	Carb.
Brandy Alexander Parfait, 1 serving	(307)	(21.5)
Bittersweet Chocolate Mousse, 1 serving	(234)	(10.1)

Snack

	Cal.	Carb.
Empanada, 1 serving	(80)	(3.0)

PAN AM

Entrees

	Cal.	Carb.
Beef Bourguignonne		
800 pounds beef cubes, 20 gallons red wine, 70 gallons brown veal stock, 10 pounds shallots, 115 pounds onions, 96 1-pound cans button mushrooms, 40 pounds trower roux, 4 pounds stabilizer, 4 pounds beef extract, 12 oz. caramel color, 2 oz. red color, 2 pounds salt, 1 pound MSG, 1 oz. thyme, 6 pounds butter, 4 gallons shortening. Serves 2,000 passengers	839966	31179.1
1 portion	450	15.6
Bird Of Paradise (Chicken)		
600 pounds sliced chicken, 65 gallons chicken stock, 4 gallons soy sauce, 15 pounds sugar, 10 pounds shallots, ½ gallon lime juice, 43 oz. oyster sauce, 1 pound salt, 1 pound MSG, 9 oz. caramel color, ½ oz. ginger, 15 pounds dehydrated black mushrooms, 72 pounds snowpeas, 30 pounds waterchestnuts, 3 pounds butter, 22½ gallons stabilizer. Serves 1,800 passengers	746734	56798.5
1 portion	(415)	(31.6)
Breast of Chicken Chilindron, 1 portion	(347)	(6.6)
Grenadins of Veal Niçoise, 1 portion	(590)	(14.1)
Poached Salmon Steak in Champagne Sauce, 1 portion	(644)	(5.1)
Roast Breast of Duckling Cointreau, 1 portion	(347)	(69.4)
Stuffed Trout Sylvia, 1 portion	(1133)	(50.8)

TAP (Air Portugal)

	Cal.	Carb.
DINNER MENU #1		
Appetizer: 1½ oz. smoked salmon (lox), 2 pumpernickel rounds, 1 tablespoon cream cheese	(146)	(7.3)
Entrée: 7 oz. (5.1 oz. cooked) short rib of beef, 1½ oz. sauce provençale, ½ oz. tomato concassee, 1 mushroom slice, 2 oz. hash brown potatoes, ½ oz. Brussels sprouts	(905)	(27.6)
Also: 1 cheese wedge, 2 French rolls, 1 cracker, 1 pat butter	(254)	(24.3)
Dessert: Apple Streusel, 2" × 3" × 1½"	(200)	(32.0)
DINNER MENU #2		
Appetizer: 2 oz. chicken gallantine, 2 oz. Waldorf salad, 1 tablespoon cumberland sauce, 2 orange slices	(191)	(12.0)

	UNIT Cal.	UNIT Carb.
Entrée: 6 oz. (4 oz. cooked) bottom round Boef Braise, 1½ burgundy sauce, 2 oz. macaroni shells, 2½ oz. Blue Lake beans with butter	(404)	(24.0)
Salad: 1/10 head lettuce, 2 slices tomato, 1 tablespoon French dressing	(95)	(4.0)
Also: 1 cheese wedge, 2 French rolls, 1 cracker, 1 pat butter	(254)	(24.3)
Dessert: Strudel with cheesecake, 2″ × 2″ × 1¼″	(240)	(23.8)
DINNER MENU #3		
Appetizer: 2 oz. chicken gallantine, 2 oz. Waldorf salad, 1 tablespoon cumberland sauce, 2 orange slices	(191)	(12.0)
Entrée: 5 oz. (3.3 oz. cooked) round Beef Roulada stuffed with ¼ oz. bacon, 1½ oz. ground beef, ¼ oz. onions, 1½ oz. sauce, 1½ oz. Duchess potatoes, 2 oz. broccoli fleurette	(514)	(16.9)
Salad with French dressing	(95)	(4.0)
Also: 1 cheese wedge, 2 French rolls, 1 cracker, 1 pat butter	(254)	(24.3)
Dessert: Sara Lee Cheesecake with Strawberries	(213)	(30.3)
DINNER MENU #4		
Appetizer: 2 snow crab claws, lettuce, 1 oz. cocktail sauce, 1 lemon wedge, 1 cherry tomato	(48)	(10.3)
Entrée: 4 oz. (2.7 oz. cooked) beef fillet medallions, 1½ oz. cognac cream sauce, 2 oz. cauliflower polanaise, 2 oz. Spanish rice	(337)	(13.7)
Salad: 1/10 head lettuce, 2 tomato slices	(95)	(4.0)
Also: 1 cheese wedge, 2 French rolls, 1 cracker, 1 pat butter	(254)	(24.3)
Dessert: Grand Marnier French pastry, 2″ × 3″ × 1½″	(250)	(25.0)
DINNER MENU #5		
Appetizer: 1 artichoke heart, 1 black olive, 1 stuffed olive, ½ oz. slice proscuitto, ½ oz. Genoa salami, 1 sardine	(193)	(6.8)
Entrée: Veal goulash (6 oz. veal cubes, 5 oz. cooked), 2 oz. paprika cream sauce, 2 oz. spaetzel with onion and bacon, 2½ oz. petit pois with tomato concasse	(558)	(23.5)
Salad with French dressing	(95)	(4.0)
Also: 1 cheese wedge, 2 French rolls, 1 cracker, 1 pat butter	(254)	(24.3)
Dessert: Apple strudel, 2″ × 2″ × 1½″	(245)	(25.0)
DINNER MENU #6		
Appetizer: 1¼ oz. crabmeat, ⅞ oz. baby shrimp, 3 oz. mayonnaise, ⅛ egg, ⅙ tomato, ⅛ lemon, 2 black olives	(161)	(2.9)

	UNIT Cal.	UNIT Carb.
Entrée: 5 oz. chicken breast cordon rouge, 1 oz. Burgundy sauce, 2½ oz. saffron rice, 2 oz. Belgian carrots	(449)	(39.0)
Salad with French dressing	(95)	(4.0)
Also: 1 cheese wedge, 2 French rolls, 1 cracker, 1 pat butter	(254)	(24.3)
Dessert: Apricot slice, dough, almond paste, chopped nuts, apricot glaze, 2″ × 2″ × 1½″	(250)	(25.0)

UNITED AIRLINES

Calculations do not include appetizers, rolls and butter, or desserts.

	UNIT Cal.	UNIT Carb.
Baked Pork Chop With Walnut Dressing, Ginger Sauce, 1 serving	(432)	(14.2)
Baked Rocky Mountain Trout With Seafood Stuffing, 1 serving	(802)	(5.8)
Beef Stew, Old Fashioned, 1 serving	(388)	(22.0)
Beef Wellington, Individual, Madeira Sauce, 1 serving	(750)	(47.5)
Biscuits Benedict, 1 serving	(701)	(15.4)
Breast of Chicken Teriyaki, 1 serving	(446)	(20.6)
California Seafood Stew, 1 serving	(253)	(7.4)
Cheese Blintzes With Strawberry Sauce, 1 serving	(267)	(30.5)
Cioppino, 1 serving	(485)	(31.1)
Coq Au Vin, 1 serving	(504)	(8.5)
Crêpes Rios Oso, 1 serving	(440)	(58.2)
Garden Fresh Quiche, 1 serving	(395)	(24.5)
Honey Glazed Pork Chops Sesame, 1 serving	(539)	(60.3)
Island Barbecued Pork Chops, 1 serving	(883)	(32.1)
Lasagne Napoletana, 1 serving	(748)	(66.5)
Monte Cristo Sandwich, 1 sandwich	(468)	(26.1)
Roast Duckling à L'Orange, 1 serving	(691)	(24.4)
Roasted Chicken Athena, 1 serving	(425)	(6.2)
Roasted Rock Cornish Game Hen, Madeira Wine Sauce, 1 serving	(834)	(22.0)
Roasted Turkey With Apple-Cornbread Dressing, 1 serving	(945)	(11.4)
Seafood Newburg, 1 serving	(247)	(10.7)
Veal Scallopini a'Limone, 1 serving	(520)	(9.4)
Waterchestnut Meat Balls, 1 meat ball	(48)	(1.8)

40 CAMPERS' FOODS •

SEIDEL'S TRAIL PACKETS

Breakfast Foods

(Some items are also available in 2- and/or 6-portion packets.)

	ENTIRE PACKAGE		1 OZ., BY WT.		1 SUGGESTED PORTION		1 CUP	
	Cal.	Carb.	Cal.	Carb.	Cal.	Carb.	Cal.	Carb.
CEREALS								
Jiffy Hot Cereal, 4-portion pack, 7 oz. net wt.	680	120.0	97.1	17.14				
1 portion, reconstituted: add 8 fl. oz. (1 cup) water (yield: approx. 8 fl. oz.)			(21.3)	(3.75)	170	30.0	170	30.0
Jiffy Hot Oatmeal, 4-portion pack, 6 oz. net wt.	612	112.0	102.0	18.67				
1 portion, reconstituted: add 6 fl. oz. (¾ cup) water (yield: approx. 6 fl. oz.)			(25.5)	(4.67)	153	28.0	204	37.4
EGGS								
Scrambled Egg Mix, 4-portion pack, 4½ oz. net wt.	580	24.0	128.9	5.33				
1 portion, reconstituted: add 3½ fl. oz. (approx. ⅓ cup) water (yield: approx. 4½ fl. oz.)			(32.2)	(1.33)	145	6.0	258	10.7
Scrambled Egg 'n' Chip Mix, 4-portion pack, 5 oz. net wt.	652	28.0	130.4	5.60				
1 portion, reconstituted: add 3½ fl. oz. (approx. ⅓ cup) water (yield: approx. 4½ fl. oz.)			(36.2)	(1.56)	163	7.0	290	12.4
Western Omelet Mix, 4-portion pack, 4½ oz. net wt.	580	24.0	128.9	5.32				
1 portion, reconstituted: add 3½ fl. oz. (approx. ⅓ cup) water (yield: approx. 4½ fl. oz.)			(32.2)	(1.33)	145	6.0	258	10.7
PANCAKES, FRENCH TOAST, AND SYRUPS								
French Toast Mix, 4-portion pack, 6 oz. net wt.	600	120.0	100.0	20.00				
1 portion, reconstituted: add 3 fl. oz. (⅜ cup) water (yield: approx. 4 fl. oz.)			(37.5)	(7.50)	150	30.0	300	60.0
Pancake Mix, 4-portion pack, 11 oz. net wt.	1308	220.0	118.9	20.00				
1 portion, reconstituted: add 4 fl. oz. (½ cup) water (yield: approx. 6 fl. oz.)			(54.5)	(9.17)	327	55.0	436	73.3
Pancake Mix, Buttermilk, 4-portion pack, 11 oz. net wt.	1124	220.0	102.2	20.00				
1 portion, reconstituted: add 4 fl. oz. (½ cup) water (yield: approx. 6 fl. oz.)			(46.8)	(9.17)	281	55.0	375	73.3
Pancake Syrup Mix, Berry, 4-portion pack, 8 oz. net wt.	904	224.0	113.0	28.00				
1 portion, reconstituted: add 1 fl. oz. (⅛ cup) water (yield: approx. 2 fl. oz.)			(75.3)	(18.67)	226	56.0	904	224.0
Pancake Syrup Mix, Maple, 4-portion pack, 8 oz. net wt.	904	224.0	113.0	28.00				
1 portion, reconstituted: add 1 fl. oz. (⅛ cup) water (yield: approx. 2 fl. oz.)			(75.3)	(18.67)	226	56.0	904	224.0

Dinners With Meat

(Some items are also available in 2- and/or 6-portion packets.)

	ENTIRE PACKAGE		1 OZ., BY WT.		1 SUGGESTED PORTION		1 CUP	
	Cal.	Carb.	Cal.	Carb.	Cal.	Carb.	Cal.	Carb.
BEEF								
Beef 'n' Gravy with Noodles Mix, 4-portion pack, 12 oz. net wt.	1324	172.0	110.3	14.33				
1 portion, reconstituted: add 12 fl. oz. (1½ cups) water (yield: approx. 12½ fl. oz.)			(26.5)	(3.44)	331	43.0	212	27.5
Beef Hash Mix, 4-portion pack, 9¼ oz. net wt.	1040	144.0	112.4	15.57				
1 portion, reconstituted: add 10 fl. oz. (1¼ cup) water (yield: approx. 10 fl. oz.)			(26.0)	(3.60)	260	36.0	208	28.8
Beef Stew, 4-portion pack, 11½ oz. net wt.	1232	168.0	107.1	14.61				
1 portion, reconstituted: add 12 fl. oz. (1½ cups) water (yield: approx. 12 fl. oz.)			(25.7)	(3.50)	308	42.0	205	28.0
Beef Stroganoff Mix, 4-portion pack, 13 oz. net wt.	1532	172.0	117.8	13.23				
1 portion, reconstituted: add 12 fl. oz. (1½ cups) water (yield: approx. 13 fl. oz.)			(29.5)	(3.31)	383	43.0	236	26.5
Spaghetti Beef Dinner Mix, 4-portion pack, 12 oz. net wt.	1140	192.0	96.0	16.00				
1 portion, reconstituted: add 12 fl. oz. (1½ cups) water (yield: approx. 12 fl. oz.)			(23.8)	(4.00)	285	48.0	190	32.0
Veg-A-Rice Beef Dinner, 4-portion pack, 10 oz. net wt.	1132	164.0	113.2	16.40				

	ENTIRE PACKAGE Cal.	ENTIRE PACKAGE Carb.	1 OZ., BY WT. Cal.	1 OZ., BY WT. Carb.	1 SUGGESTED PORTION Cal.	1 SUGGESTED PORTION Carb.	1 CUP Cal.	1 CUP Carb.
1 portion, reconstituted: add 10 fl. oz. (1¼ cups) water (yield: approx. 10 fl. oz.)			(28.3)	(4.10)	283	41.0	226	32.8
CHICKEN								
Chicken à la King Mix, 4-portion pack, 9½ oz. net wt.	1072	108.0	112.8	11.37				
1 portion, reconstituted: add 12 fl. oz. (1½ cups) water (yield: approx. 10½ fl. oz.)			(25.5)	(2.57)	268	27.0	204	20.1
Chicken Noodle Dinner Mix, 4-portion pack, 13 oz. net wt.	1336	208.0	102.8	16.00				
1 portion, reconstituted: add 12 fl. oz. (1½ cups) water (yield: approx. 12½ fl. oz.)			(26.7)	(4.16)	334	52.0	214	33.3
HAM								
Noodle 'n' Ham Dinner Mix, 4-portion pack, 12 oz. net wt.	920	164.0	76.7	13.67				
1 portion, reconstituted: add 11 fl. oz. (1⅜ cups) water (yield: approx. 12 fl. oz.)			(19.2)	(3.42)	230	41.0	153	27.3
Potato 'n' Ham Dinner Mix, 4-portion pack, 11½ oz. net wt.	1164	216.0	101.2	18.80				
1 portion, reconstituted: add 14 fl. oz. (1¾ cups) water (yield: approx. 12 fl. oz.)			(24.3)	(4.50)	291	54.0	194	36.0
TURKEY								
Turkey Dumpling Dinner Mix, 4-portion pack, 10 oz. net wt.	1180	160.0	118.0	16.00				
1 portion, reconstituted: add 10 fl. oz. (1¼ cups) water (yield: approx. 12 fl. oz.)			(24.6)	(3.33)	295	40.0	197	26.7

Meatless Dinners

(Some items are also available in 2- and/or 6-portion packets.)

	ENTIRE PACKAGE Cal.	ENTIRE PACKAGE Carb.	1 OZ., BY WT. Cal.	1 OZ., BY WT. Carb.	1 SUGGESTED PORTION Cal.	1 SUGGESTED PORTION Carb.	1 CUP Cal.	1 CUP Carb.
Macaroni 'n' Cheese Mix, 4-portion pack, 12 oz. net wt.	1292	216.0	107.7	18.00				
1 portion, reconstituted: add 12 fl. oz. (1½ cups) water (yield: approx. 11 fl. oz.)			(29.4)	(4.91)	323	54.0	235	39.3
Spaghetti Mix with Tomato, 4-portion pack, 10 oz. net wt.	920	192.0	92.0	19.20				
1 portion, reconstituted: add 12 fl. oz. (1½ cups) water (yield: approx. 11 fl. oz.)			(20.9)	(4.36)	230	48.0	167	34.9
Veg-A-Rice Chicken Style, 4-portion pack, 10 oz. net wt.	1040	212.0	104.6	21.20				
1 portion, reconstituted: add 10 fl. oz. (1¼ cups) water (yield: approx. 10 fl. oz.)			(26.0)	(5.30)	260	53.0	208	42.4

Vegetables

(Some items are also available in 2- and/or 6-portion packets.)

	ENTIRE PACKAGE Cal.	ENTIRE PACKAGE Carb.	1 OZ., BY WT. Cal.	1 OZ., BY WT. Carb.	1 SUGGESTED PORTION Cal.	1 SUGGESTED PORTION Carb.	1 CUP Cal.	1 CUP Carb.
Carrots, Diced, 4-portion pack, 2½ oz. net wt.	292	68.0	116.8	27.20				
1 portion, reconstituted: add 7 fl. oz. (⅞ cup) water (yield: approx. 4½ fl. oz.)			(16.2)	(3.78)	73	17.0	130	30.2
Corn Mix, Cream Style, 4-portion pack, 4 oz. net wt.	632	108.0	158.0	27.00				
1 portion, reconstituted: add 3½ fl. oz. (approx. ½ cup) water (yield: approx. 4½ fl. oz.)			(35.1)	(6.00)	158	27.0	281	48.0
Corn, Mexicali, 4-portion pack, 3 oz. net wt.	288	56.0	96.0	18.67				
1 portion, reconstituted: add 6 fl. oz. (¾ cup) water (yield: approx. 4 fl. oz.)			(18.0)	(3.50)	72	14.0	144	28.0
Mixed Vegetables in Sauce, 4-portion pack, 3 oz. net wt.	380	72.0	126.7	24.00				
1 portion, reconstituted: add 5 fl. oz. (⅝ cup) water (yield: approx. 4 fl. oz.)			(23.8)	(4.50)	95	18.0	190	36.0
Peas & Carrots, 4-portion pack, 3 oz. net wt.	280	60.0	93.3	20.00				
1 portion, reconstituted: add 7 fl. oz. (⅞ cup) water (yield: approx. 4 fl. oz.)			(17.5)	(3.75)	70	15.0	140	30.0
Peas & Onions, 4-portion pack, 6 oz. net wt.	596	112.0	99.3	18.67				
1 portion, reconstituted: add 6 fl. oz. (¾ cup) water (yield: approx. 4 fl. oz.)			(37.3)	(7.00)	149	28.0	298	56.0
Peas, Sweet, 4-portion pack, 4 oz. net wt.	372	68.0	93.0	17.00				
1 portion, reconstituted: add 9 fl. oz. (1⅛ cups) water (yield: approx. 3 fl. oz.)			(31.0)	(5.67)	93	17.0	248	45.3
Potato Mix, Instant Mashed, 4-portion pack, 4¾ oz. net wt.	444	96.0	93.5	20.21				
1 portion, reconstituted: add 5 fl. oz. (⅝ cup) water (yield: approx. 5 fl. oz.)			(22.2)	(4.80)	111	24.0	178	38.4
Potatoes Au Gratin, 4-portion pack, 6 oz. net wt.	620	108.0	103.3	18.00				
1 portion, reconstituted: add 5 fl. oz. (⅝ cup) water (yield: approx. 5 fl. oz.)			(31.0)	(5.40)	155	27.0	248	43.2
Potatoes, Diced, 4-portion pack, 5½ oz. net wt.	600	136.0	109.1	24.73				
1 portion, reconstituted: add 8 fl. oz. (1 cup) water (yield: approx. 7½ fl. oz.)			(20.0)	(4.53)	150	34.0	160	36.3

Gravy

(Some items are also available in 2-portion packets.)

	ENTIRE PACKAGE Cal.	ENTIRE PACKAGE Carb.	1 OZ., BY WT. Cal.	1 OZ., BY WT. Carb.	1 SUGGESTED PORTION Cal.	1 SUGGESTED PORTION Carb.	1 CUP Cal.	1 CUP Carb.
Brown Gravy Mix, 4-portion pack, 2 oz. net wt.	460	60.0	230.0	30.00				
1 portion, reconstituted: add 4 fl. oz. (½ cup) water (yield: approx. 4 fl. oz.)			(28.8)	(3.75)	115	15.0	230	30.0

Soups

(Some items are also available in 2-portion packets.)

	ENTIRE PACKAGE Cal.	ENTIRE PACKAGE Carb.	1 OZ., BY WT. Cal.	1 OZ., BY WT. Carb.	1 SUGGESTED PORTION Cal.	1 SUGGESTED PORTION Carb.	1 CUP Cal.	1 CUP Carb.
BEEF								
Beef Vegetable Soup, 4-portion pack, 3 oz. net wt.	588	88.0	196.0	29.33				
1 portion, reconstituted: add 12 fl. oz. (1½ cups) water (yield: approx. 10 fl. oz.)			(14.7)	(2.20)	147	22.0	118	17.6
CHICKEN								
Chicken Noodle Soup, 4-portion pack, 3 oz. net wt.	584	92.0	194.7	30.67				
1 portion, reconstituted: add 12 fl. oz. (1½ cups) water (yield: approx. 12 fl. oz.)			(12.2)	(1.92)	146	23.0	98	15.4

Desserts

(Some items are also available in 2- and/or 6-portion packets.)

	ENTIRE PACKAGE Cal.	ENTIRE PACKAGE Carb.	1 OZ., BY WT. Cal.	1 OZ., BY WT. Carb.	1 SUGGESTED PORTION Cal.	1 SUGGESTED PORTION Carb.	1 CUP Cal.	1 CUP Carb.
COBBLER MIX								
Blueberry Cobbler Mix, 4-portion pack, 6½ oz. net wt.	708	160.0	108.9	24.62				
1 portion, reconstituted: add 3 fl. oz. (⅜ cup) water (yield: approx. 4½ fl. oz.)			(39.3)	(8.89)	177	40.0	315	71.1
Cherry Cobbler Mix, 4-portion pack, 6½ oz. net wt.	708	160.0	108.9	24.62				
1 portion, reconstituted: add 3 fl. oz. (⅜ cup) water (yield: approx. 4½ fl. oz.)			(39.3)	(8.89)	177	40.0	315	71.1
Raspberry Cobbler Mix, 4-portion pack, 6½ oz. net wt.	708	160.0	108.9	24.62				
1 portion, reconstituted: add 3 fl. oz. (⅜ cup) water (yield: approx. 4½ fl. oz.)			(39.3)	(8.89)	177	40.0	315	71.1

	ENTIRE PACKAGE		1 OZ., BY WT.		1 SUGGESTED PORTION		1 CUP	
	Cal.	Carb.	Cal.	Carb.	Cal.	Carb.	Cal.	Carb.
CREME DESSERT								
Butterscotch Creme Dessert, 4-portion pack, 5½ oz. net wt.	580	132.0	105.5	24.00				
1 portion, reconstituted: add 4 fl. oz. (½ cup) water (yield: approx. 5 fl. oz.)			(29.0)	(6.60)	145	33.0	232	52.8
Chocolate Creme Dessert, 4-portion pack, 5½ oz. net wt.	580	124.0	105.5	22.55				
1 portion, reconstituted: add 4 fl. oz. (½ cup) water (yield: approx. 5 fl. oz.)			(29.0)	(6.20)	145	31.0	232	49.6
PUDDINGS								
Chocolate Instant Pudding, 4-portion pack, 6 oz. net wt.	620	128.0	103.3	21.33				
1 portion, reconstituted: add 4 fl. oz. (½ cup) water (yield: approx. 5 fl. oz.)			(31.0)	(6.40)	155	32.0	248	51.2
Quick Rice Pudding Mix, 4-portion pack, 7 oz. net wt.	772	152.0	110.3	21.71				
1 portion, reconstituted: add 4 fl. oz. (½ cup) water (yield: approx. 5 fl. oz.)			(38.6)	(7.60)	193	38.0	309	60.8
Toasted Coconut Instant Pudding, 4-portion pack, 6 oz. net wt.	620	132.0	103.3	22.00				
1 portion, reconstituted: add 4 fl. oz. (½ cup) water (yield: approx. 5 fl. oz.)			(31.0)	(6.60)	155	33.0	248	52.8
Vanilla Instant Pudding, 4-portion pack, 6 oz. net wt.	600	136.0	100.0	22.67				
1 portion, reconstituted: add 4 fl. oz. (½ cup) water (yield: approx. 5 fl. oz.)			(30.0)	(6.80)	150	34.0	240	54.4
Beverages								
(Some items are also available in 2- and/or 6-portion packets.)								
FRUIT FLAVORS								
Cherry Beverage Mix, 4-portion pack, 6 oz. net wt.	656	164.0	109.3	27.33				
1 portion, reconstituted: add 12 fl. oz. (1½ cups) water (yield: approx. 13 fl. oz.)			(12.6)	(3.15)	164	41.0	101	25.2
Grape Beverage Mix, 4-portion pack, 6 oz. net wt.	656	164.0	109.3	27.33				
1 portion, reconstituted: add 12 fl. oz. (1½ cups) water (yield: approx. 13 fl. oz.)			(12.6)	(3.15)	164	41.0	101	25.2
Orange Beverage Mix, 4-portion pack, 6 oz. net wt.	656	164.0	109.3	27.33				
1 portion, reconstituted: add 12 fl. oz. (1½ cups) water (yield: approx. 13 fl. oz.			(12.6)	(3.15)	164	41.0	101	25.2
Pink Lemonade Mix, 4-portion pack, 5 oz. net wt.	656	136.0	131.2	27.20				
1 portion, reconstituted: add 12 fl. oz. (1½ cups) water (yield: approx. 13 fl. oz.)			(12.6)	(2.62)	164	34.0	101	20.9
Punch Beverage Mix, 4-portion pack, 6 oz. net wt.	656	164.0	109.3	27.33				
1 portion, reconstituted: add 12 fl. oz. (1½ cups) water (yield: approx. 13 fl. oz.)			(12.6)	(3.15)	164	41.0	101	25.2
MILK BASE								
Choco Malt Kwik Shake Mix, 4-portion pack, 9 oz. net wt.	936	184.0	104.0	20.44				
1 portion, reconstituted: add 12 fl. oz. (1½ cups) water (yield: approx. 13 fl. oz.)			(18.0)	(3.54)	234	46.0	156	30.6
Cocoa Mix, Sweet Milk, 4-portion pack, 8 oz. net wt.	856	180.0	107.0	22.50				
1 portion, reconstituted: add 12 fl. oz. (1½ cups) water (yield: approx. 13 fl. oz.)			(16.5)	(3.46)	214	45.0	132	27.7
Non-Fat Instant Dry Milk, 4-portion pack, 5 oz. net wt.	516	72.0	103.2	14.40				
1 portion, reconstituted: add 8 fl. oz. (1 cup) water (yield: approx. 8 fl. oz.)			(16.1)	(2.25)	129	18.0	129	18.0
Vanilla Kwik Shake Mix, 4-portion pack, 8 oz. net wt.	788	164.0	98.5	20.50				

	ENTIRE PACKAGE		1 OZ., BY WT.		1 SUGGESTED PORTION		1 CUP	
	Cal.	Carb.	Cal.	Carb.	Cal.	Carb.	Cal.	Carb.
1 portion, reconstituted: add 12 fl. oz. (1½ cups) water (yield: approx. 13 fl. oz.)			(15.2)	(3.15)	197	41.0	121	25.2
Fruits								
(Some items are also available in 2- and/or 6-portion packets.)								
Apple Sauce Mix, 4-portion pack, 4 oz. net wt.	424	100.0	106.0	25.00				
1 portion, reconstituted: add 6 fl. oz. (¾ cup) water (yield: approx. 5 fl. oz.)			(21.2)	(5.00)	106	25.0	176	40.0
Apple, Stewed, Mix, 4-portion pack, 5 oz. net wt.	544	128.0	108.8	25.60				
1 portion, reconstituted: add 4 fl. oz. (½ cup) water (yield: approx. 5 fl. oz.)			(27.2)	(6.40)	136	32.0	218	51.2
Apricot Slices, 4-portion pack, 4 oz. net wt.	416	96.0	104.0	24.00				
1 portion, reconstituted: add 3 fl. oz. (⅜ cup) water (yield: approx. 2½ fl. oz.)			(41.6)	(9.60)	104	24.0	333	76.8
Fruit Mix, 4-portion pack, 4 oz. net wt.	388	92.0	97.0	23.00				
1 portion, reconstituted: add 3 fl. oz. (⅜ cup) water (yield: approx. 3½ fl. oz.)			(27.7)	(6.57)	97	23.0	222	52.6
Peach Slices, 4-portion pack, 4 oz. net wt.	392	92.0	98.0	23.00				
1 portion, reconstituted: add 3 fl. oz. (⅜ cup) water (yield: approx. 3 fl. oz.)			(32.7)	(7.67)	98	23.0	261	61.3
Whole Prunes, 4-portion pack, 3½ oz. net wt.	392	92.0	112.0	26.29				
1 portion, reconstituted: add 3 fl. oz. (⅜ cup) water (yield: approx. 2½ fl. oz.)			(38.0)	(9.20)	95	23.0	304	73.6
Baking Mixes								
(Some items are also available in 2- and/or 6-portion packets.)								
Biscuit Mix, 4-portion pack, 14 oz. net wt.	1548	252.0	110.6	18.00				
1 portion, reconstituted: add 1½ oz. (approx. ⅛ cup) water (yield: approx. 4 fl. oz.)			(96.8)	(15.75)	387	63.0	774	126.0
Brownie Mix, 4-portion pack, 8 oz. net wt.	1000	164.0	125.0	20.50				
1 portion, reconstituted: add 1 fl. oz. (⅛ cup) water (yield: approx. 2 fl. oz.)			(125.0)	(20.50)	250	41.0	1000	164.0
Corn Bread Mix, 4-portion pack, 12 oz. net wt.	1328	220.0	110.7	18.33				
1 portion, reconstituted: add 1½ fl. oz. (approx. ⅛ cup) water (yield: approx. 4 fl. oz.)			(83.0)	(13.75)	332	55.0	664	110.0
Gingerbread Mix, 4-portion pack, 8 oz. net wt.	956	172.0	119.5	21.50				
1 portion, reconstituted: add 1 fl. oz. (⅛ cup) water (yield: approx. 2½ fl. oz.)			(95.6)	(17.20)	239	43.0	765	137.6
Instant Spreads								
(Some items are also available in 2- and/or 6-portion packets.)								
Cheese Spread Mix, 4-portion pack, 4 oz. net wt.	468	40.0	117.0	10.00				
1 portion, reconstituted: add 1 fl. oz. (⅛ cup) water (yield: approx. 2 fl. oz.)			(58.5)	(5.00)	117	10.0	468	40.0
Grape Spred-Itt, 4-portion pack, 3 oz. net wt.	322		110.7					
1 portion, reconstituted: add 1 fl. oz. (⅛ cup) water (yield: approx. 1½ fl. oz.)			(55.3)		83		443	
Peanut Butter Honey Spred, 4-portion pack, 4½ oz. net wt.	716	32.0	159.1	7.11				
1 portion, reconstituted: add ¾ fl. oz. (approx. ⅛ cup) water (yield: approx. 1¾ fl. oz.)			(102.3)	(4.57)	179	8.0	819	36.6
Raspberry Spred-Itt, 4-portion pack, 3 oz. net wt.	332		110.3					

	ENTIRE PACKAGE		1 OZ., BY WT.		1 SUGGESTED PORTION		1 CUP	
	Cal.	Carb.	Cal.	Carb.	Cal.	Carb.	Cal.	Carb.
1 portion, reconstituted: add 1 fl. oz. (1/8 cup) water (yield: approx. 1½ fl. oz.)			(55.3)		83		443	
Vegetable Shortening, 4-portion pack, 2 oz. net wt.	500		250.0					
1 portion, ½ oz.			(250.0)		125		2000	
Four-Portion Meal Units								
BREAKFAST								
Breakfast #1: Peach Slices, Jiffy Hot Cereal, Pancake Mix, Maple Syrup Mix, Sweet Milk Cocoa, Vegetable Shortening	3740	836.0			935	209.0		
1 portion, reconstituted					935	209.0		
Breakfast #2: Jiffy Hot Cereal, French Toast Mix, Melbette Toast, Maple Syrup Mix, Sweet Milk Cocoa, Vegetable Shortening	4256	784.0			1064	196.0		
1 portion, reconstituted					1064	196.0		
Breakfast #3: Freeze Dried Orange Juice Drink, Jiffy Hot Oatmeal, Scrambled Egg Mix, Vegetable Shortening, Sweet Milk Cocoa	2808	436.0			702	109.0		
1 portion, reconstituted					702	109.0		
Breakfast #4: Apple Sauce Mix, Buttermilk Pancake Mix, Maple Syrup Mix, Orange Juice Drink, Vegetable Shortening	3464	664.0			866	166.0		
1 portion, reconstituted					866	166.0		
Breakfast #5: Jiffy Hot Oatmeal, Pancake Mix, Berry Flavored Syrup Mix, Vegetable Shortening, Sweet Milk Cocoa	4180	736.0			1045	184.0		
1 portion, reconstituted					1045	184.0		
Breakfast #6: Fruit Mix, French Toast Mix, Melbette Toast, Berry Syrup Mix, Sweet Milk Cocoa, Vegetable Shortening	3424	756.0			856	189.0		
1 portion, reconstituted					856	189.0		
Breakfast #7: Freeze Dried Orange Juice Drink, Sugar Frosted Flakes, Instant Non-Fat Dry Milk, Raisins	1768	380.0			442	95.0		
1 portion, reconstituted					442	95.0		
LUNCHES								
QUICK NO-COOK								
Lunch #1: Canned Meat (Beef), Crackers, Vanilla Instant Pudding, Raisins, Pink Lemonade Beverage, Mixing Bag	3456	504.0			864	126.0		
1 portion, reconstituted					864	126.0		
Lunch #2: Cheese Spread, Crackers, Chocolate Instant Pudding, Raisins, Vanilla Kwik Shake, Mixing Bag	2984	452.0			746	113.0		
1 portion, reconstituted					746	113.0		
Lunch #3: Canned Meat (Pork), Crackers, Raspberry Spred-Itt, Toasted Coconut Instant Pudding, Grape Beverage, Mixing Bag	3476	440.0			869	110.0		
1 portion, reconstituted					869	110.0		

	ENTIRE PACKAGE		1 OZ., BY WT.		1 SUGGESTED PORTION		1 CUP	
	Cal.	Carb.	Cal.	Carb.	Cal.	Carb.	Cal.	Carb.
Lunch #4: Chicken Salad in Tin, Peanut Butter Honey Spread, Crackers, Chocolate Instant Pudding, Punch Beverage, Mixing Bag	3420	452.0			855	113.0		
1 portion, reconstituted					855	113.0		
Lunch #5: Peanut Butter Honey Spread, Grape Spred-Itt, Crackers, Raisins, Choc-o-Malt Kwik Shake, Mixing Bag	3092	444.0			773	111.0		
1 portion, reconstituted					773	111.0		
LUNCH OR DINNER								
HOT MEALS								
Hot Meal #1: Spaghetti Dinner with Tomato Sauce, Sweet Peas, Peach Slices, Choc-o-Malt Kwik Shake	2620	496.0			655	134.0		
1 portion, reconstituted					655	134.0		
Hot Meal #2: Vegetable Beef Soup, Veg-A-Rice (Chicken Style) Dinner, Apple Sauce Mix, Punch Beverage	2708	564.0			677	141.0		
1 portion, reconstituted					677	141.0		
Hot Meal #3: Macaroni 'n Cheese, Peas & Carrots, Fruit Mix, Cherry Beverage	2616	532.0			654	133.0		
1 portion, reconstituted					654	133.0		
HOT SUPPER WITH MEAT								
Supper #1: Beef Hash, Apple Sauce Mix, Butterscotch Creme Dessert, Sweet Milk Cocoa	2900	556.0			725	139.0		
1 portion, reconstituted					725	139.0		
Supper #2: Spaghetti Beef Dinner, Mixed Vegetables in Sauce, Stewed Apple Mix, Punch Beverage	2728	556.0			682	139.0		
1 portion, reconstituted					682	139.0		
Supper #3: Chicken à la King, Mashed Potatoes, Diced Carrots, Chocolate Instant Pudding, Pink Lemonade	3084	536.0			771	134.0		
1 portion, reconstituted					771	134.0		
Supper #4: Noodle Soup (Chicken Style), Potato 'n' Ham Dinner, Vanilla Instant Pudding, Sweet Milk Cocoa	3204	624.0			801	156.0		
1 portion, reconstituted					801	156.0		
Supper #5: Chicken Noodle Dinner, Peas and Carrots, Toasted Coconut Instant Pudding, Punch Beverage	2892	564.0			723	141.0		
1 portion, reconstituted					723	141.0		
Supper #6: Mixed Vegetables in Sauce, Beef Stroganoff with Noodles, Vanilla Instant Pudding, Sweet Milk Cocoa	3276	544.0			819	136.0		
1 portion, reconstituted					819	136.0		
Supper #7: Turkey Dumpling Dinner, Fruit Mix, Toasted Coconut Instant Pudding, Sweet Milk Cocoa	3096	572.0			774	143.0		
1 portion, reconstituted					774	143.0		

41 MESS—THE ARMY •

REVEILLE

Bacon

	ENTIRE RECIPE Cal.	ENTIRE RECIPE Carb.	1 SERVING Cal.	1 SERVING Carb.
Bacon Slices, grilled 15-pound bacon slab (yield: approx. 4.5 pounds) 100 servings	(12105)	(64.5)		
1 serving: 3 slices (approx. 0.7 oz.)			(121)	(0.6)

Egg Dishes

	ENTIRE RECIPE Cal.	ENTIRE RECIPE Carb.	1 SERVING Cal.	1 SERVING Carb.
SCRAMBLED EGGS 20 pounds (200 eggs) slightly beaten fresh eggs, 3 cups melted bacon fat or shortening, 2⅛ cups nonfat dry milk, 6 tablespoons salt (yield: approx. 26 pounds) 100 servings	(32763)	(244.5)		
1 serving: ½ cup			(328)	(2.4)
OMELETS				
Plain Omelet 20 pounds (200) fresh eggs, 1½ quarts melted shortening, 1¾ cups nonfat dry milk, ½ cup salt, 2 teaspoons black pepper (yield: approx. 12½ quarts) 100 servings	(28344)	(218.6)		
1 serving: 1 omelet			(283)	(2.2)
Bacon Omelet, same as Plain Omelet, but add 6 pounds crisp chopped bacon; 1 serving: 1 omelet	(33200)	(240.0)	(332)	(2.4)
Cheese Omelet, same as Plain Omelet, but add 3 quarts shredded or ground processed cheddar cheese; 1 serving: 1 omelet	(35600)	(280.0)	(356)	(2.8)
Ham Omelet, same as Plain Omelet, but add 4 pounds chopped canned ham; 1 serving: 1 omelet	(33500)	(220.0)	(335)	(2.2)
Mushroom Omelet, same as Plain Omelet, but add 2 quarts sliced canned mushrooms sautéed in 2 cups butter or margarine; 1 serving: 1 omelet	(30600)	(260.0)	(306)	(2.6)

Breakfast Breads

	ENTIRE RECIPE Cal.	ENTIRE RECIPE Carb.	1 SERVING Cal.	1 SERVING Carb.
English Muffins 13¾ quarts sifted hard wheat flour, 4½ cups shortening, 2½ cups (12) fresh eggs, 2⅛ cups nonfat dry milk, scant cup granulated sugar, 9 tablespoons active, dry yeast, 2¼ tablespoons salt (yield: approx. 100 muffins) 100 servings	(31570)	(5580.0)		
1 serving: 1 muffin			(316)	(55.8)
French Toast 200 slices sliced dry bread, 1 quart shortening (for greasing), 12½ pounds slightly beaten fresh eggs, 3½ cups granulated sugar, 1¾ cups nonfat dry milk, 1½ tablespoons salt (yield: approx. 200 slices) 100 servings	(44159)	(5588.1)		
1 serving: 2 slices			(442)	(55.9)
Griddle Cakes 9 pounds sifted hard wheat flour, 1¾ quarts (35) beaten fresh eggs, 4 cups melted shortening, 1⅛ cups baking powder, 4⅓ cups nonfat dry milk, 3½ cups granulated sugar, 4½ tablespoons salt (yield: approx. 200 cakes) 100 servings	(22425)	(4122.9)		
1 serving: 2 cakes			(224)	(41.2)

LUNCH and DINNER

Appetizers

	ENTIRE RECIPE Cal.	ENTIRE RECIPE Carb.	1 SERVING Cal.	1 SERVING Carb.
Shrimp Cocktail 12 pounds beheaded, peeled, deveined shrimp, 6 pounds (1½ gallons) fresh, shredded lettuce, 1 quart tomato catsup, 2 cups finely chopped fresh celery, 1 cup lemon juice, ¼ cup prepared horseradish, 1 tablespoon salt, 1 teaspoon hot sauce (yield: approx. 21¼ pounds) 100 servings	(7965)	(408.5)		
1 serving: 4 shrimp plus 1 tablespoon sauce (approx. 3.4 ounces)			(80)	(4.1)
Spiced Fruit Cup 13 pounds 8 ounces canned fruit cocktail, 2½ quarts fruit juice, 5 pounds (2¼ quarts) oranges, 4 pounds fresh, unpared, diced, eating apples (1 gallon), 2 cups brown sugar, 2 teaspoons nutmeg, 1 teaspoon cinnamon (yield: approx. 3.1 gallons) 100 servings	(8032)	(2040.6)		
1 serving: ½ cup			(80)	(20.4)
Stuffed Celery 6 pounds celery, 3 pounds Cheddar cheese, 12 oz. pimentos, 1 cup salad dressing, 1 tablespoon Worcestershire sauce (yield: approx. 10 pounds 4 ounces) 100 servings	(6967)	(189.0)		
1 serving: two stalks			(70)	(1.9)
Cottage Cheese Stuffed Celery 6 pounds celery, 2 pounds cottage cheese, 4 tablespoons catsup, 2 tablespoons horseradish, 2 teaspoons dry onions (yield: 8 pounds 4 ounces) 100 servings	(1537)	(158.7)		
1 serving: two stalks			(15)	(1.6)
Peanut Butter Stuffed Celery 6 pounds celery, 2 cups peanut butter, 1½ cups honey (yield: approx. 8 pounds 2 ounces) 100 servings	(4806)	(567.2)		
1 serving: two stalks			(48)	(5.7)

	ENTIRE RECIPE Cal.	ENTIRE RECIPE Carb.	1 SERVING Cal.	1 SERVING Carb.
Tomato Juice Cocktail, Seasoned 4⅓ gallons canned tomato juice, 1 cup lemon juice, ½ cup chili sauce, ½ cup granulated sugar, ½ cup minced onions, 4 tablespoons prepared horseradish, 4 tablespoons Worcestershire sauce, 4 tablespoons fresh, minced parsley, 2 tablespoons celery salt, 1½ tablespoons salt, 3 bay leaves (yield: approx. 4½ gallons) 100 servings	(3944)	(1161.4)		
1 serving: 6 fl. oz.			(39)	(11.6)

Soups

	ENTIRE RECIPE Cal.	ENTIRE RECIPE Carb.	1 SERVING Cal.	1 SERVING Carb.
Bean Soup 6 pounds dry white beans, 6¼ gallons ham stock, 1¼ quarts shredded fresh carrots, 1 quart finely chopped dry onions, 3 cups sifted hard wheat flour, 4½ tablespoons salt, 2 teaspoons black pepper (yield: approx. 6¼ gallons) 100 servings	(9652)	(1502.3)		
1 serving: 1 cup			(97)	(15.0)
Chicken Gumbo Soup 4½ gallons hot chicken stock, 12 pounds 12 oz. crushed canned tomatoes, 1½ quarts round cut frozen okra, 4½ cups chopped fresh sweet pepper, 3 cups chopped fresh celery, 4½ cups chopped dry onions, 2⅔ cups hard wheat flour, 2 cups parboiled rice, 2 cups butter or margarine, 4½ tablespoons salt, 1½ teaspoons crushed dry garlic, 2 teaspoons ground paprika, 2 teaspoons black pepper, 1 teaspoon ground thyme, 5 bay leaves (yield: approx. 6¼ gallons) 100 servings	(10177)	(1068.6)		
1 serving: 1 cup			(102)	(10.7)
Cream of Tomato Soup 9¼ gallons canned tomato paste, 8¾ cups nonfat dry milk, 1 quart hard wheat flour, 2 cups butter or margarine, 1 cup granulated sugar, 2 cups finely chopped dry onions, 1½ cups ground fresh celery, 1½ cups chopped fresh parsley, 9 tablespoons salt, 1 teaspoon black pepper, ½ teaspoon ground cloves, 2 bay leaves (yield: approx. 6¼ gallons) 100 servings	(11963)	(2011.7)		
1 serving: 1 cup			(120)	(20.1)
Manhattan Clam Chowder 1½ gallons chopped clams, 3 gallons clam broth and water, 1½ gallons crushed canned tomatoes, 4 pounds 8 ounces diced fresh white potatoes, 2 cups chopped bacon, 1½ quarts chopped dry onion, 1½ quarts diced fresh celery, 4½ cups chopped fresh sweet peppers, 4½ cups diced fresh carrots, 4½ tablespoons salt, 1 tablespoon black pepper, 2 teaspoons ground thyme (yield: approx. 6¼ gallons) 100 servings	(8212)	(1013.0)		
1 serving: 1 cup			(82)	(10.1)
Minestrone Soup 4 gallons beef stock or water, 3 quarts macaroni, 6 cups drained canned kidney beans, 3 quarts canned tomatoes, 1½ quarts chopped fresh carrots, 1½ quarts chopped fresh celery, 1½ quarts chopped dry onions, 1¼ quarts chopped fresh cabbage, 1¼ quarts chopped fresh white potatoes, 1 quart drained canned green beans, 2 cups chopped fresh parsley, 2 cups butter or margarine, 4½ tablespoons salt, 1 tablespoon black pepper, 4 teaspoons minced dry garlic, 4 bay leaves (yield: approx. 6¼ gallons) 100 servings	(11032)	(1453.0)		
1 serving: 1 cup			(110)	(14.5)
Oyster Stew 3 gallons oysters with liquid, 2¾ quarts nonfat dry milk, 1¼ quarts butter or margarine, 6 tablespoons salt, 2 teaspoons black pepper (yield: approx. 6¼ gallons) 100 servings	(12449)	(1116.5)		
1 serving: 1 cup			(124)	(11.2)
Pepper Pot Soup 5 gallons beef or chicken stock, 1 gallon chopped dry white potatoes, 1½ quarts sliced fresh celery, 4½ cups chopped fresh sweet peppers, 1½ cups chopped dry onions, 1 cup chopped canned pimientos, 2 cups hard wheat flour, 2 cups butter or margarine, 6 tablespoons salt, 2 teaspoons black pepper (yield: approx. 6¼ gallons) 100 servings	(7426)	(912.8)		
1 serving: 1 cup			(74)	(9.1)
Split Pea Soup 4 gallons ham stock or water, 9 pounds dry split peas, 2¼ quarts finely diced bacon, 1 cup bacon fat, 1 cup sifted hard wheat flour, 1 quart finely chopped dry onions, 3 cups grated fresh carrots, ¼ cup celery salt, 3 tablespoons salt, 1 teaspoon black pepper, 4 bay leaves (yield: approx. 6¼ gallons) 100 servings	(20740)	(2908.7)		
1 serving: 1 cup			(207)	(29.1)
Vegetable Soup 5 gallons beef stock, 12 pounds 12 ounces canned tomatoes, 3½ quarts chopped fresh cabbage, 2 quarts chopped fresh white potatoes, 1½ quarts diced fresh carrots, 1½ quarts chopped dry onions, 1½ quarts chopped fresh celery, 1½ cups chopped fresh sweet peppers, ½ cup salt, 1 tablespoon black pepper (yield: approx. 6¼ gallons) 100 servings	(4182)	(898.8)		
1 serving: 1 cup			(42)	(9.0)

Meats

BEEF (also see HAMBURGERS)

	ENTIRE RECIPE Cal.	ENTIRE RECIPE Carb.	1 SERVING Cal.	1 SERVING Carb.
Beef Balls Stroganoff 30 pounds ground beef, 1⅓ cups dry nonfat milk, 6 pounds sliced, drained canned mushrooms, 1¼ gallons sour cream, 5 tablespoons monosodium glutamate, 5½ tablespoons salt, 1½ tablespoons black pepper, 4 tablespoons dehydrated garlic (yield: approx. 200 meat balls plus 15⅔ cups sauce) 100 servings	(33661)	(414.2)		
Beef Pot Pie 30 pounds diced boneless beef, 6 pounds chopped fresh white potatoes, 6 pounds fresh, chopped carrots, 12 pounds 4 ounces canned tomato juice, 3 pounds dry, finely chopped onions, 2 cups melted shortening, 1 pound 2 ounces hard wheat flour, ¾ cup salt, 2 tablespoons black pepper, plus 100 baking powder biscuits (yield: approx. 6¼ gallons) 100 servings	(52733)	(3161.2)		
1 serving: 1 cup plus 1 biscuit			(527)	(31.6)
Beef Stew 30 pounds diced boneless beef, 1 pound chopped dry onions, 6 quarts fresh, chopped carrots, 4 quarts fresh celery rings, 8 pounds diced, fresh, white potatoes, 1 quart hard wheat flour, 3 quarts canned green peas, 10½ ounces salt, 1 tablespoon black pepper (yield: approx. 6¼ gallons) 100 servings	(34312)	(1594.2)		
1 serving: 1 cup			(343)	(15.9)
Chile Con Carne 24 pounds ground beef, 8 pounds dry kidney or pinto beans, 19 pounds 2 ounces canned tomatoes, 1½ quarts chopped onions, 1¼ cups chili powder, 1 cup salt, ½ cup ground paprika, 6-8 cloves chopped dry garlic, 10 tablespoons monosodium glutamate, 1 teaspoon cayenne powder (yield: approx. 6¼ gallons) 100 servings	(35485)	(3229.8)		
1 serving: 1 cup			(355)	(32.3)
Corned Beef Mulligan 18 pounds cubed canned corned beef, 8 pounds diced fresh white potatoes, 8 pounds cooked, drained, frozen peas, 6 pounds 6 ounces canned tomatoes, 1 quart tomato catsup, 3 pounds chopped fresh celery, 2 pounds chopped dry onions, 1 pound 2 ounces chopped fresh sweet peppers, 1 pound 4 ounces melted shortening, 1 tablespoon monosodium glutamate, 4 teaspoons black pepper, 4 teaspoons salt (yield: approx. 6¼ gallons) 100 servings	(30025)	(1352.2)		
1 serving: 1 cup			(300)	(13.5)
El Rancho Stew 30 pounds diced boneless beef, 1 gallon quartered dry onions, 1 gallon fresh cut carrots, 20 pounds fresh white cut potatoes, 2 pounds 8 ounces frozen peas, 1 cup hard wheat flour, 6 ounces salt, ½ cup monosodium glutamate, 3 tablespoons black pepper (yield: approx. 7.8 gallons) 100 servings	(35587)	(1794.7)		
1 serving: 1¼ cups			(356)	(17.9)
Meat Loaf 30 pounds ground beef, 1 pound 4 ounces beaten whole eggs, 2 gallons broken dried bread, 1 quart finely chopped dry onions, 3 cups finely chopped fresh celery, 1 cup finely chopped fresh sweet peppers, 1 cup melted shortening, 9 tablespoons salt, 2 tablespoons black pepper (yield: approx. 8 loaves, each 18″ × 26″) 100 servings	(28183)	(557.5)		
1 serving: 1 slice (approx. 4 ounces)			(282)	(5.6)
Sloppy Joe 30 pounds ground beef, 7 pounds 2 ounces tomato catsup, 4 quarts dry, chopped onions, 1 pound prepared mustard, 2 cups brown sugar, ¾ cup salt, 3 cups vinegar, plus 100 sandwich buns (yield: approx. 6¼ gallons excluding buns) 100 servings	(36449)	(2966.7)		
1 serving: ½ cup plus 1 sandwich bun			(365)	(29.7)

	ENTIRE RECIPE Cal.	ENTIRE RECIPE Carb.	1 SERVING Cal.	1 SERVING Carb.
Yankee Pot Roast				
60 pounds beef carcass (yield: 40 pounds, boned), 6 pounds 6 ounces canned tomatoes, 2½ quarts dry, chopped onions, 2 quarts diced fresh carrots, 1 pound melted shortening, 3 ounces monosodium glutamate, 2 tablespoons black pepper, 6 ounces salt, 2 cloves chopped dry garlic (yield: approx. 28 pounds) 100 servings	(56204)	(455.3)		
1 serving: 2 slices (approx. 6½ ounces)			(562)	(4.6)
HAMBURGERS				
Beefburgers, Grilled				
30 pounds ground beef, 1 gallon dry breadcrumbs, ⅝ cup nonfat dry milk, 2 tablespoons black pepper, 9 tablespoons salt (yield: approx. 200 beefburgers, 3 ounces each) 100 servings	(23961)	(893.9)		
1 serving: 2 beefburgers			(240)	(8.9)
Cheeseburgers				
30 pounds ground beef, 12 pounds 8 ounces processed Cheddar cheese, 1 gallon dry breadcrumbs, ⅝ cup nonfat dry milk, 2 tablespoons black pepper, 9 tablespoons salt (yield: approx. 200 beefburgers, 3 ounces each, plus 2 slices cheese) 100 servings	(46524)	(1012.7)		
1 serving: 2 cheeseburgers			(465)	(10.1)
FRANKFURTERS				
Baked Frankfurters With Sauerkraut				
25 pounds of frankfurters, 26 pounds sauerkraut (yield: approx. 200 frankfurters plus 3.1 gallons sauerkraut) 100 servings	(35957)	(658.1)		
1 serving: 2 frankfurters plus ½ cup sauerkraut			(360)	(6.6)
Simmered Frankfurters				
25 pounds of frankfurters boiled in 2½ gallons water (yield: approx. 200 frankfurters) 100 servings	(33825)	(177.5)		
1 serving: 2 frankfurters			(338)	(1.8)
Sweet and Sour Frankfurters				
16½ pounds whole canned frankfurters, 1½ quarts finely chopped sweet cucumber pickles, 12 ounces dehydrated onion soup, 4½ ounces prepared mustard, 9 ounces brown sugar, ¾ cup cornstarch, 1½ cup lemon juice (yield: approx. 200 frankfurters plus 1½ gallons sauce) 100 servings	(25180)	(706.7)		
1 serving: 2 frankfurters plus ¼ cup sauce			(252)	(7.1)
PORK				
Baked Ham				
30 pounds precooked boneless pork ham, trimmed; 2 quarts brown sugar, 1½ quarts vinegar, 2 cups dry breadcrumbs, 1 ounce whole cloves (yield: approx. 27 pounds) 100 servings	(32182)	(1760.4)		
1 serving: 2 slices (approx. 4 oz.)			(322)	(17.6)
Glazed Ham Chunks				
36 pounds 4 ounces canned ham chunks, 1⅓ quarts brown sugar, 1 cup vinegar (yield: approx. 6¼ gallons) 100 servings	(35972)	(1252.9)		
1 serving: 1 cup			(360)	(12.5)
Ham à la King				
15 pounds cooked boneless ham cubed, trimmed; 2 pounds drained canned sliced mushrooms, 2 quarts nonfat dry milk, 1 pound 8 ounces sifted hard wheat flour, 4½ cups chopped fresh sweet peppers, 14 ounces chopped canned pimientoes, 3½ pounds butter or margarine, 3 tablespoons salt (yield: approx. 4⅔ gallons) 100 servings	(33508)	(1274.0)		
1 serving: ¾ cup			(335)	(12.7)
Roast Fresh Ham				
41 pounds boneless pork ham, trimmed; ¾ cup salt, 2 tablespoons black pepper (yield: approx. 27 pounds) 100 servings	(22099)	(0.0)		
1 serving: 2 slices (approx. 4 oz.)			(221)	(0.0)
Roast Pork				
39 pounds boneless pork loin, trimmed; 8 ounces salt, 1 ounce black pepper (yield: approx. 25 pounds) 100 servings	(24453)	(0.0)		
1 serving: 2 slices (approx. 4 oz.)			(245)	(0.0)
Sweet & Sour Pork				
32 pounds diced boneless pork, 12 pounds canned bean sprouts, 3 quarts canned pineapple chunks or tidbits, 1¾ gallons fruit juice and water, 1½ quarts vinegar, 3 cups soy sauce, 2¼ quarts granulated sugar, 6 cups corn starch, 2 quarts sliced fresh sweet peppers, 1 pound slightly beaten whole eggs, 1 pound shortening, 4 cloves or crushed dry garlic, 6 ounces salt (yield: approx. 6¼ gallons) 100 servings	(41482)	(3648.3)		
1 serving: 1 cup			(415)	(36.5)
PORK SAUSAGES				
Grilled Sausage Links				
12 pounds precooked frozen pork and beef sausage (yield: 200 links, approx. 10 pounds) 100 servings	(18240)	(120.0)		
1 serving: 2 links (approx. 1.5 oz.)			(182)	(1.2)
Grilled Sausage Patties				
25 pounds bulk pork sausage shaped into patties (yield: approx. 100 patties, 8¾ pounds) 100 servings	(25350)	(0.0)		
1 serving: 1 patty (approx. 3 oz.)			(254)	(0.0)
LAMB				
Barbecued Lamb Chops				
35 pounds boneless lamb chops (100 chops, approx. 5½ ounces each), 1½ gallons canned tomato juice, 1 cup tomato catsup, 1 quart vinegar, 1½ quarts chopped dry onions, ½ cup shortening, 1 pound 4 ounces brown sugar, 1 cup Worcestershire sauce, 4 tablespoons brown mustard, 1 tablespoon chili powder, 1 tablespoon ground paprika (yield: 100 chops) 100 servings	(39458)	(1116.3)		
1 serving: 1 chop			(395)	(11.2)
Grilled Lamb Chops				
35 pounds boneless lamb chops (100 chops, approx. 5½ ounces each), ½ cup salt, 1 tablespoon black pepper (yield: approx. 100 chops) 100 servings	(34100)	(0.0)		
1 serving: 1 chop (approx. 3.4 oz.)			(341)	(0.0)
Roast Lamb				
39 pounds partially thawed boneless lamb roast, 8 cloves dry garlic, ½ cup salt, 1½ tablespoons black pepper (yield: approx. 25 pounds) 100 servings	(34593)	(0.0)		
1 serving: 2 slices (approx. 4 oz.)			(346)	(0.0)
VEAL				
Roast Veal				
60 pounds veal sides (41 pounds veal, boneless), 9 ounces salt, 2 tablespoons black pepper (yield: approx. 25 pounds) 100 servings	(34194)	(0.0)		
1 serving: 2 slices (approx. 4 oz.)			(341)	(0.0)
Vealburgers				
31 pounds ground veal, 5 quarts broken dry bread, 2¼ quarts finely chopped dry onions, 2 cups beaten fresh eggs, ⅔ cup salt, 2 tablespoons black pepper (yield: approx. 31¼ pounds) 100 servings	(29270)	(523.9)		
1 serving: 2 veal patties, 5 oz.			(293)	(5.2)
Veal Parmesan				
35 pounds partially thawed sliced boneless veal (taken from 60-pound veal side), 2 quarts dry bread crumbs, 1 pound 8 ounces beaten fresh eggs, 6¼ quarts tomato sauce, 1 pound 6 ounces grated Parmesan cheese, 1 quart hard wheat flour, ¾ cup nonfat dry milk, ½ cup salt, 1 tablespoon black pepper, 2 dry minced garlic cloves (yield: approx. 40 pounds) 100 servings	(40308)	(1240.5)		
1 serving: 1 slice plus 2 tablespoons sauce (approx. 5 oz.)			(403)	(12.4)
RABBIT				
Fried Rabbit				
50 pounds ready-to-cook rabbit, cut into pieces; 3 quarts hard wheat flour, 1 gallon dry breadcrumbs, 1⅓ cups nonfat dry milk, 1 pound 4 ounces beaten fresh eggs, 9 tablespoons salt, 2 tablespoons garlic salt, 1½ tablespoons black pepper (yield: approx. 37½–50 pounds) 100 servings	(37667)	(2021.3)		
1 serving: 6–8 oz. of rabbit pieces			(377)	(20.2)

Poultry

	ENTIRE RECIPE Cal.	ENTIRE RECIPE Carb.	1 SERVING Cal.	1 SERVING Carb.
CHICKEN				
Baked Chicken				
65 pounds whole broiler-fryer chicken, 1 pound butter or margarine, ¾ cup salt, 4 tablespoons black pepper (yield: approx. 100 quarter chickens) 100 servings	(32075)	(412.5)		
1 serving: ¼ chicken			(321)	(4.1)
Barbecued Chicken				
50 pounds cut up broiler-fryer chicken, 1 quart finely chopped dry onions, 1 quart vinegar, 7 pounds 2 ounces tomato catsup, 3 cups brown sugar, 2 cups Worcestershire sauce, 1 pound melted butter or margarine, ¾ cup prepared mustard, 6 tablespoons salt, 1 teaspoon black pepper (yield: approx. 200 chicken pieces) 100 servings	(20934)	(1556.0)		
1 serving: 2 pieces of chicken			(209)	(15.6)

	ENTIRE RECIPE		1 SERVING	
	Cal.	Carb.	Cal.	Carb.
Chicken à la King				
45 pounds whole broiler-fryer chicken, 1 quart melted chicken fat, butter or margarine; 2 quarts hard wheat flour, 13 ounces nonfat dry milk, 5 pounds chopped fresh celery, 1 pound chopped dry onions, 1 pound chopped fresh sweet peppers, 1¾ cups chopped canned pimientos, 9 ounces salt, 9 tablespoons monosodium glutamate, 2 tablespoons black pepper, 9 bay leaves (yield: approx. 6¼ gallons) 100 servings	(25448)	(1069.4)		
1 serving: 1 cup			(254)	(10.7)
Chicken Cacciatore				
50 pounds cut up broiler-fryer chicken, 9 pounds 8 ounces canned tomatoes, 2 quarts sliced dry onions, 3 cups chopped fresh sweet peppers, 2 cups salad oil, 10½ cups hard wheat flour, 1 quart shortening, 12–16 cloves minced dry garlic, 2¼ tablespoons chili powder, 2 teaspoons ground oregano, 50 ounces salt, 2 tablespoons pepper, 5 bay leaves (yield: approx. 200 pieces chicken plus 2 gallons sauce) 100 servings	(31284)	(1490.8)		
1 serving: 2 pieces chicken plus ⅓ cup sauce			(313)	(14.9)
Fried Chicken				
50 pounds cut up broiler-fryer chicken, 3¾ quarts hard white flour, ¾ cups salt, 3 tablespoons black pepper, 1 tablespoon ground paprika (yield: approx. 200 pieces chicken) 100 servings	(35075)	(1426.5)		
1 serving: 2 pieces of chicken			(351)	(14.3)
CHICKEN OR TURKEY				
Chicken or Turkey Pot Pie				
45 pounds whole broiler-fryer chicken or 45 pounds ready-to-cook turkey, 3 quarts diced fresh white potatoes, 3 quarts diced fresh carrots, 1 quart melted butter or margarine, 3 gallons chicken stock, 6 pounds 8 ounces drained canned peas, 2 quarts hard wheat flour, 2 teaspoons celery salt, 1 tablespoon black pepper, 12 ounces salt, 9 tablespoons monosodium glutamate, 9 bay leaves (yield: approx. 6¼ gallons) 100 servings	(22492)	(1568.6)		
1 serving: 1 cup plus topping			(225)	(15.7)
Chicken or Turkey Salad				
45 pounds whole broiler-fryer chicken or 45 pounds ready-to-cook turkey, 12 pounds chopped fresh celery, 4 pounds trimmed, fresh lettuce, 1 pound 8 ounces chopped fresh sweet pepper, 1 cup lemon juice, 1½ quarts salad dressing, 9 tablespoons monosodium glutamate, 9 bay leaves (yield: approx. 6¼ gallons) 100 servings	(20875)	(673.5)		
1 serving: 1 cup			(209)	(6.7)
DUCK				
Roast Duck				
100 pounds ready-to-cook duck (25 4-pound ducks), 6 tablespoons salt, 2 teaspoons black pepper (yield: approx. 62 pounds) 100 servings	(59599)	(0.0)		
1 serving: 1 quarter duck (approx. 10 oz.)			(596)	(0.0)
TURKEY				
Roast Turkey				
65 pounds ready-to-cook turkey, 2 cups butter or margarine, ¾ cup salt, 4 tablespoons black pepper (yield: approx. 25 pounds sliced) 100 servings	(33793)	(0.0)		
1 serving: 3 slices (approx. 4 oz.)			(338)	(0.0)

Fish

	ENTIRE RECIPE		1 SERVING	
	Cal.	Carb.	Cal.	Carb.
Baked Fish Portions				
25 pounds frozen fish portions, 1½ quarts melted butter or margarine, 4 tablespoons ground paprika (yield: 25 pounds) 100 servings	(19275)	(0.0)		
1 serving (approx. 4 oz.)			(193)	(0.0)
Baked Stuffed Fish				
30 pounds thawed fish fillets, 2¼ gallons cracker crumbs, 4½ cups chopped dry onions, 3 cups chopped fresh celery, 2½ cups melted butter or margarine, ¾ cups lemon juice, 3 tablespoons salt, 2 tablespoons ground paprika, 2 tablespoons ground thyme (yield: 28 pounds fish plus 1½ quarts dressing) 100 servings	(41093)	(3385.4)		
1 serving: 4½ oz. fish plus 1 tablespoon dressing			(411)	(33.9)
Creole Shrimp				
20 pounds raw, peeled, deveined, frozen shrimp; 7 pounds 12 ounces canned tomato paste, 2¼ cups cornstarch, 4¼ quarts chopped fresh celery, 2⅛ quarts chopped dry onion, 1¾ quarts sliced fresh sweet pepper, 3 cups canned mushrooms, 1 quart melted butter or margarine, 1 cup salt, ¼ cup dehydrated garlic, 4 tablespoons black pepper, 1 tablespoon hot sauce, 1 teaspoon baking soda (yield: approx. 6¼ gallons) 100 servings	(23499)	(1269.7)		
1 serving: 1 cup			(235)	(12.7)
Deep Fat Fried Fish				
30 pounds thawed fish fillet, 2 pounds 4 ounces hard wheat flour, 1½ quarts dry breadcrumbs, ½ cup nonfat dry milk, 2 pounds beaten fresh eggs, 3½ ounces salt, 1 tablespoon pepper (yield: 28 pounds fish) 100 servings	(30225)	(1115.1)		
1 serving: 4½ oz. fish			(302)	(11.2)
Fried Oysters				
24 pounds oysters (16 pounds shelled oysters), 3¾ quarts hard wheat flour, 1 quart beaten fresh eggs, 5 pounds 8 ounces cracker crumbs, ½ cup nonfat dry milk, 4½ teaspoons salt, 1 teaspoon black pepper (yield: 600–700 oysters) 100 servings	(23755)	(3358.4)		
1 serving: 6–7 oysters			(238)	(33.6)
Oven Fried Fish				
30 pounds thawed fish fillets, 3 quarts dry breadcrumbs, 2 pounds melted butter or margarine, 6½ ounces nonfat dry milk, ½ cup salt (yield: 28 pounds fish) 100 servings	(30059)	(676.4)		
1 serving: 4½ oz. fish			(301)	(6.8)
Salmon Loaf				
20 pounds canned salmon, 2 cups butter or margarine, 3 quarts bread crumbs, 1 quart eggs, 1 quart chopped fresh celery, 1 quart chopped dry onions, 3 tablespoons salt, ½ tablespoon pepper, 2 cups lemon juice (yield: 8 loaves, 18″ × 24″ ea. 24 pounds) 100 servings	(27391)	(710.4)		
1 serving: 1 slice (approx. 4 oz.)			(274)	(7.1)
Salmon Salad				
20 pounds canned salmon, 42 chopped hard cooked eggs, 6 quarts chopped fresh celery, 4 pounds trimmed fresh lettuce, 1½ cups chopped sweet cucumber pickles, ½ cup salt, 3 pounds salad dressing (yield: 4¼ gallons) 100 servings	(30228)	(744.0)		
1 serving: ⅔ cup			(302)	(7.4)
Shrimp Salad				
20 pounds raw, peeled, deveined frozen shrimp, 8 pounds chopped fresh celery, 4 pounds trimmed fresh lettuce, 1 quart salad dressing, 1 cup lemon juice, 8 ounces salt, 2 teaspoons black pepper (yield: 3.1 gallons) 100 servings	(16968)	(734.4)		
1 serving: ½ cup			(170)	(7.3)

Vegetables

	ENTIRE RECIPE		1 SERVING	
	Cal.	Carb.	Cal.	Carb.
Baked Beans				
37½ pounds canned white beans with pork and tomato sauce, 1¾ quarts chopped bacon, 1½ quarts chopped dry onions, 2 pounds 8 ounces brown sugar, 1½ cups tomato catsup, ¾ cup prepared mustard (yield: approx. two 18″ × 24″ roasting pans) 100 servings	(34120)	(5485.2)		
1 serving: ¾ cup			(341)	(54.9)
Boston Baked Beans				
16 pounds lima, white or kidney beans; 2½ quarts chopped bacon, 1⅓ quarts brown sugar, 1 quart molasses, ½ cup vinegar, 9 tablespoons salt (yield: approx. two 18″ × 24″ roasting pans) 100 servings	(36045)	(5187.6)		
1 serving: 1 cup			(360)	(51.9)
Baked Beans, Italian Style				
8 pounds white, lima, pinto, or kidney beans; 1 gallon bean liquid and water, 5 pounds 13 ounces canned tomato paste, 1½ quarts finely diced fresh celery, 1 quart chopped dry fresh onion, 1 cup chopped fresh parsley, 1 cup salad oil, 2 cups grated Parmesan cheese, 3 tablespoons salt, 1 tablespoon granulated sugar, 1 teaspoon ground oregano, 1 teaspoon black pepper, ½ teaspoon ground thyme, 5 minced dry garlic cloves (yield: approx. one 18″ × 24″ roasting pan) 100 servings	(17925)	(2835.8)		
1 serving: ½ cup			(179)	(28.4)
Baked Hubbard Squash				
29 pounds halved hubbard squash, 2¼ cups shortening, 1 cup brown sugar, 4½ tablespoons salt, 1 teaspoon black pepper (yield: approx. 11 pounds) 100 servings	(9390)	(1205.3)		
1 serving: 1 piece (approx. 1¾ oz.)			(94)	(12.1)
Baked Potatoes				
55 pounds fresh white potatoes, 2 cups meat drippings or melted shortening, 100 servings	(18085)	(3201.0)		
1 serving: 1 potato			(181)	(32.0)
Cabbage, Fried				
20 pounds coarsely shredded cabbage, 2 cups melted butter or margarine, ½ cup salt, 1 tablespoon black pepper (yield: approx. 3⅛ gallons) 100 servings	(4710)	(486.4)		
1 serving: ½ cup			(47)	(4.9)

	ENTIRE RECIPE		1 SERVING	
	Cal.	Carb.	Cal.	Carb.
Carrots, Lyonnaise 20 pounds fresh cut carrots, 3 cups chopped dry onions, ½ cup finely chopped fresh parsley, ½ cup granulated sugar, 2 cups butter or margarine, 1½ tablespoons salt, 1 teaspoon black pepper (yield: approx. 3⅛ gallons) 100 servings	(8233)	(1022.4)		
1 serving: ½ cup			(82)	(10.2)
French Fried Potatoes 45 pounds french fry cut fresh white potatoes, cooked; 360 pounds fat, 3 tablespoons salt (yield: approx. 3⅛ gallons) 100 servings	(30096)	(3660.5)		
1 serving: ½ cup			(301)	(36.6)
Harvard Beets 26 pounds canned beets, 2¾ quarts reserved liquid and water, 2¼ cups granulated sugar, 1½ cups vinegar, 1 cup cornstarch, 1 cup butter or margarine, 3 tablespoons salt, 1 tablespoon whole cloves (yield: approx. 3⅛ gallons) 100 servings	(8138)	(1518.1)		
1 serving: ½ cup			(81)	(15.2)
Hashed Brown Potatoes 3½ gallons white potatoes, 1 quart melted shortening, 3 tablespoons salt, 2 teaspoons black pepper (yield: approx. 4⅛ gallons) 100 servings	(19335)	(2619.0)		
1 serving: ⅔ cup			(193)	(26.2)
Home Fried Potatoes 45 pounds fresh white potatoes (35 pounds when peeled), 1 quart melted drippings or shortening, 3 tablespoons salt, 2 teaspoons black pepper (yield: approx. 4⅛ gallons) 100 servings	(19335)	(2619.0)		
1 serving: ⅔ cup			(193)	(26.2)
Mashed Potatoes made from fresh potatoes 45 pounds fresh white potatoes (35 pounds when peeled), 2¼ cups nonfat dry milk, 1 pound butter or margarine, ½ cup salt (yield: approx. 4.7 gallons) 100 servings	(14284)	(2767.0)		
1 serving: ¾ cup			(143)	(27.7)
Mashed Potatoes made from instant potato mix 3 quarts instant white potatoes, 1 pound butter or margarine, 2¾ cups nonfat dry milk, 4½ tablespoons salt, 2 teaspoons black pepper (yield: approx. 4⅛ gallons) 100 servings	(12947)	(5180.0)		
1 serving: ⅔ cup			(129)	(51.8)
O'Brien Potatoes 35 pounds cubed fresh white potatoes, 3 cups finely chopped fresh sweet peppers, 1 cup finely chopped canned pimientos, 1 cup melted shortening, 4½ tablespoons salt, 1 teaspoon black pepper (yield: approx. 4⅛ gallons) 100 servings	(12920)	(2479.8)		
1 serving: ⅔ cup			(129)	(24.8)
O'Brien Summer Squash 20 pounds sliced fresh summer squash, 1½ quarts chopped bacon, 3 cups chopped fresh sweet peppers, 1 cup chopped canned pimiento, 6 tablespoons granulated sugar, 6 tablespoons salt, 1 teaspoon black pepper (yield: approx. 3⅛ gallons) 100 servings	(4197)	(535.5)		
1 serving: ½ cup			(42)	(5.4)
Peas, Buttered 12½ pounds dehydrofrozen peas, 2 cups melted butter or margarine, 2 tablespoons salt, 2 teaspoons black pepper (yield: approx. 3⅛ gallons) 100 servings	(7978)	(726.3)		
1 serving: ½ cup			(80)	(7.3)
Potatoes au Gratin 45 pounds fresh white potatoes (34 pounds when peeled), 4⅓ cups nonfat dry milk, 3 cups hard wheat flour, 1½ pounds melted butter or margarine, 3 tablespoons salt (yield: approx. 2 18" × 24" roasting pans) 100 servings	(17479)	(3190.0)		
1 serving: 1 cup			(175)	(31.9)
Sweet Potatoes, Candied 22½ pounds canned sweet potatoes, 1¼ gallons brown sugar, 2 cups butter or margarine, 2 fresh unpeeled thinly sliced oranges, 2½ tablespoons salt (yield: approx. 3 18" × 25" sheet pans) 100 servings	(27604)	(6127.6)		
1 serving: 2–3 pieces (approx. 4 oz.)			(276)	(61.3)
Succotash, Buttered 10 pounds frozen lima beans, 10 pounds frozen whole grain corn, 2 cups melted butter or margarine, 1 cup chopped fresh parsley, 6 tablespoons salt, 2 teaspoons black pepper (yield: approx. 3⅛ gallons) 100 servings	(12216)	(1784.1)		
1 serving: ½ cup			(122)	(17.8)
Tomatoes, Scalloped 25½ cups canned tomatoes, 1½ pounds toasted bread cubes, 2 cups butter or margarine, 3 cups cornstarch, 2¼ cups granulated sugar, 3 tablespoons salt, 2 tablespoons whole cloves, 1½ tablespoons brown mustard (yield: approx. 3⅛ gallons) 100 servings	(10005)	(1290.6)		
1 serving: ½ cup			(100)	(12.9)
Tomatoes, Stewed 25½ pounds crushed canned tomatoes, 2 cups granulated sugar, 1 cup butter or margarine, ½ cup chopped dry onions, 4½ tablespoons salt, 1 teaspoon black pepper (yield: approx. 3⅛ gallons) 100 servings	(5864)	(893.8)		
1 serving: ½ cup			(59)	(8.9)
White Turnips and Bacon 20 pounds sliced fresh turnips, 2¼ quarts chopped bacon, 6 tablespoons salt, 1½ teaspoons black pepper (yield: approx. 3⅛ gallons) 100 servings	(5467)	(609.1)		
1 serving: ½ cup			(55)	(6.1)

Pasta

	Cal.	Carb.	Cal.	Carb.
Baked Beef With Noodles 30 pounds diced, boneless beef, 1½ gallons dry noodles, 1 quart melted shortening, 1½ quarts sifted hard wheat flour, 3½ gallons beef stock, 1 pound tomato catsup, 2 cups dry bread crumbs, 4 ounces salt, 2 tablespoons black pepper (yield: 7.8 gallons) 100 servings	(47066)	(2368.6)		
1 serving: 1¼ cups			(471)	(23.7)
Baked Lasagne 6½ pounds ground beef, 4 pounds minced dry onions, 1¾ cups salad oil, 12 pounds 12 ounces crushed canned tomatoes, 17½ pounds canned tomato paste, 6 pounds lasagne noodles, 6½ pounds cottage cheese, 3 pounds 8 ounces mozzarella cheese, 1 pound 14 ounces grated Parmesan cheese, 2 pounds 13 ounces slightly beaten fresh eggs, 1½ ounces salt, 1 tablespoon pepper, 2 cups minced fresh parsley, 1 ounce ground oregano, 2 tablespoons ground thyme, 3 tablespoons cayenne pepper (yield: approx. 65 pounds) 100 servings	(39706)	(3781.9)		
1 serving: 1 piece approx. 6" × 9"			(397)	(37.8)
Spaghetti With Meat Balls 30 pounds ground beef, 6½ quarts dry breadcrumbs, 1 pound fresh eggs, 3 pounds 8 ounces finely chopped dry onions, 1½ cups melted shortening, 4 ounces granulated sugar, 11 ounces salt, 2 tablespoons ground thyme, 18–24 cloves of dry chopped garlic, 1 tablespoon ground oregano, 1 tablespoon cayenne pepper, 6 bay leaves, plus 12 pounds dry spaghetti (yield: 200 meat balls, 100 cups cooked spaghetti and 66 cups spaghetti sauce) 100 servings	(56163)	(6736.0)		
1 serving: 2 meat balls with 1 cup of spaghetti and ⅔ cup of sauce			(562)	(67.4)

Pizza

	Cal.	Carb.	Cal.	Carb.
4¾ quarts sifted hard wheat flour, 12 pounds 12 ounces crushed canned tomatoes, 3 pounds 4 ounces canned tomato paste, 2¼ quarts ground natural Cheddar cheese, 2 cups grated Parmesan cheese, 9 tablespoons salad oil, ¼ cup active, dry yeast, 2 tablespoons granulated sugar, 1½ tablespoons ground oregano, 2½ tablespoons salt, 2½ teaspoons black pepper (yield: approx. four 18" × 26" sheet pans) 100 servings	(18871)	(2241.4)		
1 serving: 1 piece			(189)	(22.4)

DESSERTS

Cakes

	Cal.	Carb.	Cal.	Carb.
Chocolate Cake 3⅓ quarts sifted soft wheat flour, 4¼ cups shortening, 2¼ quarts granulated sugar, 1 quart cocoa, 1⅓ cups nonfat dry milk, 1 quart (20) fresh eggs, 4 tablespoons baking powder, 2¾ tablespoons baking soda, 2¼ tablespoons salt, 4 tablespoons vanilla (yield: approx. two 18" × 26" sheet pans) 100 servings	(22809)	(3113.3)		
1 serving: 1 slice			(228)	(31.1)

	ENTIRE RECIPE Cal.	ENTIRE RECIPE Carb.	1 SERVING Cal.	1 SERVING Carb.
Devil's Food Cake 3⅓ quarts sifted soft wheat flour, 3¾ cups shortening, 3½ cups (18) fresh eggs, 2¼ quarts granulated sugar, ¼ quart vinegar, 2½ cups cocoa, 1⅓ cups nonfat dry milk, 4½ tablespoons baking soda, 2¼ tablespoons salt, 4 tablespoons vanilla (yield: approx. two 18″ × 26″ sheet pans) 100 servings	(21579)	(3064.3)		
1 serving: 1 slice			(216)	(30.6)
Fruit Shortcake 6 quarts sifted hard wheat flour, 20 pounds fresh or frozen fruit, 1¼ quarts shortening, 2 cups melted butter or margarine, 2¼ cups granulated sugar, 1½ cups nonfat dry milk, ¾ cup baking powder, 2 tablespoons salt (yield: approx. two 18″ × 26″ pans) 100 servings	(33904)	(4719.0)		
1 serving: 1 biscuit with fruit and topping			(339)	(47.2)
Ginger Bread 4½ quarts sifted soft wheat flour, 3 cups shortening, 2½ cups (12) fresh eggs, 1 quart molasses, 3 pounds granulated sugar, 4 tablespoons ground ginger, 2 tablespoons ground cinnamon, 2¼ tablespoons baking powder, 2¼ tablespoons baking soda, 1½ tablespoons salt (yield: approx. two 18″ × 26″ sheet pans) 100 servings	(21438)	(3534.0)		
1 serving: 1 slice			(214)	(35.3)
Jellyroll 5 quarts jelly, 3 quarts sifted soft wheat flour, 1½ quarts (30) fresh eggs, 3 pounds granulated sugar, 1 pound powdered sugar, 2¼ tablespoons baking powder, 2¼ teaspoons salt, 4 tablespoons vanilla (yield: approx. five 18″ × 26″ sheet pans) 100 servings	(26121)	(5980.1)		
1 serving: 1 slice			(261)	(59.8)
Peanut Butter Cake 3⅓ quarts sifted soft wheat flour, 3½ cups shortening, 1½ quarts (30) fresh eggs, 2½ pounds peanut butter, ¾ cup nonfat dry milk, 2 quarts brown sugar, 4 tablespoons vanilla (yield: approx. two 18″ × 26″ sheet pans) 100 servings	(26220)	(2626.3)		
1 serving: 1 slice			(262)	(26.3)
Pound Cake 4½ quarts sifted soft wheat flour, 1½ quarts shortening, 1½ quarts (30) fresh eggs, 4 pounds of granulated sugar, 10½ tablespoons nonfat dry milk, 1¾ tablespoons baking powder, 2 tablespoons salt, 4 tablespoons vanilla (yield: approx. two 18″ × 26″ sheet pans) 100 servings	(27719)	(3267.0)		
1 serving: 1 slice			(277)	(32.7)
Sponge Cake 3 quarts sifted soft wheat flour, 1½ quarts (30) fresh eggs, 3 pounds granulated sugar, 2¼ tablespoons baking powder, 2¼ teaspoons salt, 4 tablespoons vanilla (yield: approx. two 18″ × 26″ pans) 100 servings	(12080)	(2323.8)		
1 serving: 1 slice			(121)	(23.2)
Upside Down Cake 15 pounds 11 ounces yellow cake batter, 9 pounds canned peaches, drained solids only; 1½ pounds butter or margarine, 2 quarts brown sugar (yield: approx. two 18″ × 26″ pans) 100 servings	(32853)	(5463.4)		
1 serving: 1 slice			(329)	(54.6)

Pies

	ENTIRE RECIPE Cal.	ENTIRE RECIPE Carb.	1 SERVING Cal.	1 SERVING Carb.
Apple Pie 1¾ gallons dehydrated apples, 17 pie shells, 1½ cups melted butter or margarine, 2 cups cornstarch, 2¼ quarts granulated sugar, 6 tablespoons lemon juice, 2 tablespoons ground cinnamon, 2 tablespoons ground nutmeg, 1 tablespoon salt (yield: approx. 17 pies) 100 servings	(49389)	(6478.6)		
1 serving: ⅙ of pie			(494)	(64.8)
Blueberry Pie 25½ pounds water-packed canned blueberries, 17 pie shells, 1 gallon granulated sugar, 1 gallon berry juice, 4 tablespoons lemon juice, 3½ cups pregelatinized starch, 1 tablespoon salt (yield: approx. 17 pies) 100 servings	(52276)	(7913.4)		
1 serving: ⅙ of pie			(523)	(79.1)
Butterscotch Cream Pie 17 pie shells, 1½ quarts (30) slightly beaten fresh eggs, 1 quart butter or margarine, 8½ pounds brown sugar, 5½ cups nonfat dry milk, 1 quart cornstarch, 2½ tablespoons salt, 6 tablespoons vanilla (yield: approx. 17 pies) 100 servings	(47494)	(6523.0)		
1 serving: ⅙ of pie			(475)	(65.2)
Cherry Pie 4 pounds dehydrated cherries, 17 pie shells, 8 pounds granulated sugar, 2 gallons cherry juice, 1 pound 4 ounces pregelatinized starch, 1 teaspoon salt (yield: approx. 17 pies) 100 servings	(40892)	(7223.0)		
1 serving: ⅙ of pie			(409)	(72.2)
Chocolate Cream Pie 17 pie shells, 1½ pounds butter or margarine, 1¼ quarts (24) slightly beaten fresh eggs, 1 quart cocoa, 1¾ quarts nonfat dry milk, 3 quarts granulated sugar, 4¾ cups cornstarch, 1½ tablespoons salt, 4 tablespoons vanilla (yield: approx. 17 pies) 100 servings	(33534)	(3699.3)		
1 serving: ⅙ of pie			(335)	(37.0)
Lemon Meringue Pie 17 pie shells, 1 pound butter or margarine, 1 quart (20) slightly beaten fresh eggs, 5½ quarts granulated sugar, 4¼ quarts lemon juice, 1 cup grated lemon rind, 5½ cups pregelatinized starch, 3 tablespoons salt (yield: approx. 17 pies) 100 servings	(41646)	(6879.4)		
1 serving: ⅙ of pie			(416)	(68.8)

Gelatins, Puddings, and Custards

	ENTIRE RECIPE Cal.	ENTIRE RECIPE Carb.	1 SERVING Cal.	1 SERVING Carb.
Baked Coconut Custard Same as Baked Custard, but add 1 pound sweetened, prepared coconut and omit nutmeg (yield: approx. four 12″ × 20″ steam table pans) 100 servings	(13962)	(1678.2)		
1 serving: ½ cup			(140)	(16.8)
Baked Custard 3 quarts (60) slightly beaten fresh eggs, 1¾ quarts nonfat dry milk, 1½ quarts granulated sugar, 4 tablespoons vanilla, 1 tablespoon ground nutmeg, 2¼ tablespoons salt (yield: approx. four 12″ × 20″ steam table pans) 100 servings	(12393)	(1635.6)		
1 serving: ½ cup			(124)	(16.4)
Baked Rice Pudding 1¾ quarts dry rice, 1½ quarts (24) slightly beaten fresh eggs, 2 pounds 8 ounces raisins, 3 cups melted butter or margarine, 4⅓ cups nonfat dry milk, 4½ cups granulated sugar, 3 tablespoons vanilla, 2¼ tablespoons salt (yield: approx. four 12″ × 20″ steam pans) 100 servings	(22177)	(3345.9)		
1 serving: ⅔ cup			(222)	(33.5)
Bread Pudding 3½ gallons day old bread, 2 cups melted butter or margarine, 1½ quarts (30) slightly beaten fresh eggs, 1½ quarts granulated sugar, 4 tablespoons vanilla, 1 tablespoon ground nutmeg, 1½ tablespoons salt, 2¼ quarts raisins (yield: approx. three 12″ × 20″ steam table pans) 100 servings	(20791)	(3453.6)		
1 serving: ⅔ cup			(208)	(34.5)
Butterscotch, Chocolate, and Vanilla Puddings 8¾ cups nonfat dry milk plus one of the following: 6 pounds butterscotch pudding dessert powder (yield: approx. three 12″ × 20″ steam table pans) 100 servings	(11501)	(2401.0)		
1 serving: ½ cup			(115)	(24.0)
6 pounds chocolate pudding dessert powder (yield: approx. three 12″ × 20″ steam table pans) 100 servings	(13908)	(3078.0)		
1 serving: ½ cup			(139)	(30.8)
4 pounds 8 ounces vanilla pudding dessert powder (yield: approx. three 12″ × 20″ steam table pans) 100 servings	(11956)	(2456.0)		
1 serving: ½ cup			(120)	(24.6)
Fruit Gelatin 4½ pounds gelatin base dessert powder, 13 pounds canned fruit, solids and liquids (yield: approx. three 12″ × 20″ steam table pans) 100 servings	(12350)	(3027.4)		
1 serving: ⅔ cup			(124)	(30.3)

Other Desserts

	ENTIRE RECIPE Cal.	ENTIRE RECIPE Carb.	1 SERVING Cal.	1 SERVING Carb.
Baked Apples 39 pounds (100) whole fresh eating apples, 1 cup butter or margarine, 1 gallon granulated sugar, 2 teaspoons ground cinnamon, 1 teaspoon salt (yield: approx. 100 apples) 100 servings	(23072)	(5569.6)		
1 serving: 1 apple			(231)	(55.7)

	ENTIRE RECIPE Cal.	ENTIRE RECIPE Carb.	1 SERVING Cal.	1 SERVING Carb.
Banana Splits 17 pounds (50) bananas, 2 cups canned orange juice, 3¼ gallons ice cream, 3¼ quarts ice cream sauce, ½ gallon whipped topping, 2 cups chopped nuts, 1 pound 12 ounces maraschino cherries (yield: approx. 100 banana splits) 100 servings	(33648)	(5431.0)		
1 serving: 1 split			(336)	(54.3)
Cranberry Crunch 4 pounds 10 ounces whole or jellied cranberry sauce, 2 quarts sifted hard wheat flour, 3 cups butter or margarine, 1¾ quarts brown sugar, 7½ cups rolled oats, 1¾ teaspoons baking soda, 1⅔ teaspoons baking powder (yield: approx. two 18″ × 26″ sheet pans) 100 servings	(24699)	(5018.5)		
1 serving: one piece			(247)	(50.2)
Stewed Prunes 4¾ quarts dry prunes, 2¼ cups granulated sugar, 3 slices fresh lemon (yield: approx. 3 gallons) 100 servings	(8915)	(2386.6)		
1 serving: ½ cup			(89)	(23.9)

BREADS

	ENTIRE RECIPE Cal.	ENTIRE RECIPE Carb.	1 SERVING Cal.	1 SERVING Carb.
Date Nut Bread 7½ quarts sifted hard wheat flour, 3 cups shortening, 3 cups (15) eggs, 1¼ quarts granulated sugar, 2¾ cups brown sugar, 3½ cups nonfat dry milk, ½ cup baking powder, 1½ tablespoons baking soda, 4½ tablespoons salt, 1½ cups chopped pitted dates, 1 quart chopped nuts (yield: approx. 16 loaves) 100 servings	(31921)	(5019.1)		
1 serving: 2 slices			(319)	(50.2)
French Bread 9 quarts sifted hard wheat flour, 6 tablespoons shortening, ½ cup granulated sugar, ¼ cup dry active yeast, 4½ tablespoons salt (yield: approx. 12 loaves) 100 servings	(15870)	(3152.1)		
1 serving: 2 slices			(159)	(31.5)
Garlic Bread, Toasted 12 loaves of French bread made as above cut to 200 slices, covered with 1½ quarts melted butter or margarine and 8 cloves minced garlic (yield: approx. 12 loaves) 100 servings	(27422)	(3159.3)		
1 serving: 2 slices			(274)	(31.6)
Raisin Bread 6¾ quarts sifted hard wheat flour, ¾ cup shortening, ¾ cup granulated sugar, 1⅓ cups nonfat dry milk, 6½ tablespoons dry active yeast, 3¾ tablespoons salt, 2 tablespoons ground cinnamon, 1 tablespoon lemon flavoring, 2¼ quarts raisins (yield: approx. 12 loaves) 100 servings	(17973)	(3643.0)		
1 serving: 2 slices			(180)	(36.4)
Rye Bread 2¾ quarts medium rye flour, 6¼ quarts hard sifted wheat flour, ½ cup shortening, ½ cup granulated sugar, ⅓ cup whole caraway seeds, 5⅔ tablespoons salt, 6 tablespoons dry active yeast (yield: approx. 12 loaves) 100 servings	(16099)	(3172.4)		
1 serving: 2 slices			(161)	(31.7)
White Bread 7¾ quarts sifted hard wheat flour, ¾ cup shortening, ¾ cup granulated sugar, 1¾ cups nonfat dry milk, ¼ cup dry active yeast, 4½ tablespoons salt (yield: approx. 8 loaves) 100 servings	(15746)	(2975.9)		
1 serving: 2 slices			(157)	(29.8)
Whole Wheat Bread 1¼ quarts wheat base, 6½ quarts sifted hard wheat flour, ¾ cup shortening, ¾ cup granulated sugar, 1¾ cups nonfat dry milk, ¼ cup dry active yeast, 4½ tablespoons salt (yield: approx. 8 loaves) 100 servings	(13934)	(2938.7)		
1 serving: 2 slices			(139)	(29.4)
BUNS AND BISCUITS				
Baking Powder Biscuits 2½ gallons sifted hard wheat flour, 7½ cups shortening, 2⅛ cups nonfat dry milk, 1 cup baking powder, 4½ tablespoons salt (yield: approx. 200 biscuits) 100 servings	(30299)	(3681.9)		
1 serving: 2 biscuits			(303)	(36.8)
Hot Cross Buns 9 quarts hard wheat flour, 3¾ cups shortening, 3½ cups (18) eggs, 1 quart granulated sugar, 1¼ cups nonfat dry milk, 1½ cups dry active yeast, ⅓ cup grated lemon rind, 1½ quarts raisins (yield: approx. 100 buns) 100 servings	(24191)	(5048.6)		
1 serving: 3-oz. bun			(242)	(50.5)

SANDWICHES

	ENTIRE RECIPE Cal.	ENTIRE RECIPE Carb.	1 SERVING Cal.	1 SERVING Carb.
Bacon, Lettuce & Tomato Sandwiches 12 pounds of bread cut to 200 slices, 10 pounds bacon, 1 quart softened butter or margarine, 1 quart salad dressing, 12 pounds sliced tomatoes, 5 pounds trimmed lettuce (yield: approx. 100 sandwiches) 100 servings	(39270)	(3849.7)		
1 serving: 1 sandwich			(393)	(38.5)
Baked Bean Sandwiches 12 pounds of bread cut to 200 slices, 1 quart softened butter or margarine, 15 pounds 8 ounces canned white beans with pork and tomato sauce, 3 cups chili sauce, 3 cups chopped fresh celery, 2½ cups minced dry onions, 1 cup chopped sweet cucumber pickles (yield: approx. 100 sandwiches) 100 servings	(33223)	(4601.5)		
1 serving: 1 sandwich			(332)	(46.0)
Cheese and Bologna Sandwiches 12 pounds of bread cut to 200 slices, 1 quart softened butter or margarine, 1 quart prepared mustard, 6 pounds 4 ounces sliced processed Cheddar cheese, 8 pounds bologna, 4 pounds trimmed lettuce (yield: approx. 100 sandwiches) 100 servings	(47251)	(3601.7)		
1 serving: 1 sandwich			(473)	(36.0)
Cheese Sandwiches, Grilled 12 pounds of bread cut to 200 slices, 1 quart softened butter or margarine, 12 pounds 8 ounces sliced processed Cheddar cheese (yield: approx. 100 sandwiches) 100 servings	(44426)	(3075.9)		
1 serving: 1 sandwich			(444)	(30.8)
Corned Beef Sandwiches 12 pounds of bread cut to 200 slices, 1 quart softened butter or margarine, 1 quart prepared mustard, 16 pounds cooked corned beef, 4 pounds trimmed lettuce (yield: approx. 100 sandwiches) 100 servings	(52850)	(3414.3)		
1 serving: 1 sandwich			(529)	(34.1)
Peanut Butter and Jelly Sandwiches 12 pounds of bread cut to 200 slices, 1 quart softened butter or margarine, 7 pounds 2 ounces peanut butter, 12 pounds jelly (yield: approx. 100 sandwiches) 100 servings	(51265)	(5850.0)		
1 serving: 1 sandwich			(513)	(58.5)
Peanut Butter and Honey Sandwiches Same as Peanut Butter & Jelly above, but substitute jelly with 3 pounds honey (yield: approx. 100 sandwiches) 100 servings	(46601)	(4703.6)		
1 serving: 1 sandwich			(466)	(47.0)
Sardine Sandwiches 12 pounds of bread cut to 200 slices, 1 quart softened butter or margarine, 1 pound 4 ounces tomato catsup, 2¼ cups vinegar, 9 pounds sardines (yield: approx. 100 sandwiches) 100 servings	(32393)	(3151.7)	(324)	(31.5)
Sausage and Cold Cut Sandwiches 12 pounds of bread cut to 200 slices, 1 quart softened butter or margarine, 1 quart salad dressing, 10 pounds 9 ounces sliced fresh tomatoes, 2 pounds trimmed lettuce, plus one of the following:				
12½ pounds bologna (yield: approx. 100 sandwiches) 100 servings	(44106)	(3440.8)		
1 serving: 1 sandwich			(441)	(34.4)
Or 11 pounds Cervelat (yield: approx. 100 sandwiches) 100 servings	(50812)	(3365.7)		
1 serving: 1 sandwich			(508)	(33.7)
Or 16 pounds liver sausage (yield: approx. 100 sandwiches) 100 servings	(50594)	(3412.0)		
1 serving: 1 sandwich			(506)	(34.1)
Or 12½ pounds ham loaf (yield: approx. 100 sandwiches) 100 servings	(41569)	(3280.8)		
1 serving: 1 sandwich			(416)	(32.8)
Or 12½ pounds New England Brand sausage (yield: approx. 100 sandwiches) 100 servings	(50594)	(3941.2)		
1 serving: 1 sandwich			(506)	(39.4)
Or 11 pounds salami (yield: approx. 100 sandwiches) 100 servings	(50757)	(3284.1)		
1 serving: 1 sandwich			(508)	(32.8)

BEVERAGES

	ENTIRE RECIPE Cal.	ENTIRE RECIPE Carb.	1 SERVING Cal.	1 SERVING Carb.
Fruit Punch 8 quarts canned grapefruit juice, 2 quarts lemon juice, 3 quarts canned pineapple juice, 2¼ quarts granulated sugar (yield: approx. 8 gallons) 100 servings	(11114)	(2906.8)		
1 serving: 10 fl. oz.			(111)	(29.1)

	ENTIRE RECIPE		1 SERVING	
	Cal.	Carb.	Cal.	Carb.
Hot Cocoa or Chocolate Milk 2 pounds cocoa, 5 pounds nonfat dry milk, 2 quarts granulated sugar, 1½ teaspoons salt, 1¾ tablespoons vanilla (yield: approx. 6¼ gallons) 100 servings	(16826)	(3265.4)		
1 serving: 8 fl. oz.			(168)	(32.7)
Lemonade 1 quart frozen concentrated lemon juice (or the juice of 24 pounds lemons), 1 gallon granulated sugar (yield: approx. 8 gallons) 100 servings	(14159)	(3769.0)		
1 serving: 10 fl. oz.			(142)	(37.7)

	ENTIRE RECIPE		1 SERVING	
	Cal.	Carb.	Cal.	Carb.
Pineappleade 12 quarts canned pineapple juice, ½ cup lemon juice, 2 quarts granulated sugar, ½ teaspoon salt (yield: approx. 8 gallons) 100 servings	(12308)	(3149.6)		
1 serving: 10 fl. oz.			(123)	(31.5)
Tea Punch 2 cups loose black tea, 2¼ quarts granulated sugar, 3 quarts canned orange and grapefruit juice, 2 quarts lemon juice (juice of 12 pounds lemons), 3 quarts canned pineapple juice (yield: approx. 8 gallons) 100 servings	(10102)	(2640.8)		
1 serving: 10 fl. oz.			(101)	(26.4)

42 THE BOY SCOUTS—A DAY AT CAMP PHILMONT •

PHILMONT SCOUT RANCH & EXPLORER BASE
Cimarron, New Mexico

	1 SERVING Cal.	1 SERVING Carb.	1 OZ., BY WT. Cal.	1 OZ., BY WT. Carb.
MENU, DAY 1, THURSDAY				
BREAKFAST				
2 (to 3) slices (approx. 4.6 oz.) fresh French toast, assuming 2 slices	(442)	(55.8)	(96.1)	(12.13)
Approx. 1½ oz. fresh butter	305	0.2	203.0	0.11
Approx. 1½ oz. syrup made from scratch	(107)	(27.6)	(71.4)	(18.43)
4 slices (approx. 0.81 oz.) frozen-convenience crisp bacon	(136)	(0.7)	(168.1)	(0.90)
1 bowl (approx. 1 oz. dry) dry cereal (any one of several kinds)	(110)	(24.0)	(110.0)	(24.00)
1 pint fresh whole milk (this includes milk to be used for cereal above)	(300)	(22.8)		
1 fresh orange (approx. 5.5 oz.)	(60)	(14.5)	(10.9)	(2.64)
Unlimited cocoa (or choice of coffee or tea), assuming 1 cup of cocoa	(222)	(34.9)		
LUNCH				
8-fl.-oz. bowl (approx. 7 oz. by wt.) fresh jumbo salad	(282)	(4.7)	(40.3)	(0.67)
1½ slices Sausage and Cheese Pizza (approx. 7 oz.)	(477)	(43.2)	(68.1)	(6.17)
Approx. 3 oz. canned green beans	(20)	(4.4)	(6.8)	(1.48)
1 pint fresh whole milk	(300)	(22.8)		
Unlimited punch (or choice of coffee or tea), assuming 1 cup of punch	(120)	(29.3)		
DINNER				
4 oz. cured old fashioned ham	(206)	(3.5)	(51.6)	(0.88)
1 ladle (approx. 1 oz.) fruit glaze made from scratch	(75)	(20.1)	(74.5)	(20.13)
1 #12 dipper (approx. 4 oz.) canned sweet potatoes	(125)	(30.2)	(31.2)	(7.56)
Approx. 3 oz. canned mixed vegetables	(37)	(6.8)	(12.2)	(2.25)
8-fl.-oz. bowl (approx. 7 oz. by wt.) fresh tossed salad	(282)	(4.7)	(40.3)	(0.67)
2 slices (approx. 2 oz.) bread	(150)	(26.0)	(75.0)	(13.00)
Margarine: assuming 2 tablespoons	204	0.2	204.0	0.11
1 pint fresh whole milk	(300)	(22.8)		
1 piece (approx. 2″ × 2″, approx. 2½ oz.) pecan cake made from mix	(263)	(42.5)	(105.0)	(17.00)
Unlimited punch (or choice of coffee or tea), assuming 1 cup of punch	(120)	(29.3)		
("Snacks" are not mentioned on this menu plan.)				
TOTAL FOR DAY	(4643)	(471.0)		

43 FOODS FOR SPACE TRAVEL •

	UNIT Cal.	UNIT Carb.	1 OZ., BY WT. Cal.	1 OZ., BY WT. Carb.
NASA SPACE FLIGHTS				
Cereals				
Cereal, apricot, compressed, 6 cubes per typical serving, 1.3 oz.	168	24.6	131.3	19.22
Cereal, strawberry, compressed, 6 cubes per typical serving, 1.3 oz.	171	24.9	133.6	19.45
Cereal, sugar-coated corn flakes and toasted oats, dehydrated, typical serving, 0.85 oz.	91	18.7	107.1	22.00
Meats				
Bacon and egg, bite-size, freeze-dried, typical serving, 1 oz.	178	4.4	171.6	4.24
Beef and gravy, bite-size, freeze-dried, typical serving, 1.27 oz.	160	3.1	126.0	2.44
Beef pot roast, bite-size, freeze-dried, typical serving, 0.92 oz.	119	3.7	129.3	4.02
Beef/vegetables, bite-size, freeze-dried, typical serving, 0.85 oz.	98	6.9	115.3	8.12
Canadian bacon, applesauce, bite-size, freeze-dried, typical serving, 1 oz.	127	11.0	125.4	10.86
Chicken and gravy, bite-size, freeze-dried, typical serving, 0.85 oz.	92	4.9	108.2	5.76
Chicken and vegetables, bite-size, freeze-dried, typical serving 0.70 oz.	75	8.2	107.1	11.71
Pork sausage patties, bite-size, freeze-dried, typical serving, 1.5 oz.	223	3.7	148.4	2.46
Shrimp cocktail, bite-size, freeze-dried, typical serving, 1 oz.	118	10.0	113.5	9.62
Spaghetti/meat sauce, bite-size, freeze-dried, typical serving, 0.60 oz.	70	5.0	117.4	8.39
Vegetables				
Corn, bite-size, freeze-dried, typical serving, 0.95 oz.	105	21.5	110.3	22.58
Peas, bite-size, freeze-dried, typical serving, 0.78 oz.	81	14.8	104.4	19.07
Fruits				
Applesauce, bite-size, freeze-dried, typical serving, 1.2 oz.	139	32.9	112.6	26.65
Apricot, compressed, 8 cubes per typical serving, 1.95 oz.	284	31.1	145.6	15.95
Coconut, compressed, 6 cubes per typical serving, 1.24 oz.	206	15.7	166.1	12.68
Fruit cocktail, bite-size, freeze-dried, typical serving, 0.78 oz.	79	21.1	101.3	27.05
Peaches, bite-size, freeze-dried, typical serving, 0.88 oz.	88	23.4	100.0	26.59
Pineapple, compressed, 8 cubes per typical serving, 1.98 oz.	283	33.7	142.9	17.02

	UNIT Cal.	UNIT Carb.	1 OZ., BY WT. Cal.	1 OZ., BY WT. Carb.
Strawberry, compressed, 8 cubes per typical serving, 1.99 oz.	283	33.7	142.2	16.93
Salads				
Chicken, bite-size, freeze-dried, typical serving, 1.46 oz.	224	2.7	153.4	1.85
Potato, bite-size, freeze-dried, typical serving, 1.03 oz.	142	15.7	137.9	15.24
Salmon, bite-size, freeze-dried, typical serving, 1.51 oz.	246	1.8	162.9	1.19
Tuna, bite-size, freeze-dried, typical serving, 1.56 oz.	224	5.6	143.6	3.59
Soups				
Corn chowder, dehydrated, typical serving, 1.98 oz.	252	37.5	127.3	18.94
Potato, dehydrated, typical serving, 1.73 oz.	218	34.1	126.0	19.71
Sandwiches				
Beef, bite-size, freeze-dried, typical serving, 1.02 oz.	124	4.4	121.6	4.31
Cheese, bite-size, freeze-dried, typical serving, 1.07 oz.	158	5.6	147.7	5.23
Chicken, bite-size, freeze-dried, typical serving, 1.08 oz.	20	6.8	18.2	6.30
Bakery Items				
Brownies, dehydrated, 6 per typical serving, 1.56 oz.	241	22.0	154.5	14.10
Date fruitcake, dehydrated, 4 per typical serving, 2.07 oz.	262	32.8	126.6	15.85
Gingerbread, dehydrated, 6 per typical serving, 1.44 oz.	183	23.5	127.1	16.32
Pineapple fruitcake, dehydrated, 4 per typical serving, 2.02 oz.	233	33.7	115.3	16.68
Puddings				
Apricot, dehydrated, typical serving, 2.47 oz.	300	59.4	121.5	24.05
Banana, dehydrated, typical serving, 2.47 oz.	282	64.0	114.2	25.91
Butterscotch, dehydrated, typical serving, 2.47 oz.	311	58.0	125.9	23.48
Chocolate, dehydrated, typical serving. 2.47 oz.	307	56.0	124.3	22.67
Beverages				
Cocoa, dehydrated, typical serving, 1.48 oz.	190	31.7	128.4	21.42
Grapefruit, dehydrated, typical serving, 0.74 oz.	83	20.4	112.2	27.57
Orange, dehydrated, typical serving, 0.74 oz.	83	20.6	112.2	27.84
Orange-grapefruit, dehydrated, typical serving, 0.74 oz.	83	20.7	112.2	27.97
Tea with sugar, dehydrated, typical serving, 0.29 oz.	37	7.8	132.0	27.86
Missile-aneous Snacks				
Bacon squares, bite-size, compressed, 8 per typical serving, 1.47 oz.	180	0.4	122.4	0.27
Cinnamon toast, bite-size, freeze-dried, typical serving, 0.49 oz.	56	11.5	114.3	23.47
Peanut, compressed, 6 cubes per typical serving, 1.32 oz.	206	15.2	156.1	11.52
Toasted bread, compressed, 6 cubes per typical serving, 1.18 oz.	161	19.8	136.6	16.79

44 THREE FRUGAL REPASTS •

	UNIT Cal.	UNIT Carb.
AIR		
1 breath	0	0
1 roomful (15′ long × 12′ wide × 9′ high, 1620 cubic feet)	0	0
POSTAGE STAMPS (United States)		
Flat adhesive (usually on stamps of only 1 color):		
Regular size	0.07	0.02
Commemorative size	0.14	0.04
Shiny adhesive (usually on multi-colored stamps):		
Regular size	0.007	0.002
Commemorative size	0.014	0.004
WATER (tap water, United States)		
1 teaspoon	(0.00005)	
1 fluid oz.	(0.0003)	
1 cup	(0.002)	
1 pound	(0.005)	
1 liter	(0.01)	
1,000 liters	(10)	

PART IV

EPILOGUE

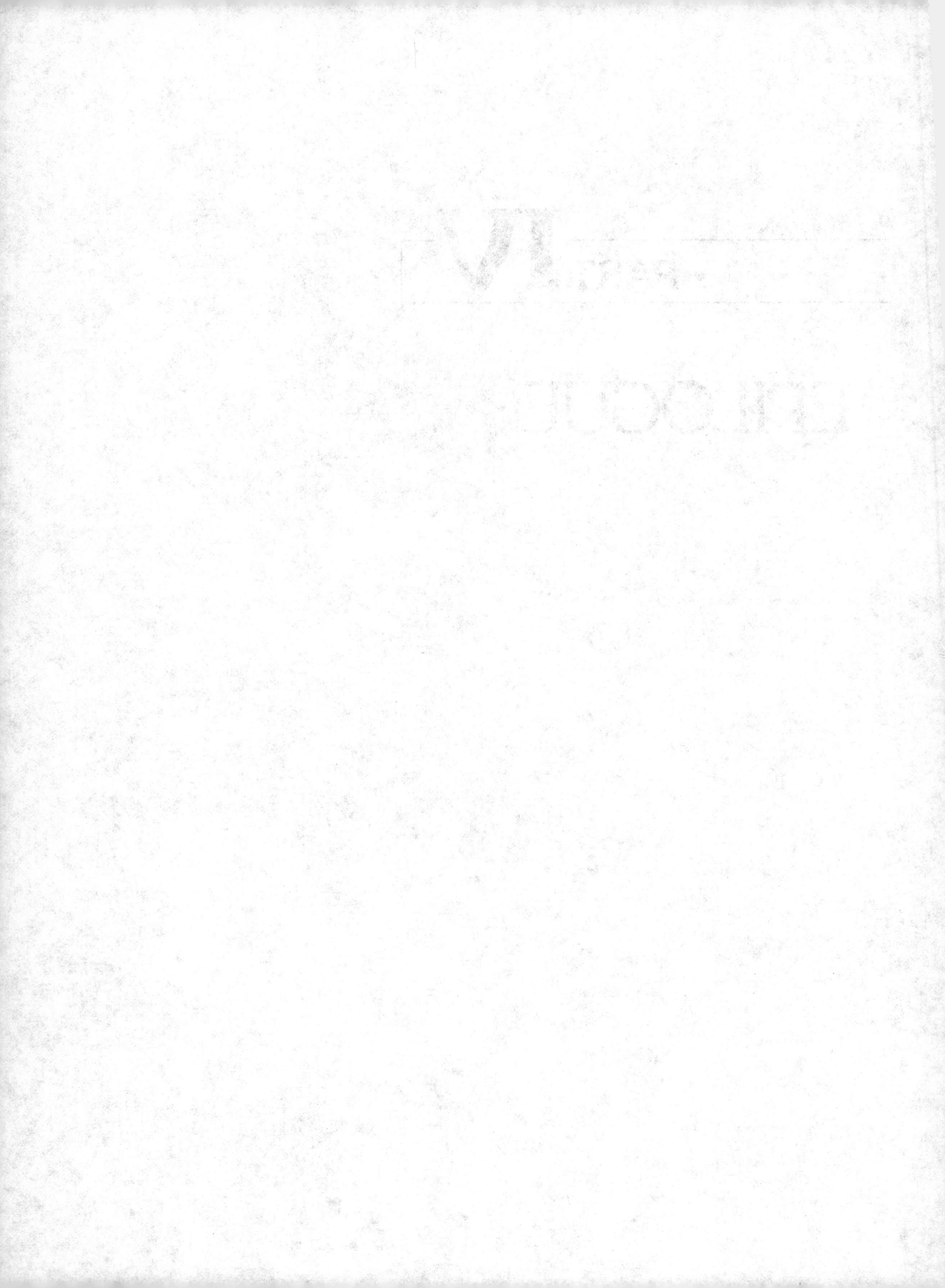

· EPILOGUE

Is it possible that being slim, like Melba toast, coasts along on reputation?

One day, when I was fat, I happened to say to a friend, "I think I'm going on a diet." His face registered concern: "I might like you better the way you are," he said.

Dear friend, you may have touched upon the collective aesthetic consciousness of us all: When I was fat, people would say, "You look like a Renoir," or "You look like you stepped out of a Titian." People would ask, "Do you pose for Soyer? For Alexander Dobkin? For Will Barnet?"

A curator at the Met once asked, "Did you model for Rubens in a former life?"

Now—after all these months of dieting—I haven't once been compared to art. Not once have I been likened to a Renoir. Not once have I been asked if Soyer, or Dobkin, or Barnet, ever painted me.

Now what people ask is, "Do you do commercials?"

• PART V

BIBLIOGRAPHY

no. 102, Agricultural Research Service, U.S. Department of Agriculture, revised Sept. 1975.

Pecot, R. K., C. M. Jaeger, and B. K. Watt. *Proximate Composition of Beef from Carcass to Cooked Meat: Method of Derivation and Tables of Values.* Washington, D.C.: U.S. Department of Agriculture, Consumer and Food Economics Research Division, Agricultural Research Service, November 1972.

Pellet, P. M., and Sossy Shadarevian. *Food Composition Tables for Use in the Middle East.* Beirut: American University of Beirut, 1970.

Posati, L. P. *Composition of Foods—Poultry Products, Raw, Processed, Prepared.* Washington, D.C.: Agriculture Handbook no. 8-5, Consumer and Food Economics Institute, U.S. Department of Agriculture, revised August 1979.

Posati, L. P., and M. L. Orr. *Composition of Foods—Dairy and Egg Products, Raw, Processed, Prepared.* Washington, D.C.: Agriculture Handbook no. 8-1, Consumer and Food Economics Institute, U.S. Department of Agriculture, revised November 1976.

Rambaut, Paul C., et al. "Nutrition and Responses to Zero Gravity." *Federation Proceedings,* vol. 36, no. 5 (April 1977): 1678–1682.

Rambaut, P. C., and Malcolm C. Smith. "Nutrition Support of Space Shuttle Crews." *Nutrition Today* (July/Aug. 1977): 6–11, 28–30.

Randoin, L., P. Le Gallic, J. Causeret, and G. Duchene. *Les Rations Alimentaires Equilibrées.* Paris: Editions Jacques Lanore, n.d.

Reeves III, J. B., and J. L. Weihrauch. *Composition of Foods—Fats and Oils, Raw, Processed, Prepared.* Washington, D.C.: Agriculture Handbook no. 8-4, Consumer and Food Economics Institute, U.S. Department of Agriculture, revised June 1979.

"Refrigeration: Storage Conditions on Quality of Frozen Fish." *Commercial Fisheries Review,* vol. 14 (1) (Jan. 1952): 17.

"Research in Service Laboratories." *Commercial Fisheries Review,* vol. 16(4) (1954): 12.

"Research in Service Laboratories." *Commercial Fisheries Review,* vol. 16(7) (1954): 20.

Root, Waverley. *Food—An International and Visual History and Dictionary of the Foods of the World.* New York: Simon and Schuster, 1980.

Setna, S. B., et al. "Nutritive Values of Some Marine Fishes of Bombay." *The Indian Journal of Medical Research,* vol. 32, (Oct. 1944): 171–176.

Shimizu, Kay. *Sushi at Home.* Tokyo: Shufunotomo Co., 1984.

Sidwell, V.D., P. R. Foncannon, N. S. Moore, and J. C. Bonnet. *Composition of the Edible Portion of Raw (Fresh or Frozen) Crustaceans, Finfish, and Mollusks, I. Protein, Fat, Moisture, Ash, Carbohydrate, Energy Value, and Cholesterol.* Washington, D.C.: MFR Paper 1043, From *Marine Fisheries Review,* vol. 36, no. 3, March 1974.

Simony, Kirsten. *Fodevare og Ernaeringstabeller of Rich, Ege.* Copenhagen: Nyt Nordisk Forlag Arnold Busck, 1978.

Smith, Malcolm C., "Feeding the New Military Man." *Activities Report: Proceedings of the 26th Annual Meeting,* vol. 24, no. 2 (April 18–19, 1972): 77–80.

Smith, M. C., P. C. Rambaut, and C. R. Stadler. 'Skylab Nutritional Studies." *NASA,* (n.d.): 193–97.

Smith, M. R., W. F. McCaughey, and A. R. Kemmerer. "Effects of Honey." *Journal of Apicultural Research,* 8(2):99–110 (1969). Department of Agricultural Biochemistry, University of Arizona, Tuscon.

Sohn, Bernard I., et al. "Composition of Commercially Important Fish From New England Waters." *Commercial Fisheries Review,* vol. 23(2) (Feb. 1961): 7–10.

Stadler, Connie R., et al. "Skylab Menu Development." *Journal of the American Dietetic Association,* vol. 62, no. 4 (April 1973): 390–393.

Standal, Bluebell R., David R. Bassett, Purification B. Policar, and Margaret Thom. *Fatty Acids, Cholesterol, and Proximate Composition of Certain Prepared and Unprepared Foods in Hawaii.* Research Bulletin 146, Hawaii Agricultural Experiment Station, University of Hawaii, Honolulu, May 1975.

Szczygla, Dr. A. *Tabele Skladu i Wartosci Odzywczych Producktow Spozywcyzch.* Warsaw: Panstwowy Zaklad Wydawnictwo Lekarskich, 1972.

Thomas, S., Margaret Corden. *Metric Tables of Composition of Australian Food.* Canberra: Commonwealth Department of Health, Australian Government Publishing Service, 1977.

Thurston, Claude E., et al. "Composition of Certain Species of Fresh-Water Fish. II. Comparative Data for 21 Species of Lake and River Fish." *The Journal of Science and Food,* vol. 24 (1959): 493–502.

Tohyama, Heihachiro. *Sushi Cook Book.* Tokyo: Joie, Inc., 1983.

Trade Publications Ltd. *New Zealand Food Export Review.* Aukland, 1978.

Tsuda, Nobuko. *Sushi Made Easy.* Tokyo: John Weatherhill, 1982.

United States Department of Agricultural Marketing Service. *How to Buy Food.* Agricultural Marketing Service, Home and Garden Bulletin nos. 141, 143, 144, 157, 167, 177, 191, 193, 198, and 201. U.S. Department of Agriculture, 1967–1972.

United States Department of Agriculture. *Cheese Varieties and Descriptions.* Washington, D.C.: U.S. Department of Agriculture, Agricultural Research Service, n.d.

United States Department of Agriculture. *Food and Your Weight.* Washington, D.C.: Agricultural Research Service, U.S. Department of Agriculture, n.d.

United States Department of Agriculture. *Lamb in Family Meals.* Washington, D.C.: U.S. Department of Agriculture, Agricultural Research Service, Home and Garden Bulletin no. 124, revised Feb. 1974.

United States Department of Agriculture. *Physical and Chemical Properties of Extracted (Liquid) Honey of Average Compositon.* Washington, D.C.: Production and Marketing Administration, Special Commodities Branch, Honey Section, n.d.

United States Department of Agriculture. *Pork in Family Meals—A Guide for Consumers.* Washington, D.C.: U.S. Department of Agriculture, Home and Garden Bulletin no. 160, revised July 1977.

United States Department of Agriculture. *Vegetables in Family Meals: A Guide for Consumers.* Washington, D.C.: Prepared by Agricultural Research Service, Home and Garden Bulletin no. 105, revised Jan. 1975.

United States Department of Health, Education and Welfare. *A Selected Bibliography of East Asian Foods and Nutrition Arranged According to Subject Matter and Area.* U.S. Government Printing Office, Dec. 1972.

United States Department of Health, Education and Welfare, and Food and Agriculture Organization of the United Nations. *Food Composition Table for Use in East Asia.* Bethesda, Dec. 1972.

Vemury, M., and H. Levine. *Beliefs and Practices That Affect Food Habits in Developing Countries.* Ann Arbor: Nutrition Planning Information Service, Document #533, n.d.

Watt, B. K., and A. L. Merrill. *Composition of Foods.* Washington, D.C.: U.S. Department of Agriculture, Agricultural Handbook no. 8, revised Dec. 1963.

Watt, B. K., and A. L. Merrill. *Composition of Foods, Raw, Processed, Prepared.* Washington, D.C.: Consumer Food Economics Institute, Agricultural Research Service, U.S. Department of Agriculture, Oct. 1975.

Wenkam, N. S., and C. D. Miller. *Composition of Hawaii Fruits.* Honolulu: Hawaii Agricultural Experiment Station, University of Hawaii, College of Tropical Agriculture, 1965.

Whedon, Donald G., et al. "Mineral and Nitrogen Metabolic Studies, Experiment M071." *The Skylab Life Sciences Symposium.* Lyndon B. Johnson Space Center (Aug. 27–29, 1974): 353–371.

Woon, A. J. *Tables of Representative Values of Foods Commonly Used in Singapore.* Singapore: Department of Social Medicine and Public Health, University of Singapore, 1969.

We Leung, Woot-Tsuen. *Food Composition Table for Use in Latin America.* Bethesda: National Institute of Health, n.d.